5th Edition
Fully Colored

A Complete NBE Centric Approach

FMGE Solutions
for MCI Screening Examination

50+ Clinical Pattern Qs with Explanations
2 Model Papers with 2 Sets of OMR Sheet on Real Time Exam Pattern for Self-evaluation

Deepak Marwah
Director
Medicine Buster Classes

Siraj Ahmad
Faculty
Dr Marwah Test Series and Trapezium Health Care

CBS
Dedicated to Education

CBS Publishers & Distributors Pvt Ltd
• New Delhi • Bengaluru • Chennai • Kochi • Kolkata • Mumbai
• Hyderabad • Nagpur • Patna • Pune • Vijayawada

A Complete NBE Centric Approach

FMGE Solutions
for MCI Screening Examination

ISBN: 978-93-89261-96-7

Copyright © Authors and Publishers

Fifth Edition: 2020

Fourth Edition: 2019

All rights reserved. No part of this book may be reproduced or transmitted in any form or by any means, electronic or mechanical, including photocopying, recording, or any information storage and retrieval system without permission, in writing, from the authors and the publishers.

Published by **Satish Kumar Jain** and produced by **Varun Jain** for

CBS Publishers & Distributors Pvt Ltd
4819/XI Prahlad Street, 24 Ansari Road, Daryaganj, New Delhi 110 002, India.
Ph: 23289259, 23266861, 23266867   Website: www.cbspd.com
Fax: 011-23243014
e-mail: delhi@cbspd.com; cbspubs@airtelmail.in.
Corporate Office: 204 FIE, Industrial Area, Patparganj, Delhi 110 092
Ph: 4934 4934   Fax: 4934 4935
e-mail: productioncbspd@gmail.com; bhupesharora@cbspd.com

DISCLAIMER

This book contains questions based on topics asked in previous years' MCI Screening Exams. Often repeated topics and sub-topics have been included for students' benefit. We do not claim that these questions are exact or similar to the questions asked in MCI Exams. If any such similarity is found, it is purely coinicidental and by chance.

Branches

- **Bengaluru:** Seema House 2975, 17th Cross, K.R. Road,
  Banasankari 2nd Stage, Bengaluru 560 070, Karnataka
  Ph: +91-80-26771678/79   Fax: +91-80-26771680
  e-mail: bangalore@cbspd.com
- **Chennai:** No. 7, Subbaraya Street, Shenoy Nagar, Chennai 600 030, Tamil Nadu
  Ph: +91-44-42032115   Fax: +91-44-42032115
  e-mail: chennai@cbspd.com
- **Kochi:** 68/1534,35,36-Power House Road, Opp. KSEB, Cochin-682018, Kochi, Kerala
  Ph: +91-484-4059061-62-64-65   Fax: +91-484-4059065
  e-mail: kochi@cbspd.com
- **Kolkata:** No. 6/B, Ground Floor, Rameswar Shaw Road, Kolkata-700014 (West Bengal), India
  Ph: +91-33-2289-1126, 2289-1127
  e-mail: kolkata@cbspd.com
- **Mumbai:** 83-C, Dr E Moses Road, Worli, Mumbai-400018, Maharashtra
  Ph: +91-22-24902340/41   Fax: +91-22-24902342
  e-mail: mumbai@cbspd.com

Representatives

- Hyderabad   +91-9885175004
- Pun e   +91-9623451994
- Patna   +91-9334159340
- Vijaywada   +91-9000660880

Printed at: Magic International Pvt. Ltd. Greater Noida, UP, India

Dedicated to

My Loving wife **Renuka**

Dr Deepak Marwah

My adorable daughter Sarah S. Ahmad

"Your smile, when I see you after a long, exhaustive day, is the purest form of opioid."

and

My Loving wife **Dr Sadia H. Ahmad**

Dr Siraj Ahmad

Preface to 5th Edition

Dear Students,

We convey our sincere regards and thanks to all our readers for the huge response to the previous edition of FMGE Solutions and also for making it the best book for FMGE aspirants. In order to improvise further we are coming up with the fifth edition of the book.

Here once again we are providing you the best text for your preparation in most updated form possible, keeping in mind the structure and level of examination at present. Medical Council of India (MCI) screening examination has always been a tough nut to crack because the examination pattern is very unpredictable ranging from single one liner to long case-based questions. Keeping that in mind we have added multiple additional image-based questions as per the recent pattern and another separate section for clinical-pattern questions.

Your preparation level should start from the basics and then gradually it should reach the maximum height. The preparation should be started from the very beginning and with perseverance, and thankfully, persistence is a great substitute for talent.

"A river cuts through the rock, NOT because of its power but because of its persistence".

As we have mentioned earlier also *"hard work beats talent, when talent doesn't work hard"*. This examination does not test your talent rather it tests your dedication, your hard work, your capacity to sit for 12 to 14 hours per day. We have seen all of you studying the same matter with similar dedication, but only a handful of people taste the success of crossing the boundary line. Oftentimes the most talented ones are also left behind. Ever wondered what is the thing that separates the winners from the rest of the population? The reasons can be many. But here we could enumerate a few:

First and foremost is: **The faith and belief that you can do it**. It is said, *"if you have acquired this belief that you can do it, your half of the journey is done."* Now the question arises, is it just enough to believe that you can do it? The answer is NO. In addition to this belief, you also need to show the consistency and willpower to challenge what comes next. You will have to work accordingly.

The second is: *"The extra mile they ran."* After your full-day exhaustive classes it is practically impossible to reach home and sit with the notes once again for the next one hour. But dear friends, this is what differentiates the winners from the rest of the population. They show this toughness, aggressiveness and willpower to run that extra mile on the same evening. It is this attitude that brings them one step closer to victory every day. Therefore it is advisable to all of you: rejuvenate yourself after all the tiredness and do the revision of the day-work in the evening itself. *"This is your battle, push yourself for one more step, no one else is going to do it for you, the success lies right there."*

The willingness to explore the new and to accept the challenge. Remember, *"if it doesn't challenges you, it won't change you,"* and *"old ways won't open new doors."*

As the level of examination has been most unpredictable, you will have to accept the challenge and be ready to learn the new things that come along. Remember, the percentage of repeated questions in the examination is very less but *"the topics are often repeated"*. Hence, your analytical and reading skills will determine your score. In the book, the explanation section contains more information than the number of questions in each topic. Therefore we would suggest you to read all the explanations in detail at least three to four times including the **"Extra Mile"** boxes which are an add-on and golden points.

At the end of the book we have also included a separate section of **"Key Points,"** which will be your most important revision tool in last few days of revision and 2 sets of model papers along with OMR sheet for self evaluation before examination.

Last but not the least, is **the proper strategy and time management**. Remember, you get only five to six months for your preparation and in this duration, you have to finish the classes of all nineteen subjects. Besides, you have to revise these subjects and appear in the tests, which certainly is a lot of work in a very short span of time. Hence, you are advised to finish the first reading in first three to four months. In the fourth and fifth months your revision should start. Whenever you start your revision, remember to do two or three subjects per day, *for example, one clinical/ major subject + one paraclinical/preclinical + one minor subject*. You should be in continuous touch with the dry subjects like Anatomy, Biochemistry and Microbiology as well. Give at least 2 hours every day on these subjects alternatively and follow them religiously on priority basis.

"The key is NOT to prioritize what's on your schedule, but to schedule your priorities."

One more point which we would like to highlight here is, keep yourself away from negative thoughts or negative people, it somehow degrades your confidence level from within. Only you have the right and power to do this task.

"Your mind is a powerful thing, when you fill it with positive thoughts, your life will start to change."

Every possible effort has been made to bring this book in the best shape possible. However, if you come across any typographical errors, queries or suggestions, please write us on: **marwahmedicine@gmail.com/sirajahmad9@ gmail.com**

With these words we would like to extend our best wishes to all our readers across the globe.

Deepak Marwah

Siraj Ahmad

Acknowledgements

We would like to thank all our readers across the globe and the people who helped and motivated us in moulding and shaping this book. Besides, our thanks are also due to:

- Our parents whose prayers and blessings have given us the strength to keep working.
- All our students in India and abroad for their continuous feedback—appreciation and criticism—which helped us shaping this book
- All our previous batch students of test and discussion batch and regular batch for their valuable contributions to the book. You all have been a constant source of motivation for us as well because you have made us work harder every day.
- Our teachers whose valuable lessons and teachings are always with us at each and every step.
- Dr Yusuf Tyagi, MS, Orthopaedics, for his priceless suggestions and round-the-clock availability in shaping this book.
- Dr Manoj Kumar Bhoomigari, MS, Anatomy, for his worthy support and contribution.
- Dr Sravan, MD, Paediatrics, for his impressive support in paediatrics section and for all his continuous support.
- Dr Mona Lisa, MS, Anatomy AFMC, for her remarkable contribution in anatomy section
- Dr Prashant Agrawal, MD, psychiatry, PGI Chandigarh for his valuable suggestions and contributions to psychiatry section.
- Dr Asma, MD (PSM), for her phenomenal contribution and support in shaping and moulding this book
- Dr Deepanshu Goyal, Prepladder for all your efforts in promotion of the book.

Not to forget the constant feedbacks and support of our colleagues:

- Dr Ankit Goel, MD Psychiatry
- Dr Naveen Porwal MD (Physiology), KGMU Lucknow
- Dr Sushant Soni, MD Pathology
- Dr Pawan, MS, General Surgery
- Dr Sonam Pruthi, MD Pathology
- Dr S Sazawal (Baltimore, John Hopkins, USA)
- Dr Shrikant, Gulbarga
- Dr Niraj Singh, Kolkata
- Dr Sinagaram, MD Pediatrics, Chennai
- Dr Pallavi Pradeep, MD, Medicine (Res), USA
- Dr Cinderella B, Medical Officer, Ranchi
- Dr Nikita, MD (Radiology)
- Dr Arshad Ansari, MD
- Dr Shanthan V, MD
- Dr Sadia H. Ahmad, MD Obstetrics and Gynecology (Res), for putting up all the efforts and for your round-the-clock availability in bringing up this book. It was next to impossible without your dedicated efforts.
- Dr Bushra Sufiyan Khan, MD Pharmacology; most disciplined and a wonderful colleague-cum-guide for all her suggestions and feedback from time to time.
- Dr Nida Rizvi, Dr Shamshi Azmi, MD Pharmacology, for all the timely intervention that was needed in shaping up this book.

FMGE Solutions Screening Examination

- Dr Sulthan Al Rashid, MD Pharmacology (Res), for being a wonderful friend and for all his help and availability throughout the journey.
- Dr Prerna Singh, Dr Aparajita for all their dedication and making themselves available in the hour of need and not to forget for endless cups of coffee.
- Dr Prashant, MD (Psychiatry) for his valuable support and expert opinion on the subject
- Dr Saleem, MD (Preventive Medicine, Res) and Dr Shahnawaz, MS (For being cool and supportive friends).
- Md Raza for being the most effective and best friend one can ever pray for.
- Mr David Pillai and Mr Kadwin Pillai, Transworld Educare, Pune for being a potent source and inspiration and motivation, and for all their constant support in shaping the book.
- All our students of Transworld educare, Pune (to mention some Dr Balaji, Dr Thirumalai, Dr Venkat, Dr Phillip and Ms Anshjeet Kaur Brar) for their continuous feedback and appraisal of the book.
- Dr Deepika (BSMU), Dr Himanshu Pandya, Dr Madhu Hundi, Dr Shailika Sharma (Davao Medical School, Philippines), Dr Sarona Sharma (Guangxi Medical School, China), Dr Asif Siddiqui (BSMU, Ukraine), Dr Mukul, Dr Suman Roy, Dr Arka Das (Guanghzou, China), Dr Pankaj Patle, Dr Vishnupriya, Dr Md Ibrahim Khan, Dr Ulfat Jahan, Dr Rahi Shoib, Dr Tanu, Dr Anindya, Dr Pradeep, Dr Avik, Dr Nikita Mahant, Dr Preksha, Dr Sukirty, Dr Sagar, Dr Angelo, Dr Balaji, Dr Aparajita, Dr Lokesh, Dr Sudarshan Subramani, Dr Avnish, Dr Preeti Gaonkar, Dr Zeeshan, Dr Nimit, Dr Sylvia, Dr Nandha, Dr Roshan, Dr Urwashi, Dr Naresh, Dr Gayathri Priyanka, Dr Stephen, Dr Paul and all others who showed interest and feedbacks about the previous edition which helped us in improvising.
- Our office staff members, Mr Soumen, Mr Naveen, Mr Alam, Ms Shweta, Ms Prachi, Mr Manish, Mr Abhishek, Mr Sandeep, Mr Krishna for their true efforts in completion of this book.

No words can describe the role of all Medical Graduate Students in India and abroad, with whom we have ever interacted, in helping me to give this book its final shape.

Our special thanks to **Mr Satish Kumar Jain** (Chairman) and **Mr Varun Jain** (Managing Director), M/s CBS Publishers and Distributors Pvt Ltd for providing me the platform in bringing out the book. We have no words to describe the role, efforts, inputs and initiatives undertaken by **Mr Bhupesh Arora**, (Vice President - Publishing and Marketing, PGMEE and Nursing Division) for helping and motivating me.

We sincerely thank the entire CBS team for bringing the book colorful with utmost care and presentation. We thank Dr Mrinalini Bakshi *(Editorial Head and Content Strategist)* for her editorial support and Ms Nitasha Arora *(Production Head & Content Strategist)*, Dr Anju Dhir *(Senior Scientific Coordinator/Editor)*, Mr Nitish Dubey *(Senior Editor)*, Mr Shivendu Pandey *(Editor)* and all the production team members Mr Ashutosh Pathak, Mr Chaman Lal, Mr Prakash Gaur, Mr Phool Kumar, Mr Bunty Kashyap, Ms Tahira Parveen, Ms Babita Verma, Mr Chander, Mr Raju Sharma, Mr Manoj Chaudhary, Mr Vikram Chaudhary, Mr Manoj Malakar, Mr Arun Kumar and Ms Manorama for devoting laborious hours in designing and typesetting of the book.

From the Publisher's Desk

We request all the readers to provide us their valuable suggestions/errors *(if any)* at:

feedback@cbspd.com

so as to help us in further improvement of this book in the subsequent editions.

Contents

Clinical Pattern Questions .... *xi*

1. ANATOMY   **1-107**
Questions (Explained, Board Review and Image-Based Questions) 1-24
Answers with Explanations 25-107

2. PHYSIOLOGY   **108-169**
Questions (Explained, Board Review and Image-Based Question) 108-124
Answers with Explanations 125-169

3. BIOCHEMISTRY   **170-224**
Questions (Explained and Board Review Questions) 170-180
Answers with Explanations 181-224

4. PHARMACOLOGY   **225-320**
Questions (Explained and Board Review Questions) 225-243
Answers with Explanations 244-320

5. PATHOLOGY   **321-405**
Questions (Explained, Board Review and Image-Based Questions) 321-345
Answers with Explanations 346-405

6. MICROBIOLOGY AND PARASITOLOGY   **406-453**
Questions (Explained and Board Review Questions) 406-417
Answers with Explanations 418-453

7. FORENSIC MEDICINE   **454-491**
Questions (Explained, Board Review and Image-Based Question) 454-462
Answers with Explanations 463-491

8. PREVENTIVE AND SOCIAL MEDICINE (PSM)   **492-575**
Questions (Explained, Board Review and Image-Based Questions) 492-513
Answers with Explanations 514-575

9. MEDICINE   **576-702**
Questions (Explained, Board Review and Image-Based Questions) 576-611
Answers with Explanations 612-702

FMGE Solutions Screening Examination

10. SURGERY — 703-809
Questions (Explained, Board Review and Image-Based Questions) 703-733
Answers with Explanations 734-809

11. PEDIATRICS — 810-855
Questions (Explained and Board Review Questions) 810-821
Answers with Explanations 822-855

12. OBSTETRICS AND GYNECOLOGY — 856-961
Questions (Explained, Board Review and Image-Based Questions) 856-878
Answers with Explanations 879-961

13. ENT — 962-1013
Questions (Explained, Board Review and Image-Based Questions) 962-975
Answers with Explanations 976-1013

14. ORTHOPEDICS — 1014-1059
Questions (Explained, Board Review and Image-Based Questions) 1014-1025
Answers with Explanations 1026-1059

15. OPHTHALMOLOGY — 1060-1119
Questions (Explained, Board Review and Image-Based Questions) 1060-1075
Answers with Explanations 1076-1119

16. DERMATOLOGY — 1120-1166
Questions (Explained, Board Review and Image-Based Questions) 1020-1136
Answers with Explanations 1137-1166

17. ANESTHESIA — 1167-1190
Questions (Explained, Board Review and Image-Based Questions) 1167-1173
Answers with Explanations 1174-1190

18. PSYCHIATRY — 1191-1213
Questions (Explained and Board Review Questions) 1191-1196
Answers with Explanations 1197-1213

19. RADIOLOGY — 1214-1250
Questions (Explained, Board Review and Image-Based Questions) 1214-1227
Answers with Explanations 1228-1250

KEY POINTS — 1251-1338

MODEL TEST PAPER-I — 1339-1360

MODEL TEST PAPER-II — 1361-1381

Clinical Pattern Questions

FMGE Solutions Screening Examination

1. **A 25-year-old tall thin man comes to your OPD with complaints of dragging sensation in groin and scrotum on left side. On examination in standing position impulse of coughing is present. His scrotum feels like a bag of worms and supine position leads to reduction of the tortuous swelling. Which is correct about this condition?**
   a. USG abdomen to look for tumor of Adrenals
   b. Unilocular acquired retention cyst
   c. Urgent aspiration
   d. Excision via scrotal approach

   Ans. (d) Excision via scrotal approach
   Ref: SRB: 5th ed. pg. 1076
   - The clinical finding of bag of worms feeling in scrotum points to Varicocele. It leads to dilatation and tortuosity of pampiniform plexus of veins and testicular veins. It is more common on left side.
   - The leading cause is idiopathic but can occur due to left sided renal cell cancer with tumor thrombus in left renal vein leading to obstruction to venous flow of left testicular vein.
   - Venous doppler should be done for scrotum and groin and since it is mentioned as a tortuous swelling, excision of veins should be done.

2. **Middle aged male presents with a scrotal swelling which has been present for previous 6 months. It shows positive fluctuation and the surgeon can get above the swelling. Which of the following is not to be done in the patient?**
   a. Lord's plication
   b. Jaboulay's procedure
   c. Aspiration
   d. Evacuation and Eversion

   Ans. (c) Aspiration
   Ref: SRB: 5th ed. pg. 1072
   The clinical presentation is of a hydrocele. The key word is that surgeon can get above the swelling. The surgeries for hydrocele are-
   - Subtotal excision of sac
   - Jaboulay's Operation
   - Evacuation and Eversion
   - Lord's plication
   - Sharma and Jhawers Technique (After excision, the sac with the testis is placed in newly created pocket between the fascial layers of the scrotum).

3. **A 25-year-old male presents with inability to place back the retracted preputial skin over the glans. The glans is edematous, swollen with severe pain and tenderness. Which is initial management of this condition?**
   a. Dorsal slit to relieve edema
   b. Urgent circumcision
   c. Injection of lignocaine in swollen part to reduce pain
   d. Part elevation and local dressing

   Ans. (a) Dorsal slit to relieve edema
   Ref: SRB: 5th ed. pg. 1061
   The key word in the question in inability to push back the preputial skin over the glans penis post intercourse indicating development of Paraphimosis.

   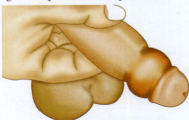

   Manual reduction should be tried. If it fails, initial dorsal slit is made to reduce edema and compression. Antibiotics and analgesics are given. Circumcision is done after 3 weeks.

4. **A 35-year-old alcoholic has presented with 2 episodes of hematemesis. On examination his pulse rate is 100/min with BP of 90/60 mm Hg. Per abdomen examination shows spleen palpable 3 cm below costal margin. Which is true about this patient?**
   a. Elevated CRP and Low C3
   b. Most common site of bleeding is First part of duodenum
   c. Urgent Elective intubation of patient
   d. The increased portal vein pressure should be lowered with octreotide

   Ans. (d) The increased pressure of portal vein pressure should be lowered with octreotide
   Ref: CMDT 2019 pg. 627
   - The presence of splenomegaly with hematemesis points to etiology of portal hypertension. Hence after stabilization of patients with fluids, octreotide should be started to lower the pressure in portal vein.
   - The leading cause of hematemesis is peptic ulcer disease *but* this patient is having portal hypertension leading to vomiting of blood.

5. **A pregnant lady was admitted with diagnosis of PIH for monitoring and bed rest. In supine position which of the following is a complication of the below representation?**

   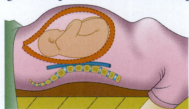

   a. Abdominal aorta syndrome
   b. Supine vena cava syndrome
   c. Ascending aorta syndrome
   d. Superior vena cava syndrome

Ans. (b) Supine vena cava syndrome

Ref: William Obstetrics pg. 1369

The image shows the developing baby compressing the IVC of the mother. This will lead to reduced venous return and development of dizziness and hypotension in the mother. This is called supine hypotension syndrome or supine vena cava syndrome.

6. A 25-year-old primigravida has presented in obstructed labor. On examination she is exhausted and has a tender uterus with a groove felt per abdomen as shown in the image. Fetal parts are not felt. What is the diagnosis?

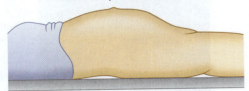
Normal shape of the abdomen

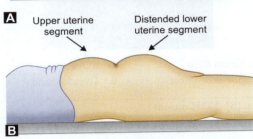
A — Upper uterine segment; Distended lower uterine segment
B

a. Constriction ring b. Retraction ring
c. Abruptio placentae d. Cervical dystocia

Ans. (b) Retraction ring

Ref: Dutta 8th ed. pg. 421

The presence of an exhausted patient with a tender uterus favours diagnosis of retraction ring. Please note that constriction ring is *only revealed during CS in first stage, forceps application during second stage and during manual removal in 3rd stage.*

Pathological retraction ring	Constriction ring
Occurs in prolonged 2nd stage	Occurs in the 1st, 2nd or 3rd stage
Always between upper and lower uterine segments	At any level of the uterus
Rises up	Does not change its position
Felt and seen abdominally	Felt only vaginally
The uterus is tonically retracted, tender and the fetal parts cannot be felt	The uterus is not tonically retracted and the fetal parts can be felt
Maternal distress and fetal distress or death	Maternal and fetal distress may not be present
Relieved only by delivery of the fetus	May be relieved by anesthetics or antispasmodics

7. The following instrument is used for performing aspiration of uterine cavity within _____ days of a missed period in a woman with previously normal cycle

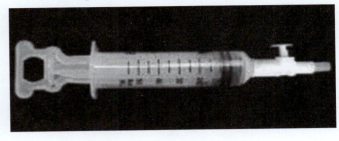

a. 14 days b. 28 days
c. 42 days d. 72 days

Ans. (a) 14 days

Ref: Datta: 8th ed. pg. 646

The image shows 50 ml syringe used for performing menstrual regulation. After cervical dilatation, Karman cannula is inserted and attached to the syringe for aspiration. The cannula is rotated, pushed in and out with gentle strokes. This method is used within 14 days of a missed period in a woman with a previous normal cycle.

8. A 25-year-old lady is undergoing the following procedure for an unplanned conception. The maximum pressure generated during the procedure is?

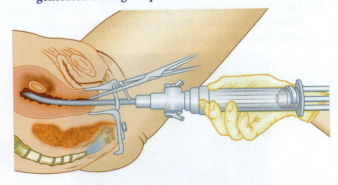

a. 100–200 mm Hg b. 200–400 mm Hg
c. 400–600 mm Hg d. 600–800 mm Hg

Ans. (c) 400–600 mm Hg

Ref: Datta 8th ed. pg. 646

The image shows suction evacuation being performed. The pressure of suction is raised to 400–600 mm Hg. The end-point of the suction evacuation procedure is when the cannula is gripped by a contracted uterus with a grating sensation.

9. During the following procedure, optimum interval between uterine incision and delivery should be less than _____ seconds.

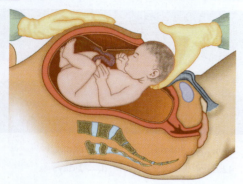

a. 30 seconds
b. 45 seconds
c. 60 seconds
d. 90 seconds

Ans. (d) 90 seconds

Ref: Datta, 8th ed. pg. 673

The image shows LSCS being performed, with the head being delivered by hooking fingers carefully between the lower uterine flap. The head is delivered by elevation and flexion using the palm as fulcrum and the *optimum time between the uterine incision and delivery should be less than 90 seconds.*

10. The following patient presented to the OPD with history of hair loss. There was no erythema, scarring or scratching. Diagnosis is?

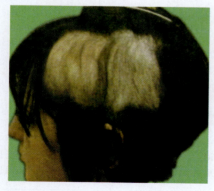

a. Trichotillomania
b. Alopecia Areata
c. Telogen Effluvium
d. Tinea infection

Ans. (a) Trichotillomania

Ref: Rook's Textbook of Dermatology, 9th ed. pg. 86

- In Trichotillomania, the hairs are plucked from fronto-parietal region and a *bizarre angular pattern of hair loss* is produced.
- Telogen effluvium develops when hair follicles go into telogen or resting face prematurely. It is related to stress like chronic illness, depression and pregnancy. It is more common in women
- Alopecia areata has a *clear demarcation* without any signs of inflammation or exclamation mark hair.

11. A child has been brought with the following scalp lesion with history of itching in scalp and hair loss for past 2 months. Which of the following is useful for diagnosis of this patient?

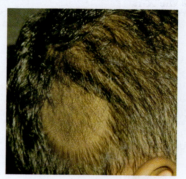

a. Gram stain
b. KOH mount
c. Slit Skin smear
d. Tzanck smear

Ans. (b) KOH mount

Ref: Fitzpatrick's Dermatology, 8th ed. pg. 2284-85

The image shows *black dot sign* classical of tinea capitis. The hairs are damaged due to endothrix infection and break easily.

12. The following image shows?

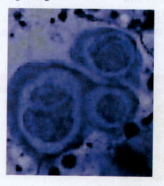

a. Acanthocyte
b. Acantholytic cell
c. Sezary cells
d. Clue cells

Ans. (b) Acantholytic cell

Ref: IAVDL Colour Atlas of Dermatology pg. 565

The image shows multinucleate giant cell with peripheral rim of cytoplasm. This is an acantholytic cell (Tzanck cell) which is a large rounded keratinocyte.

Clinical Pattern Questions

Primary acantholysis	Secondary acantholysis
• Pemphigus • Staphylococcal scalded skin syndrome • Darier disease • Hailey-Hailey disease	Seen in viral infection like herpes

13. A 10-year-old child presents with fever and wound with discharging pus from right thigh for 4 months. Given below is the X-ray of the patient. Identify the marked area.

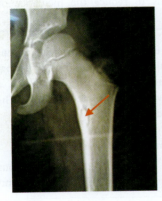

a. Sequestrum
b. Cloacae
c. Involucrum
d. Woven bone

Ans. (a) Sequestrum

Ref: Essential Orthopaedics, Maheshwari 5th ed. pg. 172

- The image shows a radio-dense area (marked by blue arrow) than the surrounding bone. Between the marked devitalized irregular bone fragment and normal bone is a radiolucent rim of granulation tissue.
- Involucrum is the *subperiosteal* reactive bone and hence, is ruled out due to location.

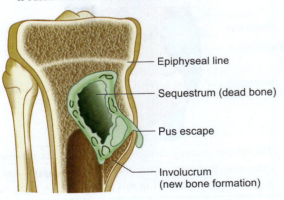

14. A 4-year-old boy fell on outstretched hand. X-ray is shown below. Which blood vessel is most commonly affected?

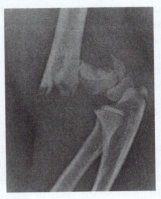

a. Ulnar artery
b. Radial artery
c. Brachial artery
d. Cubital vein

Ans. (c) Brachial artery

Ref: Essential Orthopaedics, Maheshwari 5th ed. pg. 97

The image shows displaced supracondylar fracture of humerus and the spike of proximal segment can easily traumatize the brachial artery.

15. An elderly patient slipped in the bathroom and sustained injury over the hip joint. X-ray is shown below. Her attitude of leg will be?

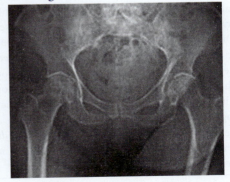

a. Shortened, abducted and externally rotated
b. Shortened and abducted
c. Lengthened and internally rotated
d. Flexed and adducted and internally rotated

Ans. (a) Shortened, abducted and externally rotated

Ref: Essential Orthopaedics, Maheshwari 5th ed. pg. 134

The image shows fracture of neck of femur on right side. This is commonly seen due to trivial trauma in older patients. Minimal limb shortening can be seen with limb showing flexion, abduction and external rotation.

FMGE Solutions Screening Examination

16. A 40-year-old male complains of hot flushes each time he bathes. Hb: 20%gm, Platelet: 1,89,000/mm³, WBC: 30,000/mm³, Investigation revealed JAK2 mutation. What is the most likely diagnosis?
    a. Progressive massive fibrosis
    b. Chronic myeloid leukaemia
    c. Polycythemia vera
    d. Essential thrombocytosis

Ans. (c) Polycythemia vera

Ref: Harrison 20th ed. pg. 734

The clinical diagnosis of polycythemia is based on presence of JAK 2 mutation with elevated cell counts and *characteristic aquagenic pruritus*. The elevated basophils produce histamine which leads to intense pruritus, after exposure to water.

17. A patient with thalassemia with a need of recurrent transfusion, develops transfusion reaction like fever and chills. What can be done to the blood to decrease the rate transfusion reactions?
    a. Leucocyte depletion   b. Antibiotics
    c. Deglycerolization   d. Washed RBCs

Ans. (a) Leucocyte depletion

Ref: Wintrobe' Clinical Hematology: 13th ed. pg. 554

- In setting of recurrent transfusions, the donor leucocytes increase the risk of development of febrile nonhemolytic transfusions as well as graft versus host disease.
- Of the methods available to reduce the number of WBC in blood products, washing of red cells, freezing and deglycerolization are effective and yield a product with short shelf life. Modern generation of leukoreduction filters and apheresis machines can provide greater than 4 log reduction of WBC.
- Leukoreduction of blood products should produce blood products with residual WBC <5 X 10⁶ per unit (99.9 percent or log 3 reduction).

18. A CKD patient had to undergo dialysis. His Hb was 5.2 gm% so two blood transfusions were to be given. First bag was completed in 2 hours. Second was started and midway he developed shortness of breath, hypertension. Vitals: BP 180/120 mm Hg and pulse rate 110/min. What is the cause?
    a. Allergy
    b. Transfusion related circulatory overload
    c. TRALI
    d. FNHTR

Ans. (b) Transfusion related circulatory overload

Ref: Harrison 20th ed. pg. 814

- This CKD patient has developed severe anemia which is a compensated heart failure state. *The patient was given first unit of blood in two hours instead of standard four hours and he is already in compensated heart failure.*
- The acute decompensation due to volume overloading that has subsequently occurred will result in pulmonary edema and shortness of breath. This presentation is called as transfusion associated circulatory overload.
- Ideally patients of CKD should be given erythropoietin injections to reduce the incidence of having severe anemia.

19. A 57-year-old man presents with sudden onset of severe and central chest pain radiating to the back. ECG shows ST segment elevation in lead V1-V6, I, aVL. The chest X-ray shows a widened mediastinum. The diagnosis is:
    a. Aortic dissection
    b. Acute cor pulmonale
    c. Acute myocardial infarction
    d. Acute Pericarditis

Ans. (a) Aortic dissection

Ref: CMDT 2019 pg. 496

The ECG finding of ST Elevation prompts diagnosis of Myocardial infarction. But the CXR showing mediastinal widening is the key word which favors diagnosis as tear in the aorta.

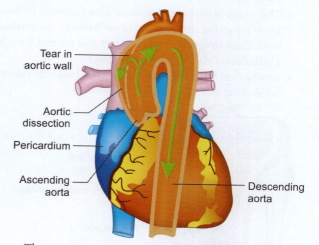

The answer is aortic dissection which exhibits a retrograde extension that can affect the coronary artery and can explain the resultant MI in this patient.

Clinical Pattern Questions

20. A 43-year-old 190 cm man post a flight to Chennai presents with left-sided chest discomfort and dyspnea. On chest X-ray, there is a small area devoid of lung markings in the apex of the left lung. Diagnosis is?
    a. Spontaneous pneumothorax
    b. Myocardial infarction
    c. Acute cor pulmonale
    d. Aortic dissection

Ans. (a) Spontaneous pneumothorax

Ref: CMDT 2019 pg. 325

Spontaneous pneumothorax occurs from a rupture of an apical pleural bleb and is associated with tall, young males and is also seen with *aeroplane ascent.*

21. A 52-year-old businessman with nephrotic syndrome after a non-stop flight from New York to New Delhi presents with sudden onset of breathlessness, hemoptysis, and chest pain. He is brought into Casualty in shock. His chest X-ray is normal. The ECG shows sinus tachycardia. The diagnosis is:
    a. Pneumothorax   b. Myocardial infarction
    c. Pulmonary embolism d. Aortic dissection

Ans. (c) Pulmonary embolism

Ref: CMDT 2019 pg. 312

- Long distance air travel is contraindicated in patients with hypercoagulable state. Patients of nephrotic syndrome have a hypercoagulable state. This patient has developed pulmonary embolism. *Pulmonary embolism leads to Sinus tachycardia. The small clots obstructing the small blood vessels of lungs cannot be seen in CXR. Hence the CXR is normal.*
- Choice A on CXR will show Deep sulcus sign and absent vascular shadows. Choice C will show bat wing pulmonary edema. Choice D will show pulmonary edema and widened mediastinum.

22. A 42-year-old man presents with central, crushing chest pain that radiates to the jaw. The pain occurred while jogging around the local park. The pain was alleviated with rest. The ECG is normal. Diagnosis is?
    a. Angina pectoris   b. Acute Pericarditis
    c. STEMI   d. NSTEMI

Ans. (a) Angina pectoris

Ref: CMDT 2019 pg. 369

The patient is having chest pain on jogging which is a presentation of chronic stable Angina. It is aggravated by cold, by anxiety, and by exercise. In the case of a normal resting ECG, an exercise ECG should be obtained. All other choices present with chest pain on rest.

23. A 53-year-old woman with ovarian tumor presents with breathlessness and right-sided chest pain. The chest X-ray shows obliteration of the right costophrenic angle. Diagnosis?
    a. Pleurisy
    b. Pericarditis
    c. Myocardial infarction
    d. Parapneumonic effusion

Ans. (a) Pleurisy

Ref: CMDT 2019 pg. 323

Ovarian tumor (Fibroma and thecoma) can be associated with a right-sided pleural effusion (Meigs syndrome). The obliteration of CP angle on X-ray is another pointer for pleural involvement of this patient.

24. A 32-year-old man involved in a high-speed Road traffic accident is found unconscious at the scene. He is breathing spontaneously. In Accident and emergency, the ECG monitor now shows an irregular rhythm and no P, QRS, ST, or T waves. The rate is rapid. Which is the best management of this patient?
    a. CPR until a defibrillator is present
    b. IV adrenaline
    c. Urgent Echo guided pericardiocentesis
    d. IV amiodarone

Ans. (a) CPR until a defibrillator is present

Ref: CMDT 2019 pg. 411

The patient is in ventricular fibrillation and needs an urgent CPR to maintain blood flow to the brain in ratio of 30:2.

FMGE Solutions Screening Examination

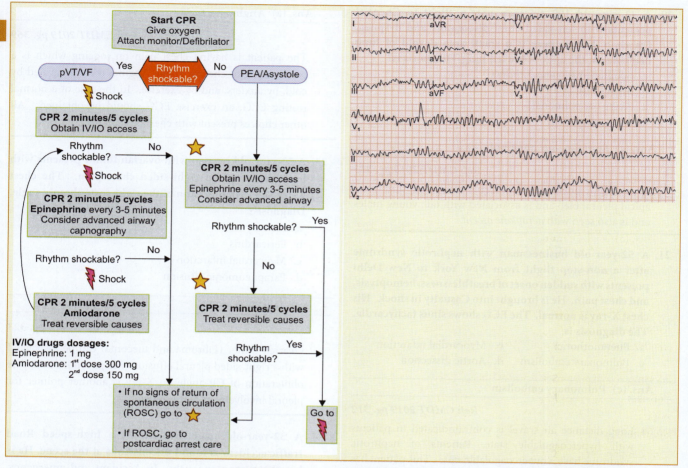

FIGURE: AHA ACLS cardiac arrest algorithm

25. **A 53-year-old man presents to Casualty with severe chest pain. He has a history of angina. ECG shows ST elevation of 4 mm in leads V_1 and V_4. Thrombolysis has been done but pain and ECG findings are persisting 90 minutes after start of thrombolysis. What is the best management of this patient?**

    a. Rescue PCI
    b. Primary PCI
    c. Delayed PCI
    d. IV Abciximab

Ans. (a) Rescue PCI

Ref: CMDT 2019 pg. 386

The patient is having failure of thrombolysis. In case of failure of thrombolysis, rescue PCI is performed. Primary PCI is done for STEMI. Delayed PCI is done for NSTEMI and hence are ruled out.

26. **A 42-year-old pedestrian has been struck by a speeding car driven by a juvenile. She is brought into emergency wearing a pneumatic anti-shock garment for an extensive injury to her pelvis which is distorted. She is intubated with fluids running via two grey color cannulas. Her current blood pressure is 100/60 mm Hg. Which is the next step in management of this patient?**

    a. Transfuse O negative blood and apply external fixator
    b. Start Packed RBC and perform exploratory laparotomy
    c. Start Packed RBC and perform decompressive hemicraniectomy
    d. Start vasopressors and perform pelvic drainage of blood

Ans. (a) Transfuse O negative blood and apply external fixator

Ref: CMDT 2019 pg. 507-8

This patient's chief concern will be massive blood loss. No delay should be taken to crossmatch blood. Ideally O negative Blood should be transfused immediately. The blood pressure may be misleading, as she is wearing an anti-shock garment. An external fixator applied by the surgeons will aid in pelvic fracture stabilisation and stem blood loss.

Clinical Pattern Questions

27. **A 10-year-old boy with smoke inhalation is brought into Casualty with worsening stridor. A face mask with 100% oxygen is covering his face, but his oxygen saturation continues to fall. What is next step in management of this patient?**
    a. Emergency tracheostomy
    b. Hyperbaric oxygen therapy
    c. Urgent intubation with positive pressure ventilation
    d. Extracorporeal membrane oxygenation

Ans. (a) Emergency tracheostomy

Ref: CMDT 2019 pg. 316

Due to hot smoke probably both the nasopharynx and oropharynx are compromised, and a tracheostomy to achieve an airway is essential. Choice B is used for management of carbon monoxide poisoning which may be considered in this patient but would be performed after tracheostomy has failed to relieve symptoms of this patient.

28. **A 4-year-old asthmatic child is brought to casualty. She is not speaking and has fast shallow breathing with pulsus paradoxus. ABG shows respiratory acidosis. What is the next best step in management of this patient?**
    a. Urgent endotracheal intubation
    b. Hyperbaric oxygen therapy
    c. MDI with salbutamol and corticosteroids
    d. Terbutaline subcutaneous with aminophylline drip

Ans. (a) Urgent endotracheal intubation

Ref: CMDT 2019 pg. 256

The child is having impending respiratory arrest due to severe exacerbation of asthma. Carbon dioxide narcosis will necessitate elective intubation and ventilation.

	Mild	Moderate	Severe	Respiratory arrest imminent
Symptoms				
Breathlessness	While walking	At rest, limits activity	At rest, interferes with conversation	While at rest, mute
Talks in	Sentences	Phrases	Words	Silent
Alertness	May be agitated	Usually agitated	Usually agitated	Drowsy confused
Sings				
Respiratory rate	Increased	Increased	Often >30/minute	>30/minute
Body position	Can lie down	Prefers sitting	Sits upright	Unable to recline
Use of accessory muscles; suprasternal retraction	Usually not	Commonly	Usually	Paradoxical thoracoabdominal movement
Wheeze	Moderate, often only end expiratory	Loud; throughout exhalation	Usually loud; throughout inhalation and exhalation	Absent
Pulse/minute	<100	100–120	>120	Bradycardia
Pulsus paradoxus	Absent <10 mm Hg	May be present 10–25 mm Hg	Often present >25 mm Hg	Absence suggests respiratory muscle fatigue

29. **A 13-year-old known asthmatic presents with severe wheezing and a respiratory rate of 40. Her pulse rate is 120. What is the next best step in management of this patient?**
    a. Oxygen and nebulized salbutamol
    b. Oxygen and Metered dose inhaler of salmeterol
    c. Oxygen and intravenous Aminophylline
    d. Oxygen and Intravenous magnesium sulphate

Ans. (a) Oxygen and nebulised salbutamol

Ref: CMDT 2019 pg. 256

An acute asthmatic attack is treated initially with oxygen and salbutamol. If necessary IV hydrocortisone is added.

30. **A 33-year-old cyclist is struck by a car in a head-on collision and arrives intubated to emergency department. Upon arrival, his Glasgow Coma Scale is 3. He has fixed and dilated pupils with absent gag reflex and with absence of spontaneous breathing efforts. EEG shows isolated bursts along a flat line. What is the next step in management of this patient?**
    a. Pronounce the patient as brain dead
    b. Do urgent craniotomy
    c. Do urgent ventriculostomy
    d. Do urgent Burr hole surgery

FMGE Solutions Screening Examination

Ans. (a) Pronounce the patient as brain dead

Ref: Bailey and Love, 26th ed. pg. 1418

A Glasgow Coma Scale of 3 is the lowest score possible with absent gag reflex and light reflex, no breathing efforts. If indicate brain-stem death. This is further confirmed by flat line on EEG.

American Academy of Neurology (AAN) guidelines for brain death in adults require one neurologic examination and one apnea test. Pediatric brain death guidelines from the American Academy of Pediatrics, Child Neurology Society, and Society of Critical Care medicine require two different physicians to conduct two neurologic examinations and two apnea tests, separated by an observation period.

AAN Guidelines for Brain Death in Adults

Clinical evaluation (prerequisites)	Clinical evaluation (neurologic assessment)	Ancillary tests	Documentation
Establish irreversible and proximate cause of come	The following must be assessed	Ordered only if	Time of death is documented
Achieve normal core temperature	Coma	Clinical examination cannot be performed	A checklist is filled out, signed, and dated
Achieve normal systolic blood pressure	Absence of brainstem reflexes	Apnea testing is inconclusive or aborted	
Perform one neurologic examination	Apnea		

31. A 62-year-old man is brought to Accident and emergency following assault to the head. He has a face mask and reservoir bag delivering 15L/min of oxygen, a stiff cervical collar and is attached to an intravenous drip. He has no spontaneous eye opening except to pain, makes incomprehensible sounds, and does not obey commands. He demonstrates flexion withdrawal to painful stimuli. On suction, he has no gag reflex. What is the next best step in management of this patient?
    a. Intubate the patient
    b. Urgent decompressive hemicraniectomy
    c. Urgent NCCT head
    d. Give mannitol and perform burr hole surgery

Ans. (a) Intubate the patient

Ref: AHA 2015 Guidelines

A GCS of 8 or less or absence of a gag reflex are both indications for urgent intubation. The patient has sustained head injury and after securing his airway, imaging would be performed to asses nature of CNS injury.

32. A 17-year-old girl presents with fever, odd behaviour, purpura, and conjunctival petechiae. Her lumbar puncture reveals Gram-negative cocci. Best treatment of this patient is?
    a. Ceftriaxone with vancomycin
    b. Ampicillin with gentamycin
    c. Ceftriaxone with dexamethasone
    d. Piperacillin with tazobactam

Ans. (a) Ceftriaxone with vancomycin

Ref: CMDT 2019 pg. 1305

The clinical diagnosis is Meningococcal meningitis and empirical ceftriaxone is started with vancomycin.

Indication	Antibiotic
Preterm infants to infants <1 month	Ampicillin + cefotaxime
Infants 1–3 months	Ampicillin + cefotaxime or ceftriaxone
Immunocompetent children >3 months and adults <55	Cefotaxime, ceftriaxone, or cefeprime + vancomycin

Contd...

Clinical Pattern Questions

Indication	Antibiotic
Adults >55 and adults or any age with alcoholism or other debilitating illnesses	Ampicillin + cefotaxime, ceftriaxone or cefepime + vancomycin
Hospital-acquired meningitis, post-traumatic or postneurosurgery meningitis, neutropenic patients, or patients with impaired cell-mediated immunity	Ampicillin + ceftazidime or meropenem + vancomycin

33. A 22-year-old woman presents with a plethora of signs and symptoms. She complains of arthralgia, depression, alopecia, fits, oral ulceration, and facial rash. She is found to have proteinuria and a normocytic normochromic anaemia. What is the best test for her diagnosis?
    a. Anti-Nuclear antibody
    b. Anti-Smith antibody
    c. Anti-Ribosomal P antibody
    d. Anti-Topoisomerase Antibody

Ans. (a) Anti-Nuclear antibody

Ref: CMDT 2019 pg. 855

The clinical diagnosis of patient is Systemic lupus erythematosus and diagnosis is based on positive ANA.

34. A 67-year-old hypertensive man presents with lower abdominal pain and back pain. An expansive abdominal mass is palpated lateral and superior to the umbilicus. What is the best investigation for this patient?
    a. X-ray KUB
    b. Ultrasound abdomen
    c. Coronary angiography
    d. Intravenous Pyelography

Ans. (b) Ultrasound abdomen

Ref: CMDT 2019 pg. 492

The presentation is suggestive of abdominal aortic aneurysm. The size should be evaluated by ultrasound and surgical repair is advisable if the aneurysm is greater than 5.5 cm in diameter as it can exhibit spontaneous rupture.

35. An 83-year-old woman suffering from rheumatoid arthritis presents with severe epigastric pain and vomiting. She also complains of shoulder tip pain. What investigation should be done in the emergency room?
    a. USG chest
    b. Serum electrolytes
    c. Upper GI endoscopy
    d. Erect chest X-ray

Ans. (d) Erect chest X-ray

Ref: CMDT 2019 pg. 640

Steroid usage for rheumatoid arthritis puts this woman at risk for a perforated peptic ulcer. Hence an urgent Erect CXR should be done to look for gas under diaphragm.

36. A 42-year-old woman with benign ovarian tumor presents with ascites and breathlessness. CXR is performed. The clinical diagnosis is?

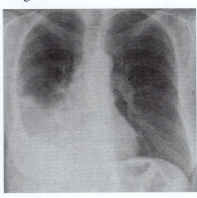

    a. Meigs syndrome
    b. Dressler syndrome
    c. Budd-Chiari syndrome
    d. Cholangiocarcinoma

Ans. (a) Meigs syndrome

Ref: CMDT 2019 page 323

- The CXR shows presence of right sided pleural effusion along with history of ascites and a benign ovarian tumor. This a triad seen in Meigs syndrome.
- Choice B is seen in post MI patients
- Choice C leads to acute onset ascites and right upper quadrant pain
- Choice D leads to obstructive jaundice and cachexia.

37. A 25-year-old woman develops nausea, vomiting, and abdominal pain. On examination, she has tender hepatomegaly and ascites. She was recently started on oral contraceptives. The clinical diagnosis is?
    a. Budd-Chiari syndrome
    b. Acute viral hepatitis
    c. Portal hypertension
    d. Acute cholecystitis

Ans. (a) Budd–Chiari syndrome

Ref: CMDT 2019 page 726

Budd-Chiari syndrome occurs from thrombosis of the major hepatic veins and has been associated with oral contraceptives. The main diagnostic features are

- Right upper quadrant pain and tenderness
- Ascites
- Imaging studies show occlusion/absence of flow in the hepatic vein(s) or inferior vena cava
- Clinical picture is similar in sinusoidal obstruction syndrome but major hepatic veins are patent.

FMGE Solutions Screening Examination

38. A 42-year-old woman presents with ascites. On examination, she has large 'a' wave in JVP and a low volume pulse. She has history of rheumatic fever. Clinical diagnosis is?

a. Right ventricular hypertrophy due to pulmonary artery hypertension
b. Right ventricular failure due to tricuspid regurgitation
c. Left heart failure due to mitral stenosis
d. Left heart failure due to aortic regurgitation

Ans. (a) Right ventricular hypertrophy due to pulmonary artery hypertension

Ref: CMDT 2019 pg. 347

- The most common valvular lesion in rheumatic etiology is mitral stenosis. Long standing mitral stenosis leads to pulmonary edema and resultant Pulmonary artery hypertension. This will lead to compensatory right ventricular hypertrophy.
- Choice B is ruled out as it leads to large V wave in JVP.
- Choice C is ruled as mitral stenosis does not lead to left heart but right heart enlargement
- Choice D does not lead to ascites, and instead leads to collapsing pulse.

39. A 52-year-old woman presents with exertional fatigue and ascites. She is noted to have a rapid, irregular pulse rate. The chest X-ray reveals a small heart with calcification seen on the lateral view. The 12-lead ECG demonstrates low QRS voltage. Clinical diagnosis is?

a. Rheumatic pancarditis
b. Constrictive pericarditis
c. Restrictive cardiomyopathy
d. Acute cor pulmonale

Ans. (b) Constrictive pericarditis

Ref: CMDT 2019 page 441

The presence of rapid irregular pulse points to presence of atrial fibrillation. The CXR finding of calcification narrows down the diagnosis to constrictive pericarditis. The impaired filling of ventricles explains the ascites. Since the left side of heart also receives less blood it can explain presence of exertional fatigue. Low voltage ECG occurs due to calcification impairing the flow of current to recording electrodes.

40. A 34-year-old female presents with hypertension, pinched facies and progressive dysphagia with decreased tone of lower esophageal sphincter (LES) The clinical diagnosis is?

a. Scleroderma   b. Hiatus hernia
c. Rolling hernia   d. Diffuse esophageal spasm

Ans. (a) Scleroderma

Ref: CMDT 2019 page 323

- Pinched facies with hypertension points to presence of scleroderma. The tone of LES is reduced in scleroderma due to fibrosis.
- Choice B and C can lead to GERD but it does not have other features like systemic hypertension.
- Choice D presents with chest pain and dysphagia and is hence ruled out.

41. A 70-year-old man presents with a 16-week history of progressive dysphagia, and recurrent pneumonia episodes. He also has palpable stony hard neck nodes on examination. Diagnosis is?

a. Carcinoma of the esophagus
b. Achalasia Cardia
c. Diffuse esophageal spasm
d. Zenker's diverticulum

Ans. (a) Carcinoma of the esophagus

Ref: Bailey and Love, 26ᵗʰ ed. page 1004

Esophageal cancer presents with mechanical symptoms, principally dysphagia, but sometimes also regurgitation. The main feature for malignancy in this case is stony hard consistency of neck Lymph nodes.

42. A 70-year-old man presents with regurgitation of food, dysphagia, halitosis, and a sensation of 'lump in the throat'.

a. Pharyngeal pouch
b. Carcinoma esophagus
c. Diffuse esophageal spasm
d. Esophageal Dysmotility

Ans. (a) Pharyngeal pouch

Ref: Bailey and Love, 26ᵗʰ ed. page 1018

The key word is regurgitation of food with dysphagia which is seen with Pharyngeal pouch. When it is small, symptoms largely reflect only in-coordination with predominantly pharyngeal dysphagia. As the pouch enlarges, it tends to fill with food on eating, and the fundus descends into the mediastinum. This leads to halitosis and esophageal dysphagia.

43. A 63-year-old man recently treated for renal tuberculosis presents with weight loss, diarrhea, hypoglycemia, hypotension, and is noted to have hyperpigmented buccal mucosa, palmar and hand creases. Which investigation is most suitable for this clinical presentation?

a. Serum iron and ferritin
b. Serum copper and ceruloplasmin
c. Plasma ACTH and cortisol
d. Gene XPERT and Intravenous pyelography

Ans. (c) Plasma ACTH and cortisol

Ref: CMDT 2019 page 323

- The key finding of hyperpigmentation of buccal mucosa, palmar and sole creases point to etiology of Addison disease. The leading cause of Addison's disease in India is tuberculosis.
- The presence of hypotension indicates hypoaldosteronism in Addison's disease. Simultaneous mention of hypoglycemia indicates cortisol deficiency.
- Choice B is done in case of hemochromatosis and bronze diabetes
- Choice C is done in case of Wilson disease
- Choice D is done in for diagnosis of tuberculosis

44. **A 66-year-old man presents with a sudden onset of diabetes, anorexia, weight loss, epigastric pain with radiation to back. Next best investigation for this patient is?**
    a. Ultrasound of abdomen
    b. CT abdomen
    c. Enteroclysis
    d. Triple contrast barium enema

Ans. (b) CT abdomen

Ref: Bailey and Love: 26th ed. page 1137

- The clinical history of epigastric pain radiating to back points to pancreatic etiology. This patient may have developed pancreatic cancer. Sudden onset of diabetes in the elderly is also suggestive. *The best imaging modality to image chronic pancreatitis or pancreatic malignancy is CT abdomen.*
- Choice A is ruled out as gas shadows of stomach obscure ultrasound view of pancreas.
- Choice C is fluoroscopic intubation-infusion small-bowel examination which is used to evaluate for small bowel pathology while this patient has pancreatic lesion
- Choice D is ruled out as it used for large bowel evaluation.

45. **A 53-year-old woman presents with weight loss, increased appetite, sweating, palpitations, and preference for cold weather, hot, moist palms, and tremors. What is the best investigation for the clinical diagnosis of this patient?**
    a. TSH levels   b. Autoimmune panel
    c. Plasma catecholamines d. Plasma Cortisol

Ans. (a) TSH levels

Ref: CMDT 2019 page 1139

This patient presents with classic signs and symptoms of hyperthyroidism. The increased Basal metabolic rate and calorigenesis explain the symptoms of the patient. These patients have highly suppressed TSH levels. The highlights of hyperthyroidism are:

- Sweating, weight loss or gain, anxiety, palpitations, loose stools, heat intolerance, fatigue, menstrual irregularity.
- Tachycardia; warm, moist skin; stare; tremor.
- **Graves disease:** Majority have a palpable goiter (sometimes with bruit); ophthalmopathy.
- Suppressed TSH in primary hyperthyroidsim; usually increased T_4, FT_4, T_3, FT_3.

46. **A 69-year-old man is noted to have a glucose level of 600mg% and a Na of 163 mmol/L. pH of blood is normal. There is no previous history of Diabetes mellitus. What is best management for this patient?**
    a. Insulin sliding scale and 5% dextrose
    b. Insulin sliding scale and 0.9% normal saline
    c. Insulin sliding scale and 3% saline
    d. Insulin sliding scale and 0.45% saline

Ans. (b) Insulin sliding scale and 0.9% normal saline

Ref: CMDT 2019, page 323

- The blood sugar of 600 mg% leads to increased plasma osmolality and resultant fluid shift across the brain leading to loss of consciousness.
- The clinical diagnosis is nonketotic hyperosmolar coma.
- It occurs in patients with mild or occult diabetes, and most patients are typically middle-aged to elderly.
- It is characterized by severe hyperglycemia in the absence of significant ketosis, with hyperosmolality and dehydration.

47. **A patient tested positive for MTB on sputum CBNAAT. He did not come again to the hospital despite multiple reminders. Today he presents with massive hemoptysis and is alarmed. What is the next best step for this patient?**
    a. Urgent coagulation studies
    b. Perform multi slice CT scan chest
    c. Schedule a flexible fibre optic biopsy
    d. Urgent rigid bronchoscopy and prophylactic balloon tamponade

Ans. (b) Perform multi slice CT scan chest

Ref: CMDT 2019, page 26-27

Multislice computed tomography is the diagnostic imaging modality that yields most information on the cause and site of hemoptysis.

FMGE Solutions Screening Examination

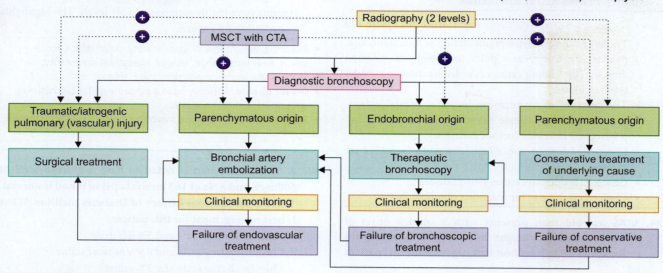

48. A 45-year-old smoker presents with sudden onset unrelenting chest pain with loss of peripheral pulses. BP measured in both arms is different. First differential diagnosis is?
    a. Mirizzi syndrome
    b. Aortic dissection
    c. Viral pericarditis
    d. Spontaneous pneumothorax

Ans. (b) Aortic dissection

Ref: CMDT 2019, page 28

The clinical presentation of chest pain with loss of peripheral pulses points to diagnosis of aortic dissection. The antegrade progression of tear leads to unequal BP between left and right arms.

49. A patient develops chest pain after bout of vomiting with subcutaneous emphysema. Comment on the diagnosis.

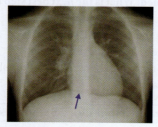

    a. Eventration of diaphragm
    b. Hampton hump
    c. Pneumomediastinum
    d. Water bottle heart

Ans. (c) Pneumomediastinum

Ref: Bailey and Love, 26th edition, page 992

The CXR shows continuous diaphragm sign. The presence of vomiting, chest pain and subcutaneous emphysema points to Mackler's triad of Boerhaave's syndrome. The rupture of esophagus due to vomiting against a closed glottis leads to contents of esophagus to spill over into mediastinum. This leads to chemical mediastinitis and pneumomediastinum.

50. A 70-year-old woman has a progressive neurological disorder resulting in degeneration of the anterior horn cells throughout her spinal cord and brainstem. Which of the following abnormal movements is she most likely to exhibit?
    a. Asterixis
    b. Chorea
    c. Fasciculations
    d. Gait Apraxia

Ans. (c) Fasciculations

Ref: Ganong 25th edition, Page 240

- The lesion at anterior horn cells of spinal cord leads to lower motor neuron lesion of spinal cord. It causes twitching of muscles leading to fasciculations.
- Choice A is seen in hepatic and uremic encephalopathy
- Choice B is seen in basal ganglia damage
- Choice D is seen in frontal lobe damage.

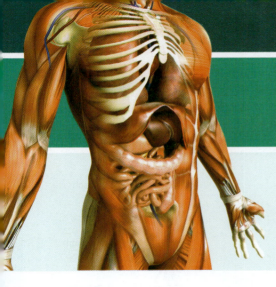

Anatomy

MOST RECENT QUESTIONS 2019

1. An injury to the shown area can lead to fracture of which bone?

   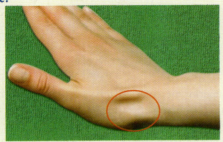

   a. Scaphoid   b. Lunate
   c. Trapezium   d. Hamate

2. Identify the marked muscle tendon in the diagram

   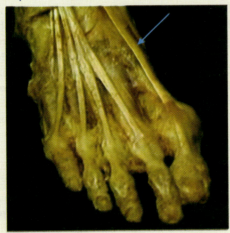

   a. Flexor hallucis longus
   b. Extensor hallucis longus
   c. Extensor digitorum longus
   d. Tibialis anterior

3. Which muscle originates from medial epicondyle of humerus?
   a. Supinator   b. Pronator teres
   c. Pronator quadratus d. Brachioradialis

4. Killian dehiscence is formed due to:
   a. Superior constrictor muscle
   b. Inferior constrictor muscle
   c. Middle pharyngeal constrictor muscle
   d. Esophageal fibres

5. Glossopharyngeal nerve supplies which of the following gland?
   a. Parotid gland   b. Submandibular gland
   c. Sublingual gland   d. Lacrimal gland

6. Failure of closure of rostral neuropore at 25th day leads to:
   a. Rachischisis   b. Spina bifida
   c. Anencephaly   d. Hydranencephaly

7. A patient presents with hypothenar muscle wasting and loss of sensation of medial one and a half digits. Which nerve is involved?
   a. Ulnar nerve
   b. Median nerve
   c. Radial nerve
   d. Musculocutaneous nerve

8. Identify the muscle marked in the diagram:

   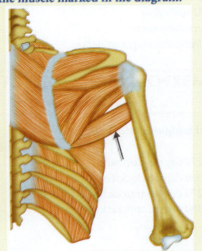

   a. Teres major   b. Teres minor
   c. Infraspinatus   d. Supraspinatus

FMGE Solutions Screening Examination

9. Deep inguinal ring is formed in:
    a. Transversus abdominis
    b. Transversalis fascia
    c. External oblique aponeurosis
    d. Internal oblique aponeurosis
10. Inguinal ligament is formed due to:
    a. External oblique aponeurosis
    b. Transversus abdominis
    c. Internal oblique aponeurosis
    d. Inguinal muscle
11. Abduction at the hip joint is done by:
    a. Gluteus maximus
    b. Obturator internus
    c. Quadratus femoris
    d. Gluteus medius
12. Inferior scapular angle is at which level?
    a. T4
    b. T6
    c. T8
    d. T2
13. Testicular artery is a branch of:
    a. Common iliac artery
    b. Abdominal aorta
    c. Internal iliac artery
    d. External iliac artery
14. Flexion, adduction and medial rotation of arm is done by which muscle?
    a. Pectoralis minor
    b. Pectoralis major
    c. Subclavius
    d. Serratus Anterior
15. Upper lateral cutaneous nerve of arm is a branch of:
    a. Radial nerve
    b. Ulnar nerve
    c. Axillary nerve
    d. Musculocutaneous nerve

EMBRYOLOGY HISTOLOGY AND OSTEOLOGY

16. Fetal midgut rotates in IUL:
    (Recent Pattern Question 2018-19)
    a. 270 degree clockwise
    b. 360 degree clockwise
    c. 270 degree anticlockwise
    d. 360 degree anticlockwise

17. Rotation of mid gut loop occurs around:
    (Recent Pattern Question 2018-19)

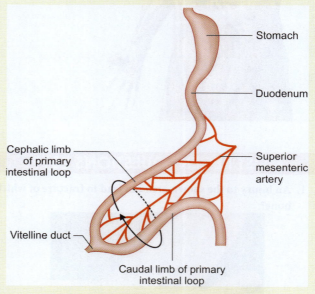

    a. Superior mesenteric artery
    b. Inferior mesenteric artery
    c. Middle-colic artery
    d. Superior rectal artery
18. Neural crest cell migration is due to:
    (Recent Pattern Question 2018)
    a. Heparin   b. Heparan sulfate
    c. Hyaluronic acid   d. Dermal sulfate
19. Which of the following is the derivative of ultimobranchial body?
    (Recent Pattern Question 2018)
    a. Thyroid   b. Parafollicular 'C' cells
    c. Capsule of thyroid d. 2nd branchial pouch
20. Which of the following is the derivative of tumor from Rathke's pouch?
    (Recent Pattern Question 2018)
    a. Meningioma   b. Craniopharyngioma
    c. Ependymoma   d. Low grade glioma
21. Hardest bone of the body is?
    (Recent Pattern Question 2017)
    a. Head of humerus b. Calcaneum
    c. Tibial condyle   d. Osseus labyrinth
22. Which of the following structure is derived from umbilical artery?
    (Recent Pattern Question 2017)
    a. Ligamentum arteriosum b. Medial umbilical ligament
    c. Ligamentum venosum   d. Ligamentum teres
23. Labia majora is homologous to _____ in a male.
    (Recent Pattern Question 2017)
    a. Glans penis   b. Scrotum
    c. Corpus cavernosa d. Shaft of penis

ANATOMY

Anatomy

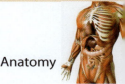

24. Morula cell stage has how many cells?
    (Recent Pattern Question 2017)
    a. 8
    b. 16
    c. 32
    d. >64

25. Umbilical cord has: *(Recent Pattern Question 2017)*
    a. One artery, two veins and umbilical artery going to fetus
    b. One artery, two veins and umbilical artery going to placenta
    c. Two arteries and one vein, umbilical artery supplying towards fetus
    d. Two arteries and one vein, umbilical vein supplying towards fetus

26. In the Umbilical cord which of the following structure does not get obliterated during fetal life?
    (Recent Pattern Question 2017)
    a. Vitelline duct
    b. Vitelline vessels
    c. Allantois
    d. Umbilical vessels

27. What is correct about embryogenesis?
    (Recent Pattern Question 2017)
    a. Branchial cleft: Mesoderm
    b. Branchial arch: Ectoderm
    c. Branchial pouch: Endoderm
    d. All are correct

28. Superior vena cava is derived from:
    (Recent Pattern Question 2017)
    a. Aortic arch
    b. Pharyngeal arch
    c. Cardinal vein
    d. Vitelline vein

29. Arch of aorta is derived from:
    (Recent Pattern Question 2017)
    a. 2nd aortic arch
    b. 3rd aortic arch
    c. 3rd pharyngeal arch
    d. 4th pharyngeal arch

30. Common carotid artery is derived from:
    (Recent Pattern Question 2017)
    a. 2nd aortic arch
    b. 3rd pharyngeal arch
    c. 4th pharyngeal arch
    d. 6th pharyngeal arch

31. Stylohyoid ligament is derived from:
    (Recent Pattern Question 2017)
    a. 1st branchial arch
    b. 2nd branchial arch
    c. 1st branchial pouch
    d. 2nd branchial pouch

32. Sphenomandibular ligament is derived from which branchial arch? *(Recent Pattern Question 2017)*
    a. 1
    b. 2
    c. 3
    d. 4

33. Which of the following is a derivative of 2nd branchial arch? *(Recent Pattern Question 2017)*
    a. Stylophyoid ligament
    b. Sphenomandibular ligament
    c. Spine of sphenoid
    d. Greater cornu of hyoid

34. Lesser cornu of hyoid bone is derived from which arch?
    a. 1st mandibular arch
    b. 2nd branchial arch
    c. 3rd branchial arch
    d. 4th branchial arch

35. Superior portion of hyoid bone is derived from which branchial arch?
    a. I
    b. II
    c. III
    d. IV

36. All of the following muscles are derived from 6th branchial arch EXCEPT:
    a. Lateral cricoarytenoid
    b. Posterior cricoarytenoid
    c. Interarytenoid
    d. Cricothyroid

37. Which of the following does not develop from branchial pouch?
    a. Superior parathyroid
    b. Inferior parathyroid
    c. Thymus
    d. Thyroid

38. The auricle develops from:
    a. 1st branchial cleft
    b. 1st branchial arch
    c. 1st, 2nd and 3rd branchial arch
    d. 1st and 2nd branchial arch

39. Inferior parathyroid gland develops from:
    (Recent Pattern Question 2017)
    a. Branchial arch 3rd
    b. Branchial arch 4th
    c. Branchial pouch 3rd
    d. Branchial pouch 4th

40. Tonsil is derived from? *(Recent Pattern Question 2017)*
    a. 1st pouch
    b. 2nd pouch
    c. 3rd pouch
    d. 4th pouch

41. Which of the following is not derived from 1st pharyngeal pouch?
    a. Middle ear
    b. Eustachean tube
    c. Tympanic membrane
    d. Palatine tonsils

42. External auditory canal is formed from:
    (Recent Pattern Question 2017)
    a. Ventral part of 1st cleft
    b. Dorsal part of 1st cleft
    c. Ventral part of 2nd cleft
    d. Dorsal part of 2nd cleft

43. Lower 1/3 of vagina is formed by:
    (Recent Pattern Question 2017)
    a. Mesonephric duct
    b. Paramesonephric duct
    c. Sinovaginal bulb
    d. Mesoderm of mullerian duct

44. Hypoblast forms: *(Recent Pattern Question 2017)*
    a. Notochord
    b. Apical ligament of atlas
    c. Endoderm
    d. Prochordal plate

45. First organ to attain functional maturity is:
    (Recent Pattern Question 2017)
    a. CVS
    b. CNS
    c. GIT
    d. Lungs

46. Gastrulation occurs in which week of embryonic development? *(Recent Pattern Question 2017)*
    a. Week 1
    b. Week 2
    c. Week 3
    d. Week 4

FMGE Solutions Screening Examination

47. **First germ layer to be formed is:**
    a. Ectoderm *(Recent Pattern Question 2017)*
    b. Endoderm
    c. Mesoderm
    d. All of them develop simultaneously

48. **Notochord is formed by:** *(Recent Pattern Question 2017)*
    a. Nucleus pulposus   b. Epiblast
    c. Hypoblast   d. Myeloblast

49. **Homeobox gene is responsible for:**
    (Recent Pattern Question 2017)
    a. Segmental organization of embryo in craniocaudal direction
    b. Proper organization along dorsal ventral axis
    c. Stimulation for lengthening of limbs
    d. All of the above

50. **Chromaffin cells are derived from:**
    (Recent Pattern Question 2017)
    a. Neural crest   b. Surface ectoderm
    c. Neuroectoderm   d. Endoderm

51. **Pancreas is derived from:** *(Recent Pattern Question 2017)*
    a. Foregut   b. Midgut
    c. Hindgut   d. Notochord

52. **Proximal umbilical artery forms:**
    (Recent Pattern Question 2017)
    a. Superior vesical artery   b. Median umbilical fold
    c. Lateral umbilical fold   d. Ligamentum teres

53. **Ligamentum teres is a remnant of:**
    a. Ductus venosus   b. Ductus arteriosus
    c. Hypogastric artery   d. Umbilical vein

54. **Remnant of ductus venosus will be:**
    a. Ligamentum teres   b. Ligamentum venosum
    c. Ligamentum arteriosum   d. Falciform ligament

55. **Left horn of sinus venosus forms:**
    (Recent Pattern Question 2017)
    a. Coronary sinus   b. Smooth part of right atrium
    c. Superior vena cava   d. Inferior vena cava

56. **Stapedial artery is derived from which aortic arch:**
    (Recent Pattern Question 2017)
    a. 1   b. 2
    c. 3   d. 4

57. **Fossa ovalis is a remnant of:**
    (Recent Pattern Question 2017)
    a. Septum primum   b. Septum secondum
    c. Bulbus cordis   d. Conus

58. **In a fetus, testis lies at superficial inguinal ring at:**
    (Recent Pattern Question 2017)
    a. 6th month   b. 7th month
    c. 8th month   d. 9th month

59. **Pons is derived from:** *(Recent Pattern Question 2017)*
    a. Metencephalon   b. Mylencephalon
    c. Mesencephalon   d. Prosencephalon

60. **Glomerulus is derived from:**
    (Recent Pattern Question 2017)
    a. Metanephros   b. Mesonephros
    c. Ureteric bud   d. Urogenital sinus

61. **Prostate gland is derived from:**
    (Recent Pattern Question 2017)
    a. Urogenital sinus   b. Urogenital folds
    c. Labioscrotal swelling   d. Gubernaculum

62. **Collecting duct is derived from:**
    a. Ureteric bud   b. Mesonephros
    c. Metanephros   d. Allantois

63. **Synovial fluid is produced by:**
    (Recent Pattern Question 2017)
    a. Type A synoviocytes   b. Type B synoviocytes
    c. Type C synoviocytes   d. Type D synoviocytes

64. **Blue color cartilage is:** *(Recent Pattern Question 2017)*
    a. Hyaline   b. Elastic
    c. Fibrocartilage   d. Synchondrosis

65. **Tyson's glands are:** *(Recent Pattern Question 2017)*
    a. Apocrine glands   b. Holocrine gland
    c. Eccrine gland   d. Endocrine gland

66. **Fecal fistula at the umbilicus is due to:**
    a. Persistent urachus   *(Recent Pattern Question 2017)*
    b. Persistent vitellointestinal duct
    c. Raspberry tumor
    d. Sister Joseph nodules

67. **Failure of fusion of maxillary and medial nasal process leads to:** *(Recent Pattern Question 2017)*
    a. Cleft lip   b. Cleft palate
    c. Bifid uvula   d. Deviated nasal septum

68. **Ribs develop from:** *(Recent Pattern Question 2017)*
    a. Endothoracic fascia   b. Para-axial mesenchyme
    c. Deep intercostal fascia   d. Superficial intercostal fascia

69. **Pituitary develops from:** *(Recent Pattern Question 2017)*
    a. Posterior neural ridge   b. Rathke pouch
    c. Neural crest   d. Neural plate

70. **What is true about spermatogenesis?**
    a. It takes 74 days
    b. Takes place in spermatic cord
    c. Meiosis occurs only after secondary spermatocyte
    d. Spermatid is formed from spermatozoa

71. **Which of the following has the largest size?**
    a. Spermatogonium
    b. Primary spermatocyte
    c. Secondary spermatocyte
    d. Spermatozoa

72. **Spermatogonium to spermatozoon transformation takes place in:**
    a. 64 days   b. 74 days
    c. 84 days   d. 94 days

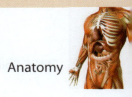

Anatomy

73. Sperm acquires motility in:
    a. Seminiferous tubule   b. Fallopian tube
    c. Epididymis   d. Spermatic cord
74. All the following statements about seminal vesicles are true EXCEPT:
    a. Stores the spermatozoa
    b. Actively depends on the level of testosterone
    c. Secretion has abundant fructose
    d. Lined by pseudostratified columnar epithelium
75. At what stage of embryonic development does an embryo normally begin to implant in the endometrium?
    a. Blastocyst   b. Four-cell stage
    c. Morula   d. Trilaminar embryo
76. Embryo term is used till:
    a. 12 weeks after LMP   b. 10 weeks after fertilization
    c. 10 weeks after LMP   d. 8 weeks of fertilization
77. Fetal stage is termed:
    a. From the day of implantation
    b. From 6th week of gestation
    c. From 8th week of gestation
    d. From 10th week of gestation
78. Which is not a derivative of midgut:
    a. Appendix   b. Jejunum
    c. Ascending colon   d. Descending colon
79. Which of the following artery mainly supplies hind gut?
    a. Celiac trunk   b. Superior mesenteric artery
    c. Inferior mesenteric artery d. Rectal artery
80. Adrenal medulla is derived from:
    a. Ectoderm   b. Endoderm
    c. Mesoderm   d. Neural crest
81. Germ cells develop from:
    a. Yolk sac   b. Surface ectoderm
    c. Coelomic endoderm   d. Trophoblastic layer
82. How may many ossification centres are there for the hyoid bone?
    a. 5   b. 4
    c. 6   d. 3
83. Trigone of urinary bladder develops from:
    a. Endoderm   b. Ectoderm
    c. Mesoderm   d. None
84. What are the vessels in umbilical cord?
    a. 1 artery, 2 veins   b. 2 arteries, 1 vein
    c. 1 artery, 1 vein   d. 2 arteries, 2 veins
85. What is the content of umbilical cord?
    a. 2 arteries, 1 vein   b. 2 veins, 1 artery
    c. 2 arteries, 2 veins   d. 1 artery, 1 vein
86. Testosterone in male is secreted from:
    a. Leydig cell   b. Sertoli cell
    c. Seminal vesicle   d. Epididymis

87. Gall bladder is lined by:
    a. Ciliated columnar cells
    b. Brush bordered columnar epithelium
    c. Striated columnar epithelium
    d. Pseudostratified columnar cells
88. Hassall's corpuscles are found in:
    a. Liver   b. Spleen
    c. Kidney   d. Thymus
89. Malphigian corpuscles are seen in:
    a. Thyroid   b. Kidney
    c. Neurons   d. Liver
90. Cord of billroth is seen in:
    a. Liver   b. Spleen
    c. Kidney   d. Thymus
91. T cells are derived from:
    a. Tonsils   b. Thymus
    c. Thalamus   d. Thyroid

UPPER LIMB

92. Identify the marked bone:
    (Recent Pattern Question 2018-19)

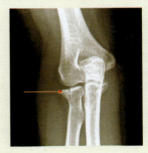

    a. Capitulum   b. Olecranon
    c. Trochlea   d. Radial head
93. Retraction of scapula at sternocleidomastoid joint is by:
    (Recent Pattern Question 2018-19)
    a. Serratus anterior   b. Trapezius
    c. Suprascapularis   d. Deltoid muscle
94. Winging of scapula is due to paralysis of:
    (Recent Pattern Question 2018-19)
    a. Nerve to trapezius
    b. Nerve to serratus anterior
    c. Nerve to latissimus dorsi
    d. Nerve to pectoralis major
95. In a patient with Fracture of upper radius and ulna at the insertion of pronator teres muscle, which movement is restricted:
    (Recent Pattern Question 2018-19)
    a. Pronation   b. Supination
    c. Hyperpronation   d. Hyperabduction

96. Which of the following is the insertion of the shown muscle? *(Recent Pattern Question 2018-19)*

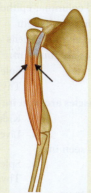

   a. Radial tuberosity
   b. Olecranon process
   c. Radial head
   d. Medial malleolus

97. Coracoid process of the scapula is: *(Recent Pattern Question 2018)*
   a. Pressure epiphysis
   b. Traction epiphysis
   c. Atavistic epiphysis
   d. Aberrant epiphysis

98. Which of the following is *not* a component of carpal tunnel? *(Recent Pattern Question 2018)*
   a. Ulnar nerve
   b. Median nerve
   c. Flexor digitorum superficialis
   d. Flexor digitorum profundus

99. Which structure passes through Guyon's canal? *(Recent Pattern Question 2018)*
   a. Ulnar nerve
   b. Median nerve
   c. Radial nerve
   d. Flexor carpi radialis

100. Which is the nerve root of Biceps jerk? *(Recent Pattern Question 2017)*
   a. C5-C6
   b. C6-C8
   c. C7-C8
   d. C8-T1

101. Angle of humeral torsion is _____ degrees? *(Recent Pattern Question 2017)*
   a. 15
   b. 35
   c. 135
   d. 164

102. Which carpal bone has a hook? *(Recent Pattern Question 2017)*
   a. Capitate
   b. Lunate
   c. Hamate
   d. Pisiformis

103. Which is the 1st carpal bone to ossify? *(Recent Pattern Question 2017)*
   a. Capitate
   b. Lunate
   c. Hamate
   d. Pisiformis

104. Which is not a part of proximal row of carpal bones? *(Recent Pattern Question 2017)*
   a. Scaphoid
   b. Lunate
   c. Triquetral
   d. Hamate

105. Which is the most commonly fractured carpal bone?
   a. Hamate
   b. Lunate
   c. Scaphoid
   d. Capitates

106. Articulation of pisiform bone is with:
   a. Triquetral
   b. Lunate
   c. Scaphoid
   d. Trapezoid

107. Middle trunk of branchial plexus is formed of: *(Recent Pattern Question 2017)*
   a. C6, C7
   b. C7, C8
   c. C8, T1
   d. C7

108. Regimental band anaesthesia is due to lesion of: *(Recent Pattern Question 2017)*
   a. Musculocutaneous nerve
   b. Axillary nerve
   c. Long thoracic nerve
   d. Spinal accessory nerve

109. Screwing movement in upper limb is possible with: *(Recent Pattern Question 2017)*
   a. Brachioradialis
   b. Anconeus
   c. Supinator
   d. Pronator teres

110. Radial artery ends as: *(Recent Pattern Question 2017)*
   a. Superficial palmar arch
   b. Deep palmar arch
   c. Both of above
   d. Profunda brachii artery

111. The largest bursa in the body is: *(Recent Pattern Question 2017)*
   a. Prepatellar bursa
   b. Infrapatellar bursa
   c. Subacromial bursa
   d. Trochanteric bursa

112. Which is the nerve passing through medial epicondyle?
   a. Ulnar
   b. Radial
   c. Median
   d. Posterior interosseus

113. Anastomosis of subscapular artery are formed by all EXCEPT:
   a. Transverse cervical artery
   b. Suprascapular artery
   c. 1st part of subclavian artery
   d. 2nd part of axillary artery

114. Which structure is present in the anatomical snuff box?
   a. Ulnar artery
   b. Radial artery
   c. Median nerve
   d. Radial nerve

115. Anatomical snuff box contains:
   a. Axillary nerve
   b. Radial artery
   c. Brachial artery
   d. Ulnar artery

116. The medial boundary of the anatomical snuffbox is formed by the:
   a. Ext. pollicis brevi
   b. Ext Carpi radialis longus
   c. Extensor pollicis longus
   d. Ext Carpi radialis brevis

117. Surgical neck fracture leads to all EXCEPT:
   a. Teres major palsy
   b. Teres minor palsy
   c. Weakness of abduction
   d. Deltoid muscle palsy

118. Which of the following artery is affected in anterior shoulder dislocation?
   a. Radial
   b. Axillary
   c. Median
   d. Ulnar

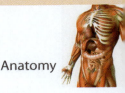

Anatomy

119. Which among the following muscles receives Dual Nerve supply?
    a. Flexor digitorum profundus
    b. Flexor digitorum superficialis
    c. Palmaris longus
    d. Extensor carpi radialis
120. All of the following structures are passing deep to flexor retinaculum EXCEPT:
    a. Flexor pollicis longus
    b. Flexor digitorum superficialis
    c. Palmaris longus
    d. Flexor digitorum profundus
121. Which structure passes superficial to flexor retinaculum?
    a. Ulnar nerve
    b. Median nerve
    c. Flexor digitorum superficialis
    d. Flexor digitorum profundus
122. Root value to axillary nerve:
    a. C5, C6   b. C6, C7, C8
    c. C5, C6, C7   d. C5-T1
123. Musculocutaneous nerve arises from which cord:
    a. Medial cord   b. Lateral cord
    c. Anterior cord   d. Posterior cord
124. Root of radial nerve:
    a. C6, C7, T1   b. C5, C6, C7, T1
    c. C5, C6, C7, C8, T1 d. C4, C5, C6, C7, C8, T1
125. Winging of scapula is due to damage of:
    a. Axillary nerve   b. Long thoracic nerve
    c. Median nerve   d. Ulnar nerve
126. Winging of scapula is due to paralysis of:
    a. Serratus anterior muscle
    b. Latissimus dorsi muscle
    c. Rhomboidus major muscle
    d. Pectoralis major muscle
127. Winging of scapula is due to paralysis of:
    a. Serratus anterior muscle b. Latissimus dorsi muscle
    c. Rhomboid major muscle   d. Pectoralis major muscle
128. 'Dropped shoulder' occurs due to paralysis of:
    a. Teres minor   b. Deltoid
    c. Teres major   d. Trapezius
129. Trapezius muscle is attached to all structures EXCEPT:
    a. First rib   b. Clavicle
    c. Scapula   d. Occiput
130. All of the following show ulnar nerve injury EXCEPT:
    a. Clawing of medial 2 digits b. Abductor pollicis palsy
    c. Adductor pollicis palsy   d. Weak grip
131. Pointing finger injury is due to injury of which nerve?
    a. Radial nerve   b. Ulnar nerve
    c. Median nerve   d. Axillary nerve
132. Claw hand is due to:
    a. Median nerve   b. Ulnar nerve
    c. Median and ulnar both d. Radial nerve

133. Ape thumb deformity is due to injury of which nerve:
    a. Radial nerve   b. Ulnar nerve
    c. Median nerve   d. Axillary nerve
134. Compression of which of the following nerves lead to carpal tunnel syndrome:
    a. Ulnar nerve   b. Median nerve
    c. Radial nerve   d. Both A and B
135. Median nerve supplies all EXCEPT:
    a. Abductor pollicis longus
    b. Pronator quadratus
    c. Flexor pollicis longus
    d. Flexor carpi radialis
136. All are muscles of rotator cuff EXCEPT:
    a. Teres major   b. Teres minor
    c. Infraspinatous   d. Supraspinatous
137. Most common injured muscle in rotator cuff is:
    a. Supraspinatous muscle b. Infraspinatous muscle
    c. Teres minor   d. Subscapularis
138. In a man lifting up a suitcase, downward dislocation of glenohumeral joint is prevented by:
    a. Deltoid   b. Latissimus dorsi
    c. Coracobrachialis   d. Supra spinatous
139. Short head of biceps is innervated by:
    a. Musculo cutaneous nerve
    b. Radial nerve
    c. Axillary nerve
    d. Median nerve
140. Muscle which covers both elbow and shoulder joint:
    a. Biceps
    b. Biceps brachialis
    c. Coracobrachialis
    d. Long head of triceps brachii
141. Which one of the following is a multipennate muscle?
    a. Tibialis anterior b. Deltoid
    c. Tibialis posterior d. Latissimus dorsi
142. Fracture of shaft of humerus leads to:
    a. Radial nerve injury
    b. Ulnar nerve injury
    c. Median nerve injury
    d. Musculocutaneous nerve injury
143. Posterior wall of axilla is formed by all EXCEPT:
    a. Teres major   b. Subscapularis
    c. Supraspinatus   d. Latissimus dorsi
144. Location of level III axillary lymph node in relation to pectoralis minor is:
    a. Anterior   b. Posterior
    c. Superior   d. Inferior
145. Supination and pronation of upper limb is due to:
    a. Wrist joint   b. Radioulnar joint
    c. Elbow joint
    d. Carpometacarpal joint

146. Medial border of cubital fossa is formed by:
    a. Pronator teres
    b. Brachioradialis
    c. Supinator
    d. Brachialis
147. All are contents of the cubital fossa EXCEPT:
    a. Ulnar artery
    b. Median nerve
    c. Brachial artery
    d. Ulnar nerve
148. All are contents of cubital fossa EXCEPT:
    a. Median nerve
    b. Ulnar nerve
    c. Biceps tendon
    d. Brachial artery
149. Boundary of triangle of auscultation is formed by all EXCEPT:
    a. Scapula
    b. Trapezius
    c. Serratus anterior
    d. Latissimus dorsi

LOWER LIMB

150. Tibial and common peroneal nerve supplies:
     (Recent Pattern Question 2018-19)
    a. Adductor magnus muscle
    b. Adductor longus muscle
    c. Gracilis muscle
    d. Biceps Femoris muscle
151. Which of the following muscle is supplied by obturator nerve:
     (Recent Pattern Question 2018-19)
    a. Gluteus medius
    b. Obturator internus
    c. Sartorius
    d. Adductor brevis
152. Which of the following muscle is evertor of foot:
     (Recent Pattern Question 2018-19)
    a. Tibialis anterior muscle
    b. Tibialis posterior
    c. Peroneus longus muscle
    d. Extensor digitorum longus
153. Most common nerve damaged in leg:
     (Recent Pattern Question 2018)
    a. Common peroneal nerve
    b. Femoral nerve
    c. Sciatic nerve
    d. Tibial nerve
154. Femoral triangle base is formed by:
     (Recent Pattern Question 2018)
    a. Medial border of sartorius
    b. Inguinal ligament
    c. Medial border of adductor longus
    d. Iliacus
155. Medial compartment of thigh is supplied by which nerve?
     (Recent Pattern Question 2018)
    a. Tibial nerve
    b. Obturator nerve
    c. Femoral nerve
    d. Common peroneal

156. First web space of foot is supplied by:
     (Recent Pattern Question 2018)
    a. Common peroneal nerve
    b. Superficial peroneal nerve
    c. Deep peroneal nerve
    d. Sural nerve
157. Which bone in foot is not attached by any muscle?
     (Recent Pattern Question 2017)
    a. Talus
    b. Calcaneum
    c. Metatarsals
    d. Fibula
158. Which muscle originates from anterior superior iliac spine?
     (Recent Pattern Question 2017)
    a. Iliofemoral ligament
    b. Sartorius
    c. Vastus lateralis
    d. Vastus medialis
159. Tibialis posterior muscle is supplied by which nerve?
     (Recent Pattern Question 2017)
    a. Posterior tibial nerve
    b. Deep peroneal nerve
    c. Femoral nerve
    d. Sural nerve
160. Adductor canal lateral boundary is formed by:
     (Recent Pattern Question 2017)
    a. Adductor longus
    b. Rectus medialis
    c. Vastus lateralis
    d. Vastus medialis
161. Which is true about origin of Femoral nerve root value?
    a. Anterior division of L2, L3, L4 ventral rami
    b. Anterior division of L1, L2, L3 ventral rami
    c. Posterior division of L2, L3, L4 ventral rami
    d. Posterior division of L1, L2, L3 ventral rami
162. Which is the muscle marked as A in the femoral triangle?
     (Recent Pattern Question 2017)

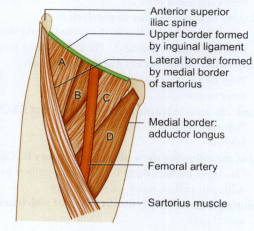

    a. Iliacus
    b. Psoas major
    c. Pectineus
    d. Adductor longus

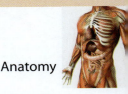

Anatomy

163. Biceps femoris does which of the following function? *(Recent Pattern Question 2017)*
    a. Adduction of knee
    b. Flexion of knee
    c. Extension of knee
    d. Abduction of knee

164. Chief extensor of thigh at hip joint is supplied by:
    a. Inferior gluteal nerve *(Recent Pattern Question 2017)*
    b. Superior gluteal nerve
    c. Sciatic nerve
    d. Peroneal nerve

165. Which of the following muscles is an evertor of foot? *(Recent Pattern Question 2017)*
    a. Peroneus tertius
    b. Tibialis anterior
    c. Extensor hallicus longus
    d. Extensor digitorum longus

166. What is the nerve supply of popliteus muscle? *(Recent Pattern Question 2017)*
    a. Tibial nerve
    b. Popliteal nerve
    c. Common peroneal nerve
    d. Deep peroneal nerve

167. Which is not a cause of positive trendelenburg sign? *(Recent Pattern Question 2017)*
    a. Paralysis of gluteus maximus
    b. Congenital dislocation of hip
    c. Un-united fracture of neck
    d. Coxa vara

168. Which of the following nerve injury leads to positive trendelenberg test?
    a. Inferior gluteal
    b. Obturator
    c. Tibial
    d. Superior gluteal nerve

169. Trendelenburg test is done for:
    a. Gluteus medius, minimus
    b. Gluteus maximus, minimus
    c. Gluteus maximus, medius
    d. Gluteus maximus, medius, minimus

170. Capsule of knee joint is supplied by: *(Recent Pattern Question 2017)*
    a. Genital branch of genitofemoral nerve
    b. Femoral branch of genitofemoral nerve
    c. Genicular branch of obturator nerve
    d. Femoral branch of obturator nerve

171. Fabella is present in: *(Recent Pattern Question 2017)*
    a. Medial head of gastrocnemius
    b. Lateral head of gastrocnemius
    c. Adductor magnus
    d. Adductor longus

172. Which is the nerve supply of soleus muscle?
    a. Tibial nerve *(Recent Pattern Question 2016)*
    b. Common peroneal nerve
    c. Superficial peroneal nerve
    d. Deep peroneal nerve

173. What is true about iliotibial tract?
    a. Thickening of fascia lata *(Recent Pattern Question 2016)*
    b. Gluteus medius is inserted into it
    c. Insertion at medial aspect of tibia
    d. Runs along the medial aspect of thigh

174. Which muscle is responsible for sitting to standing position? *(Recent Pattern Question 2016)*
    a. Gluteus medius
    b. Gluteus maximus
    c. Gluteus minimus
    d. Tensor fascia lata

175. All are branches of femoral artery EXCEPT:
    a. Superficial epigastric artery
    b. Superficial circumflex artery
    c. Inferior epigastric artery
    d. Descending genicular artery

176. Gluteus maximus is inserted on:
    a. Lesser trochanter
    b. Gluteal tuberosity
    c. Iliotibial tract
    d. Iliac crest

177. Iliotibial band has insertion of all of the following muscles EXCEPT:
    a. Tensor fasciae latae
    b. Gluteus maximus
    c. Gluteus minimus
    d. Vastus lateralis

178. Which is the longest muscle of the body:
    a. Sartorius
    b. Extraocular muscle
    c. External oblique
    d. Popliteal muscle

179. Which of the following muscles has attachment on the capsule of hip joint?
    a. Sartorius
    b. Rectus femoris
    c. Vastus lateralis
    d. Vastus medialis

180. This muscle is part of hamstrings muscle:
    a. Semimembranous
    b. Gracilis
    c. Short head of biceps femoris
    d. Sartorius

181. Gluteus medius is supplied by:
    a. Superior gluteal nerve
    b. Inferior gluteal nerve
    c. Nerve to obturator internus
    d. Nerve to quadratus femoris

182. Which of the following nerve supplies gluteus maximus?
    a. Superior gluteal nerve
    b. Inferior gluteal nerve
    c. Anterior gluteal nerve
    d. Posterior gluteal nerve

183. Which is the nerve supplying gamellus inferior muscle?
    a. Nerve to obturator internus
    b. Nerve to obturator externus
    c. Nerve to quadratus femoris
    d. Ventral rami to S1 and S2

184. All of the following structures pass through lesser sciatic foramen EXCEPT:
    a. Pudendal nerve
    b. Internal pudendal vessels
    c. Nerve to obturator internus
    d. Nerve to obturator externus

185. All of the structures pass through lesser sciatic foramen EXCEPT:
    a. Pudendal artery
    b. Pudendal nerve
    c. Nerve to obturator internus
    d. Nerve to obturator externus

FMGE Solutions Screening Examination

186. Which is the main extensor of knee?
    a. Biceps femoris   b. Quadriceps femoris
    c. Semitendinosus   d. Semimembranosus
187. Which muscle is responsible for unlocking of knee?
    a. Popliteus   b. Quadriceps femoris
    c. Semitendinosus   d. Semimembranosus
188. Which of the following bone has no muscle attachment?
    a. Navicular   b. Calcaneum
    c. Talus   d. Cuboid
189. In injury to the neck of fibula, which of the following nerve is usually injured?
    a. Superficial peroneal nerve
    b. Deep peroneal nerve
    c. Common peroneal nerve
    d. Tibial nerve
190. Medial border of Hesselbach's triangle is formed by:
    a. Linea alba   b. Linea semilunaris
    c. Inferior epigastric artery   d. Conjoint tendon
191. Poupart's ligament forms which border of hesselbach's triangle:
    a. Anterior   b. Posterior
    c. Superior   d. Inferior
192. All of the following are true about lateral cutaneous nerve EXCEPT:
    a. Supplies skin over the lateral skin of thigh
    b. Supplies skin over the medial aspect of thigh
    c. Arises from L2 and L3
    d. It is a purely sensory nerve
193. What is the nerve Root value of superior gluteal nerve?
    a. $L_{4,5}, S_1$ b. $L_{4,5}, S_1, S_2$
    c. $L_{4,5}, S_1, S_2, S_3$ d. L_5, S_1, S_2
194. Root value of the posterior cutaneous nerve of the thigh:
    a. S_1, S_2 b. S_1, S_2, S_3
    c. S_2, S_3 d. S_2, S_3, S_4
195. Root value of sciatic nerve is:
    a. $S_1 S_2 S_3$ b. $L_4 L_5 S_1 S_2 S_3$
    c. $L_1 L_2 L_3$ d. $L_2 L_3 L_4$
196. Nerve root of pudendal nerve is:
    a. $S_1 S_2 S_3$ b. $S_2 S_3 S_4$
    c. S_3-S_4 d. S_2-S_3

THORAX AND ABDOMEN

197. Which of the following structure is present over the mediastinal surface of right lung:
    (Recent Pattern Question 2018-19)
    a. Azygos vein   b. Right thoracic duct
    c. Aorta   d. Trachea
198. Which of the following structures is not found in superior mediastinum:
    a. Pulmonary trunk   b. Thymus
    c. Left intercostal artery   d. Arch of aorta
199. Which of these is true about bronchopulmonary segment?   *(Recent Pattern Question 2018)*
    a. Nonresectable
    b. Spherical in shape
    c. Artery is intersegmental
    d. Pulmonary veins are intersegmental
200. Left anterior descending artery is a branch of:
    (Recent Pattern Question 2018)
    a. Right coronary artery   b. Left coronary artery
    c. Ascending aorta   d. Coronary sinus
201. VAN (vein, artery, nerve) sequence is present in intercostal space at: *(Recent Pattern Question 2017)*
    a. Upper border of rib   b. Middle border of rib
    c. Lower border of rib
    d. Middle portion of intercostal space
202. Anterior group of lymph node runs along:
    (Recent Pattern Question 2016)
    a. Internal mammary artery   b. Cephalic vein
    c. Lateral thoracic vein   d. Subscapular vein
203. Which of the following rib is known as floating rib?
    (Recent Pattern Question 2017)
    a. 8   b. 9
    c. 10   d. 11
204. Which is not a true rib:
    a. 5th   b. 6th
    c. 7th   d. 8th
205. Xiphoid process unites with the body at age of _____ years?   *(Recent Pattern Question 2017)*
    a. 10   b. 20
    c. 30   d. 40
206. Which structures passes though foramen of langer?
    (Recent Pattern Question 2017)
    a. Inguinal canal   b. Tail of spence
    c. CN V3   d. CN VII
207. Sappey's plexus drains?   *(Recent Pattern Question 2017)*
    a. Breast   b. Thyroid
    c. Adrenal   d. Porta hepatis
208. Lingula is which part of lung?
    (Recent Pattern Question 2017)
    a. Left lower lobe   b. Left upper lobe
    c. Right lower lobe   d. Right upper lobe
209. Which muscle is involved in violent expiratory efforts?
    (Recent Pattern Question 2017)
    a. Diaphragm   b. Latissimus dorsi
    c. External oblique   d. Internal intercostal
210. Right coronary artery supplies all EXCEPT:
    a. Right atrium
    b. Posterior part of interventricular septum
    c. Anterior interventricular groove
    d. SA node
211. Base of the heart is formed by:
    a. RA   b. RV
    c. LA   d. LV

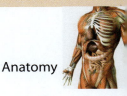

Anatomy

212. All of these form right heart border EXCEPT?
   a. SVC
   b. IVC
   c. Right atrium
   d. Right ventricle
213. What is the length of trachea?
   a. 5 cm
   b. 10 cm
   c. 20 cm
   d. 25 cm
214. What is the diameter of trachea?
   a. 0.5 cm
   b. 2 cm
   c. 3 cm
   d. 5 cm
215. Most commonly foreign body lodges in which part of esophagus?
   a. Where it crosses the aortic arch
   b. Cricopharyngeus
   c. Where it is crossed by left bronchus
   d. Where it pierces the diaphragm
216. Which is not an accessory muscle of respiration?
   a. Sternocleidomastoid
   b. Scalaneus
   c. Erector spinae
   d. None
217. 75% respiration is due to:
   a. Diaphragm
   b. Internal intercostals
   c. Intercostals
   d. Serratus anterior
218. Which is the motor supply of diaphragm?
   a. Phrenic nerve
   b. Thoracodorsal nerve
   c. Intercostals
   d. Sympathetic nerves
219. Intercostal veins drain into:
   a. Left subclavian vein
   b. Internal jugular vein
   c. Azygous vein
   d. Inferior vena cava
220. All of the following drain into azygos vein EXCEPT:
   a. Hemi-azygos vein
   b. Posterior intercostal vein
   c. Left superior intercostal vein
   d. Right superior intercostal vein

ABDOMEN

221. Identify the branch originating from Celiac trunk:
   (Recent Pattern Question 2018-19)

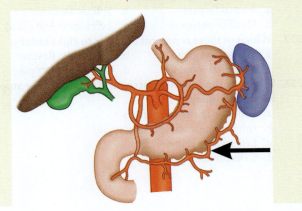

   a. Splenic artery
   b. Left gastric artery
   c. Left Gastroepiploic Artery
   d. Left renal artery
222. Pancreas tail present in:
   (Recent Pattern Question 2018-19)
   a. Gastrosplenic ligament
   b. Splenorenal ligament
   c. Hepatogastric ligament
   d. Gastroduodenal ligament
223. Sternum attached to scapula via:
   (Recent Pattern Question 2018-19)
   a. Manubrium
   b. First rib
   c. Second rib
   d. Clavicle
224. Vasa Brevia is the name of:
   (Recent Pattern Question 2018-19)
   a. Long gastric arteries
   b. Short gastric arteries
   c. Duodenal arteries
   d. Renal arteries
225. Identify the part of duodenum marked below:
   (Recent Pattern Question 2018)
   a. 1st part
   b. 2nd part
   c. 3rd part
   d. 4th part

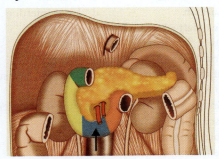

226. Cords of billroth in spleen are found in:
   (Recent Pattern Question 2018)
   a. White pulp
   b. Trabecular zone
   c. Red pulp
   d. Mantle zone
227. Which is the water shed area of inferior mesenteric artery and internal iliac artery? *(Recent Pattern Question 2017)*
   a. Griffith's point
   b. Sigmoid colon
   c. Ano rectal junction
   d. Sudeck's point
228. Portal vein starts at level of____?
   (Recent Pattern Question 2017)
   a. L2
   b. L3
   c. L4
   d. L5
229. Which is not a derivative of dorsal mesogastrium?
   (Recent Pattern Question 2017)
   a. Greater omentum
   b. Gastrosplenic ligament
   c. Gastro-phrenic ligament
   d. Coronary ligament

230. Which of the following is not a part of pancreatic bed?
    (Recent Pattern Question 2017)
    a. Splenic vein   b. Right suprarenal gland
    c. Aorta   d. Left crus of diaphragm
231. Smallest branch of celiac artery is:
    (Recent Pattern Question 2017)
    a. Right gastric artery b. Splenic artery
    c. Left gastric artery   d. Cystic artery
232. Constriction of diaphragm will not cause constriction of which opening: (Recent Pattern Question 2016)
    a. Aortic opening   b. Esophageal opening
    c. IVC opening   d. Thoracic duct aperture
233. Identify the intestinal segment:

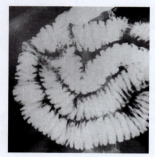

    a. Ileum   b. Jejunum
    c. Caecum   d. Large intestine
234. Shape of left adrenal gland:
    a. Oval   b. Semilunar
    c. Triangular   d. Trapezoid
235. All of the following form boundary of Left supra renal gland EXCEPT:
    a. Greater sac of stomach forms anterior border
    b. Psoas major forms posterior border
    c. Spleen forms anterolateral border
    d. Left kidney forms inferior border
236. What is the weight of adrenal gland?
    a. 4 gram   b. 8 grams
    c. 10 grams   d. 15 grams
237. Aortic hiatus pierces diaphragm at what level?
    a. T 8   b. T10
    c. T11   d. T12
238. Structures passing through aortic opening in diaphragm are all EXCEPT:
    a. Aorta   b. Azygous vein
    c. Thoracic duct   d. Vagus nerve
239. Right phrenic nerve passes through this diaphragmatic opening:
    a. Aortic opening   b. Caval opening
    c. Esophageal opening   d. Phrenic nerve opening
240. Structures passing through esophageal opening are all EXCEPT:
    a. Esophagus   b. Phrenic nerve
    c. Vagus nerve   d. Gastric artery branches
241. Which of the following structure does not pass through diaphragm?
    a. Aorta   b. IVC
    c. Esophagus   d. Cisterna chyli
242. All of the following vessels are valveless EXCEPT:
    a. Inferior vena cava   b. Superior vena cana
    c. Pulmonary vein   d. Internal jugular vein
243. All of the following are valveless EXCEPT:
    a. Internal jugular vein b. Portal vein
    c. Superior vena cava   d. Inferior vena cava
244. All are muscular arteries EXCEPT?
    a. Aorta   b. Femoral artery
    c. Popliteal artery   d. Splenic artery
245. Inferior vena cava is formed at which level:
    a. L2   b. L3
    c. L4   d. L5
246. Portal vein forms at which vertebral level?
    a. L1   b. L5
    c. S1   d. S5
247. Brunner glands are seen in:
    a. Duodenum   b. Esophagus
    c. Cardia of stomach   d. Small intestine
248. Brunner's gland in the duodenum secretes:
    a. Mucinus alkaline   b. Acid
    c. Pepsin   d. Gastrin
249. All of the following form visceral relation of spleen EXCEPT:
    a. Fundus of stomach   b. Left kidney
    c. Splenic flexure of colon d. Duodenum
250. Which of the following forms the posterior wall of kidney?
    a. Latissimus dorsi   b. Quadratus lumborum
    c. Transverse abdominis d. External Oblique
251. Which of the following is not in anterior relationship with left kidney?
    a. Jejunal flexure   b. Splenic flexure
    c. Head of pancreas   d. Left suprarenal gland
252. Which of these is present anterior to right kidney:
    a. Suprarenal gland   b. Right colic flexure
    c. Intestinal looping   d. Duodenum 2nd part
253. Which is the following structure will affect or stop the ascent of kidney?
    a. Superior mesenteric artery
    b. Inferior mesenteric artery
    c. Left splenic vein
    d. Celiac trunk

Anatomy

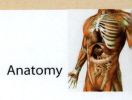

254. Kidney cortex contains:
    a. Loop of henle
    b. Pyramids
    c. Collecting tubule and duct
    d. Calyces

255. All are in close association with 3rd part of duodenum EXCEPT:
    a. Pancreas
    b. Transverse colon
    c. Sigmoid colon
    d. Stomach

256. Which is the longest part of duodenum?
    a. First part
    b. Second part
    c. Third part
    d. Fourth part

257. Which of the following is dermatome of umbilicus:
    a. T8
    b. T10
    c. T12
    d. L1

258. Commonest position of the appendix is:
    a. Paracoecal
    b. Retrocoecal
    c. Pelvic
    d. Subcoecal

259. Which is the least common position of appendix?
    a. Retroceacal
    b. Preileal
    c. Postileal
    d. Pelvic

260. All are tributaries of portal vein EXCEPT:
    a. Left gastric vein
    b. Right gastric vein
    c. Inferior pancreatoduodenal vein
    d. Superior mesenteric vein

261. Which are the correct boundaries of Calot triangle?
    a. Cystic artery, liver, right hepatic duct
    b. Cystic duct, liver, common hepatic duct
    c. Cystic duct, liver, cystic artery
    d. Common bile duct, cystic duct, liver

262. Superior boundary of calot's triangle is formed by:
    a. Hepatic duct
    b. Superior surface of liver
    c. Inferior surface of liver
    d. Cystic duct

263. All of the structures pass through Calot's triangle EXCEPT:
    a. Portal vein
    b. Cystic artery
    c. Right hepatic artery
    d. Lymph node of Lund

264. Structures at the transpyloric plane include all EXCEPT:
    a. Fundus of gall bladder
    b. Termination of portal vein
    c. Hilum of kidneys
    d. Pylorus of stomach

265. Which is true regarding portal venous system?
    a. Whole system is valve less
    b. Valves are present at the junction of superior mesenteric artery and splenic artery
    c. Valves are present in the intrahepatic system
    d. There are about 10-12 valves along the entire course

266. Chief cells are found in which area of stomach?
    a. Fundus
    b. Pit
    c. Neck
    d. Body

267. Average weight of spleen in adult:
    a. 5 ounce
    b. 7 ounce
    c. 14 ounce
    d. 21 ounce

268. Which is the most mobile part of rectum?
    a. Upper 1/3rd
    b. Middle 1/3rd
    c. Lower 1/3rd
    d. Lower 2/3rd

269. What is the length of rectum:
    a. 5 cm
    b. 12 cm
    c. 15 cm
    d. 20 cm

270. Which of the following is not in posterior relationship to rectum:
    a. Sacral vertebra
    b. Superior rectal artery
    c. Seminal vesicles
    d. Middle rectal artery

271. Opening of anal epithelium is made up of:
    a. Squamous cell
    b. Columnar
    c. Transitional
    d. Cuboidal

272. The puborectalis covers anorectal angle:
    a. Completely
    b. Anteriorly
    c. Posteriorly
    d. Laterally

273. All of the following arteries supply pancreas EXCEPT:
    a. Gastroduodenal artery
    b. Superior mesenteric artery
    c. Inferior mesenteric artery
    d. Pancreatic branch of splenic artery

274. Fundus of stomach is supplied by which of the following artery:
    a. Celiac trunk
    b. Splenic artery
    c. Left gastric artery
    d. Left gastroepiploic artery

275. Which of the following is *not* a ventral branch of abdominal aorta?
    a. Gonadal artery
    b. Celiac trunk
    c. Superior mesenteric artery
    d. Inferior mesenteric artery

276. Which of the following is a branch of external iliac artery?
    a. Femoral artery
    b. Deep circumflex artery
    c. Inferior epigastric artery
    d. Gonadal artery

NEUROANATOMY, HEAD AND NECK

277. Which branch of facial nerve supplies muscles of lower lip? *(Recent Pattern Question 2018-19)*
    a. Temporal branch
    b. Cervical branch
    c. Buccal branch
    d. Mandibular branch

278. Lower lip blood supply: *(Recent Pattern Question 2018-19)*
    a. Angular artery
    b. Lateral nasal artery
    c. Labial artery
    d. Greater palatine artery

279. Landmark of facial nerve in parotid gland: *(Recent Pattern Question 2018-19)*
    a. Tragal pointer
    b. Anterior belly of digastric muscle
    c. Helical point
    d. Suprameatal triangle

FMGE Solutions Screening Examination

280. Trismus is due to spasm of which muscle?
    (Recent Pattern Question 2018-19)
    a. Orbiculis   b. Lateral pterygoid
    c. Mentalis   d. Medial pterygoid

281. Accessory muscle of mastication:
    (Recent Pattern Question 2018-19)
    a. Risorius   b. Orbicularis oris
    c. Buccinator   d. Platysma

282. Parotid duct opens into:
    (Recent Pattern Question 2018-19)
    a. First mandibular molar
    b. First maxillary pre-molar
    c. Second mandibular molar
    d. Second maxillary molar

283. Mammillary body projects via:
    (Recent Pattern Question 2018-19)
    a. Thalamus   b. Corpus callosum
    c. Pituitary gland d. Fornix

284. Which structure connects the Broca's area and Wernicke area?
    (Recent Pattern Question 2018-19)
    a. Arcuate fasciculus
    b. Anterior commissure
    c. Corpus callosum
    d. Fornix

285. The function of superior rectus muscle is:
    (Recent Pattern Question 2018)
    a. Elevation, intorsion, abduction
    b. Elevation, intorsion, adduction
    c. Depression, extortion, abduction
    d. Depression, extortion, adduction

286. The nerve passing through cavernous sinus:
    (Recent Pattern Question 2018)
    a. Optic nerve b. Olfactory
    c. Abducens   d. Facial

287. The blood supply of abdominal part of esophagus:
    (Recent Pattern Question 2018)
    a. Bronchial vein and arch of aorta
    b. Right gastric artery and inferior phrenic nerve
    c. Left gastric artery and inferior phrenic nerve
    d. Pulmonary trunk

288. Skin over parotid is supplied by:
    (Recent Pattern Question 2018)
    a. Retroauricular nerve b. Greater auricular nerve
    c. Greater occipital nerve d. Facial nerve

289. Deepest nuclei of cerebellum is:
    (Recent Pattern Question 2018)
    a. Putamen   b. Lentiform
    c. Caudate   d. Fastigii

290. Which cranial nerve supplies lateral rectus muscle?
    (Recent Pattern Question 2017)
    a. Trochlear   b. Trigeminal
    c. Abducens   d. Glossopharyngeal

291. Blood supply of spinal cord is _____ spinal arteries?
    a. 1 anterior and 2 posterior *(Recent Pattern Question 2017)*
    b. 2 anterior and 1 posterior
    c. 2 anterior and 2 posterior
    d. 1 anterior and 1 posterior

292. Anterior 2/3rd of spinal cord is supplied by:
    a. Anterior choroidal artery *(Recent Pattern Question 2017)*
    b. Anterior communicating artery
    c. Anterior cerebral artery
    d. Anterior spinal artery

293. Which muscle is attached to the temporal bone?
    (Recent Pattern Question 2017)
    a. Stapedius muscle   b. Postauricular muscle
    c. Tensor tympani muscle d. Digastric muscle

294. Ipsilateral deviation of tongue occurs due to which intact tongue muscle?
    (Recent Pattern Question 2017)
    a. Palatoglossus   b. Styloglossus
    c. Genioglossus   d. Pharyngoglossus

295. Arteria thyroidea ima originates from:
    (Recent Pattern Question 2017)
    a. External carotid artery   b. Thyrocervical trunk
    c. Vertebral artery   d. Arch of aorta

296. Thyroid gland is situated at the level of:
    (Recent Pattern Question 2017)
    a. C4-C8   b. C4-T1
    c. C5-T1   d. C6-T2

297. How many lobes are present in cerebellum?
    (Recent Pattern Question 2017)
    a. 2   b. 4
    c. 6   d. 8

298. Which is the smallest lobe of cerebellum?
    (Recent Pattern Question 2017)
    a. Flocculonodular lobe   b. Lingular lobe
    c. Pyramidal lobe   d. Archicerebellum

299. Vertebral artery is derived from:
    (Recent Pattern Question 2017)
    a. First part of subclavian artery
    b. Second part of subclavian artery
    c. Third part of subclavian artery
    d. Fourth part of subclavian artery

300. Which of the following is a branch of 3rd part of subclavian artery? *(Recent Pattern Question 2017)*
    a. Thyrocervical trunk
    b. Dorsal scapular artery
    c. Vertebral artery
    d. Internal thoracic artery

301. Cavernous sinus is a collection of venous sinuses on either side of pituitary. Which of the following does not pass through the wall of the cavernous sinus?
    a. CN III   *(Recent Pattern Question 2017)*
    b. CN V2
    c. Post ganglionic sympathetic fibers
    d. Internal carotid artery

ANATOMY

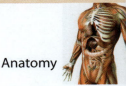

302. Anterior inferior cerebellar artery is a branch of:
 (Recent Pattern Question 2017)
 a. Subclavian artery
 b. Vertebral artery
 c. Basilar artery
 d. Middle cerebral artery

303. Smallest branch of external carotid artery is:
 a. Superior thyroid artery *(Recent Pattern Question 2017)*
 b. Ascending pharyngeal artery
 c. Facial artery
 d. Maxillary artery

304. Subarachnoid space extends up to:
 (Recent Pattern Question 2017)
 a. Lower border L1
 b. Upper border L1
 c. Upper border of S2
 d. Lower border of S2

305. Skin over angle of mandible is supplied by:
 (Recent Pattern Question 2017)
 a. Greater auricular nerve
 b. Posterior auricular nerve
 c. Greater occipital nerve
 d. Lesser occipital nerve

306. Which of the following cranial nerve carries parasympathetic fibers? *(Recent Pattern Question 2017)*
 a. CN 1
 b. CN 2
 c. CN 3
 d. CN 4

307. Which of the following cranial nerve is a pure sensory nerve? *(Recent Pattern Question 2017)*
 a. CN 3
 b. CN 5
 c. CN 8
 d. CN 9

308. Leptomeninges is formed by:
 (Recent Pattern Question 2017)
 a. Dura mater and Arachnoid
 b. Arachnoid and pia mater
 c. Dura and pia mater
 d. Dura, arachnoid and pia matter

309. Sylvian fissure separates: *(Recent Pattern Question 2017)*
 a. Temporal lobe from occipital lobe
 b. Temporal lobe from frontoparietal areas
 c. Temporal lobe from opposite frontal lobe
 d. Temporal lobe from cerebellum

310. Superior vena cava is formed by fusion of_____:
 (Recent Pattern Question 2017)
 a. Internal and external jugular veins
 b. Subclavian and internal jugular veins
 c. Left and right brachiocephalic veins
 d. Left and right common iliac veins

311. A patient was hit in the eye with a tennis ball. Following this blunt eye injury he developed a hyphema. Which blood vessel is the source of bleeding?
 (Recent Pattern Question 2017)
 a. Circulus iridis major
 b. Hyaloid artery
 c. Anterior ciliary arteries
 d. Retinal artery

312. Which is these is a Bi-condylar joint?
 (Recent Pattern Question 2017)
 a. TM joint
 b. Atlanto-occipital
 c. Interphalangeal
 d. Inter-meta-tarsal joint

313. Which structure is not transmitted by foramen ovale?
 (Recent Pattern Question 2017)
 a. Middle meningeal artery
 b. Accessory meningeal artery
 c. Lesser petrosal nerve
 d. Emissary vein

314. Maxillary nerve is transmitted via:
 (Recent Pattern Question 2017)
 a. Foramen ovale
 b. Foramen rotundum
 c. Foramen lacerum
 d. Foramen spinosum

315. Foramen transversarium is found at:
 (Recent Pattern Question 2017)
 a. Anterior cranial fossa
 b. Middle cranial fossa
 c. Posterior cranial fossa
 d. Cervical vertebra

316. Nerve carrying taste sensation from anterior 2/3rd of tongue is called: *(Recent Pattern Question 2017)*
 a. Arnold nerve
 b. Jacobson nerve
 c. Criminal nerve of grassi
 d. Nerve of wrisberg

317. Which of the following areas of the brain is not a primary sensory cortex? *(Recent Pattern Question 2017)*
 a. 1
 b. 2
 c. 3
 d. 4

318. Which is a part of limbic system:
 (Recent Pattern Question 2017)
 a. Corpus callosum
 b. Pineal gland
 c. Cingulate gyrus
 d. Tegmentum

319. Nucleus ambiguus is composed of:
 (Recent Pattern Question 2017)
 a. Sensory to 9, 10, 11 cranial nerve nucleus
 b. Motor to 9, 10, 11 cranial nerve nucleus
 c. Sensory to 7, 9, 10 cranial nerve nucleus
 d. Motor to 7, 9, 10 cranial nerve nucleus

320. IInd cranial nerve is: *(Recent Pattern Question 2017)*
 a. Optic nerve
 b. Abducens nerve
 c. Trigeminal nerve
 d. Occulomotor nerve

321. Lower one-third of auricle is supplied by:
 a. Auriculotemporal nerve
 b. Vagus nerve
 c. Greater auricular nerve
 d. Greater retrasal nerve

322. All are related to facial nerve EXCEPT:
 a. Maxillary process
 b. Stylomastoid foramen
 c. Posterior belly of diagstric muscle
 d. Parotid gland

323. Parotid duct opens:
 a. Opposite to lower 1st molar tooth
 b. Opposite to lower 2nd molar tooth
 c. In floor of mouth
 d. In relation with upper 2nd molar tooth

FMGE Solutions Screening Examination

324. Which of the following is not a test for integrity of 7th and 9th nerve:
    a. Position of uvula
    b. Palate symmetry
    c. Deviation of tongue
    d. Taste sensation of anterior 2/3rd of tongue
325. Opening of mouth is caused by:
    a. Lateral pterygoid   b. Medial pterygoid
    c. Temporalis   d. Masseter
326. Sensory supply to anterior 2/3rd of tongue given by:
    a. Facial nerve   b. Trigeminal nerve
    c. Hypoglossal nerve   d. Glossopharyngeal nerve
327. Taste sensation is not carried by:
    a. CN V   b. CN VII
    c. CN IX   d. CN XI
328. Taste sensation from mucosal membranes of oral side of tongue is carried by:
    a. Lingual nerve   b. Vagus nerve
    c. Hypoglossal nerve   d. Glossopharyngeal nerve
329. What is the site of lesion affecting cranial nerve VI, VII and VIII?
    a. Pons
    b. Midbrain
    c. Medulla
    d. Junction between pons and medulla
330. Which of the following cranial nerve decussate within the brain?
    a. Optic   b. Occulomator
    c. Trochlear   d. Trigeminal
331. Ptosis is due to:
    a. 3rd CN palsy   b. 4th CN palsy
    c. 5th CN palsy   d. 6th CN palsy
332. Muller muscle is supplied by which nerve?
    a. Facial nerve   b. Sympathetic nerve
    c. Trigeminal nerve   d. Vagus nerve
333. Which muscle is not supplied by cranial nerve III?
    a. Superior oblique   b. Superior rectus
    c. Inferior oblique   d. Medial rectus
334. Which cranial nerve has the largest intracranial course?
    a. Vagus nerve   b. Oculomotor nerve
    c. Trochlear nerve   d. Abducens nerve
335. Which of the following nerve is known as criminal nerve of grassi?
    a. Hypoglossal nerve   b. Trigeminal nerve
    c. Thyroglossal nerve   d. Vagus nerve
336. Which nerve pierces the thyroid gland?
    a. Superior laryngeal nerve b. Inferior laryngeal nerve
    c. Recurrent laryngeal nerve d. Posterior laryngeal nerve
337. All of the following structures pass through superior orbital fissure EXCEPT:
    a. Inferial ophthalmic vein b. Lacrimal nerve
    c. Trigeminal nerve   d. Nasociliary nerve

338. Which cranial nerve is not transmitted by superior orbital fissure? *(Recent Pattern Question 2017)*
    a. 2   b. 3
    c. 4   d. 5
339. Which is the following structure passes through the lateral part of superior orbital fissure?
    a. Superior ophthalmic vein
    b. Inferior ophthalmic vein
    c. Abducent nerve
    d. Nasociliary nerve
340. All these nerves pass through superior orbital fissure EXCEPT?
    a. Mandibular nerve   b. Abducens nerve
    c. Trochlear nerve   d. Oculomotor nerve
341. Which of the following structure passes through inferior orbital fissure?
    a. Infraorbital nerve   b. Infraorbital artery
    c. Both   d. None
342. Which of the following causes injury to cranial nerve 3rd, 4th and 1st branch of CN 5?
    a. Sphenoid bone tumor   b. Parotid gland tumor
    c. Petrous bone tumor   d. Acoustic neuroma
343. What is the root value of phrenic nerve?
    a. C2, C3, C4   b. C4, C5, T1
    c. C3, C4, C5   d. C5, T1, T2
344. Which of the following is the most common congenital anomaly?
    a. Cleft lip
    b. Cleft palate
    c. Cleft lip and cleft palate both
    d. None
345. Which is the dangerous layer of scalp?
    a. Subcutaneous layer
    b. Musculoapneurotic layer
    c. Loose subaponeurotic layer
    d. Periosteum layer
346. Which of the following layer of scalp is made up of a tough layer of dense fibrous tissue:
    a. Subcutaneous layer
    b. Musculoaponeurotic layer
    c. Loose subaponeurotic layer
    d. Galea aponeurotica
347. Medial wall of orbit is formed by which bone:
    a. Lesser wing of sphenoid
    b. Frontal process of maxilla
    c. Greater wing of sphenoid
    d. Arterial and posterior ethmoidal canals
348. Which of the following nerve supplies the muscles of palate?
    a. Hypoglossal nerve   b. Greater palatine nerve
    c. Glossopharyngeal nerve d. Trigeminal nerve

Anatomy

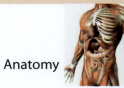

349. Safety muscle of tongue is?
   a. Genioglossus   b. Palatoglossus
   c. Styloglossus   d. Hyoglossus
350. Safety muscle of larynx is:
   a. Aryepiglotticus   b. Cricoarytenoid
   c. Thyroarytenoid   d. Posterior cricoarytenoid
351. At the end of C6 which is not true:
   a. Trachea bifurcates   b. Pharynx ends
   c. Esophagus begins   d. Larynx ends
352. Which muscle of larynx is supplied by external laryngeal nerve?
   a. Cricothyroid   b. Lateral Cricoarytenoid
   c. Thyroarytenoid   d. Posterior cricoarytenoid
353. Which one of the following muscle is supplied by the glossopharyngeal nerve?
   a. Sternohyoid   b. Stylopharyngeus
   c. Styloglossus   d. Stylohyoid
354. Which muscle is supplied by the glossopharyngeal nerve?
   a. Stylopharyngeus   b. Palatopharyngeus
   c. Glossopharyngeus   d. Salpingopharyngeus
355. Adult larynx extends between cervical spine:
   a. C_7 to T_1 b. C_2 to C_3
   c. C_3 to C_4 d. C_3 to C_6
356. Anterior fontannel corresponds to all EXCEPT:
   a. Frontal bones   b. Coronal suture
   c. Lambdoid suture   d. Saggital suture
357. Which is not a T.M. joint ligament?
   a. Temporomandibular   b. Sphenomandibular
   c. Stylomandibular ligament
   d. Tympanomandibular
358. What is the location of Hyoid bone in terms of cervical vertebral level:
   a. C2   b. C3
   c. C4   d. C5
359. What is the level of Isthmus of the thyroid gland across tracheal ring?
   a. 3rd to 5th   b. 2nd to 4th
   c. 5th to 6th   d. 2nd to 3rd
360. Which of the following artery supplies parathyroid glands?
   a. Superior thyroid artery   b. Inferior thyroid artery
   c. Common carotid artery   d. Middle thyroid artery
361. Which of the following is not a part of lower motor neuron?
   a. Anterior nerve root   b. Peripheral ganglia
   c. Peripheral nerve   d. Anterior horn cells
362. All of the following are pneumatic bones EXCEPT:
   a. Maxilla   b. Frontal
   c. Mandible   d. Ethmoid
363. Which of the following is a pneumatic bone?
   a. Tibia   b. Frontal bone
   c. Clavicle   d. Femur

364. Gustatory cortex is situated in:
   a. Superior temporal gyrus   b. Inferior frontal gyrus
   c. Superior frontal gyrus   d. Inferior parietal gyrus
365. Optic radiation arises from:
   a. Superior colliculus   b. Inferior colliculus
   c. Lateral geniculate body   d. Medial geniculate body
366. All of the following are features of Horner's syndrome EXCEPT:
   a. Ptosis   b. Miosis
   c. Heterochromia iridis   d. Exophthalmos
367. Maximum contribution to the floor of orbit is by which bone?
   a. Maxillary   b. Zygomatic
   c. Sphenoid   d. Palatine
368. Angular vein infection causes thrombosis in:
   a. Cavernous sinus   b. Suprasaggital sinus
   c. Transverse sinus   d. Inferior petrosal sinus
369. Left spinal leminiscus contains which fibers?
   a. Left sided pain, touch, temperature
   b. Left sided position, vibration sense
   c. Right sided pain, touch, temperature
   d. Right sided position, vibration sense
370. All of the following muscles are attached to the apex of orbit EXCEPT:
   a. Superior oblique   b. Superior rectus
   c. Medial rectus   d. Inferior oblique
371. Which nerve helps in looking laterally and downward:
   a. Abducent   b. Trochlear
   c. Trigeminal   d. Occulomotor
372. All of the following are parts of nasal septum EXCEPT:
   a. Septal cartilage   b. Lateral cartilage
   c. Crest of maxilla
   d. Peripendicular plate of ethmoid
373. Which is not a part of basal ganglia?
   a. Caudate nucleus   b. Thalamus
   c. Lenticular nucleus   d. Globus pallidus
374. Cerebellar cortex contains:
   a. Pyramidal cells   b. Purkinje cells
   c. Stromal cells   d. Kupffer cells
375. Cerebellar connection to other parts of the brain is projected through which cell?
   a. Golgi cells   b. Basket cells
   c. Purkinje cells   d. Oligodendrocytes
376. In adults, the spinal cord normally ends at:
   a. Lower border of L1   b. Lower border of L3
   c. Lower border of L5   d. Lower border of S1
377. The spinal cord in infants ends at the level of:
   a. L1   b. L2
   c. L3   d. L4
378. Which nerve passes from paraphyrangeal space?
   a. VI   b. VII
   c. VIII   d. X

FMGE Solutions Screening Examination

379. Which of the following tracts is seen in the posterior column of spinal cord?
    a. Lateral spinothalamic tract
    b. Fasciculus gracilis
    c. Rubrospinal tract
    d. Posterior spinocerebellar
380. Which is the most prominent spinous process?
    a. T1
    b. C7
    c. C6
    d. L5
381. The movement at the following joint permits a person to say NO by head movement:
    a. Atlanto-occipital joint
    b. Atlanto-axial joint
    c. C2-C3 joint
    d. C3-C4 joint
382. In epidural lumbar puncture, all of these structures are pierced EXCEPT:
    a. Posterior longitudinal ligament
    b. Ligamentous flavum
    c. Interspinous ligament
    d. Supraspinous ligament
383. 'Chassaignac's tubercle' is:
    a. Erb's point
    b. Carotid tubercle on C6 vertebra
    c. Found on first rib
    d. Medial condyle of humerus

PELVIS AND PERINEUM

384. The patient is having bleeding from haemorrhoids. Which of the following artery is the source of bleeding?
    (Recent Pattern Question 2018-19)
    a. Superior rectal vein
    b. Superior rectal artery
    c. Middle rectal artery
    d. Middle rectal vein
385. Blood supply of bulb of the penis:
    a. Scrotal artery   *(Recent Pattern Question 2018)*
    b. Superficial pudendal artery
    c. Bulbourethral artery
    d. Bulbocavernosus artery
386. Cremasteric muscle nerve supply:
    a. Ilioinguinal nerve   *(Recent Pattern Question 2018)*
    b. Iliohypogastric nerve
    c. Genital branch of genitofemoral nerve
    d. Femoral nerve
387. Which of the following is the artery for endometrial blood supply?   *(Recent Pattern Question 2018)*
    a. Endometrial artery
    b. Myometrial artery
    c. Spiral artery
    d. Cervical artery
388. Alcock's canal transmits: *(Recent Pattern Question 2017)*
    a. Pudendal nerve
    b. Epididymis
    c. CN VIII
    d. Fallopian tube
389. Posterior superior iliac spine is at which level?
    (Recent Pattern Question 2016)
    a. S1
    b. S2
    c. L1
    d. L2
390. Coccyx has how many vertebra:
    (Recent Pattern Question 2016)
    a. 1
    b. 2
    c. 3
    d. 4
391. Muscles of the perineal body include all of the following EXCEPT:
    a. External anal sphincter
    b. Iliococcygeus
    c. Superficial transverse perinei
    d. Bulbocavernosus
392. Structures forming perineal body are all EXCEPT:
    a. Levator ani muscle
    b. Bulbospongiosus
    c. Deep transverse perinei
    d. Ischiococcygeus
393. Pelvic diaphragm is made of all EXCEPT:
    a. Iliococcygeus
    b. Ischiococcygeus
    c. Pubococcygeus
    d. Puborectalis
394. Which is true regarding prostate gland?
    a. Only glandular tissue
    b. Glandular tissue covered with transitional epithelium
    c. Glandular tissue and fibromuscular stroma
    d. Entire gland is composed of collagen
395. What is the normal weight of uterus?
    a. 20 g
    b. 40 g
    c. 60 g
    d. 100 g
396. What is the position of normal uterus?
    a. Anteverted, extended
    b. Anteverted, Anteflexed
    c. Retroverted, extended
    d. Retroverted, anteflexed
397. All of the following statements are true EXCEPT:
    a. Cervix is lined by stratified squamous epithelium
    b. Cervix is lined by transitional epithelium
    c. It gets its blood supply from uterine artery
    d. Vagina is lined by nonkeratinized stratified squamous epithelium.
398. Transitional epithelium is seen in:
    a. Gallbladder
    b. Urinary bladder
    c. Thyroid gland
    d. Stomach
399. Ovarian artery is a branch of:
    a. Abdominal aorta
    b. Internal iliac artery
    c. External iliac artery
    d. Inferior mesenteric artery
400. Left testicular vein drains into:
    a. Inferior vena cava
    b. Left renal vein
    c. Right renal vein
    d. Femoral vein
401. Left gonadal vein drain into:
    a. Left renal vein
    b. Right renal vein
    c. Inferior vena cava
    d. Pampiniform plexus
402. Right ovarian vein drains into:
    a. IVC
    b. Right renal vein
    c. Hemi azygos vein
    d. Inferior mesenteric vein
403. Which of the following is *not* a branch of internal iliac artery?
    a. Superior rectal artery
    b. Middle rectal artery
    c. Superior gluteal artery
    d. Inferior vesicle artery

Anatomy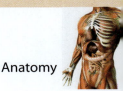

404. Which of the following is a direct branch of Inferior mesenteric artery?
    a. Superior rectal artery   b. Middle rectal artery
    c. Inferior rectal artery   d. Inferior epigastric artery
405. All of these drain into internal iliac lymph nodes EXCEPT:
    a. Ovaries   b. Uterus
    c. Rectum   d. Bladder
406. What is the lymphatic drainage of glans of penis?
    a. Superficial inguinal nodes
    b. Deep inguinal nodes
    c. Paraaortic nodes   d. Internal iliac nodes
407. What is the length of male urethra?
    a. 10 cm   b. 15 cm
    c. 20 cm   d. 30 cm
408. Urinary bladder is supplied by which branches of lumbar plexus?
    a. L1 & L2   b. L2 & L3
    c. L3 & L4   d. L2, L3 & L4
409. Efferent cremastric reflex is carried by:
    a. Illioinguinal nerve   b. Genitofemoral nerve
    c. Iliohypogastric nerve   d. Pudendal nerve
410. Cremasteric reflex is elicited by stroking on which aspect of thigh skin?
    a. Anterior   b. Posterior
    c. Medial   d. Lateral
411. All of the following are contents of the spermatic cord EXCEPT:
    a. Ductus deferens
    b. Testicular artery
    c. Pampiniform plexus of veins
    d. Ilioinguinal nerve
412. Which of the following artery is *not* a content of spermatic cord?
    a. Cremasteric artery   b. Deferential artery
    c. Internal iliac artery   d. Testicular artery

BOARD REVIEW QUESTIONS

413. Nerve supplying area between Great toe and 2nd toe:
    (Recent Pattern Question 2018-19)
    a. Deep peroneal nerve   b. Superficial peroneal nerve
    c. Sural nerve   d. Saphenous nerve
414. Retraction of scapula is by which fibre
    (Recent Pattern Question 2018-19)
    a. Upper fibre of trapezius
    b. Middle fibre of trapezius
    c. Lower fibre of trapezius
    d. Upper and Lower fibre of trapezius
415. Area around umbilicus is supplied by this spinal nerve:
    (Recent Pattern Question 2018-19)
    a. T8   b. T9
    c. T10   d. T12
416. Adam's apple seen in males because of:
    (Recent Pattern Question 2018-19)
    a. Laryngeal ring   b. Hyoid bone
    c. Thyroid cartilage   d. Cricoid cartilage
417. CNS development begins in which intrauterine week?
    a. 5 weeks   b. 6 weeks
    c. 3 weeks   d. 2 weeks
418. Double arch aorta arises from:
    a. Right 6th aortic arch   b. Left 6th aortic arch
    c. Right 4th aortic arch   d. Left 1st aortic arch
419. Urachus fistula is a remnant of?
    a. Yolk sac   b. Allantois
    c. Chorion   d. Amnion
420. Three layers of embryo are formed at what age?
    a. 8 days   b. 12 days
    c. 16 days   d. 21 days
421. Uterus develops from:
    a. Paramesonephric ducts   b. Sinovaginal bulbs
    c. Metanephricblastema   d. Urogenital folds
422. Elastic cartilage is found in:
    a. Tracheal cartilage   b. Auricular cartilage
    c. Articular disc   d. Bronchi
423. Third coronary artery is:
    a. Left anterior descending   b. Left anterior descending
    c. Conus artery   d. Vieussen's artery
424. Cardiac end of stomach lies at which rib?
    a. 8th rib   b. 7th rib
    c. 9th rib   d. 10th rib
425. Sensory supply of palatine tonsil is by which cranial nerve?
    a. IXth   b. Xth
    c. XIth   d. VIIth
426. Recurrent laryngeal nerve lies in relation to:
    a. Superior thyroid artery   b. Inferior thyroid artery
    c. Superior thyroid vein   d. Inferior thyroid vein
427. Which is not a connective tissue?
    a. Blood   b. Bone
    c. Cartilage   d. Muscle/Tendon
428. What is the function of Genioglossus?
    a. Retraction of tongue   b. Protruding tongue
    c. Diverges to the same side   d. All of the above

FMGE Solutions Screening Examination

429. Palatopharyngeus is supplied by which nerve?
    a. Vagus nerve
    b. Cranial accessory nerve
    c. Hypoglossal nerve
    d. Spinal accessory nerve
430. Blood supply of medial surface of cerebral hemisphere is from:
    a. Anterior cerebral artery
    b. Posterior cerebral artery
    c. Middle cerebral artery
    d. Vertebral artery
431. VonEbner glands are mainly present in:
    a. Palate
    b. Buccal mucosa
    c. Tongue
    d. Posterior pharyngeal wall
432. Which bone has no muscle attachment?
    a. Talus
    b. Navicular
    c. Calcaneum
    d. Cuboid
433. Alderman's nerve is:
    a. Tympanic branch of Glossopharyngeal nerve
    b. Auricular branch of vagus nerve
    c. Branch of vestibulocochlear nerve
    d. Nerve from carotid body to glossopharyngeal nerve
434. What is torus aorticus?
    a. Bulge in the atria
    b. Bulge in aorta
    c. Aortic wall tear
    d. Septal defect
435. Vein of Mayo is seen at:
    a. Saphenous junction
    b. Pylorus
    c. Colon
    d. Brain
436. Left testicular vein drains into:
    a. Left renal vein
    b. Inferior vena cava
    c. Common iliac vein
    d. Internal iliac vein
437. Where is fascia of Waldeyer's seen?
    a. Between prostate and rectum
    b. Between rectum and sacrum
    c. Between rectum and pouch of Douglas
    d. Between bladder and vas
438. Maxillary artery develops from:
    a. 1st arch
    b. 3rd arch
    c. 4th arch
    d. 5th arch
439. Root value of phrenic nerve is:
    a. C2, C3, C4
    b. C3, C4, C5
    c. C4, C5, T1
    d. C5, T1, T2
440. Lateral horn of the spinal cord is seen at which level?
    a. Thoracic
    b. Lower lumbar
    c. Sacral
    d. Cervical
441. Pisiform bone articulates with:
    a. Triquetral
    b. Lunate
    c. Scaphoid
    d. Trapezoid
442. The muscle of hand that contains a sesamoid bone is:
    a. Flexor pollicisbrevis
    b. Flexor pollicislongus
    c. Opponenspollicis
    d. Adductor pollicis
443. Lymphatic drainage of testis is?
    a. External iliac nodes
    b. Internal iliac nodes
    c. Pre & para aortic nodes
    d. Superficial inguinal node
444. Trachea is lined by?
    a. Simple columnar
    b. Pseudostratified columnar
    c. Simple cuboidal
    d. Stratified squamous, nonkeratinized
445. Medial arch of foot is made up of:
    a. Deltoid ligament
    b. Spring ligament
    c. Short plantar ligament
    d. Long plantar ligament
446. Constrictions of esophagus when measured from upper incisors are present at:
    a. 15 cm, 20 cm, 40 cm
    b. 15 cm, 25 cm, 40 cm
    c. 20 cm, 30 cm, 40 cm
    d. 30 cm, 40 cm, 60 cm
447. Maximum amount of CSF is found in:
    a. Ventricular system
    b. Subarachnoid space
    c. Epidural space
    d. Subpial space
448. Which of the following is not a branch of 1st part of maxillary artery?
    a. Middle meningeal artery
    b. Accessory meningeal artery
    c. Inferior alveolar artery
    d. Greater palatine artery
449. Short gastric artery is a branch of:
    a. Splenic artery
    b. Left gastroduodenal artery
    c. Left gastroepiploic artery
    d. Portal vein
450. Gartner cyst is a remnant of:
    a. Mesonephric duct in female
    b. Mesonephric duct in males
    c. Paramesonephric duct in males
    d. Paramesonephric duct in females
451. Which organ is derived from both mesoderm and ectoderm?
    a. Kidney
    b. Suprarenal
    c. Urinary bladder
    d. None
452. Outer cell mass gives rise to:
    a. Embryo proper
    b. Trophoblast
    c. Syncytiotrophoblast
    d. None
453. Genital ridge develops from:
    a. Paraxial mesoderm
    b. Lateral plate mesoderm
    c. Intermediate mesoderm
    d. None
454. Which of the following is true about horseshoe kidney?
    a. Fused at upper pole, lies in pelvis
    b. Fused at lower pole, lies in pelvis
    c. Fused at upper pole, lies in front of L1
    d. Fused at lower pole, lies in front of L4
455. Simple squamous epithelium is seen in:
    a. Blood vessel
    b. Thyroid folicle
    c. Esophagus
    d. Hard palate

Anatomy

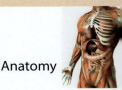

456. Costochondral joint is example of:
    a. Fibrous joint
    b. Primary cartilaginous joint
    c. Secondary cartilaginous joint
    d. Synovial joint
457. Hyoid bone is at which vertebral levels:
    a. C1 to C3   b. C2 to C5
    c. C3 to C6   d. C4 to C7
458. Posterosuperior iliac spine is at the level of:
    a. L5   b. S1
    c. S2   d. S3
459. Most posterior structure seen in root of lung is:
    a. Bronchus
    b. Superior pulmonary vein
    c. Inferior pulmonary vein
    d. Pulmonary artery
460. Most prominent spinous process is of:
    a. C2   b. C5
    c. C6   d. C7
461. Right tracheobranchial angle is:
    a. 10-15 degrees   b. 25-30 degrees
    c. 40-50 degrees   d. 80-90 degrees
462. Middle meningeal artery passes through which foramen:
    a. Foramen rotundum   b. Foramen spinosum
    c. Foramen ovale   d. Jugular foramen
463. Arrange coverings on peripheral nerve from inner to outer?
    a. Endoneurium, epineurium, perineurium
    b. Endoneurium, perineurium, epineurium
    c. Perineurium, endoneurium, epineurium
    d. Epineurium, endoneurium, perineurium
464. Nerve supply of deltoid is:
    a. Axillary   b. Musculocutaneous
    c. Median   d. Radial
465. Nerve supply of obturator is by:
    a. L1–L3   b. L4–S1
    c. L5–S2   d. S1–S3
466. Lymphatic drainage of glans penis is by:
    a. Superficial inguinal lymph nodes
    b. Deep inguinal lymph nodes
    c. Internal iliac lymph nodes
    d. Preaortic nodes
467. Preauricular sulcus is seen in:
    a. Mandible   b. Maxilla
    c. Skull   d. Pelvis
468. Cribroform plate is a part of:
    a. Ethmoid   b. Maxilla
    c. Nasal   d. Frontal
469. Ligament preventing the displacement of humerus is:
    a. Coracoclavicular   b. Coracohumeral
    c. Coracoacromial   d. Glenohumeral

470. Anterior cerebral artery supplies which part of brain:
    a. Anterior   b. Lateral
    c. Medial   d. Posterior
471. Korner's septum is seen in?
    a. Petrosquamous suture
    b. Temporosquamous suture
    c. Petromastoid suture
    d. Frontozygomatic suture
472. Third tubercle of femur provides attachment to:
    a. Gluteus maximus   b. Gluteus medius
    c. Gluteus minimis   d. Piriformis
473. Muscle which helps in protrusion and upper movement of tongue is:
    a. Palatoglossus   b. Hyoglossus
    c. Genioglossus   d. Stylogossus
474. Which of the following has a single ossification centre only?
    a. Clavicle   b. Carpals
    c. Metacarpals   d. Metatarsals
475. Which of the following is the muscle of third pharyngeal arch?
    a. Stylohyoid   b. Mylohyoid
    c. Cricothyroid   d. Stylopharyngeus
476. Morula reaches uterus on:
    a. 3rd day after fertilization   b. 4th day after fertilization
    c. 6th day after fertilization   d. 8th day after fertilization
477. Testis are developed from:
    a. Genital ridge   b. Genital tubercle
    c. Wolffian duct   d. Gubernaculum
478. Common carotid artery is formed by:
    a. 2nd arch   b. 3rd arch
    c. 4th arch   d. 6th arch
479. Palatine tonsil develops from:
    a. 1st pharyngeal arch   b. 1st pharyngeal pouch
    c. 2nd pharyngeal arch   d. 2nd pharyngeal pouch
480. Neural tube completely closes at what intrauterine age?
    a. 10 days   b. 20 days
    c. 25 days   d. 27 days
481. Tympanic membrane develops from:
    a. Mesoderm   b. Endoderm
    c. Ectoderm   d. All three germ layers
482. Horse shoe kidney is due to prevention of ascent by:
    a. Superior mesenteric artery
    b. Inferior mesenteric artery
    c. Supernumerary arteries
    d. Ureters
483. Skin over femoral triangle is supplied by:
    a. Iliohypogastric nerve
    b. Ilioinguinal nerve
    c. Genitofemoral nerve
    d. Lateral femoral cutaneous nerve

484. Vertebral level of body of sternum is:
    a. T 3 to T 4
    b. T 4 to T 5
    c. T 5 to T 7
    d. T 5 to T 9
485. Ligaments for anteroposterior stability of knee are:
    a. Cruciate ligaments
    b. Medial collateral ligament
    c. Lateral collateral ligament
    d. Patellar ligaments
486. Which structure passes through greater sciatic foramen?
    a. Superior gluteal nerve and vessels
    b. Tendon of obturator internus
    c. Anterior cutaneous nerve of thigh
    d. Semimembranosus tendon
487. Which structure passes through both greater and lesser sciatic foramen?
    a. Nerve to quadrates femoris
    b. Superior gluteal nerve
    c. Nerve to obturator internus
    d. Piriformis muscle
488. Sacrotuberous ligament is pierced by:
    a. Nerve to obturator internus
    b. Inferior gluteal artery
    c. Superior gluteal artery
    d. Sciatic nerve
489. Lesser petrosal is a branch of:
    a. Occulomotor nerve
    b. Abducens nerve
    c. Facial nerve
    d. Glossopharyngeal nerve
490. Middle piece of sperm tail is made up of:
    a. Golgibody
    b. Centriole
    c. Mitochondria
    d. Lysosome
491. Third part of duodenum is crossed by:
    a. Portal vein
    b. Hepatic artery
    c. Bile duct
    d. Superior mesenteric artery
492. Innervation of lower one fourth of vagina is done by:
    a. Pudendal nerve
    b. Pelvic splanchanic nerve
    c. Lumbar splanchanic nerve
    d. Hypogastric nerve

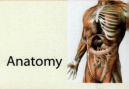

Anatomy

IMAGE-BASED QUESTIONS

493. Which part of brain presents in Turkish saddle shaped space in cranium?

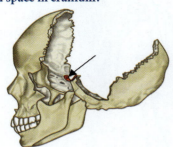

a. Pituitary
b. Frontal lobe
c. Hypothalamus
d. Basal ganglia

494. Which nerve is involved in this presentation?

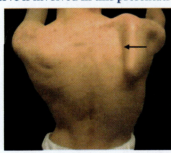

a. Long thoracic Nerve
b. Musculocutaneous nerve
c. Lateral anterior thoracic nerve
d. Thoracodorsal nerve

495. Name the ligament:

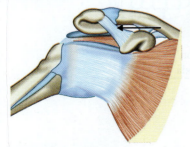

a. Coraco-acromial ligament
b. Acromio-clavicular ligament
c. Coraco-Humeral Ligament
d. Sterno-clavicular Ligament

496. Which nerve is marked by an arrow in the vicinity of popliteal fossa?

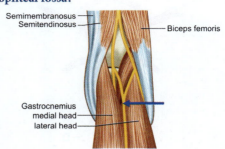

a. Common peroneal neve
b. Deep peroneal nerve
c. Sural nerve
d. Sciatic nerve

497. A patient complains of pain in the distribution shown below. All are true about the condition except:

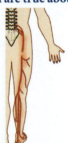

a. Sciatic Nerve is involved b. Pain worse on standing
c. Straight Leg raising leading to pain in opposite leg indicates disc herniation
d. Nerve originates from nerve roots L5-S2

498. Which of the following is branch of external carotid Artery?

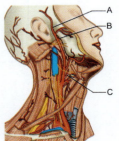

a. A
b. B
c. C
d. All of the above

499. The blockage of which of the following blood vessel will lead to medial medullary syndrome?

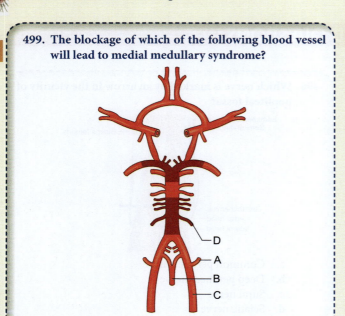

a. A b. B
c. C d. D

500. What is the insertion of shown muscle: (2018)

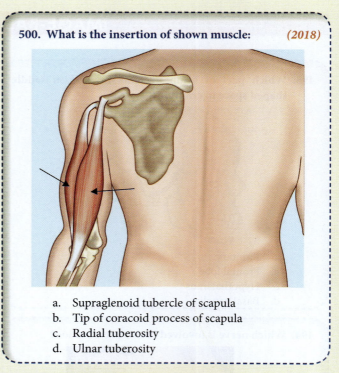

a. Supraglenoid tubercle of scapula
b. Tip of coracoid process of scapula
c. Radial tuberosity
d. Ulnar tuberosity

501. The marked area in skull represents: (2018)

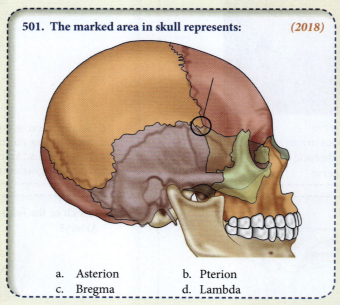

a. Asterion   b. Pterion
c. Bregma   d. Lambda

Answers to Image-Based Questions are given at the end of explained questions

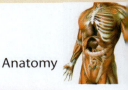

Anatomy

ANSWERS WITH EXPLANATIONS

MOST RECENT QUESTIONS 2019

1. **Ans. (a) Scaphoid**
   - The floor of the anatomical snuff box is formed by the scaphoid bone. An injury to this area increases the suspicion of scaphoid fracture

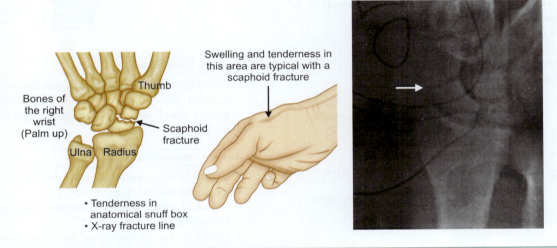

2. **Ans. (b) Extensor hallucis longus**
   - The shown tendon is extensor hallucis longus.
   - **Origin:** Anterior surface of fibula and the adjacent interosseous membrane
   - **Insertion:** Base of dorsal center of distal phalanx of great toe
   - **Function:** Dorsal flexion and eversion of foot and extension of toes.
   - **Innervation:** Deep peroneal nerve (L4, L5, S1)

FMGE Solutions Screening Examination

3. **Ans. (b) Pronator teres**
   - Among given options pronator teres originates from medial epicondyle.
   - Pronator teres muscle (from anterior arm, superior group of muscle):
     - **Action**: Pronates and flexes forearm
     - **Origin**: Medial epicondyle of humerus, coronoid process of ulna
     - **Insertion**: Lateral surface of radius
   - **Muscles originating from medial epicondyle of humerus:**
     - Pronator teres
     - Flexor carpi radialis
     - Palmaris longus
     - Flexor carpi ulnaris

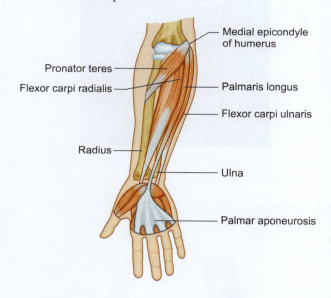

4. **Ans. (b) Inferior constrictor muscle**
   - Killian's dehiscence is a potential gap between thyropharyngeus oblique fibres and transverse fibres of cricopharyngeus muscle.
   - These two muscles thyropharyngeus and cricopharyngeus are collectively called inferior constrictor muscle.
   - There are 3 pharyngeal circular/constrictor muscles namely: Superior, Middle, Inferior.
   - This Killian's dehiscence is also the site for development of Zenker's diverticulum.

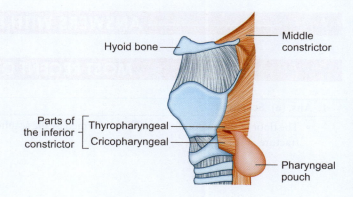

5. **Ans. (a) Parotid gland**
   - All the glands in the face (like submandibular, sublingual, lacrimal gland) are supplied by facial nerve except parotid gland, which is supplied by glossopharyngeal nerve.

6. **Ans. (c) Anencephaly**
   - Cranial (rostral) neuropore closes by day 25
   - Caudal neuropore closes by day 28
   - Failure of cranial neuropore to close at day 25 results in anencephaly
   - Failure of caudal neuropore to close results in spina bifida.

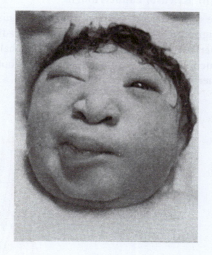

Anatomy

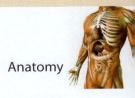

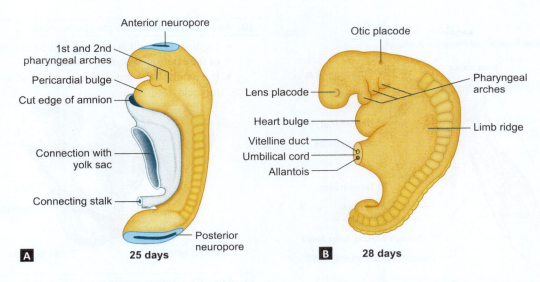

---

7. **Ans. (a) Ulnar nerve**
   - The shown course of nerve is of ulnar nerve
   - Please refer the image below

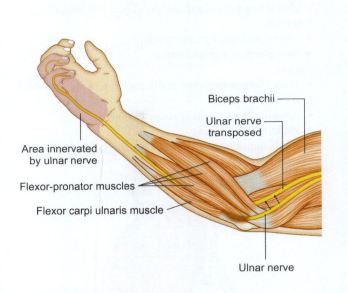

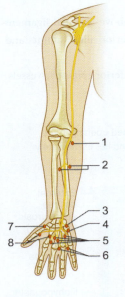

Ulnar nerve

Distribution of the motor branches
1. Flexor carpi ulnaris
2. Flexor digitorum profundus ulnar portion
3. Hypothenar muscles: abductor, short flexor, opponens of little finger
4. Palmaris brevis
5. All dorsal and palmar interossei
6. Ulnar lumbricals
7. Deep head of flexor pollicis brevis
8. Adductor pollicus

---

8. **Ans. (a) Teres major**
   - The shown muscle in the image is teres major.
   - Origin-Inferior angle of scapula
   - Insertion-Intertubecular sulcus of humerus
   - Action
     - Extends arm at shoulder joint
     - Assist in adduction and medial rotation of arm at shoulder joint
   - Nerve supply
     - Lower subscapular nerve

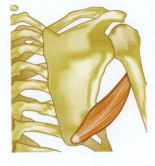

Explanations

FMGE Solutions Screening Examination

> **Extra Mile**
> Identify the deep muscles of shoulder in image

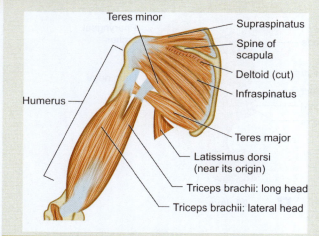

9. Ans. (b) Transversalis fascia

- **Deep inguinal ring** is an oval opening formed in transversalis fascia.
- It lies about 0.5 inch (1.3 cm) above inguinal ligament midway between anterior superior iliac supine and symphysis pubis.
- Medial to deep inguinal ring is inferior epigastric vessels.

> **Extra Mile**
> - Superficial inguinal ring: A triangular shaped opening in the aponeurosis of external oblique muscle and lies immediately above and medial to pubic tubercle.

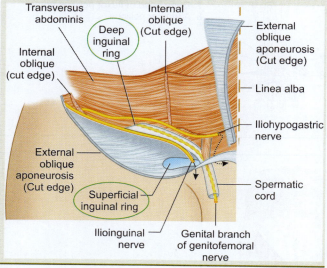

10. Ans. (a) External oblique aponeurosis

- Inguinal ligament is a fibrous, thickened, folded margin of the external oblique aponeurosis.
- It extends from anterior superior iliac spine to pubic tubercle.

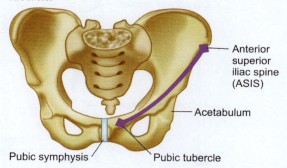

11. Ans. (d) Gluteus medius

Gluteus medius
- Posterior part covered by gluteus maximus

Origin
- Outer surface of ilium b/w iliac crest above and posterior gluteal line behind and middle gluteal line below.

Insertion
- Lateral surface of greater trochanter
- **Nerve**-superior gluteal nerve

Action
- With Gluteus minimus and tensor fascia lata-powerful abductor at hip
- Anterior fibres medially rotate the thigh
- Walking and running
- Holds opposite side of pelvis horizontally when foot is off the ground

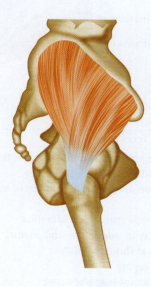

Anatomy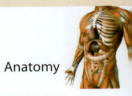

12. **Ans. (c) T8**

    - Inferior scapular angle lies at the anatomical level of T8

    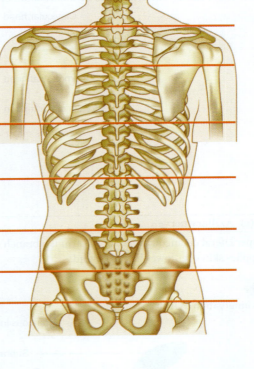

    - **C2**-First palpable SP below the occipital bone
    - **C7 or T1**–most prominent SP at base of neck (C7 will usually slide anterior from a palpating finger with cervical extension)
    - **T4**–Level with the root of the spine of scapula or apex of axillary fold
    - **T7–T8**-Level with the inferior angle of scapula

    Thoracic TP palpation rule of 3s
    - **T1–T3 TPs**: At level of corresponding SP
    - **T4–T6 TPS**: ~1/2 Segment above SP
    - **T7–T9 TPs**: At ~level of SP of vertebrae above T10–T12 have SPs that project from a position similar to T9 and rapidly regress until T12 is like T1

    - **T12**–Level with the head of the 12th rib
    - **L4**–Level with the superior border of the iliac crest
    - **PSIS and S2**–Level with the most inferior portion of the PSIS
    - **Sacral Apex**–Level with upper greater trochanter (have patient rotate hip to locate trochanter)

    SP: Spinous process, TP: Thoracic process

13. **Ans. (b) Abdominal aorta**

    - Testicular artery is a branch of abdominal aorta.
    - *Please refer the image given below:*

    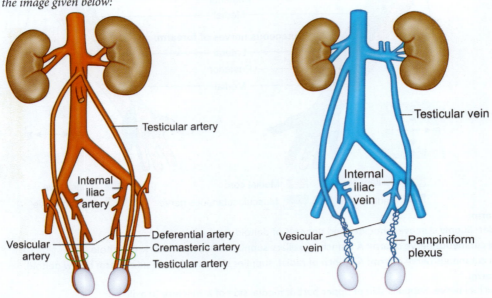

Explanations

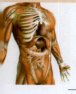

14. **Ans. (b) Pectoralis major**

   Anatomy of pectoralis major muscle:
   - **Origin:** Clavicle, sternum and costal cartilage $2^{nd} – 6^{th}$ ribs
   - **Insertion:** Lateral lip of intertubercular groove of humerus
   - **Function:** Flexion, adduction and medial rotation of arm

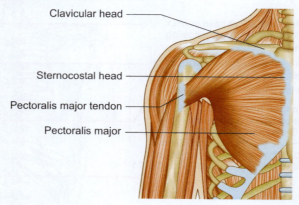

15. **Ans. (c) Axillary nerve**
    - Upper lateral cutaneous nerve of the arm is a branch of axillary nerve.
    - Supplies skin over lower half of deltoid.

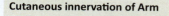

Cutaneous innervation of Arm

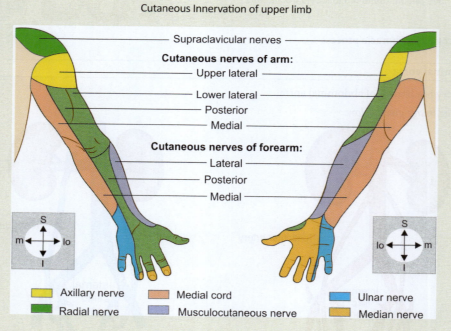

Lateral side of arm:
- Supraclavicular: Supply skin over shoulder and upper ½ of deltoid
- Upper lateral cutaneous nerve of arm: A branch of axillary supplies skin over lower ½ of deltoid
- Lower lateral cutaneous nerve of arm: A branch of radial, supplies skin over lateral side of arm below deltoid.

Medial side of arm:
- Intercostobrachial nerve: Supplies skin of upper part of medial side of arm (close to axilla)
- Medial cutaneous nerve of arm: A branch of medial cord, supplies medial side of arm below axilla.

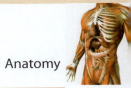

Anatomy

EMBRYOLOGY HISTOLOGY AND OSTEOLOGY

16. Ans. (c) 270 degree anticlockwise

Ref: Textbook of Clinical Embryology by Vishram Singh, P 148

- The rotation of midgut occurs when herniated intestinal loop returns back to the abdominal cavity.
- It begins at the end of third month of intrauterine life
- The primary intestinal loop rotates around an axis formed by the superior mesenteric artery, which divides the midgut loop into 2 segments:
  - **Proximal (prearterial) segment-** present cranially
    - Give rise to: Distal half of duodenum, Jejunum, Ileum except its terminal part
  - **Distal (postarterial) segment-** present caudally
    - Give rise to terminal part of ileum, Cecum, appendix, ascending colon, proximal 2/3rd of transverse colon.
- In order to return to abdominal cavity, the midgut loop undergoes anticlockwise rotation of 90° thrice → total rotation of 270°.
  - The first 90° rotation occurs outside abdominal cavity (within umbilicus), remaining 2 rotations in abdominal cavity

Stepwise midgut rotation

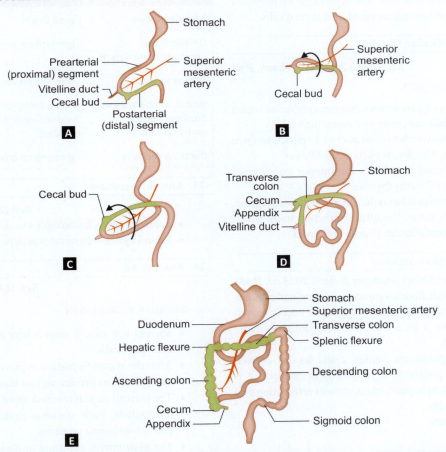

FIGURES: Rotation of midgut loop as seen in left side view. A. Primitive loop before rotation; B. Anticlockwise 90° rotation of midgut loop while it is in the extraembryonic celom in the umbilical cord; C. Anticlockwise 180° rotation of midugt loop as it is withdrawn into the abdominal cavity; D. Descent of cecum takes place later; E. Intestinal loops in final position.

17. Ans. (a) Superior mesenteric artery

Ref: Gray's Anatomy 41st ed. P 1054

Rotation of Midgut Loop
- Midgut loop has 2 ends: Cranial end and caudal end.
- The primary intestinal loop rotates around an axis formed by the superior mesenteric artery

Refer to above explanation for more detailed explanation

18. Ans. (c) Hyaluronic acid

Ref: Gray's Anatomy, E-book, 41st ed. P 188

- Hyaluronic acid and chondroitin sulfate are present in the migration pathways of neural crest cells.
- Hyaluronic acid is synthesized by the neural crest cells, ectoderm, somites and neural tube cells.
- The role of hyaluronic acid is to expand the extracellular spaces and facilitate migration of neural crest cells.

19. Ans. (b) Parafollicular 'C' cells

Ref: Gray's Anatomy E-book. P 61

ENDODERMAL POUCHES
- **1st pouch:** Dorsal part forms tubotympanic recess which forms the middle ear cavity and eustachian tube.
- **2nd pouch:** Joins with ventral part of 1st pouch to form palatine tonsil. Also forms parts of middle ear.
- **3rd pouch:** Dorsal part forms the inferior parathyroid gland and ventral forms thymus.
- **4th pouch:** Dorsal part forms the superior parathyroid gland.
  - Ventral part forms the ultimobranchial body which forms the parafollicular C-cells of thyroid.

20. Ans. (b) Craniopharyngioma

Ref: Gray's Anatomy E-Book 2015 ed. P 431

- In embryogenesis Rathke's pouch is an evagination at the roof of the developing mouth in front of buccopharyngeal membrane. It gives rise to anterior pituitary (adenohypophysis).
- Craniopharyngioma are benign cystic lesions derived from Rathke's pouch, most frequently in children. It is associated with hypopituitarism, growth retardation and diabetes insipidus.
- **Clinical features:**
  - Raised ICT
  - Presents before 20 years of age
  - Visual field abnormalities
  - Weight gain
  - Cranial nerve damage
- **Investigation:** MRI is superior to CT.

21. Ans. (d) Osseus labyrinth

Ref: Gray's Anatomy, 41st ed. pg. 644

- Osseous labyrinth is considered as hardest bone of the body. It is embedded in petrous part of temporal bone, which is also known as "rock bone".
- **American edition of British encyclopedia states:** *"The labyrinth of the ear is formed of cochlea, 3 semicircular canals and a small cavity known as vestibulum into which cochlea and semicircular canal opens. These parts are formed of the hardest bone in body, almost equal in solidity to ivory and petrous portion of temporal bone."*

22. Ans. (b) Medial umbilical ligament

Ref: Langman Embryology, pg. 148

Fetal structure	Adult structure
Foramen Ovale	Fossa Ovalis
Umbilical vein (intra-abdominal part)	Ligamentum teres
Ductus venosus	Ligamentum venosum
Umbilical arteries and Proximal part of umbilical artery	Medial umbilical ligaments Superior vesicular artery (supplies bladder)
Ductus arteriosus	Ligamentum arteriosum

23. Ans. (b) Scrotum

Ref: D.C. Dutta, 8th ed. pg. 1

- Labia majora is homologous to scrotum in male.
- Round ligament terminates at upper border of labia majora

24. Ans. (b) 16

Ref: D.C. Dutta, 8th ed. pg. 22

MORULA FORMATION
- Morula is a 16 cell stage where embryo is enclosed in zona pellucida.
- After the zygote formation, typical mitotic division of the nucleus occurs producing two blastomeres.
- The two cell stage is reached *approximately 30 hours* after fertilization. Each contains equal cytoplasmic volume and chromosome numbers.
- The blastomeres continue to divide by binary division through 4, 8, 16 cell stage until a cluster of cell is formed which is called *morula*, resembling a mulberry. As the total volume of the cell mass is not increased and the zona pellucida remains intact, the morula after spending

Anatomy

about 3 days in the uterine tube *enters the uterine cavity through the narrow uterine ostium (1 mm) on the 4th day in the 16–64 cell stage.*

25. Ans. (d) Two arteries and one vein, umbilical vein supplying towards fetus

"Remember 2AV"

- Umbilical cord is the structure which connects mother to fetus and acts as a bridge for transfer of blood and other nutrients from mother to baby.
- It contains *2 arteries and one vein*. Arteries carry deoxygenated blood from fetus to mother while *vein carries oxygenated blood from mother towards fetus.*
- Cord contains Wharton's jelly and the structures embedded in this are:
  - 2 arteries and 1 vein
  - Allantois and
  - Remains of vitellointestinal duct

26. Ans. (d) Umbilical vessels

Ref: Textbook of Human Embroyology, pg. 56

- As the amniotic cavity enlarges, it obliterates the chorionic cavity and covers the connecting stalk and gets reflected at the region of **primitive umbilical ring** (amino-ectodermal junction).
- The primitive umbilical region gradually gets crowded and contains: (i) connecting stalk having allantois, umbilical vessels (two arteries and one vein), (ii) yolk stalk (vitelline duct) along with vitelline vessels, and (iii) the canal connecting the intraembryonic and extraembryonic cavities.
- All these structures finally give rise to primitive umbilical cord. A part of the yolk sac which lies in the chorionic cavity later shrinks and gets obliterated.
- Initially when the abdominal cavity is too small, and the loops of intestine grow very fast, some of them get pushed into the extraembryonic space in the umbilical cord. This is called **physiological umbilical hernia.**
- By the end of the third month, the abdominal cavity enlarges and the loop of intestine returns into the abdomen and the extraembryonic cavity of umbilical cord gets obliterated.
  - *The structures of the umbilical cord, i.e., vitelline duct, vitelline vessels and allantois also get obliterated and are converted into* **Wharton's jelly.** *The only structures which remain functional in Wharton's jelly are the umbilical vessels.*

Extra Mile

- Obliterated umbilical artery gives rise to medial umbilical ligament
- Obliterated umbilical veins give rise to ligamentum teres

27. Ans. (c) Branchial pouch: Endoderm

Ref: Netter's Essential Histology, 2nd ed. pg. 355

The branchial apparatus is composed up of branchial clefts, arches and pouch

Branchial **C**lefts	Ectoderm
Branchial **A**rches	Mesoderm
Branchial **P**ouches	Endoderm

28. Ans. (c) Cardinal vein

Ref: Langman's essential medical Embroyology pg. 57

- During early embryonic development (through 4th week), paired cardinal veins drain the body. *Anterior cardinal* veins drain the head and upper limb buds, while *posterior cardinal veins* drain the body. Both the anterior and posterior veins on each side unite at the common cardinal veins that flow into the sinus venosus and ultimately into the common atrium (Image).
- Anterior cardinal veins are retained. An anastomosis between the two forms the left brachiocephalic vein, and anterior segments from both form the jugular system for the head and neck (Image).
- Most of the posterior segment on the left disappears except for that forming the left superior intercostal vein, whereas the right posterior segment forms the superior vena cava.

Extra Mile

Defects of SVC Development

- **Double inferior vena cava** occurs when the left supracardinal vein persists, thereby forming an additional inferior vena cava below the level of the kidneys.
- **Left superior vena cava** occurs when the left anterior cardinal vein persists, forming a superior vena cava on the left side. The right anterior cardinal vein abnormally regresses.
- **Double superior vena cava** occurs when the left anterior cardinal vein persists, forming a superior vena cava on the left side. The right anterior cardinal vein also forms a superior vena cava on the right side.

FMGE Solutions Screening Examination

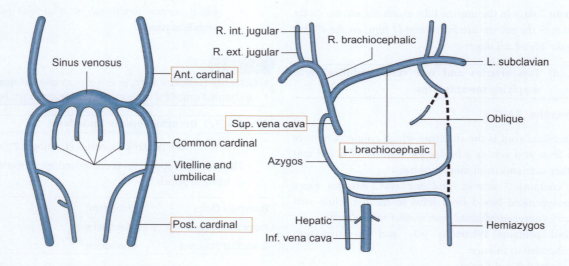

29. Ans. (d) 4th pharyngeal arch

Ref: *Gray's Anatomy, 41st ed. pg. 607*

DERIVATIVES OF THE PHARYNGEAL ARCHES

Arch number	Arch name	Embryonic cartilage	Cartilage derivative	Muscle	Nerve	Artery
1	Mandibular	Quadrate Meckel's	Incus Malleus Anterior ligament of malleus Spine of sphenoid Sphenomandibular ligament Genial tubercle of mandible	Tensor tympani Muscles of mastication Mylohyoid Anterior belly of digastric Tensor veli palatine	Trigeminal (V) Mandibular division	First aortic arch artery (transitory)

2	Hyoid	Reichert's	• Stapes
			• Styloid process of temporal bone
			• Styloid process of temporal bone
			• Stylohyoid ligament
			• Lesser horn and upper part of body of hyoid bone
				• Stapedius
				• Stylohyoid muscle
				• Facial muscles, include.
				    ▪ Buccinator
				    ▪ Platysma
				    ▪ Posterior belly digastric
					Facial (VII)	Stapedial artery (transitory)

3	Third		Greater horn and lower part of body of hyoid bone	Stylopharyngeus	Glossopharyngeal (IX)	**Common carotid artery**
4	Fourth		Thyroid cartilage Corniculate cartilage Cuneiform cartilage	Pharyngeal and extrinsic laryngeal muscles, levator veli palatini	Vagus (X) Pharyngeal branch	• Proximal part of subclavian artery on the right • **Arch of aorta** between origins of left common carotid and left subclavian arteries
6	Sixth		Arytenoid cartilages	Intrinsic laryngeal muscles	Vagus (X) Recurrent laryngeal branch	Part between the pulmonary trunk and dorsal aorta becomes ductus arteriosus on left, disappears on right

Anatomy

30. Ans. (b) 3rd pharyngeal arch

Ref: Gray's Anatomy, 41st ed. pg. 607

- The common carotid and first part of internal carotid artery is derived from **3rd pharyngeal arch**
- The common carotid arteries differ on the right and left sides with respect to their origins. **On the right**, the common carotid arises from the brachiocephalic artery as it passes behind the sternoclavicular joint.
- **On the left**, the common carotid artery comes directly from the arch of the aorta in the superior mediastinum. The right common carotid, therefore, has only a cervical part whereas the left common carotid has cervical and thoracic parts.

31. Ans. (b) 2nd branchial arch

Ref: Gray's Anatomy, 41st ed. pg. 449

- The stylohyoid ligament is a fibrous cord extending from the tip of the styloid process to the lesser cornu of the hyoid bone. It gives attachment to the highest fibres of the middle pharyngeal constrictor and is intimately related to the lateral wall of the oropharynx. Below, it is overlapped by hyoglossus.
- The ligament is derived from the cartilage of the **second branchial arch,** and may be partially calcified.

32. Ans. (a) 1

Ref: Gray's Anatomy, 41st ed. pg. 607
Refer to table of Q. 12

33. Ans. (a) Stylophyoid ligament

Ref: Gray's Anatomy, 41st ed. pg. 607
Refer to table of Q. 12

34. Ans. (b) 2nd branchial arch

*Ref: Inderbir Singh's Embroyology, 9th ed. pg. 116-117,
7th ed. pg. 119-120*

- At first there are 6 arches. The 5th arch disappears.
- *Upper half and lesser cornu of hyoid bone is derived from 2nd arch.*
- *Lower half and greater of hyoid bone is derived from 3rd arch.*
- Palatine tonsil derived from 2nd branchial pouch.

35. Ans. (b) II

Ref: I.B. Singh, 9th ed. pg. 116
Refer to table of Q. 12

36. Ans. (d) Cricothyroid

Ref: I.B. Singh, 9th ed. pg. 116

- Cricothyroid muscle is derived from fourth branchial arch. It is the only intrinsic laryngeal muscle not derived from 6th branchial arch
- **Nerve supply:** Superior laryngeal nerve

37. Ans. (d) Thyroid

Ref: I.B. Singh, 9th ed. pg. 116-17

- Superior parathyroid is derived from 4th branchial pouch
- Inferior parathyroid and thymus develop from 3rd branchial pouch
- *Most of the thyroid gland develops from thyroglossal duct (endodemal duct at foramen cecum).*

38. Ans. (d) 1st and 2nd branchial arch

Ref: P.L. Dhingra, 6th ed. pg. 11

- The auricle develops from fusion of mesenchyme of **1st and 2nd branchial arch**.
- External ear canal develops from the ectoderm of 1st branchial cleft.
- Tympanic membrane is derived from all the three germ layers contributed by 1st pharyngeal/ branchial arch.

39. Ans. (c) Branchial pouch 3rd

Ref: Netter's Essential Histology, 2nd ed. pg. 227

- **THI**rd branchial pouch forms the **TH**ymus and **I**nferior parathyroid glands.
- Fourth branchial pouch forms superior parathyroid glands and ultimobranchial body.
- Aberrant development of third and fourth branchial pouches results in *Di-george syndrome*. It leads to thymic and inferior parathyroid gland hypoplasia. The infant develops recurrent pneumonia episodes and hypocalcemia.
- 2nd branchial pouch forms tonsils.
- 1st branchial pouch *ventral* part forms tongue
- 1st branchial pouch *dorsal* part forms tubotympanic recess, Eustachian tube, middle ear cavity and inner part of Eustachian tube.

40. Ans. (b) 2nd pouch

Ref: Netter's Essential Histology, 2nd ed. pg. 227

Tonsil is derived from 2nd branchial pouch.

41. Ans. (d) Palatine tonsils

*Ref: I.B. Singh, 9th ed. pg. 1118; Fundamental Anatomy
By Walter Carl Hartwig, pg. 185*

- First pharyngeal pouch is located between 1st and 2nd pharyngeal arch
- **Palatine tonsil is a derivative of 2nd pharyngeal pouch**
- Eustachean tube, Middle ear, mastoid antrum and tympanic membrane is derived from 1st pharyngeal pouch.

Explanations

42. Ans. (b) Dorsal part of 1st cleft

Ref: Netter's Essentials of Human Embryology, 3rd ed. pg. 235

- The dorsal part of 1st cleft forms the *external auditory canal* while the *ventral part of first cleft obliterates.*
- The 2nd to 4th clefts form temporary cervical sinuses and failure to obliterate leads to branchial cleft cyst.

43. Ans. (c) Sinovaginal bulb

Ref: Human Ebroyology: The Ultimate USMLE step 1, pg. 45

- In females, the paired embryonic paramesonephric duct forms the uterine tubes, uterus, cervix and superior part of vagina.
- The **lower 3rd of vagina** develops from **sinovaginal bulbs**, which are paired evaginations of the wall of the urogenital sinus.
- At around 15 weeks of embroyologic development, the **mullerian system** which forms the **upper 2/3rd of vagina**, fuses with the invaginating cloaca or **urogenital sinus to form the lower 1/3rd of vagina.**
- These two parts of vagina, i.e. paramesonephric duct part and sinovaginal bulb part canalize to form a single, complete vaginal canal.

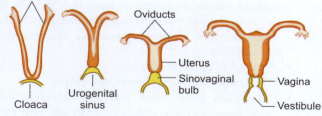

44. Ans. (d) Prochordal plate

Ref: Netter's Clinical Anatomy, 3rd ed. pg. 39

- Hypoblast and epiblast are 2 germ layers in the second week of embryonic development.
- The *hypoblast* gives rise to prochordal plate which is the future site of mouth and forms the cranio-caudal axis.
- Notochord is formed by *epiblast* cells.
- Epiblast is also the source of all three germ layers.
- *First germ layer* to be formed is the *endoderm.*[Q]
- *Remnants of notochord* are nucleus pulposus and apical ligament of atlas.

45. Ans. (a) CVS

Ref: Netter's Clinical Anatomy, 3rd ed. pg. 35

- CVS is the first fully functional organ system in fetus and first to attain maturity from functional perspective.

46. Ans. (c) Week 3

Ref: Netter's Clinical Anatomy, 3rd ed. pg. 39

- Gastrulation is defined as formation of 3 germ layers in 3rd week of embryonic development.
- The 3rd week of development is also called stage of trilaminar germ disk.
- *Gastrulation begins* with formation of primitive streak by proliferation of epiblast cells near the caudal end of embryonic disk. Primitive disc regresses by fourth week.

47. Ans. (b) Endoderm

Ref: Netter's Atlas of Embryology, 2012 ed. pg. 47

- Epiblast is the source of all three germ layers and *endoderm* is the *first germ layer* to be formed.

48. Ans. (b) Epiblast

Ref: Netter's Atlas of Neurosciences, 3rd ed. pg. 126

- Notochord is formed by epiblast cells and it provides central axis to the embryronic disc. It induces the overlying ectodermal cells to become neuro-ectodermal cells and form the neural tube.

49. Ans. (a) Segmental organization of embryo is craniocaudal direction

Ref: Netter's Atlas of Human Embryology, 2012 ed. pg. 10

- *Homeobox (HOX) gene* is involved in *segmental organization of embryo in cranio-caudal* direction. The mutation in gene leads to formation of appendages in wrong locations.
- *Sonic hedge-hog gene* is involved in patterning in *A-P axis.* The mutation in this gene leads to holoprosencephaly.

50. Ans. (a) Neural crest

Ref: Netter's Atlas of Neurosciences, 3rd ed. pg. 133

Derivatives of neural crest (mnemonic: **N.O.P.E**)
- Mela**N**ocytes
- Schwa**N**n cells
- Adrenal medulla (Chromaffi**N** cells)
- **O**dontoblasts
- **P**arasympathetic ganglia of gut
- **P**arafollicular cells of thyroid
- **P**ia and arachnoid matters
- **E**ndocardial cushions and aortopulmonary septum in heart

Anatomy

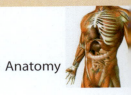

Extra Mile

Derivatives of neuroectoderm:
- All CNS neurons astrocytes, oligodendrocytes, ependymocytes, neurohypophysis and pineal gland.

51. Ans. (a) Foregut

Ref: Netter's Clinical Anatomy, 3rd ed. pg. 207

Derivatives of Foregut
- Part of mouth including the tongue to 2nd part of duodenum (up to major duodenal papilla)
- Liver, pancreas, biliary channels
- Respiratory system

Derivative of Midgut
- From 2nd part of duodenum to right 2/3rd of transverse colon

Derivatives of Hindgut
- From left 1/3rd of transverse colon to upper part of anal canal
- Part of urogenital system derived from the primitive urogenital sinus

52. Ans. (a) Superior vesical artery

Ref: Netter's Atlas of Human Embryology, 2012 ed. pg. 86

Structure name	Derivative
Obliterated umbilical artery	Medial umbilical ligament
Proximal part of umbilical artery	Superior vesical artery
Inferior epigastric artery	Lateral umbilical fold
Left umbilical vein	Ligamentum teres
Right umbilical vein	Disappears
Ductus venosus	Ligamentum venosum
Urachus	Median umbilical ligament
Vitello-intestinal duct	Meckel's diverticulum

53. Ans. (d) Umbilical vein

Ref: Langeman's, 8th pg. 264, 259

Please refer to above explanation.

54. Ans. (b) Ligamentum venosum

Ref: Langeman's, 8th pg. 264, 259

55. Ans. (a) Coronary sinus

Ref: Netter's Atlas of Human Embryology: 2012 ed. pg. 96

Heart tube embryonic derivatives

Embryonic structure	Gives rise to
Proximal 1/3rd of bulbus cordis	Primitive trabeculated left ventricle
Middle 1/3rd of bulbus cordis	Right and left ventricular outflow tract
Distal 1/3rd of bulbus cordis (truncus arteriosus)	Ascending aorta and pulmonary trunk
Left horn of sinus venosus	Coronary sinus
Right horn of sinus venosus	Smooth part of right atrium
Right common cardinal nerve and right anterior cardinal nerve	SVC (superior vena cava)

56. Ans. (b) 2

Ref: Netter's Atlas of Human Embryology: 2012 ed. pg. 88

- There are six pairs of aortic arches which develop in cephalo-caudal direction.
- The 5th aortic arch completely disappears whereas 1st and 2nd disappear partially.
- *The stapedial artery is derived from the 2nd aortic arch.*
- Inferior alveolar artery is derived from the 1st aortic arch.

57. Ans. (a) Septum primum

Ref: Netter's Clinical Anatomy, 3rd ed. pg. 113

- *Fossa ovalis* is the remnant of **septum primum**.
- *Foramen ovale* is opening between the upper and lower limbs of **septum secundum**.
- This is a very closely worded question, so get the perspectives right.

58. Ans. (c) 8 months

Ref: Netter's Clinical Anatomy, 3rd ed. pg. 325

Descent of testis

3rd month	Iliac fossa
7th month	Deep inguinal ring
7th month	Transits through inguinal canal
8th month	Superficial inguinal ring
9th month	Enters the scrotum

59. Ans. (a) Metencephalon

Ref: Netter's Atlas of Neurosciences, 3rd ed. pg. 136

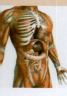

Parts of developing brain

[Diagram showing: Prosencephalon → Telencephalon, Diencephalon; Mesencephalon → Mesencephalon, Metencephalon; Rhombencephalon → Metencephalon, Myelencephalon; Spinal cord]

Myelencephalon	Medulla oblongata
Metencephalon	*Pons, cerebellum and 4th ventricle*
Mesencephalon	Midbrain and aqueduct of slyvius
Diencephalon	Thalamus, hypothalamus and *3rd ventricle*
Telencephalon	Cerebral hemispheres and lateral ventricles

60. Ans. (a) Metanephros

Ref: Netter's Atlas of Human Embryology: 2012 ed. pg. 162

- Metanephros forms the definitive adult kidney. *It gives rise to renal parenchyma*. The nephrons form PCT, DCT, Henle's Loop and glomerulus.
- *Ureteric bud* gives rise to *collecting parts of the kidney* which is pelvis of kidney, major and minor calyces with collecting tubules.
- *Urogenital sinus* develops into bladder, urethra and allantois.

61. Ans. (a) Urogenital sinus

Ref: Netter's Atlas of Human Embryology: 2012 ed. pg. 159

Genital Homologues in Male and Female

Choice number	Male	Female
A: Urogenital Sinus	• Corpus spongiosum • Bulbourethral glands of Cowper • Prostate gland	• Vestibular bulbs • Vestibular glands of bartholin • Urethral and paraurethral glands of skene
B: Urogenital Folds	Ventral shaft of penis (penile urethra)	Labia minora
C: Labio-scrotal Swelling	Scrotum	Labia majora
D: Gubernaculum	Gubernaculum testis	Ovarian and round ligaments

62. Ans. (a) Ureteric bud

Ref: I.B. Singh, 9th ed. pg. 252

- During the fifth week of gestation, the mesonephric duct develops an outpouching, the ureteric bud, near its attachment to the cloaca. This bud, also called the metanephrogenic diverticulum, grows posteriorly and towards the head of the embryo.
- *The elongated stalk of the ureteric bud, called the metanephric duct, later forms the ureter.* As the cranial end of the bud extends into the intermediate mesoderm, it undergoes a series of branchings to form the collecting duct system of the kidney. It also forms the major and minor calyces and the renal pelvis.

63. Ans. (b) Type B synoviocytes

Ref: Netter's Essential Histology, 2nd ed. pg. 156

Type A synoviocytes	Type B synviocytes
• Resemble *macrophages* and contain extensive golgi apparatus	• Specialised *fibroblasts producing synovial fluid* and contain abundant Rough endoplasmic reticulum

64. Ans. (a) Hyaline

Ref: Netter's Essential Histology, 2nd ed. pg. 133

Hyaline cartilage is blue colored while *elastic cartilage is yellow* and *fibrocartilage is white*.

Extra edge

Hyaline cartilage
The most abundant and common cartilage
All long bones are pre-formed in hyaline cartilage except clavicle.
Types (**Mnemonic** L.A.N.C.E.T- T.B) 1. **L**arynx (Arytenoid lower end, cricoid) 2. **A**rticular cartilage 3. **N**asal cartilage 4. **C**ostal cartilage 5. **E**mbryonic cartilage 6. **T**racheal cartilage 7. **T**hyroid cartilage 8. **B**ronchial cartilage

65. Ans. (b) Holocrine gland

Ref: Netter's Essential Histology, 2nd ed. pg. 259

- Tyson glands are located on external surface of prepuce and are holocrine glands.

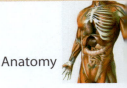

Anatomy

- Holocrine glands are characterised by *disentigration of entire cell which discharges its secretions.*
- The holocrine glands are found everywhere except palms and soles.
- Sebaceous glands are usually associated with hair follicles except in following locations
  - **Eyelids:** Glands of zeis and meibomian glands
  - **Nipple and areola:** Montgomery tubercle
  - **Tyson glands:** Prepuce

66. Ans. (b) Persistent vitellointestinal duct

Ref: Kulkarni Clinical Anatomy, 2nd ed. pg. 590

Urinary fistula at umbilicus	Persistent urachus
Faecal fistula at umbilicus	Persistent vitellointestinal duct
Raspberry tumor	Umbilical adenoma
Sister joseph nodule	Metastatic adenocarcinoma at umbilicus

67. Ans. (a) Cleft lip

Ref: Bailey and Love, 26th ed. pg. 634

The formation of *primary plate* is due to *fusion of maxillary and medial nasal processes.* Defective formation leads to cleft lip.

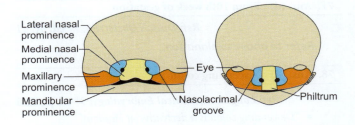

- The formation of *secondary plate* is due to *fusion of lateral palatine process, nasal septum and median palatine process.* Defective formation leads to cleft palate.

68. Ans. (b) Para-axial mesenchyme

Ref: Gray's Anatomy, 41st ed. pg. 212

- The axial skeleton, vertebrae and ribs are derived from paraxial mesenchyme
- The skull is derived from paraxial mesenchyme and neural crest mesenchyme
- The skeletal elements in the limbs are derived from somatopleuric mesenchyme, which forms the limb buds.

69. Ans. (b) Rathke pouch

Ref: Hypothalamic-pituitary Development: Genetic and Clinical Aspect, pg. 2-3

- The anterior pituitary and intermediate lobe of pituitary develops from Rathke's pouch, which is initially derived from the anterior neural ridge, adjacent to cells in the neural plate.
- Neural plate contributes to ventral diencephalon.
- **Posterior lobe** of pituitary develops from the **infundi-bulum,** an evagination of the ventral diencephalon.

70. Ans. (a) It takes 74 days

Ref: Textbook of Human Embroyology, pg. 24

- **Spermatogenesis** - Process of formation of spermatozoa from primitive germ cell (spermatogonia)
- **Spermiogenesis** - Formation of spermatozoa from spermatid.
- Spermatogenesis begins at-puberty (oogenesis begins intrauterine life)
- Spermatogenesis continues-throughout life (oogenesis-stops at menopause)
- **Average time**-74 days
- **Site**- seminiferous tubule
- **Sperm size**- 55-65 μm
- **Parts**- head, neck, middle piece, principal piece, end piece.
- **Acquire motility in**- epididymis.

71. Ans. (b) Primary spermatocyte

Ref: I.B. Singh, 9th ed. pg. 14-15

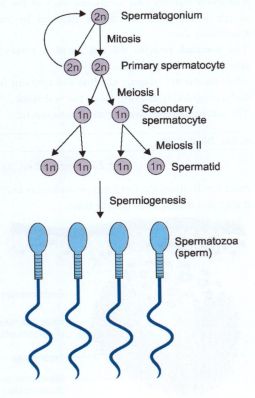

- Please refer to the image given about how spermatogonium undergoes mitotic division and forms primary spermatocyte, which further forms secondary spermatocyte and spermatid after first and 2nd meiotic division respectively.
- Microscopically primary spermatocyte is largest in size among all.
- **The formation of spermatogonium to spermatozoa takes around 74 days.**

72. Ans. (b) 74 days

Ref: I.B. Singh, 9th ed. pg. 14-15

Please refer to above explanation.

73. Ans. (c) Epididymis

Ref: I.B. Singh, 9th ed. pg. 15

74. Ans. (a) Stores the spermatozoa

Ref: I.B. Singh, 9th ed. pg. 15

- Seminal vesicles are two lobulated sacs, situated between the bladder and rectum.
- Each vesicles is about **5 cm long**, and is directed upwards and laterally and is lined by pseudostratified columnar epithelium.
- The lower narrow end forms the duct of the seminal vesicle which joins the ductus deferens to form the ejaculatory duct.
- **The seminal vesicles do not form a reservoir for spermatozoa.**
- Their secretion is slightly alkaline and contains fructose and a coagulating enzyme called the vesiculase.
- The secretion depends on level of testosterone.

75. Ans. (a) Blastocyst

Ref: I.B. Singh, 9th ed. pg. 43-44

- After fertilization, the fertilized ovum begins to divide as it migrates through the uterine tube.

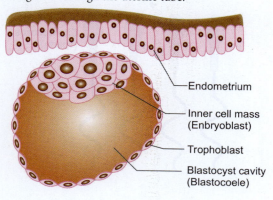

- It undergoes cleavage till a 16 cell stage and is called morula.
- Cells of morula differentiate into an inner cell mass which is completely surrounded by an outer layer of cells, which further gives rise to a structure called trophoblast.
- It reaches the blastocyst stage (approximately 110 cells) on about day 5 and it enters the uterus on about day 6.
- Implantation normally begins on day 6 with the syncytiotrophoblast of the embryonic pole of the blastocyst eroding into the endometrium.

76. Ans. (d) 8 weeks of fertilization

Ref: Dutta's Obstetrics, 7th ed. pg. 41

The prenatal period can be divided into

Period	Product (known as)	Extends
• Ovular/Germinal	Ovum	1st 2 weeks after ovulation
• Embryonic	Embryo	From fertilization (2nd week of gestation) to 8th week of development after fertilization (10th week AOG)
• Fetal	Fetus	From 8th week of fertilization (10th week AOG) till delivery

77. Ans. (d) From 10th week of gestation

Ref: Dutta's Obstetrics, 7th ed. pg. 41

Refer to above explanation.

78. Ans. (d) Descending colon

Ref: Langman's Medical Embryology, 9th ed. pg. 298

- "Descending colon is a derivative of Hindgut"

Part	Part in adult	Gives rise to	Arterial supply
Foregut	Esophagus to first 2 sections of the duodenum	Esophagus, stomach, duodenum (1st and 2nd parts), liver, gallbladder, pancreas, spleen, superior portion of pancreas	Celiac trunk
Midgut	Lower duodenum, to the first two-thirds of the transverse colon	Lower duodenum, *jejunum*, ileum, cecum, *appendix*, *ascending colon*, and first 2/3rd of the transverse colon	Branches of the superior mesenteric artery
Hindgut	Last third of the transverse colon, to the upper part of the anal canal	Last third of the transverse colon, *descending colon*, rectum, and upper part of the anal canal	Branches of the inferior mesenteric artery

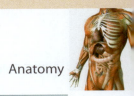

Anatomy

79. **Ans. (c)** Inferior mesenteric artery

Ref: Langman's Medical Embryology, 9th ed. pg. 298

80. **Ans. (d)** Neural crest

Ref: Keith L. Moore, 5th ed. pg. 318

- The adrenal cortex derives from mesoderm and secretes corticosteroids and androgens
- The adrenal medulla derives from **neural crest cells** and secretes catecholamines (mostly epinephrine).

81. **Ans. (a)** Yolk sac

Ref: I.B. Singh, 9th ed. pg. 252

- Umbilical vesicle (Yolk sac) attains full development and is large at *32 days (4–5 weeks)*. It can be observed sonographically early in 5th week.
- By 10 weeks, it shrinks to pear shaped 5 mm in diameter and after 20 weeks it is not visible.
- Although umbilical vesicle contains no yolk, it's essential because:
  - Site of origin of primordial germ cells is *endodermal lining of wall of umbilical vesicle.*
  - In 3rd week blood first develops in vascularized extraembryonic mesoderm covering the wall of umbilical vesicle, and continues to form there until hemopoietic activity begins in liver during 6th week
  - Endoderm which is derived from epiblast, gives rise *to epithelium of trachea, bronchi, lungs and digestive tract (form primordial gut in 4th week).*

82. **Ans. (c)** 6

Ref: Internet Source

- Hyoid bone has a body, two greater and two lesser cornua or horns.
- The hyoid bone develops from 2nd & 3rd pharyngeal arches, the lesser cornu from 2nd the greater cornu from 3rd and body from fused ventral, ends of both.
- Ossification proceeds from 6 centers i.e. a pair for body and one for each conu. Ossification begins in the greater cornu towards the end of intrauterine life, in body shortly after birth and in lesser cornu around puberty.

83. **Ans. (c)** Mesoderm

Ref: BDC, Vol-2 pg. 382

- *Trigone of bladder is formed by the absorption of mesonephric ducts and is mesodermal in origin.*

84. **Ans. (b)** 2 arteries, 1 vein

Ref: I.B. Singh, 9th ed. pg. 59

Refer to Explanation of Question 25

85. **Ans. (a)** 2 arteries, 1 vein

Ref: I.B. Singh, 9th ed. pg. 59

Just a repeat question, from a different exam.

86. **Ans. (a)** Leydig cell

Ref: I.B. Singh, 9th ed. pg. 14-16

- **Leydig cell** secretes testosterone
- **Sertoli cells** help in maturation of spermatozoa
- **Epididymis:** store sperm
- **Seminal vesicle:** Secretes thick alkaline fluid.

87. **Ans. (b)** Brush bordered columnar epithelium

Ref: BDC, 6th ed. vol. II pg. 288-89

MICROVILLI

- When microvilli are of same height & arranged regularly, they are termed as **striated** border, as observed in small intestine.
- *If they are of irregular height, they will constitute the **brush border** as seen in **gall bladder** and proximal convoluted tubules of kidney - (Gray's anatomy).*

88. **Ans. (d)** Thymus

Ref: Gray's, 41st ed. pg. 619

- **Corpuscle** means any small body.
- **Hassall's corpuscles** are spherical or ovoid bodies *found in the medulla of the thymus,* composed of concentric arrays of epithelial cells which contain keratohyalin and bundles of cytoplasmic filaments.

Extra Mile

Some Other Known Corpuscles
- **Lamellated corpuscle** a type of large encapsulated nerve ending found throughout the body, concerned with perception of sensations.
- **Malpighian corpuscles:** Found in Nephrons (kidney) and in spleen (white pulp)
- **Meissner's corpuscle:** A type of medium sized encapsulated nerve ending in the skin, chiefly in the palms and soles.
- **Paciniform corpuscles** a type of rapidly adapting lamellated corpuscles responding to muscle stretch and light pressure.
- **Red corpuscle:** Red Blood Cells
- **White corpuscle:** White Blood Cells

89. **Ans. (b)** Kidney

Please refer to above explanation

FMGE Solutions Screening Examination

90. Ans. (b) Spleen

Ref: BDC, 6th ed. vol. II pg. 297

The **Cords of Billroth** are also known as **splenic cords** or **red pulp cords**. They are found in the red pulp of the spleen between the sinusoids consisting of fibrils and connective tissue cells with a large population of monocytes and macrophages. *These cords contain half of the human body's monocytes.*

91. Ans. (b) Thymus

Ref: BDC, 6th ed. vol. II pg. 147

T cells originate in the bone marrow but mature in the thymus. So, T stands for 'Thymus'.
- Thymus and bone marrow are primary lymphoid organs.
- Lymph node and spleen are secondary lymphoid organs.

UPPER LIMB

92. Ans. (d) Radial head

Ref: Gray's Anatomy 41st ed. P 839

- The arrow here points towards radial head.
- The radial head articulates with humeral capitulum

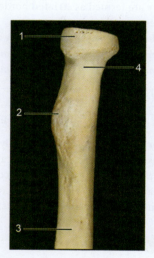
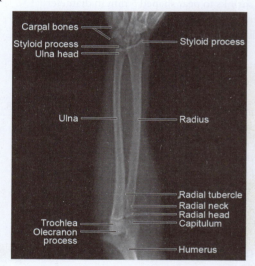

FIGURE: The proximal end of the left radius, anterior view. Key 1. head; 2. radial tuberosity; 3. shaft; 4. neck

93. Ans. (b) Trapezius

Ref: Gray's Anatomy 41st ed. P 810, 786.e1

- **Protraction:** Involves moving the scapula away from midline (Abduction)
- **Retraction:** Involves moving the scapula towards the midline (Adduction) and is done by middle part of trapezius and Rhomboids muscle

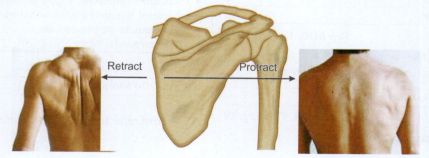

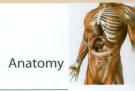

Anatomy

Muscles of Scapular Stabilization:
- **Trapezius:**
  - Retraction (middle part)
  - Elevation (superior part)
  - Depression (Inferior part)
  - Upward rotation (superior + middle)
- **Rhomboid:** Retraction
- **Levator scapulae:** Elevation
- **Serratus anterior and Pectoralis major:** Protraction

94. Ans. (b) Nerve to serratus anterior

Ref: Gray's Anatomy 41st ed. P 819

- Winging of scapula is due to paralysis of **serratus anterior muscle**.
- **Nerve supplying serratus anterior muscle:** Long thoracic nerve (C5, 6, 7). Therefore long thoracic nerve palsy can also lead to winging of scapula.
- **Vascular supply:** Serratus anterior is supplied by **superior** and **lateral thoracic arteries**, and by branches from the thoracodorsal artery after it divides in latissimus dorsi.

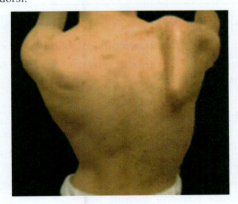

FIGURE: Winging of scapula

95. Ans. (a) Pronation

Ref: Gray's Anatomy 41st ed. P 846-48

- Pronator teres muscle is involved in pronation of forearm, by rotating the radius medially on the ulna.
- Proximally movements at the humeroradial joint and distally at radioulnar joints pronate and supinate the hand.
- In pronation, the radius turns anteromedially and obliquely across the ulna.
  - Proximal end remains lateral to the ulna while its distal end lies medially and the interosseous membrane becomes spiralled.
- If there is fracture at this pronator muscle insertion area → it may be detached → Forearm acquired supination.
- The movement pronation is restricted.

96. Ans. (a) Radial tuberosity

Ref: Gray's Anatomy 41st ed. P 824

- The shown muscle in the image is biceps brachii.
- It has two proximal heads (hence the name). Their attachments are:
  - **Short head:** Tip of coracoid process
  - **Long head:** Supraglenoid tubercle of scapula
- **Insertion:**
  - Radial tuberosity and fascia of forearm via bicipital aponeurosis
- **Innervation:** Musculocutaneous nerve (C5, C6)
- **Action:** Supination of forearm and flexion of shoulder joint

97. Ans. (c) Atavistic epiphysis

Ref: Clinical Anatomy, Kulkarni 2nd ed. P 73

TYPES OF EPIPHYSIS

- **Pressure:** Seen at the end of long bones subjected to pressure. E.g. Femur, head of humerus, condyles of tibia and femur.
- **Traction:** Formed due to pull of muscles. E.g. Mastoid process, tibial tuberosity, tubercles, trochanters.
- **Atavistic:** Functional in lower animals. Degenerated in humans e.g. Coracoid process of scapula, os trigonum of talus
- **Aberrant:** It is an extra epiphysis. E.g. Proximal end of 1st metacarpal bone.

98. Ans. (a) Ulnar nerve

Ref: Gray's Basic Anatomy E-book, P 399

Carpal Tunnel Anatomy
- Posterior border
  - Carpal bones
- Anterior border
  - Transverse carpal ligament
- Boundaries
  - Proximally—pisiform and tubercle of navicular
  - Distally—hook of hamate and tubercle of trapezium
- Contents
  - Flexor digitorum superficialis
  - Flexor digitorum profundus
  - Flexor pollicis longus
  - Median nerve

99. Ans. (a) Ulnar nerve

Ref: Gray's Anatomy review E-book, P 336

FMGE Solutions Screening Examination

Clinical Correlates: Guyon's Canal Syndrome

- Guyon's canal (ulnar tunnel) is formed by the pisiform, hook of the hamate, and pisohamate ligament, deep to the palmaris brevis and palmar carpal ligament and transmits the ulnar nerve and artery.
- Guyon's canal syndrome is an entrapment of the ulnar nerve in the Guyon's canal.
- **Symptoms:** Pain, numbness, and tingling in the ring and little fingers, followed by loss of sensation and motor weakness.
- **Rx:** Surgical decompression of the nerve.

---

100. Ans. (a) C5-C6

Ref: Gray's Anatomy, 41st ed. pg. 792

- **Biceps jerk (C5, 6)** The elbow is flexed to a right angle and slightly pronated. A finger is placed on the biceps tendon and struck with a percussion hammer; this should elicit flexion and slight supination of the forearm.

> **Extra Mile**

- **Triceps jerk (C6–8)** The arm is supported at the wrist and flexed to a right angle. Triceps tendon is struck with a percussion hammer just proximal to the olecranon; this should elicit extension of the elbow.
- **Radial jerk (C7, 8)** The radial jerk is a periosteal, not a tendon reflex. The elbow is flexed to a right angle and the forearm placed in the mid pronation/supination position. The radial styloid is struck with the percussion hammer. This elicits contraction of brachioradialis, which causes flexion of the elbow.

---

101. Ans. (d) 164

Ref: Vishram Singh, vol-1: 2nd ed. pg. 22

- Angle of humeral torsion is 164 degrees in contrast to femoral torsion of 15 degrees.
- The angle of humeral torsion is due to *angulation between the long axis of articular surface of the upper and lower ends of humerus.* This is because the upper end appears to have rotated laterally

---

102. Ans. (c) Hamate

Ref: Kulkarni Clinical Anatomy, 2nd ed. pg. 80

The largest carpal bone is capitate and the carpal bone with Hook is Hamate.

Extra edge

- **P**roximal row of carpals (Lateral to Medial): **S**caphid, **L**unate, **T**riquetral and **P**isiform
- Distal row of carpals: Trapezium, Trapezoid, Capitate and Hamate Pisiform bone is a *sesamoid* bone lying in the tendon of *flexor carpi ulnaris.*
- Mnemonics to remember carpal bones *"She Looks Too Pretty, Try To Catch Her"*

---

103. Ans. (a) Capitate

Ref: Kulkarni Clinical Anatomy, 2nd ed. pg. 80

- The carpal bones are cartilaginous at birth. Capitate is the first bone to ossify at 1 year and pisiform the last one to ossify at 12 years.

> **Extra Mile**

- Scaphoid is boat-shaped. Its neck or waist subdivides the scaphoid into proximal and distal segments. A tubercle projects from its lateral side. It lies in the floor of anatomical snuff-box, where it can be palpated.
- Lunate is shaped like lunar crescent (shape of half moon).
- Triquetral is pyramidal in shape.
- Pisiform is pea-shaped. It is a sesamoid bone in the tendon of flexor carpi ulnaris.
- Trapezium is quadrilateral and bears a crest and groove (for lodging tendon of flexor carpi radialis). It takes part in the first carpometacarpal joint, which imparts unique mobility to human thumb.
- Trapezoid is irregular like a baby's shoe.
- Capitate bears a big head. It is largest carpal bone.
- Hamate has a hook-shaped process.

---

104. Ans. (d) Hamate

Ref: Kulkarni Clinical Anatomy, 2nd ed. pg. 80

Proximal row of carpals (Lateral to Medial): **S**caphoid, **L**unate, **T**riquetral and **P**isiform.

---

105. Ans. (c) Scaphoid

Ref: BDC, 6th ed. vol. I pg. 26

- The scaphoid is a BOAT SHAPED carpal bone and has a tubercle in its lateral side.
- Scaphoid bone is the most commonly fractured carpal bone.
- Lunate (crescent shaped) is the 2nd most commonly fractured carpal bone.
- Scaphoid fracture is usually caused by a fall on an outstretched hand with the weight landing on the palm.
- Scaphoid bone forms the floor of the anatomical snuff box.
- It articulates with the following bones: radius, lunate, capitate, trapezium, and trapezoid.

---

106. Ans. (a) Triquetral

Ref: BDC, 6th ed. vol. I pg. 25; Snell's 8th ed. pg. 402

PISIFORM

- It is a sesamoid bone in the tendon of flexor carpi ulnaris.
- *Its dorsal surface presents a smooth, oval facet, for articulation with the triquetral*
- The palmar surface is rounded and rough, and gives attachment to the transverse carpal ligament, and to the Flexor carpi ulnaris and Abductor digiti quinti.

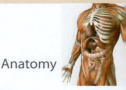

Anatomy

107. Ans. (d) C7

Ref: Kulkarni Clinical Anatomy, 2nd ed. pg. 18

- Brachial plexus is composed of anterior rami of spinal nerves C5 to T1.
- C5 and C6 join to form the *upper* trunk
- Root C7 forms the *middle* trunk
- Root C8 and T1 join to form the *lower* trunk

108. Ans. (b) Axillary nerve

Ref: Kulkarni Clinical Anatomy, 2nd ed. pg. 30

The damage to axillary nerve leads to regimental badge anaesthesia.

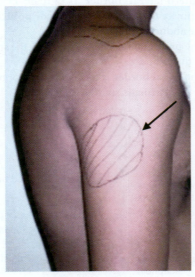

Axillary nerve injury leads to *deltoid* and *teres minor* paralysis. The manifestations are:
- *Loss of rounded contour of shoulder*
- Sensory loss in skin covering lower part of deltoid.
- Loss of abduction from 15° to 90° is due to deltoid paralysis.

109. Ans (b) Anconeus

Ref: Kulkarni Clinical Anatomy, 2nd ed. pg. 73

- The screwing movement is due to action of muscle aconeus.
- The anconeus muscle is a small triangular muscle located at the elbow. It *originates* at the *dorsal side of the lateral epicondyle* of the humerus and *inserts* at the *olecranon of ulna*.
- It is *supplied by* motor branch of *radial nerve (C6-C8)* which arises at the radial sulcus of the humerus.

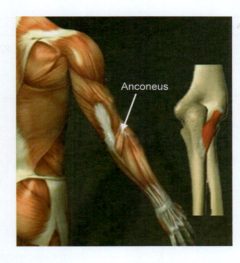

110. Ans (b) Deep palmar arch

Ref: Kulkarni Clinical Anatomy, 2nd ed. pg. 20

- *Radial* artery ends as **deep palmar arch** while the *ulnar* artery ends as **superficial palmar arch**.
- Branches of branchial artery which *terminates* as *radial and ulnar* artery:
  - Muscular artery
  - Profunda brachii artery (accompanies the radial nerve in spiral groove)
  - Superior and inferior ulnar collateral artery

111. Ans (c) Subacromial bursa

Ref: Kulkarni Clinical Anatomy, 2nd ed. pg. 48

The subacromial bursa is the *largest bursa* of the body

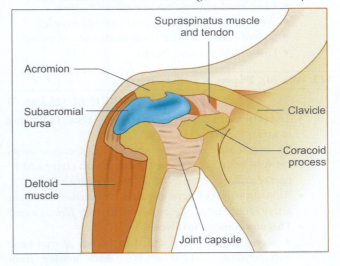

112. Ans. (a) Ulnar

Ref: BDC, 6th ed. vol. I pg. 93; Gray, 822,29,37

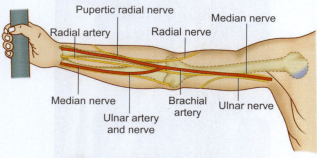
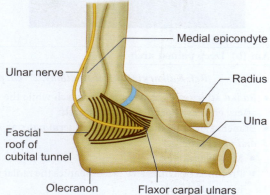

- Nerve passing through medial epicondyle is ulnar nerve. Very often when we hit our elbow on any surface, the current like feeling in arm, is due to ulnar nerve injury.
- **Medial epicondyle fracture causes injury to ulnar nerve.**
  - Ulnar nerve palsy causes partial claw hand.
  - **Claw hand**-sensory loss of medial 1 ½ digits.
  - Weakness of grip (paralysis of intrinsic muscle)
  - Loss of flexion of MCP (lumbricals and interossei)
  - Loss of adduction of thumb

113. Ans. (d) 2nd part of axillary artery

Ref: BDC, 6th ed. vol. I pg. 73

- The extreme mobility of shoulder may result in kinking of axillary artery.
- To compensate this, an arterial anastomosis exists between branches of 1st part of subclavian artery and 3rd part of axillary artery (NOT 2nd part axillary artery).
- It also provides collateral circulation when the subclavian artery is obstructed *(Eg: by a cervical rib or fibrous band)*
- **This anastomosis involves:**
  - *Suprascapular artery and deep branch of transverse (superficial) cervical arteries*- **both arising from thyrocervical trunk of 1st part of subclavian artery**
  - *Subscapular artery & its circumflexscapular branch (arising from 3rd part of axillary artery).*

114. Ans. (b) Radial artery

Ref: BDC, 6th ed. vol. I pg. 122; Gray's 41st ed. pg. 790

- The anatomical snuffbox is formed by the tendons of extensor polloicis longus and brevis, and abductor pollicis longus.
- It has the radial artery running in the floor of the snuffbox, and the radial nerve passing to the dorsum of the hand.
- **Boundaries of snuff box:**
  - **Postero-medial border** is the tendon of the extensor pollicis longus.
  - **Antero-lateral border** is a pair of parallel and intimate tendons of the **extensor pollicis brevis** and the **abductor pollicis longus.**
  - The **proximal border** is formed by the styloid process of the radius.
  - The **distal border** is formed by the approximate apex of the schematic snuffbox isosceles.

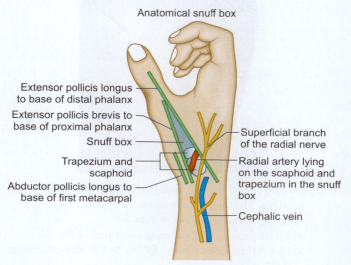

115. Ans. (b) Radial artery

Ref: BDC, 6th ed. vol. I pg. 22, 5th ed. pg. 102

Please refer to above explanation.

116. Ans. (c) Extensor pollicus longus

Ref: Gray's 41st ed. pg. 790

117. Ans. (a) Teres major palsy

Ref: BDC, 4th ed. Vol. I / 62, 171; Gray's 41st ed. /831-33

- Axillary nerve (C5, C6) is injured due to surgical neck fracture or due to shoulder dislocation.

Anatomy

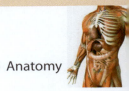

Motor injury	Sensory injury
• Deltoid muscle palsy: loss of rounded contour of shoulder • Weakness of abduction • Teres minor palsy	• Lateral cutaneous nerve of arm • Sensory loss over lower half of deltoid *(regimental batch area)*

Note: Teres Major is supplied by lower subscapular nerve.

118. Ans. (b) Axillary

Ref: Gray's 41st ed. pg. 831e-2; Keith L. Moore 5th ed. pg. 760

- Anterior shoulder dislocation can cause injury to axillary nerve
- Axillary nerve passes inferior to the humeral head and winds around the surgical neck of the humerus. The axillary nerve is usually injured during fracture of this part of the humerus.
- It may also be damaged during dislocation of the glenohumeral joint and by compression from the incorrect use of crutches.

119. Ans. (a) Flexor digitorum profundus

Ref: Gray's, 41st ed. pg. 851

- **Composite** or **hybrid muscles** are those muscles which have more than one set of fibers but perform the same function and are usually supplied by different nerves for different set of fibers
- The muscles of the anterior compartment are innervated mostly by the median nerve, but one and a half muscles are innervated by the ulnar nerve which are FLEXOR CARPI ULNARIS and HALF OF FLEXOR DIGITORUM PROFUNDUS.

OTHER HYBRID/COMPOSITE MUSCLES

- **Adductor magnus**: Adductor part is innervated by **OBTURATOR NERVE** whereas the Hamstring part is innervated by **SCIATIC NERVE**
- **Biceps femoris**: Its long head is supplied by the **TIBIAL BRANCH OF SCIATIC NERVE** whereas the short head is supplied by the **COMMON PERONEAL NERVE**. This reflects the composite derivation from the flexor and extensor musculature.
- **Pectineus**: Its anterior set of fibers are supplied by the femoral nerve, whereas posterior set of fibers are supplied by the obturator nerve.
- **Iliopsoas**: It is a composite muscle performing flexion at the hip.

120. Ans. (c) Palmaris longus

Ref: BDC, 6th ed. vol. I pg. 113

- Palmaris longus passes **superficial** to flexor retinaculum.
- **Structures Deep to flexors retinaculum:**
  - Flexor digitorum superficialis (FDS)
  - Flexor digitorum profundus (FDP)
  - Flexor pollicis longus (FPL)
  - Flexor carpi radialis
  - *Median nerve*
- **Structures Superficial to flexor retinaculum:**
  - **Palmaris longus**
  - *Ulnar nerve and artery*
  - Palmar cutaneous branches of median and ulnar nerves

121. Ans. (a) Ulnar nerve

Ref: BDC, 6th ed. vol. I pg. 113

- Ulnar nerve passes above (superficial) to flexor retinaculum especially the palmar cutaneous branch of ulnar nerve.

122. Ans. (a) C5, C6

Ref: BDC, 6th ed. vol. I pg. 55-56; Clinical Anatomy By Harold Ellis, 11th ed. pg. 189-190

Brachial Plexus in a Nutshell
- Five *roots* derived from the anterior primary rami of C5, 6, 7, 8 and T1; link up into:
- Three *trunks* formed by the union of
  - C5 and 6 (upper);
  - C7 alone (middle);
  - C8 and T1 (lower)

Which split into:
- Six *divisions* formed by each trunk dividing into an anterior and posterior division; which link up again into:
- Three *cords*
  - A lateral, from the fused anterior divisions of the upper and middle trunks;
  - A medial, from the anterior division of the lower trunk;
  - A posterior, from the union of all three posterior divisions.

Division is remembered as "RTDC"
"*The roots* lie between the anterior and middle scalene muscles. *The trunks* traverse the posterior triangle of the neck. *The divisions* lie behind the clavicle. *The cords* lie in the axilla"

The cords continue distally to form the main nerve trunks of the upper limb thus:
- The lateral cord continues as the *musculocutaneous nerve*;
- The medial cord, as the *ulnar nerve*;
- The posterior cord, as the *radial nerve* and the *axillary nerve*;
- A cross-communication between the lateral and medial cords forms the *median nerve*.

Note
- 5 BRANCHES of Posterior cord and their root nerve:
  - Upper subscapular Nerve **(C5, C6)**
  - Lower subscapular Nerve **(C5, C6)**

FMGE Solutions Screening Examination

- Nerve to latissimus dorsi (C6, 7, 8)
- **AXILLARY NERVE (C5, C6)** → *SUPPLIES DELTOID AND TERES MINOR*
- Radial nerve (C5 To T1)

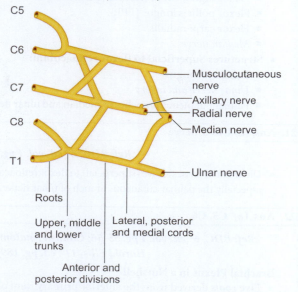

123. Ans. (b) Lateral cord

Ref: BDC, 6th ed. vol. I pg. 55-56

124. Ans. (c) C5, C6, C7, C8, T1

Ref: BDC, 6th ed. vol. I pg. 55-56

125. Ans. (b) Long thoracic nerve

Ref: BDC, 6th ed. vol. I pg. 55-56;
3rd ed. Vol. I pg. 45-50; 180,181

- Winging of scapula is due to damage of long thoracic nerve due to paralysis of serratus anterior muscle.
- **Serratus anterior** helps in *vertical overhead abduction* (assisted by trapezius), *forward punch* (assisted by pectoralis minor) & *forced inspiration*.
- Its paralysis leads to winging of scapula.
- Nerve Supply of Serratus anterior- **Long Thoracic Nerve** (Nerve of Bell) (C5, C6, C7)
- *Action of Serratus anterior muscle*
  - Rotates the scapula so that glenoid cavity is raised upward & forward- Helps in *Vertical over head abduction* (in this action *assisted by Trapezius muscle*).
  - Draws the scapula forward around the thoracic wall so *paralysis leads to winging of scapula*.
  - Also used when arm is pushed forward in horizontal position as in *forward punch* (helped by *Pectoralis minor in this action*).
  - Steadies the scapula during weight carrying.
  - Helps in *forced inspiration* (Accessory muscle of inspiration).
  - Because of greater pull exerted on the inferior angle, inferior angle passes laterally and forward and the glenoid cavity is raised upward & forward; in this action the muscle is assisted by trapezius.

126. Ans. (a) Serratus anterior muscle

Ref: Gray's Anatomy, 41st ed. pg. 819

- Winging of scapula is due to paralysis of **serratus anterior muscle**.
- **Nerve supplying serratus anterior muscle: Long thoracic nerve (C5, 6, 7)**. Therefore long thoracic nerve palsy can also lead to winging of scapula.
- **Vascular supply:** Serratus anterior is supplied by **superior** and **lateral thoracic arteries**, and by branches from the thoracodorsal artery after it divides in latissimus dorsi.

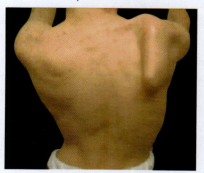

FIGURE: Winging of scapula

127. Ans. (a) Serratus anterior muscle

Ref: BDC, 6th ed. vol. I pg. 55-56;
3rd ed. Vol. I pg. 45-50; 180,181

128. Ans. (d) Trapezius

Ref: Gray's, 41st ed. pg. 817

Dropped Shoulder and Winged Scapula
- The position of the scapula on the posterior wall of thorax is maintained by the tone and balance of the muscles attached to it.
- If one of these muscles is paralyzed, the balance is upset, as in dropped shoulder, which occurs with paralysis of the trapezius or winged scapula caused by paralysis of serratus anterior.

Anatomy

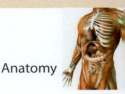

129. Ans. (a) First rib

Ref: Gray's, 41st ed. pg. 816-817

- Origin of trapezius muscle is from:
  - External occipital protruberance
  - Superior nuchal line
  - Ligament nuchae,
  - C_1 spine and
  - Spines of T_1 to T_{12} vertebrae.
- Insertion of trapezius muscle is on lateral third of clavicle (upper fibers), medial border of acromion process (middle fibers), and upper margin of spine of scapula (lower fibers).

130. Ans. (b) Abductor pollicis palsy

Ref: BDC, 6th ed. vol. I pg. 109-110, 120

- In ulnar nerve palsy grip is weak due to paralysis of intrinsic muscles *(all interossei, lateral 3rd & 4th lumbricals, hypothenar and adductor pollicis muscles)*.
- Sensory supply of ulnar nerve is medial 1½ fingers.
- *Abductor pollicis is supplied by median nerve.*
- **Finger drop** i.e. loss of extension of metacarpophalangeal joint is seen in Radial & Posterior interosseous nerve palsy

Signs of Ulnar Nerve palsy *(remembered as BCDEF)*

- **Book test/Fromet sign:** While holding the book between thumb and rest of hand, there is overaction of flexor pollicis longus due to adductor pollicis nerve palsy.
- **Claw hand:** Clawing of medial 2 digits
- **Card test:** for testing palmar interossei, i.e. adduction of fingers. *(PAD)*
- **aDDuctor pollicis paralysis:** Adduction of thumb lost
- **Egawa's test:** To test dorsal interossei i.e. abduction of fingers *(DAB)*.
- **Froment sign**

> **Extra Mile**
> - In low ulnar nerve palsy forearm muscles are spared but the clawing is more (as compared to high ulnar n. palsy) this phenomenon is known as **ulnar paradox**.
> - Lower the lesion, more the clawing.

131. Ans. (c) Median nerve

Ref: BDC, 6th ed. vol. I pg. 126-127, Vol-1 pg. 109,159; Clinical anatomy, Vishram Singh / 58

- Median nerve is the main nerve of the front of the forearm. It also supplies the muscles of thenar eminence.
- Median nerve aka *labourer's nerve* as it supplies most of the long muscles of the front of forearm.

> **Extra Mile**
> - *Deformities that may occur due to median nerve paralysis:*
>   - Carpal tunnel syndrome
>   - Pointing index finger
>   - Ape thumb deformity aka ape hand deformity
>   - Claw hand (median + ulnar)
> - *Deformities that may occur due to radial nerve paralysis*
>   - Wrist drop
>   - Saturday night palsy
> - *Deformities that may occur due to ulnar nerve paralysis*
>   - Ulnar claw hand
>   - Cubital tunnel syndrome

132. Ans. (c) Median and ulnar both

Ref: BDC Vol-1 pg. 109,159; Clinical anatomy, Vishram Singh/ 58

Please refer to above explanation

133. Ans. (c) Median nerve

Ref: BDC Vol-1 Pg. 109,159; Clinical anatomy, Vishram Singh/ 58

- Median nerve is the main nerve of the front of the forearm. It also supplies the muscles of thenar eminence.
- The ape hand deformity or ape thumb deformity of hand is due to paralysis of thenar muscles which is supplied by median nerve.

Presenting Feature of Ape Thumb Deformity

- Thumb is laterally rotated and adducted
- Loss of thenar eminence
- Loss of opposition of thumb

134. Ans. (b) Median nerve

Ref: BDC, 6th ed. vol. I pg. 126

- Median nerve is the main nerve of the front of the forearm. It also supplies the muscles of thenar eminence.
- Carpal tunnel syndrome occurs as a result of compression of the median nerve. The median nerve runs from your forearm through a passageway in the wrist (carpal tunnel) to the hand. It provides sensation to the palm, side of the thumb and fingers, with the exception of the little finger. It also provides nerve signals to move the muscles around the base of the thumb

135. Ans. (a) Abductor pollicis longus

Ref: BDC, 6th ed. vol. I pg. 126-128

- Median nerve is formed by combination of lateral cord (C5, 6, 7) and medial cord (C8, T1)
- Median nerve is the main nerve of the front of the forearm. It also supplies the muscles of thenar eminence.

FMGE Solutions Screening Examination

All the muscles of anterior compartment of forearm is innervated by Median Nerve except: FLEXOR CARPI ULNARIS, HALF OF FLEXOR DIGITORUM PROFUNDUS.

- Muscles of the extensor compartment are innervated by Radial Nerve. **Abductor Pollicis Longus belongs to this group of muscles.**

136. Ans. (a) Teres major

Ref: BDC, 6th ed. vol. I pg. 68-69, 73

- The rotator cuff is a group of tendons and muscles in the shoulder, connecting the upper arm (humerus) to the shoulder blade (scapula). The rotator cuff tendons provide stability to the shoulder; the muscles allow the shoulder to rotate.

The Muscles in the Rotator Cuff Include
- Teres minor
- Infraspinatus
- Supraspinatus
- Subscapularis

- Each muscle of the rotator cuff inserts at the scapula, and has a tendon that attaches to the humerus. Together, the tendons and other tissues form a cuff around the humerus. **Mnemonic: SITS** [Supraspinatous, Infraspinatous, Teres minor, Subscapularis].
Teres major is not a part of rotator cuff muscles.

137. Ans. (a) Supraspinatous muscle

Ref: BDC, 6th ed. vol. I pg. 68-69

- Four of the Intrinsic shoulder muscles collectively forms the Rotator cuff muscles.
- Injury or disease may damage the musculotendinous rotator cuff, producing instability of the glenohumeral joint. Trauma may tear or rupture one or more of the tendons of the SITS muscles; and **supraspinatus** is most commonly involved.

138. Ans. (c) Coracobrachialis

Ref: Gray's, 41st ed. pg. 819-821

- The coracobrachialis is an elongated muscle in the superomedial part of the arm. The coracobrachialis helps flex and adduct the arm and stabilize the glenohumeral joint.
- With the deltoid and long head of the triceps, it serves as a shunt muscle, resisting downward dislocation of the head of the humerus, as when carrying a heavy suitcase.
- The median nerve and/or the brachial artery may run deep to the coracobrachialis and be compressed by it.
- Nerve supply 2 Musculocutaneous nerve.

139. Ans. (a) Musculo cutaneous nerve

Ref: BDC, 6th ed. vol. I pg. 88

- Short head of biceps comes under anterior compartment of arm. All the muscles of the anterior compartment of arm are innervated by musculo-cutaneous nerve.
- Posterior compartment muscles are innervated by radial nerve.

140. Ans. (d) Long head of triceps brachii

Ref: BDC, 6th ed. vol. I pg. 96-97

- The **triceps brachii muscle** is the large muscle on the avoid back of the upper limb.
- It originates from the infraglenoid tubercle of scapula and inserts at the elbow joint in olecranon process of ulna.
- It is the muscle principally responsible for extension of the elbow joint (straightening of the arm).

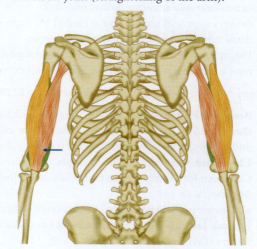

Since it has 3 heads, all of them have different origin:
- **Long head:** Infraglenoid tubercle of scapula
- **Lateral head:** Above the radial sulcus
- **Medial head:** Below the radial sulcus
Insertion: Olecranon process of ulna

141. Ans. (b) Deltoid

Ref: Gray's Anatomy, 41st ed. pg. 113

Unipennate	• Extensor digitorum longus • Flexor pollicis longus • Soleus
Bipennate	• Rectus femoris • Dorsal interossei • Gastrocnemius
Multipennate	• Deltoid
Circumpennate	• Tibialis anterior

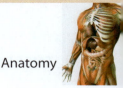

Anatomy

142. Ans. (a) Radial nerve injury

Ref: BDC, 6th ed. vol. I pg. 98

- Radial nerve gets injured in cases of humerus shaft fracture.
- Ulnar nerve injury may take place when there is damage to medial epicondyle of humerus and in cases of tardive ulnar palsy.
- Median nerve damage can be secondary to compression (for ex- carpal tunnel syndrome), which may lead to gun stock deformity, ape thumb deformity.

Extra Mile

- **Median nerve aka labourer's nerve** as it supplies most of the long muscles of the front of forearm.
- **Ulnar nerve aka musician's nerve** as it controls the fine movements of hand.

143. Ans. (c) Supraspinatus

Ref: BDC, 6th ed. vol. I /47; Gray's Anatomy, 39th ed/ 841

Boundaries of Axilla

- Anterior wall: Pectoralis major, Pectoralis minor, Clavipectoral fascia
- *Posterior wall: Subscapularis, Teres major, Latissimus dorsi*
- Medial wall: First 4 ribs & their associated intercostal muscles, Serratus anterior
- Lateral wall: Intertubercular (bicipital groove), Biceps tendon.

144. Ans. (c) Superior

Ref: Clinical Anatomy, 11th ed. pg. 160-161

The axillary lymph nodes (some 20–30 in number) drain not only the lymphatics of the breast, but also those of the pectoral region, upper abdominal wall and the upper limb, and are arranged in five groups:

- **Anterior**—lying deep to pectoralis major along the lower border of pectoralis minor;
- **Posterior**—along the subscapular vessels;
- **Lateral**—along the axillary vein;
- **Central**—in the axillary fat;
- **Apical** *(through which all the other axillary nodes drain)*—immediately behind the clavicle at the apex of the axilla above pectoralis minor and along the medial side of the axillary vein.

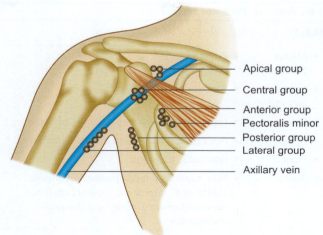

Clinicians and pathologists often define metastatic axillary node spread simply into three levels:
- Level I—nodes inferior to pectoralis minor
- Level II—nodes behind pectoralis minor
- Level III—nodes above pectoralis minor.

145. Ans. (b) Radioulnar joint

Ref: BDC, 6th ed. vol. I pg. 153-154; Clinically Oriented Anatomy by Keith, Moore, 5th ed/ 865

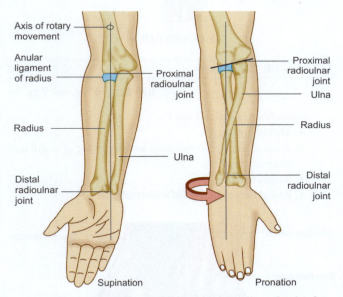

- During supination radius rotates laterally and palm faces anteriorly
- During pronation, radius rotates medially and palm faces posteriorly
- This movement takes place around distal radioulnar joint.

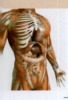

FMGE Solutions Screening Examination

146. Ans. (a) Pronator teres

TABLE: Cubital fossa boundaries

• Medial boundary	• Pronator teres
• Lateral boundary	• Brachioradialis
• Base	• Line joining the two epicondyles of humerus
• Apex	• Point joining lateral and medial boundaries
• Floor	• Brachialis, supinator
• Roof	• Skin, superficial fascia *(containing medial cubital vein, lateral and medial cutaneous nerve of forearm)*, deep facia, bicipital aponeurosis

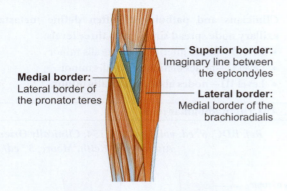

Cubital fossa (Left hand)

147. Ans. (d) Ulnar nerve

Ref: BDC, 6th ed. vol. I pg. 94

Contents of Cubital Fossa
- Median nerve
- Brachial artery *(termination and beginning of radial and ulnar arteries)*
- Biceps tendon
- Radial nerve and Radial collateral artery

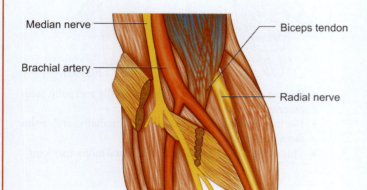

148. Ans. (b) Ulnar nerve

Ref: BDC, 6th ed. vol. I pg. 94

149. Ans. (c) Serratus anterior

Ref: Gray's, 41st pg. 749

- **Triangle of auscultation is bounded by:**
  - **Medially:** Trapezius
  - **Laterally:** Scapula
  - **Inferiorly:** Latissimus dorsi

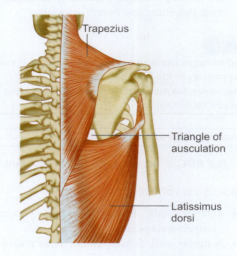

LOWER LIMB

150. Ans. (d) Biceps Femoris muscle

Ref: Gray's Anatomy 41st ed. P 1324.e2

- The posterior compartment includes semitendinosus, semimembranosus and biceps femoris
  - *Note:* Biceps femoris is the only muscle of the thigh that is attached distally to the fibula, and has no tibial attachment
- Biceps femoris muscle is supplied by tibial and common peroneal nerve.
- While in posterior descent, sciatic nerve is crossed by the long head of biceps femoris and divides it into the tibial and common fibular (peroneal) nerves proximal to the knee.
- The short head of biceps femoris is supplied by the lateral (common fibular/peroneal) component.
- Long head of biceps femoris is supplied by tibial component.

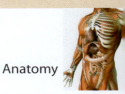

Anatomy

TABLE: Movement, muscles and segmental innervation in the lower limb

Joint	Movement	Muscle	Innervation
HIP	Flexion	Psoas major	Spinal nn. L1–3
		Iliacus	Femoral n.
		Pectineus	Femoral n. or accessory obturation n.
		Rectus femoris	Femoral n.
		Adductor longus	Obturator n.
		Sartorius	Femoral n.
	Extension	Gluteus maximus	Inferior gluteal n.
		Adductor magnus	Obturator and tibial nn.
		Semitendinosus, semimembranosus, biceps femoris	Tibial and common fibular nn.
	Medial rotation	Iliacus	Femoral n.
		Gluteus medius and minimus	Superior gluteal n.
		Tensor fasciae latae	Superior gluteal n.
	Lateral rotation	Superior and interior gemelli	Nerve to obturator internus and nerve to quadratus femoris, respectively
		Quadratus femoris	Nerve to quadratus femoris
		Piriformis	Nerve to piriformis
		Obturator internus	Nerve to obturator internus
		Obturator externus	Obturator n.
		Sartorius	Femoral n.
	Adduction	Gracilis	Obturator n.
		Adductor longus	Obturator n.
		Adductor magnus	Obturator and tibial nn.
		Adductor brevis	Obturator n.
		Pectineus	Femoral n. or accessory obturator n.
	Abduction	Tensor fasciae latae	Superior gluteal n.
		Gluteus medius and minimus	Superior gluteal n.
		Piriformis	Nerve to piriformis

151. Ans. (d) Adductor brevis

Ref: Gray's Anatomy 41st ed. P 1364

- Adductor brevis is muscle of medial compartment of thigh. Muscles of this compartment are:
- **Muscles:**
  - Adductor longus
  - Adductor brevis
  - Adductor magnus (Adductor portion)
  - Gracilis
- **Action**

Adduction of HIP joint

- **Nerve supply:**

Obturator nerve

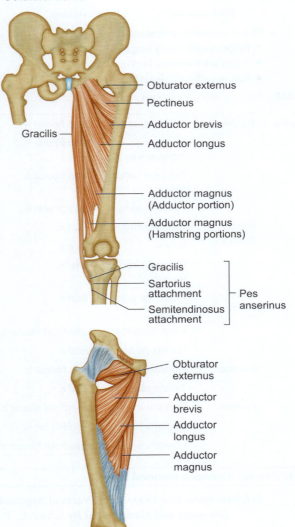

FMGE Solutions Screening Examination

152. Ans. (c) Peroneus longus muscle

Ref: Gray's Anatomy 41st ed. P 1324.e2

- Eversion of foot is the movement of foot when side of the sole is turned out laterally.

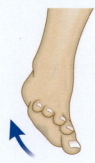
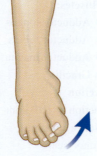

Foot eversion   Foot inversion

- Muscles causing eversion:
  - Peroneus/Fibularis longus
  - Peroneus/Fibularis brevis
  - Peroneus/Fibularis tertius

TABLE: Ankle muscles, its actions and nerve supply

Ankle	Dorsiflexion	Tibialis anterior	Deep fibular n.
		Extensor digitorum longus	Deep fibular n.
		Extensor hallucis longus	Deep fibular n.
		Fibularis tertius	Deep fibular n.
	Plantar flexion	Gastrocnemius	Tibial n.
		Soleus	Tibial n.
		Flexor digitorum longus	Tibial n.
		Flexor hallucis longus	Tibial n.
		Fibularis longus	Superficial fibular n.
		Tibialis posterior	Tibial n.
	Inversion	Tibialis anterior	Deep fibular n.
		Tibialis posterior	Tibial n.
	Eversion	Fibularis longus	Superficial fibular n.
		Fibularis tertius	Deep fibular n.
		Fibularis brevis	Superficial fibular n.

153. Ans. (a) Common peroneal nerve

Ref: Neuromuscular Diseases: A Practical Approach to Diagnosis and Management By Schwartz, P 134

- **Book states:** *"In leg the common peroneal nerve is most often affected nerve".* Nerves may be damaged at the time of fracture or afterwards from the effects of movement or of reduction of a dislocation.
- Iatrogenic injuries occur from penetrating injury to nerves. These usually occur during intramuscular injection of drugs, for example, a sciatic nerve injury may occasionally follow drug injections into the buttock. The femoral nerve is also vulnerable in the thigh. Attempted cannulation of veins or arteries, especially in the antecubital fossa where the median nerve is vulnerable, may cause a severe nerve injury.

154. Ans. (b) Inguinal ligament

Ref: Gray's Basic Anatomy E-book, P 280

FEMORAL TRIANGLE

A triangular depressed area situated in the upper part of the medial aspect of the thigh just below the inguinal ligmanent.

BOUNDARIES

Superiorly (base): The inguinal ligament
Laterally: Medial border of sartorius
Medially: Medial border of adductor longus
Apex: Continuous with adductor canal
Anterior wall: Fascia lata
Posterior wall: Consists of iliopsoas, pectineus and adductor longus from lateral to medial side.

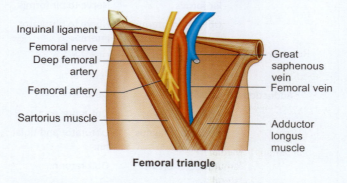

Femoral triangle

155. Ans. (b) Obturator nerve

Ref: Gray's Basic Anatomy E-book, P 205

Obturator nerve is a branch of lumbar plexus.
Related to ala of sacrum.
Forms the lateral boundary of ovarian fossa.
Emerges out of the obturator foramen and divides into anterior and posterior.

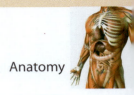

Anatomy

Branches of Obturator Nerve

A. Anterior division: Gives off:
- **Muscular branches to 3 muscles:** Adductor longus, adductor brevis and gracilis
- **Articular branch** to the hip joint
- **Cutaneous branch** to the skin of the medial side of the thigh.

B. Posterior division: Gives off:
- **Muscular branches** to 2 muscles
- Obturator externus and adductor magnus (pubic part)
- **Articular branch** to the knee joint.

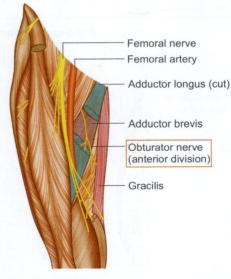

---

156. Ans. (c) Deep peroneal nerve

Ref: Anatomy of Foot and Ankle, pg. 12

Nerve	Motor Innervation	Sensory Distribution
Common peroneal (L4, L5, S1, S2)	Deep and superficial peroneal	Articular branches to knee; anterolateral aspect proximal leg (via lateral sural nerve)
Deep peroneal	Tibialis anterior, EDL, EHL, peroneus tertius Lateral branch: EDB	**Medial branch:** Dorsal first web space lateral hallux, medial second toe. **Lateral branch:** Tarsal and metatarsal joints
Superficial peroneal	Peroneus longus and brevis	Anterolateral distal two thirds of leg; dorsum of foot and toes

157. (a) Talus

Ref: Snell's Clinical Anatomy, pg. 354

Ref states: "Numerous important ligaments are attached to talus, but no muscles are attached to this bone"

Extra Mile

SUPERFICIAL GROUP OF MUSCLES IN THE POSTERIOR COMPARTMENT OF LEG (SPINAL SEGMENTS IN BOLD ARE THE MAJOR SEGMENTS INNERVATING THE MUSCLE)

Muscle	Origin	Insertion	Innervation	Function
Gastrocnemius	Medial head-posterior surface of distal femur just superior to medial condyle; lateral head-upper posterolateral surface of lateral femoral condyle	Via calcaneal tendon, to posterior surface of calcaneus	Tibial **nerve [S1, S2]**	Plantar flexes the foot and the knee
Plantaris	Inferior part of lateral supracondylar line of femur and oblique popliteal ligament of knee	Via calcaneal tendon, to posterior surface of calcaneus	Tibial nerve **[S1, S2]**	Plantar flexes the foot and the knee
Soleus	Soleal line and medial border of tibia; posterior aspect of fibular head and adjacent surfaces of neck and proximal shaft; tendinous arch between tibial and fibular attachments	Via calcaneal tendon, to posterior surface of calcaneus	Tibial **nerve [S1, S2]**	Plantar flexes the foot

Explanations

FMGE Solutions Screening Examination

158. Ans. (b) Sartorius

Ref: Gray's Anatomy, P 630

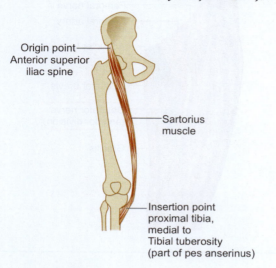

- The **anterior superior iliac spine** is a bony projection of the iliac bone and an important landmark of surface anatomy.
- It provides attachment for the inguinal ligament, and sartorius muscle.

159. (a) Posterior tibial nerve

Ref: Mac Glamry's Textbook of Foot and Ankle Surgery, pg. 196

- Posterior tibial muscle is supplied by L5, S1 (posterior tibial nerve)
  - *Action*: Inversion of the foot at the ankle.
  - *Test*: The patient holds his foot in the inverted position while the examiner pushes outward toward eversion.
- Anterior tibial muscle is supplied by L4, 5 (deep peroneal nerve)
  - *Action*: Dorsiflexion of the foot at the ankle.
  - *Test*: The patient dorsiflexes the foot and the examiner try to push the foot downward towards plantar extension.

160. (d) Vastus medialis

Ref: Gray's Anatomy, 41st ed. pg. 1319, 1339

- Adductor canal is also known as subsartorial canal or *hunter's canal*.
- It is an intramuscular space situated below the Sartorius muscle in anteromedial aspect of the distal 2/3rd of the thigh.

Boundary

- **Anterolaterally** by vastus medialis
- **Posteromedially** by adductor longus and adductor magnus.
- Its anteromedial boundary *(often referred to as the roof)* is a strong and dense fascia that extends from the medial surface of vastus medialis to the medial edge of the adductors longus and magnus, overlapping in its stride the femoral vessels in the adductor canal.

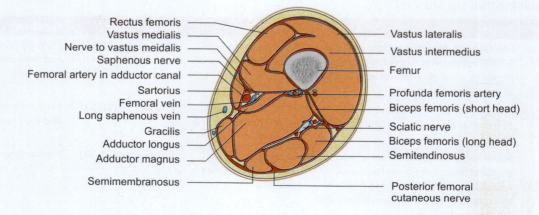

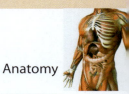

Anatomy

Contents of adductor canal:
- Femoral artery and its branch, descending genicular artery
- Femoral vein
- Saphenous nerve
- Nerve to vastus medialis

161. Ans. (c) Posterior division of L2, L3, L4 ventral rami

Ref: Gray's Anatomy, 41st ed. pg. 1322

- The femoral nerve is the nerve of the anterior compartment of the thigh.
- It arises from the **posterior divisions of the second to fourth lumbar ventral rami**, descends through psoas major and emerges on its lateral border to pass between it and iliacus.

Table: Root values
- Femoral nerve (L2–4)
- Obturator nerve (L2–4)
- Sciatic nerve (L4, L5, S1–3)
- Tibial nerve (L4, L5, S1–3)
- Common fibular nerve (L4, L5, S1, S2)
- Gluteal nerves (L4, L5, S1, S2)

162. Ans. (a) Iliacus

Ref: Netter's Clinical Anatomy, 3rd ed. pg. 191

Boundaries of femoral triangle
Upper border formed by: Inguinal ligament
Lateral border formed by: Sartorius
Medial border formed by: Lateral border of adductor longus

Contents of femoral triangle
A = Iliacus
B = Psoas major
C = Pectineus
D = Adductor longus

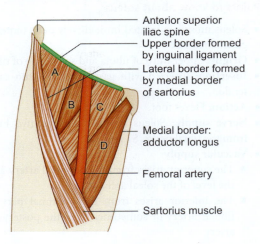

163. Ans. (b) Flexion of knee

Ref: Netter's Clinical Anatomy, 3rd ed. pg. 288

- Biceps femoris is present in posterior compartment of thigh and forms hamstrings. It is responsible for flexion of knee.
- The other hamstrings are semitendinosus and semimembranosus. All these muscles originate from the ischial tuberosity and are innervated by tibial part of sciatic nerve (L5, S1 and S2).

164. Ans. (a) Inferior gluteal nerve

Ref: Netter's Clinical Anatomy, 3rd ed. pg. 279-280

- The chief extensor of thigh at hip joint is gluteus maximus and helps in rising from sitting position.
- It is supplied by inferior gluteal nerve (L5, S1, S2). (mnemonic: M.I.G- 512)
- Gluteus medius are minimus are powerful abductor of thigh and are supplied by superior gluteal nerve (L4, 5, S1).

165. Ans. (a) Peroneus tertius

Ref: Kulkarni Clinical Anatomy, 2nd ed. pg. 864

- Peroneus tertius in an evertor of foot.
- Tibialis anterior muscle is an invertor of foot.
- Dorsiflexors of foot are-
  - Tibialis anterior
  - Extensor hallucis longus
  - Extensor digitorum longus
  - Peroneus tertius

166. Ans. (a) Tibial nerve

Ref: Kulkarni Clinical Anatomy, 2nd ed. pg. 832

- **Origin:** Anterior part of the popliteal groove on lateral surface of lateral femoral condyle

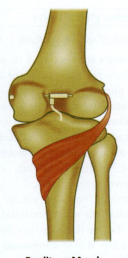

Popliteus Muscle

FMGE Solutions Screening Examination

- **Insertion:** Posterior surface of tibia in a fan-like fashion, just superior to the popliteal line
- **Action:** Rotates knee medially and flexes the leg on the thigh
- **Innervation:** Tibial nerve (L4, L5, S1)
- **Arterial supply:** Medial inferior genicular branch of popliteal artery and muscular branch of posterior tibial artery

167. Ans. (a) Paralysis of gluteus maximus

Ref: Maheswari Orthopaedics, 5th ed. pg. 135

- When a person stands on one leg, the tendency of unsupported side to sag down is *counteracted* by *gluteus medius and minimus*. These two muscles form the abductor mechanism of hip.

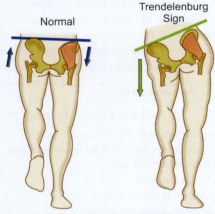

- In case the *abductor mechanism is defective*, unsupported side of the pelvis drops and is called *Positive Trendelenburg sign*. It is seen in:
  - Paralysis of gluteus medius and minimus
  - Congenital dislocation of Hip
  - Ununited fracture
  - Coxa vara

168. Ans. (d) Superior gluteal nerve

Ref: BDC 6th ed. vol. II / 68-69, 70; Keith L. Moore 5th ed./619-621

- **Trendelenburg's sign** is found in people with weak or paralyzed abductor muscles of the hip, namely gluteus medius and gluteus minimus.
- **Superior gluteal** nerve, if injured, paralyses the 3 muscles: **gluteus medius**, **gluteus minimus** and tensor fascia latae and hence leads to positive **Trendelenberg test**.
- These 3 muscles, especially the gluteus medius raises the unsupported hip during walking, which otherwise will be pulled down by the gravity.
- In Trendelenberg test this action of gluteus medius (superior pelvic tilt of contralateral hip) is absent and we actually observe that there is a downward drop of the unsupported hip- due to unopposed action of gravity.
- This leads to Lurching gait in the patient.

Extra Mile
- Trendelenburg test becomes positive in congenital dislocation of hip/ long standing fracture of neck of femur.
- Inferior gluteal nerve supplies gluteus maximus.

169. Ans. (a) Gluteus medius, minimus

Ref: BDC 6th ed. vol. II / 69-70; Keith L. Moore 5th ed. / 619-621

Please refer to above explanation.

170. Ans. (c) Genicular branch of obturator nerve

Ref: Netter's Atlas of Neurosciences, 3rd ed. pg. 194

- The capsule of knee joint is supplied by genicular branch of *obturator nerve* which pierces the oblique popliteal ligament.
- The *genitofemoral nerve* mediates the *cremasteric reflex*.

171. Ans. (b) Lateral head of gastrocnemius

Ref: Kulkarni Clinical Anatomy, 2nd ed. pg. 580

- Fabella is a small sesamoid bone present in tendon of origin of lateral *head of gastrocnemius*.

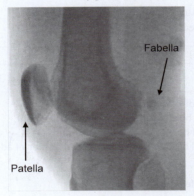

172. Ans. (a) Tibial nerve

Ref: Gray's Anatomy, 41st ed. pg. 1324e1-e2

Points to know about soleus:

- Soleus muscle is located immediately deep (anterior) to gastrocnemius.
- **Origin:** Upper third of fibula and soleal line of tibia.
- **Insertion:** inserted with gastrocnemius into calcaneal tendon.
- **Action:** Flexes foot.
- **Nerve supply:** Soleus is innervated by two branches from the tibial nerve, S1 and S2.
- **Vascular supply:**
  - The superior arises from the popliteal artery at about the level of the soleal arch, and
  - The inferior arises from the proximal part of the fibular artery or sometimes from the posterior tibial artery.

Anatomy

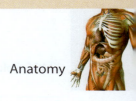

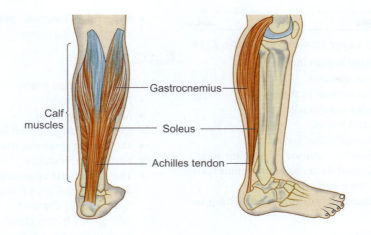

Extra Mile

TABLE: The movements and muscles tested to determine the location of a lesion in the lower limb

Movement	Muscle	Upper motor neuron	Spinal nerve level	Reflex	Nerve
Hip flexion	Iliopsoas	++	L1, 2		Femoral
Hip adduction	Adductors	+	L2, 3	(+)	Obturator
Hip extension	Gluteus maximus		L5, S1		Inferior gluteal
Knee flexion	Hamstrings	+	S1		Sciatic
Knee extension	Quadriceps femoris		L3, 4	++	Femoral
Ankle dorsiflexion	Tibialis anterior	++	L4		Deep fibular
Ankle eversion	Fibularis longus and fibularis brevis		L5, S1		Superficial fibular
Ankle inversion	Tibialis posterior		L4, 5		Tibial
Ankle plantar flexion	**Gastrocnemius/ soleus**	+	S1, 2	++	**Tibial**
Great toe extension	Extensor hallucis longus		L5		Deep fibular

---

173. Ans. (a) Thickening of fascia lata

Ref: Gray's Anatomy, 41st ed. pg. 1337-38

- The iliotibial tract is a **thickened portion of the deep fascia of the thigh (fascia lata)**. This tract runs from the lateral aspect of the iliac crest to Gerdy's tubercle and produces the flattened appearance of the lateral thigh.
- The attachment on Gerdy's tubercle is on the **anterior aspect of the lateral condyle** that is usually approximately **1 cm inferior to the joint** line and about 2 cm superolateral to the tibial tuberosity.
- The upper end of the tract splits into two layers, where it encloses and anchors tensor fasciae latae and receives, posteriorly, most of the tendon of **gluteus maximus.**

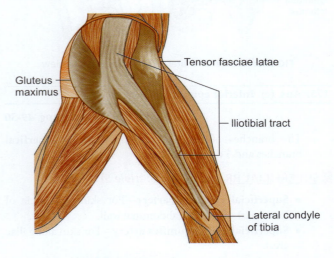

FIGURE: Important muscles of the limb

174. Ans. (b) Gluteus maximus

Ref: Grays Anatomy, 41st ed. pg. 1318

The muscles of the gluteal region include:
- Three named gluteal muscles and
- The deeper short lateral rotators of the hip joint

Gluteus maximus lies most superficially
- **Origin:** Iliac, sacrum and coccyx
- **Insertion:** Gluteal tuberosity, iliotibial band
- **Function:** It is a powerful extensor of the hip joint, acting more often to extend the trunk on the femur than to extend the limb on the trunk.
- Therefore **used for changing position from sitting to standing.**

Gluteus medius and minimus
- **Attachment:** Proximally to the outer surface of the ilium and distally to the greater trochanter of the femur
- **Function:**
  - They are **abductors of the hip**;
  - Their most important action is to stabilize the pelvis on the femur during locomotion, and they are helped in this function by tensor fasciae latae.

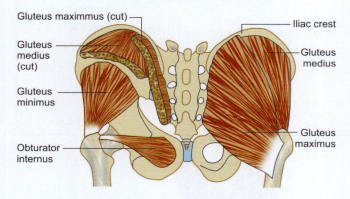

FIGURE: Gluteal and lateral rotators, posterior view

175. Ans. (c) Inferior epigastric artery

Ref: BDC, 6th ed. vol. II pg. 49-50

The branches of the femoral artery are: **3 superfical** branches and **5 deep branches**

SUPERFICIAL BRANCHES (*Mn: triple S*)

- **Superficial epigastric artery**—For skin and fascia of lower part of anterior abdominal wall.
- **Superficial iliac circumflex artery**—For skin along iliac crest.
- **Superficial external pudendal artery**—For skin of external genital organ.

DEEP BRANCHES

Mnemonic: *Deep branches: Put My Dog Down Please!*
- *Profunda Femoris*
- *Muscular Branches*
- *Deep external pudendal branches*
- *Descending genicular arteries*
- *Perforating Branches*
- The **superficial epigastric artery** *arises* from the front of the femoral artery about 1 cm. below the inguinal ligament. It distributes branches to the superficial subinguinal lymph glands, the superficial fascia, and the integument; it anastomoses with branches of the inferior epigastric artery
- The **superficial iliac circumflex artery** the smallest of the cutaneous branches. It divides into branches which supply the integument of the groin, the superficial fascia, and the superficial subinguinal lymph glands
- The **superficial external pudendal artery** *arises* from the medial side of the femoral artery to be distributed to the integument on the lower part of the abdomen, the penis and scrotum in the male, and the labium majus in the female, anastomosing with branches of the internal pudendal artery.
- The **deep external pudendal artery** in male supplies to the integument of the scrotum and perineum and in the female to the labium majus.
- **Muscular branches** are supplied by the femoral artery to the Sartorius, Vastus medialis, and Adductores.
- The **profunda femoris artery** (*profunda femoris*) is a large vessel *arising* from the lateral and back part of the femoral artery. The terminal part of the profunda is sometimes named the **fourth perforating artery**.

176. Ans. (c) Iliotibial tract

Ref: BDC, 6th ed. vol. II pg. 68

- Gluteus maximus:
  - **Origin: iliac crest**, posterior gluteal line of ilium and area above and behind it, sacrum, coccyx, sacrotuberous ligament.
  - **Insertion:** Gluteal tuberosity and iliotibial tract.
  - Major 3/4th part inserted into iliotibial tract.
  - 1/4th part inserted into Gluteal tuberosity.

177. Ans. (c) Gluteus minimus

Ref: BDC, 6th ed. vol. II pg. 67-68

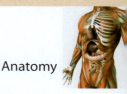
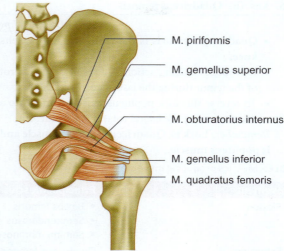

- Iliotibial band is the thickened band of fascia lata. It receives insertion of three muscles:
  - Tensor fasciae latae
  - Gluteus maximus
  - Few fibers of vastus lateralis

178. Ans. (a) Sartorius

Ref: BDC, 6th ed. vol. II pg. 53

- Sartorius muscle is the longest muscle of the body.
- It is also known as tailor's muscle (Sartor = tailor)

179. Ans. (b) Rectus femoris

Ref: BDC, 6th ed. vol. II pg. 54

- **Rectus femoris arises by two tendons**: One, the anterior or straight head, from the anterior inferior iliac spine; the other, the posterior or reflected head, from a groove above the brim of the acetabulum and the capsule of hip joint.
- The two unite at an acute angle, and are inserted into the base of the patella.

180. Ans. (a) Semimembranous

Ref: BDC, 6th ed. vol. II pg. 83

Hamstring muscles are
- Semimembranosus
- Semitendinosus
- Long head of biceps femoris and
- Ischial head of adductor magnus.

181. Ans. (a) Superior gluteal nerve

- Gluteus medius and minimus are supplied by superior gluteal nerve whereas gluteus maximus is supplied by inferior gluteal nerve.

Extra Mile

TABLE: Important muscles and their nerve supply

Nerve supply	Muscle
• Superior gluteal nerve	• Gluteus medius • Gluteus minimus • Tensor fascia lata
• Inferior gluteal nerve	• Gluteus maximus
• Nerve to obturator internus	• Obturator internus • Gamellus superior
• Nerve to quadratus femoris	• Gamellus inferior • Quadratus femoris

182. Ans. (b) Inferior gluteal nerve

Ref: BDC, 6th ed. vol. II pg. 69;
Gray's Anatomy 40th ed. pg. 1384

183. Ans. (c) Nerve to quadratus femoris

Ref: BDC, 6th ed. vol. II pg. 69;
Grays Anatomy 40th ed. pg. 1384

- Quadratus femoris and gamellus inferior muscle are arranged together. Nerve which is bifurcating to supply quadratus femoris muscle, supplies gamellus inferior muscle as well

Extra Mile

- Nerve supply of piriformis: Ventral rami to S1 and S2
- Nerve supply of obturator externus muscle: Posterior division of obturator nerve

184. Ans. (d) Nerve to obturator externus

Ref: BDC, 6th ed. vol. II pg. 74

Mnemonic to Remember this Often Asked Question

N. to obturatour internus	Not
Tendon of obturatour internus.	Tonight
Pudendal vessels and nerve.	Please

185. Ans. (d) Nerve to obturator externus

186. Ans. (b) Quadriceps femoris

Ref: BDC, vol II pg. 155

- Quadriceps femoris is the main and only extensor of knee.
- It produces locking action as a result of medial rotation of the femur during the last stage of extension.
- To reverse this lock popliteus muscle comes into action and does so by the lateral rotation of femur

Remember: **Lock is: Quadriceps femoris muscle and, Key is popliteus muscle.**

TABLE: Muscles producing movements at the knee joint

Movement	Principal muscles
A. Flexion	• Biceps femoris • Semitendinosus • Semimembranosus
B. Extension	Quadriceps femoris
C. Medial rotation of flexed leg	• Popliteus • Semimembranosus • Semitendinosus
D. Lateral rotation of flexed leg	• Biceps femoris

> **Extra Mile**

- **Quadriceps femoris incudes:** Rectus femoris, Vastus Lateralis, Vastis Medialis, Vastus Intermedius.
- Rectus femoris is also known as **"kicking muscle"**

187. Ans. (a) Popliteus

Ref: BDC, vol II pg. 155

Please refer to above explanation

188. Ans. (c) Talus

Ref: BDC, 6th ed. vol. II pg. 30

- *Talus has no muscle attachment.*
- Talus also has a precarious blood supply because blood enters it distally ie. Retrograde blood supply.
- *Remember incus in ear also has no muscle attachment.*

189. Ans. (c) Common peroneal nerve

Ref: BDC 6th ed. vol. II pg. 29; Snell's Anatomy, pg. 273

Common peroneal nerve is palpated against the neck of the fibula. It is a superficial nerve hence; it is unprotected as compared to tibial nerve. It may be injured in the fracture of neck of the fibula or due to a pressure of a tightly applied plaster cast. It is also affected in leprosy where it gets thickened and tender.

Clinical significance

Common peroneal nerve injury causes paralysis of dorsiflexors of the ankle joint and the evertors of the foot supplied through its superficial and deep perosneal nerve branches respectively. The paralysis of the muscles may result in **'foot drop'**, where the patient walks on his toes.

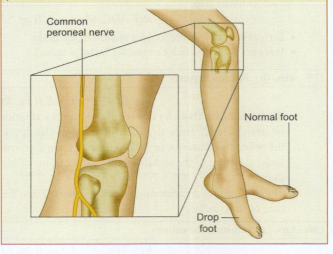

190. Ans. (b) Linea semilunaris

Ref: Gray's, 41st edn pg.1080-81; Keith L Moore clinical Anatomy, 4th ed. pg.193-4

HESSELBACH'S TRIANGLE

- **Medial border:** Lateral margin the rectus sheath, also called linea semilunaris
- **Superolateral border:** Inferior epigastric vessels
- **Inferior border:** Inguinal ligament, sometimes referred to as Poupart's ligament.

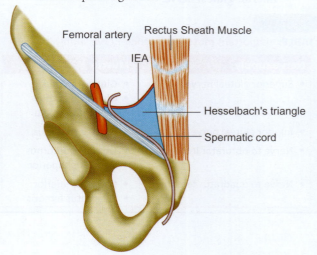

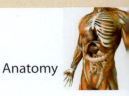

Anatomy

191. Ans. (d) Inferior

Ref: Gray's, 41st pg. 1080-81

192. Ans. (b) Supplies skin over the medial aspect of thigh

Ref: Clinical Anatomy, 11th ed. pg. 251

- The femoral nerve supplies the skin of the medial and anterior aspects of the thigh via its medial and intermediate cutaneous branches.
- The lateral aspect is supplied by the *lateral cutaneous nerve of the thigh* (L2–3).
- As its name suggests, it is purely sensory.
- It arises from L2 and L3, travels downward lateral to the psoas muscle, crosses the iliacus muscle (deep to fascia), passes either through or underneath the lateral aspect of the inguinal ligament, and finally travels onto innervate the lateral thigh.

193. Ans. (a) $L_{4,5}, S_1$

Ref: BDC, 6th ed. vol. II pg. 173

Nerve	Root valve
Sciatic nerve	$L_{4,5} S_{1,2,3}$
Tibial nerve	$L_{4,5}, S_{1,2,3}$
Common peroneal nerve	$L_{4,5} S_{1,2}$
Superior gluteal nerve	$L_{4,5}, S_1$
Inferior gluteal nerve	$L_5, S_{1,2}$
Nerve to quadratus femoris	$L_{4,5}, S_1$
Nerve to obturatus internus	$L_5, S_{1,2}$
Superior gemellus	$L_{4,5}, S_1$
Inferior gemellus	$L_{4,5}, S_{1,2}$
Posterior cutaneous nerve of thigh	$S_{1,2,3}$
Pudendal nerve	$S_2 S_3 S_4$
Perforating cutaneous nerve	$S_{2,3}$

194. Ans. (b) S_1, S_2, S_3

Ref: BDC, 6th ed. vol. II pg. 173

195. Ans. (b) $L_4 L_5 S_1 S_2 S_3$

Ref: BDC, 6th ed. vol. II pg. 173-74

196. Ans. (b) $S_2 S_3 S_4$

Ref: BDC, 6th ed. vol. II pg. 173-174

THORAX AND ABDOMEN

197. Ans. (a) Azygos vein

Ref: Gray's Anatomy 41st ed. P 955

Mediastinal Surface of Right Lung

On the mediastinal surface of the right lung, you find these structures:

- **Azygos vein** and **its arch** (posterior and over the root of the lung).
- **Vagus nerve** posterior to the root of the lung.
- **Esophagus** posterior to the root.
- **Phrenic nerve** anterior to the root of the lung.
- **Cardiac impression:** Related to right atrium.
- **Below hilum and in front of pulmonary ligament:** Groove for IVC.

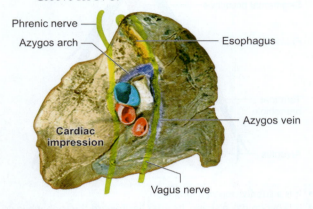

198. Ans. (c) Left intercostal artery

Ref: Gray's anatomy 41st ed. P 976

- The superior mediastinum lies between the manubrium sternum anteriorly and the upper four thoracic vertebrae posteriorly, and is bounded laterally by the mediastinal pleura.
- It accommodates the thymus, trachea, esophagus, aortic arch, pulmonary trunk, brachiocephalic trunk, left common carotid and subclavian arteries (the vertebral artery sometimes arises from the aortic arch between them), the internal thoracic arteries, the left superior intercostal, hemiazygos, internal thoracic and inferior thyroid veins, and numerous lymph nodes, including those from the tracheobronchial, paratracheal and brachiocephalic groups.

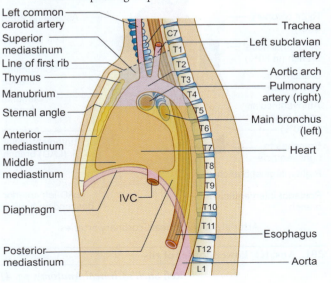

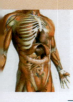

FMGE Solutions Screening Examination

199. Ans. (d) Pulmonary veins are intersegmental

Ref: Gray's Basic Anatomy E-book, P 87

Characteristics of Bronchopulmonary Segments

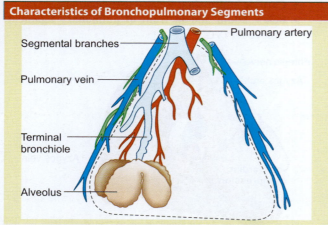

- It is a subdivision of a lung lobe.
- It is pyramidal in shape, its apex lies toward the root, while its base lies on the lung surface.
- It is surrounded by connective tissue septa.
- It has a segmental. bronchus, a segmental artery, lymph vessels, and autonomic nerves.
- The segmental vein lies in the intersegmental CT septa between the segments.
- A diseased segment can be removed surgically, because it is a structural unit.

200. Ans. (b) Left coronary artery

Ref: Gray's Anatomy Review E-book, P 80

Left anterior descending artery is a branch of left coronary artery.

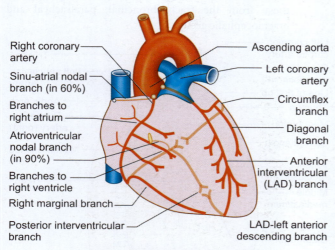

Arterial supply of heart coronary arteries

201. Ans. (c) Lower border of rib

Ref: Snell's Clinical Anatomy, pg. 41

- There are 11 **intercostal spaces** within the thoracic wall. The spaces are filled in by 3 layers of intercostal muscles and their related fasciae and are bounded superiorly and inferiorly by the adjacent ribs.
- The **costal groove** *is located along the inferior border of each rib* (upper aspect of the intercostal space) and provides protection for the vein which is most superior and the nerve which is inferior in the groove (VAN).

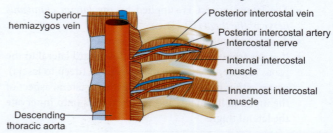

202. Ans. (c) Lateral thoracic vein

Ref: Anand's Human Anatomy for Students, pg. 148

- The lymphatics of upper limb are arranged in superficial and deep lymphatic vessels
- *Superficial lymphatics:* These run along cephalic vein and basilic vein. Vessels running along cephalic vein drain into infraclavicular and apical group of lymph nodes. Vessel along the basilic vein drain into supratrochlear group of lymph nodes.
- *Deep lymphatic vessels:* These run along the radial, ulnar and brachial arteries. They drain into lateral group of axillary lymp nodes.
- *Axillary group of lymph nodes:* They are 20 to 30 in number and are divided into five groups.

1. **Anterior group:** Lie along lateral thoracic vein
2. **Posterior group:** Lie along subscapular vein
3. **Lateral group:** Lie along axillary vein.
4. **Central group:** Are embedded in the fat of axilla
5. **Apical group:** Lie at the apex of the axilla, medial to axillary vein

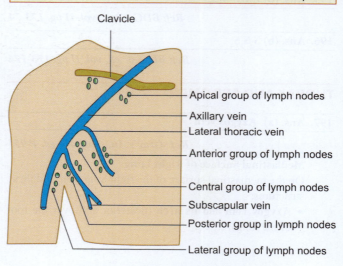

FIGURE: Axillary group of lymph nodes

Anatomy

203. Ans. (d) 11

Ref: Netter's Clinical Anatomy, 3rd ed. pg. 89

- The 11th and 12th ribs are *floating ribs* as they are free at their ends.
- The 8th, 9th and 10th ribs are *false ribs* as they are joined to form cartilage of rib immediately above.
- The first 7 pair of ribs are *true ribs*.

204. Ans. (d) 8th

Ref: BDC, 6th ed. Vol 1 pg. 196-97

- **True ribs:** Ribs directly articulating with sternum through costal cartilage. **They are ribs 1 to 7**
- **False ribs:** Ribs that do NOT articulate directly with sternum. **Ribs 8 to 12th.**

205. Ans. (d) 40

Ref: Netter's Clinical Anatomy, 3rd ed. pg. 90

- The xiphoid process unites with the body at about 40 years.
- The manubrio-sternal joint persists as cartilaginous throughout life.
- The body is completely ossified by 25 years.

206. Ans. (b) Tail of Spence

Ref: Kulkarni Clinical Anatomy, 2nd ed. pg. 182

- The *axillary tail of spence of breast* pierces the *deep fascia* through the *foramen of langer* and comes to lie in the axilla.

207. Ans. (a) Breast

Ref: Kulkarni Clinical Anatomy, 2nd ed. pg. 11

- The lymphatic plexus below the areola is the *Sub-areolar plexus of sappey*.
- 75% of breast lymphatics drain to axillary lymph nodes.

Extra Mile
Quadrant wise breast lymphatic drainage

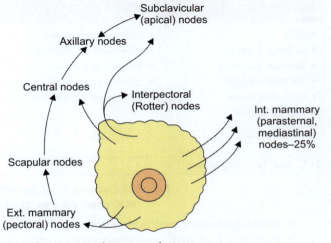

There is a quadrant-wise drainage:

- **Lateral quadrant:** Axillary nodes and supraclavicular through the pectoral, interpectoral and deltopectoral.
- **Medial quadrant:** Parasternal nodes.
- **Lower quadrant:** Inferior phrenic (abdominal) nodes.

208. Ans. (b) Left upper lobe

Ref: Kulkarni Clinical Anatomy, 2nd ed. pg. 943

- Left upper lobe is divided into apical lobe and lingular lobe.

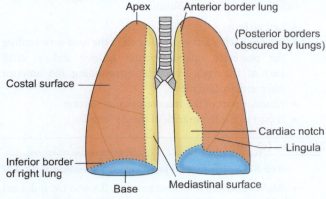

- *The Lingula is a part of the Left upper lobe of lung*
- It forms left cardiac border.

209. Ans. (b) Latissimus dorsi

Ref: Kulkarni Clinical Anatomy, 2nd ed. pg. 38

- *Latissimus dorsi* is supplied by thoracodorsal nerve. It *takes part in violent expiratory efforts*.
- *Serratus anterior* muscle is supplied by long thoracic nerve of bell. It *takes part in laboured inspiration*.

210. Ans. (c) Anterior interventricular groove

Ref: BDC's Human Anatomy, 6th ed. Vol: 1 pg. 264-65

- The entire heart is supplied by two coronary arteries, arising from the ascending aorta. They run in coronary sulcus.
- Anterior interventricular groove is supplied by left coronary artery.

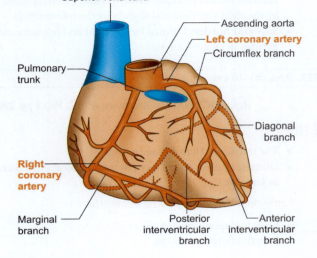

FMGE Solutions Screening Examination

Right Coronary Artery Supplies

- Right atrium
- A large part of right ventricle EXCEPT the area surrounding the anterior interventricular groove
- Posterior part of interventricular septum, and
- Whole of the conducting system of the heart except a branch of the AV bundle.

Left Coronary Artery Supplies

- Left atrium
- A large part of left ventricle except the area surrounding the posterior interventricular groove and a small part of the right ventricle surrounding the anterior interventricular groove.
- Anterior part of the Interventricular septum
- A part of the left branch of the AV bundle.

211. Ans. (c) LA

Ref: BDC, 6th ed. vol. I pg. 253; Snell's Anatomy, pg. 137

- **Right ventricle** is located between RA and LV. It doesn't form any boundary of heart
- **Right atrium** forms the right border
- **Left atrium** is located posteriorly. Forms the base of heart
- **Left ventricle** forms the left border. Apex is formed by LV.

212. Ans. (d) Right ventricle

Ref: BDC, 6th ed. vol. I pg. 253; Keith L. Moore 5th ed. pg. 147

BORDERS OF HEART

- **Right border** (slightly convex): Formed by the right atrium, SVC and the IVC.
- **Left border (nearly horizontal):** Formed by the left ventricle and slightly by the left auricle.
- **Inferior border** (oblique, nearly vertical), formed mainly by the right ventricle and slightly by the left ventricle.
- **Superior border:** Formed by the right and left atria and auricles in an anterior view.

213. Ans. (b) 10 cm

Ref: BDC's Human Anatomy, 6th ed. Vol: 1 pg. 280

TRACHEA

- The trachea is **10 to 15 cm** in length
- Diameter varies: About **2 cm in males** and about **1.5 cm in females.**

Some Important Lengths to Remember

- Length of esophagus 25 cm
- Length of ureters- 25 cm
- Length of male urethra- 20 cm
- Length of female urethra- 4 cm
- C- shaped rings in trachea- 16–20

214. Ans. (b) 2 cm

Ref: BDC, 6th ed. vol. I pg. 280

Please refer to above explanation

215. Ans. (b) Cricopharyngeus

Ref: BDC, 6th ed. vol. I pg. 282

- The first constriction present at the root of the neck is bounded by Cricopharyngeus muscle. Foreign body most commonly lodges here because of its strong constriction.

The Esophagus Shows 4 Constrictions at the Following Levels

1. At its beginning, **15 cm** from the **incisor teeth**
2. Where it is crossed by the aortic arch, **22.5 cm** from the **incisor teeth**
3. Where it is crossed by the left bronchus, **27.5 cm** from the **incisor teeth**
4. Where it pierces the diaphragm **37.5 cm** from the **incisor teeth.**

▶ **Extra Mile**

- Most common foreign body which lodges in esophagus is food particle.

216. Ans. (d) None

Ref: Snell Anatomy 7th ed. pg. 499; BDC, 6th ed. vol. I /180

- All the given options are accessory muscles of respiration.
- Muscles used for forceful breathing are accessory muscles of respiration.

Accessory muscle for inspiration	Accessory muscle for expiration
- SCM - Serratus anterior - Serratus posterior - Pectoralis major - Pectoralis minor - Erector spinae - Scalene	- Internal intercostals - Innermost intercostals - Transverse thoracis - Lattissimus dorsi - Abdominal muscle

217. Ans. (a) Diaphragm

Ref: Snell Anatomy, 7th ed. pg. 499; BDC 6th ed. vol. I pg. 212-13

- Diaphragm is major respiratory muscle
- Inspiration is an active process and requires contraction of inspiratory muscles.

- During quiet breathing expiration is a passive process.
- During inspiration all the 3 dimensions of the thoracic cavity expand
  - **Vertical-75% (by diaphragm)**
  - AP 25% (external intercostals and internal intercostals)
  - Transverse
  - Increase in vertical diameter is brought about by downward movement of diaphragm—which account for 70% of the thoracic expansion.

218. Ans. (a) Phrenic nerve

Ref: BDC, 6th ed. Vol 1 pg. 192

NERVE SUPPLY OF DIAPHRAGM

- **Motor supply:** Phrenic nerve
- **Sensory supply:**
  - Peripheral part: Lower 6 intercostal nerves
  - Central part: Phrenic nerve

219. Ans. (c) Azygous vein

Ref: BDC 6th ed. vol. I / 221-222; Keith L. Moore 5th ed. / 105

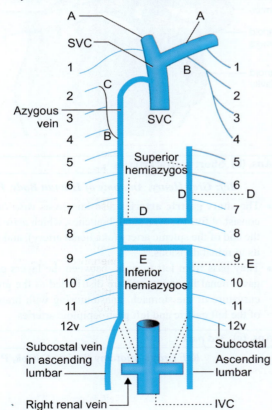

POSTERIOR INTERCOSTAL VEINS

- One in each of the 11 spaces

- **On the right:**
  - 1st drains into Rt. innominate vein (A)
  - 2nd, 3rd & sometimes the 4th unite to form Rt. Superior Intercostal vein (B) which drains into azygos vein.
  - From 5th to 11th & subcostal veins drain into azygos vein (C).
- **On the left:**
  - 1st drains into Lt. innominate vein (A)
  - 2nd, 3rd & sometimes the 4th join to form Lt. Superior intercostal vein which drains into Lt innominate vein vein (B)
  - 5th, 6th, 7th & 8th form *superior hemiazygos vein* to azygos vein (D)
  - 9th, 10th, 11th & subcostal form *inferior hemiazygos veins drain* to azygos vein (E).

220. Ans. (c) Left superior intercostal vein

Ref: BDC 6th ed. vol. I / 221-222; Keith L. Moore 5th ed. / 105

- The right superior intercostal vein is typically the final tributary of the azygos vein, before it enters the SVC.
- The left superior intercostal vein, however, usually empties into the *left brachiocephalic vein*.

ABDOMEN

221. Ans. (c) Left Gastroepiploic Artery

Ref: Gray's Anatomy 41st ed. P 1116

- The shown artery in the image is left gastroepiploic artery, the largest branch of splenic artery.
- **Origin and course:** Arises near splenic hilum and runs anteroinferiorly between the layers of the gastrosplenic ligament into the upper gastrocolic omentum → descends and anastomose with right gastroepiploic artery.
- **Size:** Up to 8 cm long (longer than right gastroepiploic artery)
- Supplies gastric fundus and body.

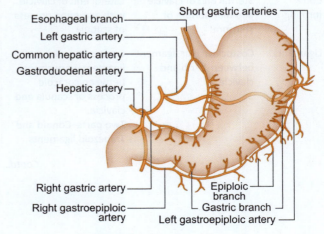

FIGURE: Arteries around stomach

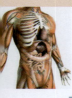

FMGE Solutions Screening Examination

222. Ans. (b) Splenorenal ligament

Ref: Gray's Anatomy 41st ed. P 1181

- Most lateral and narrowest portion of pancreas is pancreatic tail
- **Length:** 1.5 – 3.5 cm
- Lies between layers of splenorenal ligament

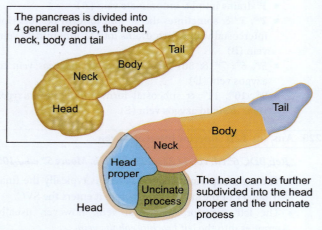

223. Ans. (d) Clavicle

Ref: Gray's Anatomy 41st ed. P 799-800

- Clavicle/collar bone is the connection between sternum and scapula
- **Sternal/Medial end:** Attaches to manubrium of sternum and first coastal cartilage
- **Acromial end/Lateral end:** Attaches to acromion on scapula → supports shoulder

	Sternoclavicular joint	Acromioclavicular joint
Type	Saddle type of synovial joint	Plane type of synovial joint
Bone forming	Sternal end of clavicle and manubrium of sternum	Lateral end of clavicle with acromion process of scapula
Ligaments	Costoclavicular ligament between 1st rib and clavicle	Coracoclavicular ligament—very strong— between coracoid process of scapula and clavicle. Two parts—Conoid and Trapezoid ligaments

224. Ans. (b) Short gastric arteries

Ref: Grey Henry, Anatomy of Human Body, P 606

- The **short gastric arteries** also known as *vasa brevia* consist of five to seven small branches, which *arise* from the end of the splenic artery (aka lienal artery), and from its terminal divisions.
- They pass from left to right, between the layers of the gastrolienal ligament, and are distributed to the greater curvature of the stomach, anastomosing with branches of the left gastric and left gastroepiploic arteries

225. Ans. (c) 3rd part

Ref: Gray's Anatomy Review E-book, P 183,

Contd...

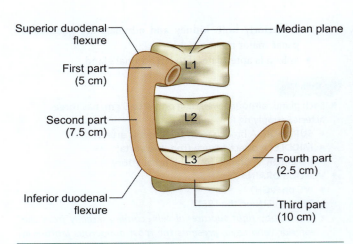

Derivatives of Dorsal Mesogastrium
Greater omentum
Gastrosplenic ligament
Gastrophrenic ligament
Lienorenal ligament
Derivatives of Ventral Mesogastrium
Lesser omentum
Falciform ligament
Coronary ligament
Right and left triangular ligament

226. Ans. (c) Red pulp

Ref: General Anatomy E-book, P 170

The **Cords of Billroth** *also* known as **red pulp cords or splenic cord** are found in the red pulp of the spleen between the sinusoids, consisting of fibrils and connective tissue cells with a large population of monocytes and macrophages.

The white pulp consists of thick layer of lymphocytes surrounding the arteries that have left the trabeculae. They form a periarterial sheath which contains mainly T cells. The sheaths expand to form well developed lymphoid nodules called malphigian nodules.

227. Ans. (d) Sudeck's point

Ref: Yamada's Textbook of Gastroenterology, Vol I, P 104

- **Watershed area:** It is the medical term referring to regions of the body that receive dual blood supply from the most distal branches of two large arteries.
- **Griffith's critical point:** A potential watershed area present between superior and inferior mesenteric arterial system. It is located at the splenic flexure.
- **Sudeck's point:** Located at the watershed area between inferior mesenteric artery and internal iliac artery. This point is located near the rectosigmoid junction.

228. Ans. (a) L2

Ref: Netter's Clinical Anatomy, 3rd ed. pg. 202

- Portal vein starts at level of *L2 vertebra* and is formed by *junction of superior mesenteric vein and splenic vein*. It is *8 cm* long and lies behind the neck of pancreas.
- Normal portal vein pressure is *5–10 mm Hg*.

229. Ans. (d) Coronary ligament

Ref: Netter's Clinical Anatomy, 3rd ed. pg. 205

230. Ans. (b) Right suprarenal gland

Ref: Vishram singh Anatomy: Volume 2: 2nd ed. pg. 97

Structures forming the pancreatic bed

- Splenic vein
- Aorta and superior mesenteric artery
- Left renal vessels and left kidney
- Left supra-renal gland
- Left crus of diaphragm

> **Extra Mile**

Structures forming the tonsillar bed	
1.	Buccopharyngeal fascia
2.	Superior constrictor muscles
3.	Palatopharyngeus
4.	Glossopharyngeus Nerve
5.	Pharyngo-basiliar fascia

231. Ans. (c) Left gastric artery

Ref: Netter's Clinical Anatomy, 3rd ed. pg. 181

The branches of celiac artery are:

- **Common hepatic artery** which gives rise to
  - Right gastric artery
  - Cystic artery
  - Right and left hepatic artery
  - Gastroduodenal artery
- **Left gastric artery:** *Smallest* branch of celiac artery and runs along the lesser curvature of stomach
- **Splenic artery** is the *largest* branch of celiac artery and gives rise to:
  - Pancreatic branches
  - Short gastric branches
  - Left gastroepiploic artery

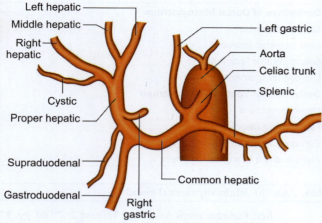

- Posteriorly both kidney and adrenals are guarded by psoas major muscle.
- Spleen is anterolateral to left adrenal gland.

> **Extra Mile**
>
> - Each gland, although weighing only **4 to 6 gm,** has three arteries supplying it:
>   - **SUPERIOR**: A branch from the phrenic artery;
>   - **MIDDLE**: A direct branch from the aorta;
>   - **INFERIOR**: A branch from the renal artery.
> - **VENOUS DRAINAGE:**
>   - IVC on RIGHT
>   - RENAL VEIN on the LEFT.
>   - *The stubby right suprarenal vein, coming directly from the inferior vena cava, presents the most dangerous feature in performing an adrenalectomy.*

236. Ans. (a) 4 gram

Ref: BDC, 6th ed. vol. II pg. 326

237. Ans. (d) T12

Ref: BDC, 6th ed. vol. II pg. 333

- Diaphragm has several openings for the passage of structures from thorax to abdomen.

TABLE: Main openings in the diaphragm and their levels

Opening	Level	Structure Passing
AORTIC OPENING- osseoaponeurotic opening (not a true opening) *Str passing: "Remember ATA"*	T12	• Aorta • Thoracic duct • Azygous vein
ESOPHAGEAL OPENING- lies in muscular part of diaphragm	T10	• Esophagus • Gastric or vagus nerve • Esophageal branch of left gastric artery
VENA CAVAL OPENING- lies in central tendon of diaphragm	T8	• Inferior vena cava • Right phrenic nerve branches

> **Extra Mile**
>
> - Only motor nerve to diaphragm- PHRENIC NERVE (C3, C4, C5)
> - It is the principle muscle of inspiration

> **Extra Mile**
>
> Structures and level of piercing in diaphragm: *(Mn: I ate, 10 Eggs, At 12)*
> - IVC: T8
> - Esophagus: T10
> - Aorta: T12

238. Ans. (d) Vagus nerve

Ref: BDC, 6th ed. vol. II pg. 333

FMGE Solutions Screening Examination

Branches of superior mesenteric artery	Branches of inferior mesenteric artery
Supplies all derivatives of mid gut from major duodenal papilla to right 2/3rd of transverse colon	Superior rectal artery Sigmoid artery Left colic artery

232. Ans. (c) IVC opening

- IVC passes through **tendon opening** and tendon is noncontracting part of muscle. Therefore constriction of diaphragm will not cause constriction of IVC.

233. Ans. (b) Jejunum

Ref: BDC, 6th ed. vol. II pg. 264

- Jejunum has valvulae conniventes, which are spaced regularly, concentrically giving a ladder effect.
- **Ileum:** Featureless or very thin valvulae coniventes
- **Caecum:** Rounded gas shadow in right liac fossa
- **Large bowel:** Haustral folds, spaced regularly.

234. Ans. (b) Semilunar

Ref: BDC, 6th ed. vol. II pg. 326

- Left adrenal gland is **crescenteric/semilunar**
- Right adrenal gland is **pyramidal in shape**
- The average weight of adrenal **gland: 4-6 g**

235. Ans. (a) Greater sac of stomach forms anterior border

Ref: Clinical Anatomy, 11th ed. pg. 151

- The suprarenal glands cap the upper poles of the kidneys and lie against the crura of the diaphragm.
- *The left is related anteriorly to the stomach across the lesser sac,* the right lies behind the right lobe of the liver and tucks medially behind the inferior vena cava.

239. **Ans. (b)** Caval opening

   Ref: BDC, 6th ed. vol. II pg. 333

240. **Ans. (b)** Phrenic nerve

   Ref: BDC, 6th ed. vol. II pg. 333, 5th ed. pg. 336

241. **Ans. (d)** Cisterna chyli

   Ref: Clinically Oriented Anatomy by Keith, Moore, 5th ed. pg. 387; Gray's Anatomy 40th ed. pg. 180
   - The **cisterna chyli** is a normal anatomical structure seen as saccular area of dilatation in the lymphatic channels that is located in the **retrocrural space,** usually to the immediate right of the abdominal aorta. It originates at the level of L1/2 vertebral body and extends 5-7 cm in the caudocephalad axis.
   - **Thoracic duct originates from the chyle cistern in the abdomen and ascends through the aortic hiatus in the diaphragm.** Thoracic duct ascends in the posterior mediastinum among the thoracic aorta on its left, the azygos vein on its right, the esophagus anteriorly, and the vertebral bodies posteriorly. At the level of the T4, T5, or T6 vertebra, the thoracic duct crosses to the left, posterior to the esophagus, and ascends into the superior mediastinum.
   - **Note:** *Although thoracic duct derives from cisterna chyli, it is the thoracic duct that passes through diaphragm and not the cisterna chyli.*

242. **Ans. (a)** Inferior vena cava

   Ref: Gray's 41st ed. pg. 1021, 1027, 1167
   - *Most of the venous system has valves to prevent backflow of blood in order to maintain venous return.*
   - IVC has only one valve present at the junction where it drains into right atrium. This valve is named **Eustachean valve**
   - *The besian valve is present in coronary sinus.*
   - Veins contain valves to help keep blood flowing toward the heart at all times.
   - Veins which are valveless can be remembered as: **IPSS**
     - Internal juglar vein
     - Pulmonary vein, Portal vein
     - Superior vena cava
     - Sinuses of brain

243. **Ans. (d)** Inferior vena cava

   Ref: Gray's, 41st ed. pg. 127-128; Repeat question
   Please refer to above explanation

244. **Ans. (a)** Aorta
   - Aorta is an elastic artery with diameter ~ 25 mm.
   - Systemic arteries can be subdivided into two types- muscular and elastic-according to the relative compositions of elastic and muscle tissue in their tunica media as well as their size and the makeup of the internal and external elastic lamina.
   - The larger arteries (>10 mm diameter) are generally elastic and the smaller ones (0.1-10 mm) tend to be muscular.

245. **Ans. (d)** L5

   Clinically Oriented Anatomy by Keith, Moore, 5th ed / 340
   - The IVC begins anterior to **the L5 vertebra** by the union of the common iliac veins.
   - This union occurs approximately 2.5 cm to the right of the median plane, inferior to the bifurcation of the aorta and posterior to the proximal part of the right common iliac artery.
   - Renal vein at the level of **L1**
   - **Portal veins form at L1**
   - Hepatic veins form at **T8**

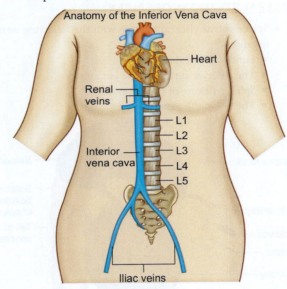

246. **Ans. (a)** L1

   Ref: Clinically Oriented Anatomy by Keith, Moore, 5th ed. pg. 340

247. **Ans. (a)** Duodenum

   Ref: BDC, 5th ed. Vol II pg. 268
   - Brunner's gland is found in duodenum above sphincter of oddi.
   - Main function of these glands is to produce mucus rich alkaline secretion which protects duodenum from gastric acidic contents.
   - It also facilitates activation of intestinal enzymes which helps in absorption.

248. Ans. (a) Mucinus alkaline

Ref: BDC, 5th ed. Vol II pg. 268

- Brunner's glands are also known as duodenal glands.
- These are small compound tubuloacinar glands which secrete mucus that protects duodenum from gastric acidic contents.
- They also facilitate activation of intestinal enzymes which helps in absorption.

Extra Mile

- The gastric glands situated in the fundus and body of stomach contain parietal/oxyntic cells which secrete acid, mucus, pepsin and other digestive enzymes.

249. Ans. (d) Duodenum

Ref: BDC, 6th ed. vol. II pg. 303

VISCERAL RELATIONS OF SPLEEN

- Spleen forms visceral relation with the following nearby organs:
  - Fundus of the stomach
  - The anterior surface of the left kidney
  - Splenic flexure of the colon and
  - The tail of the pancreas

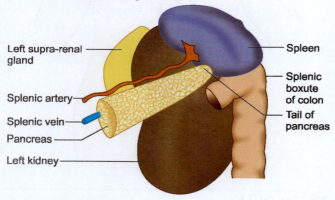

250. Ans. (b) Quadrotus lumborum

Ref: BDC, 6th ed. vol. II pg. 313-314

- The kidneys are reddish brown and measure approximately 10 cm in length, 5 cm in width, and 2.5 cm in thickness.
- **Superiorly:** The kidneys are associated with the diaphragm, which separates them from the pleural cavities and the 12th pair of ribs.
- **Posterior surfaces** of the kidney are related to **the quadratus lumborum muscle.** The subcostal nerve and vessels and the iliohypogastric and ilioinguinal nerves descend diagonally across the posterior surfaces of the kidneys.
- **Anterior surface** The kidneys are associated with liver, duodenum, ascending colon and supra renal glands.
- *The right kidney is separated from the liver by the hepatorenal recess.* **The left kidney is related to the stomach, spleen, pancreas, jejunum, and descending colon**

251. Ans. (c) Head of pancreas

Refer to above explanation.

252. Ans. (c) Intestinal looping

Ref: BDC, 6th ed. vol. II pg. 313-314

THE RELATIONS OF THE RIGHT KIDNEY

- **Anteriorly**—suprarenal gland, liver, second part of duodenum, right colic flexure
- **Posteriorly**—diaphragm, 12th rib, costodiaphragmatic recess of the pleura, psoas muscle, quadratus lumborum muscle, transversus abdominis muscle

THE RELATIONS OF THE LEFT KIDNEY

- **Anteriorly**—suprarenal gland, spleen, stomach, pancreas, left colic flexure, coils of jejunum
- **Posteriorly**—diaphragm, costodiaphragmatic recess of the pleura, 11th and 12th rib, psoas muscle, quadratus lumborum muscle, transversus abdominis muscle.

253. Ans. (b) Inferior mesenteric artery

Ref: Gray's, 41st ed. pg. 1206

The embryonic kidneys are close together in the pelvis. In approximately 1 in 600 fetuses, the inferior poles (rarely, the superior poles) of the kidneys fuse to form a horseshoe kidney. This U-shaped kidney usually lies at the level of **L3-L5 vertebrae** because the root of the **inferior mesenteric artery** prevents normal ascent of the abnormal kidney. Horseshoe kidney usually produces no symptoms; however, associated abnormalities of the kidney and renal pelvis may be present, obstructing the ureter.

254. Ans. (c) Collecting tubule and duct

Ref: BDC, 6th ed. vol. II pg. 315-16

- **The kidney consists of an outer renal cortex and an inner renal medulla that contains the renal pyramids which drain into → Calyx → Pelvis.**
- Cortex forms a continuous smooth outer zone with a number of projections (cortical columns) that extend down between the pyramids.
- It contains the renal corpuscles and the renal *tubules except for parts of the loop of Henle* which descend into

Anatomy

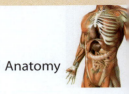

the renal medulla. *It also contains blood vessels and cortical collecting ducts.*
- The renal cortex is the part of the kidney where ultrafiltration occurs.

255. Ans. (c) Sigmoid colon

Ref: BDC, 6th ed. vol. II pg. 261

- Third part of duodenum extends in the right and left upper quadrant. Organs like pancreas, transverse colon, stomach, right kidney are also in the same quadrants and in close association with the duodenum while Sigmoid colon is present in the left lower quadrant, hence has no association with duodenum.
- **Doudenum is 25 cm long and is divided into the following four parts:**
  - First or superior part- 5cm
  - Second descending part- 7.5 cm
  - Third or horizontal part – **10 cm** (longest part)
  - Fourth or ascending part- 2.5 cm (shortest part)
- **Course of third part of duodenum**
  - This part is about 10 cm long.
  - It extends from L1 to L3.
  - It is *retroperitoneal and fixed.*
  - **Visceral relations**
    - *Anteriorly,* Superor mesenteric vessels and Root of mesentery
    - *Posteriorly,* right ureters, right psoas major, right testicular or ovarian vessels, Inferior vena cava, abdominal aorta with origin of inferior mesenteric artery
    - *Superiorly:* Head of the pancreas with uncinate process.
    - *Inferiorly:* Coils of jejunum.

256. Ans. (c) Third part

Ref: BDC, 6th ed. vol. II pg. 261

257. Ans. (b) T10

Ref: BDC, 6th ed. vol. II pg. 198

- Dermatome of umbilicus is at T10.
- **T10 segment also supplies to:**
  - Appendix: T9 - T10
  - Stomach: T6 – T10
  - Testis/Ovary: T10
  - Intestine: T9 –T11

258. Ans. (b) Retrocoecal

Ref: BDC, 6th ed. vol. II pg. 269-70

- **Most common position of vermiform appendix is retrocaecal,** (12 O'clock- 65%) followed by pelvic (4 O'clock position).

TABLE: Types of appendix and their relative position

Appendix	Position	Prevalence /comment
Retrocaecal	12 O' clock	**65%; most common**
Pelvic	4 O' clock	30%; 2nd most common
Subcaecal	6 O' clock	2.5%; points towards midinguinal point
Preileal	2 O' clock or splenic	1 %; points towards spleen & lie infront of ileum
Postileal	2 O' clock or splenic	**0.5%;** point towards spleen & lie behind ileum
Paracolic	11 O' clock	

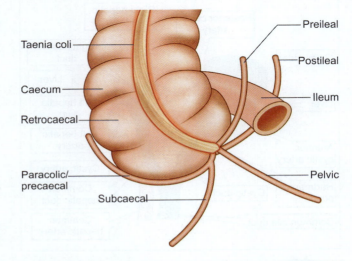

259. Ans. (c) Postileal

Ref: BDC, 6th ed. vol. II pg. 269-70

260. Ans. (c) Inferior Pancreatoduodenal vein

Tributaries of Portal Vein

1. Left Gastric vein
2. Right Gastric vein
3. Superior Pancreatoduodenal vein
4. Splenic vein
5. Superior mesenteric vein
6. Inferior mesenteric vein
7. Cystic vein

> **Extra Mile**
>
> - Hepatic portal vein is a blood vessel that conducts blood from GIT and spleen to the liver.
> - *Liver receives 75% of its blood through hepatic portal vein, and the remainder from hepatic artery proper.*
> - Note: blood leaves the liver to the heart in the hepatic vein.

FMGE Solutions Screening Examination

261. Ans. (b) Cystic duct, liver, common hepatic duct

Ref: Gray's Anatomy, 41st ed. pg. 1175

The Calot's Triangle Aka Hepatobiliary Triangle or Cystohepatic Triangle.

- Boundaries (Cystic duct, Liver, Common hepatic duct):
  - **Medial:** Common hepatic duct
  - **Infero-lateral:** Cystic duct
  - **Superior:** *Inferior surface of liver*
- **Content of Calot triangle** –Cystic artery.

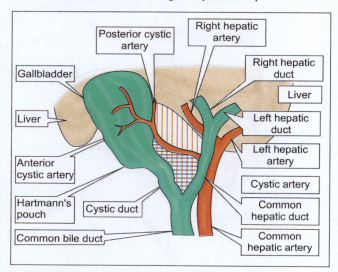

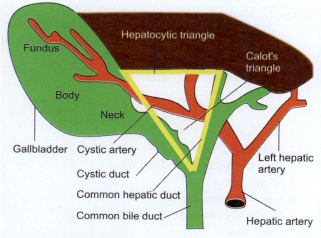

262. Ans. (c) Inferior surface of liver

Ref: Gray's Anatomy, 39th ed. pg. 1229

Please refer to above explanation

263. Ans. (a) Portal vein

Ref: Gray's Anatomy, 41st ed. pg. 1175

Contents of Calot's Triangle

- Cystic artery (Main)
- Right hepatic artery
- Lymph node of Lund

264. Ans. (b) Termination of portal vein

- The kidneys occupy the epigastric, hypochondriac lumbar and umbilical regions
- Vertically they extend from the upper border of twelfth thoracic vertebra to the centre of the body of third lumbar vertebra.
- The right kidney is slightly lower than the left and the left kidney is a little nearer to the median plane than the right.
- The transpyloric plane passes through the upper part of the hilus of the right kidney; and through the lower part of the hilus of the left kidney.

Structures at the Level of Transpyloric Plane

- Origin of superior mesenteric artery.
- Origin of portal vein.
- Hilum of left kidney.
- Origin of renal artery.
- Termination of spinal cord.
- Level of duodenojejunal flexure

265. Ans. (a) Whole system is valve less

Ref: BDC, 4th ed. Vol. II/268-71, Gray's 39th ed / 1218-19

- In adults, the portal vein and its tributaries have no valves.
- In fetal life and for a short postnatal period valves are demonstrable in its tributaries, but they usually get atrophied.
- Rarely some persist in an atrophic form into adulthood.

266. Ans. (a) Fundus

Ref: Gray's, 41st ed. pg. 1120

- Chief cells are usually **fundal** in position.
- Chief (Peptic) cells are the source of digestive enzymes like pepsin and lipase.
- These cells are cuboidal with round nucleus and contain lots of zymogen granules.
- **Parietal/Oxyntic cells** produce HCl and the intrinsic factor.
- These cells are oval with centrally placed nucleus.
- They are mainly located in the apical half of the **body** of gland, reaching as far as the **neck**.
- Surface mucus cells are distributed in the **gastric pit-**region of the gastric mucosa.

Anatomy

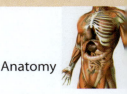

- Mucus neck cells are abundant in the neck region as the name is also suggesting.
- Neuroendocrine cells are situated mainly in the deeper / basal parts of the glands, along with the chief cells.

Also know: Gastric cells secretion
Goblet cell: Mucus (protect stomach lining)
Parietal cell: Gastric acid (HCL), intrinsic factor
Chief cell: Pepsinogen
D cell: Somatostatin
G cell: Gastrin
ECL cell: Histamine

267. Ans. (b) 7 ounce

Ref: BDC, 6th ed. vol. II pg. 294

- On an average the spleen is 1 inch or 2.5 cm thick, 3 inches or 7.5 cm broad, 5 inches or 12.5 cm long *and 7 ounces in weight.*

Some Must Know Weights
- Weight of liver: 1.5 kg.
- Weight of thyroid gland: 25 gm
- Weight of prostate: **8 gm.**

268. Ans. (c) Lower 1/3rd

Ref: BDC, 6th ed. vol. II pg. 407-408

ANATOMY OF RECTUM

- This is continuous with the sigmoid colon at the midpiece of the sacrum.
- It has a length of about **12 cm.**
- It descends along the **sacro-coccygeal concavity** as the **sacral flexure.**
- It eventually joins the **anal canal** at the **anorectal junction,** 2 to 3 cm in front of the **coccygeal tip.**
- The bend at this point is known as the **perineal flexure of the rectum.**
- The rectum is covered by **peritoneum:**
  - **UPPER 1/3rd:** on anterior surface and sides ,
  - **MIDDLE 1/3rd:** anterior surface
  - **LOWER 1/3rd: not covered by peritoneum** →thus making it more mobile.
- The lower part of the rectum is dilated as the **rectal ampulla.**
- The upper part has **3 transverse rectal folds** (upper and lower on the left, the middle on the right).
- The upper part of the rectum above the middle fold may contain faeces, but the lower part only contains faeces in **chronic constipation** or **during the call to defecate.**
- The rectum ends antero-inferior to the tip of the coccyx, immediately before a sharp posteroinferior angle (**the anorectal flexure of the anal canal**) that occurs as the gut perforates the pelvic diaphragm (levator ani). The roughly **80°degree anorectal flexure** *is an important mechanism for fecal continence, being maintained during the resting state by the tonus of the puborectalis muscle and by its active contraction during peristaltic contractions if defecation is not to occur.*
- With the flexures of the **rectosigmoid junction superiorly and the anorectal junction inferiorly, the rectum has an S shape when viewed laterally.**

269. Ans. (b) 12 cm

Ref: BDC, 6th ed. vol. II pg. 407-408

270. Ans. (c) Seminal vesicles

Ref: BDC, 6th ed. vol. II pg. 408

- **Rectum** is a 12 cm structure which is in conitunation of sigmoid colon and terminates at anal canal.

TABLE: Relationship of rectum

	Anterior	Posterior	Laterally
Males	• Base of bladder • **Seminal vesicles** • Rectovesical pouch • Ileum • Ductus deferens • Terminal ureter • Prostate gland	• S3-S5 vertebrae • Coccyx • Median sacral artery and vein • Middle rectal artery • Superior rectal artery and vein	• Sigmoid colon • Ileum • Pelvic plexuses • Coccygeus muscle • Levator ani muscle
Females	• Uterus • Vagina • Rectouterine pouch • Ileum • Sigmoid colon	Same as for male	Same as for male

271. Ans. (a) Squamous cell

Ref: Keith L. Moore, 5th ed. pg. 447-48

- The anal canal is divided into three parts. The zona columnaris is the upper half of the canal and is lined by simple columnar epithelium. The lower half of the anal canal, below the pectinate line, is divided into two zones separated by **Hilton's white line.**
- The two parts are the zona hemorrhagica and zona cutanea, *lined by stratified squamous non-keratinized and stratified squamous keratinized,* respectively.

272. Ans. (c) Posteriorly

Ref: Gray's, 41st ed. pg. 1148, 1153

Refer to above explanation.

FMGE Solutions Screening Examination

273. Ans. (c) Inferior mesenteric artery

Ref: BDC, vol II pg. 286-287

- **Superior pancreatoduodenal artery** from gastroduodenal artery and the **inferior pancreatoduodenal from superior mesenteric artery** supplies the head of the pancreas.
- Pancreatic branch of splenic artery also supplies the neck, body and tail.
- Inferior mesenteric artery supplies the left one third of transverse colon, the descending colon, sigmoid colon, rectum and upper part of anal canal.

274. Ans. (b) Splenic artery

Ref: Clinically Oriented Anatomy by Keith, Moore, 5th ed. pg. 252-253

- The stomach has a rich arterial supply arising from the celiac trunk and its branches.
- Most blood is supplied by anastomoses formed along the lesser curvature by the right and left gastric arteries, and along the greater curvature by the right and left gastro-omental arteries.
- Fundus of the stomach is supplied by splenic artery mainly.
- **Branches of splenic artery:**
  - Posterior gastric
  - Short gastric arteries
  - Left gastroepiploic artery
- Out of the three, the fundus of stomach is supplied by short gastric artery and left gastroepilpoic artery. But major contribution is by short gastric arteries.
- *This was a controversial question, but given these choices the best answer is splenic artery.*

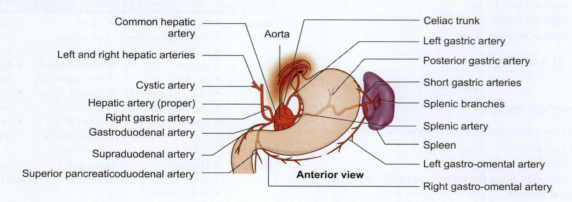

Anterior view

275. Ans. (a) Gonadal artery

Ref: Gray's, 41st ed. pg. 1047

Ventral Branches of Abdominal Aorta and Level
- Celiac trunk - T_{12}
- Superior mesenteric artery - L1
- Inferior mesenteric artery - L3

Paired/Lateral Branches of Abdominal Aorta
- Inferior phrenic artery
- Middle suprarenal artery
- Renal arteries

Testicular or Ovarian Artery
- Four paired lumbar arteries

Branches of External Iliac Artery
- Inferior epigastric artery
- Deep circumflex iliac artery
- Femoral artery

276. Ans. (d) Gonadal artery

Ref: Clinically Oriented Anatomy by Keith, Moore, 5th ed. pg. 252-253

NEUROANATOMY, HEAD AND NECK

277. Ans. (d) Mandibular branch

Ref: Gray's Anatomy 41st ed. P 502

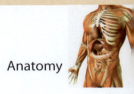

Anatomy

Branches of facial nerve on face:

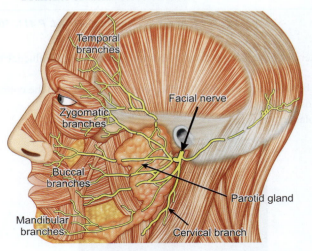

- **Temporal branch:** Aka frontal branch; supplies muscles of forehead and orbicularis oculi muscle
- **Zygomatic branch:** Supplies upper cheek and orbicularis oculi muscle
- **Buccal branch:** Emerges from anterior border of parotid gland below parotid duct to supply buccinator and muscles of upper lip and nostril.
- **Mandibular branch:** Emerges from anterior border of parotid gland to supply muscles of **lower lip**.
- **Cervical branch:** Emerges from lower border of parotid gland, it descends in the neck to supply platysma muscle + depressor anguli oris muscle.
- **Book states:** *"There are two marginal mandibular branches. They run forward under platysma towards angle of mandible. The branches supply risorius and the muscles of the lower lip and chin, and filaments communicate with the mental nerve"*

- Orbicularis oris muscle is also supplied by mandibular branch of facial nerve

278. Ans. (b) Labial nasal artery

Ref: Gray's Anatomy 41st ed. P 498

- External carotid artery gives rise to facial artery branch, which has several branches over face.
- *Superior labial*–supplies to upper lip and antero-inferior part of nasal septum.
- *Inferior labial*–supplies to lower lip.
- *Lateral nasal*–to the ala and dorsum of nose.
- *Angular*–supplies the lacrimal sac and orbicularis oculi.

279. Ans. (a) Tragal pointer

Ref: Gray's Anatomy 41st ed. P 412

Surgical Landmark of Parotid Gland

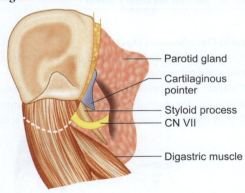

- **Tympano-mastoid suture in posterior canal wall:** 5–8 mm medial mastoid segment of facial nerve
- **Digastric ridge in mastoid tip:** Leads antero-medially to mastoid segment of facial nerve
- **Groove between mastoid and bony EAC meatus:** Bisected by facial nerve
- **Tragal pointer:** 1 cm antero-infero-medial is facial nerve
- **Root of styloid process:** Lateral to it lies facial nerve
- **Superior border of posterior belly of digastric:** Superior and parallel to it lies facial nerve

280. Ans. (d) Medial pterygoid

Ref: Gray's Anatomy 41st ed. P 552

- **Trismus/Lock jaw** is painful reflex muscle spasm. It occurs due to spasm of muscle of mastication and leads to inability to open the oral cavity
- Trismus occurs due to involvement of masseter or medial pterygoid muscle or due to sub mucosal fibrosis.
- **Note:** Infection of pterygomandibular region can cause trismus, which usually affects medial pterygoid muscle.

281. Ans. (c) Buccinator

Ref: Gray's Anatomy 41st ed. P 495

- It is a thin quadrilateral muscle of cheek, occupies the interval between maxilla and mandible.
- It compresses the cheek against the teeth and gums during mastication and assists the tongue in directing the food between teeth.

Classically the muscles of mastication are:
- *Masseter*
- *Medial Pterygoid*
- *Lateral Pterygoid*
- *Temporalis*

Accessory muscles of mastication
- *Anterior belly of digastric*
- *Mylohyoid muscle*
- *Geniohyoid muscle*
- *Buccinator*

FMGE Solutions Screening Examination

282. Ans. (d) Second maxillary molar

Ref: Gray's Anatomy 41st ed. P 411, 505

Parotid Duct/Stensen Duct
- It is a 5 cm long duct of parotid gland that originates from anterior border of upper part of parotid gland by the confluence of two main tributaries.
- **Course:** It then passes horizontally across masseter, midway between angle of mouth and zygomatic arch. Down the course it also crosses through buccal fat and buccinators muscle opposite the crown of upper third molar tooth.
- It then opens on a small papilla opposite the second upper molar crown.

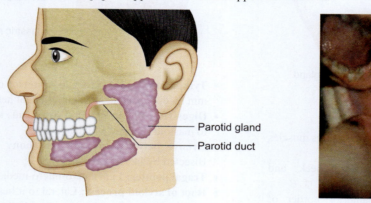

283. Ans. (d) Fornix

Ref: Gray's Anatomy 41st ed. P 356

- The mammillary bodies are hemispherical, pea-sized eminences, lying side by side, anterior to the posterior perforated substance, each with nuclei enclosed in fascicles of fibres derived largely from the fornix.

The *fornix* is a white matter structure leaving the *hippocampus* that projects mainly to the *mammillary bodies* (hypothalamus) which, in turn, mainly projects to the *thalamus* via mammillothalamic tracts.

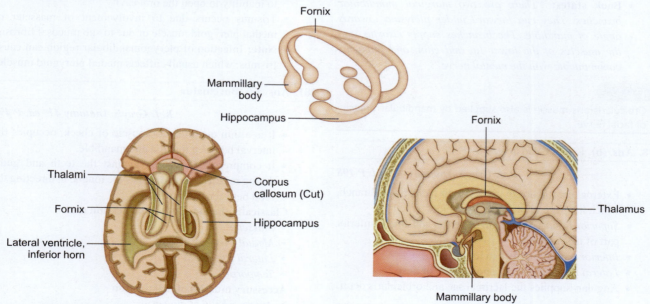

- Mammillary body is important for recollective memory.
- **Note:** Damage to mammillary bodies due to thiamine deficiency, is important in pathogenesis of Wernicke-Korsakoff syndrome.

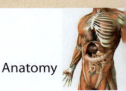

Anatomy

284. Ans. (a) Arcuate fasciculus

Ref: Gray's Anatomy 41st ed. P 391, 393

- Arcuate fasciculus is a white matter tract which connects broca's area and wernicke's area through the temporal, parietal and frontal lobes.
- It allows coordinated, comprehensive speech.
- **Note:** If damaged → Conduction Aphasia (auditory comprehension and speech articulation is present, but patient finds it difficult to repeat the heard speeches)

Extra Mile

1. **Uncinate fasciculus** connects frontal to temporal lobe
2. **Superior longitudinal fasciculus:** Connects the frontal, occipital, parietal, and temporal lobes
3. **Arcuate fasciculus:** Connect gyri in frontal to temporal lobes
4. **Inferior longitudinal fasciculus:** Connects occipital to temporal pole
5. **Cingulum:** Connects frontal and parietal lobes to the parahippocampal gyrus and adjacent temporal gyri

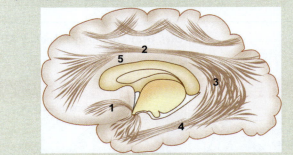

285. Ans. (b) Elevation, intorsion, adduction

Ref: Gray's Anatomy E-book: 41st ed. P 673

Muscle	Primary function	Secondary function	Tertiary function
SR	Elevation	Intorsion	Adduction
IR	Depression	Extortion	Adduction
SO	Intorsion	Depression	Abduction
IO	Extortion	Elevation	Abduction

- All superiors are intorters
- All rectus are adductors (except lateral rectus)
- All obliques are abductors

286. Ans. (c) Abducens

Ref: Textbook of Clinical Neuroanatomy 2015 ed. P 191

Abducens nerve passes through cavernous sinus. Other nerves like CN III, IV, V1 and V2 run in the wall of cavernous sinus.

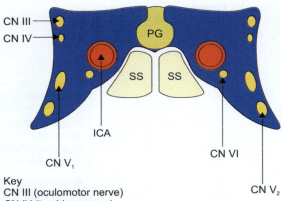

Key
CN III (oculomotor nerve)
CN IV (trochlear nerve)
CN VI (abducent nerve)
ICA (internal carotid artery)
CN V$_1$ (ophthalmic branch of the trigeminal nerve)
CN V$_2$ (maxillary branch of the trigeminal nerve)
PG (pituitary gland)
SS (sphenoidal sinus)

Cavernous sinus

287. Ans. (c) Left gastric artery and inferior phrenic nerve

Ref: Gray's anatomy for students E-Book. P 222

Blood Supply of the Esophagus

- The upper third of the esophagus is supplied by the interior thyroid artery
- The middle third by branches from the descending thoracic aorta
- The lower third by branches from the left gastric artery
- The veins from the upper third drain into the inferior thyroid veins, from the middle third into the azygos veins, and from the lower third into the left gastric vein, a tributary of the portal vein.

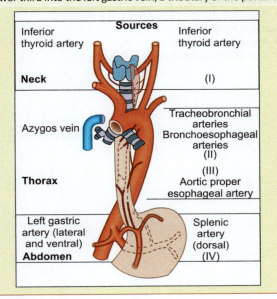

288. Ans. (b) Greater auricular nerve

Ref: Gray's Clinical Neuroanatomy E-book, P 315

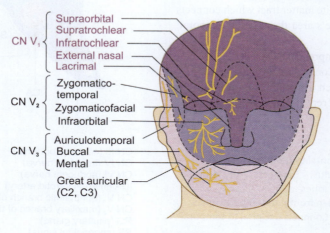

Sensory nerves of the face

289. Ans. (d) Fastigii

Ref: Gray's Anatomy E-book, P 337

- Cerebellar nuclei is deep seated nuclei.

Cerebellar Nuclei (Nuclei = Deep Cluster of Neurons)

- **Dentate nucleus**
  - Largest, communicates through cerebellar peduncle
  - Carries information important for coordination of limb movements (along with the motor cortex and basal ganglia)
- **Emboliform nucleus** (medial side of the nucleus dentatus)
  - Regulates movements of ipsilateral extremity
- **Globose nucleus**
  - Regulates movements of ipsilateral extremity
- **Fastigial nucleus**
  - Regulates body posture
  - It is related to the flocculonodular lobe

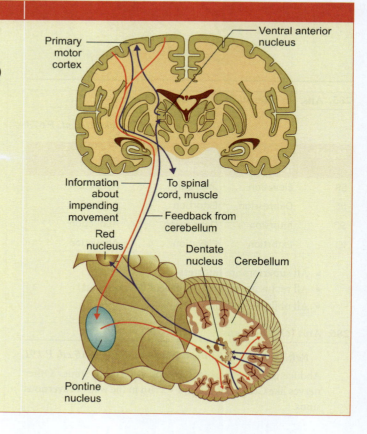

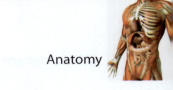

Anatomy

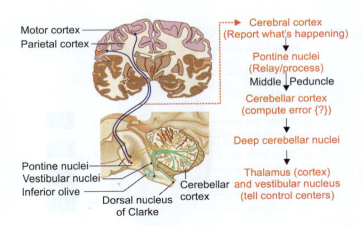

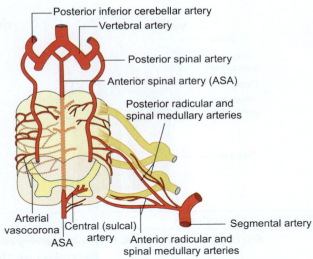

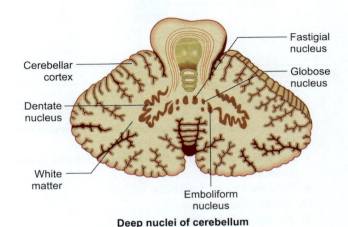

Deep nuclei of cerebellum

---

290. Ans. (c) **Abducens**

- All the extraocular muscles are supplied by CN III except lateral rectus and superior oblique.
- Lateral rectus supplied by—CN VI
- Superior oblique supplied by—CN IV

Remember- LR6; SO$_4$

---

291. Ans. (a) **1 anterior and 2 posterior**

Ref: Gray's Anatomy, 41st ed. pg. 770

- The spinal cord and its roots and nerves are supplied with blood by both longitudinal and segmental vessels.
- Three major longitudinal vessels, **a single anterior and two posterior spinal arteries** *(each of which is sometimes doubled to pass on either side of the dorsal rootlets)* originate intracranially from the vertebral artery and terminate in a plexus around the conus medullaris.

---

292. Ans. (d) **Anterior spinal artery**

Ref: Netter's Clinical Anatomy, 3rd ed. pg. 83-84

- The anterior 2/3rd of spinal cord is supplied by a single median anterior spinal artery which is a branch of vertebral artery.
- The posterior 1/3rd is supplied by posterior spinal arteries (branches of verterbral artery).
- Radicular arteries supply the neve roots of spinal cord. Additional arterial supply is via the **anterior and posterior segmental medullary arteries**—small vessels which enter via the nerve roots. The largest anterior segment medullary artery is the artery of **Adamkiewicz**. It arises from the interior intercostal or upper lumbar arteries and supplies the inferior 2/3rd of the spinal cord.

---

293. Ans. (b) **Postauricular muscle**

Ref: Gray's Anatomy, 41st ed. pg. 628

- Each temporal bone consists of four components: the squamous, petromastoid and tympanic parts and the styloid process.
- The squamous part has a shallow mandibular fossa associated with the temporomandibular joint. The petromastoid part is relatively large; its petrous portion houses the auditory apparatus and is formed of compact bone.
- The **auricularis posterior** consists of two or three fleshy fasciculi that arise by short aponeurotic fibres from the mastoid part of the temporal bone and insert into the ponticulus on the eminentia conchae.

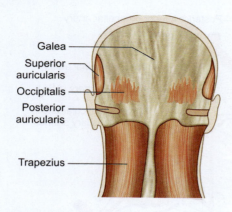
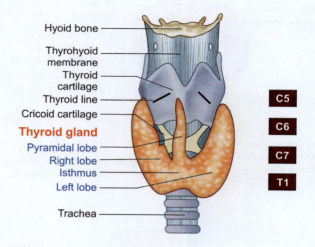

294. Ans. (c) Genioglossus

Ref: Lippincott's Illustrated, Review of Anatomy and Embryology, pg. 214

- All the intrinsic and extrinsic muscles of the tongue are innervated by hypoglossal nerve (CN XII) except the palatoglossus muscle which is innervated by vagus nerve (CN X).
- If there is damage to ipsilateral CN XII, it produces the dysarthria and fasciculations within the tongue musculature.
- The ipsilateral deviation of tongue is due to unopposed muscular contraction of contralateral **genioglossus muscle**.
- **Mn**: *"The tongue licks the wound"* (this will help you remember that the tongue deviates to the ipsilateral side in a lower motor lesion of CN XII)

295. Ans. (d) Arch of aorta

Blood Supply of Thyroid Gland
- Superior thyroid artery is first anterior branch of external carotid artery and enters the gland near superior pole as a large anterior superficial branch and a smaller posterior branch.
- Inferior thyroid artery, a branch of thyrocervical trunk of subclavian artery passes behind the carotid sheath running medially reaching the posterolateral aspect of the gland.
- Thyroidea ima artery, a branch of aorta or brachiocephalic artery enters the isthmus or lower pole of one of the lateral lobes (3%).
- Tracheal and oesophageal branches serve blood supply to retained thyroid gland after thyroidectomy.

296. Ans. (c) C5-T1

- Thyroid gland is located in anterior triangle of the neck and weighs 20 grams. Gland lies against C5 to T1 vertebra.
- Isthmus extends from 2–4th tracheal rings

297. Ans. (c) 6

Ref: Netter's Atlas of Neurosciences, 3rd ed. pg. 247

- There are *2 cerebellar hemispheres* with each divided into *3 lobes*, thus making 6 lobes in all.
- The anterior is separated from middle lobe by *fissure primura*.
- There are 4 pairs of cerebellar nuclei.
- **D:** Nucleus Dentatus
- **E:** Nucleus emboliformis
- **F:** Nucleus fastigii
- **G:** Nucleus globosus

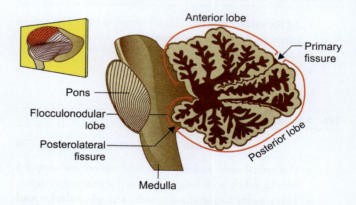

298. Ans. (a) Flocculonodular lobe

Ref: Netter's atlas of Neurosciences, 3rd ed. pg. 409

- The flocconodular lobe is the *smallest lobe*.

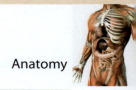

Anatomy

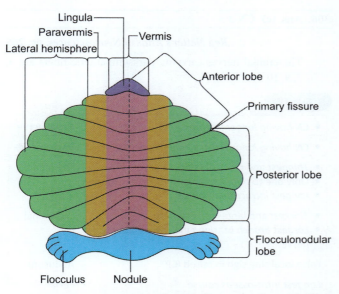

- Most *primitive part* of cerebellum is archi-cerebellum and most *recent part* is neo-cerebellum.

299. Ans. (a) First part of subclavian artery

Ref: Netter's atlas of neurosciences, 3rd ed. pg. 110

- Subclavian artery is divided into three parts by **scalaneus anticus muscle (Mn: VIT CD)**

Branches from 1st part	Branches from 2nd part	Branches from 3rd part
• Vertebral artery	• No branch on left side	• Dorsal scapular branch
• Internal thoracic artery	• Gives costocervical trunk on right side	
• Thyrocervical trunk		
• Costocervical branch on left side		

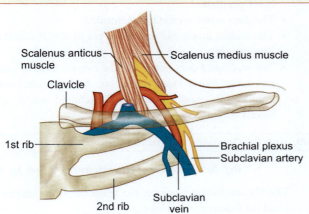

300. Ans. (b) Dorsal scapular artery

Ref: Netter's Clinical Anatomy, 3rd ed. pg. 504

- Dorsal scapular artery is a branch of 3rd part of subclavian artery.

301. Ans. (d) Internal carotid artery

Ref: Netter's Clinical Anatomy, 3rd ed. pg. 420

- The free floating structure in cavernous sinus is cranial nerve VI and internal carotid artery.
- The cranial nerves III, IV, V1, V2 and post ganglionic fibers pass through the wall of the cavernous sinus.

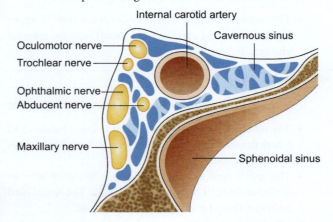

302. Ans. (c) Basilar artery

Ref: Netter's Clinical Anatomy, 3rd ed. pg. 426

Branches of Basilar artery (mnemonic: P.A.L.S)	Branches of Vertebral artery
• **P**osterior cerebral artery • **P**ontine artery • **A**nterior inferior cerebellar artery • **L**abyrinthine artery • **S**uperior cerebellar artery	• Post inferior cerebellar artery *(largest branch)* • Anterior spinal artery *(single artery and runs in anterior median fissure)* • *Posterior Spinal Artery* • *Basilar Artery*

303. Ans. (b) Ascending pharyngeal artery

Ref: Netter's Clinical Anatomy, 3rd ed. pg. 487

- The smallest branch of external carotid artery is the ascending pharyngeal artery.

FMGE Solutions Screening Examination

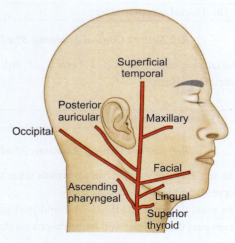

- The common carotid artery divides at the level of upper border of thyroid cartilage(C4 Level) into the internal and external carotid artery.

304. Ans. (d) Lower border of S2

Ref: Netter's Clinical Anatomy, 3rd ed. pg. 420

- The subarachnoid space extends up to *lower border of S2* where the dura fuses with filum terminale and obliterates the subarachnoid space.
- The *spinal cord* extends from *upper border of atlas* to *lower border of L1* or upper border of L2. The spinal cord ends in a sharp tip called conus medullaris.
- The *conus* is continuous with *filum terminale*, which is a fine connective tissue element which descends up to the dorsum of the *first coccygeal ligament*.

305. Ans. (a) Greater auricular nerve

Ref: Netter Atlas of Neurosciences, 3rd ed. pg. 176

The skin of face is supplied by trigeminal nerve branches except for small area over the parotid gland and angle of mandible which is supplied by greater auricular nerve (C2, C3).

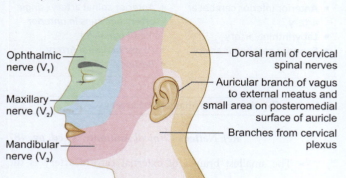

306. Ans. (c) CN 3

Ref: Netter's Atlas of Neurosciences, pg. 265

The cranial nerves carrying parasympathetic fibers are 3, 7, 9, 10.

Extra Mile

• CN having longest intraosseous course	Facial nerve
• CN having longest extracranial coursel	Vagus nerve
• *Thinnest* and most slender cranial nerve • Only one to *originate from the dorsal surface* • *Longest intracranial course*	Trochlear
• *Thickest* and largest cranial nerve • *Largest branch* of trigeminal is mandibular nerve.	Trigeminal
False localising sign in raised ICP	Abducens
Longest intra-osseus course	Facial
Cranial nerve with both motor and sensory components	5, 7, 9, 10

307. Ans. (c) CN 8

Ref: Netter's Atlas of Neurosciences, pg. 265

- Cranial nerve 3 is pure motor nerve and performs ocular movement.
- Cranial nerve 5 performs mastication and is sensory to face.
- Cranial nerve 9 is a mixed nerve and carries taste from posterior 1/3rd of tongue and performs swallowing with help of stylopharyngeus.
- CN 8th is pure sensory. Associated with hearing and balancing

308. Ans. (b) Arachnoid and pia mater

Ref: Netter's Clinical Anatomy, 3rd ed. pg. 25

- *Meninx* implies all three layers—dura, arachnoid and inner pia matter.
- The dura mater is called *pachymeninx*.
- The middle arachnoid and inner pia matter is called as *leptomeninges*.
- The arachnoid does not follow the convolutions of brain and looks like a loose fitting sac. Multiple arachnoid granulations pass through subarachnoid space and blends with pia matter.

309. Ans. (b) Temporal lobe from fronto-parietal areas

Ref: Netter's Atlas of Neurosciences, 3rd ed. pg. 52

The Slyvian fissure separates the temporal lobes inferiorly from the fronto-parietal lobes.

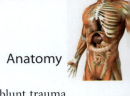

Anatomy

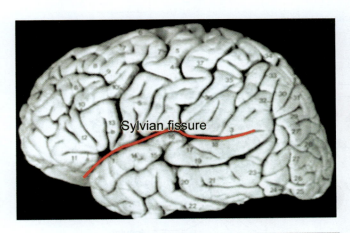

310. Ans. (c) Left and right brachiocephalic veins

Ref: Atlas of Human Anatomy, 6th ed. pg. 59

- *Superior vena cava is formed* by junction of *2 brachiocephalic veins* and has No valves.
- *Inferior vena cava* is formed by union of *2 common iliac veins.*
- *Portal vein* is formed by union of superior mesenteric vein and splenic vein.
- *External jugular vein* is formed by union of *posterior division of retromandibular vein and posterior* auricular vein.

311. Ans. (a) Circulus iridis major

Ref: Parson' Diseases of the Eye, 22nd ed. pg. 13

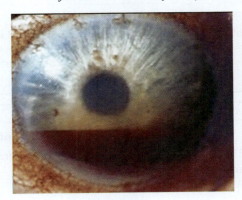

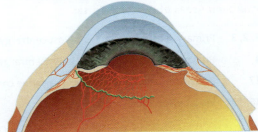

- The source of bleeding in hyphaema with blunt trauma to eye is circulus iridis major.

312. Ans. (a) TM joint

Ref: Kulkarni Clinical Anatomy, 2nd ed. pg. 24

TM joint	Bi-condylar joint
Atlanto-occipital joint	Ellipsoid joint/bi-axial joint
Interphalangeal joint	Hinge joint/uniaxial joint
Inter-metatarsal joint	Plane joint

Extra edge

- **Bi-condylar joints:** Knee joint and temporomandibular joint
- **Pivot joint/Trochoid joint:** Superior and inferior radioulnar joint, median atlanto-axial joint

313. Ans. (a) Middle meningeal artery

Ref: Netter's Clinical Anatomy, 3rd ed. pg. 460

Structures transmitted via foramen ovale (M.A.L.E.)
- **M**andibular nerve-V3
- **A**ccessory meningeal artery
- **L**esser petrosal nerve
- **E**missary vein

Extra edge

Foramen rotundum	Maxillary nerve V2
Foramen Lacerum	Internal carotid artery Lesser petrosal nerve Greater petrosal nerve Deep petrosal nerve
Foramen spinosum	Middle meningeal artery Nervus spinosus (Meningeal Branch of mandibular nerve) Posterior trunk of middle meningeal vein
Carotid canal	Internal carotid artery Venous and sympathetic plexus around the artery

Since lots of questions are asked on the topic of base of skull, students are expected to memorise this diagram by drawing it yourself.

FMGE Solutions Screening Examination

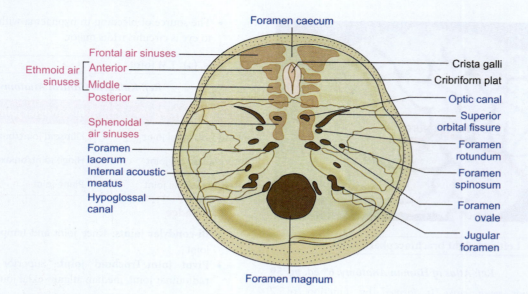

314. Ans. (b) Foramen rotundum

Ref: Netter's Clinical Anatomy, 3rd ed. pg. 352

Trigeminal nerve branches transmitted via—

V1 (Ophthalmic nerve)	Superior orbital Fissure
V2 (Maxillary nerve)	Foramen Rotundum
V3 (Mandibular nerve)	Foramen Ovale

315. Ans. (d) Cervical vertebra

Ref: Kulkarni Clinical Anatomy, 2nd ed. pg. 330

- Foramen transversarium is found only in cervical vertebra and transmits the vertebral artery.
- Another feature peculiar to cervical vertebra is bifid spinous process which is absent in C7 and has a small body.

Extra edge

Flexion and extension of neck	Atlanto-occipital joint
Rotational movement of neck	Atlanto-axial joint

316. Ans. (d) Nerve of wrisberg

Ref: Netter's Atlas of Human Anatomy, 5th ed. pg. 62

Nerve and its Details

Arnold nerve (choice A)	Auricular branch of vagus (alderman nerve)
Jacobson nerve (choice B)	Tympanic branch of glossopharyngeal nerve
Criminal nerve of grassi (choice C)	Branch of right posterior vagus that passes to left behind oesophagus ending in gastric cardia. It is cut in highly selective vagotomy to avoid recurrent peptic ulceration
Nerve of wrisberg (choice D)	Sensory component of facial nerve which carries taste sensation from anterior 2/3 of tongue

Extra Mile

Vidian nerve	Nerve of pterygoid canal
Nerve of latarjet	Branch of anterior gastric nerve and supplies the pylorus. It is left intact in highly selective vagotomy so that the function of gastric emptying remains intact.

317. Ans. (d) 4

Ref: Netter's Atlas of Neurosciences, 3rd ed. pg. 53

- The primary sensory cortex lies in the post central gyrus and is area 1, 2, 3
- Area 4 is the primary voluntary cortex.

Brodmann Areas of Cerebral Cortex

1, 2, 3	Primary sensory cortex lies in Post central gyrus
4	Primary voluntary cortex lies in precentral gyrus
17	Primary visual cortex and lies in calcarine cortex
18, 19	Visual association cortex

Contd...   *Contd...*

Anatomy

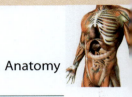

22	Wernicke's area (Superior Temporal lobe)
41	Primary auditory area
44, 45	Broca area (inferior frontal gyrus)

318. Ans. (c) Cingulate gyrus

Ref: *Netter's Correlative Imaging of Neuroanatomy, pg. 147*

The limbic system is composed of following contents:
- Cingulate gyrus
- Hippocampus
- Fornix
- Mammillary bodies

The limbic system manages the emotional behaviour, sexual behaviour and food habits.

319. Ans. (b) Motor to 9, 10, 11 cranial nerve nucleus

Ref: *Netter's Atlas of Neurosciences, 3rd ed. pg. 251*

The cells in nucleus ambiguus contain *motor neurons* concerned with three cranial nerves
1. Rostral pole = *Glossopharyngeal*
2. Middle part = *Vagus*
3. Caudal pole = *Spino-accessory*

- Axons arising from nucleus ambiguus pass laterally and slightly ventrally to exit the medulla just dorsal to the inferior olive.
- These axons then course with the three cranial nerves: IX (glossopharyngeal), X (vagus) and XI (spinoaccessory) to innervate the striated muscles of the soft palate, pharynx, larynx, and upper part of the esophagus.

320. Ans. (a) Optic nerve

Ref: *Gray's Anatomy, 41st ed. pg. 310*

- The cranial nerves are individually named and numbered, using Roman numerals, in a rostro-caudal sequence, reflecting their order of attachment to the brain. They are named as follows:

TABLE: Cranial nerves

CN number	CN name	Attachment/Comments
I	Olfactory nerve	Arises from the olfactory epithelium in the nasal cavity and terminates directly in cortical and subcortical areas of the frontal and temporal lobes
II	Optic nerve	The axons of the optic nerve (II) pass into the optic chiasma, where medially positioned axons decussate; all of the axons emerge as the optic tract, which terminates in the lateral geniculate nucleus of the thalamus
III	Occulomotor nerve	Arise in, and are attached to, the midbrain.
IV	Trochlear nerve	
V	Trigeminal nerve	Attaches to the pons, medial to the middle cerebellar peduncle.
VI	Abducens nerve	Attaches to the brainstem at, or close to, the pontomedullary junction.
VII	Facial nerve	
VIII	Vestibulocochlear N.	
IX	Glossopharyngeal N.	Attached to the medulla
X	Vagus nerve	
XI	Spinal accessory nerve	Arises from cervical levels C1–C5/C6, enters the cranium through the foramen magnum and then exits via the jugular foramen, together with the glossopharyngeal and vagus nerves.
XII	Hypoglossal nerve	Attached to the medulla

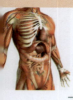

321. Ans. (c) Greater auricular nerve

Ref: Dhingra, 6th ed. pg. 4

Nerve supply of Auricle/Pinna
- **Lateral Surface**
  - Greater auricular nerve (most part)
  - Auriculotemporal nerve (supplies anteriorly, Tragus, some part of helix)
  - CN- X and CN- VII (Concha)
- **Medial Surface**
  - Upper 1/3 by Lesser occipital N.
  - *Lower 2/3 by Greater Auricular N.*
  - Concha/Root of auricle by Auricular br. Of vagus N. + Facial nerve

322. Ans. (a) Maxillary process

Ref: BDC, Vol-3 pg. 355-356

- The facial nerve leaves the skull by passing through the **stylomastoid foramen.**
- Branches and Distribution:
  - Within the facial canal:
    - **Greater petrosal nerve**- *to the eye (lacrimal gland)*
    - **The nerve to the stapedius**- *to the stapedius muscle in middle ear*
    - **The chorda tympani**- *to the tongue*
  - At its exit from the stylomastoid foramen it gives out branches to Posterior auricular, **Digastrics** and stylohyoid.
  - It has terminal branches within the **parotid gland** also like**,** temporal, Zygomatic, Buccal, Marginal mandibular and Cervical.

323. Ans. (d) In relation with upper 2nd molar tooth

Ref: Clinical Anatomy by Systems by Richard S. Snell / 55

Gland	Type of Gland	Duct	Duct opening
Parotid	Serous	Stensons duct	Vestibule of mouth opposite second upper molar
Sub-mandibular	Mixed but predominantly serous	Whartons duct	On the floor of mouth on summit of sublingual papilla at the side of frenulum of tongue
Sublingual	Mixed but predominantly mucus	Bartholins duct	On the floor of mouth on summit of sublingual papilla

324. Ans. (c) Deviation of tongue

- Facial nerve gives sensory supply to tongue.

- Chorda tympani nerve is a sensory branch of facial nerve (CN VII) which gives taste sensation of anterior 2/3rd of tongue.
- Glossopharyngeal nerve (CN IX) gives the taste sensation from posterior 2/3rd of tongue.
- Motor supply to tongue is by hypoglossal nerve (CN XII). Injury to hypoglossal nerve paralyzes ipsilateral half of tongue.
- If CN XII is functioning normally, tongue protrudes evenly in midline.
- If CN XII is paralyzed: When tongue is protruded, its tip deviates towards the paralyzed side because of unopposed action of genioglossus muscle on the normal side of tongue.(TDS)

325. Ans. (a) Lateral pterygoid

Ref: Gray's, 41st ed. pg. 507-508

- The primary function of the lateral pterygoid muscle is to pull the head of the condyle out of the mandibular fossa along the articular eminence to protrude the mandible.
- **The effort of the lateral pterygoid muscles acts in helping lower the mandible and open the jaw** whereas uniltral action of a lateral pterygoid produces contralateral excursion (a form of mastication), usually performed in concert with the medial pterygoids.
- Unlike the other three muscles of mastication, the lateral pterygoid is the only muscle of mastication that assists in depressing the mandible i.e. opening the jaw. At the beginning of this action it is assisted by the digastric, mylohyoid and geniohyoid muscles.

326. Ans. (a) Facial nerve

Ref: BDC, 5th Ed. vol. III pg. 252-253

- Basically, facial nerve supplies the taste sensation of anterior 2/3rd of the tongue, but since this option is given with this question, the best suited option is facial nerve.

According to BDC

- Sensory supply of anterior 2/3rd of the tongue is by facial nerve (CN VII).
- *Its lingual branch is for general sensation.*
- *Corda tympani branch is for taste*
- **Sensory supply for posterior 1/3rd** - glossopharyngeal nerve/ CN IX (general and taste sensation both).
- **Posterior most or valeculla** is supplied by vagus nerve (internal laryngeal branch).

327. Ans. (d) CN XI

Ref: BDC, 5th ed. Vol-III pg. 252-253

- Sensory supply of anterior 2/3rd of the tongue is by facial nerve (CN VII).

- Its lingual branch is for general sensation.
- Corda tympani branch is for taste
- Sensory supply for posterior 1/3rd - glossopharyngeal nerve/ CN IX (general and taste sensation both).
- Posterior most or valeculla is supplied by vagus nerve (*internal laryngeal branch*).

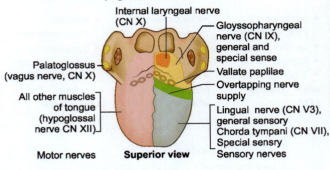

328. Ans. (a) Lingual nerve

Please refer to above explanation

329. Ans. (a) Pons

Ref: BDC, 6th ed. Vol-III pg. 364, 70, 71

- CN 3rd and 4th cranial nerve attach to midbrain
- CN 5th, 6th, 7th, and 8th attach to Pons
- CN 9th, 10th, 11th and 12th from medulla
- Vestibular component of vestibulocochlear nerve (CN 8th) arises from junction of pons and medulla.

> **Extra Mile**
> - Acoustic neuroma is most common cerebellopontine angle tumor.
> - Earliest CN involved is CN 5th, which is followed by 8th, 9th, 10th, 7th and 6th.

330. Ans. (c) Trochlear

Ref: BDC, 6th ed. Vol-II pg. 364

TROCHLEAR (IV) NERVE

- **Smallest cranial nerve** (*Keith Moore -1137*)
- **Most slender cranial** nerve (Snell-335)
- Only nerve to emerge from dorsal (posterior) surface of brain stem (mid brain)
- Passes anteriorly around the brain stem, running the longest intracranial (subarachnoid) course
- Nerve crosses the midline within the midbrain, emerges from its dorsal aspect and immediately decussates with the nerve of opposite side
- It supplies superior oblique, the only extra ocular muscle that uses pulley/trochlea to redirect its line of action

331. Ans. (a) 3rd CN palsy (oculomotor)

Ref: BDC 6th ed. Vol-III pg. 361-62

- Eyelid is comprised of 4 muscles:

TABLE: Muscles, their innervation and function

Muscle	CN innervation	Function
LPS	III	Opens the eyelid
Muller's muscle	T1 (NOT a CN; sympathetic nerve)	Opens eyelid when LPS tired
Frontalis	VII	Closes the eyelid
Orbicularis oculi	VII	Closes the eyelid

- CN III palsy leads to drooping of eyelid (Ptosis).
- CN VII palsy may also cause ptosis.

> **Extra Mile**
> - All the extraocular muscles are supplied by CN III except lateral rectus and superior oblique.
> - Lateral rectus supplied by- CN VI
> - Superior oblique supplied by- CN IV
> Remember– LR6; SO4

332. Ans. (b) Sympathetic nerve

Ref: BDC, 6th ed. Vol-III pg. 74

Please refer to above explanation

333. Ans. (a) Superior oblique

Ref: BDC, 6th ed. Vol-III pg. 360-62

- Remember the mnemonics LR6 SO4 and all other by CN III
- Superior oblique is supplied by CN IV (trochlear nerve).
- Refer to above answer for more detailed explanation.

334. Ans. (c) Trochlear nerve

Ref: BDC 6th ed. Vol-III pg. 362

- **Trochlear nerve** is the only cranial nerve to emerge dorsally from the brain stem.
  - *It has the longest intracranial course* and it is the most slender cranial nerve in terms of axon contents.
- Largest cranial nerve: Trigeminal N. (CN 5th)
- CN which has most extensive distribution beyond head and neck: Vagus Nerve (CN 10th).
- Most frequently paralyzed CN: Facial Nerve (CN 7th)- due to wide intraosseous course.
- Pure sensory CN: CN 1, 2, 8

FMGE Solutions Screening Examination

- Pure motor CN: CN 3, 4, 6, 11, 12
- Mixed CN: CN 5, 7, 9, 10

335. Ans. (d) Vagus nerve

Ref: BDC, 6th ed. Vol-III pg. 379-81

- The "criminal nerve" of Grassi is the first gastric branch of the posterior vagus nerve. This nerve may branch proximal or distal to the celiac division of the posterior vagus nerve.
- The importance of this nerve is during Truncal vagotomy, since failure to transect the nerve of Grassi proximal to its origin will result in an incomplete vagotomy.

336. Ans. (c) Recurrent laryngeal nerve

Ref: BDC, Vol: 3 pg. 171, 172, 173, 176.

- It is recurrent laryngeal nerve that pierces the thyroid gland.

Must know about Thyroid

- The gland consists of 2 lobes that are joined to each other by the isthmus
- The gland extends against vertebrae C5, C6, C7 and T1
- It weighs about 25 g.
- The thyroid gland is supplied by the superior and inferior thyroid arteries.
    - The superior thyroid artery is the first anterior branch of the external carotid artery.
    - The inferior thyroid artery is a branch of thyro cervical trunk
- Nerve supply
    - Nerves are derived mainly from the middle cervical ganglion and partly also from the superior and inferior cervical ganglia.
- It is made of following two types of Secretory cells
    - Folicular cells lining the follicles of the gland secrete T3 and T4.
    - Parafollicular cells (C cells) are fewer and lie in between the follicles. They secrete thyrocalcitonin.

Extra Mile

What is the function of thyrocalcitonin?
- It promotes deposition of calcium salts in skeletal and other tissues, and tends to produce hypocalcaemia.

337. Ans. (c) Trigeminal nerve

Ref: Gray's 41st ed. pg. 667, BDC, 6th ed. Vol-III pg. 206-7

TABLE: Structures passing through superior orbital fissure

Superior orbital fissure		
Upper part/ Lateral	Middle part (through tendinous ring)	Lower/Medial part
• Superior Opthalmic vein • Lacrimal nerve • Frontal nerve • Trochlear nerve Mn – "Superior LFT"	• Nasociliary nerve • Occulomotor nerve • Abducent nerve Mnemonic –"NOA"	• Inferior Opthalmic vein • Sympathetic nerves around internal carotid artery Mn: Inferior sympathy

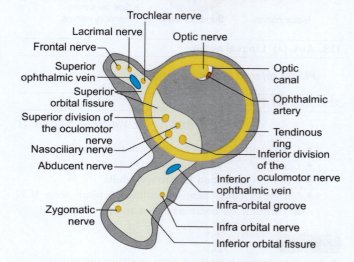

Extra Mile

Structures passing through Inferior orbital fissure
- Zygomatic branch of maxillary nerve
- Infraorbital nerve & vessels
- Rami of Pterygoid ganglion
- Communicating vein b/w inferior ophthalmic & pterygoid plexus of veins.

Mn-"ZIPC"

338. Ans. (a) 2

Ref: Netter's Clinical Anatomy, 3rd ed. pg. 442

Structures transmitted via the superior orbital fissure
- Cranial nerve III, IV, V1 (ophthalmic nerve) and VI
- Inferior ophthalmic vein

The optic nerve is transmitted via the optic canal. The optic canal transmits optic nerve, ophthalmic artery and central retinal vein.

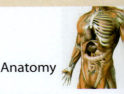

Anatomy

339. Ans. (a) Superior ophthalmic vein

Ref: Gray's, 41st ed. pg. 667

340. Ans. (a) Mandibular nerve

Ref: Keith L. Moore, 5th ed. pg. 899

341. Ans. (c) Both

Ref: Gray's, 41st ed. pg. 667

342. Ans. (a) Sphenoid bone tumor

Ref: Gray's Anatomy, pg. 801-805

TABLE: CN injury and their cause

Cranial Nerve	Usual cause
CN III, IV, first division of V	Invasive sphenoid bone tumor
CN VII, VIII	Petrous bone tumor
CN V, VII, VIII	Acoustic neuroma, Meningioma
CN IX, X, XI, XII	Parotid gland and carotid body tumor and Metastasis

343. Ans. (c) C3, C4, C5

Ref: Grey's, 38th ed. pg. 1265

TABLE: Phrenic nerve

Root value	Anterior primary rami of C3, C4, C5 (chiefly C4) Mnemonic. "C3,4,5 keeps the diaphragm alive
Relations	Front of scalenus anterior and behind prevertebral fascia in neck Behind brachiocephalic vein and front of subclavian artery in thorax entry Passes in front of hilum of lung **Rt. Phrenic:** Pass through vena caval opening (T8) **Lt. phrenic:** Muscular part of diaphragm
Supply	Motor: Diaphragm Sensory: Pleura diaphragmatic, pericardium (fibrous & parietal), coronary and falciform ligament of liver, IVC, adrenals and gallbladder.

344. Ans. (c) Cleft lip and cleft palate both

Ref: Clinical Anatomy, Vishram Singh, pg. 306

- The cleft lip and palate are the most common congenital anomalies of the head and neck, occurring in 1 per 750 live births.

345. Ans. (c) Loose subaponeurotic layer

Ref: BDC, 6th ed. Vol-III pg. 61-63

The 5 layers of scalp can be remembered as **SCALP**:

- **Skin:** Consist of hair follicles, sebaceous gland and sweat glands.
- Sub **C**utaneous layer: Contains blood vessels, nerves of the scalp
- **A**poneurotic layer aka **galea aponeurotica.** It is a tough layer of dense fibrous tissue which runs from the frontalis muscle anteriorly to the occipitalis posteriorly
- **L**oose subaponeurotic tissue containing the emissary veins and allowing free movement of layers 1 to 3 as a unit. *Layer 4 is a "dangerous area"* because it allows spread of infection even, by way of the emissary veins, to intracranial structures.
- **P**ericranium, is the periosteum of the skull bones providing nutrition.

346. Ans. (d) Galea aponeurotica

Ref: BDC, 6th ed. Vol-III pg. 61-63

347. Ans. (b) Frontal process of maxilla

Ref: BDC, 6th ed. Vol-III pg. 28

Orbit wall	Formed by
• Medial wall Mn – "uSMLE"	Sphenoid (body), Maxilla (frontal process), Lacrimal bone, Ethmoid (orbital plate)
• Lateral wall Mn – "ZyGS"	Zygomatic (frontal process) Greater wing of Sphenoid
• Roof	Frontal bone and Lesser wing of sphenoid
• Floor Mn – "Pa Ma Zy"	Palatine (orbital process), Maxilla, Zygomatic

348. Ans. (d) Trigeminal nerve

Ref: Gray's, 41st ed. pg. 315-16, 20-21

- Muscles of soft palate are supplied by pharyngeal plexus (of cranial accessory & vagus nerves) and mandibular division (V2) of trigeminal nerve.
- General sensation by lesser palatine branch of maxillary division (V2) of trigeminal nerve & glossopharyngeal nerve.
- Secretomotor parasympathic post ganglionic fibers through lesser palatine nerves (pterygopalatine ganglion) & otic ganglion.
- *Taste by facial nerve (through lesser palatine nerve)*
- Hard palate is supplied by greater palatine & nasopalatine branches of maxillary nerve in place of lesser palatine nerve. All 3 (greater, lesser & naso) palatine nerves pass through pterygopalatine ganglion.
- Palate is supplied by trigeminal (maxillary, mandibular), facial, glossopharyngeal, cranial accessory & vagus nerves.

FMGE Solutions Screening Examination

349. Ans. (a) Genioglossus

Ref: BDC, 5th ed. pg. 252

- Genioglossus is a fan shaped, *bulkiest muscle of tongue.*
- It is originated from upper genial tubercle of mandible and inserted into tip of tongue and into hyoid bone.
- **Function** -It retracts and depresses the tongue. It is also known as life saving muscle because it pulls the posterior part of tongue forwards and protrudes the tongue forwards.

Extra Mile

- **MOTOR:** All the extrinsic and intrinsic muscles of tongue are supplied by hypoglossal nerve EXCEPT palatoglossus, which is supplied by the cranial root of accessory nerve through the pharyngeal plexus.
- **SENSORY:** Anterior 2/3rd by facial nerve (lingual branch); posterior 1/3rd glossopharyngeal.
Posterior most or valeculla is supplied by vagus nerve.

350. Ans. (d) Posterior cricoarytenoid

Ref: Dhingra, 5th pg. 300

- Posterior cricoarytenoid is the most important muscle of the larynx as it is the only abductor of vocal cord.
- Paralysis of posterior cricoarytenoid will lead to adduction of vocal cord, which may lead to dyspnea resulting in death.

351. Ans. (a) Trachea bifurcates

Ref: BDC, 6th ed. Vol.II pg. 280-81

- Trachea *begins* at lower border of cricoid cartilage opposite to the *lower border of C6 vertebra.*
- Trachea extends up to upper border of T5
- Tracheal bifurcation (carina) is at T4-T5 level.
- Length of trachea is 10-12 cm
- Thyroid cartilage is over 3, 4 & 5 tracheal rings

At C6 vertebral level: *Landmark is Cricoid cartilage*
- Larynx ends; Trachea begins
- Pharynx ends; Esophagus begins
- Inferior thyroid artery crosses posterior to carotid sheath.
- Middle cervical sympathetic ganglion behind inferior thyroid artery
- Inferior laryngeal nerve enters the larynx.
- Vertebral artery enters the transverse foramen of C6.

352. Ans. (a) Cricothyroid

Ref: BDC, Vol: 3 pg. 242, 244

- All intrinsic muslces of the larynx are supplied by the recurrent laryngeal nerve except cricothyroid which is supplied by external laryngeal nerve.

- Recurrent laryngeal nerve supplies posterior cricoarytenoid, lateral cricoarytenoid, transverse and oblique arytenoids, aryepiglotticus, thyroarytenoid, thyroepiglotticus muscle.

Extra Mile

TABLE: MUST KNOW about laryngeal muscles movements

Movement	Muscles
Abduction of vocal cords	Posterior cricoarytenoids only
Adduction of the vocal cords	Lateral cricoarytenoids and transverse arytenoids, thyroarytenoid
Tensor of vocal cords	Cricothyroid
Relaxor of vocal cord	Thyroarytenoid
Elevation of larynx	Thyrohyoid, mylohyoid
Depression of larynx	Sternothyroid, sternohyoid

353. Ans. (b) Stylopharyngeus

Ref: Gray, 39th ed. pg. 584

- All the muscles of pharynx are supplied by pharyngeal plexus except the stylopharyngeus muscle, which is supplied by glossopharyngeal nerve.

Extra Mile

- All the muscles of soft palate are also supplied by pharyngeal plexus EXCEPT the tensor veli palatine muscle, which is supplied by Nerve to medial pterygoid (Branch of mandibular nerve).

354. Ans. (a) Stylopharyngeus

Please refer to above explanation

355. Ans. (d) C_3 to C_6

Ref: Gray, 41st ed. pg. 586

- In adult male at rest, larynx lies at the level of the bodies of C_3 to C_6 vertebra. Although it is somewhat higher in adult females and children.
- In infants between 6-12 months, the tip of epiglottis (the highest part of the larynx) is a little above the junction of the dens and body of axis (C_2) vertebrae.

356. Ans. (c) Lambdoid suture

Ref: Gray, 41st ed. pg. 418-419

- Anterior fontanel is formed by frontal bone and parietal bone. It is diamond shaped and closes at 18 months.
- Posterior fontanel is formed by parietal bone and occipital bone. It is triangular shaped and closes immediately after birth or within 2–3 months.

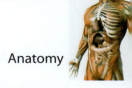

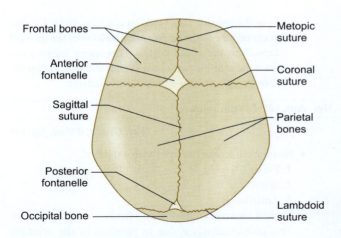

357. Ans. (d) Tympanomandibular

Ref: Gray's, 41st ed. pg. 541

TABLE: Ligaments of TM Joint

Main	Accessory
Fibrous capsule	Sphenomandibular
Lateral or Temporo mandibular	Stylomandibular

358. Ans. (b) C3

Ref: Gray's Anatomy, 39th ed. pg. 444, 634

- The hyoid bone may be felt a few centimeters below and behind the chin, especially if the neck is extended. It may be palpated between finger and thumb and moved from side to side.
- **The hyoid bone lies approximately at the level of the third cervical vertebra.**

359. Ans. (b) 2nd to 4th

Ref: Gray's, 41st ed. pg. 470

- Thyroid gland lies against C_5, C_6, C_7 & T_1 vertebra
- Isthmus extends from 2nd to 4th tracheal ring
- Each lobe extends from middle of thyroid cartilage to 4th/5th tracheal ring.

360. Ans. (b) Inferior thyroid artery

Ref: Gray's, 41st ed. pg. 472

- Both upper & lower parathyroid glands are supplied by the inferior thyroid artery

Vascular Supply and Lymphatic Drainage of Parathyroid Gland

- Inferior thyroid arteries provide primary blood supply to posterior aspect of thyroid gland and parathyroid glands (which are situated there in posterior aspect of thyroid gland).
- Parathyroid veins drain into thyroid plexus of veins of thyroid gland & trachea.
- Lymphatics drain with those of thyroid into deep cervical lymph nodes & paratracheal lymph nodes.

Innervations and Functions
- Since the gland is hormonally regulated, the nerve supply is sympathetic vasomotor, vaso constrictor and not secreto motor.
- Parathyroid activities regulated by variations in blood calcium level: It is inhibited by a rise in calcium levels and stimulated by a fall in calcium level.

> **Extra Mile**
> - The superior parathyroid glands usually lie at the level of inferior border of cricoids cartilage.
> - The inferior glands are usually within thyroid fascia 1 cm below the inferior thyroid arteries behind the lower poles.
> - Color of thyroid gland: deep red color
> - Color of parathyroid gland: Brownish yellow color

361. Ans. (b) Peripheral ganglia

Ref: Gray's, 41st ed. pg. 231, 303

Lower motor neuron (LMN): It consists of-
- Anterior horn cells or homologous cells in brainstem
- Anterior spinal nerve root
- Peripheral nerve

362. Ans. (c) Mandible

Ref: Gray's, 38th ed. pg. 431

- **Pneumatic Bone:** Some cranial bones have air filled cavities for making skull light weight, resonance of voice & air conditioning.
- Maxilla, Mastoid, Ethmoid, Sphenoid & Frontal bones are pneumatic bones.

TABLE: Types of bone

Sesamoid bones	Pneumatic bone (Mn: It has Maximum Spherical Front Mass)	Membranous (Dermal) bone
• Patella • Pisiform • Fabella	• Ethmoid • Maxilla • Sphenoid • Frontal • Mastoid (temporal)	• Skull vault bones • Facial bones

363. Ans. (b) Frontal bone

Ref: Gray, 38th ed. pg. 436

- Pneumatic bones are bones which contain air filled cavities for making the skull light weight, and aid resonance of voice and air conditioning. These include: Frontal, Ethmoid, Maxilla, Sphenoid and mastoid.

FMGE Solutions Screening Examination

> **Extra Mile**
> - **Sesamoid bones** are patella, pisiform and fabella.
> - **Membranous (dermal) bones** are skull vault bones and facial bones.

364. Ans. (d) Inferior parietal gyrus

Ref: Gray's, 41st ed. pg. 313

- The sense of taste (SVA-special visceral efferent) is transduced by gustatory hair (**neuroepithelium**), taste buds and is conveyed via **three** of the twelve cranial nerves.
  - The facial nerve carries taste sensations from the anterior two thirds of the tongue (**excluding** the circumvallate papillae) and **soft palate**.
  - The glossopharyngeal nerve carries the taste sensations from the posterior one third of the tongue (**including** the circumvallate papillae) and,
  - A branch of the vagus nerve carries some taste sensations from the back of the oral cavity (i.e. posterior-most tongue, pharynx and epiglottis).
- Impulses generated by the gustatory taste hairs on the superior surface of the tongue, travel from the tongue to medulla oblongata, to the thalamus, *ending up in the gustatorial area of the cortex of the parietal lobe (inferior gyrus) of the cerebrum.*
- The axons from these cranial nerves ascend in the spinal cord without crossing over. These fibers terminate in the medulla, ventral posterior medial (VPM) nucleus of the thalamus, and then project to the somatosensory cortex within the brain.
- Thus, a lesion of the nucleus tractus solitarius (NTS) or **solitario-thalamic tract** results in loss of taste from the ipsi-lesional, the same side as the lesion, half of the tongue.

365. Ans. (c) Lateral geniculate body

- The optic radiation also known as **geniculo-calcarine tract** is a collection of axons from relay neurons in the *lateral geniculate nucleus* of the thalamus carrying visual information to the visual cortex (also called striate cortex) along the calcarine fissure. There is one such tract on each side of the brain.
- A distinctive feature of the optic radiations is that they split into two parts on each side:
  - The fibers from the inferior retina must pass into the temporal lobe by looping around the inferior horn of the lateral ventricle. These fibers, which carry information from the superior part of the visual field, are called Meyer's loop. A lesion in the temporal lobe that results in damage to Meyer's loop causes a characteristic loss of vision in a superior quadrant.
  - The fibers from the superior retina (carrying fibres from the inferior visual field) travel straight back to the occipital lobe in the **retrolenticular** limb of the internal capsule to the visual cortex. They carry information from the inferior part of the visual field and, taking the shorter path, are less susceptible to damage.

366. Ans. (d) Exophthalmos

Ref: Gray's, 41st ed. pg. 469

- Horner syndrome presents with a triad of:
  1. Ptosis
  2. Miosis
  3. Anhydrosis
- There is apparent **enophthalmos** (and not exophth-almos). This enophthalmus is due to paralysis of the **orbitalis** muscle of the orbit, which normally keeps the eyeball prominent. Its nerve supply is sympathetic –T1 and when paralyzed leads to appearance of sunken eyeball.
- Most cases are idiopathic, but it could be due to brainstem lesions, carotid dissection, or neoplasm compressing upon the sympathetic chain (E.g., Pancoast tumor).
- Symptoms of horner's syndrome are secondary to sympathetic nerve (T1) lesion.

367. Ans. (a) Maxillary

Ref: Gray's Anatomy, 39th ed. pg. 477, 479

- The maxillae are the largest of the facial bones, other than the mandible, and jointly form the whole of the upper jaw. Each bone forms the greater part of the floor and lateral wall of the nasal cavity, and of the floor of the orbit
- *"Orbital surface of maxilla is smooth and triangular, and forms most of the floor of the orbit"*
- **The seven bones that articulate with orbit are:**
  - Frontal bone (Roof)
  - Lacrimal bone (Medial wall of orbit)
  - Ethmoid bone (Medial wall of orbit)
  - Maxillary bone (Floor of orbit)
  - Palatine bone (Floor of orbit)
  - Sphenoid bone (Lateral wall of orbit)
  - Zygomatic (Lateral wall of orbit)

> **Extra Mile**
> - *Maxilla is also the most common fracture of orbital floor.*
> - The floor (inferior wall) is formed by the orbital surface of maxilla, the orbital surface of Zygomatic bone and the orbital process of palatine bone.

Note: The nasal bone does not form part of the orbit.

368. Ans. (a) Cavernous sinus

Ref: Gray's Anatomy, 40th ed. Ch; 29

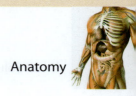

Anatomy

- The upper most segment of the facial vein, above its junction with the superior labial vein, is also called the angular vein.
- Any infection of the mouth or face can spread via the angular veins to the cavernous sinuses resulting in thrombosis.

369. Ans. (c) Right sided pain, touch, temperature

Ref: Gray's, 41st ed. pg. 299, 309

- First order neuron carrying pain, touch, temperature enter the spinal cord, relay in same side.
- Second order neurons cross over to other side and travel up in anterior and lateral spino-thalamic tract and enter the medulla.
- Same fibers are now known as spinal lemniscus and they relay at thalamus. *So spinal lemniscus on the left contain pain touch temperature from right side of the body.*

370. Ans. (d) Inferior oblique

Ref: Gray's, 41st ed. pg. 671, Gray's, 39th ed. pg. 693

- All the rectus muscles are attached to the orbital apex.
- Aside from rectus muscles, superior oblique also attaches to orbital apex, while inferior oblique has no attachment with orbital apex.

371. Ans. (b) Trochlear

Ref: Gray's, 41st ed. pg. 671

- Superior oblique muscle is supplied by trochlear nerve.
- Its actions are: aBBduct, Intort & Depress ("BID") eye in primary position.

372. Ans. (b) Lateral cartilage

Ref: Gray's, 41st ed. pg. 560

Nasal septum is an osseocartilagenous structure contributed by

Part of septum	Main structure	Contributory structures
Bony septum	• Vomer • Ethmoid (perpendicular plate)	• Nasal spine of frontal bone • Nasal crests of maxillary, nasal & palatine bones • Rostrum & crest of sphenoid
Cartilaginous septum	• Septal cartilage	• Inferior nasal cartilage (Septal process)

373. Ans. (b) Thalamus

Ref: Textbook of Neuroanatomy pg. 82,83

Basal ganglia include following nuclei-
- Caudate nucleus
- Putamen
- *Globus pallidus*
- Subthalamic nucleus
- Substantia nigra

Lenticulate nucleus = putamen + globus pallidus

Function of basal ganglia—Planning and programming of movements.

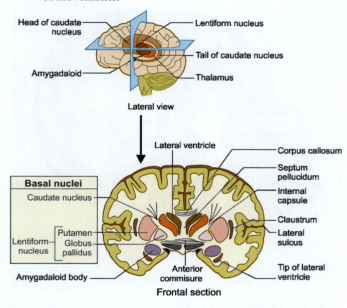

374. Ans. (b) Purkinje cells

Ref: Gray's, 41st ed. pg. 335-336

- The cerebellar cortex contains five types of neurons: Purkinje, Granule, Basket, Stellate and Golgi Cells.

375. Ans. (c) Purkinje cells

Ref: Gray's, 41st ed. pg. 335-336

- The axons of purkinje cells are the only output through cerebellar cortex.
- However, it should be kept in mind that the output from the cerebellum is through deep nuclei, and purkinje cells axons generally pass to deep nuclei.

376. Ans. (a) Lower border of L1

Ref: IB Singh, 8th ed. pg. 31

- Spinal cord begins at foramen magnum and, in adults, ends at lower border of L1.
- In newborn, spinal cord ends at L3 vertebrae.

377. Ans. (c) L3

Ref: IB Singh, 8th ed. pg. 31

378. Ans. (d) X

Ref: BDC, 5th ed. vol 3 pg. 78

FMGE Solutions Screening Examination

Parapharyngeal space contains
- Carotid vessel
- Jugular vein
- Last 4 cranial nerves (9,10,11,12)
- Sympathetic chain

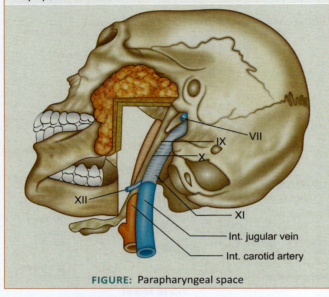

FIGURE: Parapharyngeal space

379. Ans. (b) **Fasciculus gracilis**

Ref: Gray's, 41st ed. pg. 296-97, 311

NERVE PATHWAYS
- **Posterior**-Fasciculus gracilis, fasciculus cuneatus
- **Lateral**-Lateral spinothalamic, anterior and posterior spinocerebellar, spino-olivary, spinotectal
- **Anterior**-Anterior spinothalamic

380. Ans. (b) **C7**

Ref: BDC, 5th ed Vol. III pg. 43

- The C7 vertebra is also known as the vertebra prominens because of its long spinous process.
- Atypical cervical vertebra are: 1, 2, and 7 (atlas, axis and vertebra prominens respectively)

381. Ans. (b) **Atlanto-axial joint**

Ref: Gray's, 38th ed. pg. 521

- **Atlanto-occipital (between skull and C1)** joint permits *nodding of head* (as when indicating approval or yes)
- **Atlantoaxial joint** permits the head to be **turned from side to side** i.e. rotation (as indicating disapproval, the NO movement).

382. Ans. (a) **Posterior longitudinal ligament**

Ref: Gray's, 38th ed. pg. 512; Keith Moore, 4th ed. pg. 483

- Structures pierced during lumbar puncture (from outside in) are:- Skin → subcutaneous tissue → Supraspinous & interspinous ligament → Ligament flavum → Duramater → Arachnoid mater.

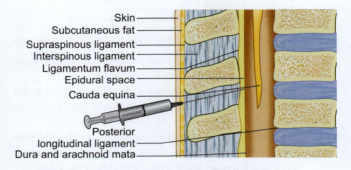

383. Ans. (b) **Carotid tubercle on C6 vertebra**

Ref: Gray's, 41st ed. pg. 414, Color Atlas of Human Anatomy, pg. 446

- Chassaignac's tubercle (carotid tubercle) is the other name of anterior tubercle of transverse process of C6 vertebra.
- It is the longest tubercle of Cervical (C6) Vertebra.

PELVIS AND PERINEUM

384. Ans. (a) **Dilatation of Superior rectal vein**

Ref: Gray's Anatomy 41st ed. P 1153, 1158

- Source of bleeding in haemorrhoids are usually the internal haemorrhoids which are symptomatic anal cushions and lie in 3, 7 and 11 o' clock position *(left-lateral, right-posterior and right-anterior quadrants of the wall of the canal)*.
- **Book states:** *"the cushions help to seal the anal canal and contribute to the maintenance of continence to flatus and fluid. The anal cushions are important in the pathogenesis of haemorrhoids."*
  - Haemorrhoids develop due to degeneration of the supporting connective tissue of anal cushion.
  - This degeneration causes downward displacement of cushions and abnormal venous dilatation.
- The superior haemorrhoidal veins draining the upper half of the anal canal above the dentate line, pass upwards to become the rectal veins: these unite to form the **superior rectal vein**, which later becomes the **inferior mesenteric vein**.
- In the middle anal canal, there are 6–10 vertical mucosal folds and the anal columns. These columns mainly contain the superior rectal vein, artery and some middle and inferior rectal vessels.

Anatomy

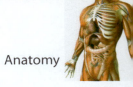

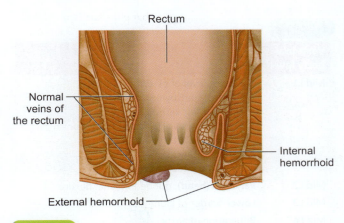

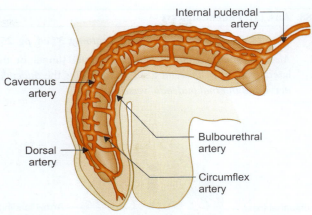

- **Extra Mile**
- Dilated veins in the subepithelial tissue below the dentate line contribute to an external haemorrhoidal venous plexus

385. Ans. (c) Bulbourethral artery

Ref: Gray's Anatomy for Students E-book, P 516

- Blood supply to the skin of the penis is from the left and right superficial external pudendal arteries, which arise from the femoral artery.
  - The superficial external pudendal arteries branch into dorsolateral and ventrolateral branches, which collateralize across the midline.
  - In addition, branches in the skin form an extensive subdermal vascular plexus.
- The blood supply to the ventral penile skin is based on the posterior scrotal artery, a superficial branch of the deep internal pudendal artery.
- The blood supply to deep structures of the penis is derived from a continuation of the internal pudendal artery, after it gives off the perineal branch. Three branches of the internal pudendal artery flow to the penis, as follows:
- **Bulbourethral artery:** Artery of the bulb passes through the deep penile (Buck) fascia to enter and supply the bulb of the penis and penile (spongy) urethra.
- The dorsal artery travels along the dorsum of the penis between the dorsal nerve and deep dorsal vein and gives off circumflex branches that accompany the circumflex veins; the terminal branches are in the glans penis.
- **Cavernosal artery:** Deep penile artery is usually a single artery that arises on each side and enters the corpus cavernosum at the crus and runs the length of the penile shaft, giving off the helicine arteries, which are an integral component of the erectile process.

386. Ans. (c) Genital branch of genitofemoral nerve

Ref: Gray's Anatomy Review E-book, P 221

- The **cremaster muscle** is a muscle that covers the testis and the spermatic cord.
- The cremaster muscle is supplied by the cremasteric artery which is a branch of inferior epigastric artery.
- The cremaster muscle is innervated from the genital branch of the genitofemoral nerve. It receives distinctly different innervation and vascular supply in comparison to the internal oblique.

387. Ans. (c) Spiral artery

Ref: Gray's Anatomy E-book, P 172

- Spiral artery, a branch of radial artery, chiefly supplies endometrium.
- Endometrium and myometrium are supplied mainly by ovarian and uterine artery.

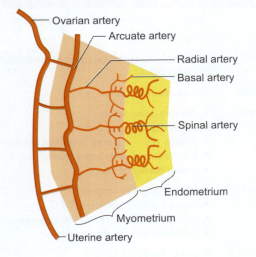

388. Ans. (a) Pudendal nerve

Ref: *Netter's Clinical Anatomy, 3rd ed. pg. 252*

Alcock's canal/pudendal canal is a fascial tunnel in the lateral wall *of ischiorectal fossa and* contains the *pudendal nerve and internal pudendal vessels.*

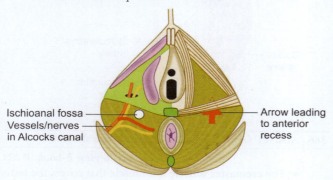

389. Ans. (b) S2

Anatomic level of some important structures:
- Posterior Superior Iliac Spine (PSIS): S2
- Anterior Superior Iliac Spine (ASIS): S1
- Pylorus and Celiac trunk: L1
- Inferior mesenteric artery: L3
- Umbilicus: Between L3 and L4

> **Extra Mile**

TABLE: Vertebral body level as landmark for the viscera *(Table extracted from Gray's Anatomy 41st ed.)*

Vertebral body level	Viscera
C6	Cricoid cartilage, start of oesophagus
C7-T1	Lung apex
Upper T4	Aorta reaches vertebral column; medial part of scapular spine
T4-5 disk	Sternal plane/angle of Louis
Upper T5	• Tracheal bifurcation • Concavity of aortic arch • Azygos vein—superior venacava junction • Bifurcation of pulmonary trunk • Upper border of heart
Upper T8	• Inferior angle of scapula • Lower border of heart • Inferior vena cava crosses diaphragm • Central tendon of diaphragm
Upper T11	• Lower border of lung • Cardia of stomach • Upper border of kidney

> **Extra Mile**

Vertebral body level	Viscera
Mid L1	• Lowest level of pleura • Pylorus; transpyloric plane • Hilum of left kidney • Origin of renal arteries and superior mesenteric artery • Pancreas **(neck)** • Spinal cord termination
Mid L2	Pancreas **(head)**; duodenojejunal flexure
Mid L3	Lower border of kidney
Mid L4	Bifurcation of aorta
Mid L5	Formation of inferior vena cava

390. Ans. (d) 4

Ref: *Gray's Anatomy, 41st ed. pg. 729*

- The coccyx is a small, **asymmetrical**, triangular bone of the spine, the distal most.
- It usually **consists of four fused rudimentary vertebrae**, although the **number varies from three to five**, and the first is sometimes separate.
- The bone is directed downwards and ventrally from the sacral apex.

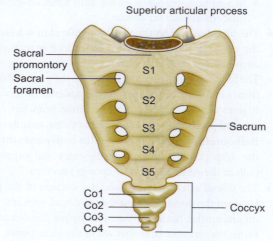

FIGURE: Coccyx, anterior view

391. Ans. (d) Bulbocavernosus

Ref: *BDC Vol II pg. 429-32; Keith Moore, 7th ed. 493-32*

STRUCTURES FORMING PERINEAL BODY

- Levator Ani (Pubo and Iliococcygeus)
- Bulbo- Spongiosus

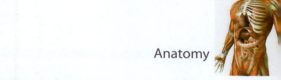

Anatomy

- Superficial and Deep Transverse perinei
- Sphincters i.e. External anal sphincter and sphincter urethrae

Clinical Significance

In episiotomy all muscles of perineal body except two sphincter (i.e. sphincter urethrae and external anal sphincter) are cut

UROGENITAL DIAPHRAGM

- Sphincter urethrae
- Deep Transverse Perinei
- Perineal membrane (Inferior fascia of urogenital diaphragm)
- Superior fascia of urogenital diaphragm

PELVIC DIAPHRAGM: TRUE PELVIC FLOOR

- Levator anii
  - Muscles (Iliococcygeus and Pubococcygeus)
- Ischiococcygeus

392. Ans. (d) Ischiococcygeus

Refer to above explanation

393. Ans. (d) Puborectalis

Refer to above explanation

394. Ans. (c) Glandular tissue and fibromuscular stroma

Ref: Gray's Anatomy, 39th ed. pg. 1302

- The anterior part of the prostate is composed mainly of fibromuscular stroma, which is continuous with detrusor fibers.
- Toward the apex of the gland, this fibromuscular tissue blends with striated muscle from the levator.
- Pubosprostatic ligaments also blend with this area.

395. Ans. (c) 60 g

Ref: William's OB, 23rd ed. Ch 1

- *William's states* "In nonparous women, the uterus averages *50 to 70 g*, whereas in parous women it averages *80 g or more*"
- Since this question is asking just the normal weight of uterus, 60 gm is most appropriate given the option.

UTERUS

- **Shape**- pyriform
- **Size**- 7.5 cm long × 5 cm broad × 2.5 cm thick
- **Weight**- 60 g
- **Position**- 90 degree with the long axis of vagina
- *Angulation*- *anteverted, anteflexed*

396. Ans. (b) Anteverted, anteflexed

Ref: Gray's, 41st ed. pg. 1294

397. Ans. (b) Cervix is lined by transitional epithelium

Ref: Gray's, 41st ed. pg. 295

- The epithelial lining of cervix is varied. Ectocervix is composed of non keratined stratified squamous epithelium and endocervix is composed of simple columnar epithelium.
- Blood supply of cervix-descending cervical branch of uterine artery.

> **Extra Mile**
>
> - **Size of cervix**- 2.5 cm *(25 mm)*
> - MC site of cervical CA is squamocolumnar junction.
> - **Lining of vagina:** Nonkeratinized stratified squamous epithelium *(same as mouth, tongue, pharynx, esophagus, cornea and conjunctiva)*
> - **Lining of urinary pathway:** Transitional epithelium

398. Ans. (b) Urinary bladder

Ref: Gray's, 41st ed. pg. 1261

Please refer to above explanation

> **Extra Mile**
>
> - **Gallbladder:** Columnar epithelium with brush border (microvilli are irregularly placed)
> - **Thyroid:** Cuboidal epithelium
> - **Stomach:** Columnar epithelium

399. Ans. (a) Abdominal aorta

Ref: Clinically Oriented Anatomy by Keith, Moore, 5th ed. pg. 387; Gray's Anatomy, 40th ed. Ch. 62

- The ovarian artery/testicular arises from the abdominal aorta.
- The ovarian arteries are branches of the abdominal aorta and originate below the renal arteries. That's the reason it is sometimes also referred as *"water under the bridge"*
- The ovarian veins emerge from the ovary as a plexus (pampiniform plexus) in the mesovarium and suspensory ligament.
- **Abdominal aorta divides into right and left common iliac artery at the level of L4 *(Gray's),*** which further divides into internal and external iliac arteries supplying the organs of pelvis.
- **Length of right iliac artery:** 5 cm^Q
- **Length of left iliac artery:** 4 cm^Q

400. Ans. (b) Left renal vein

Ref: BDC, Vol: 2 pg. 236

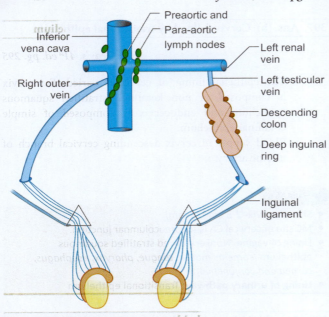

VENOUS DRAINAGE OF TESTIS

- The veins emerging from the testis form the pampiniform plexus.
- Out of this plexus finally one vein forms in each side:
  - **On the right side:** Drains into the inferior vena cava
  - **On the left side:** Drains into the left renal vein.
- Femoral vein drains into external iliac vein.
- **Remember:** IVC is on right side, so the right side testicular vein drains here."
- And left side testicular vein drains into left renal vein.

401. Ans. (a) Left renal vein

Ref: BDC, Vol. II pg. 236

Please refer to above explanation

402. Ans. (a) IVC

Ref: BDC, 6th ed./ Vol. II pg. 236

The right gonadal vein (ovarian/testicular) and the right adrenal vein both directly drain into inferior vena cava. In contrast the left adrenal and left gonadal veins drain into left renal veins, which then drains into inferior vena cava.

Extra Mile
- The hemiazygos receive the venous drainage from the lateral body wall on the left side of the thorax and abdomen. No visceral organs drain directly to azygos or hemiazygos veins.
- Inferior mesenteric vein receives venous drainage from the lower part of the intestinal tract

403. Ans. (a) Superior rectal artery

Ref: Gray's, 41st ed. pg. 1224-25

- Common iliac artery bifurcates into internal and external iliac artery at the level of sacroiliac joint.
- Length of internal iliac artery: ~4 cm.

Mnemonic to Remember the Branches of the Internal Iliac Artery

- *I Love Going Places In My Very Own Underwear!*

Mnemonic

- **I**: iliolumbar artery
- **L**: lateral sacral artery
- **G**: gluteal (superior and inferior) arteries
- **P**: (internal) pudendal artery
- **I**: inferior vesicle (uterine in females) artery
- **M**: middle rectal artery
- **V**: vaginal artery
- **O**: obturator artery
- **U**: umbilical artery
- Also, the first three arteries (iliolumbar, lateral sacral and superior gluteal arteries) are all branches of the posterior trunk of the internal iliac artery, whilst the remainder are branches of the anterior trunk.
- **Superior rectal artery is a branch of inferior mesenteric artery.**
- **Inferior epigastric artery is a branch of external iliac artery.**

404. Ans. (a) Superior rectal artery

Ref: Gray's, 41st ed. pg. 1088, 1138

Branches of Inferior Mesenteric Artery

- **Left colic artery:** supplies descending colon
- **Sigmoid artery:** supplies sigmoid colon
- **Superior rectal artery:** terminal branch of IMA
- Marginal branches

Note

- **Middle rectal artery:** branch of internal iliac artery (anterior branch)
- **Inferior rectal artery:** branch of internal iliac artery
- **Inferior epigastric artery:** branch of external iliac artery

405. Ans. (a) Ovaries

Ref: Gray's, 41st ed. pg. 1304

- The **internal iliac lymph nodes** surround the internal iliac artery and its branches (the *hypogastric vessels*), and receive the lymphatics corresponding to the distribution of the branches of it.
- They receive lymphatics from all the pelvic viscera, from the deeper parts of the perineum, including the

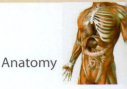

Anatomy

membranous and cavernous portions of the urethra, and from the buttock and back of the thigh.
- *It does not receive lymph from the ovary, testis, or superior half of the rectum*.
- The gonads drain to the paraaortic lymph nodes, while the superior half of the rectum drains to the pararectal lymph nodes.

406. Ans. (b) Deep inguinal nodes

Ref: Gray's, 41st ed. pg. 1284

- Glans Penis drained by → Deep Inguinal and external iliac nodes.
- Rest of the Penis → Internal Iliac nodes

407. Ans. (c) 20 cm

Ref: BDC, 5th ed. Vol II pg. 378

- Male urethra is 18-20 cm long that extends from the internal urethral orifice in the bladder to the meatus at the end of penis.
- It is divided into 4 segments:
  - Prostatic urethra
  - Membranous urethra
  - Bulbar urethra
  - Penile urethra

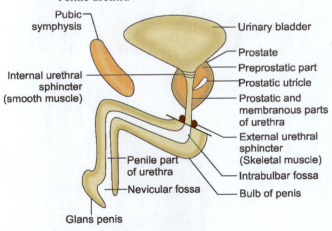

408. Ans. (a) L1 & L2

Ref: Gray's, 41st ed. pg. 1259-60284

NERVE SUPPLY OF URINARY BLADDER

- They consist of both sympathetic and parasympathetic components, each of which contains both efferent and afferent fibres.
- Parasympathetic fibres arise from the second to the fourth sacral segments of the spinal cord and enter the pelvic plexuses on the posterolateral aspects of the rectum as the pelvic splanchnic nerves or nervi erigentes.
- **The sympathetic fibres are derived from the lower three thoracic and upper two lumbar segments of the spinal cord.**

409. Ans. (b) Genitofemoral nerve

Ref: Clinically Oriented Anatomy by Keith, Moore, 5th Ed, /223

CREMASTERIC REFLEX

Efferent: genital branch of genitofemoral nerve
Afferent: Femoral branch of genitofemoral nerve

- Contraction of the cremaster muscle is elicited by lightly stroking the skin on the medial aspect of the superior part of the thigh with an applicator stick or tongue depressor.
- **The ilioinguinal nerve supplies this area of skin**. The rapid elevation of the testis on the same side is the cremasteric reflex. This reflex is extremely active in children
- A hyperactive cremasteric reflex may simulate undescended testes.

410. Ans. (c) Medial

Ref: Clinically Oriented Anatomy by Keith, Moore, 5th Ed / 223

- Cremasteric reflex is elicited by lightly stroking the skin on the **medial aspect of the superior part of the thigh** with an applicator stick or tongue depressor.

411. Ans. (d) Ilioinguinal nerve

A simplified description of the **contents of spermatic cord** in the male are:
- **3 Arteries:** Cremasteric artery, deferential artery, **testicular artery**
- **3 Nerves:** Genital branch of the genitofemoral nerve (L1/2), autonomic and visceral afferent fibres. *Remember ilioinguinal nerve is outside the spermatic cord but travels next to it.*
- **3 Fascial layers:** External spermatic, cremasteric, and internal spermatic fascia.
- **3 other structures: Pampiniform plexus of vein,** Vas deferens **(ductus deferens),** Testicular Lymphatics

Clinical significance: The spermatic cord is sensitive to torsion, in which the testicle rotates within its sac and blocks its own blood supply. Testicular torsion may result in irreversible damage to the testicle within hours. A collection of serous fluid in the spermatic cord is named 'funiculocele'. The contents of the abdominal cavity may protrude into the inguinal canal, producing an indirect inguinal hernia.

412. Ans. (c) Internal iliac artery

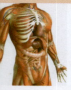

ANSWERS TO BOARD REVIEW QUESTIONS

413. Ans. (a) Deep peroneal nerve
- The deep fibular (peroneal) nerve runs through extensor digitorum longus and down the interosseous membrane. Then it crosses the tibia and enters the dorsum of the foot.
- It innervates the muscles in the anterior compartment of the leg and the dorsum of the foot.
- It also supplies a small region of skin between the first (big) and second toes

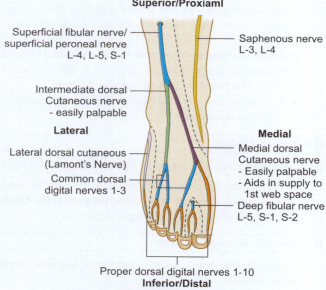

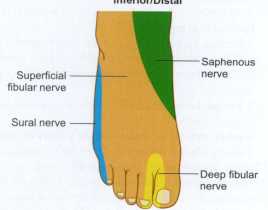

414. Ans. (b) Middle fibre of trapezius
- Retraction of scapula is done for middle fibres of trapezius muscles

Muscles of Scapular Stabilization
- Trapezius:
  - Retraction (M)
  - Elevation (S)
  - Depression (I)
  - Upward rotation (S, M)
- Rhomboid—retraction
- Levator scapular—elevation
- Pectoralis major—protraction
- Serratus anterior—Protraction

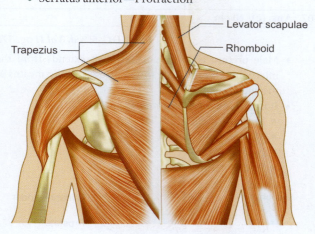

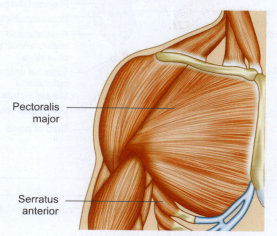

415. Ans. (c) T10
- Dermatome of area around umbilicus is supplied by T10
- Area around umbilicus is supplied by T4

Anatomy

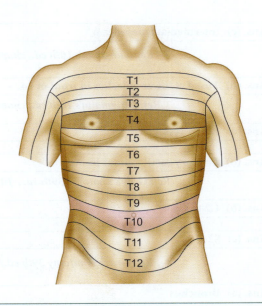

416. Ans. (c) Thyroid cartilage
- The thyroid cartilage in males are more prominent and longer than females, giving rise to adam's apple.

417. Ans. (c) 3 weeks
Ref: Langmann's, 10th ed ch: 17

418. Ans. (c) Right 4th aortic arch
Ref: High-yield Embryology Ronald W. Dudek 4thed page 41, Embryology for Medical Students By SudhirSant 2nded page 121, Langmann's 10th ed ch: 12, Human Embryology 8 Ed By Singh / 228

419. Ans. (b) Allantois
Ref: Grey's anatomy 40th ed ch: 9

420. Ans. (d) 21 days
Ref: Langmann's Embryology 10th ed ch:5

421. Ans. (a) Paramesonephric ducts
Ref: Langman 10th ed page 243

422. Ans. (b) Auricular cartilage
Ref: Basic Histology, Carlos & Jose, 11th edCh: 7 Cartilage, Textbook of human histology 4th ed/ 92-94

423. Ans. (c) Conus artery
Ref: Gray's Anatomy 40th ed Ch:56

424. Ans. (b) 7th rib
Ref: Essentials of Anatomy I.B singh 2nd ed. pg. 304

425. Ans. (a) IXth
Ref: Gray's Anatomy 40th ed Ch: 33

426. Ans. (b) Inferior thyroid artery
Ref: Gray's Anatomy 39th ed / 558

427. Ans. (d) Muscle/Tendon
Ref: Human Biology by Cecie Starr, Beverly McMillan Ch: 4 p: 70

428. Ans. (b) Protruding tongue
Ref: Gray's Anatomy 39th edCh: 32, Keith L Moore 4thed table 7.11

429. Ans. (b) Cranial accessory nerve
Ref: Gray's Anatomy 40th edCh: 33

430. Ans. (a) Anterior cerebral artery
Ref: Gray's Anatomy 39th edCh: 17

431. Ans. (c) Tongue
Ref: Thieme Atlas of Anatomy: Head and Neuroanatomy by Michael Schunke, Erik Schulte, Udo Schumacher, Lawrence M. Ross, Edward D. Lamperti p 104

432. Ans. (a) Talus
Ref: Keith L. Moore

433. Ans. (b) Auricular branch of vagus nerve
Ref: Human Anatomy by A. Halim p 192

434. Ans. (a) Bulge in the atria
Ref: Clinical 1 Anatomy for Students: Problem solving approach by Neeta. V. Kulkarn p. 190

435. Ans. (b) Pylorus
Ref: Master of Surgery: Volume 2 p 836

436. Ans. (a) Left renal vein
Ref: Gray's Anatomy 39th ed p 1307

437. Ans. (b) Between rectum and sacrum
Ref: BDC 4th ed vol-2 380

438. Ans. (a) 1st arch
Ref: Appendix-6 for "Brachial arches" & its derivatives

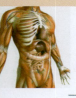

439. Ans. (b) C3, C4, C5
Ref: Gray's Anatomy 38th ed/ 1265

440. Ans. (a) Thoracic
Ref: Textbook of Medical Physiology by Khurana/ 916

441. Ans. (a) Triquetral
Ref: Snell's 8th ed / 402

442. Ans. (d) Adductor pollicis
Ref: Gray's Anatomy 39th ed / 918, 1523

443. Ans. (c) Pre & para aortic nodes
Ref: Anatomy of Abdomen and Lower Limb by Vishramsingh / 71

444. Ans. (b) Pseudostratified columnar
Ref: Appendix-10 for some Important Epithelium Linings

445. Ans. (b) Spring ligament
Ref: Gray's Anatomy 39th ed p 1512, Keith L. Moore 4th ed/400, different google books resources

446. Ans. (b) 15 cm, 25 cm, 40 cm
Ref: P L Dhingra 4th edn p 64, Keith L. Moore 4th ed/109

447. Ans. (b) Subarachnoid space
Ref: Gray's Anatomy 39th ed Ch: 16 / 294

448. Ans. (d) Greater palatine artery
Ref: Grant's Atlas of Anatomy 12thed p 670-671, THIEME Atlas of Anatomy by Michael schuenke, Erik Schulte, Udo Schumacher, Lawrence Ros /100

449. Ans. (a) Splenic artery
Ref: Gray's Anatomy 39th ed p 1146

450. Ans. (a) Mesonephric duct in female
Ref: Langman 10/th ed. / 183,184

451. Ans. (b) Suprarenal
Ref: Langman's Embryology 10th ed. chapter 6

452. Ans. (b) Trophoblast
Ref: Langman's Embryology 10th ed., p 38, Langman's Medical Embryology 12th / 37-40

453. Ans. (c) Intermediate mesoderm
Ref: Langman's 10th ed., chapter 15

454. Ans. (d) Fused at lower pole, lies in front of L4
Ref: Langmann's 10th ed., chapter 15

455. Ans. (a) Blood vessel

456. Ans. (b) Primary cartilaginous joint
Ref: Gray's anatomy 39th ed. / 103-104

457. Ans. (b) C2 to C5

458. Ans. (c) S2
Ref: Gray's Anatomy 39th ed./ 1425

459. Ans. (a) Bronchus
Ref: Gray's Anatomy 39th ed. / 561

460. Ans. (d) C7
Ref: Gray's Anatomy 39th ed. /746

461. Ans. (b) 25–30 degrees
Ref: Ballenger's Otorhinolaryngology: Head and Neck Surgery 17th / 963

462. Ans. (b) Foramen spinosum
Ref: Grant's Atlas of Anatomy 12th ed. / 670-671

463. Ans. (b) Endoneurium, perineurium, Epineurium
Ref: Gray Anatomy 39th ed. / 56

464. Ans. (a) Axillary
Ref: Grant's Atlas of Anatomy 12th ed. / 524

465. Ans. (c) L5–S2
Ref: Grant's Atlas of Anatomy 12th ed./ Table 5.6

466. Ans. (b) Deep inguinal lymph nodes
Ref: Keith L Moore /227, 263

467. Ans. (d) Pelvis
Ref: Parikh 6/e, p 2.28, Gray's anatomy 39th ed. / 1426

468. Ans. (a) Ethmoid
Ref: Gray's Anatomy 39th ed/ 474

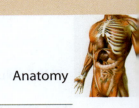

Anatomy

469. Ans. (c) Coracoacromial

Ref: BRS Anatomy 5/e, pg 25, Keith L Moor 4/e, p 479, Gray's Anatomy 39th ed. /832, Anatomy, Combined 2nd ed. by S. Mitra / 4.83

470. Ans. (c) Medial

Ref: Gray's Anatomy 39th ed. chapter 17

471. Ans. (a) Petrosquamous suture

Ref: Dhingra 5/th ed./8

472. Ans. (a) Gluteus maximus

Ref: Gray's Anatomy 39th ed./1433

473. Ans. (c) Genioglossus

Ref: Gray's Anatomy 39th ed., Chapter 32, Keith L moor 4th ed. /table 7.11

474. Ans. (b) Carpals

Ref: Gray's Anatomy 39th ed. /102

475. Ans. (d) Stylopharyngeus

Ref: Appendix-6 "Branchial arches

476. Ans. (b) 4th day after fertilisation

Ref: Langman's Embryology 10th ed/p 38, Langman's Medical Embryology 12th ed/ 37-40

477. Ans. (a) Genital ridge

Ref: Ganong's 22/e, chapter 23, Langman's Embryology 9th ed. / 239

478. Ans. (b) 3rd aortic arch

Ref: High-yield Embryology Ronald W. Dudek 4/e, p 41, Embryology for Medical Students by Sudhir Sant 2/e, p 121, Langmann's 10th ed. , chapter 12, Human Embryology 8/e, by Singh p 228

479. Ans. (d) 2nd pharyngeal pouch

Ref: Langmann's 10th ed. / 263

480. Ans. (d) 27 days

Ref: Langmann's Embryology 10th ed. , pg 285, High yield Embryology Ronald w. Dudek, 4th ed. /100

481. Ans. (d) All three germ layers

Ref: Langman's Medical Embryology 12th ed. / 326

482. Ans. (b) Inferior mesenteric artery

Ref: Langmann's 10th ed. , chapter 15, Teaching Atlas of Urologic Imaging edited by Robert A. older, matthew J. Bassignani, M.D./ 8

483. Ans. (c) Genitofemoral nerve

Ref: Gray's Anatomy 40th ed / 1080

484. Ans. (d) T 5 to T 9

Ref: Gray's Anatomy 40th ed./ chapter 54

485. Ans. (a) Cruciate ligaments

Ref: Gray's Anatomy 40th ed. chapter 82

486. Ans. (a) Superior gluteal nerve and vessels

Ref: Grays Anatomy 40th ed., Chapter 40

487. Ans. (c) Nerve to obturator internus

Ref: Gray's Anatomy 40th ed., chapter 80

488. Ans. (b) Inferior gluteal artery

Ref: Gray's Anatomy 40th ed., chapter 80

489. Ans. (d) Glossopharyngeal nerve

Ref: Gray's Anatomy 39th ed. / 659

490. Ans. (c) Mitochondria

Ref: IB singh 5/e, p 22, Gray's Anatomy 39th ed. / 1308, Guyton 12th ed. /975

491. Ans. (d) Superior mesenteric artery

Ref: Gray's Anatomy 40th ed. chapter 66

492. Ans. (a) Pudendal nerve

Ref: Gray's Anatomy 40th ed. chapter 77

FMGE Solutions Screening Examination

ANSWERS TO IMAGE-BASED QUESTIONS

493. Ans. (a) Pituitary

494. Ans. (a) Long thoracic nerve

Nerve involved	Muscle
Long thoracic Nerve	Serratus anterior
Musculocutaneous Nerve	Coracobrachialis muscle
Lateral anterior thoracic Nerve	Pectoralis major muscle
Thoracodorsal Nerve	Latissimus Dorsi

495. Ans. (a) Coraco-acromial ligament

The image shows a ligament *extending* from the coracoid process to the acromion process.

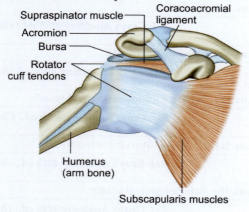

496. Ans. (c) Sural nerve

The image shows sural nerve

497. Ans. (d) Nerve originates from nerve roots L5-S2

- The image shows pain in the distribution of sciatic nerve which can occur due to disc prolapse. Such pain is worsened on standing.
- Arterial claudication pain is worsened on walking.
- The sciatic nerve originates from lumbosacral plexus L4-S3
  - Tibial division
    - Originates from anterior preaxial branches of L4, L5, S1, S2, S3
  - Peroneal division
    - Originates from postaxial branches of L4, L5, S1, S2

498. Ans. (d) All of the above

Mnemonic for Branches for External Carotid Artery

Some **a**natomists **l**ike **f**reaking **o**ut **p**oor **m**edical **s**tudents
S : superior thyroid artery

A : ascending pharyngeal artery
L : lingual artery
F : facial artery
O : occipital artery

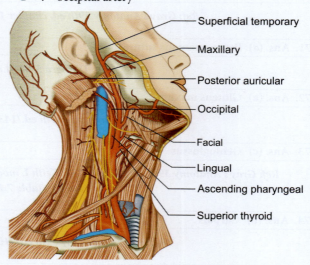

P : posterior auricular artery
M : maxillary artery
S : superficial temporal artery

499. Ans. (b) B

The following diagram and its branches should be remembered.

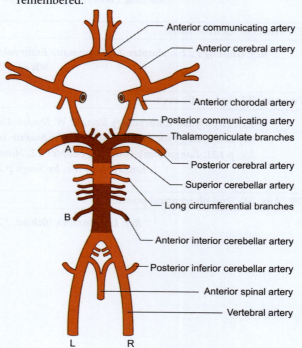

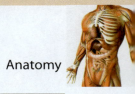

Anatomy

500. Ans. (c) Radial tuberosity

- The shown muscle in the image is biceps brachii muscle which is inserted at radial tuberosity and at fascia of forearm.

Biceps Brachii
- **Origin**
- **Short head:** Tip or coracoid process of scapula
  Long head: Supraglenoid tubercle of scapula
- **Insertion:** Tuberosity or radius and fascia of radius and fascia of forearm via bicipital aponeurosis
- **Action:** Supinates forearm and, when it is supine, flexes forearm
- **Innervation:** Musculocutaneous nerve (C5 and **C6**)

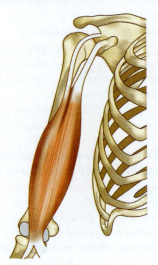

501. Ans. (b) Pterion

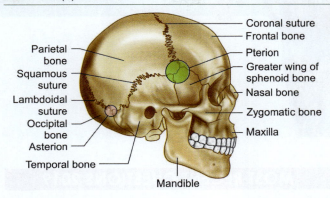

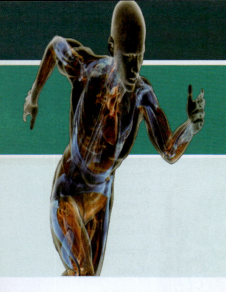

Physiology

MOST RECENT QUESTIONS 2019

1. **What is the cause of dicrotic notch?**
   a. Passive filling of blood in ventricles
   b. Rapid ejection phase
   c. Peripheral resistance
   d. Isovolumic contraction

2. **Why is sugar added to ORS?**
   a. Enhance acceptability   b. Enhance salt absorption
   c. Enhance shelf life   d. Enhance taste

3. **Which of the following is correct about Isovolumeteric relaxation?**
   a. AV valves are closed
   b. Corresponds to QT interval
   c. C wave of JVP
   d. Semilunar valves open

4. **Adequate oxygen delivery at cellular level is present in which type of hypoxia?**
   a. Histotoxic   b. Hypoxic
   c. Stagnant   d. Anaemic

5. **If radius of a vessel is doubled then the blood flow is increased by?**
   a. 8 times   b. 16 times
   c. 32 times   d. 256 times

6. **Normal anion gap value is___ mmol/L?**
   a. 4–6   b. 6–12
   c. 12–24   d. 24–50

7. **Comment on the breathing pattern of a patient with prolonged inspiratory spasms that resemble breath holding?**
   a. Biot breathing   b. Apneustic breathing
   c. Cheyne stokes breathing   d. Kussmaul breathing

CELL AND NERVE-MUSCLE PHYSIOLOGY

8. **Which of the following is not seen in Intracellular Fluid?** *(Recent Pattern Question 2018-19)*
   a. Calcium   b. Magnesium
   c. Potassium   d. Protein

9. **Which of the following is not a calcium binding protein?** *(Recent Pattern Question 2018-19)*
   a. Calbindin   b. Calmodulin
   c. Troponin   d. Clathrin

10. **Inverse stretch reflex is mediated via** *(Recent Pattern Question 2018-19)*
    a. Golgi tendon   b. Muscle spindle
    c. Unmyelinated C fibers   d. Dorsal Column

11. **Organelle having DNA is____?** *(Recent Pattern Question 2018-19)*
    a. Mitochondria   b. Golgi complex
    c. SER   d. RER

12. **Delivery of stimulus above threshold intensity leads to a constant amplitude of AP and is known as:**
    a. All or none law   *(Recent Pattern Question 2018-19)*
    b. Electrotonic potential
    c. Absolute refractory period
    d. Relative refractory period

13. **Which is correct about malignant Hyperthermia in adults?** *(Recent Pattern Question 2018)*
    a. Increase Calcium Transport via L type calcium channels in T-tubule
    b. Increase Calcium Transport via T type calcium channels in T-tubule
    c. Decrease Calcium Transport via L type calcium channels in T-tubule
    d. Decrease Calcium Transport via T type calcium channels in T-tubule

14. **Which of the following ion plays a role in exocytosis?** *(Recent Pattern Question 2018)*
    a. Sodium   b. Potassium
    c. Calcium   d. Magnesium

15. **Dense bodies are found in smooth muscle at which of the following sites?** *(Recent Pattern Question 2018)*
    a. A band   b. Z line
    c. M line   d. H band

16. **Which of the following is not a molecular motor?** *(Recent Pattern Question 2018)*
    a. Dynein   b. Kinesin
    c. Myosin   d. Actin

Physiology

17. Which is correct about function of antiporter?

a. Both molecules go in *(Recent Pattern Question 2018)*

b. One molecule goes in and other molecule goes out

c. Both molecules go out

d. One molecule goes in and two exit out

18. Which of these is true about SGLT1?

(Recent Pattern Question 2018)

a. Secondary active transport of glucose in brain

b. Secondary active transport of glucose in intestine

c. Secondary active transport of in prostate

d. Secondary active transport of glucose in rods and cones

19. Which of the following has maximum smooth muscle as compared to wall thickness?

(Recent Pattern Question 2018)

a. Respiratory bronchiole b. Alveoli

c. Terminal bronchiole d. Alveolar ducts

20. During a 100 m sprint which of the following is used by the muscle for meeting energy demands?

(Recent Pattern Question 2018)

a. Phosphofructokinase b. Phosphocreatine

c. Glucose 1-phosphate d. Creatine phosphokinase

21. Golgi tendon is innervated by which nerve fibre?

(Recent Pattern Question 2017)

a. Ia b. Ib

c. II d. III

22. Pain and temperature is carried by:

(Recent Pattern Question 2017)

a. Anterior spinothalamic tract

b. Lateral spinothalamic tract

c. Dorsal column pathway

d. Ventral column pathway

23. SGLT1 is located on: *(Recent Pattern Question 2017)*

a. Brain b. Liver

c. Intestine d. RBC

24. Steroid synthesis occurs in which organelle?

a. Lysosome *(Recent Pattern Question 2017)*

b. Smooth endoplasmic reticulum

c. Rough endoplasmic reticulum

d. Lysozyme

25. Fiber mainly affected by local anesthesia:

(Recent Pattern Question 2017)

a. A beta b. A delta

c. B fibers d. C fibres

26. Which is true about rheobase?

(Recent Pattern Question 2017)

a. Minimum time required to produce action potential

b. Maximum time required to produce action potential

c. Minimum strength of stimulus to produce action potential

d. Maximum strength of stimulus to produce action potential

27. Which of these sends K$^+$ inside cells:

(Recent Pattern Question 2016)

a. Insulin b. Glucagon

c. TSH d. FSH

28. Placenta to fetus glucose is transported by:

(Recent Pattern Question 2016)

a. Endocytosis b. Active transport

c. Facilitated diffusion d. Simple diffusion

29. During excitatory synaptic transmission all are true EXCEPT: *(Recent Pattern Question 2016)*

a. Release Ach b. Calcium influx increase

c. Decrease K efflux d. Increase chloride influx

30. Maximum excitation of cell occurs in which phase?

(Recent Pattern Question 2016)

a. Depolarization b. Hyperpolarization

c. After hyperpolarization d. Repolarization

31. Which is true about paracrine communication?

a. Action across synaptic cleft

b. Directly from cell to cell

c. By diffusion in interstitial fluid

d. By circulating body fluids

32. The electrogenic Na/K ATPase plays a critical role in cellular physiology by?

a. Using energy in ATP to extrude 3 Na$^+$ out of cells in exchange for taking two K$^+$ into the cell

b. Using energy in ATP to extrude 3K$^+$ out of cells in exchange for taking Na$^+$ into the cell

c. Using the energy in moving Na$^+$ into the cell or K$^+$ outside the cell to make ATP

d. Using energy in moving Na$^+$ outside of cell or K$^+$ inside the cell to make ATP

33. All of the following are calcium binding proteins in muscles EXCEPT?

a. Troponin I

b. Calmodulin

c. Dystrophin

d. Calcineurin

34. Which of the following is a *correct* statement?

a. Desmosomes help to attach the cells to basal lamina

b. Hemi-desmosomes help to attach cells to each other

c. Tight junctions permit passage of some solutes between cells

d. Gap junctions prevent the movement of proteins in the plane of cell membrane

35. All are true about body fluids and electrolytes EXCEPT?

a. Intracellular fluid constitutes 40% of body weight

b. Interstitial fluid constitutes 15% of body weight

c. Insensible losses are 400-800 ml per day

d. Chloride inside cells is more than outside cells

36. Motor neuron of spinal cord is?

a. Unipolar cell b. Bipolar cell

c. Pseudo-unipolar cells d. Multi-polar cells

FMGE Solutions Screening Examination

37. A person after Saturday night partying falls asleep with one arm under the head. When he awakens the arm is weak and it tingles and hurts. True reason for this is?
    a. A fibers are more susceptible to hypoxia than B fibers
    b. A fibers are more sensitive to pressure than C fibers
    c. C fibers are more sensitive to pressure than A fibers
    d. Motor fibers are more affected by sleep than sensory fibers

38. All are true about cardiac muscle EXCEPT?
    a. Phase 1 of depolarization is due to opening of voltage gated sodium channels
    b. Phase 2 of depolarization is due to slow opening of voltage gated calcium channels
    c. Phase 3 of repolarization is due to K⁺ efflux
    d. Tetany of cardiac muscle is never seen

39. Which of the following is responsible for skeletal muscle relaxation?
    a. Dystrophin   b. Tropomyosin
    c. Myosin   d. Actin

40. Which of the following is a unique feature of smooth muscle?
    a. Tetany
    b. Plasticity
    c. Excitation contraction coupling
    d. Not recalled

41. All are second messengers EXCEPT?
    a. cAMP   b. DAG
    c. IP3   d. Guanylyl cyclase

42. Transport of Na⁺ with sugar from enterocytes is example of?
    a. Diffusion
    b. Active transport
    c. Facilitated diffusion
    d. Secondary active transport

43. Permeability of which of the following ion leads to resting membrane potential?
    a. Chloride   b. Potassium
    c. Sodium   d. Calcium

44. Decrease extracellular calcium leads to?
    a. Decrease excitability of nerves
    b. Decrease membrane stability of nerves
    c. Increase amount of depolarization needed
    d. Increase amount of repolarization

45. Which of the following is a neurotransmitter at pre-ganglionic area?
    a. ATP   b. Epinephrine
    c. Norepinephrine   d. Acetylcholine

46. Resting membrane potential of RODS?
    a. –70 mV   b. –50 mV
    c. –40 mV   d. –30 mV

47. RMP of RBC?
    a. –90 mV   b. –70 mV
    c. –60 mV   d. –12 mV

48. Nerve fibers first affected in case of hypoxia?
    a. A fibers   b. B fibers
    c. C fibers   d. D fibers

49. Fastest conducting nerve fiber is?
    a. Alpha   b. Beta
    c. Gamma   d. Epsilon

50. Which of the following fiber is preganglionic:
    a. Myelinated A alpha and A delta
    b. Unmyelinated A beta and A gamma
    c. Myelinated B fibres
    d. Unmyelinated C fiber

51. True about neuropraxia:
    a. Neuronal degeneration
    b. Disruption of conduction
    c. Disrupted axon and sheath
    d. Structural change of nerve

52. Exchange between lung capillaries and alveoli is?
    a. Facilitated diffusion   b. Passive diffusion
    c. Filtration   d. Active transport

53. Which of the nerve fiber carry pain:
    a. A-Alpha   b. A-Beta
    c. A-Gamma   d. C-fibers

54. Tickling and itching is carried by which pathway?
    a. Lateral spinothalamic tract
    b. Anterior spinothalamic tract
    c. Posterior spinothalamic tract
    d. Dorsal column

55. All of the following muscle bands are covered by actin filament EXCEPT?
    a. A band   b. H band
    c. I band   d. Z band

RENAL PHYSIOLOGY

56. Glucose is absorbed from?
    (Recent Pattern Question 2018-19)
    a. Upper part of PCT   b. Ascending limb of LOH
    c. Cortical Collecting duct d. Medullary collecting duct

57. Correct about solute excretion in water diuresis?
    (Recent Pattern Question 2018-19)
    a. First increases then decreases
    b. First decreases and then increases
    c. Increased all through
    d. Remains unchanged

58. Pressure diuresis lowers arterial pressure because it?
    a. Lowers blood volume *(Recent Pattern Question 2017)*
    b. Lowers renal release of renin
    c. Lowers systemic vascular resistance
    d. Causes renal vasodilation

Physiology

59. Thiazide diuretics act on: *(Recent Pattern Question 2017)*
   a. PCT mainly
   b. DCT mainly
   c. Loop of henle
   d. All part of tubule

60. Maximum vitamin C concentration is seen in?
   (Recent Pattern Question 2017)
   a. Adrenal
   b. Liver
   c. Kidney
   d. Lung

61. Normal GFR is:
   a. 25 mL/min
   b. 50 mL/min
   c. 125 mL/min
   d. 90 mL/min

62. Which cells in the kidney are involved in acid secretion?
   a. Lacis cells
   b. Principal cells
   c. Intercalated cells
   d. Granular cells

63. Macula densa is responsible for?
   a. Tubulo-glomerular feedback
   b. Glomerulo-tubular feedback
   c. Reno-renal reflex
   d. Maintaining filtration fraction

64. All of the following increase vasopressin secretion EXCEPT?
   a. Vomiting
   b. ECF volume shrinkage
   c. Alcohol
   d. Tumor

65. Which of the following is the principal buffer in plasma?
   a. Haemoglobin
   b. Carbonic acid
   c. Compounds containing histidine
   d. H_2PO_4

66. Which cells in the kidney produce 1,25 dihydroxy-cholecalciferol?
   a. Granular cells
   b. Proximal convoluted tubule cells
   c. Mesangial cells
   d. Peritubular cells

67. Percentage of GFR to renal plasma flow:
   a. 20%
   b. 38%
   c. 50%
   d. 60%

68. Which of the following combination is true about hormone and its site of action in renal tubules?
   a. Aldosterone in collecting ducts
   b. Angiotensin in distal tubule
   c. ANP in loop of Henle
   d. ADH in proximal tubule

69. Aldosterone acts at:
   a. Collecting duct
   b. Glomerulus
   c. Proximal convoluted tubule
   d. Loop of Henle

70. CO_2 is mainly transported in blood in which form:
   a. Dissolved form
   b. HCO_3
   c. Carbamino compound
   d. Gas form

71. The tubuloglomerular feedback is mediated by:
   a. Sensing of water concentration in the macula densa
   b. Sensing of Na⁺ concentration in macula densa
   c. Sensing of sugar concentration in macula densa
   d. Sensing of NaCl concentration in macula densa

72. In proximal convoluted tubule H⁺ is exchanged for?
   a. HCO_3^-
   b. K⁺
   c. Cl⁻
   d. Na⁺

73. Osmotic diuretics act on?
   a. PCT mainly
   b. DCT mainly
   c. Ascending limb of loop of henle
   d. Collecting duct

74. HCO_3 is absorbed through?
   a. PCT
   b. DCT
   c. Loop of Henle
   d. Collecting duct

75. RAAS mechanism is mainly regulated by:
   a. Beta stimulation
   b. Alpha blocker
   c. Aldosterone antagonism
   d. Na⁺ K⁺ ATPase

76. Osmotic difference in renal calyx is maintained by?
   a. Water
   b. Sodium
   c. HCO_3
   d. Ammonia

77. 25(OH) cholecalciferol is converted to 1,25-dihydroxy-cholecalciferol in:
   a. Skin
   b. Lung
   c. Liver
   d. Kidney

78. Water is maximally reabsorbed in?
   a. Collecting duct
   b. Loop of Henle
   c. Distal convoluted tubule
   d. Proximal convoluted tubule

GASTROINTESTINAL PHYSIOLOGY

79. Esters of fat-soluble vitamins are digested by:
   (Recent Pattern Question 2018-19)
   a. Pancreatic lipase
   b. Cholesterol Esterase
   c. Colipase
   d. Carboxypeptidase

80. Enterokinase is an activator of:
   (Recent Pattern Question 2018-19)
   a. Trypsinogen
   b. Trypsin
   c. Chymotrypsin
   d. Antitrypsin

81. Histamine is secreted by:
   (Recent Pattern Question 2018-19)
   a. Enterochromaffin cell
   b. Parietal cell
   c. Oxyntic cell
   d. Chief cell

82. Colipase is an enzyme found in _____?
   (Recent Pattern Question 2018)
   a. Saliva
   b. Bile
   c. Pancreatic juice
   d. Succus entericus

83. Parietal cell secretes *(Recent Pattern Question 2016)*
   a. Pepsin
   b. Mucin
   c. Acid
   d. Gastrin

111

Questions

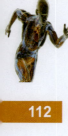

FMGE Solutions Screening Examination

84. Function of secretin is? *(Recent Pattern Question 2016)*
    a. Relax pyloric sphincter
    b. Increase gastric acid secretion
    c. Increase gastric motility
    d. Bicarbonate secretion from pancreas

85. D xylose absorption test is used to assess which of the following conditions: *(Recent Pattern Question 2016)*
    a. Colon cancer   b. PUD
    c. Celiac disease   d. Ulcerative colitis

86. A 41-year-old patient presented with chronic diarrhea from last 3 months. A D xylose absorption test will reveal which of the following: *(Recent Pattern Question 2016)*
    a. Carbohydrate malabsorption due to mucosal disorder
    b. Carbohydrate malabsorption due to chronic pancreatitis
    c. Fat malabsorption due to mucosal disorder
    d. Fat malabsorption due to chronic pancreatitis

87. All of the following are false about gastric juice secretion EXCEPT?
    a. 20% in gastric phase   b. 70% in cephalic phase
    c. 70% in gastric phase   d. 20% in intestinal phase

88. Hydrochloric acid is produced by?
    a. G-cell   b. D-cell
    c. Oxyntic cells   d. Chief cells

89. Which of the following statements is true about gastric emptying?
    a. Increased by Secretin
    b. Decreased by Cholecystokinin
    c. Decreased by Gastrin
    d. Increased by GIP

90. Gastric emptying is maximum affected by:
    a. Lipids   b. Amino acid
    c. Carbohydrates   d. Fiber

91. All are correct about stomach EXCEPT:
    a. Parietal cells secrete intrinsic factor
    b. Pylorus has more acid secreting cells
    c. Lots of goblet cells are present in mucous lining
    d. Chief cells secrete pepsinogen

92. Starch is hydrolyzed in the mouth by:
    a. Mucin   b. Ptyalin
    c. Pancreatic amylase d. Lipase

93. Fecal mass is mainly derived from:
    a. Undigested food   b. Digested food
    c. Intestinal secretion d. Intestinal absorption

94. Most sensitive taste sensation is:
    a. Salt   b. Bitter
    c. Sweet   d. Acid

95. D cells of Islet of Langerhans of pancreas secrete?
    a. Insulin   b. Glucagon
    c. Gastrin   d. Somatostatin

96. The rate of absorption of sugars by the small intestine is highest for?
    a. Pentose   b. Disaccharides
    c. Hexoses   d. Polysaccharides

97. Chymotrypsinogen is activated into chymotrypsin by?
    a. Trypsin
    b. Pepsin
    c. Enterokinase
    d. Bile salts

98. Enterogastric reflex is stimulated by all, EXCEPT?
    a. Alkaline content of small intestine
    b. Hyper-osmolality of chime
    c. Distension of duodenum
    d. Intense pain

99. Transporter of iron into enterocytes is?
    a. Ferroportin
    b. Transferrin
    c. Hepcidin
    d. Divalent metal transporter

100. All are functions of CCK EXCEPT?
    a. Gall bladder contraction
    b. Contraction of sphincter of oddi
    c. Stimulation of pancreatic secretion
    d. Inhibits gastric emptying

101. CCK is produced by?
    a. Neuro-endocrine cells in the gut
    b. Entero-endocrine cells in the gut
    c. Interstitial cells of Cajal
    d. Hepatocytes

102. All are principal digestive enzymes produced by exocrine pancreas EXCEPT?
    a. Trypsinogen   b. Lipase
    c. Lactase   d. Amylase

103. All are correct about somatostatin hormone EXCEPT?
    a. Paracrine action in GIT
    b. Produced by D cells
    c. Growth hormone inhibiting hormone
    d. Gastro-ileal reflex

104. Incorrect about bilirubin?
    a. Conjugation by UDPq Glucorornyl transferase in liver
    b. Breakdown by glucoronidase in gut to increase free pool of unconjugated bilirubin
    c. Normally excreted in urine
    d. Can cross blood brain barrier

105. Initiation of basic electrical Rhythm of intestine is by?
    a. Interstitial cells of Cajal
    b. Entero-chromaffin cells
    c. Auerbach plexus
    d. Meissner plexus

Physiology

ENDOCRINE AND REPRODUCTIVE PHYSIOLOGY

106. Sperm remains in epididymis for _____ hours?
(Recent Pattern Question 2018-19)
a. 24
b. 48
c. 72
d. 96

107. All are Glucogenic hormones except?
(Recent Pattern Question 2018-19)
a. ADH
b. Glucagon
c. Thyroxine
d. Glucocorticoids

108. Active form of Vitamin D3 is:
(Recent Pattern Question 2018-19)
a. Calcitriol
b. Calciferol
c. Calcidiol
d. Ergocalciferol

109. Inhibin-A is produced by?
(Recent Pattern Question 2018-19)
a. Sertoli cell
b. Leydig cell
c. Hilus cell
d. Placenta

110. Which hormone receptor has 4 subunits and 2 units for tyrosine kinase receptor binding?
(Recent Pattern Question 2018-19)
a. Insulin
b. Glucagon
c. T3
d. ADH

111. Name the hormone marked on the picture:
(Recent Pattern Question 2018-19)
a. Inhibin A
b. Inhibin B
c. Progesterone
d. DHEAS

112. The blood levels of 1,25 dihydroxycholecalciferol is positively regulated by: *(Recent Pattern Question 2018)*
a. PTH
b. Calcium
c. Magnesium
d. 25 OH cholecalciferol

113. Which acts on intracellular receptor:
(Recent Pattern Question 2016)
a. TSH
b. FSH
c. Glucagon
d. Epinephrine

114. During spermatogenesis Sertoli cells secrete
(Recent Pattern Question 2016)
a. FSH
b. LH
c. Inhibin
d. Testosterone

115. Somatostatin is secreted by:
a. Alpha cells
b. Beta cells
c. Gamma cells
d. Delta cells

116. Adrenal medulla secretes all EXCEPT?
a. Cortisol
b. Epinephrine
c. Nor epinephrine
d. Dopamine

117. Adrenal medulla secretes:
a. Neuro hormones
b. Cortisol
c. Aldosterone
d. Vasopressin

118. All of the following are actions of cortisol EXCEPT:
a. Increase blood amino acid
b. Decrease liver amino acid
c. Decrease blood amino acid
d. Increase liver amino acid

119. Milk ejection is facilitated by:
a. Prolactin
b. Oxytocin
c. Growth hormone
d. ACTH

120. Which of the following promotes formation of growth hormone?
a. Cortisol
b. REM sleep
c. Glucose
d. Glucagon

121. Prolactin secretion is *not* stimulated by:
a. Levodopa
b. Sleep
c. Estrogen
d. Pregnancy

122. TSH is produced by:
a. Anterior pituitary
b. Post pituitary
c. Hypothalamus
d. Thyroid gland

123. T4 to T3 conversion in peripheral tissues done by?
a. Thyroxine peroxidase
b. D1 Deiodinase
c. D2 Deiodinase
d. D3 Deiodinase

124. Which of the following is a negative feedback hormone?
a. ACTH
b. Growth hormone
c. TSH
d. GnRH

125. True statement about Melatonin are all EXCEPT:
a. Secreted by pituitary gland
b. Secreted by pineal gland
c. Associated with sleep mechanism
d. Can be used to treat jet lag

126. Separation of first polar body occurs at the time of:
a. Menstruation
b. Ovulation
c. Fertilization
d. Implantation

127. Sperm head contains:
a. Axoneme
b. Mitochondria
c. Nucleus
d. None

128. Sertoli cell secretes which hormone:
a. Testosterone
b. Inhibin.
c. LH
d. FSH

FMGE Solutions Screening Examination

129. All are true about capacitation EXCEPT:
    a. Changes that occur in sperm to penetrate ova
    b. Occurs in female genital tract
    c. Occurs in male genital tract
    d. Sperm loses its cholesterol content in the process
130. Defect in leptin leads to:
    a. Obesity   b. Anorectic
    c. Both   d. None
131. GLUT receptor on pancreas is?
    a. GLUT 1   b. GLUT 2
    c. GLUT 4   d. GLUT 5
132. Insulin increases glucose uptake in?
    a. Small intestine b. Skeletal muscle
    c. RBC   d. Kidney
133. Diagnosis of ovulation can be done by all EXCEPT?
    a. Study of cervical mucus
    b. Rise in basal body temperature in the second half of cycle
    c. Endometrial histology
    d. Measuring Serum progesterone on day 14 of the cycle
134. Release of which one of the following hormones is an example of neuroendocrine secretion?
    a. Growth hormone   b. Cortisol
    c. Oxytocin   d. Thyroxine
135. All are true about testosterone EXCEPT?
    a. Produced by Leydig cells
    b. Produced from Androstenedione secreted by adrenal cortex
    c. Carbon 17 steroid
    d. Secretion under control of LH
136. Correct about menstrual cycle?
    a. Proliferative phase by progesterone
    b. Secretory phase by Estrogen
    c. Superficial 1/3rd of endometrium is shed
    d. Menstrual blood is predominantly arterial
137. Inhibin regulates?
    a. FSH   b. LH
    c. GnRH   d. Testosterone
138. All hormones peak at term EXCEPT?
    a. Estriol   b. Progesterone
    c. Prolactin   d. hCG
139. Spinnbarkeit refers to?
    a. Cervical mucus   b. Uterine gland thickness
    c. Cervical os appearance d. Proliferation of breast alveoli

RESPIRATORY PHYSIOLOGY

140. Transpulmonary pressure is the difference between?
    (Recent Pattern Question 2017)
    a. The bronchus and atmospheric pressure
    b. Pressure in alveoli and intrapleural pressure
    c. Atmosphere and intrapleural pressure
    d. Atmosphere and intraalveolar pressure
141. Respiratory quotient of the brain is?
    (Recent Pattern Question 2017)
    a. 0.6–0.7   b. 0.7–0.8
    c. 0.8–0.9   d. 0.9–1.0
142. Mean pulmonary artery pressure:
    a. 25 mm Hg   b. 8 mm Hg
    c. 16 mm Hg   d. 20 mm Hg
143. pO$_2$ pressure at sea level:
    a. 140   b. 150
    c. 160   d. 180
144. Which is correct regarding lungs in an upright posture?
    a. V/Q ratio is high at the apex of the lung
    b. V/Q ratio is low at the apex of the lung
    c. V/Q ratio is equal at apex and base
    d. None of the above
145. Which of the following statement is true about functional residual capacity?
    a. Tidal volume + Volume Expired forcefully
    b. Volume remaining after forced expiration
    c. Tidal volume + Volume inspired forcefully
    d. Volume remaining after normal expiration
146. Production of Surfactant is by:
    a. Alveolar macrophages   b. Type I Pneumocytes
    c. Type II Pneumocytes   d. Clara cells
147. Bronchial secretions contain?
    a. Immunoglobulin G   b. Immunoglobulin M
    c. Immunoglobulin A   d. Immunoglobulin E
148. Peripheral chemoreceptors are stimulated by?
    a. CO$_2$ b. Hydrogen ions
    c. pH   d. Oxygen
149. The main danger during deep sea diving is due to?
    a. Oxygen and nitrogen   b. Oxygen only
    c. Nitrogen only   d. CO$_2$ and nitrogen
150. At high altitude acclimatization happens due to?
    a. Increased hemoglobin content and RBC
    b. Increased reticulocyte index
    c. Decreased pulmonary ventilation
    d. Decreased ability of tissues to use oxygen.
151. Which of the following is true about hypoxic hypoxia?
    a. Due to inadequate carrying capacity
    b. Due to inability to utilize oxygen
    c. Due to inadequate gas exchange
    d. Due to slow circulation
152. Over-inflation of lung is prevented by?
    a. Chemo-receptor   b. Hering-Breuer reflex
    c. Surfactant   d. Clara cells
153. Oxygen hemoglobin dissociation curve shifts to right in all of the following conditions EXCEPT:
    a. Hyperthermia   b. Decreased pH
    c. Decreased H$^+$ d. Increase CO$_2$

Physiology

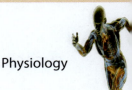

154. PCO$_2$ increase leads to:
    a. Shift of Oxy-Hb dissociation curve to left
    b. Shift of Oxy-Hb dissociation curve to right
    c. Shift of Oxy-Hb dissociation curve upwards
    d. Shift of Oxy-Hb dissociation curve downwards

155. S shaped curve of oxygen hemoglobin dissociation curve is due to?
    a. Atmospheric pressure decreases affinity of O$_2$ binding with Hemoglobin
    b. Binding of oxygen to hemoglobin decreases affinity of Hb for CO$_2$
    c. Falling of pH decreases oxygen affinity for Hemoglobin
    d. Binding of oxygen molecule increases affinity of binding other oxygen molecule

156. Which of the following is not responsible for causing a right shift of the oxygen dissociation curve:
    a. Increased carbon dioxide
    b. Temperature
    c. Exercise
    d. Alkalosis

157. Pulmonary Chemo-reflex is characterized by?
    a. Reflex bradycardia
    b. Rise in blood pressure
    c. Reflex tachycardia
    d. Pulmonary oligaemia

158. What will happen to respiration if both vagi are cut?
    a. Becomes slow and deep
    b. Becomes fast and shallow
    c. Increase in depth of respiration
    d. Increase in rate of breathing

159. "Obstructive sleep apnea" is defined as temporary pause in breathing during sleep lasting at least?
    a. 40 seconds   b. 30 seconds
    c. 20 seconds   d. 10 seconds

160. Damage to pneumotaxic centre will cause?
    a. Apneusis
    b. Apnea
    c. Slower breathing with greater tidal volume
    d. Faster breathing with lesser tidal volume

161. Damage to J receptors in lungs will result in?
    a. Apnea followed by Rapid shallow breathing
    b. Hyperpnea followed by rapid shallow breathing
    c. Cardiac arrest
    d. Hering Breur reflex

162. Myoglobin binds to _____ molecules of oxygen?
    a. 1   b. 2
    c. 3   d. 4

163. Normal ventilation/perfusion ratio is?
    a. 0.8   b. 1.2
    c. 1.6   d. 2.0

164. Normal respiratory minute volume is ?
    a. Tidal volume × Respiratory rate
    b. Tidal volume/Respiratory rate
    c. TLC/Respiratory rate
    d. FRC/Respiratory rate

165. Which of the following statement is true about inspiratory capacity:
    a. Tidal volume + volume expired forcefully
    b. Volume remaining after forced expiration
    c. Tidal volume + volume inspired forcefully
    d. Volume remaining after normal expiration

166. Which of the following is seen in placenta?
    a. Bohr effect
    b. Double Bohr effect
    c. Hamburger phenomenon
    d. Haldane effect

167. Cut off limit for deoxygenated hemoglobin for appearance of cyanosis is?
    a. >4 gm%   b. >5 gm%
    c. < 2 gm%   d. <4 gm%

168. Which is the site of generation of respiratory rhythm?
    a. Botzinger complex
    b. Pre-Botzinger complex
    c. Dorsal respiratory group of neurons in medulla
    d. Ventral respiratory group of neurons in medulla

CARDIOVASCULAR AND CIRCULATORY PHYSIOLOGY

169. Which is true about heart sound?
    (Recent Pattern Question 2017)
    a. First heart sound has maximum frequency
    b. First heart sound has maximum duration
    c. First heart sound is due to semilunar valve closure
    d. Second heart sound is due to AV valve closure

170. Purkinje fibers are   *(Recent Pattern Question 2016)*
    a. Nerve fibers
    b. Modified muscle fibers
    c. Modified connective tissue fibers
    d. Retinal fibers

171. Forward blood flow in the fetal venous system is in this phase   *(Recent Pattern Question 2016)*
    a. Preload   b. After load
    c. Systolic volume   d. All of the above

172. What is the reason for increased interstitial fluid?
    (Recent Pattern Question 2016)
    a. Increase hydrostatic pressure, increase oncotic pressure
    b. Decrease hydrostatic pressure, decrease oncotic pressure
    c. Increase hydrostatic pressure, decrease oncotic pressure
    d. Decrease hydrostatic pressure, increase oncotic pressure

173. All of the following statements are false EXCEPT:
    a. Right ventricle work more than left ventricle
    b. Left ventricle works more than right ventricle
    c. Both ventricle work equal
    d. Maximum ventricular filing occurs in isovolumetric contraction

174. All are true EXCEPT:
    a. SA is dominant pacemaker
    b. AV node shows fast conduction
    c. Purkinje fibres have fastest conduction
    d. AV nodal delay is 0.1 sec.

175. All of the following statements are false about stroke volume EXCEPT:
    a. Determined by after load
    b. Determined by pre-diastolic volume
    c. Decreases by increase in heart rate
    d. Increased by increase in heart rate

176. Severe HTN cut off is
    a. >140 mm Hg
    b. >150 mm Hg
    c. >160 mm Hg
    d. >170 mm Hg

177. In JVP, "a-wave" is due to:
    a. Atrial relaxation
    b. Atrial filling
    c. Atrial contraction
    d. Ventricular relaxation

178. Which of the following is true about Coronary blood flow?
    a. Stable throughout the cardiac cycle
    b. Maximum during diastole
    c. Maximum during systole
    d. Regulated by sympathetic vasodilatory activity

179. Repolarization in isolated muscle piece fiber proceeds from?
    a. Epicardium to endocardium
    b. Endocardium to epicardium
    c. Left to right
    d. Right to left

180. Sympathetic Stimulation causes all of the following, EXCEPT
    a. Increase in heart rate
    b. Increase in blood pressure
    c. Increase in total peripheral resistance
    d. Increase in venous capacitance

181. Incorrect about ECG?
    a. Normal axis of heart is −30 to +110 degrees
    b. ST segment is 0.40 seconds
    c. Holter is ambulatory recording
    d. AV nodal delay is 0.1 seconds

182. Which represent ventricular systole?
    a. Start of P to end of T wave
    b. End of P to end of T wave
    c. Middle of R to end of T wave
    d. Start of q to end of S wave

183. Dicrotic notch corresponds to?
    a. Closure of AV valves
    b. Closure of Aortic and pulmonic valves
    c. Opening of AV valves
    d. Opening of Aortic and pulmonic valves

184. Which of the following is correct about Frank starling law?
    a. Explains the increase in heart rate produced by exercise
    b. Explains the increase in cardiac output when venous return is increased
    c. Explains the decrease in heart rate in spinal shock
    d. Explains the decrease in heart rate by Valsava manoeuvre

185. Cardiac output is measured by all EXCEPT?
    a. Doppler
    b. Oscillometry
    c. Thermo-dilution method
    d. Fick's principle

186. All are true about circulating changes in exercising muscle EXCEPT?
    a. Complete flow stops on maximal tension reaching 70%
    b. Blood supply increases by 30 times between contractions
    c. Dilation of arterioles and pre-capillaries
    d. Peripheral resistance increases

187. Dromotropy is?
    a. Increase in Rate of transmission
    b. Increase in Force of contraction
    c. Increase in RMP potential
    d. Increase in action potential duration

188. Not a component of JVP?
    a. A wave bigger than V wave
    b. C wave is called as Dicrotic notch
    c. X wave is seen ventricular systole
    d. Y descent in ventricular diastole

189. Traube Hering waves are due to?
    a. Fluctuation in BP with respiration
    b. Fluctuations in JVP with respiration
    c. Fluctuation in CVP with respiration
    d. Fluctuation in ICP with respiration

190. Which of the following has maximum cross sectional area
    a. Aorta
    b. Artery
    c. Venule
    d. Arteriole

191. Normal arm to tongue circulation time is
    a. 5 seconds   b. 10 seconds
    c. 15 seconds   d. 30 seconds

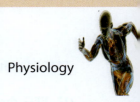

Physiology

CNS AND PNS PHYSIOLOGY

192. Resistance against passive stretch is called?
 (Recent Pattern Question 2018-19)
 a. Tone b. Spasticity
 c. Rigidity d. Paratonia

193. Which structure connects the Broca's area and Wernicke area? *(Recent Pattern Question 2018-19)*
 a. Arcuate fasciculus b. Anterior commissure
 c. Corpus callosum d. Fornix

194. Reward centre in the brain is?
 (Recent Pattern Question 2018-19)
 a. Amygdala b. Thalamus
 c. Hippocampus d. Ventral tegmental area

195. Which part of thalamus is related to motor control?
 (Recent Pattern Question 2018-19)
 a. Ventrolateral thalamus
 b. Ventral posteromedial
 c. Ventral posterolateral
 d. Superior and inferior colliculi

196. In case a small stimulus causes more pain, it is called
 (Recent Pattern Question 2018-19)
 a. Hypersensitivity b. Causalgia
 c. Hyperalgesia d. Allodynia

197. Stretch stimulus is mediated by which of the following receptors? *(Recent Pattern Question 2018)*
 a. Merkel's disc b. Meissner
 c. Pacinian d. Muscle spindle

198. During sleep which hormone is increased?
 (Recent Pattern Question 2017)
 a. Serotonin b. Dopamine
 c. GABA d. Ach

199. Which is true about sleep cycle?
 (Recent Pattern Question 2017)
 a. REM is half of sleep cycle
 b. Muscle tone is absent in REM sleep
 c. NREM is 25% of sleep cycle
 d. Muscle tone is absent in NREM sleep

200. mGluR 4 is associated with which taste?
 (Recent Pattern Question 2016)
 a. Sweet b. Sour
 c. Bitter d. Umami

201. Which cells secrete glutamate in cerebellum?
 (Recent Pattern Question 2016)
 a. Stellate cell b. Basket cells
 c. Granular cell d. Golgi cell

202. Excitatory neurotransmitter of brain is?
 (Recent Pattern Question 2016)
 a. GABA b. Aspartate
 c. Glutamate d. Glycine

203. Not a part of basal ganglia is?
 a. Caudate nucleus b. Corpus striatum
 c. Lenticular nucleus d. Sub-Fornical organ

204. True about GABA:
 a. Excitatory neurotransmitter
 b. Inhibitory to neuron
 c. Facilitatory neurotransmitter
 d. Stimulatory to neuron

205. Brain contains which neurotransmitter:
 a. Tyrosine b. Glutamate
 c. Serine d. Tryptophan

206. All of the following cells are present in cerebellar cortex EXCEPT:
 a. Granular cell b. Purkinje cell
 c. Golgi cell d. Bipolar cell

207. Posterior pre-frontal cortex contains which of the following areas?
 a. Wernicke's area b. Broca's area
 c. Brodmann's area d. Limbic association area

208. Broca's area is located at?
 a. Inferior frontal gyrus b. Superior temporal gyrus
 c. Inferior temporal gyrus d. Superior frontal gyrus

209. Which of the following vascular occlusion is the most common cause of hemiplegia?
 a. Basilar artery b. Vertebral artery
 c. Anterior cerebral artery d. Middle cerebral artery

210. Auditory receptor is present in:
 a. Broca's area b. Cingulate gyrus
 c. Superior temporal gyrus d. Inferior temporal gyrus

211. Damage to preoptic nuclei of brain leads to?
 a. Decrease heart rate, decrease arterial pressure
 b. Increase heart rate, increase arterial pressure
 c. Increase heart rate, decrease arterial pressure
 d. Decrease heart rate, increase arterial pressure

212. Which is the Longest duration NREM Stage?
 a. Stage 1 b. Stage 2
 c. Stage 3 d. Spread throughout

213. Teeth grinding is seen in which stage of sleep:
 a. NREM 1 b. NREM 2
 c. NREM 3 d. NREM 4

214. The alpha rhythm appearing in EEG has the following characteristic feature?
 a. Produces 20-30 waves per second.
 b. Disappear when a patient opens eyes
 c. Associated with deep sleep
 d. Replaced by slower, larger waves during REM sleep

215. Hippocampal formation includes all, EXCEPT?
 a. Dentate gyrus b. Subiculum
 c. Amygdaloid nucleus d. Entorhinal cortex

216. The inability to perceive the texture & shape an object occurs in lesion of?
 a. Lateral Spinothalamic tract
 b. Nucleus gracilis
 c. Spino-reticular tract
 d. Nucleus cuneatus

FMGE Solutions Screening Examination

217. EEG rhythm recorded from the surface of the scalp during REM sleep?
    a. Alpha
    b. Beta
    c. Delta
    d. Theta
218. Which of the following phrase adequately describes Pacinian corpuscles?
    a. A type of pain receptors
    b. Slowly adapting touch receptors
    c. Rapidly adapting touch receptors
    d. Located in the joints
219. All of the following structures have blood brain barrier EXCEPT?
    a. Optic tract
    b. Posterior pituitary
    c. Superior colliculus
    d. Basal ganglia
220. Paradoxical sleep is?
    a. Seen in obstructive sleep apnea
    b. REM sleep
    c. NRM sleep
    d. Narcolepsy
221. All are hyperkinetic movements EXCEPT?
    a. Chorea
    b. Atheotosis
    c. Akinesia
    d. Ballism
222. Glycinergic inhibitory interneuron in spinal cord is?
    a. Renhaw cell
    b. Purkinje cell
    c. Basket cell
    d. Golgi cell
223. Clonus is due to?
    a. Upper motor neuron damage
    b. Lower motor neuron damage
    c. Extrapyramidal damage
    d. Cerebellar damage
224. Clasp knife effect is seen in?
    a. Flaccidity
    b. Rigidity
    c. Spasticity
    d. All of the above
225. Rebound phenomenon is seen due to:
    a. Damage to cerebrum
    b. Damage to cerebellum
    c. Damage to extrapyramidal pathway
    d. Damage to rubrospinal pathway
226. First reflex to reappear after spinal shock?
    a. Myotactic reflex
    b. Withdrawal reflex
    c. Stretch reflex
    d. Inverse stretch reflex
227. Corpus striatum is formed by?
    a. Caudate and putamen
    b. Caudate and subthalamic nucleus
    c. Caudate and lenticular nucleus
    d. Caudate and amygdaloid nucleus
228. Inverse stretch reflex is_____?
    a. Monosynaptic reflex
    b. Bi-Synaptic Reflex
    c. Polysynaptic reflex
    d. Occurs when Ia spindle fibres are inhibited

229. Inverse stretch reflex is mediated by?
    a. Muscle spindle
    b. Golgi tendon organ
    c. Unmyelinated C fibres
    d. B fibers
230. Lowest level of Integration of Stretch reflex is at?
    a. Cerebral cortex
    b. Medulla
    c. Lower medulla
    d. Spinal Cord
231. Twitch of a single motor unit is called?
    a. Myoclonic-jerk
    b. Fasciculation
    c. Tremor
    d. Chorea
232. Not a component of light reflex?
    a. Lateral geniculate body
    b. Edinger westphal nucleus
    c. Occipital radiation
    d. Optic nerve
233. Globus pallidus and putamen are present in?
    a. Pons
    b. Thalamus
    c. Cerebellum
    d. Basal ganglia
234. Phantom limb phenomenon is due to?
    a. Weber Fechner Law
    b. Law of Projection
    c. Doctrine of specific nerve energies
    d. Bell Magendie Law

PHYSIOLOGY OF BLOOD

235. Which is correct about action of Vitamin K?
    (Recent Pattern Question 2018)
    a. γ-carboxylation of glutamic acid residues to clotting factor 2, 7, 9 and 10
    b. β-carboxylation of glutamic acid residues to clotting factor 2, 7, 9 and 10
    c. α-carboxylation of asparatic acid residues to clotting factor 2, 7, 9 and 10
    d. γ-carboxylation of aspartic acid residues clotting factor 2, 7, 9 and 10
236. One hemoglobin molecule can carry how many oxygen molecules? *(Recent Pattern Question 2017)*
    a. 1
    b. 2
    c. 3
    d. 4
237. Bilirubin is synthesised from *(Recent Pattern Question 2016)*
    a. Amino acid
    b. Hemoglobin
    c. Myoglobin
    d. WBCs
238. During intrauterine life, *hepatic stage* of erythropoiesis starts at?
    a. 2nd week
    b. 5th week
    c. 12th week
    d. 18th week
239. The biochemical role of vitamin K in the post-translational modification of clotting factors is by?
    a. Glycosylation
    b. Carboxylation
    c. Acetylation
    d. Phosphorylation
240. All are true about serum EXCEPT?
    a. Lacks clotting factors
    b. Higher serotonin content
    c. Does not clot
    d. Constitutes 5% of body weight

Physiology

241. All of the following proteins are synthesized by the liver EXCEPT:
    a. Haptoglobin   b. Antithrombin-III
    c. Von wilebrand factor d. Hemopexin

242. During second trimester of pregnancy, erythropoiesis occurs in the fetus primarily in?
    a. Liver   b. Spleen
    c. Red bone marrow   d. Lymph nodes

243. Which one of the following is NOT a function of albumin?
    a. Osmoregulation   b. Solubilization of glucose
    c. Transport of hormones d. Transport of bilirubin

244. Which of the following is major mechanisms causing heat loss from a normal person when the environmental temperature is 21°C?
    a. Conduction   b. Convection
    c. Radiation   d. Evaporation

245. Shivering is caused by?
    a. Stimulation of fibers coming from anterior hypothalamus
    b. Stimulation of fibers coming from posterior hypothalamus
    c. Stimulation of fibers coming from intermediate lobe of hypothalamus
    d. Stimulation of median eminence

246. Which of the following plasma proteins is not synthesized primarily in liver?
    a. Angiotensinogen   b. C-reactive protein
    c. Angiotensin converting enzyme
    d. Fibrinogen

247. Normal plasma osmolality (in mOsm/kg) is:
    a. 100-125   b. 200-225
    c. 275-300   d. 300-325

248. The chief intracellular ion in our body is?
    a. K+   b. Na+
    c. Ca"   d. Mg"

249. Half-life of serum albumin is?
    a. 10 days   b. 21 days
    c. 36 days   d. 60 days

250. Serum bilirubin is composed of?
    a. Conjugated plus direct reacting bilirubin
    b. Conjugated plus indirect reacting bilirubin
    c. Conjugated plus indirect reacting plus delta bilirubin
    d. Conjgated plus direct reacting plus delta bilirubin

251. Peyer's patches are seen in?
    a. Stomach   b. Duodenum
    c. Ileum   d. Jejunum

252. Oxytocin will not do the following action?
    a. Milk production
    b. Milk let down
    c. Contraction of myoepithelial cells
    d. Vasoconstriction

253. Rough and smooth texture of surface can be detected by:
    a. Merckel's disc   b. Pacinian corpuscle
    c. Ruffini's end organ d. Meissner's corpuscles

254. All are true about hormone and their mechanisms except?
    a. Insulin: increase tyrosine kinase activity
    b. ANP: increase cGMP levels in cells
    c. Thyroid hormone: stimulate nuclear receptors
    d. Angiotensin II: increase cAMP levels in cells

255. GM-CSF can stimulate all cell lines EXCEPT?
    a. Granulocyte   b. Megakaryocyte
    c. Erythrocyte   d. Monocyte

256. Mechanism of action of Nitric oxide is through which second messenger?
    a. cAMP   b. cGMP
    c. PIP   d. IP3/DAG

BOARD REVIEW QUESTIONS

257. Interleukin involved in anaphylaxis?
    a. IL-1   b. IL-4
    c. IL-6   d. IL-11

258. Purkinje cells are?
    a. Unipolar cells   b. Bipolar cells
    c. Pseudo-unipolar cells d. Multipolar cells

259. Flickering of eyelids is?
    a. Myotonia   b. Myokymia
    c. Myoclonus   d. Myaesthenia

260. IPSP (inhibitory post synaptic potential) is produced by?
    a. Chloride transport   b. Sodium transport
    c. Potassium transport d. Calcium transport

261. Young Helmhotz theory deals with?
    a. Color vision
    b. Saccades
    c. Pursuit movements
    d. Detect of shape and texture of object

262. Dicrotic notch corresponds to?
    a. Closure of AV valves
    b. Closure of Aortic and pulmonic valves
    c. Opening of AV valves
    d. Opening of Aortic and pulmonic valves

263. Para haemophilia is deficiency of?
    a. Factor 5   b. Factor 7
    c. Factor 8   d. Von wilebrand disease

264. Sounds of korotkoff are heard during?
    a. BP recording   b. Lung auscultation
    c. Cardiac auscultation d. ICP monitoring

265. Which of the following has the highest cross sectional area in the body
    a. Arteries   b. Arterioles
    c. Capillaries   d. Venules

266. Membrane fluidity is increased by:
    a. Stearic acid   b. Palmitic acid
    c. Cholesterol   d. Linoleic acid

267. RMP of RBC is mainly due to:
    a. K leak channels   b. Na-K pump
    c. Na leak channels   d. Cl- leak channels
268. Number of ATP required for myosin head detachament:
    a. 1   b. 1.5
    c. 2   d. 2.5
269. Optimum length corresponds to sarcomere length:
    a. 2–2.2 µm   b. 3–3.2 µm
    c. 5–5.5 µm   d. 10–100 µm
270. Windkessal effect is seen in:
    a. Large elastic vessel   b. Capillaries
    c. Capacitance vessel   d. Venules
271. Duration of 2nd heart sound:
    a. 0.15 sec   b. 0.12 sec
    c. 0.10 sec   d. 0.08 sec
272. Resting membrane potential of rods
    a. –70 mV   b. –50 mV
    c. –40 mV   d. –30 mV
273. The most susceptible fibre to hypoxia is
    a. A   b. B
    c. C   d. All are equally sensitive
274. Burning pain is carried by which type of fibres
    a. A alpha   b. A delta
    c. A beta   d. C
275. Permeability of which of the following ion leads to resting membrane potential:
    a. Chloride   b. Potassium
    c. Sodium   d. Calcium
276. Glucose linked uptake transporter present on sperms?
    a. GLUT 2   b. GLUT 3
    c. GLUT 4   d. GLUT 5
277. Which of the following is the principal buffer in interstitial fluid?
    a. Haemoglobin
    b. Carbonic acid
    c. Albumin
    d. Compounds containing histidine
278. Damage to pneumotaxic centre will cause?
    a. Apneusis
    b. Apnea
    c. Slower breathing with greater tidal volume
    d. Faster breathing with lesser tidal volume
279. Myoglobin binds to _____ molecules of oxygen?
    a. 1   b. 2
    c. 3   d. 4
280. Normal ventilation/perfusion ratio is
    a. 0.8   b. 1.2
    c. 1.6   d. 2.0
281. Normal respiratory minute volume is
    a. Tidal volume X respiratory Rate
    b. Tidal volume/ Respiratory Rate
    c. TLC/ Respiratory Rate
    d. FRC/ Respiratory Rate

282. Guardian angel against obesity?
    a. Adiponectin   b. Leptin
    c. Ghrelin   d. Pro-opiomelanocortin
283. Vitamin D is synthesized in
    a. Proximal tubule kidney   b. Lacis cells kidney
    c. Granular cells kidney   d. Distal tubule kidney
284. Growth in fetal period is determined by?
    a. IGF-1   b. IGF-2
    c. Insulin d. Growth Hormone
285. Clonus is due to
    a. Upper motor neuron damage
    b. Lower motor neuron damage
    c. Extrapyramidal damage
    d. Cerebellar damage
286. Clasp knife effect is seen in
    a. Flaccidity   b. Rigidity
    c. Spasticity   d. All of the above
287. Corpus striatum is formed by?
    a. Caudate and putamen
    b. Caudate and subthalamic nucleus
    c. Caudate and lenticular nucleus
    d. Caudate and subthalamic nucleus
288. Inverse stretch reflex is_____?
    a. Monosynaptic reflex
    b. Bi-Synaptic Reflex
    c. Polysynaptic reflex
    d. Occurs when Ia spindle fibres are inhibited
289. Inhibin regulates?
    a. FSH   b. LH
    c. GnRH   d. Testosterone
290. Hormone with shortest half life?
    a. Corticosterone   b. Renin
    c. Aldosterone   d. Nor-epinephrine
291. SAN is innervated by
    a. Nucleus ambiguus
    b. Nucleus tractus solitarius
    c. Edinger westphal nucleus
    d. Celiac ganglion
292. Peyers patches are seen in
    a. Stomach   b. Duodenum
    c. Ileum   d. Jejunum
293. Most sensitive taste sensation is
    a. Salt   b. Bitter
    c. Sweet   d. Sour
294. HCO_3 is absorbed through
    a. Cortical collecting duct
    b. Medullary collecting duct
    c. PCT
    d. DCT
295. Herring breuer reflex is an increase in:
    a. Duration of inspiration   b. Depth of inspiration
    c. Duration of expiration   d. Depth of expiration

Physiology

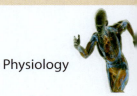

296. **Gastric emptying is maximum affected by:**
 a. Lipids
 b. Amino acid
 c. Carbohydrates
 d. Fiber
297. **Mean pulmonary capillary pressure:**
 a. 25 mm Hg
 b. 7 mm Hg
 c. 16 mm Hg
 d. 20 mm Hg
298. **Glucagon is secreted by:**
 a. Alpha cells
 b. Beta cells
 c. Gamma cells
 d. Delta cells
299. **Which of the following contains C-18**
 a. Testosterone
 b. Estrogen
 c. Androgen
 d. Progesterone
300. **Corpus luteum is maintained by**
 a. Progesterone
 b. LH
 c. FSH
 d. Estrogen
301. **Sertoli cells play a key role in which of the following process**
 a. Spermiogenesis
 b. Testosterone secretion
 c. Secretion of seminal fluid
 d. Gonadogenesis
302. **Capacitance of sperms takes place in**
 a. Seminiferous tubules
 b. Epididymis
 c. Vas deferens
 d. Uterus
303. **Intrauterine growth of fetus is affected by all EXCEPT**
 a. Growth hormone
 b. Insulin
 c. Thyroxine
 d. Glucocorticoids
304. **Fuel for sperm motility**
 a. Glucose
 b. Fructose
 c. Fatty acids
 d. Prostatic acid phosphatase
305. **ACE is produced by**
 a. Lung endothelium
 b. Liver sinusoids
 c. Alveolar macrophages
 d. Kupffer cells
306. **Paneth cells are seen in**
 a. Crypts of lieberkuhn
 b. Submucosa of appendix
 c. Carcinoid tumor
 d. Lungs
307. **K⁺ concentration is maximum in**
 a. Saliva
 b. Rectal secretions
 c. Bile
 d. Semen
308. **Hamburger effect is**
 a. Chloride shift in RBC
 b. CO_2 shift in RBC
 c. Binding of oxygen to Hb in alveoli
 d. Binding of carbon dioxide to Hb in Tissue
309. **Windkessel effect is**
 a. Elastic recoil of blood vessels
 b. Critical closing volume of lungs
 c. Autoregulation in heart
 d. Starling forces
310. **CCK causes all EXCEPT**
 a. Gall bladder contraction
 b. Inhibit gastric emptying
 c. Enhance small intestine motility
 d. Enhance small intestine secretions
311. **Faeces contain?**
 a. Undigested plant fiber
 b. Bacteria
 c. Water
 d. All
312. **Chymotrypsinogen is activated into chymotrypsin by**
 a. Trypsin
 b. Pepsin
 c. Fatty acids
 d. Bile salts
313. **Most important stimulant for bile secretion is**
 a. Cholecystokinin
 b. Secretin
 c. Bile acid
 d. Bile salt
314. **Bilirubin is derived from**
 a. Myoglobin
 b. Hemoglobin
 c. Muscle
 d. Cholesterol
315. **Best test for GFR is with**
 a. Inulin
 b. Hippuric acid
 c. Creatinine
 d. PAH
316. **Elimination of waste product from a normal person requires minimal amount of urine of**
 a. 100 mL
 b. 500 mL
 c. 800 mL
 d. 2000 mL
317. **Which one of the following acts as second messenger**
 a. Mg^{++}
 b. Cl^-
 c. Ca^{++}
 d. PO_4
318. **Delta cells of pancreas secretes**
 a. Glucagon
 b. Insulin
 c. Somatostatin
 d. Pancreatic polypeptide
319. **Malphigian corpuscles are seen in**
 a. Skin
 b. Kidney
 c. Brain
 d. Spleen
320. **Fecal mass is mainly derived from**
 a. Undigested food
 b. Digested food
 c. Intestinal secretion
 d. Intestinal absorption
321. **The main danger during deep sea diving is due to**
 a. Oxygen and nitrogen
 b. Oxygen only
 c. Nitrogen only
 d. CO_2 and nitrogen
322. **Oculo-cardiac reflex leads to**
 a. HR decreased
 b. HR increased
 c. Apnea
 d. Hyperpnea
323. **Time taken for sperm to reach fallopian tube**
 a. Minutes
 b. 6 hrs
 c. 12 hrs
 d. 24 hrs
324. **Area outside blood brain barrier is?**
 a. Anterior pituitary
 b. Neurohypophysis
 c. Basal ganglia
 d. Optic chiasma
325. **RMP of skeletal muscle is**
 a. –50 mV
 b. –60 mV
 c. –70 mV
 d. –90 mV

326. **Minimum strength of current stimulus to produce a response**
    a. Rheobase
    b. Chronaxie
    c. All or none law
    d. Utilization time
327. **Most abundant AA in brain?**
    a. Glutamate
    b. Glycine
    c. Asparate
    d. Lysine
328. **System which consist of Ammon's Horn is?**
    a. Olfactory system
    b. Auditory system
    c. Limbic system
    d. Vestibular system
329. **Ability to identify objects by touching without looking at them is called as?**
    a. Stereognosis
    b. Kinesthetic proprioception
    c. Synthetic sense
    d. Allodynia
330. **Which is a polysynaptic reflex?**
    a. Light reflex
    b. Corneal reflex
    c. Withdrawal reflex
    d. Gag reflex
331. **Receptor for inverse stretch reflex?**
    a. Golgi tendon organ
    b. Intra-fusal Fiber
    c. Extra-fusal Fiber
    d. Alpha motor neuron
332. **Righting reflexes are mediated by?**
    a. Cortex
    b. Midbrain
    c. Pons
    d. Medulla
333. **Basal ganglia does not include?**
    a. Caudate nucleus
    b. Lenticular nucleus
    c. Thalamus
    d. Globus pallidus
334. **All cross BBB EXCEPT?**
    a. Insulin
    b. Carbon dioxide
    c. Urea
    d. Bilirubin
335. **Blood brain barrier is formed by?**
    a. Foot processes of astrocytes and endothelial cells
    b. Foot processes of oligodendrocytes and endothelial cells
    c. Foot process of microglia and endothelia cells
    d. Foot process of glial cells and endothelial cells
336. **Incorrect about brown Sequard syndrome?**
    a. Hemi-section of spinal cord
    b. Contralateral loss of proprioception
    c. Contralateral loss of pain and temperature
    d. Brisk knee jerk on the side of lesion
337. **In JVP, "a-wave" is due to**
    a. Atrial relaxation
    b. Atrial filling
    c. Atrial contraction
    d. Ventricular relaxation
338. **All of the following statements are false EXCEPT**
    a. Right ventricle work more than left ventricle
    b. Left ventricle work more than right ventricle
    c. Both ventricle work equal
    d. None
339. **True about nerve fibre 'C' is?**
    a. Most susceptible to Hypoxia
    b. Unmyelinated
    c. Preganglionic autonomic
    d. Not for temp. & pain sense
340. **True about Renshaw cell inhibition is**
    a. Acts on collateral sensation
    b. Increases by local anaesthetics
    c. Has memory for spinal cord
    d. Inhibition of feed back propogation
341. **Calmodulin activates**
    a. Muscle phosphorylase
    b. Protein kinase
    c. 2, 3 DPG
    d. Glucokinase
342. **Autoregulation means**
    a. Maintains the perfusion
    b. Maintains Blood pressure
    c. Regulated by local metabolites
    d. Well developed in the skin
343. **Lewis triple response is mediated by**
    a. Histamine
    b. Axon reflex
    c. Injury to endothelium
    d. None of the above
344. **True about lipid bilayer of cell wall**
    a. Asymmetrical arrangement of cell wall component
    b. Lateral diffusion of ions
    c. Symmetrical arrangement of cell wall components
    d. Not made up of amphipathic lipids
345. **Clathrin is used in**
    a. Receptor mediated endocytosis
    b. Exocytosis
    c. Cell to cell adhesion
    d. Plasma membrane
346. **D_2O (Deuterium oxide) is used to measure volume of**
    a. Blood
    b. Total body water
    c. Extracellular fluid
    d. Intracellular fluid
347. **Which of these is not a part of extracellular matrix**
    a. Laminin
    b. Fibronectin
    c. Integrins
    d. Collagen
348. **All of the following metabolic functions occur in the mitochondria, EXCEPT**
    a. Beta oxidation of fatty acids
    b. Biosynthesis of fatty acids
    c. Protein synthesis
    d. Citric acid cycle
349. **A band which disappears on muscle contraction is**
    a. I
    b. H
    c. A
    d. Z
350. **Stimulation of post ganglionic sympathetic neurons leads to all EXCEPT**
    a. Fast EPSP
    b. Slow EPSP
    c. Fast IPSP
    d. Very slow EPSP
351. **Fine, irregular contraction of individual fibers called**
    a. Fasciculations
    b. Fibrillation
    c. Tics
    d. Spasm

Physiology

352. Best method to increase, the muscle strength is
  a. Isometric exercise
  b. Isotonic exercise
  c. Aerobic isotonic exercise
  d. Electrical stimulation

353. Strychnine acts by
  a. Exciting all the excitatory synapses in the cord
  b. Blocking inhibitory synapses
  c. Being incorporated as substitute transmitter in monoaminergic synapses
  d. Directly exciting the skeletal muscle fibrosis

354. Fick's Law of Diffusion indicates
  a. Active diffusion along concentration gradient
  b. Passive diffusion along concentration gradient
  c. Active diffusion against concentration gradient
  d. Passive diffusion against concentration gradient

355. Warfarin inhibits following coagulation factors
  a. II, V, VII, IX
  b. II, VII, IX, X
  c. II, V, IX, X
  d. II, IX, X, XIII

356. Von willebrand factor is secreted by
  a. Liver
  b. Kidney
  c. Vascular endothelium
  d. Adrenals

357. Effect of fetal hemoglobin on O_2 dissociation
  a. Right shift
  b. Left shift
  c. No effect
  d. May be right to left

358. Auditory receptor present in
  a. Broca's area
  b. Cigulate gyrus
  c. Superior temporal gyrus
  d. Inferior temporal gyrus

359. Cardiac index is
  a. Cardiac output/Body surface area
  b. Cardiac output/Blood pressure
  c. Cardiac output/End diastolic BP
  d. Cardiac output X Heart rate

IMAGE-BASED QUESTION

360. Which of the following is QT interval?

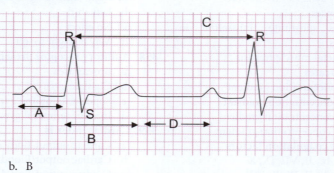

a. A
b. B
c. C
d. D

Answer to Image-Based Question is given at the end of explained question

Physiology

ANSWERS WITH EXPLANATIONS

MOST RECENT QUESTIONS 2019

1. Ans. (c) Peripheral resistance

Ref: Ganong 26th ed. P 530

Dicrotic notch is seen in pulse tracing after closing of aortic valve. The peripheral resistance generates an aberration in tracing while the aortic valves are closing. In simple words it is the pressure exerted by the vascular tree back upon the aortic valve.

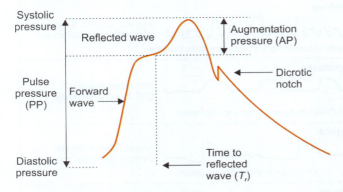

2. Ans. (b) Enhance salt absorption

Ref: Ganong 25th ed. P 478

In diarrhoea only salt is lost but sugar is added as it helps to absorb salt and sugar by process of symport. The transporter in the gut is SGLT-1.

3. Ans. (a) AV valves are closed

Ref: Ganong 25th ed. P 539

Isovolumetric relaxation is characterised by initiation of relaxation of heart and venous return is initiated. The blood will however not enter into ventricles since *Atrioventricular valves are closed*.

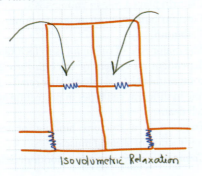

Choice B, QT interval corresponds to ventricular contraction and relaxation.
Choice C, c wave of JVP occurs in Isovolumetric contraction
Choice D, Semilunar valves opening occurs in ejection phase of cardiac cycle.

4. Ans. (a) AV valves are closed

Ref: Ganong, 25th ed. P 651

- Histotoxic hypoxia refers to a reduction in ATP production by the mitochondria *due to a defect in the cellular usage of oxygen while the delivery to tissues is normal*. The problem lies with extraction.
- Choice B, Hypoxic hypoxia occurs when the PO_2 of arterial blood falls. This could occur because inspired PO_2 is lower than normal (high altitude) or it could be due to a respiratory problem (e.g., hypoventilation, diffusion impairment caused by pulmonary oedema)
- Choice C, Stagnant hypoxia in terms of oxygen transport there is a decreased blood flow/hypoperfusion and thus the problem resides with the cardiovascular system.
- Choice D will have low delivery due to shortage of oxy-Hb values

5. Ans. (b) 16 times

Ref: Ganong: 26th ed. P 563

- The influence of lumen diameter on resistance is dramatic. This is because resistance is inversely proportional to the radius of the blood vessel (one-half of the vessel's diameter) raised to the fourth power ($R = 1/r^4$).
- This means, that if an artery or arteriole constricts to one-half of its original radius, the resistance to flow will increase 16 times. And if an artery or arteriole dilates to twice its initial radius, then resistance in the vessel will decrease to 1/16 of its original value and flow will increase 16 times.

6. Ans. (b) 6–12

Ref: Harrison 20th ed. page 316

Normal anion gap is Sodium minus sum of chloride and bicarbonate.

$$\text{Anion gap} = Na^+ - (Cl^- + HCO_3^-)$$

It is approximately 6-12 mmol/L with average of 10 mmol/L

7. Ans. (b) Apneustic breathing

Ref: Ganong: 25th ed. Page 656

FMGE Solutions Screening Examination

Prolonged inspiratory spasm that resemble breath holding is called apneusis. It occurs in case of damage to pneumotaxic centre with cut vagi.

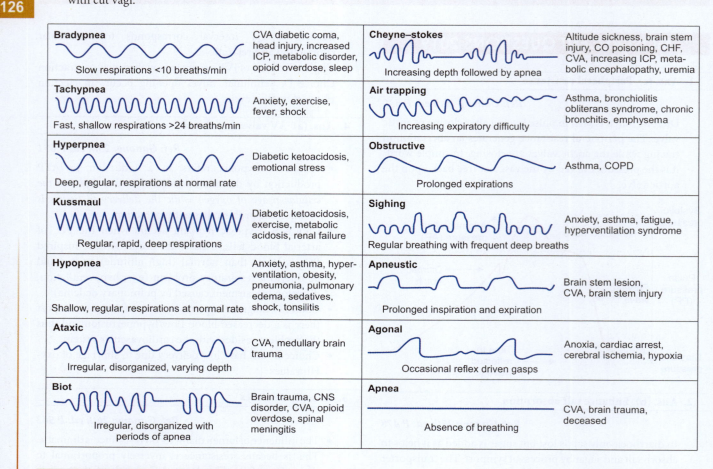

CELL AND NERVE-MUSCLE PHYSIOLOGY

8. Ans. (a) Calcium

Ref: Ganong 25th ed. page 5

- Potassium, magnesium, and phosphate are the three most common electrolytes in the ICF.

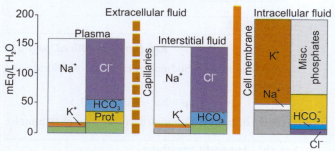

- Intracellular fluid is the place where most of the fluid in the body is contained (40% body weight).

- Magnesium is the second most important intracellular cation after potassium. Less than 1% of total body magnesium is found in red blood cells. It is distributed principally between the bone, muscle, and soft tissues.

9. Ans. (d) Clathrin

Ref: Ganong 25th edition. page 56

- Clathrin plays a role in endocytosis.
- Calcium binding proteins are troponin, Calmodulin, at Calbindin.
- The major role of *calbindin* is to facilitate the vitamin D dependent movement of calcium through the cytosolic compartment of the intestinal or renal cell. It also plays a role in different cell types in protecting against apoptotic cell death
- *Troponin* is a calcium binding protein involved in contraction of skeletal muscle.
- *Calmodulin* plays a role in smooth muscle contraction.

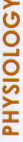

Physiology

> **Extra Mile**
> Calcineurin is a phosphatase that inactivates calcium channels by dephosphorylating them. It also plays a role in activating T cells and is inhibited by immunosuppressants.

10. Ans. (a) Golgi tendon

Ref: Ganong 25th ed. pg. 232

- Up to a certain point, harder a muscle is stretched the stronger it will contract. However when the tension becomes great enough, contraction ceases and muscle relaxes. This relaxation in response to strong stretch is called inverse stretch reflex.
- The receptor for the same is called Golgi tendon organ. It is a net like connection of knobby nerve findings amongst the fascicles of a tendon.
- There are 3-25 muscle fibers per Golgi tendon organ.
- The fibres from Golgi tendon organ make up I_b group of myelinated rapidly conducting sensory nerve fibers.

11. Ans. (a) Mitochondria

Ref: Ganong 25th edition. page 36

Mitochondria have their own genome and contain DNA. Human mitochondrial DNA has a circular double stranded molecule containing 16,500 base pairs compared to a billion in nuclear DNA. Mitochondria are derived from ovum, their inheritance is maternal. Since the repair mechanism of DNA is poor, mutation rate for mitochondrial DNA is 10 times more than nuclear DNA.

12. Ans. (a) All or none law

Ref: Ganong 25th edition. page 92

- The action potential fails to occur if stimulus is subthreshold. It occurs with constant amplitude regardless of strength of stimulus if the stimulus provided is above the threshold intensity. This is called as "All or none law".
- Anodal current producing hyperpolarization is called electrotonic potential. The magnitude of response decreases as the distance between the stimulating and recording electrodes is increased.
- During Absolute refractory period no stimulus irrespective of strength will excite the nerve. However during relative refractory period, the stronger stimuli can cause excitation.

13. Ans. (a) Increase Calcium Transport via L type calcium channels in T-tubule

Ref: Harrison 19th edition, P 40-41

- The pathophysiology of malignant hyperthermia involves dysregulation of calcium transport primarily caused by abnormal functioning of Excitation contraction coupling.
- *The EC complex is localized to the T-tubules/Sarcoplasmic reticulum of skeletal muscle.*
- The T-tubule *consists of pentameric L-type Calcium channel* (DHPR) which is a voltage gated calcium channel.
- It is triggered by inhalation of volatile inhalational agents and NM blocking agent succinylcholine.
- Clinical manifestation is intraoperative hyperthermia, respiratory acidosis, hyperkalemia and DIC.
- DOC for management is Dantrolene sodium.

> **Extra Mile**
>
> **Basic difference between T & L type Ca++ channels**
>
> | L-type Ca++ Channels | T-type Ca++ Channels |
> |---|---|
> | • Long lasting | • Short acting |
> | • Also known as DHP receptors | • T for "transient" |
> | • HVA (High voltage activated receptors) | • LVG (Low voltage Gated) |
> | • Found in
  ▪ Skeletal muscle
  ▪ Smooth muscle
  ▪ Bone (osteoblasts)
  ▪ Ventricular myocytes (responsible for prolonged action potential in cardiac cell; also termed DHP receptors)
  ▪ Dendrites and dendritic spines of cortical neurons | • Found in
  ▪ Neurons
  ▪ Cells that have pacemaker activity
  ▪ Bone (osteocytes) |

14. Ans. (c) Calcium

Ref: Ganong 25th edition, P 46

- *Exocytosis is a calcium dependent process* where vesicles containing material for export are targeted to the cell membrane.
- This area of fusion then breaks down leaving the contents of vesicle outside the cell membrane intact.
- The reverse of exocytosis is called as *endocytosis* and is mediated by the protein *Clathrin*.

15. Ans. (b) Z line

Ref: Ganong 25th ed. P 115

- Choices A and D are ruled out as bands are not present in smooth muscles.
- Smooth muscles lack visible cross striations. Actin and myosin are present and they slide on each other to produce contractions.

FMGE Solutions Screening Examination

- *Instead of Z lines, smooth muscles contain dense bodies in the cytoplasm* and are attached to cell membrane. They act by binding alpha actinin to actin filaments.

Smooth muscles are different from cardiac fibers due to the following reasons:

1. Absence of striations
2. Presence of dense bodies at site of Z lines
3. Absent troponins
4. Less extensive sarcoplasmic reticulum
5. Energy generation via glycolysis and few mitochondria

Actin and myosin contractile proteins are not organized into sarcomeres; instead the fibers attach to the dense bodies under the cell membrane

16. Ans. (d) Actin

Ref: Ganong 25th ed. P 39

Molecular motors are involved in movement of proteins, organelles and cell parts to all parts of the cell. There are three super families of molecular motors.

1. Kinesin
2. Dynein
3. Myosin

These molecular motors connect to cargo at one end and actin filaments forming microtubules at the other end.

> **Extra Mile**

Functions of actin

1. Cellular contraction
2. Cell migration
3. Cell signaling
4. Backbone for muscle contraction

17. Ans. (b) One molecule goes in and other molecule goes out

Ref: Ganong 25th ed. P 48

Uniport	Transport only one substance
Symport	More than one substance
Antiport	Exchange substance one for the other

> **Extra Mile**

- Na-H antiporter in distal convoluted tubule
- The malfunction of this antiporter leads to inability to absorb salt leading to salt wasting. The inability to excrete Hydrogen ions leads to metabolic acidosis called Renal tubular acidosis type 1.

18. Ans. (b) Secondary active transport of glucose in intestine

Ref: Ganong Physiology: 25th ed. P 432

SGLT 1 is located in GIT and SGLT 2 in proximal convoluted tubules of kidney.

> **Extra Mile**

Type of SGLT	Major sites	Functions: transport of
SGLT 1	Small intestine, heart, trachea, kidney (S3)	Na, glucose galactose
SGLT 2	Kidney (S1, S2)	Na, glucose
SGLT 3	Small intestine, uterus, lung, thyroid, testis	Na
SGLT 4	Small intestine, kidney, liver, stomach, lung	Glucose, mannose
SGLT 5	Kidney	Unknown
SGLT 6	Spinal cord, kidney, brain, small intestine	Myoinositol, glucose

19. Ans. (c) Terminal bronchiole

Ref: Ganong 25th ed. P 623

The cellular transition from conducting airways to alveoli (shown below in the image) and the amount smooth muscle decreases progressively.

Between two close options the answer is terminal bronchiole as respiratory bronchiole is more distal and has less cartilage.

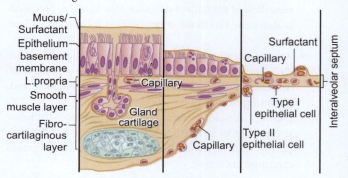

20. Ans. (b) Phosphocreatinine

Ref: Ganong 25th ed. P 108–109

During a 100 meter sprint that takes about 10 seconds anaerobic synthesis of ATP occurs. This supply comes from Phosphocreatine.

Distance covered	Contribution from anaerobic pathways
100 meter dash	85%
2 mile race	20%
Long distance race 60 minutes	5%

ENERGY SOURCES IN WORKING MUSCLES

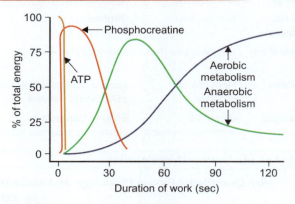

COMPARISON BETWEEN SYSTEMS

Characteristic	ATP-PC*	Lactic acid	Aerobic
Fuel/s	ATP stores and Phosphocreatine	Glycogen	CHO, Fats Then Protein
ATP production per molecule of energy source	Less than 1	Approx. 2	Glucose = 38 Fats = 460
Speed/rate of ATP production	Small amounts instantly	Limited amounts rapidly	Unlimited amount slowly
Intensity	Maximal effort	Near maximal (85–95%)	Sub-maximal (<85%)
Duration	0–10 secs	30 secs–2 minutes	5 minutes +
Oxygen requirements	Nil	Nil	O_2 required

ATP-Phosphocreatine

21. Ans. (b) Ib

GOLGI TENDON ORGAN is embedded within the musculotendinous junction (90%) and in the tendon itself (10%).
- **They are stimulated by:** Increased tension at muscle tendon
- **Afferent:** Ib fiber (myelinated).
- Mediates inverse stretch reflex

Extra Mile

Reflex	Afferent fiber	Stimulus	Response
Golgi tendon reflex	Ib	Muscle contraction	Relaxation of the muscle
Stretch reflex	Ia	Muscle is stretched	Contraction of the muscle
Flexor – withdrawal reflex	II, III, and IV	Pain, touch	Ipsilateral flexion, contralateral extension

- Group III/IV afferent fibers are afferent arm of cardiovascular ventilatory reflex responses which are mediated in nucleus tractus solitarius and ventrolateral medulla. They facilitate central fatigue and are important in endurance sports.

22. Ans. (b) Lateral spinothalamic tract

SOMATOSENSORY PATHWAYS

- **Dorasal column pathway:** This carries pressure, vibration, proprioception, fine touch and two-point discrimination.
- **Anterior spinothalamic tract:** This carries crude touch and pressure (less role).
- **Lateral spinothalamic tract:** This carries pain and temperature.

23. Ans. (c) Intestine

Ref: Ganong, 25th ed. pg. 478; Harper 30th ed. pg. 518

	Major site of expression	Proposed functions
SGLT1	Intestine and kidney	Glucose reabsorption in intestine and kidney
SGLT2	Kidney (PCT)	Low affinity and high selectivity for glucose
SGLT3	Small intestine, skeletal muscle	Glucose activated Na^+ channel

Extra Mile

- SGLT2 inhibitors, also called *gliflozins*, are used in the treatment of type 2 diabetes.
- Examples include dapagliflozin, canagliflozin and empagliflozin.

FMGE Solutions Screening Examination

24. Ans. (b) Smooth endoplasmic reticulum

- The smooth endoplasmic reticulum is continuous with the rough endoplasmic reticulum and does not contain any ribosomes. Although it has several functions, the **sER** is specialized for the production of **s**teroid hormones in cells of the adrenal cortex.
- Remember that cholesterol is the main precursor for steroid hormones produced in the adrenal cortex and the gonads.

25. Ans. (b) A delta

Ref: Ganong, 25th ed. pg. 95

Susceptibility order of nerve fibers are as follows:
- **Pressure:** Aα > Aβ > Ag > Aδ > B > C
- **Local anesthetic:** Susceptibility order Aγ & Aδ>> Aα & Aβ>> B>> C
- **Hypoxia:** Susceptibility order B > A > C
- **Paresthesias** (inappropriate sensations such as burning or prickling) usually seen when A-delta is involved.

26. Ans. (c) Minimum strength of stimulus to produce action potential

- **Rheobase:** The *minimum strength* of a stimulus, which is able to produce AP in an excitable tissue (e.g. Nerve, muscle), regardless of the duration it takes.
- **Utilization time:** Minimum *time (duration)* for which *the rheobase* has to be applied for excitation of tissue.
- **Chronaxie:** Minimum *time (duration)* for which a stimulus *double the rheobase* has to be applied for excitation of tissue.

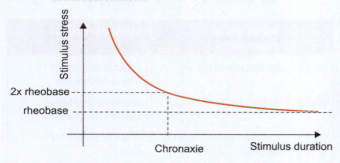

27. (a) Insulin

Ref: Quantitative Human Physiology; An Introduction. pg. 191-92

Insulin has two major roles: Sends glucose and potassium both intracellular, thereby decreasing their level (i.e. hypoglycaemia and hypokalemia).

28. Ans. (c) Facilitated diffusion

Ref: Quantitative Human Physiology; An Introduction. pg. 126-27

Since the transport of glucose to placenta is via GLUT, it is called a facilitated transfer of glucose.

	Simple diffusion	Facilitated diffusion
Energy	Not required	Not required
Carrier molecule	Not involved	Involved
Saturation	Not saturable (No Tm)	Saturable (has a Tm)
Follows	Fick's law of diffusion	Enzyme-substrate kinetics of Michaelis menten
Example:	O_2 and CO_2 exchange in alveoli	Glucose transport by glucose transporters (GLUT)

29. Ans. (d) Increase chloride influx

Ref: Quantitative Human Physiology; An Introduction. pg. 259-60

1. Action potential reaches axon terminal
2. Calcium channels open
3. Ca^{2+} causes vesicles to release neurotransmitter
4. Neurotransmitter crosses synapse
5. Neurotransmitter binds to neuroreceptors
6. Trigger signal in post-synaptic neuron

FIGURE: Summary of neurotransmission

- Most essential step in neurotransmission: Depolarization of neurons at pre-synapse

TABLE: Concept of EPSP and IPSP

EPSP (Excitatory post-synaptic potential)	IPSP (Inhibitory post-synaptic potential)
Excitatory Neurotransmitter: Glutamate and Aspartate	**Inhibitory Neurotransmitter: GABA and Glycine**
Due to influx of Calcium, Na^+ and closure of K^+ channel	Due to influx of Chloride (Cl^-) and efflux of K^+
• Fast EPSP: Na^+ and Ca^+ Influx ▪ Latency: 0.5 ms • Slow EPSP: K^+ channel closure ▪ Latency: 100 - 500 ms • Late slow EPSP: K^+ channel closure ▪ Latency: 1–5 sec	• FAST IPSP: Cl^- entry ▪ Latency: 0.5 ms • Slow IPSP: K^+ efflux/ closure of channel ▪ Latency: 100–500 ms

30. Ans. (c) After hyperpolarization

Ref: Quantitative Human Physiology;
An Introduction, pg. 215-16

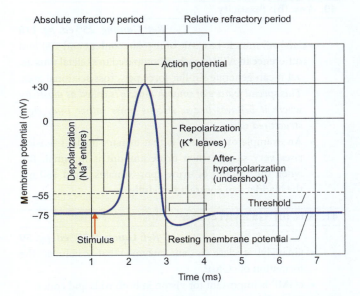

- Maximum excitation is seen after hyperpolarization state. In this phase cell is ready for another action potential, **given just the threshold stimulus.**
- Cell is in absolute refractory phase in depolarization phase. In this phase no matter how much stimulus is given, there will be no further AP.
- During repolarization phase, cell is in relative refractory phase. Action potential may ensue, if a **higher strength** of stimulus is provided.

31. Ans. (c) By diffusion in interstitial fluid

Ref: Ganong, 25th ed. pg. 752

Modalities of Communication Between Cells

Action across synaptic cleft	Synaptic transmission
Directly from cell to cell	Gap junctions
By diffusion in interstitial fluid	Paracrine and autocrine
Endocrine	By circulating body fluids

32. Ans. (a) Using energy in ATP to extrude 3 Na⁺ out of cells in exchange of taking two K⁺ into the cell

- Na⁺ K⁺ ATPase catalyse the hydrolysis of ATP to adenosine diphosphate and uses energy to extrude three Na⁺ from the cell and take two K⁺ into the cell for each molecule of ATP hydrolyzed.
- It is therefore said to have a coupling ratio of 3:2
- Its activity is inhibited by Ouabain and related digitalis glycosides which are used for CHF.
- Active transport of sodium and potassium is a major energy consuming process in the body. In body it accounts for 24% of energy utilized by cells and 70% of energy utilized by neurons.

Hormones increasing Na-K ATPase activity are
- Thyroid hormones
- Aldosterone
- Insulin

33. Ans. (c) Dystrophin

Ref: Ganong, 25th ed. pg. 56

Calcium binding proteins are:
- Troponin = Involved in contraction of skeletal muscle and cardiac muscle.
- Calmodulin = Helps in phosphorylation of myosin and muscle contraction
- Calbindin = Vitamin D dependant Calcium binding proteins
- Calcineurin = Calmodulin activated protein which inactivates Ca⁺⁺ channels and *plays role in activating T Cells*. Immunosuppressive drugs can inhibit it.

34. Ans. (c) Tight junctions permit passage of some solutes between cells

Ref: Ganong, 25th ed. pg. 41

- Desmosomes help to hold the cells together. Hence choice A is wrong
- Hemi-desmosomes and focal adhesions attach cells to basal lamina. Hence choice B is wrong
- Gap junction is a cytoplasmic tunnel for diffusion of small molecules <1000 Da between two neighbouring cells. Hence choice D is wrong.
- *The function of tight junctions is:*
  1. Passage of some ions and solutes in between adjacent cells called as para-cellular pathway.
  2. Prevent movement of proteins in the plane of membrane.

35. Ans. (d) Chloride inside cells is more than outside cells

Ref: Ganong, 25th ed. pg. 5 & 9

Composition of Body Fluids and Electrolytes into Compartments

Intracellular fluid	40%
Interstitial fluid	15%
Blood, plasma	5%

FMGE Solutions Screening Examination

Concentration of ions inside/outside mammalian spinal motor neurons in mEq/dl

Ions	Inside cell	Outside cell
Chloride	9	125
Potassium	150	5.5
Sodium	15	150

36. Ans. (d) Multipolar cells

Ref: Ganong, 25th ed. pg. 87

Unipolar cells	Invertebrate cells
Bipolar cells	Bipolar cells of retina
Pseudo-unipolar cells	Ganglion cell of dorsal root
Multi-polar cells	Motor neuron of spinal cord Pyramidal cell of hippocampus Purkinje cell of cerebellum

37. Ans. (b) A Fibers are more sensitive to pressure than C fibers

Ref: Miller's Anesthesia, P 77, 922

Susceptibility to	Most susceptible	Intermediate	Least susceptible
Pressure	A	B	C
Local anesthesia	$A\gamma > A\delta > A\alpha$	B	C
Hypoxia	B	A	C

38. Ans. (a) Phase 1 of depolarization is due to opening of voltage gated sodium channels

Phase 0	Rapid depolarization due to opening of voltage sensitive sodium channels
Phase 1	*Rapid repolarization* due to *closure of sodium channels* and opening of one type of K channels
Phase 2	Plateau phase due to slow and prolonged opening of voltage gated calcium channels
Phase 3 and 4	Final repolarization to RMP is due to closure of Ca^{++} channels and a slow delayed increase of K$^+$ efflux

Since cardiac muscle remains in refractory period until phase 4, tetanic contractions which can occur in skeletal muscle cannot occur in cardiac muscle.

39. Ans. (b) Tropomyosin

Ref: Ganong, 25th ed. pg. 101

- Tropomyosin acts as a relaxing protein at rest by covering the sites where myosin binds to action

- Dystrophin is a sarcolemmal protein providing calcium input to sarcoplasmic reticulum. This Ca^{++} is useful in coupling of actin-myosin complex.

40. Ans. (b) Plasticity

Ref: Ganong, 25th ed. pg. 118

- Smooth muscle has 20% of myosin content and 100 fold difference in ATP use when compared to skeletal muscle, yet it can generate similar force per cross sectional area. *This special feature of smooth muscle is called as plasticity where it behaves like a viscous mass rather than rigid structured tissue.*
- An example of plasticity is that urinary bladder tension rises very slowly when urine amount is minimal. But when the amount of urine approximates about 150 ml, the bladder can contract forcefully.

41. Ans. (d) Guanylyl cyclase

Ref: Ganong, 25th ed. pg. 59

- Guanylyl cyclase is an enzyme that catalyses the formation of cGMP.
- cGMP is important for vision in both rods and cones.
- Second messengers bring about short term changes by altering enzyme function, triggering exocytosis and can also lead to alteration of transcription of various genes
- *Examples of secondary messengers*
  - cAMP: Produced by action of adenyl cyclase enzyme and stimulates protein kinase A which catalyses phosphorylation of proteins and altering there activity. For example *cholera toxin increases cAMP levels whereas pertussis toxin inhibits it.*
  - IP3: Inositol phosphate diffuses into endoplasmic reticulum and triggers calcium release.
  - DAG: Diacyglycerol works with IP3.

42. Ans. (d) Secondary active transport

Ref: Ganong, 25th ed. pg. 48 & 51

Secondary active transport	Luminal membrane of mucosal cells in small intestine contain a symport that transports glucose into the cell only if sodium binds to protein and transported into cell at the same time
Active transport	Glucose movement from ECF into cytoplasm of the cell *requires carriers and utilises energy* and is called as active transport.
Facilitated diffusion	When *carrier proteins move substances* in the *direction of their chemical or electrical gradients, no energy input is required* and the process is called as facilitated diffusion

Physiology

43. Ans. (b) Potassium

Ref: Ganong, 22nd ed. BRS Physiology, 4th ed. pg. 11

Ionic Basis of Nerve Resting Membrane Potential

- **RMP:** Resting membrane potential is potential difference across the cell membrane in millivolts, *which is by convention –70 mV.*
- RMP is established by diffusion potential that results from concentration differences of permeable ions.
- Resting membrane potential (–70 mV) is close to equilibrium potential of K^+ and Cl^- (both-85 mV) and far from the equilibrium potential of Na^+ (+65 mV). *That means at rest the nerve membrane is more permeable to K^+ than Na^+*
- Na+ is actively transported out of neurons and other cells and K^+ is actively transported into cells, *but because K^+ permeability at rest is greater than Na+ permeability, K^+ channels maintain the resting membrane potential.*

44. Ans. (b) Decrease membrane stability of nerves

Ref: Ganong's, 22nd ed. chapter 2.

- A *decrease in extracellular Ca^{++} concentration increases the excitability of nerve* and muscle cells by decreasing the amount of depolarization necessary to initiate the action potential.
- Conversely, an increase in extracellular Ca^{++} concentration "stabilizes the membrane" by decreasing excitability.

45. Ans. (d) Acetylcholine

Ref: Ganong's, 25th ed. pg. 259, 266

- Acetylcholine is released at the nerve terminal of all preganglionic neuron, postganglionic parasympathetic ganglion and a few postganglionic sympathetic ganglion(e.g.: Sweat gland and sympathetic vasodilator fibres).

The remaining sympathetic postganglionic neuron release norepinephrine.

46. Ans. (c) –40 mV

- *In the dark, the resting membrane potential (RMP) of photoreceptors is –40 mV unlike other* neural receptors where the RMP is about –70 to –80 mV. This is due to dark current'.
- In the dark, the Na^+ channels in the outer segment of photoreceptors are open as they bind with cGMP. So, Na^+ enters into the cell decreasing the RMP.

47. Ans. (d) –12 mV

- Skeletal muscle cells: –95 mV
- Smooth muscle cells: –50 mV
- Astrocytes: –80/–90 mV
- Neurons: –70 mV
- Erythrocytes: −10 to −12 mV

48. Ans. (b) B fibers

Ref: Miller's Anesthesia p. 77

- In case of hypoxia, first nerve fibre affected is B fibres.
- Nerve fibres in decreasing order of susceptibility in different situations:
  - **Pressure:** A-B-C *(fibre A is most susceptible followed by B and then C in case of Pressure)*
  - **Local anesthetics:** A-B-C *(fibre A is most susceptible followed by B and C in case of LA)*
  - **Hypoxia: B-A-C** *(fibre B is most susceptible followed by A and then C in case of Hypoxia)*
- *Remember: A and B fibres are Myelinated and C fibres are unmyelinated.*

49. Ans. (a) Alpha

Ref: Ganong, 25th ed. pg. 95, Miller's Anesthesia pg. 77

Group		Myelination	Conduction velocity (m/s)	Function
Erlanger and Gasser	Lloyd & Hunt			
A α	I	Heavily myelinated	70–120 maximum	Proprioception Motor supply to skeletal muscle (extrafusal to muscle spindle)
A β	II	Myelinated	25–70	Touch, kinesthetic sense, pressure
A γ	-	Slightly myelinated	15–30	Motor supply to intrafusal muscle fibres (muscle spindle)
A δ	III	Partially myelinated	5–30	Pain, temperature, pressure, touch (cold/font sharp pain)
B	–	Partially myelinated	3–14	Preganglionic autonomic fibres
C	IV	Un-myelinated	0.2–2	Pain, temperature pressure, post-ganglionic autonomic fibres (Hot temp/slow, visceral pain)

FMGE Solutions Screening Examination

50. Ans. (c) Myelinated B fibres

Ref: Ganong, 25th ed. pg. 94

- Myelinated B fibres are preganglionic, autonomic.
- Unmyelinated C fibres are postganglionic.
- Refer to the table in above explanation.

51. Ans. (b) Disruption of conduction

Ref: Maheswari Orthopedics, 3rd ed. pg. 51

Neuropraxia *refers to physiological disruption of conduction only*. No anatomical disruption is seen.
- Both axon and sheath are intact.
- **No structural change** or **degeneration** occurs in case of neuropraxia.
- Neuronal degeneration is seen in:
  - Crush nerve injury
  - Fetal development
  - Senescence

Extra Mile

Axontemesis
- Axon and myelin sheath disrupted but endoneural perineurium and epineurium sheath is intact.
- Neural degeneration present

Neurontemesis
- Complete division of nerve
- Axon & neural tube (i.e. perineurium, epineurium, and endoneural sheath) are divided.
- Neural degeneration present.

52. Ans. (b) Passive diffusion

Ref: Ganong's 25th ed. pg. 634-635

- Exchange of oxygen and CO_2 across the lung capillary and alveoli is passive diffusion.
- Diffusion of O_2 occur from alveoli to capillary (towards the pressure gradient), and diffusion of CO_2 is in opposite direction *(from capillary to alveoli)*.
- Facilitated diffusion requires special carrier proteins.

Extra Mile

- Rate of diffusion is directly proportional to:
  - Pressure gradient
  - Surface area of respiratory membrane
  - Solubility of gas
- Rate of diffusion is inversely proportional to:
  - Thickness of respiratory membrane
  - Molecular weight of gas

53. Ans. (d) C-fibers

Ref: Ganong, 25th ed. pg. 94; Guyton Physiology, 11th ed. pg. 576-577

- **Pain** is carried by A δ and C fibres

- **General classification of Nerve Fibers**
  - In the general classification, the fibers are divided into types A, B and C.
    - Type A fibers are further subdivided into α, β, γ, and δ fibers.
  - Type A fibers are the typical large and medium-sized myelinated fibers of spinal nerves.
  - Type B fibres are Myelinated, Pre-ganglionc autonomic.
  - Type C fibers are the small unmyelinated nerve fibers that conduct impulses at low velocities.

Nerve Fibre Type and Function

Fiber type	Function
A fiber	
α	Proprioception; Somatic motor
β	Touch, pressure, motor
γ	Motor to muscle spindle
δ	Pain, cold, touch
B fiber	Preganglionic Autonomic
C fiber	
Dorsal root	Pain, temperature, reflex responses
Sympathetic root	Postganglionic sympathetic

54. Ans. (b) Anterior spinothalamic tract

Ref: Guyton, 12th ed. pg. 573-74

- *Fibres* for crude touch (itch and tickle): C- Fibre
- *Pathway* for crude touch: Anterior spinothalamic tract
- Pathway for pain and temperature: Lateral spinothalamic tract
- Pathway for proprioception, fine touch, vibration, joint position is be: Posterior column/Dorsal column.

55. Ans. (b) H band

Ref: Ganong's, 25th ed. pg. 101

- *The area between two adjacent Z lines is called a sarcomere*
- The thick filaments, which are about twice the diameter of the thin filaments, are made up of myosin; the thin filaments are made up of actin, tropomyosin and troponin
- *The lighter H bands in the center of the A bands are the regions where, when the muscle is relaxed, the thin filaments do not overlap the thick filaments.*
- The Z lines transect the fibrils and connect to the thin filaments. If a transverse section through the A band is examined under the electron microscope, each thick filament is seen to be surrounded by six thin filaments in a regular hexagonal pattern.
- Here is a quick reminder of all the structures involved in muscle contraction:
  - **Myofibril:** A cylindrical organelle running the length of the muscle fibre, containing actin and myosin filaments.

- **Sarcomere:** The functional unit of the myofibril, divided into I, A and H bands.
- **Actin:** A thin, contractile protein filament, containing 'active' or 'binding' sites.
- **Myosin:** A thick, contractile protein filament, with protrusions known as myosin heads.
- **Tropomyosin:** An actin-binding protein which regulates *muscle relaxation*.
- **Troponin:** A complex of three proteins, regulating muscle contraction.

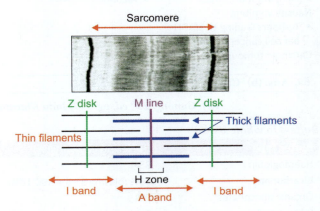

RENAL PHYSIOLOGY

56. Ans. (a) Upper part of PCT

Ref: Ganong 25th edition. page 680

Glucose, amino acids and bicarbonate are absorbed along with sodium in early portion of proximal tubule. Essentially all of the glucose is reabsorbed and no more than few mg will reappear in urine. The renal threshold for glucose is the plasma level at which glucose appears in the urine. For venous blood is blood level of 180 mg/dL.

57. Ans. (d) Remains unchanged

Ref: Ganong 25th edition. page 686-687

Water diuresis is increased urine flow rate after drinking water. The increased water intake leads to development of reduced secretion of ADH from the neurohypophysis. This decreases the water permeability of collecting duct and distal tubule leading to increased water loss initially followed by constant water load being excreted. *However, there is no change in urinary excretion of solutes in water diuresis unlike osmotic diuresis which leads to increase of urine flow as well as excretion of solutes.*

Comparison of water and osmotic diuresis

Water diuresis	Osmotic diuresis
Increased urine flow rate (No change in urine excretion of solutes)	Increases urine flow rate as well as the excretion of solutes
Causes: • Excess ingestion of water • Lack of ADH • Defect in ADH receptors in Distal segment of nephron (nephrogenic diabetes insipidus)	Causes: • Increase plasma glucose level (DM) • Increase level of poorly reabsorbed solutes/anions • Diuretic drugs (Lasix)
Diuresis is mainly due to decrease in water reabsorption in distal segment of nephron. No change to the water reabsorbed proximally	Diuresis is mainly due to decrease in reabsorption of solute in PCT or LOH. Decrease solute reabsorption results in decrease in water reabsorption proximally as well as distally

58. Ans. (a) Lowers blood volume

- Pressure diuresis lowers arterial pressure by lowering blood volume and, thereby, lowering cardiac output.
- All of the other choices do lower arterial pressure, but are not caused by pressure diuresis.

59. Ans. (b) DCT mainly

Diuretic class	Drugs	MOA	Site of action
Osmotic diuretic	Mannitol	Inhibit water and solute reabsorption	All part of tubule, **but mainly proximal tubule**
Loop diuretics	Furosemide Torsemide	Inhibit Na$^+$-K$^+$-2Cl$^-$ co-transport	Thick ascending loop of henle
Thiazide diuretic	Hydrochlorothiazide Benzthiazide Chlorthalidone Indapamide	Inhibit Na$^+$- Cl$^-$ co-transport	Distal tubule
K$^+$ sparing diuretic	Spironolactone Triamterene Amiloride	Decrease Na$^+$ reabsorption Decrease K$^+$ secretion	Collecting tubule
Carbonic anhydrase inhibitor	Acetazolamide	Inhibit H$^+$ secretion and HCO$_3$ reabsorption, which reduces Na$^+$ reabsorption	Proximal tubule

FMGE Solutions Screening Examination

60. Ans. (a) Adrenal

Ref: Modern Nutrition in Health and Disease, pg. 913

VITAMIN C CONTENT OF HUMAN TISSUES

Organ/Tissue	Vitamin C Concentration	Organ/Tissue	Vitamin C Concentration
Pituitary gland	40–50	Lungs	7
Adrenal gland	30–40	Skeletal muscle	3–4
Eye lens	25–31	Testes	3
Liver	10–16	Thyroid	2
Brain	13–15	Cerebrospinal fluid	3.8
Pancreas	10–15	Plasma	0.4–1
Spleen	10–15	Saliva	9.07–0.09
Kidneys	5–15		

61. Ans. (c) 125 ml/min

Ref: Ganong's Physiology, 23rd ed. pg. 646

- Normal GFR in a healthy person is 125 ml/min. It is best calculated by insulin clearance.

62. Ans. (c) Intercalated cells

Ref: Ganong, 25th ed. pg. 672

Lacis cells	Are cells that lie between macula densa (Sensor for distal tubule) and renin secreting granular cells
Principal cells	Seen in epithelium of collecting ducts and are involved in sodium absorption and vasopressin mediated water re-absorbtion
Intercalated cells	Seen in collecting ducts and distal tubules and are concerned with acid secretion and HCO_3 transport.
Granular cells	Seen in JG apparatus and secrete renin

63. Ans. (a) Tubulo-glomerular feedback

Ref: Ganong, 25th ed. pg. 682

Tubulo-glomerular feedback	Mantains the constancy of load delivered to distal tubule and the sensor for this response is macula densa
Glomerulo-tubular feedback	Decrease in GFR promotes solute reabsorption in proximal tubule and thick ascending limb of Henle
Reno-renal Reflex	Increase in ureteral pressure in one kidney leads to decrease in efferent nerve activity to contralateral kidney. This permits an increase in excretion of sodium and water
Filtration fraction	Ratio of GFR to renal plasma flow with normal fraction of 0.16-0.20. In hypotension GFR is lesser than renal plasma flow because of efferent arteriolar constriction

64. Ans. (c) Alcohol

Ref: Ganong, 25th ed. / Table 38-1 pg. 696

Factors Affecting Vasopressin Secretion

Increased vasopressin secretion	Decreased vasopressin secretion
• Increased effective osmotic pressure of plasma • Decreased ECF volume • Pain, emotion, stress Nausea vomiting • Tumours leading to SIADH- oat cell cancer of lung, Carcinoid tumours	• Decreased effective osmotic pressure of plasma • Increased ECF volume • Alcohol

65. Ans. (b) Carbonic acid

Ref: Ganong, 25th ed. pg. 717; Indu Khurana

Buffers in whole blood

Buffer Type	Buffering capacity (%)
Haemoglobin	35%
Bicarbonate	53% (plasma 35% + RBC 18%)
Organic phosphates	3%
Plasma protein	7%
Inorganic	2%

Most abundant buffer in the body is proteins.
Most important buffer in the body is bicarbonate.

66. Ans. (b) Proximal convoluted tubular cells

Ref: Contemporary Nephrology, 1st ed. pg. 164 and Indu Khurana

Granular cells	Produce renin
Proximal convoluted cells	Contain 1 alpha hydroxylase that is essential to produce vitamin D_3
Mesangial cells	Regulate RBC leakage
Peritubular cells	Produce erythropoietin

67. Ans. (a) 20%

Ref: Guyton's Physiology, 11th ed. pg. 316

- *GFR Is About 20 Per Cent of the Renal Plasma Flow.*
- In an average adult GFR is about 125 ml/min, or 180 L/day.
- Renal plasma flow is 650 ml/min
- The *filtration fraction* is calculated as follows: GFR/Renal plasma flow
- Therefore $\frac{125 \text{ ml/min}}{650 \text{ ml/min}} = 0.2$
- The fraction of the renal plasma flow that is filtered (the filtration fraction) averages about 0.2; this means that about 20 per cent of the plasma flowing through the kidney is filtered through the glomerular capillaries.

Physiology

Extra Mile

- The entire plasma volume is only about 3 liters, whereas the GFR is about 180 L/day, the entire plasma can be filtered and processed about 60 times each day.

---

68. Ans. (a) Aldosterone in collecting ducts

Ref: Guyton, 10th ed. pg. 290, 304

Hormones and their site of Action

Hormones	Site of action in kidney
Angiotensin II	Constricts afferent arterioles, helps to reduce GFR
Aldosterone	Cortical collecting duct & distal tubules
ADH	Medullary collecting duct
ANP	Collecting duct

---

69. Ans. (a) Collecting duct

Ref: Ganong, 23rd ed. pg. 648

- Aldosterone is secreted from adrenal cortex.
- Action of aldosterone is localized to distal tubule and collecting duct.
- Mechanism: Stimulates Na^+K^+ ATPase at basolateral end, which generate gradient for movement of sodium ion from apical membrane causing an increase in sodium reabsorption.

---

70. Ans. (b) HCO_3

Ref: Ganong, 25th ed. pg. 641-44

- CO_2 is transported in blood in 3 forms:
    1. **As HCO_3-** CO_2 is **mainly transported** in bicarbonate form ~ 70%. When CO_2 diffuses into RBC, it reacts chemically with water and with help of enzyme carbonic anhydrase it is converted into $HCO_3^- + H^+$
    $CO_2 + H_2O \rightarrow HCO_3 + H^+$

2. **As dissolved CO_2:** 6–7% of CO_2 transport
3. **As carbamino compound of Hb and other plasma proteins:** 20% of CO_2 transport.

---

71. Ans. (d) Sensing of NaCl concentration in macula densa

Ref: Guyton, 11th ed. pg. 323-324

- To perform the function of auto regulation, the kidneys have a feedback mechanism known as tubulo-glomerular feedback which links changes in sodium chloride concentration at the macula densa (tubular component) with the control of renal arteriolar resistance.
- **Macula densa**
    - It is the short segment of renal tubule *at the end of thick ascending limb* & continues into distal tubule.
    - It contains *specialized group of epithelial cells* in the distal tubule *that comes in contact with the efferent and particularly afferent arteriole.*
    - Juxta glomerular apparatus consists of macula densa (in DCT) and JG cells in afferent & efferent arterioles.
    - The macula densa senses the changes in sodium chloride concentration
    - The Na^+ and Cl^- enter the macula densa cells via the $Na^+ –K^+ –2Cl^-$ cotransporter.

---

72. Ans. (d) Na^+

Ref: Guyton Physiology, 11th ed. pg. 55

- Sodium-hydrogen counter-transport occurs in several tissues.
- An important example is in the proximal tubules of the kidneys, where sodium ions move from the lumen of the tubule to the interior of the tubular cell, while hydrogen ions are counter transported into the tubule lumen.

---

73. Ans. (a) PCT mainly

Ref: Renal Physiology, 5th ed. pg. 168

Diuretic class	Drugs	MOA	Site of action
Osmotic diuretic	Mannitol	Inhibit water and solute reabsorption	All part of tubule, *but mainly proximal tubule*
Loop diuretics	Furosemide Torsemide	Inhibit $Na^+-K^+-2Cl^-$ co-transport	Thick ascending loop of henle
Thiazide diuretic	Hydrochlorthiazide Benzthiazide Chlorthalidone Indapamide	Inhibit $Na^+- Cl^-$ co-transport	Distal tubule
K+ sparing diuretic	Spironolactone Triamterene Amiloride	Decrease Na^+ reabsorption Decrease K^+ secretion	Collecting tubule
Carbonic anhydrase inhibitor	Acetazolamide	Inhibit H^+ secretion and HCO_3 reabsorption, which reduces Na^+ reabsorption	Proximal tubule

Explanations

74. Ans. (a) PCT

Ref: Ganong, 25th ed. pg. 713

- 80-90% of bicarbonate is reabsorbed in PCT.
- Absorption of HCO_3 is indirect (due to secretion of H^+ by PCT)
- $H^+ + HCO_3 \rightarrow H_2CO_3 \rightarrow H_2O + CO_2 \rightarrow CO_2$ diffuses into epithelial cell and generate HCO_3 ion which is then reabsorbed.

Extra Mile

- **PCT reabsorbs:** Na^+, Cl, HCO_3, PO_4, K^+, Glucose and amino acid
- **PCT secretes:** H^+ ion, organic acid and bases (oxalate, urate)
- PCT is highly permeable to water.

75. Ans. (a) Beta stimulation

Ref: Harrison, 19th ed. pg. 1613

- The Renin-Angiotensin-Aldosterone System (RAAS) contributes to the regulation of arterial pressure primarily via the vasoconstrictor properties of angiotensin II and the sodium-retaining properties of aldosterone.

There are Three Primary Stimuli for Renin Secretion

1. Decreased NaCl transport in the distal portion of the thick ascending limb of the loop of Henle.
2. Decreased pressure or stretch within the renal afferent arteriole (baroreceptor mechanism)
3. **Sympathetic nervous system stimulation of renin-secreting cells via β1 adrenoreceptors.**

Conversely, RAAS can be Inhibited by

- Increased NaCl transport in the thick ascending limb of the loop of Henle
- Increased stretch within the renal afferent arteriole
- β1 receptor blockade.

76. Ans. (b) Sodium

Ref: Ganong, 22nd ed. pg. 717

- Hyperosmolarity at renal medulla is due to counter current mechanism acting at loop of henle.
- Maximum osmotic gradient is 1200–1400 mOsm/L found in the inner part of medulla at pelvic tip.
- Prime driving force (initiating event) for the countercurrent multiplier system is active reabsorption of Na^+ from thick ascending limb.
- **Renal medullary hyperosmolarity is due to:**
  1. **NaCl** (most important factor causing hyperosmolarity)
  2. Urea
  3. Potassium

77. Ans. (d) Kidney

Ref: Ganong, 23rd ed. pg. 674

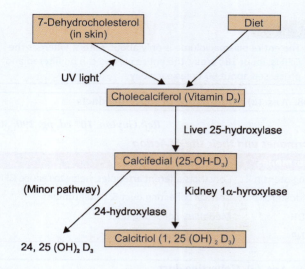

78. Ans. (d) Proximal convoluted tubule

Ref: Ganong, 25th ed. pg. 680, 683

About 2/3rd of filtered water is reabsorbed in the proximal convoluted tubule along with salt absorption. Other molecules absorbed here are bicarbonate, glucose, amino-acids and phosphate.

GASTROINTESTINAL PHYSIOLOGY

79. Ans. (b) Cholesterol Esterase

Ref: Ganong, 25th ed. pg. 482

Cholesterol esterase is a pancreatic lipase activated by bile acids. It causes the following actions

- Hydrolysis of cholesterol esters
- Hydrolysis of esters of fat-soluble vitamins
- Hydrolysis of phospholipids

Most of the fat digestion begins in the duodenum and pancreatic lipase is the most important enzyme. Colipase is activated by trypsin and allows lipase to remain associated with droplets of dietary lipid even in the presence of bile acids.

80. Ans. (a) Trypsinogen

Ref: Ganong, 25th ed. pg 479

- Trypsinogen is converted to active enzyme trypsin by enterokinase when the pancreatic juice enters into the duodenum. Enterokinase contains 41% polysaccharide and this high polysaccharide content prevents the enterokinase from getting digested.
- The trypsin, chymotrypsin and elastase act at interior peptide bonds in the peptide molecules and are called as endopeptidases.

Physiology

81. Ans. (a) Enterochromaffin cell

Ref: Ganong, 25th ed. pg. 457

Enterochromaffin cell is responsible for histamine and serotonin secretion. Chief cells produce pepsinogen.

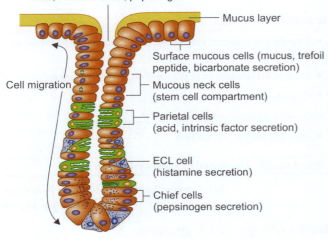

82. Ans. (c) Pancreatic juice

Ref: Ganong, 25th ed. pg. 461

- *Colipase* is secreted in pancreatic juice in inactive form. It is activated in intestinal lumen by trypsin.
- *Lingual lipase* is secreted by Von Ebner's glands.
- *Intestinal lipase* is secreted in succus entericus. Succus entericus is secreted by small intestine and has a pH of 8.3.

TABLE: Enzymes involved in fat digestion

Area	Juice	Enzyme	Substrate
Mouth	Saliva	Lingual lipase	Triglycerides
Stomach	Gastric juice	• Gastric lipase (weak lipase)	• Triglycerides
		• Pancreatic lipase	• Triglycerides
		• Cholesterol ester hydrolase	• Cholesterol ester
		• Phospholipase A	• Phospholipids
Small intestine	Pancreatic juice	• Phospholipase B	• Lysophospholipids
		• Colipase	• Facilitates action of pancreatic lipase
		• Bile-salt-activated lipase	• Phospholipids
			• Cholesterol esters
Small intestine	Succus entericus	Intestinal lipase	Triglycerides

83. Ans. (c) Acid

Ref: Quantitative Human Physiology; An Introduction. pg. 705

Gastric Cells and their Secretion

Cells	Location in stomach	Their secretion
Parietal cell/Oxyntic cell	Body	HCl and intrinsic factor
Chief cells/Peptic cell	Body	Pepsinogen
G cells	Antrum	Gastrin
Mucus neck cells	Oxyntic glands	Mucus

84. Ans. (d) Bicarbonate secretion from pancreas

Ref: Quantitative Human Physiology; An Introduction, pg. 711-712

TABLE: Important differences between GIT hormones (Gastrin, CCK, Secretin, GIP)

	Gastrin	CCK	Secretin	GIP
Site	Main site: G cells (antrum)	I-cells of the proximal two-thirds of small intestine	S-cells: Upper small intestine	K-cells: Proximal intestinal crypts
Actions	**Major:** • Stimulate acid and pepsin secretion • Stimulate gastric motility • Act as growth factor to stimulate mucosal proliferation	**Major:** • Stimulate pancreatic acinar cell enzyme secretion • Stimulate GB contraction • Relaxes sphincter of oddi • Inhibits gastric acid secretion and gastric emptying • Pyloric sphincter contraction	• **Major:** Secretion of HCO_3 from biliary and pancreatic ductular cell and Brunner gland. • Inhibit gastric acid secretion • Stimulate pyloric sphincter • Increases bile flow • Augments the action of CCK	**Major:** Stimulate insulin release from pancreas
Major stimulus	Peptides **(most potent)** Distension of stomach Calcium GRP (gastrin releasing peptides)	Peptides **(most potent)** Fatty acid (BUT NOT TG)	Acid **(most potent)** Digestive protein	Glucose, fat and amino acid

85. Ans. (c) Celiac disease

Ref: Methods in Disease: Investigating the Gastrointestinal Tract by Victor R Preddy pg. 43

- **D-xylose absorption test** is a medical test performed to diagnose conditions that present with malabsorption of the proximal small intestine *due to defects in the integrity of the gastrointestinal mucosa.*
- D-xylose is a monosaccharide, or simple sugar, that **does not require enzymes** for digestion prior to absorption. Its absorption requires an intact mucosa only.
- In this test, the patient ingests D-xylose *(a nondigestible but absorbable carbohydrate)* by mouth, and then the urinary D-xylose is measured.
- Urine excretion below certain levels *(depending on the amount of D-xylose ingested)* implies poor absorption of D-xylose and, therefore, disease of the small intestine.
- Alternatively, a blood level of xylose is measured 2 hours after the D-xylose is taken by mouth. Low levels in the blood imply poor absorption. Abnormal D-xylose tests are most frequently associated with disorders of the small intestine **such as celiac sprue.**
- Malabsorbtion can also occur in pancreatic insufficiency, **but D-xylose test should be normal.**

86. Ans. (a) Carbohydrate malabsorption due to mucosal disorder

Ref: Methods in Disease: Investigating the Gastrointestinal Tract by Victor R Preddy pg. 43

- Xylose is a pentose sugar and is absorbed directly from intestinal nucosa.
- D xylose will reveal carbohydrate malabsorption due to mucosal disorder, **but in malabsorption due to pancreatic disease, the D-xylose test should be normal.**
- Due to high false positives and ease of obtaining small intestinal biopsy after endoscopy, intestinal biopsy is the preferred method.

87. Ans. (c) 70% in gastric phase

Ref: Ganong's, 22nd ed. pg. 484

- Indirect asking for true statement

Phases of Gastric Acid Secretion

- **Cephalic phase:** *Accounts for 20% of secretion* and occurs when food is not even in mouth. It is stimulated by sight or smell of food. The impulses originate in cortex and reach the glands by dorsal motor nuclei and then through vagus nerves.
- **Gastric phase:** *It accounts for around 70% of secretion* and occurs when food reaches stomach. It Occurs by vago gastric reflexes, enter entero reflexes by gastrin.
- **Intestinal phase:** Remaining 10% is produced when food is especially in duodenum. It is caused by reflex feed back.

88. Ans. (c) Oxyntic cells

Ref: Ganong, 23rd ed. pg. 431-32

Secretion in Stomach

- **Oxyntic cell (parietal cell)** secretes: HCl and intrinsic factor of castle
- Chief cell (zymogen or peptic cell) secrete: pepsinogen
- G cell secrete: Gastrin
- D cell secrete: Somatostatin
- ECL cells secrete: Histamine

89. Ans. (b) Decreased by cholecystokinin

Ref: Ganong Review of Medical Physiology, 22nd ed. pg. 484-86

Factors Affecting Gastric Emptying

Decrease emptying	Increase emptying
Cholecystokinin Secretin GIP (Gastric inhibitory peptide) Somatostatin Hyperosmolality of duodenal contents	Carbohydrate rich food leaves stomach in few hours. Protein rich food leaves more slowly & *emptying is slowest after fat rich meal.*

90. Ans. (a) Lipids

Ref: Ganong Review of Medical Physiology, 23 ed. Chapter 28

- *The presence of fat in the small intestine is the most potent inhibitor of gastric emptying, resulting in relaxation of the proximal stomach and diminished contractions of the distal, "gastric grinder" - when the fat has been absorbed, the inhibitory stimulus is removed and productive gastric motility resumes.*
- If the fluid is hypertonic or acidic or rich in nutrients such as fat or certain amino acids, the rate of gastric emptying will be considerably slower and non-exponential.
- Indeed, the rate of gastric emptying of any meal can be predicted rather accurately by knowing its nutrient density.
- Nutrient density is sensed predominantly in the small intestine by osmoreceptors and chemoreceptors, and relayed to the stomach as inhibitory neural and hormonal messages that delay emptying by altering the patterns of gastric motility.

Physiology

91. Ans. (b) Pylorus has more acid secreting cells

Ref: Ganong, 25th ed. pg. 457

- Pylorus is mostly populated with mucus-secreting cells.

GASTRIC GLANDS

- They can be divided into three groups—the pyloric, principal (in the body and fundus) and cardiac glands.

A. Pyloric Glands

- Pyloric glands are mostly *populated with mucus-secreting cells*, parietal cells are few and chief cells scarce. In contrast, neuroendocrine cells are numerous, especially G cells, which secrete gastrin when activated by appropriate mechanical stimulation (causing increased gastric motility and secretion of gastric juices).

B. Principal Glands

- Located in body and fundus
- *Contain distinct cell types: Chief, parietal, mucous neck, stem and neuroendocrine*
1. **Chief cells:** Source of pepsinogen, rennin and lipase. Contain zymogens, contain abundant RNA and hence intensely basophilic
2. **Parietal (oxyntic) cells:** Are the source of gastric acid and intrinsic factor.
3. **Neuroendocrine cells:** Synthesize a number of biogenic amines and polypeptides important for the control of motility and glandular secretion. In the stomach they include cells designated as G cells secreting gastrin, D cells (somatostatin), and ECL (enterochromaffin-like) cells (histamine).

C. Cardiac Glands

- *Mucus-secreting cells predominate* and parietal and chief cells are few.

92. Ans. (b) Ptyalin

Ref: Guyton's Physiology, 11th ed. pg. 793

- Saliva contains two major types of protein secretion:
  - **Serous secretion**- contains ptyalin, an enzyme for digesting starches.
  - **Mucus secretion**

Gland	Secretion	Content	Function
Parotid gland	Serous type	Ptyalin	Digest starches
Submandibular gland	Serous and mucous type	Mucin	Lubricating and for surface protective purposes
Buccal gland	Only mucus	Mucin	Lubricating

- Saliva has a pH between 6.0 and 7.0, a favorable range for the digestive action of ptyalin.
- But before food and its accompanying saliva become completely mixed with the gastric secretions, as much as 30 to 40% of the starches will have been hydrolyzed mainly to form *maltose*.
- *In small intestine the remaining starch Digestion takes place by Pancreatic Amylase*. Pancreatic secretion is almost identical in its function with the α-amylase of saliva but is several times more powerful.
- Hence, within 15 to 30 minutes after the chyme empties from the stomach into the duodenum and mixes with pancreatic juice, nearly all the carbohydrates will have become digested.

93. Ans. (a) Undigested food

Ref: Ganong, 25th ed. pg. 502

- Fecal mass is derived from undigested food.
- Feces are the particles of waste matter that is left over after the body has processed and absorbed nourishment from the foods we eat.
- It contains water, dietary fiber, inorganic salts, dead cells, bacteria, and anything the body cannot or will not absorb.

94. Ans. (b) Bitter

Ref: Ganong, 25th ed. pg. 224

- There are 5 types of taste sensations commonly recognized by humans. Sweet, umami, salty, sour, and bitter.
- None of these tastes are elicited by single chemical. Also, there are different thresholds for detection of taste that differ among chemicals. **The taste having lowest threshold will be most sensitive** (please refer to table)

Taste	Substance	Threshold for tasting
Salty	Sodium chloride	0.01 M
Sweet	Sucrose	0.01 M
Umami	Glutamate	0.0007 M
Sour	Hydrochloric acid	0.09 M
Bitter	Quinine	0.000008 M

95. Ans. (d) Somatostatin

Ref: Ganong, 25th ed. pg. 154

Somatostatin is found in the D cells of pancreatic islets. It inhibits the secretion of insulin, glucagon, and pancreatic polypeptide and may act locally within the pancreatic islets in a paracrine fashion.

FMGE Solutions Screening Examination

96. Ans. (c) Hexoses

Ref: Harrison, 19th ed./Table 26.1 pg. 477

- Hexoses are absorbed most rapidly; Amongst hexoses, glucose and galactose are absorbed more rapidly than others.
- Mannose and pentose are absorbed more slowly.

97. Ans. (a) Trypsin

Ref: Ganong's Physiology, 23rd ed. ch. 27

- *Trypsin converts chymotrypsinogens into chymotrypsins and other proenzymes into active enzymes.* Trypsin can also activate trypsinogen; therefore, once some trypsin is formed, there is an auto-catalytic chain reaction.
- Trypsin, the chymotrypsins, and elastase act at interior peptide bonds in the peptide molecules and are called **endopeptidases**.
- The powerful protein-splitting enzymes of the pancreatic juice are *secreted as inactive proenzymes.*
- *Trypsinogen is converted to the active enzyme trypsin by enterokinase when the pancreatic juice enters the duodenum.*
- *Enterokinase contains 41% polysaccharide,* and this high polysaccharide content apparently *prevents it from being digested itself* before it can exert its effect.

98. Ans. (a) Alkaline content of small intestine

Ref: Guyton's, 11th ed. pg. 776, 784-90

Enterogastric reflex inhibits stomach secretions and motility based on the signals from small intestine and colon.

Enterogastric reflex is stimulated by
Duodenal acidic pH
Duodenal distension
Duodenal hypertonicity
Sympathetic stimulation
Intense pain
Increased osmolality of gastric chime
Inhibited by –
Parasympathetic stimulation
Increased volume and fluidity of gastric content

99. Ans. (d) Divalent metal transporter

Ref: Ganong, 25th ed. pg. 484

- All iron absorption occurs in the duodenum.
- *Transport of iron into the enterocytes occurs via divalent metal transporter 1 (DMT1)*

- Some is stored in form of ferritin and the rest is transported out of enterocytes by basolateral transporter called ferroportin 1
- In plasma Fe2+ is converted to Fe3+ and bound to transport protein transferrin

Transferrin saturation	35%
Plasma iron	110-130 mg/dl

100. Ans. (b) Contraction of Sphincter of oddi

Ref: Ganong, 25th ed. pg. 479

Functions of CCK

- CCK mediates digestion in the small intestine by *inhibiting gastric emptying* and decreasing gastric acid secretion.
- It *stimulates the acinar cells of the pancreas* to release digestive enzymes which catalyze the digestion of fat, protein, and carbohydrates.
- CCK also causes the increased production of hepatic bile
- Stimulates the *contraction of the gall bladder*
- *Relaxation of the Sphincter of Oddi* (Glisson's sphincter), resulting in the delivery of bile into the duodenum.
- Site of CCK release is epithelial cells in the mucosal lining of the small intestine (mostly in the duodenum and jejunum)
- The presence of fatty acids and/or certain amino acids in the chyme entering the duodenum is the greatest stimulator of CCK release.

101. Ans. (b) Entero-endocrine cells in the gut

Ref: Ganong, 25th ed. pg. 470,500

- Site of CCK release is epithelial cells called as I *cells* in the mucosal lining of the small intestine (mostly in the duodenum and jejunum)

102. Ans. (c) Lactase

Ref: Ganong, 25th ed. pg. 461

The enzymes produced by exocrine pancreas are:

1. Trypsinogen
2. Chymotrypsinogens
3. Elastase
4. Carboxypeptidase A and B
5. Colipase
6. Pancreatic lipase
7. Pancreatic alpha amylase
8. Phospholipase A2

Lactase is produced by *cells of intestinal mucosa* to breakdown lactose.

Physiology

103. Ans. (d) Gastro-ileal reflex

Ref: Ganong, 25th ed. pg. 502

- When the food leaves the stomach, caecum relaxes and the passage of chyme through ileocaecal valve increases. This is called as gastro-ileal reflex and is mediated via vagal action.
- Somatostatin is a *growth hormone inhibiting hormone* isolated from hypothalamus and is secreted as paracrine by D cells in pancreatic islets.

Actions of Somatostatin

1. Inhibits VIP, GIP, secretin and motilin
2. Inhibits GH release
3. Inhibits gastric acid secretion and motility
4. Inhibits gall bladder contraction

104. Ans. (c) Normally excreted in urine

Ref: Ganong, 25th ed. pg. 511

- Bilirubin excretion in the urine is seen in obstructive jaundice when conjugated bilirubin regurgitates back into the blood stream since it cannot be excreted secondary to obstruction. This bilirubinuria seen in obstructive jaundice leads to mustard yellow discoloration of the urine. Hence bilirubin in urine indicates a pathology.
- The conjugated bilirubin in normal people is broken down by an enzyme by name of beta-glucuronidase to form unconjugated bilirubin. This is called as enterohepatic cycle. Choice B is correct
- *Conjugation of bilirubin occurs in liver and in case of defective conjugation (Criggler najar syndrome) the levels of unconjugated bilirubin increases to level that it crosses the blood brain barrier and leads to kernicterus. Choice A and D are correct.*

105. Ans. (a) Interstitial cells of Cajal

Ref: Ganong, 25th ed. pg. 496

The basal electrical rhythm is initiated by *interstitial cells of Cajal* which are *stellate mesenchymal parenchymal cells* that send long multiple branched processes into the intestinal smooth muscle.

ENDOCRINE AND REPRODUCTIVE PHYSIOLOGY

106. Ans. (a) 24

Ref: Guyton, 13th ed. pg. 1023

The sperms acquire motility in epididymis and remain there for 18-24 hours. It involves activation of unique set of proteins called CatSper. CatSper forms an alkaline sensitive calcium channel that becomes more active as the sperms go to acidic vagina. The capacitation occurs in female genital tract.

107. Ans. (a) ADH

Ref: Ganong, 25th ed. pg. 442

Glucagon, thyroxine, cortisol and growth hormone increase blood sugar levels and are glucogenic. ADH regulates water re-absorption via the collecting duct.

108. Ans. (a) Calcitriol

Ref: Ganong, 25th ed. pg. 378

The active metabolite of vitamin D3 is produced in kidney and is called calcitriol or 1,25 dihydroxycholecalciferol. The cells of proximal convoluted tubule produce an enzyme by name of 1 alpha hydroxylase that converts 25 hydroxycholecalciferol into 1,25 dihyroxycholecalciferol.

109. Ans. (d) Placenta

Ref: Ganong, 25th ed. pg. 409, 425:

- *Inhibin A is produced by placenta and corpus luteum.* It is used in quadruple screening for prenatal detection of down Syndrome.
- *Inhibin B inhibits FSH in both males and females. It is produced by Sertoli cells in male and granulosa cells in female.*

110. Ans. (a) Insulin

Ref: Ganong, 25th ed. pg. 434

Insulin receptor is a tetramer made of two alpha and two beta glycoprotein proteins. The alpha subunits bind insulin and are extracellular while beta subunits have tyrosine kinase activity. The growth promoting anabolic effects of insulin are mediated by phosphatidyl inositol kinase pathway.

111. Ans. (b) Inhibin B

Ref: Ganong, 25th ed. pg. 409

The image shows feedback regulation of ovarian function. The marking X is of inhibin B which plays an *inhibitory* role in release of FSH from the anterior pituitary.

In contrast oestrogen from theca interna plays an inhibitory role in control of release of LH and GnRH.

112. Ans. (a) PTH

Ref: Harrison 19th edition, P. 2464

- For formation of active form of vitamin D3, proximal convoluted tubule of kidney is the main site.

- The major inducers of activity of 1-α-hydroxylase are PTH and phosphate.
- The repressors of activity of 1-α-hydroxylase are FGF23, calcium and 1,25 (OH)2D.
- The main concept is that 25 hydroxy D regulates its own enzyme 25 hydroxylase activity and 1,25(OH)2 D regulates its own enzyme 1 α Hydroxylase. The two *do not* regulate each others activity.

113. Ans. (a) TSH

Receptors for Hormones

- **Membrane receptor:** They mainly bind peptide hormones and catecholamines
- **Nuclear receptor:** Bind small molecules that can diffuse across the cell membrane, such as steroids and vitamin D.

Note:
- *Guyton states:* "*Amino acid derivatives and peptide hormones interact with cell surface membrane receptors.*"
- *Steroids,* **thyroid hormones***, vitamin D and retinoids are lipid soluble and interact with intracellular nuclear receptors.*

TABLE: Receptors and their respective hormones

Nuclear receptors (Mn: TOAD)	Thyroxine Estrogen Vitamin A Vitamin D
Cytoplasmic receptors	All steroids except Estrogen
Cell membrane via G protein stimulation	All others like ACTH, LH, FSH, GH

114. Ans. (c) Inhibin

Ref: Ganong Physiology, 24th ed. pg, 419 and 420; Guyton's Physiology, 11th ed. pg. 1007

- The walls of the seminiferous tubules are **lined by primitive germ cells and Sertoli cells.**
- **Maturation** of spermatozoa takes place in deep folds of the cytoplasm of the sertoli cells.
- Mature spermatozoa are released from the Sertoli cells and become free in the lumens of the tubules. **The sertoli cells secrete androgen binding protein (ABP), inhibin, and MIS.**
- Inhibin inhibits follicle-stimulating hormone (FSH) secretion.
- Inhibin has a strong direct effect on the anterior pituitary gland to inhibit the secretion of FSH and possibly a slight effect on the hypothalamus to inhibit secretion of GnRH.

Extra Mile

- **Testosterone,** secreted by the *Leydig cells*
- **Luteinizing hormone**—by anterior pituitary gland, stimulates the Leydig cells to secrete testosterone.
- **FSH**—also by the anterior pituitary gland, stimulates the *Sertoli cells*; essential for spermatogenesis.

115. Ans. (d) Delta cells

Ref: Guyton's Physiology, 11th ed. pg. 961

- The human pancreas has 1 to 2 million islets of Langerhans cells
- These islets contain three major types of cells: *alpha*, *beta*, and *delta* cells
- **Beta cells**—60% of all the cells of the islets, lie mainly in the middle of each islet and secrete *insulin* and *amylin*.
- **Alpha cells**—about 25% of the total islets- secrete *glucagon*.
- **Delta cells**—about 10% of the total islets- secrete *somatostatin*.

Extra Mile

The hormones secreted act as control of secretion of some hormones by other hormones:
- Insulin inhibits glucagon secretion
- Amylin inhibits insulin secretion
- Somatostatin inhibits both insulin and glucagon secretion.

In addition to these, somatostatin has other functions:
- It decreases the motility of the stomach, duodenum, and gallbladder.
- It decreases both secretion and absorption in the gastrointestinal tract.

Doing so, somatostatin has following effects:
- It extends the time period over which the food nutrients are absorbed into the blood.
- By inhibiting insulin and glucagon secretion, it prevents rapid utilization of nutrients by the tissues.

Remember: Somatostatin is also known as *growth hormone inhibitory hormone,* which is also secreted in the hypothalamus and suppresses anterior pituitary gland growth hormone secretion.

116. Ans. (a) Cortisol

Ref: Ganong, 22nd ed. ch. 20

- *Cortisol is secreted by adrenal cortex not medulla.*
- Norepinephrine, epinephrine, and dopamine are secreted by the adrenal medulla.

117. Ans. (a) Neuro-hormones

Ref: Lange Medical Physiology by Ganong, ch. 20

Adreno-medullary hormones are *catecholamines* secreted from the adrenal medulla by chromaffin cells, neurosecretory cells connected to the central nervous system.

The synthesis, storage (in chromaffin cells) and release of *catecholamines is co-regulated by synaptic input from their respective pre-synaptic sympathetic neurons, as well as hormonal and local inputs.* The adreno-medullary hormones are:
1. Epinephrine
2. Norepinephrine
3. Dopamine

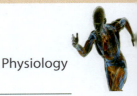

Physiology

118. Ans. (c) Decrease blood amino acid

Ref: Berne & Levy's Physiology, 5th ed. pg. 909 and chapter 20: Lange medical physiology by Ganong 23rd ed.

- *Cortisol raises the free amino acids in the serum. It does this by inhibiting collagen formation, decreasing amino acid uptake by muscle, and inhibiting protein synthesis.*
- Glucocorticoids promote protein degradation and inhibit entry of amino acids in tissues (Primarily Branch chain amino acids).
- Glucocorticoids also lead to utilization of amino acids by promoting gluconeogenesis directly and by permissive effect on Growth hormone.

119. Ans. (b) Oxytocin

TABLE: Hormones from Anterior Pituitary

Hormones	Major functions
Growth hormone	Stimulates protein synthesis and overall growth of most cells and tissues
TSH	Stimulates synthesis and secretion of thyroid hormones (T3 & T4)
Adrenocorticotropic hormone (ACTH)	Stimulates synthesis and secretion of adrenocortical hormones (cortisol, androgens, and aldosterone)
Prolactin	Promotes development of the female breast and *secretion of milk*
Follicle-stimulating hormone (FSH)	Causes growth of follicles in the ovaries and sperm maturation in sertoli cells of testes
Luteinizing hormones (LH)	Stimulates testosterone synthesis in Leydig cells of testes; stimulates ovulation, formation of corpus luteum, and estrogen and progesterone synthesis in ovaries

TABLE: Hormones from Posterior Pituitary

Antidiuretic hormone (ADH)/Vasopressin	Increase water reabsorption by the kidneys and cause vasoconstriction and increased blood pressure
Oxytocin	***Stimulates milk ejection*** from breasts and uterine contractions

120. Ans. (d) Glucagon

- GH secretion is regulated by GHRH released from hypothalamus in a pulsatile fashion.
- Large burst of secretion occurs at night during the onset of deep sleep (NREM sleep).

Stimuli that increase secretion of GH	Stimuli that decreases secretion of GH
• Hypoglycemia • Exercise • Fasting • Protein meals • Stress • **Glucagon** • Estrogens, androgens, L-dopa and alpha adrenergics	• Sleep • Glucose • Cortisol • FFA • GH

121. Ans. (a) Levodopa

Ref: Ganong's, 23rd ed. pg. 333

TABLE: Factors affecting Prolactin secretion

Increase prolactin	Decrease prolactin
• Sleep • Pregnancy; Estrogen • Opioids • TRH • Phenothiazines	• L-Dopa • Apomorphine • Bromocriptine related ergot derivative

122. Ans. (a) Anterior pituitary

Ref: Guyton Physiology 11th ed. pg. 907

- Thyroid stimulating hormone is secreted by anterior pituitary after getting stimulus by TRH (thyrotropin releasing hormone) from hypothalamus.

123. Ans. (b) D_1 Deiodinase

Ref: Harrison, 18th ed./Figure 341-1

- Deiodination is the foremost pathway of thyroid hormone metabolism.
- Three iodothyronine deiodinases (D1-D3) are identified as *seleno cysteino-containing membrane proteins with their active enzymatic sites located in the cytoplasm.*
- D1 and D2 convert T4 to T3.
- D3 has only inner ring deiodination activity and inactivates T4 and T3 to rT3 and T2, respectively

124. Ans. (c) TSH

Ref: Guyton & Hall Textbook of Physiology, 11th ed. pg. 939 and chapter 18: Lange medical physiology by Ganong

Increased thyroid hormone in the body fluids decreases secretion of TSH by the anterior pituitary. When the level

FMGE Solutions Screening Examination

of thyroid hormone secretion rises to about 1.75 times the normal, the rate of TSH secretion falls essentially to zero. Almost all this feedback depressant effect occurs even when the anterior pituitary has been separated from the hypothalamus.

125. Ans. (a) Secreted by pituitary gland

Ref: Ganong's 24th ed. pg. 278; Guyton pg. 1009-1010

- Melatonin is *secreted by pineal[Q] gland*. Its synthesis and *secretion is increased remarkably in the dark period of the day* and maintained at low levels in the daylight.
- It is associated with sleep mechanism.
- *Melatonin based drugs can be used to treat jet lag and insomnia in elderly.*
- It also acts as inhibitor of gonadotropic hormone secretion and the gonads become inhibited and even partly involuted.

126. Ans. (b) Ovulation

Ref: Guyton Physiology, 11th ed. pg. 1027

- While still in the ovary, the ovum is in the primary oocyte stage.
- *Right before it is released from the ovarian follicle*, its nucleus divides by meiosis and a *first polar body is expelled from the nucleus of the oocyte.*
- The primary oocyte then becomes the secondary oocyte.
- In this process, each of the 23 pairs of chromosomes loses one of its partners, which becomes *incorporated in a polar body that is expelled.*
- This leaves 23 unpaired chromosomes in the secondary oocyte. It is at this time that the ovum, still in the secondary oocyte stage, is ovulated into the abdominal cavity.

127. Ans. (c) Nucleus

Ref: Guyton Physiology, 11th ed. pg. 997- 998

- Each spermatozoon is composed of a head and a tail
- *The head comprises the condensed nucleus* of the cell with only a thin cytoplasmic and cell membrane layer around its surface.
- Golgi apparatus form a thick cap called the acrosome which is on the outside of the anterior two thirds of the head.
- The tail of the sperm, called the flagellum, has three major components:
  - A central skeleton constructed of 11 microtubules, collectively called the axoneme
  - A thin cell membrane covering the axoneme
  - A collection of mitochondria surrounding the axoneme in the proximal portion of the tail (called the body of the tail)

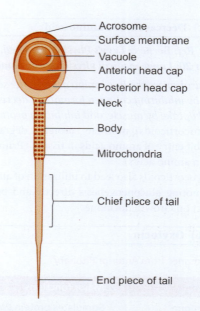

128. Ans. (b) Inhibin

Ref: Ganong Physiology, 24th ed. pg. 419 and 420; Guyton's Physiology, 11th ed. pg. 1007

- The walls of the seminiferous tubules are lined by primitive germ cells and Sertoli cells.
- Maturation of spermatozoa takes place in deep folds of the cytoplasm of the sertoli cells.
- Mature spermatozoa are released from the Sertoli cells and become free in the lumens of the tubules. *The sertoli cells secrete* **androgen binding protein** (ABP), **inhibin**, and **MIS**.
- *Inhibin inhibits follicle-stimulating hormone (FSH) secretion.*
- Inhibin also has a strong direct effect on the anterior pituitary gland to inhibit the secretion of FSH and possibly a slight effect on the hypothalamus to inhibit secretion of GnRH.

> **Extra Mile**
> - *Testosterone*, secreted by the *Leydig cells*
> - *Luteinizing hormone*- Secreted by anterior pituitary gland, stimulates the Leydig cells to secrete testosterone.
> - *FSH*- also secreted by the anterior pituitary gland, stimulates the *Sertoli cells*; essential for spermatogenesis.

129. Ans. (c) Occurs in male genital tract

- Capacitation is a process which makes spermatozoa to undergo the physical changes necessary to fertilize an egg in female genital tract.
- Spermatozoa in male genital tract are exposed to floating vesicles from seminiferous tubules which contain large amount of cholesterol that cover up the sperm acrosome, which make the membrane tough.

Physiology

- *After ejaculation,* the sperm deposited in vagina swim away from cholesterol vesicle upward into the uterine cavity and hence lose excess cholesterol and *membrane of the head of sperm becomes weaker, which makes the penetration in ova easy.*

130. Ans. (a) Obesity

Ref: Guyton Physiology, 11th ed. pg. 871

- Leptin gives a sensation of satiety.
- In case it is defective, person develops irresistible eating tendency, which may lead to obesity.
- *Hypothalamus senses energy storage* through the actions of *leptin,* a peptide hormone *released from adipocytes,* which once released in the circulation occupies its receptors in hypothalamus especially POMC neurons of arcuate nuclei.
- Mutations that render Fat cells unable to produce leptin or mutations that cause defective leptin receptors in the hypothalamus leads to marked hyperphagia and ultimately morbid obesity occurs.

131. Ans. (b) GLUT 2

Transporter	Function	Site of action
SGLT1	Absorption of glucose	Small intestine, renal tubules
SGLT2	Absorption of glucose	Renal tubules
Facilitated diffusion		
GLUT1	Basal glucose uptake	Placenta, blood-brain barrier, brain, red cells, kidneys, colon
GLUT2	B-cell glucose sensor; transport out of intestinal and renal epithelial cells	B cells islets, liver, epithelial cells of small intestine, kidneys
GLUT3	Basal glucose uptake	Brain, placenta, kidneys
GLUT4	Insulin – stimulated glucose uptake	Skeletal and cardiac muscle, adipose tissue, other tissues
GLUT5	Fructose transport	Jejunum, sperm
GLUT6	Unknown	Brain, spleen and leukocytes
GLUT7	Glucose 6-phosphate transporter in endoplasmic reticulum	Liver

132. Ans. (b) Skeletal muscle

- Insulin increases glucose uptake in skeletal muscle.
- Insulin dependent glucose transportation is mediated by GLUT4 which is expressed in skeletal muscles, cardiac muscles and adipose tissue.
- Both GLUT1 and GLUT4 are expressed in skeletal muscle but GLUT4 is main glucose transporter in the tissue.
- GLUT 1 mediates *basal* glucose uptake, whereas GLUT 4 mediates *insulin stimulated* glucose uptake.

133. Ans. (d) Measuring serum progesterone on day 14 of the cycle

Study of cervical mucus	• Estrogen makes the mucus thinner and more alkaline, a change that promotes the survival and transport of sperms. • Progesterone makes it thick, tenacious, and cellular. • The mucus is thinnest at the time of ovulation, and its elasticity, or spinnbarkeit, increases such that by mid-cycle, a drop can be stretched into a long, thin thread that may be 8-23 cm or more in length. • In addition, it *dries in an arborizing, fern-like pattern* when a thin layer is spread on a slide. • After ovulation and during pregnancy, it becomes thick and fails to form pattern.
Basal body temperature	• A convenient and reasonably reliable indicator of the time of ovulation is a change, usually a rise in the basal body temperature. The rise starts 1-2 days after ovulation. • A surge in LH secretion triggers ovulation and ovulation normally occurs about 9 hours after the peak of the LH surge at mid-cycle. The ovum lives for approximately 72 hours after it is extruded from the follicle, but it is fertilizable for a much shorter time than this.
Endo-metrial histol-ogy	• At the end of menstruation, new endometrium regrows under the influence of estrogens. • The endometrium increases rapidly in thickness from the fifth to 14th day of the menstrual cycle. • As the thickness increases, the uterine glands are drawn out so that they length but they do not become convoluted or secrete to any degree. • These endometrial changes are called proliferative, and this part of the menstrual cycle is sometimes called the *proliferative phase*. It is also called the pre-ovulatory or follicular phase of the cycle. • After ovulation, the endometrium becomes highly vascularized and slightly edematous under the influence of estrogen and progesterone from the corpus luteum. The glands become coiled and tortuous and they begin to secrete a clear fluid, consequently, this phase of the cycle is called the *secretory or luteal phase.*

Explanations

134. Ans. (c) Oxytocin

Ref: Ganong, 25th ed. pg. 313

- Oxytocin and vasopressin are typical neural hormones, ie, hormones secreted into the circulation by nerve cells.
- They are secreted from the nerve endings of the supra-optic and paraventricular nuclei of the hypothalamus. These endings are located in the posterior pituitary.

135. Ans. (c) Carbon 17 steroid

Ref: Ganong, 25th ed. pg. 421

- *Testosterone is a C19 steroid with hydroxyl group at 17 position*
- The synthesis occurs from cholesterol in the leydig cells and is formed from androstenedione secreted by adrenal cortex.
- The secretion of testosterone is under the control of LH and the mechanism by which LH stimulates leydig cells involves increased formation of cAMP. This cyclic AMP promotes conversion of cholesterol to pregnenolone and testosterone eventually.

136. Ans. (d) Menstrual blood is predominantly arterial

Ref: Ganong, 25th ed. pg. 401

Proliferative phase by progesterone (Choice A)	Incorrect	It is due to estrogen and endometrial thickness increases from 5th to 14th days of menstrual cycle.
Secretory phase by estrogen (Choice B)	Incorrect	It is due to progesterone and when corpus luteum regresses, there is coiling of spiral arteries.
Superifical 1/3rd of endometrium is shed (Choice C)	Incorrect	Whole of the endometrium except basal layer is shed
Menstrual blood is predominantly arterial (Choice D)	Correct	The menstrual blood is predominantly arterial with only 25% being venous and contains prostaglandins and fibrinolysin.

137. Ans. (a) FSH

Ref: Ganong, 25th ed. pg. 425

Inhibin is a factor of testicular origin that inhibits FSH secretion.

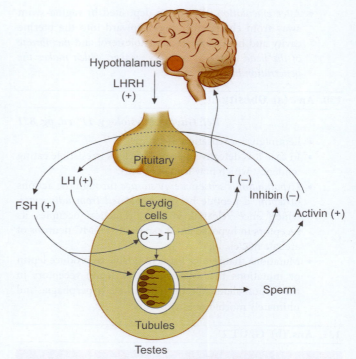

Testosterone from the testis regulates LH secretion.

138. Ans. (d) hCG

Ref: Ganong, 25th ed. /Table 22.5 pg. 412:

Hormone	Time of peak secretion
hCG	First trimester
Relaxin	First trimester
hCS (human chorionic Somatotropin)	Term
Estradiol	Term
Estriol	Term
Progesterone	Term
Prolactin	Term

139. Ans. (a) Cervical mucus

Ref: Ganong 25th ed. pg. 402

- The cervical mucus is thinnest at time of ovulation and its elasticity or spinnbarkeit increases such that by mid-cycle one drop can be stretched into a long, thin thread that may be 8-12cm or more in length.
- *It dries on a slide in an arborizing fern like pattern.*
- After ovulation it becomes thick and fails to form the fern pattern.

Physiology

RESPIRATORY PHYSIOLOGY

140. Ans. (b) Pressure in alveoli and intrapleural pressure

- Transpulmonary pressure is the difference between *intrapulmonary* (also known as intraalveolar or airway) pressure and *intrapleural pressure*

141. Ans. (d) 0.9–1.0

- Respiratory quotient (RQ) is the ratio in the steady state of the volume of carbon dioxide produced to the volume of oxygen consumed per unit time.
- RQ of the brain is 0.97–0.99; this is *because the principal fuel for the brain is carbohydrates.*

142. Ans. (c) 16 mm Hg

Ref: Guyton's Physiology, 11th ed. pg. 162

- Pulmonary artery systolic pressure averages about 24 mm Hg and diastolic pressure 8mm Hg, with *a mean pulmonary arterial pressure of only 16 mm Hg.*
- The mean pulmonary capillary pressure averages only 7 mm Hg.
- Mean pressure in the aorta is high, averaging about 100 mm Hg.

143. Ans. (c) 160

- At sea level the atmosphere exerts a total pressure of 760 mm Hg. Since the atmosphere is 21% O_2 (by volume), the partial pressure of oxygen (pO_2)= 0.21 × 760 = 160 mm Hg.
- The partial pressure of CO_2 (pCO_2) at sea level is 0.23 mm Hg.

144. Ans. (a) V/Q ratio is high at the apex of the lung

Ref: Ganong, 24th ed. pg. 636-37

- The ratio of pulmonary ventilation to pulmonary blood flow for the whole lung at rest is about 0.8.
- There is marked difference in this ventilation /perfusion ratio in various parts of the normal lung as a result of the effect of gravity.
- The ventilation/perfusion ratios are high in the upper portions of the lungs.
- In an upright posture ventilation (V) is high and perfusion (Q) is low at the apex of lung.
- While on the other hand ventilation is low and perfusion is high at the base of lung.

145. Ans. (d) Volume remaining after normal expiration

Ref: Ganong, 25th ed. pg. 629

LUNG VOLUME

Tidal volume (T.V) N = 500 ml	Air that moves in or out of the lung with each normal inspiration or expiration
Inspiratory reserve volume (IRV) N = 3300 ml	The air inspired with a maximal inspiratory effort in excess of tidal volume
Expiratory reserve volume (ERV) N = 1000 ml	The air expelled with a maximal expiratory effort in excess of tidal volume
Residual volume (RV) N = 1200 ml	The amount of air remaining in the lungs even after forced expiration

LUNG CAPACITIES

Inspiratory capacity (I.C) = (TV + IRV) N = 3800 ml	Total amount of air that can be breathed in.
Vital capacity; VC = TV + IRV + ERV N = 4800 ml	Maximum amount of air that can be expelled out force fully after a maximal (deep) inspiration
Functional residual capacity FRC = ERV + RV N = 2200 ml	It is the volume of air remaining in the lung after normal expiration (after normal tidal expiration)
Total lung capacity TLC = TV + IRV + ERV + RV N = 6000 ml. (4.2-6 lit)	The amount of air present in the lung after a maximal inspiration. This is the maximum volume to which the lungs can be expanded.

146. Ans. (c) Type II Pneumocytes

Ref: Guyton, 11th ed pg. 474,

- The smaller type II pneumocytes are often more numerous than type I pneumocytes, but they contribute less than 10% of the surface area.
- They are rounded cells which protrude from the alveolar surface, particularly at the angles between alveolar profiles.
- In the human lung they are often associated with interalveolar pores of Kohn. Their cytoplasm contains numerous characteristic secretory lamellar bodies, which they can recycle.
- Ultrastructurally, the lamellar bodies are comprised of concentric whorls of phospholipid-rich membrane, the precursors of alveolar surfactant.
- *"Surfactant is stored in lamellar bodies and secreted in the form of tubular myelin (unrelated to myelin of the nervous system) by type II pneumocytes.* It is recycled by type II pneumocytes, or cleared (phagocytosed) by alveolar macrophages.
- Clara cells of the bronchiolar epithelium serve as progenitor cells. They are nonciliated cuboidal epithelial cells in terminal bronchioles.

FMGE Solutions Screening Examination

147. Ans. (c) Immunoglobulin A

Ref: Ganong, 24th ed. pg. 77-78

- The activated B cells proliferate and transform into memory B cells and plasma cells.
- The plasma cells secrete large quantities of antibodies into the general circulation known as immunoglobulins.

Immunoglobulins	Function
IgG	Complement activation
IgA	Localized protection in external secretions (tears, intestinal secretions, etc)
IgM	Complement activation^Q
IgD	Antigen recognition by B cells
IgE	Reagin activity; releases histamine from basophils and mast cells

148. Ans. (d) Oxygen

Ref: Ganong 25th ed. Table 36. 1 pg. 657 & 659 and Guyton's, 11th ed. pg. 516

- The ultimate goal of respiration is to maintain proper concentration of oxygen, carbon dioxide and hydrogen ions in the tissues.
- Excess carbon dioxide or excess hydrogen ions in the blood mainly act directly on the respiratory centre.
- Oxygen, in contrast, does not have a significant direct effect on the respiratory center of the brain in controlling respiration.
- Instead oxygen acts almost entirely on peripheral chemoreceptors located in the carotid and aortic bodies, and these in turn transmit appropriate nervous signals to the respiratory center for control of respiration by detecting O_2 level in blood.

▶ **Extra Mile**

Central Chemoreceptors
- More powerful, less rapid than peripheral chemoreceptor
- Highly sensitive to changes in $PaCO_2$ or H^+
- $PaCO_2$: most important stimulus for central chemoreceptor.
- High $PaCO_2$ stimulates respiratory center which then increases alveolar ventilation and vice versa.

149. Ans. (a) Oxygen and nitrogen

Ref: Ganong's, 22nd ed. Chapter 37

Potential problems associated with exposure to increased barometric pressure under water:
- **Oxygen toxicity:** Lung damage, Convulsions
- **Nitrogen narcosis:** Euphoria, Impaired performance
- **High-pressure nervous syndrome:** Tremors, somnolence
- **Decompression sickness:** Pain, Paralysis
- **Air embolism:** Sudden death

150. Ans. (a) Increased hemoglobin content and RBC

Ref: Guyton's Physiology, 11th ed. pg. 539-541

- **Acclimatization:** Adaptation to new temperature or altitude so that hypoxia causes lesser effect to body.
- At high altitude there is low oxygen. When a person remains exposed to low oxygen, the hematocrit rises slowly from a normal value of 40–45 to an average of about 60.

▶ **Extra Mile**

- A person remaining at high altitudes for days, weeks, or years becomes more and more *acclimatized* to the low pO_2.
- The principle means by which acclimatization comes about are:
  - **Increased** pulmonary ventilation
  - **Increased** numbers of RBC.
  - Increased diffusing capacity of the lungs.
  - increased vascularity of the peripheral tissues, and
  - **Increased** ability of the tissue cells to use oxygen despite low PO_2

- And an increase in hemoglobin concentration from normal of 15 g/dL to about 20 g/dL.
- In addition, the blood volume also increases, often by 20 to 30 per cent.

151. Ans. (c) Due to inadequate gas exchange

Ref: Ganong, 25th ed. pg. 651

- Hypoxic hypoxia is due to *inadequate gas exchange*, in which the oxygen content of arterial blood and PO_2 are reduced. Example: COPD, High altitude.

Types of Hypoxia and causes

Type of hypoxia	Pathophysiology	Example
Anemic Hypoxia	Due to reduced oxygen carrying capacity	Anemia (Reduced RBC, Reduced Hb); CO poisoning
Hypoxic Hypoxia	Due to Inadequate gas exchange	High altitude Respiratory disease (COPD)
Histotoxic Hypoxia	Inability of cells to utilize available O_2	Cyanide poisoning
Stagnant Hypoxia	Due to slow circulation	Circulatory Shock Congestive heart failure

152. Ans. (b) Hering Breur Reflex

Ref: Ganong, 25th ed. pg. 662

- Hering- Breuer reflex is reflex *triggered to prevent over inflation of lung*.
- Smooth muscles of lung have pulmonary stretch receptors which respond to excessive stretching of lung during large inspirations.

- The reflex limits the tidal volume while increasing the respiratory frequency
- Hering Breur inflation reflex is increase in duration of expiration produced by steady lung inflation.
- Hering breur deflation reflex is a decrease in duration of expiration produced by steady lung deflation.
- Surfactant prevents collapse of the lung.

153. Ans. (c) Decreased H⁺

Ref: Ganong, 25th ed. pg. 640-641

OXYGEN HEMOGLOBIN DISSOCIATION CURVE

- Oxygen- hemoglobin dissociation curve is sigmoid 'S' shaped because *binding of one oxygen molecule to heme increases the affinity of second heme molecule for oxygen and so on.*

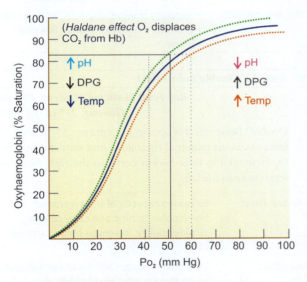

Factors affecting affinity of Hb for oxygen and causing the shift of curve are:

Left shift	Right Shift
• This means the *affinity of oxygen to Hb is increased and oxygen is bound more tightly to hemoglobin*	• This means the affinity of O_2 to Hb is decreased which *favours release of oxygen to tissue.*
• Factors leading to left shift are:	• Factors leading to right shift are:
▪ Alkalosis or ↑pH	▪ Acidosis or ↓ pH
▪ ↓ pCO_2 (CO_2 content of blood)	▪ ↑ pCO_2 (CO_2 content of blood)
▪ ↓ Temperature (Hypothermia)	▪ ↑ Temperature (Hypothermia)
▪ ↓ 2,3 DPG	▪ ↑ 2,3 DPG

154. Ans. (b) Shift of Oxy-Hb dissociation curve to right

Ref: Ganong's Physiology, 23rd ed. pg. 611 and Ganong, 25th ed. pg. 640-41

Refer to the above question. Increased carbon dioxide in blood will lead to respiratory acidosis, and shift curve to right.

155. Ans. (d) Binding of oxygen molecule increases affinity of binding other oxygen molecule

Ref: Ganong's, 23rd ed. pg. 610

- S-shape of O_2-Hb dissociation curve is formed when one oxygen molecule (among the 4 that is supposed to bind with Hb) binds with a hemoglobin molecule with greatest affinity and this binding increases affinity of other heme molecule to bind oxygen.
- Fall in pH due to increase pCO_2, decreases oxygen affinity of Hb. This phenomenon is known as **Bohr's effect.**
- Binding of O_2 to Hb reduces affinity of Hb to CO_2. This phenomenon is known as **Haldane effect.**

156. Ans. (d) Alkalosis

Ref: Ganong, 25th ed. pg. 640-41

Refer to above explanation

157. Ans. (a) Reflex bradycardia

Ref: Ganong, 25th ed. pg. 662

Pulmonary Chemo-Reflex Consists of:[Q]
1. Apnea followed by Rapid breathing
2. Bradycardia
3. Hypotension

It is caused by Stimulation of J receptors by intravenous or intra-cardiac administration of chemicals like capsaicin.

158. Ans. (c) Increase in depth of respiration

Ref: Ganong, 25th ed. pg. 656

Manifestation after both vagi are cut	Stretching of the lungs during inspiration initiates impulses in afferent pulmonary vagal discharges. These impulses inhibit inspiratory discharge. Hence after Vagotomy the impulses inhibiting inspiratory discharge are absent and this will result in *increase of depth of respiration.*
Manifestation after Pneumotaxic center is damaged	Pneumotaxic center is dorsal pons which contains neurons active in active inspiration and expiration. When this area is damaged *respiration will become slower and tidal volume greater.*
Manifestation after both vagi are cut along with damage to Pneumotaxic center	If vagi are cut after damage to pneumotaxic centre, *apneusis*[Q] (Prolonged inspiratory spasms that resemble breath holding) will develop

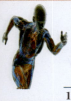

FMGE Solutions Screening Examination

159. Ans. (d) 10 seconds

Ref: Harrison, 18th ed. pg. 2186

- Apneas are defined in adults as breathing pauses lasting >10 secs. and hypopneas as events > 10 secs in which there is continued breathing but ventilation is reduced by at least 50% from the previous baseline during sleep.
- Obstructive sleep apnea/hypopnea syndrome is defined as the coexistence of unexplained excessive daytime sleepiness with at least five obstructed breathing events per hour of sleep.
- **Epworth sleepiness score** is used to assess the severity of the problem.

160. Ans. (c) Slower Breathing with greater tidal volume

Ref: Ganong, 25th ed. pg. 656

- Pneumotaxic center is dorsal pons which contains neurons active in active inspiration and expiration.
- When this area is damaged respiration will become slower and tidal volume greater.

161. Ans. (a) Apnea followed by rapid shallow breathing

Ref: Ganong, 25th ed. pg. 592

- Since the C fiber endings are close to pulmonary vessels, they are called as J (Juxta-capillary) receptors.
- They are stimulated by hyperinflation of the lung.
- Activation of chemo-sensitive vagal C fibers in the cardio-pulmonary region causes profound bradycardia, hypotension and apnea followed by rapid shallow breathing. This is called as pulmonary chemo-reflex.

Hering breuer reflexes are mediated by vagal afferent activity is mediated by slowly adapting receptors and causes shortening of inspiration.

- *Hering Breur inflation reflex is an* increase in duration of expiration produced by steady lung inflation
- *Hering Breur deflation reflex* is a decrease in duration of expiration produced by marked deflation of lung.

162. Ans. (a) 1

Ref: Ganong, 25th ed. pg. 641

Myoglobin is an iron containing pigment found in skeletal muscle and binds to 1 rather than 4 mol of O_2.

- The lack of cooperative binding is reflected in myoglobin dissociation curve which is rectangular hyperbola.
- The steepness of the curve shows that oxygen is released at low pO_2 values like at exercise.

163. Ans. (a) 0.8

Ref: Ganong, 25th ed. pg. 636

Ventilation = 4.2 L/min

Perfusion = 5.5 L/ min blood flow
Ventilation/perfusion ratio = 0.8

164. Ans. (a) Tidal volume × Respiratory rate

Ref: Ganong, 25th ed. pg. 629

RMV: Respiratory minute volume: 500 mL × 12 breaths/min = 6 L

165. Ans. (c) Tidal volume + Volume inspired forcefully

Functional residual Capacity	It represents the volume of air remaining in the lungs after expiration of a normal breath.
Inspiratory capacity	It is the maximum amount of air inspired from end expiratory level.
Vital lung capacity	Maximum amount of air expired from fully inflated lung.
Total lung capacity	Inspiratory reserve volume + Tidal volume + Expiratory reserve volume+ Residual volume

166. Ans. (b) Double Bohr Effect

Ref: Fetal Medicine 1st ed. pg. 403 and Ganong, 25th ed. pg. 641-2

Double[Q] Bohr Effect is seen in placenta as CO_2 liberated by fetus enters the maternal circulation and shifts the maternal O_2 Hemoglobin dissociation curve to the right but shifts fetal curve to the left.

Haldane effect	Increased capacity of deoxygenated hemoglobin to bind and carry carbon dioxide leading to venous blood carrying CO_2.
Bohr effect	Decrease in oxygen affinity of hemoglobin when there is a fall in pH of blood.
Hamburger phenomenon	It is also called chloride shift. • When RBC's take up carbon dioxide, it is converted into bicarbonate inside the RBC • This bicarbonate is negatively charged and leaves the RBC via anion exchanger[Q] 1 /Band 3 protein. • In return chloride enters the RBC. • Hence there is gain of osmotic molecule inside the RBC leading to entry of water into the cell leading the RBC to swell up.

167. Ans. (b) >5 gm%

Ref: Ganong, 25th ed. pg. 642

Cyanosis appears whenever the magnitude of reduced hemoglobin level of blood in capillaries is >5 gm%.

168. Ans. (b) Pre-botzinger complex

Ref: Ganong, 25th ed. pg. 656

Prebotzinger complex- located between nucleus ambiguous and lateral reticular nucleus on either side of medulla is the site of generation of respiratory rhythm.

CARDIOVASCULAR AND CIRCULATORY PHYSIOLOGY

169. Ans. (b) First heart sound has maximum duration

Heart sound	Frequency	Duration	Associated event
First heart	25–45 Hz	0.15 sec	Closure of A-V valves—onset of ventricular systole
Second heart sound	50 Hz	0.12 sec	Closure of semilunar valves—onset of ventricular diastole
Third heart sound	Low	0.1 sec	First rapid filling phase of ventricular diastole
Fourth heart sound	Below 20 Hz	0.1 sec	Last rapid filling phase of ventricular diastole due to atrial contraction

170. Ans. (b) Modified muscle fibers

- Purkinje fibers are **modified myocardial muscle fibres** (NOT nerve fibers) that lead from the A-V node through the A-V bundle into the ventricles.
- These fibers have functional characteristics that are quite **the opposite of those of the A-V nodal fibers** *(except for the initial portion of these fibers where they penetrate the A-V fibrous barrier)*
- **Purkinje fibers are very large fibres**, larger than AV nodal fibers and even larger than the normal ventricular muscle fibers.
- Hence they transmit **action potentials at a velocity of 1.5 to 4.0 m/sec**, which is about **6 times** that in the usual ventricular muscle and **150 times that in some of the A-V nodal fibres.**
- This allows almost instantaneous transmission of the cardiac impulse throughout the entire remainder of the ventricular muscle.

171. Ans. (b) After load

Ref: Current Obstetric and Gynecology by Mukherjee pg. 52

- In the normal fetuses, blood flow in the ductus venosus is always antegrade throughout the cardiac cycle.

Forward flow in the venous system is a function of cardiac compliance, contractility and afterload.
- The typical waveform of fetal blood flow in the venous vessels consists of 3 phases related to the cardiac cycle *(on Doppler)*:
  - **Peak S wave:** Corresponds to ventricular systole
  - **Peak D wave:** Corresponds to early diastole
  - **Peak A wave:** Corresponds to atrial contraction.

172. Ans. (c) Increase hydrostatic pressure, decrease oncotic pressure

- Starling's hypothesis states that the fluid movement due to filtration across the wall of a capillary is dependent on the balance between the hydrostatic pressure gradient and the oncotic pressure gradient across the capillary.

The four Starling's forces are:

1. Hydrostatic pressure in the capillary (Pc)
2. Hydrostatic pressure in the interstitium (Pi)
3. Oncotic pressure in the capillary (pc)
4. Oncotic pressure in the interstitium (pi)

The balance of these forces allows calculation of the net driving pressure for filtration.

Net Driving Pressure = [(Pc - Pi) - (pc - pi)]

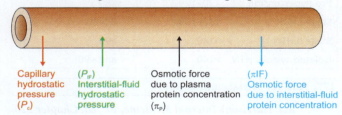

173. Ans. (b) Left ventricle works more than right ventricle

Ref: Guyton Physiology, 11th ed. pg. 110

- Right ventricular external work output is normally about *one sixth the work output of the left ventricle* because of the six-fold difference in systolic pressures that the two ventricles pump.

174. Ans. (b) AV node shows fast conduction

175. Ans. (c) Decreases by increase in heart rate

Ref: Ganong, 25th ed. pg. 570-71

- *Basically it is asking here about the TRUE statement among the given choices.*
- Stroke volume is indirectly proportional to heart rate
- Stroke volume = cardiac output/heart rate
- *As the heart rate increases, stroke volume decreases.*
- After load is determined by peripheral resistance. Therefore, it has nothing to do with stroke volume determination.

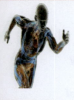

FMGE Solutions Screening Examination

- Stroke volume depends upon end diastolic volume (NOT pre-diastolic volume)

176. Ans. (d) >170 mm Hg

Ref: Harrison's, 19th ed. pg. 1616

TABLE: Guidelines for threshold values between normal and high blood pressure

	Clinic measurement (mm Hg)	Home measurement (mm Hg)
Optimal control	<140/85	<130/80
Mild hypertension	140-150/90-100	135-145/85-95
Moderate hypertension	150-170/100-110	145-165/95-105
Severe hypertension	>170/110	>165/105

The question mentioned was severe hypertension, however if the grading of hypertension is asked, then answer must be according to this table:

BP classification	Systolic mm Hg	Diastolic, mm Hg
Normal	<120	and <80
Pre-hypertension	120–129	<80
Stage I HTN	130–139	80–89
Stage II HTN	>140	>90
Isolated systolic HTN	>140	and <90

177. Ans. (c) Atrial contraction

Ref: Harrison's Internal Medicine, 17th ed. Chapter 220, PE of CVS.

NORMAL JVP WAVEFORM

- Classically three upward deflections and two downward deflections have been described.
- **The "a" wave corresponds to right Atrial contraction** and ends synchronously with the carotid artery pulse. The peak of the 'a' wave demarcates the end of atrial systole.
- **The 'c' wave corresponds to right ventricular contraction** causing the tricuspid valve to bulge towards the right atrium.
- **The 'x' descent** follows the 'a' wave and corresponds to atrial relaxation and rapid atrial filling due to low pressure.
- The "x" (x prime) descent follows the 'c' wave and occurs as a result of the right ventricle pulling the tricuspid valve downward during ventricular systole.
- **The "v" wave** corresponds to venous filling when the tricuspid valve is closed and venous pressure increases from venous return – this occurs during and following the carotid pulse.
- **The "y" descent** corresponds to the rapid emptying of the atrium into the ventricle following the opening of the tricuspid valve.

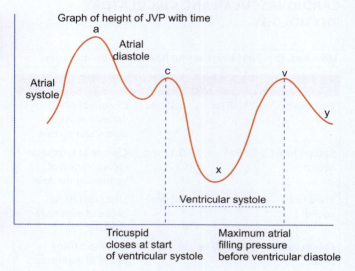

Extra Mile

About JVP

Raised JVP, Normal waveform	Raised JVP, absent pulsation:	Large 'a' wave (increased atrial contraction pressure)
Bradycardia Fluid overload Heart Failure	Superior vena cava syndrome **Cardiac Tamponade**	Tricuspid stenosis Right heart failure Pulmonary hypertension
Cannon 'a' wave (atria contracting against closed tricuspid valve)	**Absent 'a' wave (no unifocal atrial depolarization)**	**Paradoxical JVP (Kussmaul's sign: JVP rises with inspiration, drops with expiration)**
Atrial flutter Premature atrial rhythm (or tachycardia) Third degree heart block Ventricular ectopics Ventricular tachycardia	Atrial fibrillation	Pericardial effusion Constrictive pericarditis Pericardial tamponade

Physiology

- **Large 'v' wave (c-v wave):** Tricuspid regurgitation
- Slow 'y' descent: Tricuspid stenosis

178. Ans. (b) Maximum during diastole

Ref: Ganong 25th ed. pg. 611

- The Flow in coronary arteries occurs in the sub-endocardial portion of the left ventricle only during diastole, although the force is sufficiently dissipated in the more superficial portions of the left ventricular myocardium to permit some flow in this region throughout the cardiac cycle.
- Because *no blood flow occurs during systole in the sub-endocardial portion of the left ventricle, this region is prone to ischemic damage* and is the most common site of myocardial infarction.

179. Ans. (b) Endocardium to epicardium

Ref: Ganong's Physiology, 23rd ed. chapter 30

- Depolarization: From endocardium to epicardium
- Repolarization always proceeds from epicardium to endocardium leading to positive T wave in all leads.
- Depolarization of the ventricular muscle starts at the left side of the interventricular septum and moves first to the right across the mid portion of the septum.
- The wave of depolarization then spreads down the septum to the apex of the heart.
- It returns along the ventricular walls to the AV groove, proceeding from the endocardial to the epicardial surface.
- The last parts of the heart to be depolarized are the postero-basal portion of the left ventricle, the pulmonary conus, and the uppermost portion of the septum.
- In isolated myocardial fibre direction of depolarization and repolarization is same

180. Ans. (d) Increase in venous capacitance

Ref: Ganong's Physiology, 23rd ed. chapter 17

SYMPATHETIC STIMULATION

Beta 1 Receptor –

- **SA node:** Increase in heart rate
- **AV node:** Increase in conduction velocity
- **HIS Purkinje system:** Increase in conduction velocity
- **Atria:** Increase in contractility and conduction velocity
- **Ventricle:** Increase in contractility

Alpha 1 Receptor–

- Increase in total peripheral resistance leads to increase in BP.

181. Ans. (b) ST segment is 0.40 seconds

Ref: Ganong, 25th ed. pg. 524

ECG INTERVALS

PR interval	0.12-0.2 sec	Atrioventricular conduction
QRS	0.08 sec-0.1 sec	Ventricular depolarization
QT interval	0.40-0.43 sec	Ventricular action potential
ST segment		*Plateau portion of the ventricular action potential*

Normal AV nodal delay is due to slow propogation via the AV node and is 0.1 seconds.

182. Ans. (c) Middle of R to end of T wave

Ref: Ganong, 25th ed. pg. 541

Atrial systole	Beginning of P wave and peak of R wave
Ventricular systole	Middle of R wave and end of T wave
Ventricular diastole	End of T wave and beginning of next P wave

FMGE Solutions Screening Examination

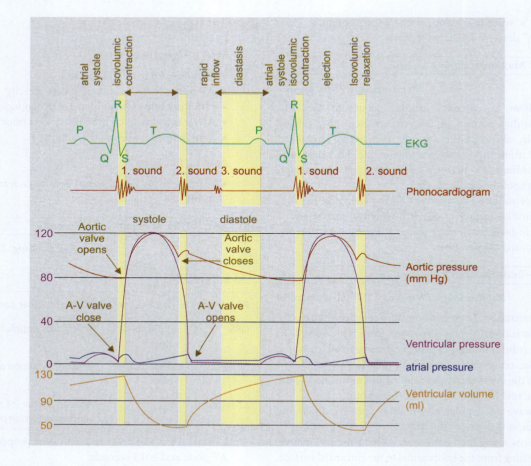

183. Ans. (b) Closure of aortic and pulmonic valves

Ref: Ganong, 25th ed. pg. 540

The Dicrotic notch is small oscillations on the falling phase of the pulse wave caused by vibrations set up when the aortic valve snaps shut.

184. Ans. (b) Explains the increase in cardiac output when venous return is increased

Ref: Ganong, 25th ed. pg. 546

- Frank starling law states that energy of contraction is directly proportional to initial length of cardiac muscle fiber.
- Hence in case of more blood coming on to the right side of the heart, the length of muscle fiber will increase and this will result in increase in force of contraction of heart.

185. Ans. (b) Oscillometry

Ref: Ganong, 25th ed. pg. 543

Doppler	Based on acoustics of sound waves
Thermodilution method	Cold Saline is injected into right atrium and temperature change in blood is recorded in pulmonary artery. The temperature change in pulmonary artery shall be inversely related to blood flow.
Fick's principle	Amount of substance taken up by an organ is equal to arterial level of substance minus the venous level of substance times the blood flow.

186. Ans. (d) Peripheral resistance increases

Ref: Ganong, 25th ed. pg. 549

- Blood flow of resting skeletal muscle is low (2-4 ml/100 gm/min)
- When the muscle contracts, it compresses the vessels and when it develops 70% of its maximal tension, blood is completely interrupted.
- Between contractions the flow is increased by 30 times
- This is due to dilatation of arterioles and precapillary sphincters cause of 10-100 times increase in open capillaries

Physiology

- *During exercise there is a net fall in peripheral resistance,* due to vasodilation in exercising muscles. Hence the SBP increases moderately and diastolic pressure remains unchanged or falls.

187. Ans. (a) Increase in rate of transmission

Ref: Ganong, 25th ed. pg. 545

Effect on heart rate = Chronotropic action
Effect on force of contraction = Inotropic action
Effect on rate of transmission = Dromotropic action

188. Ans. (b) C wave is called as dicrotic notch

Ref: Ganong, 25th ed. pg. 542

A wave	Atrial systole
C wave	Bulge of tricuspid valve into right atrium during isovolumetric contraction
X descent	Atrial relaxation
V wave	Beginning of isovolumetric relaxation
Y descent	Ventricular relaxation

Dicrotic Notch is seen in Pulse recording.

189. Ans. (a) Fluctuation in BP with respiration

Ref: Textbook of Medical Physiology, 2nd ed. pg. 435

Traube Hering Waves are oscillations in BP that occur with a frequency of 4/min, and are attributable to rhythmic oscillations in intensity of sympathetic vasomotor discharge.

TRAUBE–HERING WAVES

These are formed by fluctuation in BP synchronous with respiration. The wave shows a rise in pressure during inspiration and a fall during expiration. *These waves are produced due to change in vagal and sympathetic activity in different phases of respiration.* The vasomotor centre is stimulated during inspiration by the irradiation of impulses from the inspiratory centres which causes rise in blood pressure. Also during expiration, the intrathoracic pressure becomes less negative, therefore venous return decreases which in turn decreases cardiac output and BP.

Extra Mile

- **Traube semilunar space:** A crescentic space about 12 cm wide, just above the costal margin.
- **Traube sign:** A murmur heard in auscultation over arteries in significant aortic regurgitation.

190. Ans. (c) Venule

Ref: Ganong, 25th ed. pg. 568

- Maximum cross sectional area is of capillaries. But it is *not* given in choices.

- The second most extensive cross sectional area is of venules.
- *However the maximum of percentage of blood volume is in venules + veins and vena cava and constitutes 54% of total blood volume contained.*

Vessel	Cross sectional area	% of blood volume contained
Capillary	4500 cm²	5%
Venule	4000 cm²	54%
Arteriole	400 cm²	1%
Artery	20 cm²	8%
Aorta	4.5 cm²	2%

191. Ans. (c) 15 seconds

Ref: Ganong, 25th ed. pg. 573

The normal arm to tongue circulation time is 15 seconds and is measured by injecting a bile salt preparation into the arm vein and timing when the bitter taste will appear in the tongue of the patient.

CNS AND PNS PHYSIOLOGY

192. Ans. (a) Tone

Ref: Ganong, 25th ed. pg. 232-33

- The resistance of muscle to stretch is called tone or tonus
- *Spasticity* is found with upper motor neuron injuries and manifests as a marked resistance to the initiation of rapid passive movement. This initial resistance gives way and then there is less resistance over the remaining range of motion (clasp-knife phenomenon).
- *Rigidity* is an increase in tone that persists throughout the passive range of motion. This has been termed "lead pipe" rigidity and is common with extrapyramidal disease, especially Parkinson's disease.
- *Paratonia* is a phenomenon in which the patient is essentially unable to relax during passive movements. You will note that the resistance is irregular and generally greatest when you change the pattern of movement. Extreme paratonia is common in patients with dementia.

193. (a) Arcuate fasciculus

Ref: Ganong, 25th ed. pg. 292

Arcus Fasiciculus connects the Broca's area to Wernicke's area. It is a white matter tract and damage to this area will result in conduction aphasia where repetition will be affected.

FMGE Solutions Screening Examination

Extra Mile

Lesion at	Manifestation
Broca' area	Motor aphasia
Wernicke's area	Receptive Dysphasia
Arcuate fasciculus	Conduction aphasia

194. Ans. (d) Ventral tegmental area

Ref: Harrison, 20th ed. pg. 174

Neurons in forebrain ventral tegmental area and nucleus accumbens are involved in motivated behaviours like laughter, pleasure, addiction and fear. These areas are called reward centre. The mesocortical dopaminergic neurons that project from midbrain to nucleus accumbens and frontal cortex are also involved.

Extra Mile

Highly addictive drugs like morphine, heroin, cocaine increase the Dopamine which acts on D3 receptors in nucleus accumbens and is responsible for addictive behaviour.

195. Ans. (a) Ventrolateral thalamus

Ref: Ganong, 25th ed. pg. 270

Part of thalamus	Function
Ventrolateral and Ventro-anterior nuclei	Motor function. They receive input from basal ganglia and cerebellum and project to motor nucleus.
Medial geniculate body Lateral geniculate body	Specific sensory relay nuclei Medial geniculate relays auditory and lateral geniculate body relays motor information.
Ventral posteromedial Ventral posterolateral	Relay somatosensory information to post central gyrus

196. Ans. (c) Hyperalgesia

- Choice A, hypersensitivity is a non-specific term.
- Choice B, causalgia characterized by severe burning pain in a limb caused by injury to a peripheral nerve.
- Choice C, Hyperalgesia is heightened response to a minimal pain stimulus. Example gently pinching on arm is causing extreme pain reaction.
- Choice D, Allodynia is pain due to a stimulus that does not usually provoke pain example cold air from AC duct is causing sensation of pain

197. Ans. (d) Muscle spindle

Ref: Ganong 25th ed. Table 8.1: P 160

- The stretch stimulus is mediated by muscle spindle and tension by golgi tendon organ.
- Choice A Merkel's disc perceives touch and pressure.
- Choice B Meissner corpuscle perceives tap and flutter at 5–40 Hz.
- Choice C Pacinian corpuscle mediates deep pressure and vibration at 60–300 Hz.

Stimulus	Receptor cell types
Tap, flutter 5–40 Hz	Meissner corpuscles
Motion	Hair follicle receptors
Deep pressure, vibration 60–300 Hz	Pacinian corpuscles
Touch, pressure	Merkel cells
Sustained pressure	Ruffinil corpuscles
Stretch	Muscle spindles
Tension	Golgi tendon organ
Thermal	Cold and warm receptors
Chemical, thermal, and mechanical	Polymodal receptors or chemical, thermal, and ical nociceptors
Chemical	Chemical nociceptor
Light	Rods, cones
Sound	Hair cells (cochlea)
Angular acceleration	Hair cells (semicircular canals)
Linear acceleration, gravity	Hair cell (otolith organs)
Chemical	Olfactory sensory neuron
Chemical	Taste buds

198. Ans. (d) Ach

- **Awake state:** Increase activity of norepinephrine- and serotonin-containing neurons (locus coeruleus and raphe nuclei) and reduced level of activity in acetylcholine-containing neurons (pontine reticular formation). Reduced GABA release and increase histamine release is also there.
- **REM state:** Decrease activity of norepinephrine- and serotonin-containing neurons and increased level of acetylcholine containing neurons.

- **NREM sleep:** Increased release of GABA and reduced release of histamine.

> **Extra Mile**
> - **Serotonin: Old concept**—necessary to obtain and maintain behavioral sleep (permissive role on sleep).
> - **Serotonin; recent concept**—suggests that during waking, serotonin may complement the action of noradrenaline and acetylcholine in promoting cortical responsiveness and participate to the inhibition of REM-sleep effector neurons of the brainstem (**inhibitory** role on REM sleep).
> - **Cortical Ach:** Greatest during REM sleep > waking and reduced during non-REM (NREM) sleep.

199. Ans. (b) Muscle tone is absent in REM sleep

Physiological process	NREM (slow wave sleep)	REM (paradoxical sleep)
Time spent	75 % of total sleep duration	25% of total sleep duration
Brain activity	Decreases from wakefulness	Increases in motor and sensory areas are similar to NREM
Heart rate BP Blood flow to brain respiration	Decreases from wakefulness	Increases and varies compared to NREM
Sympathetic nerve activity	Decreases from wakefulness	Increases significantly from wakefulness
Muscle tone	**Similar to wakefulness**	**Absent in all muscle except facial and extraocular muscles**
Sexual arousal	Occurs infrequently	Greater than NREM
Dreams	Nonrecallable dream	Recallable dream (so called dream)

200. Ans. (d) Umami

Ref: Ganong, 25th ed. pg. 222

- Most taste buds on the tongue and other regions of the mouth **can detect umami taste,** irrespective of their location.
- Biochemical studies have identified the **taste receptors responsible for the sense of umami** as modified forms of **mGluR4, mGluR1** and **taste receptor type 1** (T1R1 + T1R3), all of which have been found in all regions of the tongue bearing taste buds.

201. Ans. (c) Granular cell

Ref: Barr's Human Nervous System, 9th ed. pg. 161

- The granular cells also make excitatory synapses with Purkinje cells.
- The excitatory transmitter is glutamate.
- *All other cerebellar neurons make inhibitory synapses with GABA as the transmitter.*
- The excitatory input to the cortex is modified by intra-cortical circuits that inhibit the Purkinje cells.
- The granular cells are the most numerous cerebellar interneurons with others being the golgi cells and basket cells.
- The axons afferent to the cerebellum make excitatory connections. Before reaching the cortex all the afferent axons give off collateral branches that contact the neurons in cerebellar nucleus.

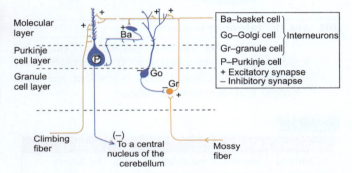

FIGURE: Neurons in the cerebellar cortex showing excitatory and inhibitory synapses. The diagram represents a longitudinally sectioned folium, with an edge on view of the dendritic tree of the Purkinje cell. Glutamatergic (excitatory) neurons are red: GABA-ergic (inhibitory) neurons are blue

202. Ans. (c) Glutamate

- The most prevalent transmitter is glutamate, which is excitatory at well over 90% of the synapses in the human brain.
- The next most prevalent is Gamma-Aminobutyric Acid, or GABA, which is inhibitory at synapses in the human brain.

203. Ans. (d) Sub-fornical Organ

- The **subfornical organ** (**SFO**), situated on the ventral surface of the fornix (the reasoning behind the organ's name), at the interventricular foramina (foramina of Monroe), is one of the circumventricular organs of the brain, meaning that it is highly vascularized and does not have a blood-brain barrier, unlike the vast majority of regions in the brain.
- The SFO is a sensory circumventricular organ responsive to a wide variety of hormones and neurotransmitters, as opposed to a secretory circumventricular organ.

FMGE Solutions Screening Examination

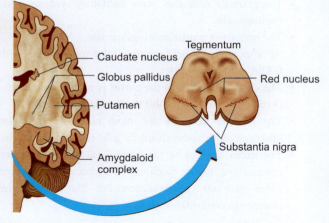

204. Ans. (b) Inhibitory to neuron

Ref: Guyton's Physiology, 11th ed. pg. 563

- GABA (gamma-aminobutyric acid) is secreted by nerve terminals in the spinal cord, cerebellum and basal ganglia. It always causes inhibition.

Extra Mile

Hormone	Source	Function
Dopamine	Neurons in substantia nigra	Inhibition
GABA	*Nerve terminals in spinal cord, baralgaylia and cerebeluar*	**Inhibition**
Glutamate	Presynaptic terminal in CNS and cerebral cortex	Excitation
Serotonin	Nuclei that originate in the median Raphe of Braine stern	Inhibition of pain pathology
Glycine	Synapses in spinal cord	Inhibition

205. Ans. (b) Glutamate

Ref: Lange Medical Physiology by Ganong, 23rd ed. ch. 15

- *Glutamate is the most abundant excitatory neurotransmitter in the vertebrate nervous system.*
- At chemical synapses, glutamate is stored in vesicles. Nerve impulses trigger release of glutamate from the presynaptic cell. Glutamate acts on ionotropic and metabotropic (G-protein coupled) receptors.
- Because of its role in synaptic plasticity, glutamate is involved in cognitive functions such as learning and memory in the brain.
- *Excitotoxicity due to excessive glutamate* release and impaired uptake occurs as part of the ischemic cascade and is associated with *stroke, autism,* some forms of intellectual disability, and diseases such as amyotrophic lateral sclerosis, lathyrism, and Alzheimer's disease.
- In contrast, *decreased glutamate release* is observed in *classical phenylketonuria*

206. Ans. (d) Bipolar cell

- Cerebellar cortex contain 5 types of neuron cells. They are:

1. Golgi cells
2. Purkinje cells
3. Basket cells
4. Granule cells
5. Stellate cells

207. Ans. (b) Broca's area

Ref: Guyton Physiology, 11th ed. pg. 717

	Location	Function
Broca's area	*Posterior* part of inferior frontal gyrus	Word formation
Limbic Association area	• Anterior pole of temporal lobe • Ventral portion of frontal lobe • Cingulate gyrus	Behavior Emotion motivation
Wernicke's area	Posterior superior temporal lobe	Language comprehension

208. Ans. (a) Inferior frontal gyrus

- Broca's area is now typically defined in terms of the pars opercularis and pars triangularis of the *inferior frontal gyrus,* represented in Brodmann's cytoarchitectonic map as areas 44 and 45 of the dominant hemisphere.
- Damage to Broca's area leads to Motor Aphasia

209. Ans. (d) Middle cerebral artery

Ref: Harrison's, 17th ed. Chapter 23

- The Middle cerebral artery is by far the largest cerebral artery and is the vessel most commonly affected by cerebrovascular accident (CVA) as it is the direct continuation of the internal carotid artery.
- The MCA supplies most of the outer convex brain surface, nearly all the basal ganglia, and the posterior and anterior internal capsules. *Hence it is most commonly affected and its occlusion most commonly leads to hemiplegia.*

210. Ans. (c) Superior temporal gyrus

Ref: Guyton's Physiology, 9th ed. pg. 658

- Auditory cortex lies principally on the supratemporal plane of the superior temporal gyrus but also extends onto the lateral side of the temporal lobe.

211. Ans. (b) Increase heart rate, increase arterial pressure

Ref: Guyton's Physiology 26th ed. pg. 733

- *Pre-optic nucleus in hypothalamus plays a role in cardiovascular regulation and it decreases heart rate and arterial pressure.*

Physiology

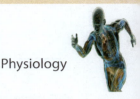

- But once this area is damaged there is no control over heart rate and arterial pressure. Hence it rises.

> **Extra Mile**
> - **Other functions of preoptic area:**
>   - It acts as temperature sensor
>   - Serve as a thermostatic body temperature control center.
>   - Increase thirst
>   - Sweating

212. Ans. (b) Stage 2

NREM 1
- NREM Stage 1 (N1 – light sleep, somnolence, drowsy sleep – 5–10% of total sleep in adults and lasts 1–7 minutes)
- This is a stage of sleep that usually occurs between sleep and wakefulness, and sometimes occurs between periods of deeper sleep and periods of REM.
- The muscles are active, and the eyes roll slowly, opening and closing moderately.
- The brain transitions from alpha waves having a frequency of 8–13 Hz (common in the awake state) to *theta waves* having a frequency of 4–7 Hz.
- Sudden twitches and hypnic jerks, also known as positive myoclonus, may be associated with the onset of sleep during N1. Some people may also experience hypnagogic hallucinations during this stage.

NREM 2
- NREM Stage 2 *(N2 – 45–55% of total sleep in adults and constitutes 10-25 minutes of initial sleep activity and progressively lengthens)*.
- In this stage, theta activity is observed and sleepers become gradually harder to awaken; the alpha waves of the previous stage are interrupted by abrupt activity called *sleep spindles* (or thalamocortical spindles) and *K-complexes*. Sleep spindles range from 11 Hz to 16 Hz (most commonly 12–14 Hz).
- During this stage, muscular activity as measured by EMG decreases, and *conscious awareness of the external environment disappears*.

NREM 3
- NREM Stage 3 *(N3 – deep sleep, slow-wave sleep – 15–25% of total sleep in adults)*:
- Formerly divided into stages 3 and 4, this stage is called slow-wave sleep (SWS) or deep sleep.
- The sleeper is less responsive to the environment; *many environmental stimuli no longer produce any reactions*.
- Slow-wave sleep is thought to be the *most restful form of sleep*, the phase which most relieves subjective feelings of sleepiness and restores the body.
- This stage is characterized by the presence of a minimum of 20% *delta waves* ranging from 0.5 Hz to 2 Hz and having a peak-to-peak amplitude >75 μV. (EEG standards define delta waves to be from 0 to 4 Hz, but sleep standards in both the original R&K, as well as the new 2007 AASM guidelines have a range of 0.5–2 Hz.)
- This is the stage in which parasomnias such as **night terrors, nocturnal enuresis, sleepwalking,** and **somniloquy occur**.

> **Extra Mile**
> **NREM Stage 4 is currently merged into stage 3 by some authors**
> - NREM stage 4 has similar attributes to stage 3, except there are a greater proportion of EEG delta waves.
> - These high voltage, slow EEG waves make up 50% or more of the record.
> - This is the deepest stage of sleep; a more intense stimulus is needed to wake someone from stage 4 sleep than any other stage of NREM sleep.
> - Children typically spend 20-25% of sleep in stages 3 and 4 slow wave sleep; this decreases to less than 10% by age 60. **Sleepwalking, sleep terrors,** and **sleep-related enuresis** episodes generally occur in stages 3 or 4, or during arousals from this stage.

213. Ans. (b) NREM 2

Ref: Ganong, 25th pg. 273-74

Bruxism: tooth grinding occurring during stage 2 of NREM period.

Nightmare
- Vivid, anxiety producing dreams during sleep.
- Patient wakes up and is able to recall the nightmare vividly.
- *Occurs in REM*.
- Treatment: REM suppressants such as tricyclic antidepressants, SSRIs, benzodiazepines.

Sleep terror (night terror)
- Arousal in the first one-third of the night.
- Invariably start with piercing scream or cry with intense panic.
- No recall on waking up the next day.
- *Occurs in NREM period (stages 3 and 4)*
- Seen especially in children, more common in boys.
- EEG is advised to rule out seizure (temporal lobe epilepsy).
- No specific treatment required

Sleep walking (somnambulism)
- Rising from bed with walking about in the first-third of the night.
- No recall on waking up the next day.
- *Occurs in **NREM period** (stages 3 and 4)*.
- Occurs between 4 and 8 years, spontaneous recovery in adolescence.

Sleep talking (Somniloquy) occurs in all stages of sleep

Sleep-related head banging (Jactatio Capitis Nocturna): rhythmic to-and-fro head rocking occurring just before or during sleep.

214. Ans. (b) Disappear when a patient opens eyes

Ref: Ganong 25th ed. / 273

- **Alpha activity** refers to activity in the range of 8–13 Hz.
- **Alpha rhythm** is 8–13 Hz activity occurring during wakefulness over the posterior head regions which is present when the eyes are closed and the patient relaxed and which is attenuated by eye opening or alerting of the patient.

FMGE Solutions Screening Examination

EEG Waves and their Significance

Band	Frequency (Hz)	Location	Normally seen in	Pathologically seen in
Delta	<4	Frontally in adults, posteriorly in children; high-amplitude waves	Adult slow-wave sleep	• Subcortical lesions • Diffuse lesions • Metabolic encephalopathy Hydrocephalus
Theta	4–7	Found in locations not related to task at hand	Drowsiness in adults (It has been found to spike in situations where as persons is actively trying to repress a response or action).	• Subcortical lesions • Metabolic encephalopathy
Alpha	8–13	Posterior regions of head, both sides, higher in amplitude on dominant side.	Relaxed/reflecting Closing the eyes	• Coma

Band	Frequency (Hz)	Location	Normally seen in	Pathologically seen in
Beta	13–30	Both sides, symmetrical distribution, most evident frontally; low-amplitude waves	**Active thinking, focus, high alert, anxious**	• Benzodiazepines
Gamma	>30	Somatosensory cortex	Displays during cross-modal sensory processing (perception that combines two different senses, such as sound and sight)	• May be associated with cognitive decline

215. Ans. (c) Amygdaloid nucleus

Ref: Ganong, 25th ed. pg. 288, Atlas of Neuroanatomy, 2nd ed. pg. 203

- The **hippocampal formation** is a compound structure in the medial temporal lobe of brain containing
  - Dentate gyrus
  - Hippocampus proper
  - Subiculum
  - Entorhinal cortex.
- Amygadala primary role in the processing of memory, decision-making, and emotional reactions, the amygdalae are considered part of the limbic system.

216. Ans. (d) Nucleus Cuneatus

Ref: Harrison, 19th ed. pg. 160 and Diagnostic Clinical Neuropsychology, 3rd ed. pg. 32

- Astereognosis is impaired or lost ability to discriminate between various forms, as well as deficits in finger localization and in graphesthesia (ability to recognize palm writing). If a lesion occurs at or above the level of the thalamus, it commonly results in astereognosis,
- Now Since Nucleus cuneatus gets information from T5 upwards including the upper limb, its lesion results in astereognosis.
- The fasciculus gracilis (graceful, like a ballerina's legs) conveys information from the lower part of the body T6 and below.
- Together the fasciculus gracilis and cuneatus are referred to as the posterior columns, because they occupy a position at the posterior of the spinal cord.
- The posterior columns travel up the ipsilateral side of the spinal cord and synapse in the nucleus gracilis and nucleus cuneatus at the level of the medulla. From there, the fibers decussate (cross over) and continue on toward the thalamus in a pathway synapses in the thalamus, and from there the information is relayed to the postcentral gyrus, known as the somatosensory cortex.

217. Ans. (b) Beta

Ref: Ganong's Physiology, 23rd ed. chapter 15

There are two kinds of sleep: Rapid eye movement (REM) sleep and non-REM (NREM) sleep.

NREM Sleep is Divided into Four Stage

A person falling asleep enters

Stage 1	The EEG begins to show a low-voltage, mixed frequency pattern. A theta rhythm (4–7 Hz) can be seen at this early stage of slow-wave sleep. Throughout NREM sleep, there is some activity of skeletal muscle but no eye movements occur
Stage 2	It is marked by the appearance of sinusoidal waves called sleep spindles (12–14 Hz) and occasional high-voltage biphasic waves called K complexes.
Stage 3	A high-amplitude delta rhythm (0.5–4 Hz) dominates the EEG waves
Stage 4	Maximum slowing with large waves is seen in stage 4

REM sleep is so named because of the characteristic eye movements that occur during this stage of sleep.

The high-amplitude slow waves seen in the EEG during sleep are periodically replaced by rapid, low-voltage EEG activity, which resembles that seen in the awake, aroused state (beta wave). For this reason, **REM sleep is also called paradoxical sleep.**

218. Ans. (c) Rapidly adapting touch receptors

Ref: Ganong, 25th ed. pg. 161; Basic Clinical Neurosciences 2nd ed. pg. 131

- When a maintained stimulus of constant strength is applied to a receptor, the frequency of the action potentials in its sensory nerve declines over time. This phenomenon is known as **adaptation or desensitization.**
- Receptors can be classified into **rapidly adapting** (phasic) receptors and **slowly adapting** (tonic) receptors.
- *Meissner and Pacinian corpuscles are examples of rapidly adapting receptors,* and Merkel cells and Ruffini endings are examples of slowly adapting receptors. Other examples of slowly adapting receptors are muscle spindles and nociceptors.

Meissner corpuscles	Tactile shapes and surfaces
Merkel disc	Tactile indentation
Hair follicle receptors	Tactile (hairy skin)
Ruffini nerve endings	Stretching
Pacinian corpuscles	Vibration
Muscle spindle	Proprioception
AS mechanical encapsulated	Pinprick
Free nerve endings	Cold/warmth

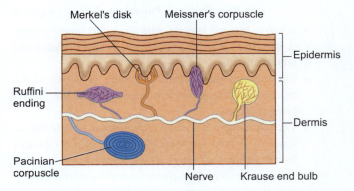

219. Ans. (b) Posterior pituitary

Ref: Ganong, 25th ed. pg. 606

List of brain structures outside the blood brain barrier called circumventricular organs:
1. Posterior pituitary and median eminence of hypothalamus
2. Area postrema (Chemoreceptor trigger zone)
3. Organum vasculosum of lamina terminalis (Osmo-receptor for vasopressin release)
4. Sub-fornical organ

All these structures have fenestrated capillaries and because of permeability are said to be outside the blood brain barrier.

220. Ans. (b) REM sleep

Ref: Ganong, 25th ed. pg. 274

- In REM sleep, the high amplitude slow waves in EEG during sleep are periodically replaced by rapid low voltage EEG activity which is identical to awake aroused state.
- Now the point is that the person is sleeping while EEG record is like that of an awake patient. Hence REM sleep is called as paradoxical sleep.

221. Ans. (c) Akinesia

Ref: Ganong, 25th ed. pg. 246

Hyperkinetic Movements and Sites of Lesion

Chorea	Lesion in Caudate nucleus
Atheotosis	Lesion in Globus pallidus
Ballism	Lesion in Sub-thalamic nucleus

222. Ans. (a) Renshaw cell

Ref: Ganong, 25th ed. pg. 233, 249

Neurons in Cerebellar Cortex

Purkinje cells	Biggest neurons in CNS
Granule cells	Innervate purkinje cells and give rise to parallel fibers
Basket cells	Located in molecular layer and receive excitatory input from parallel fibers.
Stellate cells	Same as basket cells but located more superficially
Golgi cells	Located in granular layer of cerebellum

Renshaw cell is an interneuron in spinal cord which has an inhibitory function and operates via a neurotransmitter called glycine.

FMGE Solutions Screening Examination

223. Ans. (a) Upper motor neuron damage

Ref: Ganong, 25th ed. pg. 233

Clonus is characterised by repeated rhythmic contractions of muscle subjected to sudden maintained stretch.

It is Caused by
- Increased Gamma motor neuron discharge
- Spinal cord injury causing damage to Renshaw cell which is an inhibitory inter-neuron.

Conditions in Which Clonus is seen:
1. Amyotrophic lateral sclerosis
2. Stroke
3. Multiple sclerosis
4. Spinal cord damage
5. Hepatic encephalopathy

Clonazepam and botulinum toxin is useful in management of clonus.

224. Ans. (c) Spasticity

Ref: Ganong, 25th ed. pg. 232-33

- A muscle is said to be spastic in case the resistance to stretch is high. A sequence of resistance followed by sudden decrease in resistance is when the limb is moved passively and is known as clasp knife effect since it shows similarity to closing of a pocket knife.
- Ganong also calls it the lengthening reaction since it is the response of the spastic muscle to lengthening.

225. Ans. (b) Damage to cerebellum

Ref: Ganong, 25th ed. pg. 252

- The cerebellum acts as a brake to stop a particular movement.
- In case of cerebellar lesion, the movement of the arm can be stopped and it moves in a wide arc called rebound phenomenon.

Features of Cerebellar Lesion
- Gait ataxia
- Scanning speech
- Dysmetria
- Intention tremor
- Rebound phenomenon
- Dysaidokinesia
- Nystagmus
- Pendular knee jerks

226. Ans. (b) Withdrawal reflex

Ref: Ganong, 25th ed. pg. 235

- In days following development of spinal shock patient will have low threshold for elicitation of withdrawal reflex
- Minimal noxious stimulus to arm will lead to withdrawal of one extremity and marked flexion-extension pattern of other 3 limbs.
- Later the Deep tendon reflexes become brisk
- Application of minor noxious stimulus will lead to evacuation of bladder and rectum called mass reflex.

227. Ans. (a) Caudate and Putamen

Ref: Ganong 25th ed. pg. 244

| Corpus Striatum | Caudate nucleus and putamen |
| Lenticular nucleus | Putamen and globus pallidus |

228. Ans. (b) Bi-synaptic reflex

Ref: Ganong, 25th ed. pg. 232

A Golgi Tendon Reflex/Inverse Stretch Reflex Operates as follows:
- As the tension applied to a tendon increases, the Golgi tendon organ (sensor) is stimulated.
- Nerve impulses (action potentials) arise and propagate along the 1b sensory nerve fibers into the spinal cord.
- *Within the spinal cord, the 1b sensory nerve fibers synapse and generate an IPSP (inhibitory postsynaptic potential) on the motor neurons that supply the muscles form which the fibers arise*
- The muscle relaxes and excess tension is relieved.

229. Ans. (b) Golgi Tendon organ

Ref: Ganong, 25th ed. pg. 232

Refer to the explanation of above question.

230. Ans. (d) Spinal Cord

Ref:. Ganong's Physiology, 23rd ed. chapter 9

- When a skeletal muscle with an intact nerve supply is stretched, it contracts. This response is called the **stretch reflex**.
- The stimulus that initiates the reflex is stretch of the muscle, and the response is contraction of the muscle being stretched.
- The sense organ is a small encapsulated spindle like or fusiform shaped structure called the muscle spindle, located within the fleshy part of the muscle.
- The impulses originating from the spindle are transmitted to the CNS by fast sensory fibers that pass directly to the motor neurons which supply the same muscle.
- The neurotransmitter at the central synapse is glutamate. The stretch reflex is the best known and studied monosynaptic reflex and is typified by the **knee jerk reflex**.

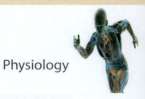

Physiology

231. Ans. (b) Fasciculation

Ref: Harrison, 18th ed. pg. 182

Fasciculation: Visible or palpable twitch within a muscle due to the spontaneous discharge of a motor unit.

Tremor: Involuntary, repetitive, oscillatory movements of a part of the body around a fixed point due to alternate contraction and relaxation of groups of muscles with their antagonists.

Chorea: Brief, rapid, jerky, explosive, Non-Repetitive, quasi-purposive involuntary movements chiefly involving face, tongue and limbs.

Myoclonic Jerk: Sudden, rapid, irregular, jerky involuntary movements of a limb due to contraction of a single muscle or a group of muscles.

232. Ans. (c) Occipital radiation

Ref: Ganong, 25th ed. pg. 190

233. Ans. (d) Basal ganglia

Ref: Ganong, 25th ed. pg. 244

234. Ans. (b) Law of Projection

Ref: Ganong, 25th ed. pg. 171

Law of projection states that irrespective of the site of application of the stimulus in the sensory pathway, the conscious perception of sensation evoked is felt at the site where receptor is present. This forms the basis of the Phantom Limb.

PHYSIOLOGY OF BLOOD

235. Ans. (a) γ-carboxylation of glutamic acid residues to clotting factor 2, 7, 9 and 10

Ref: Ganong 25th ed. P 566-67

- Vitamin K is a necessary cofactor for the enzyme that catalyses the conversion of glutamic acid residues to ϒ-carboxyglutamic acid residues.
- A total of 6 proteins involved in clotting require conversion before being released into circulation. These are factor 2, 7, 9, 10 and protein C and S.

236. Ans. (d) 4

O_2 TRANSPORT

Transport occurs via two processes:

- Hemoglobin bound O_2 (99%)
- Dissolved O_2 (1%)

Note:

- 1 Hb can carry 4 oxygen molecules.
- Molecule of oxygen bound to hemoglobin depends on saturation of Hb (SaO_2/SpO_2) with oxygen. SaO_2 depends on PaO_2

CALCULATION OF HB-BOUND O_2

In arterial blood	In venous blood
• 97% hemoglobin is saturated with oxygen, at PaO_2 of 95 mm Hg. • With this saturation, 1 g of Hb, contains 1.34 mL of O_2. • Therefore 100 mL of blood contains 20.1 mL of oxygen (when normal Hb = 15 gm%) • When hemoglobin is 100% saturated with O_2, hemoglobin binds 1.39 mL O_2 per gm of Hb [This is known as oxygen capacity (O_2cap) of Hemoglobin]	• At PvO_2 of 40 mm Hg, Hb is only 75% saturated (SO_2= 75%). • Therefore, 100 mL of venous blood would carry 14.4 mL of O_2

237. Ans. (b) Hemoglobin

Ref: Quantitative Human Physiology; An Introduction. pg. 432-33

- An average weighing adult turns over approx 6 gm of Hb daily
- 1 g of Hb yield ~35 mg of Bilirubin
- Therefore daily bilirubin formation in an adult is approx 250–350 mg

238. Ans. (c) 12th week

Ref: Diagnostic Pediatric Hematopathology By Maria A. Proytcheva 2011 ed. pg. 6

Fetal liver is the major site for erythropoeisis between 11 and 24 weeks of gestation.

	Primitive hematopoiesis	Definitive hematopoiesis
Hematopoietic site	Yolk sac and vascular endothelium	Fetal liver and fetal bone narrow Hematopoietic niches
Type of Hematopoiesis	Mostly erythroid	Multileneage Hematopoiesis
RBC Characteristics	Remain Nucleated during their entire lifespan	Enucleated RBCs
Cell Size	Macrocytic	MCV decreases with gestational age

Contd...

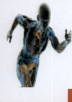

	Primitive hematopoiesis	Definitive hematopoiesis
Sensitivity to EPO	Increased	Lower sensitivity
Lifespan	Short	Increases with gestation
Hemoglobin type	Embryonic: Gower 1, Gower 2 and Portland	Fetal Hb (a_2y_2) and adult Hb ($\alpha 2 \beta 2$)

239. Ans. (b) Carboxylation

Vitamin	Action	Deficiency Symptoms	Sources
K group	Catalyze γ, carboxylation of glutamic acid residues on various proteins concerned with blood clotting	Hemorrhage	Leafy green vegetables

240. Ans. (d) Constitutes 5% of body weight

Ref: Ganong, 25th ed. pg. 561

Serum is different from plasma in the following ways:
- Fibrinogen is not present
- Factor II, V, and VIII are not present
- Higher serotonin content

Plasma constitutes 5% of body weight and choice D is wrong.

241. Ans. (c) Von Wilebrand factor

Ref: Ganong, 25th ed. pg. 563

Von wilebrand factor is synthesized by endothelial cells.

Haptoglobin	Binds and transports free hemoglobin in blood released after intravascular hemolysis
Anti-thrombin III	Protease inhibitor of intrinsic coagulation system
Hemopexin	Binds to porphyrins particularly for heme recycling.

242. Ans. (a) Liver

Sites of Haematopoiesis

Yolk sac at 2 weeks	Earliest Hemoglobin to be formed is Gower 1. This is followed by Gower 2 and finally Portland.
In fetus in liver and partly spleen.	HbF appears at 14 weeks
At birth it shifts to the bone marrow	HbA appears at 38 weeks

243. Ans. (b) Solubilization of glucose

Ref: Harper, 26th pg. 584

- Bilirubin formed in peripheral tissues is transported to the liver by plasma albumin
- Smaller amounts of cortisol and other hormones are bound to albumin.
- Half-life of albumin is 21 days.

244. Ans. (c) Radiation

Ref: Ganong, 25th ed. pg. 317

From the skin, heat is lost to the environment mainly through radiation

Body heat lost in % (at 21°C) by various means:

Radiation and conduction	70%
Vaporization of heat	27%
Respiration	2%
Urination and defecation	1%

245. Ans. (b) Stimulation of fibers coming from posterior hypothalamus

Ref: Essentials of Medical Physiology, 6th ed. pg. 362

- The hypothalamus is said to integrate body temperature information from sensory receptors (primarily cold receptors) in the skin, deep tissues spinal cord, extra-hypothalamic portions of the brain, and the hypothalamus itself.
- *The reflex responses activated by cold are controlled from the posterior hypothalamus.*
- Those activated by warmth are controlled primarily from the anterior hypothalamus.

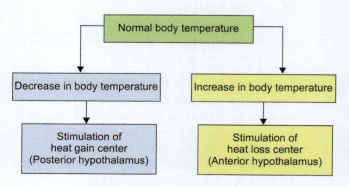

- Stimulation of the anterior hypothalamus causes cutaneous vasodilation and sweating, and lesion in this region cause hyperthermia, with rectal temperatures sometimes reaching 43°C (109.4°F).
- The threshold is >37°C for sweating and vasodilation, 36.8°C vasoconstrictions 36°C for non-shivering thermogenesis, and 35.5°C for shivering.

Physiology

246. Ans. (c) Angiotensin converting enzyme

- The lungs activate the physiologically inactive decapeptide angiotensin I to the pressor, aldosterone-stimulating octapeptide angiotensin II in the pulmonary circulation. The reaction occurs in other tissues as well, but it is particularly prominent in the lungs.
- Large amounts of the angiotensin-converting enzyme responsible for this activation are *located on the surface of the endothelial cells of the pulmonary capillaries.*

247. Ans. (c) 275–300

Ref: Ganong, 25th ed. pg. 310

Urine osmolality = 100-900 mOsm
Plasma osmolality = 275-300 mOsm

248. Ans. (a) K⁺ (Potassium)

Ref: Ganong, 25th ed. pg. 9

Normal serum potassium = 3.5–5.5 mEq/dL
Intracellular potassium = 150 mEq/dL

249. Ans. (b) 21 days

250. Ans. (c) Conjugated plus indirect reacting plus delta bilirubin

Ref: Ganong, 25th ed. pg. 511

251. Ans. (c) Ileum

252. Ans. (a) Milk production

Ref: Ganong 25th ed. / 313

253. Ans. (d) Meissners corpuscles

Ref: Ganong, 25th ed. pg. 161

Meissner corpuscles	Respond to changes in texture and slow vibrations
Merkel cells	Respond to sustained pressure and touch

Contd...

Ruffini corpuscles	Respond to sustained pressure
Pacinian corpuscles	Respond to deep pressure and fast vibration
Krause end bulb	Sense cold temperature

254. Ans. (d) Angiotensin II: Increase cAMP levels in cells

Ref: Ganong, 25th ed. pg. 53

Thyroid, steroid and retinoic acid	Act via nuclear receptors to increase the transcription of selected mRNA
Insulin	Increase tyrosine kinase activity
ANP	Increase cGMP in the cells
Angiotension II	Activate phospholipase C and produce diacyl-glycerol and Inositol phosphate IP3

255. Ans. (d) Monocyte

Ref: Ganong, 25th ed. pg. 171

GM –CSF	Erythrocyte Granulocyte Megakaryocyte
G-CSF	Granulocyte
M-CSF	Monocyte
SCF (Stem cell factor)	Erythrocyte Granulocyte Megakaryocyte Monocyte

256. Ans. (b) cGMP

Ref: Ganong, 25th ed. pg. 154

- Nitric oxide activates guanyl cyclase and it crosses cell membrane with ease. It then leads to production of cGMP.
- Nitric oxide is not stored in any vesicles like other neurotransmitters and is synthesized on demand to post

ANSWERS TO BOARD REVIEW QUESTIONS

257. Ans. (b) IL-4

258. Ans. (d) Multipolar cells

259. Ans. (b) Myokymia

260. Ans. (a) Chloride transport

261. Ans. (a) Color vision

262. Ans. (b) Closure of Aortic and pulmonic valves

263. Ans. (a) Factor 5

264. Ans. (a) BP recording

265. Ans. (c) Capillaries

266. Ans. (d) Linoleic acid

Explanations

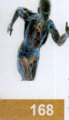

FMGE Solutions Screening Examination

267. Ans. (b) Na-K pump
268. Ans. (a) 1
269. Ans. (a) 2–2.2 μm
270. Ans. (a) Large elastic vessel
271. Ans. (b) 0.12 sec
272. Ans. (c) –40 mV
273. Ans. (b) B
274. Ans. (d) C
275. Ans. (b) Potassium
276. Ans. (d) GLUT 5
277. Ans. (b) Carbonic acid
278. Ans. (c) Slower breathing with greater tidal volume
279. Ans. (a) 1
280. Ans. (a) 0.8
281. Ans. (a) Tidal volume X respiratory rate
282. Ans. (a) Adiponectin
283. Ans. (a) Proximal tubule kidney
284. Ans. (b) IGF-2
285. Ans. (a) Upper motor neuron damage
286. Ans. (c) Spasticity
287. Ans. (a) Caudate and putamen
288. Ans. (b) Bi-Synaptic reflex
289. Ans. (a) FSH
290. Ans. (d) Norepinephrine
291. Ans. (a) Nucleus ambigus
292. Ans. (c) Ileum
293. Ans. (b) Bitter
294. Ans. (c) PCT

295. Ans. (c) Duration of expiration
296. Ans. (a) Lipids
297. Ans. (b) 7 mm Hg
298. Ans. (a) Alpha cells
299. Ans. (b) Estrogen
300. Ans. (b) LH
301. Ans. (a) Spermiogenesis
302. Ans. (d) Uterus
303. Ans. (a) Growth hormone
304. Ans. (b) Fructose
305. Ans. (a) Lung endothelium
306. Ans. (a) Crypts of lieberkuhn
307. Ans. (a) Saliva
308. Ans. (a) Chloride shift in RBC
309. Ans. (a) Elastic recoil of blood vessels
310. Ans. (d) Enhance small intestine secretions
311. Ans. (d) All
312. Ans. (a) Trypsin
313. Ans. (d) Bile salt
314. Ans. (b) Hemoglobin
315. Ans. (a) Inulin
316. Ans. (b) 500 mL
317. Ans. (c) Ca^{++}
318. Ans. (c) Somatostatin
319. Ans. (b) Kidney
320. Ans. (a) Undigested food
321. Ans. (a) Oxygen and nitrogen
322. Ans. (a) HR decreased

Physiology

169

323. Ans. (a) Minutes

324. Ans. (b) Neurohypophysis

325. Ans. (d) –90 mV

326. Ans. (a) Rheobase

327. Ans. (a) Glutamate

328. Ans. (a) Olfactory system

329. Ans. (a) Stereognosis

330. Ans. (c) Withdrawal reflex

331. Ans. (a) Golgi tendon organ

332. Ans. (b) Midbrain

333. Ans. (c) Thalamus

334. Ans. (a) Insulin

335. Ans. (a) Foot processes of astrocytes and endothelial cells

336. Ans. (b) Contralateal loss of proprioception

337. Ans. (c) Atrial contraction

338. Ans. (b) Left ventricle work more than right ventricle

339. Ans. (b) Unmyelinated

340. Ans. (d) Inhibition of feed back propogation

341. Ans. (a) Muscle phosphorylase

342. Ans. (a) Maintains the perfusion

343. Ans. (a) Histamine

344. Ans. (a) Asymmetrical arrangement of cell wall component

345. Ans. (a) Receptor mediated endocytosis

346. Ans. (b) Total body water

347. Ans. (c) Integrins

348. Ans. (b) Biosynthesis of fatty acids

349. Ans. (b) H

350. Ans. (a) Fast EPSP

351. Ans. (b) Fibrillation

352. Ans. (b) Isotonic exercise

353. Ans. (b) Blocking inhibitory synapses

354. Ans. (b) Passive diffusion along concentration gradient

355. Ans. (b) II, VII, IX, X

356. Ans. (c) Vascular endothelium

357. Ans. (b) Left shift

358. Ans. (c) Superior temporal gyrus

359. Ans. (a) Cardiac output/Body surface area

ANSWER TO IMAGE-BASED QUESTION

360. Ans. (b) B

PR interval (A)	120–200 msec and represents spread of impulse from SAN to AV node
RR interval (C)	Inversely related to heart rate
QT interval (B)	360–440 msec and represents ventricular depolarization and repolarization

Explanations

3

Biochemistry

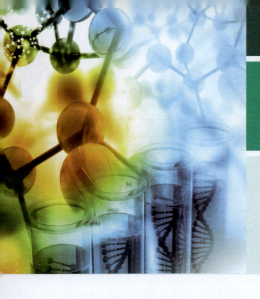

MOST RECENT QUESTIONS 2019

1. Nitric oxide is synthesized from this amino acid:
   a. Arginine b. Lysine
   c. Leucine   d. Isoleucine
2. Enzyme deficient in maple syrup urine disease:
   a. Branched chain alpha keto acid decarboxylase
   b. Methionine adenosyltransferase
   c. Fumarylacetoacetate hydrolase
   d. Tyrosine aminotransferase
3. Amino acid abundant in collagen:
   a. Glycine b. Lysine
   c. Leucine d. Isoleucine
4. Which of the following vitamin is most potent anti-oxidant?
   a. Vitamin D b. Vitamin E
   c. Vitamin K d. Vitamin B
5. Vitamin which helps in iron absorption:
   a. Vitamin A b. Vitamin B
   c. Vitamin C d. Vitamin E
6. Wernicke encephalopathy is due to deficiency of:
   a. Thiamine b. Biotin
   c. Niacin   d. Hydroxycobalamin
7. Strenuous exercise is not done in this glycogen storage disease:
   a. McArdle disease   b. Anderson disease
   c. Pompe disease   d. Von Gierke disease
8. Each of the following is a physiological uncoupler EXCEPT:
   a. 2,4 dinitrophenol   b. Thyroid hormone
   c. Unconjugated bilirubin d. Long chain fatty acid
9. In glycolysis which of the following is not involved?
   a. Pyruvate dehydrogenase b. Phosphofructokinase
   c. Glucokinase   d. Pyruvate kinase
10. First fatty acid to form in fatty acid synthesis:
    a. Palmitic acid
    b. Stearic acid
    c. Oleic acid
    d. Pantothenic acid

CARBOHYDRATE

11. Urea cycle takes place in:
    (Recent Pattern Question 2018-19)
    a. Nucleus and endoplasmic reticulum
    b. Mitochondria and Golgi apparatus
    c. Mitochondria and cytoplasm
    d. Only mitochondria
12. Which of the following is a physiological uncoupler?
    (Recent Pattern Question 2018-19)
    a. 2,4-Dinitrophenol
    b. Dinitrocresol
    c. Aspirin
    d. Unconjugated bilirubin
13. Gluconeogenesis is mainly seen in:
    (Recent Pattern Question 2018)
    a. Kidney b. Liver
    c. Spleen d. Heart
14. Glucose-6-phosphate dehydrogenase deficiency causes:
    (Recent Pattern Question 2018)
    a. Megaloblastic anemia b. Hemolytic anemia
    c. Sickle cell anemia   d. Microcytic anemia
15. Essential fructosuria is due to the deficiency of which enzyme? *(Recent Pattern Question 2017)*
    a. Aldolase A   b. Aldolase B
    c. Fructokinase d. Glucokinase
16. Identify the glycogen storage disease with exercise induced myoglobinuria: *(Recent Pattern Question 2017)*
    a. McArdle's disease
    b. Pompe's disease
    c. Von gierke disease
    d. Anderson disease
17. All of the following enzymes catalyze irreversible steps in glycolysis EXCEPT:
    a. Hexokinase b. PFK-I
    c. Enolase   d. Pyruvate kinase
18. The net ATP yield when one molecule of pyruvate is completely oxidized to CO_2 & H_2O is:
    a. 10 b. 15
    c. 18 d. 30

Biochemistry

19. Which of the following enzymes causes Substrate level phosphorylation in Glycolysis:
    a. Glyceraldehyde 3 Phosphate dehydrogenase
    b. Pyruvate kinase
    c. Phosphofructokinase
    d. Enolase

20. Glucose-6-phosphatase enzyme is absent in:
    a. Liver   b. Kidney
    c. Brain   d. Muscles

21. Which of the following doesn't occur in the mitochondria:
    a. Cori cycle   b. Urea cycle
    c. FA oxidation   d. Kreb's cycle

22. In which cells or tissue, Lactate will convert to pyruvate:
    a. Muscles   b. Liver
    c. Erythrocytes   d. Brain

23. Source of ATP in RBC cells:
    a. Fatty acid oxidation   b. Oxidative phosphorylation
    c. NADPH paroxidase   d. EMP pathway

24. In glycolysis, insulin affects all of the following enzymes EXCEPT:
    a. Phosphofructokinase
    b. Pyruvate kinase
    c. Glucokinase
    d. Hexokinase

25. Insulin is essential for entry of glucose in which of the following tissue:
    a. Most neurons in cerebral cortex
    b. Renal tubular cells
    c. Skeletal muscles   d. Mucosa of small intestine

26. All of the following metabolic pathways occur in both Cytoplasm and Mitochondria, EXCEPT:
    a. Glycolysis
    b. Gluconeogenesis
    c. Heme Synthesis
    d. Urea cycle

27. Which of the following occurs in both cytoplasm and mitochondria:
    a. Glycolysis   b. Gluconeogenesis
    c. Glycogenolysis   d. Glycogenesis

28. Gluconeogenesis is inhibited by:
    a. Insulin   b. Glucagon
    c. Glucocorticoids   d. GnRH

29. Cytoplasm to Mitochondria substrate shuttle is:
    a. Glycerophosphate shuttle b. Malate shuttle
    c. Phosphoenol pyruvate   d. Oxaloacetate

30. What is not given in fructose intolerance patient:
    a. Glucose   b. Galactose
    c. Fructose   d. Maltose

31. Aldolase is an enzyme whose substrate is
    a. Glucose -6-phosphate   b. Fructose-6-phosphate
    c. Fructose   d. Fructose-1 biphosphate

32. On weaning off from milk and addition of fruit juices, an infant had frequent attacks of vomiting and tremors. Urine reducing sugar was positive but glucose was negative. The infant is likely to have:
    a. Fructokinase deficiency
    b. Galactokinase deficiency
    c. Glucose -6- phosphatase deficiency
    d. Aldolase - B deficiency

33. An enzyme involved in the catabolism of fructose to pyruvate in the liver is:
    a. Glyceraldehydes-3-phosphate dehydrogenase
    b. Phosphoglucomutase
    c. Lactate-dehydrogenase
    d. Glucokinase

34. Which is true for glucoronidation:
    a. Water solubility is decreased
    b. Phase II reaction
    c. Phase I reaction
    d. Done by CYP enzyme

35. Glucagon receptors are NOT found in which organ:
    a. Cornea
    b. Kidney
    c. Stomach
    d. Adrenal gland

36. Sodium fluoride is a good in-vitro preservative of glucose in blood samples because it inhibits:
    a. Enolase
    b. Hexokinase
    c. Phosphofructokinase
    d. Pyruvate dehydrogenase

37. Muscle is NOT involved in which type of glycogen storage disease
    a. Type 1   b. Type 2
    c. Type 5   d. Type 7

38. Enzyme deficiency in Glycogen storage disease type V is?
    a. Glucose-6-phosphatase
    b. Acid maltase
    c. Debranching enzyme
    d. Myophosphorylase deficiency

39. Regarding HMP shunt, all of the following are true EXCEPT:
    a. Occurs in the cytosol
    b. No ATP is produced in the cycle
    c. It is active in Adipose tissue, Liver and Gonads
    d. The oxidative phase generates NADH and the Non oxidative phase generates pyruvate.

40. Pentose phosphate pathway produces:
    a. NADPH
    b. ATP
    c. Acetyl CoA
    d. ADP

Questions

FMGE Solutions Screening Examination

41. What is the composition of lugols solution?
    a. 4% iodine 10% potassium iodide
    b. 5% iodine and 10% potassium iodide
    c. 2.5% iodine and 5% potassium iodide
    d. 10% iodine and 6% potassium iodide
42. NADPH is used for:
    a. Glycolysis
    b. Lipid synthesis and glutathione reaction
    c. Krebs cycle
    d. All of the above

LIPIDS

43. **Principle building block in fatty acid synthesis:**
    (Recent Pattern Question 2018-19)
    a. Acetyl CoA   b. Palmitoyl CoA
    c. Malonyl CoA   d. Oleate
44. Ideal total cholesterol to HDL cholesterol ratio is:
    a. 1.5   b. 2.5
    c. 3.5   d. 4.5
45. Niemann's pick disease is due to deficiency of which enzyme:
    a. Sphingomyelinase   b. Hexosaminidase-A
    c. Aryl suplhatase   d. Galactosidase-A
46. Which organelle is involved in the case of sphinghomyelin deficiency:
    a. Lysosome   b. Nucleus
    c. Mitochondria   d. Cell membrane
47. The most common lysosomal storage disorder is
    a. Gaucher's disease   b. Taysach's disease
    c. Wolman disease   d. Niemann pick's disease
48. Enzyme replacement is mostly done for:
    a. Niemann pick's   b. Gangliosidosis
    c. Gaucher's disease   d. Phenylketonuria
49. Enzyme deficient in Tay-sach's disease :
    a. α galactosidase   b. Hexosaminidase A
    c. β galactosidase   d. β glucosidase
50. The enzyme is the rate limiting enzyme in cholesterol synthesis is:
    a. HMG CoA synthetase b. HMG CoA reductase
    c. HMG CoA lyase   d. Catalase
51. Main LDL receptors is:
    a. APO-A   b. APO-B-100
    c. APOc-100   d. APO-100 & APO-E
52. Receptor present in liver for uptake of LDL:
    a. Apo C   b. Apo A and Apo E
    c. Apo E and Apo B48   d. Apo B100
53. In primary familial hypercholesterolemia, there is defect in:
    a. LDL-receptors   b. Apoprotein
    c. Apoprotein B   d. VLDL

54. Which of the following has maximum cholesterol content:
    a. HDL   b. LDL
    c. VLDL   d. Chylomicrons
55. Which of the following lipoprotein transport triglyceride from liver to plasma:
    a. LDL   b. VLDL
    c. Chylomicrons   d. HDL
56. What is true regarding medium chain fatty acids:
    a. Don't require pancreatic lipase
    b. Diffuse directly into portal circulation
    c. Not deposited in adipose tissue
    d. All of the above
57. Auto oxidation is seen in:
    a. Cholesterol   b. Arachidonic acid
    c. Stearic acid   d. Palmitic acid
58. Which of the following is an Omega-3 fatty acid?
    a. Linoleic acid   b. α-Linolenic acid
    c. Oleic acid   d. Arachidonic acid
59. Which one of the following is an example of omega-3 fatty acids:
    a. Gamma Linolenic Acid b. Oleic Acid
    c. Docosahexaenoic Acid d. Palmitoleic acid
60. All of the following are derivative of omega-6 EXCEPT:
    a. Alpha linolenic acid b. Gamma linolenic acid
    c. Arachidonic acid   d. Linoleic acid
61. Ketones body production occurs in:
    a. Cytoplasm   b. Mitochondria
    c. Golgi Body   d. Nucleus
62. Which enzyme activity is increased in starvation:
    a. Pyruvate decarboxylase
    b. Pyruvate kinase
    c. Pyruvate carboxylase
    d. Pyruvate dehydrogenase
63. In 3rd day to 2nd week starvation the body depends on:
    a. Amino acid   b. Ketone bodies
    c. FA   d. Glucose
64. Which of the following is a Monounsaturated Fatty acid (MUFA):
    a. Linolenic acid   b. Oleic acid
    c. Lauric acid   d. Stearic acid
65. The product of oxidation of odd chain fatty acids is:
    a. Aceto-acetyl CoA   b. Malonyl CoA
    c. Propionyl CoA   d. Fumaryl COA
66. Beta oxidation of odd chain fatty acid produces acetyl CoA and_____?
    a. Malonyl CoA   b. Succinyl CoA
    c. Propionyl CoA   d. Methylmanoyl CoA

Biochemistry

NUCLEIC ACID

67. Which of the following X-linked condition presents as urolithiasis with gouty arthritis:

(Recent Pattern Question 2018-19)

a. Holt oram syndrome
b. Lesch nyhan syndrome
c. SCID
d. Cystic fibrosis

68. Initiator codon in prokaryotes:

(Recent Pattern Question 2018-19)

a. UAA
b. UGA
c. AUG
d. UAG

69. Correct PCR staging sequence:

(Recent Pattern Question 2018-19)

a. Denature of DNA → Extension of primer → Annealing of Primer
b. Annealing of primer → Extension of primer → DNA denature
c. Denature of DNA → Annealing of primers → Extension of primer
d. Annealing of primer → DNA denature → Extension of primer

70. Which of the following is NOT seen in DNA:

(Recent Pattern Question 2018-19)

a. Cytosine
b. Adenine
c. Guanine
d. Uracil

71. Lac operon is: *(Recent Pattern Question 2018)*

a. Repressor
b. Inducer
c. Operator
d. Activator

72. True about DNA polymerase 1:

(Recent Pattern Question 2018)

a. DNA polymerase III activity
b. 3' – 5' exonuclease activity
c. 5' – 3' exonuclease activity
d. All of the above

73. Reverse transcriptase PCR analyzes?

(Recent Pattern Question 2017)

a. DNA
b. RNA
c. Amino acid
d. Protein particle

74. Ionising radiation damages DNA by which mechanism:

(Recent Pattern Question 2017)

a. Free radical damage
b. DNA helicase damage
c. Mismatch of bases
d. Bulky adducts formation

75. X chromosome belongs to which group?

(Recent Pattern Question 2017)

a. A
b. B
c. C
d. D

76. Which is Not true about Cockayne syndrome?

(Recent Pattern Question 2017)

a. Autosomal recessive
b. DNA mismatch repair
c. Related to XP
d. Usually recurs

77. How many stop codons are seen?

(Recent Pattern Question 2017)

a. 1
b. 2
c. 3
d. 4

78. Which is true about stop codon?

(Recent Pattern Question 2017)

a. 3 codon coding for one amino acid
b. 3 codon coding for whole DNA
c. 3 codon coding for whole RNA
d. 3 codon act as terminator codon

79. Anti-codon arm is seen in *(Recent Pattern Question 2016)*

a. m-RNA
b. r- RNA
c. t-RNA
d. sn- RNA

80. Alpha helix is which structure

(Recent Pattern Question 2016)

a. Primary
b. Secondary
c. Tertiary
d. Quaternary

81. Bend of DNA is made of which amino acid

(Recent Pattern Question 2016)

a. Glycine
b. Alanine
c. Cysteine
d. Lysine

82. Enzyme involved in post-transcriptional capping at 5' end *(Recent Pattern Question 2016)*

a. 5 methyl transferase
b. 7 methyl transferase
c. 5 methyl reductase
d. 7 methyl reductase

83. Which of the following nitrogen base is not seen in RNA: *(Recent Pattern Question 2016)*

a. Adenine
b. Thymine
c. Guanine
d. Cytosine

84. Which of the following amino acid is common in Purine and pyridimines?

a. Alanine
b. Glutamine
c. Guanine
d. Uracil

85. In Pyrimidine synthesis rate limiting enzyme is:

a. Aspartate transcarbomylase
b. Carbamoyl phosphate synthetase II
c. Dihydroorotase dehydrogenase
d. OMP. Decarboxylase

86. The Watson's Crick double helix model of DNA is

a. Right handed anti parallel
b. Left handed anti parallel
c. Right handed parallel
d. Left handed parallel

87. Equal number of nucleotide bases are seen between which pair of nucleotides:

a. A≡G
b. G=T
c. G≡C
d. A=C

Questions

173

FMGE Solutions Screening Examination

88. Frame shift mutation:
    a. Substitution of amino acid
    b. Changed mRNA base at 3rd nucleotide of codon
    c. Due to stop codon
    d. Deletion of 2 bases
89. Frameshift mutation leads to cellular changes to which of the following processes
    a. Translation   b. Transcription
    c. Replication   d. Spontaneous
90. Frame shift mutation DOESN'T occur in multiples of:
    a. 2   b. 3
    c. 4   d. 5
91. Sickle cell disease is present with which mutation:
    a. Cross-linked defect   b. Base pair defect
    c. Mismatch defect   d. Base pair substitution
92. Which of the following is not a part of DNA correction mechanism:
    a. Nucleoside correction b. Pre replication
    c. Post replication   d. Base pair correction
93. 5' to 3' exonuclease activity is seen in:
    a. Proof reading   b. Repair of damaged DNA
    c. DNA synthesis   d. DNA polymerase
94. Radiation affects:
    a. RNA   b. DNA
    c. Mitochondria   d. Cytoskeleton protein
95. True about Chaperones:
    a. For misfolding of protein
    b. HSP 70 family of chaperones bind with hydrophobic amino acid
    c. HSP 60 and 70 are similar in structure
    d. Has no role in unfolding
96. DNA repair defect is seen in:
    a. Xeroderma pigmentosum b. Li-fraumani syndrome
    c. Retinoblastoma   d. None
97. DNA enzyme for aging:
    a. Telosomerase   b. Topoisomerase
    c. Telomerase   d. DNA polymerase
98. Protein synthesis occurs in which part of the cell:
    a. Smooth endoplasmic reticulum
    b. Rough endoplasmic reticulum
    c. Golgi body
    d. All of the above
99. Protein synthesis occurs in:
    a. Golgi bodies   b. Endoplasmic reticulum
    c. Mitochondria   d. Peroxisomes
100. Protein synthesized in rough Endoplasmic reticulum will first go to:
    a. Mitochondria   b. Cytosol
    c. Golgi body   d. Lysosome
101. Which of the following structure is *not affected* in protein denaturation?
    a. Primary structure   b. Secondary structure
    c. Tertiary structure   d. Quaternary structure

102. True about Lesch Nyhan Syndrome:
    a. Patient have normal intellectual capacity
    b. Pyrimidine overproduction is the cause
    c. Uric acid stones are frequently formed
    d. X- Linked dominant
103. All of the following are features of Lesch-Nyhan syndrome EXCEPT:
    a. Hyperuricaemia   b. Self-mutilation
    c. Mental retardation   d. Immunodeficiency
104. The main catabolic product/products of purine nuleotides in humans is which one of the following:
    a. Ammonia + CO_2
    b. Ammonia
    c. Uric Acid
    d. CO_2 and Water
105. Hyperuricemia occur due to all EXCEPT:
    a. Xanthine oxidase
    b. Phosphoribosyl pyrophosphate synthetase
    c. Glucose 6 phosphatase
    d. Hypoxanthine-guanine phosphoribosyl-transferase
106. Hypouricaemia is associated with deficiency of which of the following:
    a. Xanthine oxidase
    b. Von Gierke's disease
    c. Hypoxanthine guanine phosphoribosyl transferase
    d. Adenine phosphoribosyl transferase
107. The technique used for separation and detection of RNA is which one of the following?
    a. Northern Blot   b. Southern Blot
    c. Eastern Blot   d. Western Blot
108. Carrier of genetic material
    a. DNA cistrons   b. Codons of m RNA
    c. Anti-codons of t RNA   d. None
109. All of the following are true regarding cytosolic eukaryotic gene expression EXCEPT:
    a. Capping helps in attachment of mRNA to 40 S Ribosome
    b. N formyl methionine t-RNA will be the first t-RNA to come into action
    c. EF2 shifts between GDP & GTP
    d. Releasing factor releases the polypeptide chain from the P site
110. Most common RNA is
    a. t-RNA   b. m-RNA
    c. r-RNA   d. sn-RNA
111. RNA silencing is seen with:
    a. t-RNA   b. m-RNA
    c. Sn-RNA   d. mi-RNA
112. SNURPS are:
    a. Single nucleotide units for recycling of proteins
    b. Small Nuclear Ribo-nucleoproteins
    c. Small nuclear units for misfolded proteins
    d. Single nuclear unit for recycling of misfolded proteins

Biochemistry

175

113. Lac operon is classically activated by:
   a. Increased glucose concentration , increased cAMP
   b. Decreased glucose concentration, decreased cAMP
   c. Decreased glucose concentration, increased cAMP
   d. Increased glucose concentration, decreased cAMP

AMINO ACID

114. Hartnup disease can present with:
   (Recent Pattern Question 2018-19)
   a. Pellagra like symptoms   b. Nephrolithiasis
   c. Protein intolerance   d. Microcephaly

115. All of the following are derivatives of tryptophan EXCEPT: *(Recent Pattern Question 2018-19)*
   a. Melatonin   b. Serotonin
   c. Niacin   d. Creatinine

116. Prostaglandins are derived from:
   (Recent Pattern Question 2018-19)
   a. Stearic acid   b. Arachidonic acid
   c. Glutamic acid   d. Aspartic acid

117. Mental retardation is a clinical feature of:
   (Recent Pattern Question 2018-19)
   a. Alkaptonuria   b. Albinism
   c. Hawkinsinuria d. Phenylketonuria

118. Precursor of melanin synthesis:
   (Recent Pattern Question 2018-19)
   a. Tyrosine   b. Glycine
   c. Phenylalanine d. Lysine

119. Collagen contains amino acids Proline, Lysine and:
   (Recent Pattern Question 2018-19)
   a. Glycine   b. Isoleucine
   c. Cysteine   d. Methionine

120. Disulfide bonds are formed in which amino acid:
   (Recent Pattern Question 2018-19)
   a. Glycine   b. Cysteine
   c. Proline   d. Isoleucine

121. Which is not a biological derivative of tyrosine?
   (Recent Pattern Question 2018)
   a. Melanin   b. Melatonin
   c. Epinephrine d. Dopamine

122. The composition of creatine is:
   (Recent Pattern Question 2018)
   a. Glycine, arginine, methionine
   b. Glycine and histidine
   c. Glycine, glutamate, aspartate
   d. Histidine and methionine

123. All of the following are branched chain amino acids EXCEPT: *(Recent Pattern Question 2018)*
   a. Leucine   b. Lysine
   c. Isoleucine   d. Valine

124. Protein folding is done by: *(Recent Pattern Question 2017)*
   a. Chaperone   b. Endoplasmic reticulum
   c. Peroxisome d. Lysosome

125. Which is the common amino acid between urea cycle and TCA?   *(Recent Pattern Question 2017)*
   a. Asparate   b. Alanine
   c. Asparagine   d. Glutamate

126. Which amino acid is acidic? *(Recent Pattern Question 2017)*
   a. Aspartic acid   b. Valine
   c. Leucine   d. Aspartate

127. Guanidine combines with which amino acid?
   (Recent Pattern Question 2017)
   a. Tyrosine   b. Arginine
   c. Methionine   d. Proline

128. Dihydrobiopterin is used in management of which amino acid defect?   *(Recent Pattern Question 2017)*
   a. Alanine   b. Tyrosine
   c. Phenylalanine   d. Tryptophan

129. HbA1c does glycosylation with which amino acid?
   (Recent Pattern Question 2017)
   a. Arginine   b. Glutamate
   c. Valine   d. Leucine

130. Test done to check protein purity?
   (Recent Pattern Question 2017)
   a. Mass Spectrophotometry b. SDS –PAGE
   c. Western blot   d. Sanger's technique

131. LDH1 is seen in: *(Recent Pattern Question 2017)*
   a. Liver
   b. Skeletal muscle
   c. Heart
   d. Kidney

132. Non-essential amino acid *(Recent Pattern Question 2016)*
   a. Tryptophan   b. Tyrosine
   c. Arginine   d. Histidine

133. True about lysine   *(Recent Pattern Question 2016)*
   a. Deficient in pulses   b. Deficient in cereals
   c. Nonessential amino acid d. Acidic amino acid

134. Homocysteine is   *(Recent Pattern Question 2016)*
   a. Protein D alpha amino acid
   b. Protein L amino acid
   c. Non-protein alpha amino acid
   d. Seen in protein

135. Which of the following releases ammonia
   (Recent Pattern Question 2016)
   a. Aspartate dehydrogenase b. Glutaminase
   c. Adenosine deaminase   d. Aspartate synthetase

136. Carnitine is useful in transport of
   (Recent Pattern Question 2016)
   a. Aromatic amino acid   b. Aliphatic amino acid
   c. Fatty acid   d. Glucose

Questions

FMGE Solutions Screening Examination

137. PKU is due to deficiency of which enzyme:
     (Recent Pattern Question 2016)
     a. Phenylalanine reductase   b. Phenylalanine hydroxylase
     c. Tyrosine hydroxylase   d. Tyrosine reductase

138. Which protein is abundant in our body:
     (Recent Pattern Question 2016)
     a. Collagen   b. Albumin
     c. Myoglobin   d. Hemoglobin

139. Which is a niacin sparing amino acid:
     a. Tryptophan   b. Methionine
     c. Cysteine   d. Tyrosine

140. Which vitamin can be synthesized from tryptophan:
     a. Niacin   b. Riboflavin
     c. Cobalamin   d. Folic acid

141. Disease entity due to deficiency of alpha keto-decarboxylase enzyme:
     a. Hartnup's disease   b. Maple syrup disease
     c. Alkaptonuria   d. Alport syndrome

142. Limiting amino acid in maize:
     a. Niacin   b. Tyrosine
     c. Tryptophan   d. Methionine

143. In Alkaptonuria deficiency is:
     a. Phosphofructo kinase   b. HMG CoA reductase
     c. Homogentisate oxidase   d. Xanthine oxidase

144. First product of tryptophan catabolism is:
     a. Kynerunine   b. Bradykinin
     c. PAF   d. Xantheurenate

145. Urea is formed from which substrate:
     a. Arginine   b. Orginine
     c. Citrulline   d. Aspartate

146. Hydrolysis occurs at which step of urea cycle:
     a. Cleavage of Arginine
     b. Formation of Argininosuccinate
     c. Formation of citrulline
     d. Formation of ornithine

147. Polyamine like putrescine is derived from:
     a. Arginine   b. Ornithine
     c. Yohimibine   d. Arginosuccine

148. All are true about selenocystiene EXCEPT:
     a. Considered 21st Amino acid
     b. Coded by UGA
     c. Occurs in glutathione peroxidase
     d. Made of cystiene and methionine

149. Cystinuria is due to the accumulation of:
     a. Cysteine   b. Lysine
     c. Ornithine   d. Cysteine

150. Cystinuria presents with excess of
     a. Cysteine   b. Tyrosine
     c. Glutamine   d. Valine

151. Nitric oxide is synthesized from:
     a. L- arginine   b. L- citrulline
     c. Lysine   d. Tryptophan

152. Smooth muscle relaxant nitric oxide is synthesized from:
     a. Methionine   b. Cyseine
     c. Arginine   d. Ornithine

153. Carnitine is made-up of:
     a. Leusine   b. Lysine
     c. Lysine & methionine   d. Arginine

154. β alanine is a product of:
     a. Dihydrouracil   b. Carnitine
     c. Kynurenine   d. Cyano-cobalamin

155. The structural polysaccharide chitin is a polymer of which of the following:
     a. Galactosamine   b. Glucosamine
     c. N. Acetyl Galactosamine   d. N-Acetyl Glucosamine

156. The initiation of hemoglobin synthesis requires:
     a. Histidine   b. Glycine
     c. Folate   d. Iron

157. In Hartnup's disease which of the following is excreted in the urine:
     a. Ornithine   b. Glycine
     c. Tryptophan   d. Cystine

158. Intestinal flora (bacteria) digests all EXCEPT:
     a. Cellulose   b. Lignin
     c. Pectin   d. Starch

159. Amino acid which contributes to biosynthesis of purine ribonucleotide are all EXCEPT:
     a. Aspartate   b. Histidine
     c. Glutamate   d. Glycine

160. Which of the following amino acid is used in biosynthesis of purines?
     a. Alanine   b. Glycine
     c. Threonine   d. Ornithine

161. Glutathione is composed of:
     a. Glycine   b. Cycteine
     c. Glutamate   d. All of the above

162. Vitamin C is necessary in the formation of collagen. It is required for the conversion of:
     a. Proline to hydroxyproline
     b. Beta-carotene to vitamin A
     c. Glutamate to gamma-carboxyglutamate
     d. Pyridoxine to pyridoxal phosphate

163. What changes the conformation of alpha helix in collagen
     a. Methionine
     b. Proline
     c. Alanine
     d. Tyrosine

164. Used in Transamination:
     a. Pyridoxal phosphate
     b. NADPH
     c. NADP
     d. FAD

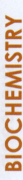

VITAMINS, MINERALS AND ENZYMES

165. Menkes disease is due to deficiency of:
(Recent Pattern Question 2018-19)
- a. Selenium
- b. Copper
- c. Chromium
- d. Manganese

166. G6PD is enzyme of: *(Recent Pattern Question 2018-19)*
- a. Mitochondria
- b. Cell membrane
- c. Golgi organ
- d. Endoplasmic reticulum

167. Inheritance pattern of G6PD:
(Recent Pattern Question 2018-19)
- a. AR
- b. AD
- c. X-linked
- d. Familial

168. Activator of trypsinogen is mainly by:
- a. Chymotrypsinogen
- b. Enteropeptidase
- c. Trypsin
- d. Hexokinase

169. Which of the following is a function of chaperone protein? *(Recent Pattern Question 2018-19)*
- a. It degrades proteins that have folded improperly
- b. It provides a template for how the proteins should fold
- c. It rescues proteins that have folded improperly and allows them to refold properly
- d. It degrades proteins that have folded properly

170. In case of cyanide poisoning, antidote of amyl nitrate is given. This is an example of:
(Recent Pattern Question 2018)
- a. Receptor antagonism
- b. Chemical antagonism
- c. Physical antagonism
- d. Physiological antagonism

171. Synthesis of type I collagen requires which vitamin?
(Recent Pattern Question 2018)
- a. Vitamin A
- b. Vitamin C
- c. Vitamin D
- d. Vitamin K

172. cAMP is formed from: *(Recent Pattern Question 2018)*
- a. AMP
- b. GMP
- c. ATP
- d. MTP

173. Among the following, which is the most effective antioxidant: *(Recent Pattern Question 2018)*
- a. Vitamin A
- b. Vitamin C
- c. Vitamin E
- d. Vitamin K

174. Selenium deficiency causes:
(Recent Pattern Question 2017)
- a. Menke's disease
- b. Wilson's disease
- c. Keshan disease
- d. Kashinbeck disease

175. Which is correct about vitamin K?
(Recent Pattern Question 2017)
- a. Shortest half life
- b. Exist in three forms
- c. All are fat soluble
- d. All are water soluble

176. Peroxidases belong to which enzyme group?
(Recent Pattern Question 2017)
- a. Oxidase-Reductase
- b. Lipase
- c. Hydrolase
- d. Transferase

177. Impaired Glucose intolerance is caused by deficiency of
(Recent Pattern Question 2016)
- a. Chromium
- b. Selenium
- c. Copper
- d. Cobalt

178. Lactate dehydrogenase enzyme requires which metal
(Recent Pattern Question 2016)
- a. Selenium
- b. Copper
- c. Magnesium
- d. Zinc

179. True about competitive inhibition with first order kinetics
(Recent Pattern Question 2016)
- a. Km increased, Vmax same
- b. Vmax increased, Km same
- c. Km same, Vmax decrease
- d. Km same, Vmax increase

180. Methylcobalamin is required for which of the following enzymes:
- a. Homocysteine deaminase
- b. Homocysteine methyl transferase
- c. Methionine synthase
- d. Methionine reductase

181. True about Riboflavin is:
- a. Deficiency causes Beri Beri
- b. Consist of flavin group which is required in oxidation-reduction reaction
- c. Pyridoxal phosphate act as a cofactor
- d. Green leafy vegetables are major sources

182. Which vitamin is associated with carboxylation reactions:
- a. Thiamine
- b. Riboflavin V
- c. Biotin
- d. Folic acid

183. In pregnancy, neural tube defect arises in the fetus due to deficiency of which of the following in the mother?
- a. Vitamin
- b. Folic Acid
- c. Vitamin A
- d. Vitamin C

184. Pellagra is due to:
- a. Utilization of tryptophan
- b. Deficiency of tryptophan
- c. Deficiency of thiamine
- d. Utilization of niacin

185. Menadione is analog of:
- a. Vitamin K
- b. Vitamin A
- c. Vitamin D
- d. Vitamin C

186. Which of the following is water soluble form of vitamin K:
- a. Menaquinone
- b. Phylloqumone
- c. Menadione
- d. Primidone

187. Water soluble form of Vitamin K
- a. Phylloquinone
- b. Menaquinone
- c. Menadione
- d. None

188. All of the following vitamins are anti-oxidants EXCEPT:
- a. Beta-carotene
- b. Ascorbic acid
- c. Vitamin E
- d. Vitamin K

189. Which of the following vitamin deficiency is seen with biliary obstruction:
- a. Vitamin K
- b. Vitamin C
- c. Vitamin B_{12}
- d. Vitamin B_2

FMGE Solutions Screening Examination

190. Of the following which is absent in eggs:
    a. Vitamin B_{12}
    b. Vitamin C
    c. Vitamin A
    d. Vitamin B_2
191. A child with alopecia, hyperpigmentation, hypogonadism and rash of genital area and mouth is likely to suffer from:
    a. Iron deficiency
    b. Zinc deficiency
    c. Calcium deficiency
    d. Copper deficiency
192. Toxicity of cholera toxin in due to which one of the following:
    a. Decrease in activity of Gi protein
    b. Decrease in activity of Gs protein
    c. ADP-ribosylation of Gs alpha sub-unit
    d. ADP-ribosylation of G1 alpha sub-unit
193. The normal pH of the human blood is which one of the following:
    a. 70-72
    b. 7.25-7.35
    c. 7.36-7.44
    d. 7.50-7.55
194. The best index for calculation of the nutritional value of protein is which one of the following:
    a. Biological Value
    b. Net protein utilization
    c. Protein digestibility
    d. Protein efficiency rates
195. Malonyl aciduria is seen in deficiency of:
    a. Vitamin B_{12}
    b. Vitamin B_2
    c. Pyridoxine
    d. Folic acid
196. Sunflower cataract is caused due to:
    a. Iron deposit
    b. Sorbitol deposit
    c. Glucose deposit
    d. Copper deposit
197. Marfan's syndrome is due to the defect in:
    a. Collagen
    b. Fibrillin
    c. Elastin
    d. Laminin
198. Conversion of norepinephrine to epinephrine:
    a. Methylation
    b. Demethylation
    c. Carboxylation
    d. Decarboxylation
199. Conversion of Norepinephrine to Epinephrine
    a. COMT
    b. MAO
    c. PENMT
    d. SAM

200. Which enzyme is used to convert phenylalanine to tyrosine:
    a. Tyrosine synthase
    b. Tyrosine hydroxylase
    c. Phenylalanine hydroxylase
    d. Phenylethanolamine methyltransferase
201. Which one of the following is a precursor of tyrosine?
    a. Epinephrine
    b. Phenylalanine
    c. DOPA
    d. Norepinephrine
202. Copper containing enzyme is:
    a. Dopamine hydroxylase
    b. Dopamine decarboxylase
    c. Dopamine carboxylase
    d. Tyrosine hydroxylase
203. Enzyme involved with copper as coenzyme
    a. Lysyl oxidase
    b. Phenylanine Hydroxyalse
    c. Alcohol dehydrogenase
    d. None of the above
204. Which of the following enzyme requires molybdenum for its activity:
    a. Cytochrome oxidase
    b. Xanthine oxidase
    c. Carbonic anhydrase
    d. Phosphogluco mutase
205. Which of the following elements is required for conversion of pro-collagen to collagen:
    a. Zinc
    b. Iron
    c. Selenium
    d. Copper
206. Which of the following ion is used in PCR?
    a. Mn^{2+}
    b. Mg^{2+}
    c. Ca^{2+}
    d. Mo
207. In Non competitive inhibition of enzyme:
    a. Decreased Km, increase Vmax
    b. Increase Km, Increase Vmax
    c. Normal Km, decrease Vmax
    d. Normal Km, increase Vmax
208. All enzymes are oxidoreductases EXCEPT:
    a. Glucokinase
    b. Peroxidase
    c. Oxidase
    d. Oxygenase

BOARD REVIEW QUESTIONS

209. Cofactor of carbonic anhydrase is?
    a. Molybdenum
    b. Zinc
    c. Copper
    d. Selenium
210. How many calories are supplied per gram of dietary fiber?
    a. 2 calories
    b. 4 calories
    c. 0 calories
    d. 10 calories
211. In the first minute, what is the main source of energy used by a person who is running?
    a. Glycogen
    b. FFA
    c. Phosphagen
    d. Glucose

212. What is not given in a fructose intolerant patient?
    a. Glucose
    b. Galactose
    c. Fructose
    d. Maltose
213. Post prandial utilization of glucose is by which enzyme?
    a. Hexokinase
    b. Glucokinase
    c. Fructokinase
    d. All of the above
214. True about competitive inhibition?
    a. Increased V_{max}
    b. Increased K_m
    c. Decreased V_{max}
    d. Decreased K_m
215. Site of protein synthesis?
    a. Nucleus
    b. Cytoplasm
    c. Peroxisomes
    d. Mitochondria

Biochemistry

216. Enzyme involved in Von Gierke disease is?
   a. Muscle glycogen Phosphorylase
   b. Glucose 6 Phosphatase
   c. Debranching enzyme
   d. Branching enzyme

217. Xanthurenic acid is produced in metabolism of?
   a. Tyrosine   b. Glycine
   c. Methiosine   d. Tryptophan

218. Ketone body production occurs in?
   a. Cytoplasm   b. Mitochondria
   c. Golgi Body   d. Nucleus

219. Which is true for glucoronidation?
   a. Water solubility is decreased
   b. Phase II reaction
   c. Phase 1 reaction
   d. Done by CYP enzymes

220. Niemann's pick disease is due to deficiency of which enzyme?
   a. Sphingomyelinase   b. Hexosaminidase-A
   c. Aryl sulphatase   d. Galactosidase-A

221. 1st product of tryptophan catabolism is?
   a. Kynurenine   b. Bradykinin
   c. PAF   d. Xanthurenate

222. Urea is formed from which substrate?
   a. Arginine   b. Pyridine
   c. Citrulline   d. Aspartate

223. Hydrolysis occurs at which step of urea cycle?
   a. Cleavage of Arginine
   b. Formation of Argininosuccinate
   c. Formation of citrulline
   d. Formation of ornithine

224. What are Aptamers?
   a. Antibodies   b. Types of m-RNA
   c. Oligonucleotides d. Ribozymes

225. Auto oxidation is seen in?
   a. Cholesterol les   b. Arachidonic acid
   c. Stearic acid   d. Palmitic acid

226. What is the composition of lugols solution?
   a. 4% iodine 10% potassium iodide
   b. 5% iodine and 10% potassium iodide
   c. 2.5% iodine and 5% potassium iodide
   d. 10% iodine and 6% potassium iodide

227. Nitric oxide is synthesized from?
   a. L-arginine   b. L-citrulline
   c. Lysine   d. Tryptophan

228. Rate limiting step in cholesterol synthesis is?
   a. HMG CoA synthetase
   b. HMG CoA reductase
   c. Thiokinase
   d. Mevalonate kinase

229. True about bile acids is?
   a. 7α hydroxylase is the rate limiting enzyme in the synthesis
   b. They are derived from cholesterol
   c. Cholic acid is primary bile acid
   d. All of the above

230. Strongest oxygen radical amongst the following is?
   a. O_2^- b. OH-
   c. H_2O_2 d. HC1O

231. LCAT activates?
   a. Apo A1   b. Apo B100
   c. Apo C-2   d. Apo C-3

232. GABA is derived from?
   a. Glycine   b. Glutamine
   c. Glutamate   d. Alanine

233. Glutamic acid is formed from which of the following amino acid?
   a. Threonine   b. Proline
   c. Alanine   d. Lysine

234. Unfolded proteins are handled by?
   a. Chaperones   b. Histones
   c. Proteases   d. Proteosomes

235. The primary role of chaperones is to help in?
   a. Protein synthesis   b. Protein degradation
   c. Protein de-naturation d. Protein folding

236. Sorting of protein molecules is performed in?
   a. Mitochondria   b. Golgi apparatus
   c. Nucleosome   d. Endosome

237. Pyruvate is converted to which substance to start gluconeogenesis?
   a. Oxaloacetate   b. Phosphenol pyruvate
   c. Cis-aconitate   d. Succinate

238. Wolman disease leads to accumulation of?
   a. Cholesterol   b. Triglycerides
   c. Sphingosides   d. Cerebrocides

239. Hydrogen sulphide acts on which complex of cytochrome oxidase?
   a. Complex I   b. Complex II
   c. Complex III   d. Complex IV

240. Succinyl CoA is formed by?
   a. Valine   b. Isoleucine
   c. Methionine   d. All of the above

241. Insulin storage in body requires which ion?
   a. Cu   b. Zn
   c. Mo   d. Se

242. All are Glucogenic amino acids EXCEPT?
   a. Valine   b. Alanine
   c. Tryptophan   d. Methionine

243. Vitamin synthesized from amino acid is?
   a. Thiamine   b. Riboflavin
   c. Biotin   d. Niacin

FMGE Solutions Screening Examination

244. Beta oxidation of fatty acids occur in?
    a. Nucleus   b. Mitochondria
    c. Cytoplasm   d. Peroxisomes
245. Glucose transport along cell membranes occurs along with?
    a. K⁺   b. Na⁺
    c. Cl⁻   d. HCO₃⁻
246. LDH isoenzymes-5 is raised in which organ injury?
    a. Lungs   b. Brain
    c. Heart   d. Liver and muscles
247. Pellagra symptoms are aggravated if diet contains?
    a. High amount of leucine
    b. High amount of lysine
    c. Low amount of leucine
    d. Low amount of lysine
248. DNA model described by Watson and crick was?
    a. Right handed parallel
    b. Left handed anti parallel
    c. Right handed anti parallel
    d. Left handed parallel
249. Enzymatic activity is measured in?
    a. mg/dl   b. microgram/litre
    c. mg/litre   d. mol/second
250. Richest source of retinoids is?
    a. Cod liver oil   b. Halibut liver oil
    c. Butter   d. Margarine
251. Which step in TCA cycle is irreversible?
    a. Succinate thiokinase
    b. Alpha ketoglutarate dehydrogenase
    c. ISO citrate dehydrogenase
    d. Aconitase
252. Succinate dehydrogenase is inhibited by?
    a. Fluoroacetate   b. Cyanide
    c. Arsenite   d. Malonate
253. Pentose pathway is essential for the production of?
    a. NAD   b. FAD
    c. NADPH   d. NADH
254. Which vitamin in large doses decreases triglyceride and cholesterol?
    a. Vit B1   b. Nicotinic acid
    c. Vit B12   d. Riboflavin
255. Which enzyme is deficient in Mc ardle's diseae?
    a. Liver phosphorylase deficiency
    b. Muscle phosphorylase deficiency
    c. Lysosomal alpha-1, 4-glucosidase deficiency
    d. G6PD deficiency

256. Source of ATP in RBCs is?
    a. Beta oxidation of fatty acids
    b. TCA cycle
    c. Anaerobic glycolysis
    d. Gluconeogensis
257. ApoE is associated with?
    a. Arginine   b. Lysine
    c. Leucine   d. Isoleucine
258. Which enzyme is deficient in Tay sachs disease?
    a. Hexosaminidase A b. Galactosidase
    c. Glucocerebrosidase d. Sphingomyelinase
259. Which is true for malate shuttle?
    a. Mitochondria to cytoplasm
    b. Cytoplasm to mitochondria
    c. Both (A) and (B)
    d. None of these
260. Oxaloacetate is formed from?
    a. Proline
    b. Glutamate
    c. Aspartate
    d. Lysine
261. Iron in haemoglobin binds with?
    a. Alanine   b. Serine
    c. Histidine   d. Glycine
262. In acute intermittent porphyria which enzyme is deficient?
    a. ALA synthase
    b. Uroporphyrinogen I synthase
    c. Uroporphyrinogen II synthase
    d. Uroporphyrinogen III synthase
263. Which of the following enzymess unwinds DNA?
    a. Ligase
    b. DNA primase
    c. Helicase
    d. DNA polymerase
264. Fluoride inhibits?
    a. Enolase   b. Aldolase
    c. Aromatase   d. None of these
265. Histidine to histamine conversion is by: (2018)
    a. Dehydrogenation b. Decarboxylation
    c. Gamma carboxylation d. Monoamino oxidase
266. Vitamin with antioxidant property: (2018)
    a. Vitamin E   b. Vitamin D
    c. Vitamin B7   d. Vitamin B9
267. Which vitamin is supplied from only animal source:
                                                      (2018)
    a. Vitamin C   b. Vitamin B₇
    c. Vitamin B₁₂   d. Vitamin D

Biochemistry

ANSWERS WITH EXPLANATIONS

181

MOST RECENT QUESTIONS 2019

1. Ans. a) Arginine

- Nitric oxide is synthesized from L-Arginine
- Reaction is catalysed from enzyme nitric oxide synthase.
- **Function:**
  - Similar in reactive oxygen species in their function
  - Potent microbial killer
  - Produced by endothelial cells and by activated macrophages

2. Ans. (a) Branched chain alpha keto acid decarboxylase

- Maple syrup urine disease is an inherited disorder characterized by the deficiency of branched-chain alpha-keto acid decarboxylase complex.
- This enzyme is required for breakdown of specific amino acid in body like valine, isoleucine and leucine.
- Due to the enzyme deficiency, these amino acid is not metabolized and hence there is accumulation in cells and body fluids → producing burnt sugar/maple syrup smelling urine.

3. Ans. (a) Glycine

- Collagen is rich in glycine and proline amino acid.
- Glycine is the smallest amino acid, present in every third position of chain, therefore it fits into the spaces where the three chains of helix comes together.
- This repeating structure, represented as (Gly-X-Y)n, is an absolute requirement for the formation of the triple helix. While X and Y can be any other amino acid, about 100 of the X positions are proline and about 100 of the Y positions are hydroxyproline. Proline and hydroxyproline confer rigidity on the collagen molecule.

4. Ans. (b) Vitamin E

- Vitamins which act as anti-oxidants are: Vitamin A, C and E (tocopherol)
- Beta Carotene (Vit A) is an anti-oxidant at low PO_2.

These antioxidants are of two types:
1. **Preventive antioxidants:** Reduce the rate of chain initiation. Includes: Catalase, EDTA, DTPA
2. **Chain breaking antioxidant:** Interfere with chain propagation. Includes: SOD, Vitamin E.

5. Ans. (c) Vitamin C

- Vitamin C reduces ferric iron to ferrous form, thereby facilitating the absorption of dietary iron from the intestine.

6. Ans. (a) Thiamine

- The active form of thiamine (Vitamin B1) is thiamine pyrophosphate which is formed by the transfer of a pyrophosphate group from adenosine triphosphate (ATP) to thiamine.
- Thiamine deficiency is diagnosed by an increase in erythrocyte transketolase activity observed on addition of TPP

Deficiency of thiamine leads to:
- **Beriberi:** A severe thiamine deficiency syndrome occurs due to intake of polished rice.
- **Wernicke-Korsakoff syndrome:** Associated with chronic alcoholism, which occurs due to dietary insufficiency or impaired dietary absorption of the vitamin. In some alcoholics there is development of Wernicke-Korsakoff syndrome, a thiamine deficiency syndrome characterized by confusion, ataxia and nystagmus with Wernicke's encephalopathy as well as memory problems, hallucination and dementia.

7. Ans. (a) McArdle disease

- **McArdle disease** is an **AR condition**, one of **the type V glycogen storage disease**.
- Enzyme deficient: Myophosphorylase enzyme
- Due to enzyme deficiency there is inability to breakdown the muscle glycogen and prevents lactate production.
- Patients usually complain of exercise intolerance and muscle pain on exercise. Therefore strenuous exercise is contraindicated.

Explanations

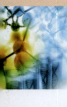

TABLE: Gycogen-storage diseases

Type	Defective enzyme	Organ affected	Glycogen in the affected organ	Clinical features
I. Von Gierke	Glucose 6-phosphatase or transport system	Liver and kidney	Increased amount; normal structure	Massive enlargement of the liver. Failure to thrive, Severe hypoglycemia, ketosis, hyperuricemia, heperlipemia
II. Pompe	α-1, 4–Glucosidase (lysosomal)	All organs	Massive increase in amount; normal structure	Cardiorespiratory failure causes death, usually before age 2
III. Cori	Amylo-1,6-glucosidase (debranching enzyme)	Muscle and liver	Increased amount; short outer branches	Like type I, but milder course
IV. Andersen	Branching enzyme (α-1,4 → α-1,6)	Liver and spleen	Normal amount; very long outer branches	Progressive cirrhosis of the liver. Liver failure causes death, usually before age 2
V. McArdle	Phosphorylase	Muscle	Moderately increased amount; normal structure	Limited ability to perform strenuous exercise because of painful muscle cramps. Otherwise patient is normal and well developed
VI. Hers	Phosphorylase	Liver	Increased amount	Like type I, but milder course
VII.	Phosphofructokinase	Muscle	Increased amount; normal structure	Like type V
VIII.	Phosphorylase kinase	Liver	Increased amount; normal structure	Mild liver enlargement. Mild hypoglycemia

Note: Types I through VII are inherited as autosomal recessives. Type VIII is sex linked.

8. Ans. (a) 2,4 dinitrophenol

- Compounds that can uncouple or delink the ETC from oxidative phosphorylation, such compounds are known as uncouplers
- As a result ATP synthesis doesn't occur.
- 2,4 Dinitrophenol is an example of chemical uncoupler.

Chemical uncouplers	
• Chemical uncouplers	• Physiological uncouplers
▪ 2, 4 dinitrophenol (has been extensively studied)	▪ Thyroid hormones
▪ Dinitrocresol	▪ Long chain fatty acids
▪ Pentachlorophenol	▪ Unconjugated bilirubin
▪ Tri fluoro carbonyl cyanide phenyl hydra zone (FCCP)	• These act as uncouplers only at high concentration
▪ Aspirin (high doses)	

9. Ans. (a) Pyruvate dehydrogenase

- The enzyme Pyruvate dehydrogenase irreversibly converts pyruvate, the end product of glycolysis, into acetyl CoA, a major fuel for the TCA cycle and the building block for fatty acid synthesis
- Thus, this enzyme pyruvate dehydrogenase is utilized in citric acid cycle and fatty acid synthesis.
- The reaction of pyruvate dehydrogenase, forming acetyl-CoA, is irreversible, and for every two carbon unit from acetyl-CoA that enters the citric acid cycle, there is a loss of two carbon atoms as carbon dioxide before oxaloacetate is reformed.
- This means that acetyl-CoA (and hence any substrates that yield acetyl-CoA) can never be used for gluconeogenesis.

10. Ans. (a) Palmitic acid

- Palmitic acid is the most common fatty acid found in animals, plant and microbes.
- Excess carbohydrates and proteins are converted to palmitic acid.
- Palmitic acid is the first fatty acid synthesized during fatty acid synthesis.
- **Note:** First step in fatty acid synthesis is transfer of acetate units from mitochondrial acetyl CoA to the cytosol.

CARBOHYDRATE

11. Ans. (c) Mitochondria and cytoplasm

Ref: Harper's Biochemistry, 30th ed. pg. 294-95

Biochemistry

Urea Cycle
- Urea is the end product of nitrogen catabolism in humans
- It takes place in both mitochondria and cytoplasm
- Some reactions of urea synthesis occur in the matrix of the mitochondrion, other reactions in the cytosol
- Synthesis of 1 mol of urea requires 3 mol of ATP plus 1 mol each of ammonium ion and of the amino nitrogen of aspartate.
- **Undergoes 5 steps in urea synthesis:**
  - Steps 1 and 2 take place in mitochondria
  - Steps 3, 4, 5 take place in cytosol

For more details please refer to mother book explanation 121

---

12. Ans. (d) Unconjugated bilirubin

- Uncouplers inhibit oxidative phosphorylation. They are hydrophobic molecules with a dissociable protein.
- They uncouple the ETC form oxidative phosphorylation
- Physiological uncouplers acts only at high dose.

Chemical Uncouplers	Physiological Uncouplers
• γ 2,4-dinitrophenol (has been extensively studied). • Dinitrocresol • Pentachlorophenol • Tri fluoro carbonyl cyanide phenylhydrazone (FCCP). • Aspirin (high doses)	• Thyroid hormones. • Long chain fatty acids. • Unconjugated Bilirubin. These act as Uncouplers only at high concentration

Extra Mile

Inhibitors of Electron Transport Chain

Inhibitors of Oxidative Phosphorylation
- **Complex I:** Rotenone
- **Complex II:** Carboxin
- **Complex III:** Antimycin A
- **Complex IV:** Cyanide, Azide, Carbon monoxide
- **ATP synthase:** Oligomycin
- **ATP-ADP translocase:** Atractyloside (a plant glycoside)

---

13. Ans. (b) Liver

Ref: Vasudevan Biochemistry 8/e. P 136

SITE OF GLUCONEOGENESIS

- **Major site of gluconeogenesis:** Liver (90%)
- **Secondary site:** Kidney cortex and in small intestine under some conditions. (10%)
- It takes place in the mitochondria and cytoplasm.
- The production of glucose is necessary for use as a fuel source by the brain, testes, erythrocytes, kidney medulla, lens and cornea of the eye and exercising muscles.

14. Ans. (b) Hemolytic anemia

Ref: Vasudevan Biochemistry, 8th ed. P 426

Extra Mile
- G6PD deficiency causes hemolytic anemia, since RBCs become susceptible to oxidative stress

Other causes of hemolytic anemias are:

FMGE Solutions Screening Examination

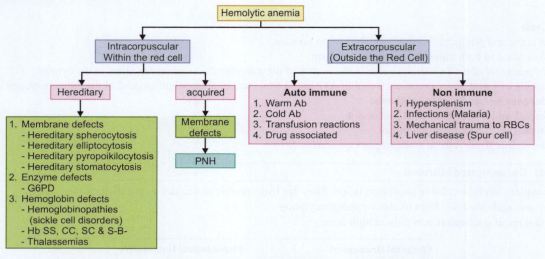

15. Ans. (c) Fructokinase

Ref: Harper, pg. 169

"Deficiencies in the enzymes of fructose and galactose metabolism lead to **essential fructosuria** and **galactosemias**."
"Lack of hepatic fructokinase causes **essential fructosuria**, and absence of hepatic aldolase B, which cleaves fructose 1-phosphate, leads to **hereditary fructose intolerance**."

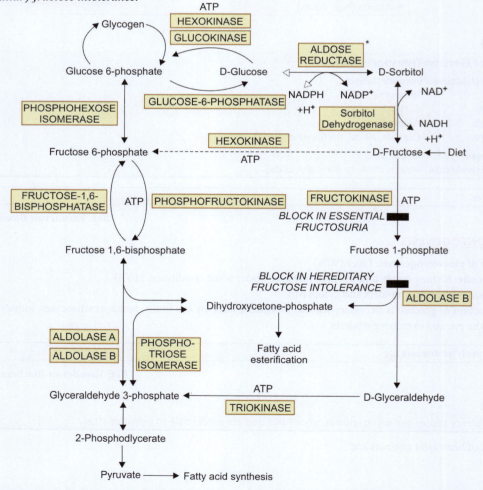

Metabolism of fructose. Aldolase A is found in all tissues, whereas aldolase B is the predominant form in liver. (*, not found in liver)

Biochemistry

16. Ans. (a) McArdle's disease

Ref: Harper's Biochemistry, pg. 145

- **Glycogen storage diseases** are a group of inherited disorders characterized by deficient mobilization of glycogen or deposition of abnormal forms of glycogen, leading to muscular weakness or even death.
- **Nelson 20th ed states**: *"Approximately 50% patients with GSD type V, report burgundy colored urine after exercise, which is a consequence of exercise-induced myoglobinuria secondary to rhabdomyolysis"*

17. Ans. (c) Enolase

Ref: Harper's Biochemistry, 30th edn. pg. 170-171

Reversible steps of glycolysis are catalyzed by	Irreversible steps of glycolysis are catalyzed by
• Phosphohexose isomerase • Aldolase • Phosphotriose isomerase • Glyceraldehyde 3-phosphate dehydrogenase • Phosphoglycerate kinase • Phosphoglycerate mutase • **Enolase**	• Glucokinase/Hexokinase • Phosphofructokinase-I • Pyruvate kinase

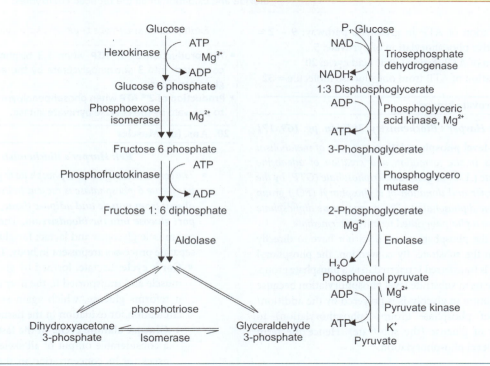

18. Ans. (a) 10

Ref: Harper's Biochemistry, 30th edn. pg. 169-170

- In glycolytic pathway, one molecule of glucose gives 2 pyruvate.
- The 2 molecules of pyruvate are further metabolized in citric acid cycle, giving out 20 ATP.
- Since the question here is asking about one molecule of pyruvate, the answer will be the half of 20, i.e. 10.
- **In simple words:** 2 molecules of pyruvate give 20 ATP. Hence one molecule will give 10 ATP.

Step	Coenzyme yield	ATP	Source of ATP
Glycolysis preparatory phase		−2	Phosphorylation of glucose and fructose 6-phosphate uses two ATP from the cytoplasm
Glycolysis pay-off phase		4	Substrate-level phosphorylation
	2 NADH (2 × 2.5)	5	Oxidative phosphorylation-Each NADH produces net 2 ATP due to NADH transport over the mitochondrial membrane

Contd...

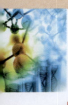

FMGE Solutions Screening Examination

Step	Coenzyme yield	ATP	Source of ATP
Oxidative decarboxylation of pyruvate	2 NADH (2 x 2.5)	5	Oxidative phosphorylation
NET ATP TILL PHOSPHORYLATION OF PYRUVATE: 5+5+4 = 14-2 = **12**		= 12	
Krebs cycle		2	Substrate-level phosphorylation
	6 NADH (6 x 2.5)	15	Oxidative phosphorylation
	2 FADH2 (2 x 1.5)	3	Oxidative phosphorylation
Total yield		32 ATP	From the complete oxidation of one glucose molecule to carbon dioxide and oxidation of all the reduced coenzymes.

- Net generation of ATP in glycolytic pathway: 9 – 2 = 7   Oxidative phosphorylation of pyruvate: **5**
- Generation of ATP during Citric acid cycle: **20**
- Net generation of ATP from one glucose molecule = **32**

19. Ans. (b) Pyruvate kinase

Ref: Harper's Biochemistry, 30th edn. pg. 169, 171

- **Substrate-level phosphorylation** is *a type of metabolism that results in the formation and creation of adenosine triphosphate (ATP) or guanosine triphosphate (GTP) by the direct transfer and donation of a phosphoryl (PO₃) group to adenosine diphosphate (ADP) or guanosine diphosphate (GDP) from a phosphorylated reactive intermediate.*
- Note that the phosphate group does not have to directly come from the substrate. By convention, the phosphoryl group that is transferred is referred to as a phosphate group.
- We use the term substrate level phosphorylation because ATP formation in glycolysis is powered by the addition/removal of phosphate groups (phosphorylation) to molecules of glucose (the substrate). Hence the term substrate-level phosphorylation.

Extra Mile

Some Important Pathways and their Rate Limiting Enzyme

Pathway	Rate limiting enzyme
Glycolysis	Phosphofructo kinase
Glycogenesis	Glycogen synthase
Glycogenolysis	Phosphorylase
Cholesterol synthesis	HMG - COA Reductase
Ketone body formation	HMG - COA synthase
Bile acid synthesis	7-a-hydroxylase
Fatty acid synthesis	Acetyl COA carboxylase
Uric acid synthesis	Xanthine oxidase

Examples of Substrate Level Phosphorylation that Occurs

- The production of 1st ATP when 1,3 bisphophoglycerate is converted into 3 phosphoglycerate by the enzyme **phosphoglycerate kinase**
- Production of 2nd ATP when phosphoenolpyruvate is converted to pyruvate by the enzyme **pyruvate kinase.**

20. Ans. (d) Muscles

Ref: Harper's Biochemistry, 30th ed. pg. 187

- The conversion of glucose 6-phosphate to glucose is catalyzed by glucose 6-phosphatase is present in liver and kidney, **but absent from muscle and adipose tissue, which cannot export glucose into the bloodstream.** Therefore in order to use muscle glycogen and lactate for gluconeogenesis two separate processes arepresent in body. They are:
  - **Cori's cycle**: Lactate, formed by glycolysis in skeletal muscle and transported to the liver and kidney where it reforms glucose, which again is available via the circulation for oxidation in the tissues.
  - **Glucose alanine cycle:** In the fasting state, there is a considerable output of all skeletal muscle, far in excess of its concentration in the muscle proteins that is catabolized. It is formed by transamination of pyruvate produced by glycolysis and glycogen, and is exported to the liver, where, after transamination back is a substrate for gluconeogenesis. This glucose-alanine cycle thus provides an indirect way of utilizing muscle glycogen to maintain blood glucose in the fasting state.

21. Ans. (a) Cori cycle

Ref: Harper's Biochemistry, 30th ed. pg. 190-191

- The Cori cycle is the only one that is not dependent on the mitochondrial enzymes. This cycle is basically the transport of lactate from the muscle to the liver to be converted via gluconeogenesis to glucose to be transported back to the muscle.

Biochemistry

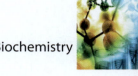

Extra Mile

Mitochondria Mn: KEBOK in all cap	Cytoplasm	Both mitochondria and cytoplasm (Mn: HUG for both)
• Kreb cycle • ETC • Bet oxidation of FA • Oxidative phosphorylation • Ketogenesis	• Glycolysis • Glycogenesis • Glycogenolysis • HMP Shunt • FA synthesis • Cholesterol synthesis • Bile acid/Salt synthesis	• Gluconeogenesis • Urea synthesis • Heme synthesis

Extra Mile

TABLE: GLUT receptors, their location and function

Receptor	Location on tissue	Function
GLUT 1	Brain, kidney, colon, placenta, RBC, retina	Glucose uptake
GLUT 2	Liver, pancreatic beta cell, small intestine, Kidney	Rapid uptake or release of glucose
GLUT 3	Brain, kidney and placenta	Glucose uptake
GLUT 4	Heart, skeletal muscles, adipose tissue	Insulin-stimulated glucose uptake
GLUT 5	Small intestine	Absorption of glucose
GLUT 6	Spleen, leukocyte	—
GLUT 7	Liver, endoplasmic reticulum	Glucose transporter in endoplasmic reticulum

22. Ans. (b) Liver

Ref: Harper's Biochemistry, 30th ed. pg. 190-191

- Each day the body has an excess production of about 1500 mmols of lactate (about 20 mmols/kg/day) which enters the blood stream and is subsequently **metabolised mostly in the liver.**
- All tissues can produce lactate under anaerobic conditions but tissues with active glycolysis produce excess lactate from glucose under normal conditions and this lactate tends to spill over into the blood. Lactate is produced from pyruvate in a reaction catalysed by lactate dehydrogenase:

Pyruvate + NADH + H⁺ <=> Lactate + NAD⁺

23. Ans. (d) EMP pathway

24. Ans. (d) Hexokinase

- **These are the enzymes of glycolysis whose action is increased by insulin (regulates positively):**
    ♦ Glucokinase
    ♦ Phosphofructokinase
    ♦ Pyruvate kinase
- **NOTE:** Insulin doesn't regulate Hexokinase

25. Ans. (c) Skeletal muscles

Ref: Harper's Biochemistry, 30th ed. pg. 191-192

- **Insulin** increases the number and activity of GLUT 4 receptor. Thereby facilitating the entry of glucose in tissues having GLUT4 receptor.
- **Tissues with abundant GLUT4 receptor are:** *Skeletal muscles, Heart and Adipose tissue*
- Thus among the given choices, skeletal muscle is the one which required for entry of glucose.

26. Ans. (a) Glycolysis

Ref: Harper's Biochemistry, 30th ed. pg. 142-144

- **Glycolysis occurs in cytoplasm.**
- **There are two major sites for gluconeogenesis, the liver and the kidneys.**
- The liver accounts for 90% of gluconeogenesis in the body and the remaining 10% occur in the kidney and other tissues of the body.
- The liver and kidneys maintain the glucose level in the blood so that the brain, muscle and red blood cells have sufficient glucose to meet their metabolic demands.

Extra Mile

Cycle occurs in both cytoplasm and mitochondria-
- Gluconeogenesis
- Urea cycle
- Heme synthesis

27. Ans. (b) Gluconeogenesis

Ref: Harper's Biochemistry, 30th ed. pg. 142-144

Please refer to above explanation

28. Ans. (a) Insulin

Ref: Harper's Biochemistry, 30th ed. pg. 191-192

- Synthesis of glucose from non-carbohydrate source is called Gluconeogenesis.

Hormonal Regulation

↑ Glucagon, epinephrine, glucocorticoids.
↓ Insulin

FMGE Solutions Screening Examination

- **Gluconeogenesis is regulated by 4 key enzymes-**
  - Pyruvate carboxylase
  - Phosphoenolpyruvate carboxylase
  - F16 bisphosphatase
  - G-6-phosphatase

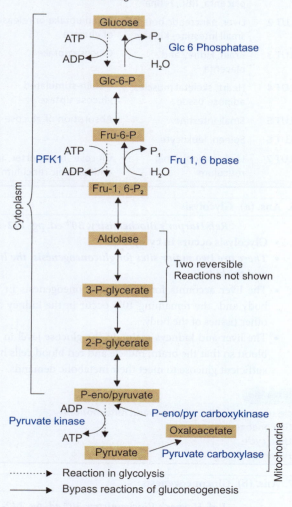

NADH which gains entry from cytosol is oxidized by mitochondrial ETC, leading to formation of 2.5 molecules of ATP.

- **Glycerophosphate shuttle:** in this mechanism, cytosolic NADH is used to reduce dihydroxyacetone phosphate to glycerol-3 phosphate which diffuse through the outer mitochondrial membrane into the inter-membrane space of the mitochondria. In this space, glycerol 3 phosphate is reoxidized to dihydroxyacetone phosphate and the reducing equivalents are transferred to FAD to form $FADH_2$. $FADH_2$ is oxidized in ETC to form 1.5 molecules of ATP.

30. Ans. (c) Fructose

Ref: Harper's Biochemistry, 30th edn. pg. 205

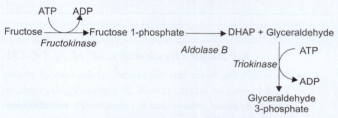

- Hereditary fructose intolerance (HFI) is an inborn error of fructose metabolism caused by a deficiency of the enzyme aldolase-B.
- In the deficiency of Aldolase B enzyme, *if fructose is ingested, it will lead to an accumulation of fructose-1-phosphate*. This accumulation has downstream effects on gluconeogenesis and regeneration of ATP.
- **Symptoms of HFI include:** Vomiting, hypoglycemia, jaundice, hemorrhage, hepatomegaly, hyperuricemia and potentially kidney failure.
- **The key identifying feature of HFI**: *Appearance of symptoms with the introduction of fructose to the diet.*
- Sucrose, sorbitol should also be restricted in diet.

31. Ans. (d) Fructose-1, biphosphate

Ref: Harper's Biochemistry, 30th ed. pg. 202-203

- **Aldolase B** is preferentially expressed in the liver, while **aldolase A** is expressed in muscle and erythrocytes and **aldolase C** is expressed in the brain. Slight differences in isozyme structure result in different activities for the two substrate molecules: Fructose 1,6-Biphosphate and fructose 1-phosphate. *Aldolase B exhibits no preference and thus catalyzes both reactions, while aldolases A and C prefer FBP.*
- **Aldolase A** is an enzyme that catalyses a reversible aldol reaction: The substrate, fructose 1,6-bisphosphate (F-1,6-BP) is broken down into glyceraldehyde 3-phosphate and dihydroxyacetone phosphate (DHAP).

29. Ans. (b) Malate shuttle

Ref: Harper's Biochemistry, 30th ed. pg. 134-135

- There are certain shuttle systems that operate for transport of reducing equivalents from cytosol into mitochondria. These shuttle systems operate because mitochondrial membrane is impermeable to cytosolic NADH produced during glycolysis. In order to gain entry of NADH into mitochondrial electron transport chain, these shuttle systems are helpful.
- **Malate shuttle (aka malate-aspartate shuttle):** it is most common and universal shuttle system. Mitochondrial

- Sucrose is composed of glucose and fructose and hence cannot be tolerated by patients of HFI.

32. Ans. (d) Aldolase - B deficiency

Ref: Harper's Biochemistry, 30th ed. pg. 202-203

- **Hereditary fructose intolerance** is an in-born error of fructose metabolism caused by a deficiency of the enzyme aldolase B. individuals affected with Hereditary fructose intolerance are asymptomatic until they ingest fructose. If fructose is ingested, the enzymatic block at aldolase B causes an accumulation of fructose-l-phosphate. This accumulation has downstream effect on gluconeogenesis and regeneration of adenosine triphosphate (ATP).
- **Symptoms:** vomiting, hypoglycemia, jaundice, hemorrhage, hepatomegaly, hyperuricemia and potentially kidney failure.

33. Ans. (c) Lactate-dehydrogenase

Ref: Harper's Biochemistry 30th ed. / 171, 321

- Excess dietary fructose can be converted to pyruvate, this then enters the Krebs cycle and emerges as citrate directed toward free fatty acid synthesis in the cytosol of hepatocytes.

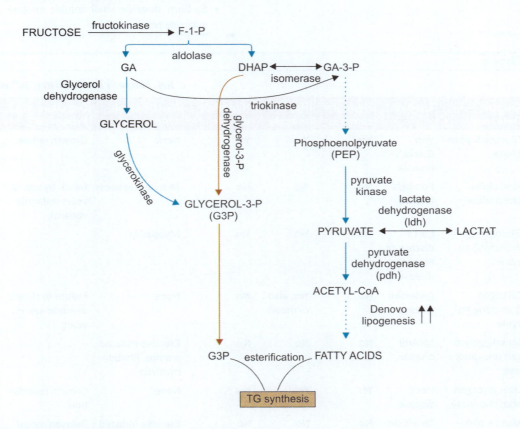

34. Ans. (b) Phase II reaction

Ref: Harper's Biochemistry, 30th edn. pg. 586

METABOLISM OF XENOBIOTICS

- **In phase 1,** the major reaction involved is hydroxylation, catalyzed by enzymes mono-oxygenases or cytochrome P450s. The reactions are:
  - Hydroxylation
  - Deamination
  - Dehalogenation
  - Desulfuration
  - Epoxidation
  - Peroxygenation
  - Reduction
- **In phase 2,** compounds produced in phase 1 are converted to various polar metabolites by conjugation

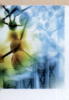

with glucuronic acid, sulfate, acetate, glutathione, or certain amino acids, or by methylation.
- The overall purpose of the two phases of metabolism of xenobiotics is to increase their water solubility (polarity) and thus excretion from the body.
  Glucuronidation: UDP Glucuronic acid is the glucuronyl donor, and a variety of glucuronosyl transferases, present in both the endoplasmic reticulum and cytosol, are the catalysts.
- **Phase II reactions are:**
  - **Glucuronidation:** is probably the most frequent conjugation reaction.
  - Sulfation
  - Conjugation with Glutathione
  - Acetylation
  - Methylation

35. Ans. (a) Cornea

Ref: Harper's Biochemistry, 30th edn. pg. 140
- Glucagon receptors are mainly expressed in liver and in kidney with lesser amounts found in heart, adipose tissue, spleen, thymus, adrenal glands, pancreas, cerebral cortex, and gastrointestinal tract.

36. Ans. (a) Enolase

Ref: Harper's Biochemistry, 30th edn. pg. 170-171
- **Enolase**, also known as phosphopyruvate hydratase, is a metallo-enzyme responsible for the catalysis of the conversion of 2-phosphoglycerate to phosphoenol pyruvate, the ninth and penultimate step of glycolysis.
- If the sample for blood glucose is kept for some time, the Red blood cells will start consuming the sugar available and hence the final report shall be lower than actual.
- Sodium flouride shall inhibit enolase and ensure an accurate result.

37. Ans. (a) Type 1

Ref: Harper's Biochemistry, 30th edn. pg. 178-179

Number	Enzyme Deficiency	Eponym	Hypogly-cemia	Hepato-megaly	Hyperlipi-demia	Muscle symptoms	Development / Prognosis	Other symptoms
GSD type I	Glucose 6-phosphate	Von Gierke's disease	Yes	Yes	Yes	None	Growth failure	Lactic acidosis, hyperuricemia
GSD type II	Acid alpha-glucosidase	Pompe's disease	No	Yes	No	Muscle weakness	Death by age -2 years (infantile variant)	Heart failure
GSD type III	Glycogen debranching enzyme	Cori's disease of Forbes's disease	Yes	Yes	Yes	Myopathy		
GSD type IV	Glycogen Branching enzyme	Andersen disease	No	Yes, also cirrhosis	No	None	Failure to thrive, death at age -5 years	
GSD type V	Muscle gklycogen phosphorylase	McArdi disease	No	No	No	Exercise induced cramps, Rhabdomyolysis		Renal failure by myoglobinuria
GSD type VI	Liver glycogen phosphorylase	Her's disease	Yes	Yes	Yes	None	Growth retardation	Haemolytic anemia
GSD type VII	Muscle phosphofructokinase	Tarui's disease	No	No	No	Exercise-induced muscle cramps and weakness	Delayed motor development, Growth retardation	
GSD type IX	Phosphorylase kinase PHKA2		Yes	Yes	Yes	None		

"Mn: Von Pump Cori And Make Her Tired"

38. Ans. (d) Myophosphorylase deficiency

Ref: Harper's Biochemistry, 30th ed. pg. 178-179

Please refer to above explanation.

39. Ans. (d) The oxidative phase generates NADH and the Non oxidative phase generates pyruvate

Ref: Harper's Biochemistry, 30th ed. pg. 198-199

- The **pentose phosphate pathway** (also called the **phosphogluconate pathway** and the **hexose monophosphate shunt**) is a process that generates NADPH and pentoses.
- There are two distinct phases in the pathway. The first is the oxidative phase, in which NADPH is generated, and the second is the non-oxidative synthesis of 5-carbon sugars. *This pathway is an alternative to glycolysis.*
- **The PPP occurs exclusively in the cytoplasm,** and is found to be most active in the liver, mammary gland and adrenal cortex in the human. The PPP is one of the three main ways the body creates molecules with reducing power, accounting for **approximately 60% of NADPH production in humans.**
- One of the uses of NADPH in the cell is to prevent oxidative stress.

40. Ans. (a) NADPH

Ref: Harper's Biochemistry, 30th ed. pg. 198-199

41. Ans. (b) 5% iodine and 10% potassium iodide

Solution	Iodine (w/v)	Potassium iodide (w/v)
Aqueous iodine (lugol's iodine)	5%	10%
Weak iodine solution (tincture of iodine)	2%	2.5%
Strong iodine solution	10%	6%

Uses of Lugol's Iodine

- During colposcopy, lugol's iodine is applied to the vagina and cervix.: Schiller's test
- Lugol's iodine may also be used to better visualize the muco-gingival junction in the mouth.
- Lugol's solution can also be used in various experiments to observe how a cell membrane uses osmosis and diffusion.
- Oxidizing germicide

42. Ans. (b) Lipid synthesis and glutathione reaction

Ref: Harper's Biochemistry, 30th ed. pg. 234-35

NADPH is Used for

- Lipid synthesis
- Cholesterol synthesis
- Fatty acid chain elongation
- Regeneration of reduced glutathione (which protects against Reactive oxygen species)

LIPIDS

43. Ans. (a) Acetyl CoA

- **Principle building block in fatty acid synthesis: Acetyl CoA**
- **Cofactors required:** NADPH, ATP, Mn^{2+} and HCO_3
- **Source of Acetyl CoA:** From mitochondria (after aerobic glycolysis and Fatty acid oxidation)
- **Site of FA synthesis:** Liver, Kidney, Brain, Lungs, Adipose tissue, Lactating breast
  - **Organelle:** Extra-mitochondrial system in cytosol
- **Enzyme:**
  - Acetyl CoA carboxylase-*rate limiting enzyme*
  - Fatty acid synthase

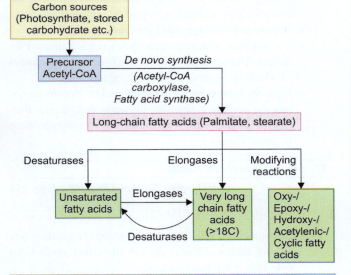

44. Ans. (c) 3.5

Ref: Harrison's, 18th ed. pg. ch 356

- The total cholesterol to HDL cholesterol ratio is a number that is helpful in predicting an individual's risk of developing atherosclerosis.
- High ratios indicate higher risks of heart attacks, low ratios indicate lower risk.
- *Ideally ratio should be kept below 4.*

45. Ans. (a) Sphingomyelinase

Ref: Harper's Biochemistry, 30th ed. pg. 250

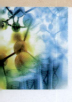

FMGE Solutions Screening Examination

- Niemann's Pick diseases are genetic diseases which are classified in a subgroup of lipid storage disorders in which harmful quantities of fatty substances, or lipids, accumulate in the spleen, liver, lungs, bone marrow, and brain.
- In the classic infantile type-A variant, a mis-sense mutation causes complete deficiency of sphingomyelinase which leads to niemann pick disease.

> **Extra Mile**
>
> **Other lysosomal storage disease and deficient enzymes**
> - **Hurler's syndrome**: Alpha-L-iduronidase deficiency
> - **Hunter's syndrome**: Iduronate-2-sulfatase deficiency
> - **Gaucher's**: β-Glucosidase deficiency
> - **Farber's disease**: Ceramidase deficiency
> - **Fabry disease**: Alpha Galactosidase-A
> - **Tay-sach's**: Hexosaminidase A deficiency
> - **Sandhoff's disease**: β-Hexosaminidase A and B
> - **Metachromatic leukodystrophy**: *arylsulfatase* A enzyme deficiency
> - *Krabbe disease*: *β-Galactosidase*

46. Ans. (a) Lysosome

Ref: Harper's Biochemistry, 30th ed. pg. 251

- Sphinghomyelin is a major neural tissue component, the core structure of which is formed by ceramide.
- *It is the only sphingholipid without sugar.*
- The common sphinghomyelin deficiency is Neiman-Pick disease. The organelle which is involved is the lysosomes which allow accumulation of sphinghomyelin.
- **Signs & symptoms of Niemen pick's**: Hepatosplenomegaly, decreased appetite, unsteady gait, ataxia, slurring of speech (due to accumulation of sphingholipids in neural tissue).

47. Ans. (a) Gaucher's disease

Ref: Harper's Biochemistry, 30th ed. pg. 251

LYSOSOMAL STORAGE DISEASE

- Lyzosomal storage disorders are a group of approximately 50 rare inherited metabolic disorders that result from defects in lysosomal function.
- Lysosomal storage disorders are caused by lysosomal dysfunction usually as a consequence of deficiency of a single enzyme required for the metabolism of lipids, glycoproteins (sugar containing proteins) or so-called mucopolysaccharides.
- **Gaucher's disease is the most common of the lysosomal storage diseases**. It is a form of sphingolipidosis (a subgroup of lysosomal storage diseases), as it involves dysfunctional metabolism of sphingolipids.
- *The disorder is characterized by bruising, fatigue, anemia, low blood platelets, and enlargement of the liver and spleen.*

48. Ans. (c) Gaucher's disease

Ref: Harper's Biochemistry, 30th ed. pg. 251

Management of Gaucher's Disease

- *Regular, intravenous enzyme therapy is currently the treatment of choice in affected patients and is highly efficacious and safe in diminishing the hepatosis and improving bone marrow involvement and hematologic findings.*
- Symptomatic management of the blood cytopenias and joint replacement continue to have important roles in management
- The bone disease is decreased but not eliminated by enzyme therapy. Adults benefit from adjunctive treatment with bisphosphonates to improve bone mass.

49. Ans. (b) Hexosaminidase A

Ref: Harper's Biochemistry, 30th ed. pg. 251

- **Tay–Sach's disease** (also known as **GM2 gangliosidosis** or **hexosaminidase A deficiency**) is a rare autosomal recessive genetic disorder.
- In its most common variant (known as infantile Tay–Sachs disease), it causes a progressive deterioration of nerve cells and of mental and physical abilities that commences around six months of age and usually results in death by the age of four.

50. Ans. (b) HMG CoA reductase

Ref: Harper's Biochemistry, 30th ed. pg. 267

- *HMG CoA reductase is the rate limiting ezyme in cholesterol synthesis.*
- HMG CoA Synthetase is involved in the formation of ketone bodies while HMG CoA lyase is involved also in the ketogenesis and also in the processing of leucine.
- Catalase on the other hand is an oxidoreductase which is involved in the connversion of hydrogen peroxide to water and oxygen.

51. Ans. (b) APO B-100

Ref: Harper's Biochemistry, 30th ed. pg. 254

- The low-density-lipoprotein (LDL) receptor is a cell-surface protein that plays an important part in the metabolism of cholesterol by mediating the uptake of LDL from plasma into cells.
- Although LDL particles bind to the LDL receptor through their apolipoprotein B (apo B) and apolipoprotein E (apo E) moieties, other apo E-containing particles, like chylomicron remnants, are not dependent on the LDL receptor for uptake into cells.
- ApoB100 levels are associated with coronary heart disease, and are even a better predictor of it than is LDL level. A simple way of explaining this observation is to use the idea that ApoB-100 reflects lipoprotein particle

Biochemistry

number (independent of their cholesterol content). In this way, one can infer that the number of ApoB100-containing lipoprotein particles is a determinant of atherosclerosis and heart disease.

> **Extra Mile**
> - Most important apoprotein in HDL: **Apo A-I**
> - Most important apoprotein in chylomicrons: **Apo B-48, E**
> - Most important apoprotein in LDL, IDL, VLDL: **Apo B-100**
> - Apo protein for IDL → **Apo B 100 and E**

52. Ans. (d) APO-B 100

> *Ref: Harper's Biochemistry, 30th ed. pg. 253-254*

53. Ans. (a) LDL-receptors

> *Ref: Harper's Biochemistry, 30th ed. pg. 275*

- **Familial hypercholesterolemia** is a genetic disorder characterized by high cholesterol levels, specifically very

high levels of low-density lipoprotein in the blood and early cardiovascular disease.

- *These patients have mutations in the LDLR gene that encodes the LDL receptor protein, which normally removes LDL from the circulation.*
- The high cholesterol levels in FH are less responsive to the kinds of cholesterol control methods that are usually more effective in people without FH (such as dietary modification and statin tablets), because the body's underlying biochemistry is slightly different. However, treatment (including higher statin doses) can often be successful.
- Heterozygous FH is normally treated with statins, bile acid sequestrants or other hypo-lipidemic agents that lower cholesterol levels.
- Homozygous FH often does not respond to medical therapy and may require other treatments, including LDL apheresis (removal of LDL in a method similar to dialysis) and occasionally liver transplantation.

54. Ans. (b) LDL

> *Ref: Harper's Biochemistry, 30th edn. pg. 254; Harper 26th ed. pg. 206*

- **Max cholesterol-** LDL
- **Max TG-** chylomicrons *(in form of triacylglycerol)*
- **Max exogenous TG-** Chylomicron
- **Max endogenous TG-** VLDL

TABLE: Lipoprotein, its source, composition, main lipid component and its apolipoprotein

Lipoprotein	Source	Composition		Main lipid component	Apo-lipoprotein
		Protein (%)	Lipid (%)		
Chylomicrons	Intestine	1-2	**98-99**	**Triacylglycerol**	A-I, A-II, A-IV, B-48, C-I, C-II, C-III, E
VLDL	Liver (intestine)	7-10	90-93	Triacylglycerol	**B-100, C-I, C-II, C-III**
IDL	VLDL	11	89	Triacylglycerol, cholesterol	B-100, E
LDL	VLDL	21	**79**	Cholesterol	B-100
HDL	Liver, intestine, VLDL, chylomicrons	32	68	Phospholipids, Cholesterol	A-I, A-II, A-IV, C-I, C-II, C-III, D, E
Albumin	Adipose tissue	99	1	Free fatty acid	

55. Ans. (b) VLDL

> *Ref: Harper's Biochemistry, 30th edn. pg. 271-272*

Lipoprotein	Transport
• HDL	Tissue → liver (good cholestrol)
• VLDL	Liver → plasma
• LDL	Liver → tissue (bad cholestrol)
• CHYLOMICRON	Intestine → plasma

56. Ans. (d) All of the above

> *Ref: Harper's Biochemistry, 30th edn. pg. 213-214*

Medium chain fatty acid contain 8-14 carbon atoms
- Examples: caproic acid (10 C), lauric acid (12C), Myristic acid (14C), Palmitic acid (16C), Stearic Acid (18C).
- They do not require prolonged digestion
- Do not require Pancreatic lipase and bile salts
- Diffuse directly into portal circulation
- Preferentially oxidized by peripheral cells and therefore do not get deposited into adipose.

Explanations

FMGE Solutions Screening Examination

57. Ans. (b) Arachidonic acid

Ref: Harper's Biochemistry, 30th edn. pg. 238-40

- Auto oxidation is any oxidation that occurs in open air or in presence of oxygen and/or radiation and forms peroxides and hydro-peroxides.
- Unsaturated fatty acids undergo auto-oxidation in presence of oxygen due to presence of highly reactive double bonds. Unsaturated fatty acids have one or more double bonds between carbon atoms.
- The carbon atoms in the chain that are bound next to either side of the double bond can occur as *cis* or *trans* configuration.
  - A cis configuration means that adjacent hydrogen atoms are on the same side of 1 double bond.
  - A trans configuration, by contrast, means that the next two hydrogen atoms are box: to opposite sides of the double bond. As a result, they do not cause the chain to bound much, and their shape is similar to straight saturated fatty acids.

58. Ans. (b) α-Linolenic acid

Ref: Harper's Biochemistry, 30th edn. pg. 214

- PUFA are carboxylic acid with hydrocarbon tails of varying length containing two or more C=C double bonds.
- There are two families of PUFA: Omega-3 and Omega-6.
- In Omega-3 PUFA, the first C=C double bond is located at carbon 3 counting from terminal or omega methyl group tail.
- In Omega-6 PUFA, the first C=C double bond is located at carbon 3 counting-from terminal or omega methyl group tail.

Remember

TABLE: Different omega families and their respective members

ω3 family	ω6 family	ω7 family	ω9 family
• Alpha linolenic • Docosahexaenoic acid (DHA) • Timnodonic • Cervonic	• Gamma linolenic • Arachidonic • Linoleic	Palmitoleic	Oleic Elaidic

59. Ans. (c) Docosahexaenoic Acid

Ref: Harper's Biochemistry, 30th edn. pg. 214

Please refer to above table.

60. Ans. (a) Alpha linolenic acid

Ref: Harper's Biochemistry, 30th edn. pg. 214

Please refer to above explanation

61. Ans. (b) Mitochondria

- Enzymes responsible for ketone body formation are associated mainly with the mitochondria.
- Under conditions like starvation, Oxidation of fatty acids occurring in mitochondria, liver produces ketone bodies. Enzyme used is: **Pyruvate carboxylase**
- Acetoacetate, 3-hydroxybutyrate (Acetoacetate continually undergoes spontaneous decarboxylation to yield acetone) and Acetone are collectively known as the ketone bodies.

62. Ans. (c) Pyruvate carboxylase

Pyruvate carboxylase plays a crucial role in:
- Gluconeogenesis
- Lipogenesis
- In the biosynthesis of neurotransmitters
- Glucose-induced insulin secretion by pancreatic islets.

63. Ans. (b) Ketone bodies

Ref: Harper's Biochemistry, 30th edn. pg. 141, 149, 227-29

- *Initially up to 24 hours glycogen stores are utilized.*
- Later it is fatty acid oxidation leading to ketone production which becomes the source of fuel.
- After 2 weeks proteins in muscles are catabolized to produce amino acids which act as substrate to produce energy.

TABLE: Source of Energy During Starvation

STAGE	I	II	III
DURATION	1st 2-3 days	Upto 2 weeks (longest)	< 1 week
Energy source	Carbohydrate	Fats	Proteins
Metabolism	Initially Glycogenolysis then gluconeogenesis	Lipolysis and **KETONE BODY formation**	Breakdown of protein

64. Ans. (b) Oleic acid

Ref: Harper's Biochemistry, 30th edn. pg. 213

- Oleic acid is a monounsaturated fatty acid.
- Polyunsaturated fatty acid are: Palmitate, stearate etc.

Extra Mile

- Essential fatty acid are:
  - **Linoleic Acid: most essential fatty acid**
  - Linolenic Acid
  - Arachidonic acid
- Richest source of essential fatty acid: Safflower oil
- Richest source of saturated fatty acid: coconut oil
- Richest source of MUFA: groundnut oil.

Biochemistry

65. Ans. (c) Propionyl CoA

Ref: Harper's Biochemistry, 30th edn. pg. 224-26

Propionyl-CoA is a coenzyme A derivative of propionic acid. There are several different ways in which it is formed:

- It is formed as a product of beta-oxidation of odd-chain fatty acids.
- It is also a product of metabolism of isoleucine and valine.
- It is a product of alpha-ketobutyric acid, which in turn is a product of digestion of threonine and methionine.

66. Ans. (c) Propionyl CoA

Ref: Harper's Biochemistry, 30th edn. pg. 224-26

- Fatty acids with an odd number of carbon atoms are oxidized by the pathway of **beta-oxidation**, producing **acetyl-CoA**, until a **three-carbon (propionyl-CoA)** residue remains.
- **Odd-chain fatty acid is the only part of a fatty acid that is glucogenic.**

NUCLEIC ACID

67. Ans. (b) Lesch nyhan syndrome

Ref: Harrison's 20th ed. P 3001

Lesch Nyhan Syndrome

- XLR condition
- Occurs due to complete deficiency of HGPRTase enzyme → accumulation of purine
- Degradation of purine → Increased uric acid
- The syndrome is characterized by hyperuricemia, nephrolithiasis, obstructive uropathy, self-mutilative behaviour, choreoathetosis, spasticity, and mental retardation.

Extra Mile

- Partial deficiency of HGPRTase enzyme → Kelley-Seegmiller syndrome.
  - Associated with hyperuricemia, nephrolithiasis, obstructive uropathy but no central nervous system manifestations.

68. Ans. (c) AUG

Ref: Lippincott's Biochemistry, 6th ed. P 457 - 458

- Initiator codon in eukaryotes: **AUG** (codes for methionine)
- Initiator codon In prokaryotes: **AUG** (codes for N-Formyl methi-onine)
- **Stop codons:**
  - **UAG:** Amber
  - **UGA:** Opal
  - **UAA:** Ochre

69. Ans. (c) Denature of DNA → Annealing of primers → Extension of primer

Ref: Lippincott's Biochemistry 6th ed. P 480 – 81

Steps in PCR cycle:

- **DNA denaturation:** DNA to be amplified is heated → to separate dsDNA into single strands
- **Annealing of primers:** separated ssDNA cooled → allowed to anneal to 2 primers
- **Extension of primer:** new chain synthesis which is complimentary to original DNA chains.

Steps	Temperature	Time (sec)
Denaturation	90-96°C	20 – 60 sec
Annealing	50-70°C	20 – 90 sec
Extension	68-75°C	10 – 60 sec

70. Ans. (d) Uracil

- Uracil is present in RNA.
- Nitrogen base pairs present in RNA: Adenine, Guanine, Uracil, Cytosine

Structure of DNA

- Double helix, right handed, anti-parallel to each other
- Two strands of DNA are held together with help of hydrogen bonds
  - 2 hydrogen bonds between A = T
  - 3 hydrogen bonds between G ≡ C
- 6 types of DNA have been described: A, B, C, D, E, Z
  - Z is left handed

Extra Mile

Important differences between DNA types:

Types of DNA	No. of base pairs per turns	Physical character	Orientation
A – DNA	11	Short and broad	Right handed
B – DNA *(MC form)*	10.5	Long and thin	Right handed
Z – DNA	12	Elongated and thin	Left handed

71. Ans. (b) Inducer

Ref: Instant Notes in Biochemistry, P 174

- Lac operon induces the production of structural genes in the absence of repressor.
- Repressor is inactivated by allolactose or simply lactose.
- In the *lac* operon, the structural genes are the *lacZ, lacY* and *lacA* genes encoding β-galactosidase, the permease and the transacetylase, respectively. They are transcribed

Explanations

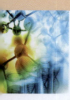

FMGE Solutions Screening Examination

to yield a single **polycistronic mRNA** that is then translated to produce all three enzymes. The existence of a polycistronic mRNA ensures that the amounts of all the gene products are regulated. Transcription occurs from a single promoter (P_{lac}) that lies upstream of these structural genes and binds RNA polymerase. Also present are an operator site (O_{lac}) between the promoter and the structural genes and a *lacI* gene that codes for the lac **repressor** protein.

72. Ans. (d) All of the above

Ref: Vasudevan Biochemistry, 7th ed. P 580

- Multiple DNA polymerase molecules engage in DNA replication. These share three important properties:
  - **Chain elongation:** Rate (in nucleotides per second) at which polymerization occurs.
  - **Processivity:** Number of nucleotides added to the nascent chain before the polymerase disengages from the template.
  - **Proofreading:** Identifies copying errors and corrects them.
- In *E. coli*, polymerase III (pol III) functions at the replication fork. Of all polymerases, it catalyzes the highest rate of chain elongation and is the **most processive**. It has 3' to 5' activity.
- Polymerase II (pol II) is mostly involved in proofreading and DNA repair. It has 3' to 5' activity.
- Polymerase I (pol I) completes chain synthesis between Okazaki fragments on the lagging strand. Eukaryotic cells have counterparts for each of these enzymes plus some additional ones.
  - **5' to 3' activity:** For repair and proofreading.
  - **3' to 5' activity:** For polymerization

Extra Mile

Classes of proteins involved in replication	
Protein	**Function**
DNA polymerases	Deoxynucleotide polymerization
Helicases	Processive unwinding of DNA
Topoisomerases	Relieve torsional strain that results from helicase-induced unwinding
DNA primase	Initiates synthesis of RNA primers
Single-strand binding proteins	Prevent premature reannealing of dsDNA
DNA ligase	Seals the single strand nick between the nascent chain and Okazaki fragments on lagging strand

A COMPARISON OF PROKARYOTIC AND EUKARYOTIC DNA POLYMERASES

E. coli	Mammalian	Function
I	α	Gap filling and synthesis of lagging strand
II	ε	DNA proofreading and repair
	β	DNA repair
	γ	Mitochondrial DNA synthesis
III	δ	Processive, leading strand synthesis

73. Ans. (b) RNA

- This technique is the PCR amplification of a reverse transcriptase product.
- It amplifies very small amount of any kind of RNA like mRNA, tRNA, rRNA and analyses the expressed mRNA sequence.
- Reverse transcriptase enzyme generates cDNA of mRNA.
- This method is used to obtain relative expression of gene in a cell.

Extra Mile

- A **real-time polymerase chain reaction**, also known as quantitative polymerase chain reaction (qPCR), monitors the amplification of a targeted DNA molecule during the PCR, i.e. in real-time, and not at its end, as in conventional PCR.

74. Ans. (a) Free radical damage

- Ionizing radiation can be divided into X-rays, gamma rays, alpha and beta particles and neutrons.
- It is a type of high-energy radiation that is able to release electrons from atoms and molecules generating ions which can break covalent bonds.
- Ionizing radiation directly affects DNA structure by inducing **DNA breaks, particularly, double stranded breaks**. Secondary effects are the generation of **reactive oxygen species** that oxidize proteins and lipids, and also induce several damages to DNA, like generation of abasic sites and single strand breaks (SSB).
- Collectively, all these changes induce cell death and mitotic failure.

Damaging agent	Defect	Repair mechanism	Associated disorder
• Ionizing radiation	• Double strand break • Single strand break • Intrastrand crosslinking • Interstrand crosslinking	• Non homologous End joining repair • Homologous repair	• SCID • Ataxia Telangiectasia • Werner Syndrome • Breast CA susceptibility • Bloom Syndrome

Biochemistry

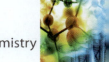

> **Extra Mile**
> - UV light creates bulky adducts and pyrimidine dimers, which is repaired by nucleotide excision repair. A defect in nucleotide excision repair can cause disorders like **Xeroderma pigmentosa, Cockayne syndrome, Trichothiodystrophy**.

75. Ans. (c) C

X chromosome belongs to group C.

Different groups of chromosomes

Groups	Chromosome
A	1–3
B	4–5
C	6–12, X
D	13–15
E	16–18
F	19–20
G	21, 22, Y

Note

> - X chromosome belongs to group C. They are submetacentric
> - Y chromosome belongs to group G. They are small acrocentric
> - The largest chromosome is chromosome 1

76. Ans. (b) DNA mismatch repair

Ref: Harrisons, 19th ed. pg. 94e.4

- **Cockayne syndrome:** Includes a number of **autosomal recessive disorders** with features such as impaired neurologic growth, photosensitivity (xeroderma pigmentosa), and death during childhood years. These disorders are caused by mutations in the genes for **DNA excision repair proteins**, *ERCC-6* and *ERCC-8*.
- **Disorder associated with mismatch repair:** Hereditary non- polyposis colon cancer

77. Ans. (c) 3

- Stop codons are a normal part of protein synthesis—they are the reason that all proteins do not go on 'forever'. During translation, it is stop codon on mRNA sequence, that *terminates the process*. Therefore they are known to act as terminator codon.
- There are three stop codons namely:
  - UAG: Amber
  - UGA: Opal
  - UAA: Ochre

> **Extra Mile**
>
> **Initiator codon:**
> - In eukaryotes: **AUG** (codes for methionine)
> - In prokaryotes: **AUG** (codes for N-Formyl methionine)
> - UGA codes for tryptophan in mitochondrial DNA.

78. Ans. (d) 3 codon act as terminator codon

Please refer to above explanation

79. Ans. (c) t-RNA

- There are three main types of RNA: tRNA, mRNA, and rRNA.
- The most abundant form of RNA is rRNA or ribosomal RNA because it is responsible for coding and producing all the proteins in cells.
- tRNA (transfer RNA): RNA which transfers amino acid from cytoplasm to ribosomal protein synthesizing machinery.
- **Secondary structure: Clover leaf shape**
- Tertiary structure: L shaped

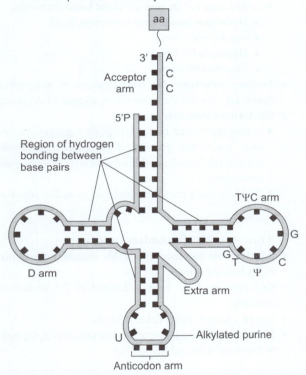

tRNA Arms

- **Acceptor arm:**
  - It is 3' end of tRNA, and has 3 unpaired nucleotide, CCA
  - It is the site of amino acid attachment
- **Anticodon arm:**
  - It has trinucleotide sequence complimentary to the codon of the amino acid, which mRNA carries.
  - Codon of mRNA and anti-codon of tRNA are antiparallel in their complimentary.
- **DHU arm/D-arm:**
  - Recognizes the specific amino acyl tRNA synthetase enzyme

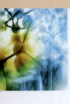

FMGE Solutions Screening Examination

- **Pseudouridine arm:**
  - Binds the charged tRNA to the ribosome
- **Variable arm/Extra arm:**
  - Most variable feature of tRNA. It differentiates the different class of tRNA.

80. **Ans. (b) Secondary**

Structural organization of amino acid can be of following types:
- **Primary structure:**
  - Linear sequence of amino acid, held together by peptide bond (a type of covalent bond).
- **Secondary structure:**
  - Folding of short ~ 3–30 residue, contiguous segment of polypeptide.
  - Joined together **by non-covalent bond** primarily.
    - **Hydrogen bond:** Most important bond
    - Vander walls force
    - Hydrophobic bond
    - Electrostatic bond
- **Tertiary structure:** 3D conformation of polypeptide. Bonds are non-covalent *(similar to secondary structure)*
- **Quaternary structure:**
  - When more than one polypeptide aggregate to form one functional protein. The spatial relationship between these polypeptide subunit is called quaternary structure.
  - Bonds are non-covalent *(similar to secondary structure)*

Alpha Helix

- It is an example of **secondary structure.**
- It is the **most common** and **stable secondary structure**. Right handed spiral
- Each turn of alpha helix is formed by 3.6 amino acyl residues.
- Size of 1 turn of alpha helix: 0.54 nm
- Proteins whose major secondary structure is alpha-helix:
  - Haemoglobin and Myoglobin

81. **Ans. (a) Glycine**

- Most abundant amino acid in bend/turn is proline > Glycine.
- Since proline is NOT given in option, glycine is our next best choice.

82. **Ans. (b) 7 methyl transferase**

Ref: PubMed

Post-transcriptional modification of mRNA:
- **7 methyl guanosine capping** at 5' end is one of the post-transcriptional modification of mRNA.
- It takes place in two steps:

	Step I	**Step II**
Step	Guanosine triphosphate is attached to 5' end of hnRNA	Methylation of guanosine triphosphate
Enzyme	Guanylyl tranferase	7 methyl transferase
Site	Nucleus	Cytoplasm

83. **Ans. (b) Thymine**

Ref: Harper's Biochemistry, 30th pg. 341, 29th ed. pg. 344

Nitrogen Bases present in RNA are-	Nitrogen Bases present in DNA are-
• Adenine	• Adenine
• Guanine	• Guanine
• Uracil	• Thymine
• Cytosine	• Cytosine

84. **Ans. (b) Glutamine**

Ref: Harper's Biochemistry, 29th ed. pg. 332

- AA for purine synthesis- glycine, aspartate, glutamine
- AA for pyrimidine synthesis- glutamine, aspartic acid (aspartate)
- Hence 2 AA are common i.e. glutamine and aspartate

85. **Ans. (b) Carbamoyl phosphate synthetase II > (A) Aspartate transcarbomylase**

Ref: Harper's Biochemistry, 30th ed. pg. 340, 353

- **Harper 27th ed p. 305 says** Aspartate transcarbomylase is the rate limiting enzyme of the pyrimidine synthesis in which case it does not make any differentiating remark between prokaryotic and eukaryotic pyrimidine synthesis.
- *"Pyrimidine synthesis is regulated by ACTase in bacteria (prokaryotes) and CPS-II in animals (eukaryotes) as there rate limiting enzymes respectively"*
- Sources of a pyrimidine:
  - Asparatic acid (NI, C4, C5, C6)
  - Amine N2 of glutamine (N3)
  - CO2 (C2)

Note: *UMP is the first pyrimidine to be synthesized.*

86. **Ans. (a) Right handed anti parallel**

Ref: Harper's Biochemistry, 30th edn. pg. 360-361

- Helical structure assumed by two strands of deoxyribonucleic acid, held together throughout their length by hydrogen bonds between bases on opposite strands, referred to as Watson-Crick base pairing. The structure is right handed anti-parallel structure.

Biochemistry

87. Ans. (c) G≡C

Ref: Harper's Biochemistry, 30th ed. pg. 360-361

Chargaff's Rules for Double stranded (ds) DNA

- In all cellular DNAs regardless of species-
  - Number of adenosine residues is equal to no. of thymidine residues (**i.e. A=T**).
  - No. of guanosine residues is equal to no. of cystidine residues (**G=C**)
- From these relationship it follows that sum of purine residues
- **A+G = T+C**
- Ratio of purine to pyrimidine is always around 1.

$$\frac{A+G}{T+C} = \sim 1$$

- The base composition of DNA generally varies from one species to another
- DNA specimens isolated from different tissues of same species have the same base composition.
- The base composition of DNA in a given species does not change with an organism's age, nutritional state or changing environment.

88. Ans. (d) Deletion of 2 bases

Ref: Harper's Biochemistry, 30th ed. pg. 417-18

Somatic Mutation Include
- **Point mutation**- (mutation of single nucleotide)
  - **Silent mutation:** If the changed base in the mRNA molecule at the third nucleotide of a codon, leads to no detectable effect.
  - **Mis-sense mutation:** Substitution of amino acid
  - **Non sense mutation:** Appearance of stop codon due to mutation
- **Frame shift mutation**-due to deletion/insertion, of one or two bases, which causes shift in reading frame. Whole reading frame is changed leading to entirely different protein molecule synthesis, called garbled protein.
- **Trinucleotide repeat mutation**-repeat more than 55 times.

89. Ans. (a) Translation

Ref: Harper's Biochemistry, 30th edn. pg. 417-418

- Frameshift mutations take place when there is an insertion or removal of 1 or 2 base pairs into the codon sequence. *When the translation of the codon takes place, as it is read in triplets, the amino acid sequence of the protein synthesized is changed which leads to a "shift" in the frame that is being translated.* But during the replicative or transcription processes there will be no problems as in the structure or stability of the DNA molecule.
- *Frameshift mutations also do not occur in multiples of 3 because in that case, only an amino acid is skipped in the translation process and the sequence is maintained.*

90. Ans: (b) 3

Ref: Harper's Biochemistry, 30th ed. pg. 417-18

- Frame-shift mutations
- *The genetic code is read in form of triplets of nucleotides which are known as codons.*
- If one or two base pairs from the code are removed or inserted, the genetic code will be misread from that change onwards, because the genetic code is not punctuated. Therefore the amino acid sequence translated from the change onwards will be completely changed. This is known as frame shift mutation.
- However *if the removal /insertion happens in multiples of three, rest of the reading frame doesn't change and hence the amino acid sequence will not change.*

91. Ans. (d) Base pair substitution

Ref: Harper's Biochemistry, 30th ed. pg. 416-17

A partial missense mutation (type of base pair substitution) glutamic acid, the normal amino acid in position 6 of the β chain, has been replaced by valine.

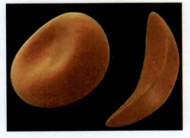

92. Ans. (a) Nucleoside correction

DNA correction has been divided into two types:
- **Pre replication repair:**
  - Most efficient form of repair
  - Done by: excision repair, photoreactivation, base replacement

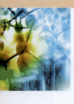

FMGE Solutions Screening Examination

- **Post replication repair:**
  - Done by: daughter strand Gap repair, error prone induced repair.

TABLE: Mechanism of Dna Repair

Mechanism	Problem	Solution
Mismatch repair	Copying errors (single base or Two -to five-base unpaired loops)	Methyl-directed strand cutting, exonuclease digestion, and replacement
Double-strand break repair	Ionizing radiation, chemotherapy, oxidative free radicals	Synapsis, unwinding, alignment, ligation
Base excision-repair	Spontaneous, chemical, or radiation damage to a single base	Base removal by N-glycosylase, abasic sugar removal, replacement
Nucleotide excision-repair	Spontaneous, chemical, or radiation damage to a DNA segment	Removal of an approximately 30-nucleotide oligomer and replacement

93. Ans. (b) Repair of damaged DNA

Ref: Harper's Biochemistry, 30th ed. pg. 389-90

Two types of exonuclease activity has been described:
- **5' to 3' exonuclease activity:** responsible for cleavage of phosphodiester bond starting from 5' end of the strand. It is considered as the error correcting activity in damaged DNA.
- **3' to 5' exonuclease activity:** responsible for cleavage of phosphodiester bond starting from 3' end of the strand. This activity provides a means for proofreading if in case any wrong base is mistakenly incorporated by DNA polymerase III during DNA synthesis.

94. Ans. (b) DNA

Ref: Harper's Biochemistry, 30th ed. pg. 724

- Radiation exposure leads to increased destruction of DNA.
- Radiation causes pyrimidine diamerisation– leading to DNA damage.

95. Ans. (b) HSP 70 family of chaperones bind with hydrophobic amino acid

Ref: Harper's Biochemistry, 30th ed. pg. 618-20, 26th ed. pg. 36-37

- **Over half of mammalian protein folding is done by Chaperone proteins.**
- Chaperones prevent aggregation, thus providing an opportunity for the formation of appropriate secondary structural elements.
- **There are 2 families of hsp:** hsp 60 and hsp 70.
- The hsp60 family of chaperones, sometimes called chaperonins, *differ in sequence and structure from hsp70 and its homologs*.
- The HSP 70 (70-kDa heat shock protein) *family of chaperones binds short sequences of hydrophobic amino acids in newly synthesized polypeptides, shielding them from solvent.*
- Hsp60 acts later in the folding process, *often together with an hsp70 chaperone*.
- Hsp 60 chaperone is donut shaped, which provides a sheltered environment in which a polypeptide can fold until all hydrophobic regions are buried in its interior, eliminating aggregation.
- **Chaperone proteins can also "rescue" proteins** that have become thermodynamically trapped in a misfolded dead end. They rescue it *by unfolding hydrophobic regions and providing a second chance to fold productively.*

96. Ans. (a) Xeroderma pigmentosum

Ref: Harper's Biochemistry, 30th ed. pg. 389-90, 28th ed. pg. 330-32

- **Xeroderma pigmentosum** is an **autosomal recessive** genetic disease which arises due to defect in DNA repair particularly of thymidine dimers.

Examples of Conditions Arising due to DNA Repair Defects:
- Xeroderma pigmentosa
- Ataxia telangiectasia
- Fanconi's syndrome
- Bloom syndrome
- HNPCC

97. Ans. (c) Telomerase

Ref: Harper's Biochemistry, 30th ed. pg. 374, 732, 26th ed. pg. 318

- The ends of each chromosome contain structures called telomeres.
- Telomeres consist of short, repeat TG-rich sequences. Human telomeres have a variable number of repeats of the sequence 5'-TTAGGG-3', which can extend for several kilobases.
- **Telomerase,** is related to viral RNA-dependent DNA polymerases (reverse transcriptases) and *is the enzyme*

responsible for telomere synthesis and thus for maintaining the length of the telomere.
- Telomere shortening has been associated with both aging and malignant transformation. Because of this reason, telomerase has become an attractive target for cancer chemotherapy and drug development.

98. Ans. (b) Rough endoplasmic reticulum

Ref: Harper's Biochemistry, 30th ed. pg. 576-77

- The surface of the rough endoplasmic reticulum is studded with protein-manufacturing ribosomes giving it a "rough" appearance.
- The ribosomes bound to ER are not a stable part of this organelle's structure as they are constantly being bound and released from the membrane.
- A ribosome only binds to the RER once a specific protein-nucleic acid complex forms in the cytosol. This special complex forms when a free ribosome begins translating the mRNA of a protein destined for the secretory pathway.
- Protein once produced from RER will go to golgi apparatus → secretory vesicles → which is further released.

99. Ans. (b) Endoplasmic reticulum

Ref: Harper's Biochemistry 30th ed. pg. 576-77

Please refer to above explanation

100. Ans. (c) Golgi Body

Ref: Ganong's Physiology, 25th ed. pg. 43-44

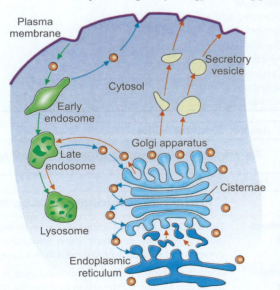

101. Ans. (a) Primary structure

Ref: Harper's Biochemistry, 30th ed. pg. 26-29, 618-19

PROTEIN DENATURATION

- In **quaternary structure** denaturation, protein sub-units are dissociated and/or the spatial arrangement of protein subunits is disrupted.
- **Primary structure**, such as the sequence of amino acids held together by covalent peptide bonds, is **not disrupted by denaturation.**
- In **secondary structure** denaturation proteins adopt a random coil as they lose all regular repeating patterns such as alpha-helices and beta-pleated sheets, and configuration.
- **Tertiary structure** denaturation involves the disruption of:
  1. **Covalent interactions** between amino acid side-chains (such as disulfide bridges between cysteine groups)
  2. **Non-covalent dipole-dipole interactions** between polar amino acid side-chains (and the surrounding solvent)
  3. **Van der Waals (induced dipole) interactions** between nonpolar amino acid side-chains.

102. Ans. (c) Uric acid stones are frequently formed

Ref: Harper's Biochemistry, 30th ed. pg. 354-55, 26th ed. pg. 300

LESCH-NYHAN SYNDROME

- It is a X- linked recessive disorder which is characterized by:
  - An overproduction hyperuricemia
  - Frequent episodes of *uric acid lithiasis*
  - Self-mutilative behavior,
  - *Mental retardation.*
- It reflects a defect in **hypoxanthine-guanine phosphoribosyl transferase, an enzyme of purine salvage.** The accompanying rise in intracellular PRPP results in purine overproduction. Mutations that decrease or abolish hypoxanthine-guanine phosphoribosyl transferase activity include deletions, frameshift mutations, base substitutions, and aberrant mRNA splicing.

103. Ans. (d) Immunodeficiency

Ref: Harper's Biochemistry, 30th edn. pg. 354-355

- **Lesch–Nyhan syndrome** is a rare inherited disorder caused by a deficiency of the enzyme hypoxanthine-guanine phosphoribosyl transferase (HGPRT), produced by mutations in the HPRT gene located on X chromosome.

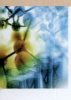

Clinical Features
- **One of the first symptoms of the disease is the presence of sand-like crystals** of uric acid in the diapers of the affected infant. *Overproduction of uric acid may lead to the development of uric acid crystals or stones in the kidneys, ureters, or bladder.* Such crystals deposited in joints later in the disease may produce gout-like arthritis, with swelling and tenderness
- **Irritability** is most often noticed along with the first signs of nervous system impairment. Within the first few years of life, extrapyramidal involvement causes abnormal involuntary muscle contractions such as dystonia, atheotosis and opisthotonus.
- **Cognitive impairment:** Affected persons have behavioral disturbances that emerge between 2 – 3 years of age. The self-injury begins with biting of the lips and tongue at the age of 3 years.

Remember
- A less severe related disease is **partial HGPRT deficiency** is known as Kelley-Seegmiller Syndrome *(Lesch-Nyhan Syndrome involves total HGPRT deficiency).* Symptoms generally involve less neurological involvement but the disease still causes gout and kidney stones.
- The prognosis for individuals with severe LNS is poor. *Death is usually due to renal failure or complications from hypotonia (PNEUMONIA), in the first or second decade of life.*

104. Ans. (c) Uric Acid

Ref: Harper's Biochemistry, 30th edn. pg. 347-357

Purines are metabolized by several enzymes:

GUANINE
- A nuclease frees the nucleotide
- A nucleotidase creates guanosine
- Purine nucleoside phosphorylase converts guanosine to guanine
- Guanase converts guanine to xanthine
- *Xanthine oxidase (a form of xanthine oxidoreductase) catalyzes the oxidation of xanthine to uric acid*

ADENINE
- A nuclease frees the nucleotide
  - A nucleotidase creates adenosine, then adenosine deaminase creates inosine
  - Alternatively, AMP deaminase creates inosinic acid, then a nucleotidase creates inosine
- Purine nucleoside phosphorylase acts upon inosine to create hypoxanthine
- *Xanthine* oxidoreductase catalyzes the biotransformation of hypoxanthine to xanthine
- *Xanthine* oxido-reductase acts upon xanthine to create uric acid

105. Ans. (a) Xanthine oxidase

Ref: Harper's Biochemistry, 30th ed. pg. 355, 120, 26th ed. pg. 300

- **Xanthine oxidase** deficiency leads to hypouricemia.
- **Hypouricemia** and increased excretion of hypoxanthine and xanthine are associated with **xanthine oxidase deficiency due to a genetic defect or to severe liver damage.**
- **Patients with a severe enzyme deficiency may exhibit xanthinuria and xanthine lithiasis**

There are at least three different inherited defects that lead to early development of severe hyperuricemia and gout:
- Glucose-6-phosphatase (G6PT) deficiency (**as seen in Von gierke's disease**)
- Severe and partial hypoxanthine-guanine phosphoribosyl-transferase (HGPRT) deficiency: (**As seen in Lesch Nyhan syndrome**)
- **Elevated** 5'-phosphoribosyl-1'-pyrophosphate synthetase (PRPP synthetase) activity.

> **Extra Mile**
>
> **DRUGS CAUSING HYPERURICEMIA:**
> **(Mn: LEAD Poisoning Causes Stone and Nephropathy)**
> - Levodopa
> - Ethcrynic acid
> - Alcohol
> - Diuretics
> - Pyrazinamide
> - Cyclosporine
> - Salicylates
> - Nicotinic acid

106. Ans. (a) Xanthine oxidase

Ref: Harper's Biochemistry, 30th ed. pg. 120, 355, 26th pg. 300

107. Ans. (a) Northern Blot

Ref: Harper's Biochemistry, 30th ed. pg. 362-63

Northern blot	The **northern blot** is a technique used in molecular biology research to study gene expression by detection of **RNA** (or isolated mRNA) in a sample.
Southern blot	A **Southern blot** is a method routinely used in molecular biology for detection of a specific DNA sequence in **DNA** samples

Contd...

Biochemistry

Eastern blot	The **eastern blot** is a biochemical technique used to analyze **protein post translational modifications (PTM)** such as **lipids, phosphomoieties and glycoconjugates.** *It is most often used to detect carbohydrate epitopes. Thus, Eastern blotting can be considered an extension of the biochemical technique of Western blotting.*
Western blot	The **western blot** (sometimes called the protein immunoblot) is a widely accepted analytical technique used to detect specific **proteins** in a sample of tissue homogenate or extract

---

108. Ans. (a) DNA cistrons

> *Ref: Harper's Biochemistry, 30th ed. pg. 359-62*

- DNA cistrons are a section of DNA that contain the genetic code for a single polypeptide and functions as a hereditary unit.

---

109. Ans. (b) N formyl methionine t-RNA will be the first t-RNA to come into action

> *Ref: Harper's Biochemistry, 30th ed. pg. 433-37*

- *Methionine t-RNA is the first t-RNA involved in eukaryotic protein synthesis.*

---

110. Ans. (c) r-RNA

> *Ref: Harper's Biochemistry, 30th ed. pg. 366-67*

- **There are three main types of RNA:** tRNA, mRNA, and rRNA.
- The most abundant form of RNA is rRNA or ribosomal RNA because it is responsible for coding and producing all of the proteins in cells.
- rRNA is found in the cytoplasm of cells and is associated with ribosomes. It takes the coded information delivered from the nucleus by mRNA and translates it so that proteins can be produced and modified.

---

111. Ans. (d) mi-RNA

> *Ref: Harper's Biochemistry, 30th ed. pg. 368, 28th ed. pg. 307-320, Lippincott 5th ed. pg. 402*

TYPES OF RNA

CODING vs NON-CODING

- **Coding RNA** – mRNA
- **Non-coding RNA** - RNA that do not encode protein. Rest all type of RNA are non coding i.e. t-RNA, r-RNA, sn RNA, sno RNA, sca RNA, mi RNA, siRNA, piRNA, etc.

miRNA

- Non-coding RNA, 21-25 nucleotide long
- Transcribed from RNA polymerase II
- All known mi RNA cause inhibition of gene expression by decreasing specific protein production via translational arrest or mRNA degradation. And thus the gene that it produces is silenced.
- Noble prize was awarded for the discovery of mi RNA in 2006.

---

112. Ans. (b) Small Nuclear Ribo-nucleoproteins

> *Ref: Harper's Biochemistry, 30th edn. pg. 365-67, 94-95, 26th edn. pg. 354*

- "SNURPS" are **small nuclear ribonucleic proteins**
- *They are RNA-protein complexes that combine with unmodified pre-mRNA and various other proteins to form a spliceosome, a large RNA-protein molecular complex with which splicing of pre-mRNA occurs.*

---

113. Ans. (c) Decreased glucose concentration, increased cAMP

> *Ref: Harper's Biochemistry, 30th edn. pg. 430-31*

- The *lac* operon aka lactose operon is an operon required for the transport and metabolism of lactose in *Escherichia coli* and some other enteric bacteria.
- **It has three adjacent structural genes,** which encodes:*(Mn: ZiYA ki GaLaThi)*
  - *lacZ* : Encodes β-ga**lact**osidase
  - *lacY* : Encodes **lact**ose permease
  - *lacA* : Encodes **th**iogalactoside transacetylase (or galactoside O-acetyltransferase)
- The *lac* operon uses a two-part control mechanism to ensure that the cell spends energy only when necessary. In the absence of lactose, the *lac* repressor stops production of the enzymes encoded by the *lac* operon.
- In the presence of glucose, the catabolite activator protein (CAP), required for production of the enzymes, remains inactive, and EIIA shuts down lactose permease to prevent transport of lactose into the cell.
- In the absence of glucose, there is an **increase in the concentration of cAMP** and this leads to the activation of the lac operon which leads to the enzyme production in order to consume the lactose present in the cells.

AMINO ACID

114. Ans. (a) Pellagra like symptoms

> *Ref: Harrison's 20th ed. P 3021*

FMGE Solutions Screening Examination

Hartnup Disease
- It is an AR condition, mainly seen due to defect in the transport of tryptophan and other neutral amino acids from the renal tubules and intestine
- **Molecular defect:** SLC6A19 gene (encode transporter protein of these amino acid)

Clinical Features:
- **MC:** Cutaneous photosensitivity
- Constant neutral aminoaciduria
- Intermittent pellagra like symptoms
- Intermittent ataxia (unsteady wide based gait)

Diagnosis: Obermeyer test (urinary test for indole compound)

Treatment: High protein diet and Nicotinic acid

> **Extra Mile**
> - **Drummond syndrome/Blue diaper syndrome:** Tryptophan transport defect lies only in intestine, NOT in kidney

Class of substance and disorder	Individual substrates	Tissues manifesting transport defect	Molecular defect	Major clinical manifestations	Inheritance
Amino acids					
Cystinuria	Cystine, lysine, arginine, ornithine	Proximal renal tubule, jejunal mucosa	Shared dibasic-cystine transporter SLC3A1, SLC7A9	Cystine nephrolithiasis	AR
Lysinuric protein intolerance	Lysine arginine, ornithine	Proximal renal tubule, jejunal mucosa	Dibasic transporter SLC7A7	Protein intolerance, hyperammonemia, intellectual disability	AR
Hartnup disease	Neutral amino acids	Proximal renal tubule, jejunal mucosa	Neutral amino acid transporter SLC6A19	Constant neutral aminoaciduria, intermittent symptoms of pellagra	AR
Brain branched-chain amino acid deficiency	Leucine, isoleucine, valine	Plasma membrane of blood brain barrier	Branched-chain amino acid transporter SLC7A5	Microcephaly, intellectual disability, seizures	AR
Citrullinemia type 2	Aspartate, glutamate, malate	Inner mitochondrial membrane	Mitochondrial aspartate/ glutamate carrier 2 SLC25413	Sudden behavioral changes with stupor, coma, hyperammonemia	AR

115. Ans. (d) Creatinine

- Tryptophan is one of the essential aromatic amino acid
- Metabolic fate of tryptophan: Metabolized by enzyme Tryptophan oxygenase (pyrrolase)
- **Derivatives of tryptophan:**
  - Niacin (Nicotinic acid)
  - Serotonin
  - Melatonin
- **Note:** Creatinine is synthesized from 3 amino acids namely: Glycine, Arginine, Methionine

116. Ans. (b) Arachidonic acid

Ref: Lippincott's Biochemistry, 6th ed. P 213

- Prostaglandin is derived from the metabolism of arachidonic acid with the help of cyclooxygenase (COX) enzyme.

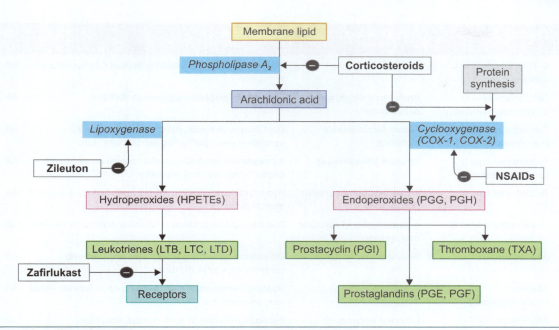

117. Ans. (d) Phenylketonuria

Ref: Harrison's 20th ed. P 3015 – 16

Phenylketonuria
- MC metabolic disorder of amino acid
- Seen due to deficiency of enzyme: Phenylalanine Hydroxylase
- Increased phenylalanine in blood → metabolized to phenylketones → excreted in urine → hence the name Phenylketonuria (PKU).
- MC organ damaged due to phenylalaninemia: Brain

Clinical Feature
- Gradual development of mental retardation (intellectual disability)
  - Infants normal at birth
- Excessive vomiting
- Autistic, choreiform movement
- Unpleasant, musty odor

Diagnosis
- Guthrie test-screening test in blood sample
- Ferric chloride test: Screening test in urine sample
- Tandem mass spectrometry: **IOC**

TABLE: Inherited disorders of Amin Acid Metabolism

Amino Acid(s)	Condition	Enzyme Defect	Clinical Findings	Inheritance
Phenylalanine	DNAJC12 Deficiency	Hydroxylase Co-chaperone	Dystonia, parkinsonism, intellectual disability	AR
	Phenylketonuria	Phenylalanine hydroxylase	Intellectual disability, microcephaly, hypopigmented skin and hairs, eczema, "mousy" odor	AR
	DHPR deficiency	Dihydroptendine reductase	Intellectual disability, hypotonia, spasticity, myoclonus	AR
	PTPS deficiency	6-Pyruvoyl-tetrahydropterin synthase	Dystonia, neurologic deterioration, seizures, intellectual disability	AR

Contd...

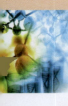

FMGE Solutions Screening Examination

Amino Acid(s)	Condition	Enzyme Defect	Clinical Findings	Inheritance
Tyrosine	GTP cyclohydrolase I deficiency	GTP cyclohydrolase I	Intellectual disability, seizures, dystonia, temperature instability	AR
	Carbinolamine dehydratase deficiency	Pterin-4α-carbinolamine dehydratase	Transient hyperphenylataninemia (benign)	AR
	Tyrosinemia type I (hepatorenal)	Fumarylacetoacetate hydrolase	Liver failure, cirrhosis, rickets, failure to thrive, peripheral neuropathy, "boiled cabbage" odor	AR
	Tyrosinemia type II (oculocutaneous)	Tyrosine transaminase	Palmoplantar keratosis, painful corneal erosions with photophobia, learning disability	AR
	Tyrosinemia type III	4-Hydroxyphenyl pyruvate dioxygenase	Hypertyrosinemia with normal liver function, occasional mental delay	AR
	Hawkinsinuria type III	4-Hydroxyphenyl pyruvate dioxygenase	Transient failure to thrive, metabolic acidosis in infancy	AD
	Alkaptonuria	Homogentisic acid oxidase	Ochronosis. arthritis, cardiac valve involvement, coronary artery calcification	AR
	Albinism (oculocutaneous)	Tyrosinase	Hypopigmentation of hair, skin, and optic fundus; visual loss; photophobia	AR
	Albinism (ocular)	Different enzymes or transporters	Hypopigmentation of optic fundus, visual loss	AR, XL
	DOPA-responsive dystonia	Tyrosine hydroxylase	Rigidity, truncal hypotonia, tremor, intellectual disability	AR

118. Ans. (a) Tyrosine

Ref: Harper's Biochemistry, 30th ed. pg. 618-20, 26th ed. P 288

- **Melanin** is pigment of skin, hair and eyes, synthesized from tyrosine in the epidermis by the melanocytes.
- **Function:** Protect underlying cells from UV rays of sun.
- **Defect in melanin production:** Albinism
- **Generalized Albinism** aka Oculocutaneous albinism (OCA) is mainly classified into 3 types:
    - **OCA 1:** Tyrosinase deficient
    - **OCA 2:** Tyrosinase positive- MC type of albinism
    - **OCA 3:** Red OCA
- **Localized albinism:** Piebaldism, Waardenburg syndrome

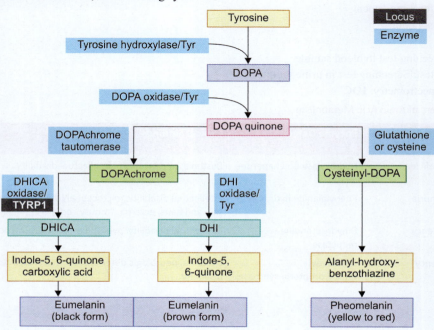

> **Extra Mile**
> - Specialized products from glycine: Creatinine, Heme, Purine nucleotide, Glutathione

119. Ans. (a) Glycine

Glycine
- In collagen every third amino acid is glycine
- Glycine is considered as the simplest amino acid
- Properties of glycine: Non-essential, Glucogenic and optically inactive amino acid
- **Acts as a conjugating agent:**
  - Conjugation of benzoic acid
  - Conjugation of bile acid
- As neurotransmitter, it has both properties excitatory and inhibitory.

Other amino acids present in collagen are: Proline, Hydroxyproline, Hydroxylysine

Lysine (K)
- An essential amino acid which is predominantly ketogenic
- It is an amino acid which is deficient in cereals
- **Functions:**
  - Important for covalent cross linking in collagen
  - Precursor of carnitine = Lysine + Methionine

120. Ans. (b) Cysteine

- –SH group of 2 cysteine in proteins can be oxidized to form a covalent disulfide bond.
- It significantly stabilizes tertiary structures of protein
- This bond plays crucial role in structures of many proteins by forming covalent links.

> **Extra Mile**
> - Amino acid that decreases ageing process: **Cysteine and Taurine**
> - Amino acid that accelerate ageing: **Homocysteine**

121. Ans. (b) Melatonin

Ref: Vasudevan Biochemistry, 8th ed. P 273

- Melatonin is released from pineal gland.

TYROSINE

- Neural cells convert tyrosine to epinephrine and norepinephrine. While dopa is also an intermediate in the formation of melanin, different enzymes hydroxylate tyrosine in melanocytes. Dopa decarboxylase, a pyridoxal phosphate-dependent enzyme, forms dopamine.
- β-oxidase then forms norepinephrine. In the adrenal medulla, phenylethanolamine-*N*-methyltransferase utilizes *S*-adenosylmethionine to methylate the primary amine of norepinephrine, forming epinephrine.

- Tyrosine is also a precursor of triiodothyronine and thyroxine.

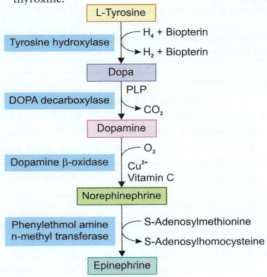

122. Ans. (a) Glycine, arginine, methionine

Ref: Vasudevan Biochemistry, 8th ed. P 269

- Creatinine is formed in muscle from creatine phosphate by irreversible, nonenzymatic dehydration and loss of phosphate.
- Glycine, arginine, and methionine all participate in creatine biosynthesis.
- Synthesis of creatine is completed by methylation of guanidinoacetate by *S*-adenosylmethionine.

123. Ans. (b) Lysine

Ref: Vasudevan Biochemistry, 8th ed, P 281-82

Based on variable side chain, amino acid can be classified into: Aliphatic amino acid and aromatic amino acid.

Aliphatic amino acid	Aromatic amino acid
It is further classified into several subtypes: - **Simple AA:** Glycine, alanine - **Branched chain AA:** Leucine, isoleucine, Valine - **Sulfur containing:** Cysteine, methionine - **With –OH group:** Serine, threonine - **With amide group:** Asparagine, glutamine - **Acidic AA:** Aspartic acid, glutamic acid - **Basic AA:** Arginine, lysine	- Histidine - Tyrosine - Tryptophan - Phenylalanine

FMGE Solutions Screening Examination

> **Extra Mile**
> - **Basic amino acid:** Histidine, arginine, lysine *(Histidine is also basic in nature, but it is aromatic)*
> - **-OH containing AA:** Threonine, serine, tyrosine
> - **Most basic amino acid:** Arginine

124. (a) Chaperone

Ref: Harper's Biochemistry, 26th ed. pg. 36-37

- Chaperone proteins participate in the *folding of over half of mammalian proteins.* The hsp70 (70-kDa heat shock protein) *family of chaperones binds short sequences of hydrophobic amino acids in newly synthesized polypeptides, shielding them from solvent.*

125. Ans. (a) Asparate

Ref: Satyanarayan Biochemistry, pg. 339

Role of Aspartate in urea cycle:
- Aspartate participates in urea cycle for condensation with citrulline to form Argino succinic acid. The reaction is catalyzed by Argino succinic acid synthetase (Asparate provides one out of the two nitrogens of urea, the other nitrogen is contributed by Glutamate).
- In the subsequent reaction, Argino succinic acid undergoes a lytic reaction to form Arginine and fumarate. Fumarate forms a link between TCA cycle and urea. Fumarate can be recycled to form oxaloacetate, through intermediate formation of malate that can be transminated to form aspartate, to get reutilized in the urea cycle

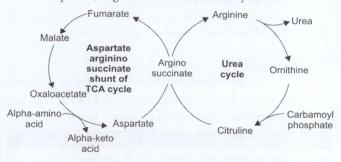

Link between TCA and urea cycle

Role of Aspartate in TCA cycle
- Oxaloacetate, the keto acid obtained from Aspartate by transamination is an intermediate of TCA cycle.
- Oxaloacetate can either be utilized in TCA cycle or be channeled to the pathway of gluconeogenesis.
- Hence asparatate is a common intermediate of TCA cycle (through oxaloacetate) and urea cycle (directly)

126. Ans. (a) Aspartic acid

Based in variable side chain, amino acid can be classified into: Aliphatic amino acid and Aromatic amino acid.

Aliphatic amino acid	Aromatic amino acid
It is further classified into several subtypes: • **Simple AA:** Glycine, Alanine • **Branched chain AA:** Leucine, Isoleucine, Valine • **Sulphur containing:** Cysteine, Methionine • **With –OH group:** Serine, Threonine • **With amide group:** Asparagine, Glutamine • **Acidic AA:** Aspartic acid, Glutamic acid • **Basic AA:** Arginine, Lysine	• Histidine • Tyrosine • Tryptophan • Phenylalanine

> **Extra Mile**
> - **Basic amino acid:** Histidine, Arginine, Lysine *(Histidine is also basic in nature, but it is aromatic)*
> - **-OH containing AA:** Threonine, Serine, Tyrosine
> - **Most basic amino acid:** Arginine

127. Ans. (b) Arginine

TABLE: Special groups present in amino acid

Special group	Amino acid
Guanidinium	Arginine
Phenol	Tyrosine
Thioether linkage	Methionine
Pyrrolidine	Proline
Benzene	Phenylalanine
Indole	Tryptophan
Thioalcohol	Cysteine
Imidazole	Histidine

128. Ans. (c) Phenylalanine

Ref: Lippincott's Biochemistry, pg. 268

Phenylketonuria (PKU), caused by a deficiency of *phenylalanine hydroxylase* and is the most common clinically encountered inborn error of amino acid metabolism (prevalence 1:11,000). **Hyperphenylalaninemia** may also be caused by deficiencies in the enzymes that synthesize or reduce the coenzyme **tetrahydrobiopterin (BH_4)**. It is important to distinguish among the various forms of hyperphenylalaninemia, because their clinical management is different. For example, a small fraction of PKU is a result of a deficiency in either *dihydropteridine (BH_2) reductase* or BH_2 *synthetase*. These mutations prevent synthesis of BH_4, and indirectly raise phenylalanine concentrations, because *phenylalanine hydroxylase* requires BH_4 as a coenzyme. BH_4 is also required for *tyrosine hydroxylase* and *tryptophan hydroxylase*, which catalyze reactions leading to the synthesis of neurotransmitters, such as serotonin and catecholamines.

Biochemistry

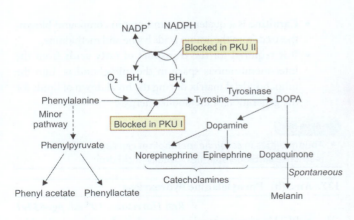

129. Ans. (c) Valine

Glycated hemoglobins arise from the non-enzymatic attachment of glucose to hemoglobin. They are formed and accumulate in the red cell in proportion to the blood glucose level. Their concentration reflects the long-term average glucose level and is thus *useful as an indicator of diabetic control.*

Types of glycated hemoglobin
- **HbA1a1:** Fructokinase 1,6 diphosphate N terminal valine
- **HbA1a2:** Glucose 6 phosphate N terminal valine
- **HbA1b:** Unknown carbohydrate N terminal valine
- **HbA1c:** Attachment of glucose to N terminal of amino acid valine

130. Ans. (b) SDS–PAGE

Ref: Harper's Biochemistry, pg. 24

- The most widely used method for determining the purity of a protein is SDS-PAGE—polyacrylamide gel electrophoresis (PAGE) in the presence of the anionic detergent sodium dodecyl sulfate (SDS)
- Electrophoresis separates charged biomolecules based on the rates at which they migrate in an applied electrical field. For SDS-PAGE, acrylamide is polymerized and crosslinked to form a porous matrix. SDS denatures and binds to proteins at a ratio of one molecule of SDS per two peptide bonds.

> **Extra Mile**
>
> - **Mass spectrometry** is considered as the method of choice for protein identification.
> - **Sanger's technique** was the first technique to determine the sequence of protein.
> - **Western blot detects** Protein by antigen-antibody interaction.
> - **Southern blot** detects DNA by DNA-DNA hybridization.
> - **Northern blot** detect RNA by RNA-cDNA hybridization.

131. Ans. (c) Heart

TABLE: Isoenzyme of LDH, its subunit, origin tissue and their respective electrophoretic activity

LDH isoenzyme	Subunit	Origin tissue	Electrophoretic activity
LDH 1	H4	Heart, RBC	Fastest
LDH 2	H3M1	Reticuloendothelial system	↓
LDH 3	H2M2	Lungs	
LDH 4	H1M3	Kidney, placenta pancreas	
LDH 5	M4	Liver and skeletal muscle	Slowest

132. Ans. (b) Tyrosine

- **TYROSINE:** nonessential AA, which is converted to Melanin, T3, T4 hormone by enzyme Tyrosinase.
  - Deficiency of Tyrosinase → Albinism
  - Deficiency of melanocyte →Vitiligo

AMINO ACIDS AT A GLANCE: Total AA = 20 in number

ESSENTIAL AA: can't be synthesized. (Mn: TV TILL 8 PM)	Semi-essential AA: can be synthesized under normal condition as per demand.	Non-Essential AA: synthesized in body readily
Threonine, Valine, Tryptophan, Isoleucine, Lysine, Leucine, Phenylanine, Methionine	Histidine Arginine	The remaining 10 AA are Non-essential (including tyrosine).

133. Ans. (b) Deficient in cereals

- Lysine is an essential amino acid.
- It is **deficient in cereals and maize.**
- It is a basic amino acid. **Basic amino acids are:**
  - Arginine
  - Lysine
  - Histidine (Aromatic)
- **Acidic amino acids are:**
  - Aspartic acid
  - Glutamic acid

Food item	Limiting Amino acids
Pulses	Methionine & cysteine
Cereals	Threonine & Lysine
Maize	Tryptophan & Lysine

FMGE Solutions Screening Examination

134. Ans. (c) Non-protein alpha amino acid

Ref: Harrisons, 19th ed. pg. 434e2

- Homocysteine is a non-protein alpha amino acid.
- It is a derived amino acid (from methionie) not seen in protein.
- Two fates of methionine
  - Derived as homocysteine
  - Derived as cysteine

TABLE: Diseases associated with homocysteine and it clinical features

Amino acid	Disease	Enzyme deficient	Clinical manifestation/ inheritance
Homo-cysteine	Homocyst-inuria— Classical	Cystathionine β-synthase	Lens dislocation, thrombotic vascular disease, intellectual disability, osteoporosis/AR
	Homocyst-inuria— Nonclas-sical	5, -1-10-Meth-ylene tet-rahydrofolate reductase	Intellectual disability, gait and psychiatric abnormalities, recurrent strokes/AR
	Homocyst-inuria	Methionine synthase	Intellectual disability, hyptonia, seizures, megaloblastic anemia/AR
	Homocyst-inuria and methyl-malonic acidemia	Vitamin B_{12} lysosomal efflux and metabolism	Intellectual disability, lethargy, failure to thrive, hypotonia, seizures megaloblastic anemia/AR

135. Ans. (b) Glutaminase

- In amino acid metabolism, there is detachment of NH_2. Since this amino group is toxic to body in free form, it is neutralized in form of glutamate by the process of transamination.
- This glutamate is converted to glutamine → which carries the ammonia to liver.
- In liver:

$$\text{Glutamine} \xrightarrow{\text{GLUTAMINASE}} \text{Glutamate}$$
$$NH_4$$

- It releases ammonia by hydrolytic cleavage and again gets converted to glutamate.
- Enzyme required here is: **Glutaminase.**

136. Ans. (c) Fatty acid

Ref: PubMed

- **Carnitine** is a quaternary ammonium compound biosynthesized from the amino acids lysine and methionine.
- It is required for the **transport of fatty acids** from the inter-membranous space in the mitochondria, into the mitochondrial matrix during the breakdown of lipids for the generation of metabolic energy.

Extra Mile

- Abnormalities in *carnitine* metabolism can cause dilated or restrictive cardiomyopathies, usually in children

137. Ans. (b) Phenylalanine hydroxylase

Ref: Harrisons, 19th ed. pg. 434e1

- PKU is an autosomal recessive disorder characterized by an increased concentration of phenylalanine and its by-products in body fluids and by severe mental retardation if untreated in infancy.
- It results from reduced activity of **phenylalanine hydroxylase.**
- The accumulation of phenylalanine:
  - Inhibits the transport of other amino acids required for protein or neurotransmitter synthesis
  - Reduces synthesis and increases degradation of myelin, and leads to inadequate formation of norepinephrine and serotonin.
- To prevent intellectual disability, diagnosis and initiation of dietary therapy must be started **before 2 weeks of age**

138. Ans. (a) Collagen

Ref: Harrisons, 19th ed. pg. 2504

- Collagen is the most abundant protein in the body.
- Harrisons states: "The first genes cloned for connective tissues were the two genes coding for **type I collagen, the most abundant protein** in bones, skin, tendons, and several other tissues.

139. Ans. (a) Tryptophan

Ref: Harper's Biochemistry 30th ed. pg. 316, 547, 5517; Food-facts and principles by N. Shakuntala, pg. 71

- Niacin can be synthesized by the bacteria of the intestinal flora and is formed in the tissues from amino acid tryptophan, which has *niacin sparing activity*. This explains why some food rich in tryptophan e.g. milk and egg, have a far greater niacin potency than would be expected from their actual content of niacin.
- In humans, deficiency of niacin results in weakness and indigestion followed by ulcerated mouth and tongue.

TRYPTOPHAN

- It is an essential amino acid, which is a precursor of melatonin, 5-HIAA and serotonin

Biochemistry

$$60 \text{ mg of tryptophan} \xrightarrow{\text{Vit B6}} 1 \text{ mg of Niacin.}$$

- In deficiency of vitamin B6, the pathyway altered and leads to formation of xanthuric acid. **Thus XAN-THURIC ACID IS THE INDEX OF VITAMIN B6 DEFICIENCY.**
- **Sulphur containing amino acid: CYSTEINE AND METHIONINE**
- **BASIC AMINO ACID:**
  - HISTIDINE
  - LYSINE
  - ARGININE (*most basic amino acid*)
- Most stable amino acid at physiologic pH: **HISTIDINE**
- **TYROSINE:** non-essential AA, which is converted to Melanin, T3, T4 hormone by enzyme Tyrosinase.
  - Deficiency of Tyrosinase → Albinism
  - Deficiency of melanocyte → Vitiligo

---

140. Ans. (a) Niacin

Ref: Harper's Biochemistry, 30th ed. pg. 557

- Niacin is synthesized from tryptophan via kynurenine and quinolinic acids as key biosynthetic intermediates.
- *Refer to above explanation for more details.*

---

141. Ans. (b) Maple syrup disease

Ref: Harper's Biochemistry, 30th ed. 309, 27th ed. pg. 257

- Branched chain amino acids are remembered as VIL (Valine, Isoleucine, **Leucine**).
- These amino acids are converted to alpha-keto acid and then undergo oxidative decarboxylation by *enzyme alpha keto-decarboxylase. Deficiency of this enzyme leads to MSUD, which is characterized by burnt sugar or maple syrup smell in urine or sometimes in ear wax also.*
- In patients with deficiency of alpha keto-decarboxylase enzyme, there is **increased concentration of valine, Isoleucine and Leucine.**
- **Management** is done by restricted dietary intake of branched chain amino acid.

> **Extra Mile**

Diseases and Deficiency
- **HARTNUP DISEASE:** TRYPTOPHAN
- **ALKAPTONURIA:** Homogentisate oxidase
- **ALPORT SYNDROME:** due to antibody against type IV collagen.

---

142. Ans. (c) Tryptophan

Ref: Harper's Biochemistry, 30th ed. pg. 281, 544

Food item	Limiting Amino acids
Pulses	**Methionine & cysteine**
Cereals	**Threonine & Lysine**
Maize	**Tryptophan & lysine**

---

143. Ans. (c) Homogentisate oxidase

Ref: Harper's Biochemistry, 30th ed. pg. 304

The defect in Alkaptonuria is lack of homogentisate oxidase. Most imp features are:

- The urine darkens on exposure to air due to oxidation of excreted homogentisate.
- Deposits called ochronosis occur in sclera, ear, nose, cheeks, intervertebral disc space. There may be calcification of inter vertebral discs.
- **Ochronosis arthritis-** affects shoulder ,hip and knee.
- **Benedicts reaction is strongly positive and gives green brown precipitate.**
- **Fehling test** reagent gives blue green colour.

---

144. Ans. (a) Kynerunine

Ref: Harper's Biochemistry, 30th ed. pg. 306-307

- Tryptophan is degraded to amphibolic intermediates via the kynurenine-anthranilate pathway. Tryptophan oxygenase (tryptophan pyrrolase) opens the indole ring, incorporates molecular oxygen, and forms N-formyl kynurenine.
- *Hydrolytic removal of the formyl group of N-formylky-nurenine, catalyzed by kynurenine formylase, produces kynurenine.*
- Since kynureninase requires pyridoxal phosphate, excretion of xanthurenate in response to a tryptophan load is diagnostic of vitamin B_6 deficiency.
- Hartnup disease reflects impaired intestinal and renal transport of tryptophan and other neutral amino acids.

---

145. Ans. (d) Aspartate

Ref: Harper's Biochemistry, 30th ed. pg. 294-95

$NH_3 + HCO_3 + Aspartate + 3ATP \rightarrow Urea + Fumarate + 2 ADP + AMP + 4 P.$

UREA CYCLE

- Urea Is the Major End Product of Nitrogen Catabolism in Humans
- Some reactions of urea synthesis occur in the matrix of the mitochondrion, other reactions in the cytosol
- *Synthesis of 1 mol of urea requires 3 mol of ATP plus 1 mol each of ammonium ion and of the amino nitrogen of aspartate.*

STEPS OF UREA METABOLISM

Step -1: Site: Mitochondria

- Carbamoyl Phosphate Synthase I Initiates Urea Biosynthesis
- Condensation of CO_2, ammonia, and ATP to form carbamoyl phosphate is catalyzed by mitochondrial carbamoyl phosphate synthase I.

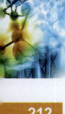

FMGE Solutions Screening Examination

- Carbamoyl phosphate synthase I, the rate-limiting enzyme of the urea cycle, is active only in the presence of its allosteric activator N-acetylglutamate
- *The step requires 2 ATPs*

Step - 2: Site: Mitochondria
- Carbamoyl Phosphate Plus Ornithine Forms Citrulline
- L-Ornithine transcarbamoylase catalyzes the reaction Next 3 steps take place in cytosol

Step -3 : Site : Cytosol
- Citrulline plus Aspartate forms Argininosuccinate
- Argininosuccinate synthase links aspartate and Citrulline via the amino group of aspartate and provides the second nitrogen of urea. The reaction requires ATP.

Step: 4 : Site : Cytosol
- Cleavage of Argininosuccinate Forms Arginine & Fumarate catalyzed by argininosuccinase.

Step: 5 : Site : Cytosol
- Cleavage of Arginine Releases Urea & Re-Forms Ornithine
- Hydrolytic cleavage of the guanidino group of arginine, catalyzed by liver arginase, releases urea
- The other product, ornithine, reenters liver mitochondria for additional rounds of urea synthesis.

146. Ans. (a) Cleavage of Arginine

Ref: Harper's Biochemistry, 30th ed. pg. 299-300
Please refer to above explanation.

147. Ans. (b) Ornithine

- Polyamines like spermine, spermidine and putrescine metabolite are produced from L-ornithine by action of ODC (ornithine decarboxylase).
- S-Adenosylmethionine, the methyl group donor for many biosynthetic processes, also participates directly in spermine and spermidine biosynthesis.

148. Ans. (d) Made of cystiene and methionine

Ref: Harper's Biochemistry, 30th ed. pg. 299-300, 295

SELENOCYSTEINE

- Considered to be the 21st proteinogenic amino acid. It exists naturally in all kingdoms of life as a building block of selenoproteins.
- It is utilized only when required for protein functions.
- **Selenocysteine is present in several enzymes** for example:
  - **Gutathione peroxidases**
  - Tetraiodothyronine 5' deiodinases
  - Thioredoxin reductases and
  - Some hydrogenases

- Selenocysteine is not coded directly in the genetic code. Instead, **it is encoded in a special way by a UGA codon**, which is normally a stop codon. Such a mechanism is called translational receding and its efficiency depends on the seleno-protein being synthesized and on translation initiation factors.
  - The UGA codon is made to encode Selenocysteine by the presence of a SECI Selement (Seleno-Cysteine Insertion Sequence) in the mRNA.

> **Extra Mile**
>
> - **Pyrrolysine is 22nd amino acid.**

149. Ans. (d) Cysteine

Ref: Harper's Biochemistry, 30th ed. pg. 301
- *The clinical disease is due to the accumulation of cysteine which forms stones.*
- **MC inborn error of AA transport**

Causes of Cysteinuria:
- Due to the defective transport in the proximal and jejunal transport of dibasic amino acids such as cysteine, lysine, arginine and ornithine.
- **Cystinuria** (cystin-lysin-uria)- kidney is not able to reabsorb mainly 4 AA- cystine, ornithine, lysine, arginine (**COLA**)- excess amount excreted in urine.

> **Extra Mile**
>
> - **Cystinosis- (**cystine storage disorder)- cystine accumulates in the lysosome in many tissue and there is generalized **aminoaciduria.**

150. Ans. (a) Cysteine

Ref: Harper's Biochemistry, 30th ed. pg. 301

151. Ans. (a) L-arginine

Ref: Harper's Biochemistry, 30th ed. pg. 314, 660-61, 26th pg. 269

- Nitric oxide, known as the *endothelium-derived relaxing factor* is biosynthesized endogenously from L-arginine, oxygen and NADPH by various nitric oxide synthase (NOS) enzymes. Reduction of inorganic nitrate may also serve to make nitric oxide.
- The endothelium of blood vessels uses nitric oxide to signal the surrounding smooth muscle to relax, thus resulting in vasodilation and increasing blood flow.

152. Ans. (c) Arginine

Ref: Harper's Biochemistry, 30th edn. pg. 314, 660-61

Biochemistry

153. Ans. (c) Lysine & methionine

Ref: Harper's Biochemistry, 30th edn. pg. 223-24

- **Carnitine** is a quaternary ammonium compound biosynthesized from the amino acid lysine and methionine.
- It is required for the transport of fatty acids from the intermembraneous space in the mitochondria, into the mitochondrial matrix during the breakdown of lipids for the generation of metabolic energy.

154. Ans. (a) Dihydrouracil

Ref: Harper's Biochemistry, 30th edn. pg. 318

- βalanine *is formed in vivo by the* **degradation of dihydrouracil and carnosine.**
- β-**Alanine** *is not used in the biosynthesis of any major proteins or enzymes. However,* It is a component of the naturally occurring peptidescarnosine and anserine and also of pantothenic acid (vitamin B_5), which itself is a component of coenzyme A. *Under normal conditions, β-alanine is metabolized into acetic acid.*
- β-Alanine is the rate-limiting precursor of carnosine, i.e. *carnosine levels are limited by the amount of available β-alanine.*

155. Ans. (d) N-Acetyl Glucosamine

Ref: Harper's Biochemistry, 30th edn. pg. 157-58

- Chitin is a long-chain polymer of *N*-acetyl-glucosamine, a derivative of glucose. Chitin's properties as a flexible and strong material make it favorable as a surgical thread. Its bio-degradibility means it wears away with time as the wound heals. Moreover, chitin has been reported to have some unusual properties that accelerate healing of wounds in humans.

156. Ans. (b) Glycine

Ref: Harper's Biochemistry, 30th ed. pg. 326-28

- Heme is synthesized in a complex series of steps involving enzymes in the mitochondrion and in the cytosol of the cell
- The first step in heme synthesis takes place in the mitochondrion. Steps in heme synthesis are:
  - **Condensation of succinyl CoA and glycine by ALA synthase to form 5-aminolevulic acid (ALA).**
  - 5 ALA is transported to the cytosol where a series of reactions produce a ring structure called coproporphyrinogen III. This molecule returns to the mitochondrion where an addition reaction produces protoporhyrin IX.
  - The enzyme ferrochelatase inserts iron into the ring structure of protoporphyrin IX to produce heme.

157. Ans. (c) Tryptophan

Ref: Harper's Biochemistry, 30th ed. pg. 308, 557; Harrison's, 19th ed. pg. 435e-2

- Hartnup disease is an **autosomal recessive** disorder caused by impaired neutral amino acid transport in the apical brush border membrane of the small intestine and the proximal tubule of the kidney.
- Patients of hartnup disease present with pellagra like skin eruptions, cerebellar ataxia, and gross aminoaciduria.
- Amino acids which are retained within the intestinal lumen due to impaired transport, are converted by bacteria to indolic compounds that can be toxic to the CNS. Amino acid like *Tryptophan is converted to indole in the intestine.*
- Following absorption, indole is converted to 3-hydroxyindole (i.e, indoxyl, indican) in the liver, where it is conjugated with potassium sulfate or glucuronic acid. Subsequently, it is transported to the kidneys for excretion (i.e, indicanuria).
- Other tryptophan degradation products which are excreted in urine are: kynurenine and serotonin.
- In these patients Tubular renal transport is also defective, contributing to gross aminoaciduria.

158. Ans. (b) Lignin

- Gut flora's primary benefit to the host is the gleaning of energy from the fermentation of undigested carbohydrates and the subsequent absorption of short chain fatty acids. *They can even digest even products like cellulose, pectin and starch.*
- **The most important of these are**: Butyrates, metabolised by the colonic epithelium; propionates by the liver; and acetates by the muscle tissue.
- Intestinal bacteria also play a role in synthesizing vitamin B and vitamin K as well as metabolising bile acids, sterols and xenobiotics.
- *The human body carries about 100 trillion microorganisms in its intestines, a number ten times greater than the total number of human cells in the body*
- Lignin or lignen is a complex polymer of aromatic alcohols known as monolignols. It is most commonly derived from wood, and is an integral part of the secondary cell walls of plants.

159. Ans. (b) Histidine

Ref: Harper's Biochemistry, 30th ed. pg. 340-42

- N1 of purine is derived from amino group of aspartate
- N3 & N9 are obtained from amide group of glutamine
- C4, C5, & N7 of the purine ring of nucleotides are contributed by glycine.

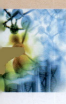

FMGE Solutions Screening Examination

160. Ans. (b) Glycine

Ref: Harper's Biochemistry 30th ed. pg. 325-27; 26th/ 264

- **Glycine** is required for the biosynthesis of **heme**, **purines** and **creatine** and is conjugated to **bile acids**.
- **Serine** is required for the **phospholipid** and **sphingosine** synthesis apart from **purines** and **thymine**.
- **S-Adenosyl methionine** (the methyl group donor) for many biosynthetic processes, also participates directly in **spermine and spermidine** synthesis.

161. Ans. (d) All of the above

Ref: Harper's Biochemistry 30th ed. pg. 22-23, 748

- *Glutathione (GSH) is a tripeptide with a gamma peptide linkage between the amine group of cysteine (which is attached by normal peptide linkage to a glycine) and the carboxyl group of the glutamateside-chain.*
- It is an antioxidant, preventing damage to important cellular components caused by reactive oxygen species such as free radicals and peroxides.

162. Ans. (a) Proline to hydroxyproline

Ref: Harper's Biochemistry, 30th ed. pg. 47, 562

- *Ascorbic acid is needed for a variety of biosynthetic pathways, by accelerating hydroxylation and amidation reactions.*
- In the synthesis of collagen, ascorbic acid is required as a cofactor for following enzymes:
  - Prolyl hydroxylase
  - Lysyl hydroxylase
- *These two enzymes are responsible for the hydroxylation of the proline and lysine amino acids in collagen.*
- *Remember, Hydroxyproline and hydroxylysine are important for stabilizing collagen by cross-linking the propeptides in collagen.*
- Clinical effects if there is defective collagen fibrillogenesis:
  - Impaired wound healing.
  - Impaired bone bormation
  - Abnormal bleeding due to fragile capillaries.

163. Ans. (b) Proline

Ref: Harper's Biochemistry, 30th ed. pg. 141, 298-99

- Proline is the amino acid which changes the conformation of the alpha helix in collagen due to the nature of proline having a cyclical structure. It also forms the ends of the beta sheets in the secondary structures.

164. Ans. (a) Pyridoxal phosphate

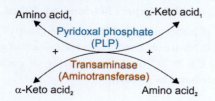

- Transamination involves reversible transfer of alpha amino group of alpha amino acid to an alpha-keto-acid to form a new amino acid and a new keto-acid.
- Enzyme catalyze this reaction is called transaminase (aminotransferase)
- All transaminase require **pyridoxal phosphate (Vit B6)** as a coenzyme
- **Example of transaminase are:**
  - Alanine transferase (ALT)
  - Aspartate transaminase (AST)
- Transamination reactions are **reversible**
- Transamination reactions occur **via ping pong mechanism** in which the 1st substrate bound and its product is realeased prior to binding of second substarte.
- Most amino acid undergo transamination **except lysine, theonine, proline, and hydroxyproline**

VITAMINS, MINERALS AND ENZYMES

165. Ans. (b) Copper

Ref: Harrison's 20th ed. P 2318

Menkes Kinky Hair Syndrome

- X-Linked metabolic disturbance of copper metabolism
- Characterized by:
  - Mental retardation
  - Hypocupremia
  - Decreased circulating ceruloplasmin
- Due to mutation in **ATP7-A gene** (copper transporting gene)
- **Cause of death:** Dissecting aneurysm or cardiac rupture (usually <5 years of age)

> **Extra Mile**
>
> - **Wilson's disease:** Copper accumulation in liver, brain; due to mutation in ATP7-B gene.
> - **Acrodermatitis enteropathica:** AR condition. Due to zinc deficiency
> - **Chromium** potentiates the action of insulin and improves lipid profile
> - **Keshan disease:** Endemic cardiomyopathy, due to dietary deficiency of selenium
> - **Kashin–Beck disease/Selenosis:** Chronic ingestion of large amount of selenium. Characterized by hair loss and nail brittleness, garlic breath odor, rash, myopathy etc.

166. Ans. (b) Cell membrane

Ref: Lippincott's Biochemistry 6th ed. P 151-152

- G6PD enzyme is located at the cell membrane. RBC membrane is one such example, and is associated with severe pathology

Biochemistry

- Location: X chromosome at q28 locus. (G6PD enzyme is X-linked gene)
- It protects the RBC from the deleterious effects of oxidizing agents by reducing themselves to NADPH.
- In deficiency of G6PD enzyme → impaired ability of RBC to form NADPH → Hemolysis

167. Ans. (c) X-Linked

Ref: Lippincott's Biochemistry 6th ed. P 151-152

- G6PD deficiency is most common disease producing enzyme abnormality in humans
- It is a X-linked disorder

168. Ans. (b) Enteropeptidase

- The pancreatic enzyme trypsinogen is activated to form trypsin with the help of enzyme enteropeptidase/enterokinase.

Activation of some pancreatic zymogens

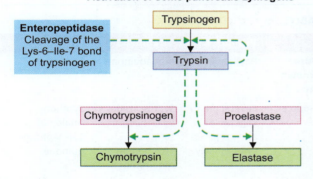

169. Ans. (c) It rescues proteins that have folded improperly and...

Ref: Harper's Biochemistry, 30th ed. pg. 618-20, 26th ed. P 36-37

- **Over half of mammalian protein folding is done by Chaperone proteins.**
- Chaperones prevent aggregation, thus providing an opportunity for the formation of appropriate secondary structural elements.
- **There are 2 families of hsp:** hsp 60 and hsp 70.
- The hsp 60 family of chaperones, sometimes called chaperonins, differ in sequence and structure from hsp 70 and its homologs.
- The HSP 70 (70-kDa heat shock protein) **family of chaperones binds short sequences of hydrophobic amino acids in newly synthesized polypeptides, shielding them from solvent.**
- **Chaperone proteins can also "rescue" proteins** that have become thermodynamically trapped in a misfolded dead end. They rescue it **by unfolding hydrophobic** regions and providing a second chance to fold productively.

> **Extra Mile**
> - Chaperones for eukaryotes: Hsp 70
> - Force favourable for protein folding: Hydrophobic interaction

170. Ans. (b) Chemical antagonism

Ref: Vasudevan Biochemistry, 8th ed. P 321

- **Chemical:** A type of antagonism where a drug counters the effect of another by simple chemical reaction/neutralization (not binding to the receptor).
- **Physiological:** Two drugs act on two different types of receptor and antagonize action of each other.
- **Competitive:** Both drugs bind to same receptor.

171. Ans. (b) Vitamin C

Ref: Vasudevan Biochemistry, 8th ed. P 481

TABLE: The vitamins

	Vitamin	Functions
A	Retinol, β-carotene	Visual pigments in the retina; regulation of gene expression and cell differentiation; β-carotene is an antioxidant
D	Calciferol	Maintenance of calcium balance; enhances intestinal absorption of Ca^{2+} and mobilizes bone mineral
E	Tocopherols, tocotrienols	Antioxidant, especially in cell membranes
K	Phylloquinone, menaquinones	Coenzyme in formation of γ-carboxyglutamate in enzymes of blood clotting and bone matrix
B_1	Thiamine	Coenzyme in pyruvate and α-ketoglutarate, dehydrogenases, and transketolase; poorly defined function in nerve conduction
B_2	Riboflavin	Coenzyme in oxidation and reduction reactions; prosthetic group of flavoproteins
Niacin	Nicotinic acid, nicotinamide	Coenzyme in oxidation and reduction reactions, functional part of NAD and NADP
B_6	Pyridoxine, pyridoxal, pyridoxamine	Coenzyme in transamination and decarboxylation of amino acids and glycogen phosphorylase; role in steroid hormone action
	Folic acid	Coenzyme in transfer of one-carbon fragments
B_{12}	Cobalamin	Coenzyme in transfer of one-carbon fragments and metabolism of folic acid
	Pantothenic acid	Functional part of CoA and acyl carrier protein; fatty acid synthesis and metabolism

Contd...

Vitamin		Functions
H	Biotin	Coenzyme in carboxylation reactions in gluconeogenesis and fatty acid synthesis
C	Ascorbic acid	Coenzyme in hydroxylation of proline and lysine in collagen synthesis; antioxidant; enhances absorption of iron

172. Ans. (c) ATP

Ref: Vasudevan Biochemistry, 8/e. P 531

- **Cyclic AMP (cAMP)** is formed from cytosolic ATP by **adenylyl cyclase**, an enzyme that is anchored in the plasma membrane
- The enzyme is inactive until bound to activated Gs_α; (by receptor-ligand stimulated acquisition of GTP and release (from $Gs_{\beta\gamma}$)
- Gi_α inhibits adenylyl cyclase

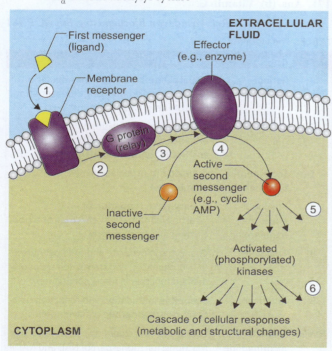

173. Ans. (c) Vitamin E

Ref: Harper's Biochemistry, 30th ed. pg. 553, 564

- *Vitamin E has many biological functions, the antioxidant function being the most important and/or best known.*
- Other functions include:
  - Enzymatic activities
  - Gene expression
  - Neurological function and
  - Cell signalling

- As an antioxidant, **vitamin E acts as a peroxyl radical scavenger,** preventing the propagation of free radicals in tissues.
- It does so by reacting with ROS to form a tocopheryl radical, which will then be reduced by a hydrogen donor (such as vitamin C) to its reduced state. As it is fat-soluble, it is incorporated into cell membranes, which protects them from oxidative damage.

174. Ans. (c) Keshan disease

- **Keshan disease** is an endemic cardiomyopathy found in children and young women of chinese regions due to dietary deficiency of selenium.
- **Kashin beck disease:** Occurs due to selenium toxicity/selenosis. It is characterized by hair loss, brittle nail, garlic breath odor, rashes, myopathy and nervous system abnormality.

175. Ans. (b) Exist in three forms

TABLE: Forms of VITAMIN K

	Vitamin K1	Vitamin K2	Vitamin K3
Also known as	Phylloquinone	Menaquinone	Menadione
Source	Several green vegetables and prepared synthetically	Synthesized by GI bacteria, supplies 50% human requirement	Synthetic, Analog of 1,4-naphtho-quinone
Solubility	Fat soluble	Fat soluble	**Diphosphate salt is Water soluble**

176. Ans. (a) Oxidase-Reductase

Oxidoreductase enzyme groups can be remembered by mnemonic DOOP
- Dehydrogenases
- Oxidases
- Oxygenases
- Peroxidases

177. Ans. (a) Chromium

Ref: Harrisons, 19th ed. pg. 96e-9

- A deficiency of chromium can cause impaired glucose tolerance.
- Physiologically, chromium potentiates the action of insulin in patients with impaired glucose tolerance, presumably by increasing insulin receptor-mediated signalling.
- Rich food sources of chromium include yeast, meat, and grain products.

Biochemistry

- **Note:**
  - **Deficiency of Selenium:** Can cause cardiomyopathy (Keshan disease)
  - **Selenium toxicity:** Can cause selenosis (Kashinbeck disease)

178. Ans. (d) Zinc

TABLE: Important minerals and their respective action as cofactor

Minerals	Function
Selenium	• Cofactor for ■ Glutathione peroxidase ■ Deiodinase ■ Thioredoxin reductase
Manganese	• Cofactor for: ■ Arginase ■ Kinase ■ Carboxylase ■ Glucosyl transferase ■ Enolase
Zinc	• Cofactor for: ■ Carbonic anhydrase ■ Alcohol dehydrogenase ■ **Lactate dehydrogenase** ■ Carboxypeptidase

179. Ans. (a) K_m increased, V_{max} same

Type of Inhibition	Km	Vmax
Competitive inhibition	INCREASED	SAME
Non-competitive inhibition	Same	DECREASED

Competitive Inhibtion: Substrate and inhibitor, both compete for same site on enzyme.

Non-competitive Inhibition: Substrate and inhibitor both bind at different sites in the enzyme.

180. Ans. (c) Methionine synthase

Ref: Harper's Biochemistry, 30th ed. pg. 558

▌CONVERSION OF HOMOCYSTEINE TO METHIONINE

- Active form in this reaction is methycobalamin. This reaction requires both methylcobalamin and folic acid. The reaction is catalyzed by methionine synthase which is a methylcobalamin dependent reaction.

$$\text{Homocysteine} \xrightarrow[\textit{Methylcobalamin + folic acid}]{\text{Methionine synthase}} \text{Methionine}$$

181. Ans. (b) Consist of flavin group which is required in oxidation-reduction reaction

Ref: Harper's Biochemistry, 30th ed. pg. 556

RIBOFLAVIN is vitamin B_2 which contains isoelloxazine ring. It gives yellow color, therefore used to fortify some foods.

- *It consists of flavin group which is required in oxidation-reduction reactions.*
- **Source:** Meat products, liver, egg, whole grain, vegetables
  - *Green leafy vegetables are major sources of folic acid (B9)*
- **Deficiency causes:** Angular stomatitis, cheilosis, dermatitis, Glossitis, geographic tongue Lesion on mouth and genitalia.

Lets summarize the other names of Vitamin B complexes:

TABLE: Vitamin B, their other names and disease entities due to deficiency

Vitamin	Other name	Deficiency causes
Vit B1	Thiamine	*Beri Beri*, *Wernicke's encephalopathy*
Vit B2	Riboflavin	Angular stomatitis, cheilosis, dermatitis, Glossitis
Vit B3	Niacin	Pellagra *(4D's- Dementia, Diarrhea, Dermatitis, Death)*
Vit B5	Pantothenic acid	Burning foot syndrome, Liener disease
Vit B6	Pyridoxine	Peripheral neuropathy, Sideroblastic anemia, Pellagra, Homocystinuria, Hartnup disease
Vit B7	Biotin	Multiple carboxylase deficiency
Vit B9	Folic acid	Megaloblastic anemia, Neural tube defect
Vit B12	Cyano-cobalamin	Megaloblastic anemia, subacute combined degeneration (SACD)

182. Ans. (c) Biotin

Ref: Harper's Biochemistry, 30th ed. pg. 560-61

- Acetyl-COA carboxylase is a biotin-depenent enzyme that catalyzes the irreversible carboxylation of acetyl-CoA to produce malonyl-CoA through its two catalytic activities, biotin carboxylase and carboxyl transferase

Explanations

FMGE Solutions Screening Examination

183. Ans. (b) Folic Acid

Ref: Harper's Biochemistry, 30th ed. pg. 299, 559-560, 26th ed. pg. 494

184. Ans. (b) Deficiency of tryptophan

Ref: Harper's Biochemistry 30th ed. pg. 546, 557, 29th ed. pg. 540

- Pellagra is seen due to deficiency of niacin (vitamin B3) aka nicotinic acid.
- **Nicotinic acid can be formed in the body from tryptophan.** 60 mg of tryptophan forms 1 mg of niacin. Henceforth, deficiency of tryptophan causes deficiency of niacin leading to pellagra.

Extra Mile

- **Deficiency of thiamine causes:** Beri-Beri, Wernicke's encephalopathy, Lactic acidosis
- **Deficiency of Vitamin B12 causes:** Pernicious anemia, Megaloblastic anemia, SCID, methymalonic acidura.
- **Deficiency of vitamin B9/Folic acid:** Megaloblastic anemia, NTD.

185. Ans. (a) Vitamin K

Ref: Harper's Biochemistry, 30th ed. pg. 554

- Menadione is the water soluble form of vitamin K.

TABLE: Forms of VITAMIN K

	Vitamin K1	Vitamin K2	Vitamin K3
Aka	Phylloquinone	Menaquinone	Menadione
Source	Several green vegetables and prepared synthetically	Synthesized by GI bacteria, supplies 50% human requirement	Synthetic, Analog of 1,4-naphtho-quinone
Solubility	Fat soluble	Fat soluble	Diphosphate salt is Water soluble

- Vitamin K Is the Coenzyme for Carboxylation of Glutamate in Postsynthetic Modification of Calcium Binding Proteins. Vitamin K Is Also Important in Synthesis of Bone Calcium Binding Proteins.
- *Dicumarol is an anticoagulant that functions as a vitamin K antagonist.*

186. Ans. (c) Menadione

Ref: Harper's Biochemistry, 30th ed. pg. 554

Please refer to above table

187. Ans. (c) Menadione

Ref: Harper's Biochemistry, 30th ed. pg. 554

188. Ans. (d) Vitamin K

Ref: Harper's Biochemistry, 30th ed. pg. 554-555

- Anti-oxidants are vitamin A, C and vitamin E (ACE). *Most important of all is vitamin E.*
- Free-radicals are formed from exposure to sunlight and pollution and also as a byproduct of cell metabolism.
- Alcohol, cigarette smoke, stress and even diet also affect the level of free-radical development in the body. Excellent antioxidants include Vitamin A, Vitamin E, Vitamin C, zinc, selenium, ginkgo biloba, grape seed extract, and green tea extract.

189. Ans. (a) Vitamin K

Ref: Harper's Biochemistry, 30th ed. pg. 5341-42, 554, 26th ed. pg. 481

Apart from **dietary inadequacy,** conditions affecting the digestion and absorption of the lipid-soluble vitamins (vitamins **A, D, E and K**) such as **steatorrhea and disorders of the biliary system,** all can lead to deficiency syndromes, including: night blindness and xerophthalmia (vitamin A); rickets in young children and osteomalacia in adults (vitamin D); neurologic disorders and anemia of the newborn (vitamin E); and hemorrhage of the newborn (vitamin K). **Vitamin K** is also important in the synthesis of bone calcium-binding proteins like osteocalcin and bone matrix Gla protein. In fact, the release into the circulation of **osteocalcin provides an index of vitamin D status.**

190. Ans. (b) Vitamin C

Ref: K. Park, 23rd ed. pg. 630

- *Eggs has all the nutrients except vitamin C and carbohydrate.*
- Eggs are also a source of folate, biotin pantothenic acid, choline, phosphorous, iodine and selenium in terms of minerals and vitamins.
- *Egg contains Avidin, which interferes with biotin absorption.*

191. Ans. (b) Zinc deficiency

Ref: Harrison's, 19th ed. pg. 96e-9

- Zinc is an essential trace nutrient required for the proper function of more than 100 enzymes and plays a crucial role in nucleic acid metabolism.
- Acrodermatitis enteropathica is an **autosomal recessive** disorder postulated to occur as a result of mutations in the *SLC39A4 gene* located on band **8q24.3.**

Biochemistry

- This protein is highly expressed in the **enterocytes in the duodenum and jejunum.** Therefore, affected individuals have a decreased ability to absorb zinc from dietary sources. Absence of a binding ligand needed to transport zinc may further contribute to zinc malabsorption.
- **Clinical manifestations include** diarrhea, alopecia, muscle wasting, depression, irritability, and a rash involving the extremities, face, and perineum. The rash is characterized by vesicular and pustular crusting with scaling and erythema.
- Features of acrodermatitis enteropathica **start appearing in the first few months of life,** if mother discontinues breast milk.

TABLE: Deficiency and toxicity of several metals

Element	Deficiency	Toxicity
Boron	No biologic function determined	Developmental defects, male sterility, testicular atrophy
Calcium	Reduced bone mass, osteoporosis	Renal insufficiency (milk-alkali syndrome)^Q nephrolithiasis, impaired iron absorption, thiazide diuretics.
Copper	Anemia, growth retardation, defective keratinization and pigmentation of hair, hypothermia, degenerative changes in aortic elastin^Q, osteopenia, mental deterioration.	Nausea, vomiting, diarrhea, hepatic failure, tremor, mental deterioration, hemolytc anemia, renal dysfunction
Chromium	Impaired glucose tolerance^Q	*Occupational;* Renal failure, dermatitis, pulmonary cancer
Fluoride	↑Dental caries^Q	Dental and skeletal flurosis^Q, osteosclerosis
Iodine	Thyroid enlargement, ↓T_4 cretinism	Thyroid dysfunction, acne-like eruptions^Q.
Iron	Muscle abnormalities, koilonychia, pica anemia, ↓work performance, impaired cognitive development, premature labor, ↑perinatal maternal death	Gastrointestinal effects, (nausea, vomiting, diarrhea, constipation), iron overload with organ damage, acute and chronic systemic toxicity, increased susceptibility to malaria, increased risk association with certain chronic diseases (e.g. diabetes)
Manganese	Impaired growth and skeletal development reproduction, lipid and carbohydrate metabolism, upper body rash	*General:* Neurotoxicity, Parkinson-like symptoms^Q *Occupational*: Encephalitis like syndrome, Parkinson like syndrome, psychosis, pneumoconiosis.
Molybdenum	Severe neurologic abnormalities	Reproductive and fetal abnormalities
Selenium	Cardiomyopathy, heart failure, striated muscle degeneration	*General:* Alopecia, nausea, vomiting, abnormal nails, emotional
Phosphorus	Rickets (osteomalacia) proximal muscle weakness, rhabdomyolysis, paresthesia, ataxia, seizure confusion, heart failure, hemolysis acidosis.	Hyperphosphatemia
Zinc	Growth retardation, ↓taste and smell alopecia, dermatitis, diarrhea, immune dysfunction, failure to thrive, gonasal atrophy, congenital malfomations.	General: Reduced copper, absorption, gastritis, sweating fever, nausea, vomiting *Occupational;* Respiratory distress, pulmonary fibrosis

192. Ans. (c) ADP-ribosylation of Gs alpha sub-unit

Ref: Harper's Biochemistry, 30th ed. pg. 250

Cholera Toxin Acts by the Following Mechanism
- The B subunit ring of the cholera toxin binds to GM1 gangliosides on the surface of target cells. Once bound, the entire toxin complex is endocytosed by the cell and the cholera toxin **A1 (CTA1) chain is released** and leads to ADP ribosylation of G_S subunit massive fluid efflux in GI lumen.
- Cholera toxin ADP-ribosylates G proteins, causing ↑cAMp and *massive fluid secretion from the lining of the small intestine, resulting in life-threatening diarrhea.*
- ADP-ribosylation is also responsible for the actions of some bacterial toxins, such as cholera toxin, diphtheria toxin, pertussis toxin, and heat-labile enterotoxin.

FMGE Solutions Screening Examination

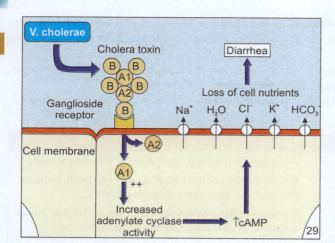

> **Extra Mile**
> - Active subunit of cholera toxin: A
> - Binding subunit of cholera toxin: B

193. Ans. (c) 7.36-7.44

Ref: Harper's Biochemistry, 30th edn. pg. 10-13

Well I think this one is too simple for an explanation. Also remember pH of urine=4.6-8.0

> **Extra Mile**
> - Values of pH going above 7.4 is alkalosis and value of pH going below 7.4 is acidosis
> - pH of Aqueous Humor - 7.2

TABLE: Conditions arising due to low and high pH

Low pH	High pH
• Metabolic acidosis	• Metabolic alkalosis
• Respiratory acidosis	• Repiratory alkalosis

194. Ans. (b) Net protein utilization

Ref: K.Park 23rd ed.

- The **net protein utilization**, or NPU, is the ratio of amino acid converted to proteins to the ratio of amino acids supplied. This figure is somewhat affected by the salvage of essential amino acids within the body, but is profoundly affected by the level of limiting amino acids within a foodstuff.
- NPU can range from 1 to 0, with a value of 1 indicating 100% utilization of dietary nitrogen as protein and a value of 0 an indication that none of the nitrogen supplied was converted to protein. Certain foodstuffs, such as eggs or milk, rate as 1 on an NPU chart.

195. Ans. (a) Vitamin B_{12}

Ref: Harper's Biochemistry 30th ed. pg. 559

- Increased methyl malonic acid levels may indicate a vitamin B_{12} deficiency. However, it is sensitive but not specific. MMA is elevated in 90-98% of patients with B_{12} deficiency.
- The coenzyme A is linked form of methylmalonic acid. Methylmalonyl-CoA, is converted into succinyl-CoA by methylmalonyl-CoA mutase, in a reaction that requires vitamin B_{12} as a cofactor.

Methylmalonyl - CoA $\xrightarrow[\text{Vitamin } B_{12}]{\text{Methylmalonyl-CoA mutase}}$ Succinyl - CoA

Methylmalonyl - CoA $\xrightarrow{\text{Methylmalonyl-CoA mutase}}$ Succinyl - CoA

- In this way, it enters the Krebs cycle, and is thus part of one of the anaplerotic reactions.

196. Ans. (d) Copper deposit

Ref: Harper's Biochemistry, 30th ed. pg. 496

- Wilson's disease is also associated with sunflower cataracts exhibited by brown or green pigmentation of the anterior and posterior lens capsule.
- *For more details about the different types of cataract, please refer to ophthalmology section.*

197. Ans. (b) Fibrillin

Ref: Harrison's, 19th ed.

- Fibrillin-1 is a major component of the microfibrils that form a sheath surrounding the amorphous elastin. It is believed that the microfibrils are composed of end-to-end polymers of fibrillin. To date, 3 forms of fibrillin have been described and mutations in the FBN1 gene cause Marfan's syndrome. This protein and its genes are found on chromosome 15.
- **Mutation in Fibrillin 1 gene (FBN 1) primarily affects: Skeletal system, Cardiovascular system and Eye.**

198. Ans. (b) Demethylation

Ref: Harper's Biochemistry, 30th ed. pg. 509-510

- Conversion of norepinephrine to epinephrine is **demethyation reaction**. It utilizes **phenylethanolamine-N-methyltransferase**.
- Epinephrine to norepinephrine conversion is called methylation.
- **Immediate precursor of tyrosine: Phenylalanine**

199. Ans. (c) PENMT

Ref: Harper's Biochemistry, 30th ed. pg. 509-510

- Phenylethanolamine N-methyltransferase (PENMT) is an enzyme found in the adrenal medulla that converts Norepinephrine (Noradrenaline) to Epinephrine (Adrenaline) cortex.
- S. Adenosyl –L- Methionine (SAM) is a required cofactor.

Biochemistry

200. Ans. (c) Phenylalanine hydroxylase

Ref: Harper's Biochemistry, 30th ed. pg. 509-510

Please refer to explanation fig.

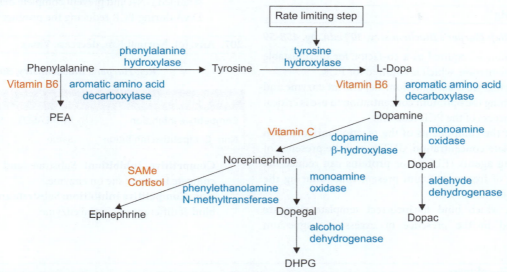

- **Phenylalanine hydroxylase:** for conversion of Phenylalanine to tyrosine conversion
- **Tyrosine hydroxylase:** for conversion of tyrosine to L-Dopa
- **Phenylethanolamine-N-methyltransferase:** for conversion of norepinephrine to epinephrine

201. Ans. (b) Phenylalanine

Ref: Harper's Biochemistry, 30th edn. pg. 509-10, 26th pg. 255, 446

202. Ans. (a) Dopamine hydroxylase

Ref: Harper's Biochemistry, 30th edn. pg. 561

- Those enzymes that require inorganic metal ions as their cofactor are termed as metalloenzymes aka cofactors.
- **Dopamine hydroxylase is a copper-containing enzyme involved in the synthesis of the catecholamines: Norepinephrine** and Epinephrine from tyrosine in the adrenal medulla and central nervous system.
- Ascorbic acid is also linked with copper containing hydroxylases such as peptidoglycine hydroxylase and dopamine hydroxylase. Dopamine decarboxylase requires pyridoxal phosphate for the conversion of L-dopa to 3,4-dihydroxyphenylethylamine.

TABLE: Metals and their Metalloenzymes

Metal	Metalloenzymes
Copper	Cytochrome oxidase, Lysyl oxidase, Dopamine Hydroxylase, ascorbic acid oxidase, Tyrosinase, Ferroxidase (Ceruloplasmin), Superoxide Dismutase
Magnesium	Hexokinase, PFK, Glucose-6-phosphatase, Kinases, Thermostable DNA polymerases, Enolase, Creatinine kinase

Contd...

Metal	Metalloenzymes
Selenium	Glutathione peroxidase
Molybdenum	Xanthine oxidase
Calcium	Lipase, Lecithinase
Iron	Cytochrome oxidase, Xanthine oxidase, Catalase, Peroxidase
Nickel	Urease

203. Ans. (a) Lysyl oxidase

Ref: Harper's Biochemistry, 30th edn. pg. 628

- Lysyl oxidase is an extracellular copper enzyme that catalyzes formation of aldehydes from lysine residues in collagen and elastin precursors.

Please refer to above table

204. Ans. (b) Xanthine Oxidase

Ref: Harper's Biochemistry, 30th edn. pg. 120

205. Ans. (d) Copper

Ref: Harper's Biochemistry, 30th edn. pg. 629-30

- Copper plays a role in collagen cross linking and is catalyzed by lysyl oxidase.

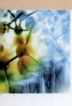

FMGE Solutions Screening Examination

- This enzyme utilizes copper as cupric ion.
- The genetic deficiency of lysyl oxidase is seen in Ehler danlos syndrome.

206. Ans. (b) Mg^{2+}

Ref: Harper's Biochemistry, 30th edn. pg. 458-59

- Magnesium is required as a co-factor for thermostable DNA polymerase, which is required for PCR.
- Taq polymerase is a magnesium-dependent enzyme and determining the optimum concentration to use is critical to the success of the PCR reaction.
- Some of the components of the reaction mixture such as template concentration, dNTPs and the presence of chelating agents (EDTA) or proteins can reduce the amount of free magnesium present thus reducing the activity of the enzyme.
- Primers which bind to incorrect template sites are stabilized in the presence of excessive magnesium concentrations and so result in decreased specificity of the reaction.
- Excessive magnesium concentrations also stabilize double stranded DNA and prevent complete denaturation of the DNA during PCR reducing the product yield.

207. Ans. (c) Normal Km, decrease Vmax

Ref: Harper's Biochemistry, 30th edn. pg. 81-82

Type of Inhibition	Km	Vmax
Competitive inhibition	INCREASED	SAME
Non- Competitive inhibition	Same	DECREASED

Competitive Inhibition: Substrate and inhibitor Both compete for same site on enzyme.

Non-Competitive Inhibition: Substrate and Inhibitor both bind at different site in the enzyme.

208. Ans. (a) Glucokinase

Ref: Harper's Biochemistry, 30th edn. pg. 61-62

- Glucokinase is an enzyme which phosphorylates the glucose to glucose 6 phosphate in the cells. It is a phosphorylase enzyme and not an oxidoreductase. *Please see below Table.*

TABLE: Enzymes according to their family

I	II	III	IV	V	VI
Oxidoreductases	**Transferases**	**Hydrolases**	**Lyases**	**Isomerases**	**Ligases**
• Dehydrogenases • Oxidases • Oxygenases • Peroxidases • Catalase	Amino transferase Methyl-transferase Phosphorylases Kinases	• Phosphatases • Phosphodiesterases • Proteases • Peptidase Lipases Nuclease, Nucleotidase, Nucleosidase	Carbonic anhydrase Aldolase Decarboxylases	RECEMASES Epimerase Mutases	Carboxylases Synthetases Synthase
Mn: DOOP–Cat	Mn: Amir Me & P-K	Mn: P4-LN	Mn: CAD	Mn: REM	

ANSWERS TO BOARD REVIEW QUESTIONS

209. Ans. (b) Zinc

Ref: Text of Biochemistry By G.P Talwar and LM Srivastava p 585, Shinde and Chatterjee 6th ed/-555

210. Ans. (a) 2 calories

Ref: Nutrition Now By Judith E. Brown p 4

211. Ans. (a) Glycogen

Ref: Guyton's 10th ed/1058

212. Ans. (c) Fructose

Ref: Harper's Biochemistry 27th ed Ch-22

213. Ans. (b) Glucokinase

Ref: Harper's 27th ed ch-18

214. Ans. (b) Increased K_m

Ref: Harper's Biochemistry 27th ed ch-8, Harper's Biochemistry 29th ed/76, 88, 85

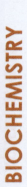

Biochemistry

215. Ans. (b) **Cytoplasm**

> *Ref: Harper's Biochemistry 27th ed ch-37*

216. Ans. (b) **Glucose 6 Phosphatase**

> *Ref: Harper's Biochemistry 27th ed ch-19*

217. Ans. (d) **Tryptophan**

> *Ref: Harper's Biochemistry 27th ed ch-29*

218. Ans. (b) **Mitochondria**

> *Ref: Harper's Biochemistry 27th ed ch:22*

219. Ans. (b) **Phase II reaction**

> *Ref: Harper's Biochemistry 27th ed ch:52*

220. Ans. (a) **Sphingomyelinase**

> *Ref: Lehininger principles of Biochemistry 4th ed / 356*

221. Ans. (a) **Kynurenine**

> *Ref: Harper's Biochemistry 27th ed ch:29*

222. Ans. (d) **Aspartate**

> *Ref: Harper illustrated biochemistry 27th ed p 246-49*

223. Ans. (a) **Cleavage of Arginine**

> *Ref: Previous question*

224. Ans. (c) **Oligonucleotides**

> *Ref: Aptamers in Bioanalysis by M. Mascini / 230*

225. Ans. (b) **Arachidonic acid**

> *Ref: Vasudevan's Biochemistry 6th ed / 77*

226. Ans. (b) **5% iodine and 10% potassium iodide**

> *Ref: Pharmaceutical chemistry-I by Dr. A.V. Kastur p 9*

227. Ans. (a) **L-arginine**

> *Ref: Guyton's physiology 22nd ed / 199*

228. Ans. (b) **HMG CoA reductase**

> *Ref: Harper Biochemistry 29/e, / 251, 254*

229. Ans. (d) **All of the above**

> *Ref: Harper's Biochemistry 28/e, chapter 26*

230. Ans. (b) **OH-**

> *Ref: Textbook of medical biochemistry by Dinesh puri 3/e, /570, 717*

231. Ans. (a) **Apo A1**

> *Ref: Harper's Biochemistry 28/e, chapter 25*

232. Ans. (c) **Glutamate**

> *Ref: Harper's Biochemistry 28/e, chapter 30*

233. Ans. (b) **Proline**

> *Ref: Harper's Biochemistry 28/e, chapter 28*

234. Ans. (a) **Chaperones**

> *Ref: Harper's Biochemistry 28/e, ch. 45, Table 45-5, & Table 45-6*

235. Ans. (d) **Protein folding**

> *Ref: Harper's 28/e, chapter 45, Table 45-5, Table 45-6*

236. Ans. (b) **Golgi apparatus**

> *Ref: Grey's anatomy 39/e, chapter 2*

237. Ans. (a) **Oxaloacetate**

> *Ref: Harper's Biochemistry 28/e, chapter 20*

238. Ans. (b) **Triglycerides**

> *Ref: Harrison's 18/e, chapter 361*

239. Ans. (d) **Complex IV**

> *Ref: Harper's Biochemistry 29/e, p 126, 127, 128*

240. Ans. (d) **All of the above**

> *Ref: Lippincott 4/e, / 261*

241. Ans. (b) **Zn**

> *Ref: Guyton 18/e, chapter 78, Cellular and molecular biology of metals by Rudolfs K. Zalups, D. James koropatnick / 196*

242. Ans. (c) **Tryptophan**

> *Ref: Lippincott's 4/e, / 261*

243. Ans. (d) **Niacin**

> *Ref: Harper's Biochemistry 28/e, chapter 44*

244. Ans. (b) **Mitochondria**

> *Ref: Lippincott's 4/e, / 194, Harper's Biochemistry 28, chapter 22*

Explanations

FMGE Solutions Screening Examination

245. Ans. (b) Na⁺

> *Ref: Ganong's 23/e, chapter 28*

246. Ans. (d) Liver and muscles

> *Ref: Biochemistry M N chatarjee 2/e, p 205, A manual of laboratory and diagnostic tests, p 429*

247. Ans. (a) High amount of leucine

> *Ref: Harrison's 18/e, chapter 24, Textbook*

248. Ans. (c) Right handed anti parallel

> *Ref: Lippincott's 4/e, chapter 29*

249. Ans. (d) mol/second

> *Ref: Textbook of biochemistry for medical students by D.M. vasudevan, Sreekumari S, Kannan Vaidyanantha 7/e, p 65, Biochemistry update by Reginald H. Gerrett, Charles M. Grishan 3/e, p 417*

250. Ans. (b) Halibut liver oil

> *Ref: Harper's Biochemistry 27/e, chapter 44, Textbook of medical biochemistry S. Ramakrishnan 3/e, p 393*

251. Ans. (b) Alpha ketoglutarate dehydrogenase

> *Ref: Harper's Biochemistry 28/e, ch-9, p 306*

252. Ans. (d) Malonate

> *Ref: Harper's Biochemistry 28/e, p chapter 9, P 306*

253. Ans. (c) NADPH

> *Ref: Harper's Biochemistry 27/e, Chapter 21*

254. Ans. (b) Nicotinic acid

> *Ref: Harper''s Biochemistry 27/e, Chapter 44*

255. Ans. (b) Muscle phosphorylase deficiency

> *Ref: Harper's Biochemistry 29/e, p 181*

256. Ans. (c) Anaerobic glycolysis

> *Ref: Harper''s Biochemistry 27/e, Chapter 51*

257. Ans. (a) Arginine

> *Ref: Protein reviews volume 4, Protein misfolding, aggregation and conformational diseases by Vladimir N. p 103*

258. Ans. (a) Hexosaminidase A

259. Ans. (a) Mitochondria to cytoplasm

> *Ref: Harrison 17/e, Table 358-1*

260. Ans. (c) Aspartate

261. Ans. (c) Histidine

> *Ref: Wintrobe's Haematology 12/e, Volume 1, p 141, Harper's 27/e, chapter 6*

262. Ans. (b) Uroporphyrinogen I synthase

> *Ref: Harper's Biochemistry 26/e, p 271-275*

263. Ans. (c) Helicase

> *Ref: Lippincott's biochemistry 3/e, p 400*

264. Ans. (a) Enolase

> *Ref: Harper 27/e, chapter 18, Textbook of practical physiology–2/e, G.K. and Pal, Pal, Pravati p-9, Manual of basic techniques for a health laboratory by Who p 69*

265. Ans. (b) Decarboxylation

> *Ref: Goodman and Gillman 13th ed. P 712*

- Histidine to histamine conversion is done by decarboxylation with the help of enzyme L-Histadine decarboxylase.

266. Ans. (a) Vitamin E

> *Ref: Harrison's 19th ed. P*

- **Harrison's states:** *"Vitamin E acts as a chain-breaking antioxidant and is an efficient pyroxyl radical scavenger that protects low-density lipoproteins and polyunsaturated fats in membranes from oxidation"*
- Vitamin E also inhibits prostaglandin synthesis and the activities of protein kinase C and phospholipase A2.
- **RDA of Vitamine E:** 15mg/day (22.5 IU)

267. Ans. (c) Vitamin B₁₂

> *Ref: Harrison's 19th ed. P 640*

- Vitamin B_{12} (Cobalamin) is synthesized solely by microorganisms.
- In humans, the only source for humans is food of animal origin, e.g., meat, fish, and dairy products.
- Vegetables, fruits, and other foods of nonanimal origin doesn't contain Vitamin B_{12}.
- Daily requirements of vitamin B_{12} is about 1–3 µg. Body stores are of the order of 2–3 mg, sufficient for 3–4 years if supplies are completely cut off.

BIOCHEMISTRY

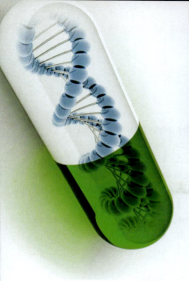

4

Pharmacology

MOST RECENT QUESTIONS 2019

1. Maximum parasympathetic outflow is by which cranial nerve?
   a. V
   b. VII
   c. IX
   d. X
2. 100% Bioavailability is seen with this route:
   a. Oral
   b. Intravenous
   c. Intramuscular
   d. Subcutaneous
3. Which among the following is shortest acting steroid?
   a. Triamcinolone
   b. Deflazacort
   c. Dexamethasone
   d. Hydrocortisone
4. Which of the following anti-epileptic drug has the highest teratogenic potential?
   a. Valproate
   b. Carbamazepine
   c. Phenytoin
   d. Lamotrigine
5. Healthy volunteers are recruited in which phase of clinical trials?
   a. Phase 1
   b. Phase 2
   c. Phase 3
   d. Phase 4
6. Long term use of which of the following drug is most likely associated with development of tremors?
   a. Propofol
   b. Salbutamol
   c. Betaxolol
   d. Timolol
7. Which of the following is a long acting bronchodilator?
   a. Salbutamol
   b. Terbutaline
   c. Adrenaline
   d. Formoterol
8. Drug of choice for neurogenic diabetes insipidus is:
   a. Terlipressin
   b. Desmopressin
   c. Chlorthalidone
   d. Conivaptan
9. Preferred drug for the treatment of ventricular tachycardia is
   a. Digoxin
   b. Diltiazem
   c. Lignocaine
   d. Propranolol
10. Drug of choice for chronic gout is
    a. Allopurinol
    b. Febuxostat
    c. Probenecid
    d. Sulfinpyrazone
11. A female with 20 weeks pregnancy presents with fever and dysuria. A preliminary diagnosis of cystitis was made. Which of the following drugs will be safe to use for this patient?
    a. Ciprofloxacin
    b. Gentamicin
    c. Cotrimoxazole
    d. Amoxicillin
12. Insulin of choice for the treatment of diabetes mellitus is:
    a. Regular Insulin
    b. NPH insulin
    c. Insulin glargine
    d. Insulin lispro
13. Which of the following is a long acting insulin that never attains a peak concentration in plasma?
    a. Insulin lispro
    b. Insulin aspart
    c. Insulin glulisine
    d. Insulin glargine
14. Praziquantel is used for the treatment of
    a. Strongyloidiasis
    b. Trichomoniasis
    c. Schistosomiasis
    d. Rhinosporidiosis
15. A young male presents with reduced sleep, hyperactivity and elevated mood. He has a family history of mania. Which of the following drug should be used for long term treatment of this patient?
    a. Sodium valproate
    b. Lithium carbonate
    c. Carbamazepine
    d. Barbiturates
16. Drug of choice for nasal carriers of MRSA is:
    a. Vancomycin
    b. Teicoplanin
    c. Mupirocin
    d. Linezolid
17. Anti-depressant drug which is used for smoking cessation is?
    a. Venlafaxine
    b. Topiramate
    c. Bupropion
    d. Amitriptyline
18. Drug of choice for treatment of Alzheimer's disease is:
    a. Atropine
    b. Donepezil
    c. Physostigmine
    d. Fluoxetine
19. Secretion of prolactin is inhibited by:
    a. Dopamine
    b. Nor-adrenaline
    c. Adrenaline
    d. Serotonin
20. Which of the following drug is a selective COX-2 inhibitor?
    a. Ketorolac
    b. Etoricoxib
    c. Piroxicam
    d. Nimesulide

FMGE Solutions Screening Examination

GENERAL PHARMACOLOGY

21. Good practice is NOT needed in which phase of clinical trial: *(Recent Pattern Question 2018-19)*
    a. Preclinical stage   b. Phase 2
    c. Phase 3   d. Phase 4

22. Drug not given with ketoconazole: *(Recent Pattern Question 2018)*
    a. Aminoglycoside   b. Macrolide
    c. Indinavir   d. All of the above

23. Physiological antagonist of histamine is: *(Recent Pattern Question 2018)*
    a. Adenosine   b. Adrenaline
    c. Atropine   d. Acetylcholine

24. In a first order kinetics Area under curve denotes: *(Recent Pattern Question 2018)*
    a. Clearance   b. Bioavailability
    c. Volume of distribution   d. A and B both

25. Adverse drug reaction class B is? *(Recent Pattern Question 2017)*
    a. Predictable side effect   b. Bizarre effect of a drug
    c. Failure of a drug   d. Chronic side effect

26. Which of the following is *not* an example of chronic adverse drug reactions?
    a. Nitrate induced headache
    b. Glucocorticoid induced osteoporosis
    c. Chloroquine induced retinopathy
    d. Amiodarone deposition in cornea

27. After oral administration the fraction of drug reaching the systemic circulation in unchanged form is: *(Recent Pattern Question 2017)*
    a. Elimination   b. Distribution
    c. Bioavailability   d. Metabolism

28. Pharmacovigilance is:
    a. Monitoring generic drugs
    b. Monitoring drug efficacy
    c. Monitoring ethical drug
    d. Monitoring adverse effects of drugs

29. Pharmacovigilence is done for:
    a. Pharmacy companies
    b. To monitor potency and efficacy
    c. To monitor adverse effects of drugs
    d. Monitoring ethical drug

30. 100% bioavailiability is seen with which route
    a. Oral   b. Intravenous
    c. Rectal   d. Subcutaneous

31. True about zero order kinetics:
    a. Rate of elimination is independent of plasma concentration
    b. Rate of elimination is dependent on plasma concentration
    c. Clearance of drug is always constant
    d. Half life of drug is constant

32. All drugs are metabolized by acetylation EXCEPT:
    a. Phenytoin   b. Isoniazid
    c. Procainamide   d. Hydralazine

33. Which of the following drug is metabolized by acetylation:
    a. Phenytoin   b. Isoniazid
    c. Salbutamol   d. Haloperidol

34. Which of the following G-proteins is a receptor for Photons:
    a. G_s b. G_i
    c. Gt_1 d. G_q

35. Glucagon acts via
    a. cAMP   b. cGMP
    c. Cytoplasmic Ca+   d. Intracellular K+

36. True about highly ionized drug:
    a. Can cross the placental barrier
    b. Well absorbed from intestine
    c. Accumulates in cellular lipids
    d. Excreted mainly by kidneys

37. Which of the following drug is an enzyme inducer:
    a. Rifampicin   b. Isoniazid
    c. Ketokonazole   d. Erythromycin

38. All are enzyme inhibitors EXCEPT:
    a. Carbamazipine   b. Cimetidine
    c. Valproate   d. Ketoconazole

39. Which is the best way to manage a patient present with aspirin poisoning:
    a. Make urine acidic with NH_4Cl^-
    b. Make urine alkaline with $NaHCO_3$
    c. Treat with N-acetyl cysteine
    d. Do gastric lavage

40. All of the following work on nuclear receptor EXCEPT:
    a. Glucocorticoids   b. Vitamin A
    c. Vitamin D   d. Thyroxine

41. All of the following work on nuclear receptors EXCEPT:
    a. Vitamin D   b. Androgen
    c. Estrogen   d. Vitamin A

42. Which of the following doesn't act via intracellular receptor:
    a. Leutenizing hormone   b. Androgen
    c. Estrogen   d. Vitamin A

43. Which of the following drug require therapeutic dose monitoring?
    a. Phenytoin   b. Warfarin
    c. Metformin   d. Propanolol

44. Duration of sub-acute toxicity study with animals:
    a. 3 months   b. 6 months
    c. 1 year   d. 1 ½ years

45. For knowing the acute toxicity of a drug, the drug micro doses should be tested on:
    a. Two different species   b. On rabbit, one rodent
    c. Two rabbits   d. Two rodents

46. Category X drugs are all EXCEPT:
    a. Warfarin   b. Methotrexate
    c. Alprazolam   d. Simvastatin

Pharmacology

47. Number of patients in Phase II clinical trial:
    a. 10–100   b. 200–400
    c. 1000–2000   d. 2000–4000
48. Patients are first enrolled in this phase of clinical trial:
    a. Phase 0   b. Phase I
    c. Phase II   d. Phase III
49. Pharmacoepidemiology is this phase of clinical trial:
    a. Phase 0   b. Phase II
    c. Phase IV   d. Phase V
50. Which of the following is *not* a prodrug:
    a. Levodopa   b. Lisinopril
    c. Carbimazole   d. Prednisolone
51. All are prodrug EXCEPT:
    a. Aspirin   b. Levodopa
    c. Dipivefrin   d. Captopril
52. True statement about orphan drugs:
    a. Drugs used for orphans
    b. Drugs used for rare disease
    c. Easily available drugs
    d. Drugs with excessive financial benefits
53. What happens to drug after expiry date:
    a. Company is not responsible after expiry date
    b. Maximum expiry to 3 years from manufacture date
    c. Product changes to toxic products
    d. Decrease in efficacy

AUTONOMIC NERVOUS SYSTEM

54. Drug of choice for motion sickness:
    (Recent Pattern Question 2018-19)
    a. Promethazine   b. Ondansetron
    c. Cyclizine   d. Domperidone
55. Mechanism of action of alpha Methyl-dopa:
    (Recent Pattern Question 2018-19)
    a. Alpha 1 agonist   b. Alpha 2 agonist
    c. Alpha 1 antagonist   d. Alpha 2 antagonist
56. Which of the following is the action of Pilocarpine?
    (Recent Pattern Question 2018-19)
    a. Active mydriatic   b. Passive mydriatic
    c. Active miotic   d. Passive miotic
57. Which of the following agents scan cause recurrent fall in elderly patient with postural hypotension:
    (Recent Pattern Question 2018-19)
    a. Methoxamine   b. Prazosin
    c. Metformin   d. Acarbose
58. Most sensitive test for organophosphate poisoning:
    (Recent Pattern Question 2018-19)
    a. Plasma acetylcholinesterase
    b. OP level in blood
    c. OP level in urine
    d. OP level in lavage

59. In a 2-year-old child refractive error test is done with:
    (Recent Pattern Question 2018-19)
    a. 1% atropine ointment   b. 1% atropine eye drop
    c. Tropicamide 0.5%   d. Eucatropine 5%
60. Ritodrine is a: *(Recent Pattern Question 2018)*
    a. β2 agonist   b. β2 antagonist
    c. α1 agonist   d. α1 antagonist
61. Esmolol is a short acting beta blocker because:
    (Recent Pattern Question 2018)
    a. It has more plasma protein binding
    b. Its plasma hydrolysis by esterases is rapid
    c. It has high lipid solubility
    d. It has high oral bioavailability
62. Correct about pralidoxime are all EXCEPT:
    a. It is given slow IV   *(Recent Pattern Question 2018)*
    b. Given effectively in carbamate poisoning
    c. It does not cross blood brain barrier
    d. Reactivates the AChE enzyme
63. Drug of choice for diabetic diarrhea:
    (Recent Pattern Question 2018)
    a. Duloxetine   b. Clonidine
    c. Domperidone   d. Alosetron
64. Botulinum toxin acts on: *(Recent Pattern Question 2017)*
    a. Inhibition of release of neurotransmitter
    b. Post synaptic block
    c. At synapse
    d. Reuptake inhibitor
65. Botulinum toxin acts by:
    a. Postsynaptic acetylcholine receptor blocker
    b. Presynaptic inhibition of release of acetylcholine
    c. GABA mimetic
    d. GABA antagonist
66. Botulinum toxin decreases transmission across nerve terminals. It is an example of:
    a. Depolarizing blockade   b. Competitive blockade
    c. Presynaptic blockade   d. Postsynaptic blockade
67. A farmer presented in OPD clinic with sweating, lacrimation, pin-point pupils with a heart rate of 40/min. Possible diagnosis:
    a. Dhatura poisoning
    b. Organophosphate poisoning
    c. Atropine poisoning
    d. Cocaine poisoning
68. A 45 year male presents with delirium, increased body temperature, dryness, dilated pupils and HR 130/min. Possible diagnosis:
    a. Carbamate poisoning
    b. Organophosphate poisoning
    c. Atropine poisoning
    d. Cocaine poisoning
69. Anticholinergic side effect is:
    a. Salivation   b. Dryness
    c. Incrased GIT motility   d. Sweating

FMGE Solutions Screening Examination

70. Neostigmine used in all EXCEPT:
    a. Myasthenia Gravis   b. Curare poisoning
    c. Snake bite   d. OP poisoning
71. Action of M2 receptor is seen at? *(Recent Pattern Question 2017)*
    a. Sphincter dilatation
    b. Sympathetic nerve
    c. Parasympathetic nerve
    d. Tachycardia
72. Methacholine acts mainly as:
    a. M1 agonist   b. M2 agonist
    c. 1 antagonist   d. M2 antagonist
73. Tripitramine acts as:
    a. M1 agonist   b. M2 agonist
    c. M1 antagonist   d. M2 antagonist
74. Alpha bungaratoxin acts at:
    a. Muscarinic receptor agonist
    b. Muscarinic receptor antagonist
    c. Nicotinic ganglion agonist
    d. Neuromuscular junction
75. All of the following side effects are seen with ipratropium bromide, EXCEPT: *(Recent Pattern Question 2017)*
    a. Urinary incontinence b. Dryness of mouth
    c. Irritation in trachea d. Bad taste
76. Mechanism of action of aminophylline in bronchial asthma: *(Recent Pattern Question 2017)*
    a. Decreasing phosphodiesterase activity
    b. Direct action on smooth muscles
    c. Releasing catecholamines
    d. Stabilizing membrane of mast cells
77. Increased urinary frequency is best managed by *(Recent Pattern Question 2016)*
    a. Oxybutynin   b. Imipramine
    c. Alfuzosin   d. Bethanechol
78. Which of the following drug is used in urinary retention: *(Recent Pattern Question 2016)*
    a. Bethanechol   b. Finasteride
    c. Oxybutynin   d. Letrozole
79. Which of the following sympathetic receptors acts as vasoconstriction and vasodilatation:
    a. Alpha 1 and Alpha 2 b. Alpha 1 and Beta 1
    c. Alpha 1 and Beta 2   d. Beta 1 and Beta 2
80. Bronchial calibre is reduced by: *(Recent Pattern Question 2016)*
    a. Beta 2 receptor stimulation
    b. Stimulation of sympathetic fibre
    c. Stimulation of parasympathetic fiber
    d. Alpha 2 receptor stimulation
81. In contrast to epinephrine, norepinephrine does the following:
    a. Increase BP, bradycardia b. Increase BP, tachycardia
    c. Decrease BP, bradycardia d. Decrease BP, tachycardia

82. Dobutamine mainly act at this receptor:
    a. Beta 1   b. Beta 2
    c. Alpha 1   d. Alpha 2
83. Midodrine is used in:
    a. Hypertension   b. Orthostatic hypotension
    c. Increasing cardiac output d. Decongestant
84. Tachyphylaxis is seen with:
    a. Dopamine   b. Salbutamol
    c. Propranolol   d. Haloperidol
85. Longest acting beta adrenergic blocker?
    a. Atenolol   b. Sotalol
    c. Nadolol   d. Esmolol
86. Which of the following drug does *not* produce hypotension during/followed by surgery?
    a. Esmolol   b. Nadolol
    c. Propanolol   d. Metoprolol
87. A hypertensive patient who is on beta blockers develops bradycardia and start to sweat whenever he takes the medication. Which beta blocker is *not* the probable cause of his condition:
    a. Atenolol   b. Acebutalol
    c. Metoprolol   d. Nadolol
88. All of the following beta blockers have intrinsic sympathomimetic activity EXCEPT:
    a. Celiprolol   b. Propanolol
    c. Pindolol   d. Acebutalol
89. β blocker with intrinsic sympathomimetic activity:
    a. Nadolol   b. Atenolol
    c. Alprenolol   d. Propanolol
90. Beta-adrenoceptor blocking agent that should be avoided in patients with renal failure is:
    a. Atenolol   b. Metoprolol
    c. Propranolol   d. Esmolol
91. Which of the following beta blocker is vasodilator:
    a. Metoprolol   b. Atenolol
    c. Propranolol   d. Carvedilol
92. Which of following is a non selective alpha blocker?
    a. Prazosin   b. Tolazoline
    c. Terazosin   d. Doxazosin
93. Drug with a first dose effect:
    a. Yohimbine   b. Verapamil
    c. Dopamine   d. Prazosin
94. Irreversible alpha-1 adrenoreceptor antagonist:
    a. Prazosin   b. Clonidine
    c. Isoprenaline   d. Phenoxybenzamine
95. All of the following drugs cause mydriasis EXCEPT:
    a. Pilocarpine   b. Epinephrine
    c. Atropine   d. Phenylephrine
96. All of the following drugs can cause mydriasis EXCEPT:
    a. Atropine   b. Phenylephrine
    c. Phentolamine   d. Cocaine

Pharmacology

97. **Shortest acting mydriatics:**
   a. Atropine
   b. Homatropine
   c. Tropicamide
   d. Cyclopentolate

98. **Treatment of choice for scorpion bite:**
   a. Anti-venin
   b. Insulin
   c. Steroids
   d. Atropine

99. **Which of the following drug is used for treating overactive bladder:**
   a. Pirezepine
   b. Tolterodine
   c. Bethanechol
   d. Alfuzosin

100. **Mechanism of action of Oxybutynin?**
   a. Cholinergic
   b. Anticholinergic
   c. Adrenergic
   d. Selectively inhibits M2 receptor

101. **Miotic agent used in glaucoma:**
   a. Methacholine
   b. Pilocarpine
   c. Cevimeline
   d. Bethanechol

CNS AND PNS

102. **Which of the following is an opioid receptor?**
   (Recent Pattern Question 2018-19)
   a. Epsilon
   b. Sigma
   c. Gamma
   d. Delta

103. **A violent manic patient should not be treated with:**
   (Recent Pattern Question 2018-19)
   a. Benzodiazepines
   b. Cognitive therapy
   c. Atypical antipsychotics
   d. Quetiapine

104. **All are morphine effects EXCEPT:**
   (Recent Pattern Question 2018)
   a. Miosis
   b. Delayed gastric emptying
   c. Respiratory depression
   d. Hyperalgesia

105. **Drug of choice for akathisia:**
   (Recent Pattern Question 2018)
   a. Lithium
   b. Fluoxetine
   c. Propranolol
   d. Haloperidol

106. **Which is the drug preferred for sleep onset insomnia?**
   (Recent Pattern Question 2017)
   a. Larazepam
   b. Lorazepam
   c. Ramelteon
   d. Ritanserin

107. **Which of the following is an atypical antipsychotic?**
   (Recent Pattern Question 2017)
   a. Clozapine
   b. Chlorpromazine
   c. Thioridazine
   d. Haloperidol

108. **Lipodystrophy is caused by which of the following?**
   (Recent Pattern Question 2017)
   a. Thioridazine
   b. Fluphenazine
   c. Prochlorphenazine
   d. Clozapine

109. **In which drug extra pyramidal side effect is not seen?**
   a. Haloperidol
   b. Carbamazapine
   c. Chlorpromazine
   d. Fluphenazine

110. **Drug of choice of neuroleptic malignant syndrome:**
   a. Lorazepam
   b. Propranolol
   c. Dantrolene
   d. Benzhexol

111. **Akathisia is best treated by:**
   a. Lithium
   b. Fluoxetine
   c. Propanolol
   d. Haloperidol

112. **Which drug has least extrapyramidal symptoms?**
   a. Haloperidol
   b. Clozapine
   c. Fluphenazine
   d. Chlorpromazine

113. **Which drug has least extrapyramidal symptoms?**
   a. Aripiprazole
   b. Loxapine
   c. Fluphenazine
   d. Chlorpromazine

114. **Anti-emetic with Extrapyramidal side effect:**
   a. Cyclizine
   b. Mozapride
   c. Prochlorperazine
   d. Ondensetron

115. **Antipsychotic which can cause cataract:**
   a. Clozapine
   b. Thioridazine
   c. Chlorpromazine
   d. Quetipaine

116. **Atypical antipsychotic with maximum risk of hyperprolactinemia:**
   a. Risperidone
   b. Aripiprazole
   c. Olanzapine
   d. Sertindole

117. **Which of the following ICU sedation drug causes neuroleptic malignant syndrome:**
   a. Midazolam
   b. Lorazepam
   c. Diazepam
   d. Haloperidol

118. **Treatment for anxiety attack:**
   (Recent Pattern Question 2016)
   a. α-blockers
   b. Diazepam
   c. Barbiturates
   d. Bupropion

119. **Which of the following anaesthetic agent leads to increase in ICT** *(Recent Pattern Question 2016)*
   a. Thiopentone
   b. Ketamine
   c. Propofol
   d. Sevoflurane

120. **True about Benzodiazepine:**
   a. It is GABA mimetic
   b. It is GABA facilitator
   c. Not a safe drug
   d. Powerful enzyme inducer

121. **Diazepam acts by:**
   a. GABA mimetic action
   b. Exciting CNS
   c. GABA facilitator
   d. By increasing duration of channel

122. **Antidote of benzodiazepine overdose:**
   a. Flupenthixol
   b. Fluoxetine
   c. Fluvoxamine
   d. Flumazenil

123. **Drug of choice for ADHD:**
   a. Amphetamine
   b. Methylphenidate
   c. Pemoline
   d. Modafinil

Questions

229

FMGE Solutions Screening Examination

124. Methylphenidate is used for:
    a. Attention deficit disorder
    b. Alzheimer's disease
    c. Seizure disorder
    d. Obsessive compulsive disorder
125. Rivastigmine is given in:
    a. Depression   b. Alzheimer's disease
    c. Schizophrenia   d. OCD
126. Which of following is not used for the prophylaxis of migraine
    a. Propanolol   b. Topiramate
    c. Verapamil   d. Ethosuximide
127. In treatment of Parkinsonism carbidopa is used along with levodopa because:
    a. It increases the half life of levodopa by inhibiting its metabolism
    b. It inhibits levopda excretion
    c. It inhibits peripheral dopa decarboxylase
    d. It inhibits central dopa deaminase
128. On-Off phenomenon seen during levodopa therapy is due to:
    a. Toxicity of drug
    b. As a mild and known side effect of drug
    c. Short half life of drug
    d. Long half life of drug
129. Antiviral drug amantadine is approved for:
    a. Achizophrenia   b. Depression
    c. Alzheimer's disease   d. Parkinsonism
130. Ergot derivative used for Parkinson's disease:
    a. Emmenagogue   b. Benzhexol
    c. Bromocriptine   d. Ropinirole
131. Anti-Parkinson drug that has the potential to cause retro-peritoneal fibrosis is:
    a. Pramipexole   b. Bromocriptine
    c. Ropinirole   d. Levodopa and carbidopa
132. Selegiline acts by:
    a. MAO-A inhibition b. MAO-B inhiition
    c. COMT inhibition
    d. Dopamine receptor stimulator
133. Which of the following anti epileptic drug act by inhibiting voltage gated sodium channel?
    a. Levetiracetam   b. Lamotrigine
    c. Ethosuximide   d. Perampanel
134. True statement about lamotrigine:
    a. It acts by blocking NMDA type of glutamate receptors
    b. It is a DA agonist used in Parkinson's disease
    c. It has Broad spectrum of anti-seizure activity
    d. It doesn't have any adverse side effects
135. Drug of choice for absence seizure:
    a. Lamotrigine   b. Sodium valproate
    c. Trimethadione   d. Ganoxolone
136. Drug preferred in generalized tonic clonic seizure:
    a. Phenytoin   b. Na+ Valproate
    c. Carbamazepine   d. Diazepam

137. A 30-year-old female with partial seizure. Drug of choice:
    a. Clonazepam   b. Carbamazepine
    c. Phenobarbitone   d. Lamotrigine
138. Reversible alopecia, weight gain, tremor, Hepatotoxicity is the major side effect of which of the following anti epileptic drug:
    a. Valproate   b. Lamotrigine
    c. Zonisamide   d. Phenytoin
139. Which of the following anti epileptic drug causes gum hypertrophy:
    a. Phenytoin   b. Valproate
    c. Topiramate   d. Vigabatrin
140. Phenytoin therapy may lead to which of the following:
    a. Microcytic anemia b. Thrombosis
    c. Hypercalcemia   d. Folic acid deficiency
141. Vigabatrin acts by:
    a. GABA receptor inhibitor
    b. Glutamate receptor inhibitor
    c. GABA transaminase inhibitor
    d. GABA transport inhibitor
142. The recently approved antiepileptic drug lacosamide acts by:
    a. Inhibiting synaptic vesicular protein
    b. Inhibing CRMP protine
    c. Inhibing GABA metabolism
    d. Inhibing glutamate release
143. A patient with recent onset primary generalized epilepsy, develops drug reaction and skin rash and neutropenia due to phenytoin sodium. The most appropriate course of action is:
    a. Shift to sodium valproate
    b. Shift to clonazepam
    c. Shift to ethosuximide
    d. Restart phenytoin after 2 weeks
144. The antiepileptic drug which causes weight loss:
    a. Valproate   b. Vigabatrin
    c. Topiramate   d. Felbamate
145. Drug of choice in acute poisoning of morphine:
    a. Naloxone   b. Naltrexone
    c. Nalmefene   d. Methadone
146. Giving intrathecal opioid leads to which side effect?
    (Recent Pattern Question 2017)
    a. Anaphylaxis   b. Pruritus
    c. Hypotension   d. Cardiac arrest
147. All of the following are anti smoking drugs EXCEPT:
    a. Bupropion   b. Buspirone
    c. Clonidine   d. Vareniciline
148. First line therapy in smoking dependence:
    a. Nicotine replacement gum
    b. Rimonabant
    c. Naloxone
    d. Acute cessation

Pharmacology

149. Ebstein anomaly is known teratogenic effect due to this drug:
    a. Clozapine   b. Phenytoin
    c. Lithium   d. Lamotrogine
150. Which of the following is SSRI:
    a. Desipramine   b. Clomipramine
    c. Fluvoxamine   d. Imipramine
151. Venlafaxine comes under which class of drugs:
    (Recent Pattern Question 2018)
    a. Selective serotonin reuptake inhibitor
    b. Serotonergic noradrenergic reuptake inhibitor
    c. Tricyclic antidepressant
    d. Serotonin receptor antagonist
152. Most common side effect of SSRI:
    a. Delayed ejaculation   b. Nausea
    c. Weight gain   d. Insomnia
153. Scopolamine is used mostly in:
    a. Hyperemesis gravidarum b. Vomiting
    c. Constipation   d. Motion sickness
154. Disulphiram acts by competitive inhibition of which enzyme?
    a. Alcohol dehydrogenase   b. Aldehyde dehydrogenase
    c. Alcohol carboxylase   d. Aldehyde carboxylase
155. Mechanism of action of ethanol in methyl alcohol poisoning:
    a. Competitively inhibits alcohol Dehydrogenase
    b. Selectively inhibits catalase
    c. Competitively inhibits lactate dehydrogenase
    d. Competitive inhibition of acetaldehyde dehydrogenase
156. All of the following drugs are used in detoxification therapy of chronic alcoholism EXCEPT:
    a. Acamprosate   b. Naltrexone
    c. Disulfiram   d. Flumazenil

ANTIMICROBIAL AGENTS

157. Drug of choice for Enterococcus faecalis:
    (Recent Pattern Question 2018-19)
    a. Cephalexin   b. Tetracycline
    c. Azithromycin   d. Ampicillin
158. Dose of oseltamivir for prophylaxis of swine flu in a child aged 3-5 months? *(Recent Pattern Question 2018-19)*
    a. 3 mg/kg/day twice daily   b. 5 mg/kg/day twice daily
    c. 10 mg/kg/day twice daily
    d. 15 mg/kg/day twice daily
159. Which of the following agent is used for prophylaxis of meningococcal meningitis in pregnancy?
    (Recent Pattern Question 2018-19)
    a. Ceftriaxone   b. Rifampicin
    c. Ciprofloxacin   d. Penicillin G

160. Which of the following is a bacterial protein synthesis inhibitor? *(Recent Pattern Question 2018-19)*
    a. Ceftriaxone   b. Streptomycin
    c. Nevirapine   d. Indinavir
161. In a pregnant female which drug is strictly contraindicated? *(Recent Pattern Question 2018-19)*
    a. Streptomycin   b. Isoniazid
    c. Cephalosporins   d. Penicillin
162. A female patient was treated with antibiotics for chlamydia induced UTI, suddenly presents again with itching/pruritus, vaginal discharge, burning micturition. Which drug should be given?
    (Recent Pattern Question 2018-19)
    a. Ceftriaxone   b. Azithromycin
    c. Moxifloxacin   d. Amphotericin B
163. CYD-TDV Vaccine is used for which of the following infections? *(Recent Pattern Question 2018-19)*
    a. Dengue   b. Malaria
    c. Yellow fever   d. Japanese encephalitis
164. DOC for management of visceral Leishmaniasis:
    (Recent Pattern Question 2018-19)
    a. Parenteral Sodium stibogluconate
    b. Liposomal Amphotericin B
    c. Miltefosine
    d. Pentamidine
165. Drug of choice for UTI:
    (Recent Pattern Question 2018-19)
    a. Fosfomycin   b. Trimethoprim
    c. Ampicillin   d. β- lactams
166. The drug pyronaridine is: *(Recent Pattern Question 2018)*
    a. Antifungal   b. Antimalarial
    c. Anti-HIV   d. PPI drugs
167. Empirical drug of choice for treatment of meningococcal meningitis is: *Recent Pattern Question 2018)*
    a. Cefoxitin   b. Ceftriaxone
    c. Cefotetan   d. Gentamicin
168. Drug *not* used in CMV retinitis:
    (Recent Pattern Question 2018)
    a. Acyclovir   b. Foscarnet
    c. Ganciclovir   d. Cidofovir
169. Resistance to ciprofloxacin is due to:
    (Recent Pattern Question 2018)
    a. Transduction   b. Transformation
    c. Conjugation   d. Mutation
170. Which of the following aminoglycoside is cochleotoxic:
    (Recent Pattern Question 2018)
    a. Kanamycin   b. Streptomycin
    c. Gentamycin   d. Minocycline
171. Following antibiotics inhibit cell wall formation EXCEPT:
    a. Cephalosporin   b. Clindamycin
    c. Cycloserine   d. Vancomycin

FMGE Solutions Screening Examination

172. Which of the following drug acts at 50s ribosome:
    a. Stremptomycin   b. Tetracycline
    c. Quinpristin   d. Demeclocycline
173. All of the following penicllins are acid resistant EXCEPT:
    a. Carbenicillin   b. Cloxacillin
    c. Ampicillin   d. Amoxicillin
174. Drug of choice for listeria
    a. Trimethoprim-sulfamethoxazole
    b. Ampicillin
    c. Chloramphenicol   d. Azithromycin
175. Which of the following drug can cause grey baby syndrome
    a. Tetracycline   b. Chloramphenicol
    c. Vancomycin   d. Clindamycin
176. Which of the following antimicrobial agent can result in ototoxicty, nephrotoxicity and redneck syndrome?
    a. Methicillin   b. Vancomycin
    c. Tetracycline   d. Chloramphenicol
177. DOC for antibiotic induced colitis:
    a. Clindamycin   b. Metronidazole
    c. Vancomycin   d. Ceftriaxone
178. Vancomycin is used orally for treatment of
    a. Hepatic encephalopathy
    b. Pseudomembranous colitis
    c. Staphylococcal food poisoning
    d. None of the above
179. All of the following drugs are used in MRSA infection EXCEPT:
    a. Vancomycin   b. Rifampicin
    c. Linezolid   d. Nafcillin
180. MRSA is resistant to:
    a. Vancomycin   b. β lactams
    c. Linezolid   d. Meropenems
181. Drug which is absolutely contraindicated in pregnancy is:
    a. Ceftriaxone   b. Chloramphenicol
    c. Penicillin   d. Erythromycin
182. All antibiotics are safe in pregnancy EXCEPT:
    a. Ciprofloxacin   b. Azithromycin
    c. Ampicillin   d. Cefotaxime
183. Drug of choice for gonorrhea:
    a. Azithromycin   b. Erythromycin
    c. Cefuroxime   d. Ceftriaxone
184. Which of the following is a second generation cephalosporin?
    a. Cefaclor   b. Cephalexin
    c. Ceftriaxone   d. Cefepime
185. Which of the following β lactams doesn't show cross allergy:
    a. Ampicillin   b. Cefotaxim
    c. Doripenem   d. Aztreonam
186. aa-tRNA synthetase inhibitor:
    a. Mitomycin- C   b. Mupirocin
    c. Metronidazole   d. Methenamine Mandelate
187. The preferred treatment option for primary syphilis is:
    a. Injection Benzathine penicillin 2.4 million units IM single dose
    b. Injection Benzathine penicillin 2.4 million units IM once a week for 3 weeks
    c. Cap. Doxycycline 100 mg orally twice a day for 2 weeks
    d. Tab. Azithromycin 2 gm single dose
188. Drug of choice for trachoma:
    a. Ceftriaxone   b. Azithromycin
    c. Erythromycin   d. Clarithromycin
189. Side effect of sulfonamide:
    a. Thrombocytosis   b. Sensorineural hearing loss
    c. Crystalluria   d. Phototoxicity
190. Ratio of Trimethoprim and Sulfamethoxazole in a Cotrimoxazole tablet: *(Recent Pattern Question 2016)*
    a. 2:1   b. 3:1
    c. 5:1   d. 1:5
191. Drug of choice for brucellosis:
    a. Chloramphenicol   b. Erythromycin
    c. Doxycycline   d. Cefuroxime
192. Drug of choice for dermatitis herpetiformis:
    a. Dapsone   b. Rifampicin
    c. Ketokonazole   d. Azithromycin
193. Drug used in dermatitis herpetiformis are all EXCEPT:
    a. Acyclovir   b. Colchicine
    c. Dapsone   d. Tetracycline
194. Which of the following is not a protease inhibitor?
    a. Atazanavir   b. Ritonavir
    c. Abacavir   d. Indinavir
195. Reverse transcriptase inhibitor zidovudine is given for:
    a. HIV   b. HBV
    c. HCV   d. All of the above
196. All drugs are used in AIDS EXCEPT:
    a. Abacavir   b. Ritonavir
    c. Acyclovir   d. Tenofovir
197. Mechanism of action of maraviroc:
    a. Cyt P 450 inhibitor   b. GP 41 inhibitor
    c. CCR5 inhibitor   d. GP 120 inhibitor
198. NRTI which has maximum tendency to cause peripheral neuropathy
    a. Zidovudine   b. Stavudine
    c. Lamivudine   d. Didanosine
199. NOT a fast acting anti- malarial drug:
    a. Mefloquine   b. Chloroquine
    c. Artemisinin   d. Pyrimethamine
200. Drug of choice for schistosomiasis:
    a. Praziquantel   b. Metronidazole
    c. Albendazole   d. Ivermectin
201. Drug of choice for fasciola hepatica:
    a. Praziquantel   b. Triclabendazole
    c. Ivermectin   d. Albendazole

Pharmacology

202. Drug of choice for neurocysticercosis:
a. Praziquantel   b. Triclabendazole
c. Ivermectin   d. Albendazole

203. Drug of choice for Taenia Solium:
a. Praziquantel   b. Triclabendazole
c. Ivermectin   d. Albendazole

204. Scabies oral drug of choice:
a. Permethrin   b. Benzyl Benzoate
c. Ivermectin   d. Lindane

205. Drug of choice for scabies
a. Ivermectin   b. Permethrin
c. Sulfur   d. Benzylv benzoate

206. Drug of choice for tetanus:
a. Metronidazole   b. Penicillin
c. Erythromycin   d. Clindamycin

207. Drug of choice for filariasis:
a. Metronidazole   b. Praziquantel
c. Ciprofloxacin   d. Ivermectin

208. What is the recommended dose of DEC in filariasis?
(Recent Pattern Question 2017)
a. 2 mg/kg   b. 6 mg/kg
c. 10 mg/kg   d. 20 mg/kg

209. Which drug is given in combination with DEC for massive reduction of filariasis?
(Recent Pattern Question 2017)
a. Albendazole   b. Streptomycin
c. Pyrimethamine   d. Tinidazole

210. Mechanism of action of amphotericin B:
a. Cell wall synthesis inhibitior
b. Alters permeability of fungal cell wall
c. Protein synthesis inhibitor
d. Act as antibody for fungus

211. To reduce Amphotericin B toxicity, it is given?
(Recent Pattern Question 2017)
a. With aminoglycoside
b. Give intravenous with saline
c. With 5% dextrose
d. Liposomal preparation

212. NOT an adverse effects of amphotericin-B?
(Recent Pattern Question 2017)
a. Thrombocytopenia   b. Renal damage
c. Cholelithiasis   d. Hepatic damage

213. Most serious side effects of amphotericin B:
a. Hepatic damage   b. Renal damage
c. Cardiotoxicity   d. Hypochromic anemia

214. Which of the following drugs causes acute kidney injury with hypomagnesemia:
a. Cyclophosphamide
b. Ceftriaxone
c. Amphotericin-B
d. Vancomycin

ANTITUBERCULAR AGENTS

233

215. Isoniazid is NOT given in:
(Recent Pattern Question 2017)
a. Renal disease   b. Liver disease
c. Diabetes mellitus   d. Hypertension

216. If somebody develops resistance to INH, patient will develop simultaneously resistance to which drug?
(Recent Pattern Question 2017)
a. Streptomycin   b. Rifampicin
c. Ethambutol   d. Pyrazinamide

217. ATT Drug that kills slowly or intermittently dividing bacteria:
a. Isonizid
b. Rifampicin
c. Pyrazinamide
d. Streptomycin

218. True statement about action of ethambutol:
a. Exclusive agent against extracellular bacilli
b. Selectively tuberculocidal agent
c. Increase the permeability of cell wall
d. More active on slowly multiplying bacilli

219. Anti TB drug causing optic neuritis:
a. Isoniazid   b. Rifampicin
c. Pyrazinamide   d. Ethambutol

220. Which of the following anti TB drug is *not* bactericidal
a. Rifampicin   b. Isoniazid
c. Pyrazinamide   d. Ethambutol

221. Which of the following anti tubercular drug requires dose adjustment in renal failure:
a. Isoniazid   b. Rifampicin
c. Pyrazinamide   d. Ethambutol

222. Isoniazid dosage in infants
a. 5 mg/kg PO qday   b. 10-15 mg/kg PO qday
c. 300 mg BID   d. 300 mg once a week

223. RNA transcription is blocked by this ATT:
a. Rifampicin   b. Streptomycin
c. Chloroamphenicol   d. INH

224. In patients on isoniazid, which vitamin deficiency is more likely to be seen?
a. Vitamin B9   b. Vitamin B12
c. Vitamin B6   d. Vitamin B3

225. Anti TB drug causing depression & suicidal tendency:
a. Kanamycin   b. Cycloserine
c. Streptomycin   d. Capreomycin

226. ATT contraindicated in pregnant women
a. Isoniazid   b. Rifampicin
c. Streptomycin   d. Ethambutol

227. Which anti TB drug is contraindicated throughout the pregnancy:
a. Rifampicin   b. Streptomycin
c. Isoniazid   d. Ethambutol

Questions

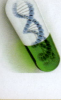

FMGE Solutions Screening Examination

228. Ototoxicity caused by:
    a. Vancomycin   b. Streptomycin
    c. Ampicillin   d. Rifampicin
229. Dose for tuberculin test:
    a. 1 TU   b. 2 TU
    c. 2.5 TU   d. 5 TU
230. ATT drug causing hypothyroidism:
    a. Isoniazid   b. Ethambutol
    c. PAS   d. Rifampicin
231. ATT drug causing hyperuricemia:
    a. Isoniazid   b. Pyrazinamide
    c. Streptomycin   d. Rifampicin

ANTICANCER DRUGS

232. DOC of anal cancer: *(Recent Pattern Question 2018-19)*
    a. Gefitinib   b. Eflorinitib
    c. 5FU   d. Cisplatin
233. Pemetrexed MOA is: *(Recent Pattern Question 2018)*
    a. RNA synthesis inhibitor
    b. Dihydrofolate reductase inhibitor
    c. Dopamine agonist
    d. Folate antagonist
234. Folinic acid used in: *(Recent Pattern Question 2018)*
    a. Methotrexate toxicity   b. Cisplatin toxicity
    c. Vincristine toxicity   d. 5FU toxicity
235. Which Radiosensitizer drug is used in head and neck surgery? *(Recent Pattern Question 2017)*
    a. Paclitaxel   b. Cisplatin
    c. Amikacin   d. Mitomycin-C
236. Which anticancer drug inhibits dihydrofolate reductase? *(Recent Pattern Question 2017)*
    a. Vincristine   b. Methotrexate
    c. Paclitaxel   d. Cisplatin
237. Which drug will be preferred in imatinib resistant CML? *(Recent Pattern Question 2017)*
    a. Nilotinib   b. Infliximab
    c. Hydroxyurea   d. Gefitinib
238. Breast cancer chemotherapeutic agent that causes osteoporosis:
    a. Letrozole   b. Nafarelin
    c. Tamoxifen   d. Leuprolide
239. A 40-year-old lady with breast cancer has undergone MRM and is on Tamoxifen for 1 year. She now presents with bleeding per vaginum 4-5 times. What is the probable cause:
    a. Bleeding disorder   b. Endometrial cancer
    c. Ovarian cancer   d. Cervical cancer
240. All are alkylating agents used in chemotherapy EXCEPT:
    a. Melphalan   b. Busulfan
    c. Cladribine   d. Cyclophosphamide

241. All are example of alkylating agents EXCEPT?
    a. Bleomycin   b. Busulfan
    c. Procarbazine   d. Melphalan
242. Alkylating agent used in chemotherapy:
    a. Mechlorethamine   b. Procarbazine
    c. Cyclophosphamide d. All of the above
243. True about Cyclophosphamide
    a. Antimetabolites   b. Alkylating agent
    c. Platinum compound d. Topoisomerase inhibitors
244. Which of the following drug is a *not* a purine analogue:
    a. 6 Mercaptopurine b. Cladribine
    c. Cytarabine   d. Fludarabine
245. Mercaptopurine is –
    a. Purine analogue
    b. Nucleoside analogue
    c. Pyrimidine analogue
    d. Anti tumor antibiotics
246. First line chemotherapy for cancer cervix:
    a. Cyclophosphamide b. Lomustine
    c. Vincristine   d. Cisplastin
247. Drug of choice for CML
    a. Imatinib mesylate
    b. Fludarabine
    c. Al trans retinoic acid (for AML 3)
    d. Methotrexate
248. Mechanism of action of Aspirin
    a. Inhibit PGI2 formation
    b. Inhibit TXA2 formation
    c. Stimulate TXA2 formation
    d. Stimulate platelet aggregation
249. Methotrexate mechanism of action:
    a. Inhibit dihydrofolate reductase
    b. Stimulate dihydrofolate reductase
    c. Inhibit tetrahydrofolate reductase
    d. Stimulate tetrahydrofolate reductase
250. Antidote for methotrexate toxicity:
    a. Folic acid   b. Folinic acid
    c. Vitamin B   d. Thymine
251. Which of the following is *not* used in treatment for Multiple myeloma:
    a. Melphalan   b. Thalidomide
    c. Zolendronic acid d. Methotrexate
252. Most emetogenic anti CA drug:
    a. 5 FU   b. Methotrexate
    c. Cisplatin   d. All
253. Most widely used anti CA drug:
    a. 5 FU   b. Methotrexate
    c. Cisplatin   d. All
254. Which of the following anti neoplastic drug commonly causes hepatotoxicity:
    a. 6-mercaptopurine b. 5- flurouracil
    c. Doxorubicin   d. Etoposide

255. Hemorrhagic cystitis is caused by:
    a. Procarbazine   b. Cisplatin
    c. Doxorubicin   d. Cyclophosphamide
256. *Not* used in treatment protocol of hodgkin's lymphoma
    a. Vincristine   b. Vinblastine
    c. Bleomycin   d. Adriamycin
257. Cardiomyopathy is caused by
    a. Actinomycin D   b. Doxorubicin
    c. Mitomycin C   d. Mitoxantrone
258. Which of the following anticancer drug causes hemolytic uremic syndrome:
    a. Vincristine   b. Vinblastine
    c. Cisplatin   d. Mitomycin C
259. Chemoradiation was given to a patient. Which drug given will reduce toxicity caused by radiotherapy?
    a. Vitamin A   b. Gemcitabine
    c. Amifostine   d. Actinomycin D

CARDIOVASCULAR SYSTEM

260. Gemfibrozil is: *(Recent Pattern Question 2018)*
    a. HMG CoA inhibitor
    b. PPAR-α activator
    c. Inhibit cholesterol synthesis
    d. Inhibit cholesterol absorption
261. Mechanism of action of statins is by:
                            (Recent Pattern Question 2018)
    a. Competitive inhibition   b. Noncompetitive inhibition
    c. Uncompetitive   d. Irreversible inhibition
262. Drug of choice for cardiogenic shock:
                            (Recent Pattern Question 2018)
    a. Dopamine   b. Dobutamine
    c. Digoxin   d. Digitoxin
263. Which of the following condition precipitate Digoxin toxicity?   *(Recent Pattern Question 2017)*
    a. Hypokalemia   b. Hyperkalemia
    c. Hypernatremia   d. Hyperphosphatemia
264. All are true statement about digitalis action EXCEPT:
    a. Increases cardiac contraction
    b. Pumps sodium inside cell in exchange of Ca+
    c. Increases intracellular calcium
    d. Causes bradycardia
265. In a patient with PIH, with BP 150/90, what will be the management   *(Recent Pattern Question 2016)*
    a. Rest   b. Labetalol
    c. Diuretics   d. CCB
266. Which of the following is not a mechanism of action of Antihypertensive agents?
    a. Blockade of alpha adrenergic receptors
    b. Blockade of ATP sensitive K+ channels
    c. Blockade of Noradrenaline release
    d. Blockade of beta adrenergic receptors

267. Drug not useful in emergency condition in pregnancy:
    a. Nifedipine   b. Labetalol
    c. Ritodrine   d. Phenobarbitone
268. Which of the following antihypertensive is contraindicated in pregnancy:
    a. Beta blockers   b. ACE inhibitors
    c. Methyldopa   d. Ca channel blockers
269. All of the following antihypertensive drugs are given in pregnancy EXCEPT:
    a. Methyldopa   b. Labetalol
    c. Captopril   d. Nifedipine
270. The drug of choice in scleroderma induced hypertensive crisis is:
    a. ACE inhibitors
    b. Angiotensin receptor blockers
    c. Beta blockers
    d. Sodium nitroprusside
271. Drug of choice in supra ventricular tachycardia
    a. Adenosine   b. Verapamil
    c. Metoprolol   d. Lignocaine
272. Drug of choice for Paroxysmal Supraventricular Tachycardia
    a. Digitalis   b. Adenosine
    c. Adrenaline   d. Verapamil
273. A Patient who is on anti hypertensive drug develops dry cough. Which of the following drug might be responsible for the condition:
    a. Diuretics
    b. ACE inhibitors
    c. Calcium channel blockers
    d. Beta blockers
274. All of the following are true about MOA of anti hypertensive drugs EXCEPT:
    a. Act by Na+ K+ ATPase inhibition
    b. Thiazide Diuretics
    c. Alpha adrenergic blockade
    d. Beta adrenergic blockade
275. Mechanism of action of statins:
    a. Inhibit HMG CoA synthase
    b. Stimulate HMG CoA reductase
    c. Inhibit HMG CoA reductase
    d. Stimulate HMG CoA synthase
276. *Not* a hypolipidemic drug:
    a. Simvastatin   b. Fenofibrate
    c. Somatostatin   d. Fluvastatin
277. All of the following anti-arrhythmic drugs are from class Ic EXCEPT:
    a. Encainide   b. Hecainide
    c. Tocainide   d. Propafenone
278. Which of the following is an L-type calcium channel blocker:
    a. Nifedipines   b. Amlodipines
    c. Diltiazem   d. All of the above

FMGE Solutions Screening Examination

279. **Drug that leads to glucose intolerance:**
   a. Hydrochlorthiazide   b. ACE inhiitors
   c. Verapamil   d. Sulfonylureas

280. **Which of the following drug has uricosuric action:**
   a. Losartan   b. Allopurinol
   c. Enalapril   d. Ramipril

281. **Angiotensin receptor blockers which attenuate platelet aggregation:**
   a. Telmisartan   b. Losartan
   c. Valsartan   d. Irbesartan

282. **Which of the following anti-hypertensives are contraindicated together:**
   a. CCB & Nitrates   b. Nitrates and β blockers
   c. CCB and β blockers   d. CCB and ARB

283. **A diabetic patient with hypertension, which drug is preferred:**
   a. ACE inhibitor   b. Beta blockers
   c. CCB   d. Diuretics

HORMONES AND AUTOCOIDS

284. **Mechanism of action of Exenatide:** *(Recent Pattern Question 2018-19)*
   a. SGLT inhibitor   b. GLP-1 Analogue
   c. DPP4 inhibitor   d. AMP kinase inhibitor

285. **Most potent analgesic:** *(Recent Pattern Question 2018-19)*
   a. COX-2 inhibitor   b. Remifentanil
   c. Morphine   d. Sufentanil

286. **Paracetamol causes:** *(Recent Pattern Question 2018-19)*
   a. Renal failure   b. Pancreatic toxicity
   c. Neurotoxicity   d. Hepatotoxicity

287. **What is the impact on foetus in case of Indomethacin used in third trimester?** *(Recent Pattern Question 2018-19)*
   a. PDA   b. Early closure of PDA
   c. VSD   d. ASD

288. **Purpose of adding zinc with insulin:** *(Recent Pattern Question 2018-19)*
   a. Make the insulin more rapid acting
   b. Provide stability in insulin molecule
   c. Increase the risk of insulin resistance
   d. Prevent insulin from causing hypoglycemia

289. **Half-life of parathormone:** *(Recent Pattern Question 2018-19)*
   a. 4 minutes   b. 10 minutes
   c. 30 minutes   d. 1 hour

290. **Zileuton is:** *(Recent Pattern Question 2018)*
   a. 5-lipoxygenase inhibitor
   b. Cyclooxygenase inhibitor
   c. Phospholipase inhibitor
   d. Leukotriene receptor antagonist

291. **Which of the following leads to obesity:** *(Recent Pattern Question 2018)*
   a. Acarbose   b. Insulin
   c. Sitagliptin   d. Pioglitazone

292. **Alcaftadine trial used this concentration of drug:** *(Recent Pattern Question 2018)*
   a. 5%   b. 1%
   c. 0.25%   d. 2.5%

293. **Phosphodiesterase inhibitor used for erectile dysfunction?** *(Recent Pattern Question 2017)*
   a. Sildenafil   b. Amrinone
   c. Milrinone   d. Tamoxifen

294. **Which of the following is a selective estrogen receptor down-regulator:** *(Recent Pattern Question 2017)*
   a. Flutamide   b. Fulvestrant
   c. Tamoxifen   d. Clomiphene citrate

295. **FDA approved drug Bevacizumab is?**
   a. VEGF 2 inhibitor   *(Recent Pattern Question 2017)*
   b. EGF receptor inhibitor
   c. Antibody to VEGF receptor
   d. TNF alpha agonist

296. **Which of the following drug acts by inhibiting IL-2 activation?** *(Recent Pattern Question 2017)*
   a. Cycloserine   b. Cyclosporine
   c. OKT-3   d. None

297. **Frequency of urine in pregnancy is increased due to**
   a. Prostaglandins   *(Recent Pattern Question 2016)*
   b. Increased progesterone
   c. Enlarged uterus pressing on bladder
   d. Oxytocin

298. **Receptor for vasopressin in collecting duct:** *(Recent Pattern Question 2016)*
   a. V1   b. V2
   c. V3   d. Endothelium

299. **Intermediate acting insulin**
   a. Regular insulin   b. Glargine
   c. Lispro   d. NPH

300. **Which of the following insulin is rapidly acting**
   a. Insulin lispro   b. Regular insulin
   c. Insulin glargine   d. NPH

301. **Fastest acting insulin:**
   a. Insulin aspart   b. Insulin Glargine
   c. Insulin Lente   d. Insulin detemir

302. **All are true about Prolactin agonist EXCEPT:**
   a. Associated with lactation
   b. Stimulate milk production after child birth
   c. Dopamine stimulate prolactin production
   d. Dopamine inhibit prolactin production

303. **Prolactin production is controlled by:**
   a. Metoclopramide   b. Chlorpromazine
   c. Dopamine   d. None

Pharmacology

304. Which of the following drugs can cause galactorrhea:
- a. Bromocriptine
- b. Pantoprazole
- c. Metoclopramide
- d. Omeprazole

305. MOA of oral hypoglycemic agent
- a. Inhibit glucose uptake by skeletal muscle
- b. Enhance glucose uptake by skeletal muscle
- c. Stimulate glycogenolysis
- d. Stimulate gluconeogenesis

306. Antidiabetic drug of choice for obese patients
- a. Metformin
- b. Sulfonylureas
- c. Repaglinide
- d. Acarbose

307. True statement about long term use of tamoxifen:
- a. Has no effect on uterine carcinoma
- b. Increased risk of heart disease
- c. Monitoring of liver enzmes is recommended
- d. Safer in DVT patients

308. Which of the drug is not used to treat hirsutism:
- a. Flutamide
- b. Finasteride
- c. Cyproterone acetone
- d. Spirinolactone

309. The drug preferred to stop the growth of prostate in a 70 year old male with Benign hyperplasia of prostate is
- a. Spironolactone
- b. Ketoconazole
- c. Finasteride
- d. Flutamide

310. Sildenafil acts by blocking which enzyme?
- a. Phosphodiesterase 3 inhibition
- b. Phosphodiesterase 5 inhibition
- c. 5 alpha Reductase inhibition
- d. Stimulate androgen production

311. Sildenafil is a drug used for erectile dysfunction. It acts by
- a. Blocking beta-adrenoceptors
- b. Inhibiting phosphodiesterase type 5
- c. Inhibiting reuptake of serotonin and nor-adrenaline
- d. Selective serotonin reuptake inhibition

312. Side effect of latanoprost:
- a. Lacrimation
- b. Increased pigmentation of cornea
- c. Increased eye lashes hair growth
- d. All of the above

313. Drug contraindicated in glaucoma patient suffering from bronchial asthma:
- a. Timolol
- b. Betaxolol
- c. Acetazolamide
- d. Latanoprost

314. Which of following prostaglandin analogue is beneficial in glaucoma?
- a. PG D2
- b. PG E2α
- c. PG I2
- d. PG F2α

315. Olopatadine is:
- a. Mast cell stabilizer
- b. Anti- histamine
- c. Both mast cell stabilizer and anti histamine
- d. None of the above

316. Which of the following is a soft steroid:
- a. Betamethasone
- b. Dexamethasone
- c. Prednisolone
- d. Ciclesonide

317. True about febuxostat:
- a. Anti-gout and Xanthine Oxidase inhibitor
- b. Purine inhibitor
- c. Dose adjustment required in renal impairment
- d. Has uricosuric action

318. Drug given for acute gout:
- a. Aspirin
- b. Indomethacin
- c. Febuxostat
- d. Allopurinol

RENAL, GIT AND RESPIRATORY SYSTEM

319. Laxative used in hepatic encephalopathy
(Recent Pattern Question 2018-19)
- a. Lactulose
- b. Sodium picosulfate
- c. Lubiprostone
- d. Bisacodyl

320. DOC for tropical pulmonary eosinophilia:
(Recent Pattern Question 2018)
- a. Albendazole
- b. Itraconazole
- c. Corticosteroid
- d. DEC

321. DOC for nephrogenic diabetes insipidus:
(Recent Pattern Question 2018)
- a. Mannitol
- b. Spironolactone
- c. Thiazides
- d. Demeclocycline

322. True about acetazolamide
(Recent Pattern Question 2016)
- a. Increase sodium reabsorption and potassium secretion
- b. Carbonic anhydrase inhibitor
- c. Acts at ascending limb of loop of Henle
- d. Increase aqueous outflow mainly

323. True reason for avoiding diuretics in pregnancy
(Recent Pattern Question 2017)
- a. Increase vascular resistance
- b. Decrease placental circulation
- c. Causes maternal distress
- d. High risk of birth defects

324. Calcium carbonate is used for
(Recent Pattern Question 2016)
- a. Antacid
- b. Renal stone
- c. Metabolic alkalosis
- d. Renal failure

325. Drug used in renal osteodystrophy:
- a. Vitamin D
- b. Calcitriol
- c. Calcidiol
- d. All of the above

326. All of the following are potassium sparing diuretic EXCEPT:
- a. Spironolactone
- b. Triamterene
- c. Indapamide
- d. Amiloride

237

Questions

FMGE Solutions Screening Examination

327. Drug of choice for initial management of CKD:
    a. Thiazide diuretics
    b. Loop diuretics
    c. K+ sparing diuretics
    d. Osmotic diuretics
328. ACE inhibitor is contraindicated in which of the following condition:
    a. Bilateral renal artery stenosis
    b. Chronic kidney disease
    c. Post myocardial infarction
    d. Diabetes mellitus
329. Drug of choice for treatment of NSAID-induced peptic ulcer is
    a. Prostaglandin analogues like Misoprostol
    b. H2-receptor antagonists like Ranitidine
    c. Proton pump inhibitors like Omeprazole
    d. Antacids like $Mg(OH)_2$
330. All of the following are indicated in drug induced vomiting EXCEPT:
    a. Ondansetron
    b. Metoclopramide
    c. Hyoscine
    d. Chlorpromazine
331. Which of the following drug is *not* effective against chemotherapy induced vomiting?
    a. Aprepitant
    b. Hyoscine
    c. Metoclopramide
    d. Ondansetron
332. All of the following statements about treatment of diarrhea are correct EXCEPT:
    a. Anti-motility drugs are drug of choice for infective diarrhea
    b. Loperamide and diphenoxylate are opioids used as anti-motility drugs
    c. Diphenoxylate overdose can cause respiratory depression
    d. Opioids decrease peristalsis and can be used in diarrhea
333. All of the following are anti tussives EXCEPT:
    a. Codeine
    b. Dextromethorphan
    c. Ambroxol
    d. Noscapine
334. Which drug should *not* be given in acute persistent asthma
    a. Theophylline
    b. Salbutamol
    c. Salmetrol
    d. Formoterol
335. Which is *not* useful in persistent severe asthma:
    a. Slow acting β2 agonist
    b. Long acting β2 agonist
    c. Inhaled corticosteroids
    d. High flow oxygen
336. Which is most common side effect of inhaled beclomethasone dipropionate:
    a. Pneumonia
    b. Oropharyngeal candidiasis
    c. Atrophic rhinitis
    d. Pituitary adrenal suppression
337. Non-sympathomimetic Bronchodilator preferred in COPD:
    a. Ipratropium bromide
    b. Salmeterol
    c. Terbutaline
    d. Salbutamol
338. Noscapine is an:
    a. Anti-tussive
    b. Anti emetic
    c. Anti dirrheal
    d. Mucolytics
339. Cough syrup acts by inhibiting
    a. Cough center
    b. Respiratory center
    c. Breathing center
    d. Pulmonary secretion center
340. A 34-year-old man with a long history of asthma is referred to pulmonologist. The physician decides to prescribe zileuton. The mechanism of action of this drug is to:
    a. Antagonize Leukotriene D4 receptor
    b. Inhibits 5-lipoxygenase
    c. Inhibit phosphodiesterases
    d. Stimulate P_2 receptors

HEMATOLOGY AND VITAMINS

341. Coumarin necrosis occurs due to:
    (Recent Pattern Question 2018-19)
    a. Heparin
    b. Low molecular weight heparin
    c. Warfarin
    d. Clopidogrel
342. Which of the following is a Factor Xa inhibitor?
    (Recent Pattern Question 2018-19)
    a. Apixaban
    b. Argatroban
    c. Fondaparinux
    d. Bivalirudin
343. Neutropenia after chemotherapy is treated by?
    (Recent Pattern Question 2018-19)
    a. Leucovorin
    b. Filgrastim
    c. Ondansetron
    d. Darbepoetin
344. Which among the following is iron chelator:
    (Recent Pattern Question 2018)
    a. EDTA
    b. Deferoxamine
    c. BAL
    d. Dimercaprol
345. What is the mode of action of warfarin?
    a. Factor Xa inhibitor *(Recent Pattern Question 2017)*
    b. Vitamin K antagonist
    c. Activates antithrombin III
    d. Activates factor IX
346. aPTT is done for assessing?
    a. Warfarin toxicity *(Recent Pattern Question 2017)*
    b. LMW heparin
    c. Heparin toxicity
    d. Extrinsic coagulation pathway defect
347. Argatroban acts by inhibiting:
    (Recent Pattern Question 2017)
    a. Factor Xa
    b. Factor IXa
    c. Factor II
    d. Factor IV

Pharmacology

348. Anticoagulant of choice in pregnancy
(Recent Pattern Question 2016)
- a. Warfarin
- b. Vitamin K
- c. Tranexamic acid
- d. Heparin

349. Which of the following drugs is used in heparin-induced thrombocytopenia *(Recent Pattern Question 2016)*
- a. Warfarin
- b. Coumarin
- c. Lepirudin
- d. Enoxaparin

350. All of the following are true about Vitamin K EXCEPT:
- a. Required for synthesis of clotting factors
- b. Hematuria is the first manifestation of deficiency
- c. Used as first line treatment in bleeding conditions
- d. It has a water soluble form also

351. All of following are anti platelet EXCEPT:
- a. Aspirin
- b. Clopidogrel
- c. Abciximab
- d. Tranexamic acid

352. Aspirin acts by inhibiting the production of:
- a. Prostaglandin
- b. Cytokines
- c. Leukotriene
- d. Thromboxane

353. Mechanism of action of Aspirin
- a. Inhibit PGI2 formation
- b. Inhibit TXA2 formation
- c. Stimulate TXA2 formation
- d. Stimulate platelet aggregation

354. Which of the following is *not* true about Heparin function:
- a. Inhibit antithrombin 3
- b. Activate antithrombin 3
- c. Inhibit factor IIa
- d. Inhibit factor Xa

355. True about oral anticoagulant warfarin are all EXCEPT:
- a. Acts in vivo
- b. Acts both in vivo and in vitro
- c. Interferes with synthesis of Vit K
- d. Causes Hematuria

356. All of the following drugs are contraindicated in G6PD EXCEPT:
- a. Ciprofloxacin
- b. Primaquine
- c. Dapsone
- d. Sulfonamide

357. Which of the following drug will cause hemolysis in G6PD patients:
- a. Cephalosporins
- b. Ampicillin
- c. Chloroquine
- d. Erythromycin

358. Which of the following is a low molecular weight heparin:
- a. Hirudin
- b. Enoxaparin
- c. Tranexamic acid
- d. Lepirudin

359. Low molecular weight heparin affects which factor:
- a. Factor X
- b. Anti-thrombin
- c. Factor Xa
- d. Factor IX

360. All of the following are true regarding enoxaparin EXCEPT:
- a. It has higher and predictable bioavailability
- b. It act by inhibiting both factor IIa and factor Xa
- c. Monitoring is not required
- d. It has more favorable pharmacokinetics

361. Treatment of choice in severe cystic acne:
- a. Isotretinoin
- b. Tretinoin
- c. Benzoyl peroxide
- d. Azelaic acid

362. Vitamin B12 is given in severe anemia via which route:
- a. I/M
- b. IV
- c. Oral
- d. All of the above

363. Antivitamin of biotin-
- a. Vitamin B6
- b. Vitamin K
- c. Avidin
- d. None

364. The vitamin which can be used for treatment of hypercholesterolemia is:
- a. Thiamine
- b. Niacin
- c. Pyridoxine
- d. VitaminB_{12}

365. Ketamine causes:
- a. Hallucination
- b. Hypotension
- c. Myocardial depression
- d. Decrease in intracranial pressure

MISCELLANEOUS

366. IUGR is caused by which drug:
(Recent Pattern Question 2017)
- a. Methyldopa
- b. Hydralazine
- c. Propranolol
- d. Nifedipine

367. Drugs contraindicated in pregnancy are all EXCEPT?
(Recent Pattern Question 2017)
- a. Chloroquine
- b. Primaquine
- c. Tobramycin
- d. ACE inhibitor

368. *Not* true about use of silver sulfadiazine:
- a. 1% concentration
- b. Burns
- c. Safer for pregnant lady and infants
- d. Acts against staph aureus

369. Medical adrenalectomy is seen with:
- a. Vincristine
- b. Vinblastine
- c. Mitotane
- d. Methotrexate

370. Which of the following is needed for conversion of norepinephrine to epinephrine:
- a. COMT
- b. MAO
- c. PENMT
- d. SAM

BOARD REVIEW QUESTIONS

371. Which of the following is a long acting beta 2 agonist?
    a. Salbutamol
    b. Salmeterol
    c. Terbutaline
    d. Levalbuterol
372. Galantamine is used in?
    a. Alzheimer's disease
    b. Parkinson's disease
    c. Emesis
    d. Chorea
373. Half life of Digoxin is?
    a. 12 hours
    b. 24 hours
    c. 36 hours
    d. 48 hours
374. Spironolactone is the first drug to be given for?
    a. Cirrhotic edema
    b. Cardiac edema
    c. Idiopathic edema
    d. Nutritional edema
375. Side effect of Amphotericin B is?
    a. Hypocalcemia
    b. Hypokalemia
    c. Hyponatremia
    d. Hypermagnesemia
376. Mechanism of action of dantroline is?
    a. Inhibits Ca++ secretion from sarcoplasm
    b. Binds to ryanodine receptors to block release of Ca++
    c. Inhibits GABA
    d. Inhibits Gamma motor neuron
377. Inhibitors of GpIIb/ IIIa receptors is all EXCEPT
    a. Eptifibatide
    b. Tirofiban
    c. Abciximab
    d. Filgrastrim
378. Omalizumab is used for
    a. Ulcerative colitis
    b. Crohn disease
    c. Asthma
    d. Psoriatic arthritis
379. Most potent loop diuretic
    a. Bumetanide
    b. Torsemide
    c. Furosemide
    d. Ethacrynic acid
380. All are advantages of LMWH over heparin EXCEPT:
    a. Longer half life
    b. Lower risk of HIT syndrome
    c. Lower risk of osteoporosis
    d. Antidote is protamine sulfate
381. Which of the following is soft steroid?
    a. Fluticasone
    b. Budenoside
    c. Ciclesonide
    d. Mometasone
382. Lubiprostone is used for
    a. Osmotic diarrhoea
    b. Secretory diarrhoea
    c. Chronic constipation
    d. Irritable bowel syndrome
383. Drug of choice for extended spectrum bacterial lactamase is
    a. Carbenicillin
    b. Carbapenem
    c. Aztreonam
    d. Clavulanic acid
384. Most common side effect of sulphonamides?
    a. Aplastic anemia
    b. Rash
    c. SLE
    d. Haemolysis
385. All drugs act on pseudomonas EXCEPT?
    a. Vancomycin
    b. Meropenem
    c. Cefipime
    d. Ciprofloxacin
386. Bulls eye maculopathy is seen with
    a. Chloroquine
    b. Quinine
    c. Pyrimethamine
    d. Halofentrine
387. Drug of choice for falciparum malaria in pregnancy?
    a. Quinine
    b. Artesunate
    c. Choloroquine
    d. Pyrimethamine
388. c-ART therapy leading to pancreatitis
    a. Didanosine
    b. Stavudine
    c. Lamivudine
    d. Emtricitabine
389. Drug of choice for larva migrans
    a. Mebendazole
    b. DEC
    c. Albendazole
    d. Praziquental
390. Best anti- thyroid drug in pregnancy is
    a. Propyl-thiouracil
    b. Levothyroxine
    c. Carbimazole
    d. Liothyronine
391. Drug of choice in Lithium induced diabetes mellitus?
    a. Conivaptan
    b. Amiloride
    c. Indapamide
    d. Vasopressin
392. Not recommended in acute CHF
    a. Diuretic
    b. ACE inhibitor
    c. NTG
    d. Beta blocker
393. Mechanism of action of sulphonamides is
    a. Inhibiting dihydrofolate synthase
    b. Inhibiting folate synthase
    c. Inhibiting tetrahydrofolate synthase
    d. Inhibiting amino acyl transferase
394. Haemorrhagic pancreatitis is seen with?
    a. Linagliptin
    b. Valdagliptin
    c. Exenatide
    d. Liraglutide
395. Drug used in Medical adrenalectomy is?
    a. Ketoconazole
    b. Terbinafine
    c. Febuxostat
    d. Tamoxifen
396. Drug used in migraine is all EXCEPT?
    a. Onabotulinum
    b. Flunarizine
    c. Telcagepant
    d. Vigabatrin
397. Shortest acting mydriatic
    a. Atropine
    b. Tropicamide
    c. Homatropine
    d. Cyclopentolate
398. Drug of choice for POAG
    a. Lanatoprost
    b. Brimonidine
    c. Dipivefrin
    d. Brinzolamide
399. Drug of choice for steroid induced osteoporosis
    a. Zoledronate
    b. Teriparitide
    c. Gallium nitrate
    d. Strontium
400. Best Drug to reduce cell counts in Hyperleucocytosis?
    a. Hydroxyurea
    b. Anagrelide
    c. Doxorubicin
    d. Radioactive phosphorus

Pharmacology

401. **Drug of choice for acyclovir resistant herpes is?**
   a. Cidofovir
   b. Gancyclovir
   c. Valacyclovir
   d. Foscarnet

402. **Drug of choice for Heparin induced thrombocytopenia?**
   a. Protamine sulfate
   b. Vitamin K
   c. Fresh Frozen plasma
   d. Argatroban

403. **Most commonly used drug for prophylaxis of migraine is?**
   a. Sumatriptan
   b. Propranolol
   c. Valproate
   d. Flunatrizine

404. **Amount of chloride in ORS**
   a. 65 mmol/L
   b. 75 mmol/L
   c. 10 mmol/L
   d. 20 mmol/L

405. **Red man syndrome is seen with**
   a. Lincomycin
   b. Vancomycin
   c. Linezolide
   d. Carbanicilliase

406. **Macrolides are drug of choice for all EXCEPT?**
   a. Chancroid
   b. Legionella
   c. Acinetobacter
   d. Bordetella

407. **DOC for hepatitis B**
   a. Sofosbuvir
   b. Entecavir
   c. Lamivudine
   d. Pegylated interferon

408. **Vitamin deficiency leading to photosensitivity?**
   a. Niacin
   b. Riboflavin
   c. Pyridoxine
   d. B12

409. **All are PDE 3 inhibitors EXCEPT:**
   a. Amrinone
   b. Milrinone
   c. Cilostazol
   d. Cilastin

410. **Which of the following inhibits degradation of dopamine**
   a. Rasagaline
   b. Ropirinole
   c. Rotigotine
   d. Carbi-dopa

411. **Drug of choice for ethylene glycol poisoning**
   a. Ethyl alcohol
   b. Disulfiram
   c. Fomepizole
   d. Methylene blue

412. **Longest acting opioid antagonist is**
   a. Naloxone
   b. Nalmefene
   c. Naltrexone
   d. Nitrazepam

413. **Short-term treatment of insomnia is**
   a. Chloral hydrate
   b. Zolpidem
   c. Diazepam
   d. Nitrazepam

414. **Anti-parkinsonism drug leading to Raynaud phenomenon?**
   a. Bromocriptine
   b. Tolcapone
   c. Ropirinole
   d. Levodopa

415. **DOC for huntington chorea**
   a. Tetrabenzamine
   b. Riluzole
   c. Alpha interferon
   d. Beta interferon

416. **DOC for febrile seizures**
   a. Oral diazepam
   b. Intranasal midazolam
   c. Intravenous lorazepam
   d. Oral PCM

417. **Longest acting anti-arrythmia drug**
   a. Amiodarone
   b. Dronaderone
   c. Ibutilide
   d. Lidocaine

418. **All are side effects of beta blockers EXCEPT**
   a. Bradycardia
   b. Hyperglycemia
   c. Rebound hypertension
   d. Ankle edema

419. **Longest acting statin is**
   a. Simvastatin
   b. Lovastatin
   c. Atorvastatin
   d. Rosuvastatin

420. **Drug useful in Pulmonary artery hypertension**
   a. Thiazide
   b. NTG
   c. Ivabradine
   d. Milrinone

421. **Adenosine is class _____ anti arrhythmia drug?**
   a. Class I
   b. Class II
   c. Class V
   d. Class IV

422. **Drug contraindicated in pregnancy are all EXCEPT:**
   a. Diuretics
   b. ACE inhibitors
   c. CCB
   d. Sodium nitroprusside

423. **Maximum decrease in HDL is by**
   a. Vitamin A
   b. Vitamin B
   c. Vitamin C
   d. Vitamin E

424. **Mechanism of action of statin is?**
   a. Stimulation of HMG COA reductase
   b. Indirect increase of LDL receptors synthesis
   c. Inhibition of HMG COA synthase
   d. Inhibition of intestinal cholesterol absorbtion

425. **Tocolytic preferred in heart disease in mother**
   a. Nifedipine
   b. Atosiban
   c. Magnesium sulfate
   d. Oxytocin

426. **Which of the following anti-epileptic drug is a microsomal enzyme inhibitor:**
   a. Ethosuximide
   b. Sodium valproate
   c. Phenobarbitone
   d. Phenytoin

427. **Number of patients in phase II clinical trial:**
   a. Few healthy patients
   b. Around 200 patients
   c. Around 2000 patients
   d. Around 5000 patients

428. **Alkaline diuresis is done for treatment of poisoning due to:**
   a. Amphetamine
   b. Morphine
   c. Paracetamol
   d. Phenobarbitone

429. **Drugs following zero order kinetics EXCEPT:**
   a. Phenytoin
   b. Phenobarbitone
   c. Theophylline
   d. Aspirin

430. **True about orphan drugs:**
   a. Drug used for orphans
   b. They are rare drugs
   c. They are emergency drugs
   d. Drugs for rare diseases

431. **All are true about rifampicin EXCEPT:**
   a. Bacteriostatic agent
   b. Acts by inhibiting DNA dependent RNA synthesis
   c. Resistance is due to rpo-B gene
   d. Can cause staining of soft lenses

432. **ATT which can interfere with function of thyroid:**
   a. Streptomycin
   b. Para amino salicylic acid
   c. Rifampicin
   d. Isoniazid

Questions

241

FMGE Solutions Screening Examination

433. Which of the following ATT can arouse suicidal tendency:
    a. Kanamycin   b. Capreomycin
    c. Cycloserine   d. Streptomycin
434. Drug used to perform stress echo:
    a. Adrenaline   b. Adenosine
    c. Dobutamine   d. Thallium
435. Pralidoxime acts by:
    a. Stimulate Ach receptor
    b. Inhibit breakdown of Ach
    c. Block Ach receptor
    d. Reactivate Ach esterase enzyme
436. Atropine can cause all EXCEPT:
    a. Mydriasis   b. Vomiting
    c. Bradycardia   d. Sweating
437. Agonist of M2 receptor:
    a. Carbachol   b. Methacholine
    c. Bethanechol   d. Pilocarpine
438. Rate limiting enzyme for noradrenaline synthesis:
    a. Dopa D carboxylase   b. Acetylcholine esterase
    c. Tyrosine hydroxylase d. Tyrosine reductase
439. Tachyphylaxis is shown by all EXCEPT:
    a. Amphetamine   b. Tyramine
    c. Imipramine   d. Ephedrine
440. Most effective in increasing heart rate:
    a. Dopamine   b. Adrenaline
    c. Noradrenaline d. Isoprenaline
441. Beta blocker with α blocker capacity is?
    (DNB 2012-section-1)
    a. Atenolol   b. Labetelol
    c. Propanolol   d. Metoprolol
442. Drug used in the treatment for hyperprolactinemia is?
    (DNB 2012-section-1)
    a. Bromocriptine b. Methyl Dopamine
    c. Haloperidol   d. Chlorpromazine
443. Which drug inhibits absorption of cholesterol from intestine?   (DNB 2012-section-1)
    a. Resins   b. Ezetimibe
    c. Niacin   d. Orlistat
444. Modafinil is used as an adjunct in the treatment of?
    (DNB 2012-section-1)
    a. Sleep apnea syndrome b. Narcolepsy
    c. ADHD   d. Shift work disorder
445. Rizatriptan is a drug used for? (DNB 2012-section-1)
    a. Prophylaxis of migraine b. Acute migraine
    c. Cluster headache d. Chronic migraine
446. Febuxostat is used for?   (DNB 2012-section-1)
    a. HyperKalemia b. Hyperuricemia
    c. Hypernatremia d. Hypercalcemia
447. Drug withdrawn in India is? (DNB 2012-section-1)
    a. Levofloxacin b. Gatifloxacin
    c. Moxifloxacin d. Ofloxacin
448. Which of the following is a parasympatholytic agent?
    (DNB 2012-section-1)
    a. Atropine   b. Neostigmine
    c. Pyridostigmine d. Acetylcholine
449. Drug of choice for prophylaxis of TB is?
    (DNB 2012-section-1)
    a. Rifampicin   b. Isoniazid
    c. Pyrizinamide d. Streptomycin
450. Anti-tubercular drug not given in liver disease is?
    (DNB 2012-section-1)
    a. Isoniazid   b. Ethambutol
    c. Pyrizinamide d. Rifampicin
451. ACE inhibitors should not be used with?
    (DNB 2012-section-1)
    a. Amilorides   b. Calcium channel blockers
    c. Chlorthialidone d. Spironolactone
452. Drug not used in the treatment of acute asthma attack is?   (DNB 2012-section-1)
    a. Oral prednisolone b. Inhalational salbutamol
    c. Inhalational salmeterol d. IV corticosteroid
453. True about clavulanic acid is? (DNB 2012-section-1)
    a. β lactamase inhibitors
    b. Extended spectrum penicillin
    c. Gram negative bacteria
    d. Plasmid inhibitors
454. Drug of choice for diarrhea in HIV is?
    (DNB 2012-section-1)
    a. Loperamide   b. Somatostatins
    c. Octreotide   d. Codeine
455. Drugs that should be given with prescription of registered medical practitioner only are included in which schedule?
    a. Schedule C   b. Schedule E
    c. Schedule H   d. Schedule I
456. Mechanism of action of clofibrates is?
    a. Inhibit HMGCoA reductase
    b. Inhibit HMG CoA synthase
    c. Inhibit absorption of cholesterol
    d. Inhibit release of TG and LDL
457. Which of the following anticancer drug is M phase specific?
    a. Methotrexate b. Vincristine
    c. Etiposide   d. Irinotectan
458. Renal papillary necrosis is caused by?
    a. NSAID   b. Cocaine
    c. Heroin   d. Morphine
459. Anti-smoking drug is?
    a. Theophylline b. Biclutamide
    c. Salmeterol   d. Varenicline
460. Antagonist of benzodiazepine is?
    a. Naltrexone   b. Flumazenil
    c. Naloxone   d. N-Acetyl cysteine

Pharmacology

461. **Inverse agonist of benzodiazepine:**
   a. β carboline
   b. Flumazenil
   c. Naloxone
   d. N-Acetyl cysteine

462. **Sumatriptan is antagonist of?**
   a. 5HT 1A
   b. 5HT 1D
   c. 5HT 2A
   d. 5HT 4

463. **Gynaecomastia is caused by?**
   a. Flutamide
   b. Cimetidine
   c. Pyrazinamide
   d. Methotrexate

464. **Drug which can cause photosensitivity reaction is?**
   a. Streptomycin
   b. Demeclocycline
   c. Clindamycin
   d. Clofibrate

465. **Daily dose of albendazole in neurocysticercosis in children is?**
   a. 1–3 mg/kg
   b. 4 to 8 mg/kg
   c. 15 mg/kg
   d. 25 mg/kg

466. **Which of the following is an oxytocin antagonist?**
   a. Ritodrine
   b. Atosiban
   c. Isoxsuprine
   d. Methergine

467. **Drug used for treatment of malignant hyperthermia is?**
   a. Succinylcholine
   b. Dantrolene
   c. Diazepam
   d. Valproate

468. **Most common side effect of calcium channel blocker is?**
   a. Headache
   b. Constipation
   c. Diarrhoea
   d. Muscle cramps

469. **Which of the following is a cerebro selective calcium channel blocker?**
   a. Nimodipine
   b. Ziconotide
   c. Verapamil
   d. Diltiazem

470. **Drug approved for anorgasmia and premature ejaculation:**
   a. SSRI
   b. Beta blocker
   c. Alfa 2 antagonist
   d. Alfa 1 antagonist

471. **Prokinetic drug with extrapyramidal side effect is?**
   a. Cisapride
   b. Domperidone
   c. Ondansetron
   d. Metoclopramide

472. **Mechanism of action of sulfonamide is:**
   a. Inhibit bacterial cell wall synthesis
   b. Inhibit translocation of mRNA
   c. Inhibit folate synthesis
   d. Inhibit bacterial respiration

473. **Mechanism of action of tranexamic acid in controlling bleeding is?**
   a. Inhibits plasminogen
   b. Promote platelet aggregation
   c. Cause vasoconstriction
   d. Promote fibrin synthesis

474. **Most common side effect of thiazide diuretics is?**
   a. Hyperuricemia
   b. Hypermagnesemia
   c. Hypocalcemia
   d. Hypokalemia

475. **H2 blockers are given for duodenal ulcer for a period of?**
   a. 4 weeks
   b. 6 weeks
   c. 8 weeks
   d. 12 weeks

476. **Therapeutic index signifies?**
   a. Potency
   b. Toxic dose
   c. Safety
   d. Efficacy

477. **Parathormone is useful in which of the following?**
   a. Hyperparathyroidism
   b. Paget's disease
   c. Osteoporosis
   d. Osteomalacia

478. **Which insulin is never mixed with other insulins?**
   a. Lente
   b. Aspart
   c. Lispro
   d. Glargine

479. **Drug of choice for neurogenic diabetes insipidus is?**
   a. Vasopressin
   b. Terlipressin
   c. Desmopressin
   d. Pralipressin

480. **Drug which does not cause hemolysis in G6PD deficiency is?**
   a. Primaquine
   b. Dapsone
   c. Aspirin
   d. Methylene blue

481. **Which of the following is a selective alpha 2 antagonist?**
   a. Prazosin
   b. Labetalol
   c. Yohimbine
   d. Butoxamine

482. **Drug of choice for acute adrenal insufficiency is?**
   a. Oral prednisone
   b. IV Hydrocortisone
   c. IV Betamethasone
   d. IV Dexamethasone

483. **Drug of choice for absence seizure is?**
   a. Clonezapam
   b. Diazepam
   c. Phenytoin
   d. Valproate

484. **Drug of choice for Lennox gastaut syndrome:**
   a. Clonezapam
   b. Diazepam
   c. Phenytoin
   d. Valproate

485. **Mechanism of action of aspirin is?**
   a. Inhibits COX-2 preferentially
   b. Inhibits COX-1 preferentially
   c. Inhibits COX1 and COX 2 reversibly
   d. Inhibits COX1 and COX 2 irreversibly

486. **Anti tubercular drug which is exclusive for intracellular mycobacterium?**
   a. Isoniazid
   b. Rifampicin
   c. Pyrazinamide
   d. Ethambutol

487. **Antiparkinson drug known to cause pleuropulmonary is?**
   a. Bromocriptine
   b. Ropinrole
   c. Pramiprexole
   d. Amantadine

FMGE Solutions Screening Examination

ANSWERS WITH EXPLANATIONS

MOST RECENT QUESTIONS 2019

1. Ans. (d) X

- Parasympathetic outflow is from cranial nerve 3, 7, 9, 10 and sacral nerve 2, 3, 4.
- Majority of parasympathetic outflow (~75%) is from vagus nerve (CN-X)

2. Ans. (b) Intravenous

- Bioavailability is fraction of unchanged drug reaching the systemic circulation following administration by any route.
- IV route has 100% bioavailability.

TABLE: Routes of administration, bioavailability, and general characteristics

Route	Bioavailability (%)	Characteristics
Intravenous (IV)	100 (by definition)	Most rapid onset
Intramuscular (IM)	75 to ≤100	Large volumes often feasible; may be painful
Subcutaneous (SC)	75 to ≤100	Smaller volumes than IM; may be painful
Oral (PO)	5 to <100	Most convenient; first-pass effect may be important
Rectal (PR)	30 to <100	Less first-pass effect than oral
Inhalation	5 to <100	Often very rapid onset
Transdermal	80 to ≤100	Usually very slow absorption; used for lack of first-pass effect; prolonged duration of action

3. Ans. (d) Hydrocortisone

Classification of steroids

Short acting: (8 – 12 hours)	• Cortisone • Hydrocortisone
Intermediate acting (12 – 36 hours)	• Fludrocortisone • Prednisone • Prednisolone • Methylprednisolone
Long acting (36 – 72 hours)	• Triamcinolone • Dexamethasone • Betamethasone

4. Ans. (a) Valproate

Ref: Katzung 14th ed P. 427, 434

- Though all the anti-epileptics have teratogenic potential, Valproate is the most teratogenic among all.
- Treatment with valproate during first trimester is associated with increased risk of neural tube defect including spina bifida, cardiovascular, orofacial and digital abnormalities.
- First trimester exposure with valproate causes 3 fold increased risk of major congenital malformations, most commonly spina bifida (absolute risk: 6–9%).

> **Extra Mile**
> - MC congenital defect associated with phenobarbitone exposure: Cardiac defect
> - MC congenital defect associated with topiramate exposure: cleft lip and palate (10 fold increased risk)
> - Antiseizure drugs with lowest congenital defect risk: Lamotrigine and Levetiracetam
> - Antiseizure drug having maximal breast milk secretion: Lamotrigine

5. Ans. (a) Phase 1

6. Ans. (b) Salbutamol

- Salbutamol is beta-2 agonist, preferred in acute bronchial asthma attack
- Most common side effect associated with the agent is Tremor

7. Ans. (d) Formoterol

- Beta-2 agonists are well known bronchodilators. This includes:
  - Salbutamol, Terbutaline, Formoterol, Salmeterol, Indacaterol, Albuterol etc.
- Among these agents formoterol, salmeterol, Indacaterol are longer acting analogue and are preferred in prophylactic therapy of bronchial asthma and COPD.

8. Ans. (b) Desmopressin

Ref: Katzung 14th ed. P 682

- Desmopressin is a long acting synthetic analogue of vasopressin
- DOC for neurogenic/pituitary diabetes insipidus: Desmopression
- Note: Desmopressin is also used for treatment of Hemophilia A and von Willebrand disease, nocturnal enuresis.

Pharmacology

Extra Mile
- DOC for nephrogenic diabetes insipidus: Thiazide diuretics
- Conivaptan and Tolvaptan: Vasopressin receptor antagonist. DOC for SIADH (Syndrome of Inappropriate Anti Diuretic Hormone). Also approved to be used in heart failure for free water clearance and in hyponatremia.

9. Ans. (c) Lignocaine

Ref: Katzung 14th ed. P 241

- **Lidocaine** is one of the local anaesthetics having anti-arrhythmic properties (Class 1B)
- It has low incidence of toxicity and high degree of effectiveness in arrhythmias associated with acute MI.
- Used only by IV route (t1/2: 1 – 2 hours)
- **MOA:** Blocks inactivated sodium channels
- **Use:**
  - DOC for termination of ventricular tachycardia and prevention of ventricular fibrillation
  - DOC for digoxin induced arrhythmia.
- It has least cardiotoxicity among sodium channel blockers.
- **Side effect:**
  - Depress myocardial contractility (can cause hypotension in heart failure patients)
  - **MC side effect:** Neurologic- Paresthesias, tremor, nausea, light headedness, hearing disturbances, slurring of speech and seizure episodes.

10. Ans. (a) Allopurinol

Ref: Katzung 14th ed. P 661

- DOC for chronic gout/period between acute gout attacks: Allopurinol
- **MOA:** Xanthine oxidase inhibitor
- When initiating allopurinol therapy, colchicine or NSAID should be used until steady-state serum uric acid is normalized or decreased to less than 6 mg/dL and they should be continued for 6 months or longer.
- **Initial dose:** 50–100 mg/day
- **Side effect:**
  - Precipitation of gout (that's why initially given with NSAIDS or colchicine)
  - GI intolerance (N/V/D)
  - Peripheral neuritis and necrotizing vasculitis
  - Bone marrow suppression → Aplastic anemia
  - Hepatotoxicity and interstitial nephritis
  - Maculopapular rash and exfoliative dermatitis
  - Cataract

Extra Mile
- DOC for acute gout attack: Probenecid (NSAID except Aspirin)
- **Febuxostat:** Also a xanthine oxidase inhibitor. Used in patients with intolerance to allopurinol or not responding to it.
- **Uricosuric agents like Probenecid, Sulfinpyrazone, Lesinurad** can also be used in treatment of gout especially when allopurinol or febuxostat is contraindicated.

11. Ans. (d) Amoxicillin

Ref: KDT 8th ed P 1018

Class of Drugs contraindicated in pregnancy and its safer alternative

Class of drug	Contraindicated	Safer alternative
Antibacterials (systemic bacterial infections)	Cotrimoxazole, Fluoroquinolones (X), Tetracycline (X), Doxycycline (X), Chloramphenicol (X), Gentamicin, Streptomycin (X), Kanamycin (X), Tobramycin (X), Clarithromycin, Azithromycin, Clindamycin, Vancomycin, Nitrofurantoin,	Penicillin G, Ampicillin Amoxicillin-clavulanate Cloxacillin, Piperacillin Cephalosporins Erythromycin

Extra Mile
- Sulfonamides (Co-Trimoxazole) if used during pregnancy can lead to kernicterus.
- Aminoglycosides (Gentamicin): Can produce ototoxicity and nephrotoxicity
- Floroquinolones (Ciprofloxacin): Affects growing cartilage and tendon

12. Ans. (a) Regular Insulin

Ref: Katzung 14th ed. P 753

- **Regular insulin** is a short-acting, soluble crystalline zinc insulin
- Hypoglycemic effect appears within 30 minutes after subcutaneous injection, peaks at about 2 hours, and lasts for 5–7 hours.
- For very insulin-resistant subjects who would otherwise require large volumes of insulin solution, a U500 preparation of human regular insulin is available both in a vial form and a disposable pen
- **IV infusion:** used in treatment of diabetic ketoacidosis

13. Ans. (d) Insulin glargine

Ref: Katzung 14th ed. P 755

FMGE Solutions Screening Examination

- **Insulin glargine** is a soluble, "peakless" (i.e. having broad concentration plateau), long acting insulin analogue.
- Onset: 1–1.5 hours. Duration of action: 11–24 hours.

TABLE: Summary of bioavailability characteristics of the insulins

Insulin preparations	Onset of action	Peak action	Effective duration
Insulins lispro, aspart, glulisine	5–15 minutes	1–1.5 hours	3–4 hours
Human regular	30–60 minutes	2 hours	6–8 hours
Technosphere inhaled insulin	5–15 minutes	1 hour	3 hours
Human NPH	2–4 hours	Flat	~24 hours
Insulin detemir	0.5–1 hours	Flat	17 hours
Insulin degludec	0.5–1.5 hours	Flat	>42 hours

14. Ans. (c) Schistosomiasis

Ref: Katzung 14th ed. P 939

- Drug of choice for all the **flukes** (**trematodes**) is **Praziquantel** except liver fluke, where drug of choice is Triclabendazole or Bithionol.
- Drug of choice for all the **tapeworms** (**cestodes**) is **Praziquantel** except Cysticercosis and Echinococcus where drug of choice is Albendazole.
- Drug of choice for all the **Roundworms (Nematode)** is Albendazole/Mebendazole except Strongyloides, Onchocerca (DOC: Ivermectin) and Filariasis, loa-loa disease (DOC is Diethylcarbamazine).

TABLE: Drugs for the treatment of helminthic infections[1]

Infection organism	Drug of choice	Alternative drugs
Roundworms (nematodes)		
Ascaris lumbricoides (roundworm)	Albendazole or pyrantel pamoate or mebendazole	Ivermectin, piperazine
Trichuris trichiura (whipworm)	Mebendazole or albendazole	Ivermectin, oxantel pamoate drug combinations
Necator americanus (hookworm); *Ancylostoma duodenale* (hookworm)	Albendazole or mebendazole or pyrantel pamoate	
Strongyloides stercoralis (threadworm)	Ivermectin	Albendazole or thiabendazole
Enterobius vermicularis (pinworm)	Mebendazole or pyrantel pamoate	Albendazole
Trichinella spiralis (trichinosis)	Mebendazole or albendazole; add corticosteroids for severe infection	
Trichostrongylus species	Pyrantel pamoate or mebendazole	Albendazole
Cutaneous larva migrans (creeping eruption)	Albendazole or ivermectin	Thiabendazde (topical)
Visceral larva migrans	Albendazole	Mebendazole
Angiostrongylus cantonensis	Albendazole or mebendazole	
Wuchereria bancrofti (filariasis); *Brugia malayi* (filariasis); tropical eosinophilia; *Log loa* (loiasis)	Diethylcarbamazine	Ivermectin
Onchocerca volvulus (onchocerciasis)	Ivermectin	
Dracunculus medinensis (guinea worm)	Metronidazole	Thiabendazole or mebendazole
Capillaria philippinensis (intestinal capillariasis)	Albendazole	Mebendazole
Flukes (trematodes)		
Schistosoma haematobium (bilharziasis)	Praziquantel	Metrifonate
Schistosoma mansoni	Praziquantel	Oxamniquine

Contd...

Pharmacology

Infection organism	Drug of choice	Alternative drugs
Schistosoma japonicum	Praziquantel	
Clonorchis sinensis (liver fluke); *Opisthorchis* species	Praziquantel	Albendazole
Paragonimus westermani (lung fluke)	Praziquantel	Bithionol
Fasciola hepatica (sheep liver fluke)	Bithionol or triclabendazole	
Fasciolopsis buski (large intestinal fluke)	Praziquantel or niclosamide	
Heterophyes heterophyes; Metagonimus yokogawai (small intestinal flukes)	Praziquantel of niclosamide	
Tapeworms (cestodes)		
Taenia saginata (beef tapeworm)	Praziquantel or niclosamide	Mebendazole
Diphyllobothrium latum (fish tapeworm)	Praziquantel or niclosamide	
Taenia solium (pork tapeworm)	Praziquantel or niclosamide	
Cysticercosis (pork tapeworm larval stage)	Albendazole	Praziquantel
Hymenolepis nana (dwarf tapeworm)	Praziquantel	Niclosamide nitazoxanide
Echinococcus granulosus (hydatid disease); *Echinococcus multilocularis*	Albendazole	

15. Ans. (b) Lithium carbonate

Ref: Katzung 14ᵗʰ ed. P 524

- Drug of choice for mania is Lithium
- DOC for acute attack of manic episode: Atypical antipsychotics/Benzodiazepines
- Agents that can be used in treatment of Mania: *(Mn: Li ACT Val)*
  - Lithium (DOC)
  - Atypical antipsychotics
  - Carbamazepine
  - Topiramate
  - Valproate

16. Ans. (c) Mupirocin

Ref: Katzung 14ᵗʰ ed. P 1070

- Mupirocin is used for topical treatment of minor skin infection such as impetigo. It is also effective against gram positive cocci including-susceptible and methicillin-resistant strains of staph aureus.
- Intranasal mupirocin ointment is preferred for eliminating nasal carrier of S. aureus
- **MOA**: inhibits staphylococcal isoleucyl tRNA synthetase.

17. Ans. (c) Bupropion

Ref: Katzung 14ᵗʰ ed. 584

- **Book states:** "*the antidepressant Bupropion is approved for nicotine cessation therapy. It is most effective when combined with behavioral therapies*"

- **Note: Topiramate** is approved for decreasing alcohol craving, obesity.

18. Ans. (b) Donepezil

Ref: Katzung 14ᵗʰ ed. P 1063

- DOC for Alzheimer's disease: Donepezil (reversible AchEsterase inhibitor)
- Other Ach Esterase inhibitor used in treatment of Alzheimer's disease is Gallantamine, Rivastigmine.

19. Ans. (a) Dopamine

- Dopamine keeps inhibitory control over prolactin.
- This explains the reason behind hyperprolactinemia in psychotic patients who are treated with dopamine antagonists.
- Dopamine agonists (bromocriptine, cabergoline) therefore are used in treatment of hyperprolactinemia, acromegaly.

20. Ans. (b) Etoricoxib

Ref: Katzung 14ᵗʰ ed. P 323, 647

TABLE: Non-steroidal anti-inflammatory drugs classification

Selective COX-2 Inhibitor (Coxibs)	Non-selective COX-1 and 2 inhibitor
• Celecoxib	• Indomethacin
• Etoricoxib	• Ibuprofen
• Valdecoxib	• Naproxen
• Rofecoxib	• Piroxicam
• Parecoxib	• Aspirin
	• Ketoprofen

Explanations

FMGE Solutions Screening Examination

GENERAL PHARMACOLOGY

21. Ans. (a) Preclinical stage

Ref: Sharma & Sharma 3rd ed. P 101

- **Clinical Trial:** Systemic study of a new drug in human subject to generate data for pharmacological and adverse effects with an aim to determine safety and efficacy.
- The procedures followed during the trial should comply with an elaborate code known as **"Good clinical practice (GCP)"** prescribed by international conference on Harmonization.
- GCP provide details about:
  - Designing the trial
  - Collection of the data
  - Recording of information
  - Statistical analysis
  - Documentation and reporting the results of clinical trials

PRECLINICAL EVALUATION PHASE (ANIMAL STUDIES)

- Animals studies are done initially in order to define the pharmacological profile of lead compound
- Aim: Satisfy all requirements that are needed before a compound is considered fit to be tested for first in humans
- It is done according to formal operating code known as *"Good Laboratory Practices"*
- Good laboratory practices ensures reliability and reproducibility of laboratory data and minimises human errors
- Duration of preclinical study: ~2 years
- **Out of 10,000** compounds screened during preclinical phase, only 10 qualify, which are then subjected to clinical trial in humans.

22. (d) All of the above

Ref: Goodman & Gillman's 13th ed. P 90

- The common antifungal agent ketoconazole is a potent inhibitor of CYP3A4
- Therefore coadministration of ketoconazole with other CYP3A4 inhibitors like anti-HIV drug viral protease inhibitors (ritonavir, indinavir), clarithromycin, itraconazole, nefazodone, and grapefruit juice reduces the clearance of these drugs and increases its plasma concentration and the risk of toxicity. Hence these drugs are not given together.

23. Ans. (b) Adrenaline

Ref: Goodman and Gillman 13th ed. P 58

- **Physiological (Functional) antagonism** occurs when two different agents produce opposite effects by acting at the different receptors.
  - Example: action and histamine and Epinephrine at smooth muscle of bronchus. Histamine causes bronchoconstriction (by acting at H1 receptor) but epinephrine causes bronchodilation (by acting at β2 receptor).

> **Extra Mile**
>
> - **Pharmacological antagonist:** Drug binds at the receptor of agonist and produce no effect, shows no intrinsic activity.
> - **Chemical antagonist:** Agent that binds chemically with the agonist. Example: Binding of chelating agent with the meta.

24. Ans. (d) A and B both

Ref: Goodman and Gillman 13th ed. P 22

- **AUC** is the total area under the curve that describes the measured concentration of drug in the systemic circulation as a function of time (from zero to infinity) after its administration.
- AUC represents extent of absorption evaluating the bioavailability of drug from its dosage form and its clearance.

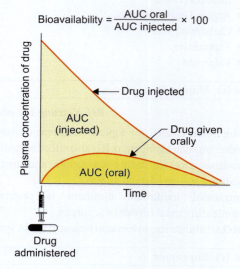

$$\text{Bioavailability} = \frac{\text{AUC oral}}{\text{AUC injected}} \times 100$$

25. Ans. (b) Bizarre effect of a drug

Ref: KD Tripathi, 7th ed. pg. 82

Pharmacology

Adverse drug reactions are classified as follows:

Type A (Predictable)	Augmented pharmacological effects: Dose dependent Side effects → at therapeutic dose Toxicity → at high dose Intolerance → toxicity at therapeutic dose
Type B (Unpredictable)	Bizarre effects: **Dose independent** Drug allergy: 4 types Anaphylaxis (type I) Blood cytolysis (type II) Complex (Ag-Ab) mediated reaction (type III) Delayed hypersensitivity (type IV) Idiosyncrasy: Abnormal effect, e.g. CNS depressants causing stimulation
Type C	**Chronic** effects: Duration dependent Adverse effects of prolonged treatment e.g. Corticosteroids causing immunosuppression
Type D	**Delayed effects:** Adverse effects long time after stopping the drug e.g. Carcinogenicity and Mutagenicity by anticancer drugs and radioisotopes
Type E	**End of treatment effects** Adverse effects due to abruptly stopping the drug e.g. withdrawal syndrome of clonidine i.e. rebound hypertension
Type F	**Failure of therapy** Ex: OCP failure Antimicrobial resistance

---

26. Ans. (a) Nitrate induced headache

Ref: KDT, 7th ed. pg. 82

Note: *Nitrate induced vasodilation and headache occur immediately, these are not chronic adverse drug reactions whereas others are example of type C or chronic ADRs.*

---

27. Ans. (c) Bioavailability

Ref: KD Tripathi, 7th ed. pg. 16

■ BIOAVAILABILITY

- Bioavailability is a measure of the fraction of administered dose of a drug that reaches the systemic circulation in the unchanged form.
- **Bioavailability of drug injected IV is 100%,** but is frequently lower after oral ingestion because—
  - The drug may be incompletely absorbed.
  - The absorbed drug may undergo first pass metabolism in the intestinal wall/liver or be excreted in bile.

---

28. Ans. (d) Monitoring adverse effects of drugs

Ref: KDT, 6th ed. pg. 79

- Pharmacovigilance is the science and activities relating to the *detection, assessment, understanding and prevention of adverse effects* or any other possible drug-related problems.
- Recently, its concerns have been widened to include herbals, traditional and complementary medicines, blood products, biologicals, medical devices and vaccines.

---

29. Ans. (c) To monitoring adverse effects of drugs

Please refer to above explanation

---

30. Ans. (b) Intravenous

Ref: Katzung Pharmacology, 10th ed. Ch 3

- Bioavailability is defined as the fraction of unchanged drug reaching the systemic circulation following administration by any route.
- In case a drug is given orally, the bioavailability shall be less than 100%. This is due to
  - Incomplete extent of absorbtion
  - First pass metabolism

TABLE: Routes of administration, bioavailability, and general characteristics

Route of Administration	General characteristics	Bioavailiabilty
Intravenous	Onset of action is fastest	100%
Intramuscular	Painful	75–100%
Subcutaneous	Lesser volumes can be given compared to intramuscular route	75–100%
Per oral	Most convenient from patients perspective MC used route	5% to <100% First pass metabolism limits blood levels
Per rectal	Less first pass metabolism than per oral	30 to <100%
Transdermal	Very slow absorbtion Lack of first pass effect Prolonged duration of action	80-100%

---

31. Ans. (a) Rate of elimination is independent of plasma concentration

Ref: Goodman & Gillman 13th ed. P 20

- In pharmacokinetics, drug's clearance, rate of elimination and half life is given by the order of kinetics i.e. by zero order kinetics or first order kinetics.

FMGE Solutions Screening Examination

Zero order kinetics Non-lnear kinetics	First order kinetics (Linear kinetics)
Constant amount of drug is eliminated per unit of time	Constant fraction of drug eliminated per unit of time
Rate of elimination is independent of plasma concentration	Rate of elimination is directly proportional to plasma concentration
Clearance is more at low concentration and less at high concentration	Clearance remains constant
Half life less at low concentration, more at high concentration	Half life is constant
Only few drugs follow zero order kinetics	Most drugs follow first order kinetics

NOTE: Drugs which follow zero order kinetics: **(WATT-Power)** Warfarin Alcohol/Aspirin Theophylline Tolbutamide Phenytoin, Propaphenone	Kinetics in a Nutshell:	
	Zero order	First order
	ROE = constant CL α 1/P.C. t1/2 α PC	ROE α P.C. CL = constant t1/2 = constant

32. Ans. (a) Phenytoin

Ref: Katzung, 11th ed. pg. 80

ACETYLATION

- Compounds having amino or hydralazine residues are conjugated with the help of N-Acetyl transferase enzyme.
  - If acetylation is slow- increased side effect
  - Fast acetylation- not effective or effectiveness decreases
  - Normal acetylation- effective
- These drugs are remembered as CHIPS-ABC drugs:
  - **Clonazepam** (sedative)
  - **Hydralazine** (anti HTN)
  - **Isoniazid** (anti TB)
  - **Procainamide** (anti-arrhythmic)
  - **Sulfonamides** (dapsone)
  - **Acebutalol, Amrinone, ASA**
  - **Benzocaine**
  - **Caffeine**
- Phenytoin hydroxylation in liver is carried out by cytochrome P 450.
- **The drugs metabolized by acetylation causes SLE.**

33. Ans. (b) Isoniazid

Ref: KDT, 6th ed. pg. 25

Please refer to above explanation

34. Ans. (c) G_{t_1}

Ref: Katzung's Pharma, 14th ed. pg. 31

TABLE: G-Proteins and their receptors and effectors

G-protein	Assicauted receptor	Effector Pathway
G_{t1}, G_{t2}	Photons (rhodopsin and color opsins in retinal rod and cone cells)	↑cGMP phospho-diesterase → ↓ ⁻cGMP (phototransduction)
Gs (stimulates membrane-bound adenylate cyclase)	β-adrenoceptors, histamine, serotonin, dopamine (D_1) receptor, Glucagon	Increased adenylyl cyclase activity → increased cAMP
Gi (inhibits membrane-bound adenylate cyclase)	$α_2$-adrenoceptors, muscarine (M_2) receptors, opioid receptors, some SHT receptors; dopamine (D_2) receptor	• Decreased adenylyl cyclase activity → decreased cAMP • Open cardiac k^+ channel → ↓ HR
$Gq/G_{12/13}$ (activates phospholipase-C)	$α_1$-adrenoceptors, muscarinic (M_1) receptor, angiotensin receptor (AT_1)	Activates phospholipase-C → ↑ IP_3, ↑DAG, ↑Ca^{2+} entry

35. Ans. (a) cAMP

Ref: Katzung, 14th ed. pg. 31

- G-protein receptor for glucagon is Gs which acts via ↑Adenylyl cyclase causing ↑ **cAMP**.
- Refer to above table for detailed explanation.

36. Ans. (d) Excreted mainly by kidneys

Ref: Katzung, 14th ed. pg. 56; KDT, 6th ed. pg. 16-17

Ionized drugs/hydrophilic drugs	Nonionized drugs/lipophilic drugs
They are water soluble	Lipid soluble
Can not cross epithelial lining	Can cross epithelial lining easily
Poor absorption from intestine	Well absorbed from intestine
Can not cross placental barrier	Can cross placental barrier
Excreted mainly by kidneys	Excreted through faeces, urine, sweat etc.

Pharmacology

> **Extra Mile**
>
> When medium is same: drugs will cross
> **Example 1:** *Acidic* drug will cross acid medium
> Acidic drugs like salicylates, barbiturates etc. are predominantly *unionized* in the acid gastric juice and are absorbed from stomach.
> **Example 2:** Basic drug will cross basic medium.
> Basic drugs like morphine, quinine etc. are highly ionized and are absorbed only after reaching small intestine when it gets basic medium.

37. Ans. (a) Rifampicin

Ref: Katzung, 14th ed. pg. 59; KDT, 6th ed. pg. 27

- **Enzyme induction** involves microsomal enzyme in liver as well as in other organ.
- It increases the rate of metabolism 2-4 fold. Therefore effect of drug decreases.
- **Enzyme inhibitors** also involves microsomal enzyme.
- It inhibits the microsomal enzyme, which decreases drug metabolism rate and increases duration of drug action.
- Let us take an example of warfarin, which is used as an anti thrombotic agent.
  - **Warfarin + enzyme inducer** = Thrombosis (warfarin metabolism increases and action of warfarin diminishes rapidly and thrombotic condition arises).
  - **Warfarin + enzyme inhibitor** = Bleeding (warfarin metabolism decreases and duration of warfarin action increases and patient develops bleeding tendency)

Drugs which are enzyme inducers and enzyme inhibitors

Enzyme inducers	Enzyme inhibitors
Griseofulvin	Phenylbutazone
Phenytoin	Erythromycin
Rifampicin	Allopurinol, Amiodarone
Smoking	Ciprofloxacin
Carbamazipine	Omeprazole
Phenobarbitone	Cimetidine
Barbiturate	Ketoconazole
DDT	Valproate
Remembered as: GPRS Cell Phone Battery Dead	Mn: PEACOCK Vala

> **Extra Mile**
>
> - Most of the anti epileptic are enzyme inducers except **VALPROATE (an inhibitor)**
> - Most of the antimicrobial are enzyme inhibitors except **GRISEOFULVIN (an Inducer)**

38. Ans. (a) Carbamazepine

Ref: Katzung, 14th ed. pg. 59

- Carbamazepine is an enzyme inducer.

Please refer to above explanation.

39. Ans. (b) Make urine alkaline with $NaHCO_3$

Ref: Katzung, 14th ed. pg. 9; KDT, 6th ed. pg. 16

- Aspirin is an acidic drug, it readily crosses any acidic medium. To treat this toxicity, make the urine alkaline with $NaHCO_3$.
- Now, this acidic drug can't be reabsorbed from the basic medium, and it readily gets excreted from the body.

> **Extra Mile**
>
> - In basic drug poisoning like amphetamine, we acidify the urine with NH_4Cl^- to change the medium, which opposes reabsorption and hence excretion.
> - N-acetyl cysteine is the DOC for paracetamol poisoning

40. Ans. (a) Glucocorticoids

Ref: Goodman & Gillman 13th ed. P 851, 809

- Ligands that act by intracellular receptors are classified into nuclear and cytoplasmic. All these ligands acts by nuclear transcription but their receptors are either present in nucleus (nuclear receptor) or in cytoplasm (cytoplasmic receptor).
- Glucocorticoids act by binding to a specific glucocorticoid receptor (GRs) that is a member of the nuclear receptor family of transcription factors.
- GRs reside predominantly in the cytoplasm in an inactive form complexed with other proteins. Steroid binding results in receptor activation and translocation to the nucleus
- The GR translocates to the nucleus and induces complex gene expression changes that lead to antiproliferative and apoptotic responses in sensitive cells.

Receptors	Ligands
Nuclear receptors present in nucleus (Mn: ROAD TRAP Fixed)	**RAR** (Retinoic acid Receptor) **Oestrogen** Vitamin **A** Vitamin **D** Thyroxine **Retinoid X receptor (RXR)** **AHR** (Aryl Hydrocarbon Receptor) **PPAR** (peroxisome proliferator-activated receptor) **PXR** (Pregnane X Receptor) **FXR** (Farnesoid X receptor)
Nuclear receptors present in Cytoplasm	All Steroids EXCEPT Oestrogen (Ex: Glucocorticoids, Androgen)
Cell membrane via G protein stimulation	All others like ACTH, LH,GH,FSH

FMGE Solutions Screening Examination

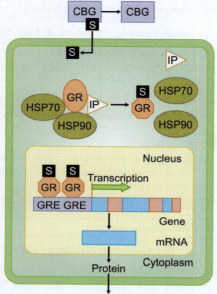

FIGURE: Intracellular mechanism of action of the GR. The figure shows the molecular pathway by which cortisol (labeled S) enters cells and interacts with the GR to change GR conformation (indicated by the change in shape of the GR), induce GR nuclear translocation, and activate transcription of target

> **Extra Mile**

(Goodman & Gillman 13th ed.) (Important)

TABLE: Nuclear receptors that induce drug metabolism

Receptor	Ligands
Aryl hydrocarbon receptor (AHR	Omeprazole
Constitutive androstane receptor (CAR)	Phenobarbital
Pregnane X receptor (PXR)	Rifampin
Farnesoid X receptor (FXR)	Bile acids
Vitamin D receptor (VDR)	Vitamin D
Peroxisome proliferator-activated receptor (PPARs)	Fibrates
Retinoic acid receptor (RAR)	*all-trans*-Retinoic acid
Retinoid X receptor (RXR)	*9-cis*-Retinoic acid

41. Ans. (b) Androgen

Ref: Goodman & Gillman 13th ed. P 851, 809

- Androgens act by binding to a specific androgen receptor (ARs) that is a member of the nuclear receptor family of transcription factors.
- ARs reside predominantly in the cytoplasm in an inactive form complexed with other proteins. Androgen binding results in receptor activation and translocation to the nucleus

Please refer to above question for detailed explanation

42. Ans. (a) Leutenizing Hormone

Ref: Goodman & Gillman 13th ed. P 851, 809

- Leutenizing hormone acts via cell membrane receptor.

43. Ans. (a) Phenytoin

Ref: Katzung, 14th ed. pg. 432; KDT, 6th ed. pg. 34-35

- Therapeutic dose monitoring (TDM) is used to monitor the effect of drug through plasma concentration.

Criteria to do TDM

- When response of drug can't be measured.

Note:
- Response of warfarin measured by INR.
- Response of metformin measured by blood glucose level.
- Response of propanolol measured by BP measurement.
- If any drug having narrow therapeutic index (unsafe drugs).
- If a drug is showing wide variation in pharmacokinetics.

Drugs in which TDM done (Remembered as: DAAALI)
- Digitalis
- Aminoglycosides (Gentamicin)
- Anti epileptics
- Anti Cancer
- Lithium
- Immuno suppressant (Cyclosporine, Tacrolimus, Sirolimus)

TABLE: Therapeutic drug range for some anti-seizure drug

Drug	Reference range
Carbamazepine	4–12
Clobazam	0.03–0.30
Ethosuximide	40–100
Phenytoin	10–20
Phenobarbital	15–40
Valproate	40–100
Lamotrigine	3–15
Levetiracetam	12–46
Oxcarbazepine	5–35
Topiramate	5–20

Pharmacology

44. Ans. (a) 3 months

Ref: Katzung's Pharmacology, 14th ed. pg. 13

Type of test	Approach
Acute toxicity	**Defined as dose that is lethal in approximately 50% of animals and is maximum tolerated dose.** It requires usually two species, two routes, single dose.
Subacute toxicity	It requires three doses and two species. **4 weeks to 3 months** may be necessary prior to clinical trial.
Chronic toxicity	It is done in Rodent and non-rodent species for 6 months or longer. Required when drug is intended to be used in humans for prolonged periods. Usually run concurrently with clinical trial.
Carcinogenic potential	**Two years, two species.** It is required when drug is intended to be used in humans for prolonged periods.
Mutagenic potential	Effects on genetic stability and mutations in bacteria (Ames test) or mammalian cells in culture
Investigative toxicology	Determine sequence and mechanisms of toxic action. Discover the genes, proteins, pathways involved. Develop new methods for assessing toxicity.

45. Ans. (a) Two different species

Ref: Katzung, 14th ed. pg. 13

Please refer to above table for explanation.

46. Ans. (c) Alprazolam

Ref: Goodman & Gillman 13th ed. 1320-21; Katzung's Pharmacology, 10th ed. Ch 60

- Alprazolam comes under "Category D" drugs
- The FDA has established five categories to indicate the potential of a drug to cause birth defects **if used during pregnancy.**
- These categories range from A to X, in increasing order of concern:

Category A	No risk in controlled human studies	Adequate and well-controlled studies have failed to demonstrate a risk to the fetus in the first trimester of pregnancy (and there is no evidence of risk in later trimesters). *Example drugs:* **Levothyroxine, Folic Acid, Magnesium Sulfate, Liothyronine**
Category B	No risk in other studies	Animal reproduction studies have failed to demonstrate a risk to the fetus and there are *no adequate and well-controlled studies in pregnant women.* **Example drugs: Metformin, Hydrochlorothiazide, Cyclobenzaprine, Amoxicillin, PPI** Should be prescribed only as needed for maternal health.
Category C	Risk not ruled out	Animal reproduction studies have shown an adverse effect on the fetus and there are no adequate and well-controlled studies in humans, but potential benefits may warrant use of the drug in pregnant women despite potential risks. **Example drugs: Tramadol, Gabapentin, Amlodipine, Trazodone, Prednisone** Prescribed in pregnancy only when benefit clearly outweighs risk.
Category D	Positive evidence of risk	There is positive evidence of human fetal risk based on adverse reaction data from investigational or marketing experience or studies in humans, but potential benefits may warrant use of the drug in pregnant women despite potential risks. **Example drugs: Lisinopril, Alprazolam, Losartan, Clonazepam, Lorazepam** Not used during pregnancy. Should be prescribed only if absolutely necessary.
Category X	Contraindicated in pregnancy	Studies in animals or humans have demonstrated fetal abnormalities and/or there is positive evidence of human fetal risk based on adverse reaction data from investigational or marketing experience, and the risks involved in use of the drug in pregnant women clearly outweigh potential benefits. **Example drugs: Atorvastatin, Simvastatin, Warfarin, Methotrexate, Finasteride** Must not be used during pregnancy or in women likely to become pregnant.

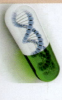

FMGE Solutions Screening Examination

47. Ans. (b) 200–400

Ref: Goodman & Gillman 13th ed. P 6

TABLE: Clinical Trials and its characteristics

Phase I first in human	Phase II first in patient	Phase III multisite trial	Phase IV postmarketing surveillance
10–100 participants	50–500 participants	A few hundred to a few thousand participants	Many thousands of participants
Usually healthy volunteers; occasionally patients with advanced or rare disease	Patient-subjects receiving experimental drug	Patient-subjects receiving experimental drug	Patients in treatment with approved drug
Open label	Randomized and controlled (can be placebo controlled); may be blinded	Randomized and controlled (can be placebo controlled) or uncontrolled; may be blinded	Open label
Safety and tolerability	Efficacy and dose ranging	Confirm efficacy in larger population	Adverse events, compliance, drug-drug interactions
1–2 years	2–3 years	3–5 years	No fixed duration
US $10 million	US $20 million	US $50–100 million	—
Success rate: 50%	Success rate: 30%	Success rate: 25%–50%	—

- Maximum drug failure occur in this phase: Phase II
- Most important phase of clinical trial: Phase III
- A new drug is launched in market after phase III

Extra Mile

- **Phase 0 trial** is microdosing study, done on normal healthy volunteers. To study the PK/PD of drug by radiolabelling and administering.
- **Phase 5** clinical trial is Pharamcoepidemiology.
- Phase 0 and 1 done on normal healthy volunteers.

48. Ans. (c) Phase II

Ref: Goodman & Gillman 13th ed. P 6

Refer to above explanation

49. Ans. (d) Phase V

Ref: Goodman & Gillman 13th ed. P 6

Refer to above explanation

50. Ans. (b) Lisinopril

Ref: KDT 6th ed. pg. 24

- Drugs that are administered and then converted to the active drug by biologic processes—inside the body are called a **prodrug**.
- If an active drug converted to another active metabolite, they are considered as prodrugs.
- All ACE inhibitors are prodrug EXCEPT **Captopril** and **Lisinopril** (Mn = **ACL**)

- **Other List of prodrugs are (MAMC-LEADS)**
  - Minoxidil, ace inhibitors, mercaptopurine, cyclophosphamide, clopidogrel
  - Levodopa, enalapril, alpha methyl dopa, dipivefrine, sulfasalazine, sulindac

51. Ans. (d) Captopril

Please refer to above explanation

52. Ans. (b) Drugs used for rare disease

Ref: Katzung, 14th ed. pg. 18

- Drugs which are developed specifically for rare diseases are called **orphan drugs.**
- These drugs are difficult to research, develop, and market due to lack of financial benefits.
- Because of this a separate law known as 'The Orphan Drug Act' was passed in 1983.
- **Examples** include deferipirone to treat iron overload in thalasemia patients, N-acetylcysteine to treat paracetamol poisoning etc.

53. Ans. (d) Decrease in efficacy

Ref: KDT pg. 73

- The food, drug and cosmetics act requires expiry date on all the drugs. Drugs used past the expiry date may lead to suboptimal therapeutic effect due to loss of efficacy.
- Drug and cosmetics act (1940) specifies the life period of drugs (mostly 1-5 years) and the conditions of storage.

Pharmacology

- The expiry of other medicines has to be specified by the manufacturer but cannot exceed 5 years.
- The expiry date doesn't mean that the medicines has actually been found to loss potency or become toxic after it, but simply the quality of the medicine is not assured after the expiry date and the manufacturer is not liable if any harm arises from the use of product.

AUTONOMIC NERVOUS SYSTEM

54. Ans. (a) Promethazine

Ref: Goodman & Gillman 13th ed. P 935

- Drugs that are used as agent of choice for motion sickness are:
  - **Antimuscarinic** agents like Hyoscine and Scopolamine
  - **H1 antagonist drugs** like Promethazine, Diphenhydramine > Buclizine, Cyclizine, etc.
- The anti-motion sickness activity of both these classes becomes more pronounced when combined with ephedrine.
- Both the class of drugs can also be used in Meniere's syndrome.

TABLE: General classification of antiemetic agents

Antiemetic class	Examples	Most effective against
5HT$_3$ receptor antagonists[a]	Ondansetron	Cytotoxic drug-induced emesis
Centrally acting Dopamine receptor antagonists	Metoclopramide	
	Promethazine	
Cannabinoid receptor agonists	Dronabinol nabilone	
Neurokinin receptor antagonists	Aprepitant	Cytotoxic drug induced emesis (delayed vomiting)
Histamine H$_1$ antagonists	Cyclizine	Vestibular emesis (Motion sickness)
Muscarinic receptor antagonists	Hyoscine (scopolamine)	

[a] The most effective agents for chemotherapy induced nausea and vomiting are the 5HT3 antagonists and metoclopramide.

55. Ans. (b) Alpha 2 agonist

Ref: Goodman & Gillman 13th ed. P 203

- Alpha methyldopa is an alpha-2 agonist acts as centrally acting sympatholytic agent

α2 agonist	Uses
Alpha methyldopa	Antihypertensive
Clonidine	Antihypertensive
Tizanidine	Sedative
Moxonidine	Analgesics
Apraclonidine Brimonidine	Glaucoma (Decrease aqueous production)
Guanfacine	Antihypertensive ADHD

56. Ans. (c) Active miotic

Ref: Goodman & Gillman 13th ed. P 1017

- Pilocarpine is one of the M$_3$ receptor agonist causing active miosis.
- To understand this concept of active and passive miosis/mydriasis, we need to know the receptors present in eye and its function:

Receptor	M3	α1	Example of drugs
Location	Sphincter pupillae Ciliary muscle	Dilator pupillae/ Radial muscle	
Agonist	Active miosis	Active mydriasis	M$_3$ agonist: Pilocarpine α1 agonist: Dipivefrin
Antagonist	Passive mydriasis	Passive miosis	M$_3$ antagonist: Atropine α1 antagonist: Prazosin

57. Ans. (b) Prazosin

Ref: Goodman & Gillman 13th ed. P 208-209

- Prazosin is one of the non-selective alpha 1 antagonists used for treatment of hypertension and BPH.
- DOC for HTN + BPH: Prazosin
- DOC for BPH: Silodosin (selective α$_{1a}$ agonist)
- **Side effect:**
  - Marked Postural hypotension (orthostatic/first dose hypotension), syncope → can cause recurrent falls. Therefore it is given at bedtime
  - Retrograde ejaculation

58. Ans. (a) Plasma acetylcholinesterase

Ref: Goodman & Gillman 13th ed. P 170

- The diagnosis of organophosphate poisoning can be made with the help of history of exposure and characteristic cholinergic signs and symptoms.
- In suspected cases of milder or chronic poisoning determination of plasma cholinesterase activities in erythrocytes and plasma establishes the diagnosis. It the most sensitive test.

FMGE Solutions Screening Examination

> **Extra Mile**
>
> - **Symptoms of organophosphate poisoning:**
>   - Salivation, Lacrimation, Urination, Diarrhea, GI distress, Emesis, Fasciculation, Bradycardia, Pin point pupil *(Mn: SLUDGE-FBP).*
> - **Antidote of OP poisoning:** Atropine (2-4 mg IV or 2 mg IM → repeated every 10–15 minutes till atropinization).
> - **AchE reactivators:**
>   - **Pralidoxime (2-PAM), Obidoxime:** Action seen peripherally only (1-2 mg IV slow infusion. If symptom persists → repeat the dose)
>   - **Diacetylmonoxime (DAM):** Action seen both peripheral and central.

59. Ans. (a) 1% atropine ointment

Ref: K.D. Tripathi 8th ed. P 131

- Atropine 1% ointment is preferred for refractive error test in children below 5 years. It is applied 24 hours and 2 hours before the procedure.
- The shorter acting agents like homatropine, tropicamide and cyclopentolate doesn't produces effective cycloplegia in children (ciliary muscle tone of child is high)
- Ointment is preferred over eye drop as there is increased risk of systemic absorption of eye drop which can cause anticholinergic side effect in child. Example: Hyperthermia, decreased secretion, tachycardia etc.

> **Extra Mile**
>
> - Cycloplegic agent of choice is adult/elderly: Tropicamide. The protein binding of esmolol is 55%.
> - For only fundoscopy/mydriasis, preferred agent is: Phenylephrine (Sympathomimetic)

60. Ans. (a) β2 agonist

Ref: Goodman & Gillman's 13th ed. P 201

- Ritodrine is a β2-selective agonist that was developed specifically as a uterine relaxant and is used in preterm labor as tocolytic agent.

Other β2 agonists are:

Short acting	Long acting	Very long acting
• Metaproterenol • Albuterol • Levalbuterol • Pirbuterol • Terbutaline • Isoetharine • Fenoterol • Procaterol	• Salmeterol • Formoterol • Arformoterol	• Indacaterol • Olodaterol • Vilanterol

61. Ans. (b) Its plasma hydrolysis by esterase's is rapid

Ref: Goodman & Gillman's 13th ed. P 216-17

- Esmolol is a β1-selective antagonist with a rapid onset and a very short duration of action (t½ = 8 minutes).
- The drug is hydrolyzed rapidly by esterase's in erythrocytes leading to its short half-life.
- Esmolol is used in urgent settings where immediate onset of β-blockade is warranted so it is given by slow intravenous injection.
- A partial loading dose (500 µg/kg over 1 minute) typically is administered, followed by a continuous infusion of the drug (maintenance dose of 50 µg/kg/min for 4 minutes).

> **Extra Mile**
>
> - The lipid solubility of esmolol is low and has no oral bioavailability so it is given via IV.
> - The protein binding of esmolol is 55%.

62. Ans. (b) Given effectively in carbamate poisoning

Ref: Sharma & Sharma 3rd ed. P 146-47

- Organophosphate poisoning causes irreversible blockade of AchE enzyme, which causes cholinergic effects on the patients.
- Symptoms are: salivation, lacrimation, urination, diarrhea, GI upset, emsesis, fasciculation, bradycardia, miosis, hypotension, restlessness, tremor, ataxia.
- Immediate management is done by atropine.
- Treatment is done by using AChE enzyme reactivating drugs along with atropine.
- AChE reactivating drugs are: Pralidoxime (PAM), obidoxime and Diacetyl=monoxime (DAM).
- Initially, atropine is injected in a dose of 2 mg IV q 10–15 minutes until muscarinic symptoms disappear.
- Thereafter pralidoxime 1–2 g is **given by slow IV infusion** over 15–30 minutes to reactivate AChE.
- Pralidoxime and obidoxime does not crosses BBB, hence cannot activate AChE inhibited in the brain. Therefore DAM which can cross BBB is used in such cases.

63. Ans. (b) Clonidine

Ref: Sleisenger and Fordtran's Gastrointestinal and Liver Disease, Volume 1; P 575

- Diabetic diarrhea is seen in middle aged type 1 poorly controlled diabetic patients and is characterized by intermittent, brown, watery and voluminous stools which is occasionally accompanied by tenesmus.
- In these patients GI adrenergic function is impaired in autonomic neuropathy. Therefore any adrenergic agonist may further stimulate the intestinal absorption of fluid and electrolytes.

Drugs used are

- **Alpha 2 adrenergic agonist: Clonidine.** Acts as adrenergic antagonist which acts by reversing the peripheral adrenergic resorptive abnormalities.
  - Because of autonomic neuropathies, these patients will not experience postural hypotension.
  - Moreover, clonidine doesn't alter diabetic control or renal function.
- **Somatostatin analogue: Octreotide.** Useful in refractory diabetic diarrhea
- **Codeine, Diphenoxylate with atropine, Loperamide:** Used for symptomatic treatment.

Extra Mile

Anti diarrheal agents

Drugs	Main uses
Tryptophan hydroxylase inhibitor: Telotristat ethyl	Severe diarrhea due to carcinoid tumors
Enkephalinase inhibitor- Racecadotril	Acute diahhrea Safe in children
Octreotide	• Severe secretory diarrhea due to GI tumors • Postgastrectomy dumping syndrome
Crofelemer (plant derived)	HIV/AIDS diarrhea
Alosetron	• Diarrhea-predominant IBS in women
Bile acid sequestrants: Cholestyramine, Colesevelam, Colestipiol	Bile salt induced diarreha
Clonidine	Diabetic diarrhea
MOR agonists • Diphenoxylate, difenoxin, Loperamide	Acute diarrhea Chronic diarrhea Traveler's diarrhea
Antibiotics—empiric therapy • Fluoroquinolone • Ciprofloxacin • Levofloxacin • Norfloxacin • Ofloxacin **Alternative antibiotics** • Azithromycin • Rifaximin	• Acute diarrhea • Traveler's diarrhea • **Azithromycin:** Preferred treatment for children with traveler's diarrhea • **Rifaxamin:** Preferred for diarrhea predominant IBS

64. Ans. (a) Inhibition of release of neurotransmitter

Ref: KD Tripathi, 7th ed. pg. 99

- Release of Ach from nerve terminals occurs in small quanta—amount contained in individual vesicles is extruded by exocytosis.

- Two toxins interfere with cholinergic transmission by affecting release:
  - **Botulinum toxin** inhibits release
  - **Black widow spider toxin** induces massive release and depletion
- **Botulinum toxin**
  - Botulinum toxin A and B are highly potent exotoxins produced by **Clostridium botulinum** that are responsible for 'botulism' (a type of food poisoning). These neurotoxic proteins cause long-lasting loss of cholinergic transmission by interacting with axonal proteins involved in exocytotic release of Ach.

65. Ans. (b) Presynaptic inhibition of release of acetylcholine

Ref: Katzung, 10th ed. Ch 27

- Botulinum toxin is a neuromuscular blocking agent which acts at neuromuscular junction by **blocking the presynaptic release of Ach vesicles.**
- Doing so, it reduces spasticity in a variety of neurologic conditions (ie, **spasmolytics**).
- **Note:** *Neuromuscular blocking drugs interfere with transmission at the neuromuscular end plate and lack central nervous system activity.*

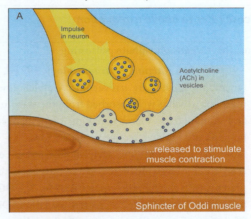
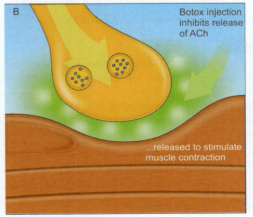

FMGE Solutions Screening Examination

Extra Mile

TABLE: MOA of drugs and their site

Drug	Site of action	MOA
Local anesthetics	Nerve axons	Block Na channels
Hemicholinium	At cholinergic nerve terminal	Blocks uptake of cholin and slows synthesis
Vesamicol	Cholinergic terminal veicle	Prevents storage, depletes
Reserpine	Adrenergic terminal vesicle	Prevents storage, depletes
Tyramine, Amphetamine	Adrenergic nerve terminals	Promote transmitter release
Bethanechol	Receptors, parasympathetic effector cells (smooth muscle, glands)	Binds and activates muscarinic receptors
Atropine	Receptors, parasympathetic effector cells	Binds muscarinic receptors; prevents activation

66. Ans. (c) Presynaptic blockade

Please refer to above explanation

67. Ans. (b) Organophosphate poisoning

Ref: Katzung Pharamacology, 14th ed. pg. 115

- Organophosphates are irreversible Acetylcholinesterase inhibitor which is well absorbed from the skin, lung, gut, and conjunctiva—thereby making them dangerous to humans and highly effective as insecticides.
- Due to inhibition of acetylcholinesterase enzyme, acetylcholine levels are increased and the patient therefore presents with cholinergic symptoms: *(Mn: SLUDGE-FB)*
- Salivation, Lacrimation, increased urination, Diarreha, GI distress, Emesis, Faciculation, Bradycardia
- DOC for this poisoning: **ATROPINE**

Extra Mile

OXIMES (Pralidoximes, Di-Acetyl monoxime) are known as AchE enzyme reactivators. These are used only in organophosphate poisoning.

Pin-point pupil is seen in poisoning with: *(Mn: POMP)*
Pontine hemorrhage, Organophosphate, Morphine and Phenol poisoning

68. Ans. (c) Atropine poisoning

Ref: Katzung Pharamacology, 14th ed. pg. 127–28

Refer to above explanation

69. Ans. (b) Dryness

Ref: Katzung'a Pharamacology, 14th ed. pg. 126

- **Anti-cholinergic agent/Muscarinic antagonists** are the class of drugs which competitively inhibit the effect of acetylcholine at muscarinic receptors. Therefore decreasing secretion from glands leading to DRYNESS.
- **Anti-cholinergic side-effect can be remembered by this mnemonic:**
  - Hot as hare- increased temperature
  - Blind as bat- mydriasis
  - Dry as bone- Dry mouth, dry eye, dry skin
  - Red as beet- Flushed face
  - Mad as hatter: Delirium

Extra Mile

- Indirect acting Cholinergic agents increases the acetylcholine level by blocking acetylcholine esterase enzyme (Ex: Organophosphate, Carbamate).
- The patient therefore will present with cholinergic symptoms: *(Mn: SLUDGE-FB)*
Salivation, Lacrimation, increased urination, Diarrhea, GI distress, Emesis, Fasciculation, Bradycardia
- DOC for this OP poisoning: **ATROPINE**

70. Ans. (d) OP poisoning

Ref: Katzung, 14th ed. pg. 115; KDT, 7th ed. pg. 111

- Neostigmine is a cholinergic agent which act by inhibiting cholinergic esterase enzyme, thereby increasing acetylcholine level at the synapse.
- Ach in eyes causes miosis
- **Uses of Physostigmine**: Atropine/Belladona poisoning
- **Uses of Neostigmine**: Myasthenia Gravis, Snake bite, Curare poisoning, post operative paralytic ileus, reversal of neuromascular blockade.
- **Uses of Rivastigmine**: Alzheimer's disease and parkinsonism
- **DOC for organo-phosphate poisoning**: Atropine

71. Ans. (c) Parasympathetic nerve

Ref: Katzung, 14th ed. pg. 127; KD Tripathi, 7th ed. P 101

Cholinergic receptors are:

- M_1: The M_1 is primarily a neuronal receptor located in ganglion cells and central neurons, especially in cortex, hippocampus and corpus striatum. It plays a major role in mediating gastric secretion, relaxation of lower esophageal sphincter (LES) caused by vagal stimulation, and in learning, memory, motor functions, etc.
- M_2: Cardiac muscarinic receptors are predominantly M_2 and mediate vagal bradycardia. Autoreceptors on cholinergic nerve endings are also M_2 subtype.

Pharmacology

- M_3: Visceral smooth muscle contraction and glandular secretions are elicited through M_3 receptors, which also mediate vasodilatation through EDRF release. Together the M_2 and M_3 preceptors mediate most of the well-recognized muscarinic actions including contraction of LES.

72. Ans. (b) M2 agonist

Ref: Katzung, 14th ed. pg. 127; KD Tripathi, 7th ed. P 101

TABLE: Muscarinic receptors

	M1	M2	M3
Site	CNS Stomach	Heart	All remaining
Func:	Gastric secretion CNS excitation	Dec HR	Increase everything
Agonist:	Oxotremorine	Methaholine	Bethanechol
Antagonist	Pirenzepine Telenzepine	Tripitramine	Tolterodine Darifenacin

73. Ans. (d) M2 antagonist

Ref: Sharma & Sharma 3rd ed. pg. 119

Refer to above explanation

74. Ans. (d) Neuromuscular junction

Ref: Sharma & Sharma 3rd ed. pg. 117

- Alpha bungaratoxin is extracted from venom of elapid snake.
- It acts by neuromuscular junction blocking, therefore producing muscular weakness, respiratory failure like symptoms.

TABLE: Nicotinic receptors

	Nn	Nm
Site	At all autonm ganglia, Adrenal medulla	NMJ
Func:	Impulse transmission NE/E secretion	Skeletal ms contraction
Agonist:	Epibatidine, Nicotine, DMPP	Ach, Sch, PTMA
Antagonist	Hexamethonium Trimethaphan	D- Tubocurarine, α- Bungaratoxin

75. Ans. (a) Urinary incontinence

- Ipratropium and Tiotropium is long acting muscarinic antagonist.
- Ipratropium bromide, given as inhalation, shows transient local side effects like dry mouth, irritation in trachea and bad taste.

- But systemic effects like urinary retention are rare because of poor absorption from GIT and lungs.

76. Ans. (a) Decreasing phosphodiesterase activity

Aminophylline and other methylxanthines act by

- Inhibiting phosphodiesterase enzyme causing – cAMP
- Blocking adenosine receptors
- Releasing Ca^{2+} from sarcoplasmic reticulum in cardiac and skeletal muscles.
- Use–Asthma, COPD, chronic bronchitis

77. Ans. (a) Oxybutynin

Ref: KD Tripathi, 6th ed. pg. 111

- Oxybutynin is a relatively M3 selective muscarinic antagonist which has preferential action on urinary bladder
- It is **indicated in overactive bladder with urinary frequency and urgency.**
- **Drugs which are used in overactive bladder:** *(remembered as: My SOFTT/BlaDder)*
  - Mirabegron (β3 agonist)
  - Solifenacin
  - Oxybutynin
  - Flavoxate, Fesoterodine $\Big\}$ (M_3 Antagonist)
  - Tolterodine, Trospium
  - Darifenacin
- **Note: Mirabegron is beta 3 agonist.** Recently approved for overactive bladder. All other drugs are parasympatholytics acting as M3 antagonist

> **Extra Mile**
> - Alfuzosin is a selective α1 blocker which is used to treat BPH.
> - Bethanechol selectively stimulates M3 receptor present on bladder. It is used in case of atonic bladder (urinary retention).

78. Ans. (a) Bethanechol

Ref: Katzung, 14th ed. pg. 109; KD Tripathi, 6th ed. pg. 111-12

- Bethanechol has mainly muscarinic action without effect on nicotinic receptors and is used to treat urinary retention secondary to general anaesthesia or diabetic neuropathy.
- Bethanechol is totally resistant to hydrolysis by AchE as well as by pseudocholinesterase and hence its t1/2 is very long.
- **Other uses of bethanechol:**
  - To reverse post op or neurogenic bladder atony.
  - To treat GI atony/post op paralytic ileus
  - To treat salivary gland malfunction (xerostomia).
- **Side effects:**
  - Hyperthyroidism, MI (due to risk of developing conduction block), peptic ulcer, asthma exacerbation.

Explanations

79. Ans. (c) Alpha 1 and Beta 2

Ref: Katzung, 14th ed. pg. 145–47

- Alpha 1 and Beta 2 receptors present at blood vessels causing vasoconstriction and vasodilatation respectively.

TABLE: Sympathetic receptors, their location, function and G protein.

Receptor	Location	Function	G-Protein
α1	BV, smooth muscle, Salivary glands	Vasoconstriction Increse secretion	Gq
α2	Presynapse Beta pancreatc cell	Brake/Inhibit NA release Decrease insulin release	Gi
β1	Heart JG cell	Inc Heart rate Renin release	Gs
β2	Lungs Smooth muscle Liver	Bronchodilatation Relaxation of smooth muscles Glycogenolysis	Gs
β3	Adipocyte Detrusor muscle	Lipolysis, thermogenesis Bladder relax	Gs

80. Ans. (c) Stimulation of parasympathetic fiber

Ref: Katzung, 14th ed. pg. 130

- Sympathetic and parasympathetic fibers present widely on the viscera, control their function.
- **Sympathetic fibers** stimulate/constrict heart (increase in HR) and inhibit/Relax all other organs (e.g. Bronchodilation, decreased GI motility, mydriasis, etc.)
    - **Receptor** of sympathetic fibres are: **β1** (present on heart mainly) and **β2** (present on lungs, muscle, liver, etc.)
    - Stimulation of β2 receptor will cause bronchodilation/Increased bronchial calibre
- **Parasympathetic fibers** inhibit/Relax heart (decreased HR) and stimulate/constrict all other organs (broncho-constriction/**reduced bronchial caliber (bronchoconstriction)**, increased GI motility, miosis, etc.)
    - **Receptors** of parasympathetic fibres are M1, M2 and M3
    - M1 is located mainly in gastric glands and CNS, M2 is located on heart and M3 is located on all other areas like eyes, glands, bladder, instestine, etc.

81. Ans. (a) Increase BP, bradycardia

Ref: Katzung, 14th ed. pg. 141–41; KDT, 6th ed. pg. 122

- Epinephrine (adrenaline) and Norepinephrine (NA) are endogenous catecholamine. These are the hormones responsible for actions like bradycardia and tachycardia by acting on their specific receptors.
- *Systolic blood pressure* (SBP) is *determined by cardiac output (β1 action)*. β1 receptors are present on heart which upon stimulation causes tachycardia.
- *Diastolic BP* (DBP) depends on the state of blood vessels. β2 receptors are present on blood vessels which upon stimulation causes vasodilation → DBP ↓
- Alpha receptors are present on vessel wall, which upon stimulation constricts vessel wall and increase total peripheral resistance → DBP ↑
- *Increased DBP stimulates* baroreceptor mediated release of ACh (reflex action) that decreases heart rate via activation of M2 receptors.
- Reduction in DBP increases central sympathetic outflow and thereby increases heart rate.
- *Note:* NA normally decreases heart rate but if given after a dose of atropine, increase in heart rate will be seen (*reflex action is abolished because of blockage of M2 receptor*).
- Adrenaline acts on α1, α2, β1, β2 receptors whereas Noradrenaline acts on α1, α2, β1. Which means.
    - Activation of adrenaline causes tachycardia (β1 action) and NO effect on DBP because action of α1 and β2 are neutralized by each other.
    - Activation of NA causes ↑DBP (due to unopposed α1 action) and reflex bradycardia.

	SBP (β1)	DBP (β2 and α1)	Heart rate Direct	Heart rate Indirect	Heart rate Net Effect
Adrenaline/ epinephrine	↑↑	–	↑	–	↑
Noradrenaline/ NE	↑↑	↑↑	↑	↓↓	↓

82. Ans. (a) Beta 1

Ref: Katzung, 14th ed. pg. 149; KDT, 6th ed. pg. 126

- Dobutamine is a relatively selective β1 agonist. Though it acts on both alpha and beta receptors, *the only prominent action of clinically employed doses is its β1 action, i.e. an increase in force of cardiac contraction and output, without significant change in HR, BP or peripheral resistance.*
- **Use:** Heart failure (*as an ionotrope*)

83. Ans. (b) Orthostatic hypotension

Ref: Katzung's Pharmacology, 14th ed. pg. 149

- Midodrine is a directly acting sympathomimetics (*selective α1 receptor agonist non catecholamines*).

Pharmacology

- Primary indication of midodrine is the **treatment of orthostatic hypotension**, typically due to impaired autonomic nervous system function.
- It may also cause hypertension when patient is supine.

Mechanism of Action

- Alpha-1 selective adrenergic agonist; increases peripheral vascular resistance; arteriolar and venous tone increases and results in a rise in sitting, standing, and supine systolic and diastolic blood pressure in patients with orthostatic hypotension.
- **Side effects:** Paresthesia, Piloerection, Pruritus, Supine hypertension, Urinary retention or urgency.
- **Orthostatic hypotension**; defined as a reduction in systolic blood pressure of at least 20 mmHg or diastolic blood pressure of at least 10 mmHg within 3 minutes of standing or head-up tilt on a tilt table. It is a manifestation of sympathetic vasoconstrictor (autonomic) failure.
- **Delayed orthostatic hypotension**; occurs beyond 3 minutes of standing; this may reflect a mild or early form of sympathetic adrenergic dysfunction.

---

84. Ans. (b) Salbutamol

Ref: Katzung 11th ed. Ch 2

- Tachyphylaxis is an acute rapid decrease in response to a drug after its administration. It can occur after an initial dose or after a series of small doses.
- Inhalation of an agonist for the beta-2 adrenergic receptor, such as **Salbutamol,** Albuterol (US), is the most common treatment for asthma. *Polymorphisms of the beta-2 receptor play a role in tachyphylaxis.*
- Increasing the dose of the drug may be able to restore the original response.
- **Drug causing tachyphylaxis: (SAD NET/*Cigarette*)**
  - Salbutamol
  - Amphetamine
  - Dobutamine
  - Nicotine
  - Ephedrine
  - Tyramine

---

85. Ans. (c) Nadolol

Ref: Katzung Pharma, 14th ed. pg. 162–166

- The β antagonists are rapidly distributed and have large volumes of distribution.
- Most β antagonists have half-lives in the range of 3–10 hours. A major exception is esmolol, which is rapidly hydrolyzed and has a half-life of approximately 10 minutes. *Therefore esmolol is the shortest acting β blocker.*
- **Nadolol** is excreted unchanged in the urine and *has the longest half-life* of any available β antagonist (up to 24 hours).

- The half-life of nadolol is prolonged in renal failure. Therefore it is contraindicated in renal failure.
- β blockers which are contraindicated in renal failure are: (*remember as ANS*)
  - Atenolol
  - Nadolol
  - Sotalol

> **Extra Mile**
>
> **"ALSO KNOW" ABOUT β BLOCKERS:**
> - β1 **receptors** are present mainly on heart. Therefore selective β 1 BLOCKERS are for cardiac condition mainly.
> - β2 **receptors** are present mainly on respiratory pathway and some on liver, uterus, bladder etc. therefore β2 stimulators are used in conditions like asthma, preterm labor, urinary incontinence etc.
> - Most cardioselective β blocker- **NEBIVOLOL**
> - Longest acting- **NADOLOL**
> - Shortest acting- **ESMOLOL**
> - β blockers which is DOC in open angle glaucoma in India-**TIMOLOL**

---

86. Ans. (a) Esmolol

Ref: KDT, 6th ed. pg. 147

- Esmolol is an ultra short acting, cardio-selective β blocker devoid of partial agonistic or membrane stabilizing effect.
- It is metabolized by pseudocholineestrase, which is abundant in our body. thereby making it least likely to cause hypotension followed by or during surgery.
- **It is used in:**
  - Terminating supraventricular tachycardia
  - Episodic atrial fibrillation or flutter
  - Arrhythmia during anaesthesia
  - To reduce BP and HR during cardiac surgery and early treatment of MI.

---

87. Ans. (b) Acebutalol

Ref: Katzung, 14th ed. pg. 166; KDT, pg. 140

- Some patients are sensitive to beta blockers. They usually develop bradycardia upon intake. Such patients are known as β-blocker sensitive patient.
- However, some beta blockers possess **Intrinsic Sympathomimetic Activity** (ISA) aka partial agonistic activity. For such sensitive patients, beta blockers with partial agonistic activity are preferred.
- These drugs themselves activate β1 or β2 receptors sub-maximally.
- **Benefits:**
  - Bradycardia and depression of contractility at rest are not prominent.
  - Withdrawal doesn't exacerbate hypertension or angina.

- **Beta Blockers With Partial Agonistic Activity**
  (Remembered as **Mn. COP Pins CAB**)
  - **C**eliprolol, **O**xprenolol, **P**enbutolol
  - **Pin**dolol
  - **C**arteolol
  - **A**cebutalol
  - **B**opindolol

88. Ans. (b) **Propanolol**

    Ref: Katzung, 14th ed. pg. 166; KDT, 6th ed. pg. 140

    Please refer to above explanation.

89. Ans. (c) **Alprenolol**

    Ref: Katzung, 14th ed. pg. 166

    Please refer to above explanation.

90. Ans. (a) **Atenolol**

    Ref: Katzung, 14th ed. pg. 179; KDT 6th ed. pg. 140 table 10.2

    Lipid insoluble β blockers: These agents are mainly excreted by kidney and are therefore contraindicated in renal failure. These have long duration of action. The drugs are:
    - Nadolol (longest acting β blockers)
    - Sotalol
    - **Atenolol**
    - Acebutolol
    - Betaxolol
    - Bisoprolol
    - Celioprolol

91. Ans. (d) **Carvedilol**

    Ref: Katzung, 14th ed. pg. 160–164; KDT, 7th ed. pg. 151
    - Carvedilol is a third generation beta blocker having blocking property of β1 + β2 + α1.
    - It produces peripheral vasodilation due to blocking property of α1 as well as L type calcium channel blocker.
    - Carvedilol also inhibits free radical induced lipid peroxidation.
    - Other third generation beta blocker having similar property is Labetalol Bucindolol.

92. Ans. (b) **Tolazoline**

    Ref: KDT, 6th ed. pg. 132
    - α1 receptor is further divided in α1A receptor (present on bladder neck and urethra) and α1B (on blood vessel)
    - **Selective α1A blocker:** TAMSULOSIN, SILODOSIN (causes relaxation of urethra and bladder neck)

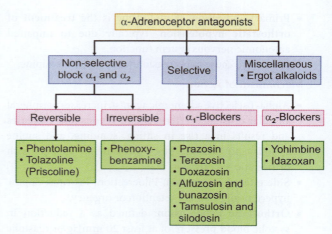

Question Forms
- Hypertensive patient with benign prostatic hyperplasia. What is the DOC: α1 **selective blocker** (PRAZOSIN/TERAZOSIN/DOXAZOSIN/ALFUZOSIN)
- **Non hypertensive patient with BPH. What is DOC:** TAMSULOSIN (selective α1A blocker)
- Side effect of selective α1 blocker: Postural Hypotension
- DOC for pheochromocytoma- PHENOXYBENZAMINE
- DOC for cheese reaction and clonidine induced rebound hypertension- PHENTOLAMINE, TOLAZOLINE

93. Ans. (d) **Prazosin**

    Ref: Katzung, 14th ed. pg. 159
    - **First dose effect** is sudden severe hypotension while changing position from lying to a standing position after first dose intake of alpha blocker, ACE inhibitor.
    - Most common class of drug for causing first dose effect: **selective alpha-1 blocker**
    - **Selective alpha-1 blocker Drugs:**
      - **Prazosin:** *Most common among all*
      - Terazosin
      - Doxazosin
      - Alfuzosin
    - Other drugs that can cause first dose effect is: Phentolamine, Tolazoline, Phenoxybenzamine.

94. Ans. (d) **Phenoxybenzamine**

    Ref: Katzung, 14th ed. pg. 170
    - **Phenoxybenzamine** binds covalently to α receptors, causing **irreversible blockade** of long duration.
    - It is DOC for pheochromocytoma
    - Examples of reversible α blocker is: Phentolamine, Tolazoline
    - **Clonidine** is α2 agonist
    - **Isoprenaline** is beta agonist (acts at β1 and β2)

Pharmacology

95. Ans. (a) Pilocarpine

Ref: Katzung, 14th ed. pg. 112

- Agents which dilate the pupillary diameter in order to facilitate fundoscopy are known as mydriatics.
- Eyes are mainly innervated by cholinergic (parasympathetic) nerves which predominantly secrete acetylcholine, which acts at circular iridis muscle causing miosis.
- Stimulation of parasympathetic system constricts pupillary diameter (miosis) while stimulation of sympathetic system dilates pupillary diameter (mydriasis).
- Anticholinergic (e.g. atropine) and sympathomimetic (e.g. phenylephrine) drugs result in mydriasis.
- Pilocarpine is a parasympathomimetic drug, which upon stimulation constricts the pupillary diameter (miosis). Used in treatment of Glaucoma.
- Atropine is a parasympatholytic drug which act as mydriatic and cycloplegic agent as well.
  - **Mydriasis:** used for fundoscopy, for full visualization of retina. Contraindicated in Glaucoma.
  - **Cycloplegic:** paralysis of ciliary muscle. Used predominantly in treatment of iridocyclitis (anterior uveitis).
- Agents like epinephrine and phenylephrine are sympathomimetic drugs, which acts at radial muscles and causes pupillary dilatation.

96. Ans. (c) Phentolamine

Ref: Katzung, 14th ed. pg. 170

- Phentolamine is an alpha blocker and can cause miosis not mydriasis *(because alpha 1 agonist in the eye causes mydriasis).*

97. Ans. (c) Tropicamide

Ref: KDT, 8th ed. pg. 130

- Agents which dilate the pupillary diameter in order to facilitate fundoscopy are known as mydriatics. These are anti-muscarinic class of drugs.

TABLE: Anti-muscarinic drugs used in ophthalmology

Drug	Duration of Effect (days)
Atropine	7–10
Scopolamine	3–7
Homatropine	1–3
Cyclopentolate	1
Tropicamide	0.25 days (6 hrs)

- These agents have mydriatic as well as cycloplegic action both.

Extra Mile

- Strongest cycloplegic is: **Atropine**
- Cycloplegic agent of choice in child: **Atropine** (child age group has strong ciliary muscles)
- Cycloplegic agent of choice in adults: **Tropicamide**

98. Ans. (a) Anti-venin

Ref: KDT, 6th ed. pg. 2748

- General time guidelines for the disappearance of symptoms after anti-venom administration are as follows:
  - **Centruroides anti-venom:** Severe neurologic symptoms reverse in 15-30 min. Mild-to-moderate neurologic symptoms reverse in 45-90 min.
  - **Non-Centruroides anti-venom:** In the first hour, local pain abates. In 6-12 hours, agitation, sweating, and hyperglycemia abate. In 6-24 hours, cardio-respiratory symptoms abate.
- Insulin administration in scorpion envenomation animal experiments has helped the vital organs to use metabolic substrates more efficiently, thus preventing venom-induced multiorgan failure, especially cardiopulmonary failure. *Unfortunately, no human studies have been conducted.*
- The use of steroids to decrease shock and edema is of unproven benefit.
- Atropine for symptomatic bradycardia.

Remember

- Scorpion venom is composed of neurotoxin cardiotoxin, nephrotoxin, hemolytic toxin, phosphodiesterases, phospholipases, hyaluronidases, glycosaminoglycans, histamine, serotonin, tryptophan, and cytokine releasers.
- *Hence the clinical effects of envenomation are neuromuscular, neuro-autonomic, or local tissue effects.*
- The main targets of scorpion venom are voltage-dependent ion channels, of which sodium channels are mainly affected.
- Alpha blocker like **Prazosin** can also be used for this purpose.

99. Ans. (b) Tolterodine

Ref: KD Tripathi, 8th ed. pg. 129

TOLTERODINE

- This M3 selective muscarinic antagonist has preferential action on urinary bladder
- It is indicated in overactive bladder with urinary frequency and urgency.

FMGE Solutions Screening Examination

> **Extra Mile**
>
> Pirenzepine is selective M1 blocker which is an antacid given for PUD.
> Alfuzosin is a selective α1 blocker which is used to treat BPH.
> Bethanechol selectively stimulate M3 receptor present on bladder. It is used in case of atonic bladder (urinary retention).

100. Ans. (b) Anticholinergic

Ref: KDT 8th ed. pg. 129

MOA oxybutynin-cholinergic-*muscarinic* receptor antagonist

- Oxybutynin is a selective M_3 receptor blocker, used to relieve bladder spasm after urologic surgery, eg, prostatectomy.
- It is also used to relieve urinary and bladder difficulties, including frequent urination and inability to control urination, by decreasing muscle spasms of the bladder.
- It competitively antagonizes the M3 subtypes of the muscarinic acetylcholine receptor.
- **M3 receptor blockers:** *Mn: MY SOFT blaDar*
    - **Solifenacin, Oxybutynin, Flavoxate, Fesoterodine, Tolterodine, Trospium and Darifenacin.**

101. Ans. (b) Pilocarpine

Ref: KDT, 8th ed. pg. 167

- **Pilocarpine** is a directly acting parasympathomimetic (cholinergic) drug which acts mainly on pupil (M3) causes miosis.
- Reduces IOP within few minutes and lasts for upto 4–8 hrs
- Hence used in Glaucoma (OAG) patients.
- **Methacholine** is a directly acting parasympathomimetic (cholinergic) drug which acts mainly on myocardium (M2) causing bradycardia. Hence used to treat tachycardia and can also be used to diagnose bronchial hyperactivity *(methacholine challenge test)*.
    - **Half life:** > 2 hours
- **Bethanechol** is directly acting parasympathomimetic (cholinergic) drug which works on bladder (M3) and is used in acute urinary retention/Atonic bladder.
    - **Half life:** ~ 2 hours
- **Cevimeline** is recently approved drug used for xerostomia in sjogren syndrome or for patients undergoing chemotherapy.

CNS AND PNS

102. Ans. (d) Delta

Ref: Goodman & Gillman 13th ed. P 358

Opioid receptors	
Opioid receptor class	**Effects**
MU_1	Euphoria, supraspinal analgesia, confusion, dizziness, nausea, low addiction potential
MU_2	Respiratory depression, cardiovascular and gastrointestinal effects, miosis, urinary retention
Delta	Spinal analgesia, cardiovascular depression, decreased brain and myocardial oxygen demand
Kappa	Spinal analgesia, dysphoria, psychomimetic effects, feedback inhibition of endorphin system

> **Extra Mile**
>
> - Sigma (σ) receptor was early identified and was thought to represent a site that accounted for the paradoxical excitatory effects of opiates.
> - Agonist binding to the σ receptor is not antagonized by naloxone, and the receptor is not classified as an opiate receptor.

103. Ans. (b) Cognitive therapy

Ref: Goodman & Gillman 13th ed. P 281-282

- For acute manic attacks, preferred agents are atypical antipsychotics, benzodiazepines, anticonvulsants (Valproate, carbamazepine), Lithium
- All atypical antipsychotics medications with the exception of clozapine, iloperidone, brexpiprazole, and lurasidone, have indications for acute mania, and doses are titrated rapidly close to or at the maximum FDA-approved dose over the first 24–72 hours of treatment. Typical antipsychotic drugs are also effective in acute mania, but often are eschewed due to the risk for EPSs.

104. Ans. (d) Hyperalgesia

Ref: Goodman & Gillman's 14th ed. pg. 363-64

- Effect of morphine is seen mainly at μ-receptor. Effect on μ-receptor depends on either supraspinal or spinal μ- receptor.
    - **Supraspinal effects:** Physical dependence, euphoria, analgesia, sedation. (PEAS)
    - **Spinal effects:** Constipation, analgesia and respiratory depression. (CAR)
- **Effect of morphine at heart:** No effect at usual dose but at high dose it can cause bradycardia and hypotension.
- **Effect of morphine at eye:** No effect if applied locally. Miosis on systemic intake. Miosis can be worsened to pin point pupil upon systemic morphine toxicity.

Pharmacology

Note: *Morphine causes analgesia. Hyperalgesia is one of the withdrawal symptoms.*

105. Ans. (c) Propanolol

Ref: KDT 8th ed. P 471

Explanation:

- **Akathisia** is an extra pyramidal symptom arise mainly due to intake of typical antipsychotics like haloperidol, fluphenazine, etc.
- It is characterized by restlessness, feeling of discomfort and constant purposeless involuntary movement from one place to another.
- **Akathisia** is the *most common* **extra pyramidal symptom.**
  DOC for akathisia: PROPRANOLOL

106. Ans. (c) Ramelteon

Ref: KD Tripathi, 8th ed. pg. 436

- The most common prescription drugs for insomnia incude: Benzodiazepines, nonbenzodiazepines, hypnotics, ramelteon as well as some anti-depressants.

> **Extra Mile**

Types of insomnia, their causes and the drugs used

Insomnia	Causes	Drugs used
Transient insomnia	Lasts less than 7 days Jet lag, Shift work, new place, overnight journey	Rapid onset and short duration of action **Triazolam:** in patients with difficulty going to sleep **Temazepam:** for insomnia caused by inability to stay asleep. Zolpidem, Zoleplon
Short term insomnia	Lasts 1-3 weeks Due to expected but self limiting problems like bereavement, pain, occupational issue.	Flurazepam, Estrazolam, Temazepam Zopiclone, Eszopiclone
Long term insomnia	Lasts > 3weeks Indicates underlying disease or a personality disorder	Flurazepam, Nitrazepam Intermittent use with a break after every 3rd day

- Benzodiazepines are first-line drugs of choice for short-term management of insomnia, especially for reducing the sleep latency (time to sleep onset).
- Among benzodiazepines, Triazolam is effective in treating individuals who have difficulty going to sleep, while temazepam is useful for insomnia caused by inability to stay asleep.
- Lorazepam, Diazepam and Midazolam is used as preanesthtic drug. It causes high degree of amnesia, has more rapid onset and shorter duration of action.
- *Recently approved Melatonin receptor agonist, Ramelteon is used for sleep onset insomnia, especially in the treatment of circadian disruptions induced by shift work and jet lag.*
- 5HT2 serotonin receptor antagonist, **Ritanserin**, has improved sleep depth and sleep quality.

107. Ans. (a) Clozapine

Ref: KD Tripathi, 7th ed. pg. 440-41

TABLE: Classification of typical vs atypical antipsychotics

Typical/Classical antipsychotics MOA: D2 receptor blocking	• **Phenothiazines:** Chlorpromazine, Thioridazine, Trifluperazine, Fluphenazine, Perphenazine • **Thioxanthenes:** Flupenthixol, Zuclopenthixol, Thiothixene • **Butyrophenones:** Haloperidol, Droperidol, Benperidol, Domperidone
Atypical Antipsychotics MOA: $5HT_{2A}$, D4, D2, α blocking	• Risperidone, Quetiapine, Aripiprazole, Clozapine, Olanzapine, Ziprasidone, Zotepine, Asenapine, Sertidole, Lurasidone

108. Ans. (d) Clozapine

Ref: KD Tripathi, 8th ed. pg. 468

Side effects of Typical vs Atypical

Typical antipsychotics	Atypical antipsychotics
Major side effect: *Extrapyramidal symptoms* • Dystonia: Earliest • Akathisia: MC • Parkinsonism • Neuroleptic malignant syndrome: Most dangerous • Perioral tremors (Rabbit syndrome) • Tardive dyskinesia	*Lipodystrophy syndrome:* metabolic side effect present with hyperglycemia, hyperlipidemia, weight gain and insulin resistance.

Explanations

FMGE Solutions Screening Examination

- Among antipsychotics, maximum risk of lipodystrophy syndrome is seen with atypical antipsychotics (MC with CLOZAPINE).
- First antisuicidal drug: Clozapine
- Other side effects of clozapine: **Sedation, Sialorhea, Agranulocytosis**
- DOC for resistant schizophrenia: Clozapine
- Atypical antipsychotics Least commonly associated with lipodystrophy syndrome are **Ziprasidone** and **risperidone**
- Typical antipsychotic with least extra pyramidal symptoms (EPS): **Thioridazine** (low potency drug)
- Atypical antipsychotic with least EPS is clozapina.

109. Ans. (b) Carbamazapine

Ref: KDT 8th ed. pg. 464

- Extra pyramidal side effect or aka Extra pyramidal symptom (EPS) is due to excess blockade of dopamine receptors in basal ganglia, leading to Parkinson like symptoms such as slow movement (bradykinesia), akathisia, stiffness and tremor.
- EPS most commonly seen with the intake of typical antipsychotics, which blocks D2 receptors.

Typical antipsychotics		Important side effect
Strong D2 blocker	Haloperidol- *has maximum risk of EPS* Droperidol	EPS Hyperprolactinemia
Weak D2 blocker	Chlorpromazine Thioridazine – *has minimum risk of EPS among typicals*	EPS Corneal opacity, Retinal Pigmentation, Decreases seizure threshold
Intermediate D2 blocker	Fluphenazine Pechlorphenazine	

Extrapyramidal Symptoms

- **Dystonia-** earliest EPS which is seen.
  - R_x for dystonia: Diphenhydramine
- **Akathisia-** most common EPS seen.
  Constant purposeless movement from one place to other.
  - *DOC for Akathisia: PROPANOLOL*
- **Neuroleptic Malignant syndrome:** Severe muscle spasm and high grade fever after intake of anti psychotics.
  - DOC for NMS: DANTROLENE
- It is most dangerous type of EPS

110. Ans. (c) Dantrolene

Ref: KDT, 8h ed. pg. 382

- DOC for NMS: Dantrolene

111. Ans. (c) Propanolol

Ref: KDT, 8th ed. pg. 471

- **Akathisia** is an extra pyramidal symptom that arises mainly due to intake of typical anti psychotics like haloperidol, fluphenazine etc.
- It is characterized by restlessness, feeling of discomfort and constant purposeless involuntary movement from one place to another without any source of anxiety.
- **Akathisia is the *most common* extra pyramidal symptom.**
- DOC for akathisia: **PROPANOLOL.**

112. Ans. (b) Clozapine

Ref: KDT 8th ed. pg. 467

- Among given option Clozapine is the only atypical antipsychotics. As discussed earlier, atypical antipsychtics has less risk of EPS development as compared to typical antipsychotics.
- Overall least risk of EPS among atypicals is: Clozapine

113. Ans. (a) Aripiprazole

Ref: KDT 8th ed. pg. 467

- Among given choice, least risk of EPS among atypicals is: ARIPIPRAZOLE.
- Typicals always has high EPS.

114. Ans. (c) Prochlorperazine

Ref: KDT 8th ed. pg. 711

- EPS most commonly seen with the intake of typical antipsychotics, which blocks D2 receptors.
- **Prochlorperazine** is a dopamine (D2) receptor antagonist that belongs to the phenothiazine class of antipsychotic agents that are **used for the antiemetic treatment of nausea and vertigo.** It is also a highly potent typical antipsychotic, 10–20× more potent than chlorpromazine.

Now lets see other options:
- **Cyclizine:** Anti-histaminics, used for nasuea and vomiting associated with motion sickness.
- **Mozapride:** is a gastroprokinetic agent that acts as a selective $5HT_4$ agonist.
- **Domperidone:** Act as anti-emetic by blocking D2 and D3 peripherally. It has no CNS side effects.

115. Ans. (d) Quetipaine

- Antipsychotic which is associated with lenticular opacity/Cataract: **Quetiapine**
- Antipsychotic associated with corneal opacity: **Chlorpromazie and Thioridazine**

Pharmacology

116. Ans. (a) Risperidone

Ref: KDT, 8th ed. pg. 469

- Atypicals with maximum risk of hyperprolactinemia is: Risperidone
- Most potent atypical antipsychotic: Risperidone
- Atypicals with least risk of EPS: Clozapine
- Atypicals that can cause cardiac arrhythmias: Sertindole, Zotepine
- **Atypicals with maximum risk of obesity: Clozapine**

117. Ans. (d) Haloperidol

Ref: KDT, 8th ed. pg. 471

Haloperidol is from typical antipsychotic class that is commonly associated with extrapyramidal symptoms like neuroleptic malignant syndrome.

118. Ans. (b) Diazepam

Ref: Katzung's, 11th ed. pg. 462-63

- Anxiety occurvs as a result of mild CNS stimulation which may occur secondary to reduction in GABAergic activity or increase in serotonin activity.
- Therefore, a drug which is used for anxiety is CNS depressant (e.g. Diazepam) or the other which is decreasing serotonin level (e.g. Buspirone, NOT Bupropion).
- **DOC for anxiety attacks: Benzodiazepines**
- **DOC for chronic anxiety disorder: SSRI (Fluoxamine)**
- Anti-serotonergic drugs take around 2 weeks for its therapeutic effect. Hence NOT preferred in acute attack of anxiety.

119. Ans. (b) Ketamine

Ref: Katzung, 11th ed. pg. 437; KDT, 6th ed. pg. 376

- Ketamine is the only intravenous anesthetic that possesses analgesic properties and produces cardiovascular stimulation.
- It causes *"dissociative anesthesia"* which is characterized by profound analgesia, immobility, amnesia and feeling of dissociation from one's own body and the surrounding.
- It has bronchodilator effect therefore considered as Induction agent of choice in asthma patient.
- **In addition it also causes:**
  - Hallucination
  - Delusion and illusion
  - Profound analgesia
- **Ketamine increases all pressures like:**
  - BP (hypertension), Heart rate, Cardiac output
  - Intracranial tension (it increases cerebral blood flow)
  - Intraocular pressure (IOP)
- It is contraindicated in intracerebral mass/haemorrhage, MI, schizophrenia, Epilepsy

MOA of Ketamine:
- It acts by blocking NMDA receptor (of glutamate).

Extra Mile

Side effect of other given options:
- **Propofol:** Apnea, Decreases BP and HR
- **Thiopentone:** Laryngospasm, Shivering & Delirium
- **Etomidate:** Adrenocortical suppression

120. Ans. (b) It is GABA facilitator

Ref: KDT, 7th ed. 402, Katzung, 11th ed. pg. 377

- GABA is an inhibitory neurotransmitter.
- Benzodiazepine helps GABA to open the chloride channel. Once Chloride enters, negativity in the neuron increases (hyperpolarized), which leads to depressed neuron.
- It is barbiturate which is GABA mimetic.

TABLE: Difference between Benzodiazepine and barbiturates

Benzodiazipine	Barbiturates
Increase FREQUENCY of GABA mediated chloride channel opening	Increase DURATION of GABA mediated chloride channel opening
GABA facilitator	GABA mimetic
Dose response curve: flat	Dose-response curve: steep
Safe drug	Unsafe drug
Non-enzyme inducer- no drug interaction	Powerful enzyme inducer; (+)drug interaction
Less amnesia	Causes strong amnesia
Antidote: FLUMAZENIL	No antidote available

121. Ans. (c) GABA facilitator

Ref: KDT, 7th ed. 402, Katzung, 11th ed. 377

122. Ans. (d) Flumazenil

- Flumazenil is antidote of benzodiazepine overdose.

123. Ans. (b) Methylphenidate

Ref: KD Tripathi, 6th ed. pg. 470-471 & 126

- **Methylphenidate** acts by releasing NA and DA in brain and is most widely used for attention deficit hyperkinetic disorder because it causes lesser tachycardia and growth retardation as compared to amphetamine.
- It is considered as DOC of ADHD
- **Modafinil**
  - Psychostimulant agent; used most commonly among night-shift (call centre) workers who need alertness and want to keep awake.
  - Increases attention span and improve accuracy compromised by fatigue and sleepiness.
- Considered as first line drug in narcolepsy.

FMGE Solutions Screening Examination

- **Pemoline**
  - It has CNS stimulant actions similar to those of methylphenidate.
  - It can also be used in ADHD, narcolepsy and excessive day-time sleepiness
  - S/E: Hepatotoxicity, thus it has limited use
- **Amphetamines**
  - It can also be used in ADHD, but not a drug of choice due to highly abusive tendency.
  - The central effects include alertness, increased concentration an attention spam, euphoria, talkativeness increased work capacity
  - Stimulate respiratory centre and Hunger centre is suppressed.

124. Ans. (a) Attention deficit disorder

Ref: KDT, 6th ed. pg. 470

- *Methylphenidate* is the preferred drug for the treatment of *attention deficit hyperkinetic disorder* (ADHD). Other drugs used for this indication are *amphetamines, atomoxetine and pemoline.* **Pemoline** has been withdrawn due to life threatening hepatotoxicity.
- Abuse of drugs like amphetamine, phencyclidine, methylphenidate, flumazenil etc. causes seizure and is NOT used for seizure disorder.
- DOC for alzheimer's disease-Donepezil
- DOC for OCD: Fluoxetine (SSRI)

125. Ans. (b) Alzheimer's disease

Ref: Katzung, 10th ed. Ch 7

- Rivastigmine is a parasympathomimetic drug used for the treatment of mild to moderate dementia of the *Alzheimer's type* and dementia due to Parkinson's disease
- **DOC for alzheimer's disorder**-Donepezil
- **DOC for OCD:** Fluoxetine
- **DOC for parkinsonism:** Levodpa + Carbidopa
- **DOC for drug induced parkinsonism:** Benzhexol (centrally acting anticholinergic)

126. Ans. (d) Ethosuximide

Ref: KD Tripathi, 6th ed. pg. 172 & 406

ETHOSUXIMIDE

- The most prominent action of ethosuximide is antagonism T type calcium channel → Thereby controlling the seizures like absence seizure. It also raises seizure threshold.
- Clinically it is effective only in absence seizures.

> **Extra Mile**
>
> **Drugs used in Prophylaxis of Migraine**
> - **β Adrenergic blockers:** Propranolol is the **most commonly used** drug for prophylaxis of migraine. It reduces frequency as well as severity of attacks in upto 70% patients. DOC for prophylaxis
> - **Tricyclic antidepressants:** amitriptyline has been most extensively tried (25–50 mg at bed time) to reduce migraine attacks.
> - **Calcium channel blockers:** Verapamil was found to reduce migraine attacks, but was judged inferior to propranolol.
> - Anticonvulsants Valproic acid and gabapentin.
> - Topiramate has recently been approved for migraine prohylaxis
> - Ethosuximide is the drug used in absent seizure. It has no role in migraine prophylaxis.

127. Ans. (c) It inhibits peripheral dopa decarboxylase

Ref: Katzung, 14th ed. pg. 495

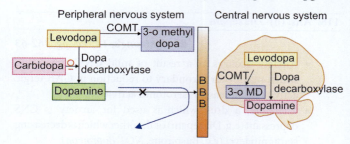

COMT = Catechol othomethyl trasferase, o MD = Ortho methyl dopa, BBB = Blood brain barrier

- In Parkinsons disease the balance between acetylcholine and dopamine (DA) is dearranged in brain.
- DA is comparatively decreased, making Ach on the higher side.
- **Principle of treatment:**
  - Either increase DA (which is the prime treatment modality), or
  - Decrease the lecel of Ach
- Levodopa can be given for treatment but it is immediately converted to DA in periphery itself by the enzyme dopa decarboxylase and causes varied side effects.
- **Note:** Dopamine cannot cross BBB but levodopa can cross it.
- Carbidopa is peripheral dopa decarboxylase inhibitor. It is always added with levodopa in treatment of Parkinsonism to avoid peripheral conversion of levodopa to carbidopa.

128. Ans. (c) Short half life of drug

Ref: Katzung, 14th ed. pg. 494

- **ON-OFF phenomenon:** unpredictable fluctuation between mobility and immobility
  - Due to very short t1/2 of Levodopa: 1-2 hrs
  - To avoid this it is used along with COMT inhibitor → Entacapone, Tolcapone

Pharmacology

129. Ans. (d) Parkinsonism

Ref: Katzung, 14th ed. pg. 501

- Amantadine is an antiviral for Infuenza A. It has been approved for treatment for Parkinson disease as well.
- Best for early stage PD or if patient not responding to L-Dopa
- **Mechanism of action**
- Facilitate DA release from presynaptic dopaminergic neuron and also Prevents DA uptake
- **Side effect:** Confusion, Hallucination, Ankle edema, Livido reticularis

130. Ans. (c) Bromocriptine

Ref: Katzung, 14th ed. pg. 498; KDT, 6th ed. pg. 167

- Ergots are derived from a fungus *Claviceps purpurea.* Important compounds are:
  - *Ergotamine*
  - *Ergometrine (ergonovine),*
  - *Ergotoxine*
  - **Bromocriptine**
  - *Methysergide and LSD.*
- These drugs possess partial agonistic and antagonistic effect at 5HT, α and dopaminergic receptors.
- Ergot derivatives *can cause dry gangrene of hand and feet as well as coronary vasospasm.*
- Ergot derivatives are highly specific for migraine pain; they are not analgesic for any other condition.
- **Bromocriptine** is extremely effective in reducing the high levels of prolactin that result from pituitary tumors and has even been associated with regression of the tumor in some cases.
- **Benzhexol** is DOC for drug induced Parkinsonism.
- **Emmenagogues** are herbs which stimulate blood flow in the pelvic area and uterus; some stimulate menstruation.
- **Ropinirole** and pramipexole is a non-ergot derivative drug, and is used in Parkinsonism.

131. Ans. (b) Bromocriptine

Ref: KDT, 6th ed. pg. 167

- **Bromocriptine** and **pergolide** are ergot derivatives and are used in Parkinsonism. All ergot derivatives can cause **retroperitoneal fibrosis,** cardiac and pleural fibrosis. They can also cause digital vasospasm leading to gangrene.
- Newer **nonergot dopamine agonists like pramipexole** and **ropinirole** do not have these limitations (these are **long acting** and **do not cause gangrene**). Adverse known side effect of these drugs is **excessive day time sleepiness**, Gambling habits, increased sexuality.

- Recently approved non ergot ROTIGOTINE is available as transdermal patch.

132. Ans. (b) MAO-B inhiition

Ref: Katzung, 14th ed. pg. 499

- After release of DA in synaptic cleft, it is metabolized either by MAO-b or by COMT (catechol-ortho methyl transferase)
- In order to prevent this metabolism following drugs can be given, which will enhance DA availability:
  - MAO-b inhibitor: Selegiline, Rasagiline, safinamide
  - COMT inhibitor: Entacapone, Tolcapone

> **Extra Mile**
>
> **Drugs stimulating DA receptor:**
> - Ergot Derivative: Bromocriptine, Cabergoline
> - Non-Ergot: Pramipexole, Ropinirole, Rotigotine *(available as transdermal patch)*

133. Ans. (b) Lamotrigine

Ref: Katzung, 14th ed. pg. 422

- Abnormal electrical activity in brain is propagated by voltage gated (VG) sodium channel, which is responsible for majority of seizure types.
- Drugs acting by inhibiting VG-Na+ sodium channel: *(Mn: Very Lame Priyanka Chopra Likes it Ruf & Top Zone)*
  - Valproate
  - Lamotrigine
  - Phenytoin
  - Carbamazepine
  - Lacosamide
  - Rufinamide
  - Topiramate
  - Zonisamide
- **Note:** In addition of VG-Na channel blocking action, these drugs also have additional action like N-type calcium channel blockage or by increasing GABAergic activity etc.

> **Extra Mile**
>
> - Ethosuximide acts by inhibiting T type VG-Ca+ channel blocking.
> - Levetiracetam acts by inhibing synaptic vesicular protein inhibition thereby increasing GABA → causing neuronal depression.
> - Glutmate receptor inhibitors:
>   - **NMDA receptor blocker:** FELBAMATE
>   - **AMPA receptor blocker:** PERAMPANEL, TELAMPANEL

FMGE Solutions Screening Examination

134. Ans. (c) It has Broad spectrum of anti-seizure activity

Ref: Lippincott's 5th ed. pg. 186; KDT 6th ed. pg. 409-410
- Lamotrigine is effective in a wide variety of seizure types, including partial seizures, generalized seizures, and typical absence seizures and in the Lennox-Gastaut syndrome.
- **MOA:** Lamotrigine acts by blocking Na+ channels, T-type Ca2+ channels and by increasing GABAergic activity.
- Lamotrigine dosages should be reduced when adding valproate to therapy unless the valproate is being added in a small dose to provide a boost to the lamotrigine serum concentration.
- **Major adverse effect:** Steven Johnson syndrome and toxic epidermal necrolysis, insomnia.
- **Other side effects:** Nausea, drowsiness, dizziness, headache, and Diplopia.

135. Ans. (b) Sodium valproate

Ref: KDT 6th ed. pg. 407-408

Uses of Sodium Valproate
- Valproic acid is the drug of choice for absence seizures.
- It is an alternative/adjuvant drug for GTCS, simple partial seizure and complex partial seizure
- Myoclonic and atonic seizures-control is often incomplete, but valproate is the drug of choice.
- Mania and bipolar illness: As alternative to lithium.
- Valproate has some prophylatic efficacy in migraine.

MOA: prolongation of Na+ channel inactivation
Augmentation of release of inhibitory transmitter GABA by inhibiting its degradation

Drugs which can be used for absence seizure:
- Sodium valproate
- Ethusuximide
- Lamotrigine
- Clonazepam.

TABLE: Drug of choice for different seizures

Seizure types	DOC
Absence seizures (petit mal) in children (<2 – 3 yr)	Ethosuximide
Absence seizures	Na+ Valproate
GTCS (Grand mal)	LAMOTRIGINE > Na+ Valproate
Focal onset/Partial seizure	Carbamazepine
Myoclonic seizures	Na+ Valproate > Lamotrigine
Tonic/Clonic seizures	Na+ Valproate
Infantile/salam seizure	ACTH
Infantile spasm associated with tuberous sclerosis	Vigabatrin
Febrile seizures	Diazepam (per rectal)
Status epilepticus	Lorazepam (I.V.)
Seizures in eclampsia	Magnesium sulphate
Seizure during pregnancy	Lamotrigine
Lennox Gastaut syndrome	Na+ Valproate

136. Ans. (b) Na+ Valproate

Ref: Katzung, 14th ed. pg. 426; KDT, 6th ed. pg. 407-408
- Given the choices the answer will be Na+ Valproate
- According to Harrison's 19th ed. the current recommendable drug of choice for GTCS is **LAMOTRIGINE > Na+ Valproate.**

137. Ans. (b) Carbamazepine

Ref: Harrison's, 19th ed. pg. 2552
- **Carbamazepine is DOC** in partial/focal seizure.
- **Harrison states:** *Carbamazepine (or a related drug, oxcarbazepine), lamotrigine, phenytoin, and levetiracetam are currently the drugs of choice approved for the initial treatment of focal seizures, including those that evolve into generalized seizures. Overall they have very similar efficacy, but differences in pharmacokinetics and toxicity are the main determinants for use in a given patient.*

TABLE: Selection of antiepileptic drug

Generalized onset tonic clonic	Focal	Typical absence	Atypical absence, myoclonic, atonic
First-line			
Lamotrigine	Lamotrigine	Valproic acid	Valproic acid
Valproic acid	Carbamazepine	Ethosuximide	Lamotrigine
	Oxcarbazepine	Lamotrigine	Topiramate
	Phenytoin		
	Levetiracetam		
Alternatives			
Zonisamide	Topiramate	Lamotrigine	Clonazepam
Phenytoin	Zonisamide	Clonazepam	Felbamate
Carbamazepine	Valproic acid		Clobazam
Oxcarbazepine	Tiagabine[a]		Rufinamide
Topiramate	Gabapentin[a]		
Phenobarbital	Lacosamide[a]		
Primidone	Exogabine[a]		
Felbamate	Phenobarbital Primidone Felbamate		

[a]As adjunctive therapy

Pharmacology

138. Ans. (a) Valproate

Ref: Katzung, 14th ed. pg. 426

TABLE: Important side effects of anti epileptic drugs

Drug	Side effect
Valpraoate	• Fulminant Hepatitis: most grave side effect • Reversible Alopecia, Hepatotoxicity, Weight Gain, Tremor, Pancreatitis, NTD, Thrombocytopenia • PCOS- gender specific side effect
Phenytoin	Gum Hypertrophy: **MC side effect** Hirsutism, Fetal hydantoin syndrome, Megaloblastic anemia
Carbamazepine	Agaranulocytosis: Most serious side effect SJS, Bone marrow suppression, confusion, Ataxia, Blurring of vision
Zonisamide	Renal stone, Amnesia, Drowsiness, wt loss
Topiramate	Renal stone, Somnolence, wt loss
Vigabatrin	Visual acuity decreased, Weight gain
Felbamate	Aplastic anemia, Hepatotoxicity

139. Ans. (a) Phenytoin

Ref: Katzung, 14th ed. pg. 418

- Gum hypertrophy is known side effect of phenytoin.

140. Ans. (d) Folic acid deficiency

Ref: Katzung, 14th ed. pg. 418-19; KDT, 6th ed. 404-405

- Phenytoin is a major epileptic drug which is effective for treatment of partial seizures and generalized tonic-clonic seizures and in the treatment of status epilepticus.
- **MOA:** Phenytoin blocks voltage-gated sodium channels by selectively binding to the channel in the inactive state and slowing its rate of recovery.
- It follows zero order kinetics.
- It can also be used as an anti-arrhythmic drug (class Ib) for the treatment of digitalis induced arrhythmia.
- Use of phenytoin during pregnancy can cause **Fetal hydantoin syndrome** characterized by: hypoplastic phalanges, cleft lip, cleft palate and microcephaly. It occurs due metabolite of phenytoin, *arene oxide.*
- **Phenytoin decreases folate absorption and increases its excretion → *Megaloblastic anemia.***
- Prolonged use of phenytoin can result in gingival hyperplasia **(gum hypertrophy).**
- It can inhibit the insulin release and can cause **hyperglycemia.**
- **Other adverse effects on long-term use include:** Hirsutism, coarsening of facial features, megaloblastic anemia (treated with folic acid), vitamin D deficiency (rickets and **osteomalacia**), vitamin K deficiency, hyperglycemia (due to inhibition of insulin release), hypersensitivity.

141. Ans. (c) GABA transaminase inhibitor

Ref: Katzung, 14th ed. pg. 431-32

- VIGABATRIN is GABAergic drug acts by inhibiting enzyme GABA transaminase.
- This enzyme inhibition causes increased level of GABA in the neuron.
- Use:
  - DOC in infantile spasm + Tuberous sclerosis
  - Simple and complex partial seizure
- Contraindicated in absence seizure, Myoclonic seizure, Pre-existing visual field defect.
- **Side effect:** Visual field defect due to peripheral retinal atrophy, weight gain, amnesia

Extra Mile

- GABA uptake transport inhibitor: TIAGABINE

142. Ans. (b) Inhibing CRMP protein

Ref: Katzung, 14th ed. pg. 417

- CRMP is Collapsing Response Mediator Protien, which causes neuronal excitotoxicity by releasing BDNF (Brain Derived Neurotropic Factor).
- The drug Lacosamide acts by inhibiting CRMP protein, thereby causing protective action against neuronal excitotoxicity.

143. Ans. (a) Shift to sodium valproate

Ref: Katzung, 14th ed. pg. 418-19; KDT 6th ed. pg. 405

Hypersensitivity reactions like rashes, DLE, lymphadenopathy and neutropenia require that phenytoin to be stopped.

144. Ans. (c) Topiramate

Ref: Katzung, 14th ed. pg. 427-28

- The only antiepileptic drug which causes weight loss: Topiramate, Zonisamide
- **MOA of topiramate:**
  - VG-Na+ channel blocker
  - Activate GABA receptor
  - Inhibit AMPA receptor *(receptor of Glutamate)*
- Use:
  - GTCS, Partial seizure
  - Maintenance therapy of alcohol withdrawal
  - LGS
  - Decreases alcohol craving
- **Side effects:** Urolithiasis, Somnolence

145. Ans. (a) Naloxone

Ref: Katzung, 14th ed. pg. 581

- In acute morphine poisoning the DOC is Naloxone (Opioid antagonist).
- It is short acting and has rapid onset of action. It is given by IV route.
- **Naltrexone**
  - It is a longer acting oral opioid antagonist.
  - Given in long term addiction therapay to prevent relapse.
- **Nalmefene:**
  - Also a naltrexone derivative. Can be given IV.
  - It is recently approved for cholestatic pruritus.

146. Ans. (b) Pruritus

Ref: https://www.ncbi.nlm.nih.gov/pubmed/8706199

- With the increasing utilization of intrathecal and epidural opioids in humans, a wide variety of clinically relevant side effects have been reported.
- The four classic side effects are *pruritus*, nausea and vomiting, urinary retention, and respiratory depression.
- Intrathecal injection has been shown to cause segmental analgesia without affecting other modalities. *It acts in the substantia gelatinosa of dorsal horn to inhibit release of excitatory transmitters from primary afferents carrying pain impulses. The action appears to be exerted through inter neurons which are involved in the 'gating' of pain impulses. Release of glutamate from primary pain afferents in the spinal cord and its postsynaptic action on dorsal horn neurons is inhibited by morphine.*

147. Ans. (b) Buspirone

Ref: Katzung, 14th ed. pg. 584; KDT, 6th ed. pg. 451

BUSPIRONE

- A new class of antianxiety drug.
- Relieves mild-to-moderate generalized anxiety
- The mechanism of anxiolytic action may be dependent on its selective partial agonistic action on 5-HT$_{1A}$ receptors.

The Following Agents can be Used as Anti-Smoking Drugs

- *Vareniciline:*
  - It is a direct acting nicotinic agonist
  - Can be used orally and has a half life of 14-20 hours.
- *Bupropion:* It acts by inhibition of neuronal reuptake of 5-HIT, NE and DA.
- *Clonidine:*
  - It is a very effective drug for reducing the withdrawal effects of nicotine.
  - It decreases the craving as well as is useful in insomnia.
- Nicotine (Gums, Patch, Inhaler)

148. Ans. (a) Nicotine replacement gum

Ref: Katzung, 14th ed. pg. 584

Treatment of smoking dependence:
- **First line:** Nicotine replacement therapy (gum, patch, inhaler).
- **Bupropion and Vareniciline** (Nicotine receptor agonist): Also first line. Considered more effective.
- **2nd line:** Clonidine and Nortryptiline
- **Rimonabant:** Cannabinoid receptor inverse agonist. Withdrawn due to increased depression and suicide risk.

149. Ans. (c) Lithium

Ref: Katzung, 14th ed. pg. 527

- Lithium is DOC in manic disorder.
- DOC for prophylaxis of mania: Lithium
- DOC for acute attack of mania: Sedative + Atypical antipsychotics
- DOC for mania in pregnancy: Atypical antipsychotics
- Side effect of lithium *(Mn: LITTH)*
  - **L:** LEUCOCYTOSIS
  - **I:** Insipidus diabetes
  - **T:** Tremors (MC side effect- Coarse tremor);
  - **T:** Teratogenic (Ebstein anomaly)
  - **H:** Hypothyroidism

> **Extra Mile**
>
> **Therapeutic Plasma concentration of Lithium**
> - Acute mania: 0.8 – 1.4 mEq/L
> - Prophylaxis: 0.5 – 0.8 mEq/L
> - Toxic plasma conc level: > 2mEq/L

150. Ans. (c) Fluvoxamine

Ref: Katzung, 14th ed. pg. 540

- SSRI are selective serotonin reuptake inhibitor. Causing increased level of only serotonin in synaptic cleft.
- DOC in mild to moderate depression
- Drugs are:
  - CITALOPRAM
  - ESCITALOPRAM: **Most specific SSRI**
  - FLUOXETINE: Longest acting (50 hrs)
  - FLUOXAMINE: Shortest acting
  - PAROXETINE
  - SERTRALINE

Pharmacology

> **Extra Mile**
>
> - **TCA: Tricyclic Antidepressant**
>   - Inhibit reuptake of serotonin, Noradrenaline (NA) and Dopamine (DA)
>   - **Drugs are:** Imipramine, Trimipramine, Desipramine, Clomipramine, Nortryptiline, Amitryptilline
> - **SNRI: Serotonergic Noradrenergic reuptake inhibitor**
>   - Inhibit reuptake of serotonin and NA
>   - **Drugs are:** Venlafaxine, Desvenlafaxine, Duloxetine, Milnacipran, Levomilnacipran

151. Ans. (b) Serotonergic noradrenergic reuptake inhibitor

Ref: Goodman & Gillman's 13th ed. P 268

- Five medications with a nontricyclic structure that inhibit the reuptake of both 5HT and NE have been approved for use in the US for treatment of depression, anxiety disorders, pain, or other specific conditions. The drugs are:
  - Venlafaxine and its demethylated metabolite desvenlafaxine
  - Duloxetine
  - Milnacipran, and
  - Levomilnacipran

Mn: Vania Duals My Love

152. Ans. (b) Nausea

Ref: Katzung, 14th ed. pg. 546

TABLE: Side effect of antidepressants

Drug	Important side effects
SSRI	**MC side effect: Nausea** Other side effects: • Delayed ejaculation: Now approved for premature ejaculation • Serotonin syndrome • Anorgasmia • Agitation, anxiety, insomnia
TCA	Sedation, weight gain, T wave flattening, QT prolongation, Postural hypotension
SNRI	Serotonin syndrome Insomnia, Tachycardia, Anxiety

153. Ans. (d) Motion sickness

Ref: Katzung's Pharma, 14th ed. pg. 135

- Scopolamine (hyoscine) is a prototypic *muscarinic receptor antagonist,* and is one of the best agents for the prevention of motion sickness.
- Scopolamine has many effects in the body including decreasing the secretion of fluids, slowing the stomach and intestines, and dilation of the pupils.
- Scopolamine is also used to relieve nausea, vomiting, and dizziness associated with motion sickness and recovery from anesthesia and surgery.

154. Ans. (b) Aldehyde dehydrogenase

Ref: Katzung, 14th ed. pg. 404; KDT, 6th ed. pg. 386

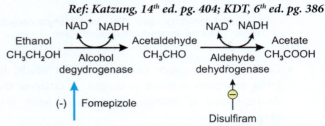

- **Disulfiram is an anti-craving agent for alcoholics. It has been used as an aversion technique in alcoholics.**
- *Disulfiram acts by inhibiting aldehyde dehydrogenase.* If a person still takes alcohol while on disulfiram treatment, alcohol is metabolized as usual, but acetaldehyde accumulates.
- This accumulation of acetaldehyde gives some distressing symptoms like **flushing, burning sensation, throbbing headache, perspiration, dizziness, vomiting, confusion** and **circulatory collapse.**
- Therefore, it is recommended only for those alcoholics who are motivated and sincerely desire to leave the habit.
- **Drugs causing disulfiram like reaction:**
  - Griseofulvin
  - Metronidazole
  - Chlorpropamide
  - Cefoperazone
  - Cefotetan
  - Trimethorprim
  - Procarbazine
  - MOXALACTAM
- **Other drugs that decrease craving for alcohol and smoking:** *(remembered as NATO)*
  - NALTREXONE
  - ACAMPROSATE
  - TOPIRAMATE
  - ONDANSETRON

> **Extra Mile**
>
> - Drug which inhibits alcohol dehydrogenase- **FOMEPIZOLE**
> - Antidote for methanol poisoning: **FOMEPIZOLE > ETHANOL**
> - Antidote for ethylene glycol poisoning: **FOMEPIZOLE**

155. Ans. (a) Competitively inhibits alcohol Dehydrogenase

Ref: Katzung, 14th ed. pg. 404; KDT, 6th ed. pg. 387

- **Ethanol** acts by competitive inhibition of alcohol dehydrogenase which block further metabolism of methanol into formaldehyde and formic acid. These products also cause retinal damage leading to subsequent blindness.

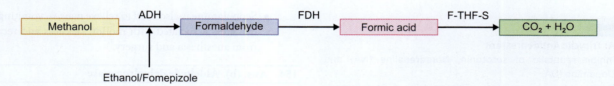

ADH: alcohol dehydrogenase: FDH : formaldehyde dehydrogenase
F-THF-S: 10-formyl tetrahydrofolate synthetase

- **Catalase** is a common enzyme found in nearly all living organisms exposed to oxygen. It catalyzes the decomposition of hydrogen peroxide to water and oxygen
- **Lactate dehydrogenase:** Dummy choice and is present in heart, RBC and is used as marker for malignancy.
- **Acetaldehyde dehydrogenase:** Converts acetaldehyde into acetic acid and is the target for disulfiram which is used to help patients quit alcohol.

Remember
- **Ethanol** is also metabolized by alcohol dehydrogenase and acts as its competitive inhibition. The enzyme's affinity for ethanol is 10-20 times higher than it is for methanol. Given via IV infusion in methanol or ethylene glycol poisoning.
- **Fomepizole** inhibits alcohol dehydrogenase. It is a stronger competitive inhibitor of ADH and, in addition, does not cause hypoglycemia or sedation.
- **Fomepizole** is relatively easier to administer than ethanol. It does not require monitoring of serum concentrations. Hence considered **as drug of choice**.

156. Ans. (d) Flumazenil

Ref: Katzung, 14th ed. pg. 404; KDT, 6th ed. pg. 385

- **Flumazenil is benzodiazepine antagonist. It has no role in alcohol detoxification.**

Alcohol Detoxification

Alcohol can produce physical and psychological dependence. In the treatment of alcohol dependence, major aim is to prevent withdrawal symptoms first and to avoid relapse of addiction thereafter.
- **Benzodiazepines** (chlordiazepoxide and diazepam) are long acting CNS depressant and are given to **prevent withdrawal.**
- **Acamprosate** is an **NMDA antagonist** that can be used for **maintenance therapy of alcohol abstinence.**
- **Naltrexone** is an opioid antagonist that can be used to reduce **alcohol craving.**
- **Disulfiram** can be used in psychologically dependent persons who are motivated to quit alcohol. It is *contraindicated in physically dependent* individuals. It produces severe distressing symptoms (like flushing, headache, vomiting, visual disturbances and mental confusion) after intake of alcohol due to accumulation of acetaldehyde.
- **Topiramate and ondansetron** can also *decrease* alcohol craving.

ANTIMICROBIAL AGENTS

157. Ans. (d) Ampicillin

Ref: Goodman & Gillman 13th ed. P 1036, 1050

- Ampicillin is considered as agent of choice in several infections like:
  - Enterococcus faecalis infection
  - Listeria infection
  - URTI (sinusitis, pharyngitis, otitis media) due to beta haemolytic streptococci
- **Other agents effective against Enterococcus faecalis:** Daptomycin, Linezolid, Tigecycline, Telavancin, Vancomycin, Carbapenems.
- **Agents effective against Enterococcus faecium:** Daptomycin, Linezolid

> **Extra Mile**
> - Enterococcus Faecium and Faecalis are highly resistant to aminoglycosides

158. Ans. (a) 3 mg/kg/day twice daily

Ref: Goodman & Gillman 13th ed. P 114

- Oseltamivir is one of the Neuraminidase inhibitor effective against influenza A and B.
- It inhibits amantadine- and rimantadine-resistant influenza A viruses and some zanamivir-resistant variants.
  - **Note:** Seasonal influenza H1N1 is resistant to oseltamivir
- **Dose required:**
  - For treatment-Adult: 75 mg twice daily for 5 days. Initiated within 48 hours of onset of illness
  - For Prophylaxis-Adult: 75 mg once daily
  - For pediatric patients dose is according to weight band (given in the table)

TABLE: Recommended dosage and duration of influenza antiviral medications for treatment of chemoprophylaxis

Antiviral agent	Use	Children	Adults
Oral oseltamivir	Treatment (5 days)	• If younger than 1 year old: 3 mg/kg/dose twice daily • If 1 yr or older, dose varies by child's weight: • 15 kg or less, the dose is 30 mg **twice** a day • >15 to 23 kg, the dose is 45 mg **twice** a day • >23 to 40 kg, the dose is 60 mg **twice** a day • >40 kg, the dose is 75 mg twice a day	75 mg twice daily
		If child is younger than 3 months old, use of oseltamivir for chemoprophylaxis is not indicated	

159. Ans. (a) Ceftriaxone

Ref: Harrison 20th edition, Page 1112

- DOC for meningococcal diseases: Penicillin G
- DOC for meningococcal meningitis: Ceftriaxone
- DOC for Prophylaxis of meningococcal meningitis: Rifampicin
- DOC for prophylaxis of H. Influenza meningitis: Rifampicin
- DOC for prophylaxis of meningococcal meningitis in pregnancy: Ceftriaxone
- DOC for listeria meningitides: Ampicillin
- **NOTE:** Rifampicin is known to cross placental barrier, hence avoided (but not contraindicated) in pregnancy.

160. Ans. (b) Streptomycin

Ref: Goodman & Gillman 13th ed. P 1039-40

- Streptomycin is one of the aminoglycosides.
- **MOA:**
  - Enters bacteria
  - Binds to 30s ribosomal unit and interferes with initiation of protein synthesis by causing the misreading and premature termination of mRNA translation.
  - This initial level interference causes accumulation of abnormal initiation complex and misreading causes insertion of incorrect amino acid in growing polypeptide chain → forming abnormal protein → Not compatible with bacterial life (Bactericidal).

- Other aminoglycosides are: Gentamicin, Tobramycin, Amikacin, Neomycin, Kanamycin, Netilmicin, Paromomycin.

USES OF AMINOGLYCOSIDES (AG)

- **Note:** AG is ineffective against anaerobes.
  - Most commonly used AG: Gentamicin
- Can be used as empirical therapy in majority of infections like UTI, hospital acquired Pneumonia, Meningitis, Peritonitis, Cystic fibrosis, sepsis.
- **Streptomycin:** DOC for tularemia, plague

SIDE EFFECT OF AG

- Ototoxicity
  - **Vestibulotoxicity:** MC due to Streptomycin and gentamicin
  - **Auditory/Cochlear dysfunction:** Irreversible, bilateral, high-frequency hearing loss. MC due to Amikacin, Neomycin, Kanamycin
    - First symptom of cochlear toxicity: High pitch tinnitus
- Nephrotoxicity
- Neuromuscular blockade (MC: Neomycin > Kanamycin)

Extra Mile

- Ceftriaxone is a third generation cephalosporin (from β Lactams class → a cell wall inhibitor).
- Nevirapine is one of the anti-retroviral drug from Non-nucleoside reverse transcriptase inhibitors class.
- Indinavir is one of the HIV protease inhibitor.

161. Ans. (a) Streptomycin

Ref: Goodman & Gillman 13th ed. P 1045; Harrison 20th edition, Page 1112

- Streptomycin is highly ototoxic (vestibulotoxic >> Cochleotoxic) and nephrotoxic drug.
- It is strictly contraindicated throughout the pregnancy.

TABLE: Drugs during pregnancy

	Drugs safe in pregnancy	Drugs contraindicated in pregnancy (Safety uncertain)
• Antitubercular	Isoniazid, Rifampicin, Pyrazinamide, Ethambutol	Streptomycin
• Antiamoebic	Diloxanide furoate, paromomycin	Metronidazole, Tinidazole, Quiniodochlor
• Antimalarial	Chloroquine, Mefloquine, Proguanil, Quinine (only in 1st trimester)	Primaquine

Contd...

FMGE Solutions Screening Examination

	Drugs safe in pregnancy	Drugs contraindicated in pregnancy (Safety uncertain)
• Antifungal	Topical: Clotrimazole, Nystatin, Tolnaftane	Amphotericin B, Fluconazole, Itraconazole, Ketoconazole, Griseofulvin
• Antiallergies	Chlorpheniramine, Promethazine	Cetirizine, Loratadine, Fexofenadine
• Anti bacterials	Penicillin G, Ampicillin, Amoxicillin-clavulanate, cloxacillin, Piperacillin, Cephalosporins, Erythromycin	Cotrimoxazole, Fluoroquinolones, Tetracycline, Doxycycline, Chloramphenicol, Kanamycin, Tobramycin, Clarithromycin, Vancomycin
• Antiviral	–	Ganciclovir, Foscarnet, Amantadine, Vidarabine, a-interferon
• Anti-retroviral	Zidovudine, Lamivudine, tenofovir, Nelfinavir, Nevirapine, Saquinavir, Efavirenz	Didanosine, Abacavir, Indinavir, Ritonavir
• Anti-diabetic	Insulin (preferably human insulin)	Sulfonylureas, metformin, Acarbose, pioglitazone, Repaglinide
• Thyroid drugs	Propylthiouracil	Carbimazole, Radioactive iodine (X), Iodide

162. Ans. (b) Azithromycin

Ref: Goodman & Gillman 13th ed. P 1017

- The patient in the given case has chlamydia induced UTI. The agent that can be preferred for management of such condition is fluroquinolones (FQ).
- **Books state:** "FQs are more efficacious than trimethoprim-sulfamethoxazole or oral B-Lactams". Moxifloxacin doesn't accumulate in urine and hence NOT approved for treatment of UTI.
- Fluoroquinolones lack activity for *Treponema pallidum* but have activity in vitro against *Chlamydia trachomatis* and *Haemophilus ducreyi*.
- This patient later presented with symptoms of sexually transmitted infection, for which the best option is Azithromycin, single dose is effective.

- **Book states:** "For chlamydial urethritis/cervicitis, a 7-day course of ofloxacin or levofloxacin is an alternative to a 7-day treatment with doxycycline or a single dose of azithromycin; other available quinolones are NOT effective in these condition"

163. Ans. (a) Dengue

Ref: Goodman & Gillman 13th ed. P 668-69

- CYD-TDV developed by Sanofi Pasteur is a recombinant tetravalent (four-serotype) live attenuated virus vaccine that was first licensed in Mexico in December 2015 for use in individuals 9–45 years of age living in endemic areas.
- However, it is given as a three-dose series on a 0–6-12-month schedule via subcutaneous route.
- It should only be given to individuals with previous history of dengue by any of the 4 serotypes.

Extra Mile

- **Malaria Vaccine:** The RTS, S vaccine is a recombinant protein-based malaria vaccine with AS01 adjuvant against *Plasmodium falciparum* only. It is the first malaria vaccine to be approved in April 2019.
  - The vaccine has been recommended by WHO for pilot introduction in selected areas of 3 African countries

164. Ans. (b) Liposomal Amphotericin B

Ref: Goodman & Gillman 13th ed. P 996

- Drug of choice for visceral leishmaniasis: Liposomal Amphotericin B.
  - **Note:** AmpB can be used even during pregnancy
  - **Side effect:** Renal toxicity, hypokalemia, hypomagnesemia
- Other agents for management of leishmaniasis:
  - **Sodium stibogluconate:** Given parenterally 20 mg/kg/day for 20 days in cutaneous disease and 28 days in visceral leishmaniasis. Due to increased resistance it has now become obsolete in India. At present oral preparation is available and shows better result.
    - **Side effect:** Pancreatitis, Hepatotoxicity, Bone marrow suppression, haemolytic anemia and renal failure
  - **Pentamidine** can be used in doses of 2–3 mg/kg IV or IM daily or every second day for 4–7 doses to treat cutaneous leishmaniasis.
    - **Side effect:** Nephrotoxic, Hypoglycemia
  - **Miltefosine:** Oral agent. Can be used in visceral and cutaneous leishmaniasis.
    - Only oral preparation available. Teratogenic → Not used in pregnancy

Pharmacology

165. Ans. (a) Fosfomycin

- Among the given choices fosfomycin is preferred agent for UTI.
- Recommendations for treatment must be considered in the context of local resistance patterns and national differences in some agents' availability.
- For example, **fosfomycin** and pivmecillinam are not available in all countries but are considered **first-line** options where they are available because they retain activity against a majority of uropathogens that produce extended-spectrum β-lactamases.
  - *Use of **fosfomycin** for UTIs (including complicated infections), particularly for infections caused by multidrug-resistant E. coli.*
- TMP-SMX was earlier recommended as the first-line agent for treatment of uncomplicated UTI, but due to increasing evidence of resistance it is less preferred.
  - ***TMP-SMX** has been recommended as first-line treatment for acute cystitis, and it remains appropriate to consider the use of this drug in regions with resistance rates not exceeding 20%*

- **UTI drugs having minimal effect on fecal flora:** Pivmecillinam, Fosfomycin, and Nitrofurantoin.
- **UTI drugs having significant effect on fecal flora:** Trimethoprim, TMP-SMX, Quinolones, and ampicillin.
  - These drugs are notably the agents for which rising resistance levels have been documented.
- Fluoroquinolones should not be used for uncomplicated cystitis unless no alternatives are available.
  - Most **fluoroquinolones** are highly effective as short-course therapy for cystitis; the exception is moxifloxacin
  - Commonly used for UTI include ciprofloxacin and levofloxacin.
- **Nitrofurantoin** remains highly active against *E. coli* and most non–*E. coli* isolates. *Proteus, Pseudomonas, Serratia, Enterobacter,* and yeasts are all intrinsically resistant to this drug.
  - Resistance to nitrofurantoin remains low compared to TMP-SMX
- In acute cystitis, β-Lactam agents generally are not preferred as well as TMP- SMX or fluoroquinolones.

TABLE: Treatment strategies for acute uncomplicated cystitis

Drug and dose	Estimated clinical efficacy, %	Estimated bacterial efficacy, %	Common side effects
Nitrofurantoin, 100 mg bid × 5–7 day	87-95	82–92	Nausea, headache
TMP-SMX, 1 DS tablet bid × 3 day	86–100	85-100	Rash, urticaria, nausea, vomiting, hematologic abnormalities
Fosfomycin, 3-g single-dose sachet	83-95	78-98	Diarrhea, nausea, headache
Pivmecillinam, 400 mg bid × 3–7 day	55–82	74–84	Nausea, vomiting, diarrhea
Fluoroquinolones, dose varies by agent; 3 day regimen	81–98	78–96	Nausea, vomiting, diarrhea, headache, drowsiness, insomnia
β-Lactams, dose varies by agent; 5–7 day regimen	79–98	74–98	Diarrhea, nausea, vomiting, rash, urticaria

166. Ans. (b) Antimalarial

Ref: Goodman & Gillman's 13th ed. P 974

- *Pyronaridine* is an antimalarial structurally related to amodiaquine.
- This drug is potent against both *P. falciparum* and *P. vivax and is very well tolerated.*
- It leads to fever resolution in 1–2 days and parasite clearance in 2–3 days.
- It is tested in clinical trials as an adjunct with artemisinin class drugs, has not yet been licensed.

167. Ans. (b) Ceftriaxone

Ref: Harrison 19th ed. P 767

- Ceftriaxone is the empirical drug of choice for treatment of meningitis. It is frequently combined with vancomycin.

168. Ans. (a) Acyclovir

Ref: Goodman & Gillman's 13th ed. P 1106-7

- Acyclovir's clinical use is limited to herpes viruses. Acyclovir is most active against HSV-1.
- Approximately half as active against HSV-2, and a tenth as potent against VZV and EBV.
- **Book states:** "*Acyclovir is ineffective therapeutically in established CMV infections, but ganciclovir is effective for CMV prophylaxis in immunocompromised patients*".
- EBV-related oral hairy leukoplakia may improve with acyclovir.
- Drugs which can be used in treatment of CMV retinitis are cidofovir, ganciclovir, foscarnet, valaciclovir.
- **DOC for CMV retinitis:** Ganciclovir

Explanations

FMGE Solutions Screening Examination

- **Fomivirsen** is active against CMV strains **resistant** to ganciclovir, foscarnet, and cidofovir. Fomivirsen is given by intravitreal injection unresponsive to other therapies.

169. Ans. (d) Mutation

Ref: Goodman & Gillman's 13th ed. P 1016

- Ciprofloxacin is one of the fluoroquinolones along with norfloxacin, ofloxacin, levofloxacin, sparfloxacin, etc.
- **MOA of quinolones:** The quinolone antibiotics target bacterial *DNA gyrase* and *topoisomerase IV*.
- The quinolones inhibit gyrase-mediated DNA supercoiling at concentrations that correlate well with those required to inhibit bacterial growth.
- **Mutations of the gene that encodes the A subunit of the gyrase** can confer resistance to these drugs.

170. Ans. (a) Kanamycin

Ref: Goodman & Gillman 13th ed. P 1044-45

- All aminoglycosides have the potential to produce reversible and irreversible vestibular, cochlear, renal toxicity and neuromuscular blockade.
- Aminoglycoside-induced ototoxicity may result in irreversible, bilateral, high-frequency hearing loss or vestibular hypofunction.
- A high-pitched tinnitus often is **the first symptom** of cochlear toxicity.
- Drugs like amikacin, neomycin and kanamycin are specifically cochleotoxic > vestibulotoxic.
- Gentamicin, streptomycin is vestiblar > cochleotoxic
- **Tobramycin:** Cochlear = Vestibular toxicity both.

171. Ans. (b) Clindamycin

Ref: KDT 6th ed. page 668

- **Lincosamide family** of antimicrobial drugs includes:
  - Clindamycin
  - Lincomycin *(It is obsolete now)*

Drugs which inhibit cell wall formation	Drugs which inhibit protein synthesis

Cycloserine
Vancomycin
 	
Fosfomycin
Beta Lactams
  Penicillin
  Cephalosporin
  Carbapenem
  Monolactams
Bacitracin
	• **T**etracycline *(tRNA inhibitor)*
	• **C**hloramphenicol *(peptide bond formation inhibitor)*
	• **M**acrolides (erythro, clarithro, azithro)
	• **C**lindamycin
	• **A**minoglycosides
	• **S**treptogramins (Quinpristin + Dalfopristin)

Remembered as: **C**ell **V**all o**F** **B**acteria	The **C**hild **M**ay **C**limb **A**mino **S**tairs

- **Clindamycin** is among the drugs which act by inhibiting protein synthesis.
- They bind to 50s subunit of ribosome resulting in bacteriostatic inhibition of bacterial protein synthesis.
- It is very effective drug against corynebacterium acne, pneumocycstis carinii and toxoplasma gondii

172. Ans. (c) Quinpristin

Ref: Sharma & Sharma 3rd ed. P 702

TABLE: Protein synthesis inhibitor drugs acting at 30s and 50s ribosomal unit

Drugs acting by inhibiting 30s ribosome	**A**minoglycoside (Streptomycin, Gentamicin, Tobramycin, Kanamycin, Amikacin) **T**etracycline (Minocycline, Demeclocyclin, Doxycycline)
Drugs acting by inhibiting 50s ribosome	**S**treptogramins (Quinpristin & Dalfopristin) **E**rythromycin (macrolides) **L**incosamides (Clindamycin) **L**inezolid **K**etolides (Telithromycin, Cethromycin) **C**hloramphenicol

Mn: Buy **AT** 30, **SELL K**aro **C**hina in 50

173. Ans. (a) Carbenicillin

Ref: Sharma & Sharma 3rd ed. P 731

- Some penicillins like Png, Procaine PnG, Benzathine PnG, Carbenicillin, Ticarcillin, Mezlocillin, Azlocillin, Piperacillin are sensitive to gastric acid degradation.
- Such penicillins are not effecrive orally, and hence are given via parenteral route.

TABLE: Acid Resistant Vs acid Labile penicillins

Acid Resistant penicillin Mn: VODCA BoTal	Acid Labile penicillin Mn: GNM Car Till MAP
• PnV • Oxacillin • Dicloxacillin • Cloxacillin • Ampicillin/Amoxycillin • Bacampicillin • Talampicillin	**Natural penicillins** • Penicillin G • Procaine PnG • Benzathine PnG **Anti-staphylococcal penicillins** • Nafcillin • Methicillin **Antipseudomonal penicillins** • Carbenicillin • Ticarcillin • Mezlocillin • Azlocillin • Piperacillin

Pharmacology

174. Ans. (b) Ampicillin

Ref: Goodman & Gillman 13th ed. P 1028; Katzung, 9th ed. pg. 1172

- First line drug of choice for listeria species is Ampicillin.
- Second line- TMP-SMZ
- The book states: "Ampicillin or penicillin G (with consideration for addition of gentamicin to both for immunosuppressed patients with meningitis) is the drugs of choice in the management of infections owing to *L. monocytogenes*. The recommended dose of penicillin G is 18–24 million units parenterally per day for at least 2 weeks."

Extra Mile

Listeria along with gropup B streptococci and E.coli is the most common cause of neonatal meningitis.
MOA of ampicillin: Inhibits cell wall synthesis during active multiplication.
First line drug of choice for neonatal meningitis- ampicillin + 3rd gen cephalosporin.
Chloramphenicol is a protein synthesis inhibitor, more specifically it inhibits formation of peptide bond between acceptor and peptide site.
- **Side effect:** Bone marrow suppression
- **Teratogenic S/E- Gray baby syndrome:** Chloramphenicol

175. Ans. (b) Chloramphenicol

Ref: KDT, 6th ed. pg. 717

Antimicrobial drugs	Side effects
Chloramphenicol	Grey baby syndrome Bone marrow suppression
Tetracycline	Teeth discoloration and bone growth suppression Phototoxicity Fanconi syndrome (in case of expired tetracycline) Vestibular dysfunction
Vancomycin	Red man/Red neck syndrome Nephrotoxic and ototoxic
Clindamycin	Pseudomembranous colitis

Extra Mile

VANCOMYCIN: drug of choice for MRSA
Vancomycin NEVER effective against Pseudomonas
β **LACTAMS** never effective against MRSA.
AMINOGLYCOSIDE never effective against Anaerobes.
Most common cause of pseudo membranous colitis: **3rd Gen. cephalosporin.**
DOC for pseudo membranous colitis: **VANCOMYCIN (Oral).**

Preferred agent in mild case of pseudomembranous colitis → Metronidazole

176. Ans. (b) Vancomycin

Ref: Katzung, 14th ed. pg. 809; Sharma & Sharma 3rd ed. P 742-43; KDT, 6th ed. pg. 732

- Vancomycin is a bactericidal drug acts by cell wall synthesis inhibitor and by damaging cell membrane integrity.
- It is exclusively active against aerobic as well as anaerobic gram positive species such as streptococcus and staphylococci including MRSA.
- Parenterally it is DOC in MRSA, Staph epideermidis infection associated with use of IV catheters or with contibuous peritoneal dialysis.
- Orally it is also effective in controlling pseudomembranous colitis not responding to metronidazole (act as local because it is poorly absorbed from GIT).
- **Side effects:**
  - Red neck syndrome (due to histamine release)
  - Ototoxicity, nephrotoxicity, skin rash, reversible neutropenia etc.

177. Ans. (b) Metronidazole

Ref: Katzung's Pharma, 10th ed. Ch 53

- Vancomycin (oral) is now considered as the drug of choice for pseudomembraneous colitis.
- Metronidazole also used for pseudomembraneous colitis in mild cases.
- Ampicillin has been associated with pseudomembranous colitis
- Ceftriaxone is DOC for typhoid/enteric fever. Should be given IV.

Extra Mile

- METRONIDAZOLE is also the drug of choice in the treatment of amebiasis, trichomoniasis, Giardiasis and extraluminal amebiasis.
- For serious pseudomembranous colitis not responding to metronidazole, DOC is Vancomycin.

178. Ans. (b) Pseudomembranous colitis

Ref: Sharma & Sharma 3rd ed. P 742-43; Katzung, 14th ed. pg. 809

Please refer to above explanation for details

179. Ans. (d) Nafcillin

Ref: KD Tripathi, 6th ed. pg. 700 & 708

- Microbes which are resistant to methicillin, are said to be MRSA. Since methicillin is not clinically used

FMGE Solutions Screening Examination

- nowadays, then if the organism is resistant to Nafcillin and Cloxacillin, they are also said to be MRSA.
- Methicillin is highly penicilinase resistant but not acid resistant.
- MRSA have emerged in many areas. These are insensitive to all penicillinase-resistant penicillins and to other β-lactams as well as to erythromycin, aminoglycosides, tetracylines, etc.
- The drug of choice for these organisms is vancomycin/linezolid, but ciprofloxacin and Rifampicin can also be used.
- Antibiotics effective against Beta lactamase producing bacteria:
  - **Beta lactamase resistant antibiotics:** Cloxacillin, Dcloxacillin, Methicillin and Nafcillin
  - **Beta lactamase inhibitors:** currently there are 3 drugs in this category (and they are added with)
    - Clavulanic acid (+ Amoxycillin)
    - Sulbactam (+ Ampicillin)
    - Tazobactam (+ Piperacillin)

180. Ans. (b) β Lactams

Ref: Sharma & Sharma 3rd ed. P 733

- No β *Lactams* are effective against MRSA, EXCEPT 5th generation cephalosporins like Ceftaroline and Ceftibiprole.
- **DOC for MRSA:** Vancomycin
- **DOC for VRSA:** Daptomycin
- Drugs used in VRSA: Quinpristin, Daptomycin, Linezolid

181. Ans. (b) Chloramphenicol

Ref: KD Tripathi, 6th ed. pg. 716 & 909

CHLORAMPHENICOL

- It is a broad-spectrum antibiotic, active against nearly the same range of organisms (gram-positive and negative bacteria, rickettsiae, mycoplasma) as tetracyclines.

Adverse Efects
- Bone marrow depression
- Hypersensitivity reactions
- Grey baby syndrome

TABLE: Choice of drugs for common problems during pregnancy

Drug class (condition)	Unsafe drugs	Safer alternative
Antibacteirals	Fluoroquinolones Tetracycline Doxycycline Chloramphenicol Streptomycin Kananmycin Tobramycin	Penicillin G; Ampicillin Amoxicillin-Clavulanate Cloxacillin, Piperacillin cephalosphorins erythromycin

Contd...

Drug class (condition)	Unsafe drugs	Safer alternative
Antitubercular	Pyrazinamide, Ethambutol Streptomycin	Isoniazid Rifampicin
Anti hypertensives	ACE inhibitors Angiotensin antagonists Diuretics Proanolol and nitroprusside	Methyldopa Hydralazine Atenolol, Metoprolol, pindolol Nifedipine
Anti thyroid drugs	Carbimazole Radio active iodine Iodide	Propylthiouracil (PTU)

182. Ans. (a) Ciprofloxacin

Ref: KDT, 6TH ed. pg. 909

- Antibiotics which are safe in pregnancy are remembered as "*PCM*":
  - Penicillin (*PnG, ampicillin etc*)
  - Cephalosporin (*cefotaxime, cefixime etc.*)
  - Macrolides (*erythromycin, azithromycin etc.*)
- *Refer above explanation table.*
- *Fluoroquinolones (Ciprofloxacin) are contraindicated in pregnancy and below 18 years patient because it effect growing bone and tendon.*

183. Ans. (d) Ceftriaxone

Ref: Katzung, 14th ed. pg. 909; KDT, 6th ed. pg. 706

- Ceftriaxone is a 3rd generation cephalosporin with long duration of action ($t^{1/2}$ - 8 hrs.) and with better CSF penetration.
- **Ceftriaxone** is highly effective in a wide range serious infections including bacterial meningitis, typhoid fever, complicated UTI's and STD's like gonorrhea.
- It is first choice drug for single dose therapy of gonorrhea if the penicillinase producing status of organism is not known.
- A single dose of 250 mg IM injection is curative in gonorrhea and in chancroid.
- Drugs which can also be given as first line in case of gonorrhea are:
  - Amoxicillin 3 g oral OR Ampicillin 3.5 g oral-for non penicillinase producing.
  - Ceftriaxone 250 mg IM or Cefuroxime 250 mg IM or Azithromycin 1 g oral single dose- for Penicillinase producing.
- TOC for Gonorrhea → VANCOMYCIN + CEFTRIAXONE

Pharmacology

184. Ans. (a) Cefaclor

Ref: Katzung, 14th ed. pg. 804

TABLE: Cephalosporin generations

Drug class	Useful antibacterial spectrum[a]
First generation Cefazolin Cephalexin monohydrate Cefadroxil Cephradine	Streptococci; *Staphylococcus aureus*; some *Proteus, E. coli, Klebsiella*
Second generation Cefaclor Cefuroxime Cefuroxime axetil Cefprozil Cefoxitin Cefotetan Cefmetazole	*Escherichia coli, Klebsiella, Proteus, Haemophilus influenzae, Moraxella catarrhalis*. Not as active against gram-positive organisms as first-generation agents
Third generation Cefotaxime Ceftriaxone Cefdinir Cefditoren pivoxil Ceftibuten Cefpodoxime proxetil Ceftizoxime	*Escherichia coli, Klebsiella, Proteus, Haemophilus influenzae, Moraxella catarrhalis, Citrobacter, Enterobacter, Serratia; Neisseria gonorrhoeae*; activity for *S. aureus, Streptococcus pneumoniae*, and *Streptococcus pyogenes* comparable to first-generation agents. Activity against *Bacteroides* spp. inferior to that of cefoxitin and cefotetan.
Antipseudomonal cephalosporins Ceftazidime	Gram negative activity similar to third generation with addition of activity against *Pseudomonas*; poor activity vs gram-positive organisms
Ceftazidime/avibactam	Expands ceftazidime's against *Pseudomonas* and multidrug-resistant Enterobactericeae, but not against gram-positives
Ceftolozame/tazobactam	Similar to ceftazidime, with enhanced activity against *Pseudomonas* and extended-spectrum β-lactamase-producing Enterobacteriaceae
Fourth generation Cefepime, cefpirome	Comparable to third generation but more resistant to some β-lactamases (especially those of *Pseudomonas* and *Enterobacter*); gram-positive activity similar to cefotaxime
Fifth generation Ceftaroline Ceftobiprole	Similar actvity to 3rd generation but with activity against methicillin resistant *Staphylococcus aureus*

185. Ans. (d) Aztreonam

Ref: KDT, 6th ed. pg. 708

- β lactams contain a β lactam ring and another one is 2nd ring.
- 4 types of β lactams based on 2nd ring:
  - Penicillins *(ampicillin)*
  - Cephalosporins *(cefotaxim)*
  - Carbapenems *(doripenem)*
  - Monobactams *(azteronam)*

- In **monolactams (azteronam)** the 2nd ring is absent, due to which it doesn't show cross allergy with other β lactams.
- Therefore it can be used in patients who are allergic to penicillins.
- It inhibits gram negative enteric bacilli, H. influenza and pseudomonas.
- It doesn't inhibit gram positive cocci or fecal anaerobes.

186. Ans. (b) Mupirocin

Ref: KDT, 6th ed. pg. 733-34

- **Aminoacyl-tRNA synthetases (aaRSs)** are enzymes that catalyze the transfer of amino acids to their cognate tRNA. They play a pivotal role in protein synthesis and are essential for cell growth and survival.
- Mupirocin, a natural product of Pseudomonas fluorescens, is the only aaRS inhibitor approved by the US Food and Drug Administration to this date.
- It is active against gram-positive cocci, including methicillin-susceptible and methicillin-resistant strains of *Staphylococcus aureus*. Mupirocin inhibits staphylococcal isoleucyl tRNA synthetase.
- Mupirocin is indicated for topical treatment of minor skin infections, such as impetigo.

> **Extra Mile**
>
> **Methenamine mandelate** is the salt of mandelic acid and methenamine and possesses properties of urinary antiseptics. It doesn't treat UTI, but it suppresses.
> **Mitomycin C** is antitumor antibiotics.
> Metronidazole, an antibiotic for anaerobes.

187. Ans. (a) Injection Benzathine penicillin 2.4 million units IM single dose

Recommended treatment for syphilis

Stage of syphilis	Treatment	Comment
Early Primary, secondary, or early latent	Benzathine penicillin G 2.4 MU, IM more	
Late latent or uncertain duration	Benzathine penicillin G 2.4 million units 1M weekly for 3 wk	
Tertiary without neurophilis	Benzathine penicillin G 2.4 million units N weekly for 3 weeks	Cerebrospinal fluid evaluation recommended in all patients
Neurosyphilis	Aqueous penicillin G 18-24 million units IV daily, given every 3-4 hours or as continuous infusion for 10-14 days	Follow treatment with benzathine penicillin G 2.4 million units 1M weekly for up to 3 weeks

188. Ans. (b) Azithromycin

Ref: KDT, 6th ed. pg. 730-31; Katzung, pg. 1172

- Azithromycin is new congener of erythromycin with expanded spectrum and improved pharmacokinetics.
- Because of its higher efficacy, better gastric tolerance and convenient once a day dosing, it is preferred over erythromycin as first line drug of choice for infections such as *(Mn: CHAL MD)*:
  - Chancroid
  - Chlamydia Trachomatis- 1 gm single dose is curative.
  - H. Influenzae
  - Atypical mycobacteria, Atypical pneumonia (by chlamydia)
  - Legionella
  - Moraxella catarrhalis
  - Donovanosis
- Erythromycin and clarithromycin are the macrolides with similar antimicrobial spectrum. But clarithromycin have action against mycobacterium avium complex (MAC), atypical mycobacteria and M. leprae, H.Influenzae, Toxoplasma gondii.

> **Extra Mile**
>
> **Spiramycin:** Given in treatment of toxoplasma gondii to prevent transmission of infection from mother to fetus.

189. Ans. (c) Crystalluria

Ref: Sharma & Sharma 3rd ed. P 715

FIGURE: Bacterial Folate synthesis and sites of action of sulfonamides and trimethoprim. Pyrimethamine also inhibits dihydrofolate reductase but preferentially of protozoa

Pharmacology

- Sulfonamides are structural analogue of PABA which enter the synthetic sequence of in place of PABA by competing with the enzyme dihydropteroic acid synthase and forms non-functional analogue of folic acid which is of no use to bacteria.
- Its growth ceases in absence of folic acid, hence these are bacteriostatic drugs.

Classification of sulfonamides:
- **Short acting** (t1/2- 6-9 hrs): Sulfacytine, Sulfadiazine, Sulfasoxazole, Sulfamethizole
- **Intermediate** (t1/2- 1 – 12 hrs): Sulfamethoxazole, Sulfamoxole
- **Long acting** (t1/2- 7 to 8 days hrs): Sulfadoxine

Side effects (Mn: Karina Cry for ASH)
- Kernicterus in neonates
- Crystalluria and renal toxicity (acetylated metabolites of drug are less soluble in acidic urine)
- **Anemia:** Hemolytic anemia in G6PD
- **SJS:** Chrct by EM, mucus ulceration of mouth and genitals
- Hypersensitivity reaction: Rash at mucocutaneous junction, eosinophilia, Drug fever seen on 7–10th day of treatment.

190. Ans. (d) 1:5

Ref: Sharma & Sharma 3rd ed. P 716;
Katzung's, 11th ed. pg. 818

- Cotrimoxazole is a combination of Trimethoprim 80 mg and sulfamethoxazole 400 mg.
- Optimal ratio **in drug combination** 1:5 – 1 Trimethoprim: 5 sulfamethoxazole)
- Ratio of cotrimoxazole **in serum** is 1:20 (1 Trimethoprim: 20 sulfamethoxazole), due to rapid metabolism of trimethoprim and slower metabolism of sulfamethoxazole the ratio changes in plasma.
- A double strength (DS) tablet contains 160 mg Trimethoprim + 800 mg sulfamethoxazole.

Uses:
- UTI
- Prostatitis (since cotrimoxazole gets concentrated in prostatic fluid)
- Typhoid
- Nocardiosis (DOC)
- Pneumocystis carinii induced pneumonia (DOC)

Extra Mile
- Alone these both the drugs shows bacteriostatic action. When combined they become bactericidal.
- **Other combination:** Sulfadoxine (500 mg) + Pyrimethamine (25 mg): ratio is 20:1
  - Curative in chloroquine resistant P. Falciparum
  - First line in toxoplasmosis

191. Ans. (c) Doxycycline

Ref: Sharma & Sharma 3rd ed. P 760

- Doxycycline is from the tetracycline class of drug.
- Tetracyclins are first line DOC in following conditions like
  - Rocky mountain spotted fever
  - Typhus fever
  - Psittacosis
  - Granuloma inguinale
  - Non-specific urethritis (ureaplasma urealyticum)
  - Lyme disease
  - Brucellosis (Brucella abortus)
  - Plague
  - Pasturella abscess

Extra Mile
- First line combination therapy for brucellosis is: Doxycycline and Rifampicin

192. Ans. (a) Dapsone

Ref: Katzung, 14th ed. pg. 1086

- **Dermatitis herpetiformis (DH)** is a chronic blistering skin condition, characterised by blisters filled with a watery fluid.
- DH is neither related to nor caused by herpes virus: the name means that it is a skin inflammation having an appearance similar to herpes.
- It characterized by intensely itchy, chronic papulovesicular eruptions, usually distributed symmetrically on extensor surfaces (buttocks, back of neck, scalp, elbows, knees, back, hairline, groin, or face).
- **Diagnosis** is confirmed by a simple blood test for IgA antibodies, and by a skin biopsy in which the pattern of IgA deposits in the dermal papillae, revealed by direct immunofluorescence, distinguishes it from linear IgA bullous dermatosis and other forms of dermatitis.
- **Treatment:** Dapsone is considered as drug of choice for DH.
- In case of intolerance to dapsone, other drugs which can be used are: Colchicine, Tetracycline, Sulfapyridine.

193. Ans. (a) Acyclovir

Ref: Katzung, 11th ed. pg.1468

Please refer to above explanation.

194. Ans. (c) Abacavir

Ref: KDT, 6th ed. pg. 773-74

- Abacavir is a NRTI

FMGE Solutions Screening Examination

Protease inhibitors (ends with "navir")	Nucleoside reverse transcriptase inhibitor (NRTI)
Indinavir Saquinavir *Ritonavir* *Atazanavir* Nelfinavir Amprenavir Lopinavir	Zidovudine Stavudine Lamivudine Didanosine Emtricitabine Zalcitabine *Abacavir*
Side effect: Lipodystrophy syndrome Minimum side effect seen with: ATAZANAVIR	**Side effect:** acute pancreatitis Peripheral neuropathy Bone marrow suppression and M.I.

Extra Mile

- NRTI which has the maximum risk of acute pancreatitis: DIDANOSINE
- NRTI which has the maximum risk of peripheral neuropathy: STAVUDINE
- **Safest NRTI:** LAMIVUDINE (minimal risk of pancreatitis and peripheral neuropathy)

195. Ans. (a) HIV

Ref: KDT, 6th ed. pg. 770

- ss Viral RNA $\xrightarrow{\text{Reverse trancriptase}}$ ds viral DNA.
- 2 class of reverse transcriptase inhibitors

Neucleoside Reverse Transcriptase Inhibitors (NRTI)	Non-Nucleoside Reverse Transcriptase Inhibitors (NNRTI)
• ZIDOVUDINE • STAVUDINE • DIDANOSINE • LAMIVUDINE • ABACAVIR • ZALCITABINE	• EFAVIRENZ • NEVIRAPINE • DELAVIRDINE Rememberd as "END"

Extra Mile

ZIDOVUDINE

- Most commonly used NRTI in the treatment of HIV
- Used as prophylaxis in needle stick injury and to decrease vertical transmission from HIV mother to fetus.
- **Side effect:** Bone marrow suppression.
- Drug of choice for decreasing vertical transmission from HIV mother to fetus: **NEVIRAPINE**
- Safest NRTI: **LAMIVUDINE**
- All NRTI's casues acute pancreatitis and peripheral neuropathy.
  ▪ Maximum risk of acute pancreatitis with: **DIDANOSINE**
  ▪ Maximum risk of peripheral neuropathy with: **STAVUDINE**
- NRTI causing aphthous ulcer in mouth: **Zalcitabine (withdrawn)**

196. Ans. (c) Acyclovir

Ref: Katzung, 14th ed. pg. 864–65

- Acyclovir is an acyclic guanosine derivative with clinical activity against HSV-1, HSV-2, and VZV. In vitro activity against Epstein-Barr virus (EBV), cytomegalovirus (CMV), and human herpesvirus-6 (HHV-6).

ANTI-RETROVIRAL DRUGS

- **Nucleoside reverse tanscriptase inhibitor:** Zidovudine, Stavudine, Lamivudine, Didanosine, Emtricitabine, Zalcitabine, *Abacavir*
- **Nucleotide reverse tanscriptase inhibitor:** *Tenofovir*
- **Protease inhibitors:** Indinavir, Saquinavir, *Ritonavir*, Atazanavir, Nelfinavir, Amprenavir, Lopinavir.

197. Ans. (c) CCR5 inhibitor

Ref: Katzung, 14th ed. pg. 872

- Maraviroc is an anti HIV drug which comes under fusion inhibitor category.
- This drug binds to the CCR5 receptor of CD4 cells and inhibits the fusion stage of virus and hence inhibits their speed of replication.
- There are two types of fusion inhibitors:

Drugs which bind to CCR5 receptor of CD4 cells	Drugs which bind to GP 41 subunit of viral envelope
Maraviroc: active against CCR5 receptor of CD4 cell	**Enfuvirtide:** Prevents entry of virus into host cell
Can be given orally	Can only be given in s.c. injection form

198. Ans. (b) Stavudine

Ref: Katzung, 14th ed. pg. 875; KDT, 6th ed. pg. 770

- NRTI's are reverse transcriptase inhibitors, which control the dsDNA formation from ssRNA
- Drugs in the category are: Zidovudine, Stavudine, Didanosine, Lamivudine, Abacavir, Zalcitabine, Emtricitabine
- All NRTI's casues acute pancreatitis, peripheral neuropathy and Lactic acidosis
  ▪ Maximum risk of acute pancreatitis with: **DIDANOSINE**
  ▪ Maximum risk of peripheral neuropathy with: **STAVUDINE**
  ▪ NRTI has maximum risk of lactic acidosis: **STAVUDINE**
  ▪ Least toxic NRTI: Emtricitabine

199. Ans. (d) Pyrimethamine

Ref: KDT, 6th ed. pg. 783

- The drugs which are erythrocytic schizontocides are used to terminate an episode of malarial fever. They can be divided into:

Pharmacology

Fast-acting high-efficacy drugs	Slow-acting high-efficacy drugs
Chloroquine, amodiaquine, quinine, mefloquine, halofantrine, lumefantrine, atovaquone, artemisinin.	*Pronguanil.* **Pyrimethamine**, *sulfonamides, tetracyclines*
They can be used singly to treat attacks of malarial fever	They are used only in combination for clinical cure

> **Extra Mile**

- DOC for malaria: **Chloroquine** (safe in pregnancy)
- DOC for cerebral malaria: **Artisunate**
- DOC for chloroquine resistant malaria: **ACT**- *artemisinin combination therapy* (artisunate+pyrimethamine + sulfadoxine)
- Fastest acting anti-malarial: **Artimisinin**.
- Safest anti-malarial: **Proguanil**
- Short term prophylaxis of malaria (<6 weeks): **Doxycycline** 300 mg OD (start 2 days before)
- Long term prophylaxis of malaria (>6 weeks): **Mefloquine** 250 mg weekly (start a week before)

200. Ans. (a) Praziquantel

Ref: Katzung, 14th ed. pg. 944; Harrison, 17th ed. pg. 1334

- **Schistosomiasis is a type of infection caused by helminth subtypes that live in fresh water, such as rivers or lakes, in subtropical and tropical regions.**
- Schistosomiasis is also known as bilharzia.
- Symptoms can develop a few weeks after someone is infected by the parasite and include flu-like symptoms, such as a high temperature (fever) above 38°C (100.4°F) and muscle aches, skin rash, cough or urinary symptoms (cystitis, hematuria)

Anti-Helminthic agents

Helminthes	Name	Drug of choice
NEMATODE	Round worm (Ascaris) Pinworm (enterobius vermicularis) Hookworm (N. Americanus, A. duodenale) Whip worm (trichuris trichura) Trichinea worm (trichinella spiralis) Guinea worm (Dracunculus medinensis)	ALBENDAZOLE/ MEBENDAZOLE
	Filarial worm (W. Bancrofti, B. Malayi)	DEC/Ivermectin
	Onchocerca volvulus Threadworms (strongyloides stercoralis)	Ivermectin

Contd...

Helminthes	Name	Drug of choice
TREMATODE	Blood fluke (schistosoma japonicum, mansoni &Hematobium) Lung fluke (paragonimus westermani) Liver fluke (fasciola Heaptica) → *DOC: **Triclabendazole/Bithionol***	**PRAZIQUANTEL** EXCEPT for fasciola Hepatica (Triclabendazole)
CESTODE	Pork tapeworm (taenia solium) Beef tapeworm (taenia saginata) Fish tapeworm (Diphyllobothrium latum) Dog tapeworm (Echinococcus granulosus) Dwarf tapeworm (Hymenolepis Nana)	**PRAZIQUANTEL/ NICLOSAMIDE**

METRONIDAZOLE is DOC for: Trichomoniasis, Giardiasis, Bacterial vaginosis, Amoebic liver disease, Hydatid disease, Cysticercosis

201. Ans. (b) Triclabendazole

Ref: Katzung, 14th ed. pg. 939

- Drug of choice for all trematodes including blood flukes like schistosoma japonicum, mansoni &Hematobium and lung flukes paragonimus westermani is Praziquantel EXCEPT Liver fluke.
- DOC for Liver fluke (fasciola Heaptica) → **Triclabendazole/Bithionol**

202. Ans. (d) Albendazole

Ref: Katzung, 14th ed. pg. 940

Drug of choice for NCC: Albendazole

203. Ans. (a) Praziquantel

Ref: Katzung, 14th ed. pg. 939

- DOC for taenia solium (pork tapeworm) and Taenia saginata (Beef tapeworm) and fish tapeworm is: **PRAZIQUANTEL**

204. Ans. (c) Ivermectin

Ref: Katzung, 14th ed. pg. 939, 1075; KDT, 6th ed. pg. 864

- Scabies is caused by an ectoparasite sarcoptes scabei. It is highly contagious. The mite burrows through the epidermis, laying eggs which form papules that itch intensely.
- Most common site of entry- finger webs.

Explanations

- **Drugs used are:**
  - **Permethrin 5%:** broad spectrum and potent insecticide, currently most efficacious.
    - It is DOC for scabies.
    - **MOA:** It causes neurological paralysis in insects by delaying depolarization.
    - Single application needed in most cases.
    - Very less toxicity; 100% cure rate.
  - **Lindane:** another broad spectrum insecticide. Efficacy lower than permethrin.
    MOA: kills lice and mites by penetrating through their chitinous cover and affecting the nervous system.
  - **Benzyl benzoate:** Oily liquid with a faint aromatic smell.
    It is applied over face and neck after a bath. A second coat is applied next day which is washed after 24 hours.
  - Crotamiton
  - Sulfur
  - **Ivermectin:** Highly effective in scabies and pediculosis as well. Oral DOC in scabies.
    - It is the only ORALLY administered drug which is used for scabies (ectoparasitosis)
    - A single dose of 0.2 mg/kg has cured almost 90–100% of population.
    - It is contraindicated in children < 5 yrs, pregnant and lactating women.

205. Ans. (b) Permethrin

Ref: Katzung, 14th ed. pg. 1075; KDT, 6th ed. pg. 864

206. Ans. (a) Metronidazole

Must know points for tetanus (8th day illness presenting with lock jaw)
- Penicillin G was considered the drug of choice, but some now consider metronidazole to be superior in this setting. Tetracycline is an alternative for patients who are allergic to penicillin or metronidazole

Tetanus immunoglobulin is used to
- Prevent tetanus and to treat patients with circulating tetanus toxin and provides passive immunity.
- Treat all patients with active tetanus, in combination with other supportive and therapeutic treatments.

207. Ans. (d) Ivermectin

Ref: KDT, 6th ed. pg. 809; Katzung, 14th ed. pg. 939
- Usually *DOC for filariasis is Diethyl carbamazine (DEC).*
- *Since DEC was not in option, the next drug which comes under first line drug for filariasis is Ivermectin.*

- IVERMECTIN is also considered as drug of choice in following conditions:
  - Strongyloidiasis
  - Onchocerciasis
- PRAZIQUANTEL is drug of choice for:
  - Tapeworm infestation (Taenia saginata, Taenia solium, H. Nana)

208. Ans. (a) 2 mg/kg

Ref: KD Tripathi, 7th ed. pg. 853

Diethylcarbamazine
- It is the first drug for filariasis caused by the nematodes *Wuchereria bancrofti* (90% cases) and *Brugia malayi*.
- Plasma *t1/2* of usual clinical doses is 4–12 hours, depending on urinary pH.
  - Acidic pH: 2 – 3 hours
  - Alkaline pH: 8 – 10 hours
- The most important action of DEC appears to be alteration of organelle membranes of the microfilariae promoting cell death.
- The recommended doses in filarisis, Loiasis and Toxocariasis are similar i.e. 50 mg on day 1, 50 mg TDS on day 2, 100 mg TDS on day 3 and then 2 mg/kg TDS for 2–3 weeks.
- It can also be used to treat tropical eosinophilia in a dose of 2 mg/kg TDS for 7 days
- Doses of DEC in chemoprophylaxis:
  - Loiasis 300 mg weekly
  - Filariasis 50 mg monthly
- Yearly treatment with a combination of DEC (2 mg/kg) and **albendazole (400 mg single dose on mass scale has brought down transmission of filariasis by reducing microfilaroma.**

209. Ans. (a) Albendazole

Ref: KD Tripathi, 7th ed. pg. 853
- Yearly treatment with a combination of DEC (2 mg/kg) and **albendazole (400 mg single dose on mass scale has brought down transmission of filariasis by reducing microfilaroma.**
- **Recent** studies have revealed that:
  - 200 mg/day for 8 weeks course of doxycycline eliminated 95% of microfilariae.
  - A combination therapy of Doxycycline and Ivermectin can cause 100% elimination of microfilarie.

210. Ans. (b) Alters permeability of fungal cell wall

Ref: Sharama & Sharma 3rd ed. P 781
- Amphotericin binds to fungal cell membrane namely ergosterol and alters the permeability of fungal cell wall by forming pores through which macromolecules like

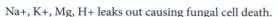

Pharmacology

Na+, K+, Mg, H+ leaks out causing fungal cell death.
- Resistance is due to replacement of ergosterol by other steol in fungal plasma membrane.
- Peak antifungal activity of the drug occurs at pH 6.0 to 7.5 and the drug is widely distributed to most tissues EXCEPT CNS.
- Plasma half life: 15 days
- Use:
  - Most commonly used to treat serious fingal infections from yeast or mould group.
  - Superficially can be given to treat candidiasis.
  - **DOC in following conditions:**
    - Invasive aspergillosis (all patients including immunocompromised)
    - Mucormycosis
    - Disseminated histoplasmosis
    - Rapidly progressive coccidiomycosis
    - Rapidly progressive blastomycosis
    - Non AIIDS cryptococcal meningitis
    - Oropharyhgeal and cutaneous candidiasis
    - Kala Azar (liposomal Amp B)

211. Ans. (d) Liposomal preparation

Ref: KD Tripathi, 7th ed. pg. 788

- Amphotericin B can be administered orally (50-100 mg QID) for intestinal moniliasis; also topically for vaginitis, otomycosis.
- **Conventional formulation of AMB (C-AMB)** For systemic mycosis, C-AMB is available as dry powder along with deoxycholate (DOC) for extemporaneous dispersion before use
- It is first suspended in **10** ml water and then diluted to 500 mL with glucose solution *(saline makes the suspension coarse and should be avoided)*.
- Initially 1 mg test dose is injected i.v. over 20 minutes. If no serious reaction follows, 0.3 mg/kg is infused over 4–8 hours daily.

Liposomal amphotericin B (small unilamellar vesicles SUV): Consists of 10% AMB incorporated in uniform sized (60-80 nM) unilamellar liposomes made up of lecithin and other biodegradable phospholipids.

The special features of these preparations are:
- They produce milder acute reaction (especially liposomal formulation) on i.v. infusion.
- They can be used in patients not tolerating infusion of conventional AMB formulation.
- They have lower nephrotoxicity.
- They cause minimal anemia.
- The liposomal preparation delivers AMB particularly to reticuloendothelial cells in liver and spleen especially valuable for Kala Azar and immunocompromised patients.

> **Extra Mile**
>
> **AMB combination regimen**
> - **Amphotericin B + Rifampin or minocycline**: The latter drugs are not themselves antifungal, but enhance the action of amphotericin B.
> - **Amphotericin B + Flucytosine**: A shorter course is needed, specially for cryptococcal meningitis, than when amphotericin is used alone.

212. Ans. (c) Cholelithiasis

Ref: Sharma & Sharma 3rd ed. P 783

Adverse Drug reactions of Amphotericin B

- The most common, most serious and long term side effect of amphotericin B is Nephrotoxicity (renal tubular necrosis)
- This nephrotoxicity presents with hypokalemia, hypomagnesemia secondary to renal tubular acidosis, azotemia and even irreversible damageif the dose exceeds 5g.
  - In order to prevent the nephrotoxicity, prior hydration with 1L of normal saline is recommended.
  - Liposomal preparation has lesser risk of nephrotoxicity
- Hypochromic normocytic anemia is common and thrombocytopenia and leukopenia although less common but has been noted.
- Intrathecal administration: Arachnoiditis and seizure
- Hepatic impairment and Jaundice
- Infusion related toxicity *(chills, tachypnea, fever, vomiting, hypotemsion, anaphylaxis)*

213. Ans. (b) Renal damage

Ref: Sharma & Sharma 3rd ed. P 783

Refer to above explanation for explanation

214. Ans. (c) Amphotericin- B

Ref: Harrison's, 18th ed. Ch. 279

- The most common, most serious and long term side effect of amphotericin B is Nephrotoxicity (renal tubular necrosis)
- This nephrotoxicity presents with hypokalemia, hypomagnesemia secondary to renal tubular acidosis, azotemia and even irreversible damageif the dose exceeds 5 g.
  - In order to prevent the nephrotoxicity, prior hydration with 1L of normal saline is recommended.
  - Liposomal preparation has lesser risk of nephrotoxicity

Note: *Cyclosporine also causes AKI with hypomagnesemia*

ANTITUBERCULAR AGENTS

215. Ans. (b) Liver disease

Ref: KD Tripathi, 7th ed. pg. 767

- INH is hepatotoxic and is avoided in pre-exisintg liver disease
- Isoniazid is an essential component of all anti-tubercular regimens. It is primarily tuberculocidal.
- Fast multiplying organisms are rapidly killed, but quiescent ones are only inhibited.
- The most common vmechanism which confers high level INH resistance is by mutation of the catalase-peroxidase (*KatG*) gene.
- INH resistance may also involve mutation in the *inhA* or *kasA* genes.

Adverse effects:

- **Peripheral neuritis** is the most important dose-dependent toxic effects (slow acetylators).
  - Pyridoxine given prophylactically (10 mg/day) prevents the neurotoxicity even with higher doses.
  - Prophylactic pyridoxine must be given to diabetics, chronic alcoholics, malnourished, pregnant, lactating and HIV infected patients, but routine use is not mandatory.
- Hepatitis, a major adverse effect of INH, (seen commonly in fast acetylators) more common in older people and in alcoholics is also a well-known side effect of the drug.
- **Other adverse effects:** Xerostomia, Allergic reactions, decrease seizure threshold.

> **Extra Mile**
> - Safest ATT in renal disease patients: Rifampicin
> - ATT which has no/least hepatotoxicity: Ethambutol and Streptomycin

216. Ans. (b) Rifampicin

Ref: KD Tripathi, 7th ed. pg. 767

- Rifampicin is considered as effective as isoniazid. This agent is active against slow and intermittently dividing bacterium (spurters).
- If someone develops resistance to INH, they are most likely to develop resistance to rifampicin as well.
- In MDR-TB, there is resistance to INH and rifampicin.

217. Ans. (b) Rifampicin

Ref: KDT 6th ed. pg. 740-44, Katzung Pharma 14th ed. pg. 845

RIFAMPICIN

- It is a tuberculocidal agent of M. tuberculosis in addition to staph. aureus, pseudomonas, proteus, legionella etc.
- It has bactericidal action of which covers all subpopulations of TB bacilli, *but acts best on slowly or intermittently dividing ones as well as on many atypical mycobacteria.*
- Both intracellular and extracellular bacilli are affected.
- **MOA:** It inhibits DNA dependent RNA synthesis
- **Resistance** of rifampicin is due to *rpoB gene*.
- **Adverse effects:**
  - Hepatotoxicity: MC/Major side effect
  - Rifampicin imparts a harmless **orange color to urine**, sweat, tears, and contact lenses *(soft lenses may be permanently stained)*.
  - Occasional adverse effects include rashes, thrombocytopenia, and nephritis.
  - It may cause cholestatic jaundice and occasionally hepatitis and flu-like symptoms.

ISONIAZID

- It is primarily tuberculocidal. *Fast multiplying organisms are rapidly killed but quiescent ones are only inhibited.*
- Acts on intracellular as well as extracellular TB bacilli and is equally active in acidic and alkaline medium.
- **MOA:** Inhibit synthesis of mycolic acid, which is a unique fatty acid component of mycobacterial cell wall.
- If given alone, resistance occurs in about 2-3 months
- **Most common mechanism of INH resistance:** Mutation of catalase-peroxidase gene > Mutation of *inh-A* gene.
- **Adverse effects:**
  - **Isoniazid-induced hepatitis** is the most common major toxic effect
  - Peripheral neuropathy is observed in 10–20% of patients
  - Neuropathy is due to a relative pyridoxine (Vit B6) deficiency. Isoniazid promotes excretion of pyridoxine, and this toxicity is readily reversed by administration of pyridoxine.
  - Central nervous system toxicity, which is less common, includes *memory loss, psychosis, and seizures.*

PYRAZINAMIDE

- It is weakly tuberculocidal. PYZ is more lethal to intracellularly located bacilli and to those at sites showing an inflammatory response.
- **MOA:** Resembles that of INH. It inhibits mycolic acid synthesis but by interacting with a different fatty acid synthase encoding gene.
- Resistance of PYZ due to mutation in *pncA gene*.
- **Adverse effects:** *Hepatotoxicity*, nausea, vomiting, drug fever, and **hyperuricemia**

ETHAMBUTOL

- Selectively tubecolostatic agent and clinically as active as streptomycin. *Fast multiplying bacilli are more susceptible as are many atypical mycobacteria.*

Pharmacology

- **MOA:** Poorly understood, but it has been found to inhibit arabinosyl transferases involved in arabinogalactan synthesis and to interfere with mycolic acid incorporation in mycobacterial cell wall.
- Resistance of ethambutol due to alteration in the drug target gene- **emb gene.**
- **Adverse effects:** *Retrobulbar neuritis, resulting in loss of visual acuity and red-green color blindness.*

▉ STREPTOMYCIN

- Tuberculocidal agent, acts only on extracellular bacilli. It penetrates the tubercular cavities but doesn't crosses the CSF. *Has poor action on acidic medium.*
- **Adverse effects:** Ototoxic and nephrotoxic.
- Resistance is due to a point mutation in either the **rpsL gene** or **rrs gene.**

218. Ans. (c) Increase the permeability of cell wall

Ref: KDT, 6th ed. pg. 742

- Ethambutol inhibits arabinosyl transferases which is involved in cell wall biosynthesis. By inhibiting this enzyme, the bacterial cell wall complex production is inhibited. **This leads to an increase in cell wall permeability.**

> **Extra Mile**
> - **ATT** acting exclusively on intracellular bacilli: Pyrazinamide
> - **ATT acting exclusively on extracellular bacilli: Streptomycin**

219. Ans. (d) Ethambutol

Ref: KDT, 6th ed. pg. 742

- **Side effect of Ethambutol:** Loss of visual acuity/colour vision, field defects due to **optic neuritis** is the most important dose and duration of therapy dependent toxicity.

> **Extra Mile**
> - Important side effects of antitubercular drugs:
> - Peripheral neuropathy (*due to vit B6 deficiency*): ISONIAZID
> - Orange color urine- RIFAMPICIN
> - Flu-like symptoms- RIFAMPICIN
> - Hyperuricemia/gout- PYRAZINAMIDE
> - Optic neuritis- ETHAMBUTOL
> - Nephrotoxic, Ototoxic, Neuromascular Junction Blocker- STREPTOMYCIN
>
> **Other important points to remember about Anti TB drugs:**
> - *First line anti TB drugs are:* **HRZE** *(Isoniazid, Rifampicin, Pyrazinamide, Ethambutol)*
> - All first line drugs are bactericidal EXCEPT- **Ethambutol** (it is bacteriostatic)
> - Most hepatotoxic ATT-**Pyrazinamide**
> - 1st line ATT with exclusive intracellular action-**Pyrazinamide**
> - 1st line ATT with exclusive extracellular action-**Streptomycin**
> - Which anti TB drugs are NOT hepatotoxic-**Ethambutol and Streptomycin.**

- It should not be used in children below 6 years of age because these young patients may not be able to report visual impairment.

220. Ans. (d) Ethambutol

Ref: KDT, pg. 742

- Ethalmbutol is selectively tuberculostatic and clinically as active as Streptomycin.

TABLE: 1st Line ATT Drugs action on bacteria and hepatoxicty

Drug	Bactericidal/ Bacteristatic	Hepatotoxicity
Isoniazid	Cidal	+
Rifampicin	Cidal	+
Pyrazinamide	Cidal	++++
Ethambutol	STATIC	- No
Streptomycin	Cidal	- No

221. Ans. (d) Ethambutol

Ref: Katzung's Pharmacology, 14th ed. pg. 846

- **Dose of Ethambutol:** 15-25 mg/kg OD dose.
- About 20% drug is excreted in feces and 50% in urine in unchanged form.
- *Ethambutol accumulates in renal failure, and the dose should be reduced by half if creatinine clearance is less than 10 mL/min.*
- **Side effect:** Most common serious adverse event is retrobulbar neuritis, resulting in loss of visual acuity and ***red green color blindness*** *(Patient develop BLUE VISION).*
  - It can also cause hyperuricemia and peripheral neuritis.
- **It is also Contraindicated** in children as they are unable to report loss of visual acuity and red-green color discrimination.

222. Ans. (a) 5 mg/kg PO qday

Ref: Katzung, 14th ed. pg. 843; KD Tripathi, 6th ed. pg. 746

TABLE: Recommended doses of antitubercular drug

DRUG	Daily dose		3 × per week dose	
	mg/kg	For >50 kg	mg/kg	For >50 kg
Isoniazid (H)	5 (4-6)	300 mg	10 (8-12)	600 mg
Rifampin (R)	10 (8-12)	600 mg	10 (8-12)	600 mg
Pyrazina-mide (Z)	25 (20-30)	1500 mg	35 (30-40)	2000 mg
Ethambutol (E)	15 (15-20)	1000 mg	30 (25-35)	1600 mg

223. Ans. (a) Rifampicin

Ref: KDT, 7th ed. pg. 768

MOA OF IMPORTANT ATT

- **Streptomycin**- inhibit protein synthesis
- **Chloroamphenicol**- inhibit protein synthesis by inhibiting transpeptidation
- **Rifampicin**- inhibit DNA dependent RNA synthesis by inhibiting RNA polymerase
- **INH & Pyrazinamide:** inhibits mycolic acid, a component of mycobacterial cell wall
- **Ethambutol:** Inhibit incorporation of mycolic acid into bacterial cell wall by inhibiting arabinosyl transferase, thus weakening the wall.

224. Ans. (c) Vitamin B6

Ref: KDT, 6th ed. pg. 740-41

- For patients who are on isoniazid; peripheral neuropathy is observed in 10–20% of patients given dosages greater than 5 mg/kg/d but is infrequently seen with the standard 300 mg adult dose.
- Pyridoxine (Vit B6), 25–50 mg/day, is recommended for those with conditions predisposing to neuropathy, an adverse effect of isoniazid.
- **Note:** *Isoniazid as a single agent is also indicated for treatment of latent tuberculosis. The dosage is 300 mg/day (5 mg/kg/day) or 900 mg twice weekly for 9 months.*

225. Ans. (b) Cycloserine

Ref: KDT, 6th ed. pg. 744; Katzung's pharma, 14th ed. pg. 847

- **Cycloserine (Cys)** is a 2nd line ATT. It is a chemical analogue of D-alanine:
- Cycloserine being cell wall inhibitior is tuberculostatic in nature and inhibits some other gram-positive bacteria, E. coli, Chlamydia also.
- **MOA:** it inhibits bacterial cell wall synthesis by inactivating the enzymes which recemize L-alanine and link two D-alanine residues.
- The dosage of cycloserine in tuberculosis is **0.5–1 g/d** in two divided doses
- **Adverse effect:** The CNS toxicity of Cys is high- sleepiness, headache, tremor, depression and **psychosis**.
- **Use:** MDK. TB

Extra Mile

- 2nd line ATT, Kanamycin, Amikacin, Capreomycin have similar side effect of ototoxicity and nephrotoxicity, same as streptomycin (1st line ATT).
- *Capreomycin, can induce electrolyte abnormalities.*

226. Ans. (c) Streptomycin

Ref: KDT, 6th ed. pg. 743-44

- Streptomycin has been assigned to pregnancy category D by the FDA.
- Streptomycin crosses the placenta; reported cord concentrations have been equal to or less than the mother's serum concentration.
- **There are reports of fetal eighth cranial nerve damage with subsequent bilateral deafness**. Most authorities, including the Centers for Disease Control and the American Thoracic Society, *discourage the use of streptomycin during pregnancy due to the risk of fetal ototoxicity.*
- Note: Streptomycin is no longer an ATT drug

227. Ans. (b) Streptomycin

Ref: KDT 6th ed. pg. 743-744

Please refer to above explanation

228. Ans. (b) Streptomycin

Please refer to above explanation.

229. Ans. (d) 5 TU

Ref: Essentials of TB Diagnosis Children, 3rd ed. pg. 325

230. Ans. (c) PAS

Ref: 2008 WHO guidelines for programmatic management or drug resistant tuberculosis

- Second line ATT like PAS (para amino salicylic acid) and ethionamide can lead to hypothyroidism. Exact mechanism is poorly understood.
- PAS also causes adverse reactions like GI upset, hepatotoxicity, Hypersensitivity.

231. Ans. (b) Pyrazinamide

Ref: Katzung, 14th ed. pg. 846; KDT, 6th ed. pg. 742

Pyrazinamide Microsomal deaminase Pyrazinoic acid (POA) → 5-hydroxypyrazinoic acid

- Pyrazinamide is hydrolyzed by microsomal deaminase to pyrazinoic acid (POA) and then hydroxylated to 5-hydroxypyrazinoic acid by xanthine oxidase for excretion by the kidneys.
- *Pyrazinamide is a first line antitubercular drug that can cause hyperuricemia (secondary to inhibition of uric acid secretion in the kidney) and hepatotoxicity.*
- This hyperuricemia leads to arthralgia due to competitive inhibition of xanthine oxidase by POA. *It should not be stopped if hyperuricemia develops*

Pharmacology

- Ethambutol also produces hyperuricemia due to interferance with urate excretion.

ANTICANCER DRUGS

232. Ans. (c) 5FU

Ref: Page 987: SRB 5th edition

Chemoradiation is the preferred treatment of anal cancer. 5FU is the preffered drug. Initially radiation is given for 3 weeks to the perenium and pelvis. This is followed by chemotherapy using 5FU and mitomycin C.

233. Ans. (b) Dihydrofolate reductase inhibitor

Ref: Goodman & Gillman's 13th ed. P 1179

- Pemetrexed is a most recent folate analogue which is avidly transported into cells via the reduced folate carrier and is converted to its metabolite (PGs- Polyglutamate) that inhibit Thymidylate synthase and glycine amide ribonucleotide transformylase, as well as DHFR. (Dihydrofolate Reductase)
- It is even more potent than methotrexate.
- Like MTX, it induces p53 and cell-cycle arrest, but this effect does not depend on induction of p21.
- **Use:** It has activity against ovarian cancer, mesothelioma, and adenocarcinomas of the lung.
- Other effects and side effects are similar to methotrexate like myelosuppression, GI toxicity. The toxicity can be attenuated with folate and vitamin B_{12} supplementation.

> **Extra Mile**
> - A newer congener, **pralatrexate**, is more effectively taken up and polyglutamated than MTX and is approved for treatment of CTCL peripheral T cell lymphoma.
> - Pramipexole is an antiparkinsonism drug which is a dopamine agonist.

234. Ans. (a) Methotrexate toxicity

Ref: Goodman & Gillman's 13th ed. P 1177

- Folic acid is an essential dietary factor which is converted to FH4 by DHFR enzyme and provide methyl groups for the synthesis of precursors of DNA.
- Folic acid analogues such as MTX interfere with FH4 metabolism, thereby inhibiting DNA replication.
- **Adverse effects:** Myelosuppression, GI toxicity.
- **Folinic acid (Leucovorin)** can reverse toxic effects; used as "rescue" in high-dose therapy.
- **Glucarpidase**, a methotrexate-cleaving enzyme, is approved to treat toxicity.

235. Ans. (a) Paclitaxel

Ref: Katzung, 14th ed. pg. 963; Cancer Medicine, 6th ed. pg. 595

TABLE: Radiosensitizers vs Radiation protection agent

Radiosensitizers	Radiation protection agent
Actinomycin	Amifostine
Gemcitabine	GM-CSF
Hydroxyurea	TL-1
Metronidazole	
Misonidazole	
5- FU	
Mitomycin	
Paclitaxel	

236. Ans. (b) Methotrexate

Ref: K.D. Tripathi, 6th ed. pg. 823

- Methotrexate is one of the oldest and highly efficacious antineoplastic drugs
- **MOA:** It inhibits dihydrofolate reductase (DHFRase)- blocking the conversion of dihydrofolic acid (DHFA) to tetrahydrofolic acid (THFA) which is an essential coenzyme required for one carbon transfer reactions in de novo purine synthesis and amino acid interconversions.
- **DHFRase inhibitors are:** methotrexate, Pemetrexed, Pralatrexate

> **Extra Mile**
> - Vincristine is a mitotic spindle formation inhibitor
> - Paclitaxel is a spindle breakdown inhibitor
> - Cisplatin is a platinum based compound.

237. Ans. (a) Nilotinib

Ref: KD Tripathi, 7th ed. pg. 870

- **Nilotinib** It is a second generation Bcr-Abl, PDGF-receptor β and c-kit receptor tyrosine kinase inhibitor with **20-50 fold higher affinity for these kinases than imatinib.** Thus, it can overcome resistance to imatinib due to Bcr-Abl mutation and is effective in chronic CML nonresponsive to imatinib.
- It is only 30% bioavailable orally, but absorption is improved by food. It is also useful in accelerated phase of CML. Thus, it is an alternative drug in imatinib non-tolerant or resistant cases of CML, and has now been used as a first-line drug as well.

238. Ans. (a) Letrozole

Ref: Katzung, 14th ed. pg. 739; KDT, 6th ed. pg. 305

- Adrenal cortex mainly produces androgen, and this androgen in females is converted to estrogen with the help of enzyme aromatase.

- Androgen $\xrightarrow{\text{Aromatase}}$ Estrogen
- Excess formation of estrogen exposes a person to develop breast CA and on the other hand also protect females from osteoporosis *(estrogen is protective in bone)*.
- A class of breast cancer drugs called aromatase inhibitors decreases the body's production of estrogen, at a level where there is nearly total estrogen deprivation in body.
- But at the same time it decreases bone mineral density and increase the risk of fractures in postmenopausal women.
- **Aromatase inhibitors include:** Letrozole, Anastrazole, and Exemestane.
- Letrozole is currently recommended as the first line therapy in case of advanced breast CA.
- **S/E:** Hot flushes, nausea, diarrhea, dyspepsia and thinning of hair and most commonly bone loss (osteoporosis)

Extra Mile

- **Tamoxifen** is a selective estrogen receptor modulator (SERM). It is beneficial in breast, bone and blood cancer.
- Side effect: Tamoxifen increases risk of endometrial CA.
- Only pulsatile exposure to GnRH induces LH/FSH secretion, while continuous exposure desensitizes pituitary which results in loss of GnRH release.

GnRH Agonist	GnRH Antagonist
Given in continuous manner for the treatment of breast CA, prostate CA, and precocious puberty. Drugs are: • Leuprolide • Nafarelin • Goserelin • Busurelin	Given in any manner/pulsatile manner for the treatment of infertility and hypogonadism. **Drugs are:** • Ganirelix • Letrorelix • Abarelix • Cetrorelix
Causes flare up reaction	Doesn't cause flare up reaction

239. Ans. (b) Endometrial cancer

Ref: KDT, 6th ed. pg. 304-5

- Tamoxifen is selective estrogen receptor modulator (SERM).
- It is having agonistic activity at uterine endometrium.

TABLE: Action of Tamoxifen

Agonistic activity	Antagonistic activity
Uterus: causes proliferation of endometrium → *can cause vaginal bleeding* as seen in the case	Breast CA
Bone: decrease resorption	Blood vessels
Lipid profile: decrease LDL without affecting HDL → decrease risk of CAD	

240. Ans. (c) Cladribine

Ref: KDT, pg. 819-20; Katzung, 14th ed. pg. 958–961

- **Alkylating agents** have cytotoxic and radiomimetic actions. They are mainly cell cycle non-specific, i.e. act on dividing as well as resting cells.
- Cross-linking of DNA appears to be of major importance to the cytotoxic action of alkylating agents, and replicating cells are most susceptible to these drugs.
- **Drugs are:**

Alkylating agents- cell cycle-nonspecific agents	Antimetabolites- cell cycle-specific agents
Nitrogen mustard • Cyclophosphamide • Ifosfamide • Mechlorethamine • *Melphalan* • Chlorambucil **Drugs acting by Methylation** • Procarbazine • Dacarbazine • Temozolomide **Nitrosoureas** • Carmustine • Lomustine • Semustine • Streptozocin **Miscellaneous** • Busulfan • Altretamine • Thiotepa • Trabectadin	**Folic acid antagonist:** Methotrexate **Purine analogues** • 6 Mercaptopurine • 6 thioguanine • Cladribine • Fludarabine *Pyrimidine analogues* • Capecitabin • Gemcitabin • Cyatarabine and 5 FU

241. Ans. (a) Bleomycin

Ref: KDT, 819-20, 26; Katzung, 14th ed. pg. 951

- **Bleomycin:** This is a mixture of closely related glycopeptides antibiotics having potent antitumour activity.
- It is highly effective in testicular tumour and squamous cell carcinoma of skin, oral cavity, head and neck, genitourinary tract and esophagus.
- **Side effect:** pulmonary fibrosis and myelosuppression.
- *Please refer to above explanation for more details of alkylating agents.*

242. Ans. (d) All of the above

Ref: KDT, pg. 819-20; Katzung, 11th ed. pg. 1280

Please refer to above explanation.

Pharmacology

243. Ans. (b) Alkylating agent

Ref: Katzung, 14th ed. pg. 951; KDT, pg. 819-820

- Cyclophosphamide is the most widely used alkylating agent.
- It is an inactive compound. Transformation into active metabolite occurs in liver, and a wide range of anti tumor action is exerted.
- It has prominent immunosuppressant property, so it has been particularly utilized in bone marrow transplantation. In other organ transplants it is employed only as a reserve drug.
- **Drugs of different category are:**

Alkylating agents	Antimetabolites	Platinum compound	Topo-isomerase inhibitors
Cyclophosphamide Ifosfamide Mechlorethamine *Melphalan Busulfan* Procarbazine **Nitrosourea** Carmustine Lomustine Semustine	**Folic acid antagonist** Methotrexate **Purine analogues** 6 Mercaptopurine 6 thioguanine **Cladribine** Fludarabine **Pyrimidine analogues** Capecitabin Gemcitabin **Cyatarabine** and 5 FU	Cisplatin Carboplatin Oxaliplatin	TOPOISOMERASE- I Irinotecam TOPOISOMERASE-II Etoposide Anthracycline Doxorubicin Daunorubicin

244. Ans. (c) Cytarabine

Ref: Katzung, 14th ed. pg. 951; KDT, 6th ed. pg. 820

- Cytarabine is pyrimidine analogue

Please refer to above explanation.

> **Extra Mile**
> - DOC for hairy cell leukemia- **CLADRIBINE**
> - DOC for CLL- **FLUDARABINE**
> - DOC for pancreatic CA- **GEMCITABINE**
> - 6 Mercaptopurine metabolized by- **XANTHINE OXIDASE**
> - DOC for choriocarcinoma- **METHOTREXATE**

245. Ans. (a) Purine analogue

Ref: Katzung, 14th ed. pg. 960; KDT, 6th ed. pg. 820

- Mercaptopurine is synthetic purine used in cancer chemotherapy.
- Use: Childhood acute leukemia.

246. Ans. (d) Cisplastin

Ref: KDT, 6th ed. 832; Katzung, 14th ed. pg. 956, 957

- Cisplatin is considered as first line chemotherapy in cervix CA and is very effective in metastatic testicular and ovarian carcinoma.
- Cisplatin is a platinum coordination complex that is hydrolyzed intracellularly to produce a highly reactive moiety which causes cross linking of DNA by platinum compound.
- The primary binding site is the N7 of guanine, but covalent interaction with adenine and cytosine also occurs.
- Cyclophospahmide, lomustine and vincristine is considered as the 2nd line drugs for the carcinoma of cervix.

> **Extra Mile**
> - Most emetogenic anti CA drug: **CISPLATIN**
> - Specific side effect of cisplatin: Nephrotoxicity and Ototoxicity.
> - Nitrosoureas like Lomustine can cross BBB and is considered as DOC for brain tumor like Glioma.
> - Most common marrow sparing anti CA drug- **VINCRISTINE**

247. Ans. (a) Imatainib mesylate

Ref: KD Tripathi, 6th ed. pg. 828 & 832

IMATINIB

- DOC for CML & GIST - Imatinib Mesylate
- It inhibits the tyrosine protein kinases in chronic myeloid leukaemia (CML) cells and and c-kit receptor found in gastrointestinal stromal tumour (GIST).
- Adverse effects are fluid retention, edema, vomiting, abdominal pain, myalgia and liver damage

TABLE: Drugs of choice for some commonly asked malignancies

Malignancy	First line drugs
Chronic Lymphatic leukaemia	Fludarabine
Chronic Myeloid leukaemia	Imatinib
Hairy cell leukemia	CLADRIBINE
Multiple myeloma	Bortezomib > Melphalan
Choriocarcinoma	Methotrexate
Prostate carcinoma	Bicalutamide/Flutamide

248. Ans. (b) Inhibit TXA2 formation

Ref: KDT, 6th ed. pg. 609; Katzung, 14th ed. pg. 620

- ASPIRIN has an antiplatelet effect by inhibiting the production of thromboxane.
- Thromboxane, normally helps in platelet aggregation.
- TXA_2 formation is suppressed even at very low doses **of aspirin.**

- PGI$_2$ is prostacyclin. Aspirin acts as prostacyclin analogue. It doesn't inhibit PGI$_2$ formation.
- TEUROTROBAN–TXA$_2$ receptor antagonist.

249. Ans. (a) Inhibit dihydrofolate reductase

Ref: Katzung, 14th ed. pg. 957; KD Tripathi, 6th ed. pg. 823

METHOTREXATE (MTX)

$$DHFA \xrightarrow{DHF\ Rase} THFA$$

- Methotrexate is a highly efficacious antineoplastic drug which inhibits dihydrofolate reductase (DHFRase) enzyme- blocking the conversion of dihydrofolic acid (DHFA) to tetrahydrofolic acid (THFA).
- This conversion is essential for formation of an essential coenzyme required for one carbon transfer reactions in denovo purine synthesis and amino acid interconversions.
- Methotrexate has cell cycle specific action kills cells in S phase; primarily inhibits DNA synthesis.

> **Extra Mile**
> Drug of choice for Mtx toxicity: FOLINIC ACID.

250. Ans. (b) Folinic acid

Ref: Katzung, 14th ed. pg. 957; KDT, 6th ed. pg. 823

- *The toxicity of Mtx can not be overcome by folic acid, because it will not be converted to the active coenzyme form.however folinic acid rapidly reverses the effect.*
- Thymidine also counteracts the Mtx toxicity.
- Refer to above explanation.

251. Ans. (d) Methotrexate

Ref: Katzung, 14th ed. pg. 955, 957; KDT, 6th ed. pg. 823

- **Methotrexate** is an antimetabolite which act by inhibiting Dihydro folate Reductase.
- It is DOC for Choriocarcinoma, and is also considered among the first line drugs in Breast CA, testicular tumors, cervix CA and osteogenic sarcoma.
- Mtx is NOT indicated in MM.
- **Melphalan** is very effective in multiple myeloma and has been used in advanced ovarian cancer.
- First line drugs of multiple myeloma: Melphalan, Prednisolone, Cyclophosphamide.
- **Thalidomide** was used previously for morning sickness but later withdrawn due to severe teratogenic effects (phocomelia).
- It has been re-introduced due to its immunomodulatory and anti-cancer properties. It has been approved for multiple myeloma and erythema nodosum leprosum and is being tried for myelodysplastic syndrome, melanoma,

Bechet disease, HIV associated ulcers and graft versus host disease.
- **Zolendronic acid:** It is a *bisphosphonate* indicated for the treatment of bony metastases and multiple myeloma.

252. Ans. (c) Cisplatin

Ref: Katzung, 14th ed. pg. 956; KDT, 6th ed. pg. 828

- **Cisplatin** is a platinum coordination complex that is hydrolyzed intracellularly to produce a highly reactive moiety which causes cross linking of DNA by platinum compound.
- It is a highly emetic drug. Antiemetics are routinely administered before infusing cisplatin.
- **DOC for cisplatin induced vomiting:** Ondansetron
- **Major s/e of cispltin:** Ototoxicity and nephrotoxicity.

253. Ans. (c) Cisplatin

Ref: Katzung 14th ed. pg. 956, 957

- **Cisplatin** is a widely used anti cancer drug.
- It has major antitumor activity in a broad range of solid tumors including
  - Non-small cell and small cell lung cancer
  - Esophageal and gastric cancer
  - Head and neck cancer and
  - Genitourinary cancers, particularly testicular, ovarian, and bladder cancer.
- When used in combination regimens with vinblastine and bleomycin or etoposide and bleomycin, cisplatin-based therapy has led to the cure of nonseminomatous testicular cancer.

> **Extra Mile**
> 5-FU is a pyrimidine analogue used in colorectal cancer. Methotrexate is considered as DOC for choriocarcinoma.

254. Ans. (a) 6-mercaptopurine

Ref: Katzung, 14th ed. pg. 960–61; KDT, 6th ed. pg. 820

- 6 mercaptopurine (6-MP) is a purine analogue which is metabolized by xanthine oxidase
- It is a competitive inhibitor of DNA.
- Allopurinol is NOT given along with 6-MP because allopurinol inhibits xanthine oxidase enzyme, which leads to increased toxicity due to accumulation of xanthine.

Anti-neoplastic drugs	Their side effect
Cyclophosphamide, ifosphamide	Hemorrhagic cystitis
Procarbazine	Disulfiram like reaction
Bleomycin, busulfan	Pulmonary fibrosis
Vincristine, vinblastine	Peripheral neuropathy
Cisplatin	Ototoxicity, Nephrotoxicity
6Mercaptopurine, 6Thioguanine	Hepatotoxicity
Doxorubicin, Daunorubicin	Cardiotoxic

Pharmacology

255. Ans. (d) Cyclophosphamide

Ref: Katzung, 14th ed. pg. 988; KDT, 6th ed. pg. 822

- **Cyclophosphamide** is a prodrug and is activated by hepatic biotransformation to aldophosphamide which is degraded to *acrolein.* This end product acrolein is responsible for hemorhagic cystitis, which is considered as the adverse side effect of cyclophosphamide.
- *This adverse effect can be controlled by Mesna (mercapto ethane sulfonic acid).*
- **Note:** Cyclophosphamide is DOC for Wegener's granulomatosis (*granulomatosis with polyangiitis*)
- *All natural anticancer products can cause bone marrow suppression EXCEPT bleomycin and vincristine.*

256. Ans. (a) Vincristine

Ref: Katzung, 14th ed. pg. 970; Harrison, 17th ed. pg. 699

Preferred regimen for Hodgkins and Non-hodgkins lymphoma

Hodgkins lymphoma (ABVD)	Non-hodgkin's lymphoma
A: Adriamycin (Doxorubicin) B: Bleomycin V: Vinblastin D: Dacarbazine	R: Rituximab C: Cyclophosphamide H: Hydroxdaunorubicin (doxorubicin) O: Oncovin (*vincristine*) P: Prednisolone

257. Ans. (b) Doxorubicin

Ref: Katzung, 14th ed. pg. 964–65; KDT, 6th ed. pg. 826-27

- **Doxorubicin** and daunorubicin are anti-tumor antibiotics. Activity of Daunorubicin is limited to acute leukemia while doxorubicin is effective in several solid tumors.
  - **MOA:** Cause breaks in DNA strands by activating topoisomerse II and generating quinolone type free radicals.
  - Doxrorubicin and daunorubicin both these antibiotics produce cardiotoxicity as a unique adverse effect.
- **Actinomycin D (Dactinomycin)** It is a very potent antineoplastic drug, highly efficacious in Wilms' tumour and rhabdomyosarcoma
  - Prominent adverse effects are vomiting, stomatitis, diarrhoea, erythema and desquamation of skin, alopecia and bone marrow depression
- **Mitoxantrone:** Recently introduced analogue of doxorubicin with lower cardiotoxicity, probably because it does not produce quinine type free radicals. Though

cardiomyopathy can occur, major toxicity is marrow depression and mucosal inflammation.
- **Mitomycin C:** This highly toxic drug is used only in resistant cancers of stomach, cervix, colon, rectum, bladder, etc
  - Bone marrow and GIT are the primary targets of toxicity.

258. Ans. (d) Mitomycin

Ref: KDT, 6th ed. pg. 827

- After 8–10 months of start of mitomycin-C treatment, the drug leads to endothelial damage
- The Renal lesions seen are similar to those seen in idiopathic HUS and include arteriolar fibrin thrombi, expanded sub-endothelial zones in glomerular capillary walls.
- HUS can be seen with: Mitomycin C, Gemcitabine

259. Ans. (c) Amifostine

Ref: Cancer Medicine 6th ed. pg. 595

TABLE: Radiosensitizers vs Radiation protection agent

Radiosensitizers	Radiation protection agent
Actinomycin Gemcitabine Hydroxyurea Metronidazole Misonidazole 5-FU Mitomycin Paclitaxel	Amifistone GM-CSF TL-1

CARDIOVASCULAR SYSTEM

260. Ans. (b) PPAR-α activator

Ref: Goodman & Gillman's 13th ed. P 6 13-14

Gemfibrozil

- Gemfibrozil, a PPARα activator, classified under hypolipidemic drugs, fibrates.
- The PPAR family is composed of three members: α, β and γ.
- PPARα is the target for the fibrate class of drugs, including the widely prescribed *gemfibrozil* and *fenofibrate*.
- Exact mechanism how the fibrates lower lipoprotein levels, or raise HDL levels, remains unclear.
- Fibrates bind to PPARα and:
  - Reduce triglycerides through PPARα-mediated stimulation of fatty acid oxidation
  - **Increased LPL synthesis** would enhance the clearance of triglyceride-rich lipoproteins.

- **Reduced expression of apo C-III** which serves as an inhibitor of lipolysis and receptor-mediated clearance, would enhance the clearance of VLDLs.
- Fibrate-mediated increases in HDL-C are due to PPARα stimulation of apo A-I and apo A-II expression, which increases HDL levels.
- Fenofibrate is more effective than gemfibrozil at increasing HDL levels.

> **Extra Mile**
> - PPARγ is the target for the thiazolidinedione class of anti-type 2 diabetic drugs, including rosiglitazone and pioglitazone. PPARγ does not induce xenobiotic metabolism.
> - Ezetimibe inhibits intestinal cholesterol absorption.
> - HMG-CoA inhibitor are statins (For example, simvastatin, rosuvastatin, etc.)

261. Ans. (a) Competitive inhibition

Ref: Goodman & Gillman's 13th ed. P 609

- Statins exert their major effect—reduction of LDL levels—through a mevalonic acid–like moiety that **competitively** inhibits HMG-CoA reductase, which is the rate limiting enzyme in the cholesterol biosynthesis.
- **Drugs are** atorvastatin, rosuvastatin, fluvastatin, lovastatin, pravastatin, simvastatin, pitavastatin.

> **Extra Mile**
> - Food increases absorption of statins
> - Statins are most active at night, so given at night except rosuvastatin and atorvastatin which are longest acting statins.

262. Ans. (b) Dobutamine

DOC for cardiogenic shock: Dobutamine

263. Ans. (a) Hypokalemia

Ref: KD Tripathi, 7th ed. pg. 496

- Digitalis increases force of cardiac contraction by a direct action independent of innervation. It selectively binds to extracellular face of the membrane associated Na^+K^+ ATPase of myocardial fibers and inhibits this enzyme.
- Inhibition of this cation pump results in progressive accumulation of Na^+ intracellularly. This indirectly results in intracellular Ca^{2+} accumulation by reversing the direction of Na-Ca+ exchanger channel, which causes ionotropic action.
- **Note:** in normal situation, Na-Ca+ exchanger pumps out Ca+ in exchange of Na+. But after bloking action of Digoxin, the direction of exchanger channel is reversed causing Pumping out Na+ in exchange with Ca+ from outside.
  - This accumulated Ca+ intracellular acts at sarcoplasmic reticulum and causes release of more calcium → Ionotropic action

- Higher serum potassium concentration inhibits digitalis binding to Na-K+ ATPase. Therefore hyperkalemia can reduce digitalis toxicity and Hypokalemia can cause digitalis toxicity.
- **Note:** Hypokalemia and hypercalcemia precipitate digoxin toxicity.
- **Action:**
  - Digitalis increases the force of contraction and decreases the heart rate due to its vagomimetic action
  - It also decreases the AV conduction, hence contraindication in WPW syndrome.
  - Causes diuresis in CHF patients
  - Causes decrease in peripheral resistance in CHF patients *(because of withdrawal of reflex sympathetic overactivity)*

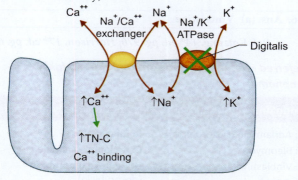

1. Inhibition of NA^+/K ATPase pump by digitalis
2. Increased NA^+ concentration inside the cell
3. Increased exchange of Na^+ for Ca^{++}
4. Increased intracellular Ca^{++}
5. Increased influx of Ca^{++} from sarcoplasmic reticulum
6. Increased contractility of cardiac muscle

264. Ans. (b) Pumps sodium inside cell in exchange of Ca+

Ref: Katzung, 14th ed. pg. 217–18

- In normal situation, Na-Ca+ exchanger pumps out Ca+ in exchange of Na+. But after bloking action of Digoxin, the direction of exchanger channel is reversed causing Pumping out Na+ in exchange with Ca+ from outside.
- This accumulated Ca+ intracellular acts at sarcoplasmic reticulum and causes release of more calcium → Ionotropic action

265. Ans. (b) Labetalol

Ref: Katzung, 14th ed. pg. 183

- CCBs and Diuretics are contraindicated in pregnancy for blood pressure management.
- In this given scenario, anti hypertensive will be started for patient's PIH management.
- Drug preferred in pregnancy induced hypertension: Labetalol (DOC)
- DOC for hypertensive emergency in pregnancy: Labetalol

Pharmacology

266. Ans. (b) Blockade of ATP sensitive K+ channels

Ref: Katzung, 14th ed. pg. 175–76

- K+ channel openers (minoxidil, diazoxide) are used as antihypertensives and not the channel blockers. Blockers of ATP sensitive K+ channels like sulfonylureas are used in diabetes mellitus.
- **Antihypertensive drugs can act by the following mechanisms:**
  - **Diuretics**: Thiazides and loop diuretics
- DOC for hypertension: Thiazide Diuretics
  - **Vasodilators: These have different mechanisms like**
    - NO releasers e.g. sodium nitroprusside and hydralazine
    - K+ channel openers e.g. minoxidil, Diazoxide
    - Ca+ channel blockers e.g. amlodipine, Nifedipine, Verapamil, Diltiazem
    - D1 agonist e.g. fenoldopam
  - **Sympathetic blockers:** These can have following mechanisms
    - Ganglion blockers e.g. trimethaphan
    - Adrenergic neuron blockers e.g. guanethidine
    - Alpha 2 agonists e.g. clonidine, alpha methyldopa
    - Receptor blockers like alpha and beta blockers
  - **Renin angiotensin system blockers:** These include:
    - Renin inhibitors e.g. Enalkiren, Remikiren
    - ACE inhibitors e.g. Enalapril, Captopril, Lisinopril
    - Angiotensin receptor blockers e.g. Losartan, Telmisartan
    - Aldosterone antagonists e.g. Spironolactone, Eplerenone

267. Ans. (a) Nifedipine

Ref: Katzung, 14th ed. pg. 203–204; KDT, pg. 323

- Nifedipine is a calcium channel blocker which is used as an alternative drug for premature labor.
- Influx of calcium ions plays an important role in uterine contractions. CCB's reduce tone of myometrium and oppose contractions.
- These drugs, especially Nifedipine can postpone labor only if started early enough.
- In emergency situation, Ritodrine (β2 selective agonist) is considered as the drug of choice to suppress preterm labor.

> **Extra Mile**
> - **Drug of choice for hypertension in pregnancy-** LABETALOL
> - **Drug of choice for epilepsy in pregnancy-** Lamotrigine
> - DOC for status eclampticus in pregnancy → phenobarbitone

268. Ans. (b) ACE inhibitors

Ref: KDT, 6th ed. pg. 553

Antihypertensive to be avoided during pregnancy	Antihypertensive safer during pregnancy
• ACE inhibitors (Ex- captopril, enelapril etc.) • Angiotensin antagonist (losartan, telmisartan) • Thiazide diuretics (Ex- hydrochlorthiazide) • Furosemide • Propanolol • Nitroprusside	• Hydralazine • Methyldopa • Atenolol • Metoprolol • *Labetalol- DOC* • Nifedipine • Prazosin and Clonidine

Drugs and their Respective Risk

- **Diuretics:** Tend to reduce blood volume; increase risk of placental infarcts, fetal wastage, still birth.
- **ACE inhibitors, AT1 antagonists:** Growth retardation and fetal damage risk.
- **Propanolol:** Causes low birth weight, neonatal hypoglycemia and bradycardia.
- **Nitroprusside:** Contraindicated in eclampsia.

269. Ans. (c) Captopril

Ref: KDT, 6th ed. pg. 553

Please refer to above explanation.

270. Ans. (a) ACE inhibitors

Ref: Katzung, 14th ed. pg. 187–188

- ACE inhibitors are drug of choice for scleroderma induced hypertensive crisis. Other important points and side effects about ACE inhibitors can be remembered as:
  - **C - Cough**
  - **A - Angioedema**
  - **P - Prodrugs** (EXCEPT captopril and Lisinopril)
  - **T - Taste disturbances**
  - **O - Orthostatic hypotension** (when combined with diuretics)
  - **P - Pregnancy** (contraindicated)
  - **R - bilateral Renal artery stenosis** (contraindicated)
  - **I - Increased K+** (contraindicated)
  - **L - Lower the formation of Ang II** (Mechanism)

271. Ans. (b) Verapamil

Ref: Katzung, 14th ed. pg. 246

- Supra ventricular tachycardia is a condition presenting as rapid heart rhythm originating at or above the AV node. SVT can be contrasted with the potentially more dangerous ventricular tachycardias- rapid rhythms that originate within the ventricular tissue.
- Calcium channel blockers have well-documented efficacy in hypertension and supraventricular tachyarrhythmias.
- SA and AV nodal tissues, which are mainly composed of slow response cells, are affected markedly by verapamil, moderately by diltiazem, and much less by dihydropyridines.

- *Thus, verapamil and diltiazem decrease atrioventricular nodal conduction and are effective in the management of supraventricular tachycardia.*

> **Extra Mile**
>
> DOC for paroxysmal supra ventricular tachycardia- **ADENOSINE**
> DOC for SVT- **VERAPAMIL**
> DOC for Atrial Fibrillation- **DIGITALIS (Digoxin, Digitoxin)**
> DOC for digitalis induced ventricular arrhythmia- **LIGNOCAINE**

272. Ans. (b) Adenosine

Ref: Katzung, 14th ed. pg. 246; KD Tripathi, 6th ed. pg. 509 & 518

- Paroxysmal supraventricular tachycardia (PSVT) is sudden onset episodes of atrial tachycardia (rate 150-200/min) with 1:1 atrioventricular conduction
- An attack of PSVT can be terminated by i.v. injection of verapamil, diltiazem, esmolol or digoxin; **but most cardiologists now prefer adenosine.**
- Adenosine has a very short t ½ in blood (~ 10 sec)
- Almost complete elimination occurs in a single passage through coronary circulation.

273. Ans. (b) ACE inhibitors

Ref: KDT, 6th ed. pg. 484

- Angiotensin converting enzyme normally helps in conversion of angiotensin I to angiotensin II, which acts as a vasoconstrictor in case of hypovolemia.
- In addition to that, ACE also helps in breakdown of bradykinin.
- When ACE inhibitors (captopril) are given, it inhibits ACE and in addition inhibits breakdown of bradykinin also, which leads to accumulation of bradykinin level in body.
- This increased level of bradykinin presents with Dry cough, rashes, urticaria and angioedema.

Other side effects of ACE inhibitors	Contraindications of ACE (–)	Safe alternative of ACE (–)
Hypotension Hyperkalemia Fetal growth retardation	Pregnancy Bilateral Renal artery stenosis Hyperkalemia	Angiotensin receptor blocker is a safe alternative in case of cough, angioedema.

> **Extra Mile**
>
> - Why ACEI is contraindicated in bilateral renal stenosis
>   - Patients with B/L renal artery stenosis or patients with single kidney having renal artery stenosis will develop renal failure if treated with ACEI.
>   - In stenosis there is reduced GFR, and body manage the adequate GFR by angiotensin II mediated efferent arteriole constriction to maintain the renal perfusion. In such patients, Inhibition of ACE can induce acute renal insufficiency.

274. Ans. (a) Act by Na+ K+ ATPase inhibition

Ref: KDT, 6th ed. pg. 540

- Thiazide and related drugs (chlorthalidone) are the diuretic of choice in uncomplicated hypertension. It acts by reducing plasma volume and by decreasing total peripheral resistance.
- Alpha receptors are present on vessel wall, which upon stimulation constricts vessel wall and increase total peripheral resistance. Alpha adrenergic blocking agents like Prazosin, terazosin, doxazosin and phentolamine inhibit the alpha receptor and decrease total peripheral resistance.
- β1 receptors are present on heart, which upon stimulation increase the heart rate. Beta adrenergic blockers like nebivolol, metoprolol, atenolol etc. are some of the beta blockers which depress myocardial contractility, and decreases the stroke volume.
- **Na+ K+ ATPase inhibition** is done by Digitalis. Digitalis however has no role in control of hypertension. It is used in congestive heart failure and atrial fibrillation.

> **Extra Mile**
>
> - Digitalis MOA in atrial fibrillation: Decreases conduction.
> - M/c side effect of digitalis: Nausea/vomiting.
> - MC cardiac side effect (arrhythmia) caused by digitalis: Ventricular Bigeminy.
> - DOC for digitalis induced arrhythmia: LIGNOCAINE

275. Ans. (c) Inhibit HMG CoA reductase

Ref: KDT 6th ed. pg. 614

- **HMG-CoA Reductase Inhibitors (statins):** This class of compound is the most efficacious and best tolerated hypolipidaemic drugs.
- **MOA:** Competitively inhibit conversion of HMG-CoA to mevalonate by the enzyme HMG-CoA reductase.
- Drugs (Statins): Lovastatin, Simvastatin, Pravstatin, Atorvasttin, Rosuvastatin

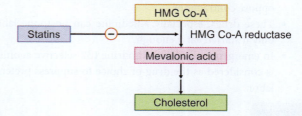

> **Extra Mile**
>
> - All statins are given at night except: Rosuvastatin, Atorvastain (can be given at anytime)
> - Major side effects of statins: Myopathy
> - Most potent statin: Pitavastain

Pharmacology

276. Ans. (c) Somatostatin

Ref: KDT, 6th ed. pg. 235

SOMATOSTATIN

- Somatostatin inhibits the secretion of GH, TSH and prolactin by pituitary, insulin and glucagon by pancreas and most importantly. It inhibits most of G.I secretions gastrin and HCl.
- It can be used in controlling esophageal varices and bleeding peptic ulcer.

- Drugs like *simvastatin*, atorvastatin, *fluvastatin*, lovastatin and rosuvastatin are statins, which are hypolipidemic drugs. They act by inhibiting HMG-CoA Reductase.
- *Fenofibrate* are from fibrates category, which has maximum triglyceride lowering activity.

Extra Mile

- Statins end with *"vastatin"*
- Maximum LDL lowering activity is by: STATINS
- Longest acting statin: ROSUVASTATIN

277. Ans. (c) Tocainide

Ref: KDT, 6th ed. pg. 511

TABLE: Anti arrhythmic drugs

Class	Actions	Drugs
I- (Na+#)	(Na+ channel blockers)	
	Ia: Na⁺+K⁺ channel blocking property	Quinidine, Procainamide, Disopyramide
	Ib: Na⁺# & K+ channel opening property	Tocainide, Lidocaine, Phenytoin, Mexiletine
	Ic: no effect on K+ channel	Flecainide, Encainide, Propafenone
II- (β#)	Antiadrenergic agents (β blockers)	Propranolol, Esmolol, (Sotalol is Class III mainly)
III- (K#)	Agents widening AP (Prolong repolarization and ERP)	Ibutilide, Sotalol, Bretylium, Amiodarone, Dronadarone, Dofetilide
IV- (Ca+#)	Calcium channel blockers	Verapamil, Diltiazem
V	Drugs with other mechanism of actions	Magnesium (**DOC** in torsades de pointes) Atropine: DOC for Bradycardia a and AV Block Digoxin Adenosine: DOC for PSVT

Note: Class IA agents also have Class III property; propranolol has Class I action as well; sotalol and bretylium have both class II and class III actions.

278. Ans. (d) All of the above

Ref: KDT 6th ed. pg. 528

TABLE: Types of calcium channel blocker

	L-Type (long lasting current)	T- Type (transient current)	N-Type (neuronal)
Locations and function	Excitation –contraction coupling in cardiac and smooth muscle SA, A-V node: conductivity Endocrine cell: Hormone release Neurons: transmitter release	Sa node- pacemaker activity "T" current and repetitive spikes in thalamic and other neurons Endocrine cells hormone release Certain arteries constriction	Only on Neurons in CNS, sympathetic and myenteric plexuses transmitter release
Blocker (drugs)	**DHP's:** Amlodipines, Nifedipine **Non- DHP:** Diltiazem, verapamil	Mibefradil, flunarizine, ethosuximide Trimethadione	ω- conotoxin

279. Ans. (a) Hydrochlorthiazide

Ref: KDT, 6th. pg. 274

Drugs causing glucose intolerance (hyperglycemia)		
Glucocorticoids Thiazides Phenytoin Pentamidine	Diazoxide Protease inhibitors β -IFN	Clozapine β adrenergic agonist Thyroid hormone Nicotinic acid

Note:
- Sulfonylureas are oral hypoglycemic agents. They cause hypoglycemia.
- ACE inhibitors also cause hypoglycemia.
- Other agents causing hypoglycemia: Quinine, Pentamidine, Octreotide, Insulin.

280. Ans. (a) Losartan

Ref: KDT, 6th ed. pg. 488

- Losartan has a uricosuric effect in hypertensive patients, and causes a decrease in serum uric acid levels by 20% to 25%.
- Losartan acts by inhibiting the urate/lactate exchanger and urate/chloride exchanger in the proximal convoluted tubule and leads to uricosuria.
- The uricosuric action of losartan is not shared by other antihypertensive agents.
- ACE inhibitors and CCBs increase uric acid excretion but the effect is modest and does not decrease serum uric acid levels.
- Diuretics have a propensity to increase serum uric acid levels and may even, rarely, provoke attacks of gout. Losartan can offset the elevations in serum uric acid levels occurring with hydrocholorothiazide or Indapamide
- Allopurinol reduces approximately 30% decrease in serum uric acid, resulting from the ability of allopurinol to inhibit xanthine oxidase, the enzyme responsible for the oxidation of purine to uric acid.

281. Ans. (b) Losartan

Ref: KDT, 6th ed. pg. 488

ANGIOTENSIN RECEPTOR BLOCKERS

- This class of anti-hypertensives developed as an alternative to ACE inhibitors, as ARB's have no action on bradykinin, causing no side effect *like cough, angioedema* as seen with ACE inhibitors.
- These are orally active AT 1 receptor antagonists which include **losartan, candesartan, valsartan, telmisartan and irbesartan.**
- **Losartan** is a competitive antagonist and inverse agonist of A-II, 10,000 times more selective for AT1 than AT2 receptor.
- It does not block any other receptor or ion channel, EXCEPT Thromboxane A2 receptor, which is responsible for its platelet anti-aggregatory property attenuation.

Extra Mile
- Telmisartan has PPAR-Y agonist action which can increase sensitivity to insulin. Therefore preferred in diabetics.

282. Ans. (c) CCB and β blockers

Ref: KDT, 6th ed. pg. 553

- Verapamil or diltiazem (CCB's) with β blockers are avoided because they may cause marked bradycardia and A-V block.
- Nitrates are used in conditions like CHF, Angina pectoris, MI, and Diffuse esophageal spasm. It can be given in combination with CCBs or β blockers.

Other antihypertensive combinations to be avoided:
- An α or β adrenergic blocker with clonidine: an apparent antagonism of clonidine action has been observed.
- **Nifedipine with diuretic:** Synergism between these two is still unproven.
- Methydopa with clonidine or any two drugs of same class.
- ACE inhibitor with ARB

283. Ans. (a) ACE inhibitor

Ref: Harrison's, 18th ed. Ch 344

- In a diabetic patient, hypertension can accelerate complications of DM, particularly cardiovascular disease and nephropathy. In these patients ACE inhibitor is preferred. It slows down the progression of diabetic nephropathy.
- *American Diabetic Association recommends that all patients with diabetes and hypertension be treated with an ACE inhibitor or an ARB.*
- Subsequently, agents that reduce cardiovascular risk (beta blockers, thiazide diuretics, and calcium channel blockers) should be incorporated into the regimen.
- While ACE inhibitors and ARBs are likely equivalent in most patients with diabetes and renal disease, the ADA notes:
  - In patients with type 1 diabetes, hypertension, and micro- or macroalbuminuria, an ACE inhibitor slowed progression of nephropathy
  - An ACE inhibitor or an ARB slowed the progression to macroalbuminuria in patients with type 2 diabetes, hypertension, and microalbumin-uria; and
  - ARB slowed the decline in GFR in patients with type 2 diabetes, hypertension, macroalbuminuria, and renal insufficiency.

HORMONES AND AUTOCOIDS

284. Ans. (b) GLP-1 Analogue

Ref: Goodman & Gillman 13th ed. P 877

- **GLP-1 analogue drugs are:** Exenatide, Liraglutide, Albiglutide, Dulaglutide, Lixisenatide
- These agents activate the GLP-1 receptor → Increased insulin biosynthesis and release

Pharmacology

- These agents are resistant to degradation by DPP4 enzyme → Has extended activity following injection.
- **Side effect:** Nausea, vomiting, Pancreatitis

TABLE: Properties of insulin secretagogues

Class Generic name	Daily Dosage (mg)	Duration of Action (hours or dosing frequency)
Sulfonylureas		
Glimepiride	1–8	24
Glipizide	5–40	12–18
Glipizide (extended release)	5–20	24
Glyburide	1.25–20	12–24
Glyburide (micronized)	0.75–12	12–24
Nonsulfonylureas (Meglitinides)		
Nateglinide	180–360	2–4
Repaglinide	0.5–16	2–6
GLP-1 Agonists		
Albiglutide	30–50	Weekly
Dulaglutide	0.75–1.5	Weekly
Exenatideb	2	Weekly
Liraglutide	0.6–1.8	Daily
Lixisenatide	0.010–0.020	Daily
Dipeptidyl Peptidase–4 Inhibitors		
Alogliptin	25	Daily
Linagliptin	5	Daily
Saxagliptin	2.5–5	Daily
Sitagliptin	25–100	12–16
Vildagliptin	50–100	Twice daily

---

285. Ans. (d) Sufentanil

Ref: Goodman & Gillman 13th ed. P 376

- Fentanyl citrate and sufentanil citrate are congeners of fentanyl and are considered as potent analgesics
- After systemic delivery:
  - Fentanyl is about 100 times more potent than morphine
  - Sufentanil is about 1000 times more potent than morphine
- Time to peak analgesic effect after IV administration: ~5 minutes
- These drugs are well known to be used as epidural analgesic.

---

286. Ans. (d) Hepatotoxicity

Ref: Goodman & Gillman 13th ed. P 696

- Paracetamol/Acetaminophen is a non-selective COX inhibitor

- **Use:** Analgesic and antipyretic agent. Preferred in patients where aspirin is contraindicated
- **Usual dose:** 325–650 mg every 4–6 hours. Maximum FDA recommended dose is 4 gm/day
- Peak plasma concentration: 30–60 minutes
- **Half-life:** 2 hours
- Metabolism of acetaminophen in liver by:
  - Hepatic conjugation with glucuronic acid (~60%),
  - Sulfuric acid (~35%),
  - Cysteine (~3%);
  - CYP mediated N-hydroxylation to form NAPQI (*N*-acetyl-*p*-benzoquinone imine)
- **Note:** NAPQI is one of the highly reactive intermediate metabolite of acetaminophen metabolism. This usually reacts with sulfhydryl groups is GSH → rendered harmless.
- In hepatotoxicity condition GSH level depleted.

SIDE EFFECTS

- The most serious acute adverse effect of over dosage of acetaminophen is a potentially fatal hepatic necrosis.
- Due to hepatotoxicity there is saturation of glucuronide and sulfate conjugation and increasing amounts undergo CYP-mediated *N*-hydroxylation to form excess of NAPQI (it accumulates due to depletion of GSH).
- The highly reactive NAPQI causes enzymatic dysfunction, produces oxidative stress and apoptosis.
- In adults hepatotoxicity may occur after ingestion of single dose of 10-15 g. Doses of 20-25 g is potentially fatal.

TREATMENT OF ACETAMINOPHEN TOXICITY:

- Activated charcoal within 4 hours of ingestion decreases absorption by 50-90%
- **N-acetylcysteine:** antidote of choice for acetaminophen toxicity. It acts by detoxifying NAPQI by:
  - Repleting GSH stores
  - Conjugate directly with NAPQI by serving as a GSH substitute

Extra Mile

In Paracetamol Toxicity:
- Liver enzyme abnormalities typically peak 72–96 hours after ingestion
- **Biopsy:** Centrilobular necrosis with sparing of the periportal area
- **Other side effects:** Renal tubular necrosis and Hypoglycemic coma

---

287. Ans. (b) Early closure of PDA

Ref: Goodman & Gillman 13th ed. P 690, 697

- Indomethacin is a potent nonselective inhibitor of COX enzyme. It is considered 20 times more potent than aspirin

- Other actions are:
  - Inhibit motility of neutrophils
  - Depress biosynthesis of mucopolysacchharides
  - COX independent vasoconstrictor effect
  - Anti-inflammatory, antipyretic and analgesic action
- An IV formulation of indomethacin is approved for closure of persistent patent ductus arteriosus in premature infants.
- The regimen involves intravenous administration of 0.1–0.25 mg/kg every 12 hours for three doses, with the course repeated one time if necessary.
- Successful closure can be expected in more than 70% of neonates treated.
- An injectable formulation of ibuprofen is an alternative for the treatment of patent ductus arteriosus.
- The agent can also cause stenosis of ductus arteriosus and oligohydramnios particularly in foetuses older than 32 weeks of gestation.

288. Ans. (b) Provide stability in insulin molecule

Ref: KD Tripathi 8th ed. P 286

- The insulin molecules namely regular human insulin and NPH insulin/lente is clear at neutral pH and exist as dimers that assemble into hexamers in the presence of two zinc ions. This provides stability in the insulin.
  - Become cloudy after adding zinc
- These hexamers are furthers stabilized by phenolic compounds like phenol and meta-cresol.
- Zinc is also necessary for proper processing, storage and secretion of insulin and also protect against Beta cell loss.
- Studies have shown that zinc manages the behaviour of amylin (a protein secreted from beta cell) to help slow down carbohydrate absorption. Unmanaged amylin can form clumps that interfere with insulin secretion.
- Since zinc is so closely tied to insulin functioning, its deficiency is associated with poor beta cell function and higher incidence of insulin resistance.

Extra Mile

Lente insulin (Insulin-zinc suspension): Two types of insulin-zinc suspensions have been produced.
- The one with large particles is crystalline and practically insoluble in water (ultralente). It is long-acting.
- The other has smaller particles and is amorphous (semilente), is short-acting. Their 7:3 ratio mixture is called 'Lente insulin' and is intermediate-acting

289. Ans. (a) 4 minutes

Ref: Sharma & Sharma 3rd ed. P 625

- Parathyroid hormone is a 84 amino acid compound which is responsible for calcium homeostasis in body.
  - Acts over osteoblast → Stimulate osteoclast → Bone resorption
- Principle factor regulating parathyroid hormone synthesis and release: Hypocalcemia
- Rapidly metabolized in liver and kidney
- Plasma half-life: 2–4 minutes

Endocrine organ	Hormones	Basic structure	Half-life
Hypothalamus	Hypothalamic releasing hormones	Small: 3 to 44 amino acid peptides	1–2 min
Pituitary	"Trophic" hormones	Large glycoproteins	20 min. – 3 hrs
Thyroid	Calcitonin	32 AA	10–30 min.
Parathyroid	PTH–parathyroid hormone	84 AA	4 min.
Pancreas	Insulin, glucagon (major)	–51 AA/29 AA	5–8 min./negligible
Adipose tissue	Leptin	167 AA	30 min.
Kidney	Renin, erythropoietin	340 AA/193 AA	15 min.
Liver	IGF-1	153 AA	12–15 hrs.
Heart	ANP/BNP	28 AA/32 AA	2 min./20 min.

290. Ans. (a) 5-lipoxygenase inhibitor

Ref: Goodman & Gillman's 13th ed. P 740-41

- In the pathway of leukotriene synthesis where phospholipase cleaves the phospholipid of cell membrane to form arachidonic acid, steroids can inhibit this particular synthesis.

$$\text{Phospholipid} \xrightarrow[(-)\text{ Steroids}]{\text{Phospholipase A2}} \text{Arachidonic acid}$$

- Further the arachidonic acid is metabolized to form leukotriene and prostaglandin with the help of 5'LOX and COX enzyme respectively.

Drugs acting at different sites:
- **PLA2 inhibitor:** Steroids
- **LOX inhibitor:** Zileuton
- **Receptor inhibitor:** Montelukast, zafirlukast, pranlukast

291. Ans. (b) Insulin

Ref: Sharma & Sharma 3rd ed. P 636

- Insulin in diabetes facilitates glucose uptake (through GLUT-4) and increases intracellular glucose oxidative metabolism.
- Insulin decreases glycogenolysis, increases lipogenesis, decreases lipolysis, increases FA synthesis and

triglyceride formation and storage. It also blunts lipolytic action if adrenaline, growth hormone and glucagon.
- Thus insulin lowers the blood glucose levels by promoting the glucose utilization and suppressing its production.

Extra Mile
- Acarbose, miglitol and voglibose is from α-glucosidase inhibitor group. Alpha glucosidase usually facilitates digestion of complex starch, oligosaccharides, monosaccharides. If they are inhibited the sugar moiety will not be absorbed, reducing the sugar level.
- **Side effect:** Flatulence, diarrhea, abdominal pain.
- Pioglitazone can cause increase in weight gain, which is attributed to fluid retention and edema.

292. Ans. (c) 0.25%
- ALCAFTADINE is a H1 receptor antagonist, and can be used for allergic conjunctivitis
- The trial done for alcaftadine used 0.25% solution.
- **The trial states:** *"When Alcaftadine was tested against placebo and olopatadine, only Alcaftadine 0.25% was shown to have a clinically significant reduction in conjunctival redness scores 7 and 15 minutes after administration"*

293. Ans. (a) Sildenafil
Ref: KD Tripathi, 7th ed. pg. 303
- Sildenafil is an orally active drug for treatment of ED. Sildenafil acts by selectively inhibiting PDE-5, causing increase in cGMP and enhancing Nitric Oxide action on corpus cavernosum.
- Amrinone and Milrinone are PDE-3 inhibitor and are also called inodilators. They are used in CHF.
- Tamoxifen is a selective estrogen receptor modulator, used in breast cancer.

294. Ans. (b) Fulvestrant
Ref: KD Tripathi, 7th ed. pg. 313
- **Fulvestrant** is the first member of a distinct class of estrogen receptor (ER) ligands called 'selective estrogen receptor down-regulators' (SERDs) or 'pure estrogen antagonists' that has been introduced for the treatment of metastatic ER positive breast cancer in postmenopausal women which has stopped responding to tamoxifen.
- In contrast to tamoxifen, it inhibits ER dimerization so that ER interaction with DNA is prevented and receptor degradation is enhanced. The ER is thus downregulated resulting in more complete suppression of ER responsive gene function. This feature along with its higher *affinity* for the ER probably accounts for its efficacy in tamoxifen resistant cases.
- Fulvestrant is administered as (250 mg) monthly IM injections in the buttock. It is slowly absorbed and has an elimination *t1/2* of more than a month.

Extra Mile
Clomiphene citrate binds to both ER-alpha and ER-beta and acts as pure estrogen antagonist
Tamoxifen is selective estrogen receptor modulator
Flutamide is selective antagonist of androgen receptor.

295. Ans. (c) Antibody to VEGF receptor
Ref: KD Tripathi, 7th ed. pg. 871
- **Bevacizumab** It is a humanized **monoclonal antibody that binds VEGF-A** and hinders its access to the VEGF receptor, interrupting angiogenic signalling.
- Combined with 5-FU, bevacizumab is used in metastatic colorectal cancer. Added to conventional chemotherapy, it improves survival in metastatic non-small cell lung cancer, breast cancer, clear cell renal carcinoma and glioblastoma. Bevacizumab is administered by IV infusion every 2–3 weeks.
- Adverse effects are–rise in BP, arterial thromboembolism leading to heart attack and stroke, vessel injury and hemorrhages, heart failure, proteinuria, gastrointestinal perforations, and healing defects.

Extra Mile
- Epidermal growth factor (EGF) receptor inhibitors are: Gefitinib and Erlotinib. Mostly used in non-small cell lung cancer
- Example of VEGF 2 receptor inhibitor is sunitinib. It is used in metastatic RCC and GIST.

296. Ans. (b) Cyclosporine
- Cyclosporine and Tacrolimus are immunosuppressants, specifically inhibit antigen stimulated activation & proliferation of helper T-cells as well as expression of various cytokines including IL-2 by inhibiting calcineurin.
- **Other immunomodulators are:**
  - **IL 1 receptor inhibitor:** Anakinra
  - **IL 6 Receptor inhibitor:** Tocilizumab
  - **Co-Stimulation inhibitor:** Abatacept, Bilatacept
  - **TNF-α inhibitor:** Adalimumab, Certolizumab, Etanercept, Infliximab, Golimumab

297. Ans. (a) Prostaglandins
Ref: Anatomy and Physiology, Ch 27, Development and Inheritance pg. 832

The text states: *"Rising estrogen and oxytocin during pregnancy, stimulate the production of prostaglandins in endometrium. These prostaglandins further stimulate smooth muscle contractions, thereby increasing frequency of urination and late in pregnancy cause spasms in uterine musculature."*

FMGE Solutions Screening Examination

298. Ans. (b) V2

Ref: Katzung's 11th ed. p-658–659

TABLE: Vasopressin receptor location and functions

Receptor	Localization	Functions	
V1a	Vascular smooth muscle Platelets Hepatocytes Myometrium	Vasoconstriction, myocardial hypertrophy Platelet aggregation Glycogenolysis Uterine contraction	
V1b*	Anterior pituitary	ACTH release	
V2	Basolateral membrane collecting tubule	Insertion of AQP2 water channels into apical membrane, induction of AQP2 synthesis	Free water reabsorption
	Vascular endothelium Vascular smooth muscle	vWF and factor 8 release Vasodilatation	
ACTH, adrenocorticotropin hormone; AQP2, aquaporin-2. *Termed V3 in some classification schemes.			
			(KI 2006)

TABLE: Hormones from posterior pituitary

Antidiuretic hormone (ADH)/ Vasopressin	Increase water reabsorption by the kidneys and cause vasoconstriction and increased blood pressure. Acts on V2 receptor. Note: V1b is also known as V3 receptor
Oxytocin	**Stimulates milk ejection** from breasts and uterine contractions

299. Ans. (d) NPH

Ref: Sharma & Sharma 3rd ed. P 641; KDT, 6th ed. pg. 259

Insulin type	Onset of action (hr.)	Duration of action (hr)
Ultrashort (Rapid Acting) Insulin Lispro Insulin Aspart Insulin Gluilisine	15 – 30 minutes	3–5 hrs
Short acting Regular insulin	30–60 minutes	6–8 hrs
Intermediate acting Insulin lente Neutral protamine hagedorn (NPH)/Isophane insulin	**1–2 hrs**	**16–20 hrs**
Long Acting Insulin Glargine Insulin Detemir Insulin Degludec	2–4 hrs	16–24 hrs Degludec: >24 hours
Inhaled insulin (Human insulin)-Liquid form	**5–10 minutes**	**3–5 minutes**

> Extra Mile

Most common side effect of insulin: hypoglycemia
DOC for Diabetic ketoacidosis (DKA): Regular insulin

Pharmacology

300. Ans. (a) Insulin lispro

Ref: KDT 6th ed. pg. 259

Please refer to above explanation.

301. Ans. (a) Insulin aspart

- Ultrashort acting insulins are the fastest acting ones.
- Onset of action within 15–30 minutes and duration of action is 3–5 hours.

302. Ans. (c) Dopamine stimulate prolactin production

Ref: KDT, 6th ed. pg. 235-236

- Prolactin is produced from anterior pituitary and is associated with lactation.
- Prolactin is under predominant inhibitory control of hypothalamus through PRIH (Prolactin Release Inhibitory Hormone), which is Dopamine that acts on pituitary lactotrope D2 receptor.
- Dopaminergic agonist like bromocriptine, DA, cabergoline decrease plasma prolactin levels and is used to treat hyperprolactinemia
- Dopaminergic antagonists like chlorpromazine halo-peridol, metoclopramide causes hyperprolactinemia by blocking D2 receptors.
- A progressive increase in prolactin occurs during pregnancy, peaking at term. After childbirth, this dopamine is inhibited and prolactin now stimulates milk production.

> **Extra Mile**
>
> *Milk production is stimulated by: Prolactin (remember production by prolactin).*
> *Milk secretion is stimulated by: Oxytocin*
> *DOC for hyperprolactinemia: Bromocriptine*

303. Ans. (c) Dopamine

Ref: KDT, 6th ed. pg. 235-236

- Prolactin is under predominant inhibitory control of hypothalamus through PRIH (Prolactin Release Inhibitory Hormone), which is **Dopamine** that acts on pituitary lactotrope D2 receptor.
- A progressive increase in prolactin occurs during pregnancy, peaking at term. After childbirth, this dopamine is inhibited and prolactin now stimulates milk production.

304. Ans. (c) Metoclopramide

Ref: KDT, 6th ed. pg. 643

- Galactorrhea is caused by increased level of prolactin.
- Normally, this prolactin is in inhibited state by Dopamine.

- Prolactin is under predominant inhibitory control of hypothalamus through PRIH (Prolactin Release Inhibitory Hormone), which is Dopamine that acts on pituitary lactotrope D2 receptor.
- Dopaminergic agonist like bromocriptine, DA and cabergoline decrease plasma prolactin levels and is used to treat hyperprolactinemia.
- Dopaminergic antagonists like chlorpromazine, halo-peridol, **metoclopramide** causes hyperprolactinemia by blocking D2 receptors.

305. Ans. (b) Enhance glucose uptake by skeletal muscle

Ref: KDT, 6th ed. pg. 267

OHA drugs	Mechanism of action
Metformin and thiazolidinediones	Inhibition of hepatic gluconeogenesis Enhance glucose uptake in skeletal muscle
Sulfonylureas and ripaglinde	Stimulate insulin release from pancreas
Acarbose	Decrease absorption of glucose from intestine

306. Ans. (a) Metformin

Ref: KDT, 6th ed. pg. 267

METFORMIN

- Metformin is an antidiabetic drug from biguanides category.
- They improve lipid profile, hence considered as DOC for DM in obese patients.
- **MOA:**
  - Increase peripheral utilization of glucose
  - Inhibit hepatic gluconeogenesis
- Metformin never causes hypoglycemia.
- Another drug from Biguanides is *Phenformin*, which is withdrawn, because it causes lactic acidosis.
- **Sulfonylureas** causes a brisk release of insulin from pancreas which stimulate the functional receptors for the intake of glucose.
  - They can cause hypoglycemia.
  - Preferred in thin patients with DM
- **Repaglinide** has same MOA as sulfonylureas, but it is short acting.
  - Used to control sudden rise of glucose after meal.
- **Acarbose** act by inhibiting G.I. absorption of sugar.
  - **s/e:** Can cause osmotic diarrhea.

> **Extra Mile**
>
> - Safest sulfonylureas: Tolbutamide (safer in elderly also)
> *Remembered as:* **MOST**- *Metformin for Obese; Sulfonylureas for Thin.*

Explanations

305

307. Ans. (c) Monitoring of liver enymes is recommended

Ref: KDT, 6th ed. pg. 304-5

- Tamoxifen is a SERM that acts as antagonist at estrogen receptors in the breast. It decreases the risk of contralateral breast cancer and is approved for primary prevention of breast cancer in women at high risk.

Adverse Effects of Tamoxifen Therapy

- Hot flashes
- Menstrual irregularities,
- Endometrial hyperplasia
- Cataract
- *Hepatotoxicity*
- Development of fatty liver: Due to an idiosyncratic reaction to a metabolite of the medication
- Steatohepatitis: Minor serum aminotransferase elevations, **monitoring of serum enzymes during long term tamoxifen therapy is often recommended.**

308. Ans. (b) Finasteride

Ref: KDT, 6th ed. pg. 294

- Hirsutism is male pattern hair growth in females. For example: Moustache, beard, chest hair.
- **Finasteride** is a 5α-reductase inhibitor. By inhibiting 5α-reductase it prevents conversion of testosterone to DHT by the type II isoenzyme, resulting in a decrease in serum DHT levels by about 65–70% and in prostate DHT levels by up to 85–90%.
- Decreasing the amount of DHT leads to increased hair regrowth and slower hair loss. Hair growth on other parts of the body is not affected by finasteride.
- **USES:** This medication is used to treat male pattern baldness (androgenetic alopecia) at the crown and in the middle of the scalp. Can also be used in treatment of BPH.
- **Flutamide:** Androgen receptor antagonist. Studies have shown that it is helpful in treatment of hirsutism. Can also be used in treatment of BPH.
- **Spironolactone:** Antialdosterone antiandrogenic compound, used in the treatment of hirsutism.
- **Cyproterone acetate:** A progestin that also has strong antiandrogenic action.

Drugs causing Hirsutism

Mn: MAD COP
- Minoxidil
- Androgen
- Dizoxide
- Cyclosporine
- OCP's
- Phenytoin

309. Ans. (c) Finasteride

Ref: Katzung 14th ed. pg. 1085

- Most of the actions of testosterone are mediated by its conversion to DHT by 5-alpha reductase. Important amongst these are growth of prostate, male pattern baldness and hirsutism in females.
- **Finasteride and dutasteride** are 5-alpha reductase inhibitors useful in the treatment of BPH, male pattern baldness and hirsutism by reducing the production of DHT.

Note: *Flutamide and Nilutamide act as antagonists of androgen receptors. These are useful for the treatment of prostatic carcinoma. Flutamide can cause gynaecomastia and reversible liver damage.*

310. Ans. (b) Phosphodiesterase 5 inhibition

Ref: KD Tripathi, 6th ed. pg. 294-295

- Sildenafil, Tadalafil and vardenafil are selective PDE-5 inhibitors effective in erectile dysfunction.
- **5α-REDUCTASE INHIBITOR**
  - **Finasteride** is competitive inhibitor of the enzyme 5α-reductase which converts testosterone into more active dihydrotestosterone responsible for androgen action in many tissues including prostate gland and hair follicles.
  - Used in treatment of BPH
- **Flutamide:** A nonsteroidal drug having specific antiandrogenic, but no other hormonal activity.
  - Used in prostate CA

Extra Mile

Tadalafil is the **longest acting** phosphodiesterase inhibitor.

311. Ans. (b) Inhibiting phosphodiesterase type 5

312. Ans. (c) Increased eye lashes hair growth

Ref: KDT, 6th ed. pg. 147

- Latanoprost is a prostaglandin analogue. It is stable long acting PGF2α derivative which is used for glaucoma.
- **MOA:** It works by increasing aqueous humor outflow.
- Other drugs act by similar mechanism: **travoprost, bimatoprost**
- Side effect:
  - Latanoprost may increase the brown pigmentation in iris (**NOT corneal pigmentation**), changing eye color to brown: Heterochromia iridis
  - It may also cause eyelashes to grow longer and thicker and darken in color
  - **Other side effects:** Stinging, burning, itching, swelling of the eye, redness of the eyelids, dry eyes.

Pharmacology

313. Ans. (a) Timolol

Ref: KDT, 6th ed. pg. 144

LATANOPROST

MOA: Increase of aqueous humor outflow

Side effects: Red eye and ocular irritation, increased iris pigmentation, and excessive hair growth of eye lashes.

- **Timolol** is a prototype of ocular β blockers. It is a non selective beta blocker (blocks β1 + β2) and has no anesthetic or intrinsic sympathomimetic activity.
- Timlol's ocular hypotesive action (20–35% fall in IOT) is smooth and well sustained.
- Lungs have β2 receptor, and if they are blocked in case of asthmatic patient, the condition worsens. Therefore non selective beta blockers are always avoided in case of asthmatic patients.
- **Betaxolol** is a β1 selective blocker, offering the advantage of less bronchopulmonary and probably less cardiac, central and metabolic side effects.
- Betaxolol is less effective in lowering IOT than timolol, because ocular beta receptors are predominantly of β2 subtype.
- **Acetazolamide** is a carbonic anhydrase inhibitor which reduces the aqueous formation by limiting generation of bicarbonate ion in ciliary epithelium.
- **Latanoprost** is a prostaglandin analogue. It is a PGF2α analogue which act by increasing uveoscleral outflow.

314. Ans. (d) PG F2α

Ref: KD Tripathi, 6th ed. pg. 146 -47

- Low concentration of $PGF_{2\alpha}$ lowers intraocular tension without inducing ocular inflammation.
- It acts by increasing unveoscleral outflow.
- Latanoprost is a $PGF_{2\alpha}$ derivative. It has shown efficacy similar to timolol and the effect is well sustained over long-term. Therefore it has become the first choice drugs of glaucoma in developed countries.

Extra Mile

- PGE_2, PGI_2 TXA_2 has no role in glaucoma treatment.
- PGE_2 cause vasodilatation in most, but not all, vascular beds.
- PGI_2 is uniformly vasodilatory and is more potent hypotensive than PGE_2
- TXA_2 consistently produces vasoconstriction.

315. Ans. (c) Both mast cell stabilizer and antihistamine

Ref: Clinical Oculor Pharmacology, 1st ed. pg. 257

- **Olopatadine hydrochloride** is an antihistamine (as well as anticholinergic and mast cell stabilizer)
- It is used as eye drop to treat itching associated with allergic conjunctivitis.

- Side effects include headache, eye burning and/or stinging, blurred vision, dry eyes, foreign body sensation, hyperemia, keratitis and taste perversion.

316. Ans. (d) Ciclesonide

Ref: KDT, 6th ed. pg. 226

- **Hard steroids may include:** Difluprednate ophthalmic emulsion, Budesonide, prednisolone, betamethasone and dexamethasone.
- **Soft steroids may include (Mn: CFL):** Ciclesonide, Fluorometholone, Loteprednol etabonate
- **Ciclesonide:** Is an inhaled corticosteroid indicated for the maintenance treatment of asthma and as prophylactic therapy in adult and adolescent patients aged 12 years and older
- The soft steroids fluorometholone and loteprednol 0.5% are ideal for treatment of an acute inflammatory episode in dry eye.

317. Ans. (a) Anti-gout and Xanthine Oxidase inhibitor

Ref: Katzung's Pharmacology, 14th ed. pg. 662 -63

- Febuxostat is a non-purine inhibitor of xanthine oxidase and thereby reduces the formation of xanthine and uric acid and is useful in management of gout.
- It is 80% absorbed following oral administration and extensively metabolized in the liver.
- All of the drug and its metabolites appear in the urine although less than 5% appears as unchanged drug. Because it is highly metabolized to inactive metabolites, no dosage adjustment is necessary for patients with renal impairment.

318. Ans. (b) Indomethacin

Ref: Katzung, 14th ed. pg. 648

- Primary gout is seen due to decreased uric acid excretion
- Secondary gout can be secondary to any cause causing hyperuricemia.
- **DOC for acute gout:** NSAID-DOC (Indomethacin), Colchicine and corticosteroids
  - **Colchicine** is fastest acting. It is NOT an anti-inflammatory drug but it specifically suppresses gout inflammation.
  - Not preferred over NSAID because of its side effects of GI upset.
- All NSAIDS can be given in acute gout EXCEPT aspirin as it competes with tubular excretion of uric acid leading to Hyperuricemia.
- **Probenecid:** Has uricosuric action
- **DOC for chronic gout:** Allopurinol

FMGE Solutions Screening Examination

RENAL, GIT AND RESPIRATORY SYSTEM

319. Ans. (a) Lactulose

Ref: Goodman & Gillman 13th ed. P 928, 940

USES OF LACTULOSE

- Constipation caused by opioids
- Idiopathic chronic constipation
- Lactulose also used to treat hepatic encephalopathy

LACTULOSE IN HEPATIC ENCEPHALOPATHY

- Impaired liver function/severe liver disease are unable to detoxify the ammonia coming from colon which is produced by colonic bacterial metabolism of fecal urea.
- The drop in luminal pH that accompanies hydrolysis to short-chain fatty acids in the colon results in "trapping" of the ammonia by its conversion to the polar ammonium ion.
- Combined with the increase in colonic transit, this therapy significantly lowers circulating ammonia levels. The therapeutic goal in this condition is to give sufficient amounts of lactulose (usually 20–30 g three to four times per day) to produce two to three soft stools a day with a pH of 5–5.5.

320. Ans. (d) DEC

Ref: Harrison's 19th ed. P 422, 1687

- Eosinophilia is the presence of >500 eosinophils per µL of blood and is common in many settings besides parasite infection.
- **Common causes of eosinophilia are:**
  - Allergic reaction to drugs (Iodides, aspirin, sulfonamides, nitrofurantoin, penicillins, and cephalosporins).
  - Allergies such as hay fever, asthma, eczema, serum sickness, allergic vasculitis, and pemphigus are associated with eosinophilia.
  - Collagen vascular disease like rheumatoid arthritis.
- Tropical eosinophilia is usually caused by filarial infection.
- Tropical eosinophilia due to *Wuchereria bancrofti* or *Brugia malayi* occurs most commonly in Southern Asia, Africa, and South America.
- **Drug of choice:** Diethylcarbamazine.

321. Ans. (c) Thiazides

Ref: Goodman & Gillman's 13th ed. P 466

- Nephrogenic DI may be congenital or acquired. Causes can be:
  - Hypercalcemia, hypokalemia, postobstructive renal failure, Li+, foscarnet, clozapine, demeclocycline, and other drugs can induce nephrogenic DI.
- Thiazide *diuretics* reduce the polyuria of patients with DI and often are used to treat nephrogenic DI.
- **DOC for central diabetes insipidus:** Desmopressin (V2 receptor agonist)
- **DOC for nephrogenic diabetes insipidus:** Thiazide diuretics.
- **DOC for lithium induced diabetes insipidus:** Amiloride

322. Ans. (b) Carbonic anhydrase inhibitor

Ref: Katzung's, 11th ed. pg. 416

- **Acetazolamide** is a carbonic anhydrase inhibitor which acts on the proximal tubule of nephron.
- **In kidney,** it inhibits H^+ secretion and HCO_3 reabsorption, which inturn reduces sodium reabsorption.
- In eye, it reduces the aqueous formation by limiting generation of bicarbonate ion in ciliary epithelium.

323. Ans. (b) Decrease placental circulation

Ref: http://www.ncbi.nlm.nih.gov/pmc/articles/ PMC 2628835

- Diuretics causes massive fluid loss via urine, which causes decreased volume and thereby decreases placental circulation. This might compromise fetal blood supply.
- Option A: Diuretics do not increase vascular resistance, instead it decreases the resistance.
- Option C: No maternal distress. However fetal stress is a possibility
- Option D: There have been few reported cases of birth defects associated with diuretic use.

324. Ans. (a) Antacid

Ref: Katzung's, 14th ed. pg. 1089

- This medication is used to treat symptoms caused by too much stomach acid such as heartburn, upset stomach, or indigestion.
- It is an antacid that works by lowering the amount of acid in the stomach.
- It can also be used in renal osteodystrophy with hyperphosphatemia, hypocalcemia and osteoporosis like conditions.
- It can cause metabolic alkalosis (Milk-alkali syndrome)

325. Ans. (d) All of the above

Ref: Katzung, 14th ed. pg. 775–776

- Vitamin D has been used in treating renal osteodystrophy
- In mild forms of malabsorption, vitamin D should suffice to raise serum levels of 25(OH)D into the normal range. Many patients with severe disease do not respond to vitamin D.
- Calcitriol and **Calcidiol** have been used successfully in treatment of renal osteodystrophy and intestinal osteodystrophy.

Pharmacology

326. Ans. (c) Indapamide

Ref: KDT, 6th ed. pg. 540

Indapamide is a thiazide diuretic

Diuretic class	Drugs	MOA	Site of action
Osmotic diuretic	Mannitol	Inhibit water and solute reabsorption	All part of tubule, but mainly proximal tubule
Loop diuretics	Furosemide, Torsemide	Inhibit Na^+-K^+-$2Cl^-$ co-transport	Thick ascending loop of henle
Thiazide diuretic	Hydrochlorthiazide, Benzthiazide, Chlorthalidone, Indapamide	Inhibit Na^+- Cl^- co-transport	Distal tubule
K+ sparing diuretic	Spironolactone, Triamterene, Amiloride	Decrease Na+ reabsorption, Decrease K+ secretion	Collecting tubule
Carbonic anhydrase inhibitor	Acetazolamide	Inhibit H+ secretion and HCO3 reabsorption, which reduces Na+ reabsorption	Proximal tubule

327. Ans. (a) Thiazide diuretics

Ref: KDT, 6th ed. pg. 540

- **Drugs under thiazide diuretics:** Hydrochlorthiazide, chlorthalidone, bendroflumethiazide, indapamide and metazolone.
- **Thiazide diuretics act on DCT by blocking Na+ Cl channel**
- In cases of initial management of CKD *(stage 1 & 2)*, thiazide diuretics is preferred and is considered as drug of choice, preferably Metazolone *(has anti-hypertensive action)*.
- Patients with stages 1 and 2 are comparatively higher than the advanced stages.
- *However, thiazide diuretics are NOT given if serum creatinine is more than 2.5 or GFR is less than 60 ml/min.*
- Thiazide diuretics have limited utility in stages 3–5 CKD, such that administration of loop diuretics, including furosemide, bumetanide, or torsemide, may also be needed. *(Harrison's 18th ed. Ch 280)*
- The combination of loop diuretics with metolazone, which inhibits the sodium chloride co-transporter of the distal convoluted tubule, can help effect renal salt excretion. Ongoing diuretic resistance with intractable edema and hypertension in advanced CKD may serve as an indication to initiate dialysis.

Indapamide is longer acting and more potent than hydrochlorthiazide. It is *effective as an antihypertensive at lower doses than those required for the diuretic effect* (due to its direct vasodilatory action). It also produces less metabolic adverse effects (hypokalemia, hyperglycemia, hyperuricemia etc.) and can be used as an antihypertensive in diabetic patients (whereas other thiazides are contra-indicated).

328. Ans. (a) Bilateral renal artery stenosis

Ref: Katzung's Pharmacology, 14th ed. pg. 188

- Patients with B/L renal artery stenosis or patients with single kidney having renal artery stenosis will develop renal failure if treated with ACEI.
- In stenosis there is reduced GFR, and body manage the adequate GFR by angiotensin II mediated efferent arteriole constriction to maintain the renal perfusion. In such patients, Inhibition of ACE can induce acute renal insufficiency.

329. Ans. (c) Proton pump inhibitors like Omeprazole

Ref: KDT, 6th ed. pg. 632

- Proton pump inhibitors (PPIs) are the drugs of choice for peptic ulcer disease (PUD) due to any etiology (even NSAID induced).
- PPIs are also the agents of choice for gastroesophageal reflux disease (GERD) and Zollinger Ellison Syndrome (ZES).
- **Misoprosotol:** Specific agent for NSAID induced ulcer.

330. Ans. (c) Hyoscine

Ref: KD Tripathi, 6th ed. pg. 641, 642, 644, 646

HYOSINE

- It is the most effective drug for motion sickness.
- Suitable only for short brisk journies.
- It act by blocking conduction of nerve impulses in the pathway leading from the vestibular apparatus to the vomiting centre and is *not effective in vomiting of other etiologies.*

ONDANSETRON

- It is considered as the drug of choice for drug induced vomiting.
- Used mainly to control cancer chemotherapy induced vomiting.
- Effective in postoperative nausea and vomiting as well.

METOCLOPRAMIDE

- It is an effective and popular drug for many types of vomiting like: Postoperative, drug induced, disease associated (especially migraine), radiation sickness, etc.

CHLORPROMAZINE

- These are from typical antipsychotic having potent antiemetic action; act by blocking D2 receptors in the CTZ.
- They have broad spectrum antiemetic action effective in:
  - Drug induced and postanaesthetic nausea and vomiting
  - Diease induced vomiting
  - Malignancy associated and cancer chemotherapy induced vomiting
  - Radiation sickness vomiting and morning sickness.

331. Ans. (b) Hyoscine

Ref: KDT, 6th ed. pg. 646-47

332. Ans. (a) Anti-motility drugs are drug of choice for infective diarrhea

Ref: KDT, 6th ed. pg. 664

- All Anti-motility drugs are contra-indicated in infective diarrhea. These are indicated only in non-infective secretory diarrhea.

Extra Mile

- Loperamide is a non-addictive over the counter anti-diarrheal drug.
- **Diphenoxylate** is an opioid but has addictive potential if used for prolonged periods. It is always given in combination **with atropine to prevent the abuse** (atropine will produce dry mouth and other anticholinergic side effects).
- Opioids are used as anti-motility drugs used in secretory diarrhea.

333. Ans. (c) Ambroxol

Ref: KDT 6th ed. pg. 214

- Ambroxol is a metabolite of bromhexine having mucolytic action.
- Antitussives are drugs that act in the CNS to raise the threshold of cough centre.
- Since antitussives aim to control rather than eliminate cough they are used only for dry unproductive cough or if cough is unduly tiring, disturbs sleep or is hazardous.

Mucolytics	Antitussives
Bromhexine Ambroxol Acetylcysteine Carbocisteine	Opioids Codeine Pholcodeine Nonopioids Noscapine Dextromethorphan Chlophedianol

334. Ans. (c) Salmetrol

Ref: KDT 6th ed. pg. 218

- β2 agonist is the drug of choice for acute attack of bronchial asthma.
- Other β2 Agonists

SABA (Short acting β2 agonist)	Salbutamol terbutaline	Used for acute attack of BA
LABA (Long acting β2 agonist)	**Salmeterol**-slow onset of action, long duration of action **Formeterol**-fast onset of action, long duration of action **Indacaterol**-fast OOA and long DOA	Used for prophylaxis of BA

- **DOC** for acute attack of asthma: SALBUTAMOL
- **Salmeterol** is the first long acting selective β2 agonist with slow onset of action. It is used as maintenance therapy and for nocturnal therapy BUT not for acute symptoms.
- **Formeterol** is fast acting and can be used in acute attack and for prophylaxis as well.
- **Theophylline** is a phosphodiesterase inhibitor. In acute attack sustained release oral form can be given.

335. Ans. (a) Slow acting β2 agonist

Ref: KD Tripathi, 6th ed. pg. 227

Pharmacology

TABLE: Treatment of choice

Severe asthma	Status asthmaticus/ refractory asthma
• Continuous symptoms; activity limitation; frequent exacerbations/ hospitalization • Regular high dose inhaled steroid + • inhaled long-acting β₂ agonist (salmeterol) twice daily • Rescue treatment with short acting inhaled β₂ agonist	• Any patient of asthma has the potential to develop acute severe asthma which may be lifethreatning. • Hydrocortisone hemisuccinate 100 mg • Nebulized salbutamol + ipratropium bromide • High flow humidified oxygen inhalation • Salbutamol/terbutaline in order to reach smaller bronchi

336. Ans. (b) Oropharyngeal candidiasis

- Most of the side effects of steroids are mainly hoarseness, orophyrangeal candidiasis, decreased growth in children with adrenal suppression.
- The plausible explanation is that since these drugs are inhaled, they avoid the first pass metabolism that orally administered steroids undergo and hence have preponderance to cause the usual manifestations of steroid toxicity.

337. Ans. (a) Ipratropium bromide

Ref: Katzung Pharmacology, 10ᵗʰ ed. Ch 10

- Ipratropium bromide is an anti-cholinergic agent/ Muscarinic antagonists which competitively inhibit the effect of acetylcholine at muscarinic receptors.
- **Ipratropium** appears to be at least as effective in patients with COPD that includes a partially reversible component. A longer-acting, selective anti-muscarinic agent, **tiotropium,** is DOC for COPD.
- **Salbutamol and terbutaline** are β2 agonist, used in acute cases of asthma.
- **Salmetrol is slow acting** β2 agonist, used for prophylaxis of asthma.

338. Ans. (a) Anti-tussive

Ref: KDT, 6ᵗʰ ed. pg. 215

- Forceful expulsion of air from lungs due to pulmonary irritation is called coughing. It can be productive or non-productive.
- **Anti-tussive** is a class of drug which *relieves coughing by suppressing cough center.* These drugs are mainly used for dry cough. Examples of anti-tussives are:
  - **Opioids:** Codeine, Phalcodeine, Ethylmorphine
  - **Non-Opioids:** NOSCAPINE, Dextromethorphan

- **Expectorants** are class of drugs that increase bronchial secretion or reduce its viscosity (mucolytics). They are mainly used in productive cough. Examples of expectorants are:
  - **Mucolytics:** Bromhexeine, Ambroxol
  - **Bronchial secretion enhancers:** Guaiphenisine, sodium or potassium citrate.

339. Ans. (a) Cough center

Please refer to above explanation.

340. Ans. (b) Inhibits 5-lipoxygenase

- Leukotrienes are biochemical mediators that contribute to asthma symptoms
  - Contracting airway smooth muscle
  - Increasing vascular permeability and mucus secretion
  - Attracting and activating airway inflammatory cells
- **Zileuton is a 5-lipoxygenase inhibitor that decreases leukotriene production,** and zafirlukast and montelukast are cysteinyl leukotriene receptor antagonists.
- They are useful to prevent asthma attacks and cause modest improvements in lung function. They lessen the need for β2-agonist rescue therapy.

HEMATOLOGY AND VITAMINS

341. Ans. (c) Warfarin

Ref: Goodman & Gillman 13ᵗʰ ed. P 593-94

- Warfarin (one of coumarin derivative) is an oral antagonist acts by antagonizing vitamin K dependent factors.
- Vitamin K dependent clotting factor: II, VII, IX, X
- Vitamin K dependent anticlotting factors: Protein C and Protein S
- Warfarin is administered as a racemic mixture of *S-* and *R*-warfarin.
- *S*-Warfarin is 3- to 5-fold more potent than *R*-warfarin and is mainly metabolized by CYP2C9.
- Because of the long t½ of coagulation factors, the anti-thrombotic action of warfarin is achieved in 4–5 days

SIDE EFFECTS

- Bleeding: Most common side effect (risk high if INR >4)
- Birth defect and abortion if administered during pregnancy (fetal warfarin syndrome)
- **Skin necrosis/Coumarin necrosis:** Can occur 3–10 days after initiation of warfarin. Usually due to protein C and S deficiency
- Purple toe syndrome-blue tinged discoloration of plantar surface and side of toes, that blanches with pressure. Can occur 3–8 weeks after initiation of therapy.

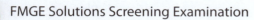

342. Ans. (a) Apixaban

Ref: Goodman & Gillman 13th ed. P 595

- Factor Xa inhibition results in reduced thrombin generation → suppression of platelet generation and fibrin formation.
- Factor Xa inhibitor drugs are: Rivaroxaban, Apixaban, Edoxaban
- Dose of apixaban: 5 mg BD
- Use:
  - Stroke prevention in patients with atrial fibrillation
  - Deep vein thrombosis, Pulmonary embolism
  - Postoperative thromboprophylaxis is patients undergoing hip/knee surgery
- Contraindicated for stroke prevention in patients with mechanical heart valve
- Side effects:
  - **Bleeding**- MC side effect. Incidence 50% lesser than warfarin induced bleeding except GI bleed.
    - (GI bleed: Apixaban, Rivaroxaban > Warfarin)
- Antidote: Andexanet Alfa, Ciraparantag

343. Ans. (b) Filgrastim

Ref: Goodman & Gillman 13th ed. P 756

- Filgrastim is G-CSF (Granulocyte Colony Stimulating Factor)
- The principal action of filgrastim is the stimulation of CFU-G to increase neutrophil production
- Forms of G-CSF are now available, including two longer-acting pegylated forms, pegfilgrastim and lipegfilgrastim.
- Use:
  - Severe neutropenia after autologous hematopoietic stem cell transplantation
  - Neutropenia after high dose cancer chemotherapy
  - Congenital neutropenia
  - Neutropenia of any other cause
- Dose: 1–20 µg/kg/day via IV or subcutaneous route
- Side effect: Mild-to-moderate bone pain

344. Ans. (b) Deferoxamine

Ref: Goodman & Gillman's 13th ed. P 63, 1314

- Iron chelating agent is: Deferoxamine

TABLE: Antidotes of different poisoning

Poisoning indication(s)	Antidote
Acetaminophen	Acetylcysteine
Organophosphorus and carbamate pesticides	Atropine sulfate
Drug-induced dystonia	Benztropine
Na+ channel blocking drugs	Bicarbonate, sodium

Contd...

Poisoning indication(s)	Antidote
Neuroleptic malignant syndrome	Dantrolene
Ca^{2+} channel blocking drugs, fluoride	Calcium gluconate or chloride
Valproate hyperammonemia	Carnitine
North American crotaline snake envenomation	Crotalidae polyvalent immune Fab
Malignant hyperthermia	Dantrolene
Iron	Deferoxamine
Cardiac glycosides	Digoxin immune Fab
Drug-induced dystonia	Diphenhydramine
Lead, mercury, arsenic	Dimercaprol (BAL)
Lead	EDTA, $CaNa_2$
Methanol, ethylene glycol	Ethanol
Methanol, ethylene glycol	Fomepizole
Benzodiazepines	Flumazenil
β adrenergic antagonists	Glucagon hydrochloride
Cyanide	Hydroxocobalamin hydrochloride
Hyperkalemia	Insulin (High dose)
Methotrexate	Leucovorin calcium
Methemoglobinemia	Methylene blue
Opioids	Naloxone hydrochloride
Sulfonylurea-induced hypoglycemia	Octreotide acetate
Carbon monoxide	Oxygen, hyperbaric
Lead, mercury, copper	Penicillamine
Anticholinergic syndrome	Physostigmine salicylate
Organophosphorus pesticides	Pralidoxime chloride (2-PAM)
Isoniazid seizures	Pyridoxine hydrochloride
Lead, mercury, arsenic	Succimer (DMSA)
Cyanide	Thisosulfate, sodium
Coumarin, indanedione	Vitamin K_1 (Phytonadione)

345. Ans. (b) Vitamin K antagonist

Ref: KD Tripathi, 7th ed. pg. 620, 621

- Warfarin and its congeners act as anticoagulants only in vivo (body), NOT in vitro (lab).
- It acts by inhibiting Vitamin K. Due to overdose, hematuria is the *first manifestation* noted.
- Dose monitoring is done by INR
- Antidote of warfarin overdose: Vitamin K

Pharmacology

346. Ans. (c) Heparin toxicity

Ref: KD Tripathi, 7th ed. P 618-620

PT (Prothrombin Time)	aPTT (Activated Partial Thromboplastin Time)
• Assess activity of extrinsic coagulation pathway. • Used when on warfarin treatment. • WePT: Warfarin for extrinsic; PT value assessed.	• Assess activity of intrinsic coagulation pathway. • Used while on heparin treatment. • *HINT: Heparin for Intrinsic; aPTT value assessed.*

347. Ans. (c) Factor II

Ref: KD Tripathi, 7th ed. pg. 620

- Direct thrombin inhibitors are a class of medication that act as anticoagulants (delaying blood clotting) by **directly inhibiting the enzyme thrombin (factor II).**
- **Argatroban** is a synthetic non-peptide compound which **binds reversibly to the catalytic site of thrombin,** but not to the substrate recognition site.
- Administered by IV infusion, it can be used in place of lepirudin for short-term indications in patients with heparin-induced thrombocytopenia.
- **Other direct thrombin inhibitors are:**
  - PARENTERAL ROUTE: **Lepirudin, Bivaluridin, Desirudin**
  - Oral rote: **Dabigatran**
- **Note:** Heparin is indirect thrombin inhibitor which acts by antithrombin 3 mediated inhibition of factor IIa and Xa.

348. Ans. (d) Heparin

Ref: KD Tripathi, 6th ed. pg. 597

- Heparin is a powerful and instantaneously acting anticoagulant, effective both in vivo and in vitro.
- It acts indirectly by *activating* plasma antithrombin III
- The heparin –AT III complex then binds to clotting factors of the intrinsic and common pathways (Xa, IIa, IXa, XIa, XIIa and XIIIa) and inactivates them.
- **Heparin is the anticoagulant of choice in pregnancy**
- Warfarin on the other hand is effective only in vivo (body). It acts by inhibiting vitamin K.

> **Extra Mile**
>
> **Heparin is monitored** by aPTT
> **Low molecular heparin inhibits** factor X_a only. It does not require monitoring because of consistent bioavailability.
> **Antidote for heparin overdose:** Protamine Sulfate.
> **Warfarin monitoring is done by:** INR
> **Antidote of warfarin overdose:** Vitamin K.
> **TOC for warfarin induced** bleeding: FFP

349. Ans. (c) Lepirudin

Ref: Katzung's, 11th ed. pg. 593-594

- Heparin is a powerful and instantaneously acting anticoagulant, effective both in vivo and in vitro.
- It acts indirectly by *activating* plasma antithrombin III
- The heparin –AT III complex then binds to clotting factors of the intrinsic and common pathways (Xa, IIa, IXa, XIa, XIIa and XIIIa) and inactivates them.
- **HIT syndrome** is a condition which arises as a potential side effect of heparin use where heparin binds with platelet factor 4 and causes thrombocytopenia *(usually seen 3–4 days after heparin use).*
- **To treat this condition, direct thrombin inhibitors are used. Drugs under direct thrombin inhibitors are: Lepirudin, bivalirudin, hirudin, dabigatran, argatroban, melagatran.**

> **Extra Mile**
>
> - Enoxaparin: It is low molecular weight heparin
> - Warfarin is oral anticoagulant, which act by inhibiting vitamin K dependent clotting factors (Factor II, VII, IX, X).

350. Ans. (c) Used as first line treatment in bleeding conditions

Ref: KDT, 6th ed. pg. 594, 595

▎ VITAMIN K

- It is a fat-soluble dietary principle required for the synthesis of clotting factors.
- *Action:* Vit. K acts as a cofactor at a late stage in the synthesis of coagulation proteins prothrombin, factors VII. IX and X.
- *Utilization:* Fat-soluble forms-absorbed from the intestine via lymph; while water-soluble forms are absorbed directly into portal blood.
- **Vitamin K has 3 forms:**
  - K1- fat soluble: Phytonadione
  - K2- fat soluble: Menaquinone, Acetomenaphthone
  - K3- water soluble: *Menadione sod. Bisulfate and Diphosphate*
- *Use:* vit K is used in prophylaxis (NOT as first line treatment)and treatment of bleeding due to deficiency of clotting factors in the following situations:
  - *Dietary deficiency*
  - *Prolonged antimicrobial therapy*
  - *Obstructive jaundice or malabsorption syndrome*
  - *Liver disease (cirohosis, viral hepatitis)*
  - *Newborns*
  - *Overdose of oral anticoagulants*
- In case of bleeding disorders, stop the anticoagulant immediately and fresh frozen plasma is recommended.

FMGE Solutions Screening Examination

351. Ans. (d) Tranexamic acid

Ref: KDT, 6th ed. pg. 608

- Antiplatelet drugs interfere with platelet function and are useful in prophylaxis of thromboembolic disorders.
- Platelets express several glycoprotein (GP) receptors on their surface like GP IIa/IIIb.
- These receptors are not exposed normally, but once exposed due to some injury they make the platelets sticky.
- Upon injury thromboxane A2 (TXA2) and ADP produced, which expose the sticky receptors (GP IIa/IIIb) that crosslinks the platelets, inducing aggregation.
- Prostacyclin (PGI2) synthesized in the intima of blood vessel is an inhibitor of TXA2. Normally, a balance between PGI2 and TXA2 is required to control thrombus formation.

TABLE: Antiplatelet drugs and their target of inhibition

Antiplatelet drugs	Target of inhibition
Aspirin	Inhibit TXA2
Clopidogrel and Ticlodipine	Inhibit ADP irreversibly by binding with P2Y12 receptor
Cangrelor, Ticagrelor	Inhibit ADP reversibly
Abciximab Tirofiban Eptifibatide	Inhibit GP IIb/IIIa

> **Extra Mile**
>
> Fibrin is associated with clotting. Agents which lyse this fibrin is known as Fibrinolytics.
> Overdose of fibrinolytic agents causes results in excessive intravascular fibrinolysis resulting in bleeding.
> **Tranexamic acid** is a specific antidote for fibrinolytic agents.
> Antifibrinolytic drugs are:
> - Epsilon Amino Caproic acid (EACA)
> - Tranexamic acid

352. Ans. (d) Thromboxane

Ref: KDT, 6th ed. pg. 609; Katzung, 9th ed. pg. 446

Thromboxane helps in platelet aggregation.
- TXA_2 formation is suppressed at very low doses of **aspirin.**
- Aspirin blocks thromboxane formation by inhibiting COX activity by enzyme COX1 and TX- synthase irreversibly.

353. Ans. (b) Inhibit TXA2 formation

Ref: KDT, 6th ed. pg. 609; Katzung 9th ed. pg. 446

Please refer to above explanation

354. Ans. (a) Inhibit antithrombin 3

Ref: KD Tripathi, 6th ed. pg. 597

- Heparin is a powerful and instantaneously acting anticoagulant, effective both in vivo and in vitro.
- It acts indirectly by *activating* plasma antithrombin III. Antithrombin mediated inhibition of factor IIa and Xa mainly.
  - The heparin –AT III complex then binds to clotting factos of the intrinsic and common pathways (Xa, IIa, IXa, XIa, XIIa and XIIIa) and inactivates them.
- Warfarin on the other hand effective only in vivo (body). it act by inhibiting vitamin K.

> **Extra Mile**
>
> Heparin is monitored by aPTT (*remembered as HINT: **Heparin-Intrinsic***)
> Low molecular heparin inhibits factor X_a only. It doesn't require monitoring because of consistent bioavailability.
> Antidote for heparin overdose: **Protamine Sulfate**.
> Warfarin monitoring is done by: **INR**
> Antidote of warfarin overdose: **Vitamin K.**

355. Ans. (b) Acts both in vivo and in vitro

- Oral anticoagulant is warfarin. It is used only in vivo (body), not in vitro (lab).
- Warfarin is not used to store blood.
- It acts by inhibiting Vitamin K. Due to overdose, hematuria is the first manifestation noted.
- Dose monitoring is done by INR.
- Antidote of warfarin overdose: Vitamin K

PT (Prothrombin Time)	aPTT (activated Partial Thromboplastin Time)
Assess activity of Extrinsic coagulation pathway	Assess activity of Extrinsic coagulation pathway.
Used when on warfarin treatment	Used while on heparin treatment.
WePT: Warfarin for extrinsic; PT value assessed.	*HINT: Heparin for Intrinsic; aPTT value assessed.*

356. Ans. (a) Ciprofloxacin

Ref: KDT, 6th ed. pg. 64

- G6PD is an enzyme present on RBC membrane provides strength to RBC which can counteract free radicals and oxidizing stress of drugs.
- In absence of G6PD enzyme, these cells can't bear the stress and results in Hemolysis.
- **Drugs causing Hemolysis in G6PD deficiency patients are:**
  - Anti malarials (Primaquine, chloroquine)
  - Antibiotic (Nitrofurantoin)

Pharmacology

- Anti emetic (Furazolidone)
- Sulfonamide (dapsone)
- Fava beans
- **Ciprofloxacin** is one of the quinolones, effective against G+ and G- including pseudomonas.
- It is contraindicated in pregnancy and children below 18 years of age because it effects growing bone and tendons.
- Ciprofloxacin is considered as oral DOC for enteric fever.
- DOC for enteric fever: Ceftriaxone

357. Ans. (c) Chloroquine

Ref: KDT 6th ed. pg. 64

Please refer to above explanation

358. Ans. (b) Enoxaparin

- Enoxaparin is a low molecular weight heparin.
- It acts by inhibiting factor Xa.
- LMWH usually doesn't need monitoring because of consistent bioavailability.
- **Drugs under LMWH:**
  - Enoxaparin
  - Dalteparin
  - Tinzaparin
  - Rabiparin

> **Extra Mile**
>
> **Hirudin along with Lepirudin** and Bivalirudin is an anticoagulant which is act by direct thrombin (factor IIa) inhibition.
> **Tranexamic acid** is an anti-fibrinolytic agent.

359. Ans. (c) Factor Xa

Ref: KD Tripathi, 6th Ed. pg. 597-598

- Low molecular heparin inhibits factor Xa mainly, having some action at factor IIa as well. It doesn't require monitoring because of consistent bioavailability.
- Heparin is a powerful and instantaneously acting anticoagulant, effective both in vivo and in vitro.
- It acts indirectly by *activating* plasma antithrombin III
- The heparin –AT III complex then binds to clotting factors of the intrinsic and common pathways (Xa, IIa, IXa, XIa, XIIa and XIIIa) and inactivates them.
- Warfarin on the other hand is effective only in vivo (body). It acts by inhibiting vitamin K.

Note

- Fondaparinaux is synthetic LMWH acts exclusively at factor Xa.

360. Ans. (b) It acts by inhibiting both factor IIa and factor Xa

Ref: KDT, 6th ed. pg. 599-600

- Low molecular weight heparin, Enoxaparin, inhibits only factor Xa whereas unfractionated heparin inhibits both factor IIa and factor Xa.

361. Ans. (a) Isotretinoin

Ref: Katzung, 11th ed. pg. 1308, 1455; KDT, pg. 854

- **13-*cis*-Retinoic acid (Isotretinoin) is an analogue of vitamin A.** It is used for the treatment of severe cystic acne
- Isotretinoin (Accutane) is a synthetic retinoid currently restricted to the treatment of severe cystic acne that is refractory to standard therapies.
- It appears to act by inhibiting sebaceous gland size and function.
- Half life- 10-20 hours.
- **Common side effect:** Hypervitaminosis A, dryness of skin and mucous membrane.
- **Teratogenic effect**: Extremely high risk of CNS, face, ear, and other malformations. Risk is equal throughout all the three trimester.

> **Extra Mile**
>
> - **Al-trans vitamin A (Tretinoin):** Effective topical agent in the treatment of acne vulgaris. It is a potent comedolytic and stimulate epidermal cell turnover, resulting in peeling.
> - **Benzoyl peroxide** is an effective topical agent in the treatment of acne vulgaris
> - MOA of benzoyl peroxide- its antimicrobial activity against *P acnes* and to its peeling and comedolytic effects.
> - **Azelaic acid** effective in the treatment of acne vulgaris.
> - MOA of azelaic acid-antimicrobial activity against *P acnes* as well as an in vitro inhibitory effect on the conversion of testosterone to dihydrotestosterone.

362. Ans. (a) I/M

Ref: KDT, 6th ed. pg. 588

VITAMIN B12

- Present in two forms: Cyanocobalamin and hydroxoco-balamin.
- Dietary sources: Liver, kidney, sea fish, egg yolk, meat and cheese.
- Only vegetable source: Legumes (pulses)
- Daily requirement: 1–2 µg/day. In cases of pregnancy and lactation: 3–5 µg/day.

Manifestation of Deficiency

- **Megaloblastic anemia**- the first manifestation.
  - Hypersegmented neutrophils and giant platelets.
- **SACD:** subacute combined degeneration of spinal cord; peripheral neuritis, paresthesias.
- **Glossitis, GI disturbance:** Damage to epithelial structures.

FMGE Solutions Screening Examination

Preparation Dose and Administration

- Cynocobalamin: 35 µg/5ml liquid; 100, 500, 1000 µg Inj.
- Hydroxycobalamin: 500, 1000 µg Inj.
- Methylcobalamin: 0.5 mg tab.
- In case of severe anemia (like pernicious anemia), Vit B12 should be given by I.M or deep s.c (but not by I.V.) injection.
- Parenteral administration is necessary to bypass the defective absorptive mechanism.
- Hydroxycobalamin has been preferred for parenteral use because of better retention.

363. Ans. (c) **Avidin**

Ref: KD Tripathi, 6th ed. pg. 876

BIOTIN

- Biotin is a sulfur containing organic acid found in egg yolk, liver, nuts and many other articles of food.
- It is well absorbed from intestine and excreted mainly unchanged in urine.
- **Avidin,** a heat labile protein in egg white, binds and prevents the absorption of biotin.

364. Ans. (b) **Niacin**

Ref: KDT, 6th ed. pg. 875

- Lipids that are liberated from adipose tissue are used to build very-low-density lipoproteins (VLDL) in the liver, which are precursors of low-density lipoprotein (LDL)
- Because niacin blocks the breakdown of fats, it causes a decrease in free fatty acids in the blood and, as a consequence, decreases the secretion of VLDL and cholesterol by the liver.
- When niacin is added to statins, it reduces carotid intima-media thickness, a marker of atherosclerosis.

365. Ans. (a) **Hallucination**

Ref: Katzung, 9th ed. pg. 1604; KDT 6th ed. pg. 376

- Ketamine is the only intravenous anesthetic that possesses analgesic properties and produces cardiovascular stimulation.
- It is pharmacologically related to the hallucinogen Phencyclidine; induces a so called *"dissociative anesthesia"* characterized by profound analgesia, immobility, amnesia and feeling of dissociation from one's own body and the surrounding.
- It causes:
    - Hallucination
    - Delusion and illusion.
    - Profound analgesia

- Ketamine increases all pressures like:
    - BP (hypertension)
    - Intracranial tension (ICT)
    - Intraocular pressure (IOP)
- It is contraindicated in intracerebral mass/hemorrhage.

MUST KNOW ABOUT KETAMINE: (*Remembered as*)

K	Kids: Can be given to kids
E	Emergence reaction: s/e occurring during recovery
T	Thalamo-cortical junction affected: Dissociative Anesthesia
A	Analgesia strongest
M	Meal: Can be given with full stomach
I	Increase: BP/IOP/ICT
N	NMDA receptor blocker
E	Excellent bronchodilator: Inducing agent of choice in asthma patient.

> **Extra Mile**
>
> **PROPOFOL** causes myocardial depression and fall in BP.

MISCELLANEOUS

366. Ans. (c) **Propranolol**

- Propranolol, a nonselective β-blocker can cause intra-uterine growth retardation.

367. Ans. (a) **Chloroquine**

Class of Drugs contraindicated in pregnancy and its safer alternative

Class of drug	Contraindicated	Safer alternative
Antibacterials (systemic bacterial infections)	Cotrimoxazole, Fluoroquinolones (X), Tetracycline (X), Doxycycline (X), Chloramphenicol (X), Gentamicin, Streptomycin (X), Kanamycin (X), Tobramycin (X), Clarithromycin, Azithromycin, Clindamycin, Vancomycin, Nitrofurantoin,	Penicillin G, Ampicillin Amoxicillin-clavulanate Cloxacillin, Piperacillin Cephalosporins Erythromycin
Antitubercular	Pyrazinamide, Streptomycin (X)	Isoniazid, Rifampicin, Ethambutol

Contd...

Pharmacology

Class of drug	Contraindicated	Safer alternative
Antimalarial	Artemether, Artesunate Primaquine (X)	Chloroquine, Mefloquine, Proguanil Quinine (only in 1st trimester), Pyrimethamine + Sulfadoxine (only single dose.)
Antihypertensives	ACE inhibitors (X), Angiotensin antagonists (X). Thiazide diuretics Furosemide, Propranolol Nitroprusside	Methyldopa, Hydralazine, Atenolol Metoprolol, Pindolol, Nifedipine Prazosin, Clonidine

368. Ans. (c) Safer for pregnant lady and infants

Ref: Wound Healing and Ulcers of the skin-Diagnosis and Therapy, pg. 154

- Silver sulfadiazine is prepared as a water soluble cream in a concentration of 1%.
- It is composed of silver nitrate and sodium sulfadiazine, both having antibacterial qualities.
- SSD is commonly used in the management of burns and cutaneous ulcers.
- It is effective against wide range of pathogenic bacteria, including staph aureus. E. Coli, proteus, enterococci and pseudomonas strain.

- **Contraindications:**
  - In G6PD patients.
  - They can cause kernicterus, hence it is contraindicated in pregnancy or during the first 2 months of life.

369. Ans. (c) Mitotane

Mitotane alters steroid peripheral metabolism, directly suppresses the adrenal cortex and alters cortisone metabolism leading to hypocortisolism.

370. Ans. (c) PENMT

Ref: KDT, 6th ed. pg. 116

- PENMT is Phenylethanolamine N- methyl transferase and is found in the cytosol of only cells of adrenal medullary cells.
- PENMT uses S- adenosylmethionine (SAMe) as a cofactor to donate the methyl group to norepinephrine, creating epinephrine.
- Epinephrine is synthesized in the medulla of the adrenal gland in an enzymatic pathway that converts the amino acid tyrosine into a series of intermediates and, ultimately, adrenaline.
- Tyrosine is first oxidized to L-DOPA, which is subsequently decarboxylated to give dopamine. Oxidation gives norepinephrine.
- The final step is methylation of the primary amine of noradrenaline by *phenylethanolamine N-methyltransferase (PNMT)* in the cytosol of adrenergic neurons and cells of the adrenal medulla (chromaffin cells).

ANSWERS TO BOARD REVIEW QUESTIONS

371. Ans. (b) Salmeterol

Ref: KDT, 6th ed. pg. 127, 128

372. Ans. (a) Alzheimer's disease

Ref: Goodman & Gillman, 11th ed. pg. 132

373. Ans. (c) 36 hours

Ref: Goodman Gillman, 11th ed. pg. 573

374. Ans. (a) Cirrhotic edema

Ref: Goodman 11th ed. ch-28

375. Ans. (b) Hypokalemia

Ref: Goodman and Gillman, 11th ed. pg. 799

376. Ans. (b) Binds to ryanodine receptors to block release of Ca++

Ref: Lippincott, 5th ed. pg. 344

377. Ans. (d) Filgrastrim

378. Ans. (c) Asthma

379. Ans. (a) Bumetanide

380. Ans. (d) Antidote is protamine sulfate

381. Ans. (c) Ciclesonide

382. Ans. (c) Chronic constipation

383. Ans. (b) Carbapenem

Explanations

FMGE Solutions Screening Examination

384. Ans. (b) Rash	409. Ans. (d) Cilastin
385. Ans. (a) Vancomycin	410. Ans. (a) Rasagaline
386. Ans. (a) Chloroquine	411. Ans. (c) Fomepizole
387. Ans. (a) Quinine	412. Ans. (c) Naltrexone
388. Ans. (a) Didanosine	413. Ans. (b) Zolpidem
389. Ans. (c) Albendazole	414. Ans. (a) Bromocriptine
390. Ans. (a) Propyl-thiouracil	415. Ans. (a) Tetrabenzamine
391. Ans. (b) Amiloride	416. Ans. (b) Intranasal midazolam
392. Ans. (d) Beta blocker	417. Ans. (a) Amiodarone
393. Ans. (b) Inhibiting folate synthase	418. Ans. (d) Ankle edema
394. Ans. (c) Exenatide	419. Ans. (d) Rosuvastatin
395. Ans. (a) Ketoconazole	420. Ans. (d) Milrinone
396. Ans. (d) Vigabatrin	421. Ans. (c) Class V
397. Ans. (b) Tropicamide	422. Ans. (c) CCB
398. Ans. (a) Lanatoprost	423. Ans. (b) Vitamin B
399. Ans. (a) Zoledronate	424. Ans. (c) Inhibition of HMG COA synthase
400. Ans. (a) Hydroxyurea	425. Ans. (b) Atosiban
401. Ans. (d) Foscarnet	426. Ans. (b) Sodium valproate
402. Ans. (d) Argatroban	427. Ans. (b) Around 200 patients
403. Ans. (b) Propranolol	428. Ans. (d) Phenobarbitone
Ref: KDT, 6th ed. pg. 172, Harrison's, 18th ed. Chapter 14	429. Ans. (b) Phenobarbitone
404. Ans. (a) 65 mmol/L	430. Ans. (d) Drugs for rare diseases
405. Ans. (b) Vancomycin	431. Ans. (a) Bacteriostatic agent
406. Ans. (c) Acinetobacter	432. Ans. (b) Para amino salicylic acid
407. Ans. (b) Entecavir	433. Ans. (c) Cycloserine
408. Ans. (a) Niacin	434. Ans. (c) Dobutamine

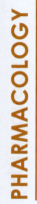

Pharmacology

435. Ans. (d) Reactivate Ach esterase enzyme

436. Ans. (d) Sweating

437. Ans. (b) Methacholine

438. Ans. (c) Tyrosine hydroxylase

439. Ans. (c) Imipramine

440. Ans. (d) Isoprenaline

441. Ans. (b) Labetelol

Ref: Appendix 107 Classiciation of alfa and beta blockers

442. Ans. (a) Bromocriptine

Ref: Goodman Gillman, 2008 pg. 973

443. Ans. (b) Ezetimibe

Ref: Harrison's, 18th ed. ch 356

444. Ans. (a) Sleep apnea syndrome

Ref: Harrison's, 18th ed. ch 27

445. Ans. (b) Acute migraine

Ref: Harrison's, 18th ed. ch 14

446. Ans. (b) Hyperuricemia

Ref: Harrison's, 18th ed. ch 333

447. Ans. (b) Gatifloxacin

Ref: http://m.medindia.net/patientinfo/drugs-drugs-banned-in-india.htm

448. Ans. (a) Atropine

Ref: KDT 6/e/ 103

449. Ans. (b) Isoniazid

Ref: KDT 6/e / 740-743

450. Ans. (c) Pyrizinamide

Ref: Harrison's 18/e, ch 161, Table 161-3, http://ww.cdc.gov/tb/

451. Ans. (a) Amilorides

Ref: Goodman Gillman 11/e, ch 30

452. Ans. (c) Inhalational salmeterol

Ref: Harrison's 18/e, p 254, Goodman and Gilman's 11/e, p 463, CMDT 2009 edition table 9-4 and 9-6

453. Ans. (a) β lactamase inhibitors

Ref: Ka Tzung 9/e, p 1064

454. Ans. (c) Octreotide

Ref: Goodman and Gillman 11/e, p 635

455. Ans. (c) Schedule H

Ref: Forensic medicine and toxicology by R.N. Karmakar, /42

456. Ans. (d) Inhibit release of TG and LDL

Ref: KDT 6/e, p 614, Harrison's 18/e, Chapter 356

457. Ans. (b) Vincristine

Ref: KDT 5/e, p 774

458. Ans. (a) NSAID

Ref: Harrison's Internal Medicine 18/e, Table 285-3, Radiology Illustrated, Uroladiology: Uroradiology by SeungHyup Ki 2/e, p 471

459. Ans. (d) Varenicline

Ref: Harrison 17/e, Chapter 390

460. Ans. (b) Flumazenil

Ref: Harrison's 17/e, Table 35-4, Goodman and Gillman's 11/e, p 270

461. Ans. (a) β carboline

462. Ans. (c) 5HT 2A

Ref: KDT 6/e, p 164-171, Harrison's 18/e, Chapter 14

463. Ans. (b) Cimetidine

Ref: Appendix-39 for "Drugs causing Gynaecomastia"

464. Ans. (b) Demeclocycline

Ref: KDT 6/e, p 83

465. Ans. (c) 15 mg/kg

Ref: Goodman Gillman 11/e, p 699, 1819, Harrison's 17/, Chapter 213, KDT 6/e, p 810, Nelson textbook of Pediatrics, 18/e, Chapter 300

Explanations

FMGE Solutions Screening Examination

466. Ans. (b) Atosiban

Ref: *Danforth's Obstetrics and Gynecology 10/e, p 175-178, Ganong's 22/e, p 243*

467. Ans. (b) Dantrolene

Ref: *Lippinott 5/e, p 344, Goodman and Gillman, p 152, 11/e*

468. Ans. (a) Headache

Ref: *Goodman and Gilman's 11/e, Chapter 31, 32*

469. Ans. (a) Nimodipine

Ref: *KDT 6/e, p 172*

470. Ans. (a) SSRI

Ref: *KDT 6/e, p 119, 12, 135*

471. Ans. (d) Metoclopramide

Ref: *KDT 6/e, p 642*

472. Ans. (c) Inhibit folate synthesis

Ref: *KDT 6/e, p 683*

473. Ans. (a) Inhibits plasminogen

Ref: *Lippincott's Pharmacology 4/e, p 265*

474. Ans. (d) Hypokalemia

Ref: *KDT 6/e, p 567*

475. Ans. (c) 8 weeks

Ref: *Mayo clinic gastroenterology and Hepatology Board review edited by Stephen Hauser 4/e, p 13, Pharmacology by George M. Brenner, Craig Stevens, 4/e, p 297*

476. Ans. (c) Safety

Ref: *KDT 7/e, p 54/55*

477. Ans. (c) Osteoporosis

Ref: *Harrison 18/e/ 3133, 3134*

478. Ans. (d) Glargine

Ref: *KDT 6/e/ 262*

479. Ans. (c) Desmopressin

Ref: *Goodman Gillman 11/e, Chapter 29, Harrison's Internal Medicine 17/e, Chapter 334*

480. Ans. (c) Aspirin

Ref: *Harrison's 18/e, Chapter 106*

481. Ans. (c) Yohimbine

Ref: *KDT 6/e, p 132*

482. Ans. (b) IV hydrocortisone

Ref: *Harrison's 18/e, Chapter 342*

483. Ans. (d) Valproate

484. Ans. (d) Valproate

Ref: *KDT 6/e, p 408*

485. Ans. (d) Inhibits COX1 and COX 2 irreversibly

Ref: *KDT 6/e, p 193, Goodman and Gillman's 11/e, p 440*

486. Ans. (c) Pyrazinamide

Ref: *Goodman Gillman's 10/e, Chapter 47*

487. Ans. (a) Bromocriptine

Ref: *Harrison 18/e, Chapter 350*

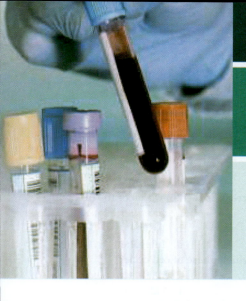

5

Pathology

MOST RECENT QUESTIONS 2019

1. Berry aneurysm most commonly occurs due to?
    a. Endothelial injury of vessel due to HTN
    b. Muscle intimal elastic lamina layer defect
    c. Endothelial layer defect
    d. Adventitia defect
2. A 45-year patient working in a factory for past 20 years presents with breathlessness. HRCT chest shows pleural thickening and fibrosis. Diagnosis is?
    a. Asbestosis
    b. Coal worker pneumoconiosis
    c. Silicosis
    d. Berylliosis
3. Most commonly observed autosomal aneuploidy leading to spontaneous abortions is?
    a. Trisomy 16   b. Trisomy 21
    c. Monosomy   d. Trisomy 18
4. Which of these is a Nephritic syndrome?
    a. Minimal change disease
    b. Membranous Glomerulopathy
    c. Post infectious Glomerulonephritis
    d. Focal segmental glomerulosclerosis
5. The following serological status is noted in a patient: HbsAg positive and HbeAg positive. Diagnosis is?
    a. Acute viral hepatitis
    b. Chronic viral hepatitis
    c. Acute viral hepatitis with infectivity
    d. Remote infection
6. Chronic viral hepatitis is seen with?
    a. HBV   b. HCV
    c. HDV   d. HEV
7. Acute auto-graft rejection occurs within?
    a. Few hours   b. < 1 month
    c. < 6 months   d. 6-12 months
8. Type II Hypersensitivity is seen in?
    a. Pernicious anaemia
    b. Serum sickness
    c. Arthus phenomenon
    d. Pathergy phenomenon
9. Which of the following is a causative agent of Farmer's Lung?
    a. Thermophilic Actinomycetes
    b. Aspergillus Fumigatus
    c. Actinobacter
    d. Aspergillus Flavus
10. Comment on the diagnosis.

    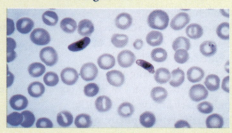

    a. Malaria   b. Hereditary spherocytosis
    c. G6PD deficiency   d. Babesia
11. Whipple's disease is caused by.
    a. Bacteria   b. Virus
    c. Protozoa   d. Helminths
12. Most common site of Brain metastasis is?
    a. Lung cancer   b. Head and neck cancer
    c. Prostate cancer   d. Breast cancer
13. Which is not seen in Tumour lysis Syndrome?
    a. Hypophosphatemia   b. Hypocalcemia
    c. Hyperuricemia   d. Hyperkalemia
14. Comment on the diagnosis for SAP normal, PTH normal, Vitamin D3 normal with elevated serum Calcium values?
    a. Vitamin D intoxication
    b. Hyperparathyroidism
    c. Multiple myeloma
    d. Nutritional rickets
15. Which of the following interfere with iron absorption?
    a. Vitamin C   b. Phytates
    c. Oxalate   d. Myoglobin
16. Most sensitive and specific marker for MI is?
    a. Troponin   b. Cytokeratin
    c. Myoglobin   d. CPK- MM

FMGE Solutions Screening Examination

17. Antecedent diagnosis of Group A streptococcal infection in Acute rheumatic fever can be made by?
    a. AS0
    b. CRP
    c. ESR elevation
    d. Low C3 levels
18. Most common anterior mediastinal tumour?
    a. Thymoma
    b. Neurofibroma
    c. Pericardial cyst
    d. Bronchogenic cyst
19. Most characteristic finding of diabetic nephropathy?
    a. Kimmelstein Wilson disease
    b. Diffuse glomerulosclerosis
    c. Focal segmental glomerulosclerosis
    d. Armani Ebstein change
20. First line of defence against tumour and virus?
    a. NK cell
    b. T cell
    c. Histiocyte
    d. Macrophage
21. Most sensitive indicator for Iron deficiency anaemia?
    a. Serum Ferrtin
    b. TIBC
    c. Percentage saturation of transferrin
    d. Bone marrow iron
22. Most common cardiac defect in Down syndrome is?
    a. Endocardial cushion defect
    b. Ventricular septal defect
    c. Perpheral pulmonic stenosis
    d. Anomalous origin of left coronary artery from pulmonary artery(A.L.C.A.P.A)
23. MC cause of atypical pneumonia?
    a. Mycoplasma pneumoniae
    b. Klebsiella pneumoniae
    c. Hemophilus influenzae
    d. Chylamydia
24. Correct about of Anaemia of chronic disease
    a. High ferritin
    b. Increased percentage of saturation of transferrin
    c. High transferrin
    d. High serum iron

CELL INJURY AND INFLAMMATION

25. Stellate granuloma is found in:
    (Recent Pattern Question 2018-19)
    a. Cat scratch disease
    b. Leprosy
    c. Coccidomycosis
    d. Histoplasmosis
26. Which proteoglycan is involved in process of healing?
    (Recent Pattern Question 2018-19)
    a. Chondroitin sulphate
    b. Dermatan sulphate
    c. Keratan sulphate
    d. Syndecan
27. Secondary healing mechanism is?
    (Recent Pattern Question 2018-19)
    a. Granuloma formation
    b. Scab formation
    c. Granulation tissue
    d. Neovascularization
28. Rolling of leucocytes on endothelial cells is mediated by:
    (Recent Pattern Question 2018)
    a. Selectins
    b. Integrins
    c. Transferrin
    d. PECAM-1
29. Liquefactive necrosis is seen in which of the following?
    (Recent Pattern Question 2018)
    a. Kidney
    b. Heart
    c. Cerebrum
    d. Intestine
30. P53 regulates which phase of cell cycle?
    (Recent Pattern Question 2018)
    a. G1S
    b. G2
    c. G2M
    d. S
31. Pro-apoptotic gene and anti-apoptotic gene belong to which gene family? *(Recent Pattern Question 2017)*
    a. p53
    b. Bcl
    c. BRAF
    d. Rb
32. Colliquative necrosis is seen in?
    (Recent Pattern Question 2017)
    a. Arthus phenomenon
    b. Malignant hypertension
    c. Tuberculoma
    d. Lung abscess
33. DNA synthesis is seen in which phase of cell cycle?
    (Recent Pattern Question 2017)
    a. Resting phase
    b. Synthetic phase
    c. Mitotic phase
    d. Premitotic phase
34. Which of the following is an opsonin?
    Recent Pattern Question 2017)
    a. C3a
    b. C3b
    c. C5a
    d. C5b
35. Councilman bodies are formed due to process of ____?
    (Recent Pattern Question 2017)
    a. Necrosis
    b. Cirrhosis
    c. Apoptosis
    d. Necroptosis
36. Stellate shaped granuloma is seen in?
    (Recent Pattern Question 2017)
    a. Sarcoidosis
    b. Cat scratch
    c. Crohn's disease
    d. Tuberculosis
37. Which of the following helps in cell to cell adhesion?
    (Recent Pattern Question 2016)
    a. Interleukins
    b. Interferons
    c. E- Cadherin
    d. Matrix metallo proteinase
38. A reversible change occurring in which a mature cell type is replaced by another mature cell, is called:
    a. Dysplasia
    b. Metaplasia
    c. Hyerplasia
    d. Hypertrophy
39. A patient who was previously with good muscle mass, now presents with decreased muscle mass. There is history of RTA which led him to be bedridden for 6 months. This decrease in muscle mass is best explained by:
    a. Metaplasia
    b. Dysplasia
    c. Hypertrophy
    d. Atrophy
40. A pregnant uterus is an example of:
    a. Metaplasia
    b. Dysplasia
    c. Atrophy
    d. Hypertrophy

Pathology

41. In individuals who donate one lobe of the liver for transplantation, the remaining organ soon grows back to its original size. This is an example of which adaptive mechanism?
    a. Hypertrophy
    b. Atrophy
    c. Hyperplasia
    d. Metaplasia

42. Apoptosis is?
    a. Internally controlled, programmed cell death
    b. Externally controlled, programmed cell death
    c. Internally controlled, programmed enzyme degradation
    d. Externally controlled, programmed karyolysis

43. All are true about apoptosis EXCEPT?
    a. Considerable apoptosis may occur in a tissue before it becomes apparent in histology
    b. Apoptotic cells appear as round mass of the intensely eosinophilic cytoplasm with dense nuclear chromatin fragments
    c. Apoptosis of cells induce inflammatory reaction
    d. Condensation of chromatin

44. All are true about apoptosis EXCEPT?
    a. Inflammation is present
    b. Chromosomal breakage
    c. Clumping of chromatin
    d. Cell shrinkage

45. Light microscopic characteristic feature of apoptosis is?
    a. Intact cell membrane
    b. Eosinophilic cytoplasm
    c. Nuclear moulding
    d. Condensation of the nucleus

46. Apoptosis is inhibited by?
    a. Bcl-2
    b. Bax
    c. Bad
    d. P53

47. In apoptosis, protein hydrolysis is due to activation of:
    a. Caspases
    b. Upases
    c. Transglutaminase
    d. Catalase

48. Caspases are associated with which of the following?
    a. Hydropic degeneration
    b. Collagen hyalinization
    c. Embryogenesis
    d. Fatty degeneration

49. Caspases are involved in?
    a. Necrosis
    b. Apoptosis
    c. Atherosclerosis
    d. Inflammation

50. Earliest feature of reversible cell injury is:
    a. Amorphous densities
    b. Ribosomal detachment
    c. Hydropic swelling
    d. Bleb formation

51. All of the following statements are true regarding reversible cell injury, EXCEPT:
    a. Diminished generation of ATP
    b. Formation of blebs in the plasma membrane
    c. Condensation of nuclear chromatin
    d. Detachment of ribosomes from the granular endoplasmic reticulum

52. Which of the following type of necrosis is most commonly associated with ischemic injury:
    a. Coagulative necrosis
    b. Casseous necrosis
    c. Liquiefactive necrosis
    d. Fat necrosis

53. Inter-nucleosomal cleavage of DNA is characteristic of?
    a. Reversible cell injury
    b. Irreversible cell injury
    c. Necrosis
    d. Apoptosis

54. Integrins include receptor EXCEPT?
    a. Fibronectin
    b. Glycoprotein on platelet surface
    c. Leukocyte adhesion molecule
    d. Platelet derived growth factor

55. Exudation of plasma and leucocytes in acute inflammation is from?
    a. Venules
    b. Capillaries
    c. Arterioles
    d. Arterioles and capillaries

56. Dystrophic calcification is seen in?
    a. Rickets
    b. Hyperparathyroidism
    c. Atheromatous plaque
    d. Vitamin A intoxication

57. Digestion of foreign material by a neutrophil or macrophage during phagocytosis is mainly due to?
    a. Complement
    b. Hydrogen peroxide
    c. Kinins
    d. Lysosomal enzymes

58. Which of the following is a peroxisomal free radical scavenger?
    a. Superoxide dismutase
    b. Glutathione peroxidase
    c. Catalase
    d. All of the above

59. Which among the following is the hallmark of acute inflammation?
    a. Vasoconstriction
    b. Stasis
    c. Vasodilation and increase in permeability
    d. Leukocyte margination

60. Which of the following is not an inflammatory mediator?
    a. Tumor necrosis factor
    b. Myeloperoxidase
    c. Interferons
    d. Interleukin

61. All of the following host tissue responses can be seen in acute infection, EXCEPT?
    a. Exudation
    b. Vasodilation
    c. Margination
    d. Granuloma formation

62. Oxygen dependent killing is done through?
    a. NADPH oxidase
    b. Superoxide dismutase
    c. Catalase
    d. Glutathione peroxidase

63. Which of the following is required for post-translational modification?
    a. Vitamin B_{12}
    b. Biotin
    c. Beta-carotene
    d. Vitamin C

64. Cell swelling is seen in all EXCEPT?
    a. Infection
    b. Malignancy
    c. Calcification
    d. Hypoxia

Questions

323

FMGE Solutions Screening Examination

65. Fat necrosis occurs at all sites EXCEPT?
    a. Pancreas   b. Liver
    c. Breast   d. Peritoneum
66. Morphological changes seen in chronic non-specific inflammation include an increase in:
    a. Neutrophils, lymphocytes and liquiefactive necrosis
    b. Neutrophils, macrophages and fibrosis
    c. Lymphocytes, plasma cells and fibrosis
    d. giant cells, macrophages and coagulative necrosis
67. Foci of granulomatous inflammation show all of the following EXCEPT?
    a. Eosinophils   b. Epithelioid cells
    c. Fibrosis   d. Lymphocytes
68. All are true about white infarcts EXCEPT?
    a. Edema is present
    b. Occurs in organs with end arterial supply
    c. Well-defined margins
    d. Coagulative necrosis

HEMODYNAMICS

69. All are true about components of Virchow's triad EXCEPT?
    a. Vasculitis   b. Stasis in veins
    c. Turbulence in artery d. Increased protein C
70. All are true about arterial thrombosis EXCEPT?
    a. Retrograde growth
    b. Line of Zahn
    c. White thrombus
    d. Complete lumen obstruction
71. Which is the most common site of arterial embolization?
    a. Brain
    b. Kidney
    c. Mesentery
    d. Lower extremities
72. Chicken fat appearance is seen in?
    a. Antemortem clots
    b. Postmortem clots
    c. Fat necrosis
    d. Fibrinoid necrosis
73. All of the following are true in respect of angioneurotic edema EXCEPT?
    a. It is caused by deficiency of complement proteins
    b. It is more common in females
    c. It manifests as pitting edema
    d. It is an autosomal dominant disorder
74. Hypersensitivity angiitis is seen in?
    a. SLE
    b. Polyarteritis Nodosa
    c. Henoch Schonlein purpura
    d. Burgers disease

NEOPLASIA

75. Which of the following is true about Anaplasia?
    (Recent Pattern Question 2018-19)
    a. Loss of cohesion between cells
    b. Loss of differentiation
    c. Change of epithelium types
    d. Benign and fully reversible
76. Cell that can form any other cell in the body is called?
    (Recent Pattern Question 2018-19)
    a. Totipotent   b. Multipotent
    c. Pluripotent   d. Lineage stem cells
77. Hyaline globules are seen in all EXCEPT:
    (Recent Pattern Question 2018)
    a. Hepatoblastoma   b. Yolk Sac tumor
    c. Teratoma   d. Hepatocellular carcinoma
78. Which is the most common tumor associated with superior vena cava syndrome?
    (Recent Pattern Question 2018)
    a. Lung cancer   b. Lymphoma
    c. Metastasis   d. Thyroid cancer
79. Which is the most common cancer which results in death? *(Recent Pattern Question 2018)*
    a. Oral cancer   b. Breast cancer
    c. Prostate cancer   d. Lung cancer
80. Which of the following shows breast necrosis and calcification? *(Recent Pattern Question 2018)*
    a. Comedo subtype of DCIS
    b. Cribriform subtype of DCIS
    c. Colloid carcinoma
    d. Lobular carcinoma in situ
81. Mucosal melanosis and hamartomatous polyps are seen in? *(Recent Pattern Question 2018)*
    a. Peutz-Jeghers syndrome
    b. Cronkhite Canada syndrome
    c. Familial adenomatous polyposis
    d. Hereditary non polyposis colonic cancer
82. Jumping gene is known as? *(Recent Pattern Question 2017)*
    a. Transposon   b. Retroposon
    c. Insertion sequence d. Integron
83. Which is correct about non-seminomatous germ cell tumour? *(Recent Pattern Question 2017)*
    a. Spreads via lymphatics
    b. Testicular contour distorted
    c. Prognosis better than germ cell tumour
    d. Radiosensitive
84. Warthin tumour is? *(Recent Pattern Question 2017)*
    a. Adenolymphoma   b. Pleomorphic adenoma
    c. Mucoepidermoid carcinoma
    d. Acinic cell carcinoma

85. Loss of polarity is a feature of?
 (Recent Pattern Question 2017)
   a. Metaplasia   b. Dysplasia
   c. Necroptosis   d. All of the above
86. L-myc leads to? (Recent Pattern Question 2017)
   a. Burkitt lymphoma   b. Neuroblastoma
   c. Oat cell cancer   d. GIST
87. Which of the following Cancer is not due to infectious etiology? (Recent Pattern Question 2017)
   a. Small cell cancer of lung   b. H.C.C
   c. Naso-pharyngeal cancer   d. MALToma
88. Most common middle mediastinal tumour?
 (Recent Pattern Question 2017)
   a. Bronchogenic cyst   b. Pericardial cyst
   c. Neurofibroma   d. Lymphoma
89. The lesion shown below is caused by?
 (Recent Pattern Question 2017)

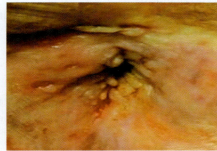

   a. HPV   b. HSV
   c. HIV   d. EBV
90. In a FAP patient which is an important CA risk
 (Recent Pattern Question 2016)
   a. Retinoblastoma
   b. Brain tumour
   c. Colorectal CA
   d. Prostate CA
91. Esophageal irradiation causes damage by
 (Recent Pattern Question 2016)
   a. Decreasing secretion   b. Glandular dysplasia
   c. Stricture formation   d. Glandular hypertrophy
92. Oncocytes are seen in all of the following EXCEPT?
   a. Pituitary   b. Thyroid
   c. Pancreas   d. Thymus
93. Tumor marker for mesotheliomas is?
   a. Desmin   b. Keratin
   c. Vimentin   d. Alpha-feto protein
94. Tongue cancer NOT seen with?
   a. Alcohol   b. Smoking
   c. Chewing tobacco   d. Apthous ulcer
95. Most radiosensitive tumour is?
   a. Ewing's sarcoma   b. Seminoma
   c. Osteosarcoma   d. Osteoid osteoma

96. Radiation exposure during infancy has been linked to which of the following carcinoma?
   a. Breast   b. Melanoma
   c. Thyroid   d. Lung
97. UV radiation has which of the following effects on the cells?
   a. Prevents formation of pyrimidine dimers
   b. Stimulates formation of pyrimidine dimers
   c. Prevents formation of purine dimers
   d. All of the above
98. The most radiosensitive cells are:
   a. Neutrophils   b. Lymphocytes
   c. Erythrocytes   d. Megakaryocytes
99. The following parasitic infections predispose to malignancies?
   a. Paragonimus westermani
   b. Guinea worm infection
   c. Clonorchiasis
   d. Ancyclostoma

IMMUNITY AND HYPERSENSITIVITY

100. Xenograft is: (Recent Pattern Question 2018-19)
   a. Graft across species
   b. Graft from same species
   c. Graft from same individual
   d. Graft from same organ
101. Which of the following is a Type 2 Hypersensitivity reaction? (Recent Pattern Question 2018-19)
   a. Chronic Kidney Rejection episode
   b. Autoimmune Hemolytic anaemia
   c. Arthus reaction
   d. Mitsuda reaction
102. Acute graft rejection occurs within?
 (Recent Pattern Question 2018-19)
   a. Minutes   b. Days to weeks
   c. >6 weeks to 6 months   d. >6 months
103. Neonatal lupus is screened by which antibody?
 (Recent Pattern Question 2018)
   a. Anti-Ro
   b. Anti-smith
   c. Antiribonucleoprotein antibody
   d. Antiphospholipid antibody
104. Class MHC 2 antigen attaches to?
 (Recent Pattern Question 2017)
   a. CD4   b. CD8
   c. CD16   d. CD34
105. Which is not an antibody mediated hypersensitivity reaction? (Recent Pattern Question 2017)
   a. Type 1
   b. Type 2
   c. Type 3
   d. Type 4

FMGE Solutions Screening Examination

106. Which is a flow cytometric B cell marker?
    (Recent Pattern Question 2017)
    a. CD 2 b. CD 3
    c. CD 7 d. CD 19
107. Caplan syndrome is characterised by?
    (Recent Pattern Question 2017)
    a. Pneumoconiosis with HLA B27
    b. Pneumoconiosis with reactive arthritis
    c. Pneumoconiosis with progressive massive fibrosis
    d. Pneumoconiosis with rheumatoid arthritis
108. HLAB27 is maximally associated with?
    (Recent Pattern Question 2017)
    a. Rheumatoid arthritis b. Ankylosing spondylitis
    c. Rieter syndrome d. Psoriasis
109. Which is the first line of defence in viral infection?
    a. B lymphocyte *(Recent Pattern Question 2017)*
    b. Macrophages c. T lymphocytes
    d. Large granular lymphocyte
110. TH1 is involved in which type of hypersensitivity?
    (Recent Pattern Question 2017)
    a. Type 1 b. Type 2
    c. Type 3 d. Type 4
111. Which of the following is an example of Type 3 hypersensitivity *(Recent Pattern Question 2016)*
    a. Asthma b. Contact dermatitis
    c. SLE d. AIHA
112. Which is true about type II hypersensitivity reaction?
    (Recent Pattern Question 2016)
    a. Immune complex mediated
    b. Antigen – antibody mediated
    c. Arthus phenomenon
    d. Granulomatous reaction
113. Highest molecular weight immunoglobulins are
    (Recent Pattern Question 2016)
    a. IgG b. IgA
    c. IgM d. IgD
114. Primary immune response is by which cell?
    a. B cell b. T cell
    c. B and T cell both d. Complement mediated
115. Steven Johnson Syndrome is seen with what kind of hypersensitivity reaction?
    a. Type 1 b. Type 2
    c. Type 3 d. Type 4
116. Patch test is what type of hypersensitivity?
    a. Type 1 b. Type 2
    c. Type 3 d. Type 4
117. Which of these is not an antigen presenting cell?
    a. Bipolar cells b. Dendritic cell
    c. Follicular dendritic cell d. Tissue macrophages
118. Which interleukin is associated with growth of natural killer cells?
    a. IL-2 b. IL-7
    c. IL-8 d. IL-13

119. In graft rejection, which type of HLA is involved?
    a. MHC class I b. MHC class II
    c. MHC class III d. MHC class IV
120. HLA-B27 is associated with?
    a. Osteoarthritis b. Sjgren syndrome
    c. Behçet disease d. Reiter's syndrome
121. Nitro-blue tetrazolium test is done for?
    a. Chronic glomerulonephritis
    b. Chronic granulomatous disorder
    c. Acute granulomatous disease
    d. Chediak Higashi syndrome
122. C1 is controlled by?
    a. Magnesium b. Manganese
    c. Phosphate d. Calcium
123. Which among the following is not an autoimmune disease?
    a. Myasthenia gravis
    b. Systemic lupus erythematosus
    c. Grave's disease
    d. Sickle cell disease
124. Tuberculin test is which type of hypersensitivity?
    a. Type 1 b. Type 2
    c. Type 3 d. Type 4

HEMATOLOGY

125. All are reduced in Iron deficiency anaemia EXCEPT:
    (Recent Pattern Question 2018-19)
    a. T.I.B.C
    b. Percentage saturation of Transferrin
    c. Hemoglobin d. Ferritin
126. Which type of anemia is seen in patients of rheumatoid arthritis? *(Recent Pattern Question 2018)*
    a. Normocytic and hypochromic anemia
    b. Microcytic and hypochromic anemia
    c. Normocytic and normochromic anemia
    d. Macrocytic anemia
127. Which of the following is the correct sequence of early erythropoiesis in a developing fetus?
    (Recent Pattern Question 2018)
    a. Yolk sac, bone marrow and liver
    b. Yolk sac, liver and bone marrow
    c. Liver, bone marrow and yolk sac
    d. Bone marrow, yolk sac and liver
128. WHO cut off for diagnosis of anemia in nonpregnant female is < _____? *(Recent Pattern Question 2018)*
    a. 07 g% b. 10 g%
    c. 11 g% d. 12 g%
129. Which of the following tests is to be done to screen a lady with family history of thalassemia?
    (Recent Pattern Question 2018)
    a. Hb A2 Levels b. NESTROFT
    c. High performance liquid chromatography
    d. P. smear and reticulocyte count

PATHOLOGY

326

Pathology

130. Which of the following is best to confirm diagnosis of thalassemia trait in a lady with positive family history of thalassemia?
   a. Elevated HbA2
   b. Reticulocytosis
   c. NESTROFT
   d. Peripheral Smear

131. Heinz bodies are composed of?
   (Recent Pattern Question 2017)
   a. DNA
   b. RNA
   c. Iron
   d. Denatured haemoglobin

132. Positive coombs test is seen in which haemolytic anaemia?
   (Recent Pattern Question 2017)
   a. SLE
   b. PAN
   c. TTP
   d. HUS

133. Arsenic is used in treatment of?
   (Recent Pattern Question 2017)
   a. A.M.L
   b. C.M.L
   c. Myeloproliferative disease
   d. A.L.L

134. Which virus leads to Aplastic Crisis?
   (Recent Pattern Question 2017)
   a. Pox virus
   b. Parvo virus B19
   c. Hepatitis A
   d. Hepatitis B

135. Which of the following will lead to X-ray appearance of crew hair cut appearance with Gamma Gandy bodies?
   (Recent Pattern Question 2017)
   a. Sickle cell anaemia
   b. Hereditary spherocytosis
   c. Acute myeloid leukemia
   d. Osteoporosis

136. Gamma gandy bodies are seen in?
   a. Portal hypertension *(Recent Pattern Question 2017)*
   b. Plasma cell dyscaria
   c. Plasma cell leukemia
   d. Primary sclerosing cholangitis

137. Rosenthal syndrome occurs due to deficiency of?
   (Recent Pattern Question 2017)
   a. Factor 2
   b. Factor 5
   c. Factor 9
   d. Factor 11

138. Which of the following is a B-cell disease
   (Recent Pattern Question 2016)
   a. Amyloidosis
   b. Multiple myeloma
   c. ALL
   d. Mycosis fungoides

139. Lacunar Reed Sternberg cell is found in which type of Hodgkin's lymphoma? *(Recent Pattern Question 2016)*
   a. Mixed cellularity
   b. Lymphocyte rich
   c. Nodular sclerosis
   d. Lymphocyte depleted

140. JAK –2 mutation is seen in?
   a. Polycythemia vera
   b. I.T.P
   c. C.M.L
   d. C.M.M.L

141. Gamma Gandy bodies contain hemosiderin and_____?
   a. Na+
   b. Ca++
   c. Mg++
   d. K+

142. The cause of the severe hemorrhage in acute promyelocytic leukemia is?
   a. Disseminated intravascular coagulation
   b. Immune complex deposits on blood vessels
   c. Thrombocytopenia
   d. Thrombocytosis

143. Which is the most common Hodgkin's lymphoma?
   a. Nodular sclerosis
   b. Mixed cellularity
   c. Lymphocyte depleted
   d. Lymphocyte rich

144. Which is the percentage of blasts in AML
   a. 8%
   b. 15%
   c. 20%
   d. 25%

145. Presence of >10% plasma cells with no lytic lesion and M protein in serum is seen in?
   a. Smoldering myeloma
   b. Multiple myeloma
   c. Monoclonal Gammopathy of unknown significance
   d. Nonsecretory myeloma

146. Langerhans cell CD marker is?
   a. CD1
   b. CD2
   c. CD4
   d. CD56

147. RBC contains?
   a. Iron
   b. Folic acid
   c. Vitamin C
   d. Biotin

148. Leucopenia is NOT seen in?
   a. New born
   b. Starvation
   c. Enteric fever
   d. Viral or protozoal infection

149. Prevalence of Burkitt's lymphoma is highest in?
   a. Australia
   b. Africa
   c. Asia
   d. America

150. Reticulocytosis is NOT seen in:
   a. Thalassemia
   b. Hereditary spherocytosis
   c. Chronic renal failure
   d. Sickle cell anemia

151. GLUT present on surface of RBC?
   a. GLUT 1
   b. GLUT 2
   c. GLUT 3
   d. GLUT 4

152. Splenectomy is useful in which of the following:
   a. Chronic ITP
   b. Sickle cell anemia
   c. Tuberculosis
   d. Good pasture syndrome

153. Extrinsic pathway of clotting factors is measured by?
   a. Prothrombin time
   b. Activated partial thromboplastin time
   c. Bleeding time
   d. Clotting time

154. Which of following viruses cause hemolysis of red blood cells?
   a. Rubella
   b. Human parvo virus B19
   c. Measles
   d. Dengue virus

155. G6PD helps in maintaining the integrity of RBC by:
   a. Controlling oxidative stress on RBC
   b. Controlling reduction stress on RBC
   c. Maintaining flexibility of cell membrane
   d. Component of electron transport chain

156. Low TIBC is seen in:
   a. Anemia of chronic disease
   b. Iron deficiency anemia
   c. Fanconi anemia
   d. Aplastic anemia

Questions

FMGE Solutions Screening Examination

157. Comment on type of anemia in peripheral smear:

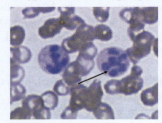

   a. Pernicious anemia
   b. Iron deficiency anemia
   c. Sickle cell anemia
   d. Hereditary spherocytosis
158. Fetal hemoglobin has features which of these?
   a. Most susceptible to denaturation by acid
   b. Resistant to denaturation by alkali
   c. By 20 weeks 90% of fetal Hb is HbF
   d. It has 2 alpha and 2 beta chains
159. Which is the life span of transfused RBC?
   a. 30 days   b. 45 days
   c. 60 days   d. 120 days
160. Schistocytes are seen in?
   a. HUS   b. HSP
   c. Abetalipoproteinemia   d. Myelofibrosis
161. All are seen in thalassemia major EXCEPT:
   a. Transfusion dependency
   b. Splenoheptatomegaly
   c. Ineffective erythropoiesis
   d. Macrocytic anemia
162. Low iron & low TIBC is seen in:
   a. Anaemia of chronic disease
   b. Sideroblastic anaemia
   c. Iron deficiency anaemia
   d. Aplastic anemia
163. Reticulocytes are stained with:
   a. Brilliant cresyl blue   b. Sudan black
   c. Warthin starry   d. Hemotoxylin-eosin stain
164. Which is the storage form of iron:
   a. Transferrin   b. Ferritin
   c. Hepcidin   d. Ferroportin
165. Which is the most common type of Hodgkin's lymphoma?
   a. Nodular sclerosis
   b. Mixed cellularity
   c. Lymphocyte predominant
   d. Lymphocyte depleted
166. Which is the most common ALL subtype?
   a. Pre B cell   b. Pre T cell
   c. T cell   d. B cell
167. All cause Reticulocytosis EXCEPT:
   a. Aplastic anemia
   b. Thalassemia
   c. Sickle cell anemia
   d. Chronic blood loss

168. Hodgkins lymphoma is caused by:
   a. EBV   b. CMV
   c. HHV6   d. HHV8
169. Which of the following leukemia almost never develops after radiation?
   a. Acute myeloblastic leukemia
   b. Chronic myeloid leukemia
   c. Acute lymphoblastic leukemia
   d. Chronic lymphocytic leukemia
170. Which is the most common defectively produced antibody in multiple myeloma?
   a. Ig G   b. Ig M
   c. Ig A   d. Ig D

CARDIOVASCULAR PATHOLOGY

171. Histopathological finding 12 hours after ischemic injury to heart is?   *(Recent Pattern Question 2018-19)*
   a. Karyorrhexis of myocytes
   b. Neocapillary invasion of myocytes
   c. Hyper-eosinophilia of myocytes
   d. Coagulation necrosis of myocytes
172. Which of the following is the correct description for type of heart lesion seen in patients of rheumatic arthritis?
                            (Recent Pattern Question 2018)
   a. Osler's nodes   b. McCallum patch
   c. Floppy valves   d. Myxomatous degeneration
173. Which is the most common cause of death in rheumatic heart disease?   *(Recent Pattern Question 2017)*
   a. Cardiac failure b. Bacterial endocarditis
   c. Mural thrombus   d. Coronary insufficiency
174. Which is the earliest histopathological change in myocardial infarction?   *(Recent Pattern Question 2017)*
   a. Stretching and waviness of fibers
   b. Neutrophilic infiltration
   c. Coagulative necrosis
   d. Fibrovascular response
175. Most common primary cardiac tumour?
                            (Recent Pattern Question 2017)
   a. Myxoma   b. Rhabdomyoma
   c. Rhabdomyosarcoma d. Angiosarcoma
176. Which is the first organ to be affected in left ventricular failure?
   a. Lungs   b. Liver
   c. Kidney   d. Brain
177. Which of the following is pathognomonic for rheumatic fever?
   a. Aschoff nodules
   b. Anitschkow cells
   c. McCallum's patch
   d. Vegetations along the cusps

Pathology

178. All are true about myocardial response and changes to myocardial infarction EXCEPT?
   a. Neutrophilic infiltrates in first 48 hours
   b. Loss of contractility within 2 minutes
   c. Reversible injury within 20–40 minutes
   d. Waviness of fibres at border of infarct

179. All are complications of atherosclerosis EXCEPT?
   a. Ulceration
   b. Thrombosis
   c. Embolism
   d. Necrosis

180. Which is incorrect about Buerger's disease?
   a. Ischemia of nerves
   b. Deep vein thrombosis
   c. Segmental inflammation
   d. Superficial thrombophlebitis

181. Why is Troponin C not used for MI diagnosis?
   a. Troponin C binds to calcium
   b. Troponin C is present in both cardiac and smooth muscle
   c. Troponin C is present in both cardiac and skeletal muscle
   d. It elevates late after onset of MI.

182. Postmortem findings of myocardial infarction are all EXCEPT:
   a. Coagulative necrosis
   b. Glycogen depletion
   c. Granulation with type 4 collagen
   d. Loss of nuclei

183. The most common primary neoplasm of the heart in adults is?
   a. Lipoma
   b. Myxoma
   c. Papillary fibroelastoma
   d. Rhabdomyoma

184. Which is the most common cardiac tumor?
   a. Myxoma
   b. Rhabdomyosarcoma
   c. angiosarcoma
   d. Metastasis

185. Which is the most common site of rhabdomyoma?
   a. Left atrium
   b. Right atrium
   c. Left ventricle
   d. Right ventricle

186. Which is the most common cardiac valve tumor?
   a. Myxoma
   b. Rhabdomyoma
   c. Papillary fibroelastoma
   d. Secondaries

187. Tree bark like calcification in chest X-ray is seen in?
   a. Syphilitic aneurysm
   b. Aorto-Arteritis
   c. Neurofibromatosis
   d. Atherosclerosis

188. Exudate in rheumatic fever is?
   a. Serous
   b. Purulent
   c. Fibrinous
   d. Myxomatous

189. Fibrinoid necrosis may be observed in all of the following, EXCEPT?
   a. Malignant hypertension
   b. Polyarteritis nodosa
   c. Diabetic glomerulosclerosis
   d. Aschoff's nodule

190. Polyarteritis Nodosa (PAN) typically involves which of the following?
   a. Large elastic arteries
   b. Small- or medium-sized muscular arteries
   c. Arterioles
   d. Capillaries

191. Medial calcification is seen in?
   a. Atherosclerosis
   b. Arteriolosclerosis
   c. Monckeberg's sclerosis
   d. Dissecting aneurysm

192. All are examples of medium vessel vasculitis EXCEPT?
   a. Classic PAN
   b. Kawasaki disease
   c. Buerger disease
   d. SLE

LUNGS

193. Curschmann spirals are characteristic of which of the following airway disease?
   a. Chronic bronchitis
   b. Emphysema
   c. Atelectasis
   d. Bronchial asthma

194. Simmond focus in tuberculosis is seen in?
   a. Brain
   b. Lungs
   c. Liver
   d. Blood vessels

195. All are true about chronic bronchitis EXCEPT?
   a. Increased Reid's index
   b. Submucosal gland hypertrophy
   c. Eosinophilic infiltration of airways
   d. Bronchorrhea

196. All are true about silicosis EXCEPT?
   a. Egg shell calcification
   b. Nodular fibrosis
   c. Bloody pleural effusion
   d. Quartz is the main form implicated in pathogenesis

197. Kveim test is used for diagnosis of?
   a. Sarcoidosis
   b. Sicca syndrome
   c. Scleroderma
   d. C.R.E.S.T. syndrome

198. Schaumann body is seen in cases of:
   a. Silicosis
   b. Asbestosis
   c. Sarcoidosis
   d. Anthracosis

199. Which is the most common clinical presentation of sarcoidosis?
   a. Pleural plaque
   b. Hilar lymphadenopathy
   c. Pulmonary fibrosis
   d. Interstitial calcification

200. Lung cancer is most commonly associated with?
   a. Silicosis
   b. Berylliosis
   c. Asbestosis
   d. Anthracosis

201. Which is the most common type of lung cancer?
   a. Small cell lung cancer
   b. Large cell lung cancer
   c. Squamous cell cancer
   d. Adenocarcinoma

FMGE Solutions Screening Examination

202. **Which is the most common lung cancer in females?**
   a. Squamous cell CA
   b. Adenocarcinoma
   c. Small cell lung CA
   d. Large cell CA

203. **Which is the most aggressive lung CA?**
   a. Squamous cell CA   b. Adenocarcinoma
   c. Small cell lung CA   d. Large cell CA

204. **Azzopardi effect is seen in:**
   a. Squamous cell CA   b. Adenocarcinoma
   c. Small cell lung CA   d. Large cell CA

205. **Which is the most common cancer associated with asbestosis?**
   a. Mesothelioma
   b. Adenocarcinoma lung
   c. Squamous cell cancer of lung
   d. Large cell cancer lung

KIDNEY

206. **Most characteristic feature of diabetic nephropathy:**
   (Recent Pattern Question 2018-19)
   a. Kimmel stein Wilson Change
   b. Armani Ebstein change
   c. Focal segmental glomerulosclerosis
   d. Membrano proliferative glomerulonephritis

207. **Fatty change is seen in?** *(Recent Pattern Question 2017)*
   a. Brain   b. Kidney
   c. Adrenal   d. Bladder

208. **The presence of sub-epithelial humps on electron microscopic examination of kidney biopsy is seen in?**
   a. PSGN   *(Recent Pattern Question 2017)*
   b. Chronic glomerulonephritis
   c. Crescentic glomerulonephritis
   d. Membranous glomerulopathy

209. **Crescent formation is seen in?**
   (Recent Pattern Question 2017)
   a. FSGS   b. MGN
   c. RPGN   d. PSGN

210. **Adult polycystic kidney disease is**
   (Recent Pattern Question 2016)
   a. Autosomal recessive   b. Autosomal dominant
   c. X-linked recessive   d. X-linked dominant

211. **Owl eye inclusions in urine are seen in?**
   (Recent Pattern Question 2016)
   a. EBV   b. HSV-1
   c. HSV-2   d. CMV

212. **Hydropic degeneration of the renal tubular epithelium occurs in?**
   a. Chronic alcoholism
   b. Carbon tetrachloride poisoning
   c. Excessive renal sodium loss
   d. Hypokalemia

213. **Podocytes are seen in?**
   a. Bowman's capsule
   b. Proximal convoluted tubule
   c. Distal convoluted tubule
   d. Collecting tubule

214. **Maximum endo-capillary proliferation is seen in:**
   a. Membranous glomerulonephritis
   b. Mesangio-proliferative glomerulonephritis
   c. Focal segmental glomerulonephritis
   d. Post streptococcal GN

215. **Wire loop lesions are seen in?**
   a. SLE   b. Diabetic nephropathy
   c. Benign nephrosclerosis d. Wegener's granulomatosis

216. **The drug which causes renal papillary necrosis is?**
   a. Acetophenetidin   b. Gentamicin
   c. Gold   d. Methicillin

217. **Which of the following statement is incorrect about ADPKD?**
   a. Autosomal dominant
   b. Chromosome 4 and 16 are involved
   c. Cysts in liver and pancreas
   d. Bilateral kidney transplantation

218. **WBC cast is seen in?**
   a. Pyelonephritis   b. Glomerulonephritis
   c. Chronic renal failure   d. Hyaline cast

219. **RBC cast is seen in?**
   a. Minimal change disease   b. Renal vein thrombosis
   c. Bladder schistomiasis
   d. Rapidly progressive glomerulonephritis

220. **Which is the most common glomerulonephritis associated with HIV?**
   a. Focal segmental glomerulosclerosis
   b. Diffuse glomerulosclerosis
   c. Membranoproliferative glomerulonephritis
   d. Crescentic glomerulonephritis

221. **Which of the following is true about complications of hemodialysis?**
   a. A beta amyloid deposition
   b. Cardiovascular complications
   c. Renal rickets   d. Metabolic acidosis

222. **Which is the most common malignant tumor of kidney:**
   a. Papillary carcinoma b. Papillary adenoma
   c. Renal cell CA   d. Wilm's tumor

223. **Which is the most common risk factor for RCC?**
   a. Urinary tract infection   b. Renal calculi
   c. Smoking   d. Hypertension

224. **Which is the RCC with best prognosis?**
   a. Clear cell CA   b. Papillary CA
   c. Medullary CA   d. Chromophobe

225. **Which is the most common type of RCC associated with dialysis?**
   a. Clear cell CA   b. Papillary CA
   c. Medullary CA   d. Chromophobe

Pathology

226. **Which is the most common type of RCC?**
   a. Papillary CA   b. Clear cell CA
   c. Medullary CA   d. Chromophobe

227. **Which of the following organ is least likely to be affected in cases of ADPKD?**
   a. Brain   b. Heart
   c. Liver   d. Lung

228. **Which is the most common organ associated with polycystic disease?**
   a. Brain   b. Heart
   c. Liver   d. Lung

229. **Which is the least common cause of death in case of polycystic disease?**
   a. Coronary heart disease   b. Infection
   c. Berry aneurysm rupture   d. Pancreatic cyst

LIVER

230. **Mallory hyaline bodies are seen in?**
   (Recent Pattern Question 2017)
   a. Acute viral hepatitis   b. Wilson disease
   c. Fulminant hepatitis   d. All of the above

231. **Conjugated hyperbilirubinemia is seen in?**
   (Recent Pattern Question 2017)
   a. Criggler Najar type 1   b. Criggler Najar type 2
   c. Gilbert syndrome   d. Dubin Johnson syndrome

232. **Pathologic changes or clinical manifestations which occur in patients with primary hemochromatosis include all of the following EXCEPT?**
   a. Congestive heart failure   b. Diabetes mellitus
   c. Testicular atrophy   d. Photosensitivity dermatitis

233. **Elevated alpha-fetoprotein is seen in all EXCEPT?**
   a. Hepatocellular cancer   b. Colonic cancer
   c. Tuberculoma   d. Pancreatic cancer

234. **Unconjugated hyperbilirubinemia is seen in:**
   a. Rotor's syndrome
   b. Crigler Najjar syndrome
   c. Dubin Johnson syndrome
   d. All of above

235. **Which of the following hereditary hyperbilirubinemia is autosomal dominant?**
   a. Dubin Johnson syndrome
   b. Rotor syndrome
   c. Crigler Najjar syndrome type I
   d. Crigler Najjar syndrome type II

236. **Which of the following hereditary hyperbilirubinemia is most fatal?**
   a. Dubin Johnson syndrome
   b. Rotor syndrome
   c. Crigler–Najjar syndrome type I
   d. Crigler–Najjar syndrome type II

237. **"Onion skin" fibrosis of bile duct is seen in:**
   a. Primary biliary cirrhosis
   b. Primary sclerosing cholangitis
   c. Extrahepatic biliary fibrosis
   d. Congenital hepatic fibrosis

238. **The complications of gallstones include all of the following EXCEPT:**
   a. Adenocarcinoma of ampulla of Vater
   b. Acute intrahepatic cholangitis
   c. Acute pancreatitis
   d. Gangrenous cholecystitis

239. **Most common tumor of liver is:**
   a. Cavernous hemangioma
   b. Hepatocellular carcinoma
   c. Adenoma
   d. Metastasis

240. **What accumulates in the space of Disse in cirrhosis?**
   a. Collagen type 1 & 4   b. Collagen type 2 & 3
   c. Collagen type 1 & 3   d. Collagen type 2 & 4

241. **Which of the following is not a function of liver?**
   a. Production of albumin
   b. Detoxification of ammonia
   c. Production of vitamin K
   d. Metabolism of drugs

242. **Which of the following is a thorium induced tumor?**
   a. Renal cell carcinoma
   b. Lymphoma
   c. Angiosarcoma of liver
   d. Astrocytoma

GASTROINTESTINAL TRACT

243. **Whipple's is disease is caused by:**
   (Recent Pattern Question 2018)
   a. Bacteroides
   b. Acinetobacter
   c. H. pylori
   d. Tropheryma whippelii

244. **Which of the following is called chronic hypertrophic gastritis?** *(Recent Pattern Question 2017)*
   a. Type A gastritis   b. Type B gastritis
   c. Menetrier's disease   d. Type AB gastritis

245. **Serpiginous ulcers with deep fissures are seen in?**
   (Recent Pattern Question 2017)
   a. Crohn's disease   b. Ulcerative colitis
   c. Neutropenic colitis   d. Amoebic dysentery

246. **Duodenal villous atrophy is seen in**
   (Recent Pattern Question 2016)
   a. Crohn's disease
   b. Ulcerative colitis
   c. Celiac disease
   d. Cystic fibrosis

FMGE Solutions Screening Examination

247. Pseudo-pancreatic cyst secretes?
    a. Lipase   b. Amylase
    c. Trypsin   d. Ptylin
248. An increased incidence of pancreatitis is associated with all of the following EXCEPT?
    a. Alcoholism   b. Cholelithiasis
    c. Chlorothiazide therapy d. Hypertension
249. Hyperplasic gastric polyps are most likely to be found in association with which one of the following conditions?
    a. Gastric carcinoma
    b. Familial polyposis syndrome
    c. Chronic gastritis
    d. Crohn's disease
250. Anti-parietal cell antibodies are found in patients with?
    a. Good-pasture syndrome b. Primary biliary cirrhosis
    c. Wegener granulomatosis d. Pernicious anemia
251. All are true about GIST EXCEPT?
    a. Most common mesenchymal tumour of GIT
    b. C-kit (CD117) positive
    c. Originate from interstitial cells of Cajal
    d. Majority seen in duodenum
252. All are true about amoebiasis EXCEPT?
    a. Flask shaped ulcers
    b. Disease affects caecum and ascending colon
    c. Anchovy pus in liver
    d. Coagulative necrosis
253. All are true about familial adenomatous polyposis EXCEPT?
    a. APC gene on chromosome 5
    b. Mutation in nucleotide excision base repair gene
    c. Colorectal cancer develops in 100% patients before the age of 30 years
    d. Prophylactic polypectomy is recommended as standard therapy
254. Which is the most likely to be associated with type A gastritis?
    a. Decreased growth of luminal bacteria
    b. Decreased chances of gastric carcinoma
    c. Decreased plasma concentration of gastrin
    d. Increased MCV of RBC
255. Which type of gastric carcinoma has the best prognosis?
    a. Linitis plastic   b. Polypoidal growth
    c. Ulcerative   d. Superficial spreading
256. All are seen in Crohn's disease EXCEPT?
    a. Poor perianal hygiene b. Stricture formation
    c. Crypt abscess
    d. Rectum is commonly involved
257. Radiation given to oesophagus will lead to?
    a. Fibrosis of oesophagus
    b. Thinning of mucosal layer
    c. Volcano ulcer in esophagus
    d. Strawberry appearance of mucosa

258. Which is the most common tumor of the spleen?
    a. Hemangioma   b. Lymphoma
    c. Angiosarcoma   d. Metastasis
259. Which is the most common site of lymphoma?
    a. Duodenum   b. Pancreas
    c. Mesenteric lymph nodes d. Stomach
260. Which of the following is not associated with Crohn's disease?
    a. Pseudo-polyps   b. Fistula
    c. Malignancy   d. Perineal sepsis
261. Which antibody is suggestive of diagnosis of ulcerative colitis?
    a. p-ANCA   b. c-ANCA
    c. a.M.A   d. a. N.A

CENTRAL NERVOUS SYSTEM

262. Which enzyme protects the brain from free radical injury?
    a. Myeloperoxidase   b. Superoxide dismutase
    c. MAO   d. Hydroxylase
263. Negri bodies are found in:
    a. Cerebellum   b. Hypothalamus
    c. Hippocampus   d. Brain stem
264. Lewy's body is seen in?
    a. Alzheimer's   b. Rabies
    c. Parkinsonism   d. Multi infarct dementia
265. Ubiquitin deposit in neurons is seen in?
    a. Huntington's chorea b. Pick's disease
    c. Cortical dementia   d. AIDS related dementia
266. Glioma Retinae is?
    a. Retinoblastoma   b. Meningioma
    c. Optic nerve glioma d. Giant cell astrocytoma

ENDOCRINE SYSTEM

267. Which of the following is correct about MEN 2 A Syndrome? *(Recent Pattern Question 2018-19)*
    a. Parathyroid adenoma
    b. Pituitary adenoma
    c. Pancreas adenoma
    d. Cavernous angioma
268. Pheochromocytoma produces all except? *(Recent Pattern Question 2018-19)*
    a. Nor-epinephrine
    b. Secretin
    c. Vasoactive intestinal polypeptide
    d. Calcitonin
269. Which of the following is not directly related to Hashimoto's thyroiditis?
    a. Hypothyroidism   b. Slow onset
    c. Neuropathy   d. Autoimmune disease

Pathology

270. **Amyloid stroma is seen with?**
   a. Papillary carcinoma Thyroid
   b. Medullary carcinoma Thyroid
   c. Follicular carcinoma Thyroid
   d. Anaplastic carcinoma Thyroid

271. **Which is the most common cause of death in a diabetic patient?**
   a. Cardiac   b. Renal
   c. Hypoglycemia   d. Infection

272. **Hyperparathyroidism is seen in all EXCEPT?**
   a. MEN I   b. MEN IIA
   c. MEN IIB   d. Parathyroid hyperplasia

273. **All are included in MEN-IIB EXCEPT?**
   a. Pheochromocytoma   b. Hyperparathyroidism
   c. Mucosal neuroma   d. Marfanoid habitus

274. **Which is incorrect about Neuroblastoma?**
   a. Most common abdominal tumor in infants
   b. X-ray abdomen shows calcification
   c. Can show spontaneous regression
   d. Urine contains 5 H.I.A.A.

275. **Which is characteristic histo-pathological feature of kidney in DM?**
   a. Nodular sclerosis   b. Fibrin cap
   c. Papillary necrosis   d. Diffuse glomerulosclerosis

276. **Psamomma bodies are seen in?**
   a. Papillary carcinoma thyroid
   b. Medullary carcinoma thyroid
   c. Follicular carcinoma thyroid
   d. Anaplastic carcinoma

277. **Orphan Annie eye nucleus is seen in?**
   a. Papillary thyroid cancer
   b. Follicular Lymphoma
   c. Hurthle cell tumor
   d. paraganglioma

278. **Which is produced by Phaeochromocytoma in M.E.N 2A Sipple syndrome?**
   a. Epinephrine   b. Nor epinephrine
   c. Dopamine   d. 5- H.I.

279. **Pseudo-myxoma peritonei occur due to?**
   a. Dysgerminoma
   b. Brenner's tumor
   c. Theca cell tumor
   d. Mucinous cystadenosarcoma

GENETICS

280. **Which of the following disease has XLR pattern of inheritance?** *(Recent Pattern Question 2018-19)*
   a. Hurler Syndrome   b. Thalassemia
   c. Hereditary Spherocytosis
   d. G6PD

281. **Consanguinity is seen with which pattern of inheritance?** *(Recent Pattern Question 2018-19)*
   a. AR   b. AD
   c. XLR   d. XLD

282. **Which of the following is regarded as outward expression of gene?** *(Recent Pattern Question 2018)*
   a. Phenotype   b. Proteomics
   c. Genotype   d. Anticipation

283. **Which of the following has a polygenic pattern of inheritance?** *(Recent Pattern Question 2018)*
   a. Diabetes mellitus
   b. Familial hypercholesterolemia
   c. G6PD
   d. Resistant rickets

284. **BRCA 1 is located on which chromosome?** *(Recent Pattern Question 2017)*
   a. Chromosome 13q21   b. Chromosome 17q21
   c. Chromosome 17q23   d. Chromosome 13q23

285. **The defect Marfan syndrome is?** *(Recent Pattern Question 2017)*
   a. Fibrillin 1   b. Fibrillin 2
   c. Fibrillin 3   d. Fibrillin 4

286. **Klinefelter syndrome genotype is?** *(Recent Pattern Question 2017)*
   a. 45XO   b. 46XXY
   c. 47XYY   d. 47XXY

287. **Which of the following is responsible for the lesion shown in the image?**

   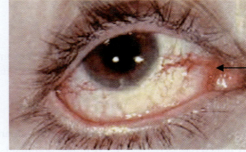

   a. 11q (14-15)   b. 11q(22-23)
   c. 13q14   d. Inv 16

288. **Which is correct about autosomal recessive condition, in case of one homozygous and one heterozygous parent?**
   a. 50% carrier and 50% affected
   b. 25% carrier and 75% affected
   c. 75% carrier and 25% affected
   d. 50% carrier and 25% affected

289. **Karyotyping is useful in diagnosis of?**
   a. Autosomal recessive disorders
   b. X-linked recessive disorders
   c. Chromosomal abnormalities
   d. Biochemical abnormalities

FMGE Solutions Screening Examination

290. Anticipation is seen in?
    a. Translocation
    b. Chromosome breaking
    c. Trinucleotide - repeat expansion
    d. Mitochondrial mutation

291. Hereditary retinoblastomas develop due to abnormality in which of the following chromosome?
    a. 13ql4
    b. 13pl4
    c. 14pl3
    d. 14ql3

292. A 22-year-old man has features of arm span greater than height, subluxed lenses, flattened and dilation of the aortic bulb. Which is the most likely diagnosis?
    a. Ehlers-Danlos syndrome
    b. Marfan syndrome
    c. Werner's syndrome
    d. Laurence-Moon-Biedl syndrome

293. Shortest chromosome is
    a. Chromosome 1
    b. Chromosome 13
    c. Chromosome 21
    d. Chromosome 22

294. Autoimmune thyroiditis is seen with?
    a. Down syndrome
    b. Marfan syndrome
    c. Louis Barr syndrome
    d. Edward syndrome

295. All are true about Lyon's hypothesis EXCEPT?
    a. Only one of X chromosomes is genetically active
    b. Only X chromosome from the mother undergoes pyknosis
    c. Inactivation occurs on 16th day of embryonic life
    d. Gene Xist causes gene silencing

296. Preferential expression of gene depending on parent of origin is called:
    a. Genomic imprinting
    b. Mosaicism
    c. Chimerism
    d. Cloning

297. All are true about F.I.S.H EXCEPT?
    a. Can detect numeric abnormalities of chromosomes
    b. Can detect complex translocation of chromosomes
    c. Can be performed on prenatal samples
    d. All of the above

298. Sickle cell anemia is:
    a. Autosomal recessive
    b. Autosomal dominant
    c. X-linked recessive
    d. X-linked dominant

299. Duchene-muscular dystrophy is:
    a. Autosomal dominant
    b. Autosomal recessive
    c. X-linked dominant
    d. X-linked recessive

300. Which of the following is autosomal recessive?
    a. Albinism
    b. Duchenne muscular dystrophy
    c. Marfan's syndrome
    d. Incontinentia pigmentia

301. Which of the following is XLR?
    a. Cystic fibrosis
    b. Haemophilia
    c. Hereditary spherocytosis
    d. Neurofibromatosis

302. Which of the following is an X-linked dominant disorder?
    a. Vitamin D resistant rickets
    b. Familial hypercholesterolemia
    c. Red green color blindness
    d. Achondroplasia

303. Which is false about Hurler syndrome?
    a. X-linked
    b. Mental retardation
    c. Joint stiffness
    d. Coarse facial features

304. Which is true about Down syndrome?
    a. Decrease in AFP
    b. Increase in AFP
    c. Increase in hCG
    d. Increased progesterone

305. Alpha feto-protein is decreased in?
    a. Down syndrome
    b. Marfan's syndrome
    c. Omphalocele
    d. Turner syndrome

306. BRCA 1 gene is located on which chromosome?
    a. Chromosome 13
    b. Chromosome 17
    c. Chromosome 19
    d. Chromosome 21

307. All are familial breast cancer gene is all EXCEPT?
    a. BRCA1
    b. P53
    c. P16
    d. PTEN

308. Klinefelter syndrome is?
    a. 47 XXXY
    b. 47XXY
    c. 47 XX
    d. 47 XY

309. Cat eye syndrome is seen with?
    a. Retinoblastoma
    b. Chromosome 22 defect
    c. Zonular cataract
    d. Cridu-chat syndrome

RESPIRATORY SYSTEM

310. Which organ is involved in Good-pasture syndrome?
    (Recent Pattern Question 2018-19)
    a. Liver
    b. Adrenals
    c. Kidney
    d. Brain

311. Not a feature of bronchial asthma:
    (Recent Pattern Question 2018-19)
    a. Thickening of bronchial wall
    b. Increase in number of goblet glands
    c. Hypertrophy of smooth muscle
    d. Increased Ig E

312. Which of the following condition is characterized by presence of hyaline deposits in alveolar walls?
    (Recent Pattern Question 2018)
    a. Interstitial lung disease
    b. Asthma
    c. Hyaline membrane disease
    d. Chronic bronchitis

313. Asthma is associated with?
    a. IL-1
    b. IL-2
    c. IL-4
    d. IL-6

Pathology

MISCELLANEOUS

314. The most abundant glycoprotein present in basement membrane is?
  a. Laminin   b. Fibronectin
  c. Collagen type 4   d. Heparan sulphate

315. All of the following are characteristically found in cases of Ochronosis EXCEPT?
  a. Alkaptonuria
  b. Arthritis
  c. Deposition of melanin-like pigment
  d. Photosensitivity

316. PAS stains all of the following EXCEPT?
  a. Glycogen   b. Lipids
  c. Fungal cell wall
  d. Basement membrane of bacteria

317. The stain used to detect amyloid is?
  a. Gram's stain   b. Congo red
  c. Oil red O   d. Reticulin stain

318. Acridine orange is a fluorescent dye used to bind:
  a. DNA and RNA   b. Protein
  c. Lipid   d. Carbohydrates

319. Which is a source of vitamin B_{12}?
  a. Animal source   b. Plant source
  c. Milk   d. Fruits

320. Which is the percentage of formalin used for histopathological preservative?
  a. 5%   b. 10%
  c. 20%   d. 40%

321. Manganese deficiency leads to?
  a. Parkinsonism
  b. Impaired skeletal growth
  c. Impaired glucose tolerance
  d. Anaemia

322. Which stain is used for fat?
  a. Oil red-O   b. Congo red
  c. Perl stain   d. PAS

323. Fluorescein stain color is –
  a. Blue   b. Pink
  c. Green   d. Red

324. Which stain is not used for lipids?
  a. Oil red O   b. Congo red
  c. Sudan III   d. Sudan black

325. Group 120 antigen on HIV surface will lead to?
  a. Fusion   b. Attachment
  c. Resistance   d. Virus entry

326. Treatment for Asymptomatic HIV is done when CD4 count is below:
  a. 200   b. 350
  c. 400   d. 500

BOARD REVIEW QUESTIONS

327. Most commonly involved organ in graft versus host disease are all EXCEPT?
  a. Gut   b. Liver
  c. Skin   d. Kidney

328. Herring bodies are seen in?
  a. Pars tuberalis   b. Pars intermedia
  c. Pars nervosa   d. All of the above

329. Sterile vegetation are seen in all EXCEPT?
  a. SLE   b. Infective endocarditis
  c. Rheumatic fever   d. Marantic endocarditis

330. Kimmelstiel wilson lesion is characteristic of?
  a. Diabetic nephropathy   b. Hypertensive nephropathy
  c. HIV nephropathy   d. Analgesic nephropathy

331. HER-2/NEU receptor gene mutation is seen in which cancer?
  a. Squamous cell carcimona
  b. Breast cancer
  c. Glioblastoma
  d. All of the above

332. Reilly bodies are seen in?
  a. Gangliosidosis   b. Behçet's disease
  c. Gaucher's disease   d. Hurler disease

333. Cigar bodies are seen in?
  a. Sporotrichosis   b. Chromoblastomycosis
  c. Mycetoma   d. Basidiomycosis

334. Histopathology of mitral valve prolapse shows what kind of change?
  a. Myxomatous   b. Fibrinoid
  c. Granulomatous   d. Fibrous

335. Thalassemia shows which kind of inheritance?
  a. Autosomal recessive   b. Autosomal dominant
  c. X-linked recessive   d. X-linked dominant

336. Range of micro albuminuria is?
  a. 10-99 mg/day   b. 20-199 mg/day
  c. 30-299 mg/day   d. 40-399 mg/day

337. Which of the following is an anti-apoptotic gene?
  a. C-myc   b. p53
  c. bcl-2   d. bax

338. Enzyme that protects the brain from free radical injury is:
  a. Myeloperoxidase   b. Superoxide dismutase
  c. MAO   d. Hydroxylase

339. Which of the following helps in generating oxygen burst in the neutrophils?
  a. NADPH oxidase   b. Superoxide dismutase
  c. Catalase   d. Glutathione peroxidase

FMGE Solutions Screening Examination

340. Heterotopic calcification occurs in
    a. Ankylosing spondylitis
    b. Reiter's syndrome
    c. Rheumatoid arthritis
    d. Gouty arthritis
341. Neutrophil secretes:
    a. Superoxide dismutase   b. Lysosomal enzyme
    c. Catalase   d. Cathepsin G
342. Liquefactive necrosis is typically seen in
    a. Ischemic necrosis of the heart
    b. Ischemic necrosis of the brain
    c. Ischemic necrosis of the intestine
    d. Tuberculosis
343. Psammoma bodies show which type of calcification?
    a. Metastatic   b. Dystrophic
    c. Secondary   d. Any of the above
344. "Russel's body" are accumulation of
    a. Cholesterol   b. Immunoglobulins
    c. Lipoproteins   d. Phospholipids
345. Dystrophic calcification is seen in
    a. Atherosclerosis   b. Paget's disease
    c. Renal osteodystrophy d. Milk-alkali syndrome
346. Nitroblue tetrazolium test is used for?
    a. Phagocytes   b. Complement
    c. T cell   d. B cell
347. Interleukin secreted by macrophages, stimulating lymphocytes is:
    a. INF alpha   b. TNF alpha
    c. IL-1   d. IL-6
348. Absolute lymphocytosis is seen in
    a. SLE   b. T.B.
    c. CLL   d. Brucellosis
349. Which complement fragments are called 'anaphylatoxins'?
    a. C3a and C3b   b. C3b and C5b
    c. C5a and C3b   d. C3a and C5a
350. First sign of wound injury is:
    a. Epithelization   b. Dilatation of capillaries
    c. Leukocytic infiltration   d. Localized edema
351. Birbeck's granules in the cytoplasm are seen in
    a. Langerhans cells   b. Mast cells
    c. Myelocytes   d. Thrombocytes
352. Virchow's triad includes all EXCEPT?
    a. Injury to vein   b. Venous thrombosis
    c. Venous stasis
    d. Hypercoagulability of blood
353. Heart failure cells are found in:
    a. Myocardium   b. Lung
    c. Liver   d. Spleen
354. White infarcts are seen in the following EXCEPT
    a. Liver   b. Kidney
    c. Spleen   d. Heart
355. Lines of Zahn are found in
    a. Thrombus
    b. Infarct tissue
    c. Postmortem clot
    d. All
356. The approximate number of genes contained in the human genome is:
    a. 40,000   b. 30,000
    c. 80,000   d. 1,00,000
357. Catastrophic variant of Ehler Danlos syndrome is
    a. I   b. II
    c. III   d. IV
358. Barr Body is not seen in:
    a. Klinefelter syndrome b. Turner syndrome
    c. Normal female   d. XXX syndrome
359. Arthus reaction is what type of hypersensitivity reaction?
    a. Localized immune complex
    b. Ag – Ab reaction
    c. Compliment mediated
    d. Ab mediated
360. What is the best method for confirming amyloidosis?
    a. Colonoscopy   b. Abdominal fat pod biopsy
    c. Rectal biopsy   d. Tongue biopsy
361. Which one of the following stains is specific for Amyloid?
    a. Periodic Acid Schiff (PAS)
    b. Alizarin red
    c. Congo red
    d. Von – Kossa
362. Antigen presenting cells are
    a. Langerhan's cell   b. Macrophage
    c. Cytotoxic T cells   d. Helper T cells
    e. B lymphocyte
363. Perforins are produced by
    a. Cytotoxic T cells   b. Suppressor T cells
    c. Memory helper T cells d. Plasma cells
    e. NK cells
364. A man develops rashes after consuming sea food. It is due to
    a. IgE mediated response b. Complement activation
    c. Cell mediated response d. None of the above
365. LE cell phenomenon is seen in
    a. Lymphocyte   b. Neutrophil
    c. Monocyte   d. Eosinophil
366. Onion peel appearance of splenic capsule is seen in
    a. SLE   b. Scleroderma
    c. RA   d. Sjogren syndrome
367. Lardaceous spleen is due to deposition of amyloid in
    a. Sinusoids of red pulp
    b. White pulp
    c. Pencillary artery
    d. Splenic trabeculae

Pathology

368. Which of the following type of hypersensitivity reaction occurs in Farmer's lung?
  a. Type I
  b. Type II
  c. Type III
  d. Type IV

369. CD3 is a marker for
  a. Monocyte
  b. T cell
  c. B cell
  d. None

370. Autoimmune hemolytic anemia is seen in
  a. ALL
  b. AML
  c. CLL
  d. CML

371. Earliest feature of correction of iron deficiency anemia is
  a. Reticulocytosis
  b. Increase in serum ferritin
  c. Increase in RBC count
  d. Increase in serum iron level immediately

372. Hypersegmented neutrophils are seen in
  a. Thalassemia
  b. Iron deficiency
  c. Megaloblastic anemia
  d. All

373. Howell Jolly bodies are seen in
  a. Alcoholics
  b. Cirrhosis
  c. Nephrotic syndrome
  d. Post splenectomy

374. Storage form of Iron in body is
  a. Ferritin
  b. Transferrin
  c. Ceruloplasmin
  d. None

375. Microcytic hypochromic anemia is seen in
  a. Hereditary spherocytosis
  b. Thalassemia major
  c. Iron deficiency anemia
  d. Pernicious anemia

376. "Pappenheimer" bodies are composed of:
  a. Copper
  b. Iron
  c. Lead
  d. Zinc

377. The most common site of Ectopic Phaeochromocytoma is:
  a. Organ of zuckerkandl
  b. Bladder filum terminate
  c. Filum terminate
  d. Celiac plexus

378. "HMB 45" is a marker for:
  a. Sarcoma
  b. Melanoma
  c. Carcinoma
  d. None of the above

379. In Nephrotic syndrome all of the following proteins are reduced EXCEPT?
  a. Transferrin
  b. Abumin
  c. Fibrinogen
  d. Cerulloplasmin

380. Arthritis "mutilans" is a feature of
  a. Dermatomyositis
  b. Psoriasis
  c. SLE
  d. Tinea versicolor

381. Marker for Hairy cell Leukemia is
  a. CD 30
  b. CD 103
  c. CD1
  d. CD4

382. "Berger Nephropathy" is due to mesangial deposition of:
  a. Fibrin and C3
  b. IgD and C3
  c. IgE and C3
  d. 1gA and C3

383. Which of the following is not Premalignant:
  a. FAP
  b. PZ syndrome
  c. Juvenile polyp
  d. Juvenile polyp syndrome

384. "Michaelis Gutmann" Bodies are seen in:
  a. Malakoplakia
  b. Nail Patella syndrome
  c. Leukoplakia
  d. Pyelonephritis

385. Which is an example of apoptosis?
  a. Council man bodies
  b. Gamma Gandy body
  c. Russel body
  d. None of the above

386. "Nut meg" liver is seen in:
  a. CVC liver
  b. Liver infarction
  c. Amyloidosis
  d. Budd chiari syndrome

387. The Common "Primary" Tumor of Heart is
  a. Rhabdomyoma
  b. Fibroma
  c. Myxoma
  d. Lipoma

388. The commonest site of diverticulosis is:
  a. Ascending colon
  b. Transverse colon
  c. Descending colon
  d. Sigmoid colon

389. "Gamma Gandy" bodies contains hemosiderin and:
  a. Na+
  b. Ca++
  c. Mg++
  d. K+

390. Chromosomes 15, 17 translocation is seen in which leukemia?
  a. APML
  b. CML
  c. CLL
  d. None of the above

391. Most common cause of Aortic Aneurysm is:
  a. Atherosclerosis
  b. Syphilis
  c. Trauma
  d. Congenital

392. APUD cells are seen in:
  a. Bronchial adenoma
  b. Bronchial carcinoid
  c. Hepatic adenoma
  d. Villous adenoma

393. Spontaneous regression though rare is seen in:
  a. Burkitt's lymphoma
  b. Wilm's tumor
  c. Neuroblastoma
  d. Melanoma

394. Immunoglobulin present in local secretions is?
  a. IgG
  b. IgA
  c. IgM
  d. IgD

395. Guardian angel against obesity is the name given to?
  a. Adiponectin
  b. Fibronectin
  c. HDL
  d. Insulin

396. LAP score is maximum in?
  a. CML
  b. AML
  c. Essential thrombocytosis
  d. Polycythemia vera

397. Hyperplasia of smooth muscle of airway is seen in?
  a. Emphysema
  b. Asthma
  c. Alveolar proteinosis
  d. Bronchiectasis

Questions

FMGE Solutions Screening Examination

398. CD marker of Angiosarcoma is?
    a. CD 10   b. CD 19
    c. CD 25   d. CD 31
399. CD marker of Langerhans histiocytosis is?
    a. CD 17   b. CD 23
    c. CD 1a   d. CD 117
400. Gene responsible for mutation of HBV is?
    a. X gene   b. S gene
    c. P gene   d. C gene
401. Michaelis gutmann bodies are found in?
    a. Malakoplakia
    b. Xanthogranulomatous pyelonephritis
    c. Nail patella syndrome
    d. Xanthelesma
402. Dohle bodies are seen in?
    a. Lysosomes   b. Endoplasmic reticulum
    c. Mitochondria   d. Toxic neutrophil granules
403. Which is the most common site of Mc Callum's patch?
    a. Right atrium   b. Left atrium
    c. Left ventricle d. Right ventricle
404. Which is the predominant cell after 72 hours of myocardial infarction?
    a. Neutrophile   b. Lymphocyte
    c. Macrophages   d. Mast cells
405. Histopathology of a lung cancer shows 'clara cells' probable diagnosis is:
    a. Squamous cell cancer   b. Bronchio alveolar cancer
    c. Large cell cancer   d. Papillary carcinoma
406. Bronchogenic carcinoma commonly metastasises to which endocrine organ?
    a. Ovaries   b. Testes
    c. Thyroid   d. Adrenals
407. Small cell cancer commonly metastasizes to
    a. Brain   b. Liver
    c. Bone   d. Kidney
408. Linitis plastica is seen in all except:
    a. Syphilis   b. Ca stomach
    c. Sarcoidosis   d. Leiomyosarcoma
409. Nesidioblastoma is due to hyperplasia of
    a. Alpha cell   b. Beta cell
    c. Acinus   d. D cells
410. Garre's osteomyelitis commonly involves:
    a. Jaw   b. Femur
    c. Ribs   d. Small bones of hand
411. Gomori's aldehyde fuchsin specifically stains
    a. Insulin   b. Glucagon
    c. Lipase   d. Amylase
412. The thinnest portion of myocardial wall is the
    a. Left ventricle b. Left atrium
    c. Right atrium   d. B and C

413. Prion includes
    a. DNA and RNA   b. Only RNA
    c. Proteins   d. Only DNA
414. Reticular pattern is seen in:
    a. Sarcoma
    b. Lymphoma
    c. Carcinoma
    d. None
415. Microdeletion is seen in?
    a. Beta Thalassemia
    b. Di George syndrome
    c. Marfan's syndrome
    d. All
416. In malignant hypertension necrosis is of which type?
    a. Caseous Necrosis
    b. Fibrinoid necrosis
    c. Liquifactive necrosis
    d. Coagulative necrosis
417. Marfan's syndrome is due to defect of?
    a. Elastin   b. Collagen
    c. Fibrillin   d. Laminin
418. Kaposi sarcoma is related to which virus?
    a. HPV 16   b. HHV-8
    c. EBV   d. CMV
419. CA 125 is used for?
    a. Follow up of ovarian cancer
    b. Diagnosis of pancreatic cancer
    c. Diagnosis of stomach cancer
    d. Diagnosis of ovarian cancer
420. Stem cells are taken from?
    a. Skin
    b. Bone marrow
    c. Oral mucosa
    d. Elementary tract
421. Ehler Danlos syndrome is due to defect in?
    a. Elastin   b. Collagen
    c. Keratin   d. Laminin
422. Interleukin responsible for pyrexia is?
    a. IL1   b. IL6
    c. INF gamma   d. IFN alpha
423. CD marker for Langerhan's Histiocytosis is?
    a. CD 17   b. CD 23
    c. CD la   d. CD 117
424. Teratozoospermia refers to?
    a. Absence of semen
    b. Absence of sperm
    c. All dead sperms in ejaculate
    d. Morphologically defective sperms
425. Rise in hemoglobin levels after one unit of whole blood transfusion is?
    a. 0.55   b. 1%
    c. 1.5%   d. 2%

426. In massive transfusion of blood, citrate toxicity is primarily due to?
    a. Hemolysis
    b. Coagulopathy
    c. DIC
    d. Direct binding to calcium
427. "Orphan Annie eye nuclei" is seen in?
    a. Papillary carcinoma of thryroid
    b. Medullary carcinoma of thyroid
    c. Anaplastic carcinoma of thryroid
    d. Follicular carcinoma of thyroid
428. Duchenne muscular dystrophy is?
    a. Autosomal recessive
    b. Autosomal dominant
    c. X linked recessive
    d. X linked dominant
429. Tuberous sclerosis is inherited as?
    a. Autosomal dominant
    b. Autosomal recessive
    c. X linked dominant
    d. X linked recessive
430. In adults, most common autoimmune disease of liver is?
    a. Autoimmune hepatitis
    b. Sclerosing cholangitis
    c. a1 antitrypsin deficiency
    d. Primary biliary cirrhosis
431. Which of the following causes malignant mesothelioma?
    a. Smoking
    b. Asbestosis
    c. Silicosis
    d. Pneumoconiosis
432. Tumor marker CA 15-3 is associated with?
    a. Ovary
    b. Breast
    c. Prostate
    d. Kidney
433. MIC-2 is a marker of?
    a. Ewing sarcoma
    b. Chronic lymphocytic leukemia
    c. Mantle Cell Lymphoma
    d. All of these
434. Ferruginous bodies are seen in?
    a. Sarcoidosis
    b. Silicosis
    c. Asbestosis
    d. Coal worker's pneumoconiosis
435. Pathology in wet lung is?
    a. Diffuse alveolar damage
    b. Surfactant deficiency
    c. Collection of pus
    d. Hemorrhage in lungs

IMAGE-BASED QUESTIONS

436. The image shows presence of?

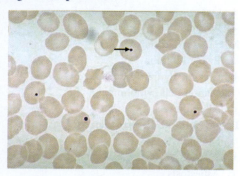

a. Howell Jolly bodies b. Heinz bodies
c. Cabot rings d. Pappenheimer's Bodies

437. Identify the cell marked

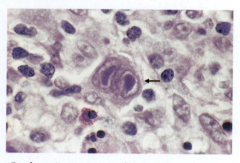

a. Orphan Annie eye nucleus
b. Reed Sternberg cell
c. Owl eye inclusions
d. Russel bodies

438. What is the diagnosis?

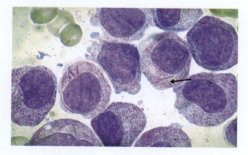

a. Lymphoblast b. Myeloblast
c. Megakaryoblast d. Normoblast

439. Identify the cell

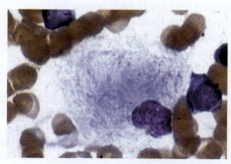

a. Gaucher cell b. Reed Sternberg cell
c. Anitschkow Cell d. Pop-corn cell

440. Spot the diagnosis

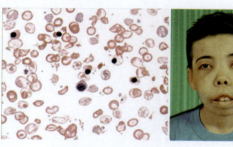

a. Iron deficiency anaemia
b. Thalassemia
c. Acute leukemia
d. Hodgkin Lymphoma

441. The following image shows

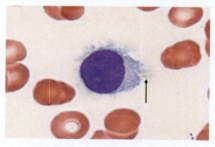

a. Hairy cell Leukaemia
b. Target cell
c. Acanthocyte
d. Pseudo-Pelger Huet anomaly

Pathology

442. The following image shows presence of:

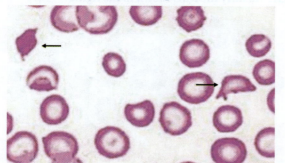

a. Target cell
b. Schistocyte
c. Sickle cell
d. Spherocyte

443. What is correct about the histopathological slide?

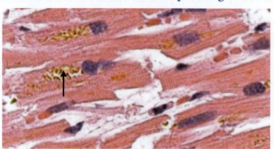

a. Lipofuscin in cardiac tissue
b. Melanin in cardiac tissue
c. Hemosiderin in kidney tubules
d. Hemopexin in hepatocytes

444. Which is true about the image shown?

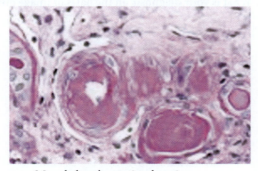

a. Monckeberg's arteriosclerosis
b. Hyaline arteriosclerosis
c. Hyperplastic arteriosclerosis
d. Fibrinoid necrosis

445. Which is true about the image shown?

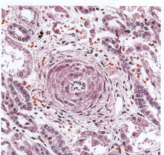

a. Hyaline arteriosclerosis
b. Hyperplastic arteriosclerosis
c. Monckeberg's arteriosclerosis
d. Fibrinoid necrosis

446. The histopathological slide shows

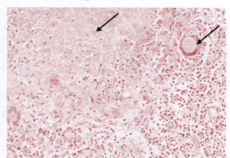

a. Coagulative necrosis
b. Liquefactive necrosis
c. Caseous necrosis
d. Fat necrosis

447. Postmortem lung specimen of a patient who developed severe respiratory distress and petechiae after fracture of shaft of femur is given below. All are true about the condition given below EXCEPT?

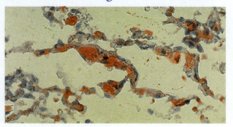

a. Oil Red O stain for fat
b. Noncardiogenic pulmonary edema
c. Gurd criteria
d. Diffuse white matter petechial hemorrhage

FMGE Solutions Screening Examination

448. Kidney biopsy depicted in the image shows

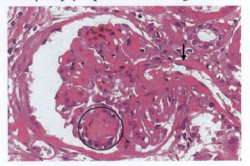

a. Focal segmental glomerulosclerosis
b. Nodular glomerulosclerosis
c. Armanni-ebstein changes
d. Membranoproliferative glomerulonephritis

449. The following liver specimen shows?

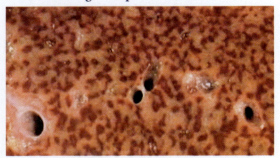

a. Postnecrotic cirrhosis
b. Dubin-Johnson syndrome
c. Miliary tuberculosis (TB)
d. Nutmeg liver

450. All are true about the marking X in histopathological specimen from a patient of fatty liver EXCEPT?

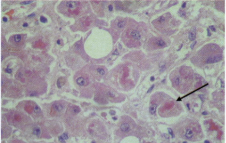

a. Eosinophilic aggregates of prekeratin
b. Intranuclear inclusions
c. Best visualised with Masson trichrome
d. Also seen in Indian childhood cirrhosis

451. Identify the RBC shown in the figure

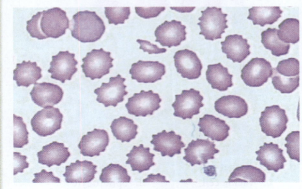

a. Acanthocyte b. Echinocyte
c. Schistocyte d. Spherocyte

452. A 6-year-old boy presents with acute abdomen and non-healing ulcer on medial malleolus. Peripheral smear is shown. The most likely cause of this condition is?

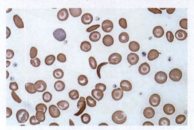

a. Trinucleotide repeat
b. Antibody to RBC membrane
c. Substitution of single amino acid base
d. Genomic imprinting

453. What is your diagnosis on the basis of image given?

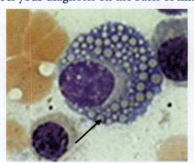

a. Langerhans cell histiocytosis
b. Plasmacytoma
c. Viral encephalitis
d. Leukemia

Pathology

454. A 45-year-old person presents with complaint of paraesthesia in hand and feet with progressive spastic weakness. On examination absent ankle jerk with Babinski sign is noted. Peripheral smear is given below. The diagnosis is

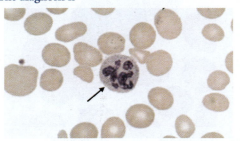

a. Lead poisoning b. Macrocytic anemia
c. Miller fisher syndrome d. Devic's disease

455. Spot the diagnosis

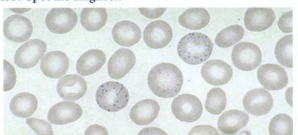

a. Lead poisoning
b. Macrocytic anemia
c. Howell-Jolly bodies
d. Heinz bodies

456. A 6-year-old child presents with lethargy and abdominal pain. Hemoglobin is 8 g% with increased serum iron and increased serum ferritin. Peripheral smear is shown. Which is correct about the image?

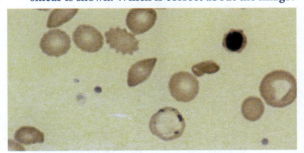

a. Pappenhiemer body b. Heinz body
c. Lead poisoning d. Howell-Jolly body

457. Which stain is preferred to diagnose these RBC inclusions seen in patients with elevated serum ferritin and serum iron?

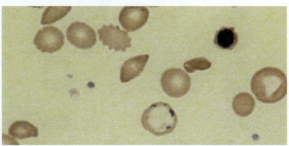

a. Perl stain b. Rubeanic acid
c. Supravital stain d. Congo red

458. The following RBC inclusion is composed of?

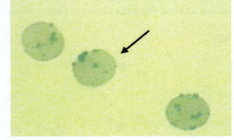

a. DNA b. RNA
c. Iron d. Denatured hemoglobin

459. The following RBC inclusions are seen in?

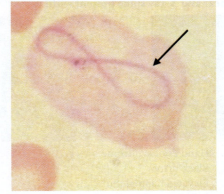

a. HbH disease b. Hemoglobin Barts
c. Pernicious anemia d. Malaria

460. The following image shows presence of?

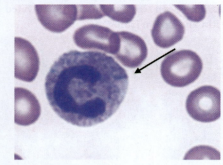

   a. Dohle bodies
   b. Toxic granules
   c. Critical green inclusions
   d. Normal inclusions

463. Identify the cell

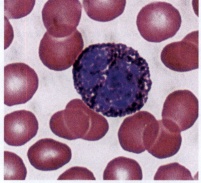

   a. Eosinophil   b. Basophil
   c. Monocyte   d. Lymphocyte

461. A 70-year-old man presents with painless cervical lymphadenopathy with progressive pallor and petechiae on ankles. Peripheral smear shows presence of?

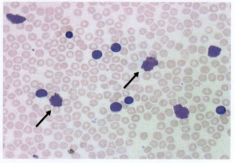

   a. Acute ITP   b. Chronic ITP
   c. CLL   d. Richter syndrome

464. Identify the cell

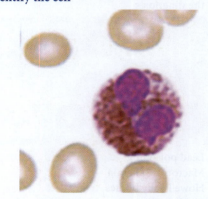

   a. Eosinophil   b. Basophil
   c. Neutrophil   d. Monocyte

462. Which will the patient with following peripheral smear and X-ray spine present with?

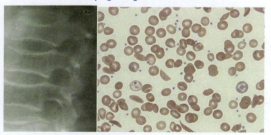

   a. Hand Foot syndrome
   b. Black urine
   c. Elevated haptoglobin
   d. Splenomegaly with gall stones

465. Name the test given

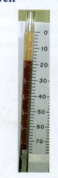

   a. Osmotic fragility   b. NESTROFT
   c. Sickling test   d. ESR measurement

466. Name the anticoagulant used in the following method?

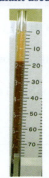

a. EDTA b. Heparin
c. Trisodium citrate d. Dalteparin

468. The image shows electrophoresis report of multiple myeloma. The spike is present in?

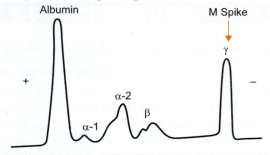

a. Alpha 1 globulin b. Alpha 2 globulin
c. Beta globulin d. Gamma globulin

467. This test is used as a screening tool for?

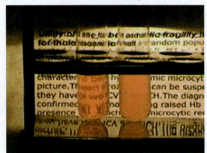

Negative   Postive

a. Hereditary spherocytosis
b. G6PD
c. Thalassemia
d. Megaloblastic anemia

469. The following image shows:

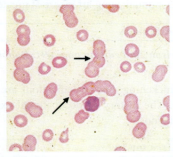

a. Microcytic hypochromic cells
b. Evidence of hemolysis
c. Sickling crisis
d. Rouleaux formation

470. Comment on the histopathological specimen

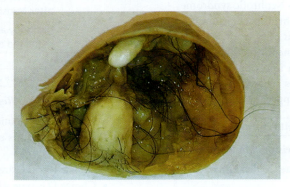

a. Teratoma b. Rhabdomyoma
c. Rhabdomyosarcoma d. Neuroblastoma

Answers to Image-Based Questions are given at the end of explained questions

FMGE Solutions Screening Examination

ANSWERS WITH EXPLANATIONS

MOST RECENT QUESTIONS 2019

1. Ans. (b) Muscle intimal elastic lamina layer defect

Ref: Harrison 20th, P 2084

As an aneurysm develops, it typically forms a neck with a dome. The length of the neck and the size of the dome vary greatly and are important factors in planning neurosurgical obliteration or endovascular embolization. The arterial internal elastic lamina disappears at the base of the neck. The media thins, and connective tissue replaces smooth-muscle cells. At the site of rupture (most often the dome), the wall thins, and the tear that allows bleeding is often ≤0.5 mm long. Aneurysm size and site are important in predicting risk of rupture. Those >7 mm in diameter and those at the top of the basilar artery and at the origin of the posterior communicating artery are at greater risk

2. Ans. (a) Asbestosis

Ref: Harrison 20th edition page 691: Robbins 9th edition, Page 1978

Pleural thickening and calcification are a feature of asbestosis. The history of occupational exposure further helps in diagnosis

3. Ans. (a) Trisomy 16

Ref: Nelson 20th edition, Page 615

The most common autosomal aneuploidy leading to spontaneous abortion is trisomy 16.

4. Ans. (c) Post infectious Glomerulonephritis) Trisomy 16

Ref: Harrison 20th edition, P 2137

- Choices A, B and D present as Nephrotic syndrome
- Post infectious Glomerulonephritis occurs after skin and throat infection with particular M types of streptococci.
- Post streptococcal glomerulonephritis due to impetigo develops 2-6 weeks after skin infection and 1–3 weeks after streptococcal pharyngitis. The renal biopsy shows subepithelial deposits which appear as humps.

5. Ans. (c) Acute viral hepatitis with infectivity

Ref: Harrison 20th edition, P 2350

- The presence of HBeAg indicates replication of virus and high infectivity of the patient.

- Choice A requires HBsAg positivity with IgM anti HbcAg positivity
- Choice B requires HBsAg positivity with IgG anti HbcAg positivity
- Choice D will have only IgG anti- HBcAg indicating past infection.

6. Ans. (b) HCV

Ref: CMDT 2019, P 698

- Most common cause of chronic viral hepatitis is Hepatitis C
- Leading cause of transfusion of associated hepatitis is Hepatitis B.
- Leading cause of fulminant viral hepatitis is hepatitis D (superinfection).
- Leading cause of Fulminant viral hepatitis in pregnancy is hepatitis E.

7. Ans. (c) <6 months

Ref: Bailey and Love: 26th edition, P 1410

Rejection Stage	Pathogenesis	Time Course
Hyperacute	Antibody mediated due to pre-existing antibodies, resulting in complement activation and thrombosis	Minutes to hours
Acute	Acute cellular rejection due to activated lymphocytes Humoral rejection due to antidonor antibodies produced after transplant	First 6 months
Chronic	Antibody and cell-mediated rejection	Months to years

8. Ans. (a) Pernicious anaemia

Ref: Robbins Pathology E-Book, P 139

- Pernicious anaemia is associated with anti-parietal cell antibodies and is an example of type 2 hypersensitivity reaction.
- Choice B and C are type 3 hypersensitivity reactions.
- Choice D is type 4 hypersensitivity phenomenon.

Extra Mile

Disease	Target Antigen	Mechanisms of Disease	Clinicopathologic Manifestations
Autoimmune hemolytic anemia	Red blood cell membrane proteins	Opsonization and phagocytosis of red blood cells	Hemolysis. anemia
Autoimmune thrombocytopenic purpura	Platelet membrane proteins (GpIIb:IIIa integrin)	Opsonization and phagocytosis of platelets	Bleeding
Pemphigus vulgaris	Proteins in intercellular junctions of epidermal cells (desmogleins)	Antibody-mediated activation of proteases, disruption of intercellular adhesions	Skin vesicles (bullae)
Vasculitis caused by ANCA	Neutrophil granule proteins. presumably released from activated neutrophils	Neutrophil degranulation and inflammation	Vasculitis
Goodpasture syndrome	Protein in basement membranes of kidney glomeruli and lung alveoli	Complement- and Fc receptor—mediated inflammation	Nephritis. lung hemorrhage
Acute rheumatic fever	Streptococcal cell wall antigen: antibody cross-reacts with myocardial antigen	Inflammation. macrophage activation	Myocarditis. arthritis
Myasthenia gravis	Acetylcholine receptor	Antibody inhibits acetylcholine binding. down-modulates receptors	Muscle weakness, paralysis
Graves disease (hyperthyroidism)	TSH receptor	Antibody-mediated stimulation of TSH receptors	Hyperthyroidism
Pernicious anemia	Intrinsic factor of gastric parietal cells	Neutralization of intrinsic factor, decreased absorption of vitamin B12	Abnormal erythropoiesis. anemia

9. Ans. (a) Thermophilic Actinomycetes

Ref: Harrison 20th edition, P 1970

Farmer's lung is a hypersensitivity pneumonitis which is caused by thermophilic actinomycetes. The same organism grows on sugarcane dust and is the antigen leading to Bagassosis.

Disease	Antigen	Source
Farming/Food Processing		
Farmer's lung	Thermophilic Actinomycetes (e.g., Saccharopolyspora rectivirgula); fungus	Grain, moldy hay, silage Sugarcane
Bagassosis	Thermophilic actinomycetes	

10. Ans. (a) Malaria

Ref: Manson Tropical diseases: 23rd edition, P 1237

The peripheral smear shows banana-shaped gametocyte of falciparum malaria.

11. Ans. (a) Bacteria

Ref: CMDT 2019, P 647

Whipple's disease is caused by Tropheryma whipelli which is an intra-cellular rod shaped gram positive bacteria found in macrophages of the gut. The lamina propria of gut harbours macrophages inside which these bacteria are demonstrated using PAS stain. The small intestinal malabsorbtion occurs in these patients leading to osmotic diarrhea. The investigation of choice is Small intestinal mucosal biopsy/ Duodenal biopsy.

FMGE Solutions Screening Examination

12. Ans. (a) Lung cancer

Ref: Bailey and Love 26th edition, P 614

The leading cause of brain metastasis is lungs > Breast>Melanoma

TABLE Tissue of origin for brain metastases (approximate).

Origin	Percentage
Lung	40
Breast	15
Melanoma	10
Renal/GU	10
Other Unknown	25

13. Ans. (a) Hypophosphatemia

Ref: Harrison 20th edition, P 519

- Hyperphosphatemia can be caused by the release of intracel¬lular phosphate pools by lysis of tumour cells.
- It produces a reciprocal depression in serum calcium, which causes severe neuromuscular irritability and tetany.
- Deposition of calcium phosphate in the kidney and hyperphos¬phatemia may cause renal failure. Potassium is the principal intracellular cation, and massive destruction of malignant cells may lead to hyperka¬lemia.
- The break-down of DNA from nucleus will produce urate crystals that will block kidney tubules and lead to urate nephropathy.

14. Ans. (c) Multiple myeloma

Ref: CMDT 2019, P 546

Vitamin D3 intoxication	Ruled out as serum vitamin D3 levels are elevated
Hyperparathyroidism	Ruled out as PTH are elevated
Multiple Myeloma	Myeloma cells produce IL-6 leading to enhanced osteoclastic activity. SAP hence remains normal while the enhanced osteoclastic activity leads to increased serum calcium values.
Nutritional rickets	Leads to low calcium and less vitamin D3 levels

15. Ans. (b) Phytates

Ref: Harrison 20th edition, P 684

Iron deficiency is a major world health problem, that is, to a great extent, caused by poor iron absorption from the diet. Several dietary factors can influence this absorption.

Absorption enhancing factors are ascorbic acid and meat, fish and poultry; inhibiting factors are plant components in vegetables, tea and coffee (e.g., polyphenols, phytates), and calcium.

16. Ans. (a) Troponin

Ref: Harrison 20th edition, P 384

Cardiac specific markers of myocardial damage include quantitative determination of CK-MB, Troponin I and Troponin T. Troponins can become elevated by 3 hours. The circulating values remain elevated up to a week.

17. Ans. (a) ASO

Ref: Nelson 20th edition, P 1333

Because other illnesses may closely resemble Acute rheumatic fever, antecedent group A Streptococcal Infection is needed whenever possible. The tests are

- Increasing or rising Anti-Streptolysin O titer or other streptococcal antibodies indicates recent streptococcal infection
- A Positive throat Culture
- A Positive Rapid group streptococcal carbohydrate antigen test in a child

Extra Mile

TABLE: Guidelines for the Diagnosis of Initial or Recurrent Attack of Rheumatic Fever (Jones Criteria, Updated 20'15)1'

Major manifestations	Minor manifestations	Supporting evidence of antecedent group a streptococcal infection
Carditis Polyarthritis Erythema marginatum Subcutaneous nodules Chorea	Clinical features: Arthralgia Fever Laboratory features: Elevated acute phase reactants: Erythrocyte sedimentation rate C-reactive protein Prolonged P-R interval	Positive throat culture or rapid streptococcal antigen test Elevated or increasing streptococcal antibody titer

18. Ans. (a) Thymoma

Ref: Bailey and Love, 26th edition, P 868

Most common anterior mediastinum tumour is thymoma. Choice B is seen in posterior mediastinum. Choice C and D are found in middle mediastinum.

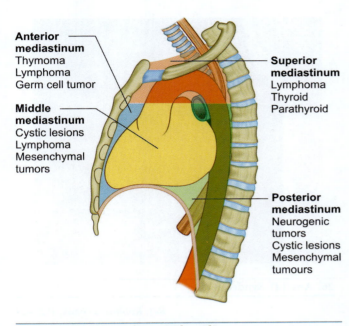

- They carry receptors for MHC class I molecules which inhibit their lytic function. When expression of class I MHC molecules is reduced on a cell surface by viral interference, inhibitory receptors on NK cells do not receive a negative signal and the targeted cells is destroyed.
- NK cells have CD16, Fc receptor that allows them to bind to opsonised cells and lyse them. This is a form of type II hypersensitivity with antibody mediated disease.

21. Ans. (a) **Serum Ferrtin**

Ref: CMDT 2019, P 512

- Low ferritin levels < 12 ng/ ml is a highly reliable indicator of reduced iron stores. Serum ferritin can increase in response to inflammation and hence normal or elevated ferritin level does not exclude diagnosis of IDA.
- As iron deficiency progresses iron levels will be less than 30 mcg/dl and transferrin levels rise to compensate.
- The elevated transferrin leads to lower saturation to < 15%.

19. Ans. (a) **Kimmelstein Wilson disease**

Ref: Robbins basic pathology, E-Book, P 781

- Nodular glomerulosclerosis is also called inter-capillary glomerulosclerosis or Kimmelstiel-Wilson disease.

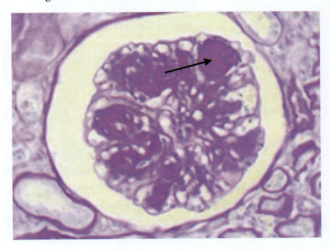

22. Ans. (a) **Endocardial cushion defect**

Ref: Nelson 20th edition, P 2165

SYNDROME	FEATURES
CHROMOSOMAL DISORDERS Trisomy 21 (Down syndrome) Trisomy 21 p (cat eye syndrome) Trisomy 18 Trisomy 13	Endocardial cushion defect, VSD, ASD Miscellaneous, total anomalous pulmonary venous return VSD, ASD, PDA, coarctation of aorta, bicuspid aortic or pulmonary valve VSD, ASD, PDA, coarctation of aorta, bicuspid aortic or pulmonary valve

23. Ans. (a) **Mycoplasma pneumoniae**

Ref: Harrison 20th edition, P 910

- Atypical bacterial pneumonia is caused by atypical organisms that are not detectable on Gram stain and cannot be cultured using standard methods.
- The most common organisms are Mycoplasma pneumoniae, Chlamydophila pneumoniae, and Legionella pneumophila. Atypical bacterial pneumonia generally is characterised by a symptom complex that includes headache, low-grade fever, cough, and malaise.
- CAP is caused by pneumococcus. If question says hospitalized patient of CAP the answer is still pneumococcus. Do not confuse with word hospital acquired pneumonia which is caused by Staphylococcus aureus.

- It presents as ovoid, spherical, laminated hyaline masses in periphery of the glomerulus. It is PAS+ and finally obliterates the glomerular tuft.
- It is specific for diabetes mellitus, membranoproliferative glomerulonephritis, light chain disease and amyloidosis.

20. Ans. (a) **NK cell**

Ref: Robbins review E-Book, P 67

- NK cells have the ability to respond without prior sensitization.

FMGE Solutions Screening Examination

Extra Mile

TABLE Microbial Causes of Community-Acquired Pneumonia, by Site of Care

Outpatients	Hospitalized Patients	
	Non-ICU	ICU
Streptococcus pneumoniae Mycoplasma pneumonlae Haemophllus influenzae	S. pneumonlae M. pneumoniae Chiamydla pneumoniae H. influenzae	S. pneumoniae Staphylococcus aureus Legionella spp. Gram-negative bacilli

24. Ans. (a) High ferritin

Ref: CMDT 2019, P 512

- Anemia of chronic disease leads to release of Hepcidin from the liver.
- Hepcidin leads to inhibition of release of iron from stores leading to stores/ ferritin being normal to increased since consumption is reduced.
- TIBC shows an inverse relation to serum ferritin always and hence is reduced.

Variable	Anemia of Chronic Disease	Iron-Deficiency Anemia
Iron	Reduced	Reduced
Transferrin	Reduced to normal	Increased
Transferrin saturation	Reduced	Reduced
Ferritin	Normal to increased	Reduced
Soluble transferrin receptor	Normal	Increased
Ratio of soluble transferrin receptor to log ferritin	Low (<1)	High (>2)
Cytokine levels	Increased	Normal

CELL INJURY AND INFLAMMATION

25. Ans. (a) Cat scratch disease

Ref: Robbins E-Book, P 462

- Cat-scratch disease is a nodal manifestation of infection by *Bartonella henselae* characterized by necrotizing granulomatous inflammation exhibiting a *characteristic stellate shape*.

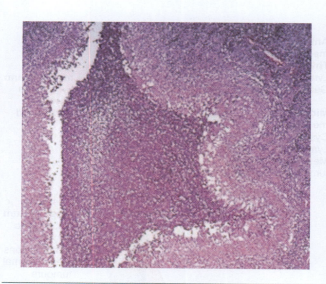

26. Ans. (d) Syndecan

Ref: Robbins E-book, P 22-23

- Choice A, B and C are Glycosaminoglycans and hence are ruled out.
- Proteoglycans have core proteins or glycoproteins with large GAG side-chains and they participate in cell-cell and cell-matrix interactions, cell proliferation, and migration associated with wound healing.
- Proteoglycans involved in wound healing are:

> - Small leucine-rich Proteoglycans
> - Glypicans
> - Versican-v3 isoform
> - Perlecan
> - Syndecans-1 and syndecans-4

27. Ans. (c) Granulation tissue

Ref: Robbins E-book, P 95

- Secondary healing is where a full-thickness wound is allowed to close and heal. It results in an inflammatory response that is more intense than with primary wound healing.
- In addition, a larger quantity of *granulation tissue is fabricated because of the need for wound closure.*
- Secondary healing results in pronounced contraction of wounds. Fibroblastic differentiation into myofibroblasts, which resemble contractile smooth muscle, is believed to contribute to wound contraction. These myofibroblasts are maximally present in the wound from the 10th – 21st days.

28. Ans. (a) Selectins

Ref: Robbins 9th ed. P 75-78

TABLE: Three phases of leucocyte recruitment at the sites of inflammation

Leukocyte adhesion to endothelium	Transmigration of diapedesis	Chemotaxis of leukocytes
• **Margination:**[Q] Leukocyte flow peripherally along endothelial surface at inflamed site (normal location—axial)	• Leukocyte migration through endothelium	• Leukocytes migration in the tissues toward the site of injury is called as chemotaxis
• **Rolling**[Q] (transient adhesion) of leucocytes to endothelium— mediated by **selectins** {leukocytes (L-selectin[Q], endothelium (E-selectin)[Q], and on platelest and endothelium (P-selectin)}[Q]	• Mediated by CD31 or **PECAM-1 (platelet endothelial cell adhesion molecule)**[Q]	**Examples:** **Exogenous chemo attractants**— bacterial products **Endogenous chemo attractants**— IL-8, C5a and leukotriene B4 (LTB4)[Q]
• **Firm adhesion**[Q] of leucocytes of endothelium— brought about by **integrins**		

29. Ans. (c) Cerebrum

Ref: Robbins 9th ed. P 41-44

Liquefactive/colliquative necrosis occurs due to digestion of dead cells and results in transformation of tissue into liquid viscous mass. The most common site involved is central nervous system.

30. Ans. (a) G1S

Ref: Robbins 9th ed. P 25-26, 292-293

- The guardian of genome mediates cell cycle arrest. It occurs in *late G1 phase* and is caused by p53 dependent transcription of CDK1.
- This prevents phosphorylation of RB essential for cells to enter G1 phase.
- Such a pause in cell cycling is welcome as it gives some breathing time for cells to repair the DNA damage.

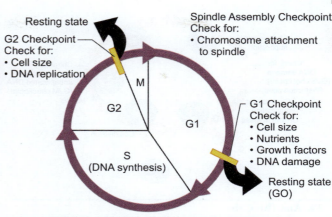

FIGURE: Various check points in cell division cycle

31. Ans. (b) Bcl

- The major mechanism of intrinsic mitochondrial pathway of apoptosis is by pro- and anti-apoptotic members of *bcl* proteins.
- Bcl protein was first detected on B cell lymphoma and hence its name.
- It is located on mitochondrial inner membrane and regulates cell growth and cell death.
- Pro-apoptotic mechanisms can damage mitochondrial membranes and allow leakage of cytochrome C into the cytoplasm. Cytochrome C is the life-line of intact mitochondria.

Growth promoter/anti-apoptotic proteins	Pro-apoptotic proteins
Bcl-2, Bcl-X and Mcl-1	Bim, Bad and Bid

32. Ans. (d) Lung abscess

Liquefaction or colliquative necrosis also occurs commonly due to ischaemic injury and bacterial or fungal infections but hydrolytic enzymes in tissue degradation have a dominant role in causing semi-fluid material. The *common examples are infarct brain and abscess cavity.*

33. Ans. (b) Synthetic phase

- Cell cycle is defined as the sequence of events that causes cell division.
- It consists of following phases:
  - G1 phase (Presynthetic growth)
  - S phase (DNA synthesis)
  - G2 (Premitotic growth), and
  - M phase (mitotic).
  - Quiescent cells that are not actively cycling are said to be in the G0 state. Cells can enter G1 either from the G0 quiescent cell pool, or after completing a round of mitosis, as for continuously replicating cells.

FMGE Solutions Screening Examination

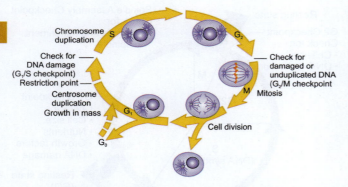

Important pathological process associated with apoptosis:

- Tumours exposed to chemotherapeutic agents
- Graft versus host disease
- Rejection episodes
- Depletion of CD4 cells in AIDS
- Prostatic atrophy after orchidectomy
- Alzheimer's disease
- MI (20% necrosis and 80% apoptosis)

Important physiological processes with apoptosis

- Organised cell destruction during formation of embryo
- Endometrial shedding, regression of lactating breast
- Involution of thymus
- Normal cell destruction followed by replacement proliferation such as intestinal epithelium

34. Ans. (b) C3b

- *The C3b molecules act as opsonins*; they bind covalently to the pathogen and thereby target it for destruction by phagocytes equipped with receptors for C3b.
- Anaphylatoxins, or complement peptides, are fragments (C3a, C4a and C5a) that are produced as part of the activation of the complement system.

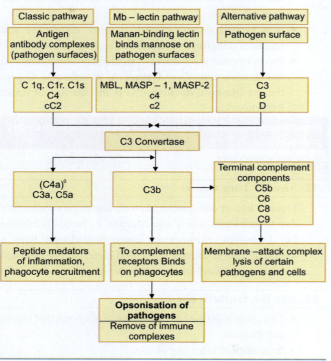

35. Ans. (c) Apoptosis

The councilman bodies are formed due to process of apoptosis in viral hepatitis.

36. Ans. (b) Cat scratch

Necrotising noncaseating granulomas are present in cat Scratch disease caused by Bartonella Henselae. The granulomas show *stellate microabscess* surrounded by palisading histiocytes.

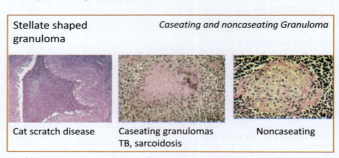

37. Ans. (c) E-cadherin

Ref: Robbin's Pathology, 9th ed. pg. 307

- Normal epithelial cells are tightly glued to each other and the ECM by a variety of adhesion molecules.
- E-cadherin, a cell surface protein, maintains intercellular adhesiveness serving to hold the cells together and relay signals between the cells.
- In several epithelial tumors, including adenocarcinomas of the colon, stomach, and breast, E-cadherin function is lost.

Pathology

Extra Mile

- TNF and IL-1 (interleukins) serve critical roles in leukocyte recruitment by promoting adhesion of leukocytes to endothelium and their migration through vessels.
- Interferons are inflammatory cytokines.
- Matrix metalloproteinase (MMP) regulate tumor invasion by:
  - Remodelling insoluble components of the basement membrane and interstitial matrix
  - By releasing ECM-sequestered growth factors.

---

38. Ans. (b) Metaplasia

Ref: Robbin's Pathology, 9ᵗʰ ed. pg. 37

- **Metaplasia** is an *adaptive response* of a cell in response to stress.
- It is a reversible change in which a *differentiated (mature) cell type is replaced by another differentiated cell type.*
- *It can be of two types:*
  - **Epithelial metaplasia**
    - ♦ **Squamous metaplasia:** MC seen in respiratory tract (in response to smoking) where columnar epithelium is replaced by squamous epithelium.
    - ♦ **Glandular metaplasia:** Metaplasia of squamous epithelium into columnar (glandular) epithelium. Example Barret's esophagus (metaplasia of stratified squamous epithelium of esophagus is replaced by intestinal-like columnar cells).
  - Connective tissue metaplasia:
    - ♦ One type of connective tissue is replaced by another.
    - ♦ **Example: Myositis ossificans.**

Extra Mile

- **Hypertrophy:** Increased cell **size** in response to increase in workload. It occurs in tissues incapable of cell division.
- **Hyperplasia:** increase in cell number in response to growth factors or hormones.
- **Atrophy:** Decrease in cell and organ size as a result of disuse or decreased nutrient supply.

---

39. Ans. (d) Atrophy

Ref: Robbin's Pathology, 9ᵗʰ ed. pg. 36

- Prolonged disuse of muscle can cause atrophy of muscle leading to decreased muscle mass in this patient (*atrophy of disuse*).

Other Causes of Atrophy can be:

- Loss of innervation (denervation atrophy)
- Diminished blood supply (ischemic/senile atrophy)
- Inadequate nutrition

- Loss of endocrine stimulation
- Pressure

---

40. Ans. (d) Hypertrophy

Ref: Robbin's Pathology, 9ᵗʰ ed. pg. 34

- **Hypertrophy refers to an increase in the size of cells,** that results in an increase in the size of the affected organ.
- The most common stimulus for hypertrophy of muscle is increased workload.
- A gravid uterus is an example of hypertrophy and hyperplasia both, but mainly hypertrophy.
- **Robbin's 9ᵗʰ ed. pg. 34 states:** "The massive physiologic growth of the uterus during pregnancy is a good example of hormone-induced enlargement of an organ that results mainly from hypertrophy of muscle fibers".
- Breast enlargement at puberty and at pregnancy is also an example of hypertrophy and hyperplasia both.

---

41. Ans. (c) Hyperplasia

Ref: Robbin's Pathology, 9ᵗʰ ed. pg. 36

- In individuals who donate one lobe of the liver for transplantation, the remaining cells proliferate so that the organ soon grows back to its original size. This is a classic example of compensatory hyperplasia.

---

42. Ans. (a) Internally controlled, programmed cell death

Ref: Robbin's Pathology, 9ᵗʰ ed. pg. 52

- Apoptosis is internally controlled, programmed cell death

Salient Features of Apoptosis:

- No inflammation
- Cell shrinkage
- Formation of apoptotic bodies

Example

- **Physiological:** Embryogenesis, organogenesis, Menstruation
- **Pathological:** Acute viral hepatitis—Councilman bodies.

---

43. Ans. (c) Apoptosis of cells induce inflammatory reaction

Ref: Robbin's Pathology, 9ᵗʰ ed. pg. 52-53

Remember Important Features of Apoptosis:

- Formation of cytoplasmic blebs and apoptotic bodies
- *Cell shrinkage:* The cells are smaller in size and the cytoplasm is dense
- *Chromatin condensation:* This is the most characteristic feature of apoptosis
- Absence of inflammation
- Gel electrophoresis of DNA shows 'step ladder pattern'.

Explanations

353

44. Ans. (a) Inflammation is present

Ref: Robbin's Pathology, 9th ed. pg. 52-55

Since in apoptosis the dead cell is rapidly cleared, before its contents have leaked out, therefore cell death by this pathway does not elicit an inflammatory reaction in the host.

45. Ans. (d) Condensation of the nucleus

Ref: Robbin's Pathology 9th ed. pg. 53-54

The Morphologic Features Characteristic of Apoptosis include:
- *Cell shrinkage*: The cell is smaller in size having dense cytoplasm and the organelles are tightly packed.
- *Chromatin condensation*: This is the *most characteristic feature of apoptosis*.
- Formation of cytoplasmic blebs and apoptotic bodies.

46. Ans. (a) Bcl-2

Ref: Robbin's Pathology, 9th ed. pg. 53-54

- Apoptosis is inhibited by anti-apoptosis genes which are mostly Bcl family genes.
  - **Example:** Bcl-2, Bcl-X, Bcl-XL
- **Pro**-apoptotic genes: they initiate and are involved in apoptosis.
  - **Example:** BAD, BIM, BAX, BAK
- P53 is a tumor suppressor gene and it causes apoptosis when there is excess DNA damage which cannot be repaired

47. Ans. (a) Caspases

Ref: Robbin's Pathology, 9th ed. pg. 53-54

- **Caspases**, or *c*ysteine-*asp*artic prote*ases* are a family of cysteine proteases that play essential roles in apoptosis, necrosis, and inflammation.
- Caspases are essential in cells for apoptosis, or programmed cell death, in development and most other stages of adult life, and have been termed "executioner" proteins for their roles in the cell.
- Some caspases are also required in the immune system for the maturation of lymphocytes.

48. Ans. (c) Embryogenesis

Ref: Robbin's Pathology, 9th ed. pg. 53-54

- Caspases are cysteine proteases and are critical for the process of apoptosis. Physiologically, apoptosis is required to eliminate the cells no longer required and to maintain a steady number of various cell populations in tissues.

- The programmed cell death (apoptosis) is required at the time of different processes in embryogenesis like implantation, organogenesis, developmental involution and metamorphosis.

49. Ans. (b) Apoptosis

Ref: Robbin's Pathology, 9th ed. pg. 53-54

Caspases are present in normal cells as inactive proenzymes and when they are activated they cleave proteins and induce apoptosis. These are cysteine proteases.

50. Ans. (c) Hydropic swelling

Ref: Robbin's Pathology, 9th ed. pg. 40

REVERSIBLE CELL INJURY
- Cell swelling

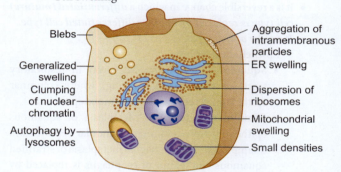

- Detachment of ribosomes from granular endoplasmic reticulum
- Dissociation of polysomes into monosomes.
- Plasma membrane blebbing, blunting, villous distortion, myelin figures, mitochondrial swelling, rarefaction.
- Nuclear disaggregation of granular and fibrillar elements.

51. Ans. (c) Condensation of nuclear chromatin

Ref: Robbin's Pathology, 9th ed. pg. 40

Refer to the explanation of the above question

52. Ans. (a) Coagulative necrosis

Ref: Robbin's Pathology, 9th ed. pg. 41-43, 50

COAGULATIVE NECROSIS
- This pattern of necrosis is typically seen in hypoxic environments, such as infarction.
- Coagulative necrosis occurs primarily in tissues such as the kidney, heart and adrenal glands.
- *Severe ischemia most commonly causes coagulative necrosis.*

Pathology

- Coagulation occurs as a result of protein denaturation, causing the albumin in protein to form a firm and opaque state.
- It is characterized by the formation of a gelatinous (gel-like) substance in dead tissues in which the architecture of the tissue is maintained, and can be observed by light microscopy.

Extra Mile

LIQUEFACTIVE NECROSIS

- It is characterized by the digestion of dead cells to form a viscous liquid mass. This is typical of bacterial, or sometimes fungal, infections because of their ability to stimulate an inflammatory response.
- The necrotic liquid mass is frequently creamy yellow due to the presence of dead leukocytes and is commonly known as pus.
- Hypoxic infarcts in the brain presents as this type of necrosis, because the brain contains little connective tissue but high amounts of digestive enzymes and lipids, and cells therefore can be readily digested by their own enzymes.

CASEOUS NECROSIS

- It can be considered a combination of coagulative and liquefactive necroses, typically caused by mycobacteria, fungi and some foreign substances.
- **The necrotic tissue appears as white and friable,** like **clumped cheese.**
- Microscopic examination shows **amorphous granular debris** enclosed within a distinctive inflammatory border. Granuloma has this characteristic.

FAT NECROSIS

- It is specialized necrosis of fat tissue, resulting from the action of activated lipases on fatty tissues such as the pancreas.
- In the pancreas it leads to acute pancreatitis, a condition where the pancreatic enzymes leak out into the peritoneal cavity, and liquefy the membrane by splitting the triglyceride esters into fatty acids through fat saponification.
- Calcium, magnesium or sodium may bind to these lesions to produce a chalky-white substance. The calcium deposits are microscopically distinctive and may be large enough to be visible on radiographic examinations. To the naked eye, calcium deposits appear as gritty white flecks.

Fibrinoid necrosis is a special form of necrosis usually caused by **immune-mediated vascular damage**. It is marked by complexes of antigen and antibodies, sometimes referred to as "immune complexes" deposited within arterial walls together with fibrin.

53. Ans. (d) Apoptosis

Ref: Robbin's Pathology, 9th ed. pg. 52-53

The inter nucleosomal cleavage of DNA into oligonucleosomes (in multiples of 180-200 base pairs) is brought about by Ca^+ and Mg^{2+} dependent endonucleases and is characteristic of apoptosis.

54. Ans (d) Platelet derived growth factor

Ref: Robbin's Pathology, 9th ed. pg. 52-53

Integrin superfamily consists of proteins that promote cell to cell, or cell to matrix adhesion. In contrast, selectins promote only cell to cell adhesion.

The Extracellular Domain Binds to:
- Matrix glycoproteins
- Adhesions molecules on other cells
- Activated complement components

55. Ans. (a) Venules

Ref: Robbin's Pathology, 9th ed. pg. 73-74

- Post capillary venules are an important point of interchange between the lumen of the vessels and the surrounding tissue.
- Moreover both vascular leakage and leucocyte exudation occur preferentially in venules in many types of inflammation.

56. Ans. (c) Atheromatous plaque

Ref: Robbin's Pathology, 9th ed. pg. 65-66

- Atheromatous plaque would have dead cells, so there is presence of dystrophic calcification.

57. Ans. (d) Lysosomal enzymes

Ref: Robbin's Pathology, 9th ed. pg. 81, 94

- The polymorphonuclear leukocyte (PMN) (Neutrophil) is particularly important in acute inflammation. The PMNs contain lysosomes.
- These granules contain several potent lytic enzymes which make it possible for these cells to destroy many types of bacteria and to liquefy the cell fragments resulting from tissue injury.
- The formation of hydrogen peroxide within neutrophils contributes to the bactericidal effect of these cells, as does the presence of superoxide, myeloperoxidase, and *halide ion*.

58. Ans. (d) All of the above

Ref: Robbin's Pathology, 9th ed. pg. 48

- Catalase is present in peroxisomes and decomposes H_2O_2 into O_2 and H_2O.
- Superoxide dismutase is found in many cell types and converts superoxide ions to H_2O_2. This group includes both manganese-superoxide dismutase, which is localized in mitochondria, and copper-zinc-superoxide dismutase, which is found in the cytosol.
- Glutathione peroxidase also protects against injury by catalyzing free radical breakdown.

Explanations

FMGE Solutions Screening Examination

59. Ans. (c) Vasodilation and increase in permeability

Ref: Robbin's Pathology, 9th ed. pg. 73

- Hallmark of acute inflammation is *increased vascular permeability* leading to the escape of protein-rich exudate into the extravascular tissue, causing edema.

60. Ans. (b) Myeloperoxidase

Ref: Robbin's Pathology, 9th ed. pg. 82-83

Myeloperoxidase (MPO) is an enzyme present in primary (or azurophilic) granules of the neutrophils. In the presence of a halide such as Cl^-, MPO converts H_2O_2 to HOCl (hypochlorous radical) during the process of respiratory burst.

61. Ans. (d) Granuloma formation

Ref: Robbin's Pathology, 9th ed. pg. 97

- Granuloma formation is characteristic of chronic granulomatous inflammation and is not seen in acute inflammation.
- Vasodilation, increase in permeability, exudation, margination, rolling etc. are seen in acute inflammation.

62. Ans. (a) NADPH oxidase

Ref: Robbin's Pathology, 9th ed. pg. 79

- The generation of reactive oxygen intermediates is due to the rapid activation of an enzyme; NADPH oxidase which is involved in oxygen dependent killing.
- Catalase, superoxide dismutase and glutathione peroxidase are free radical scavengers that prevent oxygen mediated injury.

63. Ans. (d) Vitamin C

Ref: Robbin's Pathology, 9th ed. pg. 8

- As the collagen molecule is produced, it undergoes many changes, termed post-translational modifications.
- These modifications take place in the Golgi compartment of the ER.
- Collagen, like most proteins that are destined for transport to the extracellular spaces for their function or activity, is produced initially as a larger precursor molecule called procollagen.
- Procollagen contains additional peptides at both ends that are unlike collagen. On one end of the molecule, called the amino terminal end, special bonds called disulfide bonds are formed among three procollagen chains and ensure that the chains line up in the proper alignment. This step is called registration. Once registration occurs, the three chains wrap around each other forming a string-like structure.
- One of the first modifications to take place is the very critical step of hydroxylation of selected proline and lysine amino acids in the newly synthesized procollagen protein.

64. Ans. (c) Calcification

Ref: Robbin's Pathology, 9th ed. pg. 40-41, 65

- Cellular swelling may occur due to cellular hypoxia, which damages the sodium-potassium membrane pump; it is reversible when the cause is eliminated.
- Cellular swelling is the first manifestation of almost all forms of injury to cells.
- On microscopic examination, small clear vacuoles may be seen within the cytoplasm; these represent distended and pinched-off segments of the endoplasmic reticulum.
- This pattern of non-lethal injury is sometimes called hydropic change or vacuolar degeneration.
- The ultrastructural changes of reversible cell injury include: Blebbing blunting, distortion of microvilli, loosening of intercellular attachments, mitochondrial changes, dilation of the endoplasmic reticulum.

65. Ans. (b) Liver

Ref: Robbin's Pathology, 9th ed. pg. 50-51

- In fat necrosis the enzyme lipase releases fatty acids from triglycerides.
- The fatty acids then complex with calcium to form soaps. These soaps appear as white chalky deposits.
- It is usually associated with trauma of the pancreas or acute pancreatitis.
- It can also occur in the breast, the salivary glands, neonates after a traumatic delivery but rarely in peritoneum.

66. Ans. (c) Lymphocytes, plasma cells and fibrosis

Ref: Robbin's Pathology, 9th ed. pg. 93

67. Ans. (a) Eosinophils

Ref: Robbin's Pathology, 9th ed. pg. /97

- A special form of chronic inflammation is seen in response to tissue invasion by *Mycobacterium tuberculosis*.
- Macrophages and multinucleated giant cells accumulate about the organisms, and fibrous tissue form about these small focal lesions or tubercles.
- This combination of macrophages and fibrosis is granulomatous inflammation.
- Epithelioid cells and multinucleated Langhans giant cells are present. The former are derived from macrophages and the latter by cytoplasmic fusion of macrophages.
- These lesions may heal by scarring and become calcified, or they undergo caseation necrosis.

Pathology

68. Ans. (a) Edema is present

Ref: Robbin's Pathology, 9th ed. pg. /130

White infarct	Red infarct
• Occurs in solid organs with end arterial circulation • Occurs in solid organs • Have well-defined margins • Edema is **absent**	• Occurs in organs with **dual blood supply** • Venous occlusion leads to red infarct, like in ovarian torsion • Ill-defined haemorrhagic margins • Edematous tissues

All infarcts are wedge shaped and have features of ischemic coagulative necrosis.

HEMODYNAMICS

69. Ans. (d) Increased protein C

Ref: Robbin's Pathology, 9th ed. pg. 122

Virchow's triad (in thrombosis) includes:
1. Endothelial injury
2. Stasis or turbulent blood flow
3. Hypercoagulability

Vasculitis	Vasculitis implies endothelial injury and is important for thrombus formation in coronary circulation.
Stasis in veins	Contributes to venous thrombosis
Turbulence in artery	Contributes to arterial thrombosis
Increased protein C	Protein C deficiency contributes to blood hyperviscosity whereas increased protein C would lead to bleeding

70. Ans. (d) Complete lumen obstruction

Ref: Robbin's Pathology, 9th ed. pg. 124-125

Arterial thrombus	Venous thrombus
• Associated with active blood flow leading to endothelial injury	Stasis of blood
• Grows in retrograde manner	Antegrade growth from point of attachment
• **Line of Zahn** is produced by alternating pale layers of platelets mixed with fibrin and darker layers containing more cells	Line of Zahn is absent
• **Incomplete lumen obstruction** leading to ischemia and organ infarction	Complete vessel occlusion

71. Ans. (d) Lower extremities

Ref: Robbin's Pathology, 9th ed. pg. 124-126

- *The site of arterial emboli is the heart and major site of embolization are lower extremities Brain > intestines > kidneys, etc.*
- **Most common site for venous thrombosis is deep leg veins below the knees**
- Most of pulmonary emboli arise in deep leg veins above (femoral veins) the level of the knee.

72. Ans. (b) Postmortem clots

Ref: Robbin's Pathology, 9th ed. pg. 125

- Postmortem clots may have a yellow appearance at upper end and red at the lower. These are sometimes called "chicken fat" clots. The surface is still shiny and smooth indicating a clot, not a thrombus.
- The yellow portion represents clotted plasma and the red cells have settled out and clotted at the bottom of the clot.

73. Ans. (c) It manifests as pitting edema

Ref: Robbin's Pathology, 9th ed. pg. 1162

- Angio-neurotic edema is a localized nonpitting edema involving deeper layers of the skin and subcutaneous tissue. It is an autosomal dominant clinical condition caused by **deficiency of C1 inhibitor protein** (a complement regulatory protein) and associated with elevated levels of bradykinin. It is more common in females.
- Diagnosis of hereditary angioedema is suggested by the presence of lack of pruritus and urticarial lesions, prominence of recurrent gastrointestinal attacks of colic and episodes of laryngeal edema. The levels of complement proteins C1 is normal but levels of C2 and C4 are depleted.
- Danazol is the drug which can be used for hereditary angioedema.

74. Ans. (c) Henoch Schonlein purpura

Ref: Robbin's Pathology, 9th ed. pg. 506, 510

Cutaneous small-vessel vasculitis (also known as "Cutaneous leukocytoclastic angiitis and "Hypersensitivity angiitis") is an inflammation of small blood vessels, characterized clinically by palpable purpura.

Subtypes of Small-Vessel Vasculitis Include:
- Henoch-Schonlein purpura
- Acute hemorrhagic edema of infancy
- Urticarial vasculitis
- Cryoglobulinemic vasculitis

NEOPLASIA

75. Ans. (b) Loss of differentiation

Ref: Robbins E-Book, P 192

- Anaplasia implies reversion of cells to a more primitive or undifferentiated form. In another words, there is complete loss of differentiation of normal cell.

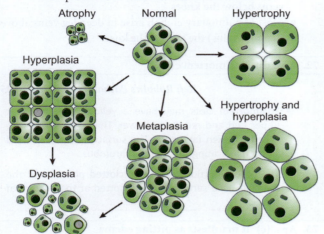

Extra Mile

Metaplasia	Dysplasia
Conversion of a mature, differentiated cell into another form of a mature cell type, often following injury or insult	Development of abnormal types of cells within a tissue, which may signify a stage preceding the development of cancer
Conversion in cell type	Change in the phenotype of cells or a tissue
Occurs in various types of tissues	Mainly occurs in the epithelium
An adaptive process that occurs due to an external stimulus	Occurs due to the alternation of genetic material
A reversible process	An irreversible process
Does not lead to the formation of cancer	May cause cancer

76. Ans. (a) Totipotent

Ref: Robbins E-book, P 25-26

- **Totipotent cells** can form all the cell types in a body, plus the extraembryonic, or placental, cells. Embryonic cells within the first couple of cell divisions after fertilization are the only cells that are totipotent.
- **Pluripotent cells** can give rise to all of the cell types of the three germ cell layers; embryonic stem cells are considered pluripotent.
- **Multipotent cells** can develop into more than one cell type, but are more limited than pluripotent cells; adult stem cells and cord blood stem cells are considered multipotent.

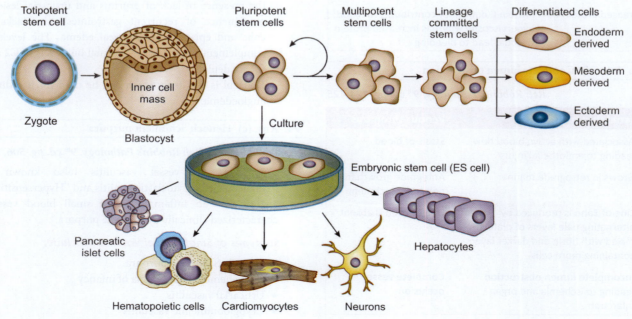

Pathology

77. Ans. (c) Teratoma

Ref: Robbins 9th ed. P 977

All tumors that produce α-fetoprotein have hyaline globules. These are eosinophilic round bodies found in following causes:

Malignant causes	Benign causes
• Yolk sac tumor	• Meningioma
• Hepatocellular carcinoma	• Pleomorphic adenoma
• Clear cell carcinoma	• α-1 anti-trypsin deficiency
• Kaposi sarcoma	
• Choroid plexus carcinoma	
• Adenoid cystic carcinoma	

78. Ans. (a) Lung cancer

Ref: Harrison 19th ed. P 1987

- SVC syndrome leads to severe reduction in venous return from head, neck and upper extremities and the causes are:

Malignant	Benign
Lung cancer	Central line catheter
Lymphoma	Pacemaker leads
Metastasis	Defibrillator leads

79. Ans. (d) Lung cancer

Ref: Harrison 19th ed. P 467

- The most common cancer leading to death in both males and females.
- The prevalence of carcinoma lung as contributor to death in males is 28% as compared to prostate cancer as 10%.
- The prevalence of carcinoma lung as contributor to death in females is 26% compared to breast cancer as 15%.

Distribution of *Cancer related deaths*

Male (%)		Female(%)	
Lung	28	Lung	26
Prostate	10	Breast	15
Colorectal	8	Colorectal	9
Pancreas	7	Pancreas	7

Extra Mile

The table given below from 19th edition of Harrison mentions prostate cancer as most common in males (27%) and breast cancer (29%) as most common in females.

Distribution of cancer incidence				
	Male		**Female**	
Sites	**%**	**Sites**	**%**	
Cancer incidence				
Prostate	27	Breast	29	
Lung	14	Lung	13	
Colorectal	8	Colorectal	8	
Bladder	7	Endometrial	6	
Melanoma	5	Thyroid	6	
Kidney	4	Lymphoma	4	
Lymphoma	4	Melanoma	4	
Oral cavity	4	Kidney	3	

80. Ans. (a) Comedo subtype of DCIS

Ref: Robbins E-book, P. 743

- The distinctive *comedo-subtype is characterized by extensive central necrosis.*
- This produces necrotic tissue with tooth paste consistency.
- Calcifications are frequently encountered in DCIS due to *calcification of necrotic tissue and are easily picked up by mammography.*
- Cribriform subtype of DCIS is a low grade tumor and hence necrosis in not seen.
- Colloid carcinoma produces abundant mucin both intracellularly and extracellularly.
- LCIS tends to be bilateral and may not be detected on mammography as it does *not* produce calcification.

81. Ans. (a) Peutz-Jeghers syndrome

Ref:Harrison 19th ed., P 240

- Peutz-Jeghers syndrome is characterized by dark brown spots on lips, buccal mucosa, nose and around eyes. There is concomitant intestinal polyposis. The most common location of polyps is in jejunum.
- It is an autosomal dominant disorder with STK11 mutation.
- The malignant potential of polyps ranges from never to rare transformation.

FMGE Solutions Screening Examination

82. Ans. (a) Transposon

- Transposons, also called jumping genes, are pieces of DNA that move readily from one site to another.
- They move either within or between the DNAs of bacteria, plasmids and bacteriophages in a manner, that plasmid genes can become part of the chromosomal complement of genes.
- Interestingly, when transposons transfer to a new site, it is usually a copy of the transposon that moves, while the original remains in situ (like photocopying).
- Transposons can code for metabolic or drug resistance enzymes and toxins. They may also cause mutations in the gene into which they insert or alter the expression of nearby genes.
- In contrast to plasmids or bacterial viruses, transposons cannot replicate independently of the recipient DNA. More than one transposon can be located in the DNA for example, resistance genes. Thus, transposons can jump from:
  - The host genomic DNA to a plasmid
  - One plasmid to another
  - A plasmid to genomic DNA.
- An *insertion sequence* is a short DNA sequence that acts as a simple transposable element. Insertion sequences have two major characteristics: they are small relative to other transposable elements (generally around 700 to 2500 bp in length) and only code for proteins implicated in the transposition activity (they are thus different from other transposons, which also carry accessory genes such as antibiotic resistance genes).

83. Ans. (b) Testicular contour distorted

TABLE: Distinguishing features of seminomatous (SGCT) and non-seminomatous (NSGCT) germ cell tumours of testis

Features	SGCT	NSGCT
Primary tumor	Large confined to testis for sufficient time, testicular contour retained	Similar at times indistinct: Testicular contour may be distorted
Metastasis	Generally to regional lymph nodes	Haematogenous spread early
Response to radiation	Radiosensitive	Radio-resistant
Serum markers	hCG: generally low levels	hCG, AFP, or both high levels
Prognosis	Better	Poor

84. Ans. (a) Adenolymphoma

- Warthin's tumour is called papillary cystadenoma lymphomatosum or adenolymphoma.
- It is a *benign tumour* of parotid comprising 8% of all parotid tumours seen in men from 4th to 7th decades of life.
- A common *wrong answer* from most candidates is pleomorphic adenoma. It is the most common tumour of the parotid.
- Most common malignant salivary gland tumour is mucoepidermoid carcinoma.

85. Ans. (b) Dysplasia

Loss of polarity implies loss of architectural orientation of cells which is seen in dysplasia.

TABLE: Differences between metaplasia and dysplasia

Feature	Metaplasia	Dysplasia
Definition	Change of one type of epithelial or mesenchymal cell to another type of adult epithelial or mesenchymal cell	Disordered cellular development may be accompanied with hyperplasia or metaplasia
Types	Epithelial (squamous columnar) and mesenchymal (osseous, cartilaginous)	Epithelial only
Tissues affected	Most commonly affects bronchial mucosa, uterine endocervix; other mesenchymal tissues (cartilage, arteries)	Uterine cervix, bronchial mucosa
Cellular changes	Mature cellular development	Disordered cellular development (pleomorphism, nuclear hyperchromasia, mitosis, loss of polarity)
Natural history	Reversible on withdrawal of stimulus	May regress on removal of inciting stimulus, or may progress higher grades of dysplasia or carcinoma in situ

86. Ans. (c) Oat cell cancer

c-myc	Burkitt's lymphoma
L-myc	Lung cancer
N-myc	Neuroblastoma
KIT (CD117)	Gastrointestinal stromal tumours

Pathology

87. Ans. (a) Small cell cancer of lung

H.C.C	Hepatitis B virus
Nasopharyngeal cancer	EBV
MALToma	*H. pylori*

88. Ans. (d) Lymphoma

TABLE: Mediastinal tumor & masses

Anterior	Middle	Posterior
• MC Thymoma • Lymphoma	• MC Lymphoma	Neurogenic tumors – neuroblastoma/ ganglioneuroblastoma/ ganglioneuroma, Schutannoma
• Metastatic CA • Thyroid lesions	• Bronchopulmonary of foregut malformations – bronchogenic cyst, oesophageal duplication • Pericardialcyst	• Lymphoma • Bronchogenic cyst • Gastroenteric hernia
• Teratoma		• Spinal tumours– PNET
• Thymic infiltration – leukaemia/ lymphoma/ histiocytosis		• Trauma–vertebral haematoma
Morgagni hernia^Q		
Lymphangioma/ haemangioma		

- MC site of mediastinal massess → Anterosuperior (59%)

89. Ans. (a) HPV

Human papillomavirus (HPV) which is the most common sexually transmitted infection, is a cause of anal dysplasia and cancer.

The approximately 40 HPV subtypes that can cause anogenital infections are divided into:

1. **Low-risk types (e.g. types 6 and 11)** that cause anal warts (condyloma acuminata)
2. **High–risk types (e.g. types 16, 18 and 33)** that can cause anal dysplasia and cancer.

HPV infection is associated with cervical, vulvar, vaginal, and penile cancers, and some patients have HPV-related dysplasia or cancer in multiple sites. Approximately 90% of anal cancers are attributable to HPV infection.

90. Ans. (c) Colorectal CA

Ref: Robbins Pathology, 9th ed. pg. 809

- Familial adenomatous polyposis (FAP) is an autosomal dominant disorder in which patients develop numerous colorectal adenomas as teenagers.
- **Robbins states: "Colorectal adenocarcinoma develops in 100% of untreated FAP patients, often before age 30 and nearly always by age 50"**
- As a result, prophylactic colectomy is the standard therapy for individuals carrying *APC* mutations. Colectomy prevents colorectal cancer, but patients remain at risk for neoplasia at other sites.
- **FAP is also associated with a variety of extraintestinal manifestations:**
  - Congenital hypertrophy of the retinal pigment epithelium
  - Gardner syndrome and
  - Turcot syndrome

91. Ans. (c) Stricture formation

Ref: Harrisons, 19th ed. pg. 532

TABLE: Some etiologic factors associated with squamous cell cancer of the esophagus

- Excess alcohol consumption
- Cigarette smoking
- Other ingested carcinogens
  - Nitrates (converted to nitrites)
  - Smoked opiates
  - Fungal toxins in pickled vegetables
- Mucosal damage from physical agents
  - Hot tea
  - Lye ingestion
  - Radiation-induced strictures
  - Chronic achalasia
- Hot susceptibility
- Esophageal web with glossitis and iron deficiency (i.e., Plummer-Vinson or Paterson-Kelly syndrome)
- Congenital hyperkeratosis and pitting of the palms and soles (i.e. tylosis palmaris et plantaris)
- Dietary deficiencies of selenium, molybdenum, zinc, and vitamin A

FMGE Solutions Screening Examination

TABLE: Some etiologic factors associated with adenocarcinoma of the esophagus

- Chronic gastroesophageal reflux
- Obesity
- Barrett's esophagus
- Male gender
- Cigarette smoking

92. Ans. (d) Thymus

- Oncocytes have been found to arise in various glandular and secretory epithelia. In the head and neck area, oncocytic change has been noted in numerous organs such as: the **salivary glands, pituitary, thyroid, parathyroid, nasal cavities, sinuses, ocular caruncle, lacrimal glands, buccal mucosa, Eustachian tube and the larynx.** They have also been **called oxyphilic cells, Askanazy cells and Hurthle cells in the thyroid gland.**
- The parotid gland is the most common site where oncocytic changes may occur, usually at the ductal or acinar cell level.

93. Ans. (b) Keratin

Ref: Robbin's Pathology, 9th ed. pg. 724

- Keratin expression is helpful in determining epithelial origin in anaplastic cancers.
- **Tumors that express keratin include** carcinomas, mesotheliomas, thymomas, sarcomas and trophoblastic neoplasms.
- Furthermore, the precise expression pattern of keratin subtypes allows prediction of the origin of the primary tumor when assessing metastases.

94. Ans. (d) Apthous ulcer

Ref: Robbin's Pathology 9th ed. pg. 728-730; Sternberg's Diagnostic Surgical Pathology, 5th ed. pg. 777

- Most cases of tongue CA are associated with lifestyle habits of smoking and drinking, tobacco chewing.
- **Most significant etiologic agent is tobacco.**
- Alcohol appears to act synergistically with tobacco as either a co-carcinogen (increasing the risk) or a promoter (decreasing the lag time) of neoplastic transformation.
- The neoplasm most often develops as an area of leukoplakia, chronic ulcer, or erythroplakia on the **lateral aspect of the middle one-third of the tongue.**

95. Ans. (a) Ewing's sarcoma

Ref: Robbin's Pathology, 9th ed. pg. 1203

HIGHLY RADIOSENSITIVE TUMOURS = W.E.L.M.S

- Wilms
- Ewing tumour
- Lymphoma

- Malignant myeloma
- Seminoma

96. Ans. (c) Thyroid

Ref: Robbin's Pathology, 9th ed. pg. 109

- The most radio-sensitive organ sites in children in the order of sensitivity are thyroid, breasts, bone marrow and brain.
- Exposure to ionizing radiation in first 2 decades predisposes a person for development of papillary CA.

97. Ans. (b) Stimulates formation of pyrimidine dimers

Ref: Robbin's Pathology, 9th ed. pg. 324-25

- The carcinogenicity of UV-B light is attributed to the formation of pyrimidine dimers in DNA. This type of DNA damage is repaired by nucleotide excision repair pathway.
- In patients with Xeroderma Pigmentosum, defective DNA repair is illustrated by appearance of high frequency of cancers.

98. Ans. (b) Lymphocytes

Ref: Robbin's Pathology, 9th ed. pg. 325-26

- The most radiosensitive blood cell is lymphocyte as it has a large nucleus.
- The least radiosensitive blood cell is platelets.

99. Ans. (c) Clonorchiasis

Ref: Robbin's Pathology, 9th ed. pg. 874-75

- **Clonorchis Sinesis:** Cholangiocarcinoma
- **Schistosoma Hematobium:** Squamous cell cancer of urinary bladder
- **Schistosoma Japonicum:** Colorectal cancer

IMMUNITY AND HYPERSENSITIVITY

100. Ans. (a) Graft across species

Ref: CMDT 2018, P 157

- Autologous graft (autograft): Within an individual, auto transplantation
- Syngeneic graft (syngraft, isograft): Identical twins, isotransplantation
- Allogeneic graft (allograft, homograft): Non-identical, allotransplantation
- Xenogeneic graft (heterologous graft, heterograft): Between species, xenotransplantation

Pathology

101. Ans. (b) Autoimmune Hemolytic anaemia

Ref: Robbins E-Book, P 135

- Choice A is type of type 4 Hypersensitivity reaction.
- Choice C is type of type 3 Hypersensitivity reaction.
- Choice D is type of type 4 Hypersensitivity reaction.

EXAMPLES OF TYPE II HYPERSENSITIVITY

Disease	Target antigen	Mechanism of disease	Clinicopathologic Manifestations
Autoimmune hemolytic anemia	Erythrocyte membrane proteins (Rh blood group antigens, I antigen)	Opsonization and phagocytosis of erythrocytes, complement mediated lysis	Hemalysis, anemia
Autoimmune thrombocytopenic purpura	Platelet membrane proteins (gplib-Illa integrin)	Opsonization and phagocytosis of platelets	Bleeding
Pemphigus vulgaris	Proteins in intercellular junctions of epidermal cells (desmoglein)	Antibody mediated activation of proteases, disruption of intercellular adhesions	Skin vesicles (bullae)
Vasculitis caused by ANCA	Neutrophil granule proteins, presumably released from activated neutrophils	Neutrophil degranulation and inflammation	Vasculitis
Goodpastere's syndrome	Non-ecellagerous NCI protein of basement membrane in glomeruli and lung	Complement and Fc receptor mediated inflammation	Nephritis, lung hemorrhage
Acute rheumatic fever	Streptococcal cell wall antigen; antibody cross reacts with myocardial antigen	Inflammation, macrophage activation	Myocarditis, arthritis

Contd...

Disease	Target antigen	Mechanism of disease	Clinicopathologic Manifestations
Myasthenia gravis	Acetylcholine receptor	Antibody inhibits acetylcholine binding and down regulates the receptors.	Muscle weakness, paralysis
Graves' disease (hyperthyroidism)	TSH receptor	Antibody mediated stimulation of TSH receptors	Hyperthyroidism
Pernicious anemia	Intrinsic factor of gastric parietal cells	Neutralization of intrinsic factor, decreased absorption of vitamin B_{12}	Abnormal erythropoiesis, anemia

102. Ans. (b) Days to weeks

Ref: Robbins E-Book, P 164

- Acute rejections appear within days or weeks and hence choice B is correct.
- Choice C is a close choice but it mentions only after 6 weeks of graft deployment while acute rejection can occur earlier as well.
- **Acute rejection is mediated by T cells and antibodies that are activated by alloantigens in the graft**. It occurs within days or weeks after transplantation, and is the principal cause of early graft failure. It also may appear suddenly months or even years later, after immunosuppression is tapered or terminated. Based on the role of T cells or antibodies, acute rejection is divided into two types, although in most rejecting grafts, both patterns are present

103. Ans. (a) Anti-Ro

Ref: Nelson 20th ed. P 1152

In SLE, Anti-Ro antibody can easily cross the placenta and damage the A-V node of the developing fetus. This leads to the baby being born with *complete heart block*. Right from day 0 of life the presentation is bradycardia and syncope. The baby may have a *malar rash* in butterfly distribution. This is called as neonatal lupus.

Antismith antibody	Most specific test for SLE
Antiribonucleoprotein antibody	Leads to psychosis in SLE
Antiphospholipid antibody	APLAS leading to recurrent abortions

104. Ans. (a) CD4

- Class I MHC antigens have loci as HLA-A, HLA-B and HLA-C. CD8+ (i.e. T suppressor) lymphocytes carry receptors for class I MHC: These cells are used to identify class I antigens on them.
- Class II MHC antigens have single locus as HLA-D. These antigens have further 3 loci: DR, DQ and DP. Class II MHC is identified by 8 cells and CD4+ (i.e. T helper) cells.
- Class III MHC antigens are some components of the complement system (C2 and C4) coded on HLA complex but are not associated with HLA expression and are not used in antigen identification.
- In view of high polymorphism of class I and Class II genes, they have a number of alleles on loci numbered serially like HLA-A 1, HLA-A 2, HLA-A3 etc.
- MHC antigens present on the cell surface help the macrophage in its function of recognition of bacterial antigen, i.e. they help of identify self from foreign and accordingly present the foreign antigen to T cells (CD4 + or CD8+) or to B cells.

105. Ans. (d) Type 4

TABLE: Comparative features of four types of hypersensitivity reactions

Feature	Type 1 (Anaphylactic, atopic)	Type 2 (Antibody – mediated, cytotoxic)	Type 3 (Immune – complex, arthus reaction)	Type 4 (Delayed T cell – mediated)
Definition	Rapidly developing immune response in a previously sensitised person	Reaction of humoral antibodies that attack cell surface antigens and cause cell lysis	Results from deposition of antigen antibody complexes of tissues	Cell-mediated slow and prolonged response
Peak action time	15–30 minutes	15–30 minutes	Within 6 hours	After 24 hours
Mediated by	IgE antibodies	IgG or IgM antibodies	IgG, IgM antibodies	**Cell mediated**
Etiology	Genetic basis, pollutants, viral infections	HLA – linked, exposure to foreign tissues/ cells	Persistence of low grade infection, environmental antigens, autoimmune process	Cutaneous antigens

106. Ans. (d) CD 19

- B cell markers are CD 19, 20, 21 and 23.
- T_H cell markers are CD 4, 3, 7, 2
- T_C cell markers are CD 8, 3, 7, 2
- NK cell markers are CD 2, 16, 56

107. Ans. (d) Pneumoconiosis with rheumatoid arthritis

- Progressive massive fibrosis of pneumoconiosis in association with *rheumatoid arthritis is known as Caplan syndrome*.
- Unlike lesions caused by progressive massive fibrosis, which congregate in the upper lobes, these lesions known as Caplan lesions tend to coalesce in the peripheral lung fields.

108. Ans. (b) Ankylosing spondylitis

Clinical Associations with HLA – B27	
Disorder	**HLA –B27 (%)**
Ankylosing spondylitis	90
Reactive arthritis (Reither's syndrome)	40–80
Juvenile SpA	70
Inflammatory bowel disease	35-75
Psoriatic arthritis With spondylitis	50
With peripheral arthritis	15
Undifferentiated SpA	70
Acute anterior uveitis	50
Aortic insufficiency, heart block	80

109. Ans. (d) Large granular lymphocyte

- *The natural killer cells are called as large granular lymphocytes and are responsible for A.D.C.C (Antibody dependant cell cytotoxicity).* This mechanism is particularly effective against viruses and tumour cells.
- NK cells are a part of natural or innate immunity and recognise antibody coated cells. Thus they bring about killing of target cells directly.

110. Ans. (d) Type 4

- *Delayed type of hypersensitivity is mediated by T cell dependant effector mechanisms involving both CD4+ TH1 cells and CD8 Cytotoxic T cells.*
- Antibodies do not play a role in type IV hypersensitivity reactions. The activated TH1 cells release Cytokines that will cause accumulation and activation of macrophages which will cause local damage.
- TH 2 cells release IL-4 and are involved in Type 1 Hypersensitivity reaction.

Pathology

111. Ans. (c) SLE

Ref: Chapter 5; Robbins, 8th ed.

TABLE: Hypersensitivity reactions

Type I (IgE mediated)	Type II (IgG, IgM and complement mediated)
• Eczema • Hay fever • Asthma atopy • Urticaria • Anaphylactic shock • Acute dermatitis • *Theobald smith phenomenon* • *Prausnitz Kustner (PK) reaction* • *Casoni's test* • *Schultz-Dale phenomenon*	• Blood transfusion reactions • Erythroblastosis fetalis • AIHA or thrombocytopenia or agranulocytosis • Pemphigus vulgaris • Good pasture syndrome • Bullous pemphigoid • Pernicious anemia • Acute rheumatic fever • *Diabetes mellitus* • *Graves disease* • *Myasthenia gravis*
Type III (IgG, IgM, complement and leucocyte mediated)	**Type IV (Cell mediated)**
• Local–Arthus reaction • Systemic-serum sickness • Schick test • Polyarteritis nodosa (PAN) • **SLE** • Acute viral hepatitis • Penicillamine toxicity • Hyperacute graft rejection • Type 2 lepra reaction (ENL) • Hypersensitivity pneumonitis • R.A • Infective endocarditis • Henoch schonlein purpura	• Tuberculin test • Lepromin test • Sarcoidosis • Tuberculosis • Contact dermatitis • Granulomatous inflammatin • Type I lepra reaction • **Patch test** • Temporal arteritis • Jones mote reaction (cutaneous basophilic HSN) • **Graft rejection** • Fairleys test • Frie's test

112. Ans. (b) Antigen – antibody mediated

Type II or Cytotoxic Hypersensitivity depends on the abnormal production of IgG or IgM directed against tissue antigens or a normal reaction to foreign antigens expressed on host cells. There are three main mechanisms of injury in Type II reactions:

- Activation of complement followed by complement mediated lysis or phagocytosis and removal by leukocytes
- Antibody dependent cellular cytotoxicity
- Inactivation of a biologically active molecule

113. Ans. (c) IgM

Ref: Ananthanarayan and Paniker's, 8th ed. pg. 100

TABLE: Immunoglobulins and their salient features

Immunoglobulins	Salient features
IgG	• **Most abundant Ig,** makes as about 80% • Marker of chronic infection • Only Ig that can cross placenta
IgA	• 2nd most abundant, 10–13% • Found in glandular secretion like saliva, tear, ileum, and mucosal secretion like bronchial secretion
IgM	• 5–8% of total Ig; aka pentameric Ig → **has highest molecular weight** • First Ig to be synthesized by fetus (20 weeks AOG) • Marker of acute infection
IgD	• Present mostly intravascular • Serve as recognition receptor for antigens
IgE	• Mostly extravascular in distribution • Highly elevated levels in case of type-I HPS reaction • Produced chiefly in the linings of respiratory and intestinal tracts

TABLE: Immunoglobulin and their effective valency

Antibody	Effective valency
• IgM	5
• IgG	2
• IgD	2
• IgE	2
• IgA	2,4

> **Extra Mile**
>
> - Ig having maximum molecular weight: **IgM**
> - First antibody produced by newborn: **IgM**
> - All immunoglobulins are heat stable except: **IgE**
> - Ig present in **breast milk: IgA**
> - Ig with **maximum half-life: IgG**
> - Ig with **minimum half-life: IgE**
> - Ig having **maximum serum concentration: IgG**
> - Ig having **least serum concentration: IgE**

114. Ans. (a) B cells

Ref: Robbin's Pathology, 9th ed. pg. 187, 191

PRIMARY COMPLEMENT IMMUNE RESPONSE

- The first exposure to a foreign antigen, a lag phase occurs in which no antibody is produced, *but activated B cells are differentiating into plasma cells.* The lag phase can be as short as 2–3 days, but often is longer, sometimes as long as weeks or months.

- The amount of antibody produced is usually relatively low.
- Over time, antibody level declines to the point where it may be undetectable.
- The first antibody produced is manily IgM (although small amounts of IgG are usually also produced).

115. Ans. (d) Type 4

Ref: Chapter 55, Harrison, 19th edition

Clinical Features of Severe Cutaneous Drug Reactions

Diagnosis	Mucosal lesions	Typical skin lesions
Stevens-Johnson syndrome	Erosions usually at two or more sites	Small blisters on dusky purpuric macules or atypical targets; rare areas of confluence; detachment ≤10% of body surface area

Diagnosis	Mucosal Lesions	Typical skin lesions
Toxic epidermal necrolysis	Erosions usually at two or more sites	Individual lesions like those seen in Stevens-Johnson syndrome; confluent erythema; outer layer of epidermis separates readily from basal layer with lateral pressure; large sheet of necrotic epidermis; total detachment of >30% of body surface area

TABLE: Classification of Adverse Drug Reactions Based on Immune Pathway

Hypersensitivity type	Key pathway	Adverse drug reaction type
Type I	IgE	Urticaria, angioedema, anaphylaxis
Type II	IgG-mediated cyto-toxicity	Drug induced hemolysis
Type III	Immune complex	Vasculitis, serum sickness, drug-induced lupus
Type IV b	T lymphocyte-mediated eosinophil inflammation	Tuberculin skin test, contact dermatitis
Type IV c	T lymphocyte-mediated cytotoxic lymphocyte inflammation	Drug-induced hypersensitivity syndrome Morbiliform eruption
Type IV d	T lymphocyte-mediated neutrophil inflammation	Acute generalized exanthematous pustulosis

116. Ans. (d) Type 4

Ref: Robbin's Pathology, 8th ed. ch. 5
Refer to Explanation of Question 99.

117. Ans. (a) Bipolar cells

Ref: Robbin's Pathology 9th ed. pg. 191-192: Pocket Companion to Robbin's Pathology, 8th ed. pg. 119

T cells cannot be activated by soluble antigens. Therefore presentation of processed antigen by **antigen presenting cells** is required for activation of T cells.

Important Antigen Presenting Cells are:
- Macrophage
- B cells
- Dendritic cells (**most potent APCs**)
- Langerhans cells

Bipolar cell is a type of neuron which has two extensions. Bipolar cells are specialized sensory neurons for the transmission of special senses. As such, they are part of the sensory pathways for smell, sight, taste, hearing and vestibular functions.

118. Ans. (a) IL-2

Ref: Robbin's Pathology, 9th ed. pg. 192-93

Salient Features of NK Cell
- Growth factor for NK cell-**IL2** (proliferate in response to IL2) and **IL-15.**
- NK cell activity is augmented by interferon
- They secrete perforin which results in formation of transmembrane pore resulting in cell death
- Cytotoxic against virus infected cells, tumour cells, transplanted foreign cells
- Its activity is neither antibody dependent nor MHC restricted.
- Component of innate immunity.
- NK cells + for-CD 16, CD56

119. Ans. (a) MHC class I

Ref: Robbin's Pathology, 9th ed. pg. 231, 232
- In transplantation immunology, the major impact in graft loss comes from the effects of HLA-B and -DR antigens
- The histocompatibility antigens [human leukocyte antigens (HLA)] are cell surface antigens that induce as response leading to rejection of allografts
- The principal physiologic function of the cell surface histocompatiblity molecules is the bind peptide fragments foreign proteins for presentation to antigen specific T cells.
- The histocompatibility antigens are encoded by a closely linked multiallelic cluster of genes: Mix histocompatibility complex (MHC) or human leukocyte antigens complex (HLA complex)

Contd...

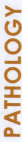

Pathology

- HLA complex of genes is located on the short arm of chromosome 6.
- It consists of three separate clusters of genes:

TABLE: HLA Complex (MHC complex)

Class I	Class II	Class III

• Comprising A, B and C loci
• Responsible for graft rejection and cell mediated cytolysis
• Found on the surface of all nucleated cells and platelets
	• 'D' region → DR, DQ, DP
	• Responsible for
	  ▪ Graft versus host response
	  ▪ Mixed leucocyte reaction
	• Found only on cells of the immune system
		Complement region encodes
		• C_2 and C_4
		• Properdin factor B
		• Heat shock protein
		• TNF – α and β
		• Enzyme 21-hydroxylase

Remember
Histocompatibility Reactions

Graft versus host disease	Host versus graft disease (Graft rejection)
• HLA class II is primarily involved • T-helper cells (CD-4)	• HLA class I is primarily involved • Cytotoxic T cell (CD-8)

120. Ans. (d) Reiter's syndrome

Ref: Robbin's Pathology, 9th ed. pg. 116, 787

In addition to its association with ankylosing spondylitis, HLA-B27 is implicated in other types of seronegative spondyloarthropathy
- Reactive arthritis (Reiter's syndrome)
- Acute anterior uveitis and iritis
- Psoriatic arthritis
- Ulcerative colitis associated spondyloarthritis

121. Ans. (b) Chronic granulomatous disorder

Ref: Robbin's Pathology, 9th ed. pg. 237-238

Nitro blue tetrazolium is used in a diagnostic test, particularly for chronic granulomatous disease. When there is an NADPH oxidase defect, the phagocyte is unable to make reactive oxygen species or radicals required for bacterial killing. As a result, bacteria may thrive within the phagocyte. The higher the blue score, the better the cell is at producing reactive oxygen species.

122. Ans. (d) Calcium

Ref: Robbin's Pathology, 9th ed. pg. 89, 238

- The initial enzyme, C1, is a complex formed through a calcium-dependent association between two reversibly interacting subunits, C1q and C1r2s2.

- In the absence of an immune response, approximately 70% of C1 exists as a complex between these two subunits.
- C1 occurs in serum as a proenzyme that tends to undergo autoactivation (in which the two subunits are bound together) but is strictly controlled by C1-inhibitor (C1-In or C1 esterase).

123. Ans. (d) Sickle cell disease

Ref: Robbin's Pathology, 9th ed. pg. 211-15, 635

- Sickle cell disease is a genetic condition which is characterized by mutation in beta globin chain of hemoglobin (**glutamic acid is replaced with valine in the 6th position of beta chain**).
- Other given choices like SLE, Grave's and MG are all autoimmune conditions.

124. Ans. (d) Type 4

Ref: Robbin's Pathology, 9th ed. pg. 208-209

HEMATOLOGY

125. Ans. (a) T.I.B.C

Ref: Robbins E- Book, P 454

Iron deficiency anaemia has all parameters reduced except Total iron binding capacity.

	Iron deficiency anemia
Hematocrit	↓ to ↓↓↓
MCV	↓ to ↓↓↓
MCHC	↓
Serum iron	↓ to ↓↓↓
Serum TIBC	Normal to ↑
Serum ferritin	↓ to ↓↓
Stainable iron in marrow	Absent
Reticulocytes	Normal to ↓

126. Ans. (c) Normocytic and normochromic anemia

Ref: Robbins 9th ed. P 652

- Rheumatoid arthritis leads to development of anemia of chronic disease.
- A more common presentation of anemia of chronic disease is normocytic normochromic anemia. In late presentation microcytic hypochromic anemia is noted.

127. Ans. (b) Yolk sac, liver and bone marrow

Ref: Robbins 9th ed. P 579-580

- Erythropoiesis starts in the yolk sac at 2 weeks of gestation and leads to production of embryonic hemoglobin.
- It shifts to liver spleen at 14 weeks of gestation and leads to production of fetal hemoglobin.
- At birth the hematopoiesis shifts to the bone marrow. The major hemoglobin at birth is fetal hemoglobin.

Explanations

FMGE Solutions Screening Examination

128. Ans. (d) 12 g%

Ref: Robbins 9th ed. P630-631

TABLE: Hemoglobin levels to diagnose anemia at sea level (g/L)±

Population	Non-anemia*	Anemia* Mild	Anemia* Moderate	Anemia* Severe
Children 6–59 months of age	110 or higher	100–109	70–99	Lower than 70
Children 5–11 years age	115 or higher	110–114	80–109	Lower than 80
Children 12–14 years of age	120 or higher	110–119	80–109	Lower than 80
Nonpregnant women (15 years of age and above)	120 or higher	110–119	80–109	Lower than 80
Pregnant women	110 or higher	100–109	70–99	Lower than 70
Men (15 years of age and above)	130 or higher	110–129	80–109	Lower than 80

129. Ans. (b) NESTROFT

Ref: Textbook of hematology Dr. Tejender singh 2nd ed. P 90-92,
Hemoglobinopathies by Anupam sachdev 1st ed. P 100

Initial screening test for diagnosis of β-thalassemia carriers is NESTROFT. The naked eye single tube osmotic fragility test is based on osmotic fragility using 0.36% buffered saline.

Procedure

- Two test tubes labeled as Buffered saline (2 mL) and distilled water 2 mL) are taken and a drop of water is added to each of tubes, which is left undisturbed for half an hour at room temperature. Following this contents of the tube are shaken and held against a white paper on which a thin black line is drawn.

Interpretation

- The line is clearly visible through the DW tube and if the same is seen in Buffered saline tube, it indicates that the test is negative.

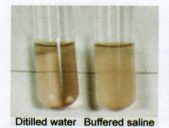

Ditilled water   Buffered saline
Positive NESTROFT

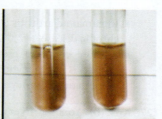

Distilled water   Buffered saline
Negative NESTROFT

Extra Mile

- Thalassemia syndrome is the most common genetic syndrome worldwide.
- IOC for thalassemia is HPLC >> Hb electrophoresis.

130. Ans. (a) Elevated HbA2

Ref: Robbins 9th ed. P 640

- Quantification of HbA2 and Hb variant via HPLC gives an accurate estimate of HbA2 levels
- Values of HbA2 >4.0% with reduced RBC indices are indicative of β-thalassemia carriers.
- The earlier cut off of HbA2 >3% must be interpreted with caution as per current guidelines.

Extra Mile

Hemoglobin	Structure	Levels at birth	Levels in adults	Comments
A	$\alpha_2\beta_2$	20–25%	97%	Reaches adult levels by 1 year of age
A$_2$	$\alpha_2\delta_2$	0.5%	2.5%	Elevated in β thalassemia trait
F	$\alpha_2\gamma_2$	75–80%	<1%	Reaches adult levels by 1 year of age
HbH	β_4	15–20% in HbH disease	NA	HbH produces heinz bodies in the erythocytes and hemolysis
HB Bart	γ_4	100% in hydrops fetalis, 15–25% in HbH disease	NA	Increase in carriers of α thalassemia trait at birth

NA = not applicable.

Pathology

131. Ans. (d) Denatured haemoglobin

Summary of Inclusions in RBCs

Howell jolly bodies	DNA
Basophilic stippling	RNA remnants
Siderotic granules/ pappenhiemer bodies	Iron
Heinz bodies	Denatured Haemoglobin

132. Ans. (a) SLE

Positive coombs test is seen in autoimmune haemolytic anaemia caused by SLE.

The remaining three choices of the question are examples of microangiopathic haemolytic anaemia.

TABLE: Causes of Microangiopathic Haemolytic Anemia

Thrombocytic thrombocytopenic purpura
Haemolytic uremic syndrome
Disseminated intravascular coagulation
Infections: gram–negative septicaemia
Snake bites
Hemolytic transfusion reactions
Obstetric complications: abruptio placentae, amniotic fluid embolism, retained dead fetus, eclampsia
Malignant hypertension
Immunologic disorders: Vasculitis
Acute glomerulonephritis
Polyarteritis nodosa
Wegner's granulomatosis
Systemic lupus erythematous
Scleroderma
Renal and hepatic allograft rejection
Disseminated carcinoma:

133. Ans. (a) A.M.L

- Arsenic trioxide is used in management of *M3 AML/ Acute Pro-myelocytic Leukemia. Also used is A.T.R.A (Al-trans- Retinoic acid).*
- Acute Pro-Myelocytic Leukemia has high risk of early hemorrhagic death due to disseminated intravascular coagulation and hyperfibrinolysis. The prognosis of APL has improved dramatically following the introduction of all-trans retinoic acid (ATRA) and its combination with anthracycline-based chemotherapy during induction and consolidation
- Arsenic trioxide and A.T.R.A are considered in frail or elderly patients. This combination can also be used in patients who are unable to tolerate anthracycline-based therapy.

134. Ans. (b) Parvo virus B19

- Hepatitis B, C and D can lead to aplastic anaemia. In contrast Parvo virus B19 leads to a transient bone marrow illness called aplastic crisis.
- Parvovirus B19 (B19V) is a single-stranded DNA virus of the family Parvo-viridae and genus Erythrovirus.
- It has a unique tropism for human erythroid progenitor cells. The virus requires the P blood antigen receptor (also known as globoside) to enter the cell.

135. Ans. (a) Sickle cell anaemia

Gamma-Gandy bodies (GGB) are siderotic nodules present in the spleen.

Causes of Gamma Gandy bodies are:

1. Portal hypertension
2. Sickle cell anaemia
3. Acquired hemochromatosis
4. Paroxysmal nocturnal hemoglobinuria
5. Angio-sarcoma.

136. Ans. (a) Portal hypertension

Refer to explanation of the question no. 88.

137. Ans. (d) Factor 11

- Rosenthal syndrome is Factor XI deficiency/Haemophilia C/Plasma thromboplastin antecedent deficiency.
- These patients will experience severe bleeding after dental extractions. FXI deficiency is inherited in an autosomal recessive pattern.

138. Ans. (c) ALL

Ref: Robbins, 9th ed. pg. 590

Acute Lymphoblastic Leukemia/Lymphoma

- **Acute lymphoblastic leukemia/lymphomas (ALLs) are neoplasms composed of immature B (pre-B) or T (pre-T)cells, which are referred to as *lymphoblasts*.**
- About 85% are B-ALLs, which typically manifest as childhood acute "leukemias."
- The less common T-ALLs tend to present in adolescent males as thymic "lymphomas."
- **ALL is the most common cancer of children.**

> **Extra Mile**

- **Multiple myeloma** is a plasma cell neoplasm commonly associated with lytic bone lesions, hypercalcemia, renal failure, and acquired immune abnormalities.
- **Amyloidosis** is a disorder characterized by the extracellular deposits of misfolded proteins that aggregate to form insoluble fibrils.
- **Mycosis fungoides/Sezary syndrome** is a disorder of helper T cells among adults. Patients present with cutaneous patches, plaques, nodules or generalized erythema.

FMGE Solutions Screening Examination

139. Ans. (c) Nodular sclerosis

Ref: Harsh Mohan, 7th ed. pg. 350

TABLE: Type of Hodgkin's lymphoma

Nodular sclerosis	Most common type of Hodgkin lymphoma	Lacunar Reed-Sternberg cell variants in a mixed inflammatory background; broad sclerotic bands of collagen usually also present	CD15+, CD30+ Reed-Sternberg cells	Most common in young adults, often arises in the mediastinum cervical lymph nodes
Mixed cellularity type	Second most common form of Hodgkin lymphoma	Frequent classic Reed-Sternberg cells in a mixed inflammatory background	CD15+, CD30+, Reed-Sternberg cells	Most common in men, more likely to present at advanced stages than the **nodular sclerosis** type EBV+in 70% of cases

140. Ans. (a) Polycyathemia vera

Ref: Robbin's Pathology, 9th ed. pg. 616

JAK-2 Mutation is seen in:
1. Polycythemia vera
2. Primary myelofibrosis
3. Essential thrombocytosis

141. Ans. (b) Ca++

Ref: Radiopaedia org.

142. Ans. (a) Disseminated intravascular coagulation

Ref: Robbin's Pathology, 9th ed. pg. 317-18, 612, 663

- Acute promyelocytic leukemia (APL) is characterized by more severe hemorrhagic phenomena than those of other acute leukemias.
- The hemorrhagic diathesis results from disseminated intravascular coagulation.
- About 40% of patients with APL have a chromosomal abnormality with translocation from the long arm of 17 to 15 (t 15q;17q)
- The patient may present with massive ecchymoses, hematuria, epistaxis, or meno-metrorrhagia.

143. Ans. (a) Nodular sclerosis

Ref: Robbin's Pathology, 9th ed. pg. 606-607; Harrison 18th ed. Chapter 110

Hodgkin's Disease
Nodular lymphocyte
Predominant Hodgkin's disease
Classical Hodgkin's disease
Nodular sclerosis Hodgkin's disease
Lymphocyte-rich classic Hodgkin's disease
Mixed-cellularity Hodgkin's disease
Lymphocyte-depletion Hodgkin's disease

144. Ans. (c) 20%

Ref: Nelson 18th ed. ch. 495

- The characteristic feature of AML is that >20% of bone marrow cells on bone marrow aspiration or biopsy touch preparations constitute a fairly homogeneous population of blast cells, with features similar to those that characterize early differentiation states of the myeloid-monocyte-megakaryocyte series of blood cells. The most common classification of the subtypes of AML is the FAB system.

TABLE: French-American-British (FAB) Classification of Acute Myelogenous Leukemia

Subtype	Common name
M1	Acute myeloblastic leukemia without maturation
M2	Acute myeloblastic leukemia with maturation
M3	Acute promyeloblastic leukemia
M4	Acute myelomonocytic leukemia
M5	Acute monocytic leukemia
M6	Erythro leukemia
M7	Acute megakaryocytic leukemia

145. Ans. (a) Smoldering myeloma

Ref: Harrison, 19th ed. pg. 715

TABLE: Diagnostic Criteria for Multiple Myeloma

MONOCLONAL Gammopathy of Undetermined Significance is defined by the presence of three criteria:
• Serum monoclonal M protein (M-protein) concentration **<3 g/dL**
• Bone marrow plasma cell concentration **<10%**
• No evidence of end organ damage
Smoldering MM is present when
• Serum M protein concentration is **>3 g/dL**
• Bone marrow plasma cell concentration is **>10%**
• No evidence of end-organ damage.

Contd...

Pathology

Symptomatic myeloma is present when
- M-protein ≥30 g/L
- Bone marrow clonal cells ≥10%
- Must have evidence of ROTI (end-organ damage) that can be attributed to the plasma cell proliferative process; manifested by CRAB (calcium, renal failure, anemia, and bone lesions).

146. Ans. (a) CD1

Ref: Robbin's Pathology, 9th ed. pg. 590

- Langerhans cells are characterized by two types of markers: an ultrastructural marker, the **Birbeck granule** and different membrane markers: **HLA-D antigens, T4 antigen, and some of the CD1 antigens.**
- These antigens which are specific for the epidermal Langerhans cells, are not expressed by the other epidermal cells. Three CD1 antigens are biochemically defined on human thymocytes, they display a glycoprotein chain non covalently attached to beta-2-microglobulin.

147. Ans. (a) Iron

Ref: Robbin's Pathology, 9th ed. pg. 631, 649

148. Ans. (d) Viral or protozoal infection

Ref: Robbin's Pathology, 9th ed. pg. 582-83

- Leucocytosis is seen with viral infections on account of increase in number of natural killer cells.

Leucopenia MNEMONIC _ VINDICATE

V- Vascular causes like MI
I- Infection like sepsis
N- Neoplasm like CLL
D-
I- DRUG INTOXICATION like lithium
C- Congenital like DOWN
A- Autoimmune like polyarteritis nodosa.
T- Trauma
E - Endocrinologic causes like cushing's disease

149. Ans. (b) Africa

Ref: Robbin's Pathology, 9th ed. pg. 588

- Globally, Burkitt lymphoma (BL) is endemic in certain regions of equatorial Africa and other tropical locations between latitudes 10° south and 10° north. Incidence in these areas of endemic disease is 100 per million children.
- Epstein-Barr virus (EBV) infection is found in nearly all areas. In endemic areas, there seems to be a correlation with the geographic distribution of endemic malaria.

- Malaria infection also probably plays a role in the pathogenesis of BL, as it can lead to inhibition of EBV-specific immune response. The exact mechanism of EBV-mediated lymphomagenesis, however, is not well understood, but evidence exists for a significant interaction between viral and cellular microRNA (miRNA) interfering with normal gene expression and translation. EBV can be detected in 25–40% of immunodeficiency-associated cases.

150. Ans. (c) Chronic renal failure

Ref: Robbin's Pathology, 9th ed. pg. 631-35, 638

- The same question was asked in different exams with different choices.
- Choices a, b, d are examples of hemolytic anemias and hence the answer by exclusion is chronic renal failure.
- CRF has low erythropoietin levels due to less production and has normocytic normochromic anaemia.

151. Ans. (a) GLUT 1

Ref: Harrison's, 19th ed. pg. 2402

Basic Rule

- **GLUT 1 and 3** = Everywhere in body (for Basal Absorption of Glucose) including RBC
- **GLUT 2** = In liver and pancreas
- **GLUT 4** = In muscle and adipose

Energy-yielding metabolism in erythrocytes depends on a constant supply of glucose from the blood plasma, where the glucose concentration is maintained at about 5 mm. Glucose enters the erythrocyte by facilitated diffusion via a specific glucose transporter, at a rate about 50,000 times greater than un-catalyzed transmembrane diffusion.

152. Ans. (a) Chronic ITP

Ref: Robbin's Pathology, 9th ed. pg. 658-59

- Splenectomy may be done in patients with chronic ITP, as platelets which have been bound by antibodies are taken up by macrophages in the spleen (which have Fc receptors).
- The procedure is potentially risky in ITP cases due to the increased possibility of significant bleeding during surgery.
- Durable remission following splenectomy is achieved in 60–65% of ITP cases, less so in older subjects. However, the use of splenectomy to treat ITP has diminished since the development of steroid therapy and other pharmaceutical remedies.

FMGE Solutions Screening Examination

Remember

Drug treatment in ITP
- *Steroids* and steroid sparing agents
- *Anti–D:* Suitable for Rh-positive, non-splenectomized patients is intravenous administration of Rho(D) immune globulin. Following administration, anti-D-coated red blood cell complexes saturate Fcγ receptor sites on macrophages, resulting in preferential destruction of red blood cells, therefore sparing antibody-coated platelets.
- *Romiplostim:* A thrombopoiesis stimulating Fc-peptide fusion protein that is administered by subcutaneous injection.
- *Eltrombopag* is an orally-administered agent with an effect similar to that of romiplostim. It too has been demonstrated to increase platelet counts and decrease bleeding in a dose-dependent manner.

153. Ans. (a) Prothrombin time

Ref: Robbin's Pathology, 9th ed. pg. 116-18

Prothrombin time	Extrinsic pathway	Factor 5/7
Activated partial thromboplastin time	Intrinsic pathway	Factor 8
Bleeding time	Platelet function and platelet count	Platelet function and count

154. Ans. (b) Human parvo virus B19

Ref: Robbin's Pathology, 9th ed. pg. 635-36

- Human parvo virus B19 is responsible for aplastic crisis that can be life threatening in cases of sickle cell anaemia and hereditarty spherocytosis. It is treated with blood transfusion.
- **Remember:** Parvovirus infection in pregnant women is associated with hydrops fetalis due to severe fetal anemia, sometimes leading to miscarriage or stillbirth. The risk of fetal loss is about 10% if infection occurs before pregnancy week 20 (*especially between weeks 14 and 20*), but minimal after then.

155. Ans. (a) Controlling oxidative stress on RBC

Ref: Robbin's Pathology, 9th ed. pg. 634

- G6PD helps in neutralizing the effect of oxidative stress on the RBC.
- Oxidative stress is induced by drugs like primaquine and hence in patients of G6PD there is accelerated hemolysis (intravascular during the hemolytic episode) resulting in hemoglobinuria and passage of shockingly black urine by the patient.

156. Ans. (a) Anemia of chronic disease

Ref: Robbin's Pathology, 9th ed. pg. 652

- In anemia of chronic disease, in response to inflammatory cytokines, the liver produces increased amounts of hepcidin.
- Hepcidin in turn causes increased internalisation of ferroportin molecules on cell membranes *which prevents release from iron stores.*
- Since stores of iron are un-utilized, serum ferritin is increased. TIBC levels are inverse of serum ferritin.
- Low serum iron and low ferritin levels with an elevated TIBC are diagnostic of iron deficiency.

157. Ans. (a) Pernicious anemia

Ref: Robbin's Pathology, 9th ed. pg. 647-648

- Since **hypersegmented neutrophils** are seen with oval RBC at 6 o'clock to neutrophils the answer is pernicious anemia.

158. Ans. (b) Resistant to denaturation by alkali

Ref: Robbin's Pathology, 9th ed. pg. 635

- Fetal blood contains fetal hemoglobin composed of **two alpha and two gamma subunits.**
- This difference in composition gives the different types of hemoglobin different chemical properties.
- Fetal hemoglobin is resistant to alkali (basic) denaturation, whereas adult hemoglobin is susceptible to such denaturation. Therefore, exposing the blood specimen to sodium hydroxide (NaOH) will denature the adult but not the fetal hemoglobin. The fetal hemoglobin will appear as a pinkish color under the microscope while the adult hemoglobin will appear as a yellow-brownish color.

159. Ans. (c) 60 days

Ref: Harrison, 18th ed. /ch. 113

- Life span of transfused RBC is **60-80** days
- Life span of fetal RBC = 100 days
- Life span of neutrophil = 6 hours
- Life span of neutrophil in tissues= 6 days
- Life span of platelets = 5–7 day
- Life span of transfused platelets = 2–3 days

160. Ans. (a) HUS

Ref: Robbin's Pathology, 9th ed. pg. 644

Characteristic of Schistocytes/Helmet Cells
- Fragmented part of a red blood cell.
- Irregularly shaped, jagged, and have two pointed ends
- Does not have central pallor.

Seen in
- Hemolytic uremic syndrome

Pathology

- Thrombotic thrombocytopenic purpura
- Disseminated intravascular coagulation
- Metallic prosthetic valves

161. Ans. (d) Macrocytic anemia

Ref: Robbin's Pathology, 9th ed. pg. 638

- Thalassemia major presents before 1 year of age with severe anemia which necessitates packed RBC transfusions every 2–3 months. The child is said to be transfusion dependent as survival is decided by RBC being transfused.
- The ineffective erythropoiesis in bone marrow results in shift of hematopoiesis to liver and the bone marrow. Hence the liver and spleen enlarge in size. But the net result is defective microcytes being produced. The type of anaemia is *microcytic hypochromic anaemia.*
- **Remember: causes of macrocytic anaemia: "ABCDEF":**
  - Alcohol + liver disease
  - B12 deficiency
  - Compensatory reticulocytosis (blood loss and hemolysis)
  - Drug (cytotoxic and AZT)/ Dysplasia (marrow problems)
  - Endocrine (hypothyroidism)
  - Folate deficieny/Fetus (pregnancy)

162. Ans. (a) Anemia of chronic disease

Ref: Robbin's Pathology 9th ed. pg. 652

Parameter	Iron deficiency anemia	Sideroblastic anemia	Anemia of chronic disease
Serum iron	Low	High	Low
Serum ferritin	Low	High	High
T.I.B.C	Increased	Decreased	Low

163. Ans. (a) Brilliant cresyl blue

Ref: Robbin's Pathology, 9th ed. pg. 631-32

- Reticulocytes are immature red blood cells, typically composing about 1% of the red cells in the human body. Reticulocytes develop and mature in the red bone marrow and then circulate for about a day in the blood stream before developing into mature red blood cells. Like mature red blood cells, reticulocytes do not have a cell nucleus. **They are called reticulocytes because of a reticular (mesh-like) network of ribosomal RNA that becomes visible under a microscope with certain stains.**
- **The most common supravital stain is performed on reticulocytes using new methylene blue or**

brilliant cresyl blue, which makes it possible to see the reticulofilamentous pattern of ribosomes characteristically precipitated in these live immature red blood cells by the supravital stains.

- By counting the number of such cells the rate of red blood cell formation can be determined, providing an insight into bone marrow activity and anemia.

164. Ans. (b) Ferritin

Ref: Robbin's Pathology, 9th ed. pg. 650

- *Ferritin is the storage and transferrin is the transport form of iron.*
- Hepcidin is released by liver in setting of anemia of chronic disease. Ferroportin is a transmembrane protein that transports iron from the inside of a cell to the outside of it.
- **Remember:** Ferroportin is inhibited by hepcidin, which binds to ferroportin and internalises it within the cell. This results in the retention of iron within cells, and a reduction in iron levels within the plasma. This is especially significant in enterocytes which are shed at the end of their lifespan where ferroportin is expressed on the basolateral membranes. The extra iron retained within them is not only prevented from entering the bloodstream but ends up being excreted into the faeces. *Hepcidin is thus the "master regulator" of human iron metabolism.*
- In the setting of anemia, low serum ferritin is the most specific lab test for iron deficiency anemia. However, it is less sensitive, since its levels are increased in the blood by infection or any type of chronic inflammation, and these conditions may convert what would otherwise be a low level of ferritin from lack of iron, into a value in the normal range. For this reason, low ferritin levels carry more information than those in the normal range. *Low ferritin may also indicate hypothyroidism, vitamin C deficiency or celiac disease.*

165. Ans. (a) Nodular sclerosis

Ref: Robbin's Pathology, 9th ed. pg. 607-610

TABLE: Types of Hodgkins lymphoma

Nodular sclerosis	*It is the most common subtype* and is composed of large tumor nodules showing scattered lacunar classical RS cells set in a background of reactive lymphocytes, eosinophils and plasma cells with varying degrees of collagen fibrosis/sclerosis

Contd...

Mixed cellularity	**Most common format seen in India;** also the most common in HIV positive patients. Biopsy shows classic Reed Sternberg cells
Lymphocyte depleted	*It is a rare subtype,* composed of large numbers of often pleomorphic RS cells with only few reactive lymphocytes which may easily be confused with diffuse large cell lymphoma. Many cases previously classified within this category would now be reclassified under anaplastic large cell lymphoma
Lymphocyte rich	Good/best prognosis
Nodular lymphocytic predominant	Expresses CD_{20}, and is classified as a form of non-classical Hodgkin's.

- Microscopic examination of the lymph node biopsy reveals complete or partial effacement of the lymph node architecture by scattered large malignant cells known *as Reed–Sternberg cells* (RSC) admixed within a reactive cell infiltrate composed of variable proportions of lymphocytes, histiocytes, eosinophils, and plasma cells.
- The Reed–Sternberg cells are identified as large often bi-nucleated cells with prominent nucleoli and an unusual $CD45^-$, $CD30^+$, $CD15^{+/-}$ immunophenotype. In approximately 50% of cases, the Reed–Sternberg cells are infected by the Epstein–Barr virus.
- Characteristics of classic Reed–Sternberg cells include large size (20–50 micrometres), abundant, amphophilic, finely granular/homogeneous cytoplasm; two mirror-image nuclei *(owl eyes)* each with an eosinophilic nucleolus and a thick nuclear membrane (chromatin is distributed close to the nuclear membrane).

166. Ans. (a) Pre B cell

Ref: Robbin's Pathology, 9th ed. pg. 590-93

- **Most common subtype of ALL is L1 according to older classification and Pre B cell variety by the latest WHO classification.**
- The recent WHO International panel on ALL recommends that the FAB classification be abandoned, since the morphological classification has no clinical or prognostic relevance. It instead advocates the use of the immunophenotypic classification:

- Acute lymphoblastic leukemia/lymphoma.
  - Synonyms: Former Fab L1/L2

Precursor B Acute Lymphoblastic Leukemia/Lymphoma. Cytogenetic Subtypes
1. t(12;21)(p12,q22)
2. t(1;19)(q23;p13)
3. t(9;22)(q34;q11)
4. t(V,11)(V;q23)

Precursor T Acute Lymphoblastic Leukemia/Lymphoma
- Burkitt's leukemia/lymphoma. Synonyms: Former FAB L3
- Biphenotypic acute leukemia

167. Ans. (a) Aplastic anemia

Ref: Robbin's Pathology, 9th ed. pg. 631

- **Aplastic anemia is characterized by destruction of bone marrow and thereby reduction in pluri-potent stem cells and their progeny.** Henceforth the production of reticulocytes is less.
- Thalassemia and sickle cells are hemolytic anemias having extra-vascular hemolysis and thereby reticulocytosis.
- In chronic blood loss the loss of RBC provoke the bone marrow to be more aggressive and release reticulocytes in circulation.
- **Remember:** Reticulocytopenia may be a result of viral Parvovirus B19 infection, which invades and destroys red blood cell precursors and halts the red cell production.

168. Ans. (a) EBV

Ref: Robbin's Pathology, 9th ed. pg. 588-90, 606

EBV	Nasopharyngeal cancer, Burkitt lymphoma, Hodgkins and non-Hodgkin lymphoma; Infectious mononucleosis (Paul Bunnel test).
CMV	CMV retinitis
HHV 6	Primary effusion lymphoma
HHV 8	Kaposi sarcoma

169. Ans. (d) Chronic lymphocytic leukemia

Ref: Robbin's Pathology, 9th ed. pg. 324-325

Cancers associated with radiation:
- ALL, AML, CML
- Thyroid cancer
- Breast cancer
- Lung cancer
- Bladder, ovarian cancer

Cancers not seen with radiation:
- CLL
- Hodgkin's lymphoma
- Prostate cancer, testis cancer and cervical cancer

Pathology

170. Ans. (a) Ig G

Ref: Robbin's Pathology, 9ᵗʰ ed. pg. 598-99

- The over production of light chains of IgG is the most common abnormality in multiple myeloma. In Waldenstrom cryoglobulinemia, IgM is overproduced.
- Most common presentation of multiple myeloma is anemia > bone pain.
- Least common presentation of multiple myeloma is hyperviscosity
- Investigation of choice for multiple myeloma is bone marrow biopsy
- Screening test for multiple myeloma is serum electro-phoresis showing M spike
- Most common cause of death in multiple myeloma is infections
- Most common cause of kidney damage in multiple myeloma is hypercalcemia.

CARDIOVASCULAR PATHOLOGY

171. Ans. (c) Hyper-eosinophilia of myocytes

Ref: Robbins E-Book, P 853

HISTOPATHOLOGICAL CHANGES AFTER MI

- First half an hour no changes are seen, which is followed by glycogen depletion and development of waviness of fibers.
- Between 12- and 24-hours H*yper-eosinophilia* of the cytoplasm of myocytes as assessed by hematoxylin-eosin staining is characteristic of myocardial damage.
- *Neutrophil infiltration* is present by 24 hours at the border areas.
- As the infarct progresses between 24 and 48 hours, *coagulation necrosis* is established, with various degrees of nuclear pyknosis, early karyorrhexis, and karyolysis.
- The myocyte striations are preserved and the sarcomeres elongate. The border areas show prominent neutrophil infiltration by 48 hours.
- At 3-5 days, the central portion of the infarct shows loss of myocyte nuclei and striations; in smaller infarcts, neutrophils invade the infarct and fragment, resulting in more *severe karyorrhexis* (nuclear dust).
- By 5-7 days, *macrophages and fibroblasts begin to appear* in the border areas.
- By 1 week, neutrophils decline and *granulation tissue is established with neo-capillary invasion* and lymphocytic and plasma cell infiltration.

172. Ans. (b) McCallum patch

Ref: Robbins 9th ed. P 557-59

- Acute rheumatic mitral valvulitis leads to chordal elongation and defective cooptation of valve leaflets.

- This leads to a posterolaterally directed jet of mitral regurgitation which is directed towards an area of fibrotic thickening on posterior left atrial wall.
- This *fibrotic thickening in left atrium is called McCallum patch.*

173. Ans. (a) Cardiac failure

Rheumatic endocarditis leads to death most commonly due to cardiac failure.

Causes of Mortality in RHD (Decreasing Incidence wise):

- CHF
- Bacterial endocarditis
- Cerebral embolism of left atrial appendage
- Coronary insufficiency

174. Ans. (a) Stretching and waviness of fibers

Time frame	Light microscopy
0–6 hours	No change, stretching and waviness of fibres
6–12 hours	Coagulative necrosis begins with neutrophilic infiltration
48–72 hours	Coagulative necrosis is complete
3ʳᵈ–7ᵗʰ day	Initiation of resorption of necrosed fibres and fibrovascular response
3ʳᵈ week	Necrosed muscles removed and in growth of fibrocollagenous tissue.

175. Ans. (a) Myxoma

- The most common primary tumour of the heart is myxoma. It constitutes 50% of all primary cardiac tumours.
- Most common site is left atrium.
- Most common tumour of heart is metastasis from lung cancer.
- Most common tumour of heart valves is papillary elastoma

176. Ans. (a) Lungs

Ref: Robbin's Pathology, 9ᵗʰ ed. pg. 529-30

- In left ventricular failure, the pooling of blood in lungs will lead to development of pulmonary edema which causes hypoxia and findings of dysnea, orthopnea, pink frothy sputum and death. Hence, lungs are immediately affected following LVF.

Explanations

FMGE Solutions Screening Examination

- Subsequently due to low BP the kidneys shall be affected and in severe LVF brain perfusion shall also be affected.

177. Ans. (a) Aschoff nodules

Ref: Robbin's Pathology, 9th ed. pg. 558

- The pathognomonic feature of rheumatic fever is *aschoff nodules*. They are the foci of eosinophilic staining collagen surrounded by *T–lymphocytes*, plasma cells and plump macrophages called Anitschkow cells.
- The Anitschkow cells have abundant cytoplasm and central round to ovoid nucleus in which chromatin has wavy ribbon fashion because of which they are called *caterpillar cells*
- The involvement of endocardium by aschoff nodules along the line of closure of valves leads to improper closure of leaflets. This leads to *leakage of blood which hits the free wall of left atria* and leads to *Macullum's patch*.

178. Ans. (c) Reversible injury within 20–40 minutes

Ref: Robbin's Pathology, 9th ed. pg. 540-41

TABLE: Evolution of Morphological Changes in MI

Time	Gross findings	Light microscopy
0–30 minutes	None	None
30 minutes–4 hours	None	Waviness of fibres at border
4–12 hours	Occasional dark mottling	Beginning of coagulative necrosis, oedema, haemorrhage
12–24 hours	Dark mottling	Ongoing coagulative necrosis, marginal band contraction necrosis and beginning of neutrophilic infiltration

TABLE: Myocardial response

Feature	Time
Cessation of aerobic respiration or onset of ATP depletion	Seconds
ATP reduced to 50% of normal	10 minutes
Irreversible cell injury	20–40 minutes
Microvascular injury	>1 hour

179. Ans. (d) Necrosis

Ref: Robbin's Pathology, 9th ed. pg. 512-15

TABLE: Complications of Atherosclerosis and their Importance

Aneurysm formation	Aortic aneurysm >5.5 cm can rupture
Calcification	Dystrophic calcification
Ulceration	Increases thrombus formation
Thrombosis	Occlusion of coronary arteries
Embolism	Erosion of plaque

180. Ans. (b) Deep Vein thrombosis

Ref: Robbin's Pathology, 9th ed. pg. 512-15; Robbins, 8th ed. pg. 517

- Buerger disease is associated with HLA B-5 and HLA-A9.
- In thromboangiitis obliterans there is acute and chronic segmental inflammation of vessels with thrombosis in the lumen
- Typically, the thrombus contains microabscesses with a central focus of neutrophils surrounded by inflammation
- Later, the inflammatory process extends into contiguous veins and nerves and in time all the arteries, veins and nerves become encased in fibrous tissue, a characteristic that is very rare with vasculitis.

181. Ans. (b) Troponin C is present in both cardiac and smooth muscle

Ref: Harrison, 19th ed. pg. 265e-7

- Troponins of cardiac origin are regulatory proteins that control the calcium mediated interaction of Actin and Myosin.
- The troponin complex consists of three subunits: Troponin T, which binds to Tropomyosin and facilitates contractions; Troponin I, which binds to Actin and inhibits Actin/Myosin interaction; and Troponin C, which binds the calcium ions.
- The amino acid sequence of the skeletal and cardiac isoforms of Troponin T and Troponin I are sufficiently dissimilar and therefore detectable by monoclonal antibody assay.
- *Troponin C is not used clinically because both cardiac and smooth muscles share Troponin C isoforms.*

Pathology

182. Ans. (c) Granulation with type 4 collagen

Ref: Robbin's Pathology, 9th ed. pg. 540-43

Time	Gross examination	Histopathology (light microscopy)
0–0.5 hours	None	None
0.5–4 hours	None	Glycogen depletion, as seen with a PAS stain Possibly waviness of fibers at border
4–12 hours	Sometimes dark mottling	Initiation of coagulation necrosis Edema Hemorrhage
12–24 hours	Dark mottling	Ongoing coagulation necrosis Karyopyknosis Hypereosinophilia of myocytes Contraction band necrosis in margins Beginning of neutrophil infiltration
1–3 days	Infarct center becomes yellow-tan	Continued coagulation necrosis Loss of nuclei and striations Increased infiltration of neutrophils to interstitium
3–7 days	Hyperemia at border Softening yellow-tan center	Beginning of disintegration of dead muscle fibers Necrosis of neutrophils Beginning of macrophage removal of dead cells at border
7–10 days	Maximally soft and yellow-tan Red-tan margins	Increased phagocytosis of dead cells at border Beginning of granulation tissue formation at margins
10–34 days	Red-gray and depressed borders	*Mature granulation tissue with type I collagen*
2–8 weeks	Gray-white granulation tissue	Increased collagen deposition Decreased cellularity
More than 2 months	Completed scarring	Dense collagenous scar formed

183. Ans. (b) Myxoma

Ref: Robbin's Pathology, 9th ed. pg. 575-76

- **MC tumor of heart:** Secondaries
- MC site of primary for cardiac secondaries: Lungs
- Most common **primary** neoplasm of heart in **adult: Myxoma**
- Most common **primary** neoplasm of heart in **child: Rhabdomyoma**
- Most common **malignant** cancer of heart in adults: Angiosarcoma
- Most common **malignant** cancer of heart in children: Rhabdomyosarcoma
- Myxoma is a soft mass, consisting of edematous connective tissue irregularly covered by thrombus, commonly attached to the endocardium by a pedicle, and hanging free into a cavity, **usually the left atrium. (MC site of myxoma: Left atrium)**
- It may block the mitral orifice, producing a murmur similar to that of mitral stenosis.
- Embolism from the surface of the neoplasm or an overlying thrombus is common.
- The papillary fibroelastoma is very rare and occurs on heart valves. **Therefore most common cardiac valve tumor is papillary fibroelastoma.**

> **Extra Mile**
> - *MC site of myxoma: Left atrium*
> - *MC site of rhabdomyoma: Left ventricle*
> - Myxoma is MC seen in **females**
> - **MC age group of myxoma:** 3rd– 6th decade

184. Ans. (d) Metastasis

Ref: Robbin's Pathology, 9th ed. pg. 575-76

Please refer to above explanation

185. Ans. (c) Left ventricle

Ref: Robbin's Pathology 9th ed. pg. 575-76

Please refer to above explanation

186. Ans. (c) Papillary fibroelastoma

Ref: Robbin's Pathology, 9th ed. pg. 575-77

Please refer to above explanation

187. Ans. (a) Syphilitic aneurysm

Ref: Harrison, 19th ed. pg. 1638

- Syphilitic aortitis, an inflammatory aortitis involving the ascending aorta, sinuses of Valsalva and the aortic valve, is observed most commonly in patients older than 50 years.

Explanations

- Syphilitic aortitis is associated with aortic insufficiency, ascending aortic aneurysms, and a positive serologic test for syphilis. In these patients, angina resulting from occlusion of the ostia of the coronary vessels also can be present.
- Calcification occurs in a linear pattern along the ascending aorta.
- On gross specimen examination, the aorta has been described as revealing a "tree-bark" appearance.

188. Ans. (c) Fibrinous

Ref: Robbin's Pathology, 9th ed. pg. 557-56

An exudate is any fluid that filters from the circulatory system into lesions or areas of inflammation.

Types of Exudate

- Purulent or suppurative exudate consists of plasma with both active and dead neutrophils, fibrinogen, and necrotic parenchymal cells. This kind of exudate is consistent with more severe infections, and is commonly referred to as pus.
- Fibrinous exudate is composed mainly of fibrinogen and fibrin. It is characteristic of rheumatic carditis, but is seen in all severe injuries such as strep throat and bacterial pneumonia. Fibrinous inflammation is often difficult to resolve due to the fact that blood vessels grow into the exudate and fill the space that was occupied by fibrin. Often, large amounts of antibiotics are necessary for resolution.
- Catarrhal exudate is seen in the nose and throat and is characterized by a high content of mucus.
- Serous exudate (sometimes classified as serous transudate) is usually seen in mild inflammation, with little protein content. Its consistency resembles that of serum, and can usually be seen in certain disease states like tuberculosis.

189. Ans. (c) Diabetic glomerulosclerosis

Ref: Robbin's Pathology, 9th ed. pg. 509-510, 558

Fibrinoid necrosis is a distinctive morphological pattern of cell injury characterized by deposition of fibrin like proteinaceous material in walls of arteries. Areas of fibrinoid necrosis appear as smudgy eosinophilic regions with obscured underlying cellular details.

Fibrinoid necrosis is seen in:
- Malignant hypertension
- Vasculitis like PAN
- Acute rheumatic fever

190. Ans (b) Small- or medium-sized muscular arteries

Ref: Robbin's Pathology, 9th ed. pg. 506-507

- PAN typically involves small- to medium-sized muscular arteries. In contrast, large arteries and the aorta are involved in Takayasu arteritis.
- Small arteries and arterioles are involved in a number of other diseases, including systemic lupus erythematosus.
- Active lesions in PAN demonstrate a neutrophilic infiltration of the involved vessel wall with thrombosis and segmental, fibrinoid necrosis. Intermittent healing produces fibrosis of the arterial wall and intimal thickening, which may lead to obstruction and infarction.
- Aneurysmal dilations may arise as a result of asymmetrical involvement. Although the lesions in PAN resemble other immune mediated vascular lesions, the exact etiology of the disorder has not been elucidated.
- PAN generally affects middle-aged men and has a poor prognosis, although steroids may be beneficial.

191. Ans. (c) Monckeberg's sclerosis

Ref: Robbin's Pathology, 9th ed. pg. 491

- Monckeberg's arteriosclerosis, also called medial calcific sclerosis, is a form of arteriosclerosis or vessel hardening, where calcium deposits form in the middle layer of the walls of medium sized vessels (the tunica media)
- It is usually more benign than other forms of arteriosclerosis because it does not cause narrowing of the lumen, but can still be associated with important medical conditions. Monckeberg's arteriosclerosis is most commonly found in the radial or ulnar arteries causing "pipestem" arteries, which will present as a bounding pulse.
- It is associated with trophic foot ulceration and peripheral artery occlusive disease.
- Its presence predicts risk of cardiovascular events and leg amputation in diabetic patients.

192. Ans. (d) SLE

Ref: Robbin's Pathology, 9th ed. pg. 506, 509-10

Large vessel vasculitis	Medium vessel vasculitis	Small vessel vasculitis
• Giant cell arteritis • Takayasu's arteritis	• Classic PAN • Kawasaki • Buerger disease	**Immune complex mediated** • SLE • HSP • Cryoglobulin vasculitis • Good pasture syndrome **Pauci- immune** • Wegener's granulomatosis • Microscopic polyangitis • Churg Strauss syndrome

Pathology

LUNGS

193. Ans. (d) Bronchial asthma

Ref: Robbin's Pathology, 9th ed. pg. 682

Findings in Bronchial Asthma in Broncho-Alveolar Lavage or in Sputum

- **Curschmann spirals**, is a finding in bronchial asthma which may result from extrusion of mucus plugs from subepithelial mucous gland ducts or bronchioles.
- **Charcot-Leyden crystals**: It is composed of an eosinophilic protein called **galectin-10.**

The other characteristic histologic findings of asthma, collectively called "airway remodeling" include:

- Airway wall thickenig
- An increase in the size of the submucosal glands and number of airway goblet cells
- Subbasement membrane fibrosis (*due to deposition of type I and III collagen*)
- Increased vascularity
- Hypertrophy and/or hyperplasia of the bronchial wall muscle

194. Ans. (c) Liver

Rich focus	Cortex of brain
Simon focus	Healed site of primary infection at lungs apex
Simmond focus	Liver
Weigart focus	Intima of blood vessels

195. Ans. (c) Eosinophilic infiltration of airways

Ref: Robbin's Pathology, 9th ed. pg. 678-679

- Chronic bronchitis is characterised by **lymphocytic infiltration** of airways coupled with submucosal gland hypertrophy
- **Reid's index** is ratio of mucus gland layer thickness to thickness of wall between epithelium and cartilage. Normal value is 0.4 and is increased in chronic bronchitis
- Bronchorrhea is due to low grade infection since the ciliated columnar epithelium and Muco-ciliary clearance is compromised.

> **Extra Mile**
> - **Earliest feature of chronic bronchitis:** Mucus hypersecretion in large airways
> - Reid index increased in chronic bronchitis (*normal = 0.4*)

196. Ans. (c) Bloody pleural effusion

Ref: Robbin's Pathology, 9th ed. pg. 688-690

- Silicosis is a nodular fibrosing disease due to inhalation of silica, and is the most common chronic occupational disease in world.
- Mostly the form implicated is Quartz.
- Involvement of upper lobes of the lungs
- **CXR:** shows presence of **egg shell calcification**
- Polarised microscopy shows presence of birefringent silica particles

197. Ans. (a) Sarcoidosis

Ref: Harrison, 19th ed. pg. 2210

The **Kveim-Siltzbach test** is a skin test used to detect sarcoidosis, where part of a spleen from a patient with known sarcoidosis is injected into the skin of a patient suspected to have the disease. If noncaseating granulomas are found (4–6 weeks later), the test is positive.

198. Ans. (c) Sarcoidosis

Ref: Robbin's Pathology, 9th ed. pg. 693

- Schaumann body is laminated concretions of calcium and protein, which is a characteristic finding of sarcoidosis.

Findings of Sarcoidosis:

- Non-necrotizing granulomas
- Asteroid body
- Schaumann body

> **Extra Mile**
> **Sarcoidosis**
> - **MC clinical presentation of sarcoidosis: Bilateral hilar lymphadenopathy (90% of cases) > Eye**
> - **Sarcoidosis MC seen in patients below 40 years (F > M)**
> - **Marker of disease activity: TNF concentration in broncho-alveolar fluid**
> - **Mikulicz syndrome:** Bilateral sarcoidosis of parotid, sub-maxillary and sublingual gland.

199. Ans. (b) Hilar lymphadenopathy

Ref: Robbin's Pathology, 9th ed. pg. 692-93

200. Ans. (c) Asbestosis

Ref: Robbin's Pathology, 9th ed. pg. 690-92

FMGE Solutions Screening Examination

- Sufferers may experience severe dyspnea (shortness of breath) and are at an increased risk for certain malignancies, including lung cancer but especially mesothelioma.
- **The most common anatomical site for mesothelioma is the pleura,** but it can also arise in the peritoneum, the pericardium or the tunica vaginalis.
- Most people who develop mesothelioma have worked in jobs where they inhaled or ingested asbestos fibers, or were exposed to airborne asbestos dust and fibers in other ways. Washing clothes of a family member who worked with asbestos also creates a risk for developing mesothelioma.
- *Unlike lung cancer, there seems to be **no** association between mesothelioma and tobacco smoking,* but smoking greatly increases the risk of other asbestos-induced cancers.

> **Extra Mile**
> - Anthracosis is a pneumoconiosis, which is seen among coal workers.
> - There is no association between anthracosis and development of tuberculosis or lung cancer.

201. Ans. (d) Adenocarcinoma

Ref: Robbin's, 9th ed. pg. 714–15

According to Robbins 9th ed. the frequency of major lung cancer and their proportion are:
- Adenocarcinoma (38%)
- Squamous cell carcinoma (20%)
- Small cell carcinoma (14%)
- Large cell carcinoma (3%)
- Other (25%)

> **Extra Mile**
> **LUNG CA**
> - MC CA overall: lung CA
> - MC CA causing death: lung CA
> - MC risk factor for lung CA: Smoking
> - Peak age for development for lung CA: 50–60's
> - MC lung cancer in females: Adenocarcinoma
> - Most aggressive type of lung CA: Small cell lung CA
> - Lung CA MC associated with paraeoplastic syndrome: Small cell lung CA
> - Lung CA associated with smoking: Squamous cell CA and small cell lung CA
> - Centrally located lung CA: Squamous cell CA and small cell lung CA
> - Peripherally located lung CA: Adenocarcinoma and large cell CA

202. Ans. (b) Adenocarcinoma

Ref: Robbin's, 9th ed. pg. 714–15

203. Ans. (c) Small cell lung CA

Ref: Robbin's Pathology, 9th ed. pg. 717

- **Small cell carcinoma** is a highly malignant tumor with a strong relationship to cigarette smoking.
- **Around** 1% occurs in nonsmokers.
- They are the most aggressive of lung tumors, metastasizing widely and are always fatal.

204. Ans. (c) Small cell lung CA

Ref: Robbin's Pathology, 9th ed. pg. 717

- **Azzopardi effect** is basophilic staining of vascular walls due to encrustation by DNA from necrotic tumor cells.
- It is seen in small cell lung carcinoma.

205. Ans. (b) Adenocarcinoma lung

Ref: Robbin's Pathology, 9th ed. pg. 690–92

- The answer has been triple checked from standard textbooks and is a denocarcinoma.
- *Mesothelioma is mentioned as associated with asbestosis but not most common.*

KIDNEY

206. Ans. (a) Kimmel stein Wilson Change

Ref: Robbins E-Book, P 781

- The characteristic finding of Diabetic nephropathy is Kimmelstein Wilson change and is also referred as nodular glomerulosclerosis.
- Most common light microscopy finding is diffuse diabetic glomerulopathy. Large acellular accumulations also may be observed within these areas. These are circular on section and are known as the Kimmelstiel-Wilson lesions/nodules.
- *Armani-Ebstein change* consists of deposits of glycogen in the tubular epithelial cells (pars straight of proximal convoluted tubule and loop of Henle).

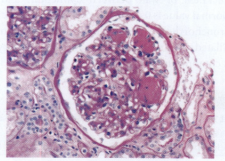

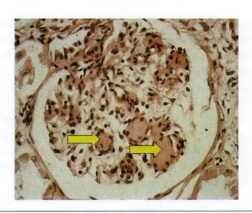

207. Ans. (b) Kidney

- *Fatty change is particularly common in the liver but may occur in other non – fatty tissues as well, e.g. in the heart, skeletal muscle, kidneys (lipoid nephrosis or minimum change disease) and other organs.*
- Fatty change, steatosis or fatty metamorphosis is the intracellular accumulation of neutral fat within parenchymal cells.
- It includes, now abandoned, terms of fatty degeneration and fatty infiltration because fatty change neither necessarily involves degeneration nor an infiltration. The deposit is in the cytosol and represents and absolute increase in the intracellular lipids.

208. Ans. (a) PSGN

- The presence of lumpy bumpy appearance due to sub-epithelial deposits is a characteristic appearance in PSGN.
- The Sub-epithelial spikes on electron microscopy are a feature of membranous glomerulopathy.

209. Ans. (c) RPGN

Type	Clinical features	Pathogenesis	Pathology LM	Pathology EM
Acute GN	Acute nephrotic syndrome	Immune complex disease (local or circulating)	Diffuse proliferation, leucocytic infiltration	Subepithelial deposits (humps)
RPGN	Acute renal failure	(i) Type I: anti GBM type (ii) Type II: Immune complex type (iii) Type III: Pauci-immune RPGN	Proliferation crescents[Q]	(i) Linear deposits along GBM (ii) Subepithelial deposits (iii) No deposits
Minimal change disease	Nephrotic syndrome (higher selective proteinuria)	Reduction of normal negative charge on GBM Cell-mediated mechanism	Normal glomeruli, lipid vacuolation in tubules	Loss of foot processes, no deposits
Membranous GN	Nephrotic syndrome	Immune complex disease (local)	Diffuse thickening of capillary wall	Subepithelial deposits (Spikes)
Membrano-Proliferative GN	Nephrotic syndrome	Type I: immune complex disease Type II: Dense deposit disease (alternate pathway activation) Type III: Rare, with systemic disease and drugs	Lobular proliferation of mesangial cells increased mesangial matrix, double contour of GBM	Type I: subendothelial deposits Type II: Dense intramembranous deposits Type III: Subendothelial and subepithelial deposits

210. Ans. (b) Autosomal dominant

Ref: *Robbin's Pathology, 9th ed. pg. 946*

- **ADPKD** is autosomal dominant—Polycystic kidney disease.
- Occurs due to mutation in PKD 1 and PKD 2 gene
- MC type of mutation: PKD 1. (80–85%)
- **Pathological feature:** Large multcystic kidney. It also involves commonly:
  - MC: Liver-Polycystic liver disease (40%)
  - Heart: Mitral valve prolapse (20–25%)
  - Brain: Berry aneurysm

211. Ans. (d) CMV

Ref: *Harsh Mohan, 7th ed. pg. 175*

Cytomegalic cells in vivo (presumed to be infected epithelial cells) are two to four times larger than surrounding cells and often contain an 8–10 μm intranuclear inclusion that is eccentrically placed and is surrounded by a clear halo, producing an "owl's eye" appearance.

FMGE Solutions Screening Examination

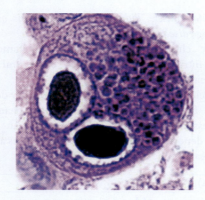

Smaller granular cytoplasmic inclusions are demonstrated occasionally. Cytomegalic cells are found in a wide variety of organs, including the salivary gland, lung, liver, kidney, intestine, pancreas, adrenal gland, and central nervous system

212. Ans. (d) Hypokalemia

Ref: Robbin's Pathology, 9th ed. pg. 1127, 1143

- Hydropic (vacuolar) degeneration results from a more severe degree of water imbibition into the cell cytoplasm.
- It occurs in some severe bacterial infections with high fever, certain types of poisoning, and hypokalemia.
- Potassium is drawn from cells and replaced by sodium and water in large amounts.
- In its most striking form, hydropic degeneration involves the renal tubular epithelium.

213. Ans. (a) Bowman's capsule

Ref: Robbin's Pathology, 9th ed. pg. 900-901

- Podocytes (or visceral epithelial cells) are cells in the Bowman's capsule in the kidneys that wrap around the capillaries of the glomerulus.
- The Bowman's capsule filters blood, holding back large molecules such as proteins, and passing through small molecules such as water, salts, and sugar, as the first step in forming urine.

214. Ans. (d) Post streptococcal GN

Ref: Robbin's Pathology, 9th ed. pg. 909-910

- PSGN is characterized by enlarged hyper-cellular glomeruli.
- There is also swelling of endothelial cells & combination of proliferation, swelling, leukocyte infiltration obliterates capillary lumen.
- Endo-capillary proliferation is also seen in MPGN

215. Ans. (a) SLE

Ref: Robbin's Pathology, 9th ed. pg. 221-225

Sub-endothelial deposits create a homogeneous thickening of the capillary wall called wire loop lesion, which can be seen by means of light microscopy when they are extensive. They usually reflect active disease.

216. Ans. (a) Acetophenetidin

Ref: Robbin's Pathology, 9th ed. pg. 423. 936t

- *Renal papillary necrosis due to acetophenetidin/phenacetin is a gradual process with slow loss of renal function.*
- The most common cause of renal papillary necrosis is diabetic glomerulopathy.

217. Ans. (d) Bilateral kidney transplantation

Ref: Robbin's Pathology, 9th ed. pg. 945-947

- The kidney transplantation is always unilateral. The left kidney is preferred for transplantation and is deployed in right iliac fossa.
- The most common extra-hepatic manifestation of polycystic kidney disease is hepatic cysts.
- ADPKD is autosomal dominant gene which is genetically heterogeneous with two genes identified: PKD1 (chromosome region 16p13.3; around 85% cases) and PKD2 (4q21; around 15% cases)

218. Ans. (a) Pyelonephritis

Causes of WBC casts	Causes of RBC Casts
• Acute pyelonephritis • Interstitial nephritis • Lupus nephritis	• Acute glomerulonephritis • Goodpasture syndrome • Lupus nephritis • Renal infarction • Right sided heart failure • Renal vein thrombosis • Polyarteritis Nodosa

219. Ans. (d) Rapidly progressive glomerulonephritis

Ref: Robbin's Pathology, 9th ed. pg. 912-915

- RBC casts are a feature of glomerular damage. Normally <3 RBC/HPF are going to leak. But in case of glomerular damage the number of RBC in urine will exceed the limit mentioned above and these RBC get impinged on tamm-horsfall protein. The resultant RBC casts can be seen under microscopic examination of urine.
- Bladder schistomiasis will cause hematuria and eosinophiluria.
- Renal vein thrombosis is a complication of severe dehydration and causes a painful enlarged kidney with hematuria.
- *Minimal change disease is the most common cause of nephritic syndrome and causes proteinuria.*

Pathology

> **Extra Mile**
>
> **Different Renal Casts and conditions where they are seen:**
> - **Hyaline cast: MC type;** seen in normal individuals in dehydration or vigorous exercise
> - **Muddy brown cast:** Seen in acute tubular necrosis
> - **Waxy casts:** Nephritic syndrome
> - **Fatty casts:** Pathognomonic for high urinary protein nephrotic syndrome.
> - **White blood cell casts:** Pyelonephritis

220. Ans. (a) Focal segmental Glomerulosclerosis

Ref: Robbin's Pathology, 9th ed. pg. 918-920

Depending on the cause, focal segmental glomerulosclerosis is broadly classified as:
- Primary, when no underlying cause is found; usually presents as nephrotic syndrome
- Secondary, when an underlying cause is identified; usually presents with kidney failure and proteinuria. *This is actually a heterogeneous group including numerous causes such as Infections such as HIV (known as HIV-Associated Nephropathy)*

Other Causes of FSGS
- Toxins and drugs such as heroin and pamidronate
- Chronic pyelonephritis
- VUR

221. Ans. (b) Cardiovascular complications

- Hypotension is the most common acute complication of hemodialysis.
- Numerous factors appear to increase the risk of hypotension, including excessive ultrafiltration with inadequate compensatory vascular filling, impaired vasoactive or autonomic responses, osmolar shifts.
- A beta 2 amyloid deposition is seen in dialysis dementia and thus rules out choice A.
- Metabolic acidosis is treated with dialysis and thus rules out choice D.
- Cardiovascular disease constitutes the major cause of death in patients with ESRD.
- Cardiovascular mortality and event rates are higher in dialysis patients than in patients post-transplantation, although rates are extraordinarily high in both populations.

222. Ans. (c) Renal cell CA

Ref: Robbin's Pathology, 9th ed. pg. 952
- Robbins 9th ed. States: "by far the **most common malignant tumor is renal cell carcinoma**, followed by Wilms tumor, which is found in children.
- Incidence of RCC is: 85%
- M > F (2:1)
- Most of the RCC are **sporadic** > AD (familial)

> **Extra Mile**
>
> **KIDNEY CA (extract from Robbins 9th ed.)**
> - MC benign tumor of kidney: Renal papillary adenoma
> - MC malignant tumor of kidney: RCC > Wilm's tumor
> - MC kidney tumor associated with tuberous sclerosis: Angiomyolipoma
> - MC type of RCC: Clear cell CA (70–80%)
> - MC type of renal CA associated with dialysis: Papillary CA
> - MC renal CA associated with sickle cell trait: Medullary CA
> - Renal CA having best prognosis: Chromophobe type

223. Ans. (c) Smoking

Ref: Robbin's Pathology, 9th ed. pg. 953

Robbins states:"Tobacco is the most significant risk factor. Cigarette smokers have double the incidence of renal cell carcinoma".

Risk factors for RCC:
- **MC risk factor: Smoking**
- **Obesity (F > M), Hypertension, asbestos exposure, CKD, tuberous sclerosis**
- **VHL (Von Hippel-Lindau syndrome):** Around half to 2/3rd of the patients with VHL develop renal cyst and bilateral RCC.

224. Ans. (d) Chromophobe

Ref: Robbin's Pathology, 9th ed. pg. 954

225. Ans. (b) Papillary CA

Ref: Robbin's Pathology, 9th ed. pg. 952-54

226. Ans. (b) Clear cell CA

Ref: Robbin's Pathology, 9th ed. pg. 952-54

227. Ans. (d) Lung

Ref: Robbins, 9th ed. pg. 946
Please refer to Explanation of Question 194.

228. Ans. (c) Liver

Ref: Robbins, 9th ed. pg. 946

229. Ans. (d) Pancreatic cyst

Ref: Robbins, 9th ed. pg. 946

Since pancreas is among the least commonly involved organs, the cause of death will also be less as compared to other mentioned conditions.

Cause of death in case of PKD *(according to Bailey 26th ed. and Robbins 9th ed.)*
- **MC cause of death:** Chronic renal failure
- Coronary/hypertensive heart disease: ~40% of cases
- Infection: 25% of cases
- Rupture of berry aneurysm: ~15% of cases

Explanations

LIVER

230. Ans. (b) Wilson disease

Mallory hyaline bodies are eosinophilic intracytoplasmic inclusions seen in peri-nuclear location with swollen and ballooned hepatocytes.

Causes of Mallory hyaline bodies are:

- Primary biliary cirrhosis
- Indian childhood cirrhosis
- Cholestatic syndrome
- Wilson disease
- Intestinal bypass surgery
- Focal nodular hyperplasia
- Hepatocellular carcinoma

231. Ans. (d) Dubin Johnson syndrome

TABLE: Causes of Hereditary Hyperbilirubinemia

Unconjugated hyperbilirubinemia	Conjugated hyperbilirubinemia
Gilbert disease (defect in ligandin leading to defective uptake of unconjugated hyperbilirubinemia)	Dubin Jonhson syndrome (Black Liver due to deposition of epinephrine).
Criggler Najar syndrome (absent UDPGT activity) Type 1 : more severe due to complete absence enzyme Type 2: less severe due to partial absence of enzyme	Rotor syndrome (Milder variant of Dubin Johnson but liver texture and color are normal).

232. Ans. (d) Photosensitivity dermatitis

Ref: Robbin's Pathology, 9th ed. pg. 650-651, 847-849

TABLE: Hereditary hyperbilirubinemias

Disorder	Inheritance	Detects in bilirubin metabolism	Liver pathology	Clinical course
Crigler-najjar syndrome type I	Autosomal recessive	Absent UGT 1A1 activity	None	Fatal in neonatal period
Crigler-Najjar syndrome type II	Autosomal dominant with variable penetrance	Decreased UGT1A1 activity	None	Generally mild, occasional kemicterus
Gilbert syndrome	Autosomal recessive	Decreased UGT1A1 activity	None	Innocuous
Conjugated hyperbilirubinemia				
Dubin-Johnson syndrome	Autosomal recessive	Impaired biliary excretion of bilirubin glucuronides due to mutation in caralicular multidrug resistance protein 2 (MRP2)	Pigmented cytoplasmic globules	Innocuous
Rotor syndrome	Autosomal recessive	Decreased hepatic uptake and storage Decreased biliary excretion	None	Innocuous
UGT1A1, Uridine diphosphate glucoronosyltransferase family, peptide A1				

PRIMARY HEMOCHROMATOSIS

In the skin, hemosiderin deposits occur in the dermis around sweat glands, and there is also an increase in melanin deposition in the epidermis.(Bronzing of skin)

- The pancreas is usually slightly enlarged, firm, and deeply pigmented. (Type 1 Diabetes Mellitus)
- The liver is usually enlarged, rusty red or ochre in color, and nodular and lobules are separated by dense fibrous tissue (Pigmentary cirrhosis)
- Restrictive cardiomyopathy

233. Ans. (c) Tuberculoma

ALPHA-FETO PROTEIN (AFP)

- It is a glycoprotein synthesized normally early in fetal life by the yolk sac, fetal liver and fetal GIT.

AFP is raised in:
- Liver cancer
- Lung cancer
- Colon cancer
- Pancreatic cancer
- Non-seminoma germ cell tumor of testis
- Cirrhosis and hepatitis
- Pregnancy

234. Ans (b) Crigler Najjar Syndrome

Ref: Robbins Pathology, 9th ed. pg. 853-54

- In **Crigler-Najjar Syndrome** due to absence of UDP glucoronyltransfersase enzyme, conjugation of bilirubin is not possible and this results in elevation of unconjugated bilirubin to very high levels in the first 24 hours of life of neonate.

Pathology

235. Ans. (d) Crigler Najjar syndrome type II

Ref: Robbins Pathology, 9th ed. pg. 853-54

236. Ans. (c) Crigler Najjar syndrome type I

Ref: Robbins Pathology, 9th ed. pg. 853-54

237. Ans. (b) Primary sclerosing cholangitis

Ref: Robbin's Pathology, 9th ed. pg. 860

PRIMARY SCLEROSING CHOLANGITIS

- Leads to obstructive jaundice leading to elevation of serum transaminases, gamma glutamyl transferase and alkaline phosphatase
- Typical onion skin fibrosis of bile ducts
- Percutaneous transhepatic cholangiography demonstrates irregularity and beading of the hepatic and common bile ducts in three patients.
  - Onion skin appearance in kidney seen in hyperplastic arteriosclerosis
  - Onion skin like lesions due to arteritis seen in Lyme's and SLE
  - Onion skin fibrosis around bile ducts seen in PSC
  - Onion skin pattern of deposition of reactive bone in ewing's sarcoma
  - Onion bulb appearance in sural nerves seen in CIDP due to recurrent demyelination and remyelination

238. Ans. (a) Adenocarcinoma of ampulla of Vater

The complications of gallstones include gangrenous cholecystitis by pressure on the mucosa and blood vessels in an acutely inflamed gallbladder

- Cholangitis by blocking the major biliary ducts and allowing bacteria to ascend into the liver
- Obstructive jaundice by blocking the common duct
- Acute pancreatitis by blocking the ampulla of Vater or a major pancreatic duct
- Gallstone ileus.

239. Ans. (d) Metastasis

Ref: Harrison, 19th ed. pg. 544

- Most common tumor of liver is metastasis
- Most common benign tumor of liver is cavernous hemangioma
- Most common cause of hepatocellular cancer is hepatitis B.

240. Ans. (c) Collagen type 1 & 3

Ref: Robbin's Pathology, 9th ed. pg. 823-824

- In cirrhosis, types I and III collagen and other ECM components are deposited in the space of Disse. In advanced fibrosis and cirrhosis, fibrous bands separate nodules of hepatocytes throughout the liver.
- In the normal liver, extracellular matrix (ECM) consisting of interstitial collagens (fibril-forming collagens types I, III, V, and XI) is present only in the liver capsule, in portal tracts, and around central veins. The liver has no true basement membrane; instead, a delicate framework containing type IV collagen and other proteins lies in the space between sinusoidal endothelial cells and hepatocytes (the space of Disse).

241. Ans. (c) Production of vitamin K

Ref: Robbin's Pathology, 9th ed. pg. 821

- **Vitamin K is produced by the bacteria of gut** and is used by liver for gamma carboxylation of factor 2/7/9/10.
  - Liver produces albumin which falls in liver cirrhosis producing ascites/edema.
  - Ammonia is combined with carbon dioxide to produce urea which in turn is excreted by the liver.
  - The cytochrome P450 is responsible for metabolism of drugs.

242. Ans. (c) Angiosarcoma of liver

Ref: Harrison, 19th ed. pg. 2027

Agents Leading to Angiosarcoma of Liver
- Arsenic
- Thorotrast (Liberates Alpha particles)
- Vinyl chloride

GASTROINTESTINAL TRACT

243. Ans. (d) Tropheryma whippelii

Ref: Harrison 19th ed. P 1092-93

- Whipple's disease is a malabsorption syndrome caused by Tropheryma whippelii. It is an intracellular bacteria found in gut macrophages.

Mnemonic: *WHIPPLE*
Weight loss
Hyperpigmentation
Infection with Tropheryma whippelii
PAS positive granules in macrophages
Polyarthritis
Lymphadenopathy
ESteatorrhea

FMGE Solutions Screening Examination

> **Extra Mile**
>
> IOC for Whipple's disease is small intestinal biopsy.
> Most common *heart valve* involved in Whipple's disease is aortic valve.
> Culture negative endocarditis is seen with duke' criteria not being satisfied.
> *CNS features* are in form of cognition defect progressive to dementia.
> MC extraintestinal manifestation of Whipple's disease is CNS feature of dementia.
> Current treatment is ceftriaxone for 2 weeks and oral doxycycline for 1 year.

244. Ans. (c) Menetrier's disease

- Menetrier's disease has chronic hypertrophic gastritis with foveolar cell hyperplasia. The rugosities of stomach are enlarged with atrophy of parietal cells.
- Type A gastritis is autoimmune gastritis and has body-fundus involvement.
- Type B gastritis is *H. pylori* related and involves the antrum. It is also called hyper-secretory gastritis.
- Type AB gastritis affects the mucosal region of A as well as B types and is overall the most common type of gastritis in all age groups.

245. Ans. (a) Crohn's disease

Serpiginous ulcers are features of Crohn's Disease. Pseudo-polyps are seen in ulcerative colitis.

Feature	Crohn's disease	Ulcerative colitis
Distribution	Segmental with skip areas	Continuous without skip areas
Location	Commonly terminal ileum and/or ascending colon	Commonly rectum, sigmoid colon and extending upwards
Extent	Usually involves the entire thickness of the affected segment of bowel wall	Usually superficial, confined to mucosal layer
Ulcers	Serpiginous ulcers may develop into deep fissures	Superficial mucosal ulcers without fissures
Pseudo-polyps	Rarely seen	Commonly present
Fibrosis	Common	Rare
Shortening	Due to fibrosis	Due to contraction of muscularis

246. Ans. (c) Celiac disease

Ref: Robbins, 9th ed. pg. 783

HPE Findings of Celiac Disease

- Biopsy specimens from the second portion of the duodenum or proximal jejunum, which are exposed to the highest concentrations of dietary gluten, are **generally diagnostic in celiac disease.**
- The histopathology is characterized by increased numbers of intraepithelial CD8+ T lymphocytes (**intraepithelial lymphocytosis**), crypt hyperplasia, and **villous atrophy.**

247. Ans. (b) Amylase

Ref: Sabiston, 19th ed. pg. 1524-1525, 1531; Schwartz, 9th ed. pg. 1200-1203; Bailey, 26th ed. pg. 1133-1134

PSEUDOPANCREATIC CYST

- A chronic collection of pancreatic fluid surrounded by a non-epithelialized wall of granulation tissue and fibrosis
- Pseudo-cysts account for 75% of cystic lesions of the pancreas.
- MC complication of chronic pancreatitis.

> - Located anywhere from the mediastinum to the scrotum
> - Found most often in the lesser sac or anterior para-renal space
> - Traumatic pseudocysts tend to occur anterior to the body of the gland
> - Chronic pancreatitis pseudocysts are commonly located within the substance of the gland

- Alcohol is the MC cause of pancreatitis related pseudo-cysts

Diagnosis
- No definitive laboratory findings are available to establish a diagnosis of pancreatic pseudocyst.
- *Elevated serum amylase and lipase concentrations may occur in half of these patients.*
- *Persistently elevated amylase after resolution of acute pancreatitis should prompt investigation for a pseudocyst.*
- CECT abdomen is investigation of choice for diagnosis of a pancreatic pseudocyst.

248. Ans. (d) Hypertension

Ref: Robbin's Pathology, 9th ed. pg. 884-86

- Acute pancreatitis is seen chiefly in males after age 40 and often associated with obesity and alcoholism.
- In about 50% of the cases, gallstones are also present.
- Pancreatitis occurs in about 10% of cases of hyperparathyroidism.

Pathology

- Long term thiazides can also contribute to development of pancreatitis.
- In some cases calculi resulting from the hypercalcemia of hyperparathyroidism develop in pancreatic ducts and lead to obstruction and inflammation.

249. Ans. (c) Chronic gastritis

Ref: Robbin's Pathology, 9th ed. pg. 763, 804

- Gastric polyps are not common.
  When they occur, they are usually hyperplastic polyps consisting of hyperplastic mucosal epithelium over an inflamed edematous stroma.
- They are most often seen in association with the chronic mucosal damage found in chronic gastritis.

250. Ans. (d) Pernicious anemia

Ref: Robbin's Pathology, 9th ed. pg. 764

- Antiparietal cell antibodies are found in patients with the autoimmune disease known as pernicious anemia.
- The antineutrophilic cytoplasmic antibodies are found in patients with Wegener granulomatosis.
- Wegener granulomatosis may also present with pulmonary and renal involvement but will have associated upper respiratory tract findings, e.g, sinusitis and sinus abscesses.

251. Ans. (d) Majority seen in duodenum

Ref: Robbin's Pathology, 9th ed. pg. 775-76

- Majority of gastrointestinal stromal tumours originate from stomach. The cell of origin is interstitial cell of Cajal which are present in muscularispropria.
- The useful marker is c-kit (CD 117) detectable in 95% of patients.
- PET scan is the imaging modality of choice
- Treatment is tyrosine kinase inhibitors like imatinib mesylate.

252. Ans. (d) Coagulative necrosis

Ref: Robbin's Pathology, 9th ed. pg. 795-96

- The typical flask shaped ulcer in amoebiasis is due to liquefactive necrosis affecting caecum and ascending colon and rectum.
- Once the infection spreads hematogenously from the gut to the liver it results in generation of liver abscess which has presence of anchovy sauce pus.

253. Ans. (d) Prophylactic polypectomy is recommended as standard therapy

Ref: Robbin's Pathology, 9th ed. pg. 809

- In FAP as many as >100 polyps may be present in colon, and anyone of these can turn malignant any day, hence

prophylactic colectomy is recommended as standard treatment.

- Most of the polyps are tubular polyps. In *attenuated FAP* (30 Polyps) are seen in proximal colon.
- The defect is in APC gene on chromosome 5, due to mutation in nucleotide excision base excision repair gene.

> **Extra Mile**
>
> - **Turcot Syndrome:** Adenomatous colonic polyposis +CNS tumours (2/3 medulloblastomas and 1/3 are gliomas)
> - **Gardener syndrome:** Intestinal polyps + Epidermal cysts + Fibromatosis + Osteomas

254. Ans. (d) Increased MCV of RBC

Ref: Robbin's Pathology, 9th ed. pg. 764

Type A gastritis is autoimmune gastritis. The antiparietal cell antibodies lead to decreased intrinsic factor production. This leads to decreased absorption of vitamin B_{12} and resultant increased MCV.

255. Ans. (d) Superficial spreading

Ref: Robbins's Pathology, 9th ed. pg. 772-73

256. Ans. (d) Rectum is commonly involved

Ref: Robbin's Pathology, 9th ed. pg. 798-99

- *Crohn's disease can lead to formation of perianal fistula which leads to poor perianal hygiene.*
- The stricture formation seen in Crohn's disease occurs due to transmural inflammation.
- Most common part of GIT involved is ileum in Crohn's disease and rectum is spared.

> **Extra Mile**
>
> - *Fecal lactoferrin* is a highly sensitive and specific marker for detecting intestinal inflammation.
> - *Fecal calprotectin* levels correlate well with histological inflammation and predict relapses and detect pouchitis.

257. Ans. (b) Thinning of mucosal layer

- The normal esophageal mucosa undergoes continuous cell turnover and renewal. Acute radiation esophagitis is primarily due to effects on the basal epithelial layer. This causes a thinning of the mucosa, which can progress to denudation.

Acute toxicity is manifested clinically as dysphagia, odynophagia, and substernal discomfort, and usually occurs within two to three weeks after the initiation of radiation therapy (RT). Patients may describe a sudden, sharp, severe chest pain radiating to the back.

FMGE Solutions Screening Examination

258. Ans. (a) Hemangioma

Ref: Robbin's Pathology, 9th ed. pg. 625

- Most common tumor of spleen is **hemangioma**
- Most common malignant tumor of spleen is **lymphoma**
- Most common malignant non-lymphoid tumor of spleen is **angiosarcoma**

259. Ans. (d) Stomach

Ref: Robbin's Pathology, 9th ed. pg. 773

- MALT lymphoma (MALToma) is a form of lymphoma involving the mucosa-associated lymphoid tissue (MALT), frequently of the stomach, but virtually any mucosal site can be afflicted. It is a cancer originating from B cells in the marginal zone of the MALT, and is also called extranodal marginal zone B cell lymphoma.
- Gastric MALT lymphoma is frequently associated (72–98%) with chronic inflammation as a result of the presence of *Helicobacter pylori*.

260. Ans. (a) Pseudo-polyps

Ref: Robbin's Pathology, 9th ed. pg. 798

- Pseudo-polyps are seen in ulcerative colitis. An **inflammatory pseudopolyp** is an island of normal colonic mucosa which only appears raised because it is surrounded by atrophic tissue (denuded ulcerative mucosa).
- It must be distinguished from inflammatory polyps, which are regions of inflamed and elevated mucosa surrounded by granular mucosa.

261. Ans. (a) p-ANCA

Ref: Robbin's Pathology, 9th ed. pg. 600

- p-ANCA, or Perinuclear Anti-Neutrophil Cytoplasmic Antibodies, show a perinuclear staining pattern. It is directed against myeloperoxidase.
- It is fairly specific, but not sensitive for ulcerative colitis, so is not useful as a sole diagnostic test. When measured together with Anti-saccharomyces cerevisiae antibodies (ASCA), p-ANCA has been estimated to have a specificity of 97% and a sensitivity of 48% in differentiating patients with ulcerative colitis from normal controls.
- It is also seen in about 50% of cases of Churg-Strauss syndrome
  - Primary sclerosing cholangitis
  - Microscopic polyangiitis
  - Focal necrotising and crescentic glomerulonephritis
  - Rheumatoid arthritis

CENTRAL NERVOUS SYSTEM

262. Ans. (b) Superoxide dismutase

Ref: Robbin's Pathology, 9th ed. pg. 48, 80

- Antioxidant enzymes include glutathione peroxidase, SOD and catalase.
- Deficiency of SOF 1 gene may result in motor neuron disorder.

263. Ans. (c) Hippocampus

Ref: Robbin's Pathology, 9th ed. pg. 277

- **Negri bodies** are eosinophilic, sharply outlined, pathognomonic inclusion bodies (2–10 μm in diameter) *found in the cytoplasm of certain nerve cells containing the virus of rabies, especially in Ammon's horn of the hippocampus.*
- They are also found in the cells of the medulla and various other ganglia. Negri bodies can also be found in the neurons of the salivary glands, tongue, or other organs. Staining with Mann's, giemsa, or Sellers stains can permit differentiation of rabies inclusions from other intracellular inclusions. With these stains, Negri bodies appear magenta in color and have small (0.2 μm to 0.5 μm), dark-blue interior basophilic granules.
- Histologic examination of tissues from clinically rabid animals show Negri bodies in about 50% of the samples; in contrast, the dFA test shows rabies antigen in nearly 100% of the samples.
- In other cases, non-rabid tissues have shown inclusions indistinguishable from Negri bodies. **Because of these problems, the presence of Negri bodies should not be considered diagnostic for rabies.**

> **Extra Mile**
>
> **Some other important bodies**
> - Lewy bodies: Parkinson's disease
> - Russel bodies: multiple myeloma
> - Mallory bodies: Alcoholism
> - Donovan bodies: Leishmaniasis
> - Heinz bodies: G-6-PD
> - Howell jolly bodies: Sickle cell anemia
> - Councilman bodies: yellow fever

264. Ans. (c) Parkinsonism

Ref: Robbin's Pathology, 9th ed. pg. 1294-95

Lewy body is an eosinophilic cytoplasmic inclusion consisting of a dense core surrounded by a halo of 10-nm-wide radiating fibrils, the primary structural component of which is alpha-synuclein. It is seen in Parkinsonism, Dementia with lewy bodies, shy dragger syndrome.

• Alzheimer disease	Hirona bodies/neurofibrillary tangles
• Rabies	Negri bodies
• Parkinsonism, dementia with lewy bodies	Lewy bodies
• Pick bodies	Picks disease

Pathology

265. Ans. (a) Huntington's chorea

Ref: Robbin's Pathology, 9th ed. pg. 1297-98

- The neuropathology of Huntington's disease consists of prominent neuronal loss and gliosis in the caudate nucleus and putamen; similar changes are also widespread in the cerebral cortex.
- *Intraneuronal inclusions containing aggregates of ubiquitin and the mutant protein huntingtin are found in the nuclei of affected neurons.*
- HD is caused by an increase in the number of polyglutamine (CAG) repeats (>40) in the coding sequence of the Huntington gene located on the short arm of chromosome 4.

266. Ans. (a) Retinoblastoma

Ref: Robbin's Pathology, 9th ed. pg. 1339; Dorland Medical Dictionary

- Glioma retinae is a congenital blastoma occurring in both hereditary and sporadic forms and is composed in tumour arising from embryonic retinal cells.
- It appears in one or both eyes in children under 5 years of age and is usually diagnosed initially by a bright white pupillary reflex (Leucocoria). It is caused by germline or somatic mutations or both, in both the alleles of retinoblastoma gene(Rb1)

ENDOCRINE SYSTEM

267. Ans. (a) Parathyroid adenoma

Ref: Harrison 20th edition, P 2747

MEN 2A is called Sipple syndrome and includes the following
- Medullary carcinoma thyroid (MC of all of these)
- Pheochromocytoma
- Parathyroid adenoma

The defect lies on chromosome 10 and *RET* proto-oncogene is responsible.

Extra Mile

MEN 2B (also known as MEN 3)	MTC (>90%) Pheochromocytoma (>50%) Associated abnormalities (40–50%) • Mucosal neuromas • Marfanoid habitus • Medullated corneal nerve fibers • Megacolon	MEN 4 (12p13)	Parathyroid adenoma Pituitary adenoma Reproductive organ tumors

268. Ans. (b) Secretin

Ref: Harrison 20th edition, P 2741

- Pheochromocytomas can produce *calcitonin, opioid peptides, somatostatin, corticotropin, and vasoactive intestinal peptide.*
- Corticotropin hypersecretion causes Cushing syndrome, and vasoactive intestinal peptide overproduction leads to watery diarrhea.
- Calcitonin is also produced by medullary carcinoma of thyroid which is related to Pheochromocytoma.

269. Ans (c) Neuropathy

Ref: Robbin's Pathology, 9th ed. pg. 1086-87

- Hashimoto's thyroiditis or chronic lymphocytic thyroiditis is an autoimmune disease in which the thyroid gland is gradually destroyed by a variety of cell and antibody mediated immune processes.
- Physiologically, antibodies against thyroid peroxidase and/or thyroglobulin cause gradual destruction of follicles in the thyroid gland. Accordingly, the disease can be detected clinically by looking for these antibodies in the blood. It is also characterized by invasion of the thyroid tissue by leukocytes, mainly T-lymphocytes. It is associated with non-Hodgkin lymphoma.

270. Ans. (b) Medullary carcinoma thyroid

Ref: Robbin's Pathology, 9th ed. pg. 1099

■ MEDULLARY CARCINOMA THYROID

- Accounts for approximately 7% of malignant tumour of thyroid
- It arises from ultimo-branchial bodies (from the parafollicular C cells derived from thyroid follicles).
- *It contains amyloid stroma*
- Familial medullary carcinomas occur in 25% of patients (Marfanoid habitus, Amyloid disease also occur in patients with familial medullary cancer).
- Medullary carcinoma occurs in association with (MEN 2A) syndrome.
- All patients with medullary carcinoma of thyroid should be screened for RET proto-oncogene.
- Medullary Carcinoma thyroid secretes calcitonin, this *does not cause hypocalcemia*

271. Ans. (a) Cardiac

Ref: Robbin's Pathology, 9th ed. pg. 1115

- *Cardiovascular insufficiency and cerebrovascular accidents are the most common causes of mortality. The*

impact of cardiovascular disease can be gauged by its involvement in as many as 80% of deaths of type 2 diabetics; in fact, diabetics have a 3 to 7.5 times greater incidence of death from cardiovascular causes than nondiabetic populations.
- The hallmark of cardiovascular disease is *accelerated atherosclerosis* of the large and medium-sized arteries (i.e., macrovascular disease).

272. Ans. (c) MEN II B

Ref: Robbin's Pathology, 9th ed. pg. 1137

MEN type 1
- Parathyroid hyperplasia or adenoma
- Islet cell hyperplasia, adenoma, or carcinoma
- Pituitary hyperplasia or adenoma
- Other, less common manifestations: foregut carcinoid, pheochromocytoma, subcutaneous or visceral lipomas

MEN IIA
- Medullary Thyroid Cancer (MTC)
- Pheochromocytoma
- Parathyroid hyperplasia or adenoma

MEN IIB
- MTC
- Pheochromocytoma
- Mucosal and gastrointestinal neuromas
- Marfanoid features

273. Ans. (b) Hyperparathyroidism

Please refer to above explanation

274. Ans. (d) Urine contains 5H.I.A.A

Ref: Robbin's Pathology, 9th ed. pg. 476

- ***Neuroblastoma (NB) is the most common extracranial solid cancer in childhood and the most common cancer in infancy.***
- Neuroblastoma is one of the few human malignancies known to demonstrate spontaneous regression from an undifferentiated state to a completely benign cellular appearance.
- *The most common location for neuroblastoma to originate (i.e., the primary tumor) is the adrenal glands.* This occurs in 40% of localized tumors and in 60% of cases of widespread disease.
- Neuroblastoma can also develop anywhere along the sympathetic nervous system chain from the neck to the pelvis.
- N-myc oncogene amplification within the tumor is a common finding in neuroblastoma. The degree of amplification shows a bimodal distribution: either 3- to 10-fold, or 100- to 300-fold. The presence of this mutation is highly correlated to advanced stages of disease
- Since it originates from chromaffin cells, in about 90% of cases of neuroblastoma, elevated levels of catecholamines or their metabolites are found in the urine or blood. Catecholamines and their metabolites include dopamine, homovanillic acid (HVA), and/or vanillyl mandelic acid (VMA)

275. Ans. (d) Diffuse glomerulosclerosis

Ref: Robbin's Pathology, 9th ed. pg. 111

- Diabetic nephropathy is a common cause of end-stage renal disease worldwide. It is characterised by diffuse or nodular glomerulosclerosis, afferent and efferent hyaline arteriolosclerosis, and tubulointerstitial fibrosis and atrophy.
- **Note-** *HPS finding of HIV nephropathy- Focal segmental glomerulosclerosis (FSGS)*

276. Ans. (a) Papillary carcinoma thyroid

Ref: Robbin's Pathology, 9th ed. pg. 1095

- Psammoma bodies are associated with the papillary histo-morphology and are thought to arise from:
  1. The infarction and calcification of papillae tips
  2. Calcification of intra-lymphatic tumor thrombi
- ***Psammoma bodies are commonly seen in certain tumors such as:***
  - **Papillary thyroid carcinoma**
  - Papillary renal cell carcinoma
  - Ovarian papillary serous cyst-adenocarcinoma
  - Endometrial adenocarcinomas (Papillary serous carcinoma ~3%-4%)
  - Meningiomas, in the central nervous system
  - Peritoneal and Pleural Mesothelioma
  - Somatostatinoma
  - Prolactinoma
  - Mesothelioma, in membranes that line body cavities

277. Ans. (a) Papillary thyroid cancer

Ref: Robbin's Pathology, 9th ed. pg. 1095-96

Orphan Annie Eye Nucleus is Seen in
- Papillary carcinoma thyroid
- Polymorphous low grade adenocarcinoma
- Hashimoto Thyroiditis
- Grave's disease
- Nodular goiter

278. Ans. (a) Epinephrine

Ref: Robbin's Pathology, 9th ed. pg. 1134-36

- *Phaeochromocytoma size <5 cm and associated with MEN 2A can produce epinephrine due to sufficient methyl transferase enzyme.*

Pathology

- However if phaeochromocytoma is >5 cm or is an extradrenal phaeochromocytoma due to absence of methyl transferase enzyme, produces only nor-epinephrine.

279. Ans. (d) Mucinous cystadenosarcoma

Ref: Robbin's Pathology, 9th ed. pg. 1027

- Pseudomyxoma peritonei (PMP) is a clinical condition caused by cancerous cells (mucinous adenocarcinoma) that produce abundant mucin or gelatinous ascites.
- The primary tumor appears to arise from the MUC2 expressing goblet cells and most commonly from these cells in the appendix. The K-Ras and p53 genes may be involved in the oncogenesis. It may be diagnosed with a range of conditions.
- *While the majority of these cases are associated with appendiceal carcinomas other conditions may also be found, including disseminated peritoneal adenomucinosis (DPAM), peritoneal carcinomas, several mucinous tumors (mucinous adenocarcinoma, mucinous cystadenoma, and mucinous cystadenocarcinoma), as well as other disease states*
- This will result in compression of organs and will destroy the function of colon, small intestine, stomach, or other organs. Prognosis with treatment in many cases is optimistic, but the disease is lethal if untreated, with death by cachexia, bowel obstruction, or other types of complications.

GENETICS

280. Ans. (d) G6PD

Ref: CMDT 2019, P 521

- Glucose-6-phosphate dehydrogenase (G6PD) deficiency is an *XLR enzyme defect* that causes episodic hemolytic anemia because of the decreased ability of red blood cells to deal with oxidative stresses. G6PD deficiency leads to excess oxidized glutathione (hence, inadequate levels of reduced glutathione) that forces hemoglobin to denature and form precipitants called Heinz bodies.

281. Ans. (a) AR

Ref: Robbins E-Book, P 246

- Marriage amongst cousins/close relatives is called as consanguinity.
- The high consanguinity rates, could induce the expression of autosomal recessive diseases, including very rare or new syndromes.

282. Ans. (a) Phenotype

Ref: Robbins 8th ed. P 136-37

Phenotype	Physical appearance ascribed to a particular genetic make-up
Proteomics	Measurement of all proteins expressed in a cell or tissue
Genotype	Genetic composition describing number of chromosomes
Anticipation	Increase in severity of disease with successive generations

283. Ans. (b) Familial hypercholesterolemia

Ref: CMDT 2017, P 1212

Disease with Polygenic Pattern of Inheritance

- Hypertension
- Diabetes mellitus
- Gout
- Schizophrenia
- Bipolar disorder

284. Ans. (b) Chromosome 17q21

- The Cytogenetic Location of BRCA1 gene is 17q21.31, which is the long (q) arm of chromosome 17 at position 21.31
- Cytogenetic Location: 13q13.1, which is the long (q) arm of chromosome 13 at position 13.1
- BRCA1- and BRCA2-associated hereditary breast and ovarian cancer syndrome (HBOC) is characterized by an increased risk for female and male breast cancer, ovarian cancer (includes fallopian tube and primary peritoneal cancers).

285. Ans. (a) Fibrillin 1

- Fibrillin is the major component of extracellular microfibrils and is widely distributed in connective tissue throughout the body.
  - *Mutations in the fibrillin-1 (FBN1) gene, on chromosome 15q21.1, have been found to cause Marfan syndrome, a dominantly inherited disorder characterised by clinically variable skeletal, ocular, and cardiovascular abnormalities.*
  - Fibrillin-1 mutations have also been found in several other related connective tissue disorders, such as severe neonatal Marfan syndrome, dominant ectopia lentis, familial ascending aortic aneurysm, isolated skeletal features of Marfan syndrome, and Shprintzen-Goldberg syndrome.

286. Ans. (d) 47XXY

287. Ans.(b) 11q(22-23)

- The image shows dilated blood vessels in the sclera which is called telangiectasia. It is seen in *Ataxia-telangiectasia.*

- The gene for ataxia-telangiectasia has been localized to band 11q22-23.
- The main abnormalities on physical examination are ocular and cutaneous telangiectasia and neurologic symptoms (ataxia and abnormal eye movements present in virtually all cases) and choreo-athetosis.

288. Ans. (a) 50% carrier and 50% affected

Ref: Harsh Mohan, 7th ed. pg. 255

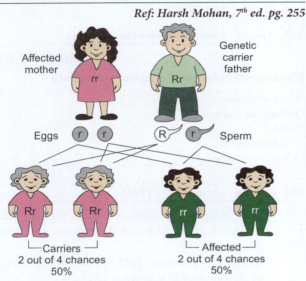

289. Ans. (c) Chromosomal abnormalities

Ref: Robbin's Pathology, 9th ed. pg. 158

Karyotyping is the study of chromosomes and is used in cytogenetics to study the chromosomal abnormalities. After arresting the cells in metaphase the chromosomes are examined to check for:
- Change in Number of chromosomes - To detect abnormalities in chromosome numbers such as aneuploidy (trisomy, tetrasomy), polyploidy.
- For detection of structural chromosomal anomalies such as translocation, deletions, inversion of chromosomes.

290. Ans. (c) Trinucleotide - repeat expansion

Ref: Robbin's Pathology, 9th ed. pg. 168

- Anticipation is a phenomenon where by the symptoms of a genetic disorder become apparent at an earlier age as it is passed to next generation. In most cases, an increased severity of symptoms is also noted.
- In triplet nucleotide repeat mutation, the DNA fragment is unstable and tends to expand further during cell division. So, in successive generations the expanded repeat increases and the manifestations of disease may worsen or may be observed at an earlier age; this phenomenon is referred to as anticipation.

291. Ans. (a) 13q l4

Ref: Robbin's Pathology, 9th ed. pg. 1339

Wilm's tumor-Aniridia complex (WAGR syndrome)	11 p 13 part of (deletion of short arm of chromosome)
Retinoblastoma	13q 14.11 (deletion of part of long arm of chromosome 13)
Prader-Willi syndrome Angelman syndrome	15q 11-13 (deletion of part of long arm of chromosome 15)
DiGeorge's syndrome Velo-Cardio-facial syndrome	22q11 (deletion of part of long arm of chromosome -22)

292. Ans. (b) Marfan syndrome

Ref: Robbin's Pathology, 9th ed. pg. 144

- The presentation in the question is of a patient with Marfan syndrome.
- Marfan syndrome is caused by a mutation in a single allele of the fibrillin gene (FBN1).
- The gene product is a major component of elastin-associated microfibrils. Long, thin extremities; ectopic lentis; and aortic aneurysms are the classical triad.
- Mutations in the FBN2 gene can also cause Marfan syndrome, but without aneurysms.

293. Ans. (c) Chromosome 21

Ref: Robbin's Pathology, 9th ed. pg. 158

- In karyotyping the image of stained chromosome pairs in metaphase stage is arranged in order of decreasing length.
- **Chromosome 21 is the smallest human chromosome**, with 48 million nucleotides, representing about 1.5 percent of the total DNA in cells
- Chromosome 1 is the largest chromosome.

294. Ans. (a) Down Syndrome

Ref: Robbin's Pathology, 9th ed. pg. 161

Autoimmune Thyroiditis is Seen with
- Down syndrome
- Turner syndrome
- Congenital rubella syndrome
  - Autoimmune thyroiditis is *not* seen with Marfan's Syndrome.
  - LouisBarr syndrome is known as ataxia telangiectasia. It characterised by deficiency of IgA with increased incidence of lympho-reticular malignancy.
  - **E**dward syndrome is **e**ighteen trisomy which is characterised by clenched hand and *overlapping of fingers* where the index finger of the neonate overlaps third finger and fifth finger overlaps the fourth finger.

Pathology

393

295. Ans. (b) Only X chromosome from the mother undergoes pyknosis

Ref: Robbin's Pathology, 9th ed. pg. 164

Lyon hypothesis is:
- Only one of the X chromosome is genetically active
- Other X chromosome which can be of paternal or maternal origin undergoes pyknosis and is rendered inactive.
- Inactivation of either paternal or maternal X chromosomes occurs at random among the cells of blastocyst by about 16th day of embryonic life
- Inactivation of X is because of a gene called Xist which causes gene silencing DNA methylation.

296. Ans. (a) Genomic imprinting

Ref: Robbin's Pathology, 9th ed. pg. 172-173

Preferential expression of an allele depending on parental origin is genomic imprinting.

- **Prader wili syndrome:** Deletion of paternal chromosome 15
- **Angelman syndrome:** Deletion of maternal chromosome 15
- **Beckwith weidmann syndrome:** have two paternal but no maternal copies of chromosome 11
- **Albright's hereditary osteodystrophy:** mutation in Gs alpha subunit leading to short stature, brachydactyl and PTH resistance only when mutation is inherited from the mother.

297. Ans. (d) All of the above

Ref: Robbin's Pathology, 9th ed. pg. 177-178

- FISH can be performed in prenatal samples, like samples obtained by amniocentesis, Cordocentesis, chorionic villus sampling or umbilical cord blood, peripheral blood lymphocytes.
- Since it does not need dividing cells, it is extremely useful for rapid diagnosis

Advantages of FISH

- Can detect numerical abonormalities of chromosomes like aneuploidy
- It can detect minor micro-deletions
- Can detect complex translocations
- For gene amplification analysis
- For mapping of recently isolated genes to their chromosomal locus

298. Ans. (a) Autosomal recessive

Ref: Robbin's Pathology, 9th ed. pg. 141

AUTOSOMAL DOMINANT

- One mutated copy of the gene in each cell is sufficient for a person to be affected by an autosomal dominant disorder.
- Autosomal dominant disorders tend to occur in every generation of an affected family.

- Associated diseases can be remembered as *"DOMINANT"*
D= Dystrophy Myotonic.
O- Ostogenesis Imperfecta.
M- Marfan's syndrome.
I- Intermittent Porphyria.
N- Noonan's Syndrome.
A- Adult Polycystic Kidney, Achondroplasia.
N- Neurofibromatosis.
T- Tuberous sclerosis.

AUTOSOMAL RECESSIVE

- Two mutated copies of the gene are present in each cell when a person has an autosomal recessive disorder.
- Autosomal recessive disorders are typically not seen in every generation of an affected family.
- **Diseases can be remembered as *"ABCDEFGH SPW"*:**
A- Albinism, Alpha 1 Antitrypsin Deficiency
B-Beta Thalassemia
C-Cystic Fibrosis, CGD, CAH
D-Deafness(SNHL), Dubin Johnson
E-Enzyme Deficiencies(Glycogen Storage And Lysosomal Storage)
F-Friedrich's Ataxia, Fanconi Anemia
G- Galactosemia
H-Hemochromatosis, Hurler syndrome
S-Sickle Cell Disease
P-Phenylketonuria
W-Wilson's disease

X-LINKED DOMINANT

- X-linked dominant disorders are caused by mutations in genes on the X chromosome.
- *Females are more frequently affected than males,* and the chance of passing on an X-linked dominant disorder differs between men and women.
- Families with an X-linked dominant disorder often have both affected males and affected females in each generation. *A characteristic of X-linked inheritance is that fathers cannot pass X-linked traits to their sons (no male-to-male transmission).*
- Ex: hypophosphatemic rickets, also called vitamin D-resistant rickets.

X-LINKED RECESSIVE

- X-linked recessive disorders are also caused by mutations in genes on the X chromosome.
- *Males are more frequently affected than females*, and the chance of passing on the disorder differs between men and women.
- Families with an X-linked recessive disorder often have affected males, but rarely affected females, in each generation.

Explanations

- A characteristic of X-linked inheritance is that fathers cannot pass X-linked traits to their sons (no male-to-male transmission).
- Diseases under this are:
  - G6PD
  - Duchenne muscular dystrophy
  - Hemophilia A

299. Ans. (d) X-linked recessive

Ref: Robbin's Pathology, 9th ed. pg. 142

300. Ans. (a) Albinism

Ref: Robbin's Pathology, 9th ed. pg. 141

301. Ans (b) Haemophilia

Ref: Robbin's Pathology, 9th ed. pg. 142

"Less hCG is Detected Clinically in A Woman"
- Lesch-Nyhan syndrome
- Hemophilia, Hunter's syndrome
- Chronic granulomatous disease
- G6PD deficiency
- Duchenne muscular dystrophy
- Color blindness
- Agammaglobulinemia
- Wiskott-Aldrich syndrome

302. Ans. (a) Vitamin D resistant rickets

Ref: Robbin's Pathology, 9th ed. pg. 142

Vitamin D resistant rickets	PHEX gene. X linked dominant
Familial hypercholesterolemia	Autosomal recessive
Red green colour blindness	X linked recessive
Achondroplasia	Autosomal dominant

303. Ans. (a) X-linked

Ref: Robbin's Pathology, 9th ed. pg. 155

- HURLER syndrome is autosomal recessive while HUNTER SYNDROME is X linked recessive
- HURLER syndrome is marked by progressive deterioration, hepatosplenomegaly, dwarfism and unique facial features. There is a progressive mental retardation, with death frequently occurring by the age of 10 years
- Hurler is due to defective IDUA gene, which has been mapped to the 4p16.3 site on chromosome 4. The gene is named IDUA because of its iduronidase enzyme protein product.

304. Ans. (a) Decrease in AFP

Ref: Robbin's Pathology, 9th ed. pg. 161, Nelson, 18th ed. ch. 81

AFP	UE3	hCG	Associated conditions
Low	Low	High	Down syndrome
Low	Low	Low	Trisomy 18 (Edward's syndrome)
High	n/a	n/a	Neural tube defects (like spina bifida that may have associated increased levels of acetylcholinesterase in the amniotic fluid), omphalocele, gastroschisis, multiple gestation triplets, or an underestimation of gestational age.

305. Ans. (a) Down syndrome

Ref: Nelson, 18th ed. ch. 81

306. Ans. (b) Chromosome 17

Ref: Robbin's Pathology, 9th ed. pg. 291

- The BRCA2 **gene** is **located** on chromosome 13 and encodes over 3000 amino acids. It appears that BRCA2 plays an important role in male breast cancer.
- *The human BRCA1 gene is located on the long (q) arm of chromosome 17*

307. Ans. (c) P16

Ref: Robbin's Pathology, 9th ed. pg. 1054-55

- Genes called BRCA1, BRCA2, TP53 or PTEN are linked with breast cancer.
- *P16 plays an important role in cell cycle regulation by decelerating cell progression from G1 phase to S phase, and therefore acts as a tumor suppressor that is implicated in the prevention of cancers, notably melanoma, oropharyngeal squamous cell carcinoma, cervical cancer, and esophageal cancer.*

308. Ans. (b) 47XXY

Ref: Robbin's Pathology, 9th ed. pg. 165

309. Ans. (b) Chromosome 22 defect

Ref: Harrison, 19th ed. pg. 83e-6

- Cat Eye Syndrome is a rare condition caused by the short arm (p) and a small section of the long arm (q) of human Chromosome 22 being present three (trisomic) or four times (tetrasomic) instead of the usual two times.

- The term "Cat Eye" syndrome was coined because of the particular appearance of the vertical colobomas in the eyes of some patients. Preauricular skin tags and/or pits constitute the most consistent features and suggest the presence of a supernumerary bisatellited marker chromosome 22 derived from duplication of the CES critical region.
- *Please do not confuse with retinoblastoma in which there is an abnormal appearance of the pupil, leukocoria, also known as amaurotic cat's eye reflex.*
- Other signs and symptoms include deterioration of vision, a red and irritated eye with glaucoma, and faltering growth or delayed development. Some children with retinoblastoma can develop a squint. Retinoblastoma presents with advanced disease in developing countries and eye enlargement is a common finding.

RESPIRATORY SYSTEM

310. Ans. (c) Kidney

Ref: Robbins E-Book, P 519

Good pasture disease is a term used to describe glomerulonephritis, with or without pulmonary hemorrhage, and the presence of circulating anti–glomerular basement membrane (anti-GBM) antibodies

311. Ans. (a) Thickening of bronchial wall

Ref: Robbin E-book, P 502-504

- Increased numbers of goblet cells (goblet cell hyperplasia) is part of airway remodelling in asthma.
- The remodelling also includes epithelial proliferation, thickening of the reticular basement membrane, increased bronchial vascularity and hypertrophy of smooth muscle and submucosal glands.
- Thickening of bronchial wall is seen in bronchiectasis.

312. Ans. (c) Hyaline membrane disease

Ref: Robbins 9th ed. P 672

The immature lungs in hyaline membrane disease show eosinophilic hyaline membranes in alveoli, alveolar ducts and terminal bronchioles.

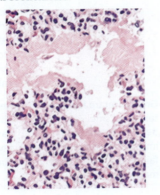

The membranes contain necrotic epithelial cells admixed with extravasated plasma proteins.

313. Ans. (c) IL-4

Ref: Robbin's Pathology, 9th ed. pg. 204

- Asthma is a chronic allergic inflammatory disease, the initiation and progression of which is dependent on the cytokines interleukin IL-4 and IL-13 acting through related receptor complexes.
- Disease pathogenesis is affected by intracellular signaling pathways that couple primarily to specific motifs within the intracellular domain of the IL-4 receptor alpha chain, a subunit that is common to the IL-4 and IL-13 receptor complexes.

314. Ans. (a) Laminin

Ref: Robbin's Pathology, 9th ed. pg. 105

Laminin is the most abundant glycoprotein in basement membranes. Type IV collagen, laminin and nidogen are present in basement membranes.

315. Ans. (d) Photosensitivity

Ref: Robbin's Pathology, 9th ed. pg. 64

- Ochronosis in its endogenous form is a rare, recessively *transmitted, congenital disorder of melanin-like pigmentation due to an inborn error in tyrosine metabolism which is due to deficiency of homogentisic acid oxidase.*
- Homogentisic acid (an intermediate in the oxidation of tyrosine) is not oxidized, so it accumulates in the extracellular fluid.
- The compound is selectively deposited in cartilage, which becomes ochre colored or black due to melanin-like pigment.
- Deposits within synovium produce ochronotic arthritis, and involvement of the intervertebral disks is seen.

316. Ans. (b) Lipids

Ref: Robbin's Pathology, 9th ed. pg. 354

PAS (periodic acid – Schiff) stain is versatile and has been used to stain many structures including glycogen, mucin, mucoprotein, glycoprotein, as well as fungi. PAS is useful for outlining tissue structures, basement membranes, glomeruli, blood vessels and glycogen in the liver.

317. Ans. (b) Congo red

Ref: Robbin's Pathology, 9th ed. pg. 257

- In biochemistry and histology, Congo red is used to stain microscopic preparations especially as a cytoplasm and erythrocyte stain.

FMGE Solutions Screening Examination

- *Apple-green birefringence of Congo red stained preparations under polarized light is indicative for the presence of amyloid fibrils.*
- *Additionally, Congo Red is used in microbiological epidemiology to rapidly identify the presence of virulent serotype 2A ShigellaFlexneri, where the dye binds the bacterium's unique lipopolysaccharide (LPS) structure*

318. Ans. (a) DNA and RNA

Ref: Harrison, pg. 150e-2

- *Acridine orange is a nucleic acid selective-fluorescent cationic dye useful for cell cycle determination.*
- It is cell-permeable, and interacts with DNA and RNA by intercalation or electrostatic attractions respectively and emits green and red right respectively.
- Acridine orange can be used in conjunction with ethidium bromide to differentiate between live and apoptotic cells.

319. Ans. (a) Animal Source

Ref: Harrison, pg. 640

Only source of vitamin B_{12} for humans is food of animal origin, e.g., meat, fish, and dairy products.

Vegetables, fruits, and other foods of non-animal origin are free from cobalamin unless they are contaminated by bacteria. Cobalamin is synthesized solely by microorganisms.

320. Ans. (b) 10%

Ref: Handbook of Histopathological and Histochemical Techniques 3rd ed. pg. 40-45

- Formalin is generally the preferred fluid for fixation and is widely used. Formalin is often sold as 37-40% aqueous Formaldehyde.
- To make a solution of 10% Formalin, nine parts of water are added to one part of 40% (aqueous) Formaldehyde.
- *Therefore, a 10% solution of Formalin is the equivalent of a 4% solution of Formaldehyde.*
- Formaldehyde is a gas produced by the oxidation of methyl alcohol, whereas 100% Formalin is a saturated solution of this gas in water.

Other Histopathological Preservatives:

- Glutaraldehyde: 25%-for electron microscopy (with osmium tetra-chloride)
- Acetaldehyde acrolein
- Mercuric chloride
- Potassium dichromate

321. Ans. (b) Impaired skeletal growth

Ref: Harrison /96e-9

- Manganese deficiency leads to impaired growth and skeletal development whereas toxicity leads to parkinsonism like features. Impaired glucose tolerance is seen with chromium deficiency.

TABLE: Deficiencies and Toxicities of Metals

Element	Deficiency	Toxicity
Manganese	Impaired growth and skeletal development, reproduction, lipid and carbohydrate metabolism; upper body rash	• Parkinsonism like symptoms • Encephalitis-like syndrome
Calcium	Reduced bone mass, osteoporosis	Renal insufficiency (milk-alkali syndrome), nephrolithiasis
Copper	Anemia, growth retardation, defective keratinisation and pigmentation of hair, degenerative changes in aortic elastin, osteopenia	Vomiting, diarrhea, hepatic failure, tremor, mental deterioration, haemolytic anemia, renal dysfunction
Chromium	Impaired glucose tolerance	Occupational: Renal failure, dermatitis
Fluoride	↑Dental caries	Dental and skeletal fluorosis, osteosclerosis
Iodine	Thyroid enlargement, ↓ T4, cretinism	Thyroid dysfunction, acne-like eruptions
Selenium	Cardiomyopathy, heart failure, striated muscle degeneration	Alopecia, nausea, vomiting, abnormal nails, emotional lability, peripheral neuropathy, lassitude, garlic odor to breath, dermatitis Occupational: Lung and nasal carcinomas
Zinc	Growth retardation, ↓ taste and smell, alopecia, dermatitis, diarrhea, immune dysfunction, failure to thrive, congenital malformations	Reduced copper absorption, gastritis, sweating, fever, nausea, vomiting

322. Ans. (a) Oil-Red O

Ref: Robbin's pathology 9th ed. /151

Oil-Red O	Fat
Congo red	Amyloid
Perl stain	Iron
PAS	Glycogen

323. Ans. (c) Green

- The color of its aqueous solution varies from green to orange as a function of the way it is observed: by reflection or by transmission
- Topical fluorescein is used in the diagnosis of corneal abrasions, corneal ulcers and herpetic corneal infections.
- Fluorescein is also used extensively in photographic retinal vasculature imaging during fundus flourescein angiography. The dye sodium fluorescein can be used either in concentration of 10% or 20% in the form of intravenous bolus injection. It is used to image retinal, choroidal, optic disc, or iris vasculature, or a combination of these. It is used diagnostically as well as in planning for many retinal laser procedures. It has a very important role in management of diabetic retinopathy, vein occlusion, and age-related macular degeneration.

324. Ans. (b) Congo red

Ref: Robbin's Pathology, 9th ed. pg. 354

Congo red is used for staining amyloid and not lipids

Stains for Lipids

- Oil red O
- Sudan black
- Sudan III and IV
- Filipin
- Schultz
- Nile blue sulfate

325. Ans. (b) Attachment

Ref: Robbin's Pathology, 9th ed. pg. 245-46

- Envelope glycoprotein GP120 (or gp120) is a glycoprotein exposed on the surface of the HIV envelope.
- The 120 in its name comes from its molecular weight of 120 kDa.
- Gp120 is essential for virus entry into cells as it *plays a vital role in attachment to specific cell surface receptors.*

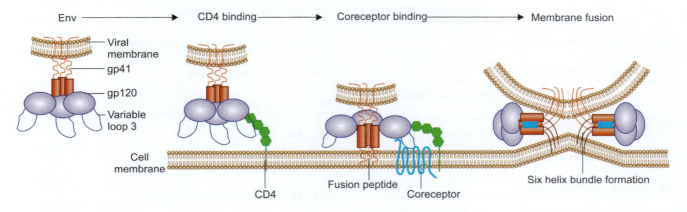

- Binding to CD4 induces the start of a cascade of conformational changes in gp120 and *gp41 that lead to the fusion of the viral membrane with the host cell membrane.*
- Gp120 is coded by the HIV *env* gene, which is around 2.5 kb long and codes for around 850 amino acids

326. Ans. (b) 350

Ref: Robbin's pathology 9th ed. /251-52

- Under the revised guidelines the treatment of AIDS patients with respect to opportunistic infections has undergone a change with H.A.A.R.T being initiated at a threshold of CD4 count <350 cells/cu.mm instead of previous 200 cells/cu.mm.

FMGE Solutions Screening Examination

ANSWERS TO BOARD REVIEW QUESTIONS

327. Ans. (d) Kidney
   Ref: Harrison's 18th ed ch-114
328. Ans. (c) Pars nervosa
329. Ans. (b) Infective endocarditis
   Ref: Robbin's 8th ed ch-12
330. Ans. (a) Diabetic nephropathy
   Ref: Robbin's 8th ed ch-24
331. Ans. (b) Breast cancer
   Ref: Robbin's 8th ed ch-7
332. Ans. (d) Hurler disease
   Ref: Pediatric Bone Marrow By Lila Penchansk / 32
333. Ans. (a) Sporotrichosis
   Ref: Lever's histopathology of skin 9th ed ch-23
334. Ans. (a) Myxomatous
   Ref: Robbin's 8th ed ch-12
335. Ans. (a) Autosomal recessive
336. Ans. (c) 30–299 mg/day
   Ref: Harrison's 118th ed ch:283
337. Ans. (c) bcl-2
338. Ans. (b) Superoxide dismutase
339. Ans. (a) NADPH oxidase
340. Ans. (a) Ankylosing spondylitis
341. Ans. (d) Cathepsin G
342. Ans. (b) Ischemic necrosis of the brain
343. Ans. (b) Dystrophic
344. Ans. (b) Immunoglobulins
345. Ans. (a) Atherosclerosis
346. Ans. (a) Phagocytes
347. Ans. (c) IL-1
348. Ans. (b) T.B.
349. Ans. (d) C3a and C5a
350. Ans. (b) Dilatation of capillaries
351. Ans. (a) Langerhans cells
352. Ans. (b) Venous thrombosis
353. Ans. (b) Lung
354. Ans. (a) Liver
355. Ans. (a) Thrombus
356. Ans. (b) 30,000
357. Ans. (d) IV
358. Ans. (b) Turner syndrome
359. Ans. (a) Localized immune complex
360. Ans. (c) Rectal biopsy
361. Ans. (c) Congo red
362. Ans. (a) Langerhan's cell
363. Ans. (a) Cytotoxic T cells
364. Ans. (a) IgE mediated response
365. Ans. (b) Neutrophil
366. Ans. (a) SLE
367. Ans. (a) Sinusoids of red pulp
368. Ans. (d) Type IV
369. Ans. (b) T cell
370. Ans. (c) CLL

Pathology

371. Ans. (a) Reticulocytosis

372. Ans. (c) Megaloblastic anemia

373. Ans. (d) Post splenectomy'

374. Ans. (a) Ferritin

375. Ans. (c) Iron deficiency anemia

376. Ans. (b) Iron

377. Ans. (a) Organ of zuckerkandl

378. Ans. (b) Melanoma

379. Ans. (c) Fibrinogen

380. Ans. (b) Psoriasis

381. Ans. (b) CD 103

382. Ans. (d) 1gA and C3

383. Ans. (c) Juvenile polyp

384. Ans. (a) Malakoplakia

385. Ans. (a) Council man bodies

386. Ans. (a) CVC liver

387. Ans. (c) Myxoma

388. Ans. (d) Sigmoid colon

389. Ans. (b) Ca++

390. Ans. (a) APML

391. Ans. (a) Atherosclerosis

392. Ans. (b) Bronchial carcinoid

393. Ans. (c) Neuroblastoma

394. Ans. (b) IgA

395. Ans. (a) Adiponectin

396. Ans. (d) Polycythemia vera

397. Ans. (b) Asthma

398. Ans. (d) CD 31

399. Ans. (c) CD 1a

400. Ans. (d) C gene

401. Ans. (a) Malakoplakia

402. Ans. (b) Endoplasmic reticulum

403. Ans. (b) Left atrium

404. Ans. (c) Macrophages

405. Ans. (b) Bronchio alveolar cancer

406. Ans. (d) Adrenals

407. Ans. (a) Brain

408. Ans. (d) Lieomyo sarcoma

409. Ans. (b) Beta cell

410. Ans. (a) Jaw

411. Ans. (a) Insulin

412. Ans. (c) Right atrium

413. Ans. (c) Proteins

414. Ans. (a) Sarcoma

415. Ans. (b) Di George syndrome

416. Ans. (b) Fibrinoid necrosis

417. Ans. (c) Fibrillin

Ref: Management of Genetic Syndromes by Suzanne B. Cassidy, Judith E. Allanson Page 513

418. Ans. (b) HHV-8

Ref: Jawetz's microbiology 24th ed ch-33 Table 33-2

419. Ans. (a) Follow up of ovarian cancer

Ref: Robbin's 8th ed ch-7

Explanations

FMGE Solutions Screening Examination

420. Ans. (b) Bone marrow

   Ref: Harrison 18th ed ch-65, 66, 67

421. Ans. (b) Collagen

   Ref: Robbin's 8th ed ch:3

422. Ans. (a) IL1

   Ref: Harrison 17th ed ch-308, Oxford journal Medical Clinical Infectious Diseases Volume 31, Issue Supplement 5 p. S178-S184

423. Ans. (c) CD la

   Ref: Rook's 8th ed p. 55.9

424. Ans. (d) Morphologically defective sperms

   Ref: Harrison 18th ed ch-346, Smith Urology 17thed p.691, http://whqlibdoc.who.int/publications/2010/9789241547789_eng.pdf

425. Ans. (b) 1%

   Ref: Textbook of Blood Banking & Transfusion Medicine 2nded by Sally V. Rudmann /451

426. Ans. (d) Direct binding to calcium

   Ref: Wintrobe's clinical hematology 11th ed ch-24

427. Ans. (a) Papillary carcinoma of thryroid

   Ref: Schwartz's Principles of Surgery 9th ed ch-38

428. Ans. (c) X-linked recessive

   Ref: Apendix 78 for "Pedigree & Inheritance"

429. Ans. (a) Autosomal dominant

   Ref: Appendix 78 for "Pedigree & Inheritance"

430. Ans. (d) Primary biliary cirrhosis

   Ref: Clinical Endocrine Oncology by Ian D. Hay, John A.H Wass /91

431. Ans. (b) Asbestosis

   Ref: Harrison 17th ed. ch-257

432. Ans. (b) Breast

   Ref: The Immunoassay Handbook edited by David Wild / 676

433. Ans. (a) Ewing sarcoma

   Ref: Diagnostic musculoskeletal surgical pathology; clinicoradiologic and cytologic correlations / 26

434. Ans. (c) Asbestosis

   Ref: Robbin's 8th ed.

435. Ans. (a) Diffuse alveolar damage

   Ref: Robbin's 8th ed. ch-15

ANWERS TO IMAGE-BASED QUESTIONS (HISTOPATHOLOGICAL SLIDE INTERPRETATION)

436. Ans. (a) Howell jolly Bodies

437. Ans. (b) Reed Sternberg cell

   The image shows presence of Reed Sternberg cell with bilobed nucleus and prominent nucleoli which lead to prominent owl eye appearance.

438. Ans. (b) Myeloblast
   - The image shows presence of Myeloblasts and you can see the Auer rods in the cytoplasm of these cells. (Arrow Marked)
   - The image shows presence of Howell-Jolly bodies— which are dense blue circular inclusions representing nuclear remnants. The presence of Howell jolly bodies implies defective splenic function.

439. Ans. (a) Gaucher cell
   - The image shows presence of an enlarged macrophage showing crumpled tissue paper appearance of cytoplasm. The cell contains undigested glucocerbroside.
   - Reed Sternberg cell is found in Hodgkin's Lymphoma
   - Anitschkow cell is seen in rheumatic fever and pop-corn cell is seen in nodular lymphocyte predominant variety of Hodgkin lymphoma.

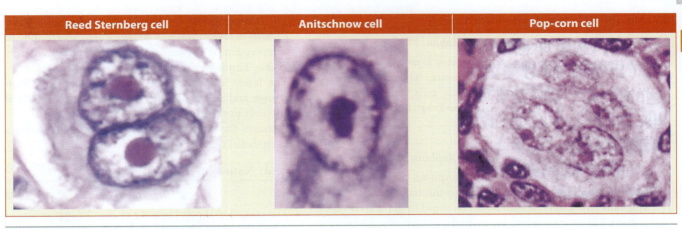

440. Ans. (b) Thalassemia

The image shows a child with prominent cheek bones due to marrow expansion. The peripheral smear shows presence of Target cells (Notice the target in the centre of RBC)

441. Ans. (a) Hairy cell Leukemia

The image shows presence of immature B cell with hairy projection on the surface.

442. Ans. (b) Schistocyte

Notice the projection on the edge of the RBC.

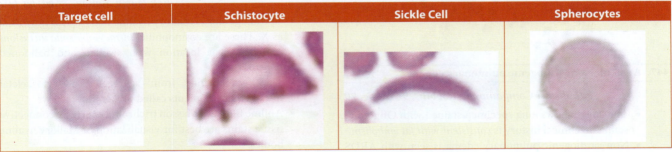

443. Ans. (a) Lipofuscin in cardiac tissue

Ref: Page 25, Harsh Mohan, 7th ed.

- The image shows presence of *wear and tear ligament* which is lipofuscin. It is a yellowish brown pigment accumulating in central part of cells around the nuclei.
- By electron microscopy it is *intralysosomal* electron dense granules in *perinuclear location*.
- It can be seen in:

  - Myocardial fibers and is associated with wasting and hence called as brown atrophy.
  - Intraneuronal in senile dementia
  - Leydig cells of testis
  - Hepatocytes

444. Ans. (b) Hyaline arteriosclerosis

Ref: Harsh Mohan, 7th ed. pg. 372

The image shows an *eosinophilic hyaline material* in tunica media and intima. The lumen of blood vessel is narrowed. This is suggestive of diagnosis of hyaline arteriosclerosis.

445. Ans. (b) Hyperplastic arteriosclerosis

Ref: Harsh Mohan, 7th ed. pg. 372

The image shows *loosely placed concentric layers* in a small artery leading to *onion skin* appearance. The presence of hyperplastic intimal smooth muscle cells with severe intimal sclerosis leads to narrowed blood vessel.

446. Ans. (a) Coagulative necrosis

Ref: Pocket Companion to Robbins, 9th ed. pg. 6

The image shows eosinophilic amorphous deposit at 12 o'clock position with surrounding infiltrate showing langhans type giant cell with nuclei arranged in horse shoe pattern. This is seen in caseous necrosis.

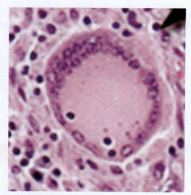

447. Ans. (b) Noncardiogenic pulmonary edema

Ref: Pocket Companion to Robbins, 9th ed. pg. 79

- The image shows lung specimen stained with Oil Red O stain and clinical history is *consistent with fat embolism*.
- Non-cardiogenic pulmonary edema is seen with ARDS and not fat embolism.
- In contrast the development of fat embolism is due to a series of biochemical cascades resulting from the mechanical insult sustained in major trauma. Release of fat emboli leads to occlusion of the microvasculature.
- Findings from noncontrast computed tomography (CT) of the head performed because of alterations in mental status may be normal or may reveal diffuse white-matter petechial hemorrhages consistent with microvascular injury.
- GURD criteria are used for diagnosis of fat embolism and one major criterion, four minor criteria, and the presence of macroglobulinemia are required for the diagnosis.

448. Ans. (b) Nodular glomerulosclerosis

Ref: Harsh Mohan, 7th ed. pg. 665

- The image shows presence of *intense eosinophilic deposits in nodular fashion all over glomerulus* leading to compression of glomerular capillaries which are hardly visible. This is seen in nodular glomerulosclerosis.
- The lesion shown is also called Kimmelstiel-Wilson change and is specific for type 1 diabetes or islet cell antibody positive diabetes.
- Armanni-Ebstein change is seen in uncontrolled diabetes in epithelial cells of proximal convoluted tubules.

449. Ans. (d) Nutmeg liver

Ref: Harsh Mohan, 7th ed. pg. 92

- The specimen shows presence of *mottled appearance of liver* where dark congestion is noted. This is diagnostic of nutmeg liver.
- Dubin-Johnson has a black liver texture and is therefore ruled out.
- Postnecrotic cirrhosis has visible scarring on surface and is therefore ruled out
- Miliary tuberculosis (TB) will show studded appearance.

450. Ans. (b) Intranuclear inclusions

Ref: Harsh Mohan, 7th ed. pg. 607

- The image shows Mallory hyaline body which is marked as X. These are eosinophilic, *intracytoplasmic inclusions* in perinuclear location with swollen and ballooned hepatocytes.
- They are formed from aggregates of cytoskeletal intermediate filaments called prekeratin.
- Aniline Blue and Masson trichrome which are connective tissue stains are best for visualization of Mallory hyaline bodies.
- Conditions that exhibit Mallory hyaline bodies are—**I WILL STAY SOBER**

- **I**ndian childhood cirrhosis
- **W**ilson disease
- **S**urgery (Intestinal bypass)
- Focal n**o**dular hyperplasia
- **B**iliary cirrhosis (primary)
- **H**epatocellular carcinoma

451. Ans. (b) Echinocyte

Ref: Oski's Pediatric Hematology, 7th ed. pg. 773

- The image shows presence of spiculated red cells with uniform projections over the entire circumference of cell. This is an echinocyte.
- In contrast acanthocytes have only few spicules of varying size that project irregularly from cell surface.

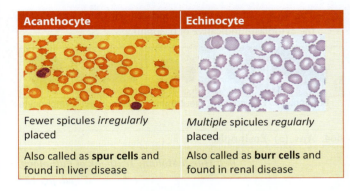

Acanthocyte	Echinocyte
Fewer spicules *irregularly* placed	*Multiple* spicules *regularly* placed
Also called as **spur cells** and found in liver disease	Also called as **burr cells** and found in renal disease

452. Ans. (c) Substitution of single amino acid base

Ref: Robbins, 8th ed. pg. 645-647

Point mutation in 6th codon of β-globin that leads to replacement of glutamate by valine residue.

453. Ans. (b) Plasmacytoma

Ref: Page 364, Harsh Mohan, 7th edition and Bone Marrow Pathology by Bain 4th ed. Page 50

The image shows presence of *Mott cells* which are plasma cells characterized by an accumulation of multiple Russell bodies, globular cytoplasmic inclusions composed of immunoglobulin.

454. Ans. (b) Macrocytic anemia

Ref: Chapter 26, Wintrobe's Hematology, 12th ed.

The image shown reveals the following findings:

- *Marked variation* in size and shape of RBC.
- *Macrocytes are seen* and have a wide central pale area. Immature RBC with bluish cytoplasm is noted in middle.
  - The combination of clinical findings and reports mentioned in the question point to diagnosis of B_{12} deficiency
  - Loss of reflexes due to an associated peripheral neuropathy in a patient who also has Babinski signs is an important diagnostic clue.

455. Ans. (a) Lead poisoning

Ref: Harsh Mohan, Textbook of Pathology, 7th ed. pg. 236

The image shows basophilic stippling of red blood cells. The causes are:

Mnemonic: **LUNATIC**
- **L**ead poisoning
- **U**nstable hemoglobin
- **N**ucleotidase deficiency
- **A**nemia due to B_{12} deficiency
- **T**halassemia
- **I**nfections
- **C**irrhosis

The closest answer Pappenheimer bodies are basophilic erythrocytic inclusions that are usually located at the periphery of the cell. They contain iron and stain with Prussian blue. Prussian blue is the stain that is used to identify that these Pappenheimer bodies are pure iron deposits, and not heme as in Heinz bodies.

456. Ans. (a) Pappenheimer body

Ref: Harsh Mohan, Textbook of Pathology, 7th ed. pg. 277

- The image shows presence of *Pappenheimer bodies* which are basophilic erythrocytic inclusions that are usually located at the periphery of the cell.
- They are composed of *ferritin aggregates* and stain on Romanowsky stain because of clumps of ribosomes which are precipitated with iron containing organelles.

457. Ans. (a) Perl stain

Ref: Harsh Mohan, Textbook of Pathology, 7th ed. pg. 98

- The image shows presence of *blue deposits called Pappenheimer bodies* and they contain iron and stain with perls' Prussian blue.
- Ferric iron deposits in tissue react with the soluble ferrocyanide in the stain, to form insoluble *Prussian blue dye* (a complex hydrated ferric ferrocyanide substance) *in situ*.

458. Ans. (d) Denatured hemoglobin

Ref: Harsh Mohan, Textbook of Pathology, 7th ed. pg. 287

- The image shows a *supra vital stain showing Heinz bodies* seen in G6PD and are composed up of denatured hemoglobin.
- *Heinz bodies*, are clinically detectable by staining with supravital dyes such as crystal violet. Removal of these inclusions by the spleen generates pitted, rigid RBCs that have shortened life spans.
- *Causes of Heinz bodies (not seen on Romanowsky stain)*

- Glucose 6 phosphatase dehydrogenase deficiency
- Glutathione synthetase deficiency
- Drugs
- Toxins
- Unstable hemoglobins

TABLE: Summary of Inclusion in RBC's

Inclusion	Composition
Howell-Jolly body	DNA
Basophilic stippling	RNA remnants
Siderotic granules/ Pappenheimer bodies	Iron
Heinz bodies	Denatured hemoglobin

459. Ans. (c) Pernicious anemia

Ref: *Clinical Hematology Turgeon, 4th ed. pg. 104*

- The image shows *Cabot ring* which may result in part from abnormalities in metabolism of both iron and arginine-rich histone that are known to occur in pernicious anemia.
- *Cabot rings are usually seen in postsplenectomy and pernicious anemia patients.*

460. Ans. (a) Dohle bodies

Ref: *Nathan and Oski Hematology of Children, 7th ed. pg. 1637*

The image shows pale blue bodies in cytoplasm of neutrophil which appears in bacterial infections. They are called Dohle bodies.

TABLE: Causes of Dohle bodies

- Infections
- Burns
- Cancer
- Massive trauma
- Prolonged use of cyclophosphamide
- May hegglin anomaly

Critical green inclusions in neutrophils are seen in severe liver disease.

461. Ans. (c) CLL

Ref: *Harsh Mohan, Textbook of Pathology, 7th ed. pg. 355-56*

- The image shows peripheral blood smear showing many *"smudge" or "basket" cells*, nuclear remnants of cells damaged by the physical shear stress of making the blood smear.
- The clinical presentation and peripheral smear favour diagnosis of CLL.

462. Ans. (a) Hand-Foot sydrome

Ref: *Harsh Mohan, Textbook of Pathology, 7th ed. pg. 294-96*

The X-ray spine shows *fish shaped vertebra* with peripheral smear showing sickle shaped RBC's. The presence of sickling crisis lead to *Hand-Foot syndrome* is characterized by painful infarcts of the digits and dactylitis.

463. Ans. (b) Basophil

Ref: *Harsh Mohan, Textbook of Pathology, 7th ed. pg. 294-96*

The image shows a white blood cell with blue granules in the cytoplasm indicative of basophil.

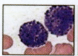
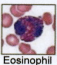
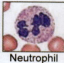
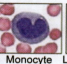
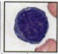

Basophil | Eosinophil | Neutrophil | Monocyte | Lymphocyte

464. Ans. (a) Eosinophil

Ref: *Harsh Mohan, Textbook of Pathology, 7th ed. pg. 129*

The image shows a white blood cell with pink granules in the cytoplasm indicative of eosinophil.

465. Ans. (d) ESR measurement

Ref: *Wintrobe's Hematology, 12th ed. pg. 16*

This method uses Wintrobe's tube, a narrow glass tube closed at the lower end only. The Wintrobe's tube has a **length of 11 cm** and **internal diameter of 2.5 mm**. It contains 0.7–1 mL of blood. The marking is 0 at the top and 10 at the bottom for ESR. This tube can also be used for PCV. The marking is 10 at the top and 0 at the bottom for PCV.

466. Ans. (a) EDTA

Ref: *Wintrobe's Hematology, 12th ed. pg. 16*

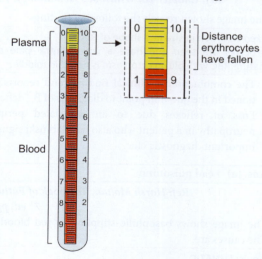

Requirements:

- Anticoagulated blood (EDTA, double oxalate)
- Pasteur pipette
- Timer
- Wintrobe's tube
- Wintrobe's stand

467. **Ans. (c) Thalassemia**

   Ref: Harsh Mohan Textbook of Pathology, 7th ed. pg. 292 and Wintrobe's Hematology, 13th ed. pg. 610

   - The image shows performance of *Naked eye single tube, osmotic fragility test*. Notice that in control sample on right side, the fine print of newspaper can be acknowledged.
   - However in the left sided sample, *osmotic fragility is reduced* leading to turbidity, leading to opacification of sample and the fine print of the newspaper cannot be read.
   - This test is a *screening test for thalassemia* following which high performance liquid chromatography is done.

468. **Ans. (d) Gamma globulin**

   Ref: Chapter 99, Wintrobe's Hematology, 12th ed.

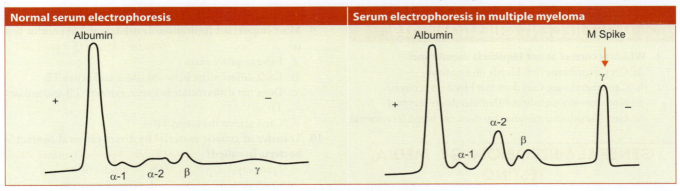

469. **Ans. (d) Rouleaux formation**

   Ref: Wintrobe's Haematology, 13th ed. pg. 593

   Rouleaux formation is associated with *increased positively charged proteins* usually fibrinogen or gamma globulins. The positively charged proteins neutralize the negatively charged RBC allowing them to form stacks in the form of stacks of four or more cells.

470. **Ans. (a) Teratoma**

   Ref: Robbins and Cotran Atlas of Pathology, 3rd ed. pg. 356

   - Teratomas are made up of a variety of parenchymal cell types representing more than 1 germ layer and often all 3 germ layer.
   - Cells differentiate along various germ lines, essentially recapitulating any tissue of the body. Examples include hair, teeth, fat, skin, muscle, and endocrine tissue.
   - Arising from totipotential cells, these tumors typically are midline or paraxial.
   - The **most common location is sacrococcygeal** (57%).
   - Because they arise from totipotential cells, they are encountered commonly in the gonads (29%).
   - The **most common gonadal location is the ovary**, although they also occur somewhat less frequently in the testes.

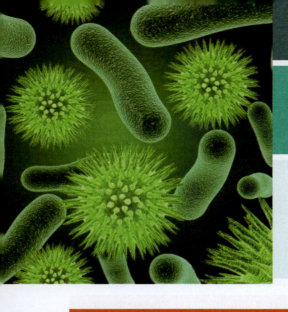

6

Microbiology and Parasitology

MOST RECENT QUESTION 2019

1. Which is correct about Diptheria membrane?
   a. Grey membrane that bleeds on removal
   b. Grey membrane that does not bleed on removal
   c. Grey pseudo-membrane that bleeds on removal
   d. Grey pseudo-membrane that does not bleed on removal

GENERAL MICROBIOLOGY, MEDIA, TESTING

2. DNA transfer in bacteria via phage is: *(Recent Pattern Question 2018-19)*
   a. Conjugation
   b. Transduction
   c. Transformation
   d. Translation

3. Sporulation occurs in this phase of bacterial growth curve: *(Recent Pattern Question 2018-19)*
   a. Stationary phase
   b. Lag phase
   c. Log phase
   d. Decline phase

4. Glutaraldehyde is used for all of the following EXCEPT: *(Recent Pattern Question 2018)*
   a. Bronchoscope
   b. Thermometer
   c. Proctoscopes
   d. Endoscopic tubes

5. Most potent disinfectant: *(Recent Pattern Question 2018)*
   a. 70% alcohol
   b. Glutaraldehyde
   c. Povidone-iodine
   d. Sodium hypochlorite

6. Sporulation is seen in which phase of bacterial growth phase? *(Recent Pattern Question 2017)*
   a. Lag phase
   b. Log phase
   c. Stationary phase
   d. Decline phase

7. Cold sterilization is done by: *(Recent Pattern Question 2017)*
   a. Steam
   b. Ionizing radiation
   c. Infra red
   d. UV

8. Metachromatic granules can be stained by *(Recent Pattern Question 2016)*
   a. Albert stain
   b. Gram stain
   c. Gram-negative stain
   d. Prussian blue

9. Most important limitation/drawback of Tuberculin test is: *(Recent Pattern Question 2016)*
   a. False negative cases
   b. Can't differentiate between latent and active TB
   c. Does not differentiate between primary TB and miliary TB
   d. Can't screen the latent TB

10. Transfer of genetic material by direct physical contact is bacteria in called? *(Recent Pattern Question 2016)*
    a. Lysogeny
    b. Transduction
    c. Conjugation
    d. Transformation

11. Lysogenic conversion is *(Recent Pattern Question 2016)*
    a. Integration of host bacterial nucleic acid to phage
    b. Integration of phage nucleic acid to host bacteria genome
    c. Bacterial mechanism to cause antigenic shift
    d. Bacterial method to acquire resistance

12. Mesophilic organism grows at *(Recent Pattern Question 2016)*
    a. – 20 to 7°C
    b. 10 to 20°C
    c. 25 to 40°C
    d. 55 to 80°C

13. Yellow bag is destroyed by *(Recent Pattern Question 2016)*
    a. Incineration
    b. Autoclave
    c. Hot air oven
    d. Steam sterilization

14. Incineration is done for *(Recent Pattern Question 2016)*
    a. Human body parts
    b. Syringes
    c. Body fluids
    d. Gloves

15. Grease, dusting powder and paraffin are sterilized by *(Recent Pattern Question 2016)*
    a. Gamma radiation
    b. Sunlight
    c. Dry heat sterilization
    d. Autoclave

16. Gram Stain is a:
    a. Simple stain
    b. Differential stain
    c. Negative stain
    d. None

17. Method of choice for sterilization of liquid paraffin:
    a. Flaming
    b. Moist heat
    c. Autoclave
    d. Hot air oven

18. Hot air oven efficiency is best checked by which bacteria:
    a. Stearothermophillus
    b. Bacillus subtilis
    c. Clostridium tetani
    d. Streptococcus

Microbiology and Parasitology

19. **Prion is best destroyed by**
   a. Autoclaving at 135 degrees
   b. Hot air oven at 160 degrees
   c. Hydrogen peroxide
   d. Sodium hypochlorite

20. **Which of the following culture medium is made by adding Agar:**
   a. Solid medium
   b. Liquid medium
   c. Selective medium
   d. Transport medium

21. **Agar is added to Broth medium:**
   a. To make the medium liquid
   b. To make the medium solid
   c. To provide extra nutrition to grow
   d. None

22. **Which of the following bacteria is isolated with Cetrimide agar?**
   a. Clostridium Perfringens
   b. Clostridium tetani
   c. Pseudomonas aeruginosa
   d. E. Coli

23. **Cetrimide agar isolates which of the following bacteria:**
   a. Clostridium perfringens
   b. Clostridium tetani
   c. Klebsiella
   d. Pseudomonas

24. **Thayer martin agar medium is for:**
   a. N. Meningitis
   b. Pseudomonas
   c. Clostridium
   d. Trypanoma pallidum

25. **Culture media for corynebacterium diphtheria:**
   a. New york media
   b. Cysteine tellurite agar
   c. Thayer martin agar
   d. Tellurite media

26. **Which of the following is best for diagnosing genital TB?**
   a. PCR
   b. Montoux
   c. LJ medium
   d. ZN staining

27. **In Robertson cooked meat media, meat color will change to:**
   a. Pink
   b. Red
   c. Blue
   d. No color change

28. **Citrate test is done for**
   a. G6PD deficiency
   b. For bacteria using glucose
   c. For bacteria using citrate
   d. For virus using citrate and glucose

29. **Mac Conkey medium is an example of:**
   a. Selective media
   b. Differential media
   c. Enriched media
   d. Transport media

30. **All of the following are examples of Indicator media EXCEPT:**
   a. Blood agar
   b. Eosin methylene blue (EMB)
   c. MacConkey (MCK)
   d. Stuart media

31. **Stain used in preparation of AFB smear:**
   a. Giemsa stain
   b. Loeffler's stain
   c. Ziehl-Neelsen stain
   d. India ink stain

32. **Weil Felix reaction is what type of agglutination reaction:**
   a. Slide agglutination
   b. Tube agglutination
   c. Passive agglutination
   d. Direct agglutination

33. **Which of the following is an example of precipitation reaction:**
   a. Coomb's Test
   b. Counter current immune-electrophoresis
   c. Weil-Felix Test
   d. Widal Test

34. **Which of the following test is an example of tube agglutination test:**
   a. Blood grouping
   b. Vibrio cholera serotyping
   c. Widal test
   d. ANA

35. **In prokaryotes, which of the following is present:**
   a. Nucleolus
   b. ER
   c. Golgi bodies
   d. Muramic acid

36. **Lancefield classification is done on the basis of:**
   a. C -substance
   b. Glycoprotein O
   c. Muramic acid
   d. Antibiotic resistance

37. **Which of the following protein is attached to surface of bacteria and phagocytized?**
   a. Antigen
   b. Antibody
   c. C-Reactive protein
   d. Propendin

38. **All of the following methods are used for the diagnosis of HIV infection in a 2 month old child EXCEPT:**
   a. DNA PCR
   b. Viral culture
   c. HIV EIisa
   d. P24 antigen assay

39. **Paul Bunnel test is used for diagnosis of:**
   a. Chicken pox
   b. Yellow fever
   c. Genital Herpes
   d. Infectious mononucleosis

BACTERIOLOGY

40. **Bacillus Anthrax is:** *(Recent Pattern Question 2018-19)*
   a. Gram positive cocci in cluster
   b. Gram positive rods with square ends
   c. Gram positive bacilli with spherical ends
   d. Gram negative cocci in cluster

41. **Which of the following is the most likely cause in a case of granuloma with positive AFB?**
   (Recent Pattern Question 2018-19)
   a. Cat scratch disease
   b. Trench fever
   c. Leprosy
   d. Syphilis

42. **Legionnaire disease causes?**
   (Recent Pattern Question 2018-19)
   a. Respiratory disease
   b. U.T.I
   c. Retroperitoneal fibrosis
   d. Acute gastroenteritis

43. **When should you perform Widal test in a case of Typhoid?** *(Recent Pattern Question 2018-19)*
   a. 1st week
   b. 2nd week
   c. 3rd week
   d. 4th week

FMGE Solutions Screening Examination

44. Which of the following is anaerobic non-acid fast bacilli? *(Recent Pattern Question 2018)*
    a. Tuberculosis b. Listeria
    c. Nocardia d. Actinomyces

45. Which of the following is a capnophilic bacteria? *(Recent Pattern Question 2018)*
    a. *Staphylococcus aureus* b. *Mycobacterium*
    c. *Clostridium* d. *Haemophilus influenzae*

46. Anton test is done for: *(Recent Pattern Question 2017)*
    a. Klebsiella b. Listeria monocytogenes
    c. Proteus mirabilis d. Nisseria

47. Diphtheria toxin acts by: *(Recent Pattern Question 2017)*
    a. Inhibiting glucose synthesis
    b. Inhibiting protein synthesis
    c. Promoting acetylcholine release
    d. Altering cyclic GMP levels

48. Tumbling motility is seen in: *(Recent Pattern Question 2017)*
    a. Listeria monocytogenes b. C. Jejuni
    c. Trichomonas d. Gonococcus

49. "Fish in stream" appearance is seen in? *(Recent Pattern Question 2017)*
    a. Hemophilus ducreyi b. Proteus
    c. Mycoplasma d. V. Cholerae

50. Pontiac fever is caused by? *(Recent Pattern Question 2017)*
    a. Rickettsia rickettsii b. Brucella
    c. Legionella d. Moraxella

51. A 30-year-old patient presented with fever, headache and vomiting. He had splenectomy few years ago. Most probable organism? *(Recent Pattern Question 2017)*
    a. Meningococcus b. Pneumococcus
    c. E. Coli d. C. Diptheriae

52. Out of 20 children that went to a party, 11 developed abdominal pain, diarrhea with nausea and vomiting around 6 hours after food intake. Most likely causative agent: *(Recent Pattern Question 2017)*
    a. Rota virus b. Staphylococcus
    c. Streptococcus d. Clostridium perfringens

53. Secondary bacterial pneumonia in a post-influenza patient is most likely due to? *(Recent Pattern Question 2017)*
    a. Staphylococcus aureus b. Moraxella
    c. Listeria d. Klebsiella

54. Corynebacterium diphtheria is *(Recent Pattern Question 2016)*
    a. Gram-positive cocci b. Gram-positive bacilli
    c. Gram-negative cocci d. Gram-negative bacilli

55. Which of the following is the most severe form of Diptheria *(Recent Pattern Question 2016)*
    a. Nasal
    b. Cutaneous
    c. Nasophyranx
    d. Laryngophyranx

56. McFadyean reaction is seen in: *(Recent Pattern Question 2016)*
    a. Yersinia pestis b. Clostridium perfringens
    c. Bacillus anthrax d. Staphylococcus aureus

57. Organism causing IV biofilm? *(Recent Pattern Question 2016)*
    a. Staph epidermis b. Acinetobacter baumannii
    c. Meningococci d. Mycobacterium

58. Staph. epidermis has become important due to
    a. Biofilm formation *(Recent Pattern Question 2016)*
    b. Virulence
    c. Wide spectrum antibiotics
    d. Novobiocin resistance

59. During examination of skin smears in leprosy test result was 1+, 2+. How many oil fields should be surveyed *(Recent Pattern Question 2016)*
    a. 10 b. 25
    c. 50 d. 100

60. In an oil immersion field 1-10 tubercle bacilli were seen per 10 field. It indicates *(Recent Pattern Question 2016)*
    a. + b. ++
    c. +++ d. Scanty

61. Which disease occurs after eating uncooked meat *(Recent Pattern Question 2016)*
    a. Bacillus anthrax b. Brucella
    c. Trichosis d. TB

62. Yersinia pestis is transmitted by *(Recent Pattern Question 2016)*
    a. Flea b. Rodent
    c. Mite d. Sandfly

63. Gram negative anaerobic bacteria use this method of gene transfer:
    a. Transduction b. Conjugation
    c. Translation d. Transformation

64. Method of bacterial gene transfer where viruses play role:
    a. Transduction b. Conjugation
    c. Translation d. Transformation

65. During the lag phase of bacterial growth curve, there is:
    a. Increase in number b. Increase in metabolic rate
    c. Increase in size d. Decreased metabolic rate

66. CLO test is done for:
    a. HPV b. Salmonella typhi
    c. HIV d. H. Pylori

67. Tumbling motility is seen in:
    a. Yersinia b. Listeria
    c. Proteus d. Pseudomonas aeruginosa

68. Which of the following is a kidney shaped bacteria:
    a. Campylobacter jejuni
    b. Corynebacterium Diphtheriae
    c. Meningococci
    d. Gonococci

Microbiology and Parasitology

69. Granuloma in lymph nodes seen is in all infections EXCEPT:
  a. TB
  b. Sarcoidosis
  c. Staph Aureus
  d. Hemophilus ducreyi

70. Which of the following organisms causes fastest food poisoning:
  a. Staph. Aureus
  b. Clostridium Perfringens
  c. Bacillus Cereus
  d. Vibrio cholerae

71. A Person ate some milk products in a party and after 6 hours started vomiting. Which organism is most likely the cause:
  a. Bacillus cereus
  b. Clostridium perfringens
  c. Staphylococcus
  d. Clostridium botulism

72. Food poisoning 2 hours after intake of food is caused by?
  a. Salmonella typhi
  b. Bacillus cereus
  c. Staphylococcus aureus
  d. Clostridium

73. How does staph aureus become resistant to methicillin:
  a. Heat shock protein
  b. Protein A
  c. Transpeptidase
  d. Protein C

74. Organism responsible for toxicity due to Chinese fried rice:
  a. Staph. Aureus
  b. B. Cereus
  c. Salmonella
  d. Shigella

75. The following are true about Bacillus Cereus induced diarrhea EXCEPT
  a. Can be transmitted by parenteral route
  b. The enterotoxins are not resistant to acidic contents of the stomach
  c. It is caused by enterotoxins
  d. It is usually associated with fried rice or chinese food which is reheated

76. Incubation period of salmonella:
  a. 7–21 days
  b. 2–5 days
  c. 14–21 days
  d. 0–60 days

77. Rice watery stool is a common indicative of which organism?
  a. Vibrio cholerae O1
  b. Vibrio cholerae O139
  c. Vibrio vulnificus
  d. Shigella

78. Which of the following is most likely cause of a child presenting with fever and diarrhea?
  a. EPEC
  b. ETEC
  c. EHEC
  d. EIEC

79. Which organism causes haemolytic uremic syndrome?
  a. Neisseria
  b. Salmonella
  c. Pseudomonas
  d. E. Coli

80. HUS is caused by:
  a. EIEC
  b. EPEC
  c. ETEC
  d. EHEC

81. Traveller's diarrhea is caused by:
  a. EIEC
  b. EPEC
  c. ETEC
  d. EHEC

82. Anti-microbials are given with which type of diarrhea:
  a. Traveller's diarrhea
  b. Rotavirus
  c. Secretory diarrhea
  d. Osmotic diarrhea

83. Which is the staphyloccocal toxin which is responsible for food poisoning?
  a. Beta Exotoxin
  b. Enterotoxin
  c. Alpha Exotoxin
  d. Toxic Shock Syndrome Toxin (TSST-1)

84. Which of the following contains single flagella?
  a. Treponema Pallidum
  b. Escherichia Coli
  c. Vibrio cholerae
  d. Heliobacter Pylori

85. Clostridium difficile can be spread through all EXCEPT–
  a. Oral - fecal route
  b. Direct
  c. Hand to hand contact
  d. Needles

86. All of the following organisms cause gas gangrene EXCEPT:
  a. Clostridium Difficile
  b. Clostridium Welchi
  c. Clostridium Septicum
  d. Clostridium Perfringens

87. Necrotizing enteritis is caused by:
  a. Clostridium tetani
  b. Clostridium difficile
  c. Clostridium perfringens
  d. Clostridium septicum

88. Gas gangrene is caused by
  a. Clostridium perfringens
  b. Bacillus cereus
  c. Helicobater pylori
  d. Treponema pallidum

89. Fournier gangrene is caused by:
  a. Cl. Welchi
  b. Proteus
  c. Streptococcus
  d. Mixed infection

90. Anchovy Sauce pus/chocolate brown pus is the clinical feature of:
  a. Amoebic liver abscess
  b. Pyogenic liver abscess
  c. Peritoneal abscess
  d. Hydatid liver

91. A patient presents with signs of pneumonia. The bacterium obtained from sputum was a Gram positive cocci which showed alpha hemolysis on sheep agar. Which of the following test will help to confirm the diagnosis:
  a. Bile solubility
  b. Coagulase test
  c. Bacitracin test
  d. CAMP test

92. Energy store of cell is:
  a. Adenosine monophosphate
  b. Adenosine diphosphate
  c. Adenosine triphosphate
  d. Adenosine quadriphosphate

93. Most common cause of Pneumatocele:
  a. Streptococcus pneumoniae
  b. Haemophilus influenza
  c. Serratia marcescens
  d. Staphylococcus aureus

94. Child presented with cystic fibrosis and Bronchorrhea. Which group of organism is appropriate causative agent:
  a. Staph. Aureus, H. influenza, Pseudomonas
  b. Streptococcus pneumonia, Klebsiella, H. Influenza
  c. H.Influenza, Klebsiella, staph aureus
  d. Strep.Pneumoniae, H.Influenza, Klebsiella

Questions

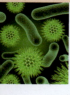

FMGE Solutions Screening Examination

95. Streptococcus pyogenes can be checked by which drug disk
    a. Bacitracin   b. Polymycin
    c. Optochin   d. None of the above
96. Chronic burrowing ulcer is caused by:
    a. Peptostreptococcus
    b. Strep.pyogenes
    c. Anaerobic streptococci
    d. Microaerophilic streptococci
97. Which of the following is common with Streptococcus infection?
    a. Cellulitis   b. Gangrene
    c. Pyoderma   d. UTI
98. All are true about Entamoeba Histolytica EXCEPT:
    a. Cyst are 4 nucleated
    b. Cyst are 8 nucleated
    c. Trophozoites colonise in the colon and rectum
    d. The chromatid bodies are stained by iron hematoxylin
99. Which of the following is a non motile bacteria –
    a. Klebsiella pneumoniae   b. Helicobacter pylori
    c. Vibrio Cholerae   d. E.Coli
100. Miliary shadow on X-Ray is seen in all EXCEPT:
    a. TB
    b. Loeffler's pneumonia
    c. Klebsiella
    d. Varicella pneumonia
101. True about Bubonic plague:
    a. An infection of the lung
    b. An infection of blood stream
    c. An infection of lymph nodes
    d. All of the above
102. Site where Neisseria Meningitidis bacteria harbour normally?
    a. Skin   b. Genitals
    c. Nasopharynx   d. Lower GIT
103. Which of the following is gram negative diplococci:
    a. Cornynebacterium Diphtheriae
    b. Neisseria Meningitidis
    c. Streptococcus pneumoniae
    d. Staphylococcus
104. Neisseria meningitidis possesses following virulent factors EXCEPT:
    a. Capsule
    b. Lipo-oligosaccharide(LOS)
    c. β lactamase
    d. IgA protease cation
105. Which one of the following microbe, found in ear discharge, has a high predilection for meningitis
    a. H. influenza
    b. Moraxella species
    c. Staphylococcus aureus
    d. Streptococcus pneumoniae
106. Which one of the following organisms is the most frequent cause of acute pyogenic meningitis in adults:
    a. Streptococcus pneumoniae
    b. Neisseria meningitis
    c. Haemophilus influenza
    d. Listeria monocytogenes
107. Meningococcal vaccine not used for:
    a. Serotype A   b. Serotype B
    c. Serotype C   d. Serotype Y
108. Air crescent sign seen in infection due to:
    a. Staphylococcus   b. Streptococcus
    c. Diphtheria   d. Aspergillus
109. Incubation period of diphtheria:
    a. 2-3 days   b. 5-7 days
    c. 14-15 days   d. 21 days
110. Calymmatobacterium is?
    a. Gram negative   b. Gram positive
    c. Acid fast   d. Non- acid fast
111. Prolonged salmonella septicemia is caused by
    a. S. Enteritidis   b. S. Typhimurium
    c. S. Typhi   d. S. Cholerae-suis
112. Draughtsman appearance of colonies is seen with?
    a. Streptococcus   b. Pneumococcus
    c. Staphylococcus   d. Menngococcus
113. A 3 yr old boy fell down and injured his leg while he was playing on ground. After a few days, there are crepitations felt from injured area, what could be the probable causative organism?
    a. Corynebacterium Diphtheriae
    b. Pseudomonas Aeruginosa
    c. Clostridium Tetani
    d. Clostridium Welchii
114. Drum stick is characteristic of:
    a. Corynebacterium diphtheriae
    b. Clostridium tetani
    c. Neisseria meningitides
    d. Strep Pneumoniae
115. Drugs indicated in MRSA infection are all EXCEPT:
    a. Vancomycin   b. Teicoplanin
    c. Linezolid   d. Imipenem
116. True about Aspergillosis?
    a. Angioinvasive
    b. Oto-mycosis
    c. Occur in asthmatics
    d. All of the above
117. Not a common cause of community acquired pneumonia EXCEPT:
    a. Staphylococci   b. Mycoplasma
    c. Chlamydia pneumonia   d. Streptococci
118. Leptospirosis is caused by :
    a. Dog urine   b. Mosquito
    c. Rat urine   d. cat urine

119. Blood culture of a patient shows growth of gram positive cocci which are catalase positive and coagulase negative. The patient was on a CVP line last week. The most likely etiological agent is?
    a. Staphylococcus aureus
    b. Staphylococcus epidermidis
    c. Streptococcus pyogenes
    d. Enterococcus faecalis
120. Which of the following parasite causes myocarditis?
    a. Trichuris trichura
    b. Ancyclostoma duodenale
    c. Taenia solium
    d. Trichenella spiralis

VIROLOGY

121. Rapid diagnosis of rabies is made with:
    (Recent Pattern Question 2018-19)
    a. Rabies virus specific antibodies
    b. Inoculation in mouse
    c. Skin biopsy with fluorescent antibody testing
    d. Corneal impression smear
122. Most common infectious cause of haemolysis:
    (Recent Pattern Question 2018-19)
    a. E. coli 0157   b. Malaria
    c. Parvovirus B19   d. Bartonella henselae
123. Which of the following virus is from Herpes virus family? *(Recent Pattern Question 2018-19)*
    a. Rubella   b. Measles
    c. Rabies   d. EBV
124. Molluscum contagiosum is a _____:
    (Recent Pattern Question 2018-19)
    a. Adenovirus   b. Flavi virus
    c. Rubi virus   d. Pox virus
125. Which of the following is an RNA virus?
    (Recent Pattern Question 2017)
    a. Hepatitis B virus   b. Hepatitis C virus
    c. Herpes virus   d. Adenovirus
126. Hand foot mouth disease is caused by:
    (Recent Pattern Question 2017)
    a. Enterobius   b. Coxsackie
    c. Adenovirus   d. Prion disease
127. Which is true about rota virus infection?
    (Recent Pattern Question 2017)
    a. Vaccine preventable disease
    b. Can be treated by saline infusion
    c. Predominates in summer season
    d. Has high mortality rate
128. Intracytoplasmic inclusion body is seen in?
    (Recent Pattern Question 2017)
    a. HSV   b. Polio
    c. Rabies   d. Yellow fever

129. A patient presented with fever, cervical lymphadenopathy and night sweats four weeks after unprotected sexual contact. Next investigation *(Recent Pattern Question 2016)*
    a. p24   b. ELISA
    c. CD4   d. HIV PCR
130. m-RNA to C-DNA is made by
    a. Reverse transcriptase   b. DNA polymerase
    c. RNA polymerase   d. DNA Ligase
131. Intracytoplasmic and Intranuclear inclusion body is seen in?
    a. Measles   b. Mumps
    c. Rabies   d. Yellow fever
132. Intra nuclear inclusion body is exclusively seen in:
    a. Rabies virus   b. Pox virus
    c. Measles virus   d. Herpes virus
133. Which among the following disease is transmitted by virus:
    a. Molluscum contagiosum   b. Taenia capitis
    c. Rhinosporodiosis   d. Impetigo
134. Molluscum contagiosum is a:
    a. Bacteria   b. Fungus
    c. Virus   d. Parasite
135. Which of the following disease acts by Reverse transcriptase action:
    a. HTLV- I   b. HIV
    c. Both A and B   d. Hepatitis C
136. Hemagglutination is caused by which organism:
    a. Influenza virus   b. Mumps
    c. Adenovirus   d. Parvovirus
137. Which of the following is not caused by virus:
    a. Rocky mountain spotted fever
    b. KFD
    c. Dengue
    d. Yellow fever
138. Most common cause of common cold/coryza is?
    a. Influenza virus   b. Adenovirus
    c. RSV   d. Rhinovirus
139. Duffy antigen is a receptor for?
    a. P. Falciparum   b. P. Ovale
    c. P. Vivax   d. P. Malariae
140. Human papilloma virus is a:
    a. RNA virus   b. DNA virus
    c. Both   d. None
141. Jarisch Herxheimer (J-H) reaction is commonly seen in
    a. Primary syphillis   b. Secondary syphilis
    c. Late congenital syphilis d. Latent syphilis
142. Intermediate host for Rabies is?
    a. Human   b. Rat
    c. Dogs   d. Cats
143. True about chicken pox:
    a. Incubation period 2-3 days.
    b. Vesicobullous rash
    c. Vesicobullous rash   d. Spare palm & sole

MYCOLOGY AND PARASITOLOGY

144. A patient presented with some unknown fungal infection. Microscopic examination revealed brown coloured spherical fungi with septate hyphae. Possible condition: *(Recent Pattern Question 2018-19)*
    a. Histoplasmosis
    b. Chromoblastomycosis
    c. Coccidiodomycosis
    d. Candida albicans

145. Which is correct about larval stage of Taenia solium? *(Recent Pattern Question 2018-19)*
    a. Larva currens
    b. Cysticercosis cellulose
    c. Cutaneous larva migrans
    d. Visceral larva migrans

146. Germ tube test is done for: *(Recent Pattern Question 2018)*
    a. Chlamydia
    b. Candida albicans
    c. Bacterial vaginosis
    d. *Neisseria gonorrhoeae*

147. Microsporum involves: *(Recent Pattern Question 2018)*
    a. Skin, hair and nails
    b. Skin and hair
    c. Skin and nails
    d. Hair and nails

148. Pulmonary eosinophilia is seen due to which of the following infection? *(Recent Pattern Question 2018)*
    a. Ancylostoma
    b. Trichinella
    c. Filaria
    d. Roundworm

149. Which parasite lives in bladder plexus? *(Recent Pattern Question 2018)*
    a. *Schistosoma*
    b. *Fasciola*
    c. *Ascaris*
    d. *Echinococcus*

150. What is true about Echinococcus Granulosus?
    a. Definitive host in humans *(Recent Pattern Question 2017)*
    b. Accidental intermediate host in humans
    c. Intermediate host in dogs
    d. Definitive host in snails

151. Which plasmodium infection has predilection for attacking old RBCs? *(Recent Pattern Question 2017)*
    a. Plasmodium Vivax
    b. Plasmodium Ovale
    c. Plasmodium malariae
    d. Plasmodium Falciparum

152. Mature spherules in sputum sample is seen in which of the following? *(Recent Pattern Question 2017)*
    a. Staphylococcus
    b. Streptococcus
    c. Coccidioidomycosis
    d. Aspergillus

153. Which parasite causes severe malabsorption syndrome *(Recent Pattern Question 2016)*
    a. Giardiasis
    b. Hook worm
    c. Ascariasis
    d. Amoebiasis

154. Definitive host of ascariasis *(Recent Pattern Question 2016)*
    a. Dog
    b. Man
    c. Pig
    d. Monkey

155. All are cestodes EXCEPT *(Recent Pattern Question 2016)*
    a. Treponema pallidum
    b. Echinococcus
    c. Taenia solium
    d. Taenia saginata

156. Kerion is a
    a. Bacteria
    b. Prion
    c. Virus
    d. Fungus

157. Which of the following method is used in the rapid identification of Candida:
    a. Culture in solid
    b. Germ tube method
    c. Growing in an animal
    d. Culture in liquid

158. KOH mount is done for:
    a. Bacterial vaginosis
    b. Candida
    c. Syphilis
    d. Chancroid

159. Lyme disease is caused by:
    a. Borrelia vincenti
    b. Borrelia Burgdorferi
    c. Borrelia Recurrentis
    d. Treponema Pertenue

160. Groove sign is seen in
    a. Chancroid
    b. Syphilis
    c. Granuloma inguinale
    d. LGV

161. Which of the following fungal infection is a leading cause of corneal ulcer?
    a. Trichophyton
    b. Aspergillus
    c. Mucor
    d. Sprothrix

162. Enterobius vermicularis commonly resides in:
    a. Duodenum
    b. Ileum
    c. Appendix and cecum
    d. Sigmoid colon

163. Which parasite multiplies in appendix and blocks lumen?
    a. Pin worm
    b. Strongyloides stercoralis
    c. Round worm
    d. Hook worm

164. All are true about Toxocariasis EXCEPT?
    a. Dogs and foxes are the host of toxocara canis
    b. Causes visceral larva migrans
    c. Causes cutaneous larva migrans
    d. Hypereosinophilia is a significant finding

165. Cutaneous larva migrans is caused by-
    a. Trichinella
    b. Ancylostoma braziliense
    c. Angiostrongylus cantonensis
    d. Toxocara canis

166. All are TRUE regarding filariasis EXCEPT:
    a. Involves lymphatic system
    b. Caused by wucheria bancrofti
    c. Man is an intermediate host
    d. DEC is used in treatment

167. A person was bitten by an infected louse and developed a disease. What is the probable diagnosis?
    a. Scrub typhus
    b. Epidemic typhus
    c. Endemic typhus
    d. Indian Tick typhus

168. Tape worm is found mainly in
    a. Liver
    b. Stomach
    c. Caecum
    d. Ileum & jejunum

169. In which stage of filariasis are microfilaria seen in peripheral blood:
    a. Acute adenolymphangitis stage
    b. Tropical eosinophilia
    c. Chyluria
    d. Elephantiasis

Microbiology and Parasitology

170. Ova in stool are not of diagnostic significance in:
   a. Ankylostoma
   b. Entrobius
   c. Strongyloides
   d. Trichuris

171. Example of Zoonoses are all EXCEPT:
   a. Plague
   b. Rabies
   c. Taeniasis
   d. Brucellosis

172. A 20 year old man presents with swelling of left lower limb and hydrocoele. All of the following may be the causative agent EXCEPT:
   a. Brugia malayi
   b. Brugia timoria
   c. Wuchereria bancrofti
   d. Onchocerca volvulus

IMMUNOLOGY AND MISCELLANEOUS

173. N. meningitis can be due to deficiency of this complement system: *(Recent Pattern Question 2018-19)*
   a. C1 – C4 deficiency
   b. C5-C9 deficiency
   c. C3 deficiency
   d. C2 deficiency

174. Classical complement activated by: *(Recent Pattern Question 2018-19)*
   a. C1
   b. C3 convertase
   c. IgA
   d. Ag – Ab complex

175. In normal immune system, the epithelioid cells are derived from: *(Recent Pattern Question 2018)*
   a. TH1
   b. TH2
   c. Macrophages
   d. TH19

176. Meningococcal meningitis is seen with which of the following complement deficiency? *(Recent Pattern Question 2018)*
   a. C1q
   b. C2
   c. C4
   d. C5

177. All of the following are true about bacteriophage EXCEPT: *(Recent Pattern Question 2017)*
   a. It is a bacteria
   b. It helps in transduction
   c. It imparts toxigenicity by lysogenic conversion
   d. It can cause drug resistanc

178. IgM is:
   a. Monomer
   b. Dimer
   c. Pentamer
   d. Tetramer

179. First antibody produced by newborn?
   a. IgA
   b. IgG
   c. IgE
   d. IgM

180. Immunoglobulin found in bronchial secretion:
   a. IgA
   b. IgG
   c. IgM
   d. IgE

181. Which of the following is used as prophylaxis in case of diphtheria:
   a. Erythromycin
   b. Ampicillin
   c. DPT vaccine
   d. DAT

182. A child presents with infective skin lesion of the leg. Culture was done which showed gram positive cocci in chains with hemolytic colonies. The test to confirm the organism is?
   a. Bile solubility
   b. Optochin sensitivity
   c. Bacitracin sensitivity
   d. Catalase +ve

183. Most common site of angioedema:
   a. Hands
   b. Lips
   c. Skin
   d. Eyelid

184. Agglutination test for typhoid is performed on which of the following:
   a. 1st week
   b. 2nd week
   c. 3rd week
   d. 4th week

185. Congenital rubella is best diagnosed by:
   a. IgM Ab against Rubella at birth
   b. IgM Ab against Rubella at 4 months of age
   c. IgG Ab against Rubella at 4 months of age
   d. IgG Ab against Rubella at birth

186. Severe combined immunodeficiency is seen with:
   a. Pre B- Cell
   b. Pre T Cell
   c. Both
   d. NK Cell

BOARD REVIEW QUESTIONS

187. Stain used in electron microscopy?
   a. 2.5% glutaraldehyde
   b. Phosphotungstic acid
   c. Safranin
   d. Coomassie blue

188. Hypogammaglobinemia causes?
   a. Chronic recurrent sinusitis
   b. Epistaxis
   c. Contractures
   d. Eczema

189. Treponema pallidum is stained during?
   a. Albert staining
   b. Giemsa stain
   c. Fontana stain
   d. ZN stain

190. Leptospirosis is caused by?
   a. Protozoa
   b. Bacteria
   c. Virus
   d. Prion

191. Nagler reaction defects?
   a. Lecithinase
   b. Perfringolysin
   c. Cytolysin
   d. Hyaluronidase

FMGE Solutions Screening Examination

192. Citron bodies are formed by?
    a. Clostridium welchii
    b. Clostridium oedematiens
    c. Clostridium septicum
    d. Clostridium histolyticum
193. Both intranuclear and intracytoplasmic inclusion bodies are seen in?
    a. CMV
    b. Herpes
    c. Measles
    d. Adenovirus
194. Donovanosis is caused by?
    a. Calymmatobacterium granulomatosis
    b. Legionella
    c. chlymadia
    d. Rickettsia
195. All are true about Antigen drift EXCEPT?
    a. Its causes pandemic
    b. Occurs due to mutation
    c. Occurs frequently
    d. Minor antigenic changes
196. Negri bodies are mainly found in?
    a. Brain stem
    b. Cortical neurons
    c. Hippocampus
    d. Spinal cord
197. Cornybacterium diphtheria is also called?
    a. Freidlander's bacillus
    b. Klebs loeffler's bacillus
    c. Fischer's bacillus
    d. Koch's bacillus
198. Whooping cough is caused by?
    a. C.dipthera
    b. B.pertussis
    c. M.catarrhalis
    d. S.pneumonea
199. Tetanus toxin acts by?
    a. Blocking gamma motor neurons
    b. Blocking muscle end plate receptor
    c. Blocking Ach release
    d. Presynaptic blocking
200. Most common initial involvement of tetanus is seen in?
    a. Face
    b. Limbs
    c. Paraspinal muscles
    d. Abdomen
201. Food poisoning that presents within 6 hours is due to?
    a. Staphylococcus
    b. Salmonella
    c. Clostridium botulinum
    d. E.coli
202. Complement synthesized by liver is?
    a. C1
    b. C5
    c. C3
    d. C4
203. Most common protozoan parasite in stool?
    a. Hook worm
    b. Pin worm
    c. Giardia
    d. Entamoeba Histolytica
204. Blood agar is
    a. Enrichment media
    b. Enriched media
    c. Selective media
    d. Transport media
205. Father of medical microbiology
    a. Louis Pasteur
    b. Robert Koch
    c. Robert whitmore
    d. Jim Morrison
206. Chinese pattern bacteria are
    a. Diptheroids
    b. Vibrio
    c. Spirochete
    d. Pleomorphic
207. Which is used for sterilization of cystoscope
    a. Glutaraldehyde
    b. Formaldehyde
    c. Isopropyl alcohol
    d. Ethylene oxide
208. First antibody to appear in intrauterine life
    a. IgM
    b. IgA
    c. IgD
    d. IgE
209. Antibody with longest half life
    a. IgM
    b. Ig
    c. IgD
    d. IgG
210. Microglia is?
    a. B cell
    b. T cell
    c. Macrophage
    d. Dendritic cell
211. Membrane attack complex is formed by all EXCEPT?
    a. C3
    b. C5
    c. C7
    d. C9
212. Colony of Streptococcus viridans resembles?
    a. Staphylococcus
    b. Streptococcus pneumoniae
    c. Enterococcus
    d. Klebsiella
213. Which organism can penetrate intact cornea?
    a. Pneumococcus
    b. Gonococcus
    c. Pseudomonas
    d. Staphylococcus
214. Medusa head colonies are seen in
    a. Bacillus anthracis
    b. Bacillus cereus
    c. C. parvum
    d. C. difficile
215. Sereny test is used for?
    a. EHEC
    b. ETEC
    c. EIEC
    d. EPEC
216. All are true about V. cholera EXCEPT?
    a. VR media is transport media
    b. Alkaline peptone water is enrichment media
    c. Selective media is bile salt agar
    d. Multi-flagellated bacteria
217. Weil felix reaction is used for diagnosis of?
    a. Infectious mononucleosis
    b. Chylamydia
    c. Rickettsia
    d. Bartonella
218. Warthin Finkeldey cells are seen in
    a. SSSS
    b. Measles
    c. Rubella
    d. Mumps
219. Most common cause of bronchiolitis in children?
    a. RSV
    b. Papova virus
    c. Adenovirus
    d. H3N1
220. Which of the following is responsible for pandemic in influenza
    a. Antigenic shift
    b. Antigenic drift
    c. Antigenic rift
    d. All of the above
221. Which is a bullet shaped virus?
    a. Rabies virus
    b. Coxsackie A
    c. Coxsackie B
    d. Polio virus

Microbiology and Parasitology

222. **Virus not transmitted by breast milk is**
   a. Hepatitis A
   b. Hepatitis B
   c. Hepatitis C
   d. HIV

223. **Pilot wheel appearance of multiple budding yeast cell is seen in?**
   a. Paracoccidioides
   b. Blastomycosis
   c. Sporothrix
   d. candida

224. **Germ tube test is positive for**
   a. Candida glabrata
   b. Candida albicans
   c. Coccidiodes immitis
   d. Rhinosporidium seeberi

225. **Which is not an opportunisitic infection in AIDS?**
   a. Crytococcus
   b. Aspergillosis
   c. Dermatophyte
   d. P. Jiroveci

226. **Sabin Feldman test is used for diagnosis of?**
   a. Toxoplasma
   b. Trypanosomiasis
   c. Kala azar
   d. Post dermal kalaazar

227. **Non bile stained eggs are seen with all EXCEPT**
   a. Necator americanus
   b. Enterobius vermicularis
   c. Hymenolepis nana
   d. Strongyloides

228. **All are seen with worm infestation EXCEPT**
   a. Perianal itching
   b. Iron deficiency
   c. Rectal prolapse
   d. Descending cholangitis

229. **Most common serological type of rota virus**
   a. Group A
   b. Group B
   c. Group C
   d. Group D

230. **Passive immunization is useful for all EXCEPT?**
   a. Measles
   b. Hepatitis A
   c. Hepatitis B
   d. Herpes simplex

231. **EB virus is associated with all EXCEPT:**
   a. Bell's palsy
   b. Hepatitis
   c. Guillain-Barre syndrome
   d. Laennec's cirrhosis

232. **Dawson disease is**
   a. SSPE
   b. Acute disseminated encephalomyelitis
   c. Neuromyelitioptica
   d. River blindness

233. **Romana's sign is seen in?**
   a. Toxoplasma
   b. Trypanosoma cruzi
   c. Loa loa
   d. Wuchereria

234. **Which of the following is not associated with Streptococcus:**
   a. Rheumatic fever
   b. Scarlet fever
   c. Acute GN
   d. Scalded skin syndrome

235. **PCR was invented by**
   a. Carry B mullis
   b. Jimmi Hendrix
   c. Van den berg
   d. Eddie van halen

236. **Gram negative cocci is?**
   a. Nisseria
   b. Helicobactor
   c. Cholera
   d. Campylobactor

237. **NK Cell activator is?**
   a. IL 1
   b. IL 10
   c. IL 12
   d. IFN-y

238. **Hand foot mouth syndrome is caused by?**
   a. Parvovirus 6
   b. Parvovirus 19
   c. Coxsackie virus A16
   d. Coxsackie virus Al9

239. **"Yellow black" granules are seen in which fungal infection?**
   a. Mucormycosis
   b. Mycetoma
   c. Aspergillosis
   d. Rhinosporidiosis

240. **Immunoglobulin in peyer's patch is?**
   a. IgM
   b. IgG
   c. IgA
   d. IgD

241. **Compound used for fixation of protozoa found in stool is?**
   a. Phenol
   b. Hypochlorite
   c. Formalin
   d. Alcohol

242. **Charcot Leyden crystal is associated with which cell?**
   a. Macrophages
   b. Eosinophils
   c. Basophils
   d. Neutrophils

243. **Which of the following is responsible for phagocytosis?**
   a. C5a
   b. C3a
   c. C3b
   d. TNF-a

244. **Which of the following acts as a chemoattractant?**
   a. C3a
   b. C3b
   c. C5a
   d. LTB4

245. **Theory of web of causation was given by?**
   a. Mc Mohan and Pugh
   b. Pettenkoffer
   c. John snow
   d. Louis Pasteur

246. **Stain used for degenerated fungi in tissue is?**
   a. PAS
   b. Gomori methenamine silver
   c. H&E
   d. Muciramine

247. **Investigation of choice for amoebiasis is?**
   a. ELISA
   b. Colonoscopy
   c. Microscopy
   d. Microscopy + ELISA

248. **Widal test is a type of?**
   a. Tube agglutination
   b. Slide agglutination
   c. Tube precipitation
   d. Slide precipitation

249. **Lepra cell are?**
   a. Histiocytes
   b. Monocytes
   c. Lymphocytes
   d. N K Cells

250. **Aschoff Body is made up of?**
   a. Fibroblast
   b. Histocytes
   c. Lymphocytes
   d. Monocytes

251. **Sterilization of fibre optic bronchoscope is done by?**
   a. Glutaraldehyde
   b. Chlorine
   c. Autoclave
   d. Phenol

252. **Gas gangrene is not caused by?**
   a. Clostridium welchi
   b. Clostridium perferenges
   c. Clostridium novyi
   d. Clostridium difficile

FMGE Solutions Screening Examination

253. Thickness of bacterial cell wall is?
   a. 0–20 nm   b. 20–80 nm
   c. 80–160 nm   d. 160–240 nm

254. Glassware sterilization is done by?
   a. Hot air oven   b. Autoclaving
   c. 5% cresol   d. Hotbath

255. Alcohol destroys bacteria by which mechanism?
   a. Protein coagulation
   b. Produce cell membrane defect
   c. Inhibits DNA synthesis
   d. Oxidation

256. MHC I is recognized by?
   a. CD 4 T cells   b. CD 8 T cells
   c. Dendritic cells   d. Macrophages

257. C3b deficiency causes?
   a. SLE
   b. Collagen vascular disorders
   c. Recurrent pyogenic infections
   d. Hereditary angioneurotic edema

258. Which is not an opsonin?
   a. C5a   b. C3b
   c. IgM   d. IgG

259. Dark field microscopy used for?
   a. Syphilis   b. Rickettsia
   c. Brucella   d. T.vaginalis

260. Chancroid is caused by?
   a. H. ducreyi   b. T.palidum
   c. Leptospira   d. None of these

261. Rickettsia is resistant to which antibiotics?
   a. Tetracyclines   b. Rifampin
   c. Penicillin   d. Doxycycline

262. Clostridium perfringens toxemia is caused by which toxin?
   a. Alpha toxin   b. Beta toxin
   c. Theta toxin   d. Delta toxin

263. Differentiating feature of Neisseria gonococcus from Neisseria meningitidis is?
   a. Lactose fermentation   b. Maltose fermentation
   c. Mennitol fermentation   d. Sucrose fermentation

264. Hemagglutination showing viruses are?
   a. Respiratory syncytial virus
   b. Influenza virus
   c. Paramyxo virus
   d. None of these

265. Most common cause of common cold is?
   a. Virus   b. Bacteria
   c. Fungus   d. Allergic

266. Intranuclear basophilic inclusion body with halo is seen in?
   a. Herpes zoster   b. Herpes simplex
   c. CMV   d. Adenovirus

267. The vector for chandipura virus is?
   a. Sandfly   b. Trombiculid mite
   c. House fly   d. Fish

268. HPV does not cause?
   a. Condyloma Lata   b. Condyloma acuminatum
   c. Common warts   d. None of these

269. Common warts are caused by?
   a. HPV 6 and 11   b. HPV 16 and 18
   c. HPV 2 and 7   d. HPV 63

270. Oral hairy leukoplakia is associated with?
   a. Cytomegalovirus
   b. Human immunodeficiency virus
   c. EBV   d. HPV

271. Which of the following are dimorphic fungi?
   a. Histoplasma   b. Dermatophytes
   c. Aspergillus   d. Cryptococcus

272. Dane particles are seen in?
   a. Hepatitis A   b. Hepatitis B
   c. Hepatitis C   d. Hepatitis D

273. Pontiac fever is caused by?
   a. Legionella   b. Mycoplasma
   c. Rickettsia   d. Salmonella

274. Scrub typhus is caused by which stage of organism?
   a. Nymph   b. Larva
   c. Pupa   d. Adult

275. What is true regarding lag phase?
   a. Period of active growth without increase in numbers
   b. Growth occurs exponentially
   c. The plateau in lag phase is due to cell death
   d. It is the 2nd phase in bacterial growth curve

276. Nakayama strain is used for which vaccine?
   a. Typhoid   b. Chicken pox
   c. Japanese encephalitis   d. Yellow fever

277. Sulphur granules in actinomycosis consist of?
   a. Monophils + neutrophils   b. Monophils + lymphocytes
   c. Eosinophils   d. Bacterial particles

278. Mycobacterium leprae can be grown on?
   a. L J medium
   b. Robertson's cooked meat medium
   c. Foot pad of mice
   d. Sabraud's agar

279. Herring bodies are found in?
   a. Neurohypophysis   b. Adenohypophysis
   c. Cerebral cortex   d. Thalamus

280. Owl eye intranuclear inclusion body is seen in?
   a. Herpes zoster   b. Herpes simplex
   c. CMV   d. EBV

281. Eosinophilic pneumonia caused by Ascaris lumbricoides is known as?
   a. Mafucci syndrome
   b. Loeffer's syndrome
   c. Primary pulmonary eosinophilia
   d. Sweet syndrome

282. Most common cause of UTI in young females is?
   a. Staph saprophyticus   b. E.coli
   c. Klebsiella   d. Proteus

Microbiology and Parasitology

283. **Inverted fir tree appearance on gelatin stab is characteristic of?**
   a. Mycoplasma
   b. Bacillus anthracis
   c. Clostridium
   d. Bacteriodes

284. **Satellitism is seen in culture of?**
   a. Campylobacter jejuni
   b. H. influenzae
   c. E.coli
   d. Beta hemolytic streptococci

285. **Which one of the following bacteria is oxidase positive?**
   a. Vibrio
   b. Pseudomonas
   c. Clostridium
   d. E.coli

286. **Which hepatitis virus is a partially single stranded, partially double stranded DNA virus?**
   a. Hepatitis A
   b. Hepatitis B
   c. Hepatitis C
   d. Hepatitis D

287. **Speed of rabies virus in axon is?**
   a. I mm per hour
   b. 3 mm per hour
   c. 5 mm per hour
   d. 7 mm per hour

288. **Mode of transmission of brucella is?**
   a. Air
   b. Water
   c. Milk
   d. Aerosol

289. **KOH wet mount can be prepared for?**
   a. Bacteria
   b. Virus
   c. Fungus
   d. Parasite

290. **Elek's gel precipitation test is seen in?**
   a. Clostridium
   b. Corynebacterium
   c. Bacteriodes
   d. Campylobacter

291. **Naegler's reaction is shown by?**
   a. Clostradium tetani
   b. Clostridium welchii
   c. Mycobacterium tuberculosis
   d. Mycobacterium leprae

292. **Chocolate agar is an example of?**
   a. Enriched medium
   b. Enrichment medium
   c. Selective medium
   d. Transport medium

293. **Skirrow's medium is used for?**
   a. Clostridium tetani
   b. Corynebacterium diphtheriae
   c. Campylobacter jejuni
   d. Helicobacter pylori

294. **Transport medium most commonly used for Vibrio cholera is?**
   a. TCBS medium
   b. Venkatraman Ramakrishna medium
   c. Sodium taurocholate medium
   d. Thayer martin medium

295. **Taxonomically chlamydia is a?**
   a. Bacteria
   b. Virus
   c. Fungus
   d. Nematode

296. **Pyoderma gangrenosum is caused by?**
   a. Streptococcus
   b. Staphylococcus
   c. Pseudomonas
   d. E.coli

297. **Germ theory of disease was proposed by?**
   a. Louis pasteur
   b. Ronald Ross
   c. Edward jenner
   d. Robert koch

298. **Microscope was invented by?**
   a. Ronald ross
   b. Robert koch
   c. Antonie van leeuwenhoek
   d. Louis pasteur

299. **Scarlet fever is caused due to?**
   a. Streptococci
   b. Staphylococci
   c. Klebsiella
   d. Proteus

300. **Influenzae virus belongs to which family?**
   a. Paramyxovirus
   b. Orthomyxovirus
   c. Bunyaviridae
   d. Togaviridae

301. **H1N1 is a type of?**
   a. SARS virus
   b. Influenza type A virus
   c. Influenza type B virus
   d. Influenza type C virus

302. **HTLV-1 causes which of the following?**
   a. Tropical spastic paraparesis
   b. Familial mediterranean fever
   c. Cutaneous T cell lymphoma
   d. Burkitt's lymphoma

303. **True about HACEK group of bacteria is?**
   a. Anaerobes
   b. Includes Coxiella burnetii
   c. Gram positive
   d. Require CO_2 for growth

304. **Proteus antigen cross react with?**
   a. Klebsiella
   b. Rickettsia
   c. Chlamydia
   d. E.coli

305. **Rapid urea breath test is positive in?**
   a. H pylori
   b. Klebsella
   c. Proteus
   d. Ureoplasma

306. **Motility difference according to the temperature changes is shown by?**
   a. Vibrio
   b. Leptospira
   c. Chlamydia
   d. Listeria

307. **Nasopharyngeal leishmaniasis is caused due to?**
   a. Leishmania braziliensis
   b. Leishmania tropica
   c. Leishmania chagasi
   d. Leishmania donovani

308. **Which viral disease is transmitted by orofecal route?**
   a. Dengue
   b. Poliovirus
   c. Hepatitis B
   d. Influenza virus

309. **Ascoli's thermoprecipitin test is done for?**
   a. Clostridium tetani
   b. Chlamydia
   c. Bacillus anthracis
   d. Cornybacterium

310. **Most common organism which can contaminate crowded army camps is?**
   a. Klebsiella
   b. E coli
   c. Neisseria meningitidis
   d. Staphylococcus

311. **Which antibody is most commonly produced in secondary immune response?**
   a. IgG
   b. IgA
   c. IgD
   d. IgM

FMGE Solutions Screening Examination

ANSWERS WITH EXPLANATIONS

MOST RECENT QUESTION 2019

1. Ans. (a) Grey pseudo-membrane that bleeds on removal

Ref: Nelson 20th ed. pg. 2018

- Development of a localized or coalescing pseudo-membrane can occur in any portion of the respiratory tract in case of Diptheria.
- The pseudomembrane is characterized by the formation of a dense, grey debris layer composed of a mixture of dead cells, fibrin, RBCs, WBCs, and organisms.
- *Removal of the membrane reveals a bleeding, oedematous mucosa*. The distribution of the membrane varies from local (e.g., tonsillar, pharyngeal) to widely covering the entire tracheobronchial tree.

GENERAL MICROBIOLOGY, MEDIA, TESTING

2. Ans. (b) Transduction

Ref: Textbook of Microbiology by Surinder Kumar, P 93 Microbiology by Ananthanarayan and Paniker, 8th ed., pg. 60

Some bacteria also transfer genetic material between cells via following ways:
- **Transduction:** Transfer of genetic material from one bacterium to another by a bacteriophage is known as transduction
  - Most widespread mechanism of gene transfer among prokaryotes
- **Transformation:** Transfer of genetic material through the agency of free DNA
- **Conjugation:** DNA is transferred through direct cell contact. Gram negative anerobes like E. Coli, Bacteroides, Porphyromonas, and Fusobacterium use this method of gene transfer

> **Extra Mile**
> - Bacteriophages are viruses that parasitize bacteria
> - Most bacteriophages carry their genetic information (the phage genome) as a length of double-stranded DNA coiled up inside a protein coat.
> - **Lysogenic conversion:** Phage DNA integrated in bacterial chromosome as prophase → replicated stably as part of host cell chromosome → transferred to daughter cell.
>   - **In other words:** *"This process by which the prophage DNA confers genetic information to a bacterium is called **lysogenic or phage conversion**."*
>   - **NOTE:** In transduction, phage acts only as a vehicle carrying bacterial genes from one cell to another but in lysogenic conversion the phage DNA itself is the new genetic element.

3. Ans. (a) Stationary phase

Ref: Microbiology by Ananthanarayan and Paniker, 8th ed. P 24

PHASES OF BACTERIAL GROWTH CURVE

LAG PHASE
- No appreciable increase in number but there is **increase in size of the cells**
- Accumulation of enzymes and metabolic intermediates
- **Maximum cell size** is obtained at the end of lag phase

LOG PHASE
- Also called **exponential phase**
- Number of cells increase exponentially
- Cells are **small and stain uniformly**
- Increase in metabolic rate

STATIONARY PHASE
- Viable **count of cells remain stationary** as an equilibrium exists between dying cells and newly formed cells
- Cells are viable and show **irregular staining** due to intracellular storage granules
- **Sporulation occurs at this stage**
- Production of antibiotics and exotoxins

PHASE OF DECLINE
- **Population** of cells **decrease** due to cell death
- **Involution forms** are common

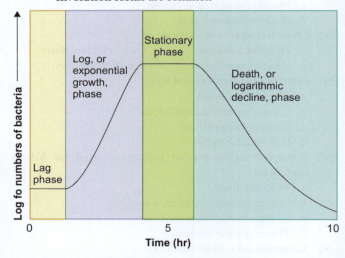

4. Ans. (b) Thermometer

Ref: Textbook of Diagnostic Microbiology, E-book, P 67

- **High level of disinfectant:** 2% glutaraldehyde for 20 minutes for all instruments coming in contact with

Microbiology and Parasitology

mucous membrane. Like bronchoscope, proctoscope, endoscopic tubes, etc.

- **Intermediate level of disinfectant:** Phenol or alcohol is used to disinfect thermometer.
- **Low level of disinfectant:** Lysol for floors and fabrics.

5. Ans. (d) Sodium hypochlorite

Ref: Textbook of Diagnostic Microbiology, E-book, P 68

- After repeated vitro studies, it is confirmed that the most potent disinfectant is hypochlorite, which disclosed the lowest minimum bactericidal concentration against various micro-organisms, when compared with iodine tincture and chlorhexidine.
- Sodium hypochlorite is proved to be efficient even at very low concentration (5% or even less) and the action is achieved very rapidly (within 30–60 minutes).

6. Ans. (c) Stationary phase

Ref: Ananthanarayan, 8th ed. pg. 24

Features of Stationary Phase

1. Viable **count of cells remain stationary** as an equilibrium exists between dying cells and newly formed cells
2. Cells are viable and show **irregular staining** due to intracellular storage granules
3. **Sporulation** occurs at this stage
4. Production of antibiotics and exotoxins is also seen at this stage.

7. Ans. (b) Ionizing radiation

Ref: Ananthanarayan's Microbiology, 8th ed. pg. 35

- Cold sterilization is a process in which sterilization is carried out at low temperature with the help of chemicals, radiations, membranes.
- Ionizing radiation such as X-rays, gamma rays and cosmic rays, cause no appreciable increase in temperature in this method, it is referred to as cold sterilization.

8. Ans. (a) Albert stain

Ref: Ananthnarayan, 9th ed. MedPub

- **Albert stain** is a type of differential stain used for staining the volutin granules also known as Metachromatic granules found in *Corynebacterium diphtheriae*.
- The name metachromatic is because of its property of changing color, i.e. *when stained with blue stain they appear red in colour. When grown in Loffler's slopes, C. diphtheriae produces large number of granules.*

> **Extra Mile**
>
> - **Stains used for C. Diphtheriae:**
>   - Ponders stain
>   - Albert stain
>   - Neisser stain
>   - Loeffler methylene blue

9. Ans. (b) Can't differentiate between latent and active TB

Ref: Harrisons, 19th ed. pg. 1114; Lange Microbiology by Jawetz, Ch 8

- The skin test with tuberculin PPD (TST) is most widely used in screening for latent tuberculosis.
- It has very low sensitivity and specificity and is **unable to discriminate between latent TB and active disease.**
- **False negative reactions** are common in immunosuppressed patients and in those with overwhelming TB.
- **False-positive reactions** may be caused by infections with non-tuberculous mycobacteria and by BCG vaccination.

10. Ans. (c) Conjugation

Ref: Textbook of Microbiology, Suirnder Kumar pg. 530

- **Lysogeny** does not affect bacterial metabolism. The prophage behaves likes segment of host chromosome and replicates synchronously by binary fission.
- **Bacterial conjugation** is the transfer of genetic material between bacterial cells by direct cell-to-cell contact and is a mechanism of **horizontal gene transfer**, like transformation and transduction, although these two other mechanisms do not involve cell-to-cell contact.
- **Transduction** is transfer of genetic material from bacteria to bacteria by bacteriophage. It was discovered by Zinder and Lederberg in *Salmonella typhimurium*. Clinically speaking it provides a way to study gene linkage.

> **Extra Mile**
>
> - **Transformation** is the genetic alteration of a cell resulting from the **direct uptake** and incorporation of exogenous genetic material (exogenous DNA) from its surroundings **through the cell membrane**.

11. Ans. (b) Integration of phage nucleic acid to host bacteria genome

Ref: PubMed

- Lysogenic conversion is characterized by **integration of the bacteriophage nucleic acid into the host bacterium's genome**.
- Once the genetic material of phage bacteria is introduced, the host bacterium continues to live and reproduce normally.
- The genetic material of the bacteriophage, called a prophage, can be transmitted to daughter cells at each subsequent cell division, and a later event (such as UV radiation or the presence of certain chemicals) can release it, causing proliferation of new phages via the lytic cycle.
- For example, a number of strains of the diphtheria bacillus acquire the capacity to form diphtheria toxin immediately after penetration of the phage into the cell and retain that capacity until the moment of the cell's dissolution (lysis).

Explanations

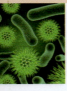

FMGE Solutions Screening Examination

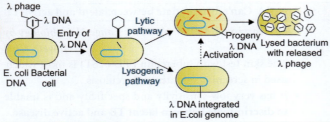

12. Ans. (c) 25 to 40°C

Ref: Ananthnarayan, 9th ed. ch-1

Organisms on the basis of their growth at different temperature:
- **Psychrophilic:** (below 20°C)
- **Psychrotrophs:** (important cause of food spoilage)
- **Mesophilic:** (25–40°C)
- **Thermophilic:** (55–80°C)

13. Ans. (a) Incineration

Ref: PubMed

Cat.	Type of Bag/ Container used	Type of waste	Treatment/ disposal options
Yellow	Non-chlorinated plastic bags — Separate collection system leading to effluent treatment system	• Human anatomical waste • Animal anatomical waste • Soiled waste • Expired or discarded medicines • Chemical waste • Micro, Bio-t and other clinical lab waste • Chemical liquid waste	Incineration of Plasma pyralysis or deep burial*
Red	Non-chlorinated plastic bags or containers	Contaminated waste (Recyclable) tubing, bottles, intravenous tubes and sets, catheters, urine bags, syringes (without needles) gloves	Auto/Micro/Hydro and then sent for recycling not be sent to landfill
White/ Trans-lucent	Puncture, leak, tamper proof containers	Waste sharps including metals	Auto or Dry Heat Sterlization followed by shredding or multilation or encapsulation
Blue	Cardboard boxes with blue colored marking	Glassware	Disinfection or auto/Micro/hydro and then sent for recycling

14. Ans. (a) Human body parts

Ref: Please refer to above explanation

15. Ans. (c) Dry heat sterilization

Ref: Ananthnarayan, 9th ed. PubMed

- Heat sterilization is considered as the most reliable method of sterilization.
- It can be done by 2 methods
  - Dry heat
  - Moist heat

Dry heat	Moist heat
Mechanism of killing: • Killing effect is due to protein denaturation, oxidative damage and the toxic effect of metabolite	**Mechanism of killing:** • Is due to protein denaturation and coagulation

Methods and its use:
• **Flaming:** for loop wire, searing spatulas
• Incineration:
  ■ Contaminated cloth
  ■ Pathological waste
  ■ Anatomical remains
• **Hot air oven**
  ■ All glass syringes and glass wares
  ■ **Liquid paraffin**
  ■ **Dusting powder**
  ■ Swabs
  ■ Scalpel, forceps, scissors
  ■ Fat and grease
	Methods and use:
	• **Pasteurization**
	  ■ Holder method
	  ■ Flash method
	• **Autoclaving (steam sterilization):** $121^0C \times 15$ min at 15 psi. Used for:
	  ■ Culture media
	  ■ Aprons, dressing
	  ■ Surgical instruments except sharps
	  ■ **Gloves**
	  ■ Catheter
	  ■ Sputum

TABLE: Radiation used for sterilization

Ionizing radiation (aka Cold sterilization)	Non-ionizing radiation
Methods: • **Photon irradiation (γ):** Most commonly used among radiation sterilization • Electron irradiation (β) **Uses:** Used for heat sensitive materials like: • Plastic disposables • Bone and tissue grafts • Adhesive dressings • **Catgut suture**	**Methods:** • **Infrared rays:** used for prepacked items like catheters and syringes • **UV Radiation:** operation theatre, Laboratories

16. Ans. (b) Differential stain

Ref: Microbiology by Ananthanarayan and Paniker, 8th ed. pg. 15

DIFFERENTIAL STAIN

- These are positive stain, which divide bacterial population into two different groups by imparting two different colors
  - **Gram Stain:** it is the **most common staining method of bacteriology**. It stains cell wall of bacteria.
    - **Gram positive** appears blue
    - **Gram Negative** appears pink/red
  - **Z-N stain** is used to distinguish acid fast bacteria and non-acid fast bacteria.
    - Presence of mycolic acid is responsible for the acid-fast nature of bacteria.

Microbiology and Parasitology

17. Ans. (d) Hot air oven

Ref: *Microbiology by Ananthanarayan and Paniker, 8th ed. pg. 31*

- **Flaming:** in this method the articles should be sterilized on the hot flame of Bunsen burner.
- **Hot air oven:** It is also called *dry heat sterilizer*.

Note: *The articles should be sterilized at the temperature 160°C for 2 hours or 150–170°C for 1 hour.*

- Glass ware like test tube, pipette, flask and glass syringes, fixed oil glycerin, liquid paraffin, propylene glycol and zinc oxide etc. can be sterilized by this method.
- **Auto clave:** this type of sterilization is done by steam heat under pressure.
  Use: Glass ware, surgical dressing, rubber, gloves, surgical instrument are sterilized by this method.

18. Ans. (b) Bacillus subtilis

Ref: *Textbook of Microbiology S. Kumar/14*

- Hot air oven is dry heat sterilization technique used most commonly to sterilize glassware and metal items.
- *Sterility check* is done for each and every lot to enhance quality of sterilization. For this purpose the *biological indicator organism bacillus subtilis is used*.
- Non pathogenic clostridium tetani can also be used to check the efficiency (*Bacillus subtilis > Non-pathogenic clostridium tetani*).
- **Note: Stearothermophillus is used to check efficiency of autoclave.**

19. Ans. (a) Autoclaving at 135 degrees

Ref: *Microbiology by Ananthanarayan and Paniker, 8th ed. pg. 32*

- Prions are best destroyed by autoclave at 135 degree for one hour.

20. Ans. (a) Solid medium

Ref: *Microbiology by Ananthanarayan and Paniker, 8th ed. pg. 39-40*

GROWING BACTERIAL CULTURES IN LIQUID NUTRIENT BROTH

- Nutrient broth is a liquid bacterial growth medium made of powdered beef extract and short chains of amino acids that have been dissolved in water.
- Liquid medium is convenient to use for growing bacteria in test tubes, and can reveal information about the oxygen requirements of bacteria growing within.
- Bacteria that require oxygen will grow close to the water's surface, and bacteria that cannot tolerate the presence of oxygen will grow at the bottom of the test tube.

GROWING BACTERIAL CULTURES ON SOLID MEDIA

- *Broth media can be made solid by adding agar*, a gel like polysaccharide extracted from red algae.
- Broth with about 1.5% agar added will be liquid when heated, but solid at room temperature, making it easy to pour into a vessel, such as a Petri dish or test tube when hot.
- The solution then becomes solid once cooled.

21. Ans. (b) To make the medium solid

- *Broth media can be made solid by adding agar*, a gel like polysaccharide extracted from red algae.
- Broth with about 1.5% agar added will be liquid when heated, but solid at room temperature, making it easy to pour into a vessel, such as a Petri dish or test tube when hot.
- The solution then becomes solid once cooled.

22. Ans. (c) Pseudomonas aeruginosa

Ref: *Microbiology by Ananthanarayan and Paniker, 8th ed. pg. 317*

- Pseudomonas is isolated from feces or other samples by using selective media such as cetrimide agar.
- E.Coli is cultured in Mac-conkey media
- Clostridium tetani grows on ordinary media and is improved by blood and serum.
- Clostridium perfringens grows on blood agar plate.

23. Ans. (d) Pseudomonas

Ref: *Microbiology by Ananthanarayan and Paniker, 8th ed. pg. 317*

- **Pseudomonas** is isolated from feces or other samples by using selective media such as cetrimide agar.

24. Ans. (a) N. Meningitis

Ref: *Microbiology by Ananthanarayan and Paniker, 8th ed. pg. 225, 227*

- Thayer martin medium is selective medium for N. Meningitis.

25. Ans. (d) Tellurite media

Ref: *Microbiology by Ananthanarayan and Paniker, 9th ed. pg. 235-236*

TABLE: Culture media used for C. Diphtheriae

Medium	Use	Time for growth
Tellurite mediun	For best for diagnosis	Days
Loeffler's serum slope	For earliest diagnosis	Hours

Explanations

26. Ans. (c) LJ medium

Ref: Harrison, 19th ed. pg. 1110

- Harrison states: "In genitourinary TB - **culture** of 3 morning urinary specimen yields a definitive diagnosis in 90% cases. LJ medium is most common solid medium used for culture."
- Prevalence of GU TB= **10-15%**
- **MC c/o**- Urinary frequency, dysuria, nocturia, hematuria, and flank or abdominal pain.
- **Diagnosis**- Culture of three morning urine specimens- definitive diagnosis in nearly 90% patient.
- **Other test**- IV pyelography, abdominal CT, MRI-may show deformities and obstructions
- **Suggestive findings**- calcifications and ureteral strictures-
- **Complication**-
  - **Female**- affects the fallopian tubes and the endometrium and may cause infertility, pelvic pain, and menstrual abnormalities.
  - **Diagnosis** requires biopsy or culture of specimens obtained by dilation and curettage.
  - **Male**- affects the epididymis, producing a slightly tender mass that may drain externally through a fistulous tract; orchitis and prostatitis may also develop.
- **Rx:** Genitourinary TB **responds well to chemotherapy.**

27. Ans. (a) Pink

Ref: Microbiology by Ananthanarayan and Paniker, 8th ed. pg. 47

- Color change in Robertson cooked meat media depends on clostridial organism:
  - **Clostridium perfringens (Saccarolytic activity):** color turns to **pink** *(Mn: P-P)*
  - If **Clostridium tetani (Proteolytic activity):** colour turns to **black**

Note: Robertson cooked meat medium is most widely used fluid medium for culture of anaerobes.

28. Ans. (c) For bacteria using citrate

Ref: Microbiology by Ananthanarayan and Paniker, 8th ed. pg. 674

- The **citrate test** detects the ability of an organism to use citrate as the sole source of carbon and energy.
- A positive diagnostic test rests on the generation of alkaline by-products of citrate metabolism. The subsequent increase in the pH of the medium is demonstrated by the color change of a pH indicator.
- The citrate test is often part of a battery of tests used **to identify gram-negative pathogens** and environmental isolates.

29. Ans. (b) Differential media

Ref: Microbiology by Ananthanarayan and Paniker, 8th ed. pg. 40

DIFFERENTIAL MEDIA (OR INDICATOR MEDIA)

- It distinguishes one microorganism type from another growing on the same media.
- This type of media is used for the detection of microorganisms and by molecular biologists to detect recombinant strains of bacteria.
- Examples of differential media include:
  - Blood agar
  - Eosin methylene blue (EMB)
  - *MacConkey (MCK)*
  - Mannitol salt agar (MSA)

Extra Mile

- **Mac Conkey agar** is a culture medium designed to grow Gram-negative bacteria and differentiate them for lactose fermentation.
- It consists of Peptone, Lactose, Agar neutral red and taurocholate shows up lactose fermenters as PINK COLONIES
- Non lactose Fermenters are colorless.

30. Ans. (d) Stuart media

Ref: Microbiology by Ananthanarayan and Paniker, 8th ed. pg. 40, 43

INDICATOR MEDIA

- It is also known as differential media which distinguishes one microorganism type from another growing on the same media.
- This type of media is used for the detection of microorganisms and by molecular biologists to detect recombinant strains of bacteria.
- Examples of differential media include:
  - Blood agar
  - Eosin methylene blue (EMB)
  - MacConkey (MCK)
  - mannitol salt agar (MSA)

TRANSPORT MEDIA

Examples of Transport Media Include

- Thioglycolate broth for strict anaerobes
- **Stuart transport medium** - a non-nutrient soft agar gel containing a reducing agent to prevent oxidation, and charcoal to neutralize
- Certain bacterial inhibitors- for gonococci, and buffered glycerol saline for enteric bacilli.
- Venkat-Ramakrishnan (VR) medium for *V. cholerae*.

Microbiology and Parasitology

31. Ans. (c) Ziehl-neelsen stain

Ref: Microbiology by Ananthanarayan and Paniker, 8th ed. pg. 352

- Z-N stain is used to distinguish acid fast bacteria and non-acid fast bacteria.
- Presence of mycolic acid is responsible for the acid-fast nature of bacteria.
- For the diagnosis and control of tuberculosis Sputum microscopy is the most reliable single method.
- Preparation of smear is from the thick purulent part of the sputum. They are the dried, heated fixed and stained by the Ziehl-Neelsen technique.
- The *smear is then covered with strong carbol fuchsin* and gently heated for 5-7 minutes, without letting the stain boil and become dry.
- *Wash the slide* with water and *decolourise* it with 20% sulphuric acid, followed by 95% ethanol for two minutes.
- Smear is then *counterstained* with Loeffler's methylene blue, 1% picric acid or 0.2% malachite green for one minute.
- Now, under the *oil immersion objective*, acid fast bacilli are seen as bright red rods while the background is blue, yellow or green depending on the counterstain used.
- At least 10,000 acid fast bacilli should be present per ml of sputum for them to be readily demonstrable in direct smears.

32. Ans. (b) Tube agglutination

Ref: Microbiology by Ananthanarayan and Paniker, 8th ed. pg. 108

TABLE: Agglutination tests and their uses

Agglutination test	Used mainly for
Direct agglutination test	Determination of blood group Bacterial agglutination test for serotyping & serogrouping. **Eg: Vibrio Cholera, Salmonella Sp.**
Slide agglutination test	Used for serotyping of salmonella **VDRL for syphillis**
Tube agglutination test	Aka standard agglutination test. Used for serological diagnosis of typhoid, brucellosis and typhus fever. **Ex: Widal Test,** *Weil felix reaction,* **and Kahn test**
Passive agglutination test	Rheumatoid factor **ANA for SLE** Antibody to Trichenella spiralis and antibody to group A strep.

33. Ans. (b) Counter current immune-electrophoresis

Ref: Microbiology by Ananthanarayan and Paniker, 8th ed. pg. 104

TABLE: Common precipitation tests and their examples

Precipitation test	Example
Ring test	**Ascoli thermoprecipitin test (anthrax)** and grouping of streptococci by **Lancefield technique**
Slide test	**VDRL test** for syphilis
Tube test	**Kahn test** for syphilis
Immuno-diffusion tests	**Elek test** for toxigenicity of diphtheria bacilli
Electroimmuno diffusion	**Counter current immune-electrophoresis** and rocket electrophoresis

34. Ans. (c) Widal test

Ref: Microbiology by Ananthanarayan and Paniker, 8th ed. pg. 108

AGGLUTINATION TEST

- It is a blood test used to identify unknown antigens.
- Blood with the unknown antigen is mixed with a known antibody and whether or not agglutination occurs helps to identify the antigen.
- *Refer to above explanation of Q 17.*

35. Ans. (d) Muramic acid

Ref: Microbiology by Ananthanarayan and Paniker, 8th ed. pg. 10, 63, 425

- All the above options except muramic acid are membrane bound organelles which are absent in prokaryotes and only present in eukaryotes.
- Muramic Acid is one of the important components of the peptidoglycan wall present in the cell wall of prokaryotic cells .

36. Ans. (a) C -substance

Ref: Microbiology by Ananthanarayan and Paniker, 8th ed. pg. 205, 673

- Lancefield classification is a grouping system for beta hemolytic bacteria based on the polysaccharide in their cell walls, C – substance (carbohydrate), which is antigenic. So this classification is serologic.

37. Ans. (b) Antibody

Ref: Microbiology by Ananthanarayan and Paniker, 8th ed. pg. 102-103

- Antibody is attached to the surface of bacteria for opsonization, which further get phagocytized.

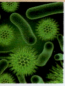 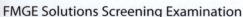

38. Ans. (c) HIV Elisa

Ref: Microbiology by Ananthanarayan and Paniker, 8th ed. pg. 570, 576

- ELISA HIV measures antibodies against the virus. These antibodies are of IgG type and can cross the placenta. Hence a baby born to HIV positive lady will test HIV positive on day 0 of life and may continue till these antibodies are cleared by the baby's immune system. The clearance may take 12-18 months and therefore Babies born to HIV lady may be false positive till the age mentioned.
- However DNA PCR or viral culture or p24 antigen positive on first few days of life is indicative of perinatal transmission rate of the virus which is 30%-

Extra Mile

- The perninatal transmission rate can be reduced by at least 50% in case single dose nevirapine given to the mother and to the baby within 72 hours. Breast feeding is indicated in baby born to HIV positive patient.

39. Ans. (d) Infectious mononucleosis

Ref: Microbiology by Ananthanarayan and Paniker, 8th ed. pg. 476

Infectious mononucleosis is diagnosed by Paul Bunnel test.

Revision of Key Points About Infectious Mononucleosis
- **Ebstein Barr virus** is causative for infectious mononucleosis.
- Infectious mononucleosis is called a **glandular fever**
- Clinical features include fever, lymphadenopathy, sore throat and presence of abnormal lymphocytes in blood.
- **Monospot test** is also used for diagnosis of infectious mononucleosis,
- Patients develop skin rash if they consume an antibiotic like **ampicillin** EBV is also **oncogenic** in nature because it causes **B cell clonal activation.**

BACTERIOLOGY

40. Ans. (b) Gram positive rods with square ends

Ref: Textbook of Microbiology by Surinder Kumar, P 282; Lange Microbiology, Ch 12

- The genus *bacillus* includes large aerobic, gram-positive rods occurring in chains.
- Principle pathogen of bacillus species is bacillus anthracis (causes anthrax).
- Anthrax is primarily a disease of herbivores—goats, sheep, cattle, horses, etc.

- In humans anthrax is acquired by:
  - Injured skin: Cutaneous anthrax
  - Mucous membrane: Gastrointestinal anthrax
  - Inhalation of spores: Inhalational anthrax (Woolsorter's disease)

Morphology:
- The typical cells, measuring 1 × 3–4 μm, have **square ends** and are arranged in long chains; spores are located in the center of the non-motile bacilli
- **Culture:** Round colonies with "cut-glass" appearance in transmitted light

Laboratory test:
- **Specimen:** Pus, Blood or sputum
- **Smear:** shows chain of large gram positive rods
- **Blood agar plates:** shows non-hemolytic gray to white colonies with rough texture and ground glass appearance.
- **Nutrient agar:** Medusa head appearance/comma shaped outgrowth from the colonies.
  - Long chain of bacilli resembles locks of matted hair under the low power microscope.
- **Gelatin stab:** Inverted fir tree appearance.

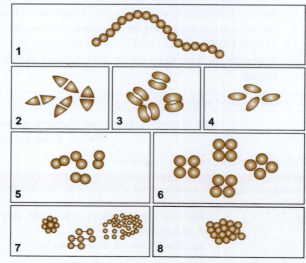

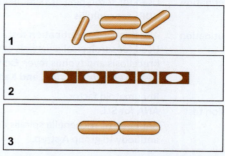

Arrangement of bacteria: A. Cocci: 1. Streptococci 2. Pneumococci 3. Gonococci 4. Meningococci 5. Neisseria catarrhalis 6. Gaffkya tetragena 7. Sarcina 8. Staphylococci; B. Bacilli: 1. Bacilli in cluster 2. Bacilli in chains (B. anthrax) 3. Diplobacilli (K. pneumoniae)

> **Extra Mile**
> - **Bacillus anthracis**
>   - It is the first pathogenic bacterium to be observed under the microscope
>   - First communicable disease shown to be transmitted by inoculation of infected blood
>   - First bacterium used for the preparation of **an attenuated vaccine** by Pasteur was *B. anthracis*.

41. Ans. (c) Leprosy

Ref: Textbook of Microbiology by Surinder Kumar, P 328

- Choice A has a stellate granuloma while choice D has a gumma. Hence both are ruled out. Choice B is a rickettsial disease
- Choice C leprosy is a chronic granulomatous disease
- A lepromatous leprosy patient develops numerous nodular skin lesions (**lepromata**) on face, ear lobes, hands, feet and less commonly trunk.
- It shows AFB positive bacilli.
- Skin Biopsy shows: Many macrophages, seen as large foamy cells packed with AFB
- **Microscopy of lepromatous leprosy**
  - Smears are stained by Ziehl-Neelsen method using 5 percent instead of 20 percent sulphuric acid for decolorization. Acid-fast bacilli (AFB) arranged in parallel bundles within macrophages

The smears are graded, based on the number of bacilli as follows:

1-10 bacilli in 100 fields	=	1+
1-10 bacilli in 10 fields	=	2+
1-10 bacilli per field	=	3+
10-100 bacilli per field	=	4+
100-1,000 bacilli per field	=	5+
More than 1,000 bacilli, clumps and globi in every field	=	6+

42. Ans. (a) Respiratory disease

Ref: Page 1138: Harrison 20th edition

- The bacterium L. pneumophila leads to legionnaire disease.
- The most common form of transmission of Legionella is inhalation of contaminated aerosols produced in conjunction with water sprays, jets or mists.
- It has 2 distinct clinical syndromes: Legionnaires disease, which most often manifests as severe pneumonia accompanied by multisystemic disease, and Pontiac fever, which is an acute, febrile, self-limited, viral-like illness

43. Ans. (b) 2nd week

Ref: page 1176: Harrison 20th edition

- Widal test should be done in *second week* of presentation of a case of typhoid. It is a serological test with patient showing H and/or O titres greater than or equal to 1:160 and typhoid-like symptoms is strongly suggestive of diagnosis of typhoid fever. *False positive widal is seen in case of malaria.*
- The criterion standard for diagnosis of typhoid fever has long been culture isolation of the organism. In the first week bone marrow culture or blood culture should be done.
- Bone marrow aspiration and blood are cultured in a selective medium (eg, 10% aqueous oxgall) or a nutritious medium (eg, tryptic soy broth) and are incubated at 37°C for at least 7 days

Basu blood culture—1st week
antibody (widal test)—2nd week
stool culture—3rd week
urine test—4th week

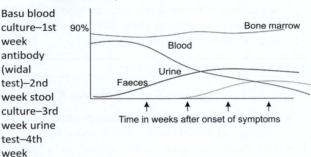

44. Ans. (d) Actinomyces

Ref: Textbook of Diagnostic Microbiology, E-book, P 505

- **Nocardia:** Aerobe, acid fast
- **Actinomyces:** Anerobe, non-acid-fast bacilli
- **Tuberculosis:** Aerobic, acid fast
- **Listeria:** Facultative anaerobe, Gram-positive, non-acid-fast

45. Ans. (d) Haemophilus influenzae

Ref: Textbook of Diagnostic Microbiology, E-book, P 14

- **Capnophilic bacteria:** Organisms which thrive on the high concentration of CO_2. They require ~5–10% of CO_2. For example, *Haemophilus influenzae, Neisseria*.
- **Facultative anaerobe:** These are capable of growing under both aerobic and anaerobic conditions. For example, *Staphylococcus aureus*.
- **Obligate anaerobe:** These organisms grow only under non-oxygen environment. Oxygen is toxic for these organisms. For example, *Clostridium*.
- **Obligate aerobe:** There is absolute requirement of oxygen for survival for this type of organism. For example, *Mycobacterium*.

FMGE Solutions Screening Examination

46. Ans. (b) Listeria monocytogenes

Ref: Ananthnarayan and Paniker's Textbook of Microbiology, 8th ed. pg. 395

- The Anton test is used in the identification of *L. monocytogenes*; instillation of a culture into the conjunctival sac of a rabbit or guinea pig causes severe keratoconjunctivitis within 24 hours.
- Experimental inoculation in rabbits causes marked monocytosis, hence the name monocytogenes. Monocytosis is a feature of human listeriosis also.

47. Ans. (b) Inhibiting protein synthesis

Ref: Ananthanarayan's Microbiology, 8th ed. pg. 234

- The diphtheria toxin causes damage to eukaryotic cells and tissues by inhibition of protein synthesis in the cells.
- Although the toxin is responsible for the lethal symptoms of the disease, the virulence of C. diphtheria cannot be attributed to toxigenicity alone, since a distinct invasive phase apparently precedes toxigenesis.

48. Ans. (a) Listeria monocytogenes

Ref: Handbook of Zoonoses, 2nd ed. pg. 322

- Listeria monocytogenes is Gram-positive, nonspore forming rod shaped bacteria with rounded ends.
- The organisms occasionally appear in a palisade arrangement, along with some V or Y forms.
- It is motile via one to six peritrichous flagella and exihibits characteristic tumbling motility.
- Tumbling motility can be seen best microscopically using cultures grown in tryptose broth incubated at 20°C. The organism is weakly motile at 37°C.

49. Ans. (d) V. Cholerae

Ref: Ananthnarayan and Paniker's Textbook of Microbiology, 8th ed. pg. 302

- In stained films of mucus flakes from acute cholera cases, the vibrios are seen arranged in parallel rows, described by Koch as the '*fish in stream*' appearance.
- "School of Fish" appearance is seen in H. ducreyi.
- Vibrios are Gram-negative, rigid, curved rods that are actively motile by means of a polar flagellum. The name 'vibrio' is derived from the characteristic vibratory motility/darting motility
- The cholera vibrio is a short, curved, cylindrical rod, about 1.5 x 0.2-0.4 µm in size, with rounded or slightly pointed ends. The cell is typically **comma shaped.**
- Aside from *V. cholera*, darting motility is also seen in Campylobacter.

50. Ans. (c) Legionella

Ref: Ananthnarayan and Paniker's Textbook of Microbiology, 8th ed. pg. 400

- Pontiac fever was named for Pontiac, Michigan, where the first case was recognized. It caused by various species of **Gram-negative bacteria in the genus** *Legionella.*
- It is a milder, non-fatal, influenza like illness with fever, chills, myalgia and headache.
- Pontiac fever resolves spontaneously and often goes undiagnosed.
- Both Pontiac fever and the more severe Legionnaire's disease are caused by the same bacteria, Leginonella Pneumophila but Pontiac fever does not include pneumonia.

> **Extra Mile**
>
> **Legionnaire's disease:**
> - Can be either epidemic or sporadic.
> - **Incubation period:** 2–10 days
> - Presents with fever, non-productive cough and dyspnea. If untreated it rapidly progresses to pneumonia.

51. Ans. (b) Pneumococcus

Ref: Ananthnarayan and Paniker's Textbook of Microbiology, 8th ed. pg. 219-220

- The pathogen that most commonly causes sepsis in patients who have undergone splenectomy, as well as in children with sickle cell disease, is S. pneumoniae (pneumococcus).
- Asplenic patients are at risk for rapidly progressive septicemia and death. Such patients should be vaccinated against pneumococci, H. influenzae type b, meningococci, and influenza virus, and if fever develops, they should receive empirical antimicrobial therapy immediately.
- Mortality among patients with post-splenectomy sepsis can be as high as 50%. Most commonly caused by *Streptococcus pneumoniae*, this infection often has a sudden onset and a fulminant course.

52. Ans. (b) Staphylococcus

Bacterial Food Poisoning

Incubation period, organism	Symptoms	Common sources
1–6 H		
Staphylococcus aureus	Nausea, vomiting, diarrhea	Ham, poultry, potato or egg salad, mayonnaise, cream pastries
Bacillus cereus	Nausea, vomiting, diarrhea	Fried rice
8–16 H		

Microbiology and Parasitology

Incubation period, organism	Symptoms	Common sources
Clostridium perfringens	Abdominal cramps, diarrhea (vomiting rare)	Beef, poultry, legumes, gravies
B. cereus	Abdominal cramps, diarrhea (vomiting rare)	Meats, vegetables, dried beans, cereals
> 16 H		
Vibrio cholerae	Watery diarrhea	Shellfish
Enterotoxigenic *Escherichia coli*	Watery diarrhea	Salads, cheese, meats, water
Enterohemorrhagic *E.coli*	Bloody diarrhea	Ground beef, roast beef, salami, raw milk, raw vegetables, apple juice
Salmonella spp.	Inflammatory diarrhea	Beef, poultry, eggs, dairy products
Campylobacter jejuni	Inflammatory diarrhea	Poultry, raw milk
Shigella spp	Dysentery	Potato or egg salad, lettuce, raw vegetables
Vibrio parahaemolyticus	Dysentery	Mollusks, crustaceans

53. Ans. (a) Staphylococcus aureus

- Staphylococcus aureus is the most common cause of postinfluenza secondary bacterial pneumonia.
- It most often affects the elderly patients.

54. Ans. (b) Gram-positive bacilli

Ref: Harrisons, 19th ed. pg. 978

- *C. diphtheriae* is a **Gram-positive bacillus that is unencapsulated, nonmotile, and nonsporulating.**
- The bacteria have a characteristic club-shaped bacillary appearance and typically form clusters of parallel rays, or *palisades*, that are referred to as **"Chinese characters."**

55. Ans. (d) Laryngopharynx

Ref: Harrisons, 19th ed. pg. 978

- Diptheria is a nasopharyngeal and skin infection caused by *Corynebacterium diphtheriae*. Toxigenic strains of *C. diphtheria* produce a protein toxin that causes systemic toxicity, myocarditis, and polyneuropathy.
- The toxigenic strains cause pharyngeal diphtheria, while the non-toxigenic strains commonly cause cutaneous disease.
- **Harrisons states:** *"Respiratory/pharyngeal form of diphtheria is from notiable diseases, while cutaneous diphtheria is NOT."*
- **Most severe form of diphtheria:** Laryngeal

56. Ans. (c) Bacillus anthrax

Ref: Harrisons, 19th ed. pg. 261e2

- **McFadyean reaction** is a special staining reaction, demonstrating a pink capsule around a blue cell, after staining with methylene blue, which is used as a presumptive diagnosis for **anthrax** in a blood smear.
- Anthrax is caused by *B. anthracis*, a Gram-positive, nonmotile, spore-forming rod that is found in soil and predominantly causes disease in herbivores such as cattle, goats, and sheep.

57. Ans. (a) Staph epidermis

Ref: Harrisons, 19th ed. pg. 145e-4

- Many bacterial, fungal, and protozoal species have the ability to grow in multicellular masses called biofilms.
- These masses are biochemically and morphologically quite distinct from the free-living individual cells referred to as *planktonic cells*.
- Growth in biofilms leads to altered microbial metabolism, production of extracellular virulence factors, and decreased susceptibility to antimicrobial agents, biocides, and host defense molecules and cells.
- **Examples of bacterial organisms forming biofilm:**
  - P. aeruginosa, staphylococci and other pathogens growing on implanted medical devices, and dental pathogens growing on tooth surfaces to form plaque
  - **S. epidermis** – on Prosthetic valve, IV catheter
  - **Strep Mutans/sanguinis** – on Dental plaques
  - **Pseudomonas** – Cystic fibrosis, contact lens
  - **Strep. viridans** – Endocarditis
  - **Non-typable H. influenza**- Otitis. Media

58. Ans. (a) Biofilm formation

- S. epidermis is a pathogenic organism which affects interventions like catheter, canula.
- It is an organism which can form biofilm.
- It is novobiocin sensitive.

59. Ans. (d) 100

Please refer the explanation for Q. 56

60. Ans. (b) ++

Ref: PubMed; http://www.hrsa.gov/hansensdisease/ diagnosis/skinsmears.html

- **Oil immersion** is a technique used to increase the resolving power of a microscope. This is achieved by immersing both the objective lens and the specimen in a transparent oil of high refractive index, thereby increasing the numerical aperture of the objective lens.

Reporting the Bacterial Index

- The results are reported on a *0 to 6+ semi-logarithmic scale* using a descriptive phrase or numerical code. This is an indicator of the total bacillary load of the patient. It falls about 1 point per year during effective treatment as dead bacilli undergo lysis and are absorbed.

Very numerous	(+6)	Over 1000 bacilli per oil immersion field
Numerous	(+5)	100 to 1000 bacilli per oil immersion field
Moderate	(+4)	10 to 100 bacilli per oil immersion field
Few	(+3)	1 to 10 bacilli per oil immersion field
Very few	(+2)	1 to 10 bacilli per 10 fields
Rare	(+1)	1 to 10 bacilli per 100 fields
None found	(NF)	No AFB seen on entire site

61. Ans. (a) Bacillus anthrax

Ref: Harrisons, 19th ed. pg. 261e-2

- **There are three major clinical forms of anthrax:**
  - Gastrointestinal, cutaneous, and inhalational.
  - **Gastrointestinal anthrax** typically results from the **ingestion of contaminated meat**.
  - **Cutaneous anthrax** typically begins as a papule following the introduction of spores through an opening in the skin. This papule then evolves to a painless vesicle followed by the development of a coal-black, necrotic eschar.
  - **Inhalational anthrax is the** form most likely to be responsible for death in the setting of a bioterrorist attack.

62. Ans. (a) Flea

Ref: Harrisons, 19th ed. pg. 1070

- Plague is a systemic zoonosis caused by *Yersinia pestis*.
- It predominantly affects small rodents in rural areas of Africa, Asia, and the Americas and is usually **transmitted to humans by an arthropod vector (the flea)**.
- Sometimes, infection follows contact with animal tissues or respiratory droplets.
  - The genus *Yersinia* comprises **gram-negative bacteria** of the family Enterobacteriaceae (gamma proteobacteria).

63. Ans. (b) Conjugation

Ref: Microbiology by Ananthanarayan and Paniker, 8th ed. pg. 60

- Some bacteria also transfer genetic material between cells via following ways:
  - **Transduction:** transfer of genetic material from one bacterium to another by a bacteriophage is known as transduction.
    - Most widespread mechanism of gene transfer among prokaryotes.
  - **Transformation:** Transfer of genetic material through the agency of free DNA
  - **Conjugation:** DNA is transferred through direct cell contact. Gram negative anerobes like E. Coli, Bacteroides, Porphyromonas, and Fusobacterium use this method of gene transfer.

64. Ans. (a) Transduction

Ref: Microbiology by Ananthanarayan and Paniker, 8th ed. pg. 61, 63

- **Transduction:** transfer of genetic material from one bacterium to another by a bacteriophage.
- *Bacteriophages are viruses* that parasites bacteria and consist of a nucleic acid core and a protein coat.

65. Ans. (c) Increase in size

Ref: Microbiology by Ananthanarayan and Paniker, 8th ed. pg. 24

PHASES OF BACTERIAL GROWTH CURVE

Lag Phase
- No appreciable increase in number but there is **increase in size of the cells**
- Accumulation of enzymes and metabolic intermediates
- **Maximum cell size** is obtained at the end of lag phase

Log Phase
- Also called as **exponential phase**
- Number of cells increase exponentially
- Cells are **small and stain uniformly**
- Increase in metabolic rate

Stationary Phase
- Viable **count of cells remain stationary** as an equilibrium exists between dying cells and newly formed cells
- Cells are viable and show **irregular staining** due to intracellular storage granules
- **Sporulation** occurs at this stage
- Production of antibiotics and exotoxins

Phase of Decline
- **Population** of cells **decrease** due to cell death
- **Involution forms** are common

Microbiology and Parasitology

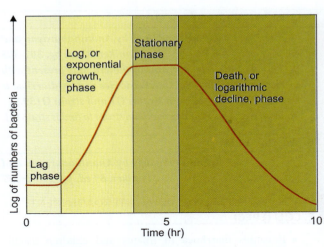

DIAGRAM: Showing bacterial curve growth curve

TABLE: Various Shapes of Bacteria

Shape	Associated bacteria
• Club Shape	Cornyebacteria
• Lanceolate	Pneumococci
• Half Moon/Lens	Meningococci
• Kidney Shape	Gonnococci
• Comma	Vibrio And Campylobacter

69. Ans. (c) Staph Aureus

Ref: Robbin's, 9th ed.

Diseases Characterized by Granulomas

- **Tuberculosis:** The granulomas of tuberculosis tend to contain necrosis ("caseating tubercules"), but non-necrotizing granulomas may also be present.
- **Leprosy:** In leprosy, granulomas are found in the skin and tend to involve nerves.
- **Sarcoidosis:** is a disease of unknown cause characterized by non-necrotizing ("non-caseating") granulomas in multiple organs and body sites, most commonly the lungs and lymph nodes within the chest cavity.
- **Hemophilus Ducreyi** causes chancre. It presents with painful genital ulcer with painful lymphadenopathy
- **Staph aureus** infections like pyoderma, abscess, HAP, food poisoning etc doesn't involve lymph nodes.

66. Ans. (d) H. pylori

Ref: Internet Source

- The rapid urease test also known as the Campylobacter like organism (CLO) test is **done for H. pylori** *in which the conversion of urea to ammonia and carbon dioxide by the urease enzyme present in the H. pylori is tested.*
- The Typhidot or dot ELISA is a test for the rapid diagnosis of S. typhi giving the separate identification of IgG and IgM antibodies whereas Widal test tests for specific antibody titres.
- Antigen tests which are EIA (Enzyme immunoassay) and Rapid HIV antibody test are used for detecting specific HIV antibodies and PCR (Polymerase Chain Reaction Test) is used for detecting genetic material of HIV.

67. Ans. (b) Listeria

Ref: Microbiology by Ananthanarayan and Paniker, 8th ed. pg. 226, 395

Listeria is the bacteria that is classically associated with **tumbling motility.**

Swarming Motility	Proteus
Gliding Motility	P. Aeruginosa, Mycoplasma
Darting Motility	Campylobacter, Vibrio Cholera
Falling Leaf Motility	Giardia
Shooting Star Motility	Vibrio
Cork Screw Motility	T. Pallidum
Lashing motility	Borrelia

68. Ans. (d) Gonococci

Ref: Microbiology by Ananthanarayan and Paniker, 8th ed. pg. 227

70. Ans. (a) Staph. aureus

Ref: Harriosn 18th ed./128, Microbiology by Ananthanarayan and Paniker, 8th ed. pg. 198

Refer to above explanation of Q. 52

71. Ans. (c) Staphylococcus

Ref: Harrison, 18th ed. pg. 128, Microbiology by Ananthanarayan and Paniker, 8th ed. pg. 198

- **Staphylococcus** causes food poisoning by enterotoxin A, due to intake of milk or milk products.
  - It is a preformed, heat stable enterotoxin, which stimulate the vagus nerve causing vomiting as main and first symptom.
  - I.P. < 6 hours
- *Outbreaks following picnics where potato salad, mayonnaise, and cream pastries have been served offer classic examples of staphylococcal food poisoning.*
- **Bacillus cereus** is an important cause of food poisoning, isolated from soil, vegetables, milk cereals, meat etc.
- It produces 2 types of food poisoning:

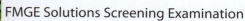
FMGE Solutions Screening Examination

Diarrhea type- main symptom	Emetic type- main symptom
• Associated with wide range of food intake including meat, puddings etc. • I.P. 8-16 hrs • Occurs due to heat labile enterotoxin	• Associated with intake of Chinese fried rice • I.P. 1-5 hrs • Due to pre-formed, heat stable toxin

- **Clostridium perfringens** causes gastroenteritis after intake of infected meat or meat products. I.P. - 8-16 hours.
- **Clostridium botulism** causes food poisoning due to consumption of canned food. I.P. 1 to 3 days.

72. Ans. (c) Staphylococcus aureus

Ref: Microbiology by Ananthanarayan and Paniker 8th ed. pg. 198, Harrison's 18th ed./Ch 128

- Among the given options staph aureus has the shortest incubation period (1-6 hrs).

Please refer to above explanation for more details

73. Ans. (c) Transpeptidase

Ref: Microbiology by Ananthanarayan and Paniker, 8th ed. pg. 197, 201-202

Resistance develops due to alteration in transpeptidase (penicillin binding protein) on which all beta lactam antibiotics act. Hence MRSA is resistant to all β-lactam antibiotics.

74. Ans. (b) B. Cereus

Ref: Microbiology by Ananthanarayan and Paniker, 8th ed. pg. 247, 654

As indicated in the table above, the common source of B. cereus is fried rice. Refer above explanation for details.

75. Ans. (a) Can be transmitted by parenteral route

Ref: Microbiology by Ananthanarayan and Paniker, 8th ed. pg. 247, 654

Please refer to explanation of Q. 38

76. Ans. (a) 7-21 days

Ref: Microbiology by Ananthanarayan and Paniker, 8th ed. pg. 293

- I.P of salmonella is 3-21 days
- **F**eatures of Typhoid-Step ladder pyrexia, Rash (rose spot) relative bradycardia, hepatospenomegaly, epistaxis
- **Complication**-Intestinal perforation and GI hemorrhage most common complication, seen during 3rd and 4th week.

77. Ans. (a) Vibrio cholerae O1

Ref: Microbiology by Ananthanarayan and Paniker, 8th ed. pg. 302-305

- Though the various strains of cholera may present with rice watery diarrhea, the classic rice watery diarrhea is usually associated with strains O1 and strain O139.
- *In these strains the more common strain to find is strain O1.*

78. Ans. (a) EPEC

Ref: Microbiology by Ananthanarayan and Paniker, 8th ed. pg. 276 & 277

ENTEROPATHOGENIC E. COLI/ENTEROADHERENT E. COLI (EPEC)

- It causes diarrhoea in infants and children usually occuring as institutional out breaks.
- In infantile enteritis, it does not produce enterotoxin, nor are they invasive,
- The bacilli are seen in to be adherent to the mucosa of the upper small intestine and cause disruption of the brush border microvilli.
- These strains can be identified by their adhesion to HEP - 2 cells.

ENTEROTOXIGENIC E. COLI (ETEC)

- **It causes traveller's diarrhoea [ETEC is the most common cause of traveller's diarrhea].**
- It produces enterotoxins. They can produce heat labile toxin (LT) or heat stable toxin or both.
- Toxin production alone may not lead to illness. The strain should first be able to adhere to intestinal mucosa.
- This adhesiveness is medicated by *fimbria! or colonisation factor antigen (CFA).*

ENTEROINVASIVE E. COLI (EIEC)

- They themselves resemble shigella and their infection resembles shigellosis (*remember : shiga like toxin is elaborated by enterohemorrhagic E. coli*).
- These strains are *non motile, do not ferment lactose or ferment it late* with acid without producing any gas.
- They produce mild diarrhoea to frank dysentry and occur in adult as well as in children.
- They have been termed enteroinvasive because they have the capacity to invade intestinal epithelial cells in vivo and penetrate HeLa or HEP - 2 cells in tissue culture.
- This ability of penetration is plasmid determined which codes for outer membrane antigens called the 'virulence marker antigen' (VMA). The detection of plasmid can be diagnostic.
- For laboratory diagnosis of EIEC, the *sereny test* used to be employed.

Microbiology and Parasitology

ENTERO-HEMORRHAGIC E. COLI OR VEROTOXIGENIC E. COLI

- These strains produce verocytotoxin (VT) or **shiga like toxin (SLT)**
- They can cause mild diarrhoea to fatal hemorrhagic colitis.
- This toxin also acts on vascular endothelium to promote the synthesis of coagulation factor VIII, vWF which triggers platelet aggregation.
- They can cause hemolytic uremic syndrome particularly in young children and the elderly.
- **0157 : H 7 is the most prominent serotype of EHEC, associated with HUS**, but 06, 026, 055, 091, 0103, 0111, 0113 and OX3 have also been associated with this syndrome.
- The primary target for V.T is vascular endothelium.
- Laboratory diagnosis of VTEC diarrhea is established by demonstration of the bacilli or VT in feces directly or in culture.

ENTEROAGGREGATIVE E COLI (EACE)

- They have been associated with persistent diarrhea, especially in developing countries.
- In vitro they appear aggregated in a 'stacked brick' formation in Hep-2 cells.

79. Ans. (d) E. Coli

Ref: Microbiology by Ananthanarayan and Paniker, 8th ed. pg. 276-77

- Hemoltic uremic syndrome (HUS) is a **type 3 hypersensitivity reaction** associated with small vessel vasculitis.
- Organisms causing HUS is E.Coli (particularly EHEC) and shigella dysentriae.

80. Ans. (d) EHEC

Ref: Ananthanaryan, 8th ed. pg. 276 & 277

Please refer to above explanation

81. Ans. (c) ETEC

Ref: Microbiology by Ananthanarayan and Paniker, 8th ed. pg. 276 & 277

Please refer to above explanation

82. Ans. (a) Traveller's diarrhea

Ref: Harrison 19th ed./727, Ananthanarayan 9/e 279

- **Anti- microbials are given for Traveller's diarrhea.**
- **Standard regimen is a 3-day course of a quinolone taken twice daily.**
- The current approach to self-treatment of travellers' diarrhea for the typical short-term traveller is to carry three once-daily doses of an antibiotic and to use as many doses as necessary to resolve the illness.

- If neither high fever nor blood in the stool accompanies the diarrhea, **loperamide** should be taken in combination with the antibiotic; studies have shown that this combination is more effective than an antibiotic alone and does not prolong illness.
- **Prophylaxis- bismuth subsalicylate-** widely used but only ~60% effective.
- For certain individuals (e.g., athletes, persons with a repeated history of travelers' diarrhea, and persons with chronic diseases), a single daily dose of a **quinolone, azithromycin, or rifaximin during travel of <1 month's duration** is 75–90% efficacious in preventing travellers' diarrhea.
- **Causes of travellers' diarrhea– Enterotoxigenic E coli is most common cause.**
- **Other causes-** Enteroaggrative E coli, Salmonella, Shigella, Vibrio, Campylobacter etc.

83. Ans. (b) Enterotoxin

Ref: Microbiology by Ananthanarayan and Paniker, 8th ed. pg. 198-199

- Enterotoxins are responsible for food poisoning and are produced when Staphylococcus Aureus grows in carbohydrate and protien foods. There are multiple types of enterotoxins (A-E, G-I, K-M) and these are usually superantigens.
- The alpha toxin is a potent hemolysin which acts on a broad spectrum of cell membranes, including RBC's.
- The beta toxin degrades spingomyelin and is also toxic for many types of cells.
- TSST-1 is the same as enterotoxin F and is therefore also a superantigen and is associated with fever, shock multisystem involvement and a desquamative skin rash.

84. Ans. (c) Vibrio cholerae

Ref: Microbiology by Ananthanarayan and Paniker, 8th ed. pg. 302-305

- Vibrio Cholerae is the organism with a single flagellum. Bacteria with a single flagellum are called monotrichous. Lophotrichous bacteria have multiple flagella located at the same end of the bacteria (or a few sites) such as Helicobacter Pylori.
- *Endoflagella are spirochetes flagella which is not external to the bacteria* but present within the cell from end to end of the cell providing rigidity to the cell and giving it the **corkscrew movement.**

Amphitrichous bacteria	A. fecalis
Peritrichous bacteria	E. Coli
Endoflagella	Spirochetes

FMGE Solutions Screening Examination

85. Ans. (d) Needles

Ref: Microbiology by Ananthanarayan and Paniker, 8th ed. pg. 251, 263, 634

- The organism is carried by about 3% of the general population and about 30% of the hospitalised patients in their gastrointestinal tract.
- It is usually transmitted by the feco-oral route and direct contact and hand to hand transmission are important modes of transmission in the hospitalized patients.
- *Clostridium difficile causes pseudomembranous colitis.*

86. Ans. (a) Clostridium Difficile

Ref: Microbiology by Ananthanarayan and Paniker, 8th ed. pg. 251, 263, 634

- Gas gangrene is myonecrosis caused by bacterial infection which can further lead to toxemia and shock. It is noticed by the black sores and crepitus caused by gas (nitrogen is the predominant gas component (74.5%), followed by oxygen (16.1%).
- **Clostridium microbes which cause gas gangrene are**:
  - Clostridium perfringens/welchi
  - Clostridium septicum
  - Clostridium Novyi
- *Clostridium Difficile causes acute enterocolitis.*
- *In a diabetic patient, the more likely pathogen of gas gangrene is Klebsiella pneumonia.*

Extra Mile

- Clostridium microbe that causes tetanus: Clostridium tetani
- Clostridium microbe that causes food poisoning:
  - **Perfringens type A-** Gastroenteritis
  - **Perfringens type C-** Necrotising enteritis
  - **Botulinum-** Botulism
  - **Difficile-** Acute colitis

87. Ans. (c) Clostridium perfringens

Ref: Microbiology by Ananthanarayan and Paniker, 8th ed. pg. 251-252

88. Ans. (a) Clostridium perfringens

Ref: Microbiology by Ananthanarayan and Paniker, 8th ed. pg. 251-52

Please refer to above explanation.

89. Ans. (d) Mixed infection

Ref: Microbiology by Ananthanarayan and Paniker, 8th ed. pg. 226, 270-75

- Fournier gangrene, is defined as a polymicrobial necrotizing fasciitis of the perineal, perianal, or genital area.
- In the majority of cases Fournier gangrene is a mixed infection caused by both aerobic and anaerobic bacteria.

Causal Agents

- Wound cultures from patients with Fournier gangrene reveal that it is a polymicrobial infection with an average of 4 isolates per case.
- *Escherichia coli is the predominant aerobe, and Bacteroides* is the predominant anaerobe that causes Fournier's gangrene
- Other common microflora include the following:
  - *Proteus*
  - *Staphylococcus*
  - *Enterococcus*
  - *Streptococcus*
  - *Pseudomonas*
  - *Clostridium*
  - *Klebsiella*

90. Ans. (a) Amoebic liver abscess

Ref: Microbiology by Ananthanarayan and Paniker, 8th ed. pg. 595, 625

AMOEBIC LIVER ABSCESS

- It is a liver abscess caused by Entamoeba histolytica
- It is common in tropical countries.
- It exists in vegetative form outside the body and is spread by the faeco-oral route.
- Presents with Pain in the right hypochondrium, fever, Profuse sweating and rigors, loss of weight etc.
- Investigation of choice: Ultrasound abdomen
- DOC: Metronidazole

91. Ans. (a) Bile solubility

Ref: Microbiology by Ananthanarayan and Paniker, 8th ed. pg. 206, 218, 219

- Organism causing respiratory tract infection (pneumonia) and alpha hemolysis is pneumococci.
- Two tests are commonly employed for distinguishing pneumococci from other alpha-hemolytic streptococci :
  1. *Optochin sensitivity*
  2. *Bile solubility*

92. Ans. (c) Adenosine triphosphate

- ATP is a nucleotide derived from adenosine that occurs in muscle tissue.
- It is the major source of energy for cellular reactions
- Energy is stored in the cell in form of ATP (Adenosine triphosphate)

Microbiology and Parasitology

93. Ans. (d) Staphylococcus aureus

Ref: Harrisons's, 19th ed.

- Pulmonary pneumatoceles are thin-walled, air-filled cysts that develop within the lung parenchyma.
- They can be single emphysematous lesions but are more often multiple, thin-walled, air-filled, cystlike cavities.
- Pneumatoceles are generally observed soon after the development of pneumonia and can be observed on the initial chest radiograph.
- *They are commonly caused by Staphylococcus Aureus.*
- Other agents also causes pneumatocele including:
  - *Streptococcus pneumonia*
  - H. Influenza,
  - E. Coli
  - Group A streptococci
  - *Serratia marcescens*
  - Klebsiella pneumoniae, adenovirus, and tuberculosis.
- Noninfectious etiologies include hydrocarbon ingestion, trauma, and positive pressure ventilation.

94. Ans. (a) Staph. Aureus, H. influenza, Pseudomonas

Ref: Harrison's, 19th ed. pg. 145e3-e5

Most common cause of pulmonary infection in Cystic fibrosis.

Age group	MC Organism
Children	Staph Aureus
Adolescent &adult	Pseudomonas aeroginosa
Overall	Pseudomonas aeroginosa

95. Ans. (a) Bacitracin

Ref: Microbiology by Ananthanarayan and Paniker, 8th ed. pg. 201, 206-07, 2012

- The various species of Streptococcus can be checked by various drug disks which is indicated as whether it is sensitive or resistant to the drug.
- S. pyogenes is bacitracin sensitive.
- S. agalactiae is bacitracin resistant.
- S. pneumoniae is inhibited by optochin.
- S. viridans is not inhibited by optochin.

96. Ans. (c) Anaerobic streptococci

Ref: Microbiology by Ananthanarayan and Paniker, 8th ed. pg. 635-36

- Chronic burrowing ulcer is also known as Meleney's synergistic hospital gangrene.
- It is caused by a mixed pattern of organisms like: *anaerobic streptococci*, coliforms, Staphyolococci, Bacteroides etc.

97. Ans. (a) Cellulitis

Ref: Microbiology by Ananthanarayan and Paniker, 8th ed. pg. 205

SKIN AND SOFT TISSUE INFECTION BY STREPTOCOCCUS

1. **Erysipelas**-diffuse infection involving the superficial lymphatics
2. **Impetigo**-superficial infection of skin (pyoderma)
3. **Cellulitis**-cellulitis is caused mainly by hemolytic streptococci. It specifically affects the dermis and subcutaneous fat.
4. **Lymphangitis**

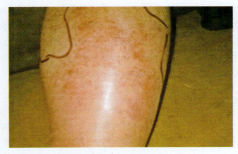

- **Gangrene**-type of ischemic necrosis
  - **Dry gangrene:** Arterial obstruction
  - **Wet gangrene:** Venous obstruction
- **Pyoderma** is most commanly caused by Staph Aureus

98. Ans. (b) Cyst are 8 nucleated

Ref: Microbiology by Ananthanarayan and Paniker, 8th ed. pg. 625, 626

- Cyst of E. histolytical is **quadri-nucleate (4 nuclei)**
- Chromatid bodies are seen as refractile oblong bars with rounded ends in prepration with normal saline and as black when stained with iron-haematoxylin.
- Trophozoites colonize cecum and ascending colon, sigmoid colon, rectum and appendix in decreasing order of frequency.

99. Ans. (a) Klebsiella pneumoniae

Ref: Microbiology by Ananthanarayan and Paniker, 8th ed. pg. 278, 707

- All the bacteria in the list except Klebsiella pneumoniae have flagella (or endoflagella) which gives them the property of motility.

100. Ans. (c) Klebsiella

Ref: Microbiology by Ananthanarayan and Paniker, 8th ed. pg. 278, 707

101. Ans. (c) An infection of lymph nodes

Ref: Microbiology by Ananthanarayan and Paniker, 8th ed. pg. 322-25

- In human beings plague occurs in three major forms:
  - **Bubonic plague:** *Infection of the lymph nodes*
  - **Pneumonic plague:** Infection of the lungs
  - **Septicemic plague:** Infection of the blood
- Bubonic Plague is caused by the bacteria *Yersinia pestis* from enterobacteriaceae family.
- Rodents, such as rats, carry the disease. It is spread by their fleas.
- People can get the plague when they are bitten by a flea that carries the plague bacteria from an infected rodent.
- After an **incubation period of 2-5 days, the lymph node** draining the site of entry of bacillus become infected
- As the plague bacillus usually enters through flea bites on the legs, the inguinal nodes are involved and hence the name "bubonic" (*bubon means groin*).

102. Ans. (c) Nasopharynx

Ref: Microbiology by Ananthanarayan and Paniker, 8th ed. pg. 224-25; K. Park 20th ed. pg. 150,151

- **N. Meningococci are capsulated *Gram negative diplococci***
- **Reservoir for N. Meningitides-**Human nasopharynx is only reservoir of meningococcus. (N.meningitidis)
- **Most important source-** carriers are the most imp source, not clinical cases.
- They are arranged in pairs with adjacent sides flattened—7 *half moon shaped.*
- **Transport medium—Stuart's medium.**
- **Blood agar, chocolate agar and Muller-Hinton agar** are the media commonly used for culturing meningococci.
- **Age group-** 3 month-5 years
- **Serotype-** total 13, out of which serotype A,B,C are most important
  - **Serotype A-** Epidemics
  - **Serotype B-** Both epidemic and local out breaks
  - **Serotype C-** Local out breaks
- Chemoprophylaxis has been suggested for close contacts.
- Is DOC for prophylaxis.
- Ceftriaxone > ciprofloxacin > Rifampicin

103. Ans. (b) Neisseria Meningitidis

Ref: Microbiology by Ananthanarayan and Paniker, 8th ed. pg. 224-25

MENINGOCOCCI

- **Meningococci are *Gram negative diplococci***
- Strep. Pneumoniae is a gram positive diplococci.
- Corynebacterium Diphtheriae is Gram positive bacillus. They are non-motile, non-sporing and non-acid fast.
- Staphylococcus are Gram positive cocci. They are also non-motile, non-spore forming, non-acid fast.

104. Ans. (c) β lactamase

Ref: Microbiology by Ananthanarayan and Paniker, 8th ed. pg. 224-26

- **Lipo-oligosaccharide (LOS)** is a component of the outer memberane of N. meningitidis which acts as an endotoxin which is responsible for septic shock and hemorrhage due to the destruction of red blood cells.
- Other virulence factors include a polysaccharide capsule which prevents host phagocytosis and aids in evasion of the host immune response; and fimbriae which mediate attachment of the bacterium to the epithelial cells of the nasopharynx.
- **Beta-lactumases are enzymes (and not virulence factors) produced by some bacteria and are responsible for their resistance to beta-lactam antibiotics like penicillins and carbapenems**

105. Ans. (d) Streptococcus pneumoniae

Ref: Dhingra, 5th ed. pg. 61, 81

- **Meningitis** is the **commonest intracranial complication** of otitis media.
- In infants and children, otogenic meningitis usually follows acute otitis media while in adults, it is due to chronic middle ear infection.
- Most common organisms in infants and children are **Streptococcus pneumonia (30%)**, H. influenza (20%), and Moraxella catarrhalis (12%). Other organisms include Strep pyogenes, Staph aureus and Pseudomonas.
- Strep. Pneumoniae is also the most common cause of pyogenic meningitis in adults.

106. Ans. (a) Streptococcus pneumoniae

Ref: Dhingra, 5th ed. pg. 61, 81

107. Ans. (b) Serotype B

Ref: Microbiology by Ananthanarayan and Paniker, 9th ed. pg. 230

- Effective vaccines prepared from purified group A, C, Y, W-135 menigococcal capsular polysaccharide.
- Immunity is group specific.
- Good immunity after single dose, in older children and adults but little value in age < 3yrs.
- Takes 10-14 days for immunity to develop.

Microbiology and Parasitology

- Vaccine may be monovalent (A or C) or polyvalent (A-C, A-C-Y)
- **There is no group B vaccine available at present.**

108. Ans. (d) Aspergillus

Ref: Microbiology by Ananthanarayan and Paniker, 8th ed. pg. 659 -660

- Air crescent sign/meniscus sign appears as crescent of air in intrapulmonary cavity.
- It is formed due to angio-invasive aspergillosis. Although indolent with few or no symptoms, fatal hemoptysis can occur.

> **Extra Mile**
>
> - **Aspergillus fumigatus** is the most common cause of aspergillosis.
> - Most common type of fungal infection of nose and paranasal sinuses is due to: Aspergillus.
> - Most common fungus causing allergy is: Aspergillus.
> - Aspergillus has septate hyphae that branch typically at 45°C (V shaped).
> - Non septate hyphae with *obtuse branching*- **Rhizopus/mucor**

109. Ans. (a) 2–3 days

Ref: Harrison's, 18th ed. Ch 138

Harrison's states: *"The incubation period for respiratory diphtheria is 2–5 days; however, disease can develop as long as 10 days after exposure"*

Types of Diphtheria Infections are

1. **Faucial (tonsillar pharyngeal)**- Commonest type, grey with white pseudomembrane and cervical lymphade-nopathy (bull neck) + toxemia
2. **Laryngeal** - Most severe form
3. **Nasal** - Mildest form
4. **Cutaneous form** - Only non toxigenic strain, punched-out ulcer
5. **Other form** - Conjuctival, otic, genital

110. Ans. (a) Gram negative

Ref: Microbiology by Ananthanarayan and Paniker, 8th ed. pg. 396-97

- **Calymmatobacterium Granulomatis** is known by another name: Klebsiella Granulomatis.
- It is non-motile bacteria containing **gram-negative,** pleomorphic rods that cause granulomatous lesions in humans, especially in the inguinal region.
- It causes **granuloma inguinale** aka Donovanosis**,** which is a contagious sexually transmitted disease occurring predominantly in tropical areas and characterized by deep purulent ulcers on or near the genital organs.

- Encapsulated bacilli called Donovan bodies (*macrophage) in which these bacilli multiply.*
- Bacteria stained at the ends, known as bipolar staining or *safety pin appearance or telephone hand appearance.*
- Granuloma inguinale is treated with streptomycin or with broad-spectrum antibiotics.

111. Ans. (d) S. Cholerae suis

Ref: Microbiology by Ananthanarayan and Paniker, 8th ed. pg. 300

- S. Cholera suis can cause septicemic disease with focal suppurative lesions, such as osteomyelitis, deep abscesses, endocarditis, pneumonia and meningitis

112. Ans. (b) Pneumococcus

Ref: Microbiology by Ananthanarayan and Paniker, 8th ed. pg. 19, 63, 193

- *Due to alpha hemolysis, colonies of pneumococci resemble colonies of Str. viridans.*
- On further incubation the colonies of pneumococci become flat with raised edges and central umbonation, so that concentric rings are seen on the surface when viewed from above seems as draughtsman appearance or Carrom coin appearance.

113. Ans. (d) Clostridium Welchii

Ref: Microbiology by Ananthanarayan and Paniker, 8th ed. pg. 643, 655, 249-54

- Clostridium Welchii is also known as Clostridium perfringens.
- It is the most common bacterial agent which causes gas gangrene.
- Gas gangrene results in tissue necrosis, putrefaction of tissues, and gas production.
- It is caused primarily by Clostridium perfringens alpha toxin, usually after a injury or trauma.
- These gases form bubbles in muscle and produce characteristic smell of decomposing tissue.
- The local spread of gases under tissue produces Crepitations when pressed on it.
- *Crepitations: sound of snow crushing*
- After rapid and destructive local spread (which can take hours), systemic spread of bacteria and bacterial toxins may result in death.

114. Ans. (b) Clostridium tetani

Ref: Microbiology by Ananthanarayan and Paniker, 8th ed. pg. 249-54

- There are species of Clostridium that bears terminal spores which appears as drumstick shaped under micro-scope.

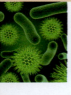

FMGE Solutions Screening Examination

- **Clostridium tetani** is a gram positive obligate anaerobe which is the causative agent of tetanus, bears spores which are spherical, terminal and twice the diameter of vegetative cells. This gives it a drumstick appearance upon viewing under microscope.

Bacteria	Appearance
• Clostridium tetani	Drumstick appearance
• Corynebacterium diphtheria	Chinese letter pattern
• Neisseria meningitides	D- shaped
• N. Gonorrhea	Kidney shaped appearance
• Strep Pneumoniae	Flame shaped appearance

115. Ans. (d) Imipenem

Ref: Harrison's 19th ed.

- Microbes which are resistant to methicillin are said to be MRSA.
- Methicillin is highly penicilinase resistant but not acid resistant.
- MRSA have emerged in many areas. These are insensitive to all penicillinase-resistant penicillins and to other β-lactams as well as to erythromycin, aminoglycosides, tetracylines, etc.
- The drug of choice for these organisms is vancomycin, but ciprofloxacin and Rifampicin can also be used.
- Drug of choice for V.R.S.A is Daptomycin > Linezolide.
- **IMIPENEM** is an extremely potent and broad-spectrum β-lactam antibiotic whose range of activity includes *gram positive cocci, Enterobacteriaceae, Ps. Aeruginosa, Listeria as well as anaerobes like Bact. Fragilis and Cl. difficile.*

116. Ans. (d) All of the above

Ref: Microbiology by Ananthanarayan and Paniker, 8th ed. pg. 613

ASPERGILLOSIS

- *Aspergillus fumigatus* is the most common cause of aspergillosis.
- Aspergillus is a mould with septate *branching* hyphae. Ability of A. fumigatus to grow at 45° C helps to distinguish it from other species.
- Mode of transmission: Inhalation of Aspergillus spores (Conidia).
- The commonest human disease caused by aspergillus is: otomycosis.
- Aspergillus infection in neutropenic patient is characterized by hyphae invasion of blood vessels, thrombosis, necrosis and hemorrhagic infarction.
- **Clinical manifestations**
  - *Allergic bronchopulmonary aspergillosis* occurs in patients with preexisting asthma or cystic fibrosis.

- *Endobronchial saprophytic pulmonary aspergillosis (Aspergilloma)* in a patient with prior chronic lung disease, such as tuberculosis, sarcoidosis, bronchiectasis or histoplasmosis
- *Invasive aspergillosis* develops as an acute pneumonic process with or without dissemination in the immuno-compromised patients (most common among patients with acute leukemia and recipient of tissue transplants.
  - CT finding: *Halo sign and crescent sign*
- *Allergic sinusitis* may take three forms :
  - A fungal ball may form.
  - Chronic fibrosing granulomatous inflammation
  - Allergic fungal sinusitis
- *Aspergillosis in AIDS*
  - Most commonly infect lung
  - CD4 +cell count is < 50/μL
  - Most common radiologic finding is bilateral diffuse or focal pulmonary infiltrates with a tendency to cavitate.

117. Ans. (a) Staphylococci

Ref: Microbiology by Ananthanarayan and Paniker, 8th ed. pg. 199-200

- *Staphylococci causes hospital acquired pneumonia.*
- **Community-acquired pneumonia** (CAP) is pneumonia acquired infectiously from normal social contact (that is, in the community).
- The most important infection in newborns is caused by *Streptococcus agalactiae*, also known as Group B Streptococcus or GBS. It causes >50% of cases of CAP in the first week of life.
- *Streptococcus pneumoniae is the most common cause of community acquired acute pneumonia in adults.* It is the most common cause of *lobar pneumonia*

Causes of Pneumonia

In Infants	In Adults
Group B Streptococcus	• Streptococcus pneumoniae
Streptococcus	• Hemophilus influenza
Pneumoniae	• Escherichia coli
Escherichia coli	• Klebsiella pneumoniae
Klebsiella pneumoniae	• Influenza, Paranifluenza and RSV virus

118. Ans. (c) Rat urine

Ref: Microbiology by Ananthanarayan and Paniker, 8th ed. pg. 381-83

- **Leptospirosis** is caused by infection with bacteria of the genus *Leptospira* and affects humans as well as other animals.

Microbiology and Parasitology

- One of the zoonotic infection, which transmits from animals to human
- Leptospirosis is transmitted by the urine of an infected animal like rat, mice or moles and is contagious as long as the urine is still moist.

> **Extra Mile**
> Doxycycline 200–250 mg once a week used as prophylaxis

119. Ans. (b) Staphylococcus epidermidis

Ref: Microbiology by Ananthanarayan and Paniker, 8th ed. pg. 655, 679

STAPHYLOCOCCUS

- Gram positive cocci, coagulase and Catalase positive: Staphylococcus aureus
- Gram positive cocci, *Coagulase negative*: Staphylococcus epidermidis and saprophyticus.
- Staph. Epidermis infect most commonly through artificial device like: IV canula, Prosthetic device, shunts and implants.
- *MCC of catheter associated blood stream infection: Staph. Epidermis*
- MC organism causing prosthetic valve endocarditits: Coagulase negative Staphylococcus.

120. Ans. (d) Trichenella spiralis

Parasitic infections associated with eosinophilic myocarditis:

PROTOZOA

- Trypanosoma cruzi (Chagas disease)
- Toxoplasma gondii (Toxoplasmosis)

METAZOA

- *Trichenella spiralis*
- Toxocara canis
- Echinococcus granulosus (Hydatid cyst)
- Schistosomiasis

VIROLOGY

121. Ans. (c) Skin biopsy with fluorescent antibody testing

Ref: Textbook of Microbiology by Surinder Kumar, P 592

Laboratory tests of rabies

IMMUNOFLUORESCENCE TEST

- Performed on samples of saliva, serum, spinal fluid, and skin biopsies of hair follicles at the nape of the neck.
- **Rabies Antigens by Immunofluorescence:**
  - MC method used for demonstration of rabies virus.

- Specimen used are corneal smears and skin biopsy (from face or neck) or saliva ante mortem, and brain post-mortem.
- **Serology**
  - Rabies antibodies can be detected in the serum and CSF of the patient by ELISA
- **RT-PCR (Reverse Transcription- Polymerase Chain Reaction)**
  - Can detect rabies virus in saliva and in skin biopsy samples

> **Extra Mile**
>
> **Laboratory Diagnosis of Rabies (in animals)**
>
> **Immunofluorescence Test**
> - Highly reliable and the best test available for the rapid diagnosis of rabies viral antigen in infected specimens.
> - Can establish diagnosis within a few hours.
> - Examination of salivary glands by immunofluorescence is useful
> - NOTE: Fluorescent antibody titers in clinical rabies have been well in excess of 1:10,000, a feature which helps to distinguish between rabies and vaccine reaction.
>
> **HPE**
> - Definitive pathologic diagnosis of rabies. Demonstration of Negri bodies in hippocampus or the spinal cord is characteristic.
> - MC used method if immunofluorescence is NOT available. A negative negri bodies doesn't rule out the infection
>
> **Corneal Test**
> - Rabies virus antigen can be detected in live animals in corneal impressions or in frozen sections of skin biopsies by the fluorescent antibody test. *A negative test doesn't rule out possibility of infection.*

122. Ans. (a) E. coli 0157

Ref: Textbook of Microbiology by Surinder Kumar, P 749

- **E. coli 0157:** H7 is the infectious cause of haemolytic uremic syndrome, Haemorrhagic colitis
- **Parvovirus B19:** Is known to cause aplastic crisis in chronic haemolytic anemia
- **Bartonella henselae:** Cat – scratch disease, Bacillary angiomatosis

> **Extra Mile**
>
> - **Ebola virus:** Ebola hemorrhagic fever
> - **Hantaan virus:** Hemorrhagic fever with renal syndrome
> - **Guanarito virus:** Venezuelan hemorrhagic fever
> - **Sabia virus:** Brazilian hemorrhagic fever

Explanations

123. Ans. (d) EBV

Ref: Textbook of Microbiology by Surinder Kumar, P 536

- Ebstein barr virus is from herpes family, HHV 4.

TABLE: Classification of human herpes viruses

Subfamily	Virus	Primary target cell	Site of latency	Mode of spread
A. Alphaherpesvirinae				
Human herpesvirus 1	Herpes simplex type 1	Mucoepithelial cell	Neuron	Close contact
Human herpesvirus 2	Herpes simples type 2	Mucoe pithelial cells	Neuron	Close contact (sexually transmitted disease)
Human herpesvirus 3	Varicella-zoster virus	Muco epithelial cells	Neuron	Respiratory and close contact
B. Betaherpesvirinae				
Human herpesvirus 5	Cytome galovirus	Monocyte, lymphocyte, and epithelial cells	Monocyte, lymphocyte,	Close contact, transfusions, tissue transplant, and congenital
Human herpesivirus 6	Herpes lymphotropic virus	T cells	T cells	Respiratory and close contact
Human herpesvirus 7	Human herpesvirus 7	T cells	T cells	
Gamma herpesvirinae				
Human herpesvirus 4	Epstein-barr virus	B cells and epithelial cells	B cell	Saliva (kissing disease)
Human herpesvirus 8	Kaposi's sarcoma-related virus	Lymphocyte and other cells		Close contact (sexual)

Extra Mile

- **Rabies** virus is from the Rhabdoviridae family (*Genus: Lyssa virus; serotype 1*)
- **Rubella** is from family Togaviridae (*Genus: Rubivirus*).
- **Measles (Rubeola)** virus is a paramyxovirus, from Morbillivirus family.

124. Ans. (d) Pox virus

Ref: Textbook of Microbiology by Surinder Kumar, P 534

- **Molluscum contagiosum** virus is a pox virus, which causes a contagious, benign epidermal tumor that occurs in humans only.
- **Lesion:** small, pink, papular, warty, pearl-like benign tumors of the face, arm, back and buttocks.

TABLE: Poxviruses causing disease in humans

Genus	Virus	Primary host	Disease
Orthopoxvirus	Variola	Humans	Smallpox (now eliminated)
	Vaccinia	Humans	Localized lesion; used for smallpox vaccination
	Buffalopox	Water buffalo	Human infections rate; localized lesion
	Monkeypox	Rodents, monkeys	Human infections rate; generalized disease
	Cowpox	Cows	Human infections rare; localized ulcerating lesion
Parapoxvirus	Orf	Sheep	Human infections rare; localized lesion
	Pseudocowpox	Cows	
	Bovine popular stomatitis	Cows	
Mollusapoxvirus	Molluscum contagiosum	Humans	Many benign skin nodules
Yatapoxvirus	Tanapox	Monkeys	Human infections rare; localized lesion
	Yabapox	Monkeys	Human infections very rare and accidental; localized skin tumors

Microbiology and Parasitology

125. Ans. (b) Hepatitis C virus

Ref: Ananthnarayan and Paniker's Textbook of Microbiology, 8th ed. pg. 545

DNA and RNA virus

DNA virus	RNA virus
• Pox virus: *largest virus* • Parvovirus: *smallest virus* • Adenovirus • Papovavirus • Hepadna virus • Herpes virus	• Rotavirus: *only double stranded RNA virus* • Orthomyxovirus • Reovirus • Bunya virus • Arena virus • Hepatitis A, C, D, E virus • Picorna, polio, coxsackie, echo and entero virus.

126. Ans. (b) Coxsackie

Ref: Ananthnarayan and Paniker's Textbook of Microbiology, 8th ed. pg. 489

Coxsackie viruses produce a variety of clinical syndromes in humans ranging from trivial to fatal infections:

1. **Herpangina (vesicular pharyngitis)** is a common clinical manifestation of coxsackie Group A infection in children. It is a severe febrile pharyngitis, with headache, vomiting and pain in the abdomen.

2. **Aseptic meningitis** may be caused by most Group A and all Group B viruses. A maculopapular rash may be present. The disease may sometimes occur as epidemic.

3. **Hand, Foot and Mouth Disease (HFMD)** was identified in 1960 as an exanthematous fever affecting mainly young children, characterized by clusters of papulovesicular lesions on the skin and oral mucosa. It occurs as sporadic cases and as outbreaks.

4. Epidemic pleurodynia or **Bornholm disease** (*so called because it was first described on the Danish island of Bornholm*) is a febrile disease with stitch-like pain in the chest and abdomen, caused by Group B viruses.

5. Myocarditis and pericarditis in the newborn, associated with high fatality may be caused by Group B viruses.

6. Fulminant diabetes and orchitis
   - **Transplacental** and neonatal transmission has been demonstrated with **Coxsackie B viruses.**

127. Ans. (b) Can be treated by saline infusion

Ref: Ananthnarayan and Paniker's Textbook of Microbiology, 8th ed. pg. 557-58

- Rotaviruses are the commonest cause of diarrhea in infants and children over the world and account for about half the cases of children hospitalized for diarrhea.

- It occurs throughout the year but **predominates in winter months,** when the virus may be detected in most of the patients. It sometimes produces large epidemics of diarrhea in winter.

- Rotavirus diarrhea is usually seen in children below the age of five years, but is **most frequent between 6 and 24 months of age**.

- Mode of spread: fecal-oral route.

- Incubation period: 2–3 days.

- Vomiting and diarrhea occur with little or no fever. Stools are usually greenish yellow or pale, with no blood or mucus. The **disease is self-limited** and recovery occurs within 5–10 days. **Mortality is low. Rehydration with O.R.S. is all the treatment needed.**

- Rotavirus vaccines are given orally before the age of 6 months.

128. Ans. (c) Rabies

- **Inclusion bodies** are nuclear or cytoplasmic aggregates of stainable substances, usually proteins. They typically represent sites of viral multiplication in a bacterium or a eukaryotic cell and usually consist of viral capsid proteins.

Examples of viral inclusion bodies

Intracytoplasmic	Intranuclear	Intracytoplasmic + Intranuclear
• **Negri bodies** in Rabies • **Guarnieri bodies** in Small pox • **Henderson-Peterson bodies** in Molluscum contagiosum	• **Cowdry type A in Herpes simplex virus** and Varicella zoster virus and Torres bodies in Yellow fever • **Cowdry type B** in Polio and adenovirus	• **Warthin finkeldey bodies** in *Measles* and SSPE.

129. Ans. (a) p24

Ref: PubMed

- This is a possible suspicion of HIV infection.
- p24 antigen is a **viral protein** that makes up most of the viral core.
- Serum concentrations of **p24 antigen are high in the first few weeks after infection**; tests sensitive to p24 antigen are therefore useful for diagnosing very early infection when antibody levels are still low.

130. Ans. (a) Reverse transcriptase

Ref: Microbiology by Ananthanarayan and Paniker, 9th ed. pg. 574-75

- cDNA is created from mRNA with use of **reverse transcriptase.** First formed is single stranded DNA and then double stranded DNA.

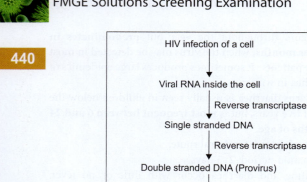

131. Ans. (a) Measles

Ref: Microbiology by Ananthanarayan and Paniker, 8th ed. pg. 444, 453

Refer to above explanation

132. Ans. (d) Herpes virus

Ref: Microbiology by Ananthanarayan and Paniker, 8th ed. pg. 444, 453

Please refer to above explanation

133. Ans. (a) Molluscum contagiosum

- Contagiosum is a viral infection of skin which is caused by a virus, *the moluscum contagiosum virus*, from pox virus family.
- The virus is contagious through direct contact.
- The virus also can be spread by sexual contact and can occur in people with compromised immune systems.

134. Ans. (c) Virus

Ref: Microbiology by Ananthanarayan and Paniker, 8th ed. pg. 443, 445

Please refer to above explanation

135. Ans. (c) Both A and B

Ref: Microbiology by Ananthanarayan and Paniker, 8th ed. pg. 569-70

- **Reverse transcriptase (RNA-directed DNA polymerase):** catalyzes the transcription of retrovirus RNA into DNA.
- Reverse transcriptase is central to the infectious nature, which causes HIV infection in humans which leads to AIDS, and
- Human T-cell lymphotrophic virus I (HTLV-I), which causes adult T-cell leukemia and tropical spastic paraparesis.

136. Ans. (a) Influenza virus

Ref: Microbiology by Ananthanarayan and Paniker, 8th ed. pg. 429

- A large number of viruses agglutinate erythrocytes from different species by the process known as Hemagglutination.
- Hemagglutination of influenza virus is due to presence of hemagglutinin spikes on the surface of virus.
- Viruses causing Hemagglutination are:
  - Influenza Virus
  - Rubella
  - RhinoVirus
  - Parainfluenza Virus
  - EnteroVIrus
  - Reo Virus
  - *Measles*
  - Coxsackie Virus
  - *Rabies*
  - Toga Virus
  - Echo VIrus

137. Ans. (a) Rocky mountain spotted fever

Ref: Microbiology by Ananthanarayan and Paniker, 8th ed. pg. 406, 408, 413

Disease	Causative agent
RMSF (Rocky Mountain Spotted Fever)	R. Rickettsii
Kyasanur forest disease	Group B togavirus (Flavivirus)
Dengue	Arbovirus 4 serotypes (Den- 1,2,3,4)
Yellow fever	Flavivirus fibricus

138. Ans. (d) Rhinovirus

Ref: Microbiology by Ananthanarayan and Paniker, 8th ed. pg. 490

- Common cold is a viral infection of the upper respiratory tract. The most commonly implicated viruses are:
  1. Rhinovirus: most common cause (30–80%), a type of Picornavirus
  2. Human coronavirus ~15%
  3. Influenza viruses 10–15%
  4. Adenoviruses 5%
  5. Other viruses include: human parainfluenza virus, human respiratory syncytial virus, and enteroviruses.

139. Ans. (c) P. vivax

Ref: Microbiology by Ananthanarayan and Paniker, 8th ed. pg. 694

- **Duffy antigen/chemokine receptor** (DARC) also known as **CD234,** is a protein that in humans is encoded by *DARC* gene.
- The Duffy antigen is located on the surface of red blood cells.

Microbiology and Parasitology

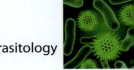

- The Duffy antigen protein is also the *receptor for the human malarial parasites Plasmodium vivax.*
- Polymorphisms in this gene are the basis of the Duffy blood group system.

Clinical Significance of Duffy Antigen

- **Asthma:** There appears to be a correlation with both total IgE levels and asthma and mutations in the Duffy antigen.
- **Malaria:** On erythrocytes the Duffy antigen acts as a receptor for invasion by the human malarial parasites *P. vivax* and *P. knowles.*
- *Duffy negative individuals whose erythrocytes do not express the receptor are believed to be resistant to merozoite invasion.*
- **HIV infection:** The absence of the DARC receptor appears to increase the susceptibility to infection by HIV. HIV-1 appears to be able to attach to erythrocytes via DARC
- **Lung transplantation:** The Duffy antigen has been implicated in lung transplantation rejection.
- **Multiple myeloma:** An increased incidence of Duffy antigen has been reported in patients with multiple myeloma compared with healthy controls
- **Pneumonia:** The Duffy antigen is present in the normal pulmonary vascular bed. Its expression is increased in the vascular beds and alveolar septa of the lung parenchyma during suppurative pneumonia.
- **Prostate cancer:** Experimental work has suggested that DARC expression inhibits prostate tumor growth. The reasons for this increased risk are not known.
- **Sickle cell anemia:** Duffy antigen-negative individuals with sickle cell anaemia tend to suffer from more severe organ damage than do those with the Duffy antigen.

140. Ans. (b) DNA virus

Ref: Microbiology by Ananthanarayan and Paniker, 8th ed. pg. 549

- **Human papillomavirus (HPV)** is a DNA virus from the papovavirus family that is capable of infecting humans.
- Usually it causes no symptoms in most people, but some types can cause warts (verrucae), while others can in a minority of cases lead to cancers of the cervix, vulva, vagina, penis, oropharynx and anus.
- HPV has been linked with an increased risk of cardiovascular disease.
- In addition, HPV 16 and 18 infections are a cause of a unique type of oropharyngeal (throat) and cervix cancer.

DNA and RNA virus

DNA virus	RNA virus
• Pox virus: *largest virus* • Parvovirus: *smallest virus* • Adenovirus • Papovavirus • Hepadna virus • Herpes virus	• Rotavirus: *only double stranded RNA virus* • Orthomyxovirus • Reovirus • Buniya virus • Arena virus • Hepatitis A, C, D, E virus • Picorna, polio, cocksackie, echo and entero virus.

141. Ans. (b) Secondary syphilis

Ref: Microbiology by Ananthanarayan and Paniker, 8th ed. pg. 378

- The Jarisch-Herxheimer reaction is classically associated with penicillin treatment of syphilis.
- It is believed to be caused by the release of endotoxin-like substances when large numbers of *Treponema pallidum* are killed by antibiotics.
- It has also been documented in tick-borne rickettsial diseases like Lyme disease and relapsing fever where the infecting organism is also a spirochete.
- The reaction can be expected *in 50% of primary syphilis, 90% of secondary syphilis, and in 25% of early latent infection,* but is very rare in late syphilis.
- It has been suggested that it is more severe in patients with HIV

142. Ans. (c) Dogs

Ref: Microbiology by Ananthanarayan and Paniker, 8th ed. pg. 112, 174, 427

143. Ans. (d) Spare palm sole

- **IP of chicken pox**-10-21 days
- Infectious period is 2 days before to 5 days after the onset of rash. The rash is maculo-papulo-vesicular rash.
- **Rash is symmetrical and centripetal**, mainly on trunk, pleomorphic, **spare palm and sole**
- *Portal of entry of virus-respiratory tract or conjunctiva*
- Rash appear on the day the fever starts

MYCOLOGY AND PARASITOLOGY

144. Ans. (b) Chromoblastomycosis

Ref: Textbook of Microbiology by Surinder Kumar, P 659

- The fungal hyphae are broken down into smaller sections/compartment by septa → septate hyphae
  - Example: Apergillus
- If there is no septation/compartment → Non-septate (Coenocytic)
  - Mucor, Zygomycetes

FMGE Solutions Screening Examination

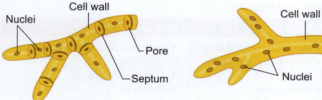

Chromoblastomycosis
- It is one of the subcutaneous mycosis.
- Characterized by: crusted, warty lesions in limbs
- **Cause:** soil inhabiting fungi of the family Dematiaceae.

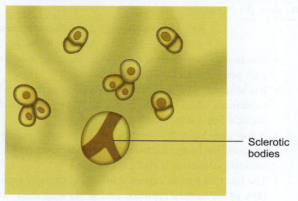

Laboratory Diagnosis
- Microscopically dark fungal elements on skin scraping or pus
- Histologically, it shows fungus having round or irregular, dark brown, yeast-like bodies with septae, called *sclerotic cells* (seen on KOH mount).

Extra Mile

Microscopic examination of some fungi
- **Tinea versicolor:** cluster of round yeast cell with short, stout hyphae which is branched or curved
- **Mycetoma:** presence of pus in draining sinus
- **Tinea Nigra:** Localized infection of the stratum corneum, particularly of the palms. It is caused by the dematiaceous fungus *Hortaea (Exophiala) werneckii*.
  - **Microscopy:** Brownish, branched, septate hyphae and budding cells
- **Histoplasmosis:** white to tan fluffy colony with septate branching hyphae
- **Aspergillus:** On direct examination of sputum with KOH or calcofluor white or in histologic sections → non-pigmented septate mycelium, with dichotomous branching.
- **Coccidiodomycosis:** large number of barrel shaped anthropores, characteristically alternate with smaller intervening empty cells.
- **Candida albicans:** Culture colonies are creamy white, smooth and with yeast odour. Identified by production of germ tube test.

---

145. Ans. (b) *Cysticercosis cellulose*

Ref: Lange Microbiology, Ch 46

- The larval stage of taenia solium is Cysticercus cellulose, which lives in pig or in humn tissues causing human cysticercosis.

Must know questions about Tenia solium:
- **Life span:** > 25 years; Cysticercus survives 5 – 6 years in human body
- **Final host:** Man
- **Intermediate host:** Pig/Man
- **Infective stage:** Cysticercus and Egg
- **Source of infection:** Consuming raw/undercooked pork
- **Inhabitation site:**
  - Adult org: In human intestine
  - Cysticercus: In tissues

146. Ans. (b) *Candida albicans*

Ref: Textbook of Diagnostic Microbiology, E-book, P 634

- A germ tube test is a diagnostic test in which a sample of fungal spores are suspended in serum and examined by microscopy. It is particularly indicated for colonies of white or cream color on fungal culture.
- A positive germ tube test is strongly indicative of *Candida albicans*. This test also helps to differentiate between *Candida albicans* and *non-albicans Candida* (germ tube test negative).

147. Ans. (b) *Skin and hair*

Ref: Textbook of Diagnostic Microbiology, E-book, P 607

- **Trichophyton:** Skin, hair, nail
- **Epidermophyton:** Skin, nail
- **Microsporum:** Skin, hair

148. Ans. (c) *Filaria*

Ref: Harrison 19th ed. P 1420

- Tropical or pulmonary eosinophilia is due to microfilaria in lung. There is no microfilaria in blood.
- It is characterized by coughing, asthmatic attacks and enlarged spleen.
- **DOC:** Diethylcarbamazine

149. Ans. (a) *Schistosoma*

Ref: Harrison 19th ed. P 605

***Schistosoma* has 3 species mainly and resides in:**
- *S. mansoni*: resides in mesenteric veins draining sigmoido-rectal region
- *S. japonicum*: resides in mesenteric veins draining the ileocecal region

Microbiology and Parasitology

- *S. haematobium*: Bladder plexus
- *Fasciola*: Liver fluke (*Fasciola hepatica*)
- *Paragonimus westermani*: Lung fluke

150. Ans. (b) Accidental intermediate host in humans

Ref: Textbook of surgical gastroenterology pg. 767, PK mission ed 2016

Human echinococcosis is a zoonotic disease that is caused by parasites, namely tapeworms of the genus *Echinococcus*.

Transmission

- *E. granulosus* requires two host types, a definitive host and an intermediate host.
- The definitive host of this parasite are dogs
- Intermediate host are most commonly sheep, however, cattle, horses, pigs, goats, and camels are also potential intermediate hosts.
- Humans can also be an *intermediate host* for *E. granulosus*, however this is uncommon and therefore *humans are considered an accidental intermediate host*.

151. Ans. (c) Plasmodium malariae

Ref: Harrison's, 19th ed. pg. 1371

- *P. vivax*, *P. ovale*, show a marked predilection for young RBCs
- *P. malariae* has predilection for old RBCs
- *P. falciparum* can invade erythrocytes of all ages and may be associated with very high levels of parasitemia.

TABLE: Characteristics of plasmodium species infecting humans

Characteristic	Finding of indicated species			
	P. falciparum	P. vivax	P. ovale	P. malariae
Duration of intrahepatic phase (days)	5.5	8	9	15
Number of merozoites released per infected hepatocyte	30,000	10,000	15,000	15,000
Duration of erythrocytic cycle (hours)	48	48	50	72
Red cell preference	Younger cell (but can invade cells of all ages)	Reticulocytes and cells up to 2 weeks old	Reticulocytes	**Older cells**
Morphology of RBC and parasites	Usually only ring forms; banana-shaped gametocytes, (Maurer dots)	Irregularly shaped large rings and trophozoites; enlarged erythrocytes; (Schuffner's dots)	Infected erythrocytes, enlarged and oval with tufted end; (James dots)	Band or rectangular forms of trophozoites common (Ziemann's dot)
Ability to cause relapses	No	Yes	Yes	No

152. Ans. (c) Coccidioidomycosis

Ref: Atlas of Infectious diseases: Fungal Infection, pg. 33

- Mature spherule in sputum sample is seen in coccidioidomycosis.
- Coccidioidomycosis may present with a syndrome of erythema nodosum, fever, and conjunctivitis. Serious complications include cavitating lung lesions or meningitis.
- *Coccidioides immitis* grows readily on routine culture media. Unlike other dimorphic fungi, colonies usually are visually apparent within 3 to 5 days. On solid media, the fungus appears as a nonpigmented mold. Unlike specimens obtained from patients. *C limitis* growing in culture is highly infectious and represents an extreme laboratory hazard.

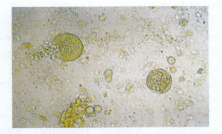

FIGURE: Potassium hydroxide (KOH) preparation of sputum. *The chitin in the spherule cell wall is resistant to digestion by KOH, whereas host cells in sputum are not*. Two mature spherules are evident in the figure, one of which has ruptured and is releasing endospores. Although KOH is not a sensitive test, the finding of spherules in a sputum specimen is diagnostic of coccidioidomycosis.

153. Ans. (a) Giardiasis

Ref: Harrisons, 19th ed. pg. 1946

Giardiasis

- **Mode of transmission:** Fecal-oral
- **Incubation period:** 7–10 days
- **Signs/symptom:**
  - Chronic diarrhea, abdominal pain, bloating, nausea, flatus due to postinfectious irritable bowel syndrome or **protein losing enteropathy**; postinfection fatigue
- **Diagnosis:** Fecal, **string test**, or duodenal aspirate microscopy; stool antigen assay
- **Treatment:** Metronidazole for ongoing infection; no specific antiparasitic therapy for postinfectious syndromes.
- **NOTE:** Hookworm infection can cause iron deficiency anemia

Important causes of Malabsorption Syndrome (Table from Harrison's 19th ed)

Impaired mucosal absorption/mucosal loss or defect

- Crohn's disease
- Amyloidosis
- Scleroderma
- Lymphoma
- Eosinophilic enteritis
- Mastocytosis
- Tropical sprue
- Celiac disease
- Collagenous sprue
- Whipple's disease
- Folate and vitamin B_{12} deficiency
- Infections—giardiasis

---

154. Ans. (b) Man

Ref: Harrisons, 19th ed. pg. 1413

- *Ascaris lumbricoides* is the largest intestinal nematode **parasite of humans**, reaching up to **40 cm** in length.
- **Humans are definitive host** of ascaris
- **Clinical disease arises** from **larval migration in the lungs** or effects of the adult worms in the intestines.
- **Clinical Features:**
  - Around, ~9–12 days after egg ingestion, patients may develop an irritating non-productive cough and burning substernal discomfort that is aggravated by coughing or deep inspiration.
  - Eosinophilia develops during this symptomatic phase and subsides slowly over weeks.
  - Chest x-rays may reveal evidence of eosinophilic pneumonitis **(Loffler's syndrome)**, with rounded infiltrates a few millimeters to several centimeters in size.
- **Treatment:** Mebendazole (DOC)

155. Ans. (a) Treponema pallidum

Ref: Harrisons, 19th ed. pg. 1146; table 245e1

- Cestodes are helminthes. **Example of cestodes:**

Cestodes	Intermediate host	Definitive host
Taenia solium	Pig	Man
Taenia saginata	Beef	Man
Echinococcus granulosus	Man, camels and sheep	Dog
Echinococcus multilocularis	Rodents and humans	Foxes, dogs and cats
H. nana	Man	Man
D. latum	Cyclops, fresh water fish	Man

Note: *Treponema pallidum* is a spirochete

156. Ans. (d) Fungus

Ref: Microbiology by Ananthanarayan and Paniker, 8th ed. pg. 605

- **Kerion** is the result of the host's response to a **fungal** ringworm infection of the hair follicles of the scalp and beard accompanied by secondary bacterial infection.
- It is usually caused by Zoophilic dermatophytes like *Trichophyton verrucosum* and *T. mentagrophytes*.
- **Treatment:** Oral Griseofulvin is the treatment of choice.

157. Ans. (b) Germ tube method

Ref: Microbiology by Ananthanarayan and Paniker, 8th ed. pg. 607-608

- A **germ tube test** is a diagnostic test in which a sample of fungal spores are suspended in serum and examined by microscopy for the detection of any germ.
- It is particularly indicated for colonies of white or cream color on fungal culture, where a *positive germ tube test is strongly indicative of Candida albicans*

158. Ans. (b) Candida

Ref: Microbiology by Ananthanarayan and Paniker, 8th ed. pg. 601; Greenwood, 16 ed. pg. 570

- For direct microscopy of tissue infected with fungus, 10% KOH is used. KOH digests cells and other tissue material, enabling fungus elements to be seen clearly.
- **Special stains for fungus-** PAS, methanamine silver
- **Culture media for fungus-**
  - Sabouraud's glucose agar (MC)
  - Corn meal agar
  - Czapek-dox medium
  - Culture medium are supplemented with chloramphenicol- to suppress bacterial contamination.
  - **Temp**- 22 to 30°C

159. Ans. (b) Borrelia burgdorferi

Ref: Microbiology by Ananthanarayan and Paniker, 8th ed. pg. 377, 379, 381

Microbiology and Parasitology

- Causal agent of lyme disease: Borrelia Burgdorferi *(I.P. 3 to 30 days)*
  - Vector: Ticks
- **Lyme disease occurs in 3 stages:**
  - **Stage 1:** Localized infection, appears an annular skin lesion (Erythema Migrans)
  - **Stage 2:** Disseminated infection, now with headache, fever, arthralgia, myalgia and lymphadenopathy.
  - **Stage 3:** Persistent infection, presents with chronic arthritis, encephalopathy, and acrodermatitis.

> **Extra Mile**
> - **Borrelia vincenti:** ulcerative gingivostomatitis or oropharyngitis (*Vincent's Angina*)
> - **Borrelia Recurrentis:** Louse borne relapsing fever
> - **Treponema carateum:** Causes Pinta
> - **Treponema Pertenue:** Causes Yaws
> - **Treponema Pallidum:** Syphilis

160. Ans (d) LGV

Ref: Microbiology by Ananthanarayan and Paniker, 8th ed. pg. 417, 420

GROOVE SIGN

- Large, hard, fixed, and extremely tender lymph nodes in the groin above and below the inguinal ligament, with a groove along the ligament characteristic of lymphogranuloma venereum.
- LGV caused by Chlamydia trachomatis
- DOC- Doxycycline.
- **DOC in pregnancy-** Erythromycin

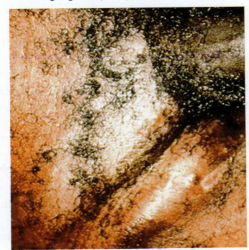

Classification of Chlamydia Trachomatis
- **A, B, Ba, C-** Trachoma conjunctivitis
- **D to K-** Inclusion conjunctivitis
- **L1, L2, L3-** LGV

> **Extra Mile**
> - Chlamydia are obligate intracellular parasites, therefore cannot be cultured on non-living artificial media. Isolation of chlamydia can be done by inoculation into:
>   - Tissue culture (cell culture, Mc coy cells)- **Most preferred.**
>   - Embryonated eggs particularly in yolk

161. Ans. (b) Aspergillus

Ref: Microbiology by Ananthanarayan and Paniker, 8th ed. pg. 613, 659-60

- Fungal infections of the cornea are secondary to injury, bacterial infection and treatment with antibacterial agents and steroids. LASIK and agricultural occupation predispose too.
- Occur most often in hot climates.
- *Aspergillus and Fusarium* are the most common isolates in fungal keratitis worldwide.

162. Ans. (c) Appendix and cecum

Ref: Manson's tropical Diseases, 22nd ed. pg. 1516

- The life cycle of Enterobius vermicularis begins with eggs being ingested. The eggs hatch in the duodenum.
- The emerging pinworm larvae grow rapidly and migrate through the small intestine towards the colon
- The male and female pinworms mate in the ileum.
- The gravid female pinworms settle in *the ileum, caecum, appendix,* and *ascending colon,* where they attach themselves to the mucosa and ingest colonic contents.

163. Ans. (c) Round worm

Ref: Manson's Tropical Diseases, 22nd ed. pg. 1516

- Older literature indicates that the pin worm is the parasite which multiples in the appendix and blocks the lumen causing appendicitis. Although new data indicates that the most common parasite in the appendix is the round worm or Ascaris lumbricoides.

164. Ans. (c) Causes cutaneous larva migrans

Ref: Manual of Family Practice, pg. 622

- Toxocara canis can cause visceral tarva migrans leading to hepatitis and pneumonitis. It can also lead to vision loss due to ocular larva migrans.
- The life cycle of Toxocara canis occurs in dogs and humans acquire the injectionas accidental hosts.

165. Ans. (b) Ancylostoma braziliense

Ref: Atlas of Clinical Microbiology Vol. II/Ch. 19

- Cutaneous larva migrans caused by Ancyclostoma braziliensie is the most common tropically acquired dermatosis. Using their proteases, larvae/penetrate through follicles, fissures or intact skin.

FMGE Solutions Screening Examination

166. Ans. (c) Man is an intermediate host

Ref: Manson's Tropical Diseases, 22nd ed. pg. 1477

For filarial parasite	For malarial parasite
• Man: Definitive host • Mosquito: Intermediate host	• Man: Intermediate host • Mosquito: Definitive host

■ LYMPHATIC FILARIASIS

- Lymphatic filariasis is caused by W. Bancrofti, B. Malayi and B. Timori.
- Man is definitive host and mosquito acts as intermediate host.
- Microfilariae resides in the blood and adult worm in the lymphatics.
- The principal pathologic changes result from inflammatory damage to the lymphatics, which is caused by adult worms and not by microfilariae.

Clinical Manifestations

1. Asymptomatic or subclinical microfilaremia
2. Acute adenolymphangitis
3. Hydrocele
4. Chronic lymphatic disease

Diagnosis

- A definitive diagnosis can be made only by detection of parasite.
- Assays for circulating antigens of W. bancrofti permit the diagnosis of microfilaremic and nonmicrofilaremic infection. Tests are:
  - ELISA
  - Rapid-format immunochromatographic card test.
  - Ultrasound in conjuction with Doppler techniques may result in the identification of motile adult worms: *Filarial dance sign*.
- **Treatment:** *Diethylcarbamazine: Drug of choice.*

167. Ans. (b) Epidemic typhus

Ref: Microbiology by Ananthanarayan and Paniker, 8th ed. pg. 410

Rickettsial Diseases

Disease	Cause	Vector
Epidemic typhus	R. Prowazeki	Louse
Endemic typhus	R. Typhii	Rat flea
Scrub Typhus	R. Tsutsugamushi	Trombiculid mite
Indian tick typhus	R. conori	Tick
RMSF	R. Ricketsii	Tick
Trench fever	Rochalimaea Quintana	Louse
Q fever	Coxiella burnetii	None but rarely soft tick

168. Ans. (d) Ileum & jejunum

Ref: Chatterjee, 12th ed. pg. 116

- Tapeworm infection can also be caused by eating raw or undercooked meat from an animal or a fish that has the larval form of the tapeworm cysts in its muscle tissue.
- Once ingested, the larvae then develop into adult tapeworms in the small intestine (jejunum and ileum).

■ TAPEWORMS

- Taenia saginata: The beef tape worm
- Taenia solium: The pork tape worm
- *Habitat of tapeworms: Small intestine (upper jejunum)*
- **Definitive host:** Man
- **Intermediate host:** Cattle (cow or buffalo) for T. Saginata Pig for T. Solium.

169. Ans. (a) Acute adenolymphangitis stage

- **Filariasis** is caused by thread-like nematodes, which are transmitted by black flies and mosquitoes.
- The adult worms, which usually stay in lymphatics, release early larval forms known as microfilariae into the host's bloodstream. Person is infective once microfilaria presents in the peripheral blood.
- This inflammatory phase is characterised by Lymphangitis, lymphadenitis and adenolymphangitis.
- It lasts for a few days, then subsides spontaneously & recurs at irregular intervals for a period of weeks to months.
- These circulating microfilariae can be taken up with a blood meal by the arthropod vector; in the vector, they develop into infective larvae that can be transmitted to a new host.
- Filariasis is diagnosed in microfilaraemic cases primarily through direct observation of microfilariae in the peripheral blood.
- **Remember:** *W. bancrofti is nocturnally periodic i.e. micro filariae are scarce in peripheral blood by day and increase at night.*

170. Ans. (c) Strongyloides

Ref: Jawetz, Melnick, & Adelberg's Medical Microbiology, 24th ed.

- Ova/egg in stool is not required for diagnosis of Strongyloides.
- In the other given cases like ankylostoma, Enterobius, and trichuris if ova/egg is seen, it indicates infestation of that parasite.

Extra Mile

- *Shape of Trichuris trichura egg: Barrel shaped*

Microbiology and Parasitology

171. Ans. (c) Taeniasis

Ref: Harrison's, 18th ed. Ch 159

- Zoonosis are infectious diseases of animals that can naturally be transmitted to humans.
- **Plague** is a systemic **zoonosis** caused by *Yersinia pestis* **(gram negative).** It predominantly affects small rodents in rural areas of Africa, Asia, and the Americas and is usually transmitted to humans by an arthropod vector (the flea).
- **Rabies** is a zoonotic infection that occurs in a variety of mammals throughout the world except in Antarctica and on some islands. Rabies virus is a member of the family Rhabdoviridae. Rabies virus is a lyssavirus that infects a broad range of animals and causes serious neurologic disease when transmitted to humans.
- **Brucellosis** is a bacterial zoonosis transmitted directly or indirectly to humans from infected animals, predominantly domesticated ruminants and swine.
- **TAENIASIS** is a tapeworm infection to humans. Taenia saginata (beef tapeworm) and Taenia Solium (pork tapeworm).

172. Ans. (d) Onchocerca volvulus

Ref: Diagnostic Medical Parasitology, 3rd ed. pg. 275, Park, 19th ed. pg. 221

- **Onchocerca volvulus** results in **river blindness** and subcutaneous nodules.
- "Lymphatic filariasis" covers infection with three closely related nematode worms - **W.Bancrofti, B. Malayi and B. timoria.**
- All three infections are transmitted to **man** by the bites of infective mosquitoes.
- All three parasites have basically similar life cycles in man- adult worms living in lymphatic vessels whilst their offspring, the microfilariae circulate in peripheral blood and are available to infect mosquito vectors when they come to feed.

> **Extra Mile**
> - **Diethylcarbamazine (DEC)** is the drug of choice for filariasis.
> - **Ivermectin** is the drug of choice for **Onchocerca volvulus**

IMMUNOLOGY

173. Ans. (b) C5-C9 deficiency

Ref: Textbook of Microbiology by Surinder Kumar, P 262

- Meningococcal disease is favoured by deficiency of the terminal complement components (C5-C9).

TABLE: Human genetic deficiencies of complement components and associated diseases

Complement deficiency	Association with disease
C1 inhibitor	Hereditary angioneurotic edema
C1r	Systemic lupus erythematosus-like disease, frequently fatal from overwhelming infection
C2	Increased susceptibility to infections
C3	Recurrent bacterial infections
C4	Systemic lupus erythematosus-like disease
C5	Recurrent infections–lupus-like disease
C6, C7, C8	Recurrent infections: Disseminated gonococcal infections
C9	Not more susceptible to disease than other individuals in the general population
Factor 1	Low C3 levels with recurrent bacterial infections

174. Ans. (d) Ag – Ab complex

Ref: Textbook of Microbiology by Surinder Kumar, P 142

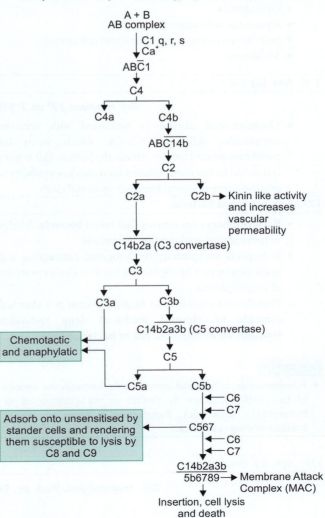

- The classical pathway is so called because it was the first one identified. Steps involved are as follows:
  - Antigen-Antibody binding: first step is the binding of C1 to the antigen-antibody complex → activation of C1s
  - Production of C3 convertase
  - Production of C5 convertase
  - Formation of membrane attack complex (MAC).

175. Ans. (c) Macrophages

Ref: Robbins Basic Pathology, E-book, P 85

- Epithelioid cells are defined as cells that resemble epithelial cells (keratinocytes). They have large oval, pale, vesicular nuclei and abundant eosinophilic cytoplasm.
- The best-known epithelioid cells are those *derived from macrophages* within granulomas, but tumor cells can also be described as epithelioid. Immunostaining may be needed to identify the type of epithelioid cell.

MOST COMMON LESIONS WITH EPITHELIOID CELLS

- Granulomas
- Squamous cell carcinoma
- Spitz nevus (spindle and epithelioid cell nevus)
- Melanoma

176. Ans. (d) C5

Ref: Harrison 19th ed. P 997

- Meningococcal disease is associated with terminal complement deficiency (C5-C9) which forms the membrane attack complex. Hence the bactericidal activity is reduced in this condition and increases susceptibility to invasive meningococcal infection *up to 600 times*.

177. Ans. (a) It is a bacteria

- **Bacteriophages are viruses that infect bacteria**. It helps in transduction and not transformation.
- **It imparts toxigenicity by lysogenic conversion e.g.** toxin production by diphtheria bacillus due to presence of prophage beta.
- Penicillinase resistance in Staphylococcus is a **classical example of plasmid mediated drug resistance transmitted by transduction or bacteriophage.**

> **Extra Mile**
>
> - Transformation is bacterial gene transfer through the agency of free DNA as shown by Griffith in the experiments of **Pneumococci with mice. Transformation plays no role in transfer of drug resistance.**

178. Ans. (c) Pentamer

Ref: Anatnayayan, 9/ed. pg. 98

Antibody	Effective valency
IgM	5
IgG	2
IgD	2
IgE	2
IgA	2,4

> **Extra Mile**
>
> - Ig having maximum molecular weight: **IgM**
> - First antibody produced by newborn: **IgM**
> - All immuniglobulin are heat stable EXCEPT: **IgE**
> - Ig present in **breast milk: IgA**
> - Ig with **maximum half life: IgG**
> - Ig with **minimum half life: IgE**
> - Ig having **maxilum serum concentration: IgG**
> - Ig having **least serum concentration: IgE**

179. Ans. (d) IgM

Ref: Microbiology by Ananthanarayan 9th ed./98-99

- First antibody produced by newborn is IgM at 20 weeks age of gestation.
- Immunoglobulin that can cross placenta: IgG_1
- Immunoglobulin that is present in breast milk: IgA

180. Ans. (a) IgA

Ref: Microbiology by Ananthanarayan and Paniker, 8th ed. pg. 100

TABLE: Immunoglobulins and their salient features

Immuno-globulins	Salient features
IgG	**Most abundant Ig,** consists of about 80% Marker of chronic infection Only Ig that Can cross placenta (IgG_1 subtype)
IgA	2nd most abundant, 10-13% Found in glandular secretion like saliva, tear, ileum, and mucosal secretion like bronchial secretion
IgM	5-8% of total Ig; aka pentameric Ig. First Ig to be synthesized by fetus (20 weeks AOG) Marker of acute infection
IgD	Present mostly intravascular Serve as recognition receptor for antigens
IgE	Mostly extravascular in distribution Highly elevated levels in case of type-I HPS reaction *Produced chiefly in the linings of respiratory and intestinal tracts*

181. Ans. (c) DPT vaccine

Ref: Microbiology by Ananthanarayan and Paniker, 8th ed. pg. 139, 143, 237-38

Microbiology and Parasitology

- DPT vaccine is most effectively used for prophylaxis and prevention of diphtheria.
- Diphtheria is caused by the bacterium Corynebacterium diphtheriae. It produces a toxin that can cause death by myocarditis.
- One type of diphtheria affects the throat and sometimes the tonsils. Another type, more common in the tropics, causes ulcers on the skin.
- Diphtheria affects people of all ages, but most often it strikes unimmunized children.
- It is transmitted from person to person through close physical and respiratory contact.
- **DOC for Diphtheria infection: Erythromycin**

182. Ans. (c) Bacitracin sensitivity

Ref: Microbiology by Ananthanarayan and Paniker, 8th ed. pg. 211-212

- Infective skin lesion with gram positive cocci in chains and hemolytic colonies suggest infection of streptococcus pyogenes.
- *A convenient method for the identification of Str. pyogenes is their sensitivity to bacitracin which is better known as: Maxted's observation.*

183. Ans. (b) Lips

Ref: Clinical oral Medicine and Pathology, 2nd ed. pg. 58
- Angioedema is the swelling of deep dermis, subcutaneous, or submucosal tissue due to vascular leakage.
- Acute episodes often involve the lip, eyes, and face; however, angioedema may affect other parts of body, including respiratory and gastrointestinal (GI) mucosa.
- Most common site of angioedema: LIPS > Tongue
- Laryngeal swelling can be life-threatening.

184. Ans. (b) 2nd week

Ref: Microbiology by Ananthanarayan and Paniker, 8th ed. pg. 654-55

- The **Widal test** is a presumptive serological test for enteric fever or undulant fever whereby bacteria causing typhoid fever are mixed with serum containing specific antibodies obtained from an infected individual.

- Typhidot is the other test used to ascertain the diagnosis of typhoid fever.
- As with all serological tests, the rise in antibody levels needed to perform the diagnosis takes *7–14 days,* which limits it applicability in early diagnosis.
- Other means of diagnosing *Salmonella typhi* (and *paratyphi*) include cultures of blood, urine and faeces.

185. Ans. (a) IgM Ab against rubella at birth

Ref: Harrison, 18th ed. pg. 1606

CONGENITAL RUBELLA DIAGNOSED BY:

- Presence of IgM against rubella
- PCR for rubella RNA
- Presence of persistent IgG beyond 1year in unvaccinated child.

Note: *IgG antibodies is transferred from mother to baby, in last over period of 6 months. Hence their presence is not diagnostic during this period.*

> **Extra Mile**

Triad of congenital rubella syndrome:
- Sensorineural hearing loss
- Cataract
- Congenital heart disease *(MC- Patent Ductus Arteriosus)*

186. Ans. (c) Both

Ref: Microbiology by Ananthanarayan and Paniker, 9th ed. pg. 174

- Severe combined immunodeficiency (SCID) syndrome has impairment of both humoral and cell mediated immunity **(B and T cell defect).**
- Inheritance pattern of SCID **is X-linked recessive > Autosomal recessive.**

Clinical Manifestation of SCID

1. Oral candidiasis in infants
2. Recurrent infection with candidia albicans, P.Carinii, CMV, varicella.
3. Organs like lymph nodes, tonsils, peyer's patches are absent.
4. Very small thymus gland
5. Poor survival rate.

ANSWERS TO BOARD REVIEW QUESTIONS

187. Ans. (b) Phosphotungstic acid

Ref: Electron Microscopy: Principles and Techniques for Biologists By John J. Bozzola, Lonnie Dee Russell pg. 139

188. Ans. (a) Chronic recurrent sinusitis

Ref: Harrison, 18th ed. ch-316

189. Ans. (c) Fontana stain

Ref: Annanthnarayan 8th ed p.374, Jawetz 24th ed. ch-25, lever's histopathology of skin 9th ed. ch-22

190. Ans. (b) Bacteria
Ref: Harrison's, 18th ed. ch-171

191. Ans. (a) Lecithinase
Ref: Ananthnaraan, 7th ed. pg. 238

192. Ans. (c) Clostridium septicum
Ref: Ananthnaraan, 8th ed. pg. 256

193. Ans. (c) Measles
Ref: Medical Virology By David O. White, Frank J. Fenner p/78

194. Ans. (a) Calymmatobacterium granulomatosis
Ref: Harrison's, 17th ed. ch-154

195. Ans. (a) Its causes pandemic
Ref: Jaweyz, 24th ed. ch-39

196. Ans. (c) Hippocampus
Ref: Harrison's 17th ed ch-188, Anantnarayan 7th ed p 539, Rabies: Scientific Basis of the Disease and Its Management by William H. Wunner, Alan C. Jackson p390.

197. Ans. (b) Klebs loeffler's bacillus
Ref: Microbiology by Ananthanarayan and Paniker 7th ed p. 231

198. Ans. (b) B. pertusis
Ref: Harrison's 18th ed ch-148

199. Ans. (d) Presynaptic blocking
Ref: Jawett 24th ed ch-14

200. Ans. (a) Face
Ref: Harrison's 18th ed ch-140
- Lock jaw is an early manifestation of tetanus.

201. Ans. (a) Staphylococcus
Ref: Harrison's 18th ed ch-141

202. Ans. (c) C3
Ref: Jawetz 24th ed ch-8

203. Ans. (d) Entamoeba Histolytica

204. Ans. (b) Enriched media

205. Ans. (b) Robert Koch

206. Ans. (a) Diptheroids

207. Ans. (a) Glutaraldehyde

208. Ans. (a) IgM

209. Ans. (d) IgG

210. Ans. (c) Macrophage

211. Ans. (a) C3

212. Ans. (b) Streptococcus pneumoniae

213. Ans. (b) Gonococcus

214. Ans. (a) Bacillus anthracis

215. Ans. (c) EIEC

216. Ans. (d) Multi-flagellated bacteria

217. Ans. (c) Rickettsia

218. Ans. (b) Measles

219. Ans. (a) RSV

220. Ans. (a) Antigenic shift

221. Ans. (a) Rabies virus

222. Ans. (c) Hepatitis C

223. Ans. (a) Paracoccidioides

224. Ans. (b) Candida albicans

225. Ans. (c) Dermatophyte

226. Ans. (a) Toxoplasma

227. Ans. (d) Strongyloides

Mnemonic: **A Hen** laid non bile stained eggs Ankylostoma duodenale

Microbiology and Parasitology

Hymenolepsis nana
Enterobius vermicularis
Necator americanus

228. Ans. (d) Descending cholangitis

229. Ans. (a) Group A

230. Ans. (d) Herpes simplex

231. Ans. (d) Laennec's cirrhosis

232. Ans. (a) SSPE

233. Ans. (b) Trypanosoma cruzi

234. Ans. (d) Scalded skin syndrome

235. Ans. (a) Carry B mullis

236. Ans. (a) Nisseria

Ref: Anantnarayan 7th ed/222

237. Ans. (c) IL 12

Ref: Jawetz 24th ed Table 8-3

238. Ans. (c) Coxsackie virus A16

Ref: Jawetz 24th ed ch-36 Table 36-3

239. Ans. (b) Mycetoma

Ref: IADVL 2nd ed p. 298, 299, Rook 8th ed/36.74

240. Ans. (c) IgA

Ref: Ananthnarayan 8th ed/99

241. Ans. (d) Alcohol

Ref: Med Lab Tech Vol-2, 2nd ed by Kanai. L Mukherjee/808

242. Ans. (b) Eosinophils

Ref: Harrison's 18th ed ch-60

243. Ans. (c) C3b

Ref: Robbin's 8th ed/59

244. Ans. (c) C5a

Ref: Robbin's 7th ed/56

245. Ans. (a) Mc Mohan and Pugh

Ref: Park 20th ed/32

246. Ans. (b) Gomori methanamine silver

Ref: Lever's histopathology of skin 10th ed p. 591-593

247. Ans. (d) Microscopy + ELISA

Ref: Harrison's 18th ed ch-109

248. Ans. (a) Tube agglutination

Ref: Textbook of Microbiology by Ananthanarayan and Paniker/299

249. Ans. (a) Histiocytes

Ref: Robbin's 8th ed ch-8, JEM vol. 43 no 2 233-239

250. Ans. (c) Lymphocytes

Ref: Robbins 7th ed/593

251. Ans. (a) Glutaraldehyde

Ref: Alcamo's Fundamentals of Microbiology: Body Systems by Jeffrey. C. Pommerville/214

252. Ans. (d) Clostridium difficle

Ref: Harrison's 18th ed ch-146

253. Ans. (b) 20–80 nm

Ref: Microbiology: Principles and exploraltions by Jacquelyn G. Black/88

254. Ans. (a) Hot air oven

Ref: Ananthnarayan 8/e/35

255. Ans. (b) Produce cell membrane defect

Ref: Ananthnarayan 8/e/40

256. Ans. (b) CD 8 T cells

Ref: Jawetz 24/e, chapter 8

257. Ans. (c) Recurrent pyogenic infections

Ref: Jawetz 24/e, chapter 8

258. Ans. (a) C5a

Ref: Robbin's 8/e, p 59, Monoclonal gammopathies and the kidney by G. Touchard p 18, Measuring immunity: Basic science and clinical practice by Michael T. lotze/148

Explanations

FMGE Solutions Screening Examination

452

259. Ans. (a) Syphilis

Ref: Annanthanarayan 8/e, p 374, Jawetz 24/e, Chapter25, Lever's histopathology of skin 9/e, chapter 22

260. Ans. (a) H. ducreyi

Ref: Fitz patricks dermatology, 6/e/2193, 2195

261. Ans. (c) Penicillin

Ref: Bergey's Manual of systematic bacteriology 2/e, p 101, Clinical pharmacology by Cynthia Webster/73

262. Ans. (a) Alpha toxin

Ref: Ananthnarayan 7/e, p 249

263. Ans. (b) Maltose fermentation

Ref: Annathnarayan 8/e, p 374, Jawetz 24/e, chapter 25

264. Ans. (b) Influenza virus

Ref: Jawetz 24/e, Various chapters

265. Ans. (a) Virus

Ref: Harrison 18/e, chapter 186

266. Ans. (c) CMV

Ref: Robbin's 8/e, chapter 8, BRS microbiology 4/e, table 4-9

267. Ans. (a) Sandfly

Ref: Textbook of microbiology and immunology by parija, p 567,Emerging epidemics, management and control by prakash S. Bisen, p 341

268. Ans. (a) Condyloma Lata

Ref: Harrison's 17/e, table 163-1

269. Ans. (c) HPV 2 and 7

Ref: Harrison's 17/e, table 163-1

270. Ans. (c) EBV

Ref: Jawetz's microbiology 24/e, chapter 33, Harepesviruses and table 48-8

271. Ans. (a) Histoplasma

Ref: Chakraborty 2/e/211

272. Ans. (b) Hepatitis B

Ref: Jawetz 24/e, chapter 35

273. Ans. (a) Legionella

Ref: BRS microbiology 4/e, p 50, Harrison's 17/e, chapter 141

274. Ans. (b) Larva

Ref: Harrison's 17/e, chapter 16

275. Ans. (a) Period of active growth without increase in numbers

Ref: Jawetz 24/e, chapter 4

276. Ans. (c) Japanese encephalitis

Ref: Appendix-46, Types of vaccine and immunization

277. Ans. (d) Bacterial particles

Ref: Jawetz's 24/e, ch.13, Harrisons medicine 18/e,/1326, 1327

278. Ans. (c) Foot pad of mice

Ref: Jawetz 24/e, chapter 24, Textbook of microbiology by surinderkumar 1/e, p 326

279. Ans. (a) Neurohypophysis

Ref: Ganong 22/e, chapter 15, Endocrine pathology: Differential diagnosis and molecular advances by Ricardo V. Lioyd, p 77

280. Ans. (c) CMV

Ref: BRS microbiology 4/e, table 4-9, Cytopathology of infectious disease by Lion pantanowitz, pam michelow, walid E. khalbuss, p 39

281. Ans. (b) Loeffer's syndrome

Ref: Harrison's 17/e, chapter 210, Thoracic imaging: pulmonary and cardiovascular radiology

282. Ans. (b) E.coli

Ref: Harrison's 17/e/1820-1823

283. Ans. (b) Bacillus anthracis

Ref: Jawetz 24/e, chapter 12

284. Ans. (b) H. influenzae

Ref: Ananthnarayan 8/e/330, jawetz 24/e, chapter 19

285. Ans. (a) Vibrio

286. Ans. (b) Hepatitis B

Ref: Jawetz 24/e, table 35-1

Microbiology and Parasitology

287. Ans. (b) 3 mm per hour

Ref: Ananthnarayan 7/e/537

288. Ans. (c) Milk

Ref: Jawetz 24/e, chapter 19

289. Ans. (c) Fungus

Ref: Harrison's 17/e, Chapter 14

290. Ans. (b) Corynebacterium

Ref: Konemans microbiology 6/e, p 801-805, Jawetz 24/e, chapter 13

291. Ans. (b) Clostridium welchii

Ref: Ananthnarayan 7/e/238

292. Ans. (a) Enriched medium

Ref: Appendix-82 for "Categories of artificial media

293. Ans. (c) Campylobacter jejuni

Ref: Jawetz 24/e, chapter 18

294. Ans. (b) Venkatraman Ramakrishna medium

Ref: Textbook of microbiology- Ananthanarayan & Paniker 7th ed/306, textbook of microbiology and immunology-parija/308

295. Ans. (a) Bacteria

Ref: Jawetz 24/e, chapter 28

296. Ans. (c) Pseudomonas

Ref: Jawetz 24/e, chapter 15, Harrison's 17/e, chapter 289

297. Ans. (a) Louis Pasteur

Ref: Park 20/e, p 5, Ananthnarayan 7/e, p 5-7, Jawetz's 24/e, chapter 34

298. Ans. (c) Antonie van leeuwenhoek

Ref: Ananthnarayan7/e/8

299. Ans. (a) Streptococci

Ref: Jawett's 24/e, chapter 15

300. Ans. (b) Orthomyxovirus

Ref: Appendix-141 for viruses classification

301. Ans. (b) Influenza type A virus

Ref: Appendix-69, Influenza a virus subtype H1N1

302. Ans. (a) Tropical spastic paraparesis

Ref: Jawetz 24/e, chapter 43, Harrison's 17/e, chapter 181, Harrison 17/e, chapter 105, Table 105-4

303. Ans. (d) Require CO_2 for growth

Ref: Harrison's 17/e, chapter 140

304. Ans. (b) Rickettsia

Ref: Harrison's 18/e, p 1042

305. Ans. (a) H pylori

Ref: Harrison's 17/e, table 144-1

306. Ans. (d) Listeria

Ref: Jawetz 24/e, chapter 13

307. Ans. (a) Leishmania braziliensis

Ref: Jawetz 24/e, chapter 46

308. Ans. (b) Poliovirus

Ref: Jawetz 24/e, chapter 36, Table 30–2

309. Ans. (c) Bacillus anthracis

Ref: Handbook of bacteriology-M.A. Gohar/260

310. Ans. (c) Neisseria meningitidis

Ref: Textbook of microbiology by R. Vasanthakumari/203

311. Ans. (a) IgG

Ref: Jawetz 24/e, chapter 8

Explanations

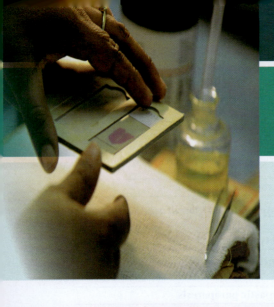

7

Forensic Medicine

MOST RECENT QUESTIONS 2019

1. **Grounds of divorce:**
   a. Sterility b. Frigidity
   c. Impotence d. Poverty
2. **IPC for causing abortion without women's consent:**
   a. 312 b. 313
   c. 314 d. 315
3. **Autopsy of stomach, incision of choice along:**
   a. Lesser curvature b. Greater curvature
   c. Vertical d. Pylorus
4. **Organ injured commonly in seat belt injury:**
   a. Mesentery b. Spleen
   c. Liver d. Lungs
5. **Before dying declaration, the role of a doctor is:**
   a. To assess compos mentis
   b. To record statement even in presence of magistrate
   c. Cross examines the person
   d. Put person under oath before declaration

IDENTIFICATION

6. **Study of birth defects is called:**
   (Recent Pattern Question 2018-19)
   a. Teratology
   b. Tetralogy
   c. Anthropology
   d. Parturitology
7. **Confirmatory test of blood stain:**
   (Recent Pattern Question 2018-19)
   a. Kastle meyer test b. Haemin crystal test
   c. Spectroscopic test d. Orthotoluidine test
8. **Gustafson method of age estimation by teeth utilizes:**
   (Recent Pattern Question 2018-19)
   a. Number of tooth
   b. Transparency of root
   c. Height and weight of teeth
   d. Structural feature of enamel

9. **Which of the following is used for biometric evaluation?**
   (Recent Pattern Question 2018)
   a. Iris b. Pupil
   c. Lens d. Cornea
10. **21st tooth erupts at:** *(Recent Pattern Question 2018)*
    a. 5 years b. 8 years
    c. 10 years d. 12 years
11. **Cephalic index 75–80 is seen in:**
    (Recent Pattern Question 2018)
    a. Mongols b. Aryans
    c. Negros d. Chinese
12. **Stack's formula for age determination from teeth is used in:** *(Recent Pattern Question 2017)*
    a. Infants
    b. Adults
    c. Between 25 and 50 years of age
    d. > 50 years of age
13. **Boyde's method is useful for age estimation of:**
    (Recent Pattern Question 2017)
    a. Dead infant b. Adult
    c. Toddler d. School going child
14. **The antero-posterior diameter of the skull is minimum in:**
    a. Brachycephaly. b. Dolicocephaly
    c. Plagicephaly d. Trigonocephaly
15. **Mongols are:**
    a. Dolicocephalic
    b. Mesaticephalic
    c. Brachycephalic
    d. Anglocephalic
16. **Palatoprints used for identification of human beings are usually taken from:**
    a. Anterior part of palate b. Posterior part of palate
    c. Lateral part of palate d. Middle part of palate
17. **Breslau's second life test detects changes in which of the following organs:**
    a. Brain
    b. Lung
    c. Heart
    d. Stomach and small intestine

Forensic Medicine

18. Raygat's test is used for testing function maturity of:
    - a. Small intestine
    - b. Kidney
    - c. Lungs
    - d. Heart

COURT OF LAW AND IPCs

19. McNaughton rule is for:
    (Recent Pattern Question 2018-19)
    - a. Civil responsibility of insane
    - b. Criminal responsibility of insane
    - c. Capacity of witness
    - d. Testamentary capacity

20. Which of the following is related to legal responsibility of insane person: *(Recent Pattern Question 2018-19)*
    - a. Hasse's rule
    - b. Curren's rule
    - c. Morrison rule
    - d. Rule of nine

21. True about summon to medical examiner for criminal case: *(Recent Pattern Question 2018-19)*
    - a. Under penalty document
    - b. Issued by magistrate
    - c. Conduct money paid along with summon
    - d. Punishable under IPC Sec 87

22. First class magistrate is selected by
    - a. State government *(Recent Pattern Question 2017)*
    - b. Chief justice of supreme court
    - c. Chief justice of high court
    - d. Governor

23. Investigation of custody death is done by:
    (Recent Pattern Question 2017)
    - a. Medical officer
    - b. Magistrate
    - c. Constable
    - d. Sub-inspector

24. Which of these following is an example of a leading question? *(Recent Pattern Question 2016)*
    - a. How did you get cuts on T-shirt
    - b. Cause of injury
    - c. Whether it is caused by knife
    - d. Size of incised wound

25. Inquest of dowry death is done by:
    - a. Magistrate
    - b. Police
    - c. Medical officer
    - d. Sub-inspector

26. Dowry death investigation is done by:
    - a. Magistrate
    - b. Sub-inspector
    - c. Police
    - d. Medical officer

27. IPC 321:
    - a. Grievous hurt
    - b. Hurt
    - c. Punishment of hurt
    - d. Voluntarily causing hurt

28. Punishment for Rape is
    - a. 5 years
    - b. 7 years
    - c. 10 years
    - d. 20 years

29. Hurt is defined by IPC:
    - a. 317
    - b. 319
    - c. 320
    - d. 321

30. Grevious hurt is defined under IPC
    - a. 320
    - b. 302
    - c. 300
    - d. 376

31. Criteria for grievous hurt are all EXCEPT:
    - a. Endanger to life
    - b. Privation to eye/sight
    - c. Permanent disfiguration of face
    - d. Injured person admitted in hospital for 21 days

32. Adultery comes under IPC section
    - a. 497
    - b. 498
    - c. 375
    - d. 376

33. Infanticide comes under which section
    - a. 83
    - b. 315
    - c. 299
    - d. 317

34. Death due to bodily injury caused by husband or his relative after marriage is punished under IPC:
    - a. 304
    - b. 304 A
    - c. 304 B
    - d. 498 A

35. Cruel behavior towards wife by husband, family members or his relatives comes under which IPC section:
    - a. 498 A
    - b. 304
    - c. 304 A
    - d. 304 B

36. Extending the hanging for pregnant women comes under which Crpc:
    - a. Section 413
    - b. Section 414
    - c. Section 419
    - d. Section 416

37. Which of the following is not illegal in India:
    - a. Bestiality
    - b. Masturbation
    - c. Buccal coitus
    - d. Indecent assault

TOXICOLOGY

38. Gastric lavage is contraindicated in:
    (Recent Pattern Question 2018-19)
    - a. Organo-phosphate poisoning
    - b. Hydrocarbons
    - c. Bicarbonate
    - d. PCM toxicity

39. Wall scraping is used in treatment of which poisoning:
    (Recent Pattern Question 2018-19)
    - a. Oxalic acid
    - b. Sulphuric acid
    - c. Carbolic acid
    - d. Phenol

Questions

FMGE Solutions Screening Examination

40. Aconite poisoning is mainly caused by:
    (Recent Pattern Question 2017)
    a. Fruit   b. Leaf
    c. Root   d. Bark

41. Heroin is which type of derivative of opium?
    (Recent Pattern Question 2017)
    a. Natural   b. Semi- natural
    c. Synthetic d. Semi-synthetic

42. Binocellate mark is seen in which snake?
    (Recent Pattern Question 2017)
    a. Cobra   b. Viper
    c. Sea scale viper d. Krait

43. Cherry red discoloration is seen in which poisoning?
    (Recent Pattern Question 2017)
    a. Nickel   b. Carbon monoxide
    c. Phosphorus d. Cyanide

44. Which of the following is a cyanide poisoning antidote
    (Recent Pattern Question 2017)
    a. Sodium dantrolene   b. Sodium thiosulfate
    c. Sodium valprotate   d. Sodium formaldehyde

45. Cyanide poisoning antidote
    (Recent Pattern Question 2017)
    a. Hydroxocobalamin b. Sodium chloride
    c. Sodium bicarbonate d. Sodium gluconate

46. Acrodynia is associated with:
    a. Lead
    b. Mercury
    c. Zinc
    d. Arsenic

47. Maximum damage to the esophagus is caused by:
    a. Acid
    b. Alkali
    c. Organophosphate
    d. Kerosene

48. In which of the following poisoning C.S.F. is required to be preserved:
    a. Alcoholic poisoning
    b. Arsenic poisoning
    c. Copper poisoning
    d. Organophosphorous poisoning

49. Which of the following is NOT used in organophosphate poisoning?
    a. Charcoal
    b. Atropine
    c. Oximes
    d. PAM

50. Gastric lavage is contraindicated in which poisoning:
    a. Kerosene
    b. Alcohol
    c. Organophosphate
    d. Lead

51. To which of following a person gets easily tolerated and addicted?
    a. Tobacco
    b. Caffeine
    c. Cannabis
    d. Alcohol

52. Antidote for phosphorus poisoning:
    a. Atropine
    b. Calcium gluconate
    c. Copper sulphate
    d. Physostigmine

53. All are true about arsenic poisoning EXCEPT:
    a. Aldrich mees line on nails
    b. Mimics tetanus
    c. Rain drop pigmentation on body
    d. Hyperkeratosis of palms and soles

54. Rain drop appearance is seen in which poisoning:
    a. Arsenic
    b. Lead
    c. Mg
    d. Tin

55. Miosis is caused by all EXCEPT:
    a. Opiates   b. Organophosphates
    c. Pontine hemorrhage d. Cyanide

56. Treatment of choice in cyanide poisoning is:
    a. Sodium chloride   b. Sodium carbonate
    c. Sodium thiosulfate d. Atropine

57. Sea snake venom is mostly:
    a. Hepatotoxic b. Neurotoxic
    c. Haemolytic   d. Myotoxic

58. Bitten by krait. Manifestation would be:
    a. Neurotoxic   b. Myotoxic
    c. Vasculotoxic d. Cardiotoxic

59. Blood alcohol level while driving mg%:
    a. 10   b. 20
    c. 30   d. 40

60. Hooch' tragedy is due to:
    a. Ethyl alcohol   b. Methyl alcohol
    c. Ethylene glycol d. Cannabis

61. Which of the following is NOT a form of cannabis:
    a. Bhang   b. Charas
    c. Cocaine d. Ganja

62. A narcotic abuse case presents with jet black tongue. The most likely cause is:
    a. Cannabis toxicity b. Alcohol poisoning
    c. LSD poisoning   d. Cocaine poisoning

63. Vitriolage can be done by which of the plant:
    a. Croton tigulum
    b. Arbus precagtorius
    c. Bhilawanol
    d. Calotropes

FORENSIC MEDICINE

456

Forensic Medicine

BURNS AND DROWNING

64. In the investigation of severe burn body, which of the following sample is taken for identification:
(Recent Pattern Question 2019)
- a. Blood
- b. Hair
- c. Teeth
- d. Bone

65. Gettler test is done in? *(Recent Pattern Question 2017)*
- a. Burn
- b. Drowning
- c. Hanging
- d. Strangulation

66. Mesohalophilic diatoms live in:
(Recent Pattern Question 2017)
- a. Brackish water
- b. Sea water
- c. Fresh water
- d. Sewer water

67. Most conclusive sign of ante-mortem death due to burns
- a. Heat hyperemia *(Recent Pattern Question 2016)*
- b. Heat fracture
- c. Presence of carboxyhemoglobin
- d. Absence of line of redness

68. Most common cause of death in drowning:
- a. Electrolyte imbalance
- b. Pneumonia
- c. Cardiac arrest
- d. Vasovagal shock

69. In case of cold water drowning death is due to
- a. Vagal stimulation
- b. Vagal inhibition
- c. Hypervolemia
- d. Ventricular fibrillation

70. Most common feature indicative of Antemortem drowing:
- a. Washerwomen feet
- b. Pugilistic attitude
- c. Clenched fist
- d. Cyanosis

71. Paltauff haemorrhage is seen in:
- a. Drowning
- b. Suffocation
- c. Throttling
- d. Burns

72. Presence of diatoms in bone marrow are characteristic of which of the following?
- a. Putrefaction
- b. Drowning
- c. Strangulation
- d. Throttling

73. Pugilistic attitude is seen in:
- a. Drowning
- b. Burns
- c. Lightening
- d. Hanging

74. Degloving injury involve:
- a. Avulsion of subcutaneous layer with fat
- b. Erosion of skin with muscle
- c. Peeling of the skin
- d. Necrosis of muscle

75. Crocodile skin is seen in:
- a. Drowning
- b. High voltage Electric burns
- c. Neck ligature
- d. High temperature water burns

76. Lichenburg flower is a classical finding in which of the following:
- a. Lightening stroke
- b. Electrical injuries
- c. Joule burn
- d. Scald burn

77. Scald burns can be caused by:
- a. Molten metal
- b. Electric burns
- c. High temperature liquids
- d. Lightening stroke

78. Which of the following is seen in antemortem burns:
- a. Decreased alkaline phosphatase
- b. Cl^- increased & albumin decreased in vesicles
- c. Presence of carbonaceous deposits in respiratory tract
- d. Dull base of blister

79. In case of burning fire in a closed room, death occurs due to:
- a. CO_2 poisoning
- b. CO poisoning
- c. Cardiac fauilre
- d. Respiratory failure

IMPOTENCY, SEXUAL PERVERSION AND SEXUAL OFFENCES

80. Lesbianism is also known as:
(Recent Pattern Question 2018)
- a. Machoism
- b. Tribadism
- c. Nymphomania
- d. Transsexualism

81. In an eligible couple, the age of woman is:
(Recent Pattern Question 2017)
- a. 18–45 years
- b. 18–49 years
- c. 21–45 years
- d. 15–49 years

82. Frotteurism is *(Recent Pattern Question 2016)*
- a. Sexual satisfaction by contact with articles of opposite sex like hanky, sandals, clothes
- b. Sexual satisfaction by rubbing the genitalia with the body of the person of opposite sex
- c. Sexual gratification by exposing one's genitalia
- d. Sexual satisfaction by watching the sexual act

83. Statutory rape is considered below the age
(Recent Pattern Question 2016)
- a. 16 years
- b. 18 years
- c. 20 years
- d. 22 years

84. Impotent quoad is seen in:
- a. Inability of the male to beget children and in the female, the inability to conceive children
- b. An individual who may be impotent with any particular woman but not with others
- c. Inability of a person to perform sexual intercourse
- d. Inability to start or maintain the sexual arousal pattern in the female

85. A posthumous child is:
- a. Still born
- b. Child born after father's death
- c. Child born after mother's death
- d. Fictitious child claimed by a women as her own

86. A female forges to have a child, whereas she doesn't have. It is:
- a. Cheating
- b. Posthumous child
- c. Suppositious child
- d. Superstitious child

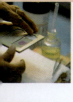

FMGE Solutions Screening Examination

87. A child who is born to an unmarried women:
    a. Posthumous child   b. Illegitimate child
    c. Suppositious child   d. Fictitious child
88. Most important cause of impotence:
    a. Male factor   b. Female factor
    c. Psychogenic   d. Anatomical
89. Which of the following is not a crime:
    a. Rape   b. Sodomy
    c. Incest   d. Indecent Assault
90. Hymen in false virgin is:
    a. Annular   b. Elastic
    c. Imperforate   d. Semilunar
91. All of the following are paraphilias EXCEPT:
    a. Bestiality   b. Frotteurism
    c. Sadomasochism   d. Bisexuality
92. Frotteurism is:
    a. Sexual satisfaction by contact with articles of opposite sex like hanky, sandals, clothes
    b. Sexual satisfaction by rubbing the genitalia with the body of the person of other sex
    c. Sexual gratification by exposing one's genitalia.
    d. Sexual satisfaction by watching the sexual act.
93. Frotteurism:
    a. Pleasure in watching intercourse
    b. Pleasure in using article of opposite sex
    c. Pleasure in touching opposite sex
    d. Pleasure in wearing opposite sex clothes
94. A person who gets satisfaction by watching others indulged in sexual activity:
    a. Voyeurism   b. Frotteurism
    c. Fetischism   d. Exihibitionism
95. A 24-year-old male is convinced to be a female, is diagnosed as:
    a. Transvestism   b. Transsexualism
    c. Homosexualism   d. Undinism
96. Incessant sexual desire in males:
    a. Satyriasis   b. Nymphomania
    c. Vaginismus   d. Quoad hoc
97. Florence test is used for
    a. Blood   b. Semen
    c. Urine   d. Albumin
98. The seminal stains shows fluorescence when examined under the filtered ultraviolet light, this property of seminal stains is due to presence of:
    a. Choline   b. Spermine
    c. Sperm   d. Enzymes
99. Identification of semen is done by:
    a. Haemochromogen Test b. Barberios Test
    c. Guaiacum Test   d. Leuco malachite green test
100. Saliva is tested by:
    a. Amylase   b. Ortho-toluidine
    c. Acid phosphatase   d. Tetra-methyl-Benzidine

INJURY/GUNSHOT INJURY/FIREARM INJURY/STAB WOUND

101. Gun powder in hand during gun-shot residue testing is collected using: *(Recent Pattern Question 2018)*
    a. Paraffin wax   b. Benzidine
    c. Acid phosphatase   d. Sulfur
102. Lacerated looking incised wounds are seen at:
    (Recent Pattern Question 2017)
    a. Cheek prominence   b. Scrotum
    c. Shin   d. Forehead
103. Yellow color of bruise is seen due to:
    (Recent Pattern Question 2017)
    a. Biliverdin in one day   b. Biliverdin in 14 day
    c. Bilirubin on 4th day   d. Bilirubin on 9th day
104. In a large bruise, color changes begins from:
    a. From the center   *(Recent Pattern Question 2017)*
    b. From the periphery
    c. All at same time
    d. Little lateral from the main site of bruise
105. Oblique bullet injury causes which type of wound
    (Recent Pattern Question 2016)
    a. Oval   b. Round
    c. Stellate   d. Keyhole
106. Teeth bite marks are which type of abrasion:
    a. Pressure Abrasion   b. Contusions
    c. Graze abrasion   d. Linear abrasion
107. Brush burn is a:
    a. Linear abrasion   b. Pressure abrasion
    c. Graze abrasion   d. Contusion
108. Whiplash injury is damage to
    a. Skull   b. Spine
    c. Rib cage   d. Long bones
109. Bruise is bluish-black in color after:
    a. 24 hour   b. 2 day
    c. Few days   d. Few months
110. True about Countre-coup injury:
    a. Injury located towards the impact
    b. Injury common in stationary head
    c. Injury common in moving head
    d. All of the above
111. Which of the following is not seen in black gun powder of Bullet:
    a. Sulphur   b. Charcoal
    c. Potassium   d. Nitrocellulose
112. True statement about Tandem bullet:
    a. Bullet that rotates in end on end during its motion
    b. Bullet which travel in irregular fashion
    c. Bullet that first hits some other object along the way
    d. Two bullets are ejected one after the other

Forensic Medicine

113. **Tailing of wound suggests:**
 a. Direction of injury
 b. Weapon used
 c. Type of wound
 d. Surface of weapon

114. **Which of the following is NOT associated with stabbing injury:**
 a. Point wound
 b. Puncture wound
 c. Perforation
 d. Chopping

115. **Tentative cuts are seen in?**
 a. Suicide
 b. Homicide
 c. Accidental cut
 d. Traumatic cut

116. **'Flaying' is seen in which type of laceration?**
 a. Split
 b. Stretch
 c. Avulsion
 d. Tears

ABORTION, THANATOLOGY AND HANGING

117. **Rule which describes the cadaveric rigidity and sequential onset of rigor mortis:** *(Recent Pattern Question 2018-19)*
 a. Curren's rule
 b. Nysten's rule
 c. Hasse's rule
 d. Durham rule

118. **Which cavity should be opened first in the suspicion of hanging?** *(Recent Pattern Question 2018)*
 a. Thorax
 b. Head
 c. Abdomen
 d. Neck

119. **Specific gravity of unrespired lung:**
 (Recent Pattern Question 2018)
 a. 0.94
 b. 1.2
 c. 0.75
 d. 1.04

120. **Respired lung weight as compared to body weight is:**
 (Recent Pattern Question 2018)
 a. 1/10
 b. 1/20
 c. 1/35
 d. 1/70

121. **Person identification can be done by:**
 (Recent Pattern Question 2017)
 a. Proctoscopy
 b. Colposcopy
 c. Chelioscopy
 d. Endoscopy

122. **A diabetic patient develops DVT and PE. Leading cause of death I(a) in medical certificate is?**
 (Recent Pattern Question 2017)
 a. Pulmonary embolism
 b. DVT
 c. DM
 d. Renal failure

123. **Which of the following is more dangerous in causing spinal damage?** *(Recent Pattern Question 2017)*
 a. Hyperextension of the neck
 b. Hyperflexion of the neck
 c. Both hyperflexion and hyperextension of the neck
 d. None can cause spinal damage

124. **Wilful MTP is allowed upto how many weeks in India**
 (Recent Pattern Question 2016)
 a. 12 weeks
 b. 20 weeks
 c. 28 weeks
 d. 32 weeks

125. **Which of the following points towards female skull differentiating from male** *(Recent Pattern Question 2016)*
 a. Mastoid bigger
 b. Prominent frontal emience
 c. Orbit square with round edges
 d. Prominent jaw

126. **All are correct about MTP EXCEPT:**
 a. Only qualified medical practitioner is allowed to perform it
 b. Medical assistant can perform in absence of gynecologist
 c. Husband's consent is not required.
 d. Can be done upto 20 weeks

127. **Which of the following statement is true about MTP:**
 a. Consent of one doctor is enough upto 14 weeks
 b. Husband's consent for MTP is must
 c. Make sure to lodge a police complaint in case of MTP due to rape
 d. Age proof is generally not required

128. **A doctor can do MTP after practicing or assisting how many MTPs:**
 a. 22
 b. 20
 c. 12
 d. 25

129. **In case of typical hanging, position of knot is at:**
 a. Occiput
 b. Angle of mandible
 c. Below the chin
 d. Side of neck

130. **On examination a dead guy was found a ligature mark on neck. According to police, the person's leg were touching the ground while hanging. You suspected death due to partial hanging. This death is due to weight of around:**
 a. 1.15 kg
 b. 2.20 kg
 c. 3.10 kg
 d. 4.50 kg

131. **A 28 year female committed suicide. On the site it was noticed that her feet was not touching the ground. Which of the following shows its suicidal and not homicidal:**
 a. Ligature mark continuous around the neck
 b. The position of the knot at the angle of mandible
 c. Saliva dribbling to the opposite side of the knot
 d. Red congested face

132. **Le-facies expression is due to**
 a. Hanging
 b. Strangulation
 c. Throttling
 d. Café coronary

133. **All are strangulation EXCEPT:**
 a. Burking
 b. Throttling
 c. Garrotting
 d. Mugging

134. **Burking is a method of:**
 a. Homicidal smothering and traumatic asphyxia
 b. Suicidal smothering and traumatic asphyxia
 c. Accidental smothering and choking
 d. Choking and traumatic asphyxia

135. **Overlying leads to death due to**
 a. Strangulation
 b. Suffocation
 c. Mugging
 d. Choking

459

Questions

FMGE Solutions Screening Examination

136. Postmortem rigidity disappears first in:
    a. Upper limbs
    b. Neck
    c. Lower limbs
    d. Eyelids
137. On postmortem examination, stiffening of muscles is observed in a burn deceased. This indicates that the person is exposed to intense heat above what temperature?
    a. 30°C
    b. 40°C
    c. 50°C
    d. 60°C
138. In asphyxia, the organ to be dissected last is:
    a. Neck
    b. Head
    c. Thorax
    d. Abdomen

FORENSIC PSYCHIATRY

139. Fodere test is done for: *(Recent Pattern Question 2017)*
    a. Bone maturity
    b. Lung maturity
    c. Heart maturity
    d. Intestinal maturity
140. Phytobezoar is:
    a. Intake of indigestible plant materials
    b. Vegetable balls
    c. Hair ball
    d. Drugs ball

BOARD REVIEW QUESTIONS

141. Cephalic index is used for determination of?
    a. Sex
    b. Race
    c. Height
    d. Stature
142. Falanga is a type of?
    a. Physical torture
    b. Sexual torture
    c. Mental torture
    d. Method of homicide
143. Telefona refers to?
    a. Pulling of hairs
    b. Beating of soles
    c. Beating on both ears
    d. Beating on head
144. Tactile hallucination is seen with?
    a. Dhatura
    b. Cocaine
    c. Cerebra thevetia
    d. None of these
145. Delirium is caused by which poison?
    a. Aconite
    b. Dhatura
    c. Morphine
    d. Kerosene
146. Fomepizole is used in which poisoning?
    a. Methyl alcohol
    b. Benzodiazepine
    c. Cyanide
    d. Phenobarbitone
147. Orderal poison is?
    a. Physostigmine
    b. Digoxin
    c. Cocaine
    d. Atropine
148. Which is not a derivative of cannabis?
    a. Heroin
    b. Charas
    c. Ganza
    d. Bhang
149. In which poisoning dialysis is not indicated?
    a. Benzodiazepine
    b. Barbiturates
    c. Aspirin
    d. Acetaminophen
150. Fusion of xiphoid process occurs at?
    a. 30 years
    b. 10 years
    c. 40 years
    d. 70 years
151. MTP act was last modified in?
    a. 2000
    b. 2003
    c. 2005
    d. 2007
152. The shape of a stab wound is due to?
    a. Edge of blade
    b. Length of blade
    c. Width of blade
    d. Strength of force
153. Tissue bridging is seen in?
    a. Stab wound
    b. Incised wound
    c. Lacerations
    d. Abrasion
154. Minimum age required for consent to donate organs as per "Transplantation of human organ act 1994" is?
    a. 16 years
    b. 18 years
    c. 21 years
    d. No age limit
155. Dicobalt EDTA is used to treat poisoning by?
    a. Cyanide
    b. Sulfuric acid
    c. Nitric acid
    d. H_2S
156. Phosphorous is preserved in?
    a. Alcohol
    b. Formalin
    c. Kerosene
    d. Water
157. Stability of a bullet is increased by?
    a. Jacketing
    b. Rifling
    c. Choke
    d. Highmass bullets
158. Fatal dose of potassium cyanide is?
    a. 30–50 mg
    b. 50–60 mg
    c. 200 mg
    d. 300 mg
159. Hatter shake is seen in which poisoning?
    a. Aluminum
    b. Mercury
    c. Lead
    d. Arsenic
160. Dialysis dementia syndrome is seen in which poisoning?
    a. Aluminium
    b. Mercury
    c. Lead
    d. Arsenic
161. Magnan's phenomenon occurs in addiction of?
    a. Alcohol
    b. Cocaine
    c. LSD
    d. Opiates
162. Saturnism is a feature of?
    a. Mercury poisoning
    b. Lead poisoning
    c. Arsenic poisoning
    d. Thallium poisoning
163. Last organ to putrefy in females is?
    a. Lung
    b. Uterus
    c. Bain
    d. Heart

Forensic Medicine

164. Most common site of diatoms test done in drowning is?
- a. Lungs
- b. Bone marrow
- c. Heart
- d. Stomach

165. Statutory rape is considered below the age of?
- a. 15 years
- b. 16 years
- c. 18 years
- d. 21 years

166. Section 509 IPC deals with?
- a. Rape
- b. Outrage of modesty of a woman
- c. Insult of modesty of a woman
- d. Criminal conspiracy

167. Dangerous weapon is related to which section of IPC?
- a. 300
- b. 302
- c. 320
- d. 324

168. Declaration of Tokyo is related to?
- a. Human experimentation
- b. Torture
- c. Euthanasia
- d. Organ transplantation

169. Maximum tissue damage is done by?
- a. Tandem bullet
- b. Ricochet bullet
- c. Dum dum bullet
- d. Wad cutter bullet

170. Dying declaration comes under?
- a. Section 32 IPC
- b. Section 32 IEA
- c. Section 60 IEA
- d. 291 CrPC

171. Permittable alcohol level in blood as per motor vehicle act 1988 is below?
- a. 30%
- b. 40%
- c. 50%
- d. 60%

172. Corpoporphyrin in urine is seen in which of the poisoning?
- a. Copper
- b. Lead
- c. Arsenic
- d. Mercury

173. Smoky stool is seen in which poisoning?
- a. Mercury
- b. Phosphorous
- c. Iodine
- d. Lead

174. Antidote for magnesium sulfate toxicity is?
- a. Calcium gluconate
- b. Penicillamine
- c. Hydrated ferric oxide
- d. Exchange resins

175. Vineyard sprayer's lung is due to?
- a. Thallium toxicity
- b. Chronic $CuSO_4$ poisoning
- c. Chronic arsenic poisoning
- d. Potassium permanganate toxicity

176. Concealment of birth comes under which IPC?
- a. 317
- b. 318
- c. 319
- d. 320

177. Postponement of death sentence of a pregnant women comes under?
- a. Section 433 A Cr.PC
- b. Section 416 CrPC
- c. Section 54 IPC
- d. Section 55 IPC

178. Virchow method of autopsy includes?
- a. Organs are removed en masse
- b. Organs are removed en block
- c. Organs are removed one by one
- d. In situ dissection combined with en block removal

179. Duret's hemorrhages are seen in?
- a. Lungs
- b. Spleen
- c. Liver
- d. Brain

180. Taches noires refers to?
- a. Postmortem staining
- b. Flaccidity of eyeball
- c. Wrinkled dusty sclera
- d. Maggot growth

181. Tache noir is seen in the eye how many hours after death?
- a. 3 to 5 hours
- b. 6 to 8 hours
- c. 12 to 14 hours
- d. 16 to 18 hours

182. Hasse's formula is used in pregnancy to?
- a. Estimate fetal age
- b. Identify fetal blood group
- c. Identify fetal sex
- d. Identify fetal congenital malformations

183. Cross examination in the court of law is for?
- a. Confusing witness
- b. To make judge understand better
- c. To protect the accused
- d. To obtain more evidence

184. Specimen containing viral particle is preserved in?
- a. NaC1 solution
- b. Formaldehyde
- c. 50% glycerine
- d. Liquid nitrogen

185. Most common type of finger print: *(2018)*
- a. Loops
- b. Whorls
- c. Composite
- d. Arches

186. Gustafson method of identification includes all EXCEPT: *(2018)*
- a. Attrition
- b. Root transparency
- c. Loss of periodontal attachment
- d. Root resorption at the base

Questions

FMGE Solutions Screening Examination

IMAGE-BASED QUESTION

187. The following picture shows?

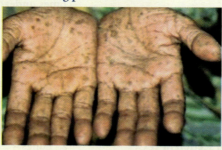

a. Lead poisoning b. Arsenic poisoning
c. Copper poisoning d. Iron poisoning

Answer to Image-Based Question is given at the end of explained questions

Forensic Medicine

ANSWERS WITH EXPLANATIONS

MOST RECENT QUESTIONS 2019

1. Ans. (c) Impotence

Ref: Forensic Medicine and Toxicology by RN Karmakar P 370

- **Impotence** can be ground for divorce. A wife can sue for marriage dissolution on grounds of husband's impotency, given that the 2 facts are proved:
  - Husband was impotent at the time of marriage
  - Husband continues is to be impotent till the filing of suit

Grounds for divorce:
- Adultery
- Cruelty
- Desertion
- Impotency
- Forced conversion of religion
- Communicable venereal diseases, incurable disease like leprosy, incurable mental disorder and insanity
- Either of spouse not alive or not seen for more than 7 years

2. Ans. (a) 312

Ref: Forensic medicine and toxicology by RN Karmakar P 532

- **IPC Section 312:** Anyone voluntarily causing miscarriage to a woman with child, other than in good faith for the purpose of saving her life is punishable by imprisonment or fine or both.
- **IPC section 313–316:** Punishment (If death during the procedure) for up to 10 years imprisonment, extending up to life and fine, where abortion was conducted without consent.

3. Ans. (b) Greater curvature

Ref: Forensic medicine and toxicology by RN Karmakar P 327-28

- Stomach autopsy is done to examine any food particle, its state of digestion, smell, color, character or presence of any foreign/suspicious body. This is very important if determining time of death is a major factor.
- For doing autopsy of stomach, double ligature is applied and the stomach is opened along greater curvature (from cardiac to pylorus).

4. Ans. (a) Mesentery

Ref: Forensic medicine and toxicology by RN Karmakar P 204

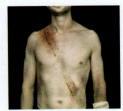

- Seat belt is usually worn diagonally across the chest, and fastened on across the opposite side, lower lateral abdominal region.
- Seat belt injury occur when there is sudden halt of a moving car. It results into following injury:
  - Abrasion, contusion and hematoma of lower abdomen
  - More commonly, laceration, avulsions or perforation of mesentery or gas filled intestine and also injury to the vertebral column, particularly lumbar vertebra
  - Rupture of abdominal organs (like liver, spleen, pancreas and cecum) due to compression.
- These injuries are collectively known as seat belt syndrome.

5. Ans. (a) To assess compos mentis

Ref: Forensic medicine and toxicology by RN Karmakar, P 259

- Dying declaration (Sec 32 IEA) is written or oral statement of a person (who is dying due to some unlawful act), relating to the cause of his death.
- The statement is recorded by magistrate, or if the condition is serious, the doctor or any other person can record the statement in absence of magistrate.
- If the person survives, he is called to give oral evidence and the dying declaration becomes useless.
- **Role of a doctor in dying declaration:**
  - Assess the condition of the patient
  - Arrange for dying declaration and send call for magistrate
  - Certify the compos mentis (mental soundness of person)- major role
  - Record dying declaration in absence of magistrate

> **Extra Mile**

Differences between dying declaration and dying deposition

Dying declaration	Dying deposition (more superior than dying declaration)
Recorded by magistrate, doctor or even a common person	Recorded only by magistrate
Person NOT put under oath (it is believed that a dying person does not lie)	Person is put under oath
Person is NOT cross examined	The person is cross examined
Accepted in India under sec 32 IEA (Indian Evidence Act)	Not accepted in India

IDENTIFICATION

6. Ans. (a) Teratology

Ref: PubMed

- Teratology is the science that studies the causes of structural, functional, behavioral and metabolic disorders present at birth (congenital malformation). It includes:
  - Size
  - Arrangement
  - Composition of any organ or part of the body
- **Classification of anomalies:**
  - **Genetic/Chromosomal:** AR, X-linked, Down syndrome, Turner syndrome
  - Teratogenic agent or environmental (~10% of congenital anomalies)
    - **Physical:** External traumatic injuries
    - Radiation/atomic explosion
    - Chemical agent like thalidomide, anticonvulsants, alcohol, smoking
    - **Infectious agents:** German measles, CMV, HSV, Syphilis
    - **Antigens:** Rh factor

7. Ans. (c) Spectroscopic test

Ref: The Essentials of FSM by KS Narayan Reddy, 31st ed. pg. 405-407

TESTS OF BLOOD STAIN

- **Spectroscopic test:** Most specific/confirmatory method for blood stain test
- **Kastle-Meyer/Phenolpthalein test:** Color produced is Pink Purple.
- **Microchemical test:** Based on RBC content of blood.
- **Takayama's test:** Hb converted to Haemochromogen crystal. Salmon pink feathery haemochromogen crystals are obtained.
- **Teichmann's Haemin crystal test:** Hb converted into Hemin/Hematin crystals. Brown rhombic haemic crystal are seen
- **Benzidine test**
  - Best preliminary test as it detects blood present in dilution of 1 in 3 lakhs.
  - **Color produced:** Deep Blue
  - *Not used because it is a potential carcinogen.*

8. Ans. (b) Transparency of root

Ref: Forensic Medicine and Toxicology by Rabindra Nath Karmakar, P 11

GUSTAFSON METHOD

- Used for age determination, when teeth eruption is complete (after age 17–25 years)

It has 6 criteria:

- **Degree of attrition:** Wear and tear due to mastication. Not very reliable
- **Degree of periodontitis:** With age → regression of gum and periodontal tissue. It can be due to disease of gum or lack of oral hygiene. So not reliable also
- Degree of secondary dentine formation
- Degree of cementum apposition (gradual thickening of cementum following changes in position of teeth at the end of root).
- Degree of root resorption
- **Degree of root transparency/translucency** (due to mineral deposition in dentine canal → gradually becomes translucent but the dentine tissue become transparent due to osteoporosis). *It is most dependable criteria.*

> **Extra Mile**
>
> - Modified Gustafson's is Daliz's formula
> - **Stack's formula:** For age estimation of infant and children from the height and weight of teeth.
> - **Boyde's method:** Age estimation from the structural feature of enamel
> - **Lamendin method:** Uses 2 criteria gingival and root transparency for age estimation. Gives better result than Gustafson's method.

9. Ans. (a) Iris

Ref: Guide to Biometric Reference Systems and Performance Evaluation, P 25

- Iris is the only internal organ available for acquisition. Its information, richness and stability make it a very suitable and efficient biometric modality.
- Iris recognition is reported as the most reliable biometrics for human recognition and it is suitable for large scale identification purposes.
- It is already being used in government programs, border or restricted areas access control.

10. Ans. (b) 8 years

Ref: Pediatric Otolaryngology, Volume 2, P 1170

- A child has a total of 20 primary teeth by age of 3 years:
  - 10 in the maxillary arch
  - 10 in the mandibular arch
- Subsequently permanent dentition starts at 6 yrs (21st Tooth). Hence choice A cannot be the answer. The correct answer is 8 yrs.

Forensic Medicine

- As the permanent teeth erupt, a mixed dentition results, giving rise to mixed dentition (*combination of primary and permanent teeth*) between ages of 6 years and 12 years.
- The early mixed dentition is characterized by the eruption of the permanent maxillary and mandibular incisors and first molar teeth, with concurrent exfoliation of their primary counterparts.
- After these teeth have erupted, dental development becomes quiescent during what is known as the intertransitional period, from age 9 to 11. During this time, no further permanent teeth erupt.
- By the age of 13 years, adolscents have 28 permanent teeth.

TABLE: Initiation and eruption timing of the permanent dentition

Tooth	Initiation (Month)	Eruption (Year)
Maxilla		
Central incisor	5–5.25 *in utero*	7–8
Lateral incisor	5–5.25 *in utero*	8–9
Canine	5.5–6 *in utero*	11–12
First premolar	Birth	10–11
Second premolar	7.5–8	10–12
First molar	3.5–4 *in utero*	10–12
Second molar	8.5–9	12–13
Third molar	3.5–4 (years)	17–25
Mandible		
Central incisor	5–5.25 *in utero*	6–7
Lateral incisor	5.25 *in utero*	7–8
Canine	5.5–6 *in utero*	9–11
First premolar	Birth	10–12
Second premolar	7.5–8	11–12
First molar	3.5–4 *in utero*	6–7
Second molar	8.5–9	11–13
Third molar	3.5–4 (years)	17–25

11. Ans. (d) Chinese

Ref: Principles of Forensic Medicine & Toxicology, 2017 ed. Bardale, P 92

Cephalic index: A number expressing the ratio of the maximum breadth of a skull to its maximum length. Range of cephalic index are as follows:

- **Dolicocephalic:** 70–75. For example, Pure Aryans, Negroes, aborigines
- **Mesaticephalic:** 75–80. For example, Europeans and Chinese
- **Brachycephalic:** 80–85. For example, Mongols
- **Hyperbrachycephalic:** >85.

12. Ans. (a) Infants

Ref: KS Narayana Reddy's 'The Essentials of Forensic Medicine and Toxicology'; 29/e, p-64-65

Stack's Method

- Stack evolved a method to know the age of infants from the weight and height of the erupting teeth of the child.
- This method can be based on both the deciduous and permanent teeth during their eruptive phase.

13. Ans. (a) Dead infant

Ref: KS Narayana Reddy's 'The Essentials of Forensic Medicine and Toxicology'; 29/e, p-64-65

Boyde's Method

- Cross-striations develop in the enamel of the teeth, till the complete formation of the enamel.
- They represent daily incremental lines.
- The age of an individual can be calculated in terms of days by counting the number of lines from the neonatal line onwards.
- Neonatal line is formed very soon after birth and can be seen in about 2–3 weeks or by electron microscopy within 1–2 days after birth.
- *It is useful* to estimate the age of a dead infant.

14. Ans. (a) Brachycephaly

Ref: KS Narayana Reddy's 'The Essentials of Forensic Medicine md Toxicology'; 29/e, p-54

Types of skull (Mn: DuMB)	Cephalic index	Race
Dolicho-cephalic (long headed)	70–75	Pure Aryans, Aborigines, Negroes
Mesaticephalic (medium headed)	75–80	Europeans and Chinese
Brachycephalic (short headed)	80–85	Mongols

Note: Cephalic index = $\dfrac{\text{Maximum breadth of skull}}{\text{Maximum length of skull}} \times 100$

Note: *Anteroposterior diameter of the skull is maximum in dolichocephalic and minimum in brachycephalic*

15. Ans. (c) Brachycephalic

Ref: KS Narayana Reddy's 'The Essentials of Forensic Medicine md Toxicology'; 29/e, p-54

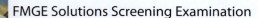

16. Ans. (a) Anterior part of palate

Ref: KS Narayana Reddy's 'The Essentials of Forensic Medicine and Toxicology'; 29/e, p-80

Palatoprints

- Harrison Allis suggested study of palate prints for identification.
- The structural details like the rugae are individual-specific and permanent **In the anterior part of the palate**
- The palatoprints can be used in the same way as fingerprints.
- **Thomas and Kurtze** have classified Palatoprints based on characteristics of rugae:
    - Primary rugae: 5 to 10 mm or >10 mm
    - Secondary rugae: 3 to 5 mm
    - Tertiary rugae-less than 3 mm

17. Ans. (d) Stomach and small intestine

Ref: KS Narayan Reddy's 'The Essentials of Forensic Medicine and Toxicology'; 26/e, p-381

Breslau's Second Life Test

- Air is swallowed into the stomach during respiration.
- The stomach and intestines are removed after tying double ligature at each end.
- They float in water if respiration has taken place, otherwise they sink.
- This is known as Breslau's second life test.
- This test is not of much value as air may be swallowed by child in attempting to free the air-passages of fluid obstruction in cases of stillbirth.
- It is useless when there is decomposition.

18. Ans. (c) Lungs

Tests for lung functional maturity/Lung chances in fetus after respiration

- **Hydrostatic test (Raygat's test):** Respired air remains in the lunge as residual air which cannot be removed after death. Hence lungs floats in water.
- **Static test or Fodere's test**—Weight of lung before (30–40 g) and after respiration (60–66 gm) is measured. The increase in weight of lung is due to increased blood flow.
- **Ploucquet's test**—weight of lung **is doubled after respiration.**
    Before respiration –1/70 of body wt.
    After respiration –1/35 of body wt.

COURT OF LAW AND IPCs

19. Ans. (b) Criminal responsibility of insane

Ref: Forensic Medicine and Toxicology by Rabindra Nath Karmakar, P 566

- McNaughton rule explains the criminal responsibility of insane, which says if a person commits crime, the person will be held guilty but considering the unsoundness of mind he/she not punished as per the verdict given by the jury of England. This theory is NOT acceptable in India.
- The Indian counterpart of McNaughton's rule is IPC Sec 84.
- According to this: *"Nothing is offence which is done by a person, who at the time of doing it, is, by reason of unsoundness of mind, incapable of knowing the nature of act or that he was doing what is either wrong or contrary to law"*

20. Ans. (b) Curren's rule

Ref: Forensic Medicine and Toxicology by Rabindra Nath Karmakar, P 566

Other Rules Regarding Fixing up Criminal Responsibility

- **Durham's rule (1954):** A person is not criminally held responsible if his unlawful act was the product of mental disease or defect.
- **Current rule (1961):** An accused person will not be criminally responsible if at the time of committing the act, he did not have the capacity to regulate his conduct to the requirement of law, as a result of mental disease or defect.
- **American law institute rest (1970):** A person is not held responsible for his criminal conduct if at the time of commission of such criminal conduct he lacks substantial capacity to appreciate the wrongfulness of his conduct to the requirement of law, resulting from mental disease or defect.
    However, repeated criminal conduct does not alone prove such abnormality
- **Irresistible impulse test (New Hampshire Doctrine):** An accused person will not be held criminally responsible, even when he knows the nature and quality of his act and that it is wrong, but he is incapable of restraining himself from committing it due to destruction of his free will to control him as a result of the mental disease.

> **Extra Mile**
>
> - **Hasse's rule:** to calculate the fetal age. As per this rule up to 5th month IUL, square root of the length of fetus is the age in months.
> - **Morrison rule:** to know the fetal length. As per this rule, after 5th month, age in lunar month multiplied by 5 is the length of fetus.

Forensic Medicine

21. Ans. (a) Under penalty document

Ref: Forensic Medicine and Toxicology by Rabindra Nath Karmakar, P 314

Summon/Subpoena (Sub = under; Poena = Penalty)

- A written document issued by court, compelling the attendance of witness for giving evidence in relation to a particular case, with a warning NOT to be absent without proper ground and after attendance not to leave the court without proper permission under penalty.
- **Two types of summons:**
  - **Subpoena Ad testificandum:** To given evidence in court
  - **Subpoena Duces Tecum:** To produce some document in the court (CrPC Sec 91)
- **Punishment for non-compliance**
  - **Civil case:** Liable to pay damages
  - **Criminal case:** Arrest warrant issued compelling attendance (CrPC 87). Later on may be ordered for punishment either in form of fine or even imprisonment (IPC Sec 174)
- **Conduct money:** Money paid to witness as expense of attending the court
  - **Civil case:** Paid along with summon
  - **Criminal case:** Not paid to witness, but court will pay the expenses as per Govt. rule
    - For government employees, paid by employer

22. Ans. (a) State Government

- **Courts of Judicial Magistrate of First Class** are at the second lowest level of the Criminal Court structure in India. According to the Section 11 of the Criminal Procedure Code, 1973 (CrPc), a Court of Judicial Magistrate of First Class may be **established by the State Government** in consultation with the High Court of the respective state at such places in the district and in any number by a notification.
- According to Section 29 of the CrPc, a Judicial Magistrate of First Class may pass a sentence of imprisonment for a term not exceeding three years, or of fine not exceeding ten thousand rupees or of both.

23. Ans. (b) Magistrate

Magistrate Inquest: Court of Trail

- Usually conducted by DM, SDM or Executive Magistrate (i.e. collector, Deputy Collector or Tahsildar)
- Magistrate inquests are usually done in following circumstances:
  - **Dowry death**, i.e. unnatural death within 7 years of marriage

- Death in prison
- Death in police custody or interrogation or during police firing
- Death in any psychiatric hospital
- Exhumation, i.e. digging out of an already buried body is also done upon order of magistrate.

24. Ans. (c) Whether it is caused by knife

Ref: Review of Forensic medicine by Sumit Seth pg. 248-49

- During a court trial, questions are put to the witness by the public prosecutor or the defence lawyer.
- A leading question is one the answer of which is desired in only YES or NO. **Examples of leading question:**
  - Whether you were present at the crime site?
  - Did you see this person at crime site?
  - Is this the knife you saw at crime site?
  - Whether the accused was holding knife or gun?
- The other options like *"how did you get cuts on T-Shirt; cause of injury, size of incised wound"* needs explanatory answer and cannot be answered in yes or no.
- Leading question can only be asked by **defence lawyer in cross examination. (Recent exam 2018)**
- A leading question is NOT allowed in chief examination by public prosecutor (*EXCEPT when the witness is hostile*)
- **NOTE:** Leading question has been classified under 141 IEA (Indian Evidence Act)

25. Ans. (a) Magistrate

Ref: The Essentials of FSM by K.S. Narayan Reddy 31st ed. pg. 5, 272

Inquest: inquiry into the cause of death
- **Police Inquest**
  - *Most common type of inquest in India*
  - Investigating officer usually is sub inspector or officer not below the rank of (senior) head constable.

Magistrate Inquest: Court of Trail

- Usually conducted by DM, SDM or Executive Magistrate (i.e. collector, Deputy Collector or Tahsildar)
- Magistrate inquests are usually done in following circumstances:
  - **Dowry deaths** i.e. unnatural deaths within 7 years of marriage
  - Death in prison
  - Death in police custody or interrogation or during police firing
  - Death in any psychiatric hospital
- Exhumation i.e. digging out of an already buried body also done upon order of magistrate.

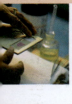

FMGE Solutions Screening Examination

Coroner's Inquest: Court of inquiry

- Coroner is an advocate, attorney, pleader, or first class magistrate with 5 years experience or metropolitan magistrate
- Coroner court is a court of inquiry & accused need not be present.
- Coroner court can't impose fine or punishment; but it can punish those guilty of contempt of his court when the offence is committed in the premises of his court (i.e. city limit only)
- *In India it was practiced in Mumbai, Kolkata. But now abolished.*

26. Ans. (a) Magistrate

Ref: The Essentials of FSM by K.S. Narayan Reddy, 31st ed. pg. 5, 272

Please refer to above explanation.

27. Ans. (d) Voluntarily causing hurt

Ref: The Essentials of FSM by K.S. Narayan Reddy, 31st ed. pg. 270-71

TABLE: Some Important IPC sections and their definitions

INDIAN PENAL CODE (IPC):
CRIMINAL PROCEDURE CODE (CrPC):

IPC Section	Definition
Sec 82	A child under 7 years is incapable of committing an offence. Not applicable to railway act.
Sec 83	A child >7 &< 12 is presumed to be mature enough to be capable of committing an offence.
Sec 84	Act of a person of unsound mind is not liable (McNaughten's rule)
Sec 85	Act of a person who's intoxicated against will.
Sec 87	A person less than 18 years cannot give valid consent to suffer any harm which may result from an act not intended or not known to cause death or grievous hurt. E.g. consent for wrestling contest
Sec 88 to 93	Legal protection to medical doctors. Sec 89 – a child < 12 years cannot give valid consent to suffer any harm which can occur by an act done in good faith or for its benefit e.g. consent for operation
Cr PC 174	Police inquest
Cr PC 176	Magistrate's inquest
Sec 179	Punishment for refusal to answer question by the police
Sec 191	Definition of perjury
Sec 193	Punishment for perjury

Contd...

IPC Section	Definition
Sec 197	Issuing false certificate (3-7 years of punishment)
Sec 201	Disappearance of evidence (2 years of punishment)
Sec 297	Trespassing of burial place, Necrophilia, Necrohagia
Sec 299	Definition of Culpable homicide
Sec 300	Murder
Sec 302	Punishment for murder/infanticide
Sec 304	Culpable homicide not amounting to murder
Sec 304 A	Causing death by negligence
Sec 304 B	Dowry death
307	Attempt to murder
308	Attempt to culpable homicide
309	Attempt to suicide
Sec 317	Exposure and Abandonment of child <12 years
Sec 318	Concealment of birth by secret disposal of dead body
Sec 319	Hurt
Sec 320	Grievous hurt
Sec 321	*Voluntarily causing hurt*
Sec 322	*Voluntarily causing grievous hurt*
Sec 323	**Punishment for voluntary causing hurt**
Sec 324	**Voluntary causing hurt by dangerous weapon/means**
Sec 325	Punishment for voluntarily causing grievous hurt
Sec 326	Punishment for voluntarily causing grievous hurt by a dangerous weapon/means
Sec 351	Assault
Sec 354	Assault to outrage the modesty of a woman.
Sec 375	Definition of rape
Sec 376	Punishment of rape
Sec 377	Unnatural sexual offence
Sec 497	Adultery

28. Ans. (b) 7 years

Ref: The essentials of FSM by KS Narayan Reddy, 31st ed. pg. 384-85

- **IPC for rape:** 375
- **IPC punishment of rape:** 376. This IPC states that whoever commits rape shall be punished with imprisonment for a term of not less than 7 years, but which may be for life or ten years plus fine.

Forensic Medicine

29. Ans. (b) 319

Ref: The Essentials of FSM by K.S. Narayan Reddy, 31ˢᵗ ed. pg. 384-85

Please refer to above table.

30. Ans. (a) 320

Ref: The Essentials of FSM by K.S. Narayan Reddy, 31ˢᵗ ed. pg. 384-85

Please refer to above table.

31. Ans. (d) Injured person admitted in hospital for 21 days

Ref: Legal Apptitude And Legal Reasoning For The Clat By Bhardwaj A. pg. 36

Section for grievous hurt: IPC 320

The book states: *"the mere fact that the injured remained in hospital for 20 days would not be enough to conclude that he was unable to follow his ordinary pursuits during that. Continuance of severe body pain for 20 days or disability to follow one's avocation for 20 days constitutes grievous hurt"*

Criteria

- Emasculation
- Permanent privation of the sight of either eye
- Permanent privation of hearing of either ear
- Privation of any joint or permanent impairment of the power of any member of joint
- Permanent disfiguration of head or face
- Fracture or dislocation of bone or tooth
- Any hurt which endangers life or which causes the sufferer to be admitted during the span of 20 days in severe body pain or unable to follow his ordinary pursuits.

32. Ans. (a) 497

Ref: The Essentials of FSM by K.S. Narayan Reddy, 31ˢᵗ ed. pg. 24

Please refer to above table.

33. Ans. (b) 315

Ref: The Essentials of FSM by K.S. Narayan Reddy, 31ˢᵗ ed. pg. 408

- **IPC Section 315 and 316** discusses the offence of foeticide and infanticide.
- If a person commits an act with the intention of preventing the child from being born alive or an act that results in the death of the child after birth, that person is committing foeticide/infanticide as long as they do not do it in the interest of the mother's health or life.

- **Section 317** states that is it a crime against children, if their mother or father expose or leave a child in a place with the intention of abandonment.
- **Sections 82 and 83** of the IPC states: a child who commits a crime and is below the age of seven is not considered to have committed a crime.
- **Section 299:** Culpable homicide

34. Ans. (c) 304-B

Ref: The Essentials of FSM by K.S. Narayan Reddy, 31ˢᵗ ed. pg. 272

Dowry Death

- Bodily injury caused by husband or relative, which lead to death comes under Dowry death and punished under IPC 304 B.
- **IPC section 304 B states:** Whenever any death of a woman is caused by any burns or bodily injury or occurs otherwise than under normal circumstances within seven years of her marriage and it is shown that soon before her death she was subjected to cruelty or harassment by her husband or any relative of her husband for, or in connection with, any demand for dowry, such death shall be called "dowry death" and such husband or relative shall be deemed to have caused her death.
- Whoever commits dowry death shall be punished with imprisonment for a term which shall not be less than **seven years and it may extend to life time imprisonment.**

35. Ans. (a) 498 A

Ref: The Essentials of FSM by K.S. Narayan Reddy, 31ˢᵗ ed. pg. 272-73

- Cruel behavior towards wife by husband or his relatives punished by IPC 498 A.
- **IPC section 498 A** states that whosoever being husband or relative subject women to cruelty shall be punished with imprisonment of upto 3 years with or without fine.

36. Ans. (d) Section 416

Ref: The Essentials of FSM by K.S. Narayan Reddy, 31ˢᵗ ed. pg. 5-6, 314-15

Section 416: If a woman sentenced to death is found to be pregnant, the High Court shall order the execution of the sentence to be postponed, and may, if it thinks fit, commute the sentence to imprisonment for life.

Section 413. Execution of order passed under Section 368: When a case submitted to the High Court for the confirmation of a sentence of death, the Court of Session receives the order of confirmation or other order of the

High Court thereon, it shall cause such order to be carried into effect by issuing a warrant or taking such other steps as may be necessary.

Section 414. Execution of sentence of death passed by High Court: When a sentence of death is passed by the High Court in appeal or in revision, the Court of Session shall, on receiving the order of the High Court, cause the sentence to be carried into effect by issuing a warrant.

Section 419. Direction of warrant for execution: Every warrant for the execution of a sentence of imprisonment shall be directed to the officer in charge of the jail or other place in which the prisoner is, or is to be, confined.

37. Ans. (b) Masturbation

Ref: The essentials of FSM by KS Narayan Reddy, 31st ed. pg. 404

- Masturbation is an offence only when practiced openly; Ex: in telephone booth, lavatories.

TOXICOLOGY

38. Ans. (b) Hydrocarbons

Ref: Harrison's 20th ed. P 3306

CONTRAINDICATION OF GASTRIC LAVAGE

- Hydrocarbon and petroleum distillate
- Caustic or corrosive poisoning-due to increased risk of gastric perforation and aspiration pneumonitis.
- Uncontrolled convulsion- due to increased risk of aspiration
- Comatose patients-compromised/unprotected airway
- Cardiac arrhythmias
- Recent upper GI surgery
- Combative patients or those who refuse- absolutely contraindicated

Extra Mile

TABLE: Contraindications of gastric lavage

Absolute contraindications	Relative contraindications
Alkali	Kerosene or volatile poisoning
Mineral acid	Strychinine
Vegetable acids	Hypothermia
Organic acids except carbolic acid	Bleeding disorder

39. Ans. (a) Oxalic acid

Ref: Forensic Medicine and Toxicology by Rabindra Nath Karmakar, P 79

- Oxalic acid is a colorless organic compound with a wide-range of use in cleaning and bleaching applications
- Oxalic Acid Poisoning is the accidental or intentional intake of oxalic acid or oxalic acid compound

SIGNS AND SYMPTOMS

- Vomiting
- Burning pain in throat, mouth
- Swelling of mouth and tongue- inability to speak clearly
- Skin burns/blister formation
- Red, watery eyes

TREATMENT

- The immediate administration of an antidote: Lime and chalk (precipitated chalk or saccharate solution of lime).
- They can be scraped off the wall, whitewashed fences, or ceilings, crushed egg shells, mixed with milk/water and given.
- Emesis to remove unabsorbed poison
- Demulcent drink to protect gastric mucosa
- IV 10% Calcium gluconate—to treat hypocalcemia

40. Ans. (c) Root

- Although entire plant is poisonous, the **root is most potent.**
- *Dry root* is conical or tapering, shows bases of the broken rootlets and shriveled with longitudinal wrinkles.
- **NO odor, Sweet taste** (mitha bish)

Mechanism of Action

- Aconitine binds with the voltage-dependent sodium-ion channels.
- Aconitine first stimulates and then paralyzes the peripheral terminations of sensory, secretory and motor nerves

41. Ans. (c) Synthetic

OPIUM/AFIM

- Heroin (brown Sugar/Junk): **Synthetic derivative of opium**
- Juice from **unripe capsule** of Papaver Somniferum (poppy) contains opioid alkaloids
- Poppy seeds are used for cooking and are non-toxic
- **Poison of choice for suicide:** As it produces painless death.
- **Pinpoint pupil,** respiratory depression.
- Marquis test: to detect opium
- **Antidote:** Naloxone sodium
- Treatment for morphine withdrawal: Methadone
- Along with routine viscera, Brain, blood and bile to be preserved.
- **Speedball** is the use of *cocaine with morphine or heroin*

42. Ans. (a) Cobra

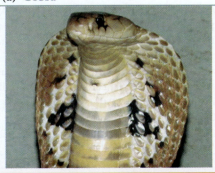

Appearance	Poisonous snakes	Nonpoisonous snakes
Habit	Nocturnal	**Not** specific
Head scales	Usually small	Usually large
	3 exceptions (Poisonous snakes with large head scales) **Pit Vipers Cobra Krait** **Pit viper** pit below the eye **Cobra** 3rd labial touches eye and nasal shields **Krait:** 4 infralabials scales below mouth and 4th being largest	
Belly scales	Large and cover the entire breadth of belly	Small, not covering the entire belly
Distal scales	Single row	Double row
Tail	Compressed	Noncompressed
Fangs	Long and canalized, like hypodermic needle	Short or small grooved
Bite mark	**Two fang marks**	**Small teeth marks**

43. Ans. (b) Carbon monoxide

- The color of livor mortis depends on the type of hemoglobin
- Normally, the lividity is bluish or purple due to the presence of deoxyhemoglobin.

Conditions	Color of lividity	Type of hemoglobin
Normal	Blue purplish	Reduced Hemoglobin
Carbon monoxide Burns	Cherry red Bright red	Carboxyhemoglobin and increased oxygen content in blood **(Anemic anoxia)**
Cyanide	Bright red	Cyanide inhibits cytochrome oxidase and decreased O_2 utilization by tissues. **(Histotoxic anoxia)** Increased oxygen content in blood

Contd...

Conditions	Color of lividity	Type of hemoglobin
Hypothermia/ Refrigeration	Pink	Oxygen retention in cutaneous blood by cold air
NaCl/Nitrite/ Nitrate/aniline Potassium chlorate	Chocolate Brown	Methemoglobin **(meth Hb)**
Septic abortion	Bronze	**Due to** Cl. Perfringens
Hydrogen sulphide	Green	**Sulfhemoglobin**

44. Ans. (b) Sodium thiosulfate

TABLE: Poisoning and their Antidote

Poisoning	Antidote/treatment
Oxalic acid (ink remover)	Calcium gluconate
Phosphorus	Copper sulphate
Organophosphorus	Atropine
Dhatura	Physostigmine
Arsenic	BAL, DMSA
Mercury	BAL, DMSA
Lead (Plumbism)	EDTA, DMSA
Alcohol	Ethyl alcohol
Opium (Afeem)	Naloxone
Heroine/Brown sugar/ Junk/ Smack	Amyl nitrite
Bhang/Ganja/Charas	Diazepam
Strychinine	Diazepam
Copper	EDTA, penicillamine desferrioxamine
Cyanide	• Hydroxocobalamin. If not available then Na^+ thiosulphate/Na^+ nitrite can be used • **GASTRIC LAVAGE:** 5% of sodium thiosulphate, sodium nitrite.

45. Ans. (a) Hydroxocobalamin

Hydrocyanic acid (Cyanide poisoning)

- CYANOGEN/PRUSSIC ACID is colorless, **odor resembling bitter almond.**
- **Cause of death in cyanide poisoning:**
    - Cytotoxic and histo-toxic anoxia.
    - Corrosive effect on the mucous membrane, when inhaled instantaneous death is the result.

Treatment

- **ANTIDOTE:** Hydroxocobalamin
- **GASTRIC LAVAGE:** 5% of sodium thiosulphate, sodium nitrite.

46. Ans. (b) Mercury

Ref: The Essentials of FSM by K.S. Narayan Reddy, 31st ed. pg. 505

FMGE Solutions Screening Examination

MERCURY POISONING (HYDRAGYRISM)

- Vapours of mercuric compounds are poisonous because it will be absorbed in the systemic circulation.
- Mercuric compounds being soluble are more poisonous than mercurous (less soluble) compounds.

Clinical Presentation of Mercury Poisoning (Remembered as MEATS)

- **Mercuria lentis:** Brownish deposition of mercury on anterior lens.
- **Membranous colitis**
- **Erethism:** Characterized by shyness, irritability, tremors, loss of memory & insomnia.
- **Acrodynia (Pink disease):** Generalized pinkish body rash starting from tips of fingers & toes
  - **Characterized by 5 P's:** Pinkish, Puffy, Painful, Paresthetic hands and feet with Peeling of skin.
- **Tremors:** Also known as *Danbury tremors, hatter's or glass-blower's shake*
- **Salivation & gingivitis:** excessive salivation associated with metallic taste, gingivitis, loosening of teeth and **blue-black line on gums.**

Extra Mile

TABLE: Different metallic poisoning and their effect on hair and skin

Poisoning	Color of Hair & Skin
Arsenic (As)	• Yellow color of skin, hair & mucous membrane • Milk rose (Brownish pigmentation)/Rain drop pigmentation • BLACK FOOT DISEASE
Copper (Cu)	• Jaundiced skin • Green-blue skin, hair & perspiration • Green – purple line on gums
Mercury (Hg)	• Blue-black line on gums with jaw necrosis and loosening of tooth • Brown deposits on anterior lens capsule (mercuria lentis) • Acrodynia (pink disease)
Lead (Pb)	• Blue stippled burtonian line on gums, especially on upper jaw.

Other Features of Mercury Poisoning

- Proximal Convoluted Tubule necrosis
- Prevalence of abortions are common
- **Minimata disease** is an organic mercury poisoning due to consumption of fish poisoned by mercury.

47. Ans. (b) Alkali

Ref: The Essentials of FSM by K.S. Narayan Reddy, 31st ed. pg. 499

- Maximum damage to the esophagus is caused by ingestion of alkali as compared to acid.

- Alkali causes Liquifactive necrosis which is more damaging than coagulative necrosis caused by acid.
- Liquifactive necrosis is caused by hydrolytic enzymes. It attracts WBC which leads to bacterial infection and Pus formation. It can cause CNS ischemia also.
- Acid causes coagulative necrosis due to coagulation of proteins. Coagulative necrosis is seen in all organs of body except brain.
- MCC of coagulative necrosis is hypoxia.

48. Ans. (a) Alcoholic poisoning

Ref: The Essentials of FSM by K.S. Narayan Reddy, 31st ed. pg. 540-41

- In case of alcohol poisoning, CSF as much as can be withdrawn is required to be preserved.
- Preservative used is Na/K- Fluride and K-Oxalate.
  - Fluoride is added to CSF for alcohol estimation.
  - It can be also be used for vitreous humor and urine if alcohol estimation is required.

Extra Mile

TABLE: Poisoning and Organ preserved

Poisoning	Organ preserved
Strychnine poisoning	Spinal cord (entire length)
Pesticides and Insecticides poisoning	Fat
CO, Cyanide, Organophosphates, Opiates, Barbiturates, Alkaloids and Strychnine poisoning (Mn: COOBAS)	Brain
Arsenic, Radium and Thalium poisoning (Mn: ART)	Bone

49. Ans. (a) Charcoal

Ref: The Essentials of FSM by K.S. Narayan Reddy, 31st ed. pg. 485-86

ORGANOPHOSPHORUS

- **Alkyl phosphate:** Malathion (bug killer)
- **Aryl phosphate:** Parathion; Diazinon (Tik 20)
- Absorbed by inhalation, through skin, mucous membrane & gastro intestinal tract.
- **MOA:** It irreversibly inhibits acetylcholine esterase enzyme, which subsequently leads to increase in acetylcholine in body and patient presents with cholinergic symptoms.

Clinical Features

- Increases all secretions of body (eg: increased sweating, salivation, urination, diarrhea, emesis).
- Stimulate bronchial asthma
- Miosis
- Bradycardia
- Irritability, confusion and fine tremors.

Forensic Medicine

Investigation
- **RBC cholinesterase:** Most popular and most commonly used.
- Plasma cholinesterase

Treatment
- **Antidote:** Atropine, Pralidoxime
- Atropine (antidote) is highly effective in counteracting peripheral muscarinic effects, and higher doses are required to antagonize CNS effects.
- It is not effective against nicotinic actions.
- Cholinesterase reactivators like DAM (Di Acetyl Monoxime), PAM (Pralidoxime iodide) action is most marked at nicotinic site.
- Oximes should be started as early as possible preferably withing 24 hours before phosphorylated enzyme has undergone aging & become resistant to hydrolysis
- Oximes do not cross BBB. It directly detoxify OPC.
- *Note: Activated charcoal is used in case of cyanide poisoning.*

---

50. Ans. (a) Kerosene

Ref: The Essentials of FSM by K.S. Narayan Reddy, 31ˢᵗ ed. pg. 551

TABLE: Contraindications of Gastric Lavage

Absolute contraindications	Relative contraindications
• Alkali	• **Kerosene or volatile poisoning**
• Mineral acid	• Strychinine
• Vegetable acids	• Hypothermia
• Organic acids **except carbolic acid**	• Bleeding disorder

---

51. Ans. (a) Tobacco

Ref: The Essentials of FSM by K.S. Narayan Reddy, 31ˢᵗ ed. pg. 577

- Among the given options, tobacco is the substance which is most commonly used in India and also persons can easily get addicted and can tolerate this agent.

---

52. Ans. (c) Copper sulphate

Ref: The Essentials of FSM by K.S. Narayan Reddy, 31ˢᵗ ed. pg. 512-13

- *White phosphorus is toxic while Red phosphorus is non-toxic*
- **Phosphorus poisoning presents with Phossy jaw, Garliky mucosa.**
- Garlicky mucosal odor is also seen in Celphos and Arsenic poisoning.
- **Antidote:** Copper sulphate

---

53. Ans. (b) Mimics tetanus

Ref: The Essentials of FSM by K.S. Narayan Reddy, 31ˢᵗ ed. pg. 501–502

Arsenic Poisoning Features
- It is the most commonly used homicidal poison.
- Presents with Haemorrhagic gastroenteritis and necrosis of intestinal mucosa.
- **It mimics Cholera NOT tetanus (*Strychinine mimics tetanus*).**
- Diarrhea accompanied by tenesumus and anal irritation.
- **Arsenic poisoning is also characterized by:**
  - Black foot disease
  - Red velvety mucosa upon PM
  - *Rain drop pigmentation on body*
  - Reinsch test or maRsh test- used to test the arsenic
- They deposited on skin, hair and nail because they contain keratin, hence it is preserved.
- Hyperkeratosis on palms and soles.
- **Fatal dose:** 0.1–0.2 gm.
- On nails specific lines seen known as: **Aldrich Mees Line**
- **Upon chronic poisoning**
  - Sensory motor polyneuropathy causing tingling, numbness and paresis
  - Encephalopathy
- **Antidote:** BAL, Succimer.

---

54. Ans. (a) Arsenic

Ref: The Essentials of FSM by K.S. Narayan Reddy, 31ˢᵗ ed. pg. 501-502

Please refer to above explanation.

---

55. Ans. (d) Cyanide

Ref: The Essentials of FSM by K.S. Narayan Reddy, 31ˢᵗ ed. pg. 588-89

HYDROCYANIC ACID (CYANIDE POISONING)
- CYANOGEN/PRUSSIC ACID is colorless, with an odor *resembling bitter almond.*
- Hydrocyanic acid, a colorless volatile liquid found in fruits like peach, plum, bitter almond.
- Cyanides (white powder) used in photography, electroplating, fumigation of ship.
- It is Cytochrome oxidase and Carbonic anhydrase inhibiter.
- **Cause of death:**
  - Cytotoxic and histo-toxic anoxia.
  - Corrosive effect on the mucous membrane, when inhaled leads to instantaneous death.

Signs and Symptoms
- Headache, giddiness, convulsion, seizure
- **Dilated & fixed pupil**
- Smell of bitter almond and froth at the mouth
- Cyanosed face, clenched jaw
- Respiratory failure leads to death

Fatal dose: 60 mg of pure acid or 60 drops of crude oil of bitter almond or 200 mg of KCN

FMGE Solutions Screening Examination

Treatment
- **ANTIDOTE:** Hydroxocobalamin.
- **GASTRIC LAVAGE:** 5% of sodium thiosulphate, sodium nitrite.

PM: BRICK RED blood due to cyano-meth Hb.
(Brain, Lung, Blood, Urine, Vomitus are preserved.)

56. Ans. (c) Sodium thiosulfate

Ref: The Essentials of FSM by K.S. Narayan Reddy, 31ˢᵗ ed. pg. 588-89

57. Ans. (d) Myotoxic

Ref: The Essentials of FSM by K.S. Narayan Reddy, 31ˢᵗ ed. pg. 524

TABLE: Snakes and their respective poisoning

Snake	Type of poisoning
Vipers	Vasculotoxic, Hemotoxic
Sea snakes	Myotoxic
Cobra, Krait	Neurotoxic

58. Ans. (a) Neurotoxic

Ref: The Essentials of FSM by K.S. Narayan Reddy 31ˢᵗ ed. / 523

Please refer to above explanation.

59. Ans. (c) 30

Ref: The Essentials of FSM by K.S. Narayan Reddy, 31ˢᵗ ed. pg. 530-40

- 30 mg%- Normal limit for drink and drive
- 80 mg%- Nystagmus
- 150 mg%- Muscle incoordination
- 400 mg%- Coma

60. Ans. (b) Methyl alcohol

Ref: Internet Source

- Methyl alcohol poisoning is referred to as HOOCH tradegy. It is converted in the body to formaldehyde which is toxic to retina, leading to blindness. Concomitant high anion gap metabolic acidosis results in mortality.
- The latest hooch tragedy was in Mumbai in June, 2015 and in Cuttack, Odissa in 2012.

61. Ans. (c) Cocaine

Ref: The Essentials of FSM by K.S. Narayan Reddy, 31ˢᵗ ed. pg. 562-63

- Cannabis and its products contain (−) D-9 TetraHydroCoannabinol (Δ9-THC).
- It is obtained from Indian hemp plant known as cannabis Sativa.
- Different parts of this plants give different products:
  - Dried leaves: **Bhang**
  - Dried female inflorescence: **Ganja**
  - Resinous extract of stem: **Charas/Hashish**
  - Marijuana/Marihuana: Other name for cannabis
- In case of cannabis abuse there is an episode of acute violent behavior for which the person claims amnesia. This is known as **Run Amok**.

Extra Mile

TABLE: Commonly abused substances and their characteristic clinical feature

Substance	Characteristic clinical feature
Cocaine	Magnus symptoms *(cocaine bugs or Tactile hallucination)* **Black tongue and teeth**
Cannabis	• Run Amok • Amotivation syndrome • Flash backs
Alcohol	• Mc-Evan's sign • Morbid jealousy
LSD	• Bad Trips • Flash backs
Amphetamine	Paranoid hallucinatory syndrome (like paranoid schizophrenia)
Phencyclidine (Angel dust)	Dissociative anesthesia

62. Ans. (d) Cocaine poisoning

Ref: The Essentials of FSM by K.S. Narayan Reddy, 31ˢᵗ ed. pg. 564-65

63. Ans. (c) Bhilawanol

Ref: The Essentials of FSM by K.S. Narayan Reddy, 31ˢᵗ ed. pg. 517

Semi carpus anacardium (*bhilawanol* or marking nut): Juice applied to the skin produces irritation, painful blisters, followed by itching and eczematous eruption. Lesions formed resemble bruise which ulcerate and slough.

Active principles: *bilawanol* and *semicarpol*
- Used by washermen as marking ink on clothes
- Used to produce artificial bruise
- Used as abortifacient by an abortion stick

BURNS AND DROWNING

64. Ans. (c) Teeth

Ref: PubMed

- In severely burnt body, dental data is most helpful in identification.

Forensic Medicine

65. Ans. (b) Drowning

- Gettler test is done to distinguish between freshwater drowning and salt water drowning.
- It is done by measuring the chloride difference of right and left side of heart. A difference of >25% is considered as significant.

66. Ans. (a) Brackish water

- Oligohalophilic diatoms live in fresh water.
- Polyhalophilic diatoms live in sea water.
- **Mesohalophilic diatoms** live in brackish water (water midway in salinity between freshwater and seawater)

67. Ans. (c) Presence of carboxyhemoglobin

Ref: *Textbook of Forensic Medicine And Toxicology: Principles And Practice by Vij, pg. 221*

TABLE: Difference between antemortem burns vs postmortem burns

Features	Antemortem Burns	Postmortem Burns
Line of redness	Present around the injured burn area	Not so
Vesicles	Contain serous fluid with **high proportion of albumin and chloride**	Contain air mostly. If fluid present it comprises of very little albumin and no chlorides
Base of blister	Red and inflamed	Dull, dry, hard and yellow
Inflammation evidence	Inflammatory edema and repair processes; (+) Leucocyte Infiltration	No such changes noticed
Presence of carbonaceous deposits/soot in the respiratory tract	**PRESENT.** *Indicates death from suffocation following antemortem burn*	Not present
Presence of Carboxyhemoglobin	Present *(its highly suggestive and diagnostic)*	Absent
Enzymatic activity	Time related **increase** in enzymatic activity: • **Immediate:** Tissue Cathepsin • **At 2 hours:** Leucine Aminopeptidase • **At 3 hours:** Acid Phosphatase • **At 4 hours:** Alkaline Phosphatase	Never noticed

68. Ans. (c) Cardiac arrest

Ref: *The Essentials of FSM by K.S. Narayan Reddy, 31st ed. pg. 339-40*

DROWNING

- In most of the cases it is accidental.

Types of Drowning

- **Wet drowning**
  - Most common form of drowning.
  - In this type water is withheld in lungs.
  - **Cause of death in wet drowning: Cardiac Arrest**
  - In fresh water death is earlier compared to sea water. Fresh water causes hemodilution and due to hemodilution there is hyperkalemia which causes ventricular fibrillation.
  - In case of sea water, death is little later, because sea water causes hemoconcentration in body, which leads to Hypernatremia and as a result death due to bradycardia.
- **Dry drowning**
  - In this type of drowning, water in not inside the lung.
  - Death is due to Reflex Laryngospasm.
- **Delayed drowning/Near Drowning**
  - This is also known as post immersion syndrome.
  - Resuscitation after drowning and death after 24 hours.
  - **Cause of death:**
    - Metabolic acidosis
    - Pneumonia
    - Electrolyte imbalance.
- **Hydrocution/Immersion syndrome**
  - Drowning in extreme cold water.
  - **Cause of death:** Vaso-vagal shock (VVS).

69. Ans. (b) Vagal inhibition

Ref: *The essentials of FSM by KS Narayan Reddy, 31st ed. pg. 342*

- **Cause of death in drowning:**
  - **Asphyxia:** cause of death in sea water drowning. Inhalation of fluid causes obstruction to the air passages which leads to respiratory and circulatory failure due to anoxia.
  - **Ventricular fibrillation: MCC of death in fresh water drowning.** Death may occur in 3-5 minutes from a combination of anoxia and electrolyte imbalance which might lead to ventricular tachycardia and fibrillation.
  - **Vagal Inhibition:** MCC of death in icy cold water, drunkenness, high emotion or excitement.
  - **Exhaustion**
  - **Injuries**

FMGE Solutions Screening Examination

> **Extra Mile**
> - Fatal period:
>   - Death in fresh water: 4–5 minutes
>   - Death in salt water: 8–10 minutes

70. Ans. (c) Clenched fist

Ref: The essentials of FSM by KS Narayan Reddy, 31st ed. pg. 344

- Presence of gravel, grass. etc firmly grasped in hand due to cadaveric spasm strongly suggest that person was alive when drowned as it indicates the struggle of person for life.

TABLE: Postmortem signs of drowning

Pathognomic Signs: indicates antemortem drowning	Non Specific signs
External • Fine copious white leathery froth from mouth, nose and air passage which increases on chest pressure. • Weeds, grass, mud etc in tightly clenched hand: a very definite sign. **Internal** • Water in stomach and intestine and middle ear • Diatoms in brain and bone marrow of long bones.	• Cutis anserine or goose skin • Washer woman hand and feet • Paltauf (subpleural, pectechial) haemorrhage • Emphysema aqousum

71. Ans. (a) Drowning

Ref: The essentials of FSM by KS Narayan Reddy, 31st ed. pg. 344

- Paltauff haemorrhage is subpleural, pectechial haemorrhage. It is shiny, pale pink or bluish red and may be minute or 3-5 cm in diameter, seen in case of drowning.
- During drowning there is more powerful inspiratory efforts which causes air entry to lungs with water and foam which makes the lungs heavy and increased pressure inside. This causes forced expiration which causes rupture of alveolar walls that may present subpleurally and is referred as paltauff haemorrhage.
- ***Paltauff haemorrhage most commonly occur in lower lobes of lung.***

> **Extra Mile**
> - Other important findings of drowning:
>   - Emphysema aquosum
>   - Oedema aquosum
>   - Diatoms (microscopic unicellular or colonial algae)
>   - Washerwomen hand/feet
>   - Cutis anserine or goose skin

72. Ans. (b) Drowning

Ref: The Essentials of FSM by K.S. Narayan Reddy, 31st ed. pg. 346

73. Ans. (b) Burns

Ref: The Essentials of FSM by K.S. Narayan Reddy, 31st ed. pg. 299

- Pugilistic attitude is seen in case of burns.
- It is also known as Boxing or fencing attitude.
- Pugilistic attitude is due to coagulation of proteins other than those affected by rigor mortis.
- It is seen in both antemortem as well as postmortem burns.

> **Extra Mile**
> - **Most common finding of antemortem drowning:** Clenched Fist.
> - In case of Lightning: Branching tree pattern seen.

74. Ans. (c) Peeling of the skin

Ref: The Essentials of FSM by K.S. Narayan Reddy, 31st ed. pg. 296-98; Internet source

An injury most commonly to an extremity or digit in which the skin and subcutaneous tissue are separated from the deeper tissue layers thereby depleting its blood supply and increasing the risk of tissue necrosis.

75. Ans. (b) High voltage Electric burns

Ref: The Essentials of FSM by K.S. Narayan Reddy, 31st ed. pg. 308-309

ELECTRICAL INJURIES

- **JOULE BURN:** contact electrical and endogenous burn.
- **CROCODILE FLASH BURN:** high voltage burn.
- Multiple lesions due to 'ARC EFFECT'.
- **Cause of Death-** ventricular fibrillation.
- Current pearls and wax drops seen on autopsy.

76. Ans. (a) Lightening stroke

Ref: The Essentials of FSM by K.S. Narayan Reddy, 31st ed. pg. 310-311

- **Lightening stroke:** It is an electrical discharge from the cloud to the earth.
- **Classical finding:** FILLIGREE BURN/ LITCHENBURG'S FLOWERS: superficial, irregular, thin resembling the branches of a tree also known as arborescent burn.

- Most common site is shoulder flanks. *(Cause is staining of tissues with Hb along the path of current.)*

77. Ans. (c) High temperature liquids

Ref: The Essentials of FSM by K.S. Narayan Reddy, 31st ed. pg. 305

Scalds: Caused by application of liquid above 60°C or steam. Skin becomes sodden and bleach. Clothes are wet but do not burn.

78. Ans. (c) Presence of carbonaceous deposits in respiratory tract

Ref: Textbook of Forensic Medicine And Toxicology: Principles And Practice by Vij pg. 221

TABLE: Difference between Antemortem burns vs Postmortem burns

Features	Antemortem Burns	Postmortem Burns
Line of redness	Present around the injured burn area	Not so
Vesicles	Contain serous fluid with **high proportion of albumin and chloride**	Contain air mostly. If fluid present it comprises of very little albumin and no chlorides
Base of blister	**Red and inflamed**	*Dull, dry, hard and yellow*
Inflammation evidence	Inflammatory edema and repair processes; (+) Leucocyte Infiltration	No such changes noticed
Presence of carbonaceous deposits/soot in the respiratory tract	**PRESENT.** *Indicates death from suffocation following antemortem burn*	Not present
Presence of Car-boxyhemoglobin	Present (its highly suggestive and diagnostic)	Absent
Enzymatic activity	Time related **increase** in enzymatic activity: **Immediate**: Tissue Cathepsin **At 2 hrs**: Leucine Aminopeptidase **At 3 hrs**: Acid Phosphatase **At 4 hrs**: Alkaline Phosphatase	Never noticed

79. Ans. (b) CO poisoning

Ref: The essentials of FSM by KS Narayan Reddy, 31st ed. pg. 582

IMPOTENCY, SEXUAL PERVERSION AND SEXUAL OFFENCES

80. Ans. (b) Tribadism

Ref: Principles of Forensic Medicine & Toxicology, 2017 ed. Bardale, P 316

- **Lesbianism/tribadism:** Gratification of sexual desire of a woman by a woman.
- **Masochism:** Pleasure on receiving painful stimulus from sexual partner.
- **Nymphomania:** Excess sexual desire in female.
- **Transsexualism:** A gender identity that is inconsistent with or not culturally associated with their assigned sex and desire to permanently transition to the gender with which they identify.

81. Ans. (d) 15–49 years

Eligible Couples

For the purpose of family welfare, an eligible couple is the one who is currently married and the wife is in the reproductive phase, i.e. of age 15–49 years. There are nearly 180 such couples per 1000 population on average in India. All these are targeted for family welfare activities. Those with two or more children are targeted for sterilization and with fewer children for spacing methods such as condom, pills and IUDs.

82. Ans. (b) Sexual satisfaction by rubbing the genitalia with the body of the person of opposite sex

Frotteurism: Rubbing the genitalia with the body of the person of other sex for sexual satisfaction.

Sexual perversion	Mode of sexual pleasure
Sadism	Pleasure in giving pain to sexual partner
Masochism	Pleasure on receiving painful stimulus from sexual partner
Bondage	Sadism + masochism are found together
Fetischism	Sexual gratification by article of opposite sex
Frotteurism	Sexual gratification by contact. **Ex: rubbing genitalia on another person**
Exhibitionism	Satisfaction in exhibition of genitals with or without mastutbation
Transvestism/ Eonism	Pleasure in wearing clothes of opposite sex

Contd...

Sexual perversion	Mode of sexual pleasure
Buccal coitus or Sin of Gomorrah	**Fellatio** is oral stimulation of penis by male or female **Cunnilingus** is oral stimulation of female genitals
Voyeurism/ Scotophilia	Also known as Peeping tom Desire to watch sexual intercourse or to observe genitals of others
Trolism	Extreme degree of voyeurism. Ex: A perverted husband enjoy watching his wife having sexual intercourse with another man.
Urolangia	Sexual excitement by sight or odor of urine or faeces.
Tribadism/ Lesbianism	Gratification of sexual desire of a women by another women
Sodomy or Buggery of Greek Love	• Anal sex • **Gerantophilia** –when passive agent is adult • **Paederasty** – when the passive agent is young boy (catamite)
Incest	Sexual intercourse with close relative
Bestiality	Sexual intercourse by a human being with a lower animal

83. Ans. (b) 18 years

Ref: https://www.ageofconsent.net/world/India

The Age of Consent in India is **18 years old**. The age of consent is the minimum age at which an individual is considered legally old enough to consent to participation in sexual activity. Individuals aged 17 or younger in India are not legally able to consent to sexual activity, and such activity may result in prosecution for **statutory rape** or the equivalent local law.

84. Ans. (b) An individual who may be impotent with any particular woman but not with others.

Ref: The Essentials of FSM by K.S. Narayan Reddy, 31st ed. pg. 357-58

- **IMPOTENCE:** inability of a person to perform sexual intercourse. *It cannot be placed as a defense for rape.*
- **STERILITY:** inability of the male to beget children and in the female, the inability to conceive children.
- **FRIGIDITY:** inability to start or maintain the sexual arousal pattern in the female.
- **QUOAD:** an individual who may be impotent with any particular woman but not with others.

85. Ans. (b) Child born after father's death

Ref: The Essentials of FSM by K.S. Narayan Reddy, 31st ed. pg. 369

- **Posthumous child**: Child born after father's death, the mother being conceived by the said father.

- **Suppositious child**: Fictitious child claimed by a women as her own, a women may pretend pregnancy & deliver and later produce a living child as her own or substitute a living male child for a dead child or for a living female child born for her.
- **Spurious or phantom child (pseudocyesis):** Usually seen in women nearing menopause or younger women with an intense desire for children.

86. Ans. (c) Suppositious child

Ref: The Essentials of FSM by K.S. Narayan Reddy, 31st ed. pg. 370; Forensic Medicine By P.V. Guhara, pg. 230

- **A suppositious child** is one produced by a women whom claims it as her own whereas in actual fact it is not her child. A women may substitute a living male child for a dead or living female child born of her or may feign pregnancy and delivery and later produce a living child.
  - *Suppositious child also known as fraudulent offspring*
- **Posthumous child** is a child born after the death of the father in a legally married couple.

87. Ans. (b) Illegitimate child

Ref: The Essentials of FSM by K.S. Narayan Reddy, 31st ed. pg. 369-70; Principles of Forensic Medicine and Toxicology By Rajesh Bardale / 364

- A child is born to a couple who are not married legally is considered to be **illegitimate or a bastard.**

Conditions for being illegitimate or bastard if:
- The child is born out of wedlock OR
- Birth of child is not within a competent period after the cessation of the relationship of a man and wife OR
- Born within wedlock when procreation by the husband is not possible because of congenital or acquired malformation or disease.

88. Ans. (c) Psychogenic

Ref: The Essentials of FSM by K.S. Narayan Reddy, 31st ed. pg. 356-58

- Impotence is inability to perform sexual acticity.
- It is applied to male only
- Most important cause of impotence is: **Psychogenic**
- *If psychogenic cause is ruled out then male factor should be tested next*
- **NOTE:** FRIGIDITY: impotency which is seen in females

89. Ans. (c) Incest

Ref: The Essentials of FSM by K.S. Narayan Reddy, 31st ed. pg. 398

- Incest is Sexual intercourse with close relative. It is not considered as crime in India.

Forensic Medicine

- Other acts like rape, sodomy and indecent actions are considered as crime in India and are punished as and according to law.
    - **Rape**: punished under IPC 376
    - **Adultery**: under IPC 497
    - **Sodomy or any other un-natural sexual activity**: punished under IPC 377
    - **Grievous hurt or Indecent assault**: punished under IPC 320.

- The presence of unruptured hymen is a presumption, BUT IS NOT AN ABSOLUTE PROOF OF VIRGINITY.
- This makes the diagnosis of virginity difficult. With an intact hymen there are: TRUE VIRGINS and FALSE VIRGIN.
- **References states**: *"Hymen may not be ruptured even after repeated acts of coitus if it is loose, lax, folded and **elastic** or thick, tough and fleshy which permits displacement, distortion and stretching without rupture"*

90. Ans. (b) Elastic

Ref: The essentials of FSM by KS Narayan Reddy, 31st ed. pg. 365-66

> **Extra Mile**
> - **MC type of hymen**: Semilunar/Crescentic.

91. Ans. (d) Bisexuality

Ref: The Essentials of FSM by K.S. Narayan Reddy, 31st ed. pg. 402-403

- **Paraphilias**: Abnormal & unorthodox sex play by using unusual objects or parts are know as paraphilia eg. Sadomasochism, Transvestism, Bestiality, Frotteurism, Homosexuality etc.
- **Bisexuality** means hermaphrodite; an individual with both ovary & testis & external genitals of both sexes.

TABLE: Different Paraphilias/Perversion

Sexual perversion	Mode of sexual pleasure
Sadism	Pleasure in giving pain to sexual partner
Masochism	Pleasure on receiving painful stimulus from sexual partner
Bondage	Sadism + masochism are found together
Fetischism	Sexual gratification by article of opposite sex
Frotteurism	Sexual gratification by contact. Ex: rubbing genitalia on another person
Exhibitionism	Satisfaction in exhibition of genitals with or without mastutbation
Transvestism/Eonism	Pleasure in wearing clothes of opposite sex
Uranism	Sexual gratification by fingering, fellatio, cunnilingus etc.
Buccal coitus or Sin of Gomorrah	**Fellatio** is oral stimulation of penis by male or female **Cunnilingus** is oral stimulation of female genitals
Voyeurism/Scotophilia	Also known as Peeping tom Desire to watch sexual intercourse or to observe genitals of others
Trolism	Extreme degree of voyeurism. Ex: A perverted husband enjoy watching his wife having sexual intercourse with another man.
Urolangia/Coprophilia	Sexual excitement by sight or odor of urine or faeces.
Tribadism/Lesbianism	Gratification of sexual desire of a women by another women
Sodomy or Buggery of Greek Love	• Anal sex • Gerantophilia –when passive agent is adult • Paederasty – when the passive agent is young boy (catamite)
Incest	Sexual intercourse with close relative
Bestiality	Sexual intercourse by a human being with a lower animal

FMGE Solutions Screening Examination

92. Ans. (b) Sexual satisfaction by rubbing the genitalia with the body of the person of other sex

Ref: The Essentials of FSM by K.S. Narayan Reddy, 31st ed. pg. 404

- **FROTTEURISM:** rubbing the genitalia with the body of the person of other sex for sexual satisfaction.
- *Refer to above explanation.*

93. Ans. (c) Pleasure in touching opposite sex

Ref: The Essentials of FSM by K.S. Narayan Reddy, 31st ed. pg. 404

Please refer to above explanation.

94. Ans. (a) Voyeurism

Ref: The essentials of FSM by KS Narayan Reddy, 31st ed. pg. 403-404

95. Ans. (a) Transvestism

Ref: The Essentials of FSM by K.S. Narayan Reddy, 31st ed. pg. 403

TRANSVESTISM/ EONISM (trans= opposite; vista = clothing): whole personality is dominated by the desire of being identified with the opposite sex.

96. Ans. (a) Satyriasis

Ref: The essentials of FSM by KS Narayan Reddy, 31st ed. pg. 357

- **SATYRIASIS:** Excessive sexual desire in males
- **Nymphomania:** Excessive sexual desire in females
- **Vaginismus** is one of the causes of female sterilization. It is spasmodic contraction of vagina due to hyperaesthesia.
- **Quoad hoc:** Individual impotent with one particular women, but NOT with others.

97. Ans. (b) Semen

Ref: The Essentials of FSM by K.S. Narayan Reddy, 31st ed. pg. 405

Tests for Detection of

Seminal Stain (*Mnemonic- "Creat Acid Fast Bacilli")*
- **Acid phosphatase test:** to detect Aspermia cases
- **BarberioS test:** to detect Spermine (yellow needle shaped spermine picrate)
- **Creatine phosphokinase test:** for old seminal stain
- **Florence test:** choline crystals of semen shows fluoroscence when examined (*Rhombotic crystals of choline iodide*)
- **Most specific test for seminal stain:** Isoenzyme LDH assay
- **For dry seminal stain:** UV rays used

Blood Benzidine test
- Best preliminary test as it detects blood present in dilution of 1 in 3 lakhs.
- Color produced: Deep Blue
- Not used because it is a potential carcinogen.

Kastle-Mayer/Phenolpthalein test- color produced is Pink Purple.

Microchemical test: Based on RBC content of blood.
- **Takayama's test:** Hb converted to Haemochromogen crystal.
  - Salmon pink feathery haemochromogen crystals are obtained.
- **Teichmann's Haemin crystal test:** Hb converted into Hemin/Hematin crystals.
  - Brown rhombic haemic crystal are seen
- **Spectroscopic test:** Most specific/confirmatory method for blood stain test
- Thin layer chromatography (TLC)
- Electrophoresis

Note: *Test to distinguish human vs. animal blood-* **Precipitin Test.**

98. Ans. (a) Choline

Ref: The Essentials of FSM by K.S. Narayan Reddy, 31st ed. pg. 405-406

Please refer to above explanation.

99. Ans. (b) Barberios Test

Ref: The Essentials of FSM by K.S. Narayan Reddy, 31st ed. pg. 405

Please refer to above explanation.

100. Ans. (a) Amylase

• Amylase	Saliva
• Ortho-toluidine	Blood
• Acid phosphatase	Semen
• Tetra-methyl-Benzidine	Blood

INJURY/ GUNSHOT INJURY/FIREARM INJURY/ STAB WOUND

101. Ans. (a) Paraffin wax

Ref: Principle of Forensic Medicine & Toxicology, 2017 ed. Bardale, P 217,

- **The basic formula for black powder:**
  - A mixture of saltpeter (potassium nitrate), charcoal and sulfur.

FORENSIC MEDICINE

480

- Later versions of gunpowder contain these same basic ingredients, but the overall chemistry evolved to include modifications that produced "smokeless gunpowder," **Cordite**, which eliminated the sulfur.
- Other advances added materials such as nitrocellulose (guncotton) and glycerol trinitrate (nitroglycerin).

• Gunshot residue, or simply GSR, is a means of testing for the presence of certain materials on the hands and clothing of a subject in hopes of determining that this individual may have discharged a firearm.

• Gunshot residue contains burned particles (potassium nitrite) and some unburned particles (potassium nitrate), and criminal investigators collected these particles by **applying melted paraffin wax to a subject's hands**. Upon removal of the wax cast, a reagent containing diphenylamine and sulfuric acid was applied to the cast. The development of blue specks was indicative of the presence of nitrates.

102. Ans. (b) Scrotum

• *Lacerated looking incised wound* is seen at area where there is loose skin. For example scrotum and axilla.
• *Incised looking lacerated wounds* are seen at area where there is bony prominences. For example forehead, shin, etc.

103. Ans. (d) Bilirubin on 9th day

Ageing or Dating of Bruise

• As bruises heal, there is a gradual destruction and removal of the extravasated blood. Color change *starts at the periphery and extends inwards to the center.*
• It follows this order:

Red (Oxyhemoglobin)
↓
Blue (Deoxyhemoglobin)
↓
Brown/violet (Hemosiderin) by day 5
↓
Green (Hematoidin/biliverdin) – day 5 to 7
↓
Yellow (Bilirubin) – after day 7

104. Ans. (b) From the periphery

• A large bruise takes longer time to heal than a smaller bruise. The color changes begin at the periphery first.
• A large old bruise may contain all possible colors seen in a bruise – from purple in the center to yellow at the edges.

105. Ans. (d) Keyhole

Ref: Forensic medicine, Clinical and Pathological aspect by Jason, Anthony and Williams. pg. 161

• If a bullet strikes the skull at an oblique, shallow angle, a characteristic defect may occur. This defect is often referred to as "keyhole defect" based on its resemblance to an old fashioned wooden door keyhole.
• **Graze wound** occurs when a bullet strikes the skin at a shallow angle and passess across the skin almost parallel to the skin surface, abrading the skin without penetrating the body. Abrasion produced is elongated, ovoid to elliptical in shape.
• **In tangential gunshot wound** bullet strikes the skin at a shallow angle, but penetrates into subcutaneous tissue, lacerating the tissue before exiting at a point separate from entry. The entry and exit wound appear as crescent shaped abrasion.

> **Extra Mile**
>
> **TABLE:** Wounds from shot gun suggesting range
>
> | Shape of wound | Distance |
> |---|---|
> | Cruciate or stellate shaped | Contact over bone |
> | Oval shaped | Up to 30 cm |
> | Rat hole wound | 30–100 cm |
> | Satellite wound | More than 2 meters |
> | Individual pellets | Over 4 meters |

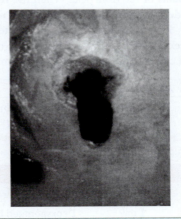

106. Ans. (a) Pressure Abrasion

Ref: The Essentials of FSM by K.S. Narayan Reddy, 31st ed. pg. 166-67

• **Abrasion:** An injury involving superficial layers of skin & is caused by friction between skin & some rough object. It is of 3 types:

FMGE Solutions Screening Examination

Scratch	Graze	Imprint/Pressure/Contact abrasion
• Produced by sharp object as pin • Direction of injury is indicated by sharp edge initially & heaped up epithelium at end	• Also known as Friction or brush burn • Produced when broad surface of skin slides against rough surface	• Also known as Patterned abrasion • Produced as a result of direct impact or pressure with some object. • **Example:** ligature mark in hanging & strangulation; nail & thumb mark in throttling; **teeth mark in biting**; tire marks in accident etc.

107. Ans. (c) Graze abrasion

Ref: The Essentials of FSM by K.S. Narayan Reddy, 31st ed. pg. 166-67

- Brush burn or friction burn is seen in graze abrasion.
- Produced when broad surface of skin slides against rough surface.

108. Ans. (b) Spine

Ref: The essentials of FSM by KS Narayan Reddy, 31st ed. pg. 246

- Fracture of spine need not injure the cord, but the cord is rarely injured without associated fractures of the vertebral column. **"Whiplash injury"** is an exception to this rule. This injury sustained commonly by the occupants of the front seat. When the vehicle comes to a sudden stop, there is forward thrust which produces acute hyperflexion but this converted into acute hyperextension as the forehead strikes the windscreen which causes injury to the cervical column.

109. Ans. (b) 2 day

Ref: The Essentials of FSM by K.S. Narayan Reddy, 31st ed. pg. 169-70

TABLE: Color Changes of Bruise according to duration and systemic causes

Color	Duration	Due to
Red	Day 0	Hemoglobin (fresh blood)
Blue	1 day	Deoxygenated hemoglobin
Bluish Black/ Dark Blue to Brown	2-4 days	Hemosiderin
Green	5-7 days	Biliverdin/Haematoidin
Yellow	7-10 days	Bilirubin
Normal color	14-15 days	Pigment removed by phagocytes

Note: *These color changes are not seen in subconjunctival hemorrhage which is being kept oxygenated by air. It is red at first then becomes yellow and finally disappears.*

110. Ans. (c) Injury common in moving head

Ref: The Essentials of FSM by K.S. Narayan Reddy 31st ed. pg. 233; Reddy's Essentials of forensic medicine & toxicology 23 ed. pg. 205

- Coup & Countre coup lesions are most commonly seen in brain.
- Remember countre coup injury this way:
  - When a body is in motion, brain is also in motion in same direction.
  - A sudden stop, puts the body in static condition, but the brain is still in motion, and hits the skull leading to injury known as coup injury, brain then again hits on the opposite side causing countrecoup injury.

TABLE: Differences between coup and countre coup injury

Coup	Countre-coup
• Means that the injury is located towards the side of impact/injury. • It results directly by the impacting force • Seen MC in stationary condition	• Means that the lesion is present in an area opposite the side of impact/injury. • It results due to sudden hitch of a moving head. • Seen MC in moving head

111. Ans. (d) Nitrocellulose

Ref: The essentials of FSM by KS Narayan Reddy, 31st ed. pg. 197-98

Gun powders can be of two types and is made of:

Black gun powder	Smokeless powder
Consists of: • Potassium nitrate 75% • Sulphur 10% • Charcoal 15%	Consists of: • *Nitrocellulose* (single base; gun cotton) • Nitroglycerine + Nitrocellulose • Nitroglycerine + Nitrocellulose + Nitroguanidine (triple base)

112. Ans. (d) Two bullets are ejected one after the other

Ref: The Essentials of FSM by K.S. Narayan Reddy, 31st ed. pg. 213

- **Tandem or Piggyback bullet** are the bullets ejected one after the other, when the first bullet having been stuck in the barrel, fails to leave the barrel & is ejected when the next bullet is fired.

Forensic Medicine

> **Extra Mile**
>
> **TABLE:** Different types of bullet movements
>
> | Term | Feature |
> |---|---|
> | Yawning Bullet | Bullet which travel in an irregular fashion instead of travelling straight and cause a key hole entry wound. |
> | Ricochet bullet | Bullet strikes some intervening object first, and then after ricocheting & rebounding from this hits the object. |
> | Dum dum Bullet | A jacketed bullet with its nose cut off to expose the core and it expands on impact |
> | Tumbling B. | One that rotates in end on end during its motion. |
> | Souvenir Bullet | A bullet left in body for long time & it gets surrounded by dense fibrous tissue |
> | Gutter wound | Bullet strikes the skull but does not enter and travel in soft tissue and form an elongated gutter like depression |
> | Bullet gaze/slap | Bullet that does not perforate the skin, but produces only friction wound |

113. Ans. (a) Direction of injury

Ref: The essentials of FSM by KS Narayan Reddy, 31st ed. pg. 178

- Tailing of wound is one of the characteristics of the incised wound which indicates the direction in which the cut was made.
- Incised wounds are deeper at the beginning as more pressure is exerted at this point (head of wound). Towards the end of the cut the wound becomes increasingly shallow, till finally as the knife leaves the tissues, the skin alone is cut. This is known as tailing of wound.

114. Ans. (d) Chopping

Ref: The essentials of FSM by KS Narayan Reddy, 31st ed. pg. 182-83

- Stab wound is produced when force is delivered along long axis of narrow or a pointed object, such as knife, dagger, sword, chisel, screw driver etc into the depth of the body.
- It can present as point wound, puncture wound or perforation.
- **Chop wound/slash wound** are deep gaping wound caused by a blow with the sharp cutting edge with a heavy weapon like axe, sword, chopper or meat cleaver.

115. Ans. (a) Suicide

Ref: The essentials of FSM by K.S. Narayan Reddy, 31st ed. pg. 180

- Tentative cuts/Hesitation marks are multiple small superficial cuts seen in cases where there is a trial of suicide.
- MC site for tentative cuts are: **Forearm**

116. Ans. (c) Avulsion

Ref: KS Narayana Reddy's 'The Essentials of Forensic Medicine and Toxicology'; 29/e, p-171

Avulsion (Shearing Laceration)

- The shearing and grinding force by a weight, such as heavy vehichle wheel passing over a limb may produce separation of the skin from the underlying tissues over a relatively large area. This is called 'flaying'.
- The underlying muscles are crushed and the bones may be fractured.
- The separated skin may show abrasions from the rotating frictional effect of the tyre, but one portion is still in continuity with the adjacent skin.

ABORTION, THANATOLOGY AND HANGING

117. (b) Nysten's rule

Ref: Forensic Medicine: Clinical and Pathological Aspects, P 101

- Nysten's rule describes that rigor mortis doesn't start in all muscles simultaneously. It can be used for rough estimation of time since death.
- The law states: *"the rigidity in humans begins in mandibular joint then in trunk and neck, followed by upper extremities and then lower extremities. It follows the same order during resolution".*
- The development of rigor mortis is thus descending.

118. Ans. (b) Head

Ref: APC Essentials of Forensic Medicine By Anil Aggarwal P. 143

- In suspected cranial injury, neck and chest should be opened first. It decompresses the CVS draining the blood in chest cavity.
- While in suspected neck trauma/hanging, **cranial cavity is opened first** to drain out blood from head. A bloodless field is thus created in the neck which prevents artifactual hemorrhages occurring in the neck.
- The **neck should be opened or dissected last** in case of death due to asphyxia/hanging.
- This is because the neck structure show marked congestion and suffusion of blood along with petechial hemorrhage in cases of asphyxia, therefore in an already congested neck it becomes sometimes difficult to distinguish a bruise on neck from congestion.
- Therefore, the neck needs to be drained of blood by opening the other structures like head, thorax, abdomen first to have a clear field devoid of artifacts.

FMGE Solutions Screening Examination

119. Ans. (d) 1.04

Ref: Guide to Forensic Medicine & Toxicology, P 157

TABLE: Difference between respired and unrespired lung

Character	Unrespired lung	Respired lung
Weight in relation to body weight	1/70	1/35
Specific gravity	1.04	0.94
Color	Uniform, reddish	Mottled/marbled appearance

120. Ans. (c) 1/35

Ref: Textbook and Principles of Forensic Medicine by Bardale, P 357:

Character	Unrespired lungs	Respired lungs
Weight in relation to body weight	1/70	1/35
Volume	Small	Large and covers the heart
Consistency	Liver like: Dense firm noncrepitant	Soft, spongy, elastic, crepitant
Extension	Up to the level of 4th and 5th rib	Up to the level of 6th and 7th rib
Specific gravity	1.04	0.94
Margin	Sharp	Rounded
Color	Uniform reddish	Mottled/marbled appearance
Air vesicle	Not inflated	Inflated
Section	Little froth less blood exudates on pressure	Abundant frothy blood exudates
Breslow life test	Whole or part sinks	Expanded
Microscopy	Cuboidal lining	Squamous epithelium
Blood vessel	Less patent	More patent

121. Ans. (c) Chelioscopy

Ref: Textbook of forensic medicine and toxicology by R N Karmakar pg. 358

Chelioscopy is the study of furrows or grooves present on the lips.

Le Moyne Snyder (1950) pointed out that the pattern of the furrows on the lips like finger prints are also individualistic and the prints left over glass, wine bottles, cup, saucer, fruit, cloth, paper, love letters may help in identification. Later on *Santosh* classified the furrows or the grooves of the lips into simple and compound types and further subdivided into 6 types.

Kazvo Suzuki and Yasvo Tsuchihashi (1970) classified lip prints as follows (Figs)

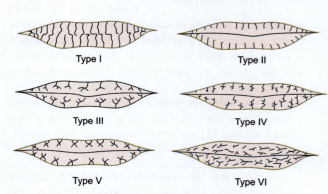

FIGURES: Types of lip-prints

- Type-I (Long vertical type)—Grooves running vertically for whole length

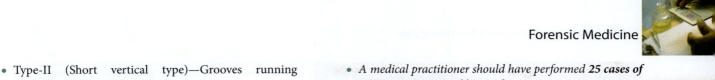

Forensic Medicine

- Type-II (Short vertical type)—Grooves running vertically for partial length
- Type-III (Branching type)—Grooves are branched.
- Type-IV (Diamond type)—Grooves are intersected
- Type-V (Reticular type)—Grooves are reticulated
- Type-VI (Non-specific type)—Irregular having no specific pattern

122. Ans. (a) Pulmonary embolism

- In death certificate, 1A is the immediate cause of death. Like in this example, diabetic patient developed DVT, which leads to pulmonary embolism. The pulmonary embolism is the immediate cause of death.
- Line 1c is known as essence of death certificate.
- Given below is an example of death certificate:

Cause of death the disease or condition thought to be the underlying cause should appear in the lowest completed line of part I		
I	(a) *Disease or condition leading **directly** to death*	Intraperitoneal hemorrhage
	(b) *Other disease or condition, if any, **leading to** I(a)*	Ruptured metastatic deposit in liver
	(c) *Other disease or condition, If any, leading to I(b)*	Primary adenocarcinoma of ascending colon
II	*Other significant conditions* **Contributing to death** *but not Related to the disease or Condition causing it*	Non–insulin dependent diabetes mellitus

The colon cancer on line I (c) led directly to the liver metastases on line I (b), which ruptured, causing the fatal hemorrhage on I (a). Adenocarcinoma of the colon is the underlying cause of death

123. Ans. (a) Hyperextension of the neck

Hyperextension is more dangerous because flexion is protected by the contraction of strong posterior neck muscles.

124. Ans. (b) 20 weeks

Medical Termination is permitted up to 20th week.

- Indications of MTP:
  - **Social:** Failure of contraceptives in a married woman.
  - **Eugenic:** Child born with serious physical or mental abnormalities
  - **Therapeutic:** If continuation of pregnancy endangers life.
  - **Humanitarian:** If pregnancy is the outcome of rape.

Important points about MTP act 1971:

- Only a qualified registered practitioner can perform it. Chief Medical Officer of district is empowered to certify that a doctor can perform it.
- A medical practitioner should have performed **25 cases of MTP** in a recognized hospital
- The operation should be performed either in a Government hospital or a place recognized by government.
- Non government institutions authorized by chief medical officer can also perform MTP.
- Consent of husband is **not** required, however written consent of the women or her guardian (if she is minor or mentally ill) is required
- Abortion can't be performed at the husband's request, if the woman is not willing.
- **No age proof is required**
- If the woman was raped, it's not necessary to lodge a police complaint
- Professional secrecy should be maintained
- If the duration of pregnancy is <12 weeks, opinion of single doctor is required
- Between 12 and 20 weeks, two doctors should consent that there is an indication.
- Termination can be performed by any of the doctor

125. Ans. (b) Prominent frontal emience

Ref: Review of Forensic medicine by Sumit Seth pg. 5–6

TABLE: Important identification differences between male and female

		Male	Female
Skull	General appearance	Larger, heavier	Smaller, lighter, smooth
	Capacity:	1500–1550 cc	Capacity: 1350–1400 cc
	Forehead:	Steeper, less rounded	Vertical, round
	Orbits	Square, relatively smaller	Rounded, relatively larger
	Frontal eminence	Small	Large
	Mastoid	Large, round, blunt	Small, smooth, pointed
	Rest all structure	Larger, broader	Relatively small, less prominent
Mandible	General	Larger and thicker	Smaller and thinner
	Chin	Square	Rounded
	Angle of body and ramus	Less obtuse (125°), prominent, everted	More obtuse, not prominent, inverted

Contd...

FMGE Solutions Screening Examination

		Male	Female
Pelvis	General	Deep funnel	Flat bowl
	Framework	Massive, tougher, narrow, tough	Less massive, smooth
	Preauricular sulcus	Not frequent, shallow, narrow	Frequent, deep, broad
	Obturator foramen	Large, OVAL with base upwards	Small, triangular with apex forward
	Greater sciatic notch	Smaller, narrower, deeper	Larger, Wider, shallower
	Subpubic angle	V shaped, 70–75°	U-shaped, 75–90°
	Corpobasal index of sacrum	More in males	Less in female

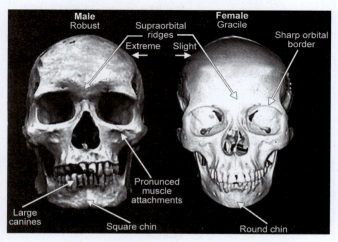

FIGURES: Comparison of male and female pelvis

FIGURES: Comparison of male and female skullls

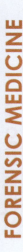

126. Ans. (b) Medical assistant can perform in absence of gynecologist

Ref: The Essentials of FSM by K.S. Narayan Reddy, 31st ed. pg. 374-75

- **Indications of MTP:**
  - **Social:** failure of contraceptives in a married woman.
  - **Eugenic:** child borne with serious physical or mental abnormalities
  - **Therapeutic:** if continuation of pregnancy endangers life.
  - **Humanitarian:** if pregnancy is the outcome of rape.

Important Points about MTP act 1971

- Only a qualified registered practitioner can perform it, Chief medical officer of district is empowered to certify that a doctor can perform it.
- *A medical practitioner should have performed 25 cases of MTP in a recognised hospital*
- The operation should be performed either in a Government hospital or a recognised place by government.
- Non government institutions authorised by chief medical officer can also perform MTP.
- *Consent of husband not required, however written consent of the woman or her guardian (If she is minor or mentally ill)*
- Abortion can't be performed at her husband's request, if the woman is not willing.
- **No age proof is required**
- If the woman was raped, it's not necessary to lodge a police complaint
- Professional secrecy should be maintained
- If the duration of pregnancy is < 12 weeks opinion of single doctor is required
- Between 12-20 weeks two doctors should consent that there is an indication.
- Termination can be performed by any of the doctor
- Termination permitted upto 20th week.

127. Ans. (d) Age proof is generally not required

Ref: The Essentials of FSM by K.S. Narayan Reddy, 31st ed. pg. 374-75

- Please read the question carefully. After reading the options of this question, we generally get a tendency to mark among option A to C.
- Please read the last option carefully, it's given as if it has no significance. But actually that's the correct answer.
- In case of MTP, age proof is not required.
- *Please refer to the previous answer for detailed explanation.*

Forensic Medicine

128. Ans. (d) 25

Ref: *The Essentials of FSM by K.S. Narayan Reddy, 31st ed. pg. 374-375*

Please refer to above explanation.

129. Ans. (a) Occiput

Ref: *The Essentials of FSM by K.S. Narayan Reddy, 31st ed. pg. 314-15*

HANGING

- A form of violent asphyxia as a result of suspension of the body by a ligature round the neck the constricting force being the weight of body.

TABLE: Type of Hanging according to position of Knot

Typical Hanging	Atypical Hanging
• Knot of ligature should be at the nape of neck on the back (Occiput). • 'V' shape above thyroid cartilage • Eg: suicide hanging	• At any site other than the nape of neck • **Most common site is near on angle of mandible** • No V-shape • Eg: Judicial hanging

130. Ans. (d) 4.50 kg

Ref: *The Essentials of FSM by K.S. Narayan Reddy, 31st ed. pg. 314-18*

- Upon hanging the death can either be cervical bone fracture or can be secondary to vascular occlusion.
- **In case of partial hanging some part of body touching the ground. Therefore weight responsible for death is weight of head, which is nearly equal to 4–5 kg.**
- There are 4 important vascular structures in neck which can bear weight of upto:
  - **Jugular vein: 2 kg**
  - Carotid artery: 5 kg
  - Tracheal artery: 15 kg
  - Vertebral artery: 20-30 kg.

TABLE: Type of Hanging according to degree of suspension

Complete hanging	Incomplete (partial) hanging
• Body is fully suspended & no part of body touches the ground • Constricting force is weight of body	• The lower part of body is in touch with ground • Weight of head acts as constricting force

131. Ans. (c) Saliva dribbling to the opposite side of the knot

Ref: *Textbook of Forensic Medicine and Toxicology: Principles and Practice by Vij/162*

TABLE: Difference between Hanging and Strangulation by ligature

Trait	Hanging	Strangulation by ligature
Manner of death	Mostly suicidal	Homicidal
Face	Pale, No petechiae	**Red congested,** marked petechiae
Bleeding	Bleeding from nose, mouth and ears not common	Common
Saliva	Often dribbles out of mouth	Very rare
Ligature	Oblique, Non-continuous, placed high up in the neck between chin and larynx	Horizontal or transverse, continuous round the neck, low down in the neck below or across the thyroid
Abrasion and Ecchymosis around the edge of ligature	Rare	Common
Larynx and trachea fracture	Rare That too in Judicial hanging	Comparatively more common

Note: Position of knot in suicidal hanging is at the nape of neck. In Judicial hanging position of knot mostly is at the angle of mandible.

132. Ans. (a) Hanging

Ref: *The Essentials of FSM by KS Narayan Reddy, 31st ed. pg. 319*

- Le facies sympathique is an expression which is seen in cases of antemortem hanging.
- When the ligature knot presses on cervical sympathetic, the eyes on the same side may remain open and its pupil dilated. This particular finding is known as le facies sympathique.

133. Ans. (a) Burking

Ref: *The essentials of FSM by KS Narayan Reddy, 31st ed. pg. 335*

- **Strangulation** is a form of asphyxia which is caused by constriction of the neck by a ligature without suspending the body. It can be several types:
  - **Bansdola:** One bamboo stick at back of neck and other at the front of neck. Both ends tied with rope which causes death of the victim.
  - **Garotting:** Victim is attacked from behind with a rope over the neck.
  - **Mugging:** Strangulation caused by holding the neck of the victim in the bend of the elbow.

- **Suffocation is** a form of asphyxia, which is caused by deprivation of oxygen, either due to lack of oxygen in environment or from obstruction of air passages at the level of nose and mouth.
- **Forms of suffocation asphyxia:**
  - **Burking** is a method of homicidal **smothering and traumatic asphyxia.**
  - **Smothering:** form of asphyxia caused by closing the external respiratory orifices either by hand or other means
  - **Gagging:** Asphyxia by forcing cloth into the mouth.
  - **Overlaying:** Asphyxia due to compression of chest. Ex: Mother overlied on infant.
  - **Choking:** Asphyxia by obstruction of air passages, usually between the pharynx and bifurcation of trachea. Almost always accidental.
  - **Café coronary:** Alcoholic who is grossly intoxicated dies while having meal. Death occurs due to sudden heart attack. High blood alcohol content anesthesizes the gag reflex.

134. Ans. (a) Homicidal smothering and traumatic asphyxia

Ref: The essentials of FSM by KS Narayan Reddy, 31st ed. pg. 335

Please refer to above explanation.

135. Ans. (b) Suffocation

Ref: The Essentials of FSM by KS Narayan Reddy, 31st ed. pg. 335

Please refer to above explanation.

136. Ans. (d) Eyelids

Ref: The Essentials of FSM by K.S. Narayan Reddy 31st ed. pg. 140-43, 147; Reddy's, 27th pg. 142

Order of appearance and disappearance (in sequence)
- Heart (left chamber in 1 hour)
- Eyelids (3-4 hours)
- Face muscles
- Neck and trunk
- Upper extremities
- Legs
- Small muscle of finger and toes (last to be affected, 11–12 hours)

> **Extra Mile**
> - Postmortem rigidity lasts for **18-36 hours in** summer and 24–48 hours in winter.
> - Postmortem rigidity disappear in the same order as that of the appearance

137. Ans. (d) 60°C

Ref: AK Gupta's 'Essentials of Forensic medicine & Toxicology' 4/e, p-96

- When temperature of flame is 65 degree Celsius or above, body is rigid with limbs flexed known as pugilistic or Fencing posture **due to coagulation of albumin constituents of muscles (Boxer's posture in defence).**
- But this is not always a true ante-mortem phenomenon as heat stiffening can occur after death due to postmortem burns.

138. Ans. (a) Neck

Ref. Forensic Medicine and Toxicology' by RN Karmakar
Bloodless dissection of neck is to be done in asphyxia.

FORENSIC PSYCHIATRY

139. Ans. (b) Lung maturity

Tests to detect infanticide:
- **Fodere test:** The lungs are ligated across the hila and separated. Weight of the lung in an infant before respiration is 30 g, after respiration it doubles. The increase in weight is due to increased flow of blood.
- **Plouquets test:** Weight of the lung is 1/70th of the total fetal weight before respiration and 1/35th of the total weight after respiration.
- **Breslau's second life test:** Test to detect air in stomach and intestine

140. Ans. (a) Intake of indigestible plant materials

- Bezoar is mass found trapped in GIT
- A **phytobezoar** is a type of bezoar, or trapped mass in the stomach, that consists of components of indigestible plant material, such as fibres, skins and seeds. It is frequently reported in patients with impaired digestion and decreased gastric motility.
- **Trichobezoar** is a bezoar formed from hair.
- **Pharmacobezoar:** are mostly tablets or semi-liquid masses of drugs, normally found following overdose of sustained-release medications.

Forensic Medicine

ANSWERS TO BOARD REVIEW QUESTIONS

489

141. Ans. (b) Race

Ref: Parikh 6th ed. / 2.26, http://en.wikipedia.org/wiki/
Cephalic_index

142. Ans. (a) Physical torture

Ref: Textbook of forensic medicine and toxicology:
Principles and practice, 5/e, By Krishan Vij / 192

143. Ans. (c) Beating on both ears

Ref: Reddy 5th ed. / 257

144. Ans. (b) Cocaine

Ref: Parikh 6th ed. 11.9

145. Ans. (b) Dhatura

Ref: Parikh 6th ed. 11.30

146. Ans. (a) Methyl alcohol

147. Ans. (a) Physostigmine

Ref:Medical Toxicology edited by Richard C. Dard
3rd ed / 567

148. Ans. (a) Heroin

Ref: Parikh 6th ed. 10.54

149. Ans. (a) Benzodiazepine

Ref: Parikh 6th ed. /11.16

150. Ans. (c) 40 years

Ref: Textbook of Forensic medicine and Toxicology:
Principles and Practice, 5/e, p 43

151. Ans. (b) 2003

Ref: Selected Topics in Obstetrics and Gynaecology-3:
For Postgraudate and by Shirish N Daftar, http://www.
rajswasthya.nic.in

152. Ans. (a) Edge of blade

Ref: Parikh 6th ed / 4.16, Oxford Handbook of forensic
Medicine by Jonathan P. Wyatt, Tim Squires,
Guy Norfolk / 135

153. Ans. (c) Lacerations

Ref: Forensic Pathology for Forensic Scientists, Police,
and Death investigators by Joseph Prahlow/305

154. Ans. (b) 18 years

Ref: Forensic Medicine: Clinical and pathological aspects
edited by Jason Payne-James Anthony Busuttil, William
Smock / 395, http://india.gov.in/allimpfrms/allacts/2606

155. Ans. (a) Cyanide

Ref: Parikh 6th ed /8.38

156. Ans. (d) Water

Ref: Parikh 6th ed /9.2

157. Ans. (b) Rifling

Ref: Parikh 6th ed / 4.34

158. Ans. (c) 200 mg

Ref: Parikh 6th ed / 8.39

159. Ans. (b) Mercury

Ref: Harrison 18/e, chapter 371

160. Ans. (a) Aluminium

Ref: Harrison 18/, chapter 371

161. Ans. (b) Cocaine

Ref: Parikh 6/e, p 11.9

162. Ans. (b) Lead poisoning

Ref: Parikh 6/e, p 9.18

163. Ans. (b) Uterus

Ref: Parikh 6/e, p 3.26

164. Ans. (b) Bone marrow

Ref: Forensic medicine and toxicology, R. N. Karmakar
154, Review of forensic medicine, Toxicoloty by gautam
biswas 2/e, p 160

165. Ans. (c) 18 years

Ref: Parikh 6/e, p 5.29

Explanations

FMGE Solutions Screening Examination

166. Ans. (c) Insult of modesty of a woman

Ref: Textbook of forensic medicine and toxicology: Principles and practice, 5/e, Krishnan vij, p 211

167. Ans. (d) 324

Ref: Textbook on the Indian penal code by Krishna deo gaur 4/e, p 587

168. Ans. (b) Torture

Ref: Ethics for doctors, Nurses and patients by H.P. Dunn P 37, World medical association website and various internet resources

169. Ans. (c) Dum dum bullet

Ref: Parikh 6/e, p 4.26, Textbook of forensic medicine and toxicology: Principle and practice 5/e, krishan vij, p 239, Forensic medicine and toxicology by R.N. Karmakar, p 157

170. Ans. (b) Section 32 IEA

Ref: Textbook of forensic medicine and Toxicology by Krishan, p 7-8, Textbook on The law of evidence-M. Monir, P 145

171. Ans. (a) 30%

Ref: Forensic medicine by P.V. Guharaj, 2/e, p 397

172. Ans. (b) Lead

Ref: Parikh 6/e, p 9.22

173. Ans. (b) Phosphorous

Ref: Parikh 6/e, p 9.2, Textbook of forensic medicine and Toxicology by Nagesh kumar rao, p 371, Modern medical toxicology by V.V. Pillary, 3/e, p 61

174. Ans. (a) Calcium gluconate

Ref: Harrison's 17/e, Chapter 346

175. Ans. (b) Chronic $CuSO_4$ poisoning

Ref: Forensic medicine and toxicology R.N. Karmakar, 3/e, p 94, Clinical immunotoxicology by David S. Newcombe, p 233

176. Ans. (b) 318

Ref: Parikh 6, p 5.87

177. Ans. (b) Section 416 CrPC

Ref: Principles of forensic medicine and toxicology by Rajesh bardale, p 3, Textbook on the Indian penal code by Krishna deo gaur, p 107

178. Ans. (c) Organs are removed one by one

Ref: Parikh 6/e/5.71, Handbook of death and dying, vol. 1, Clifton D. Bryant/530, 531, Ludwig J. Handbook of Autopsy Practice. 3/e, Totowa, NJ: Humana Press, 2002, Volmar KE. History of autopsy technique. In: Collins KA, Hutchins GM, eds. Autopsy performance and reporting. 2./e, Northfield, Ill, Col. of American Pathologister, 2003

179. Ans. (d) Brain

Ref: Esssential forensic neuropathology, p 94

180. Ans. (c) Wrinkled dusty sclera

Ref: Parikh 7/e, p 3.10, Knight's forensic pathology, 3/e, p 54

181. Ans. (a) 3 to 5 hours

Ref: Parikh 7/e, p 3.10, Knight's forensic pathology 3rd/e, p 54

182. Ans. (a) Estimate fetal age

Ref: Textbook of forensic medicine and toxicology by nageshkumar rao, p 321

183. Ans. (c) To protect the accused

Ref: Parikh 7/e, p 1.11

184. Ans. (c) 50% glycerine

Ref: Textbook of forensic medicine and toxicology: Principles and practice by vij 4/e, p 33

185. Ans. (a) Loops

Ref: Fingerprint Analysis Laboratory Workbook by Hillary Moses Daluz, P 15-16

- **Loops are the** most common type of finger print present in around 60-70% of the finger prints.
- **Whorls** are the second most common type of finger print, seen in around 30-35% of finger prints.
- **Arches** are the least common type of finger print, seen in only 5% of finger prints.
- **Fingerprint classifications are:**
  - Henry classification system
  - National Crime Information System classification period

186. Ans. (d) Root resorption at the base

Forensic Medicine

GUSTAFSON'S METHOD

- This method is based on morphological and histological changes of the teeth.
- This assessed **regressive changes** such as:
  - Amount of occlusal attrition(A)
  - Coronal secondary dentine deposition(S)
  - Loss of periodontal attachment(P)
  - Cementum apposition at the root apex(C)

- Root resorption at the apex(R)
- Dentine translucency(T)
  An + Sn + Pn + Cn + Rn + Tn = X; a total score
- Age was estimated using the formula
  Age = (11.43 + 3.63X) years
- If was found that an increase in the total score corresponds to an increase in age

---

ANSWER TO IMAGE-BASED QUESTION

187. Ans. (b) Arsenic Poisoning

Explanations

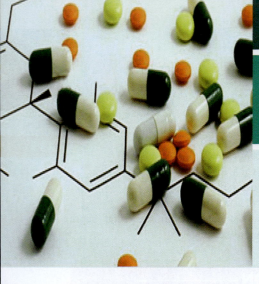

Preventive and Social Medicine (PSM)

MOST RECENT QUESTIONS 2019

1. Inertization is:
   a. Reducing organic and combustible waste to inorganic
   b. Burning biomedical waste
   c. Biomedical waste converted into non harmless
   d. To avoid water contamination
2. Amplifier host of Japanese encephalitis:
   a. Pig   b. Dogs
   c. Cats   d. Birds
3. Best index for calculation of nutrient value of protein
   a. Serum albumin concentration
   b. Arm-muscle circumference
   c. Creatinine-height index
   d. Serum transferrin level
4. Best index for measurement health indicator in society:
   a. Under 5 mortality rate
   b. Infant Mortality Rate
   c. Child death rate
   d. Maternal mortality rate
5. Which of these has the max natural source of vitamin A?
   a. Carrot   b. Halibut liver oil
   c. Cod fish oil   d. Cow milk
6. According to WHO, marker for obesity Index is:
   a. Quetelet index   b. Chandler index
   c. Pearl index   d. Sullivan's index
7. According to WHO, which one is a notifiable disease?
   a. Yellow fever   b. Polio
   c. Influenza   d. Malaria
8. Most common reported disease in post disaster period:
   a. Acute gastroenteritis
   b. Pneumonia
   c. Leptospirosis
   d. Malnutrition
9. Amount of sodium in ORS as per WHO:
   a. 65 mmol/L
   b. 75 mmol/L
   c. 20 mmol/L
   d. 100 mmol/L
10. As compared to cow milk, the protein content of human milk is:
    a. 3–4 times more than cow milk
    b. 3–4 times less than cowmilk
    c. Double than cow milk   d. Same as cowmilk
11. BCG is diluted with:
    a. NS   b. DW
    c. RL   d. Distilled water
12. Nowadays which is the most common pasteurization method?
    a. Holder (vat) method
    b. Ultra high temperature method
    c. High temperature and short time method
    d. Low temperature and long time method
13. True about Quarantine:
    a. Restriction of movement of Infected patient
    b. Restriction of movement of healthy contact of an infectious disease
    c. Movement restricted for shortest incubation period
    d. Isolation of diseased person
14. Which test is done at sub Centre during pregnancy:
    a. USG   b. Haemoglobin
    c. OGTT   d. Triple test

CONCEPT OF HEALTH AND DISEASE

15. True about PQLI   *(Recent Pattern Question 2016)*
    a. Literacy rate, birth rate, life expectancy at birth
    b. Life expectancy at 1 year, IMR, literacy rate
    c. Life expectancy at birth, income, literacy rate
    d. Soon to be replaced by GNP
16. Father of public health:
    a. Tuberculosis   b. Cholera
    c. Malaria   d. Plague
17. PQLI lies between:
    a. 0 and 1   b. 0 and 10
    c. 0 and 100   d. 1 and 10
18. Which of the following is true about Human Development Index:
    a. Maternal mortality rate   b. IMR
    c. Life expectancy-Birth   d. Life expectancy- 1 year

Preventive and Social Medicine (PSM)

19. **HDI consists of all EXCEPT:**
   a. Real GDP per capita income
   b. Life expectancy at birth
   c. Mean year of schooling and expected year of schooling
   d. Range 0 to 100

20. **Human development index value is:**
   a. 0–1
   b. 0–100
   c. Any number
   d. No number

21. **Not included in PQLI is:**
   a. Income
   b. Literacy
   c. Life expectancy at age 1
   d. Infant mortality

22. **Image of iceberg phenomenon with value of 12 cases mentioned above the surface, 20 at the surface, 50 beneath the surface. Which disease has following pattern:**
   a. Tuberculosis
   b. Measles
   c. Rabies
   d. Tetanus

23. **In iceberg phenomenon, the submerged part represents**
   a. Undiagnosed cases in community
   b. Diagnosed cases in community
   c. Clinial cases that physician sees
   d. Clinical cases that investigator sees

24. **Changes in occurrence of a disease over a long period of time:**
   a. Secular trend
   b. Cyclic trends
   c. Seasonal trends
   d. Epidemic

25. **Disease recurring after many years:**
   a. Secular trends
   b. Cyclic trend
   c. Seasonal trend
   d. Propagated epidemics

26. **A disease condition like influenza pandemics occurs every 10 years. Which trend is reflected here:**
   a. Secular trend
   b. Epidemic
   c. Seasonal trend
   d. Cyclic trend

27. **Accidents happening during weekends is:**
   a. Cyclic trends
   b. Seasonal trends
   c. Secular trends
   d. Point source epidemic

28. **Which of following defines ability of organism to cause infection:**
   a. Pathogenicity
   b. Infectivity
   c. Antigenicity
   d. Virulence

29. **In ICD-10 how many volumes are there:**
   a. 1
   b. 2
   c. 3
   d. 4

STUDY DESIGNS AND PREVENTIVE MEASURES

30. **Framingham study is:** *(Recent Pattern Question 2018)*
   a. Prospective cohort
   b. Retrospective cohort
   c. Case control study
   d. Cross sectional study

31. **Incidence can be calculated by:**
   (Recent Pattern Question 2018)
   a. Cohort study
   b. Case control study
   c. Cross sectional study
   d. Retrospective cohort

32. **Framingham heart study comes under:**
   (Recent Pattern Question 2017)
   a. Cohort
   b. Case control
   c. Cross sectional study
   d. Ecological study

33. **Framingham heart study is** *(Recent Pattern Question 2016)*
   a. Cohort
   b. Case control
   c. Interventional
   d. Cross sectional

34. **Hospital patient admission rate differs in different hospitals with different disease. This causes which type of bias?** *(Recent Pattern Question 2016)*
   a. Subject bias
   b. Investigator bias
   c. Berkesonian bias
   d. Analyser bias

35. **Fetal cardiac monitoring is a type of:**
   (Recent Pattern Question 2016)
   a. Primary prevention
   b. Secondary prevention
   c. Tertiary prevention
   d. Primordial prevention

36. **Relative risk calculation is done for:**
   (Recent Pattern Question 2016)
   a. Cohort study
   b. Case control study
   c. Cross sectional study
   d. Ecological study

37. **What is true about double blind trial?**
   a. Patient getting double treatment
   b. Patient does not know that he is a part of clinical trial
   c. Patient is getting both placebo and medication
   d. Patient does not know what is he getting

38. **Randomization is:**
   a. It brings bias in study group, therefore avoided
   b. It is the Procedure by which participants are allocated into groups usually called 'study' and 'control' group
   c. It ensures that investigator has full control over allocation of participants to study or control group
   d. It is done usually before entering in the study and then consent is taken

39. **'Primordial Prevention' means:**
   a. Preventive action taken prior to onset of disease
   b. Prevention of emergence of risk factors of the disease
   c. Prevention of disease from causing complication
   d. Early detection of disease by screening

40. **Immunization is which type of prevention?**
   a. Primordial
   b. Primary
   c. Secondary
   d. Tertiary

41. **Polio vaccine is which type of prevention:**
   a. Primary
   b. Secondary
   c. Tertiary
   d. Primordial

FMGE Solutions Screening Examination

42. All of the following are true regarding primary prevention EXCEPT:
    a. Immunization
    b. Specific protection
    c. Early diagnosis and treatment
    d. Contraceptives

43. Screening of cervical cancer is which level of prevention?
    a. Primordial   b. Primary
    c. Secondary   d. Tertiary

44. Vaccine is what level of prevention:
    a. Primordial   b. Primary
    c. Secondary   d. Tertiary

45. Tracking of blood pressure is which type of prevention:
    a. Primordial   b. Primary
    c. Secondary   d. Tertiary

46. All of the following comes under primary prevention EXCEPT:
    a. Pap smear   b. Helmets
    c. Contraception   d. Vaccines

47. PAP smear is an example of:
    a. Early diagnosis and treatment
    b. Health promotion
    c. Specific protection
    d. Disability limitation

48. Desk provided with table top to prevent neck problems is an example of:
    a. Primordial prevention
    b. Primary protection
    c. Specific protection
    d. Disability limitation

49. Patient is on psychotherapy, what is the level of prevention:
    a. Primordial   b. Primary
    c. Secondary   d. Tertiary

50. Iodized salt is given in an area endemic to goiter. Type of prevention:
    a. Health promotion   b. Specific protection
    c. Primordial prevention d. Treatment

51. IFA supplementation is an example of:
    a. Primordial   b. Specific protection
    c. Secondary   d. Tertiary

52. Tracking of BP implies:
    a. BP increase with age
    b. BP decreases with age
    c. BP of normotensive becomes hypertensive
    d. BP of hypertensive remains hypertensive

53. Best for prevention of risk factor:
    a. Primordial prevention
    b. Primary prevention
    c. Secondary prevention
    d. Tertiary prevention

EPIDEMIOLOGY, SCREENING AND VACCINES

54. Vaccine storage at level of PHC? *(Recent Pattern Question 2018-19)*
    a. Walk in freezer   b. Walk in coolers
    c. Ice line refrigerator d. Cold boxes

55. In a Baby who is on steroids, live vaccine can be given after: *(Recent Pattern Question 2018-19)*
    a. 2 weeks   b. 4 weeks
    c. 6 weeks   d. 10 weeks

56. All of the following live vaccines are contraindicated in pregnancy EXCEPT: *(Recent Pattern Question 2018)*
    a. Yellow fever   b. BCG
    c. Rubella   d. OPV

57. Food poisoning is an example of:
    a. Point source epidemic *(Recent Pattern Question 2018)*
    b. Propagated source epidemic
    c. Common source epidemic
    d. Pandemic

58. Diabetes, hypertension or CAD screening should be started after: *(Recent Pattern Question 2018)*
    a. 30   b. 35
    c. 45   d. 55

59. Neonatal tetanus prevention is best done by:
    a. Tetanus toxoid   *(Recent Pattern Question 2018)*
    b. Tetanus immunoglobulin
    c. Metronidazole
    d. Penicillin

60. True about incidence: *(Recent Pattern Question 2018)*
    a. Total number of cases in a community
    b. Number of at risk patients
    c. Number of new cases
    d. Number of deaths in community

61. Only vaccine given to adults *(Recent Pattern Question 2018)*
    a. DPT   b. dT
    c. MMR   d. OPV

62. In a case of epidemic, 3 villages are affected simultaneously with typhoid cases. Upon study it is found that one milk man is going to all these 3 villages. Identify the type of epidemic: *(Recent Pattern Question 2017)*
    a. Point source
    b. Common source, propagative
    c. Common source, multiple exposure
    d. Common source, continuous exposure

63. When some people develop a disease after exposure from a primary case, it is known as: *(Recent Pattern Question 2017)*
    a. Incidence
    b. Prevalence
    c. Lead time
    d. Secondary attack rate

Preventive and Social Medicine (PSM)

64. In situation of an epidemic, what is the medical officer's first role/first to do: *(Recent Pattern Question 2017)*
    a. Do diagnosis and submit
    b. Find out at risk population
    c. Find out about number of cases
    d. Confirm epidemic whether it exists in real

65. Net reproduction rate is defined as: *(Recent Pattern Question 2017)*
    a. Number of live birth in the reproductive age group of a female
    b. Average number of children born to a married woman
    c. Average number of girls born to a woman assuming no mortality
    d. Number of girls born to a woman during her lifetime assuming mortality

66. If net reproduction rate is desired to be 1, what should be the couple protection rate: *(Recent Pattern Question 2017)*
    a. 42
    b. 60
    c. 70
    d. 82

67. Lung cancer patients : 300 smokers and 300 nonsmokers, 10 year history taken. What can be calculated? *(Recent Pattern Question 2017)*
    a. Prevalence
    b. Incidence
    c. RR
    d. Odds ratio

68. What is the recommended dose for human rabies immunoglobulin (Ig) in 4-month-old child? *(Recent Pattern Question 2016)*
    a. 20 IU/kg
    b. 30 IU/kg
    c. 40 IU/kg
    d. 50 IU/kg

69. What is the measles vaccine dose? *(Recent Pattern Question 2016)*
    a. 0.1 cc
    b. 0.5 cc
    c. 0.01 cc
    d. 1.0 cc

70. Reconstructed Japanese encephalitis vaccine at 2–8 degrees can be stored up to how many years? *(Recent Pattern Question 2016)*
    a. 1
    b. 2
    c. 3
    d. 4

71. True about sentinel surveillance:
    a. Includes notifiable cases *(Recent Pattern Question 2016)*
    b. Done through evaluation of sub centre reports
    c. Done by anganwadi worker
    d. Increase reporting bias

72. Varicella zoster immunization is given to all EXCEPT: *(Recent Pattern Question 2016)*
    a. Contacts with varicella zoster
    b. To the newborn and pregnant female who was exposed 6 week before delivery
    c. All HIV positive patients
    d. Patients with varicella zoster

73. Father of epidemiology is:
    a. Hippocrates
    b. John Snow
    c. Ambroise Pare
    d. Rudolf Virchow

74. Father of Medicine:
    a. John Snow
    b. Edward Jenner
    c. Louis Pasteur
    d. Hippocrates

75. Which of the following set is termed as epidemiological triad?
    a. Endemic, epidemic and outbreaks
    b. Agent, host and environment
    c. Incidence, prevalence and disease load
    d. Agent, man and disease

76. In a population of 5000, number of new cases of TB is 500; old cases in the same population are 150. What is the prevalence of TB:
    a. 9%
    b. 12%
    c. 13%
    d. 18%

77. First case which comes to the notice of investigator is:
    a. Index case
    b. Initial case
    c. Primary case
    d. Secondary case

78. 1st case seen by an investigator:
    a. Index case
    b. Primary case
    c. Secondary case
    d. Generation time

79. First case in community is known as:
    a. Index case
    b. Initial case
    c. Primary case
    d. Secondary case

80. Quarantine is:
    a. Separation for the period of communicability of infected person from others
    b. Limitation of freedom of movement of well person or animals till incubation period of disease
    c. Identification of source of infection and factors influencing its spread in community
    d. Notification of disease to local health authority to put control measures on it

81. Disease seen all over the world:
    a. Endemic
    b. Epidemic
    c. Pandemic
    d. Sporadic

82. Point source epidemic is:
    a. Gradual rise and gradual fall in number of cases
    b. Sharp rise and sharp fall in number of cases
    c. Sharp rise and fall is interrupted by secondary waves
    d. Gradual rise and fall is interrupted by secondary waves

83. Period between infected host to appearance of symptoms
    a. Generation time
    b. Serial interval
    c. Communicable period
    d. Latent period

84. Period of disease initiation to disease detection is known as:
    a. Window period
    b. Generation time
    c. Lead time
    d. Latent period

FMGE Solutions Screening Examination

85. Lead time is:
    a. Time from early diagnosis to starting treatment
    b. Time from treatment to mortality
    c. Time between detection of disease through screening and its clinical symptoms
    d. Time between clinical symptom to complete treatment

86. Number of live birth per 1000 women in the reproductive age is:
    a. Net reproductive rate   b. Total fertility rate
    c. Gross reproduction rate   d. General fertility rate

87. General fertility rate:
    a. Average number of children born to a women in her reproductive life span
    b. Annual number of live births per 1000 married women during reproductive age
    c. Total number of girl child born to a female
    d. Total number of boy child born to a female

88. Average number of girls born to woman experiencing Curie pattern is denoted by:
    a. Net reproductive rate   b. Total fertility rate
    c. Gross reproduction rate   d. General fertility rate

89. Maternal mortality rate is expressed as:
    a. 1000 live births   b. 100,000 live births
    c. 1000 pregnancies   d. 100 pregnancies

90. Which of the following is true about cohort study:
    a. Disease to risk factor study
    b. Effect to cause
    c. NOT associated with attributable risk
    d. Associated with antecedent causation

91. Disadvantage of case control study when compared to cohort study:
    a. Easy to carry out   b. Rapid and inexpensive
    c. Cannot measure cause to effect
    d. Useful in rare diseases

92. Cross sectional study is associated with:
    a. Indicates prevalence   b. Incidence
    c. Positive predictive value d. Relative risk

93. Cohort study can determine all EXCEPT:
    a. Prevalence   b. Incidence
    c. Relative risk   d. Exposure

94. True statement about PPV is:
    a. It increases with prevalence
    b. It decreases with prevalence
    c. No relation with prevalence
    d. Increases incidence

95. Sensitivity is used to calculate:
    a. True negative   b. False positive
    c. True positive   d. False negative

96. Components of epidemiological triad are all EXCEPT
    a. Environment   b. Agent
    c. Host   d. Pathogenesis

97. Predictive value indicating positive test in a screening modality is calculated by:
    a. TP/TP + FP × 100   b. TN/TN + FN × 100
    c. TP/TP + FN × 100   d. TN/FP + TN × 100

98. Specificity formula:
    a. TP/TP + FP × 100   b. TN/TN + FN × 100
    c. TP/TP + FN × 100   d. TN/FP + TN × 100

99. Important "great divide year" after which the added population exceeds that of previous decade:
    a. 1957   b. 1921
    c. 1951   d. 1957

100. All are true about case control study EXCEPT:
    a. Attribute risk   b. Measurement of exposure
    c. Matching   d. Odd's ratio

101. Screening is done because of all EXCEPT:
    a. Testing for infection or disease in population or in individuals who are not seeking health care
    b. It is defined presumptive identification of un recognized disease
    c. The search for unrecognized disease or defect by means of rapidly applied test, examinations or other procedures in apparently healthy individuals
    d. This is use of clinical or laboratory tests to detect disease in individual seeking health care for other reasons

102. All of the following vaccines are contraindicated in pregnancy EXCEPT:
    a. Measles   b. Rubella
    c. BCG   d. Tetanus

103. Newborn child with HIV+ and symptomatic, which vaccine will NOT be given:
    a. Measles   b. OPV vaccine
    c. BCG   d. Live J.E.

104. Yellow fever vaccination becomes effective after how many days of vaccination:
    a. 5 days   b. 10 days
    c. 10 weeks   d. 10 months

105. All of the following are true for yellow fever EXCEPT:
    a. Caused by vector aedes
    b. Incubation period of 3-6 days
    c. One attack gives life long immunity
    d. Validity of vaccination certification begins immediately after vaccination

106. Postexposure prophylaxis schedule of rabies vaccine in a previously immunized person:
    a. Day 0, 3, 7, 14, 21, 90   b. Day 0, 3, 7, 14, 28, 90
    c. Day 0, 3   d. Day 0, 7, 28

107. Pre-exposure schedule in rabies vaccine?
    a. Day 0, 3, 7, 14, 28, 90   b. Day 0, 3, 7, 14, 21, 90
    c. Day 0, 7, 28   d. Day 0, 7, 21

108. Live attenuated vaccine can be given to:
    a. Children under 8 years   b. HIV patients
    c. Patients on steroids   d. Patients on radiation

Preventive and Social Medicine (PSM)

109. Toxoids are prepared from:
    a. Exotoxins   b. Biotoxins
    c. Both   d. None
110. Japanese encephalitis vaccine is:
    a. Live attenuated   b. Inactivated toxoid
    c. Cellular fractions   d. Combined
111. Strain of Varicella zoster vaccine is:
    a. Nakayama   b. DANISH 1331
    c. Jeryll Lynn   d. Oka
112. Reverse cold chain is used for:
    a. Transportation of vaccines to laboratory to check its potency
    b. Carrying stool samples of polio patients from Primary Health Centre (PHC) to laboratory
    c. Transportation of outdated vaccines from PHC to district hospital
    d. Transportation of vaccines from camps to sub center
113. Which of the following vaccines does not provide herd immunity:
    a. Hepatitis A   b. Rabies
    c. Measles   d. Diphtheria
114. Naranjo algorithm is used for:
    a. Environmental factors effecting drug
    b. Para-meteric based data evaluation
    c. Calculating adverse drug reaction
    d. Demographic factor affecting drugs action
115. Phase IV of clinical trial is done:
    a. To find safety and toxicity
    b. To compare with existing drugs
    c. Pre marketing surveillance
    d. Post marketing surveillance
116. At which stage of clinical trial be taken should the permission of drug control
    a. Phase 1   b. Phase 2
    c. Phase 3   d. Phase 4

COMMUNICABLE AND NONCOMMUNICABLE DISEASE

117. Identify the mosquito: *(Recent Pattern Question 2018-19)*

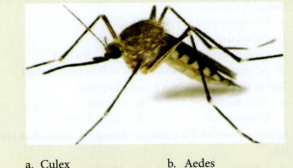

    a. Culex   b. Aedes
    c. Anopheles   d. Mansonia

118. In a case of Measles, postexposure immunoglobulin can be given within how many days after exposure:
    (Recent Pattern Question 2018-19)
    a. 3 days   b. 7 days
    c. 10 days   d. 14 days
119. In a case of Cholera period of isolation is for _____ days?
    (Recent Pattern Question 2018-19)
    a. 7 days   b. 7–14 days
    c. 3–4 weeks   d. 1–2 months
120. How much is the daily Iodine requirement of a 3–5 months old child? *(Recent Pattern Question 2018-19)*
    a. 150–200 mcg/day   b. 100–120 mcg/day
    c. 200–400 mcg/day   d. >400 mcg/day
121. Advantage of adding zinc with ORS:
    (Recent Pattern Question 2018-19)
    a. Reduces infection
    b. Antispasmodic
    c. Reduces duration of diarrhoea
    d. Enhance sodium absorption
122. Which of the following disease transmission does not require vector: *(Recent Pattern Question 2018-19)*
    a. RMSF   b. Q fever
    c. Scrub typhus   d. Trench fever
123. Correct about lepromin test:
    (Recent Pattern Question 2018-19)
    a. Differentiates from TB
    b. Example of type 2 Hypersensitivity reaction
    c. Test result can be read after 24 hours
    d. Classify the type of leprosy
124. Dose of vitamin-A to a 2-year-old child with keratomalacia? *(Recent Pattern Question 2018-19)*
    a. 1 lac IU once
    b. 1 Lac IU three times at 0,1,14 days
    c. 2 Lac IU once
    d. 2 Lac IU thrice every 6 months
125. Correct about initiating treatment in an adult patient with AIDS: *(Recent Pattern Question 2018-19)*
    a. CD4 count <200/cu.mm required for initiation of treatment
    b. CD4 count <350/cu.mm required for initiation of treatment
    c. CD4 count <500/cu.mm required for initiation of treatment
    d. No cut off of CD 4 count required for initiation of treatment
126. Cattle and sheep livestock is natural host for which of the following? *(Recent Pattern Question 2018)*
    a. Crimean-Congo fever
    b. Dengue
    c. KFD
    d. Yellow fever

127. True about chicken pox infection:
    a. Centrifugal distribution *(Recent Pattern Question 2018)*
    b. Centripetal distribution
    c. Severe prodromal symptoms
    d. Involves mainly extensor surface
128. Which is the most common clinical feature of Tularemia? *(Recent Pattern Question 2018)*
    a. Fever
    b. Headache
    c. Lymphadenopathy
    d. Diarrhea
129. Quintan fever is caused by: *(Recent Pattern Question 2018)*
    a. Rickettsia typhi
    b. Bartonella
    c. Coxiella burnetti
    d. Rickettsia conorii
130. Culex mosquito is a vector for:
    a. Chikungunya fever *(Recent Pattern Question 2018)*
    b. Dengue fever
    c. Japanese encephalitis
    d. Malaria
131. What is the color of RTI/STI kit number 6:
    (Recent Pattern Question 2017)
    a. Grey
    b. Yellow
    c. Red
    d. Black
132. Black RTI kit is used in: *(Recent Pattern Question 2017)*
    a. Urogenital infection
    b. Genital ulcer
    c. Scrotum swelling
    d. Inguinal bubo
133. Which cancer is preventable by vaccine:
    (Recent Pattern Question 2016)
    a. Ovarian CA
    b. Cervix CA
    c. Breast CA
    d. Uterus CA
134. Incubation period for cholera:
    (Recent Pattern Question 2016)
    a. 1–7 days
    b. Few hours to 5 days
    c. 2 weeks
    d. 4 weeks
135. All of the following are WHO notifiable diseases EXCEPT:
    a. Cholera
    b. Chickenpox
    c. Plague
    d. Yellow fever
136. Which of the following diseases are notifiable to WHO in Geneva under the International Health Regulations:
    a. Plague, polio and malaria
    b. Cholera, influenza and yellow fever
    c. Cholera, plague and polio
    d. Cholera, plague and yellow fever
137. Chicken pox is infective:
    a. 2 days before and 2 days after rash appearance
    b. 2 days before and 5 days after rash appearance
    c. 4 days before and 4 days after rash appearance
    d. 4 days before and 5 days after rash appearance
138. Which has lowest incubation period:
    a. Mumps
    b. Influenza
    c. Measles
    d. Chicken pox
139. Nosocomial infections are those which develop:
    a. 24 hours after hospitalization
    b. Within 48 hours of hospitalization
    c. After 48 hours of hospitalization
    d. After 7 days of hospitalization
140. Cycle that is seen in RBCs in malaria:
    a. Sexual
    b. Sporogony
    c. Exogenous
    d. Endogenous
141. Following is not caused by virus:
    a. Rocky mountain spotted fever
    b. KFD
    c. Dengue
    d. Yellow fever
142. Which of the following is transmitted by mites:
    a. Endemic typhus
    b. Epidemic typhus
    c. Trench fever
    d. Scrub typhus
143. Which of the following is not transmitted by aedes mosquito:
    a. Bancroftian filariasis
    b. Yellow fever
    c. Dengue fever
    d. Chikungunya fever
144. Subacute Sclerosing Pan Encepahalitis (SSPE) is a late complication of:
    a. Measles
    b. Mumps
    c. Rubella
    d. Chicken pox
145. Prevalence of TB in a community is estimated by:
    a. Tuberculin test
    b. AFB smear
    c. Chest X-ray
    d. Montoux test
146. Tuberculosis diagnosis in India is based on:
    a. Sputum smear microscopy
    b. Sputum culture examination
    c. Mantoux test
    d. Chest X-ray
147. XDR means extensive drug resistance to:
    a. H+R
    b. 1 Fluoroquinolone
    c. Minimum of 1 injectable drug
    d. All of the above
148. All of the following are the components of DOTS in India EXCEPT:
    a. Uninterrupted supply of drugs
    b. Political commitment
    c. Case detection with the help of X-ray chest
    d. Accountability (evaluation as well as monitoring)
149. Test to differentiate M.TB from Leprosy:
    a. AFB smear
    b. Culture
    c. Montoux test
    d. Chest X-ray
150. Sputum positive TB patients should be isolated at least for:
    a. 2 weeks
    b. 3 weeks
    c. 4 weeks
    d. 6 weeks

Preventive and Social Medicine (PSM)

151. **Sputum positive patient who should be quarantined:**
    a. Pregnant women   b. Old people
    c. Children above 6 years   d. Children below 6 years

152. **Intermediate host of Rabies is:**
    a. Man   b. Dog
    c. Cow   d. Rat

153. **Leptospirosis is transmitted by:**
    a. Fecal oral route   b. Aerosol route
    c. Infected rat's urine   d. Milk

154. **Single drug treatment recommended for Trachoma control in India is:**
    a. Azithromycin   b. Tetracycline
    c. Erythromycin   d. Penicillin

155. **Not a component of SAFE strategy for control of Trachoma:**
    a. Surgery   b. Antibiotics
    c. Facial cleanliness   d. Education

156. **Pneumonic plague transmission route:**
    a. Mice   b. Tick
    c. Inhalation   d. Flea

157. **All are true about WHO considerations regarding Dracunculosis eradication, EXCEPT:**
    a. Provision of safe drinking water like piped water and instillation of hand pumps
    b. In endemic areas step wells or by chemoradiation
    c. Education and awareness of public
    d. Control of cyclops

158. **Plague is transmitted by all EXCEPT?**
    a. X. Cheopsis
    b. X. Astia
    c. Pulex irritans
    d. Culex

159. **Antiretroviral therapy is started when CD4 count is less than:**
    a. 100   b. 200
    c. 350   d. 400

160. **Ebola virus is spread by:**
    a. Tics
    b. Inhalation from person to person
    c. Air droplet
    d. Through contact of body fluids

161. **A village affected with epidemic of cholera, what is the 1st step which should to be taken in the village to decrease the chances of death from cholera:**
    a. Safe water supply & sanitation
    b. Cholera vaccination to all individuals
    c. Primary Chemoprophylaxis
    d. Treat everyone in the village with tetracycline

162. **In cholera epidemic which step should be first taken:**
    a. Vaccination to all individuals immediately
    b. Primary chemoprophylaxis
    c. Cure with tetracycline
    d. Safe water supply and sanitation

163. **Oral cancer is caused due to:**
    a. 50-70% in India by tobacco chewing
    b. 90% in south east Asia population by tobacco chewing
    c. In central Asian district of Former Soviet Union most cases are due to smoking
    d. In eastern coastal region of Andhra Pradesh chewing betel nuts

164. **Reverse smoking causes:**
    a. Carcinoma lip   b. Carcinoma hard palate
    c. Carcinoma soft palate d. Carcinoma lung

165. **Which of the following increases the risk of lung CA:**
    a. Amount of smoking/day b. Use of filter cigarette
    c. Duration of smoking   d. All of the above

NATIONAL HEALTH PROGRAMS & POLICIES

166. **Which of the following is not correct about Urban Malaria scheme?**   *(Recent Pattern Question 2018-19)*
    a. Comprise vector control by intensive Anti-larval measure
    b. Includes all urban areas with more than 50,000 population
    c. Areas with annual parasite index of 2 are included
    d. Includes area with slide positivity of more than 10 cases per 10,000 smears

167. **Blood smear for malaria is collected by:**
                    (Recent Pattern Question 2018-19)
    a. Male MPW   b. Medical officer
    c. ASHA   d. Health assistant

168. **Sputum for AFB is collected at village level by:**
                    (Recent Pattern Question 2018-19)
    a. Medical officer   b. Anganwadi worker
    c. Health worker male   d. Health assistant

169. **Active surveillance of malaria is done by:**
                    (Recent Pattern Question 2018-19)
    a. Anganwadi workers   b. Multipurpose worker
    c. ASHA   d. Medical officer

170. **Suraksha clinic is for:** *(Recent Pattern Question 2018-19)*
    a. NVBDCP   b. RTI/STD
    c. Blood transfusion safety d. Women safety

171. **Ujjawala Scheme is for:** *(Recent Pattern Question 2018-19)*
    a. Drug abuser rehabilitation
    b. Blind persons rehabilitation
    c. Online tracking of AIDS positive patients
    d. Child trafficking

172. **Under vision 2020: in a school eye screening program, a teacher checks vision of a student will refer to which centre:** *(Recent Pattern Question 2018-19)*
    a. Service centre
    b. Training centre
    c. Centre for excellence
    d. Vision centre

173. HIV targeted intervention not done in which population? *(Recent Pattern Question 2018-19)*
    a. Migrant labourer
    b. Street children
    c. Truck driver
    d. Transgenders

174. Programs included in NRHM is/are: *(Recent Pattern Question 2018)*
    a. National vector borne disease control program
    b. Revised national tuberculosis control program
    c. Iodine deficiency disorder control program
    d. All of the above

175. Which of the following is *not* emphasized in school health services: *(Recent Pattern Question 2018)*
    a. Dental caries
    b. Infectious diseases
    c. Malnutrition
    d. Lung infections

176. Which of the following is *not* the work responsibility of ASHA: *(Recent Pattern Question 2018)*
    a. Immunization and contraception counseling
    b. Delivery at home
    c. Provide primary medical care for minor ailments
    d. Promote construction of household toilets

177. True about incentives given to ASHA worker in Janani Suraksha Yojna: *(Recent Pattern Question 2018)*
    a. 400 INR to ASHA and 1000 INR to mother in rural area in high performing states
    b. 400 INR to ASHA and 1000 INR to mother in rural area in low performing states
    c. 400 INR to ASHA and 1000 INR to mother in urban area high performing states
    d. 400 INR to ASHA and 1000 INR to mother in Urban area low performing states

178. An IQ of 55 comes in which category: *(Recent Pattern Question 2017)*
    a. Profound
    b. Mild
    c. Moderate
    d. Idiot

179. 1 male health worker, 1 female health worker should be present at each PHC. This is given by which committee?
    a. Jungalwalla committee *(Recent Pattern Question 2016)*
    b. Kartar singh committee
    c. Bhore committee
    d. Mudaliar committee

180. All are true about national mental heath program EXCEPT:
    a. Inpatient service
    b. Outpatient service
    c. Complete hospitalization
    d. Emergency service

181. Regarding mental health program, which statement is true:
    a. Started in 1951
    b. Started in 1987
    c. Started in 1987
    d. Started in 1999

182. Cafeteria approach is related with which of the following:
    a. National rural health mission
    b. National surveillance program for communicable diseases
    c. Reproductive and child health program
    d. National Vector Borne Disease Control Programme.

183. According to guidelines in AIDS control program, for a lady presenting with lower abdominal pain, the color code of kit used in treatment is?
    a. White
    b. Yellow
    c. Green
    d. Gray

184. Maximum recommended number of students in a school class room:
    a. 30
    b. 35
    c. 40
    d. 50

185. IQ level in severe mental retardation is:
    a. 50–69
    b. 40–49
    c. 20–39
    d. 21–34

186. True about national population policy 2000:
    a. Reduce MMR to <30/10,000 live births
    b. Reduce IMR to <100/10,000 live births
    c. 100% birth and death registration
    d. 100% institutional deliveries

187. True about millennium development goal 2000:
    a. Immunization coverage 85%
    b. Decrease child mortality rate
    c. Decrease maternal mortality rate
    d. Eradicate the communicable disease

188. The millennium development goals (MDG) are to be achieved by the year:
    a. 2010
    b. 2012
    c. 2015
    d. 2020

189. Which of the following is not eradicated:
    a. Leprosy
    b. Yaws
    c. Measles
    d. Polio

190. NOT included in immunization schedule:
    a. Kala-azar
    b. Polio
    c. Hepatitis
    d. BCG

191. In national vector borne disease control program which disease is not included?
    a. Malaria
    b. Yellow fever
    c. Japanese encephalitis
    d. Kala-azar

PREVENTIVE OBSTETRICS, PEDIATRICS AND GERIATRICS

192. For doctor to practise MTP minimum number of MTP to be performed is *(Recent Pattern Question 2018-19)*
    a. 10
    b. 25
    c. 50
    d. 100

Preventive and Social Medicine (PSM)

193. A 28-year-old lady (G₂P₁) does not want to conceive again immediately after first trimester abortion. Which of the following is the best method for her?
    (Recent Pattern Question 2018-19)
    a. OCP
    b. IUD
    c. Barrier method
    d. Implanon

194. How much additional calories per day is required in a pregnant lady: *(Recent Pattern Question 2018-19)*
    a. 350 kcal
    b. 550 kcal
    c. 650 kcal
    d. 520 kcal

195. Most common cause of LBW in India:
    (Recent Pattern Question 2018-19)
    a. Short gestational age
    b. Intrauterine growth retardation
    c. Maternal diabetes mellitus
    d. Genetic cause

196. According to WHO, all are true about reduced osmolarity ORS (in mmol/L) EXCEPT: *(Recent Pattern Question 2018)*
    a. Glucose – 90
    b. Na – 75
    c. Potassium – 20
    d. Citrate – 10

197. Iron required in lactation: *(Recent Pattern Question 2017)*
    a. 300 µg/day
    b. 400 µg/day
    c. 20 mg/day
    d. 100 mg/day

198. Total calories (kcal/day) required for a Female with sedentary activity: *(Recent Pattern Question 2017)*
    a. 1900
    b. 2200
    c. 2500
    d. 2800

199. Total osmolarity of reduced osmolality ORS:
    (Recent Pattern Question 2017)
    a. 215 mmol/L
    b. 220 mmol/L
    c. 225 mmol/L
    d. 245 mmol/L

200. Most common indirect cause of maternal mortality:
    a. Anemia
    b. Sepsis
    c. Hemorrhage
    d. Obstructed labor

201. Obstetric care will mostly affect:
    a. Infant mortality rate
    b. Early neonatal mortality rate
    c. Late neonatal mortality rate
    d. Perinatal mortality rate

202. Prophylactic iron and folic acid content according to RCH program during pregnancy:
    a. 500 mg iron + 100 mcg folic acid
    b. 100 mg iron + 500 mcg folic acid
    c. 100 mg iron + 100 mcg folic acid
    d. 20 mg iron + 100 mcg folic acid

203. Total amount of iron given during the pregnancy:
    a. 600 mg
    b. 800 mg
    c. 1000 mg
    d. 1200 mg

204. IFA tablet strength is:
    a. Iron 100 mg and folic acid 500 µg
    b. Iron 500 mg + folic acid 100 µg
    c. Iron 100 mg + folic acid 100 µg
    d. Iron 500 mg + folic acid 500 µg

205. Additional calorie allowance for a mother during first six months of lactation should range between
    a. 250–300 kcal
    b. 350–400 kcal
    c. 500–550 kcal
    d. 650–700 kcal

206. Registration of birth should be done:
    a. Within 15 days
    b. After 21 days
    c. Before 21 days
    d. Within 30 days

207. According to Integrated Management of Neonatal And Childhood Illness, color used in triage for home management
    a. Red
    b. Green
    c. Black
    d. Yellow

208. Best drug for diarrhea is:
    a. Cotrimoxazole
    b. Metronidazole
    c. ORS
    d. Ringer lactate

209. Exclusive breast feeding is up to:
    a. 6 weeks
    b. 6 months
    c. 9 Months
    d. 1 year

210. Infant mortality rate does not include:
    a. Post neonatal mortality
    b. Early neonatal mortality
    c. Perinatal mortality
    d. Late neonatal mortality

NUTRITION AND HEALTH

211. Waist to hip ratio that increases risk of cardiovascular disease is: *(Recent Pattern Question 2018-19)*
    a. >0.80 in male
    b. >0.80 in female
    c. >0.85 in male
    d. >0.85 in female

212. Which of the following food adulteration can lead to beriberi: *(Recent Pattern Question 2018-19)*
    a. Maize
    b. Sorghum
    c. Undermilled rice
    d. Polished rice

213. True about low glycemic index food:
    (Recent Pattern Question 2018-19)
    a. Reduced peak and rapid absorption
    b. Reduced peak and prolonged absorption
    c. High peak and fast absorption
    d. High peak and prolong absorption

214. The glycemic index for glucose is:
    (Recent Pattern Question 2018)
    a. 0.5
    b. 1
    c. 1.5
    d. 2

215. Richest source of linoleic acid? *(Recent Pattern Question 2017)*
    a. Safflower oil
    b. Palm oil
    c. Sunflower oil
    d. Corn oil

216. Plant source with highest protein:
    (Recent Pattern Question 2017)
    a. Black gram
    b. Dry peas
    c. Soyabean
    d. Bengal gram

Questions

FMGE Solutions Screening Examination

217. **What is the dose of iron folic acid given till 6-10 years?**
    (Recent Pattern Question 2017)
    a. 20 mg iron with 0.1 mg FA
    b. 20 mg iron with 0.2 mg FA
    c. 50 mg iron with 0.5 mg FA
    d. 100 mg iron with 0.5 mg FA

218. **Total calories (kcal/day) required for a male with moderate activity?** *(Recent Pattern Question 2017)*
    a. 2230   b. 2730
    c. 2900   d. 3500

219. **How many calories are there in 100 mL breast milk?**
    (Recent Pattern Question 2017)
    a. 60–65   b. 67–70
    c. 72–78   d. 100–110

220. **WRDA Vitamin B$_{12}$ in pregnancy:**
    (Recent Pattern Question 2017)
    a. 1.2 mcg   b. 1.5 mcg
    c. 0.8 mcg   d. 0.2 mcg

221. **Epidemic dropsy is caused by this toxin:**
    (Recent Pattern Question 2016)
    a. BOAA   b. Sanguinarine
    c. Alkaloid   d. Ergot

222. **In first 6 months of lactation how much extra calories are required by the lactating mother?**
    a. 150 Kcal
    b. 350 Kcal
    c. 600 Kcal
    d. 650 Kcal

223. **All of the following statements are true with regard to a reference Indian adult woman EXCEPT:**
    a. She is healthy
    b. She is between 20–39 years of age
    c. She may be engaged in 8 hours of moderately active work in a day
    d. She weighs 60 kg

224. **In Xeropthalmia, what is X1B:**
    a. Conjunctival xerosis   b. Bitot's spot
    c. Corneal xerosis   d. Corneal ulcer

225. **Secondary sign noted for xerophthalmia according to WHO:**
    a. Conjuctival xerosis   b. Corneal xerosis
    c. Bitot spots   d. Night blindness

226. **Xerophthalmia is a public health problem if bitot's spot incidence is:**
    a. 0.1%   b. 1%
    c. 0.5%   d. 5%

227. **According to prevalence criteria for determining xerophthalmia problems given by WHO, following are true for an endemic area:**
    a. Bitot spot 5% poluation of under 6 years
    b. Conjuctival xerosis 1%
    c. Conjuctival ulcers 0.05%
    d. Night blindness 1%

228. **Trace element is what percent of bodyweight:**
    a. 0.001%   b. 0.01%
    c. 0.1%   d. 1%

229. **Protein daily requirement is:**
    a. 1 g/kg   b. 2 g/kg
    c. 3 g/kg   d. 4 g/kg

230. **Which of the following vitamin is not an antioxidant:**
    a. Vitamin A   b. Vitamin B
    c. Vitamin C   d. Vitamin E

231. **All of the following vitamins are antioxidants EXCEPT:**
    a. Beta carotene   b. Vitamin B
    c. Vitamin C   d. Vitamin E

232. **Pellagra is caused by deficiency of:**
    a. Thiamine   b. Niacin
    c. Biotin   d. Ascorbic acid

233. **All are features of kwashiorkor EXCEPT:**
    a. Irritability   b. Edema in lower limb
    c. Increase appetite   d. Apathy

234. **Toxin of epidemic dropsy is:**
    a. BOAA   b. Sanguinarine
    c. Alkaloid   d. Ergot

235. **Epidemic dropsy can be due to this toxin:**
    a. BOAA   b. Sanguinarine
    c. Alkaloid   d. Ergot

236. **Epidemic dropsy is caused by:**
    a. Sanguinarine   b. Ergot
    c. Alkaloid   d. BOAA

237. **All are tests of pasteurization of milk efficiency EXCEPT:**
    a. Methylene blue reductase test
    b. Phosphatase test
    c. Standard plate count   d. Coliform count

238. **Refrigerated breast milk can be kept for:**
    a. 6 hours   b. 10 hours
    c. 12 hours   d. 24 hours

239. **Methionine is a limiting amino acid in:**
    a. Cereals   b. Maize
    c. Wheat   d. Pulses

240. **Which amino acid is deficient in pulses:**
    a. Lysine   b. Threonine
    c. Methionine   d. Cysteine

241. **What is the biological value of egg protein:**
    a. 80   b. 90
    c. 100   d. 120

242. **Vitamin D is high in:**
    a. Human Milk   b. Cow's milk
    c. Green vegetables   d. Egg

243. **Which of the following is a rich source of vitamin D?**
    a. Milk   b. Shark liver oil
    c. Halibut liver oil   d. Cod liver oil

244. **Vitamin D is found in:**
    a. Iron   b. Milk
    c. Meat   d. Fish liver oil

PREVENTIVE AND SOCIAL MEDICINE (PSM)

502

Preventive and Social Medicine (PSM)

245. **Physiologically most active form of vitamin D is:**
   a. Calciferol
   b. Calcidiol
   c. Ergocalciferol
   d. Calcitriol

246. **Most essential fatty acid is:**
   a. Linoleic acid
   b. Linolenic acid
   c. Arachidonic acid
   d. All of the above

247. **All are essential fatty acids EXCEPT:**
   a. Linoleic acid
   b. Linolenic acid
   c. Arachidonic acid
   d. Glutamic acid

248. **Hypothyroidism is associated with deficiency of:**
   a. Iron
   b. Iodine
   c. Zinc
   d. Fluorine

249. **Chronic malnutrition is assessed by:**
   a. Weight/height
   b. Height/age
   c. Weight/age
   d. Mid arm circumference

ENVIRONMENT AND HEALTH

250. **Horrock's apparatus is used for:**
   (Recent Pattern Question 2018)
   a. Measuring the hardness of water
   b. Surveillance of drinking water quality
   c. Calculating bleaching powder dose for water disinfection
   d. Calculating mid arm circumference in malnutrition

251. **Hospital infection is known as** *(Recent Pattern Question 2016)*
   a. Opportunistic infection
   b. Nosocomial infection
   c. Viral infection
   d. Health care infection

252. **For hookworm to be a major public health problem, chandler's index should be more than:**
   a. 100
   b. 200
   c. 250
   d. 300

253. **Chandler's index is:**
   a. Number of hookworm larva per gram of stool
   b. Number of hookworm eggs per gram of stool
   c. Number of hookworm per gram of stool
   d. Number of E. coli in a water sample

254. **Chandler's index is associated with:**
   a. Hook worm
   b. Pin worm
   c. Round worm
   d. Guinea worm

255. **Soiling index is used to monitor:**
   a. Water pollution
   b. Air pollution
   c. Soil pollution
   d. All of the above

256. **The indicator agents to determine fecal pollution of drinking water is:**
   a. Proteus species
   b. Coagulase-negative staphylococcus
   c. Klebsieila species
   d. E. coli

257. **In India, at least how many meters away the sanitary well should be located from likely source of contamination:**
   a. 10 meters
   b. 15 meters
   c. 50 meters
   d. 75 meters

FAMILY PLANNING AND CONTRACEPTION

258. **Highest Contraceptive failure:**
   (Recent Pattern Question 2018-19)
   a. Implant
   b. IUCD
   c. Spermicide
   d. OCP

259. **A woman from village delivers her 7th baby and she wants contraception. When is the ideal time for immediate post-partum IUD insertion?**
   (Recent Pattern Question 2018-19)
   a. Immediately after baby's expulsion
   b. Within 1 week of delivery
   c. After 6 weeks of delivery
   d. After 6 months of delivery

260. **Unmet need for contraceptive means:**
   a. Contraception desired   *(Recent Pattern Question 2018)*
   b. Sexually inactive female
   c. Family planning in those who are not using any contraception
   d. Women younger than 25 years

261. **Definition of pearl index is?** *(Recent Pattern Question 2017)*
   a. Failure rate in 100 couple
   b. Failure rate in 1000 couple
   c. Failures per 100 women years of exposure
   d. Failures per 1000 women years of exposure

262. **100 females used contraceptive for 1 year. There is 1 failure (HWY). How much is the accidental pregnancy rate?**   *(Recent Pattern Question 2017)*
   a. 0.01
   b. 1
   c. 1.5
   d. 2.0

263. **Contraceptive contraindicated during lactation is:**
   a. Combined OCP
   b. IUD
   c. Progesterone only pill
   d. None

264. **Best contraceptive for a lactating female:**
   a. Barrier
   b. Triphasic pill
   c. Combined OCP
   d. Progesterone only pill

265. **Mechanism of action of combined OCP pills:**
   a. Prevent fertilization
   b. Prevent release of ovum from ovary
   c. Prevent implantation of fertilized ovum
   d. Reduce sperm motility

266. **OCPs give protection against:**
   a. STDs
   b. Breast cancer
   c. Ovarian cancer
   d. Hepatocellular carcinoma

FMGE Solutions Screening Examination

267. Best time to screen in Breast self examination (BSE) technique is:
    a. Just before the menstruation
    b. Just after the menstruation
    c. During ovulation
    d. 2-3 days post-ovulation

268. True about pearl index:
    a. Population study   b. Family planning
    c. Contraceptive methods d. Contraceptive failure

269. Failure rate of pomoroy's technique of sterilization?
    a. 0.1%   b. 0.5%
    c. 1%   d. 5%

DEMOGRAPHY AND HEALTH

270. Death registration has to be done in:
    (Recent Pattern Question 2018-19)
    a. 7 days   b. 14 days
    c. 21 days   d. 28 days

271. Which of the following is true about population attributable risk: *(Recent Pattern Question 2018-19)*
    a. PAR = $\dfrac{\text{Incidence among exposed}}{\text{Incidence among non-exposed}}$
    b. PAR = $\dfrac{\text{Incidence among exposed} - \text{incidence among non exposed}}{\text{Incidence among exposed}} \times 100$
    c. PAR = $\dfrac{\text{Incidence among non-exposed} - \text{incidence among exposed}}{\text{Incidence among total population}} \times 100$
    d. PAR = $\dfrac{\text{Incidence among total population} - \text{incidence among non-exposed}}{\text{Incidence among total population}} \times 100$

272. In which of the following mortality is considered:
    (Recent Pattern Question 2018-19)
    a. Total fertility rate
    b. Net reproduction rate
    c. Gross reproduction rate
    d. General fertility rate

273. Birth rate reduced and death rate reduced. Population is in which stage: *(Recent Pattern Question 2017)*
    a. 1   b. 2
    c. 4   d. 5

274. Which is not a demographic indicator?
    (Recent Pattern Question 2016)
    a. Social Mobility   b. Mortality
    c. Immigration   d. Emmigration

275. Numerator of dependency ratio is:
    a. Population >10 years and <65 years
    b. Population <15 years and >65 years
    c. Population < 10 years- and >60 years
    d. Population >15 years and >60 years

276. Age pyramid of India is:
    a. Broad at base and narrow at apex
    b. Broad from base to apex
    c. Broad at apex and narrow at base
    d. Spindle shaped

277. All of the following are true regarding confounding factor EXCEPT:
    a. It is associated with exposure under investigation
    b. It is distributed equally in study & control groups
    c. It is associated both with exposure and disease
    d. It is removed by matching in case control study

278. Area under standard normal curve on area between two standard deviation on either side of mean is:
    a. 68.3%
    b. 85.2%
    c. 95.4%
    d. 99.7%

279. In a standard, normal curve, between three standard deviations on either side of mean will cover approximately
    a. 68.3% values   b. 94.2% values
    c. 95.4% values   d. 99.7% values

280. Growth curve of country like India, true is:
    a. Tapering at top   b. Tapering at bottom
    c. Bulging in middle d. Widening of base

281. Range of kuppu swami scale for upper middle class:
    a. 26-29   b. 16-25
    c. 16-26   d. 26-30

282. Blindness rate in india due to refractive errors
    a. 62.6%   b. 19.7%
    c. 5.8%   d. 6.2%

283. According to national control programme of cancer, diabetes and heart diseases, all of the following are true EXCEPT:
    a. According to WHO, Coronary Heart disease is considered as a modern epidemic i.e., a disease that affects the population, not an unavoidable attribute of ageing.
    b. According to the stroke control programme, first priority goes to control of Diabetes, elimination of smoking, prevention and management of other risk factors.
    c. Cancer is characterized by group of diseases i.e., abnormal cell growth, ability to invade adjacent tissues, distant organs, eventual death of affected person if tumor has progressed beyond the stage. The DALY's lost world wide due to cancer is 77.812.
    d. Diabetes is an "ice berg" disease. Increase in both prevalence and incidence of type 2 DM globally is associated with industrialization & socio-economic development.

Preventive and Social Medicine (PSM)

DISASTER MANAGEMENT, DISINFECTION AND BMW MANAGEMENT

284. Best method for waste disposal when suitable land available: *(Recent Pattern Question 2018-19)*
   a. Burial
   b. Dumping
   c. Controlled tipping
   d. Composting

285. Human anatomical wastes are disposed of in a _____ bag? *(Recent Pattern Question 2018-19)*
   a. Yellow
   b. Red
   c. Black
   d. Blue

286. Most important step to be taken before disaster: *(Recent Pattern Question 2018-19)*
   a. Response and rehabilitation
   b. Response and mitigation
   c. Response and preparedness
   d. Mitigation and preparedness

287. First step to be taken postdisaster: *(Recent Pattern Question 2018-19)*
   a. Response and mitigation
   b. Response and rehabilitation
   c. Reconstruction and mitigation
   d. Mitigation and preparedness

288. Which ministry will be responsible for rehabilitation postdisaster? *(Recent Pattern Question 2018-19)*
   a. Ministry of HRD
   b. Ministry of Home affairs
   c. Ministry of Agriculture
   d. Ministry of water and forest

289. In a triage black color is for: *(Recent Pattern Question 2018)*
   a. Immediate resuscitation required
   b. Ambulatory patients
   c. Unsalvageable
   d. Highest priority patients

290. Body fluids and fetuses are classified under this category of waste: *(Recent Pattern Question 2018)*
   a. Infectious waste
   b. Pathological waste
   c. Genotoxic waste
   d. Humanized waste

291. Disaster management day:
   a. 2nd week of November
   b. 2nd week of October
   c. 4th week of October
   d. 4th week of November

292. Who will be in-charge in case of disaster management:
   a. PHC
   b. Sub centre
   c. CHC
   d. District hospital

293. During massive disaster what should be done first:
   a. Search and rescue, first aid
   b. Triage
   c. Stabilization of victims
   d. Hospital treatment and redistribution of patients to hospitals if necessary

294. In a disaster management triage, patients who need surgery within 24 hours, are categorized under which color category:
   a. Red
   b. Green
   c. Blue
   d. Black

295. Which is the colour of highest priority in emergency triage:
   a. Red
   b. Yellow
   c. Black
   d. White

296. Gamma rays are used for sterilization of:
   a. Catheters
   b. Canulas
   c. Syringes
   d. All of the above

297. Autoclaving is not useful for disposal of:
   a. Surgical dressings
   b. Metallic instruments
   c. Petri dishes
   d. Liquid paraffin

298. Hot air oven can be used to sterilize all EXCEPT:
   a. Scalpels
   b. Glassware
   c. Plastic Syringes
   d. Dressings

299. Sharp wastes should be disposed in which color bag?
   a. Blue
   b. Black
   c. Red
   d. Yellow

300. Which of the following hospital waste must be discarded in Blue bag?
   a. Plastic syringe
   b. Catheter
   c. Canula
   d. All of the above

301. Category 7 on biomedical waste management contains
   a. Soiled waste
   b. Solid waste
   c. Liquid waste
   d. Incineration ash

302. Phenol co-efficient indicates
   a. Efficacy of a disinfectant
   b. Dilution of a disinfectant
   c. Quantity of a disinfectant
   d. Purity of a disinfectant

HEALTH PLANNING, CARE AND MANAGEMENT IN INDIA

303. Population covered by PHC in plains: *(Recent Pattern Question 2018-19)*
   a. 20,000
   b. 30,000
   c. 50,000
   d. 80,000

304. Which is correct about Kartar Singh Committee:
   a. No private practice *(Recent Pattern Question 2017)*
   b. Multi-purpose worker scheme
   c. ROME scheme
   d. Equal pay for equal work

Questions

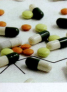

FMGE Solutions Screening Examination

305. As per norms pharmacist and lab technician are suggested per how much population?
    (Recent Pattern Question 2017)
    a. 5000   b. 10,000
    c. 15,000 d. 20,000

306. In a District hospital, the requirement of special new born care beds is?   *(Recent Pattern Question 2017)*
    a. 6   b. 10
    c. 16   d. 20

307. ASHA covers how much population in a plain?
    (Recent Pattern Question 2016)
    a. 1000   b. 2000
    c. 1500   d. 2500

308. Number of visits to be carried out by ASHA in a home delivery   *(Recent Pattern Question 2016)*
    a. 3   b. 4
    c. 6   d. 7

309. Under RNTCP, rural lab covers how much population in plains   *(Recent Pattern Question 2016)*
    a. 5000   b. 20,000-30,000
    c. 1 lakh d. 1 lakh to 5 lakh

310. Which of the following is NOT an element of PHC:
    a. Water chlorination   b. Maternal health care
    c. Sanitation   d. Equity of distribution

311. A health care system which is appropriate to everyone whether the service is needed at all in relation to essential human needs, can be accessible to everyone, available to everyone as first level of health care and the cost can be affordable by everyone is:
    a. Primary health care
    b. Secondary health care
    c. Tertiary health care
    d. Basic health care

312. All are true about principles of primary health care EXCEPT?
    a. Community participation
    b. Intersectoral co-ordination
    c. Unequitable distribution
    d. Appropriate technology

313. Not evaluated in clinical evaluation of pneumonia at PHC:
    a. Respiratory rate   b. Inability to feed
    c. Oxygen saturation   d. Chest indrawing

314. Population covered by CHC:
    a. 5000   b. 20,000
    c. 30,000 d. 100,000

315. 1st referral unit is:
    a. PHC   b. CHC
    c. Subcenter   d. District hospital

316. Beds in CHC:
    a. 20   b. 30
    c. 40   d. 60

317. National Rural Health Mission was established in:
    a. 1993   b. 1995
    c. 2005   d. 2010

318. Multipurpose worker scheme was implemented in India with the recommendation of:
    a. Bhore Committee   b. Kartar singh Committee
    c. Srivastava Committee d. Jungalwalla Committee

319. Multipurpose health worker works for _____ population
    a. 1000   b. 3000
    c. 100   d. 5000

320. Asha worker works for ___ population:
    a. 3000   b. 1000
    c. 5000   d. 400

321. All are true about ASHA are all EXCEPT:
    a. Selected by village panchayat/Gram Sabha
    b. Trained by ANM
    c. Minimum class 4 passed
    d. Comes under NRHM 2005-2012

322. ASHA is located at:
    a. Subcentre   b. PHC
    c. CHC   d. Village

323. All of the following are true about Accredited Social Health Activist (ASHA) EXCEPT:
    a. Is a mental health worker
    b. Is a basic sanitation activist
    c. Is deployed for one thousand population
    d. Arranges escort/accompanies pregnant women/children requiring admission/treatment

324. Functions of female multipurpose health worker includes:
    a. Visit 4 sub-centers/month
    b. Collection of blood sample
    c. Conduct 50% delivery
    d. Chlorination of water

325. A female multipurpose worker should be able to detect all of the following EXCEPT:
    a. Mal-presentation   b. Renal disease
    c. Anemia   d. Hydramnios

326. A female multipurpose health worker does not work in:
    a. Distribution of condoms
    b. Birth/death statistics
    c. Active malaria surveillance
    d. Immunization of mothers

327. Amount of cereals provided to children under the mid-day meals in schools is:
    a. 50 grams   b. 100 grams
    c. 150 grams   d. 75 grams

328. Mid-day meal programme provides
    a. 1/3 calories, 1/3 proteins   b. 1/3 calories, 1/2 proteins
    c. 1/2 calories, 1/3 proteins   d. 1/2 calories, 1/2 proteins

Preventive and Social Medicine (PSM)

329. **BMI obesity starts:**
    a. 25
    b. 30
    c. 35
    d. 40

330. **Body mass index is calculated by:**
    a. (Weight in kg/Height in meters^2)
    b. (Weight in kg/Height in meters^3)
    c. (Weight in kg^2)/Height in meters^2)
    d. (Weight in kg^2 × Height in meters^2)

331. **Least common cause of neonatal mortality in India:**
    a. Prematurity
    b. Birth injuries
    c. Low birth weight
    d. Asphyxia

332. **ICDS include children upto age of _____ years**
    a. 3
    b. 5
    c. 6
    d. 14

333. **Baby Friendly Hospital Initiative was launched in the year**
    a. 1981
    b. 1991
    c. 1993
    d. 1997

334. **All of the following are features of baby friendly hospitals EXCEPT:**
    a. Breast feeding is initiated within half an hour of normal delivery
    b. No pacifiers and teats are given
    c. No advertisements, promotional material or free products for infant feeding are allowed
    d. Infants are kept in the nursery for first 24 hours

335. **Which of the following seen in block:**
    a. Panchayat samiti
    b. Panchayat sabha
    c. Gram sabha
    d. Gram samiti

336. **Community development is block comprises of:**
    a. 70 villages and 70000 population
    b. 100 villages and 100000 population
    c. 500 villages and 500000 population
    d. 1000 villages and 1000000 population

OCCUPATIONAL HEALTH

337. **Green house gas includes** *(Recent Pattern Question 2016)*
    a. CO_2, ozone, methane
    b. Only ozone
    c. Ozone, methane only
    d. Methane, CO

338. **Maximum permissible dose of radiation exposure for general human beings is:**
    a. 0.5 Rad per person per year
    b. 5 Rad per person per year
    c. 50 Rad per person per year
    d. 5 Rem per person

339. **Acceptable noise level (in decibels) for Hospital wards is:**
    a. 20–35
    b. 35–45
    c. 45–55
    d. 50–60

340. **Asbsestosis is associated with which cancer:**
    a. Lung cancer
    b. Liver cancer
    c. Colon cancer
    d. Stomach cancer

341. **Mesothelioma is seen in which type of pneumoconiosis:**
    a. Anthracosis
    b. Byssinosis
    c. Asbestosis
    d. Silicosis

342. **Bagassosis is the name given to occupational disease of lung caused by inhalation of**
    a. Silica
    b. Cotton dust
    c. Sugarcane dust
    d. Asbestos

343. **All are FALSE about Lead Poisoning EXCEPT:**
    a. CPU > 100 mcg/L indicates exposure to lead
    b. Greatest source is drinking water from lead pipes
    c. Stippling of basophils is a significant finding
    d. Can cause Blue Line on gums

344. **One of the following symptoms is NOT caused by inorganic lead poising:**
    a. Anemia
    b. Insomnia
    c. Pallor
    d. Burtonian line

345. **Nausea, Vomiting, Blue line on gums, Wrist/ foot drops, Pallor, Colic are manifestations of poisoning due to:**
    a. Mercury
    b. Arsenic
    c. Organic lead
    d. Inorganic lead

346. **True about ESI act 1948:**
    a. Applicable on educational institutions also
    b. Employer : employee contribution is 1.75:4.75 %
    c. Maternity benefit for 3 months
    d. Benificiaries are those income with >15000/month

347. **According to ESI act 1948, 4.75 percent of total wage bill of employer is:**
    a. Total wages
    b. Turn over
    c. Profit
    d. Contribution

348. **Which is true about EMPLOYEE STATE INSURANCE ACT (ESI), 1948:**
    a. The employer contributes 4.75%
    b. The employee contributes 1.80%
    c. Include sickness benfit of 70% of average daily wages & is payable for 91 days
    d. Dependency benefit : pension at rate of 50% wages

349. **In which of the following management techniques, interpretation is done in terms of finding out cost effectiveness:**
    a. Cost effective analysis
    b. Cost benefit analysis
    c. System analysis
    d. Network analysis

350. **Critical path is shown by:**
    a. Time
    b. Money
    c. Man power
    d. Proper sequence

351. **In a baby ward, temperature should be:**
    a. 27–29°C
    b. 29–31°C
    c. 32–33°C
    d. 33–35°C

FMGE Solutions Screening Examination

DISINFECTION AND MISCELLANEOUS

352. In chlorination of water, the main disinfecting action is due to
   a. Hypochlorite ions   b. Hydrogen ions
   c. Hydrochloric acid   d. Hypochlorous acid

353. Residual chlorine is detected by:
   a. Horrock's test   b. Polarimeter
   c. Ortho toluidine test   d. Chromatography

354. In Nalgonda technique:
   a. Lime is added after bleaching powder
   b. Alum is added after lime
   c. Lime is added after alum
   d. Bleaching powder is added before lime

355. Hardy Weinberg law indicates all EXCEPT:
   a. States that genotype frequencies in a population remain constant or are in equilibrium from generation to generation unless specific disturbing influences are introduced
   b. Hardy Weinberg law states that population is static
   c. Factors influencing gene pool include mutation, natural selection, population movements(assertive mating), public health measures
   d. Natural selection is a process where harmful genes are not eliminated from the gene pool and genes favorable to individual are not passed onto offspring

356. Which of the following is a prospective study?
   a. 30-year-old female to check for cystic fibrosis
   b. Female > 40 years with breast lump
   c. Heel prick test for neonatal tetanus at birth
   d. Illegal immigrant screening

357. In 1935 students were admitted to a college where height and weight was taken. Based on previous data a study was conducted in 1977 in same population to determine how many will develop CAD in 1986. This study is known as:
   a. Experimental
   b. Cohort
   c. Retrospective cohort
   d. Mixed cohort

358. Biological environmental changes are recurrent. What is to be done to reduce error
   a. Standardization
   b. Excessive training of examiner
   c. Using 2 examiner
   d. Repeated measurement

BIOSTATISTICS

359. Sample registration is done:
   (Recent Pattern Question 2018)
   a. Every 3 months   b. Every 6 months
   c. Every 9 months   d. Every 12 months

360. Pictoral diagram of frequency distribution is:
   (Recent Pattern Question 2018)
   a. Histogram   b. Scatter diagram
   c. Pie chart   d. Bar chart

361. Calculate odds ratio from the given table:
   (Recent Pattern Question 2017)

	Disease	Non diseased
Exposure	33	53
Non exposed	2	27
	35	82

   a. 32   b. 8.4
   c. 88.4   d. 11.4

362. Sensitivity formula is   *(Recent Pattern Question 2016)*
   a. TP/TP + FP × 100   b. TN/TN + FN × 100
   c. TP/TP + FN × 100   d. TN/FP + TN × 100

363. A pharmaceutical company introduced a new pregnancy kit. It shows out of 100 pregnant women, 99 were positive and out of 100 non pregnant women, 90 negative. Sensitivity is   *(Recent Pattern Question 2016)*
   a. 95   b. 97
   c. 98   d. 99

364. From 1970–1995, 500 people were monitored. Exposed to smoking 400, Non-exposed 100. Out of 400 exposed 50 developed the lung cancer and out of 100 non exposed 5 developed the lung cancer. Calculate relative Risk:
   (Recent Pattern Question 2016)
   a. 1.2   b. 2.5
   c. 12.5   d. 1.5

365. In a hospital 10 babies were born in a day, each weighs 2.7 kg. what is the probable standard deviation:
   a. 0.00   b. 0.27
   c. 2.7   d. 27

366. All are true about Chi-square test EXCEPT:
   a. Non parametric test
   b. Degree of freedom is calculated by (c-1)(r-1)
   c. Used to test significance of association between two quantitative data
   d. Used for non-Gaussian distribution

367. In a 4 x 5 table for Chi-square test, what is the degree of freedom?
   a. 20   b. 16
   c. 12   d. 9

368. Correlation coefficient of 1.76 indicates
   a. Positive correlation   b. Highly positive correlation
   c. Absence of correlation d. Wrong calculation

369. Which is the best method of central tendency that is used to show quantitative variable:
   a. Mean   b. Median
   c. Mode   d. Box and whisker

370. Frequently occurring value in a series is known as
   a. Average   b. Median
   c. Mean   d. Mode

Preventive and Social Medicine (PSM)

371. A smoker states that he has been smoking for 6 years. In the first year he was taking up to 5 sticks per day only. In the next 3 years he increased it to half pack per day. In the 5th year, his habits worsened to 1 pack per day. In the last year he stated that his daily sticks consumption is 2 packs per day. Select the correct statement:
    Mean, median and mode of number of sticks are:
    a. 16, 10, 15 　　 b. 16, 10, 10
    c. 10, 10, 15 　　 d. 16, 10, 15

372. Calculate the mean & mode of the given values: 2,2,3,4,4,4,5,5,7,8,9
    a. 4 and 5 　　 b. 5 and 4
    c. 5 and 9 　　 d. 9 and 5

373. A diagnostic test for a particular disease has a sensitivity of 0.90 and a specificity of 0.80. A single test is applied to each subject in the population in which the diseased population is 30%. What is the probability that a person, negative to this test, has no disease?
    a. Less than 50% 　　 b. 70%
    c. 95% 　　 d. 72%

374. 40 out of 100 smokers and 20 out of 100 non-smokers developed lung cancer. Calculate the odd's ratio:
    a. 2.1 　　 b. 2.6
    c. 3.1 　　 d. 3.33

375. On a screening test, negative result is seen in 50% of non-diseased population and positive result in 10% healthy population. Calculate specificity:
    a. 0.5 　　 b. 0.6
    c. 0.83 　　 d. 0.9

376. According to malaria control program 2017, the goal is to reduce the annual incidence by:
    a. <1/100 　　 b. <1/1000
    c. <1/10000 　　 d. <1/100000

BOARD REVIEW QUESTIONS

377. Patient requiring immediate referral is allotted what colour code according to IMNCI colour coding?
    a. Pink 　　 b. Red
    c. Green 　　 d. Yellow

378. Which of the following procedure is not done in CHC?
    a. Abortion
    b. Blood transfusion
    c. Caesarean section
    d. Urine microscopy and culture sensitivity

379. Identification of cholera by Snow is an example of?
    a. Spot map 　　 b. Random trial
    c. Analytical design 　　 d. Experimental design

380. Random sampling is not done in?
    a. Cluster sampling 　　 b. Quota sampling
    c. Stratified sampling 　　 d. Simple random

381. Hard tick causes which of the following?
    a. Oriental sore 　　 b. KFD
    c. Tick Typhus 　　 d. Q fever

382. Radiation exposure permissible per year is?
    a. 2 rads 　　 b. 5 rads
    c. 10 rads 　　 d. 20 rads

383. Maximum iron is in which nut?
    a. Pista 　　 b. Cashew
    c. Peanut 　　 d. Walnut

384. Cyclical trend is due to?
    a. Migration 　　 b. Herd immunity
    c. Seasonal variation 　　 d. Life style modification

385. The extended sickness benefit is given for?
    a. 4 years 　　 b. 365 days
    c. 3 years 　　 d. 2 years

386. Average incubation period of typhoid is:
    a. 2-3 days 　　 b. 5-8 days
    c. 10-15 days 　　 d. 15-30 days

387. The systematic distortion of retrospective study is?
    a. Confounding 　　 b. Effect modification
    c. Recall bias 　　 d. Measurement bias

388. Duration of training of ASHA worker is?
    a. 21 days 　　 b. 23 days
    c. 30 days 　　 d. 35 days

389. Which is not true for components of DOTS?
    a. High compliance 　　 b. Given under observation
    c. Political commitment 　　 d. Accountability

390. Vitamin deficient in breast milk is?
    a. Vitamin A 　　 b. Vitamin B complex
    c. Vitamin C 　　 d. Vitamin D

391. Discarded cytotoxic medicines should be disposed in?
    a. Blue bag 　　 b. Black bag
    c. Red bag 　　 d. Yellow bag

392. Midyear population is calculated on?
    a. 1st June 　　 b. 30th June
    c. 1st July 　　 d. 31st June

393. True about "Zero base budgeting" is?
    a. Relies on data of previous budget
    b. Proceeds from resources to target
    c. Proceeds from target to resource
    d. Not a priority based budgeting

394. First disability census was done in the year?
    a. 1881 　　 b. 1951
    c. 1981 　　 d. 2001

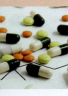

FMGE Solutions Screening Examination

395. Gas causing global warming but is not a green house gas?
    a. CO_2 b. SO_2
    c. CFC d. Ozone
396. Two variables are highly correlated when "r" is?
    a. 0 b. +0.5
    c. +1.0 d. −1.0
397. Secular trend is best demonstrated by?
    a. Line diagram b. Bar graph
    c. Stem-leaf plot d. Box and whisker plots
398. Rural health scheme was introduced by?
    a. Bhore committee b. Mukherjee committee
    c. Shrivastava committee d. Mudaliar committee
399. "Import General Manifest" comes under?
    a. Custom's Act b. Railway Act
    c. Transport Act d. Merchant Marine Act
400. Antemortem rabies diagnosis is commonly made by?
    a. Corneal scraping b. Brain biopsy
    c. Skin biopsy d. Saliva
401. Which of the following is a live attenuated bacterial vaccine?
    a. BCG vaccine b. OPV
    c. HiB vaccine d. Pertusis vaccine
402. Epidemic typhus is transmitted by?
    a. Louse b. Soft tick
    c. Hard tick d. Rat flea
403. Reference weight of Indian men and women is?
    a. 60 and 55 kg b. 60 and 50 kg
    c. 55 and 50 kg d. 50 and 45 kg
404. Age group of child under children rights is?
    a. < 10 years b. 10-15 years
    c. 15-18 years d. 18 years and younger
405. KFD is caused by?
    a. Flavivirus b. Myxovirus
    c. Alphavirus d. Phlebovirus
406. Byssinosis is most commonly seen in?
    a. Spinners b. Sugarcane industry
    c. Dyers d. Weavers
407. Lung disease seen in Coal & Rock miners?
    a. Anthracosis b. Byssinosis
    c. Bagassosis d. Silicosis
408. Goal for blindness under NPCB is to reduce prevelance of blindness in 2010 to
    a. 0.1% b. 0.3%
    c. 0.5% d. 1.0%
409. Calculate BMI if weight in kilograms is 98 and height in centimeters is 175:
    a. 28 b. 32
    c. 36 d. 40
410. Children surveyed in cluster sampling for coverage of national immunization programme?
    a. 30 cluster of 5 children b. 20 cluster of 5 children
    c. 30 cluster of 10 children d. 30 cluster of 7 children
411. Neoplasia is classified under which chapter of ICD?
    a. Chapter I b. Chapter II
    c. Chapter IV d. Chapter V
412. Risk modification in CAD is?
    a. Primordial prevention
    b. Primary prevention
    c. Secondary prevention
    d. Tertiary prevention
413. Growth rate is calculated by?
    a. Crude birth rate/Crude death rate
    b. Net reproduction-Crude death rate
    c. Total fertility rate – Crude death rate
    d. Crude birth rate-Crude death rate
414. Life span of mosquito is?
    a. 1 week b. 2 weeks
    c. 1 month d. 1 year
415. Life span of house fly is?
    a. 5 days b. 10 days
    c. 15 days d. 30 days
416. Denominator of infant mortality rate is?
    a. Per live birth b. per 100 live births
    c. Per 1000 live births d. Per lakh live births
417. Content of chlorine in bleaching powder is?
    a. 25% b. 27%
    c. 33% d. 35%
418. Two standard deviation includes what percentage of the values of distribution:
    a. 68.27% b. 86%
    c. 95.45% d. 99.73%
419. WHO funds which programme in India?
    a. RNTCP
    b. National Leprosy Eradication Programme
    c. Janani Suraksha Yojnna
    d. National old age pension plan
420. Serial interval is a measure of?
    a. Sensitivity b. Specificity
    c. Incubation period d. Positive predictive value
421. Caloric requirement to maintain BMR in a normal healthy person is?
    a. 20-30 kcal/kg/day b. 30-40 kcal/kg/day
    c. 35-40 kcal/kg/day d. 40-50 kcal/kg/day
422. Breast Feeding Week is celebrated during:
    a. 1st week of March
    b. 1st week of July
    c. 1st week of August
    d. 3rd week of September
423. World health day is celebrated on?
    a. 7 th April b. 1st July
    c. 3rd December d. 1st December
424. Perinatal mortality includes what time after birth?
    a. 7 days b. 28 days
    c. 10 months d. 1 Year

Preventive and Social Medicine (PSM)

425. Comfort zone of temperature is?
    a. 25-26.9°C
    b. 27-29°C
    c. <19°C
    d. 19-23°C
426. Average Hospital waste produced per bed per day in govt hospitals is?
    a. 1.5 - 2.0 kg
    b. 0.5 - 4.0 kg
    c. 0.5 - 2.0 kg
    d. 1.5 - 4.0 kg
427. Screening of the diseases is which type of prevention?
    a. Primordial
    b. Primary
    c. Secondary
    d. Tertiary
428. Urban malaria is caused by?
    a. Anopheles culicifacies
    b. Anopheles stephensi
    c. Anopheles fluviatilis
    d. Anopheles minimus
429. ASHA is recruited under?
    a. NRHM
    b. National urban health mission
    c. ICDS
    d. Village health system
430. JE virus life cycle in nature runs between?
    a. Pigs - Cattle
    b. Cattle-Birds
    c. Pigs-human
    d. Bird-Pigs
431. Range of flight of Ades mosquito is?
    a. 1 Km
    b. Less than 100 m
    c. 500 m
    d. 10 km
432. Bacterial indicator of recent contamination of water is?
    a. Clostridium perfringens
    b. E.coli
    c. Clostridium welchii
    d. Klebsiella

IMAGE-BASED QUESTIONS

433. The following image shows:

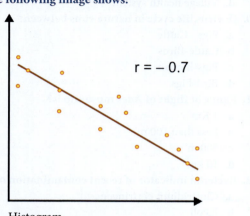

a. Histogram
b. Correlation coefficient
c. Frequency Polygon
d. Bar Diagram

434. The following image shows:

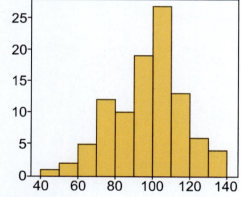

a. Histogram
b. Correlation coefficient
c. Frequency Polygon
d. Bar Diagram

435. The following image shows presence of ?

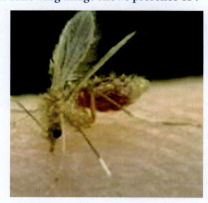

a. Sandfly
b. Aedes
c. Culex
d. Tse Tse Fly

436. The image shows presence of?

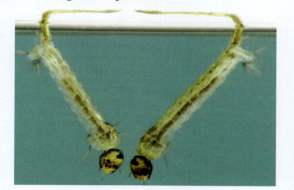

a. Aedes larvae
b. Culex larvae
c. Anopheles larvae
d. Mansonia larva

Preventive and Social Medicine (PSM)

437. Which of the following organization is shown below?

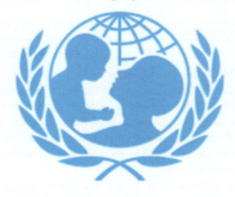

a. World health organization
b. UNICEF
c. FAO
d. World Bank

438. The following symbol shows which program of government of India?

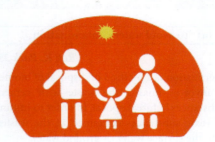

a. National Rural Health Mission
b. National urban health Mission
c. Reproductive and child Health Programme
d. A.Y.U.S.H

439. Identify:

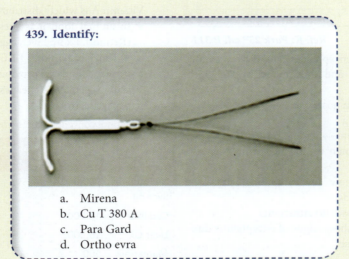

a. Mirena
b. Cu T 380 A
c. Para Gard
d. Ortho evra

Answers to Image-Based Questions are given at the end of explained questions

FMGE Solutions Screening Examination

ANSWERS WITH EXPLANATIONS

MOST RECENT QUESTIONS 2019

1. Ans. (a) To avoid water contamination

Ref: K. Park 25th ed. P 851

- Inertization is a method of disposal of biomedical waste.
- It involves mixing the waste with cement or other substances before disposal, in order to minimize the risk of toxic substances contained in the wastes migrating into the surface water or ground water.

Extra Mile

- **Incineration:** It is high temperature dry oxidation process, that reduces organic and combustible waste into inorganic incombustible matter and results in a very significant reduction of waste- volume and weight

2. Ans. (a) Pig

Ref: K. Park 25th ed. P 311

- JE is a mosquito borne encephalitis caused by a group B arbovirus (Flavivirus) and transmitted by Culicine mosquitoes.
- JE has several extrahuman hosts
  - Pig → Mosquito → Pig
  - Ardeid bird → Mosquito → Ardeid bird
- Disease transmitted to man by infected host. Man is incidental dead-end host.
- Infected pigs do not show any symptom. They are considered as amplifier host
- Cattles and Buffaloes: Mosquito attractants
- Domestic animal which shows signs of encephalitis due to JE virus infection: Horse.

3. Ans. (a) Serum-Albumin concentration

Ref: K. Park 25th ed. P 667

- To assess the state of protein nutrition, multiple tests have been suggested. These include:
  - Serum albumin concentration, Arm-muscle circumference, Creatinine-height index, Serum transferrin level.
- At present, the best measure of the state of protein nutrition is serum-albumin concentration.
  - **Normal:** >3.5 g/dL
  - **Mild malnutrition:** <3.5 g/dL
  - **Severe malnutrition:** 3 g/dL
- Serum albumin and transferrin assess the ability of liver to synthesize protein.

4. Ans. (b) Infant mortality rate

Ref: K. Park 25th ed. P 25

- IMR is the ratio of deaths under 1 year of age in a given year to the total number of live births in the same year.
- It is usually expressed as a rate per 1000 live births
- It is one of the most universally accepted indicators of health status not only of infants, but also of whole population and of the socio-economic conditions under which they live.
- In addition IMR is also a sensitive indicator of the availability, utilization and effectiveness of health care, particularly perinatal care.

5. Ans. (b) Halibut liver oil

Ref: K. Park 25th ed. P 672

Vitamin A is widely distributed in animal and plant foods.
- In animal food it is present as preformed Vitamin A (Retinol). Ex in: Liver, egg, butter, cheese, fish and meat.
  - 1 mcg of retinol = 1 RE (Retinol Equivalents)
- In plant foods as provitamins (carotenes). Ex in green leafy vegetables (cheapest source), fruits like mango, papaya, carrots

TABLE: Retinol content of some foods

Food products	Retinol Equivalents (RE) (mcg/100 gram)		
Halibut liver oil	900,000	Carrot	1,167
Cod liver oil	18,000	Spinach	607
Liver Ox	16,500	Amaranth	515
Margarine	900	Mango ripe	313
Butter	825	Papaya	118
Egg	140	Tomato	85
Cow milk	38	Orange	25

6. Ans. (a) Quetelet index

Ref: K. Park 25th ed. P 429

- For assessment of obesity, WHO has given the Body Mass Index formula, also known as Quetelet index.
- $BMI = \dfrac{\text{Weight (in kg)}}{\text{Height (in m}^2\text{)}}$

Other indices are:

- Ponderal index = $\dfrac{\text{Weight (in cm)}}{\text{Cube root of body weight (kg)}}$

Preventive and Social Medicine (PSM)

- Broca index = Height in cm — 100
- Corpulence index = $\dfrac{\text{Actual weight}}{\text{Desirable weight}}$
  - This shouldn't exceed 1.2

> **Extra Mile**
>
> - **Pearl index:** Measures contraceptive failures
> - **Chandler index:** Used for measurement of hookworm infestation as public health problem
> - **Sullivan's Index** is measurement of Disability Free Life Expectancy

7. Ans. (a) Yellow fever

Ref: K. Park 25th ed. P 904

- At the international level, following diseases are notifiable to WHO in Geneva, under the International Health Regulations (IHR).
- According to IHR, yearly data of notofocation should be detailed by age and sex,
- **Notifiable diseases are:**
  - Cholera, Plague, Yellow fever, as per WHO
  - Relapsing fever, louse borne typhus, polio, influenza, malaria, rabies and salmonellosis as per international surveillance.

8. Ans. (a) Acute gastroenteritis

Ref: K. Park 25th ed. P 858

- **Book states:** *"most commonly reported disease in post-disaster period is outbreak of gastroenteritis".*

9. Ans. (b) 75 mmol/L

Ref: K. Park 25th ed. P 247

TABLE: Composition of reduced osmolarity ORS

Constituent	Amount (mmol/L)
• Sodium	75
• Glucose, Anhydrous	75
• Chloride	65
• Potassium	20
• Citrate	10
Total	**245**

10. Ans. (b) 3–4 times less than cowmilk

Ref: K. Park 25th ed. P 591-92

- Human milk has low protein content. It is *around 3 times less than cow's milk* and lower than the most mammals.

- Vitamin D is present in human milk (earlier it was believed that human milk was deficient in Vit D)
- In human breast milk Vitamin A and C content is more than cow's milk
- Iron absorption and bioavailability of human milk is more (70%) as more compared to cow's milk (30%)
- Human milk is more rich in copper, selenium and cobalt, as compared to cow's milk.

TABLE: Comparison between breast milk during the 1st month of lactation and unprocessed cow milk

Constituent	Breast milk (g/L)	Cow milk (g/L)
Proteins	11	33
• Casein	4	28
• Soluble protiens	7	5
▪ Lactalbumin	3.5	1.5 to 1.8
▪ Beta-lactaglobulin	0	3.7
▪ Lactotransferrin	1 to 2	0.2 to 0.5
▪ Immunoglobulin	1 to 2	0.5
▪ Lysozyme	0.5	Traces
Non-protein: Nitrogenous substances	0.32	0.32
Lipids	35	35
• Linoleic acid	3.5	1
Carbohydrates	70	50
▪ Lactose	62	50
▪ Nitrogenous oligosaccharides	8	0
Minerals:	2	8
• Ca (Calcium)	0.33	1
• P (Phosphorus)	0.15	1
• Fe (Iron)	0.4 to 1.5 mg	0.3 to 0.5 mg
Vitamins		
• C60 mg	20 mg	
• D50 IU	25 IU	
Energy	640–720 kcal	650 kcal
	2670–3000 kJ	2717 kJ

11. Ans. (a) NS

Ref: K. Park 25th ed. P 213

- For reconstituting the vaccine, normal saline is recommended as diluent (distilled water can cause irritation)

Explanations

FMGE Solutions Screening Examination

- Reconstituted vaccine can be used up to 3 hours and left over should be discarded
- A satisfactory injection should produce a wheal of 5 mm in diameter.

12. Ans. (c) High temperature and Short Time method

Ref: K. Park 25th ed. P 711

- HTST method, also known as High Temperature and Short Time method.
  - Milk is rapidly heated to 72° C, held at that temperature for not less than 15 seconds and then rapidly cooled to 4°C
  - **Book states:** *"This is the most widely used method now"*
  - Large amount of milk can be pasteurized by HTST method

13. Ans. (b) Restriction of movement of healthy contact of an infectious disease

Ref: K. Park 25th ed. P 132

- **Quarantine** is defined as: *"the limitation of freedom of movement of such well persons who are exposed to communicable disease for a period of time no longer than the longest usual incubation period of the disease, in such manner as to prevent effective contact with those not so exposed."*
- **Isolation** on the other hand is separation of infected person from others for the period of communicability.

14. Ans. (b) Haemoglobin

Ref: K. Park 25th ed. P 961

- At sub-centre laboratory examinations that are given are:
  - Urine test for pregnancy confirmation
  - Haemoglobin estimation
  - Urine and albumin and sugar

CONCEPT OF HEALTH AND DISEASE

15. Ans. (b) Life expectancy at 1 year, IMR, literacy rate

Ref: K. Park, 23rd ed. pg. 17

TABLE: Comparison between PQLI and HDI

PQLI (Physical Quality of Life Index)	HDI (Human Development Index)
Literacy rate	Knowledge
Infant mortality rate	Income
Life expectancy (at 1 year)	Life expectancy (@ birth)
Range: 0 and 100	Range: 0 and +1
Value in India: 65	0.640

Extra Mile
- Range of correlation coefficient: –1 to +1

16. Ans. (b) Cholera

Ref: K. Park, 23rd ed. pg. 5

- **Father of public Health:** John Snow, identified Cholera
- Father of modern epidemiology: John Snow
- Father of Medicine/first true epidemiologist: Hippocrates.

17. Ans. (c) 0 and 100

Ref: K. Park, 23rd ed. pg. 17

Physical Quality of Life Index (PQLI)	Human Development Index (HDI)
Literacy rate	Knowledge
Infant mortality rate	Income
Life expectancy (at 1 year)	Life expectancy (@ birth)
Range: 0 and 100	Range: 0 and +1
Value in India: 65	0.640

Extra Mile
- Range of correlation coefficient: –1 to +1

18. Ans. (c) Life expectancy- Birth

Ref: K. Park, 23rd ed. pg. 17

Please refer to above table

19. Ans. (d) Range 0 to 100

Ref: K. Park, 23rd ed. pg. 17

Refer to above explanation

20. Ans. (a) 0–1

Ref: K. Park, 23rd ed. pg. 17

- The HDI value ranges between 0 to 1.
- This value for a country shows the distance that it has already travelled towards maximum possible value of 1 and also allows comparisons with other countries.

21. Ans. (a) Income

Ref: K. Park 23rd ed. pg. 17

Components/Indicators of PQLI
- Literacy rate
- Infant mortality rate
- Life expectancy at age 1 year

Preventive and Social Medicine (PSM)

22. Ans. (a) Tuberculosis

Ref: K. Park, 23rd ed. pg. 39, 135

- **Iceberg phenomenon** can be compared to a disease in community.
- **Floating tip of iceberg** (visible portion): clinical cases that physicians sees in community. It can be detected by diagnostic tests.
- **Submerged part** (hidden portion): are the latent, undiagnosed cases and carriers. It is detected by screening test by an epidemiologist.
- **Water surface** (demarcation line): demarcation between apparent and inapparent disease.
- **Iceberg phenomenon of a disease is NOT shown by:**
  - Rabies
  - Tetanus
  - Measles
  - Rubella

23. Ans. (a) Undiagnosed cases in community

Ref: K. Park, 23rd ed. pg. 39, 135; K. Park, 21st ed. pg. 37

24. Ans. (a) Secular trend

Ref: K. Park, 23rd ed. pg. 66, 21st ed. pg. 61,62

Time Distribution of Disease

- **Secular trend:** It implies changes in occurrence of a disease over a period of long time, generally several years or decade.
  - **Ex:** Polio, Diphtheria, Pertusis are the diseases which are reducing in India in fast few decades; and diseases like DM, Obesity and hypertension has increased in past few decades.
- **Epidemic:** Short term fluctuation of a Disease occur in few days, week, or months. E.g. food poisoning, Bhopal gas tragedy

Periodic Fluctuation

- **Cyclic trends:** some diseases occur in cycles spread over a period of time which means days, weeks, months, or years. Non-infectious condition may also show periodic fluctuations *ex: automobile accidents in US are more frequent on weekends, esp: Saturday.* Other examples can be measles occurring every 2-3 years, Rubella every 6–9 years, influenza pandemics at intervals of 7-10 years (due to antigenic variations)
- **Seasonal trend:** It is seasonal variation/fluctuation in occurrence of a disease. The seasonal variation of disease occurence may be related to environmental condition like humidity, rainfall, temperature.
- **Example:** Measles and varicella in early spring season, upper respiratory infection in incidence increases in winter, gastroenteritis increases in summer.

25. Ans. (a) Secular trends

Ref: K. Park, 23rd ed. pg. 66, 21st ed. pg. 62

Please refer to above explanation

26. Ans. (d) Cyclic trend

Ref: K. Park, 23rd ed. pg. 66, 21st ed. pg. 62

27. Ans. (a) Cyclic trends

Ref: K. Park, 23rd ed. pg. 65-66, 21st ed. pg. 61,62

Please refer to above explanation

28. Ans. (b) Infectivity

Ref: K. Park, 23rd ed. pg. 36

- **Infectivity:** this is ability of an infectious agent to invade and multiply (produce infection) in a host.
- **Pathogenicity:** it is the ability to induce **clinically apparent illness.**
- **Virulence:** proportion of clinical cases resulting in **severe clinical manifestation.**

29. Ans. (c) 3

Ref: K. Park, 23rd ed. pg. 49, 21st ed. pg. 47

- ICD-10 (International Classification of Diseases, 10th revision on January 1, 1993).
- ICD does uniform classification of diseases which can be used throughout the world to make accurate comparisons of morbidity and mortality data for decision making in prevention, facilitation and management of health care system.
- **ICD-10 consists of 3 volumes:**
  - **Volume-I:** contains reports of the international conference of 10th revision, classification of morphology of neoplasms, special tabulation list for mortality and morbidity, definition and nomenclature regulation.
  - **Volume-II:** Instruction manual
  - **Volume- III:** Alphabetical Index
- **Note:** there are 21 major chapters in ICD-10

STUDY DESIGNS AND PREVENTIVE MEASURES

30. Ans. (a) Prospective cohort

Ref: K. Park 23rd ed. P 80

- The Framingham heart study was initiated in 1948 by US public health service to study the relationship between number of risk factors (like BP, smoking, serum cholesterol, obesity) and subsequent development of cardiovascular disease.

FMGE Solutions Screening Examination

- Study was done in town of Framingham for 20 years in view of the slow development of heart disease.
- It is an example of prospective cohort study.

31. Ans. (a) Cohort study

Ref: K. Park 23rd ed. P 65

- Incidence and relative risk is accurately calculated by cohort study.
- It is a type of analytical or observational study used for hypothesis testing, also called TROHOC study prospective study/forward looking study/*cause to effect study*/*exposure to outcome study*/*risk factor to disease study* incidence study follow-up study.
- Prevalence is determined by cross sectional studies.

32. Ans. (a) Cohort

Ref: K. Park, 23rd ed. pg. 80

- The Framingham heart study was initiated in 1948 by US public health service to study the relationship between number of risk factors (like BP, smoking, serum cholesterol, obesity) and subsequent development of cardiovascular disease. It was a very good example of cohort study.

33. Ans. (a) Cohort

Ref: K. Park, 23rd ed. pg. 80

- The Framingham heart study was initiated in 1948 by US public health service to study the relationship between number of risk factors (like BP, smoking, serum cholesterol, obesity) and subsequent development of cardiovascular disease.

34. Ans. (c) Berkesonian bias

Ref: K. Park, 23rd ed. pg. 73-74

- Berkesonian bias is a type of study bias that arises because of the different rates of admission to hospitals for people with different diseases.
- It is termed after Dr. Joseph Berkeson who recognized this problem.

35. Ans. (b) Secondary prevention

Ref: K. Park, 23rd ed.

- Fetal cardiac monitoring is a screening test to detect any fetal distress in utero.
- All screening and diagnostic tests are secondary level of prevention.

TABLE: Levels of prevention

Level of prevention	Timing	Mode of prevention	Example
Primordial	Before emergence of risk factor	—	• Preventing obesity • Practicing healthy lifestyle
Primary	Risk factor present but no disease yet	*By health promotion and specific protection.*	• **All vaccines** • Contraceptives • Mosquito nets/repellants/DDT • Chemoprophylaxis
Secondary	When Disease has probably started	*By early diagnosis and treatment*	• All screening and diagnostic tests. • Treatment measures • BP monitoring
Tertiary	Disease in progression	*By disability limitation and rehabilitation.*	• Physiotherapy • Crutches in polio

36. Ans. (a) Cohort study

Ref: K. Park, 23rd ed. pg. 78

- Relative risk is the ratio of disease among exposed and disease among non exposed. It is also known as risk ratio.
- RR = incidence of disease among exposed/Incidence of disease among non-exposed
- It is a direct measure of strength of association between suspected cause and effect.

37. Ans. (d) Patient does not know what is he getting

Ref: K. Park, 23rd ed. pg. 83

- In **double blind trial**, neither patient nor the doctor are aware of group allocation and the treatment received. Patient is either getting placebo or the drug.
- All the clinical trials must take an informed consent regarding the same from the participants.

Preventive and Social Medicine (PSM)

Extra Mile

- **SINGLE BLIND TRIAL:** it is planned in such a way that participant is not aware whether he belong to the study group or control group.
- **TRIPLE BLIND TRIAL:** in this type of trial, the participant, the investigator and the person analyzing the data are all "blind" (not aware)
- **Note:** Double blinding is most commonly used method when blind trial is conducted.

---

38. Ans. (b) It is the procedure by which participants are allocated into groups usually called 'study' and 'control' group

Ref: K. Park, 23rd ed. pg. 82, 21st ed. pg. 78

- Randomization is "heart" of a control trial. It is a statistical procedure by which the participants are allocated into groups usually called "study" and "control" group.
- It is an attempt to eliminate bias and allow comparability.
- By doing this it is ensured that investigator has NO control over allocation of participants to study or control group. THIS REMOVES SELECTION BIAS.

---

40. Ans. (b) Primary

Ref: K. Park, 23rd ed. pg. 41, 370-73

- All vaccines/immunization are primary level of prevention.
- *BCG vaccine used for treatment of bladder CA is secondary level of prevention.*

- RANDOMIZATION is done only after the participant has entered the study, i.e. after having been qualified for the trial and has given his informed consent to participate in the study.

---

39. Ans. (b) Prevention of emergence of risk factors of the disease

Ref: K. Park, 23rd ed. pg. 41, 370

- Primordial prevention refers to prevention of development of risk factors in countries or population groups where they are yet to appear.
- For instance, adult health problems like obesity, hypertension etc. take root in childhood, when lifestyles like smoking, eating patterns, physical exercise are formed
- As part of primordial prevention, efforts are made to discourage high risk children, adolescents and young adults from adopting harmful lifestyles. The primary intervention is through individual and mass education.

Extra Mile

TABLE: Level of Prevention with their modes and example

Level of prevention	Timing	Mode of prevention	Example
Primordial	Before emergence of risk factor	–	• Practising healthy lifestyle • Preventing obesity
Primary	Risk factor present but NO disease yet	By health promotion and specific protection.	• *All vaccines* • Contraceptives • Mosquito nets/repellants/DDT • Chemoprophylaxis
Secondary	When Disease has probably started	By early diagnosis and treatment	• *All screening and diagnostic tests.* • Treatment measures • *BP monitoring*
Tertiary	Disease in progression:	By disability limitation and rehabilitation.	• Physiotherapy • Crutches in polio

---

41. Ans. (a) Primary

Ref: K. Park, 23rd ed. pg. 41, 370-74

FMGE Solutions Screening Examination

42. Ans. (c) Early diagnosis and treatment

Ref: K. Park, 23rd ed. pg. 41, 370-74

- Early diagnosis and treatment comes under secondary level of prevention.

Please refer to above explanation

43. Ans. (c) Secondary

Ref: K. Park, 23rd ed. pg. 41, 370-74

- *All screening and diagnostic tests and treatment measures come under secondary level of prevention.*
- *Refer to previous explanation.*

44. Ans. (b) Primary

Ref: K. Park, 23rd ed. pg. 41, 370-74

- All vaccines/immunization are primary level of prevention.
- *Refer to above table.*

45. Ans. (c) Secondary

Ref: K. Park, 23rd ed. pg. 41, 376

- Tracking of blood pressure helps in early diagnosis of hypertension.
- Hence comes in secondary level of prevention.

46. Ans. (a) Pap smear

Ref: K. Park, 23rd ed. pg. 41, 385

- **Primary prevention** is the action taken prior to the onset of disease which removes the possibilities of disease occurrence.
- **Modes of intervention:**
  - Health promotion
  - Specific protection
- It is applicable for "risk factors are present but disease has not yet taken place"
- *Pap smear is a screening test, which comes under secondary level of prevention.*

47. Ans. (a) Early diagnosis and treatment

Ref: K. Park, 23rd ed. pg. 41, 370

- Pap smear is a screening test for cervical cancer. It is an example of secondary level of prevention. The mode of secondary level of prevention is by early diagnosis and treatment.

48. Ans. (c) Specific protection

Ref: K. Park, 23rd ed. pg. 41, 370

- *Specific prevention of neck problem before onset of disease.*

- Desk provided with table top, probably decrease the risk of developing neck problems like cervical spondylosis etc.
- This is primary level of prevention done by specific protection.

TABLE: Levels of prevention

Level of Prevention	Timing	Mode of prevention
Primordial	Before emergence of risk factor	-
Primary	Risk factor present but NO disease yet	• Health promotion • *Specific protection*
Secondary	When probably Disease has started	• Early diagnosis • Treatment
Tertiary	Disease in progression	• Disability limitation • Rehabilitation

49. Ans. (c) Secondary

Ref: K. Park, 23rd ed. pg. 41, 370-73

- Any treatment measure comes under secondary level of prevention.
- *Refer to above explanation*

50. Ans. (b) Specific protection

Ref: K. Park, 23rd ed. pg. 41, 370-73

- Iodised salt is given in an area which has risk of developing goiter. This is a primary level of prevention done by specific protection.
- Primordial prevention is done before the emergence of risk factor.

51. Ans. (b) Specific protection

Ref: K. Park, 23rd ed. pg. 41

- IFA supplement is a chemoprophylaxis given during pregnancy for anemia. It comes under primary level of prevention which is implemented under specific protection.

52. Ans. (d) BP of hypertensive remains hypertensive

Ref: K. Park 23rd ed. pg. 374

Park 23rd/P 374 States:
If BP of a person is tracked from early childhood to adult life then those individuals whose blood pressure was initially high in the distribution, would probably continue in the same "track".

53. Ans. (a) Primordial prevention

Ref: K. Park, 23rd ed. pg. 41, 21st ed. pg. 39-40

Preventive and Social Medicine (PSM)

- Primordial level of prevention is defined as prevention of emergence or development of risk factors in countries or population groups in which disease entity is not yet appeared, or population group which are not yet exposed.

- **Modes of intervention:**
  - Individual education
  - Mass education
- *Primordial level is considered as best level of prevention for non-communicable diseases*

521

EPIDEMIOLOGY, SCREENING AND VACCINES

54. Ans. (c) Ice line refrigerator

Ref: K. Park 25th ed. P 118-19

TABLE: Cold chain equipment

Storage	Transportation
Electrical • Walk in cooler • Walk in freezer • Ice line refrigerator (ILR) • Domestic refrigerator • Deep freezer	• Refrigerated vaccine • Insulated vaccine van • Cold box • Vaccine carrier: used to carry 16-20 vials • Day carriers: used to carry 6-8 vials. Two fully frozen ice packs are used
Solar • Solar refrigerator battery drive • Solar refrigerator direct drive	**NOTE:** • The risk of cold chain failure is greatest at sub-centre and village level
Nonelectrical • Cold box • Vaccine carrier	• Therefore, vaccines are NOT stored at sub centre level and must be supplied on the day of use

TABLE: Differences between all the equipment

Equipment	Temperature	Used for storing	Installed at
Walk in cooler	Maintain + 2 to + 8°C	Store all vaccines like BCG, HepB, DPT, Pentavalent, IPV, TT	• **Govt medical store depots** • **State and regional vaccine stores**
Walk – in- freezer	(−15 to − 25°C)	• For bulk storage of OPV vaccine • Preparation of frozen ice packs for vaccine transportation	**National, regional and state vaccine stores**
Deep freezer	(−15 to − 25°C)	• Store OPV vaccine for 3 months • Freezing ice packs	District level and sub district level
Ice line refrigerator (ideal for safe storage of vaccine)	(+2 to + 8°C)	• For vaccines like OPV, BCG, Measles and JE stored at the bottom of basket • DPT, TT, Hep B, IPV, pentavalent and Diluents—kept in upper part of basket	Large size ILR: District and sub district level Small size ILR: **PHC**
Domestic refrigerator	(+2 to + 8°C)	• Placement of vaccine in the refrigerator with freezer on top is as follows: • **Top shelf:** Measles, BCG, OPV, Rota virus • **Middle shelf:** DPT, Pentavalent, TT, IPV, Hep-B, JE • **Bottom shelf:** Ice packs filled with water and in door of refrigerator	Used for storage vaccine at private clinics and nursing homes
Cold boxes	Fully frozen ice packs are used. Kept at bottom and sides	Used for transportation of vaccines.	Supplied to all **peripheral centres**

Explanations

55. Ans. (b) 4 weeks

Ref: K. Park 25th ed. P 111;
www.immunize.org/askexperts/precautions-contraindications.asp

- Book states: *"Live vaccines should not be administered to persons with immune deficiency diseases or to persons whose immune system is suppressed because of leukaemia, lymphoma, malignancy or because of therapy with corticosteroids, alkylating agent, anti-metabolites and radiation"*
- The immunosuppressive effect of corticosteroid may vary.
- As dose of 2 mg/kg or 20 mg/day for 2 weeks or more raise concern about safety of vaccination with live vaccines like MMR, varicella etc.
- It is recommended to wait for 1 month after discontinuation of steroid therapy before administering a live vaccine virus.
- **Note:** Inactivated vaccines and toxoids can be used administered to all immunocompromised patients in usual doses and schedules.

> **Extra Mile**
> - Pregnancy is also a contraindication for live vaccines.
> - When two live vaccines are required, they should be given either simultaneously at different sites or with an interval of atleast 3 weeks

56. Ans. (a) Yellow fever

Ref: K.Park 23rd ed. P 283

Contraindications of Yellow Fever Vaccines

- Children aged <9 months for routine immunization (or <6 months during an epidemic)
- Pregnant women (except during outbreak)
- People with severe egg protein allergy
- People with severe immunodeficiency caused by HIV/AIDS.

57. Ans. (a) Point source epidemic

Ref: K. Park 23rd ed. P 64-65

Types of Epidemics

- **Point source or single exposure epidemics:**
  - Sharp rise and sharp fall in number of cases
  - Clustering of cases in narrow spectrum of time
  - All cases develop within one incubation period of disease.
  - Ex: Food poisoning, measles, chicken pox, *Bhopal gas tragedy*
- **Common source, continuous or repeated exposure epidemics:**
  - Sharp rise in number of cases
  - Fall in number of cases is interrupted by secondary waves/peaks
  - **Ex: Contaminated well in a village, Sex worker in a gonorrhea outbreak**
- **Propagated epidemics:**
  - Gradual rise and gradual fall over a long time (tail off)
  - Usually infectious in origin and results from person to person transmission
  - Transmission continues till number of susceptibles is depleted or they are no longer exposed to infected individuals
  - **Ex: Hep A, Polio, HIV, Tuberculosis**

> **Extra Mile**
> - **Endemic:** Constant presence of a disease in a defined geographical area
> - **Pandemic:** Epidemic affecting a large population, occurring over a large geographical area.
> - **Sporadic:** Scattered cases. They are widely separated in space and time and show little or no connection.

58. Ans. (c) 45

Ref: K. Park 23rd ed. P 360, 395

- Diabetes, hypertension and coronary artery diseases are among the diseases with high mortality.
- **Book states:** *"CHD is responsible for 30–50%" of deaths in diabetics over the age of 40 years.*
- *"Target population for screening diabetes are those from age group 40 and above"*

59. Ans. (a) Tetanus toxoid

Ref: K. Park 23rd ed. P 311-312

- Tetanus occurring in newborn is known as neonatal tetanus. However it is acquired more commonly during the active age i.e. 5–40 years.
- Infants usually contract the disease during the birth, when delivered in a nonaseptic condition, especially when the umbilical cord is cut with the unclean instrument or when the umbilical stump is dressed with ashes, soil or cow dung.
- No age is immune unless protected by previous immunization.
- *The immunity resulting from 2 injections from tetanus toxoid is highly effective and lasts for several years.*

Prevention of Neonatal Tetanus

- **Active immunization:** Tetanus is best prevented by active immunization with tetanus toxoid. It stimulates the production of the protective antitoxin. Two preparations are available:

- **Combined vaccine:** DPT.
  - Offered routinely to infants under expanded immunization program.
  - 3 doses of vaccine given starting at 6 weeks of age in a gap of 4–8 weeks
- **Monovalent vaccine:**
  - Plain or fluid (formal) toxoid
  - Tetanus vaccine, adsorbed
- Passive immunization
  - Temporary protection can be provided by an injection of human tetanus hyperimmunoglobulin or ATS. It is the prophylactic to be used.
  - **Dose:** 250 IU for all ages.

60. Ans. (c) Number of new cases

Ref: K.Park 23rd ed. P 60

Incidence

Incidence rate is defined as "the number of NEW cases occurring in a defined population during a specified period of time". It is given by the formula:

$$\text{Incidence} = \frac{\text{Number of new cases of specific disease during a given time period}}{\text{Population at-risk during that period}} \times 100$$

For example, if there had been 500 new cases of an illness in a population of 30,000 in a year, the incidence rate would be:

= 500/30,000 × 1000
= 16.7 per 1000 per year

61. Ans. (b) dT

Ref: K. Park 23rd ed. P 162

- **Book states:** *"For immunizing children over 12 years of age and adults, the preparation of choice is dT, which is adult type of diphtheria tetanus vaccine"*
- This preparation contains no more than 2 L of diphtheria toxoid per dose, as compared to 25 L in the ordinary DPT vaccine.
- Administration of dT vaccine to adults is carried out in 2 doses at an interval of 4–6 weeks, followed by booster 6–12 months after second dose.

62. Ans. (d) Common source, continuous exposure

Ref: K. Park, 23rd ed. pg. 65

- **EPIDEMIC:** Sudden occurrence and rise of a particular health related behaviour/events which is in excess of "expected occurrence"
- **Common source, continuous or repeated exposure epidemics:**
  - Sharp rise in number of cases
  - Fall in number of cases is interrupted by secondary waves/peaks
  - **Ex: Contaminated well in a village, Sex worker in a gonorrhea outbreak**

63. Ans. (d) Secondary attack rate

Ref: K. Park, 23rd ed. pg. 100

- **Secondary attack rate** is defined as "the number of exposed persons developing the disease within the range of incubation period, following exposure to the primary case." It is given by the formula:

$$SAR = \frac{\text{No. of exposed person developing the disease within range of incubation period}}{\text{Total no. of exposed/susceptible contacts}}$$

64. Ans. (d) Confirm epidemic whether it exists in real

Ref: K. Park, 23rd ed. pg. 131

In case of investigating an epidemic, an orderly procedure or the following practical guidelines should be followed:

- **Verification of diagnosis:** It is the first step in epidemic investigation
- **Confirmation of existence of epidemic:** It is the next step to confirm if epidemic exists. It is done by comparing the disease frequencies during the same period of previous years.
- Defining the population at risk
- Rapid search for all cases and their characteristics
- Data analysis
- Hypothesis formulation
- Testing of hypothesis
- Ecological factor evaluation
- Further investigation of population at risk
- Writing the report

65. Ans. (d) Number of girls born to a woman during her lifetime assuming mortality

Ref: K. Park, 23rd ed. pg. 488-89

- **Net Reproduction Rate (NRR):** Net Reproduction Rate (NRR) is denied as the number of assuming fixed age-specific fertility and mortality rates (21).
  NRR is a demographic indicator. NRR of 1 is equivalent to attaining approximately the 2-child norm.
- **General Fertility Rate (GFR):** It is the "number of live births per 1000 women in the reproductive age-group (15-44 or 49 years) in a given year".

$$GFR = \frac{\text{Number of live births in an area during the year}}{\text{Mid-year female population age 15-44 (or 49) in the same area in same year}} \times 1000$$

FMGE Solutions Screening Examination

General fertility rate is a better measure of fertility than the crude birth rate because the denominator is restricted to the number of women in the child–bearing age, rather than the whole population. The major weakness of this rate is that not all women in the denominator are exposed to the risk of childbirth.

- **General Marital Fertility Rate (GMFR):** It is the "number of live births per 1000 married women in the reproductive age group (15–44 or 49) in a given year".

$$GMFR = \frac{\text{Number of live births in an year}}{\text{Mid-year married female population in the age-group 15-49 years}} \times 1000$$

- **Total fertility rate (TFR):** Total fertility rate represents the average number of children a woman would have if she were to pass through the women now in each age group.
- **Total marital fertility rate:** Average number of children that would be born to a married woman if she experiences the current fertility pattern throughout her reproductive span.
- **Gross reproduction rate (GRR):** Average number of girls that would be born to a woman if she experiences the current fertility pattern throughout her reproductive span (15–44 or 49 years), assuming no mortality.

66. Ans. (b) 60

Ref: K. Park, 23rd ed. pg. 493

Couple Protection Rate (CPR)

- **Couple protection rate (CPR)** is an indicator of the prevalence of contraceptive practice in the community. It is defined as the per cent of eligible couples effectively protected against childbirth by one or the other approved methods of family planning, viz. sterilization, IUD, condom or oral pills.
- Sterilization accounts for over 60% of effectively protected couples. Demographers are of the view that the **demographic goal of NRR = 1 can be achieved only if the CPR exceeds 60%.**

67. Ans. (d) Odds ratio

- The *given scenario is a retrospective study*, also known as case control study. It is better known to calculate the odd's ratio.
- Prevalence is better given by cross sectional study.
- Incidence and relative risk is accurately calculated by cohort study.

68. Ans. (a) 20 IU/kg

Ref: K. Park, 23rd ed. pg. 280

- Rabies Ig for passive immunization is administered only once, preferably at, or as soon as possible after the initiation of post exposure vaccination.
- Beyond 7th day after the first dose, rabies Ig is not indicated
- The dose of human rabies Ig is 20 IU/kg body weight.
- The dose of equine Ig and F (ab') 2 products, is 40 IU/kg body weight.

69. Ans. (b) 0.5 cc

Ref: K. Park, 23rd ed. pg. 148

- Only live attenuated vaccines are recommended for use.
- The vaccine is presented as freeze-dried product. Before use, the lyophilized vaccine is reconstituted with sterile diluent.
- **Each dose of 0.5 cc** contains $\geq$ 1000 viral infective units of the vaccine strain.

> **Extra Mile**
> - Reconstituted measles vaccine **loses 50% of its potency after 1 hour at 20°C.**
> - It **loses almost all potency after 2 hour at 37°C.**
> - The vaccine is sensitive to light, hence **kept in colored glass vials.**
> - After reconstitution, the vaccine must be **stored in the dark at 2 – 8°C and used within 4 hours.**

70. Ans. (c) 3

Ref: http://www.who.int/immunization_standards/ vaccine_quality/pq266_je_1dose_biologicale/en/; K. Park 23rd ed. pg. 481

- JE vaccine can be stored at 2–8°C for up to 3 years (shelf life)
- Similarly, Rabies vaccines prequalified by WHO, do not contain preservatives, such as thiomersal. The shelf life of these vaccines is $\geq$3 years, provided they are stored at +2 to +8°C and protected from sunlight.

71. Ans. (a) Includes notifiable cases

Ref: K. Park, 23rd ed. pg. 40

- **Surveillance** is defined as "the continuous scrutiny of the factors that determines the occurrence and distribution of disease and other conditions of ill health"
- **The main objectives of surveillance are:**
  - To provide information about new and changing trends in the health status of a population.
  - To provide timely warning of public health disasters so that intervention can be mobilized.
  - To provide feedback which may be expected to modify the policy of the system itself and lead to redefinition of objectives.

Preventive and Social Medicine (PSM)

Sentinel surveillance:
- A method to identify the "missing cases" (by usual surveillance).
- The sentinel surveillance data is extrapolated to the entire population to estimate the disease prevalence in total population.
- This system provides more valuable and detailed information that could be obtained from traditional notification system *(e.g. Subcenter reports)*.
- Advantage:
  - **Reporting bias is minimized** and feedback information to the providers is simplified
- **Done by whom?**
  - Sentinel surveillance agencies
  - Competent physicians (or institutions) in selected areas

72. Ans. (d) Patients with varicella zoster

Ref: K. Park, 23rd ed. pg. 145

Varicella Zoster Immunoglobulin (VZIG)
- VZIG given within 72 hours of exposure, has been recommended for prevention of chicken pox in exposed susceptible individuals particularly in immunosuppressed patients. These include:
  - Person with congenital cellular immunodeficiency
  - Susceptible persons receiving immunosuppressive therapy
  - Persons with HIV/AIDS
  - Susceptible and exposed persons, in particular pregnant women
  - Newborns
  - Premature infants of low birth weight
- **Note:** VZIG has no role in established disease
- **Dose of VZIG:** 12.5 units/kg up to max of 625 units
- Since VZIG appears to bind the varicella vaccine, the two should not be given together.

73. Ans. (b) John Snow

Ref: K. Park, 23rd ed. pg. 5-6

- Father of public Health: Cholera
- *Father of modern epidemiology: John Snow*
- Father of Medicine/first true epidemiologist: Hippocrates.

74. Ans. (d) Hippocrates

Ref: K. Park, 23rd ed. pg. 5-6

Refer to above answer

75. Ans (b) Agent, host and environment

Ref: K. Park, 23rd ed. pg. 33-34, Park, 19th pg. 30

A broad concept of disease causation that synthesized the basic factors of agent, host and environment (see adjacent figure)

Epidemiological triad

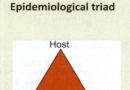

This model—agent, host and environment—has been in use for many years. It helped epidemiologists to focus on different classes of factors, especially with regard to infectious diseases

76. Ans. (c) 13%

Ref: K. Park, 23rd ed. pg. 61

- Prevalence is calculated as

$$\frac{\text{No. of new cases + no of old cases}}{\text{Total Population}} \times 100$$

- Therefore prevalence = $\frac{500 + 150}{5000} \times 100$
- Prevalence = 13%

Extra Mile
- Prevalence is a Proportion
- Incidence is a Rate

77. Ans. (a) Index case

Ref: K. Park 23rd ed. pg. 95

- **Index Case:** In epidemiology, first case of a disease in a group which is **seen** by an investigator or which brought to the attention of the clinician. *It is not always the primary case.*
- **Primary case:** *First case of communicable disease introduced into the population unit being studied.*
- **Secondary case:** All case who develop from primary case
- **Incubation period:** Entry of organism till 1st sign/symptom
- **Median incubation:** Time period for 50% case to occur

78. Ans. (a) Index case

Ref: K. Park, 23rd ed. pg. 95

Please refer to above explanation

79. Ans. (c) Primary case

Ref: K. Park, 23rd ed. pg. 95, 21st ed. pg. 91

FMGE Solutions Screening Examination

- **Index case:** First case which comes to attention of investigator.
- **Primary case:** First case of communicable disease introduced into the population unit being studies.
- **Secondary case:** Cases which arise due to contacts with primary case.

80. Ans. (b) Limitation of freedom of movement of well person or animals till incubation period of disease

Ref: K. Park, 23rd ed. pg. 120, 21st ed. pg. 111

- **QUARANTINE** is defined as **Limitation of freedom of movement of such well person or domestic animals who are exposed to a communicable disease for a longer period of time, not longer than the longest usual incubation period of the disease.** This effectively prevents the contact with those who are not exposed, thereby reduces chances of possible transmission.
- **ISOLATION** is separation for the period of communicability of INFECTED person or animals from others in order to reduce direct or indirect transmission.
- **Epidemiological investigations** Identification of source of infection and factors influencing its spread in community
- **Notification:** Notification of an infectious disease to local health authority to put control measures on it.

81. Ans. (c) Pandemic

Ref: K. Park, 23rd ed. pg. 93, 21st ed. pg. 88-89

- **Endemic:** Constant presence of a disease or an infectious agent within a given geographical area or a population group.
- **Epidemic:** Sudden occurrence and rise of a particular health related behaviour/event which is in excess of "expected occurrence".
- **Sporadic:** Scattered cases, which occur irregularly, haphazardly from time to time. These cases are few and separated widely in space and time that they show little or no connection with each other, nor a recognizable common source of infection.
- **Pandemic:** An epidemic usually affecting a large proportion of population, occurring over a wide geographic area such as a section of nation, the entire nation, a continent or the world.

82. Ans. (b) Sharp rise and sharp fall in number of cases

Ref: K. Park, 23rd ed. pg. 64, 93

Types of Epidemics

- **Point source or single exposure epidemics**
  - Sharp rise and sharp fall in number of cases
  - Clustering of cases in narrow spectrum of time
  - All cases develop within one incubation period of disease.
  - Ex: Food poisoning, measles, chicken pox, *Bhopal gas tragedy*
- **Common source, continuous or repeated exposure epidemics:**
  - Sharp rise in number of cases
  - Fall in number of cases is interrupted by secondary waves/peaks
  - Ex: Contaminated well in a village, Sex worker in a gonorrhea outbreak
- **Propagated epidemics:**
  - Gradual rise and gradual fall over a long time (tail off)
  - Results from person to person transmission
  - Transmission continues till number of susceptibles is depleted or they are no longer exposed to infected individuals
  - Ex: HIV, Tuberculosis

> **Extra Mile**
> - **Endemic:** constant presence of a disease in a defined geographical area
> - **Pandemic:** epidemic affecting a large population, occurring over a large geographical area.
> - **Sporadic:** scattered cases. They are widely separated in space and time and shows little or no connection.

83. Ans. (a) Generation time

Ref: K. Park, 23rd ed. pg. 100

- **Generation time:** The interval of time between receipt of infection by a host and a **maximal infectivity** of the host *(Generation time = Incubation period)*
- **Serial interval:** The gap in time between the onset of primary case and secondary case is called serial interval.
- **Communicable period:** Time during which an infectious agent may be transferred directly or indirectly from an infected person to another person, from an infected animal to a person or vice versa including arthropods.
- **Latent period:** The period from disease **initiation to disease detection**.

84. Ans. (d) Latent period

Ref: K. Park, 23rd ed. pg. 99, 21st ed. pg. 94

- In infectious diseases the term incubation period is used, which is equivalent to latent period in non-infectious diseases.
- **Latent period** is defined as "the period from disease initiation to disease detection"

Preventive and Social Medicine (PSM)

85. Ans. (c) Time between detection of disease through screening and its clinical symptoms

Ref: K. Park, 23rd ed. pg. 99-100

- **Lead time** is the length of time between the detection of a disease and its usual clinical presentation and diagnosis

OR

- It is the time between early diagnosis with screening, and when diagnosis would have been made without screening (through symptoms) (Image).

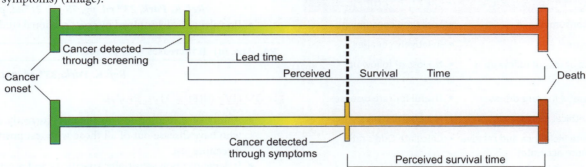

86. Ans. (d) General fertility rate

Ref: K. Park, 23rd ed. pg. 488

- **General fertility rate** is the annual number of live births per 1000 married women of child bearing age (15-49 years).
- **Total fertility rate** average number of children born to a women in her reproductive life span.
- **Gross reproduction rate** is total number of girl children born to a female. It is half of the TFR.
- **Net reproduction rate** is total number of girl children born to a female, taking into account their mortality.

87. Ans. (b) Annual number of live births per 1000 married women during reproductive age

Ref: Park's, 21st ed. pg. 451

Please refer to above explanation

88. Ans. (c) Gross reproduction rate

Ref: K. Park, 23rd ed. pg. 488-89

89. Ans. (b) 100,000 live births

Ref: K. Park, 23rd ed. pg. 25, 557

- Maternal Mortality Rate (MMR) is expressed as per 100,000 live births.
- MMR

$$= \frac{\text{No. of maternal deaths in a given year}}{\text{Total no. of live births in the same year}} \times 100,000$$

- MMR is a RATIO

- **MCC of MMR in India**: Post-partum hemorrhage
- **MC direct cause of MMR**: PPH
- **MC indirect cause of MMR**: Anemia
- **Maternal death**: Death of mother anytime during pregnancy/labor or **within 42 days** of termination of pregnancy.

90. Ans. (d) Associated with antecedent causation

Ref: K. Park, 23rd ed. pg. 75

COHORT STUDY

- Is a type of analytical or observational study used for hypothesis testing, also called as TROHOC study / prospective study/forward looking study/*cause to effect study*/exposure to outcome study/*risk factor to disease study* /incidence study/ follow up study.
- **Strength of association of prospective study is given by:**
  - **Relative risk:** incidence exposed/incidence among non exposed
  - **Attributable risk** =

    $$\frac{\text{incidence among exposed - incidence among non-exposed}}{\text{Inidence among exposed}} \times 100$$

- **Population attributable risk** =

  $$\frac{\text{incidence among total - incidence among non-exposed}}{\text{Inidence among total}} \times 100$$

- Classical example of cohort study is FRAMINGHAM HEART STUDY which is an antecedent study.
- Other examples include DOLLS AND HILLS which is an example of prospective study on smoking and lung cancer.

FMGE Solutions Screening Examination

91. Ans. (c) Cannot measure cause to effect

Ref: K. Park, 23rd ed. pg. 75-76

- "*Cause to effect*" study is done only in Cohort study. In case- control study, study is done from "*effect to cause*".

Comparison Between Cohort Study and Case Control Study

Cohort Study	Case Control study
• Time consuming	• Less time consuming
• Expensive	• Relatively cheaper
• Chance of loss of follow up is high	• No loss of follow up
• NOT useful for rare diseases	• Useful for rare diseases
• It has ethical issues	• NO ethical issues
• Calculate incidence and relative risk (more accurate)	• Calculate Odd's ratio

• Cohort study is also known as:
  ■ Prospective study
  ■ *Cause to effect study*
  ■ Exposure to outcome study
  ■ Incidence study
  ■ Follow up study
	• Case control study is also known as:
	  ■ Retrospective study
	  ■ Effect to cause study
	  ■ Outcome to exposure study
	  ■ Case reference study

92. Ans. (a) Indicates prevalence

Ref: K. Park, 23rd ed. pg. 75-77

Cross sectional study is the simplest form of observational epidemiological study which is based on single examination of a cross section of a population at one point of time , results of sample are then projected to the whole population

Advantages

- Provides prevalence of a disease
- Provides a whole picture of population at one point of time
- More useful for chronic disease

Disadvantages

- Tells about distribution of a disease rather than the etiology
- Establishment of time sequence of a disease is not possible
- Provides little information of a natural history and incidence of a disease

93. Ans. (a) Prevalence

Ref: K. Park, 23rd ed. pg. 75-77, 21st ed. pg. 71-72

- Prevalence is determined by cross sectional studies.

94. Ans. (a) It increases with prevalence

Ref: K. Park, 23rd ed. pg. 140-141

■ POSITIVE PREDICTIVE VALUE

- Ability of screening test to identify correctly all those who have disease out of all those who test positive on a screening test.
- It depends upon sensitivity, specificity and prevalence of a disease in a population
- PPV of a screening is directly proportional to prevalence of disease
- **If Prevalence of a disease increases in a population, PPV increase for the screening test.**

$$PPV = TP/TP+FP \times 100$$

- PPV α Prevalence

95. Ans. (c) True positive

SENSITIVITY: Defined as ability of a screening test to identify all those who have disease (cases/ True Posiive)

$$\text{Sensitivity} = \frac{a}{(a+c)} \times 100 = \frac{TP}{(TP+FN)} \times 100$$

96. Ans. (d) Pathogenesis

The causative factors of disease include AGENT, HOST, ENVIRONMENT. These 3 are referred as Epidemiological triad. Interaction of these 3 factors is required for development of disease.

97. Ans. (a) TP/TP + FP × 100

SENSITIVITY	$\dfrac{TP}{TP+FN} \times 100$	**PREDICTIVE VALUE OF A NEGATIVE TEST**	$\dfrac{TN}{TN+FN} \times 100$
SPECIFICITY	$\dfrac{TN}{FP+TN} \times 100$	**% OF FALSE NEGATIVES**	$\dfrac{FN}{TP+FN} \times 100$
PREDICTIVE VALUE OF A POSITIVE TEST	$\dfrac{TP}{TP+FP} \times 100$	**% OF FALSE POSITIVES**	$\dfrac{FP}{FP+TN} \times 100$

PREVENTIVE AND SOCIAL MEDICINE (PSM)

98. Ans. (d) TN/FP + TN × 100

Ref: K. Park, 23rd ed. pg. 139-140, 21st ed. pg. 113

- Specificity is defined as ability of a test to identify correctly those who do not have the disease i.e. "true negatives"

Specificity

$$= \frac{\text{True Negative}}{\text{False Positive + True Negative}} \times 100$$

99. Ans. (b) 1921

Ref: Internet Source

The year **1921** is a "**year of the great divide**" in the demographic history of India when mortality started to decline leading to acceleration in the rate of population growth. During the next three decades (1921-51) the rate of population growth continued at a level of over one per cent per annum. It is going increasingly since then. Hence the year 1921 is rightly called the demographic divide or year of great divide.

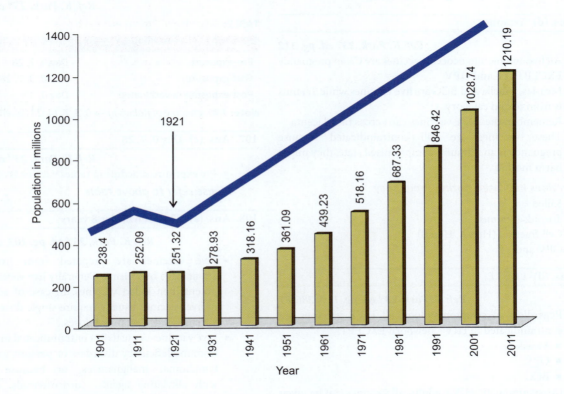

Impact of economic growth in an economy will generally have the following impact on the population:

- High birth rate and High death rate –Leads to low population growth (under-developed economy)
- *High birth rate and Low death rate: Leads to High population growth (developing economy)*
- Low birth rate and Low death rate: Leads to Low population growth (developed economy)
- In countries where children are regarded as assets, the rate of birth will be high, however due to low economic growth the health services will be poorer leading to high death rates also. E.g. India
- Once the country achieves certain level of economic growth over a period of time, the health services would become accessible to people, which would lead to high rate of birth and low rate of death.
- Once a good level of economic growth and literacy rate is achieved, the people will tend to have less children, leading to low rate of birth and low rate of death.

100. Ans. (a) Attribute risk

Ref: K. Park, 23rd ed. pg. 71-72

Case control study is often called retrospective study.

The 4 Basic Steps of Case Control Study
- Matching
- Measurement of exposure
- Selection of cases and controls

FMGE Solutions Screening Examination

- Analysis and interpretation (relative risk)

$$\text{Relative Risk} = \frac{\text{Incidence among exposed}}{\text{Incidence among non-exposed}}$$

101. Ans. (d) This is use of clinical or laboratory tests to detect disease in individual seeking health care for other reasons

Ref: K. Park, 23rd ed. pg. 135

Option D is case finding and the difference is that the examinatons or test done for an individual *who is seeking health care is case finding not a screening.*

102. Ans. (d) Tetanus

Ref: K. Park, 23rd ed. pg. 312

- All live and meningococcal vaccines are C/I in pregnancy EXCEPT: **YF and OPV**
- Measles, rubella and BCG are live vaccines while Tetanus is from toxoid category.
- Remember, these live vaccines can't cross the placenta
- These vaccines are still contraindicated because pregnancy is an immune-compromised state, they might harm mother.

Vaccines Indicated During Pregnancy
- Killed
- Toxoids (*tetanus*)
- Cell fraction (Hep A, Hep B)
- OPV and YF

103. Ans. (d) Live J.E.

Ref: K. Park, 23rd ed. pg. 119, 286-87

- Regardless of symptomatology, all LIVE vaccines are contraindicated in HIV+ newborn EXCEPT:
  - Measles
  - OPV
  - BCG
- In asymptomatic HIV+ adults, all vaccines can be given during asymptomatic phase.
- In symptomatic HIV+ adults, all live vaccines are contraindicated except: **BCG and MMR**

Extra Mile

- All vaccines are contra-indicated during epidemics EXCEPT: **MEASLES**
- All vaccines are contra-indicated post disaster EXCEPT: **MEASLES**

104. Ans. (b) 10 days

Ref: K. Park, 23rd ed. pg. 121, 283

- Yellow fever vaccine certificate becomes valid **after** 10 days of vaccination and valid upto 10 years.
- Immunity of yellow fever vaccination coverage: **10 days- lifetime 35 years.**
- Quarantine period of yellow fever: **6 days** (maximum I.P of YF)

International Travelers
- WHO recommends revaccination every 10 years

105. Ans. (d) Validity of vaccination certification begins immediately after vaccination

Ref: K. Park, 23rd ed. pg. 121, 283

106. Ans. (c) Day 0, 3

Ref: K. Park, 23rd ed. pg. 279-80

TABLE: Schedule of Prophylaxis Rabies vaccine

Types of prophylaxis	Schedule
Pre-exposure	Day 0, 7, 28
Post-exposure	Day 0, 3, 7, 28, (1/0)
Post-exposure in vaccinated	Day 0, 3

Note: *1/M schedule of Rabies Ig → 0, 3, 7, 14, 28 (Essen Regimen)*

107. Ans. (c) Day 0, 7, 28

Ref: K. Park, 23rd ed. pg. 279-80

- Pre exposure schedule in rabies vaccine is on day 0, 7, 28.

Please refer to above table

108. Ans. (a) Children under 8 years

Ref: K. Park, 23rd ed. pg. 103, 21st ed. pg. 28

- Live vaccines are prepared from live (generally attenuated) organisms. Generally live vaccines are more potent then killed vaccines. In case of administration of live vaccines usually require single dose except polio vaccine which require 3 doses.
- Live vaccines are usually contraindicated in persons with immunodeficiency disorders or persons with leukemia, lymphoma, malignancies, or because of therapy with alkylating agents, corticosteroids, radiotherapy, antimetabolite drugs.
- Pregnancy is the another contraindication unless risk of infection exceeds the risk of harm to the fetus.

109. Ans. (a) Exotoxins

Ref: K. Park, 23rd ed. pg. 105

110. Ans. (a) Live attenuated

Ref: K. Park, 23rd ed. pg. 286-87

- JE vaccine is a live attenuated vaccine. It is available in killed vaccine form also.
- **Strain**: SA 14-14-2- live
  Nakayama strain- killed
- *One dose of JE vaccine is given at 16-24 months of age.*

Preventive and Social Medicine (PSM)

531

Extra Mile

- **MC live vaccine used:** BCG
- **MC killed vaccine used:** Pertusis
- **All live vaccines are contra-indicated in pregnancy EXCEPT:** YF and OPV

Live Vaccine	Killed	Toxoids	Cell fraction	Combined
• BCG • OPV *(sabin)* • MMR • Yellow fever • Live J.E. • Live H1N1 • Live cholera	Hep A Hep B Pertusis IPV *(salk)* Rabies Meningo-coccal Killed J.E. Killed H1N1	Diph-theria Tetanus	Hep B Meningo-coccal HiB Pneumo-coccal	DPT MMR

111. Ans. (d) Oka

Ref: K. Park, 23rd ed. pg. 143

Vaccines and their Associated Strain

Vaccine	Strain
• Anti HIV	Ankara strain *(under trial)*
• Anti-malarial	Lytic cocktail (SPF 66)
• BCG	DANISH 1331
• Japanese Encephalitis	Nakayama Strain (killed) SA 14-14-2 (live)- currently used
• Killed H1N1	California strain
• Measles	Edmonston strain
• Mumps	Jeryll Lynn Strain
• Rabies	Fixed viral strain
• Rubella	RA 27/3 strain
• Varicella	**Oka strain**
• Yellow fever	17 D strain

112. Ans. (b) Carrying stool samples of Polio patients from Primary Health Centre (PHC) to laboratory

Ref: K. Park 23rd ed./109-110, 19th/99

- **WHO indicators of AFP surveillance and laboratory performance:** it has several indicators, including Stool specimens for isolation of a non-polio enterovirus (Target > 10%).
- The indicator of quality of **"reverse cold chain"** (which means that **the specimen has been maintained at <8°C during transportation from field to laboratory continuously**) and how well laboratory has been able to perform routine isolation of enteroviruses.

Revising Concept and Key Points of 'Cold Chain'

- **Cold chain** is a system of storage and transport of vaccines at low temperature from the **manufacturer to the actual vaccination site**
- The cold chain system is necessary because vaccine failure may result due to non strict temperature controls
- **Polio** is the most sensitive to heat, requiring storage at minus 20 degree °C.
- Vaccines which must be stored in the **freezer compartment** are: **polio and measles.**
- Vaccines which must be stored in the **COLD PART but never allowed to freeze** are: typhoid, DPT, tetanus toxoid, DT, BCG and diluents.

113. Ans. (b) Rabies

Ref: K. Park, 23rd ed. pg. 102, 21st ed. pg. 97

- Herd immunity is the level of resistance of a community or a group of people to a particular disease.

Vaccines which DONOT provide herd protection	Vaccines which provide herd protection	
• Tetanus • *Rabies* • Japanese encephalitis • Hepatitis B • Yellow fever	• **Diphtheria** • Pertussis • **Measles** • Mumps • **Hepatitis A** • Polio	Small pox Rubella Meningococcal vaccine Rota virus vaccine H. influenza and pneumococcal V

114. Ans. (c) Calculating adverse drug reaction

- The **Naranjo algorithm**, **Naranjo Scale**, or **Naranjo Nomogram** is a questionnaire designed by Naranjo *et al.* for determining the likelihood of whether an adverse drug reaction is actually due to the drug rather than the result of other factors.
- Probability is assigned via a score termed definite, probable, possible or doubtful. Values obtained from this algorithm are sometimes used in peer reviews to verify the validity of author's conclusions regarding adverse drug reactions. It is also called the Naranjo Scale or Naranjo Score.

Scoring
• ≥ 9 = definite ADR
• 5–8 = probable ADR
• 1–4 = possible ADR
• 0 = doubtful ADR

115. Ans. (d) Post marketing surveillance

Ref: K. Park, 23rd ed. pg. 84-85

Explanations

FMGE Solutions Screening Examination

Clinical Trials

Phase	Subjects	Purpose
• Phase 1	Healthy human volunteer	Safety and non-toxicity
• Phase 2	Patients (20–200)	Effectiveness
• Phase 3	Patients	Comparison with existing drug
• Phase 4	Patient	Long term side effects. Post marketing surveillance

- Most important phase of clinical trial: Phase 3
- A new drug is launched in market after phase 3

PHASE 4

- *Post marketing surveillance*
- Longest phase: **10–25 years**
- To study the long term side effects of a drug
- Doesn't require ethical clearance.

116. Ans. (c) Phase 3

Ref: K. Park, 23rd ed. pg. 84-85

- **Phase 1**: Human pharmacology and safety: Drugs are tested on healthy individuals (20–50 people).
  - **Main aim:** To find out maximum tolerable dose hence, dose finding study.
- **Phase 2:** Therapeutic exploration and dose ranging:
  - **Main aim:** to check the safety, efficacy of drug.
- **Phase 3:** Therapeutic confirmation/comparison:
  - **Main aim:** To confirm the safety of drug, efficacy. 'New drug application' (NDA) is submitted to the licencing authority, who if convinced give marketing permission for the drug.
- **Phase 4:** Postmarketing surveillance studies:
  - **Main aim:** To study the rare side effect caused by new drugs.

COMMUNICABLE AND NONCOMMUNICABLE DISEASE

117. Ans. (c) Anopheles

Identification features of anopheles mosquito

- Spotted wings
- When at rest, inclined at an angle of 45° to the surface
- No buzzing sound

TABLE: Difference between anopheles and Aedes mosquito

Anopheles Mosquito		Aedes Mosquito
Malaria	Diseases spread	Dengue, Yellow Fever, Chikungunya, Lymphatic filariasis
Pregnant females	Which mosquitoes bite?	Pregnant females
Night	When do they bite?	Day
With abdomen sticking upwards	Resting position	Lies parallel to resting surface
Predominantly rural	Location	Predominantly urban
Bodies of water	Breeding ground	Shallow water surfaces

118. Ans. (a) 3 days

Ref: K. Park 25th ed. P 162

- Apart from vaccine, measles can be prevented by administration of immunoglobulin early in the incubation period.
- **Dose:** 0.25 ml/kg
- It should be given within 3–4 days of exposure
- These persons who are passively immunized should be given live measles vaccine 8–12 weeks later

119. Ans. (b) 7–14 days

Ref: K. Park 25th ed. P 253

- Infection of cholera is dose dependent. Infection occurs when the number of vibrio ingested exceeds the dose that is infective for individual.
- To produce clinical disease 10^{11} organisms required.
- NOTE: An infected person can excrete 10-20 litre of fluid, which contain $10^7 – 10^9$ vibrios per ml.
- A case of cholera is infectious for a period of 10–14 days
- Convalescent carriers are infectious for 2–3 weeks.
- A chronic carrier state may last from a month up to 10 years or more.

120. Ans. (b) 100–120 mcg/day

Ref: K. Park 25th ed. P 681, PubMed

Requirement of iodine in child age group:

- **7–12 month:** 110 mcg/day
- **1–8 years:** 90 mcg/day
- **9–13 years:** 120 mcg/day
- **Adult/14–18 years:** 150 mcg/day
- **Pregnancy:** 250 mcg/day

121. Ans. (c) Reduces duration of diarrhoea

Ref: K. Park 25th ed. P 489

- For the control of diarrhoea, India is the first country to introduce low osmolarity ORS.
- As an adjunct to ORS, zinc is also added.
- Addition of zinc results in reduction of the number and severity of episodes and duration of diarrhoea.

122. Ans. (b) Q fever

Ref: K. Park 25th ed. P 328

- **Q fever** differs from other rickettsial infection. There is no arthropod involved in its transmission to man.
- **Transmission can be due to:**
  - Inhalation of infected dust contaminated by urine or faeces of diseased animal or through aerosol (*most important route: respiratory route*).
  - Through abrasion, conjunctiva or ingestion of contaminated food such as meat, milk and milk products
- **I.P.:** 2 – 3 weeks
- **Clinical feature:** Acute onset fever, chills, general malaise, headache. NO rash or local lesion. The infection can cause: pneumonia, hepatitis, encephalitis.
- **DOC:** Doxycycline

> **Extra Mile**

Rickettsial diseases, their Agents and insect vectors

Disease	Rickettsial agent	Insect Vectors
Epidemic typhus	R. prowazekii	Louse
Endemic typhus	R. typhi	Flea
Scrub typhus	R. tsutsugamushi	Mite
Indian tick typus	R. conorii	Tick
Rocky mountain spotted fever	R. rickettsii	Tick
Rickettsial pox	R. akari	Mite
Q fever	C. burnetii	
Trench fever	Rochalimaea quintana	Louse

123. Ans. (d) Classify the type of leprosy

Ref: K. Park 25th ed. P 347-48

- Lepromin test is performed by injecting 0.1 ml of lepromin in inner aspect of forearm
- Routinely, reaction is read at 48 hours and 21 days. Two types of reactions:
  - **Early reaction:** Aka **Fernandez reaction.** Reaction is evidenced by redness and induration at the site of inoculation. Size >10 mm after 48 hours is considered positive
    - **Early reaction** indicates if a person has been previously sensitized by exposure to and infection by leprosy bacilli.
    - It is described as **delayed hypersensitivity reaction (type IV)** to soluble constituents of leprosy bacilli.
  - **Late reaction: Aka Mitsuda reaction:** Become apparent 7-10 days after injection. Evaluate after 21 days. Reaction is said to be positive if there is nodule >5 mm at the site of inoculation
    - **Late reaction** is induced by bacillary component of the antigen. It indicates cell mediated immunity
- **Value of lepromin test:**
  - **Lepromin test** is NOT a diagnostic test
  - **Drawbacks:** Positives result in non-cases and negative result in lepromatous and near-lepromatous cases.
  - A useful tool in evaluating the immune status of leprosy patients (cell mediated immunity).
  - It is of considerable value in confirming the results classification and cases of leprosy on clinical and bacteriological ground.
  - In other words the test is widely used as an aid to classify the type of disease.

124. Ans. (d) 2 Lac IU thrice every 6 months

Ref: K. Park 25th ed. P 673

- The strategy to counter vitamin A deficiency is to administer a single massive dose of 200,000 IU of vitamin A in oil (retinol palmitate) orally every 6-month to preschool children (1–6 years).
- Dose is reduced to half in children In age group of 6 months to 1 year.

125. Ans. (d) No cut off of CD 4 count required for initiation of treatment

Ref: K. Park 25th ed. P 380-81

TABLE: WHEN TO START ART

When to Start in adult (>19 years old)	ART should be initiated in all adults living with HIV, regarding of WHO clinical stage and at any CD4 cell count.
	As a priority. ART should be initiated in all adults with severe or advanced HIV clinical disease (WHO clinical stage 3 or 4) and adults with a CD4 count ≤350 cells/mm³.

Contd...

FMGE Solutions Screening Examination

When to start ART in pregnant and breast-feeding women	ART should be initiated in all pregnant and breastfeeding women living with HIV, regardless of WHO clinical stage and at any CD4 cell count and continued lifelong.
When to start ART in adolescents (10-19 years of age)	ART should be initiated in all adolescents living with HIV, regardless of WHO clinical stage and at any CD4 cell count (conditional recommendation). As priority, ART should be initiated in all adolescents with severe or advanced HIV clinical disease (WHO clinical stage 3 or 4) and adolescents with a CD4 count ≤ 350 cells/mm³.
When to start ART in children younger than 10 years of age	ART should be initiated in all children living with HIV, regardless of WHO clinical stage or at any CD4 cell count. • Infants diagnosed in the first year of life • Children living with HIV 1 year old to less than 10 years old (conditional recommendation).
	As a priority, ART should be initiated in all children <2 years of age or children younger than 5 years of age with WHO clinical stage 3 or 4 or CD count ≤750 cells/mm³ or CD4 percentage <25% and children 5 years of age and older with WHO clinical stage 3 or 4 or CD4 count ≤350 cells/mm³.
Timing of ART for adults and children with TB	ART should be started in all TB patients living with HIV regardless of CD4 count. TB treatment should be initiated first, followed by ART as soon as possible within the first 8 weeks of treatment. HIV-positive TB patients with profound immunosuppression (e.g. CD4 counts less than 50 cells/mm³) should receive ART within the first two weeks of initiating TB treatment.
	ART should be started in any child with active TB disease as soon as possible and within 8 weeks following the initiation of antituberculosis treatment regardless of the CD4 cell count and clinical stage.

126. Ans. (a) Crimean-Congo fever

Ref: PubMed

- Host of Crimean-Congo hemorrhagic fever is cattle like cows and sheep.
  Crimean-Congo hemorrhagic fever (CHF) is caused by infection with a tick-borne virus (Nairovirus) in the family *Bunyaviridae*. The disease was first characterized in the crimea in 1944 and given the name Crimean hemorrhagic fever.

Extra Mile

- **Host of KFD:** Small mammals like squirrels and rats are main reservoirs. Monkeys are amplifying host.
- **Monkeys and forest mosquitoes** are the reservoir of the Yellow fever.

127. Ans. (b) Centripetal distribution

Ref: K.Park 23rd ed. P 145

TABLE: Differences between smallpox and chicken pox

Smallpox	Chicken pox
• **Incubation:** About 12 days (Range: 7–17 days)	About 15 days (Range 7–12 days)
• **Prodromal symptoms:** Severe	Usually mild
• **Distribution of rash:**	
• Centrifugal	• Centripetal
▪ Palms and soles frequently involved	▪ Seldom affected
▪ Axilla usually free	▪ Axilla affected
▪ Rash predominant on extensor surfaces and bony prominences	▪ Rash mostly on flexor surfaces
• **Characteristics of the rash:**	
▪ Deep-seated	▪ Superficial
▪ Vesicles multilocular and umbilicated	▪ Unilocular dew-drop like appearance
▪ Only one stage of rash may be seen at one time	▪ Rash pleomorphic. i.e. different stages of the rash evident at one given time, because rash appears in successive crops
▪ No area of inflammation is seen around the vesicles	▪ An area of inflammation is seen around the vesicles
• **Evolution of rash:**	
▪ Evolution of rash is slow, deliberate and majestic, passing through definite stages of macule, papule, vesicle and pustule	▪ Evolution of rash is very rapid
▪ Scabs begin to form 10–14 days after the rash appears	▪ Scabs begin to form 4–7 days after the rash appears
• **Fever:**	
▪ Fever subsides with the appearance of rash, but may rise again in the pustular stage (secondary rise of fever)	▪ Temperature rises with each fresh crop of rash

128. Ans. (c) Lymphadenopathy

Ref: Harrison's 19th ed. P 1067-68

- Tularemia is a zoonosis caused by *Francisella tularensis*.
- Humans of any age, sex, or race are universally susceptible to this systemic infection.

Preventive and Social Medicine (PSM)

- It is primarily a disease of wild animals and persists in contaminated environments, ectoparasites, and animal carriers.
- *F. tularensis* is a class A bioterrorism agent. With rare exceptions, tularemia is the only disease produced by *F. tularensis*—a small (0.2 μm by 0.2–0.7 μm), gram-negative, pleomorphic, nonmotile, non-spore-forming bacillus. Bipolar staining results in a coccoid appearance.
- **Incubation period:** 2–10

Clinical Manifestations

- Tularemia often starts with a sudden onset of fever, chills, headache, and generalized myalgias and arthralgias.

TABLE: Clinical Presentation of Tularemia

Sign or symptom	Rate of occurrence, %	
	Children	Adults
Lymphadenopathy	96	65
Fever (>38.3°C of > 101°F)	87	21
Ulcer/eschar/papule	45	51
Myalgias/arthralgias	39	2
Headache	9	5
Cough	9	5
Pharyngitis	43	–
Diarrhea	43	–

129. Ans. (b) *Bartonella*

Ref: K.Park 23rd ed. P 302

- **Quintan fever or Trench fever** (also known as "five-day fever" and "urban trench fever") is a moderately serious disease transmitted by body louse.
- It is caused by **Bartonella Quintana** (found in the stomach of the body louse).
- The disease is limited to central Europe.

131. Ans. (b) Yellow

Ref: K. Park, 23rd ed. pg. 438

- NACO has branded the STI/RTI (sexually transmitted infection/Reproductive tract infection) as "suraksha clinic" and has developed a communication strategy for generating demand for these services.
- Pre-packed STI/RTI colour coded kits have been provided for free supply to all designated STI/RTI clinics.

TABLE: RTI/STI Color kits under NACP/RCH/NRHM

STI/RTI syndromic diagnosis	Contents of the STI/RTI drug kits		
	Name of the kit prescribed	Color coding of the kit	Contents of the kits (Name of the Drugs)
Urethral Discharge (UD) Cervicitis (CD) Ano-rectal Discharge (ARD) Presumptive Treatment (PT)	Kit-1	Gray	1 tablet of Azithromycin (1 gram) 2 tablets of Azithromycin (500 mg): **If chlamydia** Cefixime 400 mg single dose: **If gonococcal**

> **Extra Mile**

- *Rickettsia conorii* causes Indian tick typhus
- *Coxiella burnetti* causes Q fever
- Epidemic typhus is caused by Louse
- *Rickettsia typhi* causes Murine typhus (flea borne typhus).

130. Ans. (c) Japanese encephalitis

Ref: K.Park 23rd ed. P 284-85

- Japanese encephalitis (JE) is a mosquito borne infection, caused by group B arbovirus (Flavivirus) and transmitted by culex mosquito.
- Disease is transmitted by man by the bite of infected mosquito. Man is incidental dead end host.
- Major host for JE: Pigs.
- Infected pigs do not show any overt symptom but circulate the virus so that mosquitoes get infected and transmit the virus to man. Therefore pigs are also considered as amplifier host.
- Cattles and buffaloes are mosquito attractants.
- **Mosquito vectors of JE:**
  - Culex tritaeniorhynchus (common)
  - Culex vishnui (common)
  - Culex gelidus

> **Extra Mile**

Disease	Vector
Chikungunya fever	Aedes mosquito
KFD	Ticks
Malaria	Anopheles mosquito
	• **An. Culicifacies:** For rural areas
	• **An. Stephensi:** For urban areas
Dengue	*Aedes aegypti*
	Aedes albopictus

Contd...

Explanations

535

FMGE Solutions Screening Examination

Contents of the STI/RTI drug kits			
STI/RTI syndromic diagnosis	Name of the kit prescribed	Color coding of the kit	Contents of the kits (Name of the Drugs)
Vaginitis (VD)	Kit-2	Green	1 table of secnidazole (2 gram)/2 tablets of secnidazole (1 gram) & fluconazole (150 mg)
Genital Ulcer-Disease Non-Herpetic (GUD-NH)	Kit-3	White	Injection Benzathine penicillin (2.4 MU) + 1 tablet azithromycin (1 gram)
Genital Ulcer-Disease Non-Herpetic (GUD-NH)- for patient allergic to penicillin	Kit-4	Blue	28 tablets/capsules of Doxycycline (100 mg) & 1 tablet of azithromycin (1 gram)
Genital Ulcer-Disease-Herpetic (GUD-H)	Kit-5	Red	21 tablets of Acyclovir (400 mg)
Lower Abdominal Pain (LAP/PID)	**Kit-6**	**Yellow**	1 tablet of cefixime (400 mg) 28 tablets of Metronidazole (400 mg) 28 tablets of Doxycycline (100 mg)
Inguinal bubo (IB)/Scrotal swelling	Kit-7	Black	42 tablets of Doxycyline (100 mg) & 1 tablet of Azithromycin (1 gram)

132. Ans. (d) Inguinal bubo

Please refer to above explanation

133. Ans. (b) Cervix CA

Ref: PubMed

- Among the given options, only cervix cancer can be prevented by vaccine.
- The most common causative agent of cervix CA is HPV (6, 11, 16, 18). HPV 16 and 18 has maximum risk.
- Vaccine is protective against either: 2, 4 or 9 types of HPV.
- Three HPV vaccines have Food and Drug Administration (FDA) approval in the US
- Cervarix *(provides protection against HPV 16, 18)* is for girls only, while Gardasil *(against 6, 11, 16, 18)* and Gardasil 9 can be used for both girls and boys. Gardasil 9 offers girls protection against more strains of HPV that can cause cervical cancer.
- The HPV vaccine is **recommended for girls and boys ages 11 or 12,** although it can be given as early as age 9. It is ideal for girls and boys to receive the vaccine before they have sexual contact and are exposed to HPV.

134. Ans. (b) Few hours to 5 days

Ref: K. Park 23rd ed. P 230

- Incubation period of cholera is **few hours** to **5 days,** but **commonly 1–2 days.**

135. Ans. (b) Chicken pox

Ref: K. Park, 23rd ed. pg. 143, 841, 21st ed. pg. 780

- **The following diseases are notifiable to WHO in Geneva:**
  - Cholera
  - Plague
  - Yellow fever

- In addition to these a few others like: Louse borne typhus, relapsing fever, Polio, Influenza, malaria, rabies and salmonellosis are subject to international surveillance.

136. Ans. (d) Cholera, plague and yellow fever

Ref: K. Park, 23rd ed. pg. 841-42, 21st ed. pg. 780

137. Ans. (b) 2 days before and 5 days after rash appearance

Ref: K. Park, 23rd ed. pg. 143

- Chicken pox is infective 2 days before appearance of rash and 5 days after rash disappearance.
- Measles is infective 4 days before appearance of rash and 5 days after rash disappearance
- *Mnemonic: rule of 25 and 45*
  - 2–5: chicken pox
  - 4–5: measles

138. Ans. (b) Influenza

Ref: K. Park, 23rd ed. pg. 153

Disease	Causative Organism	Incubation Period
Mumps	RNA Myxo Virus	14 to 21 days
Influenza	Orthomyxo Virus	18 to 72 hours
Measles (rubeola)	RNA Paramyxo Virus	10 to 14 days
Chicken pox	Human Herpes Virus 3	14 to 16 days

139. Ans. (c) After 48 hours of hospitalization

Ref: K. Park, 23rd ed. pg. 94, 359

- Nosocomial infections are hospital acquired infections.
- It is considered nosocomial if it develops **after a minimum of 48 hours of hospitalization.**
- *Most common organism responsible for nosocomial infection:* **Staph. Aureus.**

Preventive and Social Medicine (PSM)

140. Ans. (d) Endogenous

Ref: K. Park 23rd ed. pg. 255-57

TABLE: Cycle of Plasmodium in Humans

Pre-erythrocytic • Development of sporozoites in liver • Liberate merozoites known as "Cryptozoites" • No clinical sign/symptoms; sterile blood.
Erythrocytic • Parasite resides inside RBCs **(endogenous)**; passes through the stages of Trophozoite, schizont, Merozoite. • Multiplication of parasite leads to clinical signs/symptoms now
Gametogony • Few merozoites develop in RBCs of spleen and bone marrow to form gametocytes
Exo-erythrocytic • Persist in liver • Seen in P. vivax and P. ovale. • Causes relapse of vivax and ovale malaria

141. Ans. (a) Rocky mountain spotted fever

Ref: K. Park, 23rd ed. pg. 299-300

537

TABLE: Diseases, their causative agents and vectors

Disease	Causative agent	Vector
RMSF *(Rocky Mountain Spotted Fever)*	*R. Rickettsii*	Tick
Kyasanur forest disease (KFD) aka monkey disease	*Group B togavirus (Flavivirus)*	Hard tick (in India); Soft tick (outside India)
Dengue	*Arbovirus* 4 serotypes (Den-1,2,3,4)	Aedes Aegypti
Yellow fever	*Flavivirus fibricus*	Aedes Aegypti

142. Ans. (d) Scrub typhus

Ref: K. Park, 23rd ed. pg. 299-300, Park's, PSM, 20/ 262

Rickettsial Diseases, their Agents and Insect Vectors

Disease	Rickettsial agent	Insect Vectors
Epidemic typhus	*R. prowazekii*	Louse
Endemic typhus	*R. typhi*	Flea
Scrub typhus	*R. tsutsugarnushi*	Mite
Indian tick typhus	*R. conorii*	Tick
Rocky mountain spotted fever	*R. rickettsii*	Tick
Rickettsial pox	*R. akari*	Mite
Q fever	*C. burnetii*	
Trench fever	*Rochalimae aquintana*	Louse

• DOC for rickettsial infection: **Doxycycline**

143. Ans. (a) Bancroftian filariasis

Ref: K. Park, 23rd ed. pg. 270-71, Park, 20th pg. 262

Bancroftian filariasis is transmitted by Culex Mosquito.

Anopheles (Sophisticated mosquito)	Culex (nuisance mosquito)	Aedes (tiger mosquito)	Mansonoides
Malaria	• Japanese encephalitis • West nile fever • *Bancraftian filariasis* • Viral arthritis	• Yellow fever • Rift valley fever • Chikangunya fever • Dengue • Dengue haemorrhagic fever	Brugian filariasis

Explanations

144. Ans. (a) Measles

MEASLES

- Caused by RNA paramyxovirus
- **I.P.: 10–14 days.**
- Pathognomonic feature: **Koplik's spot** (on Buccal mucosa opposite 2nd molar)
- **Most common complication** of measles in **young children: Otitis Media**
- Late/rare complication of measles: **SSPE.**

> **Extra Mile**
> - Late complication of mumps: Orchitis
> - Most common late complication of chicken pox: Shingles
> - Complication of rubella infection in pregnancy: *Congenital Rubella Syndrome*
>   - **Triad of CRS**
>   - Sensorineural deafness
>   - Congenital heart defect (PDA most commonly)
>   - Cataract

145. Ans. (a) Tuberculin test

Ref: K. Park, 23rd ed. pg. 185

- **Tuberculin Test** is the only way of estimating the prevalence of infection in a community.
  - A positive test indicates past or present infection by *Mycobacterium tuberculosis.*
  - Remember: A positive tuberculin test is NOT a confirmatory diagnostic of MTB.
- **Sputum smear examination** (Z-N stain) by direct microscopy is the diagnostic choice for TB case detection.
- **Chest X-Ray** is a supportive diagnostic test for TB.
- **Montoux test** is also a screening test for TB. A positive test indicates current or past infection.

146. Ans. (a) Sputum smear microscopy

Ref: K. Park, 23rd ed. pg. 176-77

- **Sputum smear examination** (Z-N stain) by direct microscopy is the diagnostic choice for TB case detection in India.
- **Chest X-Ray** is a supportive diagnostic test for TB.
- **Montoux test** is also a screening test for TB. A positive test indicates current or past infection with any of the mycobacterium species.

147. Ans. (d) All of the above

Ref: K. Park, 23rd ed. pg. 199-200

Definition of Extensive Drug Resistance

- Resistance to both isoniazid (H) and rifampicin, and
- Resistance to 1 fluoroquinolones and
- Resistance to one 2nd line injectables out of 3 *(kanamycin, amikacin, capreomycin).*

Older Definition of XDR

- Resistance of isoniazid (H) and rifampicin both +
- Resistance to any 3rd line drugs.

> **Extra Mile**
> - Multiple drug resistance (MDR) means resistance to isoniazid (H) and rifampicin (R).

148. Ans. (c) Case detection with the help of X-ray chest

Ref: K. Park, 23rd ed. pg. 176, 188, 427, Park, 19th pg. 354

Good quality sputum microscopy and not X ray chest is one of the components of DOTS, **DOTS components**
- **Political commitment**
- **Good quality sputum microscopy**
- **Directly observed treatment**
- **Uninterrupted supply of good quality drugs**
- **Accountability**

149. Ans. (b) Culture

Ref: K. Park, 23rd ed. pg. 176-177, 183

- **Sputum smear examination** (Z-N stain) by direct microscopy to check acid fast bacilli is the diagnostic of choice for TB case detection in India.
- Lepsrosy is caused by M. Leprae and is diagnosed by clinical examination.
- *All mycobacterial infections are acid fast. So, MTB and M.Leprae can't be differentiated by AFB smear.*
- Culture has better sensitivity and M.TB infection can be differentiated from other mycobacterial infection by culture.

150. Ans. (c) 4 weeks

Ref: K. Park, 23rd ed. pg. 181-182

151. Ans. (d) Children below 6 years

Ref: K. Park, 23rd ed. pg. 182-84

- **About national TB program, if a person is smear positive for TB:**
  - All the family who is in close contact with the patient is given prophylaxis
  - Children under age 6 is given prophylaxis

Note: *India's Revised National Tuberculosis Control Programme (RNTCP) recommends screening of all household contacts of smear-positive pulmonary tuberculosis (PTB) cases for tuberculosis (TB) disease, and 6-month isoniazid preventive therapy (IPT) for asymptomatic **children aged <6 years**.*

Preventive and Social Medicine (PSM)

152. Ans. (b) Dog

Ref: K. Park, 23rd ed. pg. 276-77

- Rabies is caused by Lyssa virus type 1
- **Types of rabies virus:** Street virus and fixed virus
- **I.P.:** 4 days to 3–8 weeks or upto years in some cases
- *Intermediate host: Dog*
- **Dead end host:** Humans

Extra Mile
- *Rat bite or Human bite doesn't cause rabies.*

153. Ans. (c) Infected rat's urine

Ref: K. Park, 23rd ed. pg. 291-92

- *Leptospirosis* is caused by infection with bacteria of the genus *Leptospira* and affects humans as well as other animals.
- One of the zoonotic infection, which transmits from animals to human
- Leptospirosis is transmitted by the urine of an infected animal like rat, mice or moles and is contagious as long as the urine is still moist.

Extra Mile
- Doxycycline 200–250 mg once a week used as prophylaxis.

154. Ans. (a) Azithromycin

Ref: K. Park, 23rd ed. pg. 308-309

- Trachoma is caused by *C. Trachomatis*.
- I.P.- 5-12 days
- **SAFE** strategy used for control of trachoma
  - **S:** Surgery
  - **A:** Antibiotic
  - **F:** Face wash
  - **E:** Environment
- DOC for Trachoma: **Azithromycin** > tetracycline

Extra Mile
- Please don't confuse between SAFE strategy and Safe delivery strategy.
  - *Safe delivery strategy is used for prevention of neonatal Tetanus.*
  - Neonatal tetanus is aka 8th day disease (I.P.- 8 days)
- **DOC for Ricketsial diseases:** *Doxycycline*

155. Ans. (d) Education

Ref: K. Park, 23rd ed. pg. 308-209

Please refer to above explanation

156. Ans. (c) Inhalation

Ref: K. Park, 23rd ed. pg. 292-94

- **Pneumonic plague**, a severe type of lung infection
- It is one of three main forms of plague, all of which are caused by the bacterium *Yersinia pestis*.
- Primary pneumonic plague results from inhalation of fine infective droplets and can be transmitted from human to human without involvement of fleas or animals.

157. Ans. (b) In endemic areas step wells or by chemo radiation

Ref: K. Park, 23rd ed. pg. 245-46

WHO considerations for Dracunculosis Eradication:
- Control of Cyclops
- Provision of safe drinking water like piped water and instillation of hand pumps
- Education and awareness of public for safe drinking water
- Active search for new cases
- Niridazole, mebendazole and metronidazole are not effective in preventing transmission.

158. Ans. (d) Culex

Ref: K. Park, 23rd ed. pg. 292-93

- The commonest and most effective vector of plague is rat flea x.cheopsis.
- Others are X.Astia, X.Brasiliensis and Pulexirritans.
- Culex is a vector of lymphatic filariasis and Japanese encephalitis (*culex tritaeniorhynchus*).

159. Ans. (c) 350

Ref: K. Park, 23rd ed. pg. 343-45

- Best marker of HIV progression: CD4:CD8 ratio
- Normal CD4 count: 900-1400
- Opportunistic infection occur when CD4 count goes below: < 500
- *Anti retroviral therapy is started when CD4 count goes below: < 350 (old guidelines). The latest guidelines suggests to intiate ART in all symptomatic HIV positive patients regardless of CD4 count.*
- Single pill once a day regimen consists of dolutregravir, abacavir and lamivudine or choose 2 NRTI and 1 NNRTI combination.

160. Ans. (d) Through contact of body fluids

Ref: K. Park, 23rd ed. pg. 356

- Incubation period of ebola virus **2-21 days**
- According to WHO *"Ebola then spreads through human-to-human transmission via direct contact (through broken skin or mucous membranes) with the blood, secretions, organs or other bodily fluids of infected people, and with surfaces and materials (e.g. bedding, clothing) contaminated with these fluids."*

Explanations

161. Ans. (a) Safe water supply & sanitation

Ref: K. Park, 23rd ed. pg. 232-33

- Cholera is an acute diarrheal disease caused by *Vibrio cholerae*.
- I.P.- 1-2 days
- **First step in epidemic of cholera: Verification of diagnosis**
- **First line treatment of choice:** water and electrolyte replacement because most death in cholera is due to hypovolemic shock.
- In the given question, safe water supply and sanitation should be the 1st step to decrease mortality from cholera.

Extra Mile

- Stool appearance of cholera: *"Rice watery stool"*
- **Chemoprophylaxis of cholera:** Tetracycline 500mg BID for 5 days.
- **Drug of choice for cholera:**
  - **Adults:** Doxycycline 300 mg stat.
  - **Children:** Azithromycin 20 mg/kg, single dose
  - **Pregnant Female:** Azithromycin 1 gm, single dose

162. Ans. (d) Safe water supply and sanitation

Ref: K. Park, 23rd ed. pg. 232-33

Please refer to above explanation

163. Ans. (b) 90% in south east Asia population by tobacco chewing

Ref: Park, 21st ed. pg. 357-358

ORAL CANCER

- Most cases of oral cancer (~ 90%) in south east asia are linked to tobacco chewing and tobacco smoking.
- Alcohol and pre-cancerous lesion (like leukoplakia, erythroplakia) have also shown to increase the risk of development of oral cancer.
- In India, the most common form of tobacco chewing is betel quid which usually consist of betel leaf, areca nut, lime and tobacco.
- Cancer of oral cavity is also very prevalent in central Asian districts of Erstwhile Russian Republics, where people chew "nass" or "nasswar"- a mixture of tobacco, ashes, lime and cotton seed oil.
- In eastern coastal regions of Andhra Pradesh epidermoid carcinoma of hard palate is most common. It is linked with habit of reverse smoking of cigar *(chutta)*, i.e., smoking with burning end inside the mouth.

164. Ans. (b) Carcinoma hard palate

Ref: K. Park, 21st ed. pg. 357-58

- In eastern coastal regions of Andhra Pradesh epidermoid **carcinoma of hard palate** is most common. It is linked with habit of reverse smoking of cigar *(chutta)*, i.e., smoking with burning end inside the mouth.

165. Ans. (d) All of the above

Ref: K. Park, 21st ed. pg. 360

- Recent studies have shown that smoking increases the risk of lung cancer by 8.6% as compared to non smokers.
- **The risk is strongly related to:**
  - Number of cigarette smoked
  - Age of starting to smoke
  - Mode of smoking
  - Nicotine and tar content
  - Length of cigarette
- One study in India has proved that there is no difference between the tar and nicotine delivery of the filter and non-filter cigarettes smoked in India. Therefore a **filter gives NO protection to Indian smokers.** The "king-size" filter cigarettes deliver more tar and nicotine than ordinary cigarette.

NATIONAL HEALTH PROGRAMS & POLICIES

166. Ans. (d) Includes area with slide positivity of more than 10 cases per 10,000 smears

Ref: K. Park 25th ed. P 429, 286

- The urban malaria scheme was launched in 1971 to reduce or interrupt malaria transmission in urban areas.
- It is currently protecting 130 million population from malaria and other mosquito borne diseases
- It comprises of following methodologies:
  - Vector control by intensive antilarval measure and drug treatment
  - Prevention of mosquito breeding in domestic and peri domestic areas by using larvivorous fish in water bodies
  - Use of larvicides in water bodies
- The expert committee on malaria had recommended the inclusion of:
  - All urban areas with more than 50,000 population
  - Slide positivity rate of **5% and above**
  - Areas with annual parasitic index ≥2 per 1000 per year have been classified as high risk areas, and thereby eligible for vector control.

167. Ans. (a) Male MPW

Ref: K. Park 25th ed. P 973

Work responsibilities for health worker male/male MPW (Multi-purpose worker)

Preventive and Social Medicine (PSM)

- Malaria surveillance activities
- Collect thick and thin blood smears on glass slide from a case having fever
- Identify cases of Japanese encephalitis, filariasis, kala azar
- Identify persons 15 years and above with prolonged cough and take sputum smear and supervise the TB patients to take regular treatment (DOTS-MDT)
- Identify suspects of leprosy patients, blindness all cases including cataract suspects
- Administer vaccine under expanded program on immunization
- Spread awareness and educate public on family planning and distribution of conventional contraceptives
- Identify cases of diarrhoea, dysentery, jaundice, whooping cough, diphtheria, encephalitis, acute eye infection and notify to health assistant. Give ORS and educate community about preventive measures
- Maintain record of birth, death and other diseases like TB, leprosy, malaria cases

168. Ans. (c) Health worker male

Ref: K. Park 25ᵗʰ ed. P 973

- Collection of sputum from TB suspected patients and making smear is job responsibility of health worker-male.
- Under RNTCP they need to:
  - Identify persons >15 years with prolonged cough and haem-optysis. Take their sputum smear and refer them to PHC for further investigations.
  - Check whether all cases of TB are taking regular medication or not and motivate them to do so.
  - Assist ASHA and village health volunteers to carry out DOTS activities.

169. Ans. (b) Multipurpose worker

Ref: K. Park 25ᵗʰ ed. P 449

- Aim of malaria surveillance program:
  - Target controlled interventions in high transmission areas and assess their impact
  - Early detection of outbreaks
- The active surveillance (active case detection) is done by multipurpose worker/ANM in rural areas with blood smears
- Passive case detection is done in fever cases by ASHA/peripheral health volunteer.
- Best method of diagnosis with maximum sensitivity and specificity: Microscopy
- Method of choice for malaria diagnosis in remote areas/tribal, inaccessible rural areas: RDT kit (Rapid Diagnostic Test).

170. Ans. (b) RTI/STD

Ref: K. Park 25ᵗʰ ed. P 472

- According to STD control program, STD control is linked to HIV/AIDS control as behaviour leading to both are same
- HIV is transmitted more easily in presence of STD
- NACO, therefore has branded the Sexually Transmitted Infection (STI)/Reproductive Tract Infections (RTI) services as **Suraksha clinic, and has developed** a communication strategy for generating demand for these services.
- Prepacked STI/RTI colour coded kits are provided at all state AIDS control societies. The kits are:
  - **Kit 1:** Grey—For urethral discharge, anorectal discharge and cervicitis
  - **Kit 2:** Green—for vaginitis
  - **Kit 3:** White—for genital ulcers—non herpitic
  - **Kit 4:** Blue—for genital ulcers—non herpitic in patient allergic to penicillin
  - **Kit 5:** Red—for genital ulcers—herpitic
  - **Kit 6:** Yellow—for lower abdominal pain
  - **Kit 7:** Black—for Inguinal bubo

171. Ans. (d) Child trafficking

Ref: K. Park 25ᵗʰ ed. P 645

- In India, Ujjawala scheme was launched to combat child trafficking by the ministry of women and child development on 4ᵗʰ December 2007.
- Scheme has 5 provisions for victims trafficked for commercial sexual exploitation:
  - **Prevention:** Formation of community vigilance group, adolescents group, awareness creations and organizing work-shops
  - **Rescue:** Safe withdrawal of victims from exploitation place
  - **Reintegration:** of victims into society
  - **Rehabilitation:** By providing them safe shelter, medical care, basic amenities, legal aid, vocational training and employment
  - **Repatriation:** Provide support to cross border victims for their safe repatriation to their country of origin

172. Ans. (a) Service centre

Ref: K. Park 25ᵗʰ ed. P 474

Vision 2020: The Right to Sight

- A global initiative to reduce avoidable (preventable and curable) causes of blindness by year 2020.
- The plan has the following features:
  - Target diseases are: cataract, refractive error, childhood blindness, corneal blindness, glaucoma, diabetic retinopathy

- The proposed 4 tier structure includes:
  - Centre of excellence (20)
  - Training centres (200)
  - Service centres (2000)
  - Vision centres (20,000)
- The shown **image** depicts the proposed structure for primary, secondary and tertiary eye care (referral from base to apex)

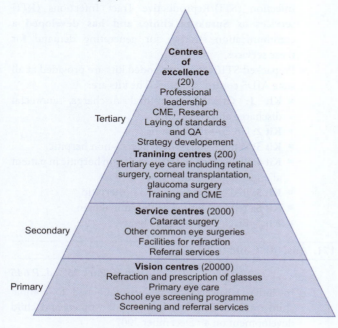

173. Ans. (b) Street children

Ref: K. Park 25th ed. P 373

Key population affected with HIV in India

- The HIV epidemic in India is driven by sexual transmission, which accounts for 86% of new infection in 2017.
- The following population is mainly affected, which needs targeted intervention:
  - **Female sex workers:** in 2017, ~1.6% were found to be living with AIDS
  - **IV drug abusers:** Major route of HIV transmission in north-east states. In 2017, 6.3% of HIV drug abusers are found to be living with AIDS
  - **Hijras/transgenders:** Prevalence in 2017 was found to be 3.1%
  - **Migrant labourers:** An estimated 7.2 million migrant workers in India, of whom 0.2% are living with HIV
  - **Truck drivers:** NACO estimated 0.2% of truck drivers are living with HIV in 2017-18. They are considered as bridge population for HIV transmission since they often have unprotected sex with high risk groups as well as their regular sex partners.

174. Ans. (d) All of the above

Ref: K.Park 23rd ed. P 449

- The main aim of NRHM is to provide accessible, affordable, accountable, effective and reliable primary health care, and bridging the gap in rural health care through creation of a cadre of Accredited Social Health Activist (ASHA).
- The mission is an instrument to integrate multiple vertical programs alongwith their funds at the district level.
- The programs integrated into NRHM are existing programs of health and family welfare including RCH II: national vector borne disease control programs against malaria, filarial, kala-azar dengue fever/DHF and Japanese encephalitis; national leprosy eradication program; revised national tuberculosis control program; national program for control of blindness; iodine deficiency disorder control program, and integrated disease surveillance project.

175. Ans. (d) Lung infections

Ref: K.Park 23rd ed. P 579

- School health services is an economical and powerful means of raising community health, especially in future generations.
- It is based on the local health problems of school child and vary from one place to another.
- **According to surveys, the main emphasis of school health fall in following categories:**
  - Malnutrition
  - Infectious diseases
  - Intestinal parasites
  - Diseases of the skin, eye and ear
  - Dental caries
- **Objectives of school health service**
  - Promotion of positive health
  - Prevention of diseases
  - Early diagnosis, treatment and follow up of defects
  - Awakening health consciousness in children
  - Provision of healthful environment

176. Ans. (b) Delivery at home

Ref: K.Park 23rd ed. P 449-450

- ASHA is a health activist in the community, who creates awareness on health. Her responsibilities are as follows:
  - Create awareness and information on nutrition, basic sanitation, hygienic practices and the need for timely utilization of health and family welfare services.
  - Counsel the women for safe delivery, breastfeeding, immunization, contraception and prevention of common infections including STI's.

Preventive and Social Medicine (PSM)

- Facilitate the services available at anganwadi, subcenter, PHC.
- Escort/accompany pregnant women and children requiring treatment/admissions to the nearest health center.
- Act as depot holder for essential provisions being made available to every habitation like ORS powder, iron and folic acid tablet, chloroquine, disposable delivery kits, OCP's, condoms etc.
- Provide primary medical care for minor ailments like diarrhea, fever and first aid for minor injuries. Also provide DOTS under RNTCP.
- To inform about the birth and death in her village or any unusual health problems/outbreaks in the community.
- To promote construction of household toilets under total sanitation campaign.

177. Ans. (d) 400 INR to ASHA and 1000 INR to mother in Urban area low performing states

Ref: K.Park 23rd ed. P 455

- The scale of assistance under the scheme from 2012–2013 for encouraging safe delivery at the health institutions is as follows:

	Rural area			Urban area		
Category	Mother's package	ASHA's package*	Total ₹	Mother's package	ASHA's package**	Total ₹
LPS	1400	600	2000	1000	400	1400
HPS	700	600	1300	600	400	1000

Abbreviations: LPS, low performing states; HPS, high performing states
* ASHA incentive of ₹600/- in rural areas includes ₹300/- for ANC component and ₹300/- for accompanying pregnant woman for institutional delivery.
** ASHA incentive of ₹400/- in urban area includes ₹200/- for ANC component and ₹200/- for accompanying pregnant woman for institutional delivery.

178. Ans. (b) Mild

Ref: K. Park, 23rd ed. pg. 582

TABLE: Categories of mental retardation

Mental Status	IQ Range
Normal IQ	>70
Mild mental retardation	50–70
Moderate MR	35–49
Severe MR	20–34
Profound MR	Below 20

179. Ans. (b) Kartar Singh Committee

Ref: K. Park, 23rd ed. pg. 874-75

- **Kartar Singh Committee:** Recommended multi-purpose worker scheme. Kartar singh committee recommended:
  - **Current ANM** to be replaced by the newly designated "female health worker" and present day basic health workers, malaria surveillance workers, family planning health assistants to be replaced by "male health workers"
- **Bhore Committee recommendation:**
  - Integration of preventive and curative services at all administrative levels
  - **Short-term program:** Each PHC should cater to a population of 40,000 with a secondary health centre to serve as a supervisory, coordinating and referral institution
  - **Long-term program aka 3 million plan:** Setting up a 75 bedded primary health unit for each 10,000 to 20,000 population; and secondary health unit with 650 bedded hospital, again regionalized around district hospital with 2500 beds
  - **Major change in medical education** which includes 3 month training in preventive and social medicine to prepare "social physicians".
- **Srivastava Committee**
  - Group on medical education and manpower.
  - Recommended bands of para-professionals and semi-professional health worker.
  - ROME (Reorientation of Medical Education) scheme.
  - Village Health Guide scheme.
  - 3-Tier rural health infrastructure
- **Jungalwalla committee**
  - Equal pay for equal work
  - No private practice
- **Mudaliar committee:** Health survey and planning committee

180. Ans. (c) Complete hospitalization

Ref: K. Park, 23rd ed. pg. 473-74

Community Mental Health Programme Include Essential Elements

- Inpatient services
- Outpatient service
- Partial hospitalization
- Emergency services
- Diagnostic services
- Pre care & after care services including foster home placement and home visiting

FMGE Solutions Screening Examination

- Education services
- Training
- Research and evaluation

181. Ans. (c) Started in 1987

Ref: K. Park, 23rd ed. pg. 473-74

- National Mental Health Program: **1982**
- National Family Planning Program: **1952**
- National Aids Control Program: **1987**
- National Anti Malaria Program: **1999**

182. Ans (c) Reproductive and child health program

Ref: K. Park, 23rd ed. pg. 452, Park, 19th ed. pg. 392

- India's family welfare program seeks to promote on a voluntary basis, responsible and planned parenthood with the "two child norm" male, female or both through **'cafeteria approach'**, that is **an independent choice of family planning methods, best suited for the couples.**

183. Ans. (b) Yellow

Ref: Parks, 21st ed. pg. 397

Color Coding System

Kit 1	Grey	Urethral and ano-rectal discharge and cervicitis
Kit 2	Green	Vaginitis
Kit 3	White	Genital ulcers
Kit 4	Blue	Genital ulcers
Kit 5	Red	Genital ulcers
Kit 6	**Yellow**	**Abdominal pain**
Kit 7	Black	Scrotal swelling

184. Ans. (c) 40

Ref: K. Park 23rd ed. / 804-805

185. Ans. (d) 21–34

Ref: K. Park, 23rd ed. pg. 582-83

Mental status	IQ Range
Normal IQ	70 and over
Mild mental retardation	50–70
Moderate MR	35–49
Severe MR	20–34
Profound MR	20 and below

186. Ans. (c) 100% birth and death registration

Ref: K Park, 23rd ed. pg. 493-94

- **National Population Policy 2000**
  - Address the unmet needs for basic reproductive and child health services, supplies and infrastructure
  - Make school education up to age 14 free and compulsory, and reduce drop outs at primary and secondary school levels to <20% for both boys and girls
  - **Reduce IMR to < 30 per 1000 live births**
  - **Reduce MMR to <100 per 100,000 live births**
  - Achieve universal immunization of children against all VPDs
  - Promote delayed marriage for girls (not <18 years and preferably >20 years)
  - **Achieve 80% institutional deliveries and 100% by trained persons**
  - Achieve universal access to information/counseling, and services for fertility regulation and contraception with a wide basket of choice
  - **Achieve 100% registration of birth, deaths, marriage & pregnancy**
  - Contain the spread of AIDS, and promote greater integration between the management of RTI and STI and the NACO.

187. Ans. (b) Decrease child mortality rate

Ref: K. Park, 23rd ed. pg. 11,27, 32, 893

MILLENNIUM DEVELOPMENT GOALS (MDGS)

- There are 8 MDGs:
  - **Goal 1:** Eradicated extreme poverty and hunger
  - **Goal 2:** universalize primary education
  - **Goal 3:** Gender equality and women empowerment
  - **Goal 4: Reduce child mortality**
  - *Goal 5: Improve maternal health*
  - **Goal 6:** Combat HIV/AIDS, malaria and other disease (Tuberculosis)
  - **Goal 7:** Ensure environmental sustainability
  - **Goal 8:** Develop global partnerships for development 3 out of 8 goals, 8 out of 18 targets required to achieve them and 18 out of 48 indicators of progress are *'directly health related'*
- **Goal 4, 5 and 6 are directly health related**
- Goal 2 and 3 *'do not pertain to health'*

188. Ans (c) 2015

Ref: K. Park, 23rd ed. pg. 27, 32, K. Park, 19th ed. pg 743

- The Millennium Development Goals (MDG) are to be achieved by the year **2015**.

189. Ans. (a) Leprosy

Ref: K. Park, 23rd ed. pg. 314-15, 22nd ed pg. 289-90

Preventive and Social Medicine (PSM)

- Leprosy has been eliminated from India, but it has not yet eradicated.
- The definition of elimination is <1 case/10,000 population.

190. Ans. (a) Kala-azar

Ref: K. Park, 21ˢᵗ ed. pg. 113

- Indian Academy of Pediatrics (IAP) approved following vaccines (Kala Azar is NOT included in schedule)
- **Following vaccines are approved by IAP:** Polio, hepatitis, BCG, DPT, Hib, MMR, TT, typhoid.

191. Ans. (b) Yellow fever

Ref: K. Park, 21ˢᵗed. pg. 380

- The National Vector Borne Disease Control Programme (NVBDCP) is implemented for the prevention and control of vector borne diseases such as: Malaria, Filariasis, kala-azar, Japanese encephalitis, Dengue and Chikunguniya.
- Yellow fever is NOT a part of NVBDCP.

PREVENTIVE OBSTETRICS, PEDIATRICS AND GERIATRICS

192. Ans. (b) 25

Ref: K. Park 25ᵗʰ ed. P 557

MTP Act 1971
- **Conditions for MTP:**
  - **Medical:** Where continuation of pregnancy might endanger mother's life
  - **Eugenic:** There is high risk of child being born with serious physical or mental abnormalities
  - **Humanitarian:** Where pregnancy is outcome of rape
  - **Socio-economic:** Social or economic environment that could lead to risk of injury to the health of mother
  - **Failure of contraceptive devices:** Where pregnancy is as a result of contraceptive method failure
- In case the woman is under 18 years or a lunatic of any age—a written consent of guardian is necessary
- **Who can perform:**
  - **If pregnancy below 12 weeks:** A registered medical practitioner having experience in OBG
  - **If >12 weeks – 20 weeks:** Opinion of two registered medical practitioner is necessary
- **Where to be performed:** Established hospitals or a place approved by government or any non-government institution after obtaining license from chief medical officer of district.

MTP Rules 1975
- **Approval of boards:** According to new rules the chief medical officer of district is empowered to certify if the doctor has necessary training in gynaecology and obstetrics to do abortions. Application to certification boards is NOT required.
- **Qualification required:**
  - If assisted an RMP of an approved institution in performance of **25 cases** of MTP or
  - 6 months of house manship in OBG or
  - MD in OBG or
  - 3 years of practice in OBG for those doctors registered before 1971 MTP Act
  - 1 year of practice in OBG for those doctors registered after 1971 MTP Act

193. Ans. (b) IUD

Ref: K. Park 25ᵗʰ ed. P 549

- The best contraceptive method post placental and post abortion is IUD
- IUD is the most effective reversible contraceptive method.
- IUD is generally contraindicated in unmotivated persons, but since in this case the patient herself doesn't wish to conceive in near future, IUD is preferred.

Advantages of IUD:
- Ease of insertion
- Prevent uterine synechiae
- Longer action and inexpensive
- Contraceptive effect is reversible by simply removal of IUD
- Free of systemic metabolic side effects as seen with pills
- No need for continuous motivation (as seen with pills or barrier method). Only a single act of motivation is required.

Ideal IUD candidate:
- In monogamous relationship
- Has borne at-least one child
- No history of PID
- Has normal menstrual period
- Willing to check the IUD tail
- Has access to follow up and treatment

Timing of insertion
- During menstruation or within 10 days of beginning of a menstrual period (diameter of cervical canal is greater)
- Can be done during the **first week after the delivery** before she leaves hospital (immediate postpartum insertion).
  - Special care required during first week as it has greater risk of perforation

- **Note:** Immediate postpartum can also be done within 10 minutes after placenta expulsion in a vaginal delivery.
- **Loop insertion:** Convenient time for loop insertion is 6–8 weeks after delivery *(postpuerperal insertion/Extended postpartum)*
- Can also be taken up immediately after first trimester abortion
  - IUD insertion after second trimester is NOT recommended → Increased risk of infection

194. Ans. (a) 350 kcal

Ref: K. Park 25th ed. P 690-91

- The energy requirement of women is increased over and above their normal requirement in following conditions:
  - **Pregnancy:** + 350 kcal/day throughout pregnancy
  - **Lactation:** + 600 kcal/day during first 6 months and +520 kcal/day during next 6 months.

Extra Mile

TABLE: Energy requirement of indians at different ages

Age group	Remarks	(kcal/day)
Man	Sedentary work	2,320
	Moderate work	2,730
	Heavy work	3,490
Woman	Sedentary work	1,900
	Moderate work	2,230
	Heavy work	2,850
	Pregnant woman	+350
	Lactation	+600
		+520
Infants	0-6 months	500
	6-12 months	670
Children	1-3 years	1,060
	4-6 years	1,350
	7-9 years	1,690

195. Ans. (b) Intrauterine growth retardation

Ref: K. Park 25th ed. P 587

Low birth weight
- Defined as birth weight of less than **2.5 kg**, regardless of gestational age
- The birth weight of an infant is the single most important determinant of its chances of survival, healthy growth and development.
- Two main groups of low birth weight:
  - **Premature born (short gestation):** MC in developed countries where population of low birth weight is less
  - **Fetal growth retardation:** MC in countries (like India) where proportion is high. It is considered as the most common cause of low birth weight in India.

Extra Mile

- Apart from birth weight, babies can be classified in 3 groups according to gestational age:
  - **Preterm:** Born before 37 weeks of gestation (<259 days)
  - **Term:** Born between 37–42 weeks (259–293 days)
  - **Post-term:** Born at 42 completed week or any time after (≥294 days)
- Preterm babies are further classified as:
  - **Extremely preterm:** (<28 weeks)
  - **Very preterm** (28 to <32 weeks)
  - **Moderate to late preterm** (32–37 weeks)
- Birth weight >4 kg is considered as overweight
- **Average birth weight in India:** 2.8 kg.

196. Ans. (a) Glucose – 90

Ref: K.Park 23rd ed. P 224

- In reduced osmolarity ORS, content of glucose is 75 mmol/L

Composition of reduced osmolarity ORS	
Reduced osmolarity ORS	**Grams/Liter**
Sodium chloride	2.6
Glucose, anhydrous	13.5
Potassium chloride	1.5
Trisodium citrate, dehydrate	2.9
Total weight	20.5
Reduced osmolarity ORS	**mmol/Liter**
Sodium	75
Chloride	65
Glucose, anhydrous	75
Potassium	20
Citrate	10
Total osmolarity	245

197. Ans. (c) 20 mg/day

Ref: K. Park, 23rd pg. 636

- **Park states:** *"Iron required during lactation is 21 mg/day"*

198. Ans. (a) 1900

Ref: K. Park, 23rd ed. pg. 634

Preventive and Social Medicine (PSM)

TABLE: Energy requirements of Indians at different ages

Age group	Remarks	(kcal/day)
Man	Sedentary work	2,320
	Moderate work	**2,730**
	Heavy work	3,490
Woman	**Sedentary work**	**1,900**
	Moderate work	2,230
	Heavy work	2,850
	Pregnant woman	+350
	Lactation	+600
		+520
Infants	0–6 months	500
	6–12 months	670
Children	1–3 years	1,060
	4–6 years	1,350
	7–9 years	1,690

199. Ans. (d) 245 mmol/L

Ref: K. Park, 23rd ed. pg. 224

Composition of reduced osmolarity ORS

Reduced osmolarity ORS	Grams/Liter
• Sodium chloride	2.6
• Glucose, anhydrous	13.5
• Potassium chloride	1.5
• Trisodium citrate, dehydrate	2.9
Total weight	**20.5**
Reduced osmolarity ORS	**mmol/liter**
• Sodium	75
• Chloride	65
• Glucose, anhydrous	75
• Potassium	20
• Citrate	10
Total osmolarity	**245**

200. Ans. (a) Anemia

- Most common Indirect cause of maternal mortality in India: Anemia
- Most common cause of maternal mortality in India: Post partum hemorrhage (PPH)
- Most common direct cause of MMR: PPH

Direct maternal mortality	Indirect maternal mortality
• It results from obstetric complication of pregnant state (pregnancy, labor and puerperium) from interventions or incorrect treatment.	• It results from previous existing disease or disease that develops during pregnancy.
• Ex: PPH, obstructed labor, sepsis	• Anemia, HTN, gestational DM, epilepsy

201. Ans. (d) Perinatal mortality rate

Ref: K. Park, 23rd ed. pg. 563-64

- **Perinatal period** is from 28th week age of gestation to 7th day of newborn life.
- Perinatal mortality rate includes late fetal deaths and early neonatal deaths.
- A better obstetric care will be able to diagnose any fetal stress which will result in early intervention, which will certainly help in delivering a healthy baby.
- Therefore an obstetric will mostly affect Perinatal mortality rate.

202. Ans. (b) 100 mg iron + 500 mcg folic acid

Ref: K. Park, 23rd ed. pg. 527

- **Adult** iron + folic acid tablet given in pregnancy: 1 tab/day × 100 days
- **Kids** iron + folic acid tablet given: 1 tab/day × 100 days per year- 0 to 5 years of age.

TABLE: Iron and Folic acid tablet content

	Iron	Folic acid
Adult tab	100 mg	500 mcg
Kids tab (1/5th)	20 mg	100 mcg

203. Ans. (c) 1000 mg

Ref: K. Park, 23rd ed. pg. 527

According to RCH program, 100 mg of elemental iron and 500 mcg of folic acid must be given to a pregnant lady for 100 days, which will be around 1000 mg iron absorbed.

- **Adult:** Iron + folic acid tablet given in pregnancy: 1 tab/day x 100 days
- **Kids:** Iron + folic acid tablet given: 1 tab/day x 100 days per year- 0 to 5 years of age.

FMGE Solutions Screening Examination

204. Ans. (a) Iron 100 mg and folic acid 500 μg

Ref: K. Park, 23rd ed. pg. 620-22

205. Ans. (c) 500-550 kcal

Ref: K. Park, 23rd ed. pg. 530-31

1st trimester	+ 150 kcal/day
3rd trimester	+300 kcal/day
Lactation	+550 Kcal/day

206. Ans. (c) Before 21 days

Ref: K. Park, 23rd ed. pg. 840-41

Registration of Some Vital Events
- Birth: before 21 days
- Death: before 21 days
- Marriage: before 30 days

207. Ans. (b) Green

Ref: Park's PSM, 21st ed. pg. 414

- According to Integrated Management of Neonatal and Childhood Illness (IMNCI), childhood morbidity and mortality is caused by diarrhea, ARI, malaria, malnutrition etc.
- Conditions are classified according to severity, and treatment action taken according to color code triage:
  - **Red:** Urgent referral after pre-referral treatments.
  - **Yellow:** treat at outpatient health facility (treat local infection, give oral drugs, advise care-taker)
  - **Green:** *Home management* (advise care-taker on how to give oral drugs, when to approach immediately, follow up etc.)

208. Ans. (c) ORS

Ref: K. Park, 23rd ed. pg. 224, 453

- WHO recommends ORS as the best measure in diarrhea for preventing the complications that may arise due to water and electrolyte loss.
- Metronidazole can be used as supportive therapy. It controls the anaerobic infection of G.I.

209. Ans. (b) 6 months

Ref: K. Park, 23rd ed. pg. 508, 530-33

Exclusive breast feeding: 0 to 6 month and should be continue upto 2 years

210. Ans. (c) Perinatal mortality

Ref: K. Park, 23rd ed. pg. 567, 19th pg. 449 fig 9

$$IMR = \frac{\text{Number of death of children less than 1 year of age in a year}}{\text{Number of live births in the same year}} \times 1000$$

Perinatal Mortality Rate (PMR)

$$PMR = \frac{\text{[Late fetal deaths (28 weeks gestation and more) + early neonatal deaths (first week) in one year]}}{\text{Live births in the same year}} \times 100$$

Perinatal Mortality Rate (PMR) =

$$\frac{\text{Late fetal deaths + Early neonatal deaths}}{\text{Late fetal deaths + live births}} \times 100$$

Where Late fetal means 28 weeks gestation or more; Early neonatal means first week

NUTRITION AND HEALTH

211. Ans. (d) >0.85 in female

Ref: K. Park 25th ed. P 429

- Waist circumference is measured at the mid-point between lower border of rib and iliac crest. It correlates closely to BMI and waist to hip ratio.
- Changes in waist circumference reflects changes in risk factor of cardiovascular disease and other chronic diseases.
- Increased risk of metabolic complications with **waist circumference:**
  - Men ≥ 102 cm
  - Women ≥ 88 cm
- Waist hip ratio is calculated by waist circumference measurement divided by hip measurement.
- **Waist hip ratio** that increases the risk of cardiovascular disease:
  - Men: > 1
  - Women: > 0.85

212. Ans. (d) Polished rice

Ref: K. Park 25th ed. P 675

- Beri-Beri occurs as a result of thiamine deficiency.
- Thiamine is usually lost from rice during process of milling, washing and cooking of rice.
- This is the reason peoples are advised to avoid highly polished rice and consume parboiled and under milled rice.
- Thiamine is also destroyed in toast and in cereals cooked with baking soda.

Preventive and Social Medicine (PSM)

Extra Mile

- Thiamine deficiency can lead to: Beri-Beri and Wernicke's encephalopathy
- Beri-Beri occur in 3 main forms:
  - **Dry Beri-Beri:** Characterized by nerve involvement (peripheral neuritis)
  - **Wet Beri-Beri:** Aka cardiac Beri-Beri. Heart involvement
  - **Infantile Beri-Beri:** Seen in infants between 2-4 months. Occur secondary to thiamine deficient mother breast feeding.

---

213. Ans. (b) Reduced peak and prolonged absorption

Ref: K. Park 25th ed. P 670

- **Glycemic index (GI)** of a food is defined by the area under 2 hours blood glucose response curve (AUC) following the ingestion of a fixed portion of test carbohydrate (usually 50 g) as a proportion (%) of the AUC of the standard (either glucose or white bread).
- Food can be of low glycemic index or high glycemic index:
  - **Low glycemic index:** Food products having soluble and insoluble fibers, which favour slow release of sugar into small intestine and slow absorption into blood (reduced peak and prolonged absorption rate).
  - **High glycemic index:** Foods with readily digestible and absorbable sugar (high peak and rapid absorption)

Classification	GI range	Examples
Low GI	55 or less	Most fruit and vegetables (except potatoes, watermelon and sweet corn), whole grains, pasta foods, beans lentils
Medium GI	56-69	Sucrose, basmati rice brown rice
High GI	70 or more	Corn flakes, baked potato, some white rice varieties (e.g jasmine), White bread, candy bar and syrupy foods.

---

214. Ans. (b) 1

Ref: K.Park 23rd ed. P 613–14

- Glycemic index (GI) of a food is defined by the area under 2 hours blood glucose response curve (AUC) following the ingestion of a fixed portion of test carbohydrate (usually 50 g) as a proportion (%) of the AUC of the standard (either glucose or white bread).
- A value of 100 represents the standard, an equivalent amount of pure **glucose**.
- Food can be of low glycemic index or high glycemic index:

- **Low glycemic index:** Food products having insoluble fibers, which favor slow release of sugar into small intestine and its absorption into blood.
- **High glycemic index:** Foods with readily digestible and absorbable sugar.

TABLE: Classification of food according to GI

Classification	GI range	Examples
Low GI	55 or less	Most fruit and vegetables (except potatoes, watermelon and sweet corn), whole grains, pasta foods, beans, lentils
Medium GI	56-69	Sucrose, basmati rice, brown rice
High GI	70 or more	Corn flakes, baked potato, some white rice varieties (e.g. jasmine), white bread, candy bar and syrupy foods.

---

215. Ans. (a) Safflower oil

Ref: K. Park, 23rd pg. 611

TABLE: Dietary Sources of EFA

Essential fatty acids	Dietary source	Percent content
Linoleic acid	Safflower oil	73
	Corn oil	57
	Sunflower oil	56
	Soyabean oil	51
	Sesame oil	40
	Groundnut oil	39
	Mustard oil	15
	Palm oil	9
	Coconut oil	2
Arachidonic acid	Meat, eggs Milk (Fat)	0.5–0.3 0.4-0.6
Linolenic acid	Soyabean oil Leafy greens	7 Varied
Eichosapentaenoic acid	Fish oil	10

---

216. Ans. (c) Soyabean

Ref: K. Park, 23rd pg. 628

549

Explanations

FMGE Solutions Screening Examination

TABLE: Nutritive value of pulses (values per 100 g)

Pulses	Energy (kcal)	Proteins (g)
Bengal gram	360	17.1
Black gram	347	24.0
Red gram	335	22.3
Soyabean	432	43.2
Green gram	348	24.5
Peas dry	315	19.7
Horse gram	321	22.0

217. Ans. (a) 20 mg iron with 0.1 mg FA

Ref: K. Park, 23rd pg. 620, 624

218. Ans. (b) 2730

Ref: K. Park, 23rd ed. pg. 634

Please refer to above explanation

219. Ans. (a) 60–65

Ref: K. Park, 23rd ed. pg. 630

TABLE: Nutritive value of milks compared (value per 100 g)

	Buffalo	Cow	Goat	Human
Fat (g)	6.5	4.1	4.5	3.4
Protein (g)	4.3	3.2	3.3	1.1
Lactose (g)	5.1	4.4	4.6	7.4
Calcium (mg)	210	120	170	28
Iron (mg)	0.2	0.2	0.3	
Vitamin C (mg)	1	2	1	3
Minerals (g)	0.8	0.8	0.8	0.1
Water (g)	81.0	87	86.8	88
Energy (kcal)	117	67	72	65

220. Ans. (a) 1.2 mcg

Ref: K. Park, 23rd ed. pg. 620

Vitamin B$_{12}$

- Vitamin B$_{12}$ is complex organo-metallic compound with a cobalt atom. The preparation which is therapeutically used is cyanocobalamin, which is relatively cheap.
- **Source:** Good sources are liver, kidney, meat, fish, eggs, milk and cheese. Vitamin B$_{12}$ is not found in foods of vegetable origin. It is also synthesized by bacteria in colon.
- **Deficiency:** Vitamin B$_{12}$ deficiency is associated with megaloblastic anaemia (pernicious anaemia), demyelinating neurological lesions in the spinal cord.

REQUIREMENT

Intake values recommended by ICMR (2010) are as below:

Population group	Per day requirement
a. Normal adults	1 mcg
b. Pregnancy	1.2 mcg
c. Lactation	1.5 mcg
d. Infants & children	0.2 mcg

221. Ans. (b) Sanguinarine

Ref: K. Park, 23st ed. pg. 658

- **Epidemic dropsy** is caused by contamination of mustard oil with Argemone oil *(seeds of argemone Mexicana seeds closely resemble that of mustard oil)*
- Toxin which is contained in argemone oil is **Sanguinarine**
- This sanguinarine interferes with oxidation of Pyruvic acid, which leads to accumulation of pyruvic acid in blood.
- This may cause non-inflammatory edema of lower limbs, diarrhea, dyspnea and even cardiac failure and death.

222. Ans. (d) 650 Kcal

Ref: D.C. Dutta, 8th ed. pg. 174

Dutta states: A healthy mother will produce **about 500–800 mL of milk a day** to feed her infant. This requires about **700 Kcal/day** for the mother, which must be made up from diet or from her body store. For this purpose a store of about 5 kg of fat during pregnancy is essential to make up any nutritional deficit during lactation.

Extra Mile

- Iron need during lactation is 1 mg/day.
- Daily requirement of calcium during pregnancy and lactation averages 1–1.5 g.

223. Ans (d) She weighs 60 kg

Ref: Park, 19th pg. 501-2

- 60 kg weight is of Indian reference man and not woman

TABLE: Summary of Indian reference man and woman

An Indian reference man	An Indian reference woman
• Between **18 and 29 years** of age	• Between **18 and 29 years** of age
• **Weighs 60 kg** • **Height = 1.73**	• **Healthy** and **weighs 55 kg.** • **Height = 1.61**
• Free from disease and physically fit for active work.	• Engaged for **8 hours** in general household work, in light industry or in other moderately active work.

Contd...

PREVENTIVE AND SOCIAL MEDICINE (PSM)

Preventive and Social Medicine (PSM)

An Indian reference man	An Indian reference woman
• Employed for 8 hours in occupation that usually involves moderate activity	• Spends 4 to 6 hours sitting or moving around only through light activity
• Spends 8 hours in bed, 4 to 6 hours sitting and moving around and 2 hours in walking and in active recreation or household duties	• Spends 2 hours in walking or in active recreation or in household duties

224. Ans. (b) Bitot's spot

Ref: K. Park, 23rd ed. pg. 615, 641

- **Xeropthalmia:** All the ocular manifestation of Vitamin A deficiency.
- First clinical sign of Vitamin A deficiency: *Conjunctival Xerosis*
- First clinical symptom of vitamin A deficiency: *Night blindness* WHO Classification of Xeropthalmia

CLASS	SIGNS
X1A	Conjunctival xerosis
X1B	Conjunctival xerosis with bitot's spot
X2	Corneal xerosis
X3A	Corneal xerosis with ulceration
X3B	Keratomalacia

225. Ans. (c) Bitot spots

Ref: K. Park, 23rd ed. pg. 606, 615, 641

- First clinical sign: conjuctival xerosis
- First clinical symptom: Night blindness
- *Refer to above table.*

226. Ans. (c) 0.5%

Ref: K. Park, 23rd ed. pg. 615, 641

Criteria and Prevalence for Determining Xerophthalmia Severity:

Criteria	Prevalence at risk
• Night blindness	>1%
• Bitot's spot	>0.5%
• Corneal xerosis/keratomalacia	>0.01%
• Corneal ulcer	>0.05%
• Serum retinol	>5%

- Refer to previous answer for WHO classification of Xerophthalmia

227. Ans. (d) Night blindness 1%

Ref: K. Park, 23rd ed. pg. 615, 641, 899

Please refer to above explanation.

228. Ans. (b) 0.01%

Ref: K. Park, 23rd ed. pg. 625

- Minerals form only 5 percent of the typical human diet but are essential for normal health and function.
- **Trace elements (or trace minerals)** are usually defined as minerals that are required in amounts between 1 to 100 mg/day by adults or make up less than 0.01 percent of total body weight.
- **Macrominerals** are defined as minerals that are required by adults in amounts greater than 100 mg/day or make up *less than 1 percent of total body weight*.
- **Ultra-trace minerals** generally are defined as minerals that are required in amounts less than 1 mg/day.

229. Ans. (a) 1 g/kg

Ref: K. Park, 21st ed. pg. 563

- According to Indian medical council recommendation the daily protein requirement is 1 g/kg body weight.
- Assessment of protein nutritional status is done by: arm muscle circumference, the creatinine-height index, serum albumin and transferrin, total body nitrogen etc.
- Best measure of the state of protein nutrition is: serum albumin concentration (should be more than 3.5 g/dL)

230. Ans. (b) Vitamin B

Ref: K. Park, 23rd ed. pg. 626

- Antioxidants are substances which are both nutrients and non-nutrients.
- These anti-oxidants reduce the toxic effects of reactive oxygen species and nitrogen species which are generated during physiological or pathological conditions and result in oxidant damage
- **Vitamins which acts as antioxidants are** *remembered as ACE*: vitamin A, C and E
- Other vitamins which acts as anti-oxidants are: Selenium, Glutathione
- **Non-nutrient products that also act as anti-oxidants are**: Plant phenols, Flavonoids, Coumarins, caffeic, benzyl isothiocyanates, gallic and ellagic acid.
- Vitamin B is not an anti-oxidant.

231. Ans. (b) Vitamin B

Ref: K. Park, 23rd ed. pg. 626

Please refer to above explanation

FMGE Solutions Screening Examination

232. Ans. (b) Niacin

Ref: K. Park, 23rd ed. pg. 619

- Pellagra is caused by deficiency of Vitamin B3 *(Niacin).*
- It is seen commonly in maize eating populations because maize is deficient in tryptophan which is usually converted to niacin.
- Therefore maize eaters develop deficiency of Niacin which ultimately leads to pellagra.
- **4 D's associated to Pellagra:**
  - Diarrhea
  - Dermatitis
  - Dememntia
  - Death
- In severe cases of pellagra *Casal's Necklace* is seen which is a scaly pigmented rash around neck, seems like necklace.

233. Ans. (c) Increase appetite

Ref: K. Park, 23rd ed. pg. 639-40

TABLE: Features of Kwashiorkor and Marasmus

Features	Marasmus	Kwashiorkor
Muscle wasting	Obvious	Hidden by fat and edema
Edema	None	Present in lower legs and face
Mental changes	Quiet and apathic	Irritable, Moaning and apathic
Weight	*Very low*	*Low to Normal*
Appetite	Good	Poor
Hepatomegaly	None	Present, due to fat deposition
Hair changes	Seldom	Sparse, silky *"flag sign"*

234. Ans. (b) Sanguinarine

Ref: K. Park, 23st ed. pg. 658

- **Epidemic dropsy is** caused by contamination of mustard oil with Argemone oil *(seeds of argemone Mexicana seeds closely resembles to that of mustard oil)*
- Toxin which is contained in argemone oil is **Sanguinarine**
- This sanguinarine interferes with oxidation of Pyruvic acid, which leads to accumulation of pyruvic acid in blood.
- This may cause non-inflammatory edema of lower limbs, diarrhea, dyspnea and even cardiac failure and death.

235. Ans. (b) Sanguinarine

Ref: K. Park, 23st ed. pg. 658

236. Ans. (a) Sanguinarine

237. Ans. (a) Methylene blue reductase test

Ref: K. Park, 23rd ed. pg. 655

There are 3 tests to check the efficiency of milk pasteurization:

- **Phosphatase test:** *Most widely used method.* Phosphatase enzyme present in raw milk is degraded upon heating. If found in pasteurized milk, it indicates inadequate pasteurization or addition of raw milk.
- **Standard plate count:** To determine the bacteriological quality of pasteurized milk. 30,000 bacterial count per ml of pasteurized milk is the standard value in most western countries.
- **Coliform count:** Coliform organisms are completely destroyed by pasteurization and therefore, their presence in pasteurized milk is an indication of improper pasteurization or post pasteurization contamination.

> **Extra Mile**
>
> - Pasteurization of milk is by following methods:
>   - **Holder Method/ vat method:** 63°C x 30 min- most commonly used method
>   - **Flash Method:** 72°C x 15 sec
>   - **UHT method (ultra high temp):** 125°C for 2–3 secs, rapidly cooled and bottled ASAP

238. Ans. (d) 24 hours

- Refrigerated milk can be kept for around 24 hours
- At Room temperature: upto 6 to 8 hour
- In Freezer: 3 months

239. Ans. (d) Pulses

Ref: K. Park, 23rd ed. pg. 628

- Pulses contain 20-25% of protein, which is considered more than eggs, fish, meat products. However the quality of protein in pulses is inferior to that of meat products.
- Soyabean contains 40% of protein
- Pulses protein are poor in **methionine** and to a lesser extent in **cysteine.**
- Amino acid rich in pulses: **Lysine**

> **Extra Mile**
>
> **TABLE:** Food products and their limiting amino acid
>
> | Food Item | Limiting Amino Acids |
> |---|---|
> | Pulses | Methionine & Cysteine |
> | Cereals | Threonine & Lysine |
> | Maize | Tryptophan & Lysine |

240. Ans. (c) Methionine

Ref: K. Park, 23rd ed. pg. 628

PREVENTIVE AND SOCIAL MEDICINE (PSM)

552

Preventive and Social Medicine (PSM)

- Pulses protein are poor in **methionine** and to a lesser extent in **cysteine.**
- Since option C and D both are correct, we have to choose single best answer and that will be Methionine. Literatures clearly states that cysteine is deficient only up to a lesser extent.

241. Ans. (c) 100

Ref: K. Park, 23rd ed. pg. 630

Biological value [BV] is a measure of the proportion of absorbed protein from a food which becomes incorporated into the proteins of the organism's body.

TABLE: Biological value of Proteins in several food products

- **Whole egg: 100**
- Cow milk: 91
- Beef: 80
- Casein: 77
- Soy: 74
- Wheat gluten: 64

242. Ans. (d) Egg

Ref: K. Park, 23rd ed. pg. 617

- Given these options, the correct answer will be egg which contains 1.25 to 1.5 µg/100 gm.

TABLE: Compare the sources of vitamin D from different dietry sources

Dietary sources	Vitamin D content (µg/100 g)
Halibut liver oil	500 – 10,000
Cod fish liver oil	200 – 750
Shark liver oil	30 – 100
Fish fat	5 – 30
Eggs	**1.25 – 1.5**
Butter	0.5 – 1.5
Milk, whole	0.1

Extra Mile

- **Richest source of Vitamin D:** Halibut fish liver oil > codfish liver oil > shark liver oil
- Human milk is a poor source of vitamin D.
- Cow's milk is poor in Vitamin C and Iron.
- Vitamin D and Vitamin B$_{12}$ has no plant source.

243. Ans. (c) Halibut liver oil

Ref: K. Park, 23rd ed. pg. 617

- **Richest source of Vitamin D:** Halibut fish liver oil > codfish liver oil > shark liver oil

244. Ans. (d) Fish liver oil

Ref: K. Park, 23rd ed. pg. 617

Please refer to above explanation

245. Ans. (d) Calcitriol

Ref: K. Park, 23rd ed. pg. 617

- Vitamin D has 3 forms:
  - D1: Calciferol
  - D2: Ergocalciferol
  - *D3: Calcitriol- most potent/active form, synthesized by sunlight. Also found in fish liver oil and animal fats*

246. Ans. (a) Linoleic acid

Ref: K. Park, 23rd ed. pg. 609-10

- **Essential fatty acid are**
  - Linoleic Acid: *most essential fatty acid*
  - Linolenic Acid
  - Arachidonic acid
  - Eicosapentanoic acid
  - DHA
- **Richest source of essential fatty acid:** Safflower oil
- **Richest source of saturated fatty acid:** coconut oil
- **Richest source of MUFA:** groundnut oil.

247. Ans. (d) Glutamic acid

Ref: K. Park, 23rd ed. pg. 609-10

Refer to previous explanation.

248. Ans. (b) Iodine

- Iodine deficiency leads to hypothyroidism which manifests as goiter.
- Due to hypothyroidism, thyroid cells try to compensate it by hyperplasia and hypertrophy of thyroid gland cells (goiter).
- Iron deficiency leads to Microcytic anemia (IDA).
- Zinc deficiency may manifest with *acrodermatitis enteropathica.*
- Fluorine deficiency/excess manifests with dental caries.

Extra Mile

- *Optimum level of fluorine in drinking water: 0.5–0.8 mg per liter.*

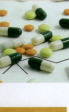

FMGE Solutions Screening Examination

249. Ans. (b) Height/age

*Ref: K. Park, 23rd ed. pg. 640;
Nelson's Pediatrics, 18th ed. Ch 43*

The nutritional indices commonly calculated for young children are:
- **Weight for height** – an index used to measure wasting or acute malnutrition; (WHAM)
- **Height for age** – an index used to measure stunting or chronic malnutrition; (HA-CM)
- **Weight for age** – an index used to measure underweight (or wasting and stunting combined). (WASW)
- **Mid arm circumference** is a specific indicator of wasting or acute malnutrition.

ENVIRONMENT AND HEALTH

250. Ans. (c) Calculating bleaching powder dose for water disinfection

Ref: K.Park 23rd ed. P 728

Book states: *"Horrock's water testing apparatus is designed to find out the dose of bleaching powder required for disinfection of water".*

251. Ans. (b) Nosocomial infection

Ref: K. Park, 23rd ed. pg. 94

- Nosocomial infection is defined as infection acquired by patient while in a hospital or other health care facility.
- Infection occurs more than 48 hours after admission
- It denotes a new disorder, unrelated to patients primary condition
- Examples: UTI, surgical wound infection.
- **Sources of infection can be:**
  - **Patients** with viral infection (measles, viral hepatitis, influenza), skin infections, UTI and respiratory infection.
  - **Hospital staff** viz doctors, nurses, ward boys
  - **Environment:** Hospital environment viz dust, bed clothes, furniture, sinks, etc.

252. Ans. (d) 300

Ref: K. Park, 23rd ed. pg. 243-44

- **Chandler's index** is also known as Endemic index.
- It is defined as average number of hookworm eggs per gram of stool for the entire community.
- >300 eggs per gram of stool denotes important public health problem.

TABLE: Interpretation of chandler's index:

Average No. of eggs/g of stool	Interpretation
• < 200	No significance
• 200–250	Potential danger
• 250–300	Minor public health problem
• >300	Major public health problem

253. Ans. (b) Number of hookworm eggs per gram of stool

Ref: K. Park, 23rd ed. pg. 243-44

- **Chandler's index** is also known as Endemic index.
- It is defined as average number of hookworm eggs per gram of stool for the entire community.
- *Refer to above table for interpretations.*

254. Ans. (a) Hook worm

Ref: K. Park, 23rd ed. pg. 243-44

Please refer to above explanation

255. Ans. (b) Air pollution

Ref: Park, 23rd ed. pg. 736

Indicators of Air Pollution
- **Smoke or Soiling index:** A known volume of air is filtered through a white filter paper under specified conditions and the stain is measured by photoelectric meter. Smoke concentration is estimated and expressed as micrograms/cubic metre of air as an average level over a period of time.
- **Sulphur dioxide** This gas is a major contaminant in many urban and industrial areas. Its concentration is estimated in all air pollution surveys. *So, it is the best indicator of air pollution*
- **Grit and dust measurement:** Deposit gauges collect grit, dust and other solids. There are analysed monthly.
- **Coefficient of haze:** A factor used, particularly in the USA in assessing the amount of smoke or other aerosol in air.
- **Air pollution index:** It is an arbitrary index which takes into account one or more pollutants as a measure of the severity of pollution

256. Ans (d) E. coli

Ref: Park, 23ed pg. 720-21

- Ideally, drinking water shouldn't contain any organism known to be pathogenic.
- The primary bacterial indicator recommended as a bacteriological indicator is the **coliform group** of organisms as a whole. These include both fecal and non-fecal organisms.
- Typical example of the fecal group is **E. coli *(single best indicator)*** and of the non-faecal group, **Klebsiella aerogens**.

PREVENTIVE AND SOCIAL MEDICINE (PSM)

Reasons why coliform organisms are chosen as indicators of fecal pollution rather than the water borne pathogens directly:

- Constant presence of coliform organisms in great abundance in human intestine. These organisms are foreign to potable water. Therefore their presence is looked upon as evidence of fecal contamination.
- They are easily detected by culture methods
- Longer survival as compared to other water borne pathogens
- They have greater resistance to the forces of natural purification, as compared to water borne pathogens

Other Indicators Include

- **Faecal streptococci:** Faecal streptococci regularly occur in faeces, but in much smaller numbers than E. coli. Their presence is regarded as important **confirmatory evidence of recent faecal pollution of water.**
- **Cl. perfringens:** They also occur regularly in faeces and their spores are capable of surviving in water for a longer time than organisms of the coliform group. So, **the presence of spores in the absence of the coliform group**, suggests that faecal contamination occurred at **some remote time.**

---

257. Ans. (b) 15 meters

Ref: K. Park, 23ʳᵈ ed. pg. 709, Park, 19ᵗʰ pg. 465

- The safe distance between the latrine and a source of water supply will depend upon the porosity of the soil, level of ground water, its slope and direction of flow. In general, it may be stated, that latrines of any kind should not be *located within 15 m (50 ft)* from a source of water supply, and should be at a lower elevation to prevent the possibility of bacterial contamination of the water supply.

FAMILY PLANNING AND CONTRACEPTION

---

258. Ans. (c) Spermicide

Ref: K. Park 25ᵗʰ ed. P 550-54

- Contraceptive failure is measured by pearl index.

$$PI = \frac{\text{Total accidental pregnancy}}{\text{Total month of exposure}} \times 1200$$

- Spermicide is a chemical method of contraception usually used with vaginal sponge. It has highest contraceptive failure (highest pearl index).
- No spermicide is effective alone for contraception, therefore they are best used with barrier methods.
- Commonly used modern spermicides are "surface – active agents" → which attach themselves to spermatozoa and inhibits oxygen uptake → Sperms killed.

- Failure rate of different forms of contraception are as follows:

Contraceptive method	Failure rate (Pearl index- per 100 women years -HWY)
OCP	0.1 – 0.5
IUCD	0.2 – 3.0 (**Mirena/LNG-20:** 0.2 per 100 women)
Subdermal implant/ Norplant	0.7
Centchroman/Saheli	1.83–2.84
Condoms	Male: 2–14 Female: 5–21
Diaphragm	6 – 12
Vaginal sponge/Today	Nulliparous: 9 – 20 Parous: 20 – 40

- **Main drawbacks of spermicide:**
  - High failure rate
  - Must be used immediately before intercourse
  - Difficulty in application
  - Lots of messiness and mild burning sensation

---

259. Ans. (b) Within 1 week of delivery

Ref: K. Park 25ᵗʰ ed. P 549

Refer to above explanation

---

260. Ans. (c) Family planning in those who are not using any contraception

Ref: K.Park 23ʳᵈ ed. P 511

- Many women who are sexually active would prefer to avoid becoming pregnant, without using any methods of contraception neither by their partner.
- These womens are considered to have an "unmet need" for family planning.
- Concept is usually applied and limited to married women only, however it can be applied to sexually active fecund women.

Unmet Need

Unmet need for family planning is defined as the percentage of women of reproductive age, either married or in a union who want to stop or delay childbearing but are not using any method of contraception.

$$\text{Unmet need for family planning} = \frac{\begin{array}{c}\text{Women of reproductive age (15–49)}\\\text{who are married or in a union and who}\\\text{have an unmet need for family planning}\end{array}}{\begin{array}{c}\text{Total number of women of reproductive}\\\text{age (15–49) who are married or in a}\\\text{union}\end{array}}$$

- **Most common reasons for unmet needs are:**
  - Inconvenient or unsatisfactory services
  - Lack of information
  - Contraceptives side effect fears
  - Opposition from husband or relatives
- According to national family health survey, it is most commonly seen in women below 20 years (almost entirely for spacing the birth).
- It is higher in rural areas than in urban areas.

261. Ans. (c) Failures per 100 women years of exposure

Ref: K. Park, 23rd ed. pg. 510

- **Pearl index** is used to measure the contraceptive efficacy/contraceptive failure.
- It is defined as the number of failures per 100 women-years (HWY) of exposure. It is given by the formula:

$$\text{Failure rate per HWY} = \frac{\text{Total accidental pregnancies}}{\text{Total months of exposure}} \times 1200$$

262. Ans. (a) 0.01

Ref: K. Park, 23rd ed. pg. 510

- Failure rate is 1 HWY; Total month of exposure is 12. We have to find out the number of accidental pregnancies.
- Putting the values in pearl index formula:

$$\text{Failure rate per HWY} = \frac{\text{Total accidental pregnancies}}{\text{Total months of exposure}} \times 1200$$

$$1 = \frac{x}{12} \times 1200$$

$$12 = 1200\,x$$

Therefore, $x = \dfrac{12}{1200} = 0.01$

263. Ans. (a) Combined OCP

Ref: K. Park, 23rd ed. pg. 503

- IUD is considered safe during lactation.
- Progesterone Only Pills (mini pills) used mainly within 72 hours of intercourse to reduce the risk of pregnancy. **Considered safe during lactation.**
- **Composition of combined OCP:** (MALA-N/MALA-D)
  - Ethinyl estradiol: 0.03 mg (30 mcg)
  - Norgesterol/Desogesterol: 0.15 mg (150 mcg)
- **Adverse effects of combined OCP**
  - Myocardial infarction
  - Thrombosis
  - Cervical CA
  - Breast CA
  - Hepatocellular adenoma

Contraindications of OCPs

Absolute contraindication	Relative contraindication
• Breast CA • History of thromboembolism • Abnormal uterine bleeding • Cardiac abnormalities	• Age > 40 years • *Lactating mothers (0-6 months)* • DM, HTN, chronic renal disease • Infrequent bleeding, Amenorrhea • Epilepsy and migraine

264. Ans. (d) Progesterone only pill

Ref: K. Park, 23rd ed. pg. 503

Please refer to above explanation

265. Ans. (b) Prevent release of ovum from ovary

Ref: K. Park, 23rd ed. pg. 501

- Combined oral contraceptive pills act by inhibiting ovulation by suppressing the release of gonadotropins.
- Continuous progesterone by OCPs which give negative feedback to GnRH, which decreases LH release and upto some extent FSH release also.
- This prevents LH surge and as a result inhibits ovulation.

266. Ans. (c) Ovarian cancer

Ref: K. Park, 23rd ed. pg. 501-502

Beneficial Effects of OCPs
- Ovarian CA
- PID
- Ectopic pregnancy
- Endometrial CA

267. Ans. (b) Just after the menstruation

Ref: K. Park, 23rd ed. pg. 389-90

- **Breast self-examination** (BSE) is a screening method used in an attempt to detect early breast cancer. The method involves the woman herself looking at and feeling each breast for possible lumps, distortions or swelling.
- **For pre-menopausal** women, the most commonly recommended time is just after the end of menstruation, because the breasts are least likely to be swollen and tender at this time.
- **For postmenopausal,** women or these having irregular cycles might do a self-exam once a month regardless of their menstrual cycle.

268. Ans. (d) Contraceptive failure

Ref: Park's PSM, 23rd ed. pg. 510

- Pearl index is used to measure the contraceptive efficacy/ contraceptive failure.
- It is defined as the number of failures per 100 women-years (HWY) of exposure.

$$PI = \frac{\text{Total accidental pregnancies}}{\text{Total months of exposure}} \times 1200$$

- Another method used to measure contraceptive failure/ efficacy is *life table analysis*.
- Life table analysis: calculates failure rates for each month of use.

269. Ans. (a) 0.1%

Ref: K. Park, 23rd ed. pg. 494-96

- Pomoroy's technique is the most popular method of ligation.
- Failure Rate: 0.1-0.3%
- *Failure rate of vasectomy: 0.15 per HWY*

DEMOGRAPHY AND HEALTH

270. Ans. (c) 21 days

Ref: K. Park 25th ed. P 903

- According to Central Birth and Death Registration Act 1969:
  - The time limit for registration of vital events like births and death is 21 days
  - Late fee is imposed in case of default
  - From October 2018, Aadhar number is must for registration of death
- **Lay reporting of health information:** Collection of information (birth and death), its use and its transmission to other levels of the health system by the non-professional health worker (like village health guide).

> **Extra Mile**
- **Registration of marriage:** Within 30 days

271. Ans. (d) $PAR = \frac{\text{Incidence among total population} - \text{incidence among non-exposed}}{\text{Incidence among total population}} \times 100$

Ref: K. Park 25th ed. P 86

- **Population – attributable risk is** incidence of disease (or death) in total population minus the incidence of disease (or death) among those who were NOT exposed to the suspected causal factor divided by incidence among total population.

- **Use:** It provides an estimate of the amount by which the disease could be reduced in that population if the suspected factor is eliminated or modified.

> **Extra Mile**
>
> $$\text{Relative risk} = \frac{\text{Incidence among exposed}}{\text{Incidence among non-exposed}}$$
>
> $$\text{Attributable risk} = \frac{\text{Incidence among exposed} - \text{incidence among non exposed}}{\text{Incidence among exposed}} \times 100$$

272. Ans. (b) Net reproduction rate

Ref: K. Park 25th ed. P 539 – 540

- **Net Reproduction Rate (NRR):** No. of daughters a new-born girl will bear during her life time *assuming fixed age specific fertility and mortality rates*.
  - It is a demographic indicator
  - NRR of 1 is equivalent to attaining approximately the 2-child norm.
  - If NRR <1, the reproductive performance of the population is said to be below replacement level.
- **Total Fertility Rate:** it is the average number of children a woman would have if she were to pass through her reproductive years bearing children at the same rates as the women now in each age group.
- **Gross Reproduction Rate:** Average number of girls that would be born to a woman if she experiences the current fertility pattern throughout her reproductive span (15–44 or 49 years), assuming no mortality.
- **General Fertility Rate:** It is the number of live birth per 1000 women in reproductive age group (15–44 or 49 years) in a given year
  - GFR =

$$\frac{\text{No. of live births in an area during a year}}{\text{Mid year female population of age 15-44 (or 49) years}} \times 1000$$

273. Ans. (c) 4

Ref: K. Park, 23rd ed. pg. 479

Demographic cycle

The history of world population since 1650 suggests that there is a demographic cycle of 5 stages through which a nation passes:

- **First stage (High stationary):** This stage is characterized by a **high birth rate and a high death rate** which cancel each other and the population remains stationary.
- **Second stage (Early expanding):** The **death rate begins to decline, while the birth rate remains unchanged**. Many countries in South Asia, and Africa

are in this phase. Birth rates have increased in some of these countries possibly as a result of improved health conditions, and shortening periods of breastfeeding.
- **Third stage (Late expanding):** The death rate declines still further, and the birth rate tends to fall. The population continues to grow because births exceed deaths. **India has entered this phase.**
- **Fourth stage (Low stationary):** This stage is characterized by a **low birth and low death rate** with the result that the population becomes stationary.
- **Fifth stage (Declining):** The population begins to decline because birth rate is lower than the death rate.

274. Ans. (d) Emmigration

Ref: K. Park 23rd ed. P 481

- Demographic characteristics provide an overview of its population size, composition, territorial distribution and changes therein and the **components of changes such as: Nativity, mortality, social mobility.**
- Demographic indicators have been divided into 2 parts:
  - **Population statistics:** Include indicators that measures the population size, sex ratio, density and dependency ratio
  - **Vital statistics:** Include indicators such as birth rate, death rate, natural growth rate, life expectancy at birth, mortality and fertility rates.

275. Ans. (b) Population <15 years and >65 years

Ref: K. Park 23rd ed. / 484

- Dependency ratio is the proportion of persons above 65 years of age and children below 15 years of age who are considered to be dependent on economically productive age group (15-64).

Dependency Ratio =

$$\frac{\text{Persons} < 15 \text{ years} + > 65 \text{ years}}{\text{Persons between 15 and 65 years}}$$

- Dependency ratio of India is 62 per 100 or 0.62. this means 62 non-earning peoples in India are dependent on 100 earning population.

276. Ans. (a) Broad at base and narrow at apex

Ref: K. Park 23rd ed. / 482

277. Ans. (b) It is distributed equally in study & control groups

Ref: K. Park 23rd ed. / 72

278. Ans (c) 95.4%

Ref: K. Park 23rd ed. /849

- The standard normal curve is a smooth, bell shaped, perfectly symmetrical curve, based on infinitely large number of observations.
- The area between 2 standard deviations on either side of the mean will cover most of the values i.e. ~95%.

The normal distribution or 'normal curve' is an important concept in statistical theory. In a normal curve :

- The area between one standard deviation on either side of the mean will include approximately 68% of values in the distribution.
- The area between two standard deviations will cover approx 95% of the values.
- The area between two standard deviations will cover approx 99.7% of the values

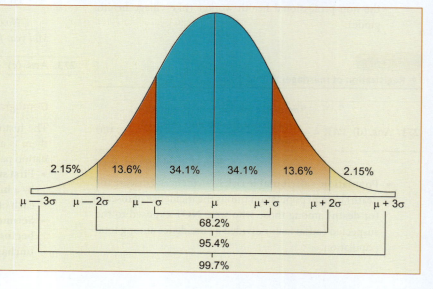

More About Standard Curve

- The standard normal curve is a smooth, **bell-shaped, perfectly symmetrical curve**
- It is based on an infinitely large number of observations.
- The **total area of the curve is 1**
- Its **mean is zero**
- Its **standard** deviation is 1
- The mean, median and mode all coincide

---

279. Ans. (d) 99.7% values

Ref: K. Park, 23rd ed. pg. 848-49

---

280. Ans. (a) Tapering at top

Ref: K. Park, 23rd ed. pg. 848-49

---

281. Ans. (b) 16-25

Ref: K. Park, 23rd ed. pg. 690

MODIFIED KUPPUSWAMI SCALE: Scale of socio-economic status of urban families, includes Education status of head, occupation status of head, Income per capita.

Total score of 3 components	Socioeconomic class
• 26–29	Upper
• 16–25	Upper-middle
• 11–15	Lower-middle
• 05–10	Upper-lower
• <5	Lower

---

282. Ans. (b) 19.7%

Ref: Park, 23rd ed. pg. 402

- According to the National survey on blindness 2001-2002 conducted in the country recognized the main causes for visual impairment and blindness are given below:

Cataract	62.6%
Refractive Errors	**19.7%**
Glaucoma	5.8%
Posterior segment pathology	4.7%
Corneal opacity	0.9%
Other causes	4.19%

---

283. Ans. (b) According to the stroke control programme, first priority goes to control of Diabetes, elimination of smoking, prevention and management of other risk factors

Ref: K. Park 23rd ed. pg. 472

According to the STROKE CONTROL PROGRAMME the *first priority goes to control of arterial hypertension which is the major cause of stroke.*

DISASTER MANAGEMENT, DISINFECTION AND BMW MANAGEMENT

284. Ans. (c) Controlled tipping

Ref: K. Park 25th ed. P 814

- **Book states**: "Controlled tipping or sanitary landfill is the most satisfactory method of refuse disposal where suitable land is available"
- **Three methods of controlled tipping:**
  - **The trench method:** Preferred where level ground is available. The refuse is compacted in long trench (6-10 feet deep, 12-36 feet wide) and covered with excavated earth.
  - **The ramp method:** Preferred where terrain in moderately sloping
  - **The area method:** Used for filling land depressions, disused quarries and clay pits. The refuse uniformly consolidated in layers up to 2-2.5 m (6-8 ft). Each layer is sealed with mud (12 inches/30 cm thick).

Extra Mile

Other methods of refuse disposal
- **Dumping:** Easy method for disposal of dry waste. Refuse is dumped (as open) in low lying areas usually as a method of land reclamation. It is the most insanitary method that creates public health hazard (WHO expert committee).
- **Incineration:** Disposal of refusal hygienically by burning or incineration. Method of choice where suitable land is NOT available. Best for hospital and industrial waste
- **Composting:** Method of combined disposal of refuse and night soil or sludge. Best and cultivation and soil. Methods of composting:
  - **Bangalore method** (Anaerobic method)
  - **Mechanical composting** (Aerobic composting)
- **Manure pits:** Done by digging manure pits by individual house hold. Preferred in rural areas where system of refuse collection and disposal is not systematic. Refuse is converted into manure in 5-6 months → used in field.
- **Burial:** Preferred for small camps. Refuse is disposed in a small trench (1.5 m wide and 2 m deep). It is covered with 20-30 cm of earth every day. Can be taken out after 6 month and used in field.

FMGE Solutions Screening Examination

285. Ans. (a) Yellow

Ref: K. Park 25th ed. P 853

TABLE: Biomedical waste management

Color Category	Type of biomedical waste	Treatment options
Yellow	• Human & Animal anatomical waste • Soiled waste (with blood, body fluid) • Expired/Discarded/cytotoxic medicine • Chemical waste • Chemical liquid waste • Discarded linen, mattress, beddings contaminated with blood or body fluids	Incineration/Deep burial Nonchlorinated chemical disinfection
Red	• Recyclable contaminated waste ▪ Disposable items such as tubes, bottles, IV sets, urine bags, syringes without needle, gloves	Autoclaving or microwaving/hydroclaving followed by shredding
White/Translucent *(puncture/leak proof container)*	• Waste sharps including metals: Needles, blades or any contaminated sharp object	Autoclaving or dry heat sterilization followed by shredding and mutilation
Blue	• Glassware: included medicine vials except those contaminated with cytotoxic waste • Metallic body implants	Disinfection (by soaking waste with detergent and sodium hypochlorite)/Autoclaving/Microwaving/Hydroclaving

286. Ans. (d) Mitigation and preparedness

Ref: K. Park 25th ed. P 857, 859

- There are 3 fundamental aspects of disaster management (as seen in disaster cycle):
  ▪ Disaster response
  ▪ Disaster preparedness
  ▪ Disaster mitigation

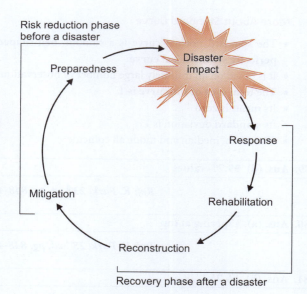

- Before the disaster the most important steps are mitigation and preparedness of disaster
- **Emergency prevention and mitigation** involves measures designed to either prevent hazard or to lessen the effect of emergencies. It also reduces the medical causalities drastically. It includes:
  ▪ Flood mitigation works
  ▪ Appropriate land use planning
  ▪ Improved building codes
  ▪ Reduction and protection of vulnerable population and structures
- **Disaster preparedness:**
  ▪ It is a long-term development activities whose goals are to strengthen the overall capacity and capability of a country to manage efficiently all types of emergency
  ▪ **Objective:** To ensure that all resources, systems are in place to provide prompt effective assistance to disaster victims thus facilitating relief measures and rehabilitation of services
- **Cornerstone of emergency preparedness programme:** Community members, resources, organizations and administration.

287. Ans. (b) Response and rehabilitation

Ref: K. Park 25th ed. P 857

- After the disaster the first step is **response in first few hours** in order to manage the mass casualties.
- This is further divided into:
  ▪ **Search, rescue and first aid** (most immediate help comes from an uninjured survivor)
  ▪ **Field care:** Most injured ones are converged spontaneously to health facilities using any form of transport

Preventive and Social Medicine (PSM)

- **Triage:** Rapidly classifying the injured on basis of severity of injury.
  - ♦ Highest priority is given to victim whose immediate or long term prognosis is dramatically affected by simple intensive care
  - ♦ **Lowest priority:** Moribund patients
  - ♦ **Most accepted triage method:** 4 colour coded system:
    - * **Red:** High priority treatment or transfer
    - * **Yellow:** Mdium priority
    - * **Green:** Ambulatory patients
    - * **Black:** Dead or moribund patients
- **Tagging:** Victims should be tagged with name, age, place of origin, triage category, diagnosis and initial treatment
- Identification and removal of dead from disaster scene
- **Rehabilitation and reconstruction:**
  - The final phase in a disaster should lead to restoration of the pre-disaster condition. This is done by:
  - **Water supply:** first priority of ensuring water quality is chlorination (increase residual chlorine level to about 0.2 – 0.5 mg/litre)
  - Food safety
  - Basic sanitation and personal hygiene
  - Vector control

288. Ans. (b) Ministry of Home affairs

Ref: K. Park 25th ed. P 862

- The overall coordination of disaster management vests with ministry of Home affairs
- Top-level decision making committee:
  - Cabinet committee on security
  - National crisis management committee
- Agency responsible for preparation of disaster management plans and its execution at national level: The National Disaster Management Authority
- Health management in a disaster is under: Ministry of Health and family welfare (a special wing under it- Emergency Medical Relief Wing)

Extra Mile

- **World disaster reduction day:** Second Wednesday of October
- **Execution of relief work in case of natural disasters:** The state government

289. Ans. (c) Unsalvageable

Ref: PubMed

- In a disaster management, categorization of victims are done on the basis of likelihood of survival.

TABLE: Triage color code and their significance

Category	Color	Remarks/steps
Category 1	**Red**	**Highest priority**—patient immediate resuscitation or life-saving surgery (0 to 6 hours)
Category 2	Yellow/blue	High possible resuscitation or life saving surgery (within 6 to 24 hours)
Category 3	Green	Ambulatory/low minor injuries; non-life threating
Category 4	Black	Dead, Moribund; least priority/unsalvagable

290. Ans. (b) Pathological waste

Ref: K.Park 23rd ed. P 789

TABLE: Classification of health care waste

Waste category	Description and examples
Infectious waste	Waste suspected to contain pathogens e.g. laboratory culture; waste from isolation wards; tissues (swabs), materials, or equipments that have been in contact with infected patients; excreta.
Pathological waste	Human tissues or fluids e.g. body parts; blood and other body fluids; fetuses.
Sharps	Sharp waste e.g. needles; infusion sets; scalpels; knives; blades; broken glass.
Pharmaceutical waste	Waste containing pharmaceuticals e.g. pharmaceuticals that are expired or no longer needed: items contaminated by or containing pharmaceuticals (bottles, boxes)
Genotoxic waste	Waste containing substances with genotoxic properties e.g. waste containing cytostatic drugs (often used in cancer therapy): genotoxic chemicals.
Chemical waste	Waste containing chemical substances e.g. laboratory reagents; film developer; disinfectants that are expired or no longer needed; solvents.
Wastes with high content of heavy metals	Batteries; broken thermometers; blood-pressure gauges; etc.
Pressurized containers	Gas cylinders, gas cartridges aerosol cans
Radioactive waste	Waste containing radioactive substances e.g. unused liquids from radiotherapy or laboratory research; contaminated glassware, packages, or absorbent paper; urine and excreta from patients treated or tested with unsealed radionucleides; sealed sources.

FMGE Solutions Screening Examination

291. Ans. (b) 2nd week of October

Ref: K. Park 23rd ed. pg. 795

- **WORLD DISASTER REDUCTION DAY:** 2ND WEDNESDAY IN MONTH OF OCTOBER
- **24TH OCTOBER:** UN DAY
- **25TH NOVEMBER:** INT'L DAY FOR ELIMINATION OF VIOLENCE AGAINST WOMEN

292. Ans. (d) District hospital

Ref: K. Park, 23rd ed. pg. 795-96

- There are 3 fundamental aspects of disaster management:
  - Disaster response
  - Disaster preparedness, and
  - Disaster mitigation
- District hospital take role in case of disasters like earth quake, flood etc.

293. Ans. (a) Search and rescue, first aid

Ref: K. Park, 23rd ed. pg. 795-97

- The management of mass casualties (massive disaster) can be further divided into:
  - Search and rescue, first aid,
  - Triage
  - Stabilization of victims,
  - Hospital treatment and redistribution of patients to hospitals if necessary.
- Foremost step for disease prevention and control in post disaster phase is chlorination of all the water bodies. Most practical and effective strategy of disease prevention is "supplying safe drinking water and proper disposal of excreta.

294. Ans. (c) Blue

Ref: K. Park, 23rd ed. pg. 795-97

- In a disaster management, categorization of victims are done on the basis of likelihood of survival.

TABLE: Triage color code and their significance

Category	Color	Remarks/Steps
Category 1	Red	**Highest priority-** patient immediate resuscitations or life-saving surgery (0 to 6 hr)
Category 2	Yellow/blue	High priority resuscitation or life saving surgery (within 6 to 24hr)
Category 3	Green	Ambulatory/ low minor injuries; non-life threating
Category 4	Black	Dead, Moribund; least priority

295. Ans. (a) Red

Ref: K. Park, 23rd ed. pg. 795-97

296. Ans. (d) All of the above

Ref: K. Park 23rd ed. pg. 127-128

- Gamma radiation is used for sterilizing plastics, syringes, swabs, culture plates, catheter, rubber, oils, greases and metal foils.

297. Ans. (d) Liquid paraffin

Ref: K. Park, 23rd ed. pg. 128

- **Autoclaving** is a method of disinfection mainly used for surgical dressings, instruments, laboratory wares, media and pharmaceutical products.
- Principle: Steam + High pressure (~ 30 psi) and temperature 121 C.
- Efficiency test of autoclaving: spores of *Bacillus Stearothermophillus*.

298. Ans. (c) Plastic syringes

Ref: K. Park, 23rd ed. pg. 127-28

HOT AIR OVEN

- Holding period of 160 C x 1 hour
- Used for forceps, glasswares, scissors, scalpels, glass syringes, swabs and few pharmaceutical products like liquid paraffin, fats, grease.

299. Ans. (a) Blue

Ref: K. Park, 23rd ed. pg. 126-28, 753

- Sharp wastes like needles, syringes, blades, scalpels, glass are disposed in blue/white translucent bag

Color coding	Biomedical waste	Treatment option
Yellow	• Human anatomical waste • Animal waste • Microbiological waste • Soiled waste	Incineration/deep burial
Red	• Microbiological waste • Soiled waste and Solid waste	Autoclave/microwave/chemical treatment
Blue/white translucent	• Sharp waste • Solid waste	Autoclave/microwave/chemical treatment and destruction/shredding
Black	• Discarded and cytotoxic meds • Incineration ash • Chemical waste (solid)	Secured landfill

300. Ans. (d) All of the above

Ref: K. Park, 23rd ed. pg. 126-28, 753

- Sharp wastes like needles, syringes, blades, scalpels, glass are disposed in blue/white translucent bag

Preventive and Social Medicine (PSM)

- Blue/white translucent bag: Sharp waste and Solid waste
- *Refer to above explanation.*

301. Ans. (b) Solid waste

Cat.	BMW	Wastes included
1.	Human Anatomical Waste	Human tissues, organs, body parts
2.	Animal waste	Animal tissues, body parts,organs,carcasses, fluids, blood
3.	Microbiology & biotechnology waste	Waste from lab cultures,stocks,specimens of microorganisms, vaccines,cellcultues ,toxins, wastes from production of biological
4.	Waste sharps	Needles, syringes,scalpels,glass,blade
5.	Discarded medication &cytotoxic drugs	Expired medicines, discarded medicines
6.	Soiled waste	Items contaminated with blood, fluids,includingcotton,dressings,linen,bandage,plasters
7.	**Solid waste**	**Disposable items (except sharps),including catheter,tubes,i.v sets**
8.	Liquid waste	Waste generated from lab,washing ,cleaning,disinfecting activities
9.	Incineration ash	Ash from incineration of any BMW
10.	Chemical waste	Chemical used in disinfection

302. Ans. (a) Efficacy of a disinfectant

HEALTH PLANNING, CARE AND MANAGEMENT IN INDIA

303. Ans. (b) 30,000

Ref: K. Park 25th ed. P 964

Health Care Unit	Population covered	
	Plain	Hilly/Tribal/Backward
CHC	120,000	80,000
PHC	30,000	20,000
MPW	5000	3000
AWW	400-800	300-800
ASHA/VHG/TBA	1000	One ASHA per habitation

304. Ans. (b) Multi-purpose worker scheme

Ref: K. Park, 23rd ed. pg. 874-75

- **Kartar Singh Committee:** Recommended multi-purpose worker scheme. Kartar Singh Committee recommended:
  - **Current ANM** to be replaced by the newly designated "female health worker" and present day basic health workers, malaria surveillance workers, family planning health assistants to be replaced by "male health workers"

305. Ans. (b) 10,000

Ref: K. Park, 23rd ed. pg. 900

TABLE: Suggested norms for health personnel

Personnel category	Norms suggested
Nurses	1 per 5000
Health worker male and female	1 per 5000 in plain 1 per 3000 in tribal and hilly areas
Trained dai	One for each village
Health assistant (male and female)	1 per 30,000 in plain 1 per 20,000 in tribal and hilly areas
Pharmacist	1 per 10,000
Lab technician	1 per 10,000
ASHA	1 per 1000

306. Ans. (c) 16

The guidelines are from India New Born Action Plan 2014

Special New Born Care Unit (SNCU)

- It should be present in all district and sub-district hospitals.
- It comprises 12 beds and 4 beds for rooming in purposes
- The unit provides care for sick newborns >1800 g and routine new born care except ventilator services.

New Born Stabilization Unit (NBSU)

- It should be present in all CHC and FRU
- It comprises 4 beds and 2 beds for rooming in purposes.
- The unit aims to stabilize the sick new-borns before referral and manage baby >1800 g with jaundice, sepsis and hypothermia.

FMGE Solutions Screening Examination

New Born Care Corner (NBCC)

- It should be present at all points where delivery will occur including PHC and subcenter.
- It comprises minimum one bed.
- Objective is to provide immediate care at birth, feeding support and immediate referral.

307. Ans. (a) 1000

Ref: Park's, 23rd ed. pg. 449-50

- ASHA is Accredited Social Health Activist.
- One ASHA works for **1000 population.**
- In tribal, hilly and desert areas, the norm is one ASHA per habitation.

Impact Indicators of ASHA

- Infant mortality rate
- Child malnutrition rate
- Number of TB/leprosy case detection as compared to previous year.

Must Know Points About ASHA

- **ASHA** must be the resident of the village preferably in the **age group of 25-45 years**.
- Minimum **education** required for ASHA: **8th pass**
- ASHA is selected by village panchayat/Gram Sabha
- ASHA comes under national Rural Health Mission (NRHM): 2005-2012
- Act as bridge between village and ANM (Auxiliary Nurse midwife)
- Training of ASHA is done by ANM and AWW for a **minimum duration of 23 days**.

308. Ans. (d) 7

Ref: Park's, 23rd ed. pg. 449-50

- ASHA will make visits to all newborns according to specified schedule up to 42 days of life. The scheduled visits are as follows:
  - **Six visits** in case of **institutional delivery**: Day 3, 7, 14, 21, 28, 42
  - **Seven visits** in case of **home delivery**: Day 1, 3, 7, 14, 28, 42
  - **Five visits** in case of **caesarean delivery** (mother discharged after 5 – 6 days): **Day** 7, 14, 21, 28, 42

309. Ans. (c) 1 lakh

Ref: K. Park, 23rd ed. pg. 428

- Designated microscopy centre (DMC): The most peripheral laboratory under RNTCP network is DMC which serves a population of around **100,000 in plains** and **50,000 in tribal and hilly areas.**

310. Ans. (d) Equity of distribution

Ref: K. Park, 23rd ed. pg. 891

- PHC is Primary Health Care outlined by Alma Ata in 1978.
- It is defined as essential health care, which is characterized by 4 A's
  - Acceptable (*it should be acceptable by everyone*)
  - Accessible (*it should be accessible by everyone*)
  - Available (*it should be available to everyone*)
  - Affordable (*it should be affordable to everyone*)

TABLE: Elements of PHC (Primary Health Care) (remembered as ELEMENTS)

E	Essential drugs
L	Locally endemic disease prevention and control
E	EPI (Expanded program of immunization)
M	MCH (Maternal and child Health care including family planning)
E	Education
N	Nutrition
T	Treatment of common ailments
S	Safe water supply and sanitation

- Equity of distribution is NOT an element of PHC, but it is one of the principles/pillars of the PHC.
- **4 Principles/Pillars of Primary Health Care:**
  - Equitable distribution
  - Community participation
  - Intersectoral coordination
  - Appropriate technology.

311. Ans. (a) Primary health care

Ref: K. Park, 23rd ed. pg. 891-92

Please refer to above explanation

312. Ans. (c) Unequitable distribution

Ref: K. Park, 23rd ed. pg. 891-92

Please refer to above explanation.

313. Ans. (c) Oxygen saturation

Ref: K. Park, 23rd ed. pg. 904-905

314. Ans. (d) 100,000

Ref: K. Park, 23rd ed. pg. 907

- **CHC** is community health Centre. It covers 120,000 population in plain areas and 80,000 population in hilly areas.

Preventive and Social Medicine (PSM)

- Since, 120,000 is not in option, 100,000 is the closest and best answer.

> **Extra Mile**
>
> - PHC is considered as *Primary level of health care* is. It is considered as *1st level of contact*.
> - CHC is considered as *secondary level of health care* and *first referral unit*.
> - *Tertiary level of health* care is delivered through medical colleges and hospitals.

Health Care Unit	Population covered	
	Plain	Hilly/Tribal/Backward
CHC	120,000	80,000
PHC	30,000	20,000
MPW	5000	3000
AWW	400-800	300-800
ASHA/VHG/TBA	1000	

315. Ans. (b) CHC

Ref: K. Park 23rd ed. pg. 907

Please refer to above explanation

316. Ans. (b) 30

Ref: K. Park 23rd ed. pg. 907

- **PHC level: 4 to 6 bed** and staff 15 and 1 MBBS and medical officer
- **CHC level: 30 beds** and 30 staff including 7 doctors MD/MS/OBS/GYNE/ PEDIA/ OPTHA/ANES/PSM
- **Sub center level: zero bed** and 3 staff. MPW *(1 male and 1 female)*/ ANM *(auxillary nurse midwife)*.

317. Ans. (c) 2005

Ref: K. Park, 23rd ed. pg. 448

- National Rural Health Mission (NRHM) was established in 2005.
- Goal of NRHM is to provide every village in the country with a trained female community health activist: **ASHA** *(Accredited Social Health Activist)*.

Other Important Health Programmes of India

- National Tuberculosis Programme (NTP): 1962
- Revised National TB Control Programme (RNTCP): 1993
- National AIDS Control Programme (NACP): 1987
- National Malaria Control Programme (NMCP): 1953
- National Leprosy Control Program: 1955
- Integrated Child Development Services scheme (ICDS): 1975

- National Programme for Control of Blindness (NPCB): 1976

318. Ans. (b) Kartar Singh Committee

Ref: K. Park, 23rd ed. pg. 874

- **Kartar Singh Committee:** Recommended multi-purpose worker scheme
- **Bhore Committee:** Health survey and development
- **Srivastava Committee**
  - Group on medical education and manpower.
  - Recommended bands of para-professionals and semi-professional health worker.
  - ROME (Reorientation of Medical Education) scheme.
  - Village Health Guide scheme.
  - 3-Tier rural health infrastructure
- Jungalwalla committee
  - Equal pay for equal work
  - No private practice

319. Ans. (d) 5000

Ref: K. Park, 23rd ed. pg. 903-904

- MPW works at sub centre level, 1 per 5000 population in plain areas and 1 per 3000 population in hilly/tribal areas.
- At present a sub centre is staffed by one female health worker known as Auxiliary Nurse Midwide (ANM) and one male health health worker known as multipurpose worker.

320. Ans. (b) 1000

Ref: K. Park, 23rd ed. pg. 449, 21st ed. pg. 407

- ASHA is Accredited Social Health Activist.
- One ASHA works for **1000 population.**
- In tribal, hilly and desert areas, the norm is one ASHA per habitation.

Impact Indicators of ASHA

- Infant mortality rate
- Child malnutrition rate
- Number of TB/leprosy case detection as compared to previous year.

> **Extra Mile**
>
> **ASHA**
> - **ASHA** must be the resident of the village preferably in the **age group of 25–45 years**.
> - Minimum **education** required for ASHA: **8TH pass**
> - ASHA is selected by village panchayat/Gram Sabha
> - ASHA comes under national Rural Health Mission (NRHM): 2005–2012
> - Act as bridge between village and ANM (Auxiliary Nurse midwife)
> - Training of ASHA is done by ANM and AWW for a **minimum duration of 23 days**.

FMGE Solutions Screening Examination

Extra Mile

- One multi-purpose worker (MPW) is for: **5000 population**
- One village health guide (VHG) is for: **1000**
- One Anganwadi worker (AWW) is for: **400-800**

321. Ans. (c) Minimum class 4 passed

Ref: K. Park, 23ʳᵈ ed. pg. 449-50, s 21ˢᵗ ed. pg. 407

- *Minimum education required for ASHA: 8ᵀᴴ pass*
- *Please refer to above explanation for more details.*

322. Ans. (d) Village

Ref: K. Park, 23ʳᵈ ed. pg. 449-50

323. Ans. (a) Is a mental health worker

Ref: K. Park, 23ʳᵈ ed. pg. 449-50

324. Ans. (c) Conduct 50% delivery

Ref: K. Park, 23ʳᵈ ed. pg. 903-904

- The Female Health Workers are expected to provide comprehensive primary health care to the community.
- The range of services they are expected to provide under Multi purpose Health Worker (MPW) scheme is very wide and encompasses promotive, preventive and curative services including conducting around 50% of deliveries, *anemic mothers and other pregnancy related issues.*
- **Visit**- At least *one visit, once in two months* to each household in the area allotted.
- *Collection of blood samples are functions of MPW male.*
- Female health workers have no role in the process of chlorination or disinfection of water.

325. Ans (b) Renal disease

Ref: K. Park, 23ʳᵈ ed. pg. 903, 196ᵗʰ pg. 754

- Renal disease cannot be picked up by a health worker unless it is responsible for alteration of the urine grossly.
- *Please refer to above explanation*

326. Ans. (c) Active malaria surveillance

Ref: K. Park, 23ʳᵈ ed. pg. 903-904

327. Ans. (d) 75 grams

Ref: K. Park, 23ʳᵈ ed. pg. 661, 20ᵗʰ 575

A Midday School Meal

Foodstuffs	g/day/child
• Cereals and millets	75
• Pulses	30
• Oils and fats	8
• Leafy vegetables	30
• Nonleafy vegetables	30

Principles of Mid Day Meal Programme

- The meal should be a *supplement and not a substitute to the home diet*
- The meal should supply at least **one-third of the total energy** requirement, and **half of the protein** need
- The cost of the meal should be *reasonably low*
- The meal should be such that it can be prepared *easily in schools*; no complicated cooking process should be involved.
- As far as possible, *locally available foods should be used*; this will reduce the cost of the meal, and the menu should be frequently changed to avoid monotony.

328. Ans. (b) 1/3 calories, 1/2 proteins

Ref: K. Park, 23ʳᵈ ed. pg. 661-62

- Mid-day meal program is also known as National Program of Nutritional Support to primary education.
- The main advantage of this program is to influence more children towards schools in order to improve the literacy.
- This meal only act as a supplement and NOT as a substitute to home diet.
- *This meal should provide 1/3 of the total calories requirement and ½ of the total protein requirement.*

329. Ans. (b) 30

Ref: K. Park, 23ʳᵈ ed. pg. 399-400

- BMI is Body Mass Index, aka Quetlet's Index.
- It is calculated as: BMI = weight (kg)/height (m)^2

Classification	BMI
Underweight	<18.5
Normal BMI	18.5–24.99
Overweight/pre-obese	25–29.99
Obesity • Grade I • Grade II • Grade III	>30.0 • 30–34.99 • 35–39.99 • ≥40

Preventive and Social Medicine (PSM)

330. Ans. (a) (Weight in kg/Height in meters^2)

Ref: K. Park, 23rd ed. pg. 399-400

331. Ans. (b) Birth injuries

Ref: K. Park, 23rd ed. pg. 564

- **Most common cause of neonatal mortality in India** is preterm birth.
- A preterm child is more likely to be low birth weight and premature, which contribute to neonatal mortality rate.
- Death due to Birth injuries are there, but it is relatively very less as compared to prematurity, low birth weight and asphyxia.

332. Ans. (c) 6

Ref: K. Park, 23rd ed. pg. 590,661, 21st ed. pg. 545, 611

- **ICDS** is Integrated Child Development Services which was started in 1975.
- This program include a strong supplementary nutrition component in form of Vitamin A prophylaxis and iron & folic acid distribution.
- The workers at village level who deliver the services are called *Anganwadi workers*.

Beneficiaries of ICDS

- Preschool children below 6 years.
- Adolescent girls 11 to 18 years old.
- Pregnant and lactating mothers.

333. Ans. (b) 1991

Ref: K. Park, 23rd ed. pg. 540-41

- The **Baby Friendly Hospital Initiative (BFHI**, is programme of the World Health Organization and UNICEF.
- *Main goal of this initiative is to improve infant and young child nutrition by promoting breast feeding.*
- This includes helping the mother *initiate breast-feeding within the **first hour** of birth in normal delivery* and 4 hours following caesarean section
- It also aims at improving the care of pregnant women, mothers and newborns at health facilities that provide maternity services for protecting, promoting and supporting breastfeeding.
- No advertisement promotional material or free products for infant feeding should be allowed in the facility.

334. Ans. (d) Infants are kept in the nursery for first 24 hours

Ref: K. Park, 23rd ed. pg. 540-541

335. Ans. (a) Panchayat samiti

Ref: K. Park, 23rd ed. pg. 881-82

- **Panchayat Samiti** is a local government body at the tahsil level in India. It works for the villages of the tahsil that together are called a **Development Block**.
- The Panchayat Samiti is the link between the Gram Panchayat and the zila parishad.

Note

- *Gram Sabha has been envisaged as the foundation of the Panchayati Raj system. A village having population not less than 1500 forms Gram Sabha and every adult of the village is member of Gram Sabha. These members of gram sabha can elect members of gram panchayat.*

336. Ans (b) 100 villages and 1,00,000 population

Ref: Park's PSM, 20 pg. 783, 784

"Under the community development programme, the rural areas of the country have been organized into Community Development Blocks —each Block comprising approximately **100 villages and a population of one lakh.**"

OCCUPATIONAL HEALTH

337. Ans. (a) CO_2, ozone, methane

Ref: Inventory of US greenhouse gas emissions and sinks, 1990-1994 By United States Environmental Protection Agency

- A **greenhouse gas** is a gas in an atmosphere that absorbs and emits radiation within the thermal infrared range. This process is the fundamental cause of the greenhouse effect.
- **The primary greenhouse gases in Earth's atmosphere** are **water vapor, carbon dioxide, methane, nitrous oxide,** and **ozone (O_3).**
- Chlorofluorocarbons (CFCs), Hydrofluorocarbons (HFCs) and other compounds such as perfluorinated carbons are also green house gases.
- Without greenhouse gases, the average temperature of Earth's surface would be about −18°C (0°F), rather than present average of 15°C (59°F).

338. Ans. (b) 5 Rad per person per year

Ref: K. Park, 23rd ed. pg. 804

- Maximum permissible radiation exposure for general population: 5 Rad (0.5 Rem) per person per year.
- Maximum permissible radiation exposure for workers: 50 Rad (5 Rem) per person per year.

FMGE Solutions Screening Examination

- Greatest source of radiation outside house: Extra-terrsetrial cosmic rays.
- Greatest source of radiation inside house: TV
- Greatest man-made source of radiation: X-ray

Extra Mile
- *Permissible sound level in hospital wards: 20–35 decibel.*
- *Maximum tolerable sound level: <85 decibel*
- *Permanent hearing loss at: >100 decibel*
- *Tympanic membrane ruptures at: 150–160 decibel.*

339. Ans (a) 20-35

Ref: K. Park, 23rd ed. pg. 741-42, 19th pg. 599

Acceptable noise levels (dBA)		
Residential:	Bed room	25
	Living room	40
Commercial:	Office	35-45
	Conference	40-45
	Restaurants	40-60
Industrial:	Workshop	40-60
	Laboratory	40-50
Educational:	Class room	30-40
	Library	35-40
Hospitals:	**Wards**	**20-35**

340. Ans. (a) Lung cancer

Ref: K. Park, 23rd ed. pg. 807

- Asbestosis occurs due to long duration (>10 years) exposure to asbestos.
- This may lead to pulmonary fibrosis, carcinoma of bronchus, mesothelioma of pleura/peritoneum and GIT cancer.

Other Important Occupational Cancer

Agent	Associated Cancer
Asbestosis	Mesothelioma
Arsenic	Skin, lung, liver CA
Benzene	Leukemia
Benzidine	Bladder CA
Silica	Lung CA
Wood dust	Nasal sinus

- *Most common occupational cancer: skin CA (75%), mainly squamous cell CA.*

341. Ans. (c) Asbestosis

Ref: K. Park, 23rd ed. pg. 807

- Pneumoconiosis occurs due to occupational exposure to dust.
- Dust particle of size 0.5 to 3 microns are most dangerous, as they can reach the interior of lungs easily.
- Most common pneumoconiosis associated with Mesothelioma and lung cancer: **Asbestosis**.
- Most common pneumoconiosis: **Silicosis**

TABLE: Other important pneumoconiosis to remember:

Disease	Exposure source
Silicosis	Silica dust
Anthracosis	Coal dust
Asbestosis	Asbestos dust
Bagassosis	Sugarcane dust (*thermoactinomyces sacchari*)
Byssinossis	Cotton fibre
Siderosis	Iron dust

342. Ans. (c) Sugarcane dust

Ref: K. Park, 23rd ed. pg. 807

343. Ans. (d) Can cause Blue Line on gums

Ref: K. Park, 23rd ed. pg. 807-808

- Lead poisoning is known as Plumbism.
- This is most commonly seen among painters, therefore also known as Painter's colic.
- *Most common source of lead poisoning: Petrol*
- Most common mode of lead poisoning: Inhalation

Clinical Finding of lead poisoning:
- *Burtonian line: Blue line on gums*
- Facial pallor: first and most consistent sign (always present).
- Lead colic: constipation/diarrhea
- Wrist drop/foot drop
- Encephalopathy

Investigation of Pb Poisoning:
- CPU: Coproporphyrin in Urine is a useful *screening test- > 150: exposure to lead*
- Amino Levulinic Acid (ALAU), lead levels in blood and urine: *diagnostic test.*
- Upon PBS, **basophilic stippling of RBC's** and *Microcytic Hypochromic anemia* seen.
- DOC for Pb poisoning: **EDTA**

344. Ans. (b) Insomnia

Ref: K. Park, 23rd ed. pg. 807-808

- Insomnia is caused by organic lead poisoning.
- Organic lead poisoning causes CNS side effects while Inorganic lead poisoning causes non-CNS side effects.

Preventive and Social Medicine (PSM)

Due to organic lead (CNS effects)	Due to inorganic lead (Non-CNS effects)
• Insomnia • Mental confusion • Headache • Delirium	• Facial pallor: *earliest and most consistent sign.* • Anemia: Microcytic Hypochromic • RBC's stippling • Burtonian Line on upper gums • Lead Colic: constipation *(or copper)* • Lead Palsy (wrist + foot drop)

345. Ans. (d) Inorganic lead

Ref: K. Park, 23rd ed. pg. 807-808

Please refer to above explanation

346. Ans. (c) Maternity benefit for 3 months

Ref: K. Park, 23rd ed. pg. 8015-16

- ESI (The Employees State Insurance) Act 1948 covers the social security and health insurance in India.
- ESI NOT applicable on: *(MERD)*
  - *Mines*
  - *Education*
  - *Railways*
  - *Defence*
- *The employer contributes 4.75% and employee contributes 1.75 % of total wage bill.*
- *It covers all employees getting wages upto 15,000 per month.*
- *Maternity benefit for a duration of 12 weeks (3 months).*
- Sickness benefits payable upto 91 days and extended sickness benefit payable for upto 2 years.

347. Ans. (d) Contribution

Ref: K. Park, 23rd ed. pg. 815-16

- The scheme is run by the contribution of the both employee and employer, and grants from central and state government.
- The employer contributes 4.75% of total wage bill. The employee contributes 1.75 % of wages.
- **Exemption:** employees getting < Rs. 70. The state government share of expenditure on medical care is 1/8 of total cost of medical care. ESI corporation share of expenditure is 7.8 of total cost of medical care.

348. Ans. (a) The employer contributes 4.75%

Ref: K. Park, 23rd ed. pg. 815-816

Please refer to above explanation.

349. Ans. (c) System analysis

Ref: K. Park, 23rd ed. pg. 872

- **Cost effective analysis** is a management technique where benefits are stated in terms of results achieved. Eg: No. of life saved.
- **Cost benefit analysis** is a management technique where benefits are stated in terms of money.
- **System analysis** is a management technique of *finding out the cost effectiveness* of the available alternatives.
- **Network analysis** is the graphic plan of all events and activities to be completed in order to reach an end objective. 2 types of network analysis technique:
  - **PERT** (Programme Evaluation And Review Technique): arrow diagram representation of event.
  - **CPM** (Critical Path Method): the longest path.

350. Ans. (a) Time

Ref: K. Park, 23rd ed. pg. 872

- **Network analysis** is the graphic plan of all events and activities to be completed in order to reach an end objective. 2 types of network analysis technique:
  - **PERT** *(Programme Evaluation and Review Technique)*: an arrow diagram representing the logical sequence in which events must take place. It aids in planning scheduling and monitoring the project.
  - **CPM** *(Critical Path Method)*: the longest path of the network. If any activity in the critical path is delayed, entire project will be delayed.

351. Ans. (b) 29-31°C

DISINFECTION AND MISCELLANEOUS

352. Ans. (d) Hypochlorous acid

Ref: K. Park, 23rd ed. pg. 714-15

CHLORINATION OF WATER

- **Disinfecting action of chlorine in water is mainly due to hypochlorous acid (HOCl).**
- Hypochlorite ions has minor role in disinfection.
- Compared to UV rays or ozone, only Chlorine has residual germicidal effect.

Extra Mile

- **Chlorine has no effect on:**
  - Bacterial spores, protozoal cysts and helminthic ova
  - Viral agents of Hepatitis A, Polio are also resistant at normal doses.
- **Horrock's apparatus:** Cl_2 demand (to measure Cl_2 required for water disinfection)

353. Ans (c) Ortho toluidine test

Ref: K. Park, 23rd ed. pg. 715, 19th pg. 578

Explanations

- **Orthotolidine arsenite test** - used for testing residual chlorine at the end of **one hour contact.**
- If the "free" residual chlorine level is less than 0.5 mg/litre, the chlorination procedure should be repeated before any water is drawn.
- Wells are best **disinfected at night** after the day's draw off.
- During epidemics of cholera, wells should be disinfected every day

Extra Mile

- **Horrock's Apparatus** is used for **estimating the chlorine demand of the well water** and calculate the amount of bleaching powder required to disinfect the well.
- Roughly, **2.5 grams of good quality bleaching powder** would be required to disinfect **1,000 litres** of water. Bleaching powder contains **33% available chlorine**
- The **hypochlorous acid** is the most effective form of chlorine for **water disinfection.**
- Chlorine acts best as a disinfectant when the **pH of water is around 7.**
- The **standard prescribed** for chloride is **200 mg/litre**
- The **maximum permissible level is 600 mg/litre**

354. Ans. (b) Alum is added after lime

Ref: K. Park, 23rd ed. pg. 714-15

- Nalgonda Technique is utilized for defluorination of water.
- Sequence of components added for defluorination is: (LAB)
  - Lime
  - Alum
  - Bleaching powder

355. Ans. (d) Natural selection is a process where harmful genes are not eliminated from the gene pool and genes favorable to individual are not passed onto offspring.

According to Hardy Weinberg law genes are passed on to the offsprings in a gene pool.

356. Ans. (a) 30-year-old female to check for cystic fibrosis

357. Ans. (d) Mixed cohort

358. Ans. (d) Repeated measurement

BIOSTATISTICS

359. Ans. (b) Every 6 months

Ref: K.Park 23rd ed. P 841

Sample Registration System (SRS)

Since civil registration is deficient in India, a Sample Registration System (SRS) was initiated in the mid-1960s to provide reliable estimates of birth and death rates at the National and State levels. The SRS is a dual-record system, consisting of continuous enumeration of births and deaths by an enumerator and an independent survey every 6 months by an investigator-supervisor. The half-yearly survey, in addition to serving as an independent check on the events recorded by the enumerator, produces the denominator required for computing rates.

The SRS now covers the entire country. It is a major source of health information.

360. Ans. (a) Histogram

Ref: K.Park 23rd ed. P 845

Histogram

It is a pictorial diagram of frequency distribution. It consists of a series of blocks (Figure). The class intervals are given along the horizontal axis and the frequencies along the vertical axis. The area of each block or rectangle is proportional to the frequency. The figure is the histogram of the frequency distribution of blood pressure in females 45–64 years.

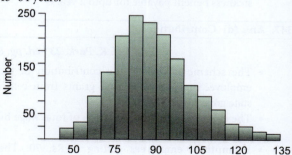

Frequency distribution of diastrolic blood pressure in females aged 45–64 years

361. Ans. (b) 8.4

Ref: K. Park, 23rd ed. pg. 65

- An odds ratio (OR) is a measure of association between an exposure and an outcome. The OR represents the odds that an outcome will occur given a particular exposure, compared to the odds of the outcome occurring in the absence of that exposure.

- $OR = \dfrac{a \times d}{b \times c} = \dfrac{33 \times 27}{53 \times 2} = \mathbf{8.4}$

362. Ans. (c) TP/TP + FN × 100

Sensitivity: Defined as ability of a screening test to identify all those who have disease (cases/ True positive)

$$\text{Sensitivity} = \dfrac{a}{(a+c)} \times 100 = \dfrac{TP}{(TP+FN)} \times 100$$

363. Ans. (d) 99

	Pregnant	Non-Pregnant
Positive test	99	10
Negative test	1	90

$$\text{Sensitivity} = \dfrac{a}{(a+c)} \times 100 = \dfrac{99}{99+1} \times 100 = \mathbf{99}$$

364. Ans. (b) 2.5

Ref: K. Park, 23rd ed. pg. 78

- RR = incidence of disease among exposed/ Incidence of disease among non-exposed

	Disease (+)	Disease (–)	Total
Exposed	50	350	400
Non- exposed	5	95	100

- Putting the value in formula = 50/400 ÷ 5/100
  = 50/400 × 100/5
  = **2.5**

365. Ans. (a) 0.00

Ref: K. Park, 23rd ed. pg. 848

- Standard deviation is the deviation from the mean value.
- 10 babies were born, each weighs 2.7 kg, which gives a mean value of 2.7, indicating there is no deviation from the mean value.
- Hence the answer will be 0 (zero)
- *Standard deviation is also known as root mean square deviation.*

366. Ans. (c) Used to test significance of association between two quantitative data

Ref: K. Park, 23rd ed. pg. 852

- Chi-square test is used to test significance of association between two *QUALITATIVE* data.
- It is used for non-Gaussian distribution.
- This test is a non-parametric test of significance.

- Degree of freedom used in chi- square test is calculated by (c-1) (r-1)

367. Ans. (c) 12

Ref: K. Park, 23rd ed. pg. 852

- **Degree of freedom:** It is the no. of observations in a dataset that can freely vary once the parameters have been estimated.
- It is used in *chi-square test and t-test.*
- *DOF: (c-1) (r-1), where c is no. of columns and r is no. of rows.*
- In the given question there are 4 columns and 5 rows.
- Therefore (4-1) (5-1) gives **12.**

368. Ans. (d) Wrong calculation

Ref: K. Park, 23rd ed. pg. 852-53

- Correlation coefficient (r) is used to find out if there is any significant relationship between two variables (e.g: x and y) or not.
- Correlation coefficient (r) tends to lie between –1.0 to +1.0 (-1 < r < +1)
  - If r = + 1: strong positive association between two variables
  - If r = 0: no association between two variables
  - If r = –1: strong negative association

369. Ans. (a) Mean

Ref: K. Park, 23rd ed. pg. 847-88

- Best measure of central tendency: **MEAN**
- Best measure of central tendency for NOMINAL data: **MODE**
- Best measure of central tendency for ORDINAL data: **MEDIAN**
- Best measure of central tendency foe metric/quantitative data: **MEAN**

370. Ans. (d) Mode

Ref: K. Park, 23rd ed. pg. 847-88

THE MODE

- The mode is the commonly occurring value in a distribution of data. It is the most frequent item or the most fashiionable" value in a series of observations. For example, the diastolic blood pressure of 20 individuals was:

85, 75 79, 71, 95, 75, 75, 77, 75, 90

71, 75, 79, 95, 75, 77, 84, 75, 81, 75

- The mode or the most frequently occurring value is 75.

371. Ans. (b) 16, 10, 10

Ref: K. Park, 23rd ed. pg. 847-88

- Patient is smoker from last 6 years.

- In the first year 5 sticks per day; in the 2nd, 3rd and 4th year it is 10 sticks per day; in 5th year 20 sticks per day and in 6th year 40 sticks per day.

  Therefore, mean = $\frac{5 + 10 + 10 + 10 + 20 + 40}{6}$

  = 15.83, which is rounded as **16**

- Median is middle value in ascending order. Since, it has two middle value,

  $\frac{10 + 10}{2} = 10$

- Mode is most repeated/frequent value, which is 10, repeated 3 times.
- *Therefore the mean, median and mode will be 16, 10, 10 respectively.*

372. Ans. (b) 5 and 4

Ref: Park, 22nd ed. pg. 789-90

Mean = $\sum \frac{X}{n}$

Therefore, mean =

$\frac{2+2+3+4+4+4+4+5+5+7+8+8+9}{13}$ = 65/13

Mean = 5

- Mode is most repeated/frequent value, which is 4, repeated 4 times.
- *Therefore the mean, mode will be 5 and 4 respectively.*

373. Ans. (c) 95%

Ref: K. Park, 23rd ed. pg. 140-141

- Assume there are 1000 people. So, there are 300 diseased people among them (as it given prevalence 30%) and the people who do not have the disease is 700. So true positive is 270 (sensitivity-90%)

False negative is 30.
True negative is 560 (specificity-80%).
False positive is 140.
Negative Predictive Value = (True Negative / True Negative + False Negative) x 100
= (560/560+30) x 100
= **94.9%**

374. Ans. (b) 2.6

Ref: K. Park, 23rd ed. pg. 73

- An odds ratio (OR) is a measure of association between an exposure and an outcome. The OR represents the odds that an outcome will occur given a particular exposure, compared to the odds of the outcome occurring in the absence of that exposure. Odds ratios are most commonly used in case-control studies.
- For example in the given case, 40 out of 100 smokers developed lung cancer and 20 out of 100 developed lung cancer. For calculating odd's ratio, we first plot this in the 4 boxes

	Disease (+)	Disease (-)
Smoker	40	60
Non-smoker	20	80

OR = $\frac{a \times d}{b \times c}$ = $\frac{40 \times 80}{60 \times 20}$ = **2.6**

375. Ans. (c) 0.83

Ref: K. Park, 21st ed. pg. 113

- The screening test shows true negative result in 50% of diseased population
- In 10% healthy population, the test shows positive result. That means 10% false positive.

  Putting this into formula:

  $\frac{\text{True negative}}{\text{False positive + True negative}} \times 100$

  $\frac{50}{10 + 50} \times 100$

  $\frac{50}{60} \times 100 = 83\% = \mathbf{0.83}$

376. Ans. (b) <1/1000

Ref: Park's 23rd ed.

Strategic action plan for malaria control in India (2012–2017)

- Malaria control is now incorporated into the health service delivery programmes under NRHM.

Objective

To achieve API **<1 per 1000** population by the end of 2017.

Goals

The national goals for strategic plan are:
- Screening all fever cases suspected for malaria *(60% through quality microscopy and 40% by rapid diagnostic test.*
- Treating all *P. falciparum* cases with full course of effective ACT and primaquine, and all *P. vivax* cases with 3 days chloroquine and 14 days primaquine.
- Equipping all health institutions (PHC level and above), especially in high-risk areas, with microcopy facility and RDT for emergency use and injectable artemisinin derivatives.
- Strengthening all district and sub-district hospitals in malaria endemic areas as per IPHS with facilities for management of severe malaria cases.

Preventive and Social Medicine (PSM)

Outcome Indicators

The outcome indicators of strategic plan are:

1. At least 80% of those suffering from malaria get correct, affordable, appropriate and complete treatment within 24 hours of reporting to the health system, by the year 2017.
2. At least 80% of those at high risk of malaria get protected by effective preventive measures such as ITN/LLIN or IRS by 2017.

3. At least 10% of the population in high-risk areas is surveyed annually (annual blood examination rate > 10%).

Impact Indicators

The impact indicators of strategic plan are:

1. To bring down annual incidence of malaria to **less than 1 per 1000 population** at national level by 2017.
2. At least 50% reduction in mortality due to malaria by the year 2017, taking 2010 level as baseline.

ANSWERS TO BOARD REVIEW QUESTIONS

377. Ans. (a) Pink

Ref: Park, 20th ed. pg. 387, OP Ghai, 7th ed. pg. 738

378. Ans. (d) Urine microscopy and culture sensitivity

Ref: www.mohfw.nic.in/NRHM/Task_grp/Task_group_IPHS.pdf

379. Ans. (a) Spot map

Ref: Park, 20th ed. pg. 63

380. Ans. (b) Quota sampling

Ref: Fundamentals of Biostatistics 2nd ed By Rastogi V.B 37

381. Ans. (c) Tick typhus

Ref: Park, 20th ed pg. 684

382. Ans. (b) 5 rads

Ref: Park, 20th ed. pg. 651

383. Ans. (a) Pista

Ref: Park, 22nd ed. pg. 583

384. Ans. (b) Herd immunity

Ref: Park, 20th ed. pg. 61

385. Ans. (d) 2 years

Ref: Park, 23rd ed. pg. 817

In addition to 91 days of sickness benefit, insured persons suffering from certain long-term diseases are entitled to extended sickness benefit for a maximum period of 2 years.

386. Ans. (c) 10-15 days

Ref: Harrison's, 18th ed. ch-15211.

387. Ans. (c) Recall bias

Ref: Park, 20th ed. pg. 68, 69

388. Ans. (b) 23 days

Ref: Park's, 22nd ed. pg. 412

389. Ans. (a) High compliance

Ref: Park's, 20th ed. ch-167

390. Ans. (c) Vitamin C

Ref: Park's, 20th ed. pg. 545

391. Ans. (b) Black bag

Ref: Park's, 20th ed. pg. 699

392. Ans. (c) 1st July

Ref: Park's, 18th ed. pg. 639

393. Ans. (c) Proceeds from target to resource

Ref: CIMA official Learning System Management According-Performance-p 209

394. Ans. (a) 1881

Ref: http://censusinida.gov.in/Data_Products/Library/ Indian_perceptive_link/History /link/censushistory. htm, http://censusindia.gov.in/Ad_Campaign/drop_inarticles/05-History_of_Census_in_India.pdf

395. Ans. (b) SO_2

Ref: www.sciencedirect.com/science/journal/00406090, Introduction to Astrobiology by C. Sivaram

396. Ans. (c) +1.0

Ref: Park's 20th ed. pg. 755

397. Ans. (a) Line diagram

Ref: Park's, 20th ed. pg. 62, 748

398. Ans. (c) Shrivastava Committee

Ref: Park's, 20th ed. pg. 778

Explanations

FMGE Solutions Screening Examination

399. Ans. (a) Custom's Act

Ref: www.cbec.gov.in/customs/cs-act/cs-act-idx.htm

400. Ans. (c) Skin biopsy

Ref: Harrison's, 18th edjaweet 24th ed.

401. Ans. (a) BCG vaccine

Ref: Appendix-46 for "Types of vaccine"

402. Ans. (a) Louse

Ref: Park textbook of preventive and social medicine 20th ed. pg. 684

403. Ans. (a) 60 and 55 kg

Ref: Park's, 20th ed. pg. 547, Park's, 21st ed. pg. 584

404. Ans. (d) 18 years and younger

Ref: Convention on the Right of the child united Nations 1989-11-20

405. Ans. (a) Flavivirus

Ref: Jawetz, 24th ed. ch-38

406. Ans. (a) Spinners

Ref: Park, 20th ed. /210

407. Ans. (a) Anthracosis

Ref: Harrison's, 18th ed. ch. 255

408. Ans. (b) 0.3%

Ref: Park, 22nd ed. pg. 405-407

409. Ans. (b) 32

Ref: Park, 20th ed. pg. 347

410. Ans. (d) 30 cluster of 7 children

Ref: http://www.who.int/vaccines-documents/DocsPDF/www592.pdf

411. Ans. (b) Chapter II

Ref: Park, 22nd ed. pg. 47

412. Ans. (b) Primary prevention

Ref: Park, 20th ed. pg. 38

413. Ans. (d) Crude birth rate-Crude death rate

Ref: Park, 20th ed. pg. 412

414. Ans. (b) 2 weeks

Ref: Park, 20th ed. pg. 674

415. Ans. (c) 15 days

Ref: Park, 21st ed. pg. 714

416. Ans. (c) Per 1000 live births

Ref: Park, 20th ed. pg. 488

417. Ans. (c) 33%

Ref: Park, 20th ed. pg. 625

418. Ans. (c) 95.45%

Ref: Park, 20th ed. pg. 751

419. Ans. (a) RNTCP

Ref: With text

420. Ans. (c) Incubation period

Ref: Park textbook, 22nd ed. pg. 96

421. Ans. (d) 40-50 kcal/kg/day

Ref: Park, 22nd ed. pg. 587

422. Ans. (c) 1st week of August

Ref: Appendix-70 FOR "Health Related Days"

423. Ans. (a) 7th April

Ref: Park 22nd ed. pg. 859

424. Ans. (a) 7 days

Ref: Park, 22nd ed. pg. 521

425. Ans. (a) 25-26.9°C

Ref: Park, 22nd ed. pg. 680

426. Ans. (b) 0.5–4.0 kg

Ref: Park, 22nd ed. pg. 735

427. Ans. (c) Secondary

Ref: Park, 22nd ed. pg. 38

428. Ans. (b) Anopheles stephensi

Ref: Park, 22nd ed. pg. 236

429. Ans. (a) NRHM

Ref: Park, 22nd ed. pg. 412

430. Ans. (d) Bird-Pigs

Ref: Park, 22nd ed. pg. 259

431. Ans. (b) Less than 100 m

Ref: Park, 22nd ed. pg. 715

432. Ans. (b) E. coli

Ref: Park, 22nd ed. pg. 669

Preventive and Social Medicine (PSM)

ANSWERS TO IMAGE-BASED QUESTIONS

433. Ans. (b) Correlation coefficient

436. Ans. (a) Aedes Larvae

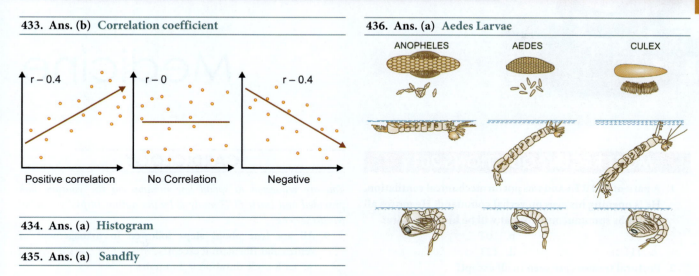

434. Ans. (a) Histogram

435. Ans. (a) Sandfly

437. Ans. (b) UNICEF

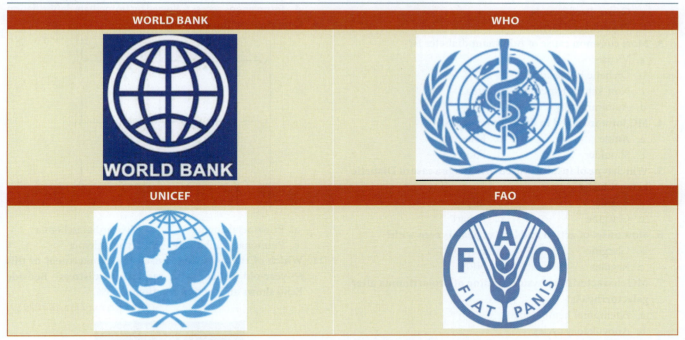

438. Ans. (a) National Rural Health Mission

439. Ans. (a) Mirena

The image shows presence of Mirena is a long acting reversible contraceptive, which contains Levonorgestrel and hence has a dual benefit of hormonal action and local action of intrauterine device.

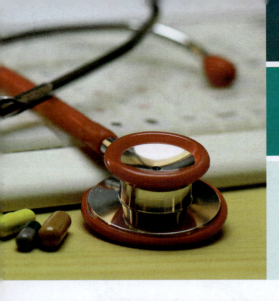

9

Medicine

MOST RECENT QUESTIONS 2019

1. A patient had RTA and was put on mechanical ventilation. He is opening his eyes on verbal command. He moves all his limbs spontaneously. What will be his GCS score?
   a. 9T
   b. 10T
   c. 11T
   d. 12T
2. Postural tremors are seen in all except?
   a. Alcohol withdrawal
   b. Essential tremors
   c. Generalized paresis
   d. Physiological tremors
3. Most common cause of fulminant diabetes is?
   a. Viruses
   b. Diabetic Ketoacidosis
   c. Non-ketotic hyperosmolar coma
   d. Autoimmunity
4. MC joint involved in diabetes is seen is?
   a. Ankle
   b. Knee
   c. Shoulder
   d. Foot
5. Which type of Insulin is used to manage a case of Diabetic ketoacidosis?
   a. Regular
   b. Lispro
   c. Glargine
   d. Aspart
6. Slow onset of action and lack of peak is seen with?
   a. Glargine
   b. Lispro
   c. Regular
   d. NPH
7. MC characteristic physical finding of prolactinoma after galactorrhea is?
   a. Bitemporal hemianopia
   b. Anovulatory cycles
   c. Amenorrhea
   d. Infertility
8. Ipsilateral 3rd nerve palsy with crossed hemiplegia is a feature of?
   a. Weber syndrome
   b. Benedikt syndrome
   c. Wallenberg syndrome
   d. Horner syndrome

CARDIOLOGY

You are requested to spend few minutes on the youtube link provided and learn ECG analysis by the author https://youtu.be/M-8Rt3e7×8g

9. All are true about steps followed in management of ventricular fibrillation except? *(Most Recent Question 2019)*
   a. CPR cycle duration is 2 minutes
   b. Chest compressions at 100-120/min
   c. Start CPR followed by immediate defibrillation
   d. Intravenous access followed by Immediate defibrillation
10. Comment on the diagnosis.

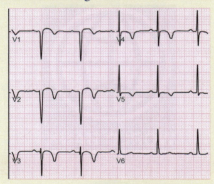

   a. Prinzmetal angina
   b. Myocardial ischemia
   c. Pulmonary embolism
   d. Hyperkalemia
11. Which of the following is used for management of this 65-year-old patient with respiratory distress? Bedside Echo shows an Ejection fraction of 35%.

(Most Recent Question 2019)

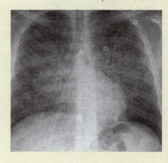

Medicine

a. Lasix, nitrates and sacubitril-valsartan
b. Lasix, norepinephrine and sacubitril-valsartan
c. Lasix, nitrates and morphine
d. Lasix, ACEI and digoxin

12. **Which of following leads to a continuous murmur?**
a. Peripheral Pulmonic stenosis
b. Severe Pulmonary artery hypertension
c. Type A aortic dissection
d. Rupture of cardiac chamber

13. **Which is true about Postural Hypotension?**
(Most Recent Question 2019)
a. Decrease in systolic blood pressure 20 mm Hg within 6 mins of postural change
b. Decrease in systolic blood pressure 20 mm Hg within 3 min of postural change
c. Decrease in diastolic blood pressure 20 mm Hg within 6 mins of postural change
d. Decrease in diastolic blood pressure 20 mm Hg within 3mins of postural change

14. **A 60-year-old female presents with left sided weakness for more than one hour and left sided facial weakness with BP of 160/100 mm Hg. CT is normal. What is the next best step?** *(Most Recent Question 2019)*
a. Start thrombolysis
b. Give loading dose of aspirin and clopidogrel
c. Only manage BP
d. No intervention required

15. **Best management of a hemodynamically stable patient with ECG showing Broad QRS complex with antidromic tachycardia is?** *(Recent Pattern Question 2018-19)*
a. Oral Verapamil
b. Oral Beta-blocker
c. Cardioversion
d. Intravenous Procainamide

16. **Which of these is not done in Wolf Parkinson White syndrome?** *(Recent Pattern Question 2018-19)*
a. Treadmill
b. Holter monitoring
c. Oral beta blocker
d. Procainamide

17. **Which of the following is not correct about defibrillation?** *(Recent Pattern Question 2018-19)*
a. Easy for untrained person
b. Decrease in success rate with delay in initiation
c. Improves prognosis
d. 1-minute gap between 2 shocks

18. **Modified Duke's criteria are used for diagnosis of?**
(Recent Pattern Question 2018-19)
a. Infective endarteritis
b. Infectious mononucleosis
c. Inflammatory myopathy
d. Infective endocarditis

19. **Which of the following shall be seen with use of a small size BP cuff?** *(Recent Pattern Question 2018-19)*
a. False elevation of BP
b. Falsely low value of BP
c. Cancels the effect of calcified arteries
d. Increases trans-arm impedance

20. **Which of the following is a cardioprotective lipid?**
(Recent Pattern Question 2018-19)
a. LDL
b. HDL
c. VLDL
d. Chylomicrons

21. **Rescue P.C.I is done for which of the following?**
(Recent Pattern Question 2018-19)
a. Persistent chest pain with ST elevation >30 minutes after thrombolysis
b. Persistent chest pain with ST elevation >60 minutes after thrombolysis
c. Persistent Chest pain with ST elevation >90 minutes after thrombolysis
d. Persistent Chest pain with ST elevation for >120 minutes after thrombolysis

22. **Which of the following condition should *not* be considered if JVP rises on deep inspiration?**
(Recent Pattern Question 2018)
a. Constrictive pericarditis
b. Restrictive cardiomyopathy
c. Complete heart block
d. Atrial fibrillation

23. **The PR interval in ECG denotes**
(Recent Pattern Question 2018)
a. Atrial depolarization only
b. Atrial depolarization with A-V conduction
c. Ventricular depolarization and ventricular repolarization
d. Atrial depolarization with atrial repolarization

24. **Which of the following is not associated with pulmonary artery hypertension?** *(Recent Pattern Question 2018)*
a. Interstitial lung disease
b. Left ventricular hypertrophy
c. Mitral stenosis
d. Cor-pulmonale

25. **A patient presents with pedal oedema with Water-hammer pulse. What is the diagnosis?**
(Recent Pattern Question 2017)
a. B_1 deficiency
b. B_3 deficiency
c. B_6 deficiency
d. B_{12} deficiency

26. **Which is correct about the ECG finding of hypo-calcemia?** *(Recent Pattern Question 2017)*
a. Prolonged QT
b. Tall tented T wave
c. Prolonged PR
d. Narrow QRS

27. **Which is the preferred bypass graft used in CABG?**
(Recent Pattern Question 2017)
a. Internal mammary artery
b. Great saphenous vein
c. Short saphenous vein
d. Gastro-epiploic artery

28. Wide fixed Split S2 is seen in?
    (Recent Pattern Question 2017)
    a. PDA   b. ASD
    c. TOF   d. VSD
29. What is the earliest change in ECG in case of hyperkalemia? *(Recent Pattern Question 2017)*
    a. Tall tented T wave
    b. Inverted P
    c. Prolonged QRS
    d. T wave inversion
30. Which rhythm disorder is shown in this ECG?
    (Recent Pattern Question 2017)

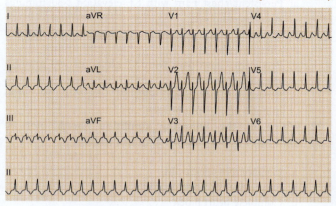

    a. Ventricular fibrillation   b. PSVT
    c. Atrial fibrillation   d. Atrial flutter
31. Which is incorrect about the ECG shown below?
    (Recent Pattern Question 2017)

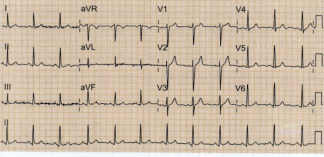

    a. QT = 0.04 sec
    b. PR = 0.16 sec
    c. QRS = 0.10 sec
    d. P wave = 0.12 sec
32. Which drug is not useful in chronic CHF?
    (Recent Pattern Question 2017)
    a. Carvedilol
    b. Ramipril
    c. Atenolol
    d. Diuretics

33. The ECG finding shown below is due to which of the following drugs? *(Recent Pattern Question 2017)*

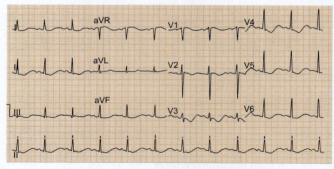

    a. Diuretics   b. A.R.B
    c. A.C.E inhibitors d. Beta blockers
34. Which of the following is correct about the image shown below? *(Recent Pattern Question 2017)*

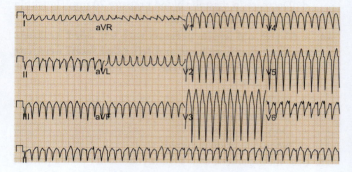

    a. Atrial fibrillation   b. Atrial flutter
    c. PSVT   d. VT
35. During CPR when is vasopressin given?
    a. Never be used   *(Recent Pattern Question 2016)*
    b. Use every 3 minutes
    c. First line drug of choice
    d. Given along with adrenaline
36. Which antiarrhythmic drug is given in post resuscitation arrhythmia? *(Recent Pattern Question 2016)*
    a. Lignocaine   b. Magnesium sulfate
    c. Amiodarone   d. Atropine
37. In JVP y descent is absent and X wave is prominent? This suggests:
    a. Restictive cardiomyopathy
    b. Cardiac tamponade
    c. Constrictive pericarditis
    d. Right ventricular failure
38. Digitalis is used in mitral stenosis when patient develops?
    a. Atrial fibrillation
    b. Right ventricular failure
    c. Acute pulmonary edema
    d. Myocarditis

Medicine

39. Murmur heard in aortic stenosis?
   a. Right 2nd intercostal, low pitch murmur
   b. Apex, low pitch murmur
   c. Left Sternal area, low pitch murmur
   d. Pan-systolic murmur, high pitch murmur
40. In coarctation of aorta, site of rib notching is?
   a. Superior to rib   b. Inferior to rib
   c. At sternum   d. At Vertebra
41. Cardiac marker earliest to rise is?
   a. CPK MB   b. LDH
   c. SAP   d. Troponin I
42. Hypotension with muffled heart sounds and congested neck veins is seen in?
   a. Cardiac tamponade
   b. Pericardial effusion
   c. Constrictive pericarditis
   d. Acute congestive heart failure
43. Which of the following is given to decrease Serum Triglycerides?
   a. Fibrates   b. Statins
   c. Ezetimibe   d. Niacin
44. In a patient there is dyspnea in upright position which is relieved in supine position. Diagnosis?
   a. Tachypnea
   b. Orthopnea
   c. Paroxysmal nocturnal dyspnea
   d. Platypnea
45. Which is the best way to differentiate between stable angina and NSTEMI?
   a. ECG
   b. Cardiac-biomarker
   c. Trans thoracic Echocardiography
   d. Multi uptake gated Acquisition scan
46. Duroziez's sign is seen in?
   a. Aortic regurgitation   b. Aortic stenosis
   c. Mitral stenosis   d. Mitral regurgitation
47. Which of the following is a diagnostic criteria for Rheumatic fever?
   a. Oral ulcer
   b. Malar rash
   c. Erythema Marginatum
   d. Morning stiffness
48. Organism leading to hospital acquired infective endocarditis?
   a. Staph aureus
   b. Klebsiella
   c. Streptococcus pneumoniae
   d. Meningococcus
49. Aetiology of Dressler syndrome is?
   a. Viral   b. Autoimmune
   c. Idiopathic   d. Toxin mediated

50. Rib notching is seen in?
   a. Coarctation of aorta
   b. Hypertension
   c. Fibromuscular dysplasia
   d. Aortic dissection
51. A female has a DBP = 100 mm Hg on two consecutive occasions. Best treatment is?
   a. Rest
   b. Sedative
   c. Anti-hypertensive drugs
   d. Error in BP machine
52. A 65-year-old male had MI one year ago. Now the same patients presents with hypertension. Which of the following drug is best suited for this patient?
   a. Clonidine   b. Thiazide
   c. Metoprolol   d. Lisinopril
53. Resistant hypertension is defined as?
   a. Resistance to 2 or more anti hypertension drugs
   b. Resistance to 3 or more anti-hypertensive drugs including thiazides
   c. Resistance to aldosterone
   d. Resistance of Angiotension II receptors
54. An 8-year-old girl, collapsed while playing and died. CXR given below. Which of the following is unlikely to be an etiology of this event?

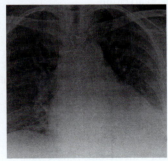

   a. Stroke   b. Cardiomyopathy
   c. Arrhythmia   d. Shock
55. If a person is having ventricular tachycardia, extra systoles appears in:
   a. P wave   b. QRS complex
   c. T wave   d. R wave
56. Internal jugular vein pressure determines pressure of:
   a. RA   b. RV
   c. LA   d. LV
57. Hyaline atherosclerosis is seen in:
   a. Benign hypertension   b. Chronic hypertension
   c. Diabetic nephropathy   d. Analgesic nephropathy
58. Mccallum patch in rheumatic heart disease is seen in?
   a. Right atrium   b. Left atrium
   c. Right ventricle   d. Left ventricle
59. Canon A wave is seen in:
   a. Atrial fibrillation   b. Complete heart block
   c. Ventricular fibrillation   d. Mobitz 1 heart block

FMGE Solutions Screening Examination

60. **Aortic dissection is seen in?**
    a. Takayasu disease   b. Atherosclerosis
    c. Syphilis aortitis   d. Marfan syndrome

61. **Incorrect about conduction system of heart:**
    a. SAN is dominant pacemaker
    b. AVN exhibits conduction delay of 0.1 sec
    c. Purkinje fibres have the slowest conduction
    d. Left fascicle divides into anterior and posterior fascicle

62. **A wave in JVP is absent in:**
    a. Atrial fibrillation   b. Heart block
    c. Tricuspid regurgitation   d. Complete heart block

63. **Canon a waves are seen in:**
    a. Atrial fibrillation   b. Junctional tachycardia
    c. Constrictive pericarditis   d. Cardiac tamponade

64. **Severe mitral stenosis is identified by:**
    a. Loud S1
    b. Loud opening snap
    c. Duration of mid-diastolic murmur
    d. Intensity of mid-diastolic murmur

65. **What would you do immediately after a cardiac arrest?**
    a. Give epinephrine   b. Check for breathing,
    c. Check for pulse   d. Chest compressions

66. **P wave in ECG is due to:**
    a. Ventricular depolarization
    b. Atrial repolarization
    c. Ventricular repolarization
    d. Atrial depolarization

67. **Initial ECG change in Hyperkalemia is?**
    a. Tall tented T waves   b. PR prolongation
    c. qRS widening   d. ST segment depression

68. **Incorrect about Dressler syndrome is?**
    a. Post MI pericarditis
    b. Post MI pleuritis
    c. Autoimmune
    d. Treatment with steroids is necessary

69. **Most common cause of aortic dissection:**
    a. Syphilis   b. Hypertension
    c. Marfan syndrome   d. Cystic medial necrosis

70. **Marker specific for myocardial infarction:**
    a. Troponin I   b. Troponin C
    c. Troponin T   d. LDH

71. **All are used for secondary prevention of MI EXCEPT:**
    a. Aspirin   b. Statins
    c. Beta blockers   d. Warfarin

72. **Reverse split S2 is seen in**
    a. Aortic stenosis
    b. Mitral stenosis
    c. Pulmonary artery hypertension
    d. Pulmonic stenosis

73. **ECG finding of Hyperkalemia:**
    a. T wave inversion   b. ST depression
    c. P pulmonale   d. Wide QRS complex

74. **Coronary artery disease is associated with all EXCEPT:**
    a. Chylamydia   b. Poor dental hygiene
    c. Smoking   d. Alcohol

75. **Pericardical cyst is seen at:**
    a. Cardiophrenic angle   b. Middle mediastinum
    c. Posterior mediastinum   d. Lingula

76. **Snow man appearance or figure of 8 appearance is seen in?**
    a. Total anomalous pulmonary venous connection
    b. Transposition of great arteries
    c. Tetralogy of fallot
    d. Tricuspid atresia

77. **Which of the following is a cause of wide pulse pressure:**
    a. Aortic stenosis   b. Aortic regurgitation
    c. Mitral stenosis   d. Tricuspid stenosis

78. **Canon a wave is seen in?**
    a. Junctional rhythm   b. Atrial fibrillation
    c. Atrial flutter   d. Ventricular fibrillation

79. **Most common cause of unilateral pedal edema?**
    a. Pregnancy   b. Lymphedema
    c. Venous insufficiency   d. Milroy disease

80. **Which of the following affects HOCM?**
    a. Systolic dysfunction   b. Diastolic dysfunction
    c. Valvular dysfunction   d. Rhythm defects

81. **According to revised guidelines of American heart association, which of the following drugs is not recommended in cardiac arrest?**
    a. Adrenaline   b. Atropine
    c. Amiodarone   d. Vasopressin

82. **A Patient presented with deficiency of thiamine. What could be possible outcome:**
    a. Delayed wound healing   b. Cardiac abnormality
    c. Memory loss   d. Gingival bleeding

83. **After intake of NSAID tablet a lady complains of difficulty in breathing and appearance of bee hives. Pulse rate is 100 and BP is 90/60 mm Hg. Diagnosis is:**
    a. Massive pulmonary embolism
    b. Neurogenic shock
    c. DIC
    d. Anaphylaxis

84. **Which is the best investigation best to confirm diagnosis of anaphylaxis?**
    a. Ig A levels   b. Ig D levels
    c. Serum tryptase   d. Serum precipitins

85. **MCC of aortic aneurysm?**
    a. Idiopathic   b. Trauma
    c. Atherosclerosis   d. Arteriosclerosis

86. **A 1-year-old male child is having a Heart Rate 40/min, BP 90/60. His serum Potassium = 6.5. What is the next best management?**
    a. Ipratropium   b. Adrenaline
    c. Sodium bicarbonate   d. Calcium chloride

Medicine

87. Mortality in primary cardiac amyloidosis develops over?
    a. 3–6 months   b. 6–12 months
    c. 12–18 months   d. 24–36 months
88. Which is best for plaque morphology in atherosclerosis?
    a. CCTA   b. Echocardiography
    c. ECG   d. Coronary angiography

NEUROLOGY

89. A 60-year-old male diabetic and hypertensive patient was found unconscious in the morning. On examination pulse rate is 120/min, BP = 160/100 mm Hg and bilateral extensor plantars are elicited. What is the next step to be done for management? *(Most Recent Question 2019)*
    a. Order CT scan
    b. Check blood glucose
    c. Give intravenous mannitol
    d. Immediately reduce BP with antihypertensives
90. Which of the following is not a feature of Parkinson disease? *(Recent Pattern Question 2018-19)*
    a. Hypophonia
    b. Freezing
    c. Rigidity
    d. Diplopia
91. Normal deep tendon reflexes with muscle weakness is seen in? *(Recent Pattern Question 2018-19)*
    a. M. Gravis   b. G.B.S
    c. Transverse myelitis d. Traumatic neuritis
92. Reversible dementia is seen in? *(Recent Pattern Question 2018-19)*
    a. Subacute combined demyelination of spinal cord
    b. Acute inflammatory demyelinating polyneuropathy
    c. Creutzfeldt Jacob disease
    d. Pick's disease
93. Extensor plantar reflex on pinching gastrocnemius muscle is called? *(Recent Pattern Question 2018-19)*
    a. Gower sign   b. Homan sign
    c. Oppenheim reflex   d. Gordon reflex
94. Which is the most common cranial nerve involved in raised ICP? *(Recent Pattern Question 2018-19)*
    a. Abducens   b. Trochlear
    c. Trigeminal   d. Facial
95. Which of the following is not seen in Horner syndrome? *(Recent Pattern Question 2018-19)*
    a. Mydriasis   b. Ptosis
    c. Anhidrosis   d. Enopthalmos
96. Painless burn in hand is seen in:
    (Recent Pattern Question 2018)
    a. SLE
    b. Syringomyelia
    c. Mononeuritis multiplex
    d. Diabetes mellitus

97. Prosopagnosia is: *(Recent Pattern Question 2018)*
    a. Inability to read   b. Inability to write
    c. Anosmia   d. Inability to recognize face
98. Wernicke's encephalopathy is due to deficiency of:
    (Recent Pattern Question 2018)
    a. Thiamine   b. B_6
    c. Niacin   d. B_{12}
99. Which of the following manifestation is seen in metabolic encephalopathy?
    (Recent Pattern Question 2018)
    a. Motor aphasia   b. Sensory aphasia
    c. Conduction aphasia d. Anomic aphasia
100. Which of these is the best for management of methanol poisoning? *(Recent Pattern Question 2018)*
    a. Acamprosate   b. Fomepizole
    c. Disulfiram   d. Naltrexone
101. All are examples of upper motor neuron lesion EXCEPT:
    (Recent Pattern Question 2018)
    a. Prion disease   b. Multiple sclerosis
    c. Anterior horn cell disease d. Tuberous sclerosis
102. What is the most common cause of meningitis in young adults? *(Recent Pattern Question 2017)*
    a. Listeria   b. Strep pneumonia
    c. Neisseria meningitis d. Group B streptococcus
103. What is seen in complete transection of spinal cord?
    a. Loss of bladder control *(Recent Pattern Question 2017)*
    b. Loss of temperature regulation
    c. Hemianaesthesia   d. Hemiparesis
104. Which of the following is not lost on the same side in hemi-section of the spinal cord half injury?
    (Recent Pattern Question 2017)
    a. Position sense   b. Thermal sense
    c. Vibration sense   d. Tactile discrimination
105. Pendular knee jerk is seen in lesion at_____?
    (Recent Pattern Question 2017)
    a. Cerebellum   b. Basal ganglia
    c. Tectum   d. Uncus
106. Unconscious proprioception is carried by?
    a. Dorsal column   *(Recent Pattern Question 2017)*
    b. Spinocerebellar pathways
    c. Anterior spinothalamic tract
    d. Rubro-spinal pathway
107. In which of the following will EMG show decremental response? *(Recent Pattern Question 2017)*
    a. M. Gravis   b. Lambert-Eaton syndrome
    c. Guillain-Barré syndrome d. Botulinism
108. Most common cause of headache?
    a. Tension headache   *(Recent Pattern Question 2016)*
    b. Cluster headache
    c. Migraine
    d. Raised intra-cranial tension

581

109. Which of the following is the correct Miller Fisher syndrome triad? *(Recent Pattern Question 2016)*
    a. Global confusion, areflexia, ataxia
    b. Ophthalmoplegia, ataxia, areflexia
    c. Ophthalmoplegia, areflexia, aphasia
    d. Global confusion, areflexia, aphasia

110. CT head of a patient shows? *(Recent Pattern Question 2016)*

    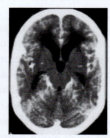

    a. Neurosarcoidosis
    b. SAH
    c. TB meningitis
    d. Intraparenchymal bleed

111. Treatment of post-lumbar puncture headache? *(Recent Pattern Question 2016)*
    a. Codeine   b. Dantrolene
    c. Caffeine   d. Diazepam

112. Best treatment for glioblastoma multiforme? *(Recent Pattern Question 2016)*
    a. Chemotherapy   b. Radiation
    c. Excision with radiation   d. Stereotactic surgery

113. Axillary freckling is seen in? *(Recent Pattern Question 2016)*
    a. Neurofibromatosis
    b. Tuberous sclerosis
    c. Ichthyosis vulgaris
    d. Von Hippel-Lindau

114. True about chorea? *(Recent Patter Question 2016)*
    a. Semi-purposive and rhythmic movements
    b. Slow and uniform movement
    c. Slow writhing movement
    d. Semi-purposive and non-repetitive, randomly distributed movements

115. Which tract damage leads to loss of pain and temperature? *(Recent Pattern Question 2016)*
    a. Lateral spinothalamic tract
    b. Ventral spinothalamic tract
    c. Lateral corticospinal pathway
    d. Dorsal column

116. Lesion of which tract leads to voluntary skilled movements? *(Recent Pattern Question 2016)*
    a. Corticospinal tract
    b. Rubrospinal tract
    c. Tectospinal tract
    d. Lateral spinothalamic pathway

117. Log roll positioning is done for?
    a. Spine injury evaluation *(Recent Pattern Question 2016)*
    b. Relieve compression on back
    c. Perform rapid sequence intubation
    d. Perform peritoneal lavage

118. Kernohan-Woltman sign is? *(Recent Pattern Question 2016)*
    a. Medial displacement of midbrain
    b. Lateral displacement of midbrain
    c. Upper displacement of pons
    d. Downward displacement of pons

119. Which is true about uncal herniation? *(Recent Pattern Question 2016)*
    a. 3rd nerve involvement   b. 4th nerve involvement
    c. 6th nerve involvement   d. 7th nerve involvement

120. Rivastigmine is given in?
    a. Parkinsonism   b. Alzheimer's disease
    c. Schizophrenia   d. Anxiety

121. A lady cannot speak but can tell by writing. Which of the following brain areas is affected?
    a. Broca's area   b. Wernicke's area
    c. Paracentral lobule   d. Insula

122. Nucleus ambiguus is located in?
    a. Medulla   b. Pons
    c. Midbrain   d. Paracentral lobule

123. Wernicke's area is located in:
    a. Superior temporal gyrus b. Inferior temporal gyrus
    c. Post-central gyrus   d. Angular gyrus

124. Glasgow coma scale = 3 indicates?
    a. Death   b. Severe disability
    c. Coma   d. Brain death

125. Glasgow coma scale score of M_4 represents?
    a. Withdrawal on flexion   b. Decorticate posturing
    c. Decerebrate posturing   d. Localise pain

126. A patient after alcoholic drink fell asleep in chair overnight with hanging arm and develops Saturday Night Palsy. Which of the following best describes the clinical manifestations?
    a. Neuropraxia   b. Axonotmesis
    c. Neurotmesis   d. Necroptosis

127. CSF glucose compared to blood glucose is of _____ concentration in blood?
    a. <30%   b. 30–60%
    c. 60–80%   d. 40–50%

128. A 32-year-old AIDS positive female presented with headaches and nuchal stiffness. On lumbar puncture examination clear CSF was obtained with leucocytes >100/cu.mm. India ink staining was positive. The most probable diagnosis is?
    a. Candida meningitis
    b. Tubercular meningitis
    c. Cryptosporidium
    d. Cryptococcus meningitis

Medicine

129. A man has acute onset of paraplegia with symmetrical bilateral areflexia. Diagnosis is:
a. Acute transverse myelitis
b. Subacute combined degenerative disorder
c. Guillian Barre syndrome
d. Poliomyelitis

130. Boxers present with:
a. Epidural hemorrhage
b. Subdural hemorrhage
c. Sub arachnoid hemorrhage
d. Intra ventricular hemorrhage

131. All of the following are causes of primary headache EXCEPT:
a. Migraine
b. Tension headache
c. Cluster headache
d. Sinusitis

132. DOC for listeria meningitis:
a. Ampicillin
b. Cefotaxime
c. Cefotriaxone
d. Ciprofloxacin

133. DOC for Herpes simplex encephalitis:
a. Acyclovir
b. Inosine prabonex
c. Intravenous immunoglobulins
d. Amphotericin B

134. SSPE is seen in?
a. Rubella
b. Mumps.
c. Measles
d. Chicken pox

135. All are seen in Horner syndrome EXCEPT:
a. Ptosis
b. Miosis
c. Hyperhidrosis
d. Enophthalmos

136. Which is not a part of lower motor neuron:
a. Anterior nerve root
b. Peripheral ganglia
c. Peripheral nerve
d. Anterior horn cell

137. Most common brain tumor?
a. Astrocytoma
b. Glioblastoma Multiforme
c. Meningioma
d. Ependymoma

138. Increased intra-cranial tension leads to?
a. Hyotension and tachycardia
b. Hypertension and tachycardia
c. Hypertension and bradycardia
d. Hypotension and bradycardia

139. In increased intracranial pressure which is the first cranial nerve to be affected first?
a. 3rd
b. 4th
c. 5th
d. 6th

140. A road traffic accident patient in the casualty is comatose with unilaterally dilated pupil. The NCCT of the patient shows a Lesion peripherally present with concavo – convex border. What is the probable diagnosis?
a. Sub-dural hematoma
b. Epi-dural hematoma,
c. Sub-arachnoid hemorrhage
d. Intra-parenchymal bleeding

141. Extradural hemorrhage on NCCT is visualized as?
a. Hyperdense biconvex
b. Hypodense biconcave
c. Hyperdense biconcave
d. Hypodense biconvex

142. The submerged part of cerebral cortex is?
a. Insula
b. Broadman area
c. Corpus callosum
d. Piriform sulcus

143. Investigation of choice for sub-arachnoid hemorrhage is:
a. NCCT
b. MRI
c. CECT
d. MRA

144. Wernicke's aphasia is characterized by all EXCEPT:
a. Non fluent speech
b. Poor comprehension
c. Poor repetition
d. Para-phasia

145. Most common benign brain tumor?
a. Meningioma
b. Oligodendroglioma
c. Ependymoma
d. Medulloblastoma

146. Lewy bodies are seen in:
a. Parkinsonism
b. Alzheimer's disease
c. Huntington chorea
d. All of above

147. Least chances of seizures are seen with?
a. Hypoglycemia
b. Hypocalcemia
c. HIV encephalopathy
d. Neuro-cysticercosis

148. A patient presents with headache and nuchal rigidity. Lumbar puncture was performed and CSF shows normal protein and normal glucose with clear CSF. Microscopic examination of CSF showed 50 lymphocytes/cu.mm with lymphocytic pleocytosis. What is the diagnosis?
a. Bacterial meningitis
b. Viral meningitis
c. TB meningitis
d. Aseptic meningitis

149. Which of the following is not seen in tubercular meningitis:
a. Evidence of old pulmonary lesions or a miliary pattern is found on chest radiography
b. Culture of CSF is diagnostic in majority of cases and remains the gold standard.
c. It is seen most often in young children but also develops in adults.
d. Cerebrospinal fluid reveals a low leukocyte count.

150. CSF finding in Gullian Barre syndrome is?
a. Normal cells with increased protein
b. Increased protein with normal cells
c. Normal cells and normal protein
d. Increased cells with low sugar

151. Which is the earliest symptom of Parkinson's disease?
a. Tremors
b. Rigidity
c. Bradykinesia
d. Chorea

152. Which of the following is not a feature of Parkinsonism?
a. Chorea
b. Recurrent falls
c. Tremors
d. Freezing

Questions

FMGE Solutions Screening Examination

153. **Earliest feature of parkinsonism?**
     a. Anosmia   b. Rigidity
     c. Postural instability   d. Freezing
154. **Which of the following is not the feature of upper motor neuron disease?**
     a. Hypotonia   b. Spasticity
     c. Weakness of muscles   d. Superficial reflex absent
155. **Incorrect about LMN defect?**
     a. Flaccid paralysis   b. Muscular hypertrophy
     c. Hypo-reflexia   d. Superficial reflex present
156. **Right 12th nerve damage leads to?**
     a. Tongue deviation to left on protrusion
     b. Tongue deviation to right on protrusion
     c. Nasal twang to voice
     d. Scanning speech defects
157. **Which of the following tests are helpful in diagnosing neural tube defect?**
     a. Acetyl choline esterase in the amniotic fluid
     b. Alpha-ketoglutarate in the amniotic fluid
     c. Glutamate in the amniotic fluid
     d. Beta hydroxyl butyrate in the amniotic fluid
158. **Protein deposited in Alzheimer's disease is?**
     a. Tau protein   b. Alpha synuclein protein
     c. Huntington protein   d. Protein 14.3.3
159. **Unilateral ptosis is not seen in?**
     a. Myasthenia gravis   b. Thyroid ophthalmopathy
     c. Marfan syndrome   d. Pancoast tumor
160. **A patient after an accident was unconscious. On physical examination there was unilateral papillary dilatation. Possible reason for the same is?**
     a. Uncal herniation   b. Tonsillar herniation
     c. Cingulate herniation   d. Transcalvarial herniation
161. **Most common site of brain hemorrhage is?**
     a. Putamen   b. Internal capsule
     c. Ventral pons   d. Cerebellum
162. **Investigation of choice for myasthenia gravis?**
     a. Single fiber E.M.G
     b. Muscle biopsy
     c. Nerve conduction velocity
     d. Anti-acetylcholine receptor antibody
163. **CSF is absorbed by:**
     a. Choroid plexus
     b. Sub-arachnoid granulations
     c. Dura matter
     d. Pia matter
164. **Incorrect about dementia pugilistica:**
     a. Seen in boxers   b. Difficulty in gait
     c. Decreased cognition   d. Nystagmus
165. **Most common cause of cerebro vascular accident:**
     a. Infarction   b. Hemorrhage
     c. Embolism   d. Aortic dissection

166. **Korsakoff psychosis is seen in:**
     a. Thiamine deficiency
     b. Riboflavin deficiency
     c. Niacin deficiency
     d. Cyanacobalamin deficiency
167. **Two point discrimination test exhibits maximum sensitivity in?**
     a. Shin   b. Toes
     c. Finger pads   d. Soles
168. **A patient presented with right sided hemiplegia while on warfarin. Which of the following will be the initial investigation of choice?**
     a. Chest X-ray   b. CT-scan
     c. MRI   d. PET-scan
169. **Hemiballismus is due to lesion in?**
     a. Ipsilateral caudate nucleus
     b. Contralateral sub-thalamic lesion
     c. Contralateral Putamen
     d. Ipsilateral sub-thalamic lesion
170. **Pontine stroke is due to involvement of?**
     a. Basiliar artery
     b. Middle cerebral artery
     c. Middle meningeal artery
     d. Anterior communicating artery
171. **Which vessel does not contribute to circle of Willis:**
     a. Middle cerebral artery   b. Anterior cerebral artery
     c. Posterior cerebral artery d. Internal carotid artery
172. **Duret hemorrhage is?**
     a. Traumatic brain haemorrhage in contre-coup injury
     b. Adrenal haemorrhage in water house friderichsen
     c. Brain hemorrhage due to tear of basiliar artery branches
     d. Petechial hemorrhages in fat embolism
173. **Which of the following is not a feature of Wernicke's encephalopathy:**
     a. Global confusion   b. Ophthalmoplegia
     c. Ataxia   d. Aphasia
174. **Broca's aphasia is characterized by:**
     a. Non-fluent aphasia   b. Word salad
     c. Anomia   d. Apraxia
175. **Which of the following cranial nerve is first compressed in unruptured berry aneurysm?**
     a. 3rd nerve   b. 4th nerve
     c. 5th nerve   d. 6th nerve
176. **Which of the following is not a test for integrity of 7th and 9th nerve:**
     a. Position of uvula   b. Palate symmetry
     c. Taste   d. Tongue protusion
177. **Cranial Nerve 8 palsy causes all EXCEPT:**
     a. Gag reflex   b. Vertigo
     c. Motion sickness   d. Tinnitus

Medicine

178. A patient is unable to solve mathematical calculations, which part of his brain is damaged?
   a. Temporal lobe
   b. Frontal lobe
   c. Parietal lobe
   d. Occipital lobe

179. Asymetrical Ptosis is seen in?
   a. Myasthenia gravis
   b. Thyroid myopathy
   c. Drug induced myopathy
   d. Duchenne's muscular dystrophy

180. Cut off for TiA definition?
   a. 12 hours
   b. 24 hours
   c. 48 hours
   d. 36 hours

181. What are nitrergic neurons:
   a. Postganglionic neurons releasing nitric oxide
   b. 1st order neurons releasing nitric oxide
   c. Post ganglionic neurons releasing substance P
   d. 1st order neurons releasing calcitonin gene related peptide

182. Stenosis of aqueduct of sylvius results in?
   a. Enlargement of lateral ventricles
   b. Enlargement of fourth ventricle
   c. Enlargement of lateral and third ventricle
   d. Enlargement of lateral and fourth ventricle

ENDOCRINOLOGY

183. An 18-year-old boy appears for army medical. On medical check-up his FBS = 120 and PP = 140 and HbA1c = 6.1%. What is the diagnosis?
   a. Impaired glucose tolerance *(Most Recent Question 2019)*
   b. Type 2 diabetes mellitus
   c. Type 1 diabetes mellitus
   d. Normal

184. Fulminant diabetes mellitus is seen in?
   (Recent Pattern Question 2018-19)
   a. Diabetic ketoacidosis
   b. Coxsackie B virus
   c. Non-Ketotic hyperosmolar coma
   d. Autoimmune pancreatitis

185. In a newly diagnosed case of sick child with Type 1 diabetes mellitus (DM), insulin was given. Which of the following will increase? *(Recent Pattern Question 2018)*
   a. pH
   b. Breathing rate
   c. Glucosuria
   d. Urine osmolality

186. All of the following syndromes are seen with obesity EXCEPT:
   a. Prader-Willi syndrome
   b. Cohen syndrome
   c. Laurence Moon-Biedl syndrome
   d. Carcinoid syndrome

187. Which of the following is associated with elevated alkaline phosphate, low calcium with low phosphate?
   (Recent Pattern Question 2018)
   a. Paget's disease
   b. Osteoporosis
   c. Primary hyperparathyroidism
   d. Vitamin D deficiency

188. Which of the following leads to development of SIADH?
   (Recent Pattern Question 2018)
   a. Head trauma
   b. Pituitary adenoma
   c. Lithium
   d. All of the above

189. Which of the following is seen in secondary thyrotoxicosis but not in Grave's disease? *(Recent Pattern Question 2017)*
   a. Lid retraction
   b. Lid lag
   c. Exophthalmos
   d. Atrial fibrillation

190. A 15-year-old Type I DM patient presents to O.P.D. When should you recommend the patient to come for follow-up visits for microvascular complications evaluation?
   (Recent Pattern Question 2017)
   a. 1 year
   b. 5 years
   c. 10 years
   d. 20 years

191. Nephrognic DI occurs due to defect in?
   a. Na-K ATPase
   b. SGLT-2
   c. Aquaporin 1
   d. Aquaporin 2

192. Which is the gene involved in pathogenesis of Type 1 Diabetes mellitus? *(Recent Pattern Question 2017)*
   a. CTLA-4
   b. ABCD1
   c. HNF-1 Alpha
   d. HNF-4 Alpha

193. Which is the most common tumour of pituitary?
   (Recent Pattern Question 2017)
   a. Non-functioning adenoma
   b. Prolactinoma
   c. ACTH producing adenoma
   d. Oncocytoma

194. Which chromosome is responsible for most common type of MODY? *(Recent Pattern Question 2017)*
   a. Chromosome 11
   b. Chromosome 12
   c. Chromosome 13
   d. Chromosome 14

195. Which is not a diabetic patient?
   (Recent Pattern Question 2016)
   a. FBS = 136 mg%
   b. 2 hour value = 180 mg%
   c. HbA1c = 7%
   d. RBS > 210 mg%

196. Cause of death in diabetic ketoacidosis?
   (Recent Pattern Question 2017)
   a. Cerebral edema
   b. Dehydration
   c. Electrolyte imbalance
   d. Central pontine myelinosis

197. Hyperpigmentation is seen with which hormone?
   a. FSH
   b. LH
   c. TSH
   d. ACTH

FMGE Solutions Screening Examination

198. Female with blood sugar of 600 mg% and sodium of 110 mEq. Insulin was given, what will happen to serum sodium levels?
    a. Sodium increase
    b. Sodium decrease
    c. Sodium unaffected
    d. Relative sodium deficiency

199. Which is most common type of Diabetic neuropathy?
    a. Sensory polyneuropathy
    b. Autonomic neuropathy
    c. Radiculopathy
    d. Myelopathy

200. Lady 45 years of age presents with decreased oestrogen level, increased testosterone and temporal hair recession. Diagnosis is?
    a. Osteoporosis
    b. Rheumatoid arthritis
    c. P.C.O.D
    d. Granulosa theca cell tumor

201. Which of the following present with hypothyroidism?
    a. Struma ovarii
    b. Grave's disease
    c. Myasthenia gravis
    d. Toxic multinodular goiter

202. Earliest finding in Diabetic nephropathy is:
    a. Shrunken kidney is hallmark
    b. Fibrin Caps
    c. Elevated Creatinine Clearance
    d. Urine albumin > 30 mg/dL

203. Which of the following is a mineralocorticoid?
    a. Cortisone
    b. Estrogen
    c. Testosterone
    d. Aldosterone

204. Which of the following is NOT a steroid?
    a. Estrogen
    b. Progesterone
    c. Relaxin
    d. Testosterone

205. Aldosterone is secreted by:
    a. Pituitary
    b. Zona glomerulosa
    c. Zona fasciculata
    d. Adrenal medulla

206. Glucose fever is related with:
    a. Glucagonoma
    b. Parathyroid adenoma
    c. Insulinoma
    d. Addison disease

207. All are seen in Addison's disease EXCEPT?
    a. Hyponatremia
    b. Hyperkalemia
    c. Hypotension
    d. Metabolic alkalosis

208. In prolactinoma most common symptom other than galactorrhea is?
    a. Bitemporal hemianopia
    b. Amennorhea
    c. Thyroid dysfunction
    d. Headache

209. Turner syndrome presents with which heart defect?
    a. Patent ductus arteriosus
    b. Atrial septal defect
    c. Coarctation of aorta
    d. Ventricular septal defect

210. Rib notching is found in all the following EXCEPT:
    a. Neurofibromatosis
    b. Coarctation of aorta
    c. Taussig bing operation
    d. Hypoparathyroidism

211. All are true about Hyperthyroidism EXCEPT:
    a. Anxiety
    b. Palpitations
    c. Tachycardia
    d. Weight gain

212. Obesity in children is seen in:
    a. Adrenal insufficiency
    b. Pseudo-hypo-parathyroidism
    c. Prader Willi syndrome
    d. Soto syndrome

213. True about obesity?
    a. Seen mostly in females
    b. Prevalence decrease upto 40 years of age
    c. No genetic predisposition
    d. Smoking is a risk factor

214. Which is the best indicator for short term control (2-3 weeks) of blood glucose?
    a. Serum fructosamine
    b. HbA1c
    c. Blood sugar
    d. Urine sugar

215. Which of the following drugs used for Diabetes Mellitus causes lactic acidosis:
    a. Phenformin
    b. Metformin
    c. Glipizide
    d. Pioglitazone

216. Best drug to be used in obese type 2 diabetes mellitus patient?
    a. Metformin
    b. Glipizide
    c. Pioglitazone
    d. Exenatide

217. Post Prandial capillary glucose should be _____ mg/dl for adequate diabetes control:
    a. <100 mg/dL
    b. <140 mg/dL
    c. <180 mg/dL
    d. <200 mg/dL

218. All are true about Diabetes insipidus EXCEPT?
    a. Low urine osmolality
    b. Dilutional Hyponatremia
    c. Water deprivation test is used for diagnosis
    d. Polyuria

219. All are correct about SIADH EXCEPT:
    a. Normal KFT
    b. Low uric acid
    c. Relative hypernatremia
    d. Normal BP with gain of water

220. Whipple's triad is useful for diagnosis of:
    a. Insulinoma
    b. Glucagonoma
    c. Somatostatinoma
    d. V.I.Poma

221. Best test for diagnosis of Carcinoid tumor:
    a. 24-hour urinary 5H.I.A.A
    b. 24-hour catecholamines
    c. 24-hour vanilymandelic acid levels
    d. 24-hour metanephrine levels

222. Which of the following is produced by carcinoid tumor?
    a. G.A.B.A
    b. Serotonin
    c. Epinephrine
    d. Nor-epinephrine

223. Most reliable marker for hypothyroidism:
    a. T3
    b. T4
    c. TSH
    d. Thyroxine binding globulin

224. Wolf Chaikoff effect is due to
    a. Iodine deficiency   b. Excessive iodine
    c. Iodine metabolism defect d. TPO enzyme deficiency
225. Which of the following is not a feature of thyrotoxicosis?
    a. Palpitation   b. Anxiety
    c. Weight loss   d. Menorrhagia
226. Proptosis not seen in?
    a. Grave's disease   b. Sarcoidosis
    c. Pituitary Apoplexy d. Myxoedema
227. All are true about Plummer Vinson syndrome EXCEPT?
    a. Glossits   b. Lower esophageal web
    c. Anemia   d. Premalignant condition
228. All of following are seen in GH deficiency EXCEPT:
    a. Hyperglycemia   b. Stunting
    c. Delayed bone age d. High pitched voice
229. Vitamin D deficiency has all EXCEPT:
    a. Hypocalcemia   b. Increased SAP
    c. Increased PTH d. Hyperphosphataemia
230. Which of the following finding shall be seen in patient with hyper-parathyroidism?
    a. Hypophosphatemia   b. Hyperphosphatemia
    c. Hypermagnesemia   d. Hypo magnesemia
231. All are features of hyper-parathyroidism EXCEPT:
    a. Increase serum calcium b. Decreased serum phosphate
    c. Diarrhea   d. Nephrocalcinosis
232. Secretory diarrhea is caused by all EXCEPT?
    a. Medullary thyroid tumor b. Carcinoid Tumor
    c. Somatostinoma   d. Glucagonoma
233. Chorionic villus sampling is done for all EXCEPT?
    a. Downs   b. Trisomy 21
    c. Phenylketonuria d. Gastrochisis
234. Congenital adrenal hyperplasia due to 11 beta hydroxy-lase deficiency presents with all EXCEPT?
    a. Metabolic acidosis b. Hypokalemia
    c. Virilization   d. Hypertension

HEMATOLOGY

235. The coagulogram of this patient shows increased Prothrombin time, activated partial thromboplastin time with platelet count of 1.2 Lacs/cu mm. The diagnosis is?
    (Most Recent Question 2019)

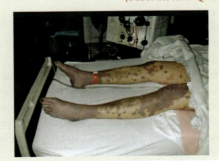

    a. Henoch-Schonlein purpura
    b. Porphyria
    c. D.I.C
    d. Acute ITP
236. Which of the following test is used for diagnosis of DIC?
    (Recent Pattern Question 2018-19)
    a. Fibrin degradation products
    b. Activated partial thromboplastin time
    c. Prothrombin time
    d. D- Dimer assay
237. In sickle cell crisis bone pain is due to:
    (Recent Pattern Question 2018)
    a. Bone infarction   b. Osteoporosis
    c. Osteomalacia   d. Periosteal reaction
238. A 35-year-old patient shows abnormal Schilling test. Antibiotics were given for 5 days which results in normalization of Schilling test. What is the diagnosis of the patient? *(Recent Pattern Question 2018)*
    a. Bacterial overgrowth syndrome
    b. Chronic pancreatitis
    c. Atrophic gastritis
    d. Ileocecal TB
239. HTLV-1 is associated with which disease:
    (Recent Pattern Question 2016)
    a. AML   b. NHL
    c. Adult T cell leukemia d. AML
240. In cobalamin deficiency which is not seen?
    a. Microcytic anemia   b. Long tract signs
    c. Loss of proprioception d. Rhomberg sign
241. Adult with progressive pallor, hyper-segmented neutrophils and MCV>100 shows?
    a. Hereditary spherocytosis b. Megaloblastic anemia
    c. Dimorphic Anemia   d. Thalassemia
242. Poikilocytosis and anisocytosis is seen in?
    a. Megaloblastic anaemia b. Iron deficiency anaemia
    c. Nutritional deficiency anaemia
    d. Thalassemia
243. 2-year-old child with ALL, which of the following has the best prognosis?
    a. Age between 1–10 years b. TLC >1 lac
    c. Petechiae   d. t(9:22)
244. Blood transfusion associated acute lung injury occurs due to?
    a. Nosocomial infections b. HLA mediated
    c. Auto-immune disorder d. Genetic susceptibility
245. Thalassemia is a:
    a. Autosomal dominant b. Autosomal recessive
    c. X-linked dominant   d. X-linked recessive
246. Low serum iron and low serum ferritin is seen in:
    a. Iron deficiency anemia
    b. Chronic kidney disease
    c. Sideroblastic anemia
    d. Fanconi anemia

FMGE Solutions Screening Examination

247. Thrombocythemia is characterized by:
    a. Platelets elevation
    b. Low platelets
    c. Neutrophilia
    d. Monocytosis
248. Schistocytes are seen in:
    a. HUS
    b. TTP
    c. DIC
    d. All of the above
249. Correct about vitamin-K deficiency is?
    a. Associated thrombocytopenia with prolonged bleeding
    b. Deficiency is rarely seen, except in infants
    c. Factor X is first to be affected
    d. Warfarin causes Vitamin K deficiency
250. Hemolytic anemia is associated with the following gall stones:
    a. Pigmented
    b. Mixed
    c. Cholesterol
    d. None
251. A 60-year-old industrial worker presents with shortness of breath for the past week. Blood withdrawn shows thick brownish red color. Diagnosis?
    a. Sickle cell anemia
    b. Hemolytic anemia
    c. Meth-hemoglobinaemia
    d. G-6-P-deficiency
252. All are true about cross-matching of blood EXCEPT:
    a. Mandatory in all cases except emergency
    b. Recipient serum is tested against donor packed cells
    c. Donor serum is tested against recipient packed cells
    d. Involves visible agglutination
253. Bleeding time is increased in all EXCEPT:
    a. Dengue hemorrhagic fever
    b. Von willebrand disease
    c. Chronic liver disease
    d. Bernard soulier syndrome
254. Blood is stored at blood bank at:
    a. +4 degree Celsius
    b. −4 degree Celsius
    c. +24 degree Celsius
    d. −60 degree Celsius
255. Which of following is a myelo-proliferative disease?
    a. Acute lymphatic leukemia
    b. Acute myeloid leukemia
    c. Chronic myeloid leukemia
    d. Chronic lymphocytic leukemia
256. Which organism causes infection after splenectomy :-
    a. H. Influenza
    b. Staph aureus
    c. E. coli
    d. Klebsiella
257. Drug of choice in chronic myeloid leukemia:
    a. Imitanib Mesylate
    b. Fludarabine
    c. Cladribine
    d. Pentostatin
258. Philadelphia chromosome refers:
    a. Long arm of chromosome 9 and long arm of chromosome 22
    b. Short arm of chromosome 9 and short arm of chromosome 22
    c. Short arm of chromosome 9 and long chromosome 22
    d. Long arm of chromosome 9 and short arm of chromosome 2
259. All are seen in Thalassemia major EXCEPT
    a. Macrocytic anemia
    b. Transfusion dependency
    c. Hepato-splenomegaly
    d. Target cells
260. Which of the following is *not* a hyper-coagulable state
    a. Pregnancy
    b. MI
    c. Abruptio-placentae
    d. Cirrhosis
261. Elective splenectomy is done in
    a. Hereditary spherocytosis
    b. G6PD
    c. Beta thalassemia
    d. Sickle cell anaemia
262. Priapism can be due to?
    a. C.M.L
    b. Myelo-fibrosis
    c. A.I.H.A.
    d. Thrombocytopenia
263. Hairy cell leukemia is
    a. B cell tumor
    b. T cell tumor
    c. NK cell tumor
    d. All of above

GASTROINTESTINAL TRACT

264. A 3-year-old child presents with steatorrhea, weight loss and features of malabsorption. Which test is done for confirmation of diagnosis? *(Most Recent Question 2019)*
    a. Small intestinal mucosal biopsy
    b. Fecal elastase
    c. Benedict's test for reducing substances
    d. Rectal mucosal suction biopsy
265. Which of the following is correct about cancer developing in Ulcerative colitis? *(Recent Pattern Question 2018-19)*
    a. Not a premalignant condition
    b. Incidence dependant on smoking history
    c. Directly related to duration of disease
    d. Increased risk in younger patients
266. Initial treatment for management of mild to moderate Crohn's disease is: *(Recent Pattern Question 2018)*
    a. Mesalamine
    b. Infliximab
    c. Budesonide
    d. Sulfasalazine
267. Which of the following is true about carcinoid tumor?
    a. Occurs along structures derived from foregut
    b. Presentation is hypertension and diaphoresis
    c. Intestinal carcinoids are of high malignant potential
    d. Best diagnosed by elevated urinary vanillylmandelic acid levels

Medicine

268. Carcinoid tumor leads to increase in levels of?
    a. 5-Hydroxy tryptamine *(Recent Patter Question 2017)*
    b. 5-Hydroxy indole acetic acid
    c. Homovanillic acid
    d. Vaniyl mandelic acid
269. Gastric cancer is caused by
    a. Squamous metaplasia *(Recent Pattern Question 2016)*
    b. Blood group O
    c. Intestinal metaplasia Type 3
    d. Intestinal hyperplasia
270. Most common site of GIST? *(Recent Pattern Question 2016)*
    a. Stomach   b. Jejunum
    c. Ileum   d. Colon
271. A lady presented with IDA and malabsorption. Most accurate test for diagnosis is?
    (Recent Pattern Question 2016)
    a. Antiendomysial antibody
    b. Anti-tissue transglutaminase antibody
    c. Antiepidermal tissue transglutaminase antibody
    d. Antimitochondrial antibody
272. A patient presents with sensory ataxia and patchy loss of papilla on tongue, the first investigation to be done is?
    a. B_{12} *(Recent Pattern Question 2016)*
    b. Punch biopsy of terminal ileum
    c. Brush biopsy of terminal ileum
    d. Serum iron studies
273. A 41-year-old patient presents with chronic diarrhoea for last 3 month. First investigation to be done?
    a. D-xylose absorption *(Recent Pattern Question 2016)*
    b. Intestinal biopsy
    c. Tissue transglutaminase antibody
    d. Schilling's test
274. Patient presents with loss of tongue papilla. Hemoglobin = 9.5 gm% and MCV = 100 fl? *(Recent Pattern Question 2016)* First investigation to be performed is?
    a. B_{12} estimation   b. Brush biopsy
    c. Folic acid levels   d. Incision biopsy
275. Cushing ulcer is seen in? *(Recent Pattern Question 2016)*
    a. Stomach   b. Duodenum
    c. Jejunum   d. Ileum
276. Most common site of carcinoid tumor is?
    a. Appendix   b. Ileum
    c. Stomach   d. Rectum
277. A 45-year-old male is brought to casualty after a night party with complaints of epigastric pain, penetrating towards back. Which is the best for diagnosis?
    a. Serum lipase   b. CPK-MB
    c. ALP   d. Gamma- GGT
278. GERD is best diagnosed by?
    a. 24 hour pH Monitoring
    b. Upper GI endoscopy
    c. Barium meal follow through
    d. Barium Swallow

279. Which cereal is not to be given in celiac sprue?
    a. Wheat   b. Maize
    c. Corn   d. Rice
280. In ulcerative colitis, which is *not* true about malignancy?
    a. Metaplasia   b. Low grade dysplasia
    c. High grade dysplasia   d. Pleomorphism
281. Iron is absorbed from:
    a. Duodenum with fast clearance
    b. Jejunum with fast clearance
    c. Ileum with low clearance
    d. Bone marrow
282. DOC for enteric fever:
    a. Ceftriaxone   b. Ciprofloxacin
    c. Amikacin   d. Cefotaxime
283. Enteric fever on fourth day is best diagnosed by:
    a. Stool test   b. Widal test
    c. Urine test   d. Blood culture
284. Which of the following is seen on the image?

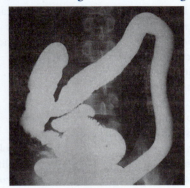

   a. Barium enema = Pipe stem colon
   b. Double contrast enema= Apple core appearance
   c. Barium enema = Pseudo-polyps
   d. Double contrast enema = Thumb printing sign
285. Which of the following is the most probable diagnosis of this X-ray abdomen?

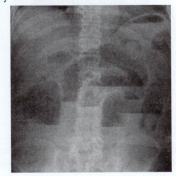

   a. Gas under diaphragm- Peritonitis
   b. Multiple air fluid level- Adhesions and bands
   c. Bird beak – Volvulus
   d. Normal X-ray PA view

286. Diagnosis:

   a. CBD dilatation on ERCP
   b. CBD dilatation on PTC
   c. Cystic duct dilation on ERCP
   d. Cystic duct ectasia on ERCP
287. IOC for G.E.R.D:
   a. 24-hour pH monitoring b. Upper G.I. endoscopy
   c. Ultrasound   d. X-ray abdomen
288. Aspirin is given in management of which cancer:
   a. Pancreatic cancer   b. Liver cancer
   c. Colon cancer   d. Stomach cancer
289. Incorrect about Zenkers diverticulum?
   a. Located in Killian triangle
   b. Regurgitation of previous day food
   c. Premalignant
   d. Dysphagia
290. Cobble stoning of colon is seen in?
   a. Crohn's disease   b. Ulcerative colitis
   c. Ischemic colitis   d. Amoebic colitis
291. Which of the following is not true about Crohn's disease?
   a. It can involve stomach and duodenum also
   b. Skip lesion
   c. All layers of intestine are involved
   d. Invasion of lymph nodes seen
292. Colon in the given picture is suggestive of:

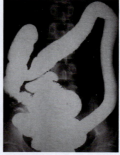

   a. Ulcerative colitis   b. Crohn's disease
   c. Diverticulosis   d. Intussusception
293. Which of the following is least likely to be seen with Crohn's disease:
   a. Skip lesions   b. Fistula
   c. Toxic megacolon   d. Transmural involvement

294. In which of the following conditions smoking is protective?
   a. Ulcerative colitis   b. Crohn's disease
   c. SLE   d. Alzheimer's
295. Barrett's esophagus causes which cancer:
   a. Adenocarcinoma   b. Squamous cell CA
   c. Carcinoid tumor   d. Esophageal leiomyoma
296. H. pylori causes all EXCEPT:
   a. Peptic ulcer   b. Maltoma
   c. Carcinoid tumor   d. Gastric CA
297. Traveler diarrhea is caused by?
   a. Campylobacter   b. Aeromonas
   c. Actinobacillus   d. Cryptosporidium

HEPATOLOGY

298. Which of the following is not a component of Child Pugh classification? *(Recent Pattern Question 2018-19)*
   a. SGOT   b. Bilirubin
   c. Albumin   d. Prothrombin time
299. Not a prehepatic cause of portal HTN?
      (Recent Pattern Question 2018-19)
   a. Budd Chiari syndrome b. Banti disease
   c. Portal vein thrombosis d. Pyelophlebitis
300. Fatty liver with hepatomegaly is seen in:
      (Recent Pattern Question 2018)
   a. Marasmus   b. Metabolic syndrome
   c. Wilson disease   d. Nutmeg liver
301. Which of the following is used for chelation of zinc in Wilson disease? *(Recent Pattern Question 2017)*
   a. Desferroxamine   b. Zinc
   c. Trientine   d. Tetrathiomolybdate
302. Which is the best investigation for Wilson disease?
      (Recent Pattern Question 2017)
   a. KF ring   b. Urine copper
   c. Serum copper   d. Liver copper
303. Steatosis is due to: *(Recent Pattern Question 2016)*
   a. Triglycerides   b. LDL
   c. VLDL   d. Cholesterol
304. Central regulator of iron metabolism is:
      (Recent Pattern Question 2016)
   a. Transferrin   b. Ferritin
   c. Ferroportin   d. Hepcidin
305. In Wilson disease, chelation is done by:
   a. Iron   b. Zinc
   c. Copper   d. Selenium
306. In hemochromatosis, all are affected EXCEPT:
   a. Hippocampus
   b. Bronze Pancreas
   c. Hyperpigmentation
   d. Restrictive cardiomyopathy

Medicine

307. Most common chronic viral illness is caused by:
- a. Hepatitis A
- b. Hepatitis B
- c. Hepatitis C
- d. Hepatitis D

308. Palmar erythema in liver failure is due to:
- a. Coagulopathy
- b. Hyperbilirubinemia
- c. Hyperammonemia
- d. Estrogen

309. A man presented with (+) fever, chills and jaundice. Diagnosis:
- a. Acute Cholecystitis
- b. Acute cholangitis
- c. Choledocholithiasis
- d. Acute viral hepatitis

310. Fulminant liver disease is defined as encephalopathy, coagulopathy developing within how many weeks?
- a. 2 weeks
- b. 3 weeks
- c. 4 weeks
- d. 8 weeks

311. Most common cause of Fulminant hepatitis in pregnancy
- a. Hep B
- b. Hep C
- c. Hep D
- d. Hep E

312. Best marker for maternal to child transfer of hepatitis B virus?
- a. HBsAg
- b. HBV DNA
- c. HBeAg
- d. IgM Anti- HBcAg

313. Spironolactone is most useful in?
- a. Cardiac Hypertrophy
- b. Cirrhotic ascites
- c. Exudative pleural effusion
- d. Renal artery stenosis

314. Raised Intra-abdominal pressure to consider abdominal compartment syndrome is?
- a. 0-12 mm Hg
- b. >12 mm Hg
- c. >20 mm Hg
- d. >30 mm Hg

315. Trans-esophageal echocardiography is better over trans-thoracic echocardiography in?
- a. Evaluation of left ventricle
- b. Evaluation of left atria and left Atrial appendage thrombus
- c. Evaluation of Pericardial fluid
- d. Evaluation of commissural fusion

316. Select the best answer from the picture of temperature charting of patient with history of constipation for over 2 weeks
- a. Enteric fever
- b. Brucellosis
- c. Relapsing fever
- d. Hodgkin lymphoma

Date	1st week							2nd week							3rd week							4th week			
Day of disease	1	2	3	4	5	6	7	8	9	10	11	12	13	14	15	16	17	18	19	20	21	22	23	24	25

Pulse	Temp.
170	108
160	107
150	106
140	105
130	104
120	103
110	102
100	101
90	100
80	99
70	98
60	97
50	96
40	95
Respirations	
Stools	

RHEUMATOLOGY

317. Most common pulmonary manifestation of SLE:
- a. Shrinking Lung syndrome
- b. Pleuritis *(Most Recent Question 2019)*
- c. Intra alveolar hemorrhage.
- d. Interstitial inflammation

318. Which of the following cannot be diagnosed without positive ANA? *(Most Recent Question 2019)*
- a. SLE
- b. Sjogren Syndrome
- c. Drug induced lupus
- d. Scleroderma

319. Correct about Rheumatoid nodules?
(Recent Pattern Question 2018-19)
- a. Tender, located on extensor surface and seen with arthritis
- b. Non-tender, located on extensor surface and seen with arthritis
- c. Non-tender, located on flexor surface and seen with arthritis
- d. Tender, located on flexor surface and seen with arthritis

320. Which of the following is the best investigation for acute gout? *(Recent Pattern Question 2018)*
- a. Serum uric acid
- b. Uric acid in synovial fluid
- c. Uric acid in urine
- d. Anti CCP antibodies

321. Which is the drug of choice for acute gout?
(Recent Pattern Question 2018)
- a. Febuxstat
- b. Probenecid
- c. Rofecoxib
- d. Naproxen

322. Pulseless disease is? *(Recent Pattern Question 2017)*
- a. Takayasu's arteritis
- b. Raynaud phenomenon
- c. Coarctation of aorta
- d. Wegener's granulomatosis

FMGE Solutions Screening Examination

323. Best Lab test for rheumatic fever?
     (Recent Pattern Question 2016)
     a. ASO   b. CRP
     c. Anti DNASe B   d. Anti phospholipid
324. What is the effect of rheumatoid arthritis on the lung?
     a. DL$_{CO}$ normal   (Recent Pattern Question 2016)
     b. CXR is normal
     c. Exudative pleural effusion
     d. Flow volume pattern showing a obstructive pattern
325. In which of causes of oral ulcer, Auto-antibodies are not seen?
     a. Behçet disease   b. SLE
     c. Pemphigus   d. Celiac disease
326. Which antibody is incriminated in causing Henoch Schonlein Purpura?
     a. IgA   b. IgG
     c. IgM   d. IgD
327. LE cells are seen in:
     a. SLE   b. Dermatomyositis
     c. Sickle cell anemia d. Scleroderma
328. Wegener's granulomatosis is diagnosed by:
     a. P-ANCA   b. c-ANCA
     c. m-ANCA   d. A.N.A
329. Antibody in Goodpasture syndrome:
     a. Lupus anticoagulant
     b. Anti-GBM antibody
     c. Anti-Ro antibody
     d. Anti- mitochondrial antibody
330. Which of the following condition does not cause multiple painful ulcers on tongue?
     a. TB   b. Sarcoidosis
     c. Herpes   d. Behçet's disease
331. Wrong about Duchenne muscular dystrophy is?
     a. Pseudo-hypertrophy of calf muscles
     b. Gower sign positive
     c. Death occurs due to pneumonia
     d. Female is symptomatic
332. Gower's sign is seen in
     a. Duchenne muscular dystrophy
     b. Congenital myopathy
     c. Gullian barre syndrome
     d. All of the above
333. Joint usually not involved in Rheumatoid arthritis?
     a. D.I.P   b. P.I.P
     c. M.C.P   d. Wrist
334. Correct about Wegener Granulomatosis is?
     a. Both lung and kidney is involved
     b. p-ANCA is positive
     c. Seen with inflammatory bowel disease
     d. Non granulomatous vasculitis
335. All are seen in rheumatoid arthritis EXCEPT:
     a. Deformities   b. Mononeuritis multiplex
     c. Peri-articular osteoporosis
     d. Sero-negative arthritis
336. Which of the following is seen in sarcoidosis:
     a. Hypercalcemia   b. Hypocalcemia
     c. Hyperphosphatemia d. Hypophosphatemia
337. Sequela of rheumatic heart disease in a 5 year old child is:
     a. Mitral stenosis b. Mitral regurgitation
     c. Tricuspid stenosis d. Tricuspid regurgitation
338. Which of the following is not a major Criteria for rheumatic fever?
     a. Carditis   b. Arthritis
     c. Syndenham chorea d. ASO titer
339. All are major criteria for rheumatic fever EXCEPT?
     a. Pancarditis   b. Chorea
     c. Deforming arthritis d. Subcutaneous nodules
340. All of the following are Jones criteria EXCEPT?
     a. Elevated ASO titers b. History of sore throat
     c. Increased PR interval d. Arthritis
341. Which one of the following is not associated with anti (Ro) SSA antibody
     a. Rheumatoid arthritis b. Sicca syndrome
     c. Sarcoidosis   d. Ankylosing spondylitis
342. Most specific test for SLE
     a. ss DNA   b. ds- DNA
     c. Anti-smith antibody d. Histone
343. Anti RO bodies are present in all EXCEPT:
     a. SLE   b. Sjogren syndrome
     c. Neonatal lupus
     d. Mixed connective tissue disorder
344. Which of the following statement is false about Hurler syndrome:
     a. X linked   b. MR
     c. Joint stiffness d. Coarse facial features
345. In Henoch schonlen purpura Ig and complement involved:
     a. IgG, C 3   b. IgA, C 3
     c. IgA, C 1   d. IgG, C 1
346. Which of these doesn't present with granulomatous Vasculitis?
     a. Polyarteritis nodosa b. Wegener's
     c. Churg strauss syndrome d. Microscopic polyangitis
347. Martel sign is seen in?
     a. Gout   b. Ankylosing spondylitis
     c. Osteoarthritis   d. Rheumatoid arthritis
348. Lady presents with joint pain in both knees and low grade fever off and on. On examination she has a rash on sun exposed parts. Clinical diagnosis?
     a. SLE   b. Rheumatoid arthritis
     c. Photo-dermatitis d. Porphyria
349. In long standing rheumatoid arthritis which will be seen?
     a. Milk alkali syndrome b. Nephrolithiasis
     c. Paradoxical aciduria d. Secondary amyloidosis
350. Rheumatoid arthritis is seen with?
     a. HLA DR3   b. HLA DR4
     c. HLA DR 27   d. HLA B 27

351. Gold is used for management of?
    a. Ankylosing Spondylitis   b. Rheumatoid arthritis
    c. Psoriatic arthritis   d. Rheumatic arthriitis

RESPIRATORY SYSTEM

352. All are true about Allergic Bronchopulmonary aspergilloma except?   *(Recent Pattern Question 2018-19)*
    a. Distal bronchiectasis
    b. Increased in bronchial gland secretions
    c. Increased Ig E
    d. Seen in asthmatics

353. On putting a Subclavian vein catheter, a patient has developed sudden onset severe respiratory distress. Clinical diagnosis is?   *(Recent Pattern Question 2018-19)*
    a. Pneumothorax   b. Sepsis
    c. A.R.D.S   d. Nosocomial pneumonia

354. Which is correct about transudative pleural effusion?   *(Recent Pattern Question 2018)*
    a. Pleural fluid protein to serum protein ratio <0.5
    b. Pleural fluid LDH to Serum LDH >0.6
    c. Pleural Fluid LDH more than 2/3 of upper reference limit for serum LDH
    d. Pleural fluid sugar to blood sugar ratio >0.5

355. Which of the following is seen in COAD?
    a. Chronic bronchitis   *(Recent Pattern Question 2018)*
    b. Follicular bronchiolitis
    c. Desquamative pneumonitis
    d. Chemical pneumonitis

356. A 26-year-old patient presents with a history suggestive of tuberculosis. On examination he has pleural effusion. All of the following parameters will be used for analysis of pleural fluid EXCEPT?   *(Recent Pattern Question 2017)*
    a. Gene XPERT   b. LDH
    c. Albumin   d. ADA

357. A 2 year malnourished child presents with fever, weight loss, tachypnea. CXR of the patient is shown below. What is the best treatment?   *(Recent Pattern Question 2017)*

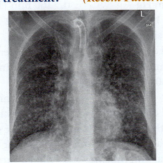

    a. A.T.T   b. A.T.T plus steroids
    c. Chloramphenicol
    d. Clarithromycin + amoxicillin

358. Leukostasis syndrome affects which organ?
     (Recent Pattern Question 2016)
    a. Liver   b. Spleen
    c. Kidney   d. Lung

359. Drainage hemothorax is done best through which space?   *(Recent Pattern Question 2016)*
    a. 2nd intercostal space   b. 5nd paravertebral space
    c. 5th midaxillary space   d. 7th midaxillary space

360. Shock lung synonym is used for?
     (Recent Pattern Question 2016)
    a. COPD   b. Alveolar proteinosis
    c. ARDS   d. HMD

361. Pneumatocele is caused by?   *(Recent Pattern Question 2016)*
    a. Staphylococcus aureus
    b. Streptococcus pyogenes
    c. Hemophilus parainfluenzae
    d. Mycoplasma pneumoniae

362. Health care associated pneumonia is treated by?
     (Recent Pattern Question 2016)
    a. Azithromycin   b. Doxycycline
    c. Levofloxacin   d. Vancomycin

363. A patient develops fracture of shaft of femur. On day 3, he develops respiratory distress and decrease SPO_2 and petechiae. Probable diagnosis is?
     (Recent Pattern Question 2016)
    a. Hypostatic pneumonia   b. Hemolytic pneumonia
    c. Crush syndrome   d. Fat embolism

364. A 30-year-old male presents with severe abdominal pain and rigidity with rebound tenderness. X-ray abdomen shows?

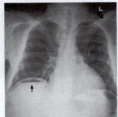

    a. Acute gastritis   *(Recent Pattern Question 2016)*
    b. DU perforation
    c. Intra-abdominal infection anaerobic
    d. Peritoneal rupture of amoebic liver abscess

365. Biot breathing is seen in?
    a. Flail chest   b. Uremia
    c. High altitude   d. Lesion in the brain

366. Which is the best test to be done for Pulmonary embolism?
    a. D Dimer Assay
    b. MRI
    c. Ventilation perfusion scan
    d. CT with IV contrast

367. Which of the following patients will not be able to respond to increased carbon dioxide levels?
    a. Narcotic over-dosage   b. Obesity
    c. Pulmonary edema   d. Type 1 respiratory failure

368. In HIV positive patient with pneumocystis jiroveci infection, which of the following is used for prevention?
    a. Azithromycin
    b. Acyclovir
    c. Levofloxacin
    d. Sulfomethoxazole+ trimethoprim
369. Pop-corn calcification is seen with?
    a. Pulmonary Hamartoma
    b. Aspergillosis
    c. Broncho-Alveolar cancer
    d. Pulmonary Embolism
370. ARDS is characterised by all EXCEPT?
    a. Decreased surfactant
    b. Alveolar transudate
    c. Decreased lung compliance
    d. pAO_2/FiO_2 ratio <200
371. A 45-year-old with trauma presents after 4 hours with cheek swelling and urine not passed. On examination crepitus is palpated with periorbital swelling. What is your diagnosis?

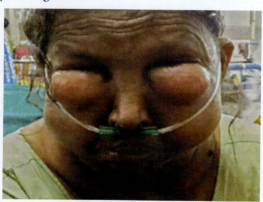

    a. Renal shut down   b. Lung laceration
    c. Gas gangrene   d. Base of skull fracture
372. All are true about Aspirin sensitive asthma EXCEPT?
    a. Nasal polyposis
    b. Treatment with inhaled corticosteroids
    c. Rhinosinusitis
    d. Increased prostaglandins
373. In a patient with COPD, best management option is?
    a. Quit smoking
    b. Bronchodilators
    c. Low flow Oxygen
    d. Mucolytics
374. In a patient with smoking history, which is important?
    a. Duration of smoking   b. Number of smoking
    c. Brand of Cigarette   d. Filter of cigarette
375. Hyperventilation leads to?
    a. Increased CO_2 b. Decreased CO_2
    c. Increased DL_{CO} d. Decreased PO_2

376. What is the diagnosis of CXR shown?

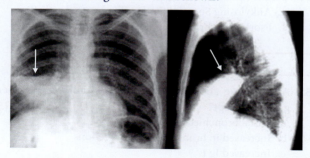

    a. Viral pneumonia
    b. Bacterial pneumonia
    c. Fungal pneumonia
    d. TB
377. Image CXR shows:

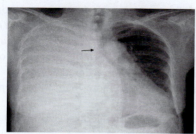

    a. Right pleural effusion   b. Left pleural effusion
    c. Left lung consolidation d. Right lung consolidation
378. Female patient with bilateral hilar lymphadenopathy and joint pain. ACE levels are elevated. Diagnosis is?
    a. Sarcoidosis   b. Silicosis
    c. Hodgkin's lymphoma   d. Non Hodgkin's lymphoma
379. Mesothelioma is most commonly caused by?
    a. Asbestosis
    b. Silicosis
    c. Anthracosis
    d. Coal workers pneumoconiosis
380. Partial pressure of oxygen in alveoli:
    a. 60 mm Hg   b. 103 mm Hg
    c. 136 mm Hg   d. 160 mm Hg
381. Which of the following is given in the maintenance of severe persistent asthma:
    a. Steroid   b. Leukotriene agonist
    c. Ipratomium bromide   d. Long acting beta2 agonist
382. Oxygen (30–50%) is *not* given in:
    a. COPD   b. Pneumonia
    c. Pleural effusion d. Severe asthma
383. Which of the following is due to chronic smoking:
    a. Centri-acinar emphysema b. Panacinar emphysema
    c. Irregular emphysema   d. Mixed variety
384. Mottling of lungs is seen in?
    a. Silicosis   b. histoplasmosis
    c. ARDS   d. Nocardia

385. Which is correct regarding the CXR?

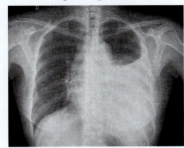

   a. Pleural thickening
   b. Segmental collapse
   c. Ellis curve
   d. Hypertranslucency
386. Diagnosis on CXR is?

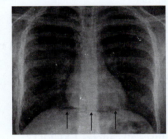

   a. Congenital diaphragmatic hernia
   b. Bochdalek hernia
   c. Pneumothorax
   d. Pneumo-mediastinum
387. CURB 65 criteria includes all EXCEPT:
   a. Age is always more than or equal to 65 years
   b. Respiratory rate more than 30/min
   c. Systolic Blood pressure is more than 90 mm Hg
   d. BUN level is more than >7 mmol/L
388. Most common type of emphysema
   a. Panacinar emphysema
   b. Irregular emphysema
   c. Centriacinar emphysema
   d. Paraseptal emphysema
389. Emphysema presents with all EXCEPT:
   a. Cyanosis
   b. Barrel shaped chest
   c. Associated with smoking
   d. Type 1 respiratory failure
390. In case of Pulmonary embolism, Right ventricle hypokinesia and decreased output, which Drug therapy is most helpful:
   a. Thrombolytic
   b. LMW heparin
   c. Warfarin
   d. Heparin
391. Best treatment for massive pulmonary embolism:
   a. Intravenous tissue plasminogen activator
   b. Heparin
   c. Pulmonary thromboembolectomy
   d. Low molecular weight heparin + warfarin
392. What is the full form of ARIA?
   a. Allergic rhinitis induced asthama
   b. Allergic rhinitis and its impact on asthma
   c. Allergy rheumatology immunology and asthma
   d. Acetylcholine receptor inducing activity

393. Pneumatocele is commonly caused by:
   a. Streptococcus pneumonia
   b. Haemophilus influenza
   c. Serratia marcescens
   d. Klebsiella pneumonia
394. Finger in glove sign is seen in?
   a. Pulmonary alveolar proteinosis
   b. Pneumocystis carinii
   c. Tuberculosis
   d. Bronchocele
395. Aspergillosis can present with all EXCEPT:
   a. Lung cavity
   b. Ear infection
   c. Normal component in sputum
   d. Rhinocerebral involvement
396. Allergic broncho-pulmonary Aspergillosis presents with all EXCEPT:
   a. Eosinophiluria
   b. Occurs in asthmatics
   c. Brownish plugs in sputum
   d. Central bronchiectasis
397. Central bronchiectasis is seen with
   a. Cystic adenomatoid malformation
   b. Cystic fibrosis
   c. Broncho carcinoma
   d. Tuberculosis
398. IOC for Bronchiectasis:
   a. HRCT scan
   b. Spiral CT
   c. Bronchoscopy
   d. Pulmonary angiography
399. Miliary shadow on X-ray is seen in all EXCEPT:
   a. Tuberculosis
   b. Loeffler's pneumonia
   c. Klebsiella
   d. Varicella pneumonia
400. TB causes all EXCEPT:
   a. Conjunctivitis
   b. Uveitis
   c. Lymphadenopathy
   d. Addison disease
401. Congenital tuberculosis affects which organ the most
   a. Brain
   b. Liver
   c. Kidney
   d. Lungs
402. Which drugs are not used in severe persistent Asthma:
   a. Short acting beta 2 agonist
   b. Oral corticosteroids
   c. Long acting beta 2 agonist
   d. Inhaled high dose Steroids
403. Most common cause of community acquired pneumonia?
   a. Pneumococcus
   b. Streptococcus pyogenes
   c. Staph. Aureus
   d. Mycoplasma
404. Unipolar flagellated organsim that causes pneumonia
   a. Pseudomonas
   b. Mycoplasma
   c. Aeromonas
   d. Klebsiella pneumonia
405. Which of the following is not true in obstructive lung disease?
   a. $FEV_1 \downarrow$
   b. $TLC \downarrow$
   c. $FVC \downarrow$
   d. Reduced timed vital capacity

FMGE Solutions Screening Examination

406. Which of the following is the common cause of respiratory failure Type 2?
    a. COPD
    b. Acute asthma
    c. ARDS
    d. Pneumonia

407. A 65-year-old lady suddenly dies 7 days after a surgery of femur fracture suddenly dies while having lunch in the ward. What would be the most likely cause:
    a. Calf vein thrombosis
    b. Pulmonary embolism
    c. Myocardial infarction
    d. Choking on food

408. A 65-year-old woman after total knee implant surgery complains of calf pain and swelling in the leg from last 2 days. Later she complains of breathlessness and dies suddenly in the ward. Probable cause?
    a. Pulmonary embolism
    b. Myocardial infarction
    c. Stroke
    d. ARDS

409. Westermark sign is seen in:
    a. Pulmonary embolism
    b. Pulmonary sequestration
    c. Pulmonary alveolar proteinosis
    d. Pneumothorax

410. Mean pulmonary artery pressure is:
    a. 15 mm Hg
    b. 8 mm Hg
    c. 25 mm Hg
    d. 10 mm Hg

411. What is not correct about smoking?
    a. Nicotine causes increase in blood sugar
    b. It reduces anxiety due to release of beta endorphins
    c. Acts a psychostimulant
    d. Acts on Alpha 2 Beta 4 nicotinic receptor

412. A 65-year-old man presented with hemoptysis and stage 3 clubbing. The probable diagnosis of the patient is?
    a. Non small cell lung Ca
    b. Small cell cancer of lung
    c. Tuberculosis
    d. Sarcoidosis

413. The following CXR shows

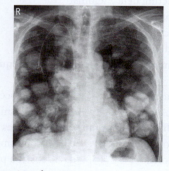

   a. Metastasis to lungs
   b. Pneumothorax
   c. Pneumatocele
   d. Bronchial adenoma

414. Look at the image of popcorn on CXR. In which condition is this seen?

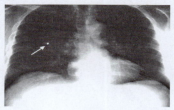

   a. TB
   b. Metastasis
   c. Pulmonary hamartoma
   d. Carcinoid tumor

415. ARDS includes all EXCEPT?
   a. Hypoxia
   b. Hypercapnia
   c. Non cardiogenic pulmonary edema
   d. Normal P.C.W.P

416. Which component of cigarette smoke is responsible for CAD?
   a. Nicotine
   b. Tar
   c. Polycyclic aromatic hydrocarbons
   d. Benzene

417. Smoking causes all cancers EXCEPT?
   a. Liver cancer
   b. Oral cancer
   c. Kidney cancer
   d. Bladder cancer

418. Water test is done for?
   a. Pneumothorax
   b. Diabetic insipidus
   c. Peritonitis
   d. Bladder injury

419. Hypersensitivity pneumonitis is consistent with the following findings EXCEPT:
   a. Decreased DLCO
   b. Precipitating antibodies to causative antigens
   c. Granuloma on lung biopsy
   d. Eosinophilic alveolitis

420. Drug of choice for treatment of type 2 Brittle Asthma is
   a. β-adrenergic agonist
   b. Inhaled corticosteroids
   c. Antileukotrines DM
   d. Subcutaneous epinephrine

421. All of the following criteria are required for diagnosis of obesity hypoventilation syndrome EXCEPT:
   a. Hypertension
   b. Sleep disorder breathing
   c. BMI ≥ 30 kg/m^2
   d. PaCO$_2$ ≥ 45 mm Hg

422. The following CXR shows

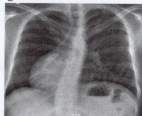

   a. Dextrocardia
   b. Pneumothorax
   c. Pneumomediastinum
   d. Pulmonary hamartoma

423. The CXR shows

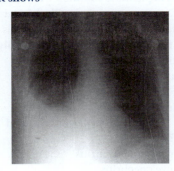

   a. Meniscus sign
   b. Consolidation lower lobe
   c. Bilateral pneumothorax
   d. Pulmonary artery hypertension

NEPHROLOGY

424. What is the most common cause of death in patients of G6PD deficiency? *(Recent Pattern Question 2018)*
   a. Low oxyhemoglobin values
   b. Acute renal failure
   c. Sequestration crisis
   d. Low oxygen affinity

425. Which of the following is correct about urinary loss in Fanconi syndrome? *(Recent Pattern Question 2017)*
   a. Bicarbonate, Uric acid and Amino-acids
   b. Bicarbonate, Chloride and Amino acids
   c. Bicarbonate, Sugar and Potassium
   d. Bicarbonate, Uric acid and Potassium

426. Which is the Gold standard investigation for Renal Artery Stenosis? *(Recent Pattern Question 2017)*
   a. DTPA
   b. MRA
   c. Doppler
   d. Contrast arteriography

427. Nephrotic syndrome is associated with?
   a. Goodpasture disease *(Recent Pattern Question 2017)*
   b. Membranoproliferative glomerulonephritis
   c. Membranous glomerulopathy
   d. Berger disease

428. Broad casts are seen in? *(Recent Pattern Question 2016)*
   a. Chronic renal failure
   b. Chronic glomerulonephritis
   c. Minimal change disease
   d. Membranous nephropathy

429. Streptococcal skin infection is followed by episode of hematuria and hypertension. All are needed for diagnosis EXCEPT? *(Recent Pattern Question 2016)*
   a. Serum C3
   b. ASO
   c. Anti DNA-ase B
   d. CRP

430. Salt losing nephritis is? *(Recent Pattern Question 2016)*
   a. Interstitial nephritis
   b. Glomerulonephritis
   c. Lupus nephritis
   d. IgA nephropathy

431. Cockroft gault formula is used for calculation of *(Recent Pattern Question 2016)*
   a. GFR
   b. Microalbuminuria
   c. Serum anion gap
   d. Urinary anion gap

432. A 70-year-old patient develops pneumonia and sepsis and has renal failure with BP 70/50. Best drug used is? *(Recent Pattern Question 2016)*
   a. Adrenaline
   b. Phenylephrine
   c. Norepinephrine
   d. Ephedrine

433. All are true about most common cause of nephrotic syndrome in children?
   a. It is not associated with hypertension
   b. Minimal change disease in children <10 year
   c. Massive Proteinuria >3.5 gm%/24 Hours
   d. Low Complement Levels

434. Drug helpful in Chronic kidney disease?
   a. Beta blocker
   b. Amlodipine
   c. ACE inhibitor
   d. Telmisartan

435. Which of the following will have a contrast nephropathy?
   a. Diabetes nephropathy
   b. Hypertension
   c. Malignant hypertension
   d. Hypertensive Glomerulosclerosis

436. Potassium excretion is caused mainly by?
   a. Spironolactone
   b. Frusemide
   c. Thiazide
   d. Aldosterone

437. ACE inhibitors are contraindicated in all EXCEPT?
   a. Bilateral renal artery stenosis
   b. Chronic renal failure
   c. Pregnancy
   d. Hyperkalemia

438. Patient on insulin in CKD stage 4. What is the dose adjustment of insulin required?
   a. Increased insulin
   b. Decreased insulin
   c. Normal insulin
   d. Add DPP-4 inhibitors

439. Which of the following helps most in nephrolithiasis?
   a. Low sodium diet
   b. Low calcium diet
   c. High sodium diet
   d. Low citrate diet

440. Absolute indication for hemodialysis is?
   a. Hypertension
   b. Hypokalemia
   c. Pericarditis
   d. Metabolic alkalosis

441. Most common cause of glomerulonephritis?
   a. P.S.G.N
   b. Diabetes mellitus
   c. Autosomal dominant Polycystic kidney disease
   d. Crescentric Glomerulonephritis

442. All are true about GFR EXCEPT?
   a. 30-40% decrease after 70 years of age
   b. Best estimated by Creatinine clearance
   c. CKD is defied as GFR < 30 ml/min/1.73 m^2 for 4 weeks
   d. GFR is dependent on height in children

FMGE Solutions Screening Examination

443. Membranous Glomerulopathy is seen in?
    a. Diabetes
    b. HTN
    c. Renal failure
    d. Malignancy
444. Positive dipstick for RBC with Red color urine and clear supernatant after centrifugation is due to:
    a. Porphyria   b. Hematuria
    c. Hemolysis   d. Rhabdomyolysis
445. RBC cast is present in:
    a. Acute tubular nephritis   b. Acute glomerulonephritis
    c. Acute Pyelonephritis   d. Acute interstitial nephritis
446. Oliguric renal failure is due to all EXCEPT:
    a. Diabetic nephropathy
    b. Fanconi syndrome
    c. Multiple myeloma
    d. Aminoglycosides
447. Which of the following Microorganism is incriminated in infection after Hemodialysis?
    a. Chlamydia   b. Gram positive
    c. Gram negative   d. Anaerobes
448. Gross hematuria is seen in:
    a. IgA nephropathy   b. Minimal change disease
    c. Chronic renal failure d. Nephritic syndrome
449. Xantho-granulomatous infection is caused by:
    a. Nephrolithiasis
    b. Urinary obstruction
    c. Proteus Mirabilis
    d. All of the above
450. Hypokalemia is seen in:
    a. RTA- I   b. RTA- II
    c. RTA- III   d. RTA- IV
451. Acute renal failure results in:
    a. Hyperkalemic alkalosis
    b. Hypokalemic alkalosis
    c. hyperkalemic acidosis
    d. Hypokalemic acidosis
452. All of the following causes acute renal failure EXCEPT:
    a. Pyelonephritis   b. Snakebite
    c. Rhabdomyolysis   d. Analgesic nephropathy
453. Which of these is correct about Struvite stones?
    a. Present in alkaline urine
    b. Most common kidney disease
    c. Are Calcium pyrophosphate stones
    d. Most common kidney stones
454. All are seen in Nephrotic syndrome EXCEPT:
    a. Atherosclerosis   b. Thrombo-embolism
    c. Hypertension   d. Lipiduria
455. Red cell cast are more common with
    a. Acute tubular necrosis b. Nephrotic syndrome
    c. Nephritic syndrome   d. Interstitial nephritis
456. Interstitial nephritis is common with
    a. NSAID   b. Black water fever
    c. Rhabdomyolysis   d. Tumor lysis syndrome
457. Which of the following does not cause Polyuria:
    a. Interstitial nephritis
    b. Hypokalemia
    c. A.D.H insufficiency
    d. Rhabdomyolysis
458. Triad of Hematuria, hypertension and edema are a feature of?
    a. Acute glomerulonephritis
    b. Acute pyelonephritis
    c. Chronic glomerulonephritis
    d. Renal cell carcinoma
459. Type of glomerulopathy in HIV positive patient is?
    a. Focal segmental glomerulosclerosis
    b. Diffuse glomerulosclerosis
    c. Membranous glomerulopathy
    d. Mesangio-proliferative glomerulonephritis
460. Hemodialysis can be performed for long periods from the same site due to?
    a. Arteriovenous fistula reduces bacterial contamination of site
    b. Arteriovenous fistula results in arterialization of vein
    c. Arteriovenous fistula reduces chances of graft failure
    d. arteriovenous fistula facilitates small bore needles for high flow rates
461. Chronic hemodialysis in ESRD patient is done?
    a. Once per week   b. Twice per week
    c. Thrice per week   d. Daily

INFECTION

462. Which of the following is a good prognosis determining step in septic shock? *(Recent Pattern Question 2018-19)*
    a. Adequate IVF
    b. Adequate vasopressor
    c. Adequate IVF plus Vasopressor
    d. Time between hypotension and introduction of antibiotic
463. Rapid diagnosis of rabies is made with?
    (Recent Pattern Question 2018-19)
    a. Skin biopsy with fluorescent antibody testing
    b. Rabies virus specific antibodies
    c. Inoculation in mouse
    d. Corneal impression smear
464. Recurrent Neisseria meningitis episodes are caused by deficiency of? *(Recent Pattern Question 2018-19)*
    a. C5-C9 deficiency
    b. IgA deficiency
    c. CD4 cell deficiency
    d. Perforin deficiency

Medicine

465. In fever of unknown origin, how many times blood sample should be drawn?
(Recent Pattern Question 2018-19)
a. 2
b. 3
c. 4
d. 5

466. A 6-year child presents with low grade fever for 7 days and on examination has enlarged cervical lymph nodes with a palpable spleen tip. He was given ampicillin followed by development of extensive rash all over the body. Diagnosis is? *(Recent Pattern Question 2018-19)*
a. Infectious mononucleosis
b. Scarlet fever
c. Kawasaki
d. Hodgkin's Lymphoma

467. Correct about initiating treatment in AIDS patient
(Recent Pattern Question 2018-19)
a. No cut off of CD4 count required for initiation of treatment
b. CD4 count < 200/cu.mm required for initiation of treatment
c. CD4 count <350/cu.mm required for initiation of treatment
d. CD4 count <500/cu.mm required for initiation of treatment

468. Which of the following is correct about differential leucocyte count in late catarrhal stage of pertussis?
(Recent Pattern Question 2018)
a. Neutropenia
b. Eosinophilia
c. Monocytosis
d. Lymphocytosis

469. Which is the drug of choice for prophylaxis of meningococcal meningitis in pregnancy:
(Recent Pattern Question 2018)
a. Penicillin
b. Ceftriaxone
c. Rifampicin
d. Ampicillin

470. In a diagnosed lepromatous leprosy patient, the treatment was started. After intake of drug skin lesions and fever develop within few days. Which type of hypersensitivity reaction leads to this manifestation?
(Recent Pattern Question 2018)
a. Type 4
b. Type 3
c. Type 2
d. Type 1

471. What is the incubation period of hepatitis B?
(Recent Pattern Question 2018)
a. 1–30 days
b. 15–45 days
c. 45–180 days
d. 2 weeks–6 months

472. Which of the following is an initial presentation of HIV infection when ART is not started?
(Recent Pattern Question 2018)
a. Primary CNS lymphoma
b. Kaposi sarcoma
c. Bacterial pneumonia
d. Extrapulmonary tuberculosis

473. The most important parameter to monitor dengue haemorrhagic fever is? *(Recent Pattern Question 2017)*
a. Platelet count
b. Haemoglobin
c. Total leucocyte count
d. Haematocrit

474. Causative agent for hand-foot-mouth disease is?
(Recent Pattern Question 2017)
a. Enterovirus
b. Cocksackie
c. Adenovirus
d. Hepatitis C

475. DOC for actinomycosis? *(Recent Pattern Question 2016)*
a. Penicillin
b. Ceftriaxone
c. Chloroamphenicol
d. Moxifloxacin

476. Best treatment for Swine flu is
(Recent Pattern Question 2016)
a. Oseltamivir
b. Indinavir
c. Abacavir
d. Zanamavir

477. Rickettsia is treated in all ages by which drug?
(Recent Pattern Question 2016)
a. Doxycycline
b. Penicillin
c. Macrolides
d. Quinolones

478. Empirical antibiotic regimen in suitable community acquired pneumonia in previously health adults?
(Recent Pattern Question 2016)
a. Amoxicillin + Clavulanate
b. Azithromycin
c. Ceftriaxone
d. Moxifloxacin

479. Mad cow disease is due to?
a. Protein misfolding
b. Bacterial
c. Viral
d. Spirochete

480. Sputum smear is diagnostic if?
a. >25 neutrophils and >10 squamous epithelial cells
b. <25 neutrophils and <10 squamous epithelial cells
c. >25 neutrophils and <10 squamous epithelial cells
d. <25 neutrophils and >10 squamous epithelial cells

481. Meningitis bacteria are normally present in?
a. Nasopharynx
b. Skin
c. Genitals
d. Lower G.I.T

482. Quadrivalent Meningococcal vaccine is not used for?
a. Serotype A
b. Serotype B
c. Serotype C
d. Serotype Y

FLUIDS AND ELECTROLYTES

483. Which of these has no role in treatment of dangerous hyperkalemia? *(Recent Pattern Question 2018)*
a. Injecting calcium chloride
b. Salbutamol
c. Hemodialysis
d. IV soda-bicarbonate

FMGE Solutions Screening Examination

484. High anion gap acidosis is seen in all EXCEPT:
    (Recent Pattern Question 2018)
    a. Lactic acidosis   b. Diarrhea
    c. Acute renal failure d. Salicylate poisoning

485. Anion gap is increased in all EXCEPT:
    (Recent Pattern Question 2018)
    a. Renal tubular acidosis   b. Diabetic ketoacidosis
    c. Acute tubular necrosis   d. Ethylene glycol poisoning

486. In which of the following condition is blood osmolality increased: *(Recent Pattern Question 2018)*
    a. Diarrhea   b. SIADH
    c. Psychogenic polydipsia d. Cerebral toxoplasmosis

487. Which is correct about a female with chronic vomiting?
    (Recent Pattern Question 2018)
    a. Hypokalemic hypochloremic metabolic alkalosis
    b. Hypokalemic hyperchloremic metabolic alkalosis
    c. Hypokalemic hypochloremic metabolic acidosis
    d. Hypokalemic hyperchloremic metabolic acidosis

488. Normal anion gap is seen in?
    (Recent Pattern Question 2017)
    a. Renal tubular acidosis b. Diabetic Keto-acidosis
    c. Hyper-alimentation   d. Acute tubular necrosis

489. Increased anion gap is seen in?
    (Recent Pattern Question 2017)
    a. Starvation   b. Renal tubular acidosis
    c. Diarrhoea   d. Fistula

490. In a patient who was brought to casualty after RTA with pulse rate 108, SBP 80. Which fluid is to be given ideally?
    a. Plasma   b. Normal saline
    c. Blood   d. 5% dextrose

491. All are seen in Hypokalemia EXCEPT?
    a. U wave in ECG   b. Tall T wave in ECG
    c. ST Depression   d. Prolonged QU interval

492. Which of the following presents with hypokalemia and metabolic acidosis?
    a. Diarrhea   b. Vomiting
    c. Nasogastric suction d. Conn's syndrome

493. Seborrheic dermatitis, cellulitis, alopecia and apathy is seen in?
    a. Pyridoxine deficiency b. Biotin deficiency
    c. Riboflavin deficiency d. Vitamin A deficiency

494. Normal anion gap is seen in:
    a. Diabetic ketoacidosis b. Chronic renal failure
    c. Renal tubular acidosis d. Methanol toxicity

495. Normal anion gap is seen in:
    a. Diabetic ketoacidosis   b. Lactic acidosis
    c. Starvation ketoacidosis d. Renal tubular acidosis

496. Widened anion gap is caused by all EXCEPT:
    a. Lactic acidosis   b. Diarrhea
    c. Diabetic keto-acidosis d. Methanol poisoning

497. Hypernatremia causes all EXCEPT:
    a. Seizure   b. Increased plasma osmolality
    c. Brain hemorrhage   d. Central pontine myelinosis

498. Chvostek's sign is elicited by:
    a. Facial nerve stimulation by tapping over the parotid
    b. BP cuff in arm for 5 minutes
    c. Tapping over extensor pollicis brevis
    d. Tapping over flexor retinaculum

499. Which can be given immediately in hemorrhagic stroke?
    a. Packed RBC   b. Colloids
    c. Blood transfusion d. Hypertonic fluids

500. Women working in hot environment & drinking lots of water without intake of salts are liable to develop
    a. Heat hyperpyrexia b. Heat cramps
    c. Heat stroke   d. Heat encephalopathy

501. Hypocalcemia will *not* lead to?
    a. Bone fractures   b. Tetany
    c. QT prolongation d. Osteoporosis

502. After Road traffic accident a patient presented to casualty with vitals showing BP of 90/60 mm Hg with heart of 56 bpm. Which kind of shock occurs?
    a. Cardiogenic   b. Neurogenic
    c. Distributive   d. Hypovolemic shock

503. Following stays least in plasma?
    a. Renin   b. Cortisol
    c. aldosterone   d. Norepinephrine

MISCELLANEOUS

504. Black Hairy Tongue is seen in? *(Most Recent Question 2019)*
    a. Elongation of filiform papillae
    b. Elongation of circumvallate papillae
    c. Carcinoma tongue
    d. Hyperplastic candidiasis

505. What is the site of intramuscular injection in gluteal area?   *(Recent Pattern Question 2017)*
    a. Upper outer   b. Upper inner
    c. Lower outer   d. Lower inner

506. Angiography of CCA is shown with an arrow mark at branch of ECA. Identify the vessel?
    (Recent Pattern Question 2017)

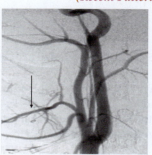

    a. Superior thyroid artery
    b. Facial artery
    c. Thyrocervical trunk
    d. Lingual artery

507. During cannulation at internal jugular vein, which is the most likely complication?
    a. Pneumothorax
    b. Ventricular tachycardia
    c. Pulmonary thrombo-embolism
    d. Arterial puncture
508. Severe combined immunodeficiency is seen with?
    a. Pre B Cell
    b. Pre T Cell
    c. Both
    d. NK Cell
509. Which of the following is *not* involved in Buerger disease?
    a. Nerve
    b. Lymphatics
    c. Small Artery
    d. Vein
510. APACHE II score involves all EXCEPT?
    a. GCS
    b. Arterial PH
    c. Mean BP
    d. Serum amylase
511. In Buerger disease which is the site of pain?
    a. Calf pain
    b. Foot pain
    c. Hand pain
    d. Thigh pain
512. Central line is not put in?
    a. External Jugular Vein
    b. Internal Jugular Vein
    c. Femoral vein
    d. Subclavian vein
513. Rectal temperature in hypothermia should be < than _____ degree Celsius?
    a. 35
    b. 35.5
    c. 36
    d. 36.5
514. Which of the following is most common cancer leading to death?
    a. Lung cancer
    b. Oral cancer
    c. Skin cancer
    d. Prostate cancer
515. All are true regarding Leptospirosis EXCEPT:
    a. Water contamination by Rat urine
    b. Jaundice
    c. Uraemia
    d. Drug of choice is ciprofloxacin
516. Defective DNA repair is seen in all EXCEPT?
    a. Xeroderma pigmentosum
    b. Fredreich's ataxia
    c. Werner syndrome
    d. Bloom syndrome
517. Which is incorrect about Paget's disease?
    a. Bone pain
    b. Elevated alkaline phosphatase
    c. Biphosphonates are used
    d. Low output cardiac failure
518. What is the etiology behind Mycosis fungoides
    a. Viral Infection
    b. Bacterial Infection
    c. Fungal Infection
    d. Malignancy
519. Chemotherapeutic agent acting as an Immunomodulator
    a. Lenalidomide
    b. Cisplatin
    c. Irinotecan
    d. Mycophenolate
520. Marker test for vertical transmission of HIV
    a. p24 antigen
    b. Serum ELISA
    c. Western blot
    d. Immunoblot
521. Case of 30 year chronic smoker male, visited your clinic with this condition. Diagnosis:

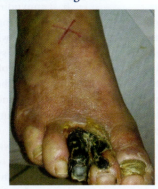

    a. Diabetic gangrene
    b. Buerger's disease
    c. Atherosclerotic plaque
    d. Septic foot
522. A 20-year-old boy after Road Traffic Accident with CT Abdomen. The patient is having abdominal distention and no urine output. Likely cause is?
    a. Spleen rupture
    b. Bladder rupture
    c. Renal shutdown
    d. Pneumothorax
523. What is shown in the image below?

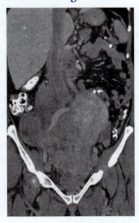

    a. CT scan
    b. MRI scan
    c. Digital X-ray
    d. Bone Scintigraphy
524. Brodie Tredelenburg test is done for?
    a. Sapheno-femoral incompetence
    b. Deep Vein thrombosis
    c. Varicose veins
    d. Superficial migratory thrombophlebitis
525. Myelin figures in necrosis is due to?
    a. Loss of glycogen
    b. Dilated mitochondria
    c. Phospholipid precipitates
    d. Pyknosis

BOARD REVIEW QUESTIONS

526. Which drug is usually not preferred in treatment of HIV with TB?
a. Efavirenz
b. Lamivudine
c. Stavudine
d. Nevirapine

527. Pancoast's triad includes all of the following EXCEPT?
a. Shoulder pain
b. Horner's syndrome
c. Hemoptysis
d. Atrophy of hand muscles

528. Most sensitive investigation for cystic fibrosis is?
a. CT scan
b. Ultrasound
c. Sweat electrolytes
d. Tomogram

529. ECG changes in Hypokalemia are?
a. Tall T wave
b. Large P wave
c. Short QT interval
d. Presence of U waves

530. Drug of choice for American trypanosomiasis is?
a. Miltefosine
b. Amphotericin
c. Antinomy
d. Nifurtimox

531. Hemiballismus is due to lesion of?
a. Contralateral thalamus
b. Contralateral subthalamus
c. Ipsilateral thalamus
d. Ipsilateral subthalamus

532. Investigation of choice for diagnosis of Epilepsy is?
a. EEG
b. CT scan
c. MRI
d. CSF investigation

533. Elevated JVP is seen in
a. Corpulmonale
b. Pneumonia
c. ARDS
d. Pleural effusion

534. Which of the following is seen in sarcoidosis:
a. Hypercalcemia
b. Hypocalcemia
c. Hyperphosphatemia
d. Hypophosphatemia

535. Sequel of rheumatic heart disease in a 5 year old child is:
a. Mitral stenosis
b. Mitral regurgitation
c. Tricuspid stenosis
d. Tricuspid regurgitation

536. Aldosterone is secreted by
a. Pituitary
b. Zonaglomerulosa
c. Zona fasciculate
d. Adrenal medulla

537. Glucose fever is seen due to:
a. Adrenal disease
b. Diabetes mellitus
c. Glucagonoma
d. Hyperthyroidism

538. Duke score is used for?
a. Infective endocarditis
b. Stable angina
c. Unstable angina
d. Esophageal varices grading

539. Priapism is called
a. Involuntary erection
b. Involuntary painful erection >2 hours
c. Persistent painful erection for >4 hours
d. Persistent non tender erection >4 hours

540. Which of the following drugs used for Diabetes Mellitus causes lactic acidosis:
a. Phenformin
b. Metformin
c. Glipizide
d. Pioglitazone

541. CURB 65 criteria include all EXCEPT:
a. Age is always more than or equal to 65 years
b. Respiratory rate more than 30/min
c. Systolic Blood pressure is more than 90 mm Hg
d. BUN level is >7 mmol/L

542. Most common type of emphysema is:
a. Panacinar emphysema
b. Irregular emphysema
c. Centriacinar emphysema
d. Paraseptal emphysema

543. Not a diagnostic criteria for rheumatoid arthritis?
a. Rheumatoid nodules
b. RA factor
c. Anti-cyclic citrullinated phospholipid antibody
d. PIP, MCP, Wrist arthritis

544. Broadbent sign is seen in
a. Acute pericarditis
b. Constrictive pericarditis
c. S.L.E
d. Libman sacks endocarditis

545. Weight gain is seen in all except
a. Hypothyroidism
b. Insulinoma
c. Type 2 diabetes mellitus
d. Carcinoid syndrome

546. Drug of choice for focal seizure is:
a. Carbamazepine
b. Valproate
c. Ethosuximide
d. Clobazam

547. Which is not a feature of SLE?
a. Serositis
b. Synovitis
c. Arthritis
d. Low complement level

548. Metabolic acidosis is seen in?
a. Raised ICT
b. Hypotension
c. Status asthmaticus
d. Conn syndrome

549. Hypokalemia is seen in:
a. RTA-1
b. RTA-2
c. RTA-3
d. RTA-4

550. Acute renal failure results in:
a. Hyperkalemic alkalosis
b. Hypokalemic alkalosis
c. Hyperkalemic acidosis
d. Hypokalemic acidosis

551. Hemolytic anemia is associated with the following gall stones:
a. Pigmented
b. Mixed
c. Cholesterol
d. None

552. Cell of origin of epileptic seizures is
a. Pyramidal cells
b. Schwann cells
c. Oligodendrocytes
d. Stellate cells

Medicine

553. **Most common tumour to metastasize to spine is**
   a. Carcinoma lung   b. Carcinoma breast
   c. RCC   d. Carcinoma prostate

554. **Bovine cough is seen in**
   a. Croup   b. Epiglottitis
   c. Foreign body   d. Laryngeal paralysis

555. **Normal anion gap is seen in:**
   a. Diabetic ketoacidosis   b. Lactic acidosis
   c. Starvation ketoacidosis d. Renal tubular acidosis

556. **Berry sign is?**
   a. Obliteration of carotid pulse
   b. Dancing carotid artery
   c. Carotid thrill
   d. Carotid artery bruit

557. **SIADH leads to?**
   a. Hyponatremia   b. Hypernatremia
   c. Hypokalemia   d. Hyperkalemia

558. **Myelopathy does not occur in**
   a. Tabes dorsalis   b. Syringomyelia
   c. Polyneuritic leprosy
   d. Sub-acute combined demyelination of cord

559. **Drug of choice for exercise induced asthma is?**
   a. Inhaled steroids   b. Salmeterol
   c. Formoterol   d. Ketotifen

560. **What is not reabsorbed from PCT of kidney:**
   a. Glucose   b. Bicarbonate
   c. Calcium   d. Phosphate

561. **Hyperkalemia is seen with**
   a. RTA 1
   b. RTA 2
   c. RTA 4
   d. Nephrogenic diabetes insipidus

562. **Most common cause of stroke is**
   a. Carotid artery atherosclerosis
   b. Hypertension
   c. Trauma
   d. Cyanotic heart disease

563. **What is not a feature of Millard gubler syndrome?**
   a. Ptosis   b. Squint
   c. Facial weakness   d. hemiparesis

564. **Most common cause of death in the world is:**
   a. CAD   b. Stroke
   c. Accident   d. Infection

565. **Bulging anterior fontanelle in a neonate with vacant stare is suggestive of diagnosis of?**
   a. Neonatal meningitis
   b. Intra-ventricular haemorrhage
   c. Hydrocephalus
   d. Status marmoratus

566. **Vascular dementia is seen in**
   a. Parkinsonism   b. Alzheimer's
   c. Lacunar stroke   d. Huntington's chorea

567. **Most common part of heart involved in carcinoid syndrome**
   a. Inflow Right side   b. Inflow left side
   c. Outflow left side   d. All of the above

568. **Which is the best test for pheochromocytoma**
   a. 24 hour urinary VMA
   b. Plasma fractionated metanephrine levels
   c. Plasma catecholamines
   d. MIBG scan

569. **IOC for Cushing syndrome**
   a. Low dose dexamethasone suppression test
   b. High dose dexamethasone suppression test
   c. Plasma ACTH
   d. Plasma CRH

570. **All of the following drugs are useful in preventing post prandial rise of sugar EXCEPT**
   a. Sitagliptin   b. Canagliflozin
   c. Acarbose   d. Repaglinide

571. **Most common type of epilepsy in children is:**
   a. Subtle seizure   b. Absence seizure
   c. Benign rolandic epilepsy d. Grand mal epilepsy

572. **What is the duration of symptoms for generalised convulsive status epilepticus**
   a. 5 minutes   b. 15 minutes
   c. 30 minutes   d. 60 minutes

573. **Word salad is a feature of**
   a. Lesion in inferior frontal gyrus
   b. Lesion in superior frontal gyrus
   c. Lesion in superior temporal gyrus
   d. Lesion in inferior temporal gyrus

574. **Most common cause of death in Subarachnoid haemorrhage is:**
   a. Rebleeding   b. Vasospasm
   c. Re-rupture   d. Dyselectrolytemia

575. **Most common site of Hemorrhagic stroke?**
   a. Parenchyma   b. Internal capsule
   c. External capsule   d. Interventricular

576. **Blast crisis is seen in?**
   a. ALL   b. AML
   c. CML   d. CLL

577. **Radiation causes all blood cancers EXCEPT?**
   a. ALL   b. AML
   c. CML   d. CLL

578. **All are features of blood cancer EXCEPT**
   a. Sternal tenderness
   b. Anemia
   c. Marrow hypoplasia
   d. Hyperleucocytosis

579. **First hormone to be supplemented in Sheehan syndrome**
   a. Cortisol   b. GH
   c. Thyroxine   d. Estrogen

603

Questions

580. Weight gain with Cushingoid appearance with proximal myopathy occurs due to?
    a. Oat cell cancer of lung
    b. Iatrogenic steroids
    c. TB of adrenals
    d. Waterhouse freidschen syndrome
581. Which is not included in the triad of Parkinsonism?
    a. Masked facies   b. Resting tremors
    c. Bradykinesis   d. Cog wheel rigidity
582. Dementia pugilistica is characterised by development of
    a. Extradural haemorrhage b. Epi-dural haemorrhage
    c. Cortical atrophy   d. Fine tremors of tongue
583. Fasciculations are seen in?
    a. Motor neuron disease   b. Stroke
    c. Paralysis agitans   d. Pseudo-tumour cerebri
584. Not involved in Gullian-Barre syndrome?
    a. Motor involvement
    b. Sensory involvement
    c. Autonomic involvement
    d. Bladder and bowel involvement
585. Heel pad thickness is measured in
    a. Myxedema
    b. Angioedema
    c. Acromegaly
    d. Marfan syndrome
586. AED stands for?
    a. Automated external defibrillator
    b. Automatic external defibrillator
    c. Automatic electrical defibrillator
    d. Automated electrical defibrillator
587. Most common cause of Hyperparathyroidism is?
    a. Parathyroid adenoma
    b. Parathyroid hyperplasia
    c. Thyroid carcinoma
    d. Medullary carcinoma thyroid
588. Ipsilateral third nerve lesion & contralateral hemiplegia is seen in?
    a. Weber syndrome   b. Parinaud syndrome
    c. Foville syndrome   d. Wallenburg syndrome
589. Whole thickness of bowel is involved with skin lesions in?
    a. Crohn's disease
    b. Ulcerative colitis
    c. Irritable bowel disease
    d. Both crohn's and ulcerative colitis
590. Most common site of ulcerative colitis is?
    a. Rectum   b. Caecum
    c. Small intestine   d. Appendix
591. Treatment of choice for Hepatorenal syndrome is?
    a. ACE inhibitors
    b. Calcium channel blockers
    c. Peritoneal dialysis
    d. Liver transplant
592. Most common cause of upper GI bleed is?
    a. Esophageal varices   b. Gastric erosion
    c. Peptic ulcer   d. Mallory weiss tear
593. Most common primary site for congenital tuberculosis is?
    a. Lungs   b. Lymph nodes
    c. Liver   d. Skin
594. Most common renal condition in HIV patient is?
    a. Membranoproliferative glomerulonephritis
    b. Focal segmental glomerulosclerosis
    c. Membranous glomerulonephritis
    d. Diffuse proliferative glomerulonephritis
595. Acute endocarditis with abscess is most commonly associated with?
    a. Listeria   b. Staphylococcus
    c. Streptococcus   d. Enterococcus
596. Early loss of bladder control is seen in?
    a. AMLS   b. Conus medullaris
    c. Caudal equine   d. Guillain barre syndrome
597. Parkinsonism is associated with which metal?
    a. Mg   b. Se
    c. Mn   d. Mo
598. CNS tumor which is most commonly associated with HIV?
    a. Lymphoma   b. Glioma
    c. Astrocytoma   d. Medulloblastomas
599. Burst suppression EEG pattern is seen in?
    a. Herpes simplex encephalitis
    b. Absence seizures
    c. Myoclonic epilepsy
    d. Hypothermia
600. Auer rods are seen in which subtype of AML?
    a. M0   b. M1
    c. M3   d. M5
601. Cystatin C is used for?
    a. Diagnosis of acute renal failure
    b. Transplant survival
    c. Sepsis
    d. Pancreatitis
602. Increased VMA is seen in?
    a. Pheochromocytoma   b. Tyrosinemia
    c. Parkinsonism   d. Phenylketonuria
603. A 20-year-old girl presents with pain in abdomen and purpuric rash all over the body, most probable diagnosis is?
    a. HUS   b. Kawasaki disease
    c. ITP   d. HSP
604. Wide fixed split S2 is seen in?
    a. ASD   b. VSD
    c. TOF   d. TAPVC
605. Which of the following is not seen in hypothyroidism?
    a. Edema   b. Cold skin
    c. Diastolic hypertension d. Atrial fibrillation

Medicine

606. Best marker of iron deficiency anemia is?
    a. Serum iron
    b. Serum ferritin
    c. Total iron binding capacity
    d. Transferrin saturation

607. Schilling test is done for?
    a. Vitamin B12 deficiency
    b. Folic acid deficiency
    c. Vitamin B6 deficiency
    d. Vitamin D deficiency

608. Burkitt's lymphoma is due to which virus?
    a. EBV   b. HTLV-1
    c. HHV-8   d. Adenovirus

609. Conventional site for taking biopsy in secondary amyloidosis is?
    a. Liver   b. Kidney
    c. Rectum   d. Abdominal fat aspirate

610. Most common cause of death in primary amyloidosis is?
    a. Respiratory failure   b. Cardiac failure
    c. Renal failure   d. Septicemia

611. Treatment for restless leg syndrome is?
    a. Ropinirole   b. Haloperidol
    c. Carbamezapine   d. Gabapentin

612. Cranial nerve most commonly involved in cranial aneurysms?
    a. 3rd nerve   b. 4th nerve
    c. 5th nerve   d. 6th nerve

613. Hemiplegia is most commonly due to Occlusion of?
    a. Middle Cerebral Artery b. Basilar artery
    c. Vertebral artery   d. Anterior cerebral artery

614. Most common site of Hypertensive intracerebral bleed is?
    a. Pons   b. Putamen
    c. Frontal lobe   d. Thalamus

615. Broca's aphasia is seen due to lesion in?
    a. Precentral gyrus   b. Inferior frontal gyrus
    c. Superior temporal gyrus d. Inferior temporal gyrus

616. Wernicke's aphasia is seen due to lesion in?
    a. Precentral gyrus   b. Inferior frontal gyrus
    c. Superior temporal gyrus d. Inferior temporal gyrus

617. Central pontine myelinolysis is seen with rapid correction of?
    a. Hypermagnesemia b. Hyponatremia
    c. Hyper kalemia   d. Hypokalemia

618. Drug of choice for acute exacerbation of ulcerative colitis is?
    a. Sulfasalazine   b. Mesalazine
    c. Steroids   d. NSAID's

619. Muller's sign is seen in?
    a. Mitral stenosis   b. Aortic stenosis
    c. Mitral regurgitation d. Aortic regurgitation

620. Restrictive cardiomyopathy is seen in?
    a. Amylodosis   b. Fatty change of heart
    c. Viral myocarditis   d. Doxorubicin toxicity

621. ASO titre is diagnostic in?
    a. SABE
    b. Rheumatoid arthritis
    c. Infective endocarditis
    d. Acute rheumatic fever

622. Acute chest syndrome is caused by?
    a. Sickle cell anemia
    b. Pneumonia
    c. Acute myocardial infarction
    d. Penetrating chest trauma

623. Enzyme missing is refsum's disease is?
    a. Sphingomyelinase
    b. Phytanoyl-CoA α-hydroxylase
    c. Alpha-galactosidase-A
    d. N-acetylglucosaminidase

624. First line drug used for painful diabetic neuropathy is?
    a. Carbamazepine   b. Duloxetine
    c. Venlafaxine   d. EMLA

625. Artery involved in 3rd cranial nerve lesion?
    a. Anterior communicating
    b. Posterior communicating
    c. Posterior cerebral
    d. Anterior cerebral

626. Dose of anti-D in idiopathic thrombocytopenic purpura?
    a. 75 mg/kg
    b. 150 mg/kg
    c. 200 mg/kg
    d. 300 mg/kg

627. Acute kidney injury in RIFLE criteria is?
    a. Urine output <0.5 ml/kg/h for >8 hours
    b. Urine output <0.5 ml/kg/h for > 12 hours
    c. Urine output <0.3 ml/kg/h for > 24 hours
    d. Anuria for > 12 hours

628. Antibody responsible for photosensitivity in SLE is?
    a. Anti-Sm   b. Anti-Ro
    c. Antihistone   d. Anti-La

629. Most common cause of renal artery stenosis above 50 years of age is?
    a. Atherosclerosis
    b. Fibromuscular dysplasia
    c. Takayasu arteritis
    d. RCC

630. Least commonly affected site in arterial thromboembolism is?
    a. Liver   b. Kidney
    c. Heart   d. Brain

631. Most common lymph node involved in Hodgkin's lymphoma is?
    a. Inguinal
    b. Cervical
    c. Axillary
    d. Subclavian

605

Questions

FMGE Solutions Screening Examination

632. Takayasu arteritis mainly affects?
   a. Pulmonary artery
   b. Celiac artery
   c. Subclavian artery
   d. SMA

633. Which among the following is true about iron deficiency anemia?
   a. Increased ferritin
   b. Increased TIBC
   c. Increased saturation
   d. Macrocytic hypochromic anemia

634. Drug of choice for Madura mycosis is?
   a. Imipenem
   b. Dapsone
   c. Itraconazole
   d. Amikacin

635. Antihypertensive used in angina pectoris is?
   a. Alpha blocker
   b. Beta blocker
   c. Calcium channel blockers
   d. ACE inhibitors

636. Most common cause of intraventricular bleed is?
   a. SDH
   b. EDH
   c. SAH
   d. Parenchymal bleed

637. FEV1/FVC is decreased in?
   a. Asthma
   b. Kyphosis
   c. Scoliosis
   d. Fibrosis

638. Most common complication of cardiac catheterization?
   a. Arrhythmia
   b. Hypertension
   c. Vascular bleeding
   d. Contrast reaction

639. Specific antibody for SLE is?
   a. Anti sm antibodies
   b. Anti-ds DNA antibodies
   c. Anti-Histone antibodies
   d. Anti Ro (SS-A) antibodies

640. Pulsus bigeminy is seen in?
   a. Digitalis
   b. Beta blockers
   c. ACE inhibitors
   d. Calcium channel blockers

641. Drug of choice in post diabetic peripheral neuropathy?
   a. Pregabalin
   b. Amitryptyline
   c. Carbamazepine
   d. Valproate

642. Judkins technique is used for?
   a. Central venous line placement
   b. Coronary arteriography
   c. Renal angiography
   d. Chest tube insertion

643. Carcinoid of heart presents as?
   a. Aortic stenosis
   b. Tricuspid regurgitation
   c. Mitral stenosis
   d. Aortic regurgitation

644. Most common mode of spread of congenital tuberculosis is?
   a. Lymphatics
   b. Hematogenous
   c. Local spread
   d. None

645. Which ion channel is affected in hypokalemic periodic paralysis?
   a. K+   b. Na+
   c. Cl-   d. Ca2+

646. Gaisbock syndrome is known as?
   a. Primary familial polycythemia
   b. High-altitude erythrocytosis
   c. Spurious polycythemia
   d. Polycythemia vera

647. In case of chest pain with pericarditis and pericardial effusion, pain is refered by?
   a. Phrenic nerve
   b. Vagus nerve
   c. Trigeminal nerve
   d. None

648. Most common cause of dilated cardiomyopathy is?
   a. Alcohol
   b. Viral infection
   c. Pregnancy
   d. Metabolic disease

649. Osborne waves in ECG is seen in?
   a. Hypothyroidism   b. Hypothermia
   c. Hypocalcemia   d. Hypercalcemia

650. Most common LMN cause of facial nerve palsy is?
   a. Trauma   b. Bell's palsy
   c. Infections   d. Vascular causes

651. Aphasia which affects the arcuate fibres is called?
   a. Global aphasia   b. Anomic aphasia
   c. Conduction aphasia   d. Broca's aphasia

652. Koenen's tumor are seen in?
   a. Neurofibromatosis
   b. Tuberous sclerosis
   c. Sturge weber syndrome
   d. Tuberculosis

IMAGE-BASED QUESTIONS

653. Test shown is:

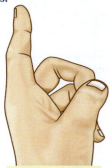

a. Card Test
b. Froment's Sign
c. Pointing index
d. Pen Test

654. Diverticulosis appearance on barium enema as shown is called:

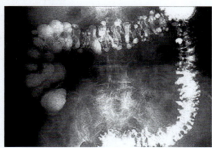

a. Saw tooth appearance
b. Cork screw appearance
c. Bird of prey appearance
d. Claw sign

655. A 65-year-old diabetic with extensive sweating and dizziness?

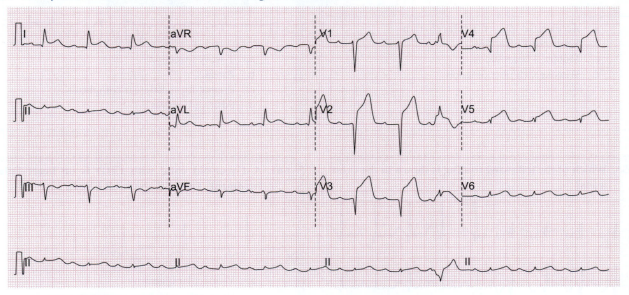

a. Hypoglycemia
b. Hypoglycemic Unawareness
c. Anterior wall MI
d. Inferior wall MI

656. A 35-year-old lady has been diagnosed as having anxiety neurosis by her psychiatrist. She came to you for second opinion. Comment on the diagnosis based on ECG?

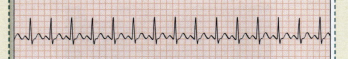

a. Sinus tachycardia
b. WPW syndrome
c. Multifocal atrial tachycardia
d. Atrial fibrillation

659. What ECG finding is shown here?

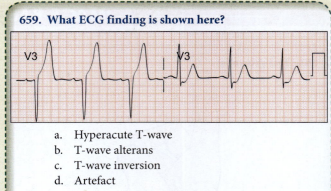

a. Hyperacute T-wave
b. T-wave alterans
c. T-wave inversion
d. Artefact

657. A 60-year-old patient is having recurrent syncopal attacks post myocardial infarction. The ECG shows?

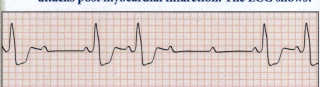

a. Accelerated idioventricular rhythm
b. Ventricular bigeminy
c. Mobitz II heart block
d. Wenckebach phenomenon

660. What ECG finding is shown here?

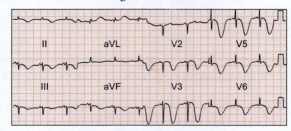

a. T-wave inversion
b. Artifact
c. Premature ventricular complexes
d. Positive U waves

658. Which of the following finding is shown in the chest leads?

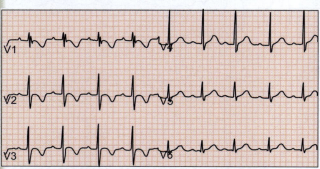

a. Myocardial ischemia
b. Myocardial injury
c. Digoxin
d. Digoxin toxicity

661. A 1-year-old child with CHD is on heart failure treatment. The ECG shows all EXCEPT?

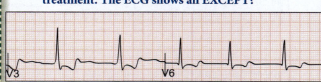

a. Ventricular bigeminy
b. Heart rate of 60 bpm approximately
c. ST depression
d. U wave

Medicine

662. A 65-year-old man is brought with complaints of breathlessness and chest pain for 18 hours. ECG was done. Which of the following is incorrect?

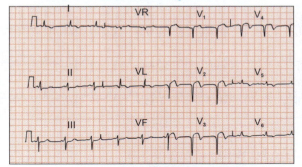

a. Normal sinus rhythm   b. Normal axis
c. ST elevation in V2-V4
d. Premature ventricular contractions

664. A 50-year-old woman with rheumatic heart disease is on medication for heart disease. She feels unwell for most part of the day. Which of the following medicine is responsible for the ECG changes shown below?

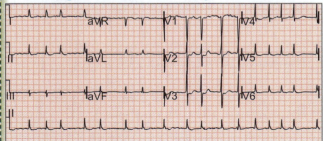

a. ACE inhibitor   b. Diuretics
c. Ivabradine   d. Digoxin

663. A 10-year-old child of valvular heart disease on heart failure treatment, has the following ECG tracing. What is the diagnosis?

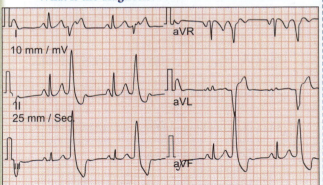

a. Tall tented T wave
b. Ventricular bigeminy
c. Non paroxysmal atrial tachycardia with irregular AV block
d. Non paroxysmal atrial tachycardia with regular AV block

665. A 25-year-old woman presents with complaints of recurrent episodes of sudden onset palpitations. What does her ECG tracings show?

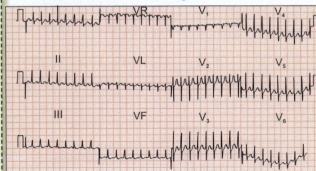

a. Atrial flutter
b. Atrial bigeminy
c. PSVT
d. Sinus tachycardia

FMGE Solutions Screening Examination

666. A 65-year-old pensioner in ESI dispensary complains of exercise intolerance. On auscultation a systolic murmur grade 3 is heard. What does the ECG show?

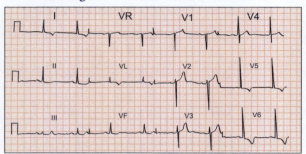

a. Normal tracing
b. Left ventricular hypertrophy
c. Atrial fibrillation
d. Left bundle branch block

667. Identify the ECG given in the figure below?

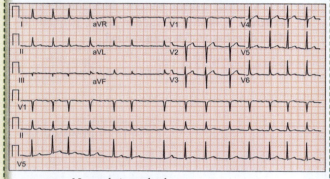

a. Normal sinus rhythm
b. Paroxysmal supraventricular tachycardia
c. Atrial fibrillation
d. Ventricular fibrillation

668. In the ECG shown below which drug will not be given?

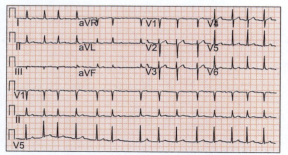

a. Amiodarone   b. Adenosine
c. Diltiazem   d. Beta blocker

669. 65-year-old elderly male has history of sweating and chest pain for last 24 hours with the following ECG. Which of the following is not given in managing the patient?

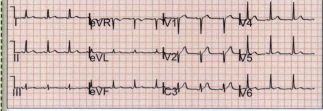

a. Aspirin
b. Statin
c. Thrombolytic therapy
d. Morphine

670. A 52-year-old male diabetic patient presents with palpitations to the AIIMS emergency. Urgent ECG was performed. What is the immediate next step in the management?

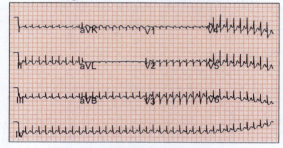

a. Electrical cardioversion
b. Amiodarone
c. Adenosine   d. Primary PCI

671. A 75-year-old male patient presents to the AIIMS emergency with retrosternal chest pain for 6 hours. The following ECG was done. What will be the primary management of the patient?

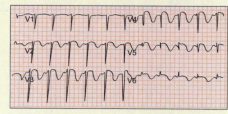

a. Primary PCI   b. Thrombolysis
c. Abciximab
d. Low molecular weight heparin

Medicine

672. For calculation of rate related (corrected) QT interval, QT interval is divided by √ X?

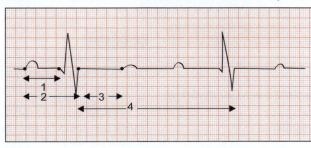

   a. 1 b. 2
   c. 3 d. 4

673. The marked part of the ECG points to which phase of cardiac action potential?

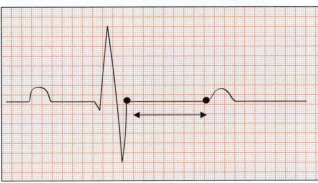

   a. Phase 0 b. Phase 1
   c. Phase 2 d. Phase 3

674. What does the following ECG show?

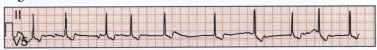

   a. Osbourne wave b. Delta wave
   c. Hockey stick sign d. Epsilon wave

Answers to Image-Based Questions are given at the end of explained questions

FMGE Solutions Screening Examination

ANSWERS WITH EXPLANATIONS

MOST RECENT QUESTIONS 2019

1. **Ans. (a) 9T**

   Ref: Harrison 20th ed. pg. 3183 and NCBI Bookshelf

   - Opening eyes on command = 3
   - Moving limbs/obeying commands = 6
   - Intubated = T
   - The total score is 9T

   The maximum score in intubated patient can be 10T and minimum as 2T.

   > **Extra Mile**
   >
   > **Glasgow coma scale- P**
   > The GCS-P is calculated by subtracting the Pupil Reactivity Sore (PRS) from the Glasgow Coma Scale (GCS) total score:
   > - GCS-p GCS - PRS
   > - The Pupil Reactivity Sore is calculated as follows:
   >
   > **Pupils unreactive to light - Pupil Reactivity Score**
   > - Both pupils - 2
   > - One pupil - 1
   > - Neither pupil - 0

2. **Ans. (c) Generalized paresis**

   Ref: 5-minute Neurology, Consult ed. pg. 32

   Postural tremor occurs when limb is positioned against gravity. It is seen in choices A, B and D. General **paresis** is a late manifestation of neurosyphilis and is characterized by delusion of grandiosity.

   Mnemonic
   P: Personality
   A: Affect
   R: Reflexes (Hyperactivity)
   E: Argyll Robertson Pupil
   S: Sensorium (hallucinations, delusions)
   I: Intellect deterioration
   S: Speech defects

   > **Extra Mile**
   >
   > Classification of tremors and their characteristics and treatment

   TABLE : Classification of tremors and their characteristics and treatment

Type of Tremor	Frequency	Occurrence	Etiology	Treatment
Postural tremor	5–9 Hz	When limb is positioned against gravity	Physiologic tremor, essential tremor, alcohol or drug withdrawal, metabolic disturbances, drug-induced tremor, psychogenic tremor	Beta blockers, primidone (Mysoline), acetazolamide (Diamox), clonazepam (Klonopin), botulinum toxin, brain gabapentin (Neurontin), deep stimulation thalamotomy
Rest tremor	3–6 Hz	When limb is fully supported against gravity and the muscles are not voluntarily activated	Parkinson's disease, multiple systems atrophy, progressive supranuclear palsy, drug-induced tremor, rubral tremor, psychogenic tremor	Levodopa- carbidopa (Sinemet), anticholinergics and other antiparkinsonian agents, deep brain stimulation, pallidotomy, thalamotomy
Action tremor+	3–10 Hz	During any type of movement	Cerebellar lesions, rubral tremor, psychogenic tremor	Wrist weights, isoniazid

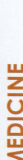

Medicine

3. Ans. (a) Viruses

Ref: Harrison 20th ed. pg. 2851

The leading cause of fulminant diabetes is viral insult that damages the beta cells of pancreas and can lead to development of type 1 diabetes mellitus.

4. Ans. (d) Foot

Ref: Harrison 20th ed. pg. 2642

- The distribution of joint involvement in diabetic neuropathy is tarsal and tarsometatarsal joints of foot.
- In tabes dorsalis knees, hips and ankles are most commonly affected
- In syringomyelia, Glenohumeral joint, elbow and wrist are involved.

Extra Mile

TABLE: Disorders associated with neuropathic joint disease

Diabetes mellitus	Amyloidosis
Tabes dorsalis	Leprosy
Meningomyelocele	Congenital indifference to pain
Syringomyelia	Peroneal muscular atrophy

5. Ans. (a) Regular

Ref: CMDT 2019, pg. 1256

- Immediately after initiation of fluid replacement, regular insulin can be given intravenously in loading dose of 0.1 unit/kg as a bolus to prime the tissue insulin receptors.
- Subsequently IV infusion of insulin at 0.1 units/kg/Hour are continuously infused or given hourly as an intramuscular injection is sufficient to replace the insulin deficit in most patients.

6. Ans. (a) Glargine

Ref: CMDT 2019, pg. 1238

Glargine is called peak-less insulin. It acts after 0.5 hour and has a flat curve with effective duration of 24 hours.

Insulin preparations	Onset of action	Peak action	Effective duration
Insulins lispro, aspart,[1] glulisine	5-15 minutes	1-1.5 hours	3-4 hours
Human regular	30-60 minutes	2 hours	6-8 hours
Human NPH	2-4 hours	6-7 hours	10-20 hours
Insulin glargine	0.5-1 hour	Flat	~24 hours
Insulin determir	0.5-1 hour	Flat	17 hours

Contd...

Insulin preparations	Onset of action	Peak action	Effective duration
Insulin degludec	0.5-1.5 hours	Flat	More than 42 hours
Technosphere inhaled insulin	5-15 minutes	1 hour	3 hours

[1]Insulin aspart formulated with niacinamide has ~10 minutes faster onset of action.

7. Ans. (a) Bitemporal hemianopia

Ref: Harrison, 20th ed. pg. 2676

Physical findings most commonly encountered in patients with hyperprolactinemia are galactorrhea and, in the case of prolactinomas, visual-field defects. Choices B, C and D are not physical findings but symptoms.

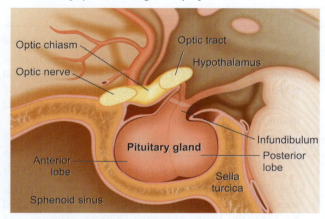

Notice the position of optic chiasma with respect to anterior pituitary in the line diagram shown here.

8. Ans. (a) Weber syndrome

Ref: Harrison 20th ed. pg. 191

Weber syndrome occurs due to occlusion of posterior cerebral artery P1 segment. It leads to compromise of oculomotor nerve and crus cerebri. Due to involvement of crus cerebri corticospinal pathway is affected. Since the corticospinal pathway crosses over at the lower border of medulla contralateral hemiplegia occurs.
Brain stem stroke always leads to crossed hemiplegia.

CARDIOLOGY

9. Ans. (d) Intravenous access followed by Immediate defibrillation

Ref: Harrison, 20th ed. pg. 2064

One cycle of CPR is for 2 minutes and chest compressions are given@100-120/min. intravenous access is done after defibrillation and not before. Hence Choice D is wrong.

FMGE Solutions Screening Examination

Ventricular fibrillation of pulseless ventricular tachycardia

Chest compressions at 100–120/min immediate defibrillation and resume CPR for 2 minutes

↓ No ROSC

2 minutes of chest compressions/ventrilation and repeat shock

↓ No ROSC

Continue chest compressions, IV or IO access, advanced airway
Epinephrine 1 mg 3–5 minutes
Repeat shock

↓ No ROSC

I.V. amiodarone 300 mg (may repeat 150 mg), continue CPR repeat shock

---

10. Ans. (b) Myocardial ischemia

Ref: Harrison, 20th ed. pg. 1680

The ECG shows heart rate of 70/min with T wave inversion noted in leads V1 to V4. This indicates possible myocardial ischemia. Choice A and D are ruled out as there is no ST elevation. Pulmonary embolism leads to $S_1Q_3T_3$ pattern and in this case limb leads are not seen.

11. Ans. (c) Lasix, Nitrates and morphine

Ref: Harrison, 20th ed. pg. 1771

The CXR shows evidence of bat wing oedema which is seen with Acute decompensated CHF which is managed by LMNOP: Lasix, Morphine, Nitrates, Oxygen and Positioning of the patient.

12. Ans. (a) Peripheral Pulmonic stenosis

Ref: Harrison, 20th ed. pg. 1674

Continuous murmurs are seen in:
- Peripheral pulmonic stenosis
- Coarctation of aorta
- Patent ductus arteriosus
- Rupture of sinus of Valsalva
- Mammary souffle
- Venous Hum

13. Ans. (b) Decrease in systolic blood pressure 20 mm Hg within 3 min of postural change

Ref: AHA clinical Cardiac Consult pg. 280

Orthostatic hypotension is defined as decrease of BP> 20 mm Hg systolic and Diastolic >10 mm Hg accompanied with symptoms of cerebral hypoperfusion.

14. Ans. (a) Start thrombolysis

Ref: Harrison, 20th ed. pg. 3081, 3087

The patient has presented with features of right sided cortical stroke leading to focal deficits on the left side. How to Interpret the normal CT head given in the question?

> Haemorrhagic stroke is ruled out
> - Most importantly *CT scan showing no haemorrhage or oedema >1/3 of MCA territory is an indication for thrombolysis* (Table 420-1 20th edition Harrison)

- In this scenario, the patient is treated as a case of ischemic stroke and managed with thrombolysis. The cut off for management of Thrombolysis is >4.5hours from symptom onset.
- *The closest choice is choice B which is used for management of Transient Ischemic attack. As per the definition of TIA symptoms resolve within 24 hours and most cases within one hour (Page 3087). TIA usually resolves before presenting to the physician.*
- Choice C, BP should not be lowered in CNS events as it mantains brain perfusion. Only if BP is >185/110 mm Hg that lowering of BP should be done before initiating thrombolysis.

15. Ans. (d) Intravenous Procainamide

Ref: Harrison, 20th ed. pg. 1741

Anti-dromic tachycardia implies conduction via the accessory pathway in Wolf Parkinson White syndrome and retrograde conduction via the bundle of His. DOC for management of acute episode in WPW is procainamide and to prevent episodes of fast conduction flecainide is given. Since patient is hemodynamically stable DC shock is ruled out.

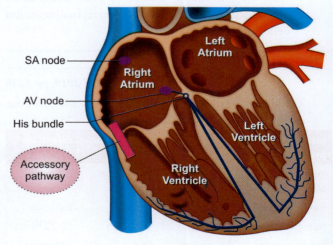

Medicine

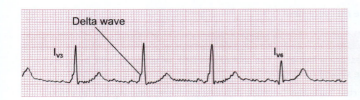

16. Ans. (a) Treadmill

Ref: Harrison, 20th ed. pg. 1742

- Wolf Parkinson White syndrome has an accessory pathway called Bundle of Kent that bypasses the normal conduction system in the heart. The faster conduction in these patients leads to complaints of tachycardia, dizzy spells and recurrent syncopal episodes.
- Choice B is correct as for these patients Holter monitoring (continuous ECG monitoring using a device worn by the patient for 24 hours) should be done to identify the tendency for arrythmias.
- Choice C is correct as Beta blockers can control the fast beating ventricular rate.
- Choice D is correct as Procainamide slows the conduction via bundle of Kent leading to current to go via normal route and termination of a tachycardia episode.

17. Ans. (d) 1-minute gap between 2 shocks

Ref: AHA 2015 Guidelines

The time lag between two Defibrillation shocks is 2 minutes during which CPR is continued at a rate of 30:2.

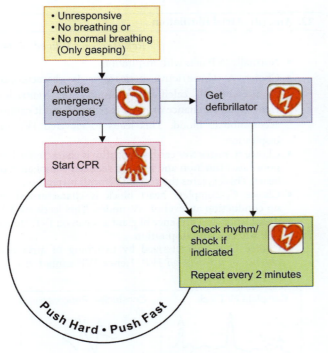

Figure: Simplified adult BLS algorithm

18. Ans. (d) Infective endocarditis

Ref: Harrison 20th ed. pg. 925

Major Criteria

- Blood culture positive for IE
  - Typical microorganisms consistent with IE from separate blood cultures
    - Viridans streptococci; *Streptococcus bovis*, HACEK group, *Staphylococcus aureus*, or
    - Community-acquired enterococci, in the absence of a primary focus
  - Microorganisms consistent with IE from persistently positive blood cultures, defined as follows:
    - At least two positive blood cultures of blood samples drawn > 12 h apart; or
    - All of three or a majority of ≥4 separate cultures of blood (with first and last sample drawn at least 1 h apart)
  - Single positive blood culture for *Coxiella burnetii* or antiphase I IgG antibody titer >1:800
- Evidence of endocardial involvement
- Echocardiogram positive for IE (TEE recommended in patients with prosthetic valves, rated at least "possible IE" by clinical criteria, or complicated IE [paravalvular abscess]; TTE as first test in other patients), defined as follows:
  - Oscillating intracardiac mass on valve or supporting structures, in the path of regurgitant jets, or implanted material in the absence of an alternative anatomic explanation; or
  - Abscess; or
  - New partial dehiscence of prosthetic valve
- New valvular regurgitation (worsening or changing or pre-existing murmur not sufficient)

Minor criteria

- Predisposition, predisposing heart condition or injection drug use
- Fever, temperature >38°C
- Vascular phenomena, major arterial emboli, septic pulmonary infarcts, mycotic aneurysm, intracranial hemorrhage, conjunctival hemorrhages, and janeway lesions
- Immunologic phenomena: Glomerulonephritis, Osler nodes, Roth's spots and rheumatoid factor
- Microbiological evidence: Positive blood culture but does not meet a major criterion as noted previously (excluding single positive cultures for coagulase-negative staphylococci and organisms that do not cause endocarditis) or serologic evidence of active infection with organisms consistent with IE
- Echocardiographic minor criteria eliminated

19. Ans. (a) False elevation of BP

Ref: AHA BP Measurement Guidelines

During BP recording the cuff should cover 80% of arm circumference. In case the BP cuff is undersized it will over estimate the BP value while an over sized cuff will under estimate the actual BP values.

FMGE Solutions Screening Examination

American Heart Association guidelines for in-clinic blood pressure measurement

Recommendation	Comments
Patient should be seated comfortably, with back supported, legs uncrossed, and upper arm bared.	Diastolic pressure is higher in the seated position, whereas systolic pressure is higher in the supine position
	An unsupported back may increase diastolic pressure; crossing the legs may increase systolic pressure
Patient's arm should be supported at heart level.	If the upper arm is below the level of the right atrium, the readings will be too high; if the upper arm is above heart level, the readings will be too low.
	If the arm is unsupported and held up by the patient, pressure will be higher.
Cuff bladder should encircle 80 percent or more of the patient's arm circumference.	An undersized cuff increases errors in measurement
Mercury column should be deflated at 2 to 3 mm per second.	Deflation rates greater than 2 mm per second can cause the systolic pressure to appear lower and the diastolic pressure to appear higher

20. Ans. (b) HDL

Ref: Harrison, 20th ed. pg. 1851

High density lipoprotein plays a role in reverse cholesterol transport from tissues and is cardioprotective in nature.

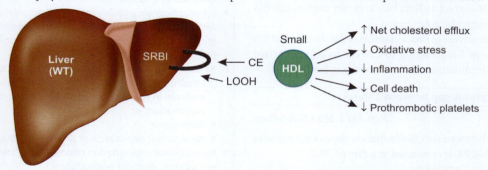

21. Ans. (c) Persistent Chest pain with ST elevation >90 minutes after thrombolysis

Ref: Harrison, 20th ed. pg. 1879

Rescue PCI should be done in case of failure of reperfusion which is defined as Persistent Chest pain and ST segment elevation >90 minutes.

> **Extra Mile**
>
> *Primary PCI* is done in cases of STEMI and should have a door to device time of less than 90 minutes.
> *Delayed PCI* is done in cases of NSTEMI and has no time guidelines unlike above subtypes.
> *PCI with drug eluting stents* is used in cases of single and double vessel disease in case of chronic stable angina.
> Window period for thrombolysis in STEMI is 12 hours

22. Ans. (d) Atrial fibrillation

Ref: Harrison 19th ed. P 444

- Normally JVP falls with inspiration.
- Choice A, Constrictive pericarditis is characterized by presence of calcification around the ventricles. Hence the compliance of heart is reduced and it cannot accommodate blood. This leads to elevated JVP on inspiration.
- Choice B, restrictive cardiomyopathy is characterized by poor heart function and leads to reduced compliance of heart. This explains the rise of JVP with inspiration.
- Choice C, complete heart block is characterized by no conduction at level of AV nodes. This leads to A:V dissociation and presence of giant a waves on JVP. Hence JVP will rise with inspiration.
- Choice D is characterized by twitching of atria and *absence of a waves on JVP*. Hence JVP cannot rise on inspiration.

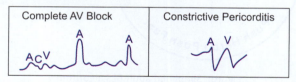

Medicine

23. Ans. (b) Atrial depolarization with A-V conduction

Ref: Harrison 19th ed. P 1451

P wave	Atrial depolarization
PR interval	Atrial depolarization and AVN conduction
Q	Septal activation
QRS	Ventricular depolarization
QT	Ventricular repolarization plus ventricular repolarization

24. Ans. (b) Left ventricular hypertrophy

Ref: Harrison 19th ed. P 1658-59

- Pulmonary artery hypertension is due to constriction of pulmonary bed secondary to chronic hypoxia.
- Interstitial lung disease leads to lung shrinkage, and mitral stenosis due to pulmonary edema leads to hypoxia. Hence PAH will develop.
- Cor-pulmonale is right sided heart failure due to pulmonary artery hypertension. Leading cause of Cor-pulmonale is COPD.

25. Ans. (a) B$_1$ deficiency

Water hammer pulse is seen in high output cardiac failure caused by wet beri-beri. The development of CHF can explain the pedal/periorbital edema of the patient.

26. Ans. (a) Prolonged QT

QT interval shows an inverse relation with values of calcium and magnesium.

Must know information about QT interval
- 360–440 msec (9–10 small, squares)
- Measured in lead II or V5 –V6

QT prolongation	QT shortening
• *Hypocalcemia* • Hypomagnesemia • Hypokalemia (prolonged QU interval) • Class IA and III drugs • Subarachnoid hemorrhage • Long QT syndrome • Romano ward syndrome	• *Hypercalcemia* • Digoxin • Congenital short QT syndrome

27. Ans. (a) Internal mammary artery

Long-term patency rates are considerably higher for internal mammary and radial artery implantations than for saphenous vein grafts. In patients with left anterior descending coronary artery obstruction, survival is better when coronary bypass involves the internal mammary artery rather than a saphenous vein.

28. Ans. (b) ASD

PDA	Narrow split S2
ASD	Wide fixed S2
TOF	Single S2
VSD	Wide variable split S2

29. Ans. (a) Tall tented T wave

The earliest ECG finding of hyperkalemia is tall tented T wave.

Serum potassium	ECG changes
5.5–6.5 mM	Tail peaked T waves
6.5–7.5 mM	Loss of P waves
7–8 mM	Wide, qRS, PR prolongation
>8 mM	Sine wave pattern

Treatment

Intervention	Lowering of potassium	During	Comments
Calcium gluconate or calcium chloride	No change in potassium levels	Effect starts in 1–3 minutes and lasts for 30–60 minutes	Reduces excitability of heart and is the drug of choice
Insulin drip (**most effective drug** to lower K$^+$ concentration)	0.5–1.5 mmol/L	4–6 hours	Redistribution of potassium by sending potassium inside cells
Parenteral or nebulized salbutamol	0.5–1.0 mmol/L	Full effect takes up to 24 hours	Sorbitol in enema omitted in post-operative patients due to increased incidence of sorbital-induced colonic necrosis
Hemodialysis		(**Most effective method** to lower potassium)	Refractory life threatening hyperkalemia failing to respond to conventional measures

Explanations

617

FMGE Solutions Screening Examination

30. Ans. (b) PSVT

- The heart rate is 150 bpm
- Axis is normal
- P waves are absent with narrow complex QRS
- ST segment depression is noted in lead II
- The diagnosis is PSVT

31. Ans. (a) QT = 0.04 sec

Normal QT interval is 360-440 milli-seconds (Average 400 msec). The QT interval is written wrongly as 0.04 seconds where as it is 0.4 seconds.

32. Ans. (c) Atenolol

ACE ⊖ are used to prevent ventricular remodelling in chronic CCF. β blockers like carvedilol metoprolol and bisoprolol reduce myocardial oxygen consumption. Atenolol is not useful in chronic CCF.

Drugs used in chronic CHF with EF <40%

Diuretics
Furosemide
Hydrochlorothiazide
Metolazone
Angiotensin converting enzyme inhibitors
Captopril
Enalapril
Lisinopril
Ramipril
Antiotensin receptor blockers
Valsartan
Candesartan
Irbesartan
Losartan
β receptor blockers
Carvedilol
Bisoprolol
Metoprolol Succinate

Contd...

Additional therapies
Spironolactone
Eplerenone
Combination of hydralazine/isosorbide dinitrate
Fixed dose of hydralazine/isosorbide dinitrate digoxin

33. Ans. (a) Diuretics

- The heart rate is about 70 bpm and axis is normal.
- P, PR interval and QRS complex is of normal duration.
- Lead II and chest lead V3 shows T wave inversion with presence of U waves suggestive of hypokalemia.
- Choice B and C lead to Hyperkalemia and tall tented T waves whereas in the ECG given the T waves are inverted.
- Choice D is ruled out as bradycardia is not present.

34. Ans. (d) Ventricular Tachycardia (VT)

The image shows a broad complex QRS suggestive of diagnosis of ventricular tachycardia.

35. Ans. (d) Given along with adrenaline

Ref: AHA 2015 Guidelines

Ventricular fibrillation or pulseless ventricular tachycardia

Immediate defibrillation within 5 minutes of onset: 60–90 seconds of CPR before defibrillation for delay ≥5 minutes

If return of circulation fails

5 cycles of CPR followed by repeat shock: repeat sequence twice, if needed

If return of circulation fails

Continue CPR, Intubate, IV Access

Epinephrine, 1 mg IV or Vasopressin, 40 units IV; follow with repeat defibrillation at maximum energy within 30–60 seconds as required; repeat epinephrine

If return of circulation fails

Epinephrine, ↑dose | Antiarrhythmics | $NaHCO_3$, 1 mEq/kg(↑K^+)

Amiodarone: 150 mg over 10 min, 1mg/min lidocaine: 1.5 mg/kg; repeat in 3–5 min

Magnesium sulfate: 1–2 g I.V.(Polymorphic VT) Procainamide: 30 mg/min, to 17 mg/kg (limited use-see text)

If return of circulation fails

Defibrillate, CPR: Drug-Shock-Drug-Shock

36. Ans. (c) Amiodarone

Ref: AHA 2015 Guidelines

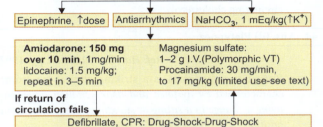

37. Ans. (b) Cardiac tamponade

Ref: Harrison, 19th ed. pg. 1573

JVP Findings

JVP Waves	Findings Constrictive pericarditis	Findings Cardiac tamponade
X wave	Prominent	Prominent
Y wave	Prominent	Absent[Q]

38. Ans. (a) Atrial fibrillation

Ref: Harrison, 19th ed. pg. 1487-88

- Beta blockers, nondihydropyridine calcium channel blockers (e.g., verapamil or diltiazem), and digitalis glycosides are useful in slowing the ventricular rate of patients with AF.
- Digitalis, because left ventricular muscle function usually is normal in mitral stenosis, the use of digitalis is of little benefit to patients in sinus rhythm. In patients in atrial fibrillation, however, digitalis is used to slow ventricular rate. A rapid ventricular rate in mitral stenosis shortens diastole, thereby reducing left ventricular filling, which, in turn, further increases left atrial pressure and reduces cardiac output. β-Blockers and diltiazem or verapamil may be added to digoxin if further heart rate control is necessary.

39. Ans. (a) Right 2nd intercostal, low pitch murmur

Ref: Harrison, 19th ed. pg. 144B

- Aortic stenosis is the most common cause of a mid-systolic murmur in an adult.
- *The murmur of AS is low to medium pitch and rasping or harsh in character.*
- It is usually loudest to the right of the sternum in the second intercostal space (aortic area) and radiates into the carotids.
- Mid-systolic murmurs begin at a short interval after S_1, end before S_2, and are usually crescendo-decrescendo in configuration.

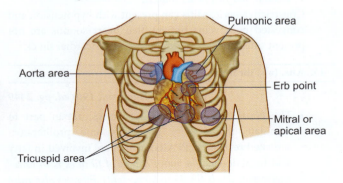

- Transmission of the mid-systolic murmur to the apex, where it becomes higher-pitched, is common (Gallavardin effect). This can cause misdiagnosis with murmurs of mitral regurgitation.

40. Ans. (b) Inferior to rib

Causes of inferior rib notching
- Arterial: Aortic coarctation, aortic thrombosis, pulmonary-oligemia/AV malformation, Blalock Taussig shunt, Tetralogy of fallot, absent pulmonary artery and pulmonary stenosis.
- Venous: AV Malfomations of chest wall, superior vena cava or other central venous obstruction.
- Neurogenic: Intercostal neuroma, Neurofibromatosis type 1, poliomyelitis.
- Osseous: Hyperparathyroidism, Thalassemia

Causes of superior rib notching
- Poliomyelitis
- Osteogenesis Imperfecta
- Neurofibromatosis
- Marfan's syndrome
- Collagen vascular disease
- Hyperparathyroidism.

41. Ans. (d) Troponin I

Ref: Braunwald, 8th ed. Table 50-4

Biomarker	Range of Times to Initial Elevation (hr)	Mean Time to Peak Elevations (Nonreperfused)	Time to Return to Normal Range
Frequently Used in Clinical Practice			
MB-CK	4–6	24 hours	48–72 hours
cTnI	3	24 hours	5–10 days
cTnT	3	12 hours–2 days	5–14 days
Infrequently Used in Clinical Practice			
Myoglobin	1–4	6–7 hours	24 hours

42. Ans. (a) Cardiac Tamponade

Ref: Harrison, 18th ed. chapter 238

Beck's triad is a collection of three medical signs associated with acute cardiac tamponade, an emergency condition wherein fluid accumulates around the heart and impairs its ability to pump blood. The signs are:
1. *Low arterial blood pressure*
2. *Distended neck veins*
3. *Distant, muffled heart sounds.*

Constrictive pericarditis can present with hypotension and congested neck veins but muffled heart sounds are not present. Auscultatory finding heard is pericardial shock.

43. Ans. (a) Fibrates

Ref: Harrison, 19th ed. pg. 2449

- The *fibrates, or fibric acid derivatives*, act in part to stimulate the activity of peroxisome proliferator-activated receptors (PPARs), which are involved in fatty acid breakdown. *The main action of fibrates is to lower triglyceride levels (by 35 to 50 percent). Fibrates also raise serum high density lipoprotein (HDL) by 15 to 25 percent. Fibrates are the drugs of choice when treating isolated elevated triglycerides.*
- *Niacin*, fibrates, and prescription omega-3 fatty acids are approved for the treatment of patients with hypertriglyceridemia.
- *Statins* (or HMG-CoA reductase inhibitors) are a class of cholesterol lowering drugs that inhibit the enzyme HMG-CoA reductase which plays a central role in the production of cholesterol.
- *Ezetimibe* inhibits the absorption of cholesterol from the small intestine and decreases the amount of cholesterol normally available to liver cells, leading them to absorb more from circulation and thus lowering levels of circulating cholesterol.

44. Ans. (d) Platypnea

Ref: Harrison, 19th ed. pg. 1992

- Platypnea-orthodeoxia is a striking clinical syndrome characterized by *dyspnea and deoxygenation accompanying a change to a sitting or standing from a recumbent position*.
- In orthopnea (reverse findings are seen) the dysnea is seen in supine position and reduces in sitting position. It is usually due to acute CHF and bilateral diaphragmatic hernia.

Causes of Platypnea

- ASD or PFO with position-dependent shunting
- Other Cardiac conditions
  - Atrial Myxoma[Q]
  - Constrictive pericarditis
  - Aortic aneurysm
- Pulmonary
  - Multiple pulmonary emboli
  - Pulmonary emphysema
  - Radiation-induced bronchial stenosis
  - Hepatopulmonary syndrome[Q]
  - Amiodarone toxicity of the lungs
  - Pulmonary A-V communications
  - Fat embolism syndrome
- Autonomic
  - Parkinson disease
  - Bilateral thoracic sympathectomy
- Abdominal
  - Hepatic cirrhosis
  - Ileus

Medicine

45. Ans. (b) Cardiac Biomarkers

Ref: Harrison, 19th ed. pg. 1580

- Cardiac markers are used in the diagnosis and risk stratification of patients with chest pain and suspected acute coronary syndrome (ACS).
- The cardiac troponins, in particular, have become the cardiac markers of choice for patients with acute coronary syndrome which includes NSTEMI.
- *However in chronic Stable angina the symptoms arise on exertion/emotion or post-prandially and have characteristic ST segment depression on exercise testing. Cardiac biomarkers are normal as no cell death occurs in this case.*

46. Ans. (a) Aortic regurgitation

Ref: Harrison, 19th ed. pg. 411

Duroziez's sign is seen in severe aortic regurgitation, *gradual pressure over the femoral artery leads to a systolic and diastolic bruit.* The systolic murmur is heard best when the proximal femoral artery is compressed and the diastolic when the distal femoral artery is compressed.

47. Ans. (c) Erythema Marginatum

Ref: Harrison, 19th ed. pg. 2149

Morning stiffness is seen in Rheumatoid arthritis, while the question is on Rheumatic fever. Erythema Marginatum is a major Jones criteria for diagnosis of Rheumatic Fever.

Revised Jones criteria (2015 update)

A. Diagnosis

For all patient populations with evidence of preceding gas infection
Initial ARF – 2 Major or 1 major plus 2 minor
Recurrent ARF- 2 Major or 1 major and 2 minor or 3 minor

B. What are major criteria?

Low-risk populations	Moderate-and high-risk population
• Carditis 　■ Clinical and/or subclinical carditis	• Carditis 　■ Clinical and/or subclinical carditis
• Arthritis 　■ Polyarthritis only	• Arthritis 　■ Monoarthritis or polyarthritis 　■ Polyarthralgia
• Chorea	• Chorea
• Erythema marginatum	• Erythema marginatum

Contd...

Revised Jones criteria (2015 update)

• Subcutaneous nodules	• Subcutaneous nodules

C. What are the minor criteria

Low-risk populations	Moderate-and high-risk population
• Polyarthraigia	• Monoarthralgia
• Fever ($\geq$38.5°)	• Fever ($\geq$38°C)
• **ESR$\geq$60 mm** in 1st hour and/or CRP $\geq$3.0 mg/d	• **ESR$\geq$30** mm/h and /or CRP $\geq$3.0
• Prolonged PR interval, after accounting for age variability (unless carditis is a major criterion) in all population	

48. Ans. (a) Staphylococcus aureus

Ref: Harrison, 19th ed. pg. 816

- Overall *S. aureus* infection is the most common cause of IE, including Prosthetic Valve Endocarditis, acute Infective Endocarditis, and IVDA(Intravenous drug Abuse) Infective Endocarditis.
- The mortality rate of *S. aureus* IE is 40-50%.

49. Ans. (b) Autoimmune

- Post-MI pericarditis following myocardial infarction is called Dressler syndrome and is an *autoimmune process.*
- *It also seen* as an unusual complication after percutaneous procedures such as coronary stent implantation, after implantation of epicardial pacemaker leads and transvenous pacemaker leads,and following blunt trauma,stab wounds,and heart puncture.

50. Ans. (a) Coarctation of aorta

Ref: Harrison, 19th ed. pg. 1525

- Coarctation of Aorta is most common cause of rib notching. It Usually involves the posterior 4th - 8th Ribs.
- *Collateral flow* bypassing the aortic constriction to reach the abdomen and lower extremities comes almost entirely from the two *subclavian arteries* via the thyrocervical, costocervical, and *internal mammary arteries* and their subdivisions to the *posterior intercostals* and then into the descending aorta.
- The large volume of blood traversing this route, and increased pulsation of the *intercostal arteries*, leads to erosion of lower border of ribs.

FMGE Solutions Screening Examination

51. Ans. (c) Anti-hypertensive drugs

Ref: Harrison, 19th ed. pg. 1622

The question is incomplete but none the less asks about diastolic hypertension which can be a presentation of essential hypertension. Hence to reduce the diastolic overload of the heart, anti-hypertensive drugs are required for this case.

Causes of Isolated Diastolic Hypertension are
- Essential hypertension
- Hypothyroidism
- Conn syndrome

52. Ans. (d) Lisinopril

Ref: Harrison, 19th ed. pg. 1623, 18th ed. ch. 247

- *ACEIs* attenuate the development of left ventricular hypertrophy, improve symptomatology and risk of death from CHF, and *reduce morbidity and mortality rates in post-myocardial infarction patients.*
- *Similar benefits in cardiovascular morbidity* and mortality rates in patients with CHF have been *observed with the use of ARBs.*
- ACEIs provide better coronary protection than do calcium channel blockers, whereas calcium channel blockers provide more stroke protection than do either ACEIs or beta blockers.

53. Ans. (b) Resistance to 3 or more anti-hypertensive drugs including thiazides

Ref: Harrison, 18th ed. chapter 247

- *Resistant hypertension* refers to patients with blood pressures persistently >140/90 mm Hg despite taking three or more antihypertensive agents, including a diuretic, in a reasonable combination and at full doses.
- Resistant or difficult-to-control hypertension is more common in patients >60 years than in younger patients.
- Resistant hypertension may be related to:
  - "Pseudoresistance" (high office blood pressures and lower home blood pressures), nonadherence to therapy
  - Identifiable causes of hypertension (including obesity and excessive alcohol intake

54. Ans. (d) Shock

Ref: Harrison, 18th ed. chapter 233 and 238

- The CXR shows increased CT ratio which points to probable diagnosis of Dilated cardiomyopathy
- Patients dilated cardiomyopathy are predisposed to development of arrhythmia.
- Since atrial fibrillation is common, embolic stroke can occur and can lead to development of sudden death.

55. Ans. (b) QRS complex

Ref: Harrison, 19th ed. pg. 1489

- The origin of premature beats/ventricular extra systoles in the ventricle at sites remote from the Purkinje network produces slow ventricular activation and a wide QRS complex that is typically >140 ms in duration.
- Ventricular premature complexes are common and increase with age and the presence of structural heart disease.

56. Ans. (a) Right atrium (RA)

Ref: Chapter 227, Harrison, 18th ed.

■ **NORMAL JVP = 5-8 CM OF WATER**

- Elevated JVP is indicative of right sided CHF
- Kussmaul sign is seen in constrictive pericarditis
- *Kussmaul sign is not seen in cardiac tamponade*
- Canon a waves are seen AV dissociation/ventricular tachycardia/junctional tachycardia

57. Ans. (a) Benign hypertension

Ref: Robbins, 8th ed. chapter 10

- **Hyaline arteriolosclerosis,** the vascular lesion associated with hypertension, is both more prevalent and more severe in diabetics.
- It takes the form of an *amorphous, hyaline thickening of the wall* of the arterioles, which causes narrowing of the lumen.
- It is encountered frequently in elderly patients, whether normotensive or hypertensive, hyaline arteriolosclerosis is more generalized and more severe in patients with hypertension.

58. Ans. (b) Left atrium

Ref: Robbins, 8th ed. Chapter 11

Mural endocardial lesions can be seen as *MacCallum* plaques in rheumatic heart disease. These plaques appear as map-like areas of thickened, roughened, and wrinkled part of the endocardium in the left atrium. They are *caused by regurgitant jets of blood flow, due to incompetence of the mitral valve.*

59. Ans. (b) Complete heart block

Ref: Harrison, 18th ed. chapter 227

- The 'a' wave reflects right atrial contraction and occurs just after the electrocardiographic P wave, preceding the first heart sound (S_1).
- The *a* wave is not present with atrial fibrillation.

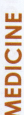

- Canon *a* wave occurs with
  - Atrioventricular (AV) dissociation/complete heart block due to right atrial contraction against a closed tricuspid valve.
  - Wide complex tachycardia like ventricular tachycardia
- A prominent *a* wave is seen in patients with reduced right ventricular compliance like Right ventricular failure.

60. Ans. (d) Marfan syndrome

Ref: Harrison, 19th ed. pg. 2512

- Etiology of an aneurysm may affect the incidence of dissections. Atherosclerosis, when advanced, typically results 4 in medial and adventitial fibrosis, which hampers the development of dissections. *Dissections are common in Marfan syndrome, idiopathic T.A.A (thoracic aorta aneurysm).*

61. Ans. (c) Purkinje fibres have the slowest conduction

Ref: Harrison, 19th ed. pg. 265e-12

- Purkinje fibers have the fastest speed of conduction of 4 metres/second.
- The dominant pacemaker is the SAN due to its automaticity and the lowest RMP of all the pacemakers.

62. Ans. (a) Atrial fibrillation

Ref: Harrison, 19th ed. pg. 1443-1444

- A wave in JVP is due to atrial contraction. In atrial fibrillation, since the atria are twitching, the power of atria is reduced to a level that a wave would be absent.
- Heart block will have large a waves.
- Tricuspid Regurgitation has absent x and large v waves.
- Constrictive Pericarditis has a large y descent.

63. Ans. (b) Junctional tachycardia

Ref: Harrison, 19th ed. pg. 1480

Atrial fibrillation	Absent 'a' waves
Junctional tachycardia	The AVN node becomes the dominant pacemaker and simultaneously depolarizes the Atria and ventricles. Hence the AV valves might not be open and hence the atria will contract against the closed AV valves resulting in very large a waves
Constricitive pericarditis	Due to impaired compliance of ventricles, rapid ventricular filling occurs leading to steep y
Cardiac tamponade	Absent ý waves

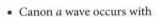

Medicine

64. Ans. (c) Duration of mid-diastolic murmur

Ref: Harrison, 19th ed. pg. 1539

- Severity of mitral Stenosis implies that the mitral valve orifice has become smaller in size. This implies that the blood will take longer time to go from left atrium to left ventricle. This implies the LENGTH Of murmur will increase.

65. Ans. (d) Chest compressions

Ref: Harrison, 19th ed. pg. 1768

- According to AHA 2015 guidelines, the basic life support entails C_A_B and a shift from ABC protocol. Therefore the first thing to be done is chest compressions@100 times per minute. The depth of sternal depression should be 2 inches (5 cm)
- ALSO remember that in Advance cardiac life support the drugs used are epinephrine, vasopressin and amiodarone. ATROPINE has been withdrawn and this is a change from 2005 guidelines.

66. Ans. (d) Atrial depolarization

ECG finding	Significance
P wave	Atrial Depolarization
QRS	Ventricular depolarization
T wave	Ventricular repolarization
U wave	Delayed repolarization of papillary muscles
PR interval	Spread of impulse from SAN to AVN
ST segment	Iso-electric segment

67. Ans. (a) Tall tented T waves

Ref: Harrison, 19th ed. pg. 310

Serum potassium > 5.5 mEq/L is associated with repolarization abnormalities:
- Peaked T waves (usually the earliest sign of hyperkalemia)

Serum potassium > 6.5 mEq/L is associated with progressive paralysis of the atria.
- P wave widens and flattens
- PR segment lengthens
- P waves eventually disappear

Serum potassium >7.0 mEq/L is associated with conduction abnormalities and bradycardia:
- Prolonged QRS interval with bizarre QRS morphology
- High-grade AV block with slow junctional and ventricular escape rhythms, followed by sine wave appearance.

FMGE Solutions Screening Examination

Serum potassium level of > 9.0 mEq/L causes cardiac arrest due to:
- Asystole
- Ventricular fibrillation

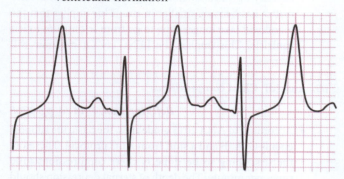

68. Ans. (d) Treatment with steroids is necessary

- Dressler syndrome is post MI pericarditis/Pleuritis and is characterized by autoimmunity causing damage to the heart. The resultant inflammation causes chest pain in these patients upto 6 weeks of a preceding myocardial inflammation. The investigations show ECG evidence of pericarditis with ST elevation with concavity in upwards direction. The CPKMM levels are normal. The treatment of these patients shall be aspirin 650 mg TID.

69. Ans. (b) Hypertension

Ref: Harrison, 19th ed. pg. 1640

- *70% cases of aortic dissection occur due to hypertension.* The tear occurs in tunica media and causes a tearing pain in the chest with maximum intensity in interscapular area. The IOC for aortic dissection is trans-esophageal echocardiography > MRI chest.
- Marfan syndrome also can present with aortic dissection, which in fact is the leading cause of death in these patients. Syphilis involves the arch of aorta and causes an aneurysm that can rupture any day.

70. Ans. (a) Troponin I

Ref: Harrison, 19th ed. pg. 1600

- The best test for diagnosis of MI is troponin I which can be quantified as value more than 0.04 ng/dl after 3 hours of onset of myocardial infarction.

Remember TROPONIN-I can be false positive in the following cases

Cardiac causes	Noncardiac causes
Cardiac contusion resulting from trauma	Pulmonary embolism

Contd...

Cardiac causes	Noncardiac causes
Cardiac surgery	Severe pulmonary hypertension
Cardio eversion	Renal failure
Endomyocardial biopsy	Stroke, subarachnoid hemorrhage
Acute and chronic heart failure	Infiltrative disease, e.g, amyloidosis
Aortic dissection	Cardiotoxic drugs

71. Ans. (d) Warfarin

Ref: AHA 2016 update: Secondary prevention of MI

- Aspirin and clopidogrel have been shown to reduce mortality due to MI.
- Statins regress atherosclerosis and β blockers due to oxygen conserving action will prevent future episode of MI.
- Warfarin is not routinely used in post MI Patients.

72. Ans. (a) Aortic stenosis

Ref: Harrison pg. 19th ed. pg. 1529

- Reverse split S2 implies aortic valve closes very late to a level that it closes after the pulmonic valve closure (Normally aortic valve closes first and then pulmonic valve).
- **This occurs in severe aortic stenosis** where the valvular obstruction makes the work of left ventricle harder. The longer ejection time leads to delayed closure of aortic valve. Due to this delayed closure the split becomes narrowed
- *In mitral stenosis loud S1 is seen. In pulmonary artery hypertension loud P2 is seen. In pulmonic stenosis single S2 is seen.*

73. Ans. (d) Wide QRS complex

Ref: Harrison, 19th ed. pg. 310

ECG Findings of Hyperkalemia

- The first ECG finding in hyperkalemia is tall tented T waves followed by slowing of depolarization of heart.
- This results in prolonged PR interval with QRS widening.
- Subsequently the P waves start becoming smaller.
- Sine wave pattern leading to ventricular fibrillation/ diastolic arrest of heart.

Medicine

74. Ans. (d) Alcohol

Ref: Harrison, 19th ed. pg. 95e-5

- Alcohol in mild amounts has been shown to have beneficial effect on heart. All of you would have heard and read about benefits of red wine.
- Studies have shown chylamydia as incriminating factor for atherosclerosis and so does poor dental hygiene.

75. Ans. (a) Cardiophrenic angle

Ref: Harrison, 19th ed. pg. 1719

Most common site of pericardial cyst is cardiophrenic angle.

> **Extra Mile**
> - *Anterior mediastinal* tumors are **thymoma, lymphoma, pheochromocytoma,**
> - *Posterior mediastinal* tumors are **neurogenic tumors** (20% of mediastinal tumors).
> - *Middle mediastinal* tumors are **pericardial cyst, bronchogenic cyst, thyroid mass, tracheal tumors.**

76. Ans. (a) Total anomalous pulmonary venous connection

Ref: Nelson, 18th ed. / ch 431

Conditions	Radiological findings
Total anomalous pulmonary venous connection	Figure of 8 or snowman heart
Transposition of great arteries	Egg on side appearance
TOF	Boot shaped heart
Ebstein anomaly	Box shaped heart

77. Ans. (b) Aortic regurgitation

Ref: Harrison, 19th ed. pg. 1534

Pulse pressure is SBP – DBP. In aortic stenosis or mitral stenosis SBP is low leading to reduction of pulse pressure. In tricuspid stenosis since the blood flow into right side of heart is reduced, so is left side inflow and therefore reduction in SBP.

Other Changes in Pulse Pressure Include
- Increased pulse pressure: Aortic regurgitation, Aortic sclerosis
- Decreased pulse pressure: Aortic stenosis, Mitral stenosis
- Increased diastolic pressure: Mitral stenosis
- Decreased diastolic pressure: Aortic regurgitation, Patent ductusarteriosus

Causes of wide pulse pressure	
• Atherosclerosis	• Anxiety
• Arteriovenous fistula	• Heart block
• Chronic aortic regurgitation	• Aortic dissection
• Thyrotoxicosis	• Endocarditis
• Fever	• Raised intracranial pressure
• Anemia	
• Pregnancy	

78. Ans. (a) Junctional rhythm

Ref: Harrison, 19th ed. pg. 1443-44

- In Junctional rhythm the inherent AV node is the dominant pacemaker that causes simultaneous activation of atria and ventricles. Normally the Atria contract before the ventricles. Therefore in JUNCTIONAL RHYTHM atria will contract against the closed tricuspid and mitral valves leading to a very large a wave referred to as canon a waves.

REMEMBER *the traditional question on canon a waves is related to complete heart block.*

JVP findings	Conditions
Absent a waves	Atrial fibrillation
Canon a waves	Complete heart block, junctional rhythm, A-V dissociation
Large a waves	Tricuspid stenosis, pulmonic stenosis, pulmonary artery hypertension.

79. Ans. (c) Venous insufficiency

Ref: Harrison, 19th ed. pg. 253

- Edema is defined as a palpable swelling caused by an increase in interstitial fluid volume. The most likely cause of leg edema in patients over age 50 is venous insufficiency.
- The most important cause of unilateral pedal edema is also venous insufficiency which must be evaluated using a Doppler exam.

80. Ans. (b) Diastolic dysfunction

Ref: Harrison, 19th ed. pg. 1568

- HOCM stands for Hypertrophic Obstructive Cardiomyopathy and is seen in young male athletes.
- Hypertrophic cardiomyopathy is characterized by diastolic dysfunction, attributed to the hypertrophy, fibrosis, and intraventricular gradient when present.
- Asymmetrical septal hypertrophy and hypertrophy of left ventricular wall leads to decrease in LV cavity size.

Clinical Features
1. Dyspnea (MC symptom)
2. Effort intolerance

3. Sub endocardial ischemia leading to angina
4. Sudden death in HOCM is seen in young male players due to ischemic *ventricular fibrillation*.
5. Narrow split S_2 is seen.

Treatment
- Propranolol (decrease heart rate, decrease O_2 consumption) and Verapamil

> **Extra Mile**
>
> **Drugs C/I in HOCM :** Furosemide, ACE Inhibitors, Digoxin, NTG as they will all decrease pre-load, which will lead to decrease flow to right and then left side of heart leading to Decreased SBP

81. Ans. (b) Atropine

Ref: AHA 2010 Guidelines; Management of Cardiac Arrest

82. Ans. (b) Cardiac abnormality

Ref: Harrison, 19th ed. pg. 96e-1t

- **Vitamin B1** deficiency causes Beri-Beri which is of two types- WET BERI-BERI having cardiac failure and DRY BERI-BERI causing CNS problems like Wernicke encephalopathy and Korsakoff psychosis.
- Gingival bleeding and delayed wound healing (choice A) is seen with scurvy. Memory loss is seen with niacin deficiency.

83. Ans. (d) Anaphylaxis

Ref: Harrison 19th ed. pg. 2116

The life-threatening anaphylactic response of a sensitized human appears within minutes after systemic exposure to specific antigen and is manifested by:
- Respiratory distress due to laryngeal edema
- Intense bronchospasm
- Vascular collapse, or by shock without antecedent respiratory difficulty.
- Cutaneous manifestations exemplified by pruritus and urticaria with or without angioedema are characteristic of such systemic anaphylactic reactions.
- Gastrointestinal manifestations include nausea, vomiting, crampy abdominal pain, and diarrhea.

84. Ans. (c) Serum tryptase

Ref: Harrison 19th ed. pg. 2116

- *Elevations of tryptase levels in serum implicate mast cell activation in a systemic reaction and are particularly informative for anaphylaxis* with episodes of hypotension during general anesthesia or when there has been a fatal outcome.
- However, because of the short half-life of tryptase, elevated levels are best detected within 4 hours of a systemic reaction

- Immunoassays using purified antigens can demonstrate the presence of specific IgE in the serum of patients with anaphylactic reactions, and intracutaneous skin testing may be performed after the patient has recovered to elicit a local wheal and flare in response to the putative antigen.

85. Ans. (c) Atherosclerosis

Ref: Harrison 19th ed. pg. 1639

- Abdominal aortic aneurysms <4.0 cm may affect 1–2% of men older than 50 years.
- *At least 90% of all abdominal aortic aneurysms >4.0 cm are related to atherosclerotic disease, and most of these aneurysms are below the level of the renal arteries.*
- Prognosis is related to both the size of the aneurysm and the severity of coexisting coronary artery and cerebrovascular disease.
- *The risk of rupture increases with the size of the aneurysm: the 5-year risk for aneurysms <5 cm is 1–2%, whereas it is 20–40% for aneurysms >5 cm in diameter (remember the percentage asked)*
- Abdominal aortic aneurysm commonly produces no symptoms. It is detected on routine examination as a palpable, pulsatile, expansile, and non-tender mass.
- Some patients complain of strong pulsations in the abdomen; others experience pain in the chest, lower back, or scrotum. Aneurysmal pain is usually a harbinger of rupture and represents a medical emergency.

86. Ans. (d) Calcium chloride

Ref: Harrison, 19th ed. pg. 312

- In a clinical setting of hyperkalemia in 1 year old child, cardiac arrhythmias associated with hyperkalemia *include sinus bradycardia, sinus arrest, slow idioventricular rhythms, ventricular tachycardia, ventricular fibrillation, and asystole.*
- Intravenous calcium serves to protect the heart while measures are taken to correct hyperkalemia.
- Calcium raises the action potential threshold and reduces excitability without changing the resting membrane potential. By restoring the difference between the resting and threshold potentials, calcium reverses the depolarization blockade caused by hyperkalemia.
- *The recommended dose of treatment of hyperkalemia is 10 mL of 10% calcium gluconate (3–4 mL of calcium chloride), infused intravenously over 2 to 3 min with cardiac monitoring.*
- The effect of the infusion starts in 1–3 min and lasts 30–60 min; the dose should be repeated if there is no change in ECG findings or if they recur after initial improvement.

87. Ans. (c) 12–18 months

Ref: Harrison, 19th ed. pg. 1567

- Amyloid involvement of the heart is seen, especially in the elderly population.

Medicine

- Recent data suggests that life expectancy has increased from 6 to 16-20 months in the most common subtype, AL amyloid.
- Gold standard diagnostic test for restrictive cardiomyopathy is right-ventricular biopsy, which demonstrates positivity for Congo Red staining.

88. Ans. (a) CCTA

Ref: Harrison, 19th ed. pg. 270e-4

- *Coronary lesions prone to rupture* and subsequent development of MI have different morphology compared with stable plaques, and *can be evaluated by CCTA* to identify vulnerable plaques before they lead to clinical events. Large plaque volume, low CT attenuation, napkin-ring sign and spotty calcification are all associated with a high risk of acute cardiovascular events in patients.
- Coronary angiography is used to detect percentage of blockage in coronary artery.

NEUROLOGY

89. Ans. (a) Order CT scan

Ref: Harrison, 20th ed. pg. 2072

- Choice C is ruled out since no features of raised ICP are given.
- Choice D is ruled out since BP lowering is done in case of CNS events if the BP >185/110 mm Hg. Moreover, CT is required for diagnosis of a CNS event. At lower BP values, reducing BP would be counterproductive and can lower Brain perfusion.
- Now we have to choose between the two choices CT scan and blood glucose.
- As per the algorithm of management of an unconscious patient, blood sugar levels should be checked first.
- In any unconscious patient of diabetes mellitus, status of blood sugar should be assessed immediately as hypoglycemia/ hyperglycemia would change the line of management.
- Once these two possibilities are ruled out then CT head is to be performed to rule out a CNS event.
- Page 2072: 20th edition of Harrison quotes "the studies most useful in diagnosis of coma are chemical-toxicologic analysis of blood and urine followed by Cranial CT/MRI, EEG and CSF examination".

90. Ans. (d) Diplopia

Ref: Harrison, 19th ed. pg. 3120

- Due to rigidity of vocal cords patient speaks slowly and cannot raise his voice. This is choice A hypophonia/soft voice.

- Choice B is correct as patient of PD cannot start a movement like a normal person.
- Choice C is correct and when it involves upper limb it is called cog wheel rigidity and lower limb involvement is called lead pipe rigidity.

Cardinal features	Other motor features	Nonmotor features
Bradykinesia Rigidity Resting Tremor Gait disturbance/ postural instability	Micrographia Masked facies Reduced eye blink Soft voice Freezing	Anosmia Mood disorders, e.g., depression Sleep disturbances Autonomic disturbances Cognitive impairment/dementia

91. Ans. (a) M. Gravis

Ref: Harrison, 20th ed. pg. 3233

- The presence of muscle weakness/fatiguability with *normal reflexes* is a feature of M. Gravis. Due to lesser number of receptors available at NMJ and rundown presynaptic release of Ach, decremental response to repetitive nerve stimulation is a *hallmark* feature of this disease.
- Guillain barre has segmental demyelination of spinal cord and presents with ascending symmetrical paralysis with areflexia.
- Transverse myelitis also presents with ascending paralysis and areflexia due to spinal cord involvement.
- Traumatic neuritis is a LMNL and leads to flaccidity and areflexia.

92. Ans. (a) Subacute combined demyelination of spinal cord

Ref: Harrison, 20th ed. pg. 152

- The question is framed to check whether the student is aware of vitamin deficiencies that lead to reversible dementia. These are B1, B12 and nicotinic acid(pellagra). Since vitamin B12 deficiency also leads to Subacute combined demyelination of spinal cord, the correct answer is choice A.
- Choice B Acute inflammatory demyelinating polyneuropathy presents as ascending symmetrical flaccid paralysis and is also called Guillain Barre syndrome.
- Choice C is a prion disease and presents as dementia with myoclonic jerks and leads to neuro-degeneration.
- Choice D leads to frontotemporal dementia with inappropriate aggressive behavior.

93. Ans. (d) Gordon reflex

Ref: Oxford Handbook of Neurology, 2nd ed. pg. 605

- Gordon reflex is an alternative method of eliciting the Balbinski sign. It presents as extensor plantar response

when the calf muscle is squeezed. The clinical sign is used to determine whether a lesion of the pyramidal tract exists. The Gordon reflex is closely associated with the Babinski, Chaddock, and Oppenheim reflexes.
- Choice A is seen in Duchene muscular dystrophy
- Choice B is seen in deep vein thrombosis
- Choice C is alternative method eliciting an extensor plantar by providing *tactile stimulus on shin*.

Alternative methods of eliciting Babinski sign

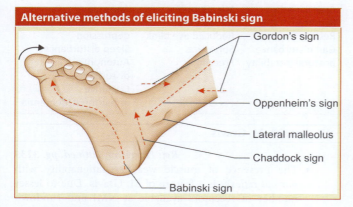

94. Ans. (a) Abducens

Ref: Harrison, 20th ed. pg. 192

The abducens nerve has the longest subarachnoid course and is therefore the most common cranial nerve involved in case of raised ICP. It is also the most common nerve involved in post lumbar puncture or spinal anesthesia.

Extra Mile
- Cranial nerve with longest intracranial route is trochlear nerve
- Only cranial nerve with crossed origin/only one with dorsal origin is trochlear nerve
- Cranial nerve with longest intra-osseous route is facial
- Cranial nerve with longest route overall is Vagus

95. Ans. (a) Mydriasis

Ref: Harrison 20th ed. pg. 541

Due to damage to sympathomimetic fibers, mydriasis cannot occur in Horner syndrome. It is usually caused by lung cancer which is then called Pancoast tumour of superior sulcus tumour.

Features of Horner syndrome : Mnemonic: SAMPLE

S	Sympathetic nerve fiber injury
A	Anhidrosis
M	Miosis
P	Ptosis
L	Loss of ciliospinal reflex
E	Enophthalmos

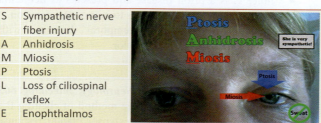

96. Ans. (b) Syringomyelia

Ref: Harrison 19th ed. 2654

- Syringomyelia is characterized by dilatation of syrinx leading to compression of lateral spinothalamic pathways.
- This leads to sensory loss in hands that leads to *painless burn* which is not appreciated by the patient.
- Muscle wasting in the lower neck, shoulders, arms and hands with asymmetric or absent reflexes in arms represents expansion of cavity in gray matter of cord.
- Diabetes mellitus leads to neuropathic ulcers involving the sole of foot.
- Mononeuritis multiplex leads to multiple peripheral neuropathies like carpal tunnel syndrome, tarsal tunnel syndrome, meralgia paresthetica occurring simul-taneously.

Extra Mile
- Expansion of syrinx can lead to involvement of descending tract of trigeminal nerve leading to cough induced headache.
- Characteristic feature of syringomyelia is dissociative anesthesia.
- IOC for syringomyelia is MRI spine

97. Ans. (d) Inability to recognize face

Ref: Harrison 19th ed. P 182

Prosopagnosia is inability to recognize familiar faces including self-image in the mirror. The affected person can identify a face as a face or a car as a car but cannot tell the person or model of car.

The *lesion* lies in occipitotemporal area.

98. Ans. (a) Thiamine

Ref: Harrison 19th ed. P 2607

Wernicke' encephalopathy is manifestation of Dry beriberi.

Extra Mile
- Clinical features are (G.O.A) Global Confusion, ophthalmoplegia and ataxia.
- 1st clinical feature to respond to IV thiamine treatment is ophthalmoplegia.
- 1st to be initiated is intravenous thiamine followed by dextrose.
- Dextrose infusion will first lead to worsening of neurological features
- Best test for thiamine deficiency is serum thiamine levels >> RBC transketolase activity

99. Ans. (d) Anomic aphasia

Ref: Harrison 19th ed. P 178

Metabolic encephalopathy leads to anomic aphasia. The presentation is difficulty in naming an object, word finding pauses, and impaired spelling.

Motor aphasia	Lesion in Broca's area
Sensory aphasia	Lesion in Wernicke's area
Conduction aphasia	Lesion in arcus fasciculus

Medicine

> **Extra Mile**
>
> Anomic aphasia is also seen in
> 1. Alzheimer's disease
> 2. Head trauma
> 3. Metabolic encephalopathy—Uremic encephalopathy, ammonia intoxication

100. Ans. (b) Fomepizole

Ref: Harrison 19th ed. P 473 e-12

Methanol causes ethanol like CNS depression and increased serum osmolality. Formic acid leads to retinal toxicity and manifests as clouding, spots and blindness.

MANAGEMENT

- Gastric aspiration
- Sodium bicarbonate
- High dose folinic acid
- Fomepizole is the DOC and helps in management of high anion gap metabolic acidosis
- Ethanol can be used in absence of fomepizole and is given via nasogastric tube
- Hemodialysis for enhancing methanol elimination and shortening duration of treatment.

101. Ans. (c) Anterior horn cell disease

Ref: Harrison: 19th ed. P 154

- Anterior horn cell disease involves motor neuron in the ventral horn of spinal cord and hence is an example of lower motor neuron disease.
- Prion particles infect the neurons and lead to corticospinal pathway damage.
- Multiple sclerosis is pure white matter disease characterized by plaques.
- Tuberous sclerosis has subependymal nodules in periventricular location. It presents as epilepsy since birth.

102. Ans. (b) Strep pneumonia

TABLE: Causative agents of meningitis age wise

Neonate	Group B streptococcus (India) Klebsiella > E. coli
Child	Pneumococcus
Adult	Pneumococcus
Adult (epidemic)	Meningococcus

103. Ans. (a) Loss of bladder control

Complete Cord Transection Syndrome

Complete cord transection syndrome results in complete loss of all sensibility and voluntary movement below the level of the lesion. It can be caused by fracture dislocation of the vertebral column, by a bullet or stab wound, or by an expanding tumor. The following characteristic clinical features will be seen after the period of spinal shock has ended:

- *Bilateral lower motor neuron paralysis and muscular atrophy in the segment of the lesion*. The result from damage to the neurons in the anterior gray column (i.e lower motor neuron) and possibly from damage to the nerve roots of the same segment.
- *Bilateral spastic paralysis below the level of the lesion*. A bilateral Babinski sign is present, and depending on the level of the segment of the spinal cord damaged, bilateral loss of the superficial abdominal and cremaster reflex occurs. All these signs are caused by an interruption of the corticospinal tract on both side of the cord.
- *Bilateral loss of the sensations below the level of the lesion*. The loss of tactile discrimination and vibratory and proprioceptive sensations is due to bilateral destruction of the ascending tracts in the posterior white column. The loss of pain, temperature, and light touch sensations is caused by section of the lateral and anterior spinothalamic tracts on both sides.
- *Bladder and bowel functions are no longer under voluntary control, since all the descending autonomic fibers have been destroyed.*

If there is a complete fracture dislocations at the L2-3 vertebral level (i.e. a level below the lower end of the cord in the adult), no cord injury occurs and neural damage is confined to the cauda equine, and lower motor neuron, autonomic, and sensory fibers are involved.

104. Ans. (b) Thermal sense

Hemisection of spinal cord is called as Brown Sequard syndrome.

Manifestation of Brown Sequard Syndrome

- *Interruption of the lateral corticospinal tracts*—Ipsilateral spastic paralysis below the level of the lesion and Babinski sign ipsilateral to the lesion (abnormal reflexes and Babinski sign may not be present in acute injury)
- *Interruption of posterior white column*—Ipsilateral loss of tactile discrimination, as well as vibratory and position sensation, below the level of the lesion
- *Interruption of lateral spinothalamic tracts*—Contralateral loss of pain and temperature sensation. This usually occurs 2–3 segments below the level of the lesion

105. Ans. (a) Cerebellum

- Pendular knee jerk is seen in cerebellar lesions
- DTR are normal in basal ganglia damage.
- Hung up reflexes are seen in chorea.
- Hung up ankle jerks are seen in hypothyroidism

FMGE Solutions Screening Examination

Must know points about cerebellar lesions

- Scanning speech: The words are broken into syllable components (Dysarthria).
- Nystagmus
- Hypotonia
- Pendular knee jerk
- Truncal ataxia:
  - Positive Romberg sign, with *eye open*
- Tests for coordination shows incoordination: There will be dysmetria and dyssynergia in the following tests:
  - Finger nose test
  - Balaney's past pointing test
  - Knee heel test
  - Dysdiadochokinesia
- Intention tremor.
- Ataxic gait (Reeling gait)

Site of lesion

- **Cerebellar vermis:** The midline structure is concerned for posture and equilibrium. Lesion at this site causes truncal and gait ataxia.
- **Cerebellar hemispheres:** The smooth conduction of movement (by co-ordinated contraction and relaxation of muscles is controlled by cerebellum. **Lesion in cerebellar hemisphere produces ipsilateral signs**.

106. Ans. (b) Spinocerebellar pathways

- *Unconscious proprioception* is the sensation of limb and joint position and range and direction of limb mediated by *(spinocerebellar pathways and serves as a back up to)* the dorsal column medial lemniscal system.
- Unconscious proprioception involves acquisition and maintenance of skilled motor activities such as walking speaking writing, swallowing, unconscious proprioception.
- *The spinocerebellar pathways, unlike the other sensory pathways follow a two-order neuronal system and do not directly project the cortex.*
- The system consists of three second order fiber tracts ventral spinocerebellar, dorsal spinocerebellar and cuneocerebellar.

107. Ans. (a) M. Gravis

- In M. Gravis, the fundamental defect is a decrease in the number of available AChRs at the postsynaptic muscle membrane. These changes result in decreased efficiency of neuromuscular transmission.
- Therefore, although ACh is released normally, it produces small end-plate potentials that may fail to trigger muscle action potentials.
- The amount of ACh released per impulse normally declines on repeated activity (termed *presynaptic rundown*).
- In the myasthenic patient, the decreased efficiency of neuromuscular transmission combined with the normal rundown results in the activation of fewer and fewer muscle fibers by successive nerve impulses and hence increasing weakness, or *myasthenic fatigue*.
- This mechanism accounts for the decremental response to repetitive nerve stimulation seen on electrodiagnostic testing.

108. Ans. (a) Tension headache

- Overall the *most common cause of headache is tension headache*.
- Episodic tension headache is usually associated with a stressful event. This headache type is of moderate intensity, self-limited, and usually responsive to non-prescription drugs.
- Chronic tension headache often recurs daily and is associated with contracted muscles of the neck and scalp. This type of headache is bilateral and usually occipitofrontal.
- Most common cause of secondary headache is systemic infection
- Rare cause of primary headache is cluster headache
- Rare cause of secondary headache is brain tumor.

109. Ans. (b) Ophthalmoplegia, ataxia, areflexia

Miller Fisher syndrome presents as:
- Rapidly evolving ataxia
- Areflexia of limbs without weakness
- Ophthalmoplegia often with pupillary paralysis

The MFS variant accounts for <5% of all cases of G.B.S and is strongly associated with antibodies to the ganglioside GQ1b.

110. Ans. (c) TB meningitis

- Contrast-enhanced computed tomography shows tuberculous meningitis demonstrating acute hydrocephalus and meningeal enhancement. Notice the dilated lateral ventricles.
- Diagnostic triad of tubercular meningitis:
  - Basal exudates
  - Infarcts
  - Hydrocephalus

Must know points for tubercular meningitis

- The combination of unrelenting headache, stiff neck, fatigue, night sweats, and fever with a *CSF lymphocytic pleocytosis and a mildly decreased glucose concentration* is highly suspicious for tuberculous meningitis.
- If there is a pellicle in the CSF or a *cobweb-like clot* on the surface of the fluid, AFB can best be demonstrated in a smear of the clot or pellicle

111. Ans. (c) Caffeine

Post-lumbar puncture headache usually resolves without specific treatment:
1. Care is largely supportive with oral analgesics like acetaminophen, nonsteroidal anti-inflammatory drugs and anti-emetics.
2. Patients may obtain relief by lying in a comfortable (especially a recumbent or head-down Trendelenburg) position.
3. For some patients, beverages with caffeine can provide temporary pain relief.
4. *For patients with persistent pain, treatment with IV caffeine (500 mg in 500 mL saline administered over 2 hours) is effective.*
5. Alternatively, an epidural blood patch accomplished by injection of 15 mL of autologous whole blood is usually effective.
6. Some clinicians reserve epidural blood patch for patients who do not respond to caffeine, while others prefer to use blood patch as initial management for unremitting post-LP symptoms.

112. Ans. (c) Excision with radiation

- These are highly infiltrative tumors, and the areas of increased T2/FLAIR signal surrounding the main tumor mass contain invading tumor cells.
- Treatment involves *maximal surgical resection followed by partial-field external beam radiotherapy (6000 cGy in thirty 200-cGy fractions)* with concomitant temozolomide, followed by 6–12 months of adjuvant temozolomide.

113. Ans. (a) Neurofibromatosis

NF-1 is diagnosed when *any two of the following seven signs* are present:
1. Six or more café au-lait macules. *Café au-lait spots are the hallmark of neurofibromatosis and are present in almost 100% of patients.*
2. *Axillary or inguinal freckling*[Q] consisting of multiple hyperpigmented areas 2–3 mm in diameter.
3. Two or more iris Lisch nodules. Lisch nodules are hamartomas located within the iris and are best identified by a slit-lamp examination.
4. Two or more neurofibromas or one plexiform neurofibroma.
5. Osseous lesion such as sphenoid dysplasia (which may cause pulsating exophthalmos) or cortical thinning of long bones with or without pseudoarthrosis.
6. Optic gliomas are present in ≈15% of patients with NF-1.
7. First degree relative with NF-1.

114. Ans. (d) Semi-purposive and non-repetitive, randomly distributed movements

Lesion	Manifestations	Lesion seen in
Chorea	State of *excessive*, spontaneous movements, *irregularly timed, non-repetitive*, randomly distributed and abrupt in character.	Caudate
Atheotosis	Because of the slowness, the movements have a writhing (i.e. squirming, twisting, or snakelike) appearance	Globus pallidus
Hemiballismus	Very severe form of chorea in which the movements have a *violent, flinging quality*. Ballism has been defined as "continuous, violent, coordinated involuntary activity involving the axial and proximal appendicular musculature such that the limbs are flung about.	Subthalamic nucleus

115. Ans. (a) Lateral spinothalamic tract

Important tracts

Posterior/Dorsal column	Joint position, vibration and pressure
Lateral spinothalamic tract	Pain and temperature
Ventral spinothalamic	Pressure, touch
Lateral corticospinal/ pyramidal pathways	Distal limb movements
Vestibulospinal and tectospinal tract	Axial and proximal limb movements

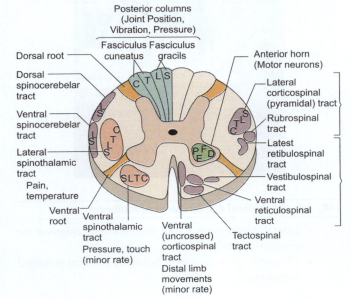

116. Ans. (a) Corticospinal tract

- The corticospinal tract (along with the corticobulbar tract) is the primary pathway that carries the motor commands that underlie voluntary movement.
- The **lateral corticospinal tract** is responsible for the control of the distal musculature and the **anterior corticospinal tract** is responsible for the control of the proximal musculature.
- A particularly important function of the lateral corticospinal tract is the fine control of the digits of the hand.
- The corticospinal tract is the only descending pathway in which some axons make synaptic contacts directly onto alpha motor neurons.
- This direct cortical innervation presumably is necessary to allow the powerful processing networks of the cortex to control the activity of the spinal circuits that direct the exquisite movements of the fingers and hands.

117. Ans. (a) Spine injury evaluation

- *Log rolling* is a method of turning patients to either inspect their backs for *spine injury evaluation* especially in sports related injuries. It will also help to put the patient on long spinal board.
- To log roll a patient, *there should be a minimum of four people. The objective is to keep the whole spine in alignment.* To achieve it the cervical spine is stabilized and the patient is moved with the neck, shoulders and pelvis kept in the same plane.

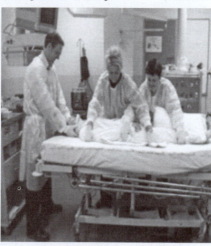

118. Ans. (b) Lateral displacement of midbrain

- Lateral displacement of the midbrain may compress the opposite cerebral peduncle
- This produces an ipsilateral Babinski's sign and ipsilateral hemiparesis
- Normally in CNS lesion the hemiparesis and Babinski sign is bilateral
- This unusual fact is called as Kernohan-Woltman sign.
- Herniation may also compress the anterior and posterior cerebral arteries as they pass over the tentorial reflections, with resultant brain infarction

119. Ans. (a) 3rd nerve involvement

Ref: Harrison, 19th ed. pg. 1772

- *Uncal transtentorial* herniation refers to impaction of the anterior medial temporal gyrus (the uncus) into the tentorial opening just anterior to and adjacent to the midbrain.
- *The uncus compresses the third nerve as it traverses the subarachnoid space, causing enlargement of the ipsilateral pupil (putatively because the fibers subserving parasympathetic pupillary function are located peripherally in the nerve).*

120. Ans. (b) Alzheimer's disease

Ref: Harrison, 19th ed. pg. 2617

- *Rivastigmine is a reversible inhibitor of both the acetylcholinesterase and butyrylcholinesterase enzymes.*
- *It is used for the treatment of Alzheimer's, as well as for the treatment of dementia associated with Parkinson's disease. This drug is available as a skin patch that provides continuous delivery of the drug over 24 hours*

121. Ans. (a) Broca's Area

Ref: Harrison, 19th ed. pg. 177

- Broca's area damage is called **expressive aphasia** (non-fluent aphasia).
- Pattern has loss of the ability to produce language (spoken or written).
- Patient has insight to his problem and is frustrated.
- *Remember: Broca is broke. Speaks broken words.*
- Damage to paracentral lobule would lead to loss of control over urination and lead to urge incontinence.
- Damage to insula leads to loss of hand eye coordination and loss of social skills.

122. Ans. (a) Medulla

Ref: Ganong, 25th ed. pg. 525

- *Nucleus ambiguus is a group of large motor neurons, situated deep in the medullary reticular formation.*
- *The nucleus ambiguus contains the cell bodies of nerves that innervate the muscles of the soft palate, pharynx, and larynx which are strongly associated with speech and swallowing.*

Medicine

633

123. Ans. (a) Superior Temporal Gyrus

Ref: Harrison, 19th ed. pg. 177

- Wernicke's area is located in the posterior section of the superior temporal gyrus (STG) in the dominant cerebral hemisphere (which is the left hemisphere in about 95% of right handed individuals and 60% of left handed individuals).
- Damage caused to Wernicke's area results in receptive, fluent aphasia. This means that the person with aphasia will be able to fluently connect words, but sentences will lack meaning.

124. Ans. (b) Severe disability

Ref: Harrison, 19th ed. chapter 370

- *Patients scoring 3 or 4 have an 85% chance of dying or remaining vegetative.*

- Glasgow come scale of <8 indicates coma.
- The minimum score in glasgow coma scale is 3 (severe disability) and maximum score is 15.

125. Ans. (a) Withdrawl on flexion

Ref: Chapter 370: Harrison, 19th ed.

Best motor response (M)	
Obeys	6
Localizes	5
Withdraws (flexion)	4
Abnormal flexion posturing	3
Extension flexion posturing	2
Nil	1

126. Ans. (a) Neuropraxia

Ref: Maheshwari, 5th ed. pg. 69

- In most cases of compressive radial neuropathy, the type of injury is a "neuropraxia" that does not involve damage to the axon.
- Neuropraxia is classified as a *transient conduction block of motor or sensory function without neuronal degeneration.* Therefore, despite decreased motor function, patients with neuropraxia are able to regain normal neurologic function within several weeks to months.
- Posture-induced radial neuropathy, known as *Saturday night palsy*, occurs because of compression of the radial nerve.

	Neurotmesis	Axonotmesis	Neurapraxia
Pathological			
Anatomical continuity	May be lost	Preserved	Preserved
Essential damage	Complete disorganisation, Schwann sheaths preserved[Q]	Nerve fibres interrupted	Selective demyellnation of larger fibres, no degeneration of axons[Q]
Clinical			
Motor paralysis	Complete	Complete	Complete
Muscle atrophy	Progressive	Progressive	Very little
Sensory paralysis	Complete	Complete	Usually much sparing
Autonomic paralysis	Complete	Complete	Usually much sparing
	Electrical phenomena		
Nerve conduction distal to the lesion	Absent	Absent	Absent
Fibrillation	Present	Present	Occasionally detectable
Recovery			
Surgical repair	Essential	Not necessary	Not necessary

127. Ans. (c) 60-80%

Ref: Harrison 18th edition, chapter 381

- The glucose level in CSF is proportional to the blood glucose level and corresponds to 60–70% of the concentration in blood.

Hypoglycorrhachia (low CSF glucose levels) can be caused by

- CNS infections
- Inflammatory conditions
- Subarachnoid hemorrhage

Explanations

FMGE Solutions Screening Examination

- Hypoglycemia
- Impaired glucose transport, increased CNS glycolytic activity
- Metastatic carcinoma.

CSF glucose levels can be useful in distinguishing among causes of meningitis as more than 50% of patients with bacterial meningitis have decreased CSF glucose levels while patients with viral meningitis usually have normal CSF glucose levels.

128. Ans. (d) Cryptococcus meningitis

Ref: Harrison 18th edition, Chapter 189

- *C. neoformans* is the leading infectious cause of *meningitis* in patients with AIDS[Q]
- It is the initial AIDS-defining illness in <2% of patients and generally occurs in patients with CD4+ T cell counts <100/μL[Q]
- Most patients present with a picture of subacute meningoencephalitis with fever, nausea, vomiting, altered mental status, headache, and meningeal signs.
- The CSF profile may be normal or may show only modest elevations in WBC or protein levels and decrease in glucose. The opening pressure in the CSF is usually elevated.
- **The diagnosis of cryptococcal meningitis is made by identification of organisms in spinal fluid with India ink examination or by the detection of cryptococcal antigen.** Blood cultures for fungus are often positive. A biopsy may be needed to make a diagnosis of CNS cryptococcoma.
- Treatment is with IV amphotericin B[Q] 0.7 mg/kg daily, or liposomal amphotericin 4–6 mg/kg daily, with flucytosine 25 mg/kg qid for at least 2 weeks and, if possible, until the CSF culture turns negative. This is followed by fluconazole 400 mg/d PO for 8 weeks, and then fluconazole 200 mg/d until the CD4+ T cell count has increased to >200 cells/uL for 6 months in response to cART.

129. Ans. (c) Gullian Barre syndrome

Ref: Harrison, 18th ed. Chapter 386

The symmetrical nature of disease favors diagnosis of Guillain-Barre syndrome. The absence of sensory symptoms also makes Transverse myelitis an unlikely diagnosis

	Poliomyelitis	Guillain-Barre syndrome	Transverse myelitis
Fever	Present; may be biphasic	May have a prodromal illness	May have a prodromal illness

Contd...

	Poliomyelitis	Guillain-Barre syndrome	Transverse myelitis
Symmetry Sensations	Asymmetric Intact; may have diffuse myalgias	Symmetrical Variable	Symmetrical Impaired below the level of the lesion
Respiratory insufficiency	May be present	May be present	May be present
Cranial nerves	Affected in bulbar and bulbospinal variants	Usually affected	Absent
Radicular signs	May be present	Present	Absent
Bladder, bowel complaints	Absent	Transient; due to autonomic dysfunction	Present
Nerve conduction	May be abnormal	Abnormal	Normal
Cerebrospinal fluid	Lymphocytic pleocytosis; normal or increased protein	Albumino-cytologic dissociation	Variable
MRI spine	Usually normal	Usually normal	Characteristic

130. Ans. (b) Subdural hemorrhage

Ref: Harrison, 18th ed. chapter 378

- Boxing is a violent sport in which every participant accepts the risk of brain damage or death. This sport has been linked to acute neurological injury and chronic brain damage. The *most common life-threatening injury encountered by its participants is subdural hematoma* (SDH), and the most feared consequence of chronic insult to the nervous system is dementia pugilistica, or punch drunkenness.

131. Ans. (d) Sinusitis

Ref: Harrison, 18th ed. chapter 14

Primary Headache		Secondary Headache	
Type	%	Type	%
Tension –Type	69	Systemic infection	63

Contd...

Primary Headache		Secondary Headache	
Migraine	16	Head injury	4
Idiopathic stabbing	2	Vascular disorders	1
Extertional	1	Subarachnoid hemorrhage	<1
Cluster	0.1	Brain tumor	0.1

132. Ans. (a) Ampicillin

Ref: Harrison, 18th ed. chapter 139

133. Ans. (a) Acyclovir

Ref: Harrison, 18th ed. chapter 381

134. Ans. (c) Measles

Ref: Harrison, 18th ed. chapter 192

135. Ans. (c) Hyperhidrosis

Ref: Harrison, 18th ed. chapter 370

Horner syndrome (Horner's syndrome) results from an interruption of the sympathetic nerve supply to the eye and is characterized by the *classic triad* of *miosis* (i.e., constricted pupil), *partial ptosis*, and *loss of hemifacial sweating* (i.e., anhidrosis)

(Mnemonic: PERFECT M.E.A.L) Clinical features of Horner syndrome

Ptosis
Miosis
Enophthalmos (pseudo)
Anhidrosis
Loss of ciliospinal reflex

■ ANATOMY OF HORNER SYNDROME

- *First-order central sympathetic fibers arise from the posterolateral hypothalamus*, descend uncrossed through the midbrain and pons, and terminate in the intermediolateral cell column of the spinal cord at the level of C8-T2 (ciliospinal center of Budge).
- *Second-order preganglionic pupillomotor fibers exit the spinal cord at the level of T1 and enter the cervical sympathetic chain*, where they are in close proximity to the pulmonary apex and the subclavian artery. (association with pancoast tumor)
- *The third-order pupillomotor fibers ascending along the internal carotid artery* enter the cavernous sinus.

136. Ans. (b) Peripheral ganglia

Ref: Harrison, 18th ed. chapter 374

Lower motor neurons are motor neurons located in either the *anterior grey column, anterior nerve roots* or the *cranial nerve nuclei of the brainstem and cranial nerves with motor function*

Lower motor neurons are classified based on the type of muscle fiber they innervate:

- Alpha motor neurons innervate extrafusal muscle fibers, the most numerous type of muscle fiber and the one involved in muscle contraction.
- Beta motor neurons innervate intrafusal fibers of muscle spindles with collaterals to extrafusal fibers
- Gamma motor neurons innervate intrafusal muscle fibers, which together with sensory afferents compose muscle spindles. These are part of the system for sensing proprioception

137. Ans. (c) Meningioma

Ref: Harrison, 18th ed. chapter 379

- Meningiomas are the most common primary brain tumor, accounting for approximately 32% of the total.
- Overall most common Brain tumour is metastases arising from hematogenous spread from a lung primary.
- The most common sources of brain metastases are lung and breast carcinomas; melanoma has the greatest propensity to metastasize to the brain, being found in 80% of patients at autopsy
- **Remember: Metastasis > meningioma>astrocytoma.**

138. Ans. (c) Hypertension and Bradycardia

Ref: Harrison, 18th ed. chapter 25

- Cushing's reflex is a *hypothalamic response* to brain ischemia wherein the sympathetic nervous system is activated which causes increased peripheral vascular resistance with a *subsequent increase in BP.*
- The *increased BP then activates the parasympathetic nervous system* via carotid artery baroreceptors, *resulting in vagal-induced bradycardia.*
- The brain ischemia that leads to cushings reflex is usually due to the poor perfusion that results from increased ICP due to head bleeds or mass lesions.
- Cushing's reflex leads to the clinical manifestation of Cushing's triad.
- *Cushing's triad = hypertension, bradycardia, and irregular respirations (Cheyne-Stokes breathing).*
- Cushing's triad signals *impending danger of brain herniation*, and thus, the need for decompression. Consider administering mannitol, hyperventilation, and elevation of the head of bed as temporizing measures

139. Ans. (d) 6th

Ref: Harrison, 19th ed. pg. 209

- In raised intracranial tension the cranial nerves afflicted are the ones which have long intracerebral courses leading to false localizing signs. *Since the 6th cranial nerves emerges straight forwards from the brainstem, while others originate obliquely, the nerve is more liable to the mechanical effects of backward brainstem displacement by ICSOL.*
- Neurological signs have been described as "false localizing" if they reflect dysfunction distant or remote.

140. Ans. (a) Sub-dural hematoma

Lesions	NCCT finding
Sub dural hematoma	Concavo-convex bleed hyper-density
Extra dural hemorrhage	Biconvex /flame shaped hyper-density
Sub arachnoid hemorrhage	Intra-ventricular bleed/blood in slyvian fissure
Intra –parenchymal bleed	Mostly a lesion or hyper-density in basal ganglia secondary to hypertension

141. Ans. (a) Hyperdense biconvex

Ref: Harrison's 17th ed. Ch 364

- **Extradural hemorrhage:** Bleeding occurs between skull and duramatter. Bleeding occurs due to the rupture of Middle meningeal artery. Lucid Interval (Consciousness between two periods of unconsciousness) exists.
- In NCCT it shows hyperdensity which has bi-convex or flame shaped appearance.
- **Treatment:** Burr hole surgery.
- **Subdural hemorrhage:** Occurs due to rupture of Cortical bridging veins. *In NCCT it shows concavo-convex or sickle shaped bleed.*

142. Ans. (a) Insula

Ref: Textbook of Anatomy Vol. 3 by Vishram singh, pg. 391

- *Insula is called Island of Reil or central lobe.*
- The word insula means hidden. *The insula is the submerged portion of cerebral cortex in the floor of lateral sulcus.*
- The insula is divided into 2 regions: Anterior and Posterior by a central sulcus. The anterior region represents 3 or 4 short gyri call *gyri brevia* and posterior region presents 1 or 2 long gyri called *gyri longa.*
- The insulae are involved in consciousness and play a role in diverse functions usually linked to emotion or the regulation of the body's homeostasis. These functions include perception, motor control, self-awareness, cognitive functioning, and interpersonal experience.

143. Ans. (a) NCCT

Ref: Harrison, 19th ed. pg. 1785

- The basic rule for intra-cranial hemorrhage is to perform NCCT.
- Remember MRI is recommended for ICH >>48 hours.
- NCCT Brain in SAH, shows accumulation of blood in slyvian fissure.
- Drug of choice for management of SAH is nimodipine 60 mg TDS for 3 weeks with complete bed rest.
- Neurosurgical consult is required in case of development of hydrocephalus.

144. Ans. (a) Non fluent speech

Ref: Harrison, 19th ed. pg. 177-178

- **Wernicke's area in the brain (Brodmann area 22) is present** in the posterior part of the superior temporal gyrus of the dominant hemisphere.
- People with (Wernicke's area damage) **receptive** aphasia are **unable to understand language in its written or spoken form, and even though they can speak with normal grammar, syntax, rate, and intonation, they cannot express themselves meaningfully using language.**
- A patient with Wernicke's aphasia can and may speak a great deal, but he or she confuses sound characteristics, **producing** "*word salad*" in extreme cases.
- **Paraphasia** is seen in people with wernicke's area damage and it presents like **a syllable from later in the word replaces a syllable from earlier in the word - "papple" for apple or "lelephone" for telephone. Similarly patient might use the word "plants" for "pants"**

> **Extra Mile**
> - Wernicke's Area is for understanding of speech = hence lesion results in receptive dysphasia
>   Broca's Area for expression = hence lesion results in non-fluent aphasia.

145. Ans. (a) Meningioma

Ref: Harrison, 19th ed. pg. 599-600

- **M**ost malignant brain tumor is Glioma (subtype – astrocytoma)
- Most common brain tumor is metastasis to brain (oat cell cancer/breast cancer/malignant melanoma)
- *Most common benign brain tumor is Meningioma*
- IOC for brain tumor is gadolinium enhanced MRI

Medicine

146. Ans. (a) Parkinsonism

Ref: Harrison, 19th ed. pg. 2606

- Lewy bodies are intra-neuronal inclusion bodies in Parkinsonism and in Dementia with lewy body (D.L.B).
- *Hirona bodies are seen in Alzheimer's disease.* **The intra-neuronal inclusions in AD are known as neurofibrillary tangles.**

147. Ans. (c) HIV encephalopathy

Ref: Harrison, 19th ed. pg. 1263

- HIV leads to asymptomatic neurocognitive impairment or HIV-associated dementia.
- Hypoglycemia can lead to neuroglucopenia and seizures
- Hypocalcemia/Tetany leads to larynospasm. The resultant hypoxia can lead to seizures.
- NCC leads to intracranial calcification and leads to seizures.

148. Ans. (b) Viral meningitis

Ref: Harrison, 19th ed. pg. 890

- T*he key word in the diagnosis of patient is lymphocytic pleocytosis.* Pleocytosis means a dimorphic cell population where first neutrophils and later lymphocytes are predominant".
- Harrison states that "**As a rule, a lymphocytic pleocytosis with a low glucose concentration should suggest fungal or tuberculous meningitis, or noninfectious disorders (e.g., sarcoid, neoplastic meningitis)".** Where as in this question CSF sugar is normal. Hence the answer is viral meningitis.
- **Viral meningitis** has typical profile of **lymphocytic pleocytosis (25–500 cells/L), a normal protein concentration (20–80 mg/dL), a normal glucose concentration,** and a normal or mildly elevated opening pressure (100–350 mm H_2O).

CSF	Normal	Acute bacterial meningitis	Tubercular meningitis	Viral meningitis	Gullian–Barre syndrome	Fungal meningitis
Pressure	50 – 180 mmH$_2$O	Increased	Increased	Increased	Normal	Elevated
Color	Clear	Turbid	Straw	Clear	Normal	Normal
Cells	0-4 lymphocytes/cu.mm	>1000	>100	>25	Normal	25-500
Sugar	2/3rd of blood sugar	Decreased	Decreased	Normal	Normal	Low
Protein	15-45 mg %	Increased	Increased	Increased	Increased (albumin-cytological disassociation)	Normal/elevated

CSF findings OF VIRAL ENCEPHALITIS IS SAME AS VIRAL MENINGITIS.

149. Ans. (d) Cerebrospinal fluid reveals a low leukocyte count

Ref: Harrison 19th ed. / 898-99

Refer to above table

- Tubercular meningitis is seen most often in young children but also develops in adults, especially those infected with HIV.
- Tubercular meningitis results from the hematogenous spread of primary or post primary pulmonary TB.
- The disease often presents subtly as headache and slight mental changes after a prodrome of weeks of low-grade fever, malaise, anorexia, and irritability.
- *In general, examination of cerebrospinal fluid (CSF) reveals a high leukocyte count (up to 1000/µL), usually with a predominance of lymphocytes but sometimes with a predominanc of neutrophils in the early stage; a protein content of 1–8 g/L (100–800 mg/dL); and a low glucose concentration.*
- Culture of CSF is diagnostic in up to 80% of cases and remains the gold standard. Polymerase chain reaction has a sensitivity of up to 80%, but rates of false-positivity reach 10%.
- Imaging studies (CT and MRI) may show hydrocephalus and abnormal enhancement of basal cisterns or ependyma.

150. Ans. (a) Normal cells with increased protein

Ref: Harrison, 19th ed. pg. 2694

Refer to above table

- The characterized feature of GBS is albumin-cytological dissociation, characterized by elevated proteins due to autoimmunity while the cell count remains perfectly normal.
- A normal CSF protein level does not rule out GBS, however, as the level may remain normal in 10% of patients. CSF protein may not rise until 1-2 weeks after the onset of weakness.
- Normal CSF cell counts may not be a feature of GBS in HIV-infected patients. CSF pleocytosis is well recognized in **HIV**-associated GBS.

FMGE Solutions Screening Examination

151. Ans. (a) Tremors

Ref: Harrison 19th ed. pg. 2609

- In the early presentation, about 70% patients experience a slight tremor in the hand or foot on one side of the body, or less commonly in the jaw or face. The tremor consists of a shaking or oscillating movement, and usually appears when a person's muscles are relaxed, or at rest, hence the term "resting tremor".
- The tremor of PD can be exacerbated by stress or excitement, sometimes attracting unwanted notice.
- Resting tremor is the earliest and most common symptom of Parkinson's disease.
- The most debilitating feature is Akinesia.
- Non motor symptoms precede motor symptoms.

152. Ans. (a) Chorea

Ref: Harrison 19th ed. pg. 2609

Chorea occurs due to lesion of caudate nucleus whereas the disease process in parkinsonism afflicts the substantia nigra.

Cardinal Features	Other Motor Features	Non motor Features

• Bradykinesia
• Rest tremor
• Rigidity
• Gait disturbance/ postural instability
	• Micrographia
	• Masked facies (Hypomimia)
	• Reduced eye blink
	• Hypo-phonia/soft voice
	• Dysph*agia*
	• *Freezing*
		• **Anosmia-earliest feature**
		• Sensory disturbances (e.g., pain)
		• Mood disorders (e.g., depression)
		• Sleep disturbances
		• **Autonomic disturba**nces
		  ■ Orthostatic hypotension
		  ■ Gastrointestinal disturbances
		  ■ Genitourinal disturbances
		  ■ Sexual dysfunction
		• Cognitive impairment/Dementia

- Parkinson's disease (PD) is the second msot common neurodegenerative disease, exceeded only by Alzheimer's disease (AD)

153. Ans. (a) Anosmia

Ref: Harrison, 19th ed. pg. 2609

Non-motor symptoms may precede motor symptoms of Parkinson's diagnosis by years. The most recognizable early symptoms include:

- Loss of sense of smell, constipation
- REM behavior disorder
- Mood disorders
- Orthostatic hypotension

Subsequently Motor Features Appear

- Tremors (resting 4-6 Hz)
- Rigidity
- Bradykinesia
- Good Response to levodopa

154. Ans. (a) Hypotonia

Ref: Ganong, 25th ed. pg. 110, 233

	LMN	UMN	Extra Pyramidal Damage
TONE	**Decreased tone**/ flaccidity	Increased spasticity	Decreased rigidity
DTR	Areflexia	Brisk reflex	Normal

Contd...

	LMN	UMN	Extra Pyramidal Damage
SPECIAL FEATURES	Fasciculations + wasting	Babinski's sign + No wasting	Chorea, atheosis, hemiballismus
Superficial reflex	Present	Absent	–
EXAMPLE	Motor neuron disease	Cerebral malaria	Punch drunk syndrome

155. Ans. (b) Muscle hypertrophy

Please refer to above explanation

156. Ans. (b) Tongue deviation to right on protrusion

Ref: Harrison, 19th ed. Ch 367

Following a lesion of the hypoglossal nucleus or nerve

- ATROPHY of the muscles of the IPSILATERAL one-half of the tongue occurs.
- FASCICULATIONS (tiny, spontaneous contractions) can be seen.
- *Upon protrusion, the tongue will deviate TOWARD the side of the lesion (i.e., same side). This is due to the* unopposed action of the genioglossus muscle on the

normally innervated side of the tongue (the genioglossus pulls the tongue forward).

- The corticobulbar input to the hypoglossal nucleus arises from motor cortex and is predominantly CROSSED. Thus, a lesion in motor cortex will result in deviation of the tongue toward the opposite side or CONTRALATERAL to the lesion.

157. Ans. (a) Acetyl choline esterase in the amniotic fluid

Ref: Nelson 18th ed. / ch. 592

- Failure of closure of the neural tube allows excretion of fetal substances (α–fetoprotein, acetylcholinesterase) into the amniotic fluid, serving as biochemical markers for a neural tube defect. Prenatal screening of maternal serum for AFP in the 16th to 18th wk of gestation is an effective method for identifying pregnancies at risk for fetuses with neural tube defects in utero.

158. Ans. (a) Tau protein

Ref: Harrison, 19th ed. pg. 172t, 175

- Pathologies and dementias of the nervous system such as Alzheimer's disease can result when *tau proteins* become defective and no longer stabilize microtubules properly.
- *Alpha synuclein protein* is seen in parkinsonism.
- *Huntington protein* is related to Huntington disease related to chromosome 4. Protein 14.3.3 is related to prion disease like variant Creutzfeldt Jakob disease.

159. Ans. (b) Thyroid ophthalmopathy

Ref: Harrison, 19th ed. pg. 2294-95

- **The question is on unilateral ptosis whereas thyroid ophthalmopathy has PROPTOSIS.**
- In myasthenia gravis, due to anti-Ach-receptor blocking antibodies there is ptosis which can be unilateral or asymmetrical which will again appear unilateral.
- Marfan syndrome has congenital Ptosis.
- Pancoast tumor causes horner syndrome in which unilateral sympathetic chain is compressed leading to Ptosis, Miosis, Anhidrosis, Enophthalmos and loss of Cilio-spinal reflex.

160. Ans. (a) Uncal herniation

Ref: Harrison, 19th ed. pg. 1772

- In uncal or mid brain herniation, the raised ICT compresses the same side third cranial nerve while it originates from Edinger -Westphal nucleus. This causes ptosis, diplopia and divergent squint. The reason for unconsciousness can be damage to reticular activating system in the midbrain.

161. Ans. (a) Putamen

Ref: Harrison, 19th ed. pg. 2582

- Most common site of brain hemorrhage is Putamen.
- Intra-parenchmal hemorrhage is most lethal and has mortality rate of 40%.
- The IOC is NCCT. For management BP must be controlled which is to maintain a target BP of 160/90.

162. Ans. (a) Single Fiber E.M.G

Ref: Harrison, 19th ed. pg. 442e-6

- *Single fiber E.M.G is the investigation of choice* for myasthenia gravis and shows a decremental response
- Anti-acetylcholine receptor blocking antibody TITER is the most specific test for diagnosis of myasthenia gravis. Also remember that *Tensilon test is a screening test* for myasthenia gravis. False positive tensilon test can be seen in motor neuron disease.

163. Ans. (b) Sub-arachnoid granulations

Ref: Harrison, 19th ed. pg. 443e-4

- *CSF is produced by the choroid villi* in the lateral ventricles and third ventricles. The CSF flows via aqueduct of slyvius to the 3rd ventricle and then via foramen of Munro to the 4th ventricle. The CSF emerges out of Foramen of Luschka and Magendie and accumulates at the base of the skull in basal cisterns.
- *This CSF is then reabsorbed via the arachnoid granulations back into the blood stream.*
- The CSF is produced at a rate of 20 mL per hour and reabsorbed at the same rate. The total amount of CSF at any point of time is 150 mL.

164. Ans. (d) Nystagmus

Ref: Harrison, 19th ed. pg. 2608

- Dementia pugilistica is seen in athletes who participate in body contact sport like martial arts, boxing etc.
- Repeated blows to the head of the athlete over entire career span of the boxer can lead to cortical damage and Parkinson like features. (*Best example to remember this is Muhammad Ali, the greatest boxer of all times, suffers from dementia pugilistica*).
- Nystagmus is not a clinical feature of this disease and is rather seen with vestibular diseases or cerebellar lesions.

165. Ans. (a) Infarction

Ref: Bringham Intensive Review of Internal Medicine 2nd ed. pg. 888

- Most common type of stroke is ischemic stroke caused by extracranial and intracranial atherosclerosis.

FMGE Solutions Screening Examination

166. Ans. (a) Thiamine deficiency

Ref: Harrison, 19th ed. pg. 2607, 2724

There are six Major Symptoms of Korsakoff's Syndrome
1. Anterograde amnesia
2. Retrograde amnesia
3. Severe memory loss
4. Confabulation
5. Minimal content in conversation
6. Lack of insight or Apathy

Thiamine is essential for the carboxylation of pyruvate and deficiency during this metabolic process is thought to cause damage to the medial thalamus and mammillary bodies of the posterior hypothalamus as well as generalized cerebral atrophy. These brain regions are all parts of the limbic system, which is involved in emotion and memory.

167. Ans. (c) Finger pads

Ref: De Jong Neurological Examination, 7th ed. pg. 542

- Two-point discrimination is the ability to discern that two nearby objects touching the skin are truly two distinct points, not one. It is often tested with two sharp points during a neurological examination and is assumed to reflect how finely innervated an area of skin is.
- The maximum sensitivity for this test is in lips and finger tips which can be remembered as the most sensitive areas in the body.

168. Ans. (b) CT-scan

Ref: Harrison, 19th ed. pg. 2582

- For evaluation of bleeding in the brain the preferred investigation is CT scan. The bleeding in the brain shows up as hyper-density on CT scan.

169. Ans. (b) Contralateral subthalamic lesion

Ref: Harrison, 19th ed. pg. 2623

Lesion	Manifestation
Caudate nucleus	Contralateral chorea
Globus pallidus	Contralateral athetosis
Sub-thalamic nucleus	Contralateral hemiballismus
Cerebellum	Ipsilateral intentional tremors
Internal capsule	Contra-lateral hemiplegia with hemi-anesthesia
Ventral pons	Locked in syndrome

170. Ans. (a) Basiliar artery

Ref: Harrison, 19th ed. pg. 2573

Basiliar artery occlusion	Pontine stroke
Middle cerebral artery	Contralateral hemiplegia
Anterior cerebral artery	Spastic paraplegia
Posterior cerebral artery	Midbrain stroke like weber syndrome
Vertebral artery	Medullary stroke

171. Ans. (a) Middle cerebral artery

Ref: Gray's Anatomy, 40th ed. pg. 246

- The Circle of Willis is a part of the cerebral circulation and is composed of the following arteries:
  - Anterior cerebral artery (left and right)
  - Anterior communicating artery
  - Internal carotid artery (left and right)
  - Posterior cerebral artery (left and right)
  - Posterior communicating artery (left and right)

  The basilar artery and middle cerebral arteries, supplying the brain, are not considered part of the circle.

172. Ans. (c) Brain hemorrhage due to tear of basiliar artery branches

Ref: Radiology Review Manual, 7th ed. pg. 234

- The classical appearance of a Duret hemorrhage is located in the midline near the ponto-mesencephalic junction.

Medicine

641

- Often however, these hemorrhages can be multiple or even extend into the cerebellar peduncles.
- Usually it is seen in patients with severe herniation for 12–24 hours prior to death

173. Ans. (d) Aphasia

Ref: Harrison, 19th ed. pg. 2724

The classic triad of symptoms found in Wernicke's encephalopathy is:

- Global Confusion
- Ophthalmo-plegia (Most commonly affecting the lateral rectus muscle).
- Ataxia

For diagnosis: Thiamine can be measured using an erythrocyte transketolase activity assay or by activation by measurement of in vitro thiamine diphosphate levels.

174. Ans. (a) Non- fluent aphasia

Ref: Harrison, 19th ed. pg. 177-78

- Broca's area is present in inferior frontal gyrus and is responsible for fluency, syntax and expression of speech and damage to this area causes loss of ability to express self and thereby development of non-fluent aphasia.
- Word salad is seen in patients with damage to Wernicke's area (Area responsible for comprehension).
- Anomia is seen in global aphasia where both Broca and Wernicke area are damaged.
- Apraxia is seen in patients with damage to non dominant parietal lobe.

175. Ans. (a) 3rd nerve

Ref: Harrison, 19th ed. pg. 1784-85

- Most common cranial nerve affected in unruptured berry aneurysm is the 3rd cranial nerve which will present as ipsilateral ptosis, and strabismus.

176. Ans. (d) Tongue protusion

Ref: Harrison, 19th ed. pg. 2537-38

Functions of the Glossopharyngeal Nerve

- Receives general sensory fibers from the tonsils, the pharynx, the middle ear and the posterior 1/3 of the tongue.
- Receives visceral sensory fibers from the carotid bodies, carotid sinus.
- Receives special sensory fibers from the posterior one-third of the tongue
- Supplies parasympathetic fibers to the parotid gland via the otic ganglion.

- Supplies motor fibers to stylopharyngeus muscle, the only motor component of this cranial nerve.
- Contributes to the pharyngeal plexus.

Testing of 9th Nerve

1. Testing the gag reflex using a wooden spatula
2. Asking the patient to swallow or cough
3. Evaluating for speech impediments.
4. Test the posterior one-third of the tongue with bitter and sour substances to evaluate for impairment of taste.

177. Ans. (a) Gag reflex

Ref: Harrison, 19th ed. pg. 2537-38

Damage to the vestibulocochlear nerve may cause the following symptoms:

- Hearing loss
- Vertigo
- False sense of motion
- Loss of equilibrium (in dark places)
- Nystagmus
- Motion sickness
- Gaze-evoked tinnitus

The gag reflex has the following pathway

- The sensory limb is mediated predominantly by CN IX (glossopharyngeal nerve)
- The motor limb by CN X (Vagus nerve).

The gag reflex involves a brisk and brief elevation of the soft palate and bilateral contraction of pharyngeal muscles evoked by touching the posterior pharyngeal wall.

178. Ans. (c) Parietal lobe

Ref: Harrison, 19th ed. pg. 209

Performing Mathematical calculations is a function of parietal lobe. Damage to the left hemisphere of this lobe will result in problems in mathematics, long reading, writing, and understanding symbols. The parietal association cortex enables individuals to read, write, and solve mathematical problems.

179. Ans. (a) Myasthenia gravis

Ref: Harrison, 19th ed. pg. 2701

- Myasthenia gravis is characterized by eye muscle weakness, ptosis and diplopia. In contrast all myopathies have proximal weakness (exception being Myotonic dystrophy).

180. Ans. (b) 24 hours

Ref: Harrison, 19th ed. pg. 2568, 17th ed. Ch. 364

- The standard definition of TIA requires that all neurologic signs and symptoms resolve within 24 hours

Explanations

regardless of whether there is imaging evidence of new permanent brain injury; stroke has occurred if the neurologic signs and symptoms last for >24 hours.

181. Ans. (b) 1st order neurons releasing nitric oxide

Ref: Vascular Medicine, 3rd ed. pg. 84

182. Ans. (c) Enlargement of lateral and third ventricle

Ref: Harrison, 19th ed. pg. 174

- Aqueduct of slyvius connects the third ventricle to the fourth one. Therefore the obstruction to this area will not only cause enlargement of third ventricle but will also dilate the lateral ventricles proximal to the obstruction.

ENDOCRINOLOGY

183. Ans. (a) Impaired glucose tolerance

Ref: Harrison, 20th ed. pg. 2850

Value given	Normal value	Interpretation
120 mg%	<100 mg%	Elevated
140 mg%	<140 mg%	Border line
6.1%	<5.6%	Elevated to Impaired glucose tolerance range

Please note that normal HbA1c is <5.6% and values of 5.7 to 6.4% is impaired glucose tolerance.

184. Ans. (b) Coxsackie B virus

Ref: Harrison, 20th ed. pg. 2851

Fulminant diabetes is an autoimmune form of diabetes which has been noted in Japan. It occurs due to viral insult to pancreas. The viruses incriminated are Coxsackie, Enterovirus and rubella.

185. Ans. (a) pH

Ref: Harrison 19th ed. P 2418

- Type 1 diabetes mellitus is characterized by insulinopenia. The low insulin levels will lead to ketoacidosis. *Hence when insulin is administered the ketone production will stop and pH of patient will rise to normal values.*
- Increase in breathing rate/Kussmaul breathing will occur with worsening of diabetic ketoacidosis. On insulin administration respiratory rate will normalize. Hence choice B is wrong.
- On insulin administration glucose levels will come back to normal and glucosuria will disappear. Hence choice C is wrong.
- Due to solute diuresis (sugar rich urine) in diabetes mellitus urine osmolality is >300 mOsm. It will normalize on treatment. Hence Choice D is wrong.

186. Ans. (d) Carcinoid syndrome

Ref: Harrison 19th ed. P 415e-2

TABLE: A comparison of syndromes of obesity—Hypogonadism and mental retardation

Feature	Prader-Willi	Laurence-Moon-Biedl	Carpenter's
Inheritance	Sporadic; two-thirds have defect	Autosomal recessive	Autosomal recessive
Stature	Short	Normal; infrequently short	Normal
Obesity	• Generalized • Moderate to severe • Onset 1–3 years	• Generalized • Early onset, 1–2 years	Truncal, gluteal
Craniofacies	• Narrow bifrontal diameter • Almond shaped eyes[Q] • Strabismus-V-shaped mouth • High-arched palate	Not distinctive	• Acrocephaly • Flat nasal bridge • High-arched palate

Medicine

187. Ans. (d) Vitamin D deficiency

> *Ref: Harrison 19th ed. P 2494 and 426e-2*

- Choice A, Paget's disease has increased bone remodeling leading to disproportionate rise of SAP with *normal* serum calcium and phosphate.
- Choice B, osteoporosis has *normal* values of calcium, phosphate and SAP.
- Choice C, primary hyperparathyroidism leads to *increase* in value of serum calcium due to increased bone resorption. The increased PTH leads to loss of phosphate in urine of patient leading to *low* phosphate levels.
- Choice D, vitamin D deficiency leads to low serum calcium values. The resultant low calcium leads to secondary increase of PTH. This increased PTH explains the urinary loss of phosphate and low phosphate levels. The increased bone turnover leads to elevated SAP. Hence in this condition *both calcium and phosphate are low and SAP is elevated.*

188. Ans. (a) Head trauma

> *Ref: Harrison 19th ed. P 2281*

Syndrome of Inappropriate Anti-Diuretic Hormone is seen with following CNS causes:

1. Head trauma
2. Amyotrophic lateral sclerosis
3. Agenesis of corpus callosum
4. *Brain abscess*
5. *Cerebral toxoplasmosis*
6. Delirium tremens
7. GBS
8. Hydrocephalus/*Tubercular meningitis*
9. Multiple sclerosis
10. *Bronchial adenoma, Ca lung, carcinoid tumor*

Note: *Important causes are italicized*

189. Ans. (d) Atrial fibrillation

> *Ref: Page 469, SRB Surgery, 5th ed.*

TABLE: Differences in primary and secondary thyrotoxicosis

	Primary (Grave's disease)	Secondary
Neck swelling	Diffuse smooth bilateral involvement	Large nodular involvement
Eye signs and exophthalmos	More common	Not seen
Cardiac features	Resting tachycardia	Atrial fibrillation
Age group	Young	Older
Presentation	Entire gland is overactive and no pre-existing goiter is present	The inter-nodular tissues are overactive and it occurs in setting of pre-existing multinodular goiter.

190. Ans. (b) 5 years

ADA recommends the following ophthalmologic examination schedule:

1. Individuals with *type 1 DM* should have an initial eye examination *within 5 years of diagnosis*
2. Individuals with *type 2 DM* should have an initial eye examination *at the time of diabetes diagnosis*
3. Women with DM who are pregnant or contemplating pregnancy should have an eye examination prior to conception and during the first trimester
4. If eye exam is normal, repeat examination in 2–3 years may be appropriate.

Screening guidelines for other complications

1. The ADA recommends *annual screening for distal symmetric neuropathy* beginning with the initial diagnosis of diabetes and annual screening for autonomic neuropathy 5 years after diagnosis of type 1 DM and at the time of diagnosis of type 2 DM.
2. An annual microalbuminuria measurement (albumin-to-creatinine ratio in spot urine) is advised in individuals with type 1 or type 2 DM *Screening for microalbuminuria should commence 5 years after the onset of type 1 DM and at the time of diagnosis of type 2 DM.*
3. Regardless of protein excretion results, the GFR should be estimated using the serum creatinine in all patients on an annual basis.

191. Ans. (d) Aquaporin 2

The defect in nephrogenic DI is in the collecting duct where V2 receptor/aquaporin-2 receptors are exhibiting resistance. An important cause of receptor resistance is lithium.

192. Ans. (a) CTLA-4

> *Ref: Harrison, 19th ed. pg. 2403*

- Polymorphism in promoter region of insulin gene, CTLA-4 contributes to susceptibility to type 1 diabetes mellitus.
- The most common cause of type 1 diabetes mellitus is autoimmunity. Most patients have DR3 and/or DR4 haplotype.
- Haplotype DQA1*0301 is strongly associated with type 1 DM
- Concordance of type 1 DM in identical twin is 40–60%
- Chances of type 1 DM if single parent has type 1 DM is only 3–4%.

193. Ans. (a) Non-functioning adenoma

> *Ref: Page 2265, Harrison:19th ed. and pg. 611: UICC Manual of Oncology, 2015 edition*

- The majority of pituitary adenomas (33–40%) are clinically non-functioning and produce no distinct clinical hypersecretory syndrome.

Explanations

643

- Most of them arise from gonadotrope cells and may secrete small amounts of alpha- and beta-glycoprotein hormone subunits or, very rarely, intact circulating gonadotropins.
- The most common secretory adenoma is prolactinoma.
- The least common secretory adenoma is TSH secreting tumours. The UICC manual of oncology 2015 edition mentions it as rare (<1%). This is followed by LH/FSH secreting tumor whose prevalence is mentioned as 1%.

194. Ans. (b) Chromosome 12

The most common type of MODY is due to defect on chromosome number 12 and the gene involved is HNF-1 alpha.

MODY, caused by mutations in:
1. HNF–4α (MODY1)
2. Glucokinase (MODY2)
3. HNF–1α (MODY3)
4. IPF–1 (MODY4)
5. HNF–1 β (MODY5)
6. Neuro D1 (MODY6)

195. Ans. (b) 2 hour value = 180 mg%

TABLE: Criteria for the Diagnosis of Diabetes Mellitus

- Symptoms of dilabetes plus random blood glucose concentration ≥11.1 mmol/L (200 mg/dL) or
- Fasting plasma glucose ≥ 7.0 mmol/L (126 mg/dL) or
- A1C > 6.5% or
- Two-hour plasma glucose ≥ 11.1 mmol/L (200 mg/dL) during an oral glucose tolerance test

196. Ans. (a) Cerebral edema

- The Major nonmetabolic complication of DKA therapy is cerebral edema, which most often develops in children as DKA is resolving.
- Precipitating events leading to D.K.A:
  1. Infection
  2. Myocardial infarction
  3. Venous thrombosis
  4. Upper gastrointestinal bleeding
  5. Acute respiratory distress syndrome

197. Ans. (d) ACTH

Ref: Harrison, 19th ed. pg. 401e-4

The precursor molecule of ACTH is pro-opio-melanocortin (P.O.M.C). This P.O.M.C breaks down to produce ACTH and MSH (melanocyte stimulating hormone). In conditions like primary addison disease P.O.M.C is elevated. The resultant increase in MSH leads to hyperpigmentation.

198. Ans. (a) Sodium increase

Ref: Harrison, 18th ed. / ch 344

- In hyperosmolar coma seen with diabetes mellitus, Serum sodium concentration is usually decreased because of the osmotic flux of water from the intracellular to the extracellular space in the presence of hyperglycemia.
- Hence *sodium* and *blood sugar follow inverse relation* in diabetes mellitus

> **Extra Mile**
>
> **Diagnostic criteria for nonketotic hyperglycaemic hyperosmotic syndrome (HHS)**
> - Profound dehydration (decreased skin turgor, postural changes in blood pressure and pulse rate)
> - Neurological symptoms (ranging from mental confusion to coma)
> - Plasma glucose levels > 600 mg/dL (36 mmol/L)
> - Plasma osmolality (Posm) >310 mOsm/kg
> - Arterial pH > 7.3
> - Plasma bicarbonate levels > 15 mmol/L
> - Normal anion gap (< 14 mEq/L)
> - Absence of ketones

199. Ans. (a) Sensory polyneuropathy

Ref: Harrison, 19th ed. pg. 2426, 2682

- *Most common form of diabetic neuropathy is distal symmetric polyneuropathy.*
- *Most frequently presents with distal sensory loss.*
- Symptoms may include a sensation of numbness, tingling, sharpness, or burning that begins in the feet and spreads proximally.
- Neuropathic Pain typically involves the lower extremities, is usually present at rest, and worsens at night.
- Physical examination reveals sensory loss, loss of ankle reflexes, and abnormal position sense.

200. Ans. (c) P.C.O.D.

Ref: Harrison 19th ed. pg. 331, 332

- Testosterone is the most important androgen in both men and women.
- In women, testosterone is produced primarily through peripheral conversion of androstenedione (50 percent) with the remainder of production concentrated in the ovary (25 percent) and adrenal cortex (25 percent).
- *In women, abnormally high levels of testosterone have been associated with hirsutism and polycystic ovary syndrome.*
- Granulosa-theca cell tumors, more commonly known as granulosa cell tumors, belong to the sex cord–stromal category.
- They commonly *produce estrogen,* and estrogen production often is the reason for early diagnosis.

Medicine

201. Ans. (c) Myasthenia Gravis

Ref: Harrison, 18th ed. chapter 386, table 386-3

Disorders associated with Myaesthenia Gravis

Disorders of the thymus: Thymoma, thymic hyperplasia	
Other autoimmune disorders: Hashimoto's thyroiditis, Graves' disease, rheumatoid arthritis, lupus erythematosus, skin disorders, family history of autoimmune disorder	

202. Ans. (d) Urine albumin > 30 mg/dL

Ref: Harrison, 18th ed. chapter 44

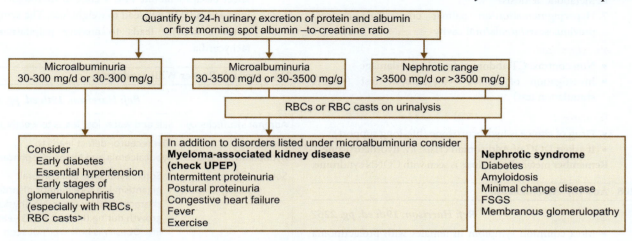

203. Ans. (d) Aldosterone

Ref: Harrison, 18th ed. chapter 277

204. Ans. (c) Relaxin

Ref: Harrison, 18th ed. chapter 338

- Relaxin is produced mainly by the corpus-luteum, and it rises to peak within 14 days of ovulation, and then declines in the absence of pregnancy, resulting in menstruation.
- In the first trimester of pregnancy, levels rise and additional relaxin is produced by the decidua.
- Peak level of Relaxin is reached during the 14 weeks of the first trimester and at delivery.
- It is known to mediate the hemodynamic changes that occur during pregnancy, such as increased cardiac output, increased renal blood flow, and increased arterial compliance. It also relaxes other pelvic ligaments. It is believed to soften the pubic symphysis.

205. Ans. (b) Zona glomerulosa

Ref: Harrison's, 18th ed. Ch 336

- Adrenal gland is divided into adrenal cortex and adrenal medulla, the cortex is further sub-divided into 3 parts, listing them from outside to inside for production of different hormones.

- **Zona Glomeruosa:** Mineralocorticoids
- **Zona Fasciculata:** Glucocorticoids
- **Zona Reticuaris:** Sex Steroids

Extra Mile

Aldosterone	: ↑Conn's ↓ Addisons
Cortisol	: ↑Cushing syndrome
Sex Sterioids hyperplasia	: ↑Congenital adrenal ↓Hypogonadism
Medulla Tumor	: Pheochromocytoma

206. Ans. (d) Addison disease

Ref: Journal, Indian Academy of Clinical Medicine, Vol. 13, No. 1 Jan-March, 2012, pg. 72-3

- *It is known that if glucose infusion is given without glucocorticoid in patients with Addison's disease, they may develop high fever (glucose fever). The exact reason is not specified in textbooks.*

FMGE Solutions Screening Examination

207. Ans. (d) Metabolic alkalosis

Ref: Harrison, 19th ed. pg. 2324

- Addison disease in India is most commonly caused by tuberculosis.

Clinical Features of Addison's
1. Hypotension
2. Salt wasting and salt craving
3. Hypotension fatigue dizziness/ pre-syncope
4. Hyponatremia
5. Hyperkalemia^Q
6. Metabolic acidosis^Q
7. Hyperpigmentation-on palmar creases/sole creases/ previous scars/areola/oral cavity

Investigations
- Non contrast CT abdomen for adrenal damage
- Investigation of choice- Cosyntropin test (ACTH stimulation test)

Treatment
- Drug of choice is hydrocortisone (life-long support)
- If asked DOC of Addisonian crisis: i.v. hydrocortisone
Remember metabolic alkalosis is seen with CONN syndrome.

208. Ans. (b) Amennorhea

Ref: Harrison, 19th ed. pg. 2267

- Most common symptom in females with prolactinoma (after galactorrhea) is menstrual - abnormalities.
- Most common symptom in men is: loss of libido followed by headache.

209. Ans. (c) Coarctation of aorta

Ref: Harrison, 19th ed. pg. 1620

The most common congenital cardiac malformations in Turner syndrome is Bicuspid Aortic valve and Coarctation of Aorta.

210. Ans. (d) Hypoparathyroidism

- The inferior notching of ribs is seen due to pulsation of collaterals in coarctation of aorta.
- Taussig bing operation is done for tetralogy of fallot and is a shunt surgery where the shunt pulsations can cause inferior rib notching.
- **Remember:** Inferior rib notching **(Roesler sign)**
1. Enlarged collateral vessels -Coarctation of the aorta
2. Interrupted aortic arch
3. Subclavian artery obstruction-Takayasu disease
4. Blalock-Taussig shunt: Involves only upper 2 rib spaces
5. AVM of the chest wall
6. SVC obstruction with enlarged venous collaterals
7. Neurogenic tumours - schwannoma (usually single)
8. Neurofibromatosis type 1 (rarely can be superior if neurofibroma is very large)
9. **Superior notching of ribs is seen in Marfan syndrome, rheumatoid arthritis, SLE and hyperparathyroidism.**

211. Ans. (d) Weight gain

Ref: Harrison, 19th ed. pg. 152

- T3 and T4 have sympatho-mimetic activity and they affect basal metabolic rate. Hence in thyrotoxicosis the increase in BMR will lead to weight loss. The sympatho-mimetic activity leads to anxiety palpitations and tachycardia.

212. Ans. (c) Prader Willi syndrome

Ref: Harrison, 19th ed. pg. 415e-4

Adrenal insufficiency	Salt and water loss leads to weight loss
Pseudo-hypoparathyroidism	PTH receptor defect leads to hypocalcemia and hyperphosphatemia
Soto syndrome	• Soto's syndrome aka cerebral gigantism is a rare genetic disorder characterized by excessive physical growth during the first 2 to 3 years of life. Obesity is however not seen. • Patients with Soto's syndrome tend to be large at birth and are often taller, heavier, and have macrocephaly.

PRADER WILLI SYNDROME

- Neonatal hypotonia with normal growth immediately after birth
- Small hands and feet, mental retardation
- Hypogonadism
- Some have partial deletion of chromosome 15 and loss of paternally expressed genes
- Hyperphagia leading to severe childhood obesity; ghrelin paradoxically elevated.

213. Ans. (d) Smoking is a risk factor

Ref: Harrison, 19th ed. pg. 2392

- The prevalence of obesity is same for men and women at 36%.
- Prevalence increases with age.
- Genetic pre-disposition plays an important role.
- Smoking predisposes to obesity.

Medicine

647

BMI (kg/m²)	Weight status	BMI percentile for children	Weight status
<18.5	Underweight	<5th percentile	Underweight
18.5–24.9	Normal weight	5th–84th percentile	Normal weight
25–29.9	Overweight	85th–94th percentile	At risk for overweight
30–34.9	Obese	≥95th percentile	Overweight
35–39.9	Moderately obese		
40–49.9	Morbid obesity		
≥50	Super morbid obesity		

214. Ans. (a) Serum fructosamine

Ref: Evidence Based Diabetes Care, 2nd ed. pg. 229

- Serum fructosamine is a retrospective test that determines fluctuations in blood sugar in the previous 2–3 weeks.
- In contrast glycosylated hemoglobin gives fluctuations in blood sugar value over the previous 6-8 weeks.
- **Also remember:** severity of bronze diabetes is determined by GLYCATED albumin.

215. Ans. (a) Phenformin

Ref: KD Tripathi 7th ed. pg. 275

- Phenformin was withdrawn from the market as it causes lactic acidosis
- Metformin is the drug of choice for management of type 2 diabetes mellitus with obesity. *Metformin also causes lactic acidosis of given in renal failure (diabetic nephropathy) patients.*
- Rosiglitazone was withdrawn as it causes coronary artery thrombosis
- Pioglitazone has a black box warning as it causes bladder cancer.

216. Ans. (a) Metformin

Ref: Harrison, 19th ed. pg. 2413-14

- Drug of choice for obese type 2 diabetes mellitus is metformin. This drug increases the peripheral utilization of sugar by sensitizing the receptors. The fall in HbA1c is 1–2%.

217. Ans. (c) < 180 mg/dL

Ref: Harrison, 18th ed. ch. 344

TABLE: Treatment goal for adults with diabetes

Parameters	Goal
HbA1C	<7%
Preprandial capillary plasma glucose	70–130 mg/dL

Contd...

Parameters	Goal
Peak post prandial capillary plasma glucose	<180 mg/dL
Blood pressure	<130/80
LIPIDS	
LDL	<70 mg/dL
HDL	>40 mg/dL in men >50 mg/dL in women
Triglycerides	<150 mg/dL

218. Ans. (b) Dilutional hyponatremia

Ref: Harrison, 19th ed. pg. 303-304

- Diabetes insipidus has either low levels of vasopressin or it is not able to act. Therefore these patients pass a large amount of dilute urine(Polyuria and resultant polydipsia develops). The result is that due to loss of water from body these patients will develop relative hypernatremia.
- *The diagnostic test is water deprivation test*

Drugs

- NEUROGENIC diabetes inspidus is treated with desmopressin nasal spray.
- Nephrogenic diabetes inspidus is treated with thiazide diuretics.
- **Remember:** Dilutional hyponatremia is seen with S.I.A.D.H.

219. Ans. (c) Relative hypernatremia

Ref: Harrison 19th ed. pg. 2280

- SIADH is characterized by gain of water and hence dilutional hyponatremia sets in. The gain of water explains low uric acid.
- Since in SAIDH most of the water is reabsorbed via the CD, the low urine output prompts a physician to possibility of renal parenchymal disorder for which KFT must be done and must be normal to consider diagnostic possibility of SIADH.

220. Ans. (a) Insulinoma

Ref: Harrison, 19th ed. pg. 569

- Whipple's triad is used for diagnosis of insulinoma. The findings seen are:
  1. Fasting hypoglycemia (sympathomimetic symptoms)
  2. Relief of symptoms with oral/IV sugar
  3. Rebound hypoglycemia
- IOC for insulinoma is 72 hour prolonged fasting test[Q]
- Imaging modality is P.E.T scan[Q]
- *Drug of choice is Octreotide > diazoxide*

Explanations

FMGE Solutions Screening Examination

221. Ans. (a) 24-hour urinary 5H.I.A.A.

Ref: Harrison, 19th ed. pg. 564-65

- 5-HIAA is the major urinary metabolite of serotonin, a ubiquitous bioactive amine. Serotonin, and consequently 5-HIAA, are produced in excess by most carcinoid tumors, especially those producing the carcinoid syndrome of flushing, hepatomegaly, diarrhea, bronchospasm, and heart disease.

222. Ans. (b) Serotonin

Ref: Harrison, 19th ed. pg. 564-65

- Argentaffin cells in Carcinoid produce 5HT derivatives like serotonin. Epinephrine and norepinephrine are produced by chromaffin cells which are seen in phaeochromocytoma.

223. Ans. (c) TSH

Ref: Harrison, 19th ed. pg. 2289

- Best test for diagnosis of hypothyroidism is T.S.H (Thyroid Stimulating Hormone).
- TSH can also be used for monitoring response to treatment.

224. Ans. (b) Excessive iodine

Ref: Harrison, 19th ed. pg. 2285, 2297

- Excess iodide transiently inhibits thyroid iodide organification, a phenomenon known as the *Wolff-Chaikoff effect.*
- Thyroid hormone synthesis becomes excessive as a result of increased iodine exposure (Jod-Basedow phenomenon which is opposite of Wolf Chaikoff effect.)
- Iodine deficiency increases thyroid blood flow and upregulates the iodine trapping, stimulating more efficient iodine uptake.
- Ingestion of excess thyroid hormone or thyroid tissue is known as thyrotoxicosis factitia. In the first and second statements of this explanation iodine intake was affected but in Throtoxicosis factitia is due to the ingestion of hormone.

225. Ans. (d) Menorrhagia

Ref: Harrison, 19th ed. pg. 2293

- Thyrotoxicosis is characterized by increased sympathomimetic action causing palpitations, anxiety and increased BMR causing weight loss. *The menstrual abnormality in Grave's disease is oligo-menorrhea.*
- REMEMBER. Weight gain with menorrhagia is seen in hypothyroidism.
- Weight gain with hirusutism with oligomenorrhea is seen in Cushing syndrome.

226. Ans. (d) Myxoedema

Ref: Harrison, 19th ed. pg. 2289

Choices	Logic
Grave's	Cytokines appear to play a major role in thyroid-associated ophthalmopathy. There is infiltration of the extraocular muscles by activated T cells; the release of cytokines such as IFN-alpha and TNF results in fibroblast activation and increased synthesis of glycosaminoglycans that trap water, thereby leading to characteristic muscle swelling
Sarcoidosis	Approximately 20% of patients with ophthalmic findings of sarcoid have soft tissue involvement of the orbit or lacrimal gland and present as a mass lesion with proptosis, ptosis, or ophthalmoplegia
Pituitary apoplexy	Pituitary adenoma if a Macro-adenoma or is associated with pituitary apoplexy can lead to Proptosis

227. Ans. (b) Lower esophageal web

Ref: Harrison, 19th ed. pg. 237

- Plummer Vinson syndrome is a premalignant condition characterized by *upper esophageal web* plus *Koilonchyia* and *iron deficiency anemia*. These patients also complain of a burning sensation on the tongue and oral mucosa, and atrophy of lingual papillae produces a smooth, shiny, red dorsum of the tongue.

228. Ans. (a) Hyperglycemia

Ref: Harrison 19th ed. pg. 2257-58

- From late in the first year until mid teens, poor growth and/or shortness is the hallmark of childhood GH deficiency.
- It tends to be accompanied by delayed physical maturation so that bone maturation and puberty may be delayed by several years.
- Severe GH deficiency in early childhood also results in slower muscular development, so that gross motor milestones may be delayed.
- Some severely GH-deficient children have recognizable, cherubic facial features characterized by maxillary hypoplasia and forehead prominence. These children have a high pitched voice and are stunted. *GH deficiency is associated with hypoglycemia.* In contrast gigantism or acromegaly is associated with impaired glucose tolerance.

229. Ans. (d) Hyperphosphataemia

Ref: Harrison 19th ed. /96e-7

- Vitamin D deficiency will lead to Hypocalcemia. This will result in secondary increase in PTH.

Medicine

- This PTH will now act on proximal convoluted tubule to *cause loss of phosphate*. The increased bone turnover will cause increase in serum alkaline phosphate.
- Important calcium/phosphate and SAP fluctuations which are asked (especially those in bold).

Condition	Rickets	Hyperparathyroidism	Osteoporosis[Q]	Paget disease	Chronic renal failure[Q]
Serum calcium	Less	Increased	**Normal**	Normal	**Less**
Serum phosphate	Less	Less	**Normal**	Normal	**Increased**
SAP	Increased	Increased	Normal	Disproportionate Increased	**Increased**
PTH	Increasing	Increased	**Normal**	Normal	**Increased**

230. Ans. (a) Hypophosphatemia

Refer to above table

231. Ans. (c) Diarrhea

Ref: Harrison, 19th ed. pg. 2342

- Hyperparathyroidism leads to increase PTH. PTH increases serum calcium by increasing dietary absorption of vitamin D3. It also ensures that the proximal convoluted tubule start loosing phosphate in urine leading to decreased serum phosphate.
- The increase serum calcium leads to deposition in kidney parenchyma forming calcium phosphate stones. The increased level of calcium also leads to constipation. Therefore abdominal pain are a feature of hyperparathyroidism. Renal Colic is due to stones and severe constipation. *Diarrhea is not seen with hypercalcemia/hyperparathyroidism.*

232. Ans. (c) Somatostinoma

Ref: Harrison, 19th ed. pg. 570

- In Secretory diarrhea, the epithelial cells' ion transport processes are turned into a state of active secretion. Now *since somatostatin is the inhibitory hormone of the GIT therefore secretory diarrhea cannot be seen* and rather constipation is seen.

234. Ans. (a) Metabolic acidosis

Causes of Secretory Diarrhea

- The most common cause of acute-onset secretory diarrhea is a bacterial infection of the gut.
- Features of secretory diarrhea include a high purging rate, a *lack of response to fasting*, and a normal stool ion gap (i.e., 100 mOsm/kg or less), indicating that nutrient absorption is intact.

Causes of Secretory diarrhea
1. Zollinger Ellison syndrome
2. VIPoma
3. Glucagonoma
4. Insulinoma

233. Ans. (d) Gastrochisis

Ref: Chapter 96: Intrauterine Diagnosis of Fetal Disease, Nelson 18th ed.

- All structural defects can be best picked up by antenatal ultrasound whereas chromosomal and genetic aberrations can be picked up by chorionic villus sampling.
- Chorionic villi are tiny finger-shaped growths found in the placenta. The genetic material in chorionic villus cells is the same as that in the baby's cells.
- During CVS, a sample of the chorionic villus cells is taken for biopsy. The chorionic villus cells are checked for problems. The procedure is generally done late in the first trimester, most often between the 10th and 12th weeks.

Ref: Harrison, 19th ed. pg. 2327

11 beta hydroxylase deficiency, is characterized by:
- Mineralocorticoid excess and hence hypertension can be seen
- *Mineralocorticoid excess leads to hypokalemia and metabolic alkalosis.*
- Glucocorticoid deficiency leads to hypoglycemia plus excess of ACTH leads to hyperpigmentation around genitals
- Excess of adrenal androgens leads to Virilization.

Variant	Gene	Impact on steroid synthesis	Diagnostic marker in serum (and urine)
21-Hydroxylase deficiency (21OHD)	*CYP21A2*	Glucocorticoid deficiency, mineralocorticoid deficiency, adrenal androgen excess	17-Hydroxyprogesterone

Contd...

Explanations

FMGE Solutions Screening Examination

Variant	Gene	Impact on steroid synthesis	Diagnostic marker in serum (and urine)
11-Hydroxylase deficiency (11OHD)	CYP11B1	Glucocorticoid deficiency, mineralocorticoid excess, adrenal androgen excess	11-Deoxycortisol
17-Hydroxylase deficiency (17OHD)	CYP17A1	Glucocorticoid deficiency, mineralocorticoid excess, androgen deficiency	11-Deoxycorticosterone
3-Hydroxysteroid dehydrogenase deficiency	HSD3B2	Glucocorticoid deficiency, mineralocorticoid deficiency, adrenal androgen excess	17-Hydroxypregnanolone

HEMATOLOGY

235. Ans. (c) D.I.C

Ref: CMDT 2019, pg. 563

As per the question:

Prothrombin time	Increased
Activated partial thromboplastin time	Increased
Platelet count	Reduced (Normal = 1.5–4.5 Lac/cu.mm)
Interpretation	Consumption of clotting factors and platelets seen in Disseminated intravascular coagulation.

- Choice A has non thrombocytopenic purpura due to complement mediated damage to blood vessels. Platelet count is normal in HSP.
- Choice B has recurrent abdominal pain with photo-sensitivity but no bleeding
- Choice D has only low platelet count with normal PT and aPTT

236. Ans. (a) Fibrin degradation products

Ref: Harrison, 20th ed. pg. 835

- Fibrin and fibrinogen degradation product (FDP) testing is commonly used to diagnose disseminated intravascular coagulation (DIC).
- The reference range of FDP levels is less than 10 mcg/mL. Level of more than 40 mg/mL is considered critical.
- Choice B and C are deranged in multiple conditions like haemophilia and chronic liver disease and hence are not diagnostic of DIC.
- Choice D, D- Dimer assay is used as a screening test for pulmonary embolism.

Fibrinolytic system and its regulation

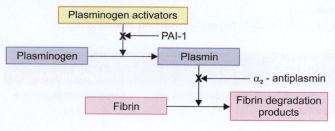

237. Ans. (a) Bone infarction

Ref: Harrison, 19th ed. P 634

- Sickle cell anemia leads to development of sickling episodes. This leads to vaso-occlusive crisis and bone infarction involving mainly long bones.
- The *hand foot syndrome* is caused by painful infarcts of digits and dactylitis.
- The vaso-occlusive crisis/painful crisis develop suddenly and lead to pain anywhere in the body lasting for weeks.
- Spleen is also destroyed by these cumulative small infarcts by 18–36 months of age.

238. Ans. (a) Bacterial overgrowth syndrome

Ref: Harrison 19th ed. P 350e-1

- Schilling test helps in determining etiology of vitamin B_{12} deficiency.
- Bacterial overgrowth syndrome occurs due to growth of *large intestinal microbiota flora* like bacteroides to *multiply in small intestine*.
- Hence after a course of antibiotics when the flora will die, normal B_{12} absorption can take place and Schilling's test will become normal.

TABLE: Differential results of the Schilling's test in several diseases associated with cobalamin malabsorption

	58Co-labeled cobalamin	With intrinsic factor	With pancreatic enzymes	After 5 days of antibiotics
Pernicious anemia	Reduced	Normal	Reduced	Reduced
Chronic pancreatitis	Reduced	Reduced	Normal	Reduced
Bacterial overgrowth	Reduced	Reduced	Reduced	Normal
Ileal disease	Reduced	Reduced	Reduced	Reduced

- In chronic pancreatitis, test will become normal with addition of pancreatic supplements.
- In atrophic gastritis, IF supplementation will normalize the Schilling's test.
- If in spite of antibiotics, IF supplementation and pancreatic enzymes the test remains abnormal, it indicates presence of ileal mucosal disease.

Medicine

239. Ans. (c) Adult T cell leukemia

Human T cell linked virus is related to development of:
- Adult T cell leukaemia
- Tropical spastic paraparesis

Clinical Picture for Adult T cell Leukemia
1. Rapidly progressive skin lesions that mimic mycosis fungoides
2. Pulmonary involvement
3. Hypercalcemia
4. Lymphocytosis with cells containing lobulated or "flower-shaped" nuclei
5. Serum levels of CD25 can be used as a tumor marker. *The cumulative lifetime risk of developing ATL is 3% among HTLV-1 infected patients*

> **Extra Mile**
>
> HTLV-I infection is transmitted in three ways:
> - Mother to child, especially via breast milk
> - Sexual activity
> - Blood via contaminated transfusions or contaminated needles. The virus is most commonly transmitted perinatally. Compared with HIV, which can be transmitted in cell-free form, HTLV-I is less infectious, and its transmission usually requires cell-to-cell contact.

240. Ans. (a) Microcytic Anemia

Ref: Harrison, 19th ed. pg. 640, 645

B12 deficiency is characterised by:
- Loss of vibratory and position sense (Rhomberg sign)
- Abnormal gait
- Dementia
- Impotence
- Loss of bladder and bowel control
- Macrocytic anemia

241. Ans. (b) Megaloblastic anaemia

Ref: Harrison, 19th ed. pg. 81e-3f

The presence of macrocytes with hyper segmented neutrophils confirms the answer as megaloblastic anaemia.

242. Ans. (b) Iron deficiency anemia

Ref: Harrison, 19th ed. pg. 627-28

- Initially the anemia is normocytic normochromic and subsequently hypochromic and microcytic. There is mild to moderate anisocytosis (variation in size) and poikilocytosis (Variation and shape).
- The long, thin elliptocytes of iron deficiency are sometimes referred to as pencil cells.
- Target cells are uncommon and anisochromasia is characteristic. There are two features that can be useful in making the distinction from thalassaemia trait.
- Subsequently there is a fall in the MCV and the MCH and, when it is measured by a sensitive technique, a fall in the MCHC as well.

243. Ans. (a) Age between 1 and 10 years

Ref: Harrison, 19th ed. pg. 699-700

Prognostic factor in acute lymphoblastic leukemia

Excellent prognosis	- t(12;21) and TEL-AML1 fusion - Hyperdiploidy and trisomy of specific chromosomes (4, 10 and 17) is associated with an excellent prognosis. - Age >1 years and <10 years
Dismal prognosis	- t(9;22) or Philadelphia chromosome and BCR-ABL fusion - Hypodiploidy with chromosome number <45 is associated with a poor prognosis - Age >10 years - WBC >50,000/cu.mm^3 - CNS leukemia at presentation

244. Ans. (b) HLA mediated

Ref: Harrison, 18th ed. Chapter 113

- Transfusion-Related Acute Lung Injury (TRALI) is a syndrome characterized by acute respiratory distress following transfusion.
- *TRALI usually results from the donor plasma that contains high-titer anti-HLA antibodies that bind recipient leukocytes.*
- The leukocytes aggregate in the pulmonary vasculature and release mediators that increase capillary permeability.
- Testing the donor's plasma for anti-HLA antibodies can support this diagnosis.
- The implicated donors are frequently multiparous women, and transfusion of their plasma component should be avoided.
- All plasma-containing blood products have been implicated including rare reports of IVIG and cryoprecipitate.
- *Symptoms of TRALI typically develop during, or within 6 hours of a transfusion.* Patients present with the rapid onset of dyspnea and tachypnea. There may be associated fever, cyanosis, and hypotension and clinical exam reveals non-cardiogenic pulmonary edema.

245. Ans. (b) Autosomal recessive

Ref: Harrison, 18th ed. Chapter 104

THALASSEMIA SYNDROMES

- The thalassemia syndromes are inherited disorders of alpha- or beta-globin biosynthesis and have autosomal recessive inheritance.
- The *most common genetic mutation* in thalassemia arises from mutations that derange splicing of the mRNA precursor or prematurely terminate translation of the mRNA
- Investigation of choice is high performance liquid chromatography

- Treatment of choice is allogenic bone marrow transplantation
- For survival in thalassemia major recurrent packed RBC transfusions are given initially.

246. Ans. (a) Iron deficiency anemia

Ref: Chapter 104: Harrison, 18th ed.

Disease	Serum iron	Serum ferritin	TIBC
Iron deficiency anemia	Decreased	Decreased	Increased
Chronic kidney disease (anemia is due to deficiency of erythropoietin)	Normal	Normal/decreased if lost in urine due to kidney pathology	Normal
Sideroblastic anemia	Increased	Increased	Decreased
Fanconi anemia (congenital aplastic anemia)	Normal	Normal	Normal

247. Ans. (a) Platelet elevation

Ref: Harrison, 18th ed. chapter 115

Essential thrombocytosis (primary thrombocythemia) is a nonreactive, *chronic myeloproliferative disorder* in which sustained megakaryocyte proliferation leads to an increase in the number of circulating platelets.

248. Ans. (d) All of the above

Ref: Harrison's, 17th ed. Ch. 109

- Schistocytes are fragmented part of a red blood cells which are typically irregularly shaped, jagged, and have two pointed ends. A true schistocyte does not have central pallor. They are sometimes referred to as **"helmet cells"**.
- The presence of schistocytes on the peripheral blood smear suggests red blood cell injury from damaged endothelium **and is a characteristic feature of microangiopathic hemolytic anemia.**

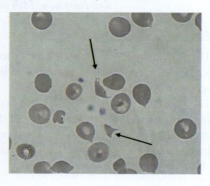

- Microangiopathic hemolytic anemia is an infrequent cause of Coombs-negative intravascular hemolytic anemia, and its causes include:
  1. *Thrombotic thrombocytopenic purpura*
  2. *Hemolytic uremic syndrome*
  3. *Disseminated intravascular coagulation*
  4. Valvular prosthesis

249. Ans. (b) Deficiency is rarely seen, except in infants

Ref: Harrison, 19th ed. pg. 96e-8

- Vitamin-K is a fat soluble compound. It promotes blood clotting by increasing hepatic biosynthesis of prothrombin and other coagulation factors.
- The best sources are green leafy vegetables, liver, cheese, butter and egg yolk. *Deficiency, usually seen only in neonates, in disorders of absorption or during antibiotic therapy is characterized by hemorrhage.*
- *Warfarin acts by inhibiting Vitamin K, and does not causes deficiency of the same.*
- Factor VII is the first to reduce, since it has shortest half life.

250. Ans. (a) Pigmented

Ref: Harrison, 19th ed. pg. 2078

- Pigmented gall stones have composition of Calcium Bilirubinate and are seen in hemolytic anemia like hereditary spherocytosis, sickle cell anemia.

251. Ans. (c) Meth-hemoglobinaemia

Ref: Harrison, 19th ed. pg. 636

- Sickle cell anemia has a pediatric presentation.
- Hemolytic anemia will cause pallor and not brown discoloration of blood.
- In G6PD in event of intravascular hemolysis the hemoglobinuria will cause a black urine. Therefore by exclusion the answer is meth-hemoglobinaemia.

252. Ans. (c) Donor serum is tested against recipient packed cells

Ref: Harrison, 19th ed. pg. 138e-2

Cross-matching blood is performed prior to a blood transfusion in order to *determine if the donor's blood is compatible with the blood of an intended recipient*, or to identify matches for organ transplantation.

253. Ans. (c) Chronic liver disease

Ref: Harrison, 19th ed. pg. 405

- Dengue hemorrhagic fever has thrombocytopenia so bleeding time is increased.
- Von wilebrand disease has deficiency of vWf which acts as an adhesive and glues the platelet to the damaged vessel wall. Hence the platelets are not able to glue on to the bleeding site and the bleeding time is increased.

Medicine

- Bernard soulier is a platelet function defect of Ib/IIa receptor defect which leads to defective platelet adhesion and thereby an increased bleeding time.
- In chronic liver disease, the clotting factor 7 (shortest half life) depletes very fast leading to prolongation of PROTHROMBIN TIME.

254. Ans. (a) +4 degree Celsius

Ref: Harrison, 19th ed. pg. 138e-6

Blood is stored in blood bank at 4 degrees Celsius. This results in decrease in metabolic rate of RBC and their cellular requirements. Hence the advantage is that the shelf life of blood in blood bank is 21–42 days. *(Average of 35 days as best answer in MCQ).*

- Cryoprecipitate is stored at minus 20 degree Celsius.
- In contrast platelets are stored in blood bank at room temperature with average of +20-24 degree Celsius.

255. Ans. (c) Chronic myeloid leukemia

Ref: Harrison, 19th ed. pg. 672

The following are Myelo-proliferative disorders:
1. Polycythemia vera
2. Chronic myeloid leukemia
3. Essential thrombocytosis
4. Myelofibrosis
5. Systemic mastocytosis
6. Chronic eosinophilic leukemia

256. Ans. (a) H. Influenza

Ref: Harrison, 19th ed. pg. 484, 652

- Spleen protects from capsulated organisms and hence protects from infection from organisms like *pneumococcus, meningococcus, hemophilus influenza.*
- *Vaccination against these organisms must be done 4 weeks before planned splenectomy.*

257. Ans. (a) Imatinib mesylate

Ref: Harrison, 19th ed. pg. 102e-3

- *Imatinib mesylate is an inhibitor of tyrosine kinase which is used for treatment of the following cancers*
  - Chronic myeloid leukemia
  - Gastro-intestinal stromal tumors
  - Systemic mastocytosis

258. Ans. (a) Long arm of chromosome 9 and long arm of chromosome 22

Ref: Harrison, 19th ed. pg. 101e-3

- The exact chromosomal defect in Philadelphia chromosome is a *translocation*, between the long arms of chromosome 22 and 9. The result is that a fusion gene is created by *juxta positioning* the Abl1 gene on chromosome 9 (region q34) to a *part of the BCR ("breakpoint cluster region") gene on chromosome 22 (region q11).*
- The significance of knowing this information is that this chromosome defect causes activation of an enzyme by the name of tyrosine kinase which provides energy to the cancer cells to divide uncontrollably.

259. Ans. (a) Macrocytic anemia

Ref: Harrison, 19th ed. pg. 637

- Thalassemia major is a hemolytic anemia where defective RBC's are produced resulting in transfusion dependency since the defective RBC's are destroyed by the spleen. *These defective RBC in blood circulation are referred to as target cells on a peripheral smear.*
- The type of anemia seen is referred to as **Microcytic Hypochromic anemia**.
- The Hematopoiesis that occurs in liver and spleen in these patients is referred to as extramedullary hematopoiesis and is responsible for spleno-hepatomegaly in these patients.

260. Ans. (d) Cirrhosis

Ref: Harrison, 19th ed. pg. 739

- In cirrhosis of the liver the production of all clotting factors will be reduced and therefore in these patients bleeding diathesis is seen.
- In pregnancy the elevated fibrinogen levels will lead to hyper-coagulable state.
- In abruption placentae the retro-placental clot formation implies the same hypercoagualability.
- In MI the preceding plaque fissure results in development of increased clotting tendency.

261. Ans. (a) Hereditary spherocytosis

Ref: Harrison, 19th ed. pg. 651

- In hereditary spherocytosis, the RBCs have a tendency to be trapped and destroyed in splenic sinusoids. The main features of this disease include anemia, reticulocytosis, jaundice, and splenomegaly. Hence elective splenectomy would be the treatment of choice for this condition.

262. Ans. (a) C.M.L.

Ref: Harrison, 19th ed. pg. 324, 634

Priapism is characterized by prolonged, painful and irreducible erection, not resulting in ejaculation. It is an emergency with a poor prognosis, as the risk of impotence is 50%.

Causes of Priapism

- Sickle cell anemia
- Chronic myelogenous leukemia, Chronic lymphocytic leukemia, and acute lymphoblastic leukemia. The hyper-leukocytosis leads to increased viscosity of blood and resultant priapism
- Drugs

FMGE Solutions Screening Examination

263. Ans. (a) B cell tumor

Ref: Harrison 19th ed. / 706

- Hairy cell leukemia is a B cell tumor disease that presents in older males.
- Usual presentation involves pancytopenia with splenomegaly.
- The malignant cells appear to have "*hairy*" *projections* on light and electron microscopy and show a characteristic staining pattern with *tartrate-resistant acid phosphatase*.
- *Bone marrow* is typically not able to be aspirated, and *biopsy shows a pattern of fibrosis*.
- Patients with this disorder are prone to unusual infections, including infection by Mycobacterium avium intracellulare, and to vasculitic syndromes.
- Hairy cell leukemia is responsive to chemotherapy with interferon, pentostatin, or *cladribine, with the latter being the usually preferred treatment*.

GASTROINTESTINAL TRACT

264. Ans. (a) Small intestinal mucosal biopsy

Ref: Harrison, 20th ed. pg. 2253

- The clinical presentation given is of malabsorbtion syndrome and is confirmed with small intestinal mucosal biopsy.
- Choice B allows the diagnosis or exclusion of pancreatic exocrine insufficiency, which can be caused by chronic pancreatitis, cystic fibrosis, pancreatic tumour.
- Choice C is done for picking up sugar in stool of osmotic diarrhea patient
- Choice D is done for Hirschsprung's disease.

265. Ans. (c) Directly related to duration of disease

Ref: Harrison, 20th ed. pg. 2275

- The risk of neoplasia in UC is increased with *duration* and *extent of disease*.
- Incidence is 2% at end of 10 years and a huge 18% at end of 30 years. The risk is 1.5-2 times higher than general population.
- Choice A is wrong as UC is a premalignant condition.
- Choice B is wrong as smoking has no bearing on development of colorectal cancer in ulcerative colitis.
- Choice D is wrong as disease should be present for long duration to lead to development of malignancy. Annual biopsy is recommended for patients with extensive colitis persisting for 10-12 years.

266. Ans. (c) Budesonide

Ref: Harrison: 19th ed. P 1963

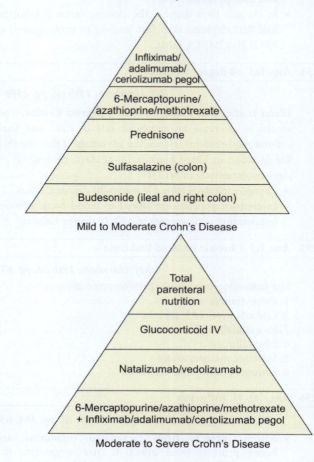

267. Ans. (a) Occurs along structures derived from foregut

Ref: Harrison 19th ed. P 537

- Carcinoid tumor can occur at sites derived from foregut, midgut and hindgut.
- The most common site is bronchus which is derived from foregut.
- In the GIT, common sites are ileum, rectum and appendix.
- Most intestinal carcinoids are asymptomatic and are of *low* malignant potential.
- Bronchial carcinoid can *present* as flushing episodes with secretory diarrhea.
- Elevated VMA levels are found in neuroblastoma and *not pheochromocytoma*^{Q}.

268. Ans. (b) 5-Hydroxyindole acetic acid

Carcinoid tumour produces 5HT derivatives like serotonin and histamine. The degradation of these leads to elevated levels of Urinary 5-Hydroxyindole acetic acid.

Investigations used for diagnosis

1. Urinary 5-HIAA levels   2. Plasma neuropeptide K   3. Serum chromogranin A

Must know points about carcinoid tumor

Name	Biologically Active Peptide(s) Secreted	Tumor location in GIT	Malignant, %	Associated with Multiple Endocrine Neoplasia	Main symptoms/signs
Carcinoid syndrome	Serotonin Tachykinins, Prostaglandins	Midgut (75–87%)^Q Foregut (2–33%) Hindgut (1–8%) Unknown (2–25%)	95–100	Rare	Diarrhea (32–84%)^Q Flushing (63–75%) Pain (10–34%) Asthma (4–18%) Heart disease (11–41%)

269. Ans. (c) Intestinal metaplasia Type 3

- Serial endoscopic examinations of the stomach in patients with atrophic gastritis have documented replacement of the usual gastric mucosa by intestinal type cells. This process of *intestinal metaplasia* may lead to cellular atypia and eventual neoplasia.
- Gastric cancer is associated with blood group A.
- Gastric adenocarcinomas may be subdivided into two categories: a *diffuse type*, in which cell cohesion is absent, so that individual cells infiltrate and thicken the stomach wall without forming a discrete mass; and an *intestinal type*, characterized by cohesive neoplastic cells that form gland like tubular structures.
- Diffuse cancers have defective intercellular adhesion, mainly as a consequence of loss of expression of E-cadherin. Intestinal-type lesions are frequently ulcerative, more commonly appear in the antrum and lesser curvature of the stomach, and are often preceded by a prolonged precancerous process, often initiated by *Helicobacter pylori* infection.

270. Ans. (a) Stomach

- Up to 70% of GIST arise in the stomach and remaining in small bowel.
- Most exhibit an exophytic growth pattern growing across the bowel wall.
- Mucosal ulceration occurs in large aggressive tumors.
- It is the *most common mesenchymal neoplasm of the gastrointestinal tract.*
- It arises from the intestinal cells of cajal which are called pacemaker cells of intestine.
- They express *cKIT (CD117)* which is a tyrosine kinase growth factor receptor
- Imatinib mesylate is used for treatment.

271. Ans. (a) Antiendomysial antibody

The clinical diagnosis is celiac sprue.
Serum antibodies seen in celiac sprue are:
- The antiendomysial antibody has the antigen recognized by the antiendomysial antibody is tTG, which deaminates gliadin.
- *Choice C, antiepidermal tissue transglutaminase antibody is seen in Dermatitis herpetiformis* which is a papulovesicular eruption caused by ingestion of gluten. It is characterized by the deposition of IgA in the dermal papillae.
- *Choice D,* antimitochondrial antibody is seen in primary biliary cirrhosis.

272. Ans. (a) B_{12}

- Cobalamin deficiency may cause a bilateral peripheral neuropathy or degeneration (demyelination) of the posterior and pyramidal tracts of the spinal cord. This explains the presence of sensory ataxia in the patient.
- The patchy loss of papillae points to diagnosis of geographical tongue consistent with vitamin B_{12} deficiency. Hence cobalamin/B_{12} estimation should be done.
- Cobalamin can measured by an automated enzyme-linked immunosorbent assay (ELISA). Normal serum levels range from 118–148 pmol/L (160–200 ng/L). In patients with megaloblastic anemia due to cobalamin deficiency, the level is usually <74 pmol/L (100 ng/L).

273. Ans. (b) Intestinal biopsy

Ref: Harrison, 19th ed. pg. 1938

- A small intestinal biopsy is essential in evaluation of a patient with documented steatorrhea or chronic diarrhea lasting for >3 months.

- Endoscopy is done and is a preferred method for obtaining biopsy material from proximal small intestinal mucosa.
- **Choice A** is ruled out due to false negative D-xylose test and ease of obtaining small intestinal biopsy after endoscopy.
- **Choice C** is used for evaluation of celiac sprue and is not the first test to be done.
- **Choice D** is not available in United States or India.

274. Ans. (a) B₁₂ estimation

- The patient has macrocytic anemia with loss of tongue papillae suggestive of vitamin B₁₂ deficiency. The loss of papillae leads to beef/y bald tongue.

275. Ans. (a) Stomach

- Cushing's ulcer is a gastroduodenal ulcer produced by elevated intracranial pressure caused by an intracranial tumor, head injury or other space-occupying lesion.
- The ulcer, usually single and deep, may involve the esophagus, stomach, and duodenum.
- Increased intracranial pressure may affect different areas of the hypothalamic nuclei or brainstem leading to overstimulation of the vagus nerve or paralysis of the sympathetic system. Both of these circumstances increase secretion of gastric acid and the likelihood of ulceration of gastroduodenal mucosa.

276. Ans. (b) Ileum

Ref: Harrison, 18th ed. Table 350-3

Site	Percentage of site
Bronchus, lung, trachea	27.9
Midgut	
Jejunum	1.8
Ileum	14.9
Meckel's diverticulum	0.5
Appendix	4.8
Colon	8.6
Liver ovary	0.4
Testis	1.0
Hindgut	<0.1
Rectum	13.6

277. Ans. (a) Serum lipase

Ref: Harrison, 19th ed. pg. 2100

- The cardinal symptom of acute pancreatitis is abdominal pain, which is characteristically dull, boring, and steady.
- *Elevated lipase levels are more specific to the pancreas than elevated amylase levels. Lipase levels remain high for 12 days. In patients with chronic pancreatitis (usually caused by alcohol abuse and question mentions that the patient is back from a party), lipase levels may be elevated in the presence of a normal serum amylase level*
- Usually, the pain is sudden in onset and gradually intensifies in severity until reaching a constant ache.
- *The pain radiates directly through the abdomen to the back in approximately one half of cases.*
- Fever (76%) and tachycardia (65%) are common abnormal vital signs; hypotension may be noted
- Abdominal tenderness, muscular guarding (68%), and distention (65%) are observed in most patients; bowel sounds are often diminished or absent because of gastric and transverse colonic ileus; guarding tends to be more pronounced in the upper abdomen
- Lipase has a slightly longer half-life and its abnormalities may support the diagnosis if a delay occurs between the pain episode and the time the patient seeks medical attention.

278. Ans. (a) 24-hour pH monitoring

Ref: Harrison 19th ed. pg. 261-2

- Ambulatory 24-hour pH monitoring is the criterion standard in establishing a diagnosis of GERD, with a sensitivity of 96% and a specificity of 95%. It quantifies the gastroesophageal reflux and allows a correlation between the symptoms of reflux and the episodes of reflux.
- However the diagnosis can be established on basis of Upper Gastrointestinal endoscopy with esophageal manometry.
- Oesophageal pH < 4.0, for 4 hrs/day is diagnostic of GERD.

279. Ans. (a) Wheat

Ref: Harrison, 19th ed. pg. 1940

- Coeliac disease is caused by a reaction to gliadin found in wheat, oats, rye and Barley. Upon exposure to gliadin, there is production of anti-tissue transglutaminase antibody which cross-reacts with small-bowel tissue, causing an inflammatory reaction.
- This leads to villous atrophy and leads to osmotic diarrhea.

280. Ans. (a) Metaplasia

Ref: Robbins, 8th ed. chapter 15

- Categories in ulcerative colitis, include indefinite for dysplasia, low-grade dysplasia, and high-grade dysplasia. It may be difficult to distinguish dysplasia from the reactive/reparative atypia that occurs after periods of disease activity.
- These diagnoses must be made with caution, because the implications for the patient are serious. Low-grade dysplasia warrants consideration for colectomy, whereas

high-grade dysplasia or carcinoma is an indication for colectomy

- Dysplasia is defined as an unequivocal neoplastic alteration of colonic epithelium. It may consist of architectural disorganization of colonic crypts, cytologic atypia (including nuclear hyperchromasia), pseudostratification, pleomorphism, clumped chromatin, and prominent nucleoli, with increased mitotic activity, particularly in the upper portion of the crypts.

281. Ans. (a) Duodenum with fast clearance

Ref: Harrison, 18th ed. Chapter 103

- *Iron absorbed from the diet from the duodenum or released from stores circulates in the plasma bound to transferrin.*
- *The turnover of transferrin-bound iron is very rapid typically 60-90 min.*
- Because almost all of the iron transported by transferrin is delivered to the erythroid marrow, the clearance time of transferrin-bound iron from the circulation is affected most by the plasma iron level and the erythroid marrow activity.
- When erythropoiesis is markedly stimulated, the pool of erythroid cells requiring iron increases and the clearance time of iron from the circulation decreases. The half-clearance time of iron in the presence of iron deficiency is as short as 10-15 minutes.

282. Ans. (a) Ceftriaxone

Ref: Harrison 19th ed. and Multiple Infectious Disease Journals

Location	Severity	First–line antibiotics	Second-line antibiotics
South-East Asia	Uncomplicated	Cefixime PO	Azithromycin PO
	Complicated	Ceftriaxone IV or Cefotaxime IV	Aztreonam IV or Imipenem IV

283. Ans. (d) Blood culture

Ref: Harrison 18th ed. Chapter 153

- The definitive diagnosis of enteric fever requires the isolation of *S.* typhi or *S.* paratyphi from blood, bone marrow, other sterile sites, rose spots, stool, or intestinal secretions.

For diagnosis in the first week

- Sensitivity of **blood culture** is only 40–80%, probably because of high rates of antibiotic use in endemic areas and the small quantities of *S. typhi* (i.e., <15 organisms/mL).

- **Bone marrow culture** is 55–90% sensitive, and, unlike that of blood culture, its yield is not reduced by up to 5 days of prior antibiotic therapy.
- Culture of **intestinal secretions (best obtained by a noninvasive duodenal string test)** can be positive despite a negative bone marrow culture.

284. Ans. (a) Barium enema- Pipe stem colon

Ref: Internal Medicine Guide 2e/36

Lead pipe appearance of colon is the classical barium enema finding in chronic ulcerative colitis. There is complete loss of haustral markings in the diseased section of colon, and the organ appears smooth walled and cylindrical.

285. Ans. (b) Multiple air fluid level- adhesions and bands

Ref: Manual of Emergency Medicine, 5th ed. pg. 247

- In X-ray you can see that due to intestinal obstruction secondary to adhesions or bands, the loops proximal to the point of obstruction will become dilated and fluid-filled and are usually greater than 2.5-3 cm in size
- Loops of small bowel in a *step-ladder* configuration from the left upper to the right lower quadrant are seen.
- Mostly fluid-filled loops of bowel may demonstrate a *string-of-beads sign* caused by the small amount of visible air in those loops

286. Ans. (a) CBD dilation on ERCP

Ref: Cleveland Internal Medicine Case Reviews, 5th ed. pg. 93

You can see the endoscope in left top half and right 5 o clock position which is radiopaque. It is advanced into D2 from where the ampulla of vater is located. The probe is advanced and dye injected which shows dilatation of whole biliary tree. A stricture is also noted proximal to which the biliary pathway is advanced.

287. Ans. (a) 24-hour pH monitoring

Ref: Harrison, 19th ed. pg. 261-62

- 24-hour pH monitoring is done for GERD.
- Components of 24-hour pH monitoring:
  - Percent total time pH < 4
  - Percent upright time pH < 4
  - Percent supine time pH < 4
  - Number of reflux episodes
  - No. of reflux episodes in 5 minutes
  - Longest reflux episode (minutes)

Remember: This method is also used for detection of *laryngoesophageal reflux* that causes asthma, laryngospasm.

288. Ans. (c) Colon cancer

Ref: Gastrointestinal Oncology, 2nd ed. pg. 24

- Aspirin has been shown to reduce the risk of colorectal cancer in latest studies in JAMA in September 2013. How it works is a matter of research but has shown a reduction in mortality.

289. Ans. (c) Premalignant

Ref: Harrison, 19th ed. pg. 1903

- **Zenker's diverticulum**, aka **pharyngoesophageal diverticulum** is a diverticulum of the mucosa of the pharynx, just above the cricopharyngeal muscle. It is a false diverticulum.
- Pharyngo-oesophageal wall herniates through the point of least resistance (known as Killian's triangle).
- Zenker diverticulum often causes clinical manifestations such as dysphagia, and sense of a lump in the neck, regurgitation, cough, halitosis, infection, involuntary gurgling noises when swallowing.

290. Ans. (a) Crohn's disease

Ref: Harrison, 19th ed. pg. 1951-52

CD is a transmural process. Endoscopically, aphthous or small superficial ulcerations characterize mild disease; in more active disease, stellate ulcerations fuse longitudinally and transversely to demarcate islands of mucosa that frequently are histologically normal.

This "cobblestone" appearance is characteristic of CD, both endoscopically and by barium radiography

Ulcerative colitis	Crohn disease
Only colon involved	Panintestinal
Continuous inflammation extending proximally from rectum	Skip-lesions with intervening normal mucosa
Inflammation in mucosa and submucosa only	Transmural inflammation
No granulomas	Noncaseating granulomas
Perinuclear ANCA (pANCA) positive	ASCA positive
Bleeding (common)	Bleeding (uncommon)
Fistulae (rare)	Fistulae (common)

291. Ans. (d) Invasion of lymph nodes seen

Ref: Harrison, 19th ed. pg. 1951

- Crohn's disease is an inflammatory bowel disease in which all the layers of intestine are involved. It involves both the small as well as large intestine.
- Most common part involved is the ileo-caecal area and skip lesions are common with normal areas interspersed. Invasion of lymph nodes is a feature of malignancy and can be easily excluded.

292. Ans. (a) Ulcerative colitis

Ref: Harrison's, 17th ed. Ch. 289

- In ulcerative colitis there is loss of haustrations, and edema of mucosa gives lead pipe appearance.

293. Ans. (c) Toxic megacolon

Ref: Harrison's, 17th ed. Ch. 289

- Crohn's disease is a chronic, recurrent disease characterized by patchy transmural inflammation involving any segment of the gastrointestinal tract from the mouth to the anus **but most common site is Ileum.**
- Crohn's disease is one of the two main forms of Inflammatory bowel disease and is also known as Granulomatous colitis.
- *Earliest manifestation is Apthous ulcers.*
- Skip lesions, stricture formation, string sign of kantor is also seen.
- **Hallmark feature of crohn's** is fistula formation.
- **Cobble stone appearance is seen** on X-ray.
- **Note:** *Toxic mega colon can be seen in Crohn's disease but more commonly is seen in Ulcerative colitis.*

294. Ans. (a) Ulcerative colitis

Ref: Harrison 19th ed. pg. 1952-53

EPIDEMIOLOGY OF IBD

	Ulcerative colitis	Crohn's disease
Male/female ratio	1:1	1.1–1.8:1
Smoking	May prevent disease	May cause disease
Oral contraceptives	No increased risk	Odds ratio 1.4
Appendectomy	Protective	Not protective
Monozygotic twins	6% concordance	58% concordance
Dizygotic twins	0% concordance	4% concordance

295. Ans. (a) Adenocarcinoma

Ref: Harrison's, 17th ed. Ch. 286

- Metaplastic columnar epithelium develops during healing of erosive esophagitis with continued acid reflux since columnar epithelium is more resistant to acid-pepsin damage than is squamous epithelium.
- The metaplastic epithelium has different epithelial types, including goblet cells and columnar cells.
- Finding intestinal metaplasia with goblet cells in the esophagus is diagnostic of Barrett's esophagus; this type of mucosa is thought to be at risk of cancer

296. Ans. (c) Carcinoid tumor

Ref: Harrison 19th ed. pg. 1039-1040

- *H. pylori* is gram negative bacteria, non sporing, micro aerophilic, extra cellular bacteria. *H. pylori* releases urease enzyme which converts urea to ammonia. Ammonia stimulates G cells of stomach which inturn stimulates parietal cells and cause secretion of Hcl à Hyperchlorydia. This acid travels into stomach & duodenum and causes **peptic ulcers.**

- H.pylori is a type I carcinogen, which, if present in stomach for long term can cause cancer called MALTOMA (Mucosa Associated Lymphoid Tumor), which is a B-type NHL.

> **Extra Mile**
> - MC site of duodenal ulcer in duodenum: D1
> - Peptic ulcer refractory to PPi treatment is seen in Zollinger Ellison Syndrome
> - IOC for *H. pylori*: Urease test (invasive procedure)
> - Urea breath test: test for eradication of infection
> - S. Elisa: Screening test for *H. Pylori*

297. Ans. (a) Campylobacter

Ref: Harrison, 19th ed. pg. 266

- Diarrhea, the leading cause of illness in travelers, is usually a short-lived, self-limited condition; however, 40% of affected individuals need to alter their scheduled activities, and another 20% are confined to bed.
- The most frequently identified pathogens causing travelers' diarrhea are
  1. Toxigenic *Escherichia coli* and Enteroaggregative *E. coli (Most common but not in choices)*
  2. In Southeast Asia *Campylobacter* infections appear to predominate
  3. *Salmonella*, *Shigella*
  4. Rotavirus
  5. Norovirus has caused numerous outbreaks on cruise ships
  6. Except for giardiasis, parasitic infections are uncommon causes of travelers' diarrhea.
- A growing problem for travelers is the development of antibiotic resistance among many bacterial pathogens. Examples include strains of *Campylobacter* resistant to quinolones and strains of *E. coli*, *Shigella*, and *Salmonella* resistant to trimethoprim-sulfamethoxazole

HEPATOLOGY

298. Ans. (a) SGOT

Ref: Harrison, 20th ed. pg. 2337

Child Pugh Classification

Points	1	2	3
Encephalopathy	None	Minimal	Advanced (coma)
Ascites	Absent	Controlled	Refractory
Bilirubin (mmol/L)	<34	34–51	>51
Albumin (g/L)	>35	28–35	<28
Prothrombin (sec)*	<4	4–6	>6

*International normalized ratio

Note: The Child-Pugh score is calculated by adding the scores for the five factors and can range from 5 to 15. The resulting Child-Pugh class can be A (a score of 5–6), B (7–9), or C (≥10). Decompensation indicates cirrhosis, with a Child-Pugh score of ≥7 (class B). This level has been the accepted criterion for listing a patient for liver transplantation

299. Ans. (a) Budd Chiari syndrome

Ref: Harrison, 20th ed. pg. 2410

Budd chiari syndrome leads to occlusion of hepatic veins and leads to post hepatic cause of portal hypertension.

Pre-hepatic causes	Hepatic causes	Post hepatic causes

Portal vein thrombosis
Splenic vein thrombosis
Massive splenomegaly (Banti's syndrome)
	Presinusoidal
	• Schistosomisis
	• Congenital hepatic fibrosis
	Sinusoidal
	• Cirrhosis–many causes
	• Alcoholic hepatitis
	Postsinusoidal
	• Hepatic sinusoidal obstruction (venoocclusive syndrome)
		Posthepatic
		• Budd-Chiari syndrome
		• Inferior vena caval webs
		• Cardiac causes
		  ▪ Restrictive cardiomyopathy
		  ▪ Constrictive pericarditis
		  ▪ Severe congestive heart failure

- Choice B, Banti's disease is fibro-congestive splenomegaly and is a pre-hepatic cause of portal HTN
- Choice C and D are also prehepatic causes of portal hypertension.

> **Extra Mile**
>
> **Clinical Features of portal Hypertension**
>
>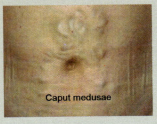
> Caput medusae
>
> ✓ **ABCDE**
> Ascites
> Bleeding (hematemesis, piles)
> Caput medusae
> Diminished liver
> Enlarged spleen

FMGE Solutions Screening Examination

300. Ans. (b) Metabolic syndrome

Ref: Harrison, 19th ed. P 2452

Metabolic syndrome is the most common cause of non-alcoholic fatty liver disease.

It is a lifestyle disease characterized by centripetal obesity, increased blood pressure, impaired glucose tolerance and hypertriglyceridemia.

CAUSES OF NONALCOHOLIC FATTY LIVER

1. *Metabolic syndrome[Q] (MC cause)*
2. Reye syndrome
3. Pregnancy
4. Drugs
5. Kwashiorkor

301. Ans. (c) Trientine

- The *drug of choice for Wilson disease* is zinc acetate but it is **not** a chelator.
- The *chelator for zinc is trientine.* Earlier d-pencillamine was used but not used new due to toxicity.
- For *initial medical therapy of patients with hepatic decompensation,* a chelator (trientine is preferred) plus zinc is recommended zinc should not, however, be ingested simultaneously with trientine, because it will chelate zinc and form therapeutically ineffective complexes; administration of the two drugs should be separated by at least one hour.
- For *initial neurologic therapy, tetrathiomolybdate* is the drug of choice because of its rapid control of free copper, preservation of neurologic function, and low toxicity. penicillamine and trientine should be avoided because they each have a high risk of worsening the neurologic condition.

302. Ans. (d) Liver copper

Investigations for Wilson disease and their relative importance

Test	Usefulness
Serum ceruloplasmin	+
KF rings	++
24-h urine Cu	+++
Liver Cu	++++

303. Ans. (a) Triglycerides

The intracellular triglyceride accumulation is expressed histologically as microvesicular steatosis.

304. Ans. (d) Hepcidin

Ref: Chapter 162, Goldman and Cecil Textbook of Medicine, 24th ed.

- Hepcidin is a 25 amino acid peptide and central regulator of iron homeostasis through its effects on iron homeostasis through its effects on intestinal absorption, macrophage recycling of iron from senescent RBC and iron metabolism from hepatic stores. Thus hepcidin affects all major sites of iron metabolism.
- Hematopoiesis occurs in marrow cords, essentially loose arrangement of cells in dilated sinus area between the arterioles that feed the bone and the venous sinus that returns blood to efferent veins. Erythropoiesis occurs in erythroid islands.

305. Ans. (b) Zinc

Ref: Harrison, 18th ed. Chapter 360

Disease status	First choice
Initial hepatic	
Hepatitis or cirrhosis without decomposition	Zinc
Hepatic decompensation	
Mild	Trientine and zinc
Moderate	Trientine and zinc
Severe	Hepatic transplantation
Initial neurologic/psychiatric	Tetrathiomolybdate and zinc
Maintenance	Zinc

306. Ans. (a) Hippocampus

Ref: Harrison, 18th ed. Chapter 357

Organs Involved in Hemochromatosis are:

- Liver (first organ to be affected) = 95%
- Excessive skin pigmentation
- Diabetes mellitus (bronze diabetes)
- Arthropathy
- Cardiac involvement (restrictive cardiomyopathy)
- Pituitary involvement (leading to hypopituitarism and hypogonadism) = mentioned in textbook as endocrine involvement.

307. Ans. (c) Hepatitis C

Ref: Harrison, 18th ed. Chapter 306

- Chronic hepatitis follows acute hepatitis C in 50–70% of cases; chronic infection is common even in those with a return to normal in aminotransferase levels after acute hepatitis C, *adding up to an 85% likelihood of chronic HCV infection after acute hepatitis C.*

308. Ans. (d) Estrogen

Ref: Harrison, 18th ed. chapter 311

- The hyperdynamic circulatory state of portal hypertension is associated with a dilated, vascular periphery. *This is driven by an excess of systemic nitric oxide and estrogen.*

Medicine

- When these telangectasias occur in the palms, it frequently manifests as a diffuse Palmar erythema.
- This is because the skin on the thenar and hypothenar prominences is thicker and the ectatic vessels are deeper within the dermis.
- Ectatic blood vessels commonly form, and are often noted atop the chest, neck and face. These are referred to as 'spider telangectasias' because they fill centrifugally (like legs of a spider) after the center is blanched.
- Palmar erythema can also be seen in pregnancy, polycythemia, thyrotoxicosis, rheumatoid arthritis, excema, psoriasis and even normal individuals

Extra Mile

Signs of Liver Cell Failure
1. The liver and spleen may be enlarged, with the liver edge being firm and nodular
2. Scleral icterus
3. Palmar erythema
4. Spider angiomas
5. Parotid gland enlargement
6. Digital clubbing
7. Muscle wasting, or the development of edema and ascites.
8. Men may have decreased body hair and gynecomastia as well as testicular atrophy, which may be a consequence of hormonal abnormalities or a direct toxic effect of alcohol on the testes.
9. In women with advanced alcoholic cirrhosis, menstrual irregularities usually occur, and some women may be amenorrheic.

309. Ans. (b) Acute cholangitis

Ref: Harrison, 18th ed. Chapter 311

Acute cholangitis	• The characteristic presentation of acute cholangitis involves biliary **pain, jaundice, and spiking fevers with chills** (Charcot's triad). • ERCP with endoscopic sphincterotomy is safe and the preferred initial procedure for both establishing a definitive diagnosis and providing effective therapy. • Blood cultures are frequently positive, and leukocy-tosis is typical.
Acute Cholecystitis	• Attack of biliary pain that progressively worsens. Approximately 60–70% of patients report having experienced prior attacks that resolved spontaneously. • As the episode progresses, however, the pain of acute cholecystitis becomes more generalized in the right upper abdomen, which may radiate to right shoulder.
Acute viral hepatitis	This is the closest differential diagnosis and is ruled out because of the following points mentioned below. • The *prodromal symptoms like* anorexia, nausea and vomiting, fatigue, malaise, arthralgias, myalgias, headache, photophobia, pharyngitis, cough, and coryza may precede the onset of jaundice by 1–2 weeks.

Cotnd...

- The nausea, vomiting, and anorexia are frequently associated with alterations in olfaction and taste.
- A *low-grade fever* between 38° and 39°C (100°–102°F) is more often present in hepatitis A and E than in hepatitis B or C, except when hepatitis B is heralded by a serum sickness–like syndrome.
- Dark urine and clay-colored stools may be noticed by the patient from 1–5 days before the onset of clinical jaundice

310. Ans. (d) 8 weeks

Ref: Harrison, 19th ed. pg. 2018

- It is sub-divided into "*fulminant hepatic failure*", which *requires onset of encephalopathy within 8 weeks* and Sub-fulminant which leads to encephalopathy after 8 weeks but before 26 weeks.
- Acute liver failure is a broad term that encompasses both fulminant and subfulminant.

311. Ans. (d) Hep E

Ref: Harrison, 19th ed. pg. 152e-2t, 0215

- Most common cause of fulminant hepatitis in pregnancy is HEV
- Most common cause of viral hepatitis in India overall = Hepatitis A
- Most common cause of blood transfusion associated hepatitis = HBV
- Most common viral hepatitis in India in children= HAV
- Most common viral hepatitis in India in adults= HEV
- Most common cause of FULMINANT hepatic failure= toxins> Hepatitis D.

312. Ans. (d) IgM anti- HbcAg

Ref: Harrison, 19th ed. pg. 2017-18

- In most cases, serologic markers of infection and antigenemia appear 1–3 mo after birth, suggesting that transmission occurred at the time of delivery; virus contained in amniotic fluid or in maternal feces or blood may be the source.
  - Most common mode of acquisition, is during delivery..
  - *HBsAg is the 1st serologic marker of infection to appear and is found in almost all infected persons; its rise closely coincides with the onset of symptoms.*
  - Because HBsAg levels fall before symptoms wane, *IgM antibody to HBcAg (anti-HBc IgM) helps to identify acute infection,* as it rises early after infection and remains positive for many months before being replaced by anti-HBc IgG, which persists for years.
  - Anti-HBc is the most valuable single serologic marker of acute HBV infection because it is present almost as early as HBsAg and continues to be present later in the course of the disease when HBsAg has disappeared

313. Ans. (b) Cirrhotic ascites

Ref: Harrison, 19th ed. pg. 286-87

- Diuretics that block aldosterone receptors in the distal convoluted tubule are preferred because of the presence of hyperaldosteronism in patients with cirrhosis.
- Spirinolactone is useful in CHF but not in hypertrophy of heart. It is also useful in transudative pleural effusion
- ACE inhibitors and CCB are used is renal artery stenosis.

314. Ans. (c) >20 mm Hg

- Intra-abdominal hypertension is defined as a pressure over 12 mm Hg in adults. However, if the pressure continues to rise over 20 mm Hg and organs begin to fail, the syndrome has now progressed to the end stage of the highly fatal process termed abdominal compartment syndrome.
- Causes of primary (acute) abdominal compartment syndrome include the following:
  - Penetrating trauma
  - Intraperitoneal hemorrhage
  - Pancreatitis
  - External compressing forces (debris from a motor vehicle collision or after a explosion)
  - Pelvic fracture
  - Rupture of abdominal aortic aneurysm
  - Perforated peptic ulcer

IAP can be easily monitored by measuring bladder pressure. Measurement of intraluminal bladder pressure

315. Ans. (b) Evaluation of left atria and left Atrial appendage thrombus

Ref: Harrison, 19th ed. pg. 270e-2

- Trans-esophageal echocardiography is better than trans-thoracic echocardiography as it is better able to evaluate the left Atrial thrombus and left Atrial appendage. Therefore in patients of atrial fibrillation of long standing duration for evaluation of clots in left atrium, trans-esophageal echocardiography is done.

316. Ans. (a) Enteric fever

Ref: Harrison, 19th ed. pg. 1050-51

Clinical features of Typhoid fever begin 7-14 days after ingestion

- Fever pattern is stepwise, characterized by a rising temperature over the course of each day that drops by the subsequent morning.
- Over the course of the first week of illness, gastrointestinal manifestations of the disease develop. These include diffuse abdominal pain and tenderness and, in some cases, fierce colicky right upper quadrant pain.
- The individual then develops a dry cough, dull frontal headache, delirium, and an increasingly stuporous malaise.
- The patient develops rose spots, which are salmon-colored, blanching, truncal, Maculo-papules usually 1–4 cm wide and fewer than 5 in number; these generally resolve within 2–5 days.

RHEUMATOLOGY

317. Ans. (a) Shrinking Lung syndrome

Ref: Harrison, 20th ed. pg. 2520

The most common lung manifestation of SLE is pleuritis with or without pleural effusion. It may respond to NSAIDS or may require steroids. Life threatening manifestations include interstitial inflammation and shrinking lung syndrome.

318. Ans. (a) SLE

Ref: Harrison, 20th ed. pg. 2518

- ANA> reference value is the first immunological manifestation mentioned in SLICC criteria for diagnosis of SLE. It is not a criterion for diagnosis of the remaining rheumatological diseases mentioned in choices b, c and d.
- This test is positive in 95% cases at the onset of disease and the remaining patients turn positive within one year of disease onset.
- ANA testing using immuno-fluorescent antibodies is more reliable than ELISA.

319. Ans. (b) Non-tender, located on extensor surface and seen with arthritis

Ref: Harrison, 20th ed. pg. 2528-2529

Rheumatic nodules are the most common extra-articular feature of rheumatoid arthritis and consists of non-tender nodules on extensor surface of joints.

Medicine

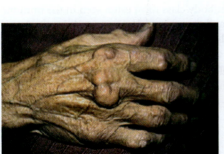
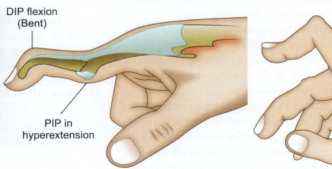

Swan neck deformity — DIP flexion (Bent), PIP in hyperextension

Boutonniere deformity

320. Ans. (b) Uric acid in synovial fluid

Ref: Harrison 19th ed. P 2223

- Since 50% of patients with acute gouty attack have normal serum uric acid levels, the best test to confirm the diagnosis is joint aspiration uric acid crystals.
- Under microscope, needle shaped MSU crystals are seen both intracellularly and extracellularly.
- With compensated polarized light, crystals are brightly birefringent with negative elongation.
- The clinical presentation is dramatic with overnight development of red inflamed 1st MTP joint.
- Anti CCP antibodies are used for diagnosis of rheumatoid arthritis.

321. Ans. (d) Naproxen

Ref: Harrison 19th ed. P 2234

- The mainstay of treatment is administration of NSAIDs. The most effective drugs are those with short half-life including indomethacin, naproxen, ibuprofen, diclofenac and celecoxib.
- Glucocorticoids are given IM or orally and are highly effective in poly-articular gout.

> **Extra Mile**
>
> NSAID contraindicated in acute gout is aspirin.

322. Ans. (a) Takayasu's arteritis

Diagnosis of Takayasu's arteritis should be suspected strongly in a patient who develops:
1. A decrease or absence of peripheral pulses, this disease is hence called pulseless disease
2. Unequal blood pressure between left and right arm
3. Arterial bruits.
   - It is an inflammatory and stenotic disease of medium- and large-sized arteries characterized by a strong predilection for the aortic arch and its branches. For this reason, it is often referred to as the *aortic arch syndrome*
   - Most common vessel involved is left subclavian artery followed by common carotid artery.
   - The diagnosis is confirmed by arteriography

> **Extra Mile**

Clinical Manifestations of Takayasu's Arteritis

Artery	Percent of arteriographic abnormalities	Potential clinical manifestations
Subclavian	93	Arm claudication, Raynaud's phenomenon
Common carotid	58	Visual changes, syncope, transient ischemic attacks, stroke
Abdominal aorta	47	Abdominal pain, nausea, vomiting
Renal	38	Hypertension, renal failure

323. Ans. (a) ASO

- Evidence of an antecedent Group A Streptococcal infection is usually based on elevated or increasing serum antistreptococcal antibody titers.
- *As most cases do not have a positive throat swab culture or rapid antigen test, serologic evidence is usually needed.*
- *The most common serologic tests are the antistreptolysin O (ASO) and anti-DNase B (ADB) titers*
- *If only a single antibody is measured (usually antistreptolysin O), only 80–85% of patients with acute rheumatic fever have an elevated titer.*

324. Ans. (c) Exudative pleural effusion

Lung Disease in Rheumatoid Arthritis
- Most common pulmonary manifestation is pleural involvement leading to pleural friction rub and effusion. This is due to inflammatory breakdown of pulmonary nodules.
- *Pleural effusions tend to be exudative with increased numbers of monocytes and neutrophils.*
- Interstitial lung disease. Pulmonary function testing shows a restrictive pattern (e.g. reduced total lung capacity) with a reduced diffusing capacity for carbon monoxide (DLCO).
- Caplan's syndrome is characterized by the development of nodules and pneumoconiosis following silica exposure.

325. Ans. (a) Behçet's disease

Ref: Harrison, 19th ed. pg. 2194
- Although Behçet's disease is classified among the vasculitides laboratory diagnostic does not include regularly autoantibodies associated with vascular manifestations of systemic autoimmune diseases.
- The autoantigens for pemphigus vulgaris and pemphigus foliaceus are desmoglein 3 and desmoglein 1, respectively.
- *The anti-desmoglein 1 antibodies in pemphigus foliaceus and anti-desmoglein 3 antibodies in pemphigus vulgaris are pathogenic.*
- *Anti-tissue transglutaminase antibodies are pathognomonic for celiac disease.*
- *Anti- nuclear antibody is seen in SLE*
- Causes of Apthous Ulcers:

> **Infections:**
> - Viral (Herpes, CMV, EBV, HIV)
> - Fungal (Candida)
> - Bacterial (Vincent's infection, syphilis)
>
> **Dermatological:**
> - Pemphigus, pemphigoid, lichen planus
>
> **Drug :**
> - Chemotherapy drugs
> - Erythema multiforme, Stevens-Johnson syndrome
>
> **Systemic diseases:**
> - Behcet's syndrome, SLE
>
> **Nutritional:**
> - Vitamin deficiency (Vitamin B and C), iron deficiency
>
> **Neoplasia:**
> - Leukemia, squamous cell carcinoma, Kaposi's sarcoma
>
> **Gastrointestinal:**
> - Crohn's disease, celiac disease
>
> **Traumatic**
> - Dentures
>
> **Chemical or thermal burns:**
> - Corrosives, hot liquids

326. Ans. (a) IgA

Ref: Harrison, 18th ed. Chapter 326
- The Presumptive pathogenic mechanism for Henoch-Schönlein purpura is immune-complex deposition.
- IgA is the antibody class most often seen in the immune complexes and has been demonstrated in the renal biopsies of these patients.
- A number of inciting antigens have been suggested including upper respiratory tract infections, various drugs, foods, insect bites, and immunizations.

327. Ans. (a) SLE

Ref: Harrison, 18th ed. chapter 319
- An LE cell is a neutrophil or macrophage that has phagocytized (engulfed) the denatured nuclear material of another cell
- LE cell testing was once performed to diagnose systemic lupus erythematous (SLE) but has been replaced for this purpose by antinuclear antibody testing.
- The LE cell reaction is positive in 50%–75% of individuals with acute disseminated lupus.
- Positive reactions are also seen in rheumatoid arthritis, chronic hepatitis (lupoid), scleroderma, dermatomyositis, polyarteritis nodosa, acquired hemolytic anemia, and Hodgkin disease.

328. Ans. (b) c-ANCA

Ref: Harrison, 18th ed. Chapter 326:
- c-ANCA = Wegener granulomatosis/Granulomatosis with angitis
- p-ANCA
  - Microscopic polyangitis
  - Primary sclerosing cholangitis
  - Churg strauss syndrome

The terminology of *cytoplasmic ANCA* (cANCA) refers to the diffuse, granular cytoplasmic staining pattern observed by immunofluorescence microscopy when serum antibodies bind to indicator neutrophils. Proteinase-3, a 29-kDa neutral serine proteinase present in neutrophil azurophilic granules, is the major cANCA antigen.

329. Ans. (b) Anti GBM antibody

Ref: Harrison, 18th ed. Chapter 283
- Patients who develop autoantibodies directed against glomerular basement antigens frequently develop a glomerulonephritis termed *antiglomerular basement membrane (anti-GBM) disease.* When they present with lung hemorrhage and glomerulonephritis, they have a pulmonary-renal syndrome called *Goodpasture's syndrome.*

> **Extra Mile**
> - Good's syndrome is a Thymoma with immunodeficiency
> - It is a cause of combined B and T cell immunodeficiency in adults.
> - The clinical characteristics of Good's syndrome are increased susceptibility to bacterial infections with encapsulated organisms and opportunistic viral and fungal infections.
> - The most consistent immunological abnormalities are hypogammaglobulinaemia and reduced or absent B cells.

Medicine

330. Ans. (b) Sarcoidosis

Ref: Harrison, 19th ed. pg. 237, 417

Painful ulcers in mouth

- Apthous ulcers
- Denture stomatitis
- Tuberculosis
- Carcinoma tongue
- Behcet disease
- Thermal burns
- Herpes
- Arsenic poisoning

331. Ans. (d) Female is symptomatic

Ref: Harrison, 19th ed. pg. 462e-5

- Duchenne's muscular dystrophy is an X-linked recessive condition where boys suffer from disease while girls are carriers. **The protein defective is dystrophin** due to defect of dystrophin gene on chromosome Xp.21.
- Boys present between 3-5 years of age with clumsy gait and history of recurrent falls. The gait is peculiar and is known as **waddling gait**. Most children become wheel chair bound by 12–15 years of age. **Gower sign** is a characteristic feature characterized by child getting up gradually.
- On physical examination pseudo-hypertrophy (called so because of the physical appearance) but actually has fat deposition around the muscles. The weakness of respiratory muscles results in **recurrent pneumonia that ultimately results in mortality.**

Investigations

1. CPK MM
2. EMG and nerve conduction velocity
3. Muscle biopsy and western blot analysis of tissue specimen

332. Ans. (a) Duchenne muscular dystrophy

Please refer above question

333. Ans. (a) D.I.P

Ref: Harrison, 19th ed. pg. 2142

- Rheumatoid arthritis characteristically causes swelling of small joints in the hand like the P.I.P, M.C.P and the wrist joint bilaterally.
- Isolated D.I.P joint involvement is seen in psoriatic arthropathy.
- D.I.P joint involvement is also seen with osteo-arthritis but the involvement is with pain at the base of thumb. Knee joint is the commonest joint involved in these patients.

334. Ans. (a) Both lung and kidney is involved

Ref: Harrison, 19th ed. pg. 2183-84

According to the American College of Rheumatology accepted classification criteria for Wegener's, two or more positive criteria have a sensitivity of 88.2% and a specificity of 92.0% of describing Wegener's.

- **Nasal or oral inflammation:**
  - Painful or painless oral ulcers or
  - Purulent or bloody nasal discharge
- **Lungs:** Abnormal chest X-ray with:
  - Nodules,
  - Infiltrates or
  - Cavities
- **Kidneys:** Urinary sediment with:
  - Microhematuria or
  - Red cell casts
- *Biopsy: Granulomatous inflammation*
  - Within the arterial wall or
  - In the perivascular area

335. Ans. (d) Sero-negative arthritis

Ref: Harrison, 19th ed. pg. 2136

- Patients of rheumatoid arthritis harbor an antibody by the name of anti – C.C.P (cycliccitrulline phosholipid antibodies).
- The rheumatoid nodules in these patients can compress on various peripheral nerves leading to mono-neuritis multiplex. The joints are damaged with peri-articular erosions and osteoporosis.
- *The characterstic joint involvement is P.I.P, M.C.P and the wrist joint bilaterally.*

Sero-negative arthritis is a broad term and included within he group are the entities psoriatic arthritis, Reiter's syndrome, enteropathic arthritis, reactive arthritis, ankylosing spondylitis, undifferentiated seronegative arthritis, Whipple's disease, arthritis associated with pustular acne, post-intestinal bypass arthritis, and several forms of HIV associated arthritis.

336. Ans. (a) Hypercalcemia

Ref: Harrison, 19th ed. pg. 313, 2208

- Hypercalcemia is seen with sarcoidosis as the granulomas present in this disease synthesize vitamin D3. This increases the amount of absorption of calcium from the intestine and leads to hypercalcemia.

337. Ans. (b) Mitral regurgitation

- In rheumatic heart disease, the damage to chordae tendinae by inflammatory aschoff nodules results in development of mitral regurgitation in pediatric presentation.
- The most common valve involvement >18 years of age is mitral stenosis
- Remember that pulmonic valve is not involved in rheumatic etiology

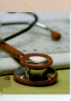

338. Ans. (d) ASO titer

Ref: Harrison, 19th ed. pg. 2151

Modified Jones Criteria

Low-risk populations	Moderate-and high-risk populations

• Carditis
  ▪ Clinical and/or subclinical carditis
	• Carditis
	  ▪ Clinical and/or subclinical carditis

• Arthritis
  ▪ Polyarthritis only
	• Arthritis
	  ▪ Monoarthritis or polyarthritis
	  ▪ Polyarthralgia

• Chorea	Chorea
• Erythema marginatum	Erythema marginatum
• Subcutaneous nodules	Subcutaneous nodules

Minor Criteria

Low-risk populations	Moderate and high-risk populations
• Polyarthralgia	Monoarthralgia
• Fever ($\geq$38.5°)	Fever (>38°C)
• ESR >60 mm in 1st hour	ESR $\geq$30 mm/h and/or CRP $\geq$3.0
• Prolonged PR interval, after accounting for age variability (unless carditis is a major criterion) in all population.	

Supporting evidence of a preceding streptococcal infection within the last 45 days	• Elevated or rising antistreptolysin O or other streptococcal antibody, or • A positive throat culture, or • Rapid antigen test for group A streptococcus, or • Recent scarlet fever

339. Ans. (c) Deforming arthritis

Ref: Harrison, 19th ed. pg. 2151

Please refer to above question

The arthritis in rheumatic arthritis is migratory polyarthritis involving the large joints and is NON erosive arthritis.

340. Ans. (b) History of sore throats

Ref: Harrison, 19th ed. pg. 2151

Refer above
- History of sore throats is not a component of Jones criteria.

341. Ans. (d) Ankylosing spondylitis

Ref: Harrison 19th ed. pg. 377e-5
- **SSA autoantibodies** (also called **anti-Ro**, or the combination **anti-SSA/Ro** or **anti Ro/SSA autoantibodies**) are anti-nuclear auto-antibodies that are associated with many autoimmune diseases, such as systemic lupus erythematosus, neonatal lupus and primary biliary cirrhosis. Also, they are often present in Sjögren's syndrome and sarcoidosis as well.
- Presence of Anti-SSA/Ro in pregnant women with SLE is associated with an increased risk of neonatal lupus Erythematosus in the child.

342. Ans. (c) Anti-smith antibody

Test Description
- ANA Screening test has sensitivity 95% not diagnostic without clinical features
- Anti-dsDNA Antibody: High specificity, sensitivity only 70% and levels are variable based on disease activity
- Anti-Sm antibody: Most specific antibody for SLE
- AntiSSA (Ro) or Anti-SSB (La) Present in 15% of patients with SLE and other connective tissue disease such as Sjögren syndrome
- Lupus anticoagulant
- Direct Russell viper venom test to screen for inhibitors in the clotting cascade in antiphospholipid antibody syndrome
- Direct Coombs test
- Anti-histone: Drug-induced lupus (e.g with procainamide or hydralazine)

343. Ans. (d) Mixed connective tissue disorder

Ref: Harrison, 19th ed. pg. 2165
- Anti-Rho or SS-A antibodies are seen in SLE, Sjogren syndrome and can be transmitted across the placenta resulting in neonatal lupus which presents as complete heart block.
- *Mixed connective tissue disorder is associated with U1 R.N.P. (Ribo-Nucleo-protein antibody).*

344. Ans. (a) X linked

Ref: Harrison's 17th ed. Ch.

Disorder	Enzyme Def:	Inheritance	Neurologic	Ophthalmologic	Hematologic	Unique features
Hurler syndrome	α-L-Iduronidase	AR	Mental retardation +	Corneal clouding	Vacuolated lymphocytes	Coarse facies, cardiovascular involvement, joint stiffness, wide spaced teeth
Hunter syndrome	Iduronate sulfatase (ET)	X-linked	Mental retardation, less in mild form	Retinal degeneration, no corneal clouding	Granulated lymphocytes	Coarse facies, cardiovascular, joint stiffness, distinctive pebbly skin lesions

Medicine

- Both have hepatosplenomegaly and skeletal dysplasia
- In Hurler syndrome, death usually occurs by 10 years because of respiratory infection and heart failure.

345. Ans. (b) IgA, C 3

Ref: Harrison, 19th ed. pg. 2190

- Henoch Schonlein purpura is a small-vessel vasculitis in which complexes of immunoglobulin A (IgA) and C3 are deposited on arterioles, capillaries, and venules.
- As with IgA nephropathy, serum levels of IgA are high in HSP.
- IgA nephropathy has a predilection for young adults while HSP is more predominant among children. Further, IgA nephropathy typically only affects the kidneys while HSP is a systemic disease.
- HSP involves the skin and connective tissues, scrotum, joints, gastrointestinal tract and kidneys.
- **Investigation:** IgA levels high, platelet count normal and skin biopsy (IOC).
- **Treatment:** Steroids

346. Ans. (d) Microscopic polyangitis

Ref: Harrison, 19th ed. pg. 2186

- MPA is characterized by pauci-immune, necrotizing, small vessel vasculitis without clinical or pathological evidence of granulomatous inflammation
- The family of vasculitic granulomatoses comprise
  1. Wegener's granulomatosis[Q]
  2. Churg-Strauss syndrome[Q]
  3. Polyarteritis nodosa[Q]
  4. Bronchocentric granulomatosis
  5. Giant cell arteritis[Q]
  6. Systemic lupus erythematosus.

347. Ans. (a) Gout

Ref: Harrison, 19th ed. pg. 2233-34

- In approximately 40% of cases, *the gouty erosions have a raised margin or lip that radiologically is referred to as Martel's hook or Martel's Sign.* No loss of bone density is expected
- The osteological signs of gout can be located on the joint surfaces, around the joint itself, or even at a distance from the joint.
- Lesions from gout have a diagnostic appearance on radiographs that radiologists refer to as a "punched out" appearance, and which can be seen as crescent-shaped erosions, with smooth, well remodelled margins, on dry bone
- Lesions vary in size, are usually rounded or oval, and may have a sclerotic border.

348. Ans. (a) SLE

Ref: Harrison, 19th ed. pg. 2126-27

The diagnosis is based on joint pain in fever with rash and photosensitivity. Rheumatoid arthritis involves the small joints symmetrically and does not have presence of Rash.

The diagnostic criteria for SLE are as follows:

- Rash Fixed erythema, over the Malar Eminences
- Erythematous circular raised patches with adherent keratotic scaling and follicular plugging; atrophic scarring may occur
- Photosensitivity Exposure to UV light causes rash
- Oral ulcers Includes oral and nasopharyngeal ulcers
- Synovitis/Non-erosive arthritis of two or more peripheral joints
- Serositis: Pleuritis or pericarditis documented by ECG or rub or evidence of effusion
- Renal disorder Proteinuria >0.5 g/day or 3+, or cellular casts
- Neurologic disorder Seizures or psychosis without other causes
- Hematologic disorder Hemolytic anemia or leukopenia
- Immunological criteria like positive CRP, low C3, ELISA cardiolipin antibody
- ANA positivity

349. Ans. (d) Secondary amyloidosis

Ref: Harrison, 19th ed. pg. 719, 723, 2458

- Reactive amyloid A (AA) amyloidosis, one of the most severe complications of RA, is a serious, potentially life-threatening disorder caused by deposition of AA amyloid fibrils in multiple organs. These AA amyloid fibrils derive from the circulatory acute-phase reactant serum amyloid A protein (SAA), and may be controlled by treatment
- The introduction of biological therapies targeting specific inflammatory mediators revolutionised the treatment of rheumatoid arthritis (RA). Targeting key components of the immune system allows efficient suppression of the pathological inflammatory cascade that leads to RA symptoms and subsequent joint destruction.
- Milk alkali syndrome occurs due to abuse of calcium containing anta-acids leading to hypercalcemia

350. Ans. (b) HL ADR 4

Ref: Harrison, 19th ed. pg. 372e-1

HLA allele	Diseases with increased risk
HLA-B27[Q]	Ankylosing spondylitis Post-gonococcal arthritis Acute anterior uveitis
HLA-B47	21-hydroxylase deficiency
HLA-DR2[Q]	Systemic lupus erythematosus
HLA-DR3	Autoimmune hepatitis Primary Sjogren syndrome Diabetes mellitus type 1 Systemic lupus erythematosus

Contd...

FMGE Solutions Screening Examination

HLA allele	Diseases with increased risk
HLA-DR4[Q]	Rheumatoid arthritis Diabetes mellitus type 1
HLA-DR3 and – DR4[Q] combined	Diabetes mellitus type 1
HLA-DQ2 and HLA-DQB	Celiac disease

351. Ans. (b) Rheumatoid arthritis

Ref: Harrison, 19th ed. pg. 2144-45

- *Minocycline, gold salts, enicillamine, azathioprine, and cyclosporine have all been used for the treatment of RA with varying degrees of success; however, they are used sparingly now due to their inconsistent clinical efficacy or unfavorable toxicity profile.*

Drugs used in Rheumatoid arthritis

1. Hydroxychloroquine–preferred in pregnancy
2. Lefluonomide
3. Methotrexate–preferred drug
4. Abatacept
5. Anakinra
6. Rituximab

RESPIRATORY SYSTEM

352. Ans. (a) Distal bronchiectasis

Ref: Harrison 20th ed. pg. 1535

Allergic bronchopulmonary aspergilloma is related to development of *Central bronchiectasis*.
It is seen in asthmatics and is associated with increase of IgE.

Predisposing conditions
- Bronchial asthma, cystic fibrosis

Obligatory criteria
- Elevated serum total IgE levels (>1000 IU/ml)
- Elevated serum IgG and/or IgE against A. *fumigatus*

Other criteria (at least three of five)
- Immediate type I reaction to A. *fumigatus* antigen
- Presence of serum A. *fumigatus* precipitins
- Transient and/or permanent chest radiographic opacities
- Eosinophil count >1000 cells/*ml* in peripheral blood
- Central bronchiectasis on HRCT chest

353. Ans. (a) Pneumothorax

Ref: Harrison, 20th ed. pg. 853

Leading cause of respiratory distress post subclavian central line access is puncture of lung leading to traumatic pneumothorax.

COMPLICATIONS OF CENTRAL VENOUS CATHETERIZATION

Immediate
- Bleeding
- Arterial puncture
- Arrhythmia
- Air embolism
- Thoracic duct injury (with left SC or left IJ approach)
- Catheter malposition
- Pneumothorax or hemothorax

Delayed
- Infection
- Venous thrombosis, pulmonary emboli
- Catheter migration
- Myocardial perforation
- Nerve injury

354. Ans. (a) Pleural fluid protein to serum protein ratio <0.5

Ref: Harrison 19th ed. P 1716

To differentiate between exudative and transudative pleural effusion, the following criteria known as *Light's criteria* is used:

1. Pleural fluid protein/serum protein >0.5
2. Pleural fluid LDH/Serum LDH >0.6
3. Pleural fluid LDH more than 2/3rd the upper normal limit for serum

Exudative pleural effusion meets at least one of the given criteria while transudative meets none.

355. Ans. (a) Chronic bronchitis

Ref: Harrison 19th ed. 1701

- Chronic obstructive airway disease leads to development of damage to ciliated columnar epithelium. The resultant stasis promotes low grade infection leading to bronchorrhea. This manifestation is called chronic bronchitis.
- Follicular bronchiolitis is due to hyperplasia of bronchial associated lymphoid tissue (BALT) seen due to collagen vascular disease and immune deficiency states. It mainly involves the lower lobes of lung.
- Desquamative pneumonitis is interstitial lung disease in smokers. It leads to development of pulmonary fibrosis.
- Chemical pneumonitis is due to aspiration of stomach acid and is also known as Mendelson syndrome.

356. Ans. (c) Albumin

- Pleural effusion in TB could be a presentation of primary TB due to sub-pleural location of Gohn's focus or can present as extra-pulmonary TB.
- Gene XPERT is a nucleic acid amplification based test which in a matter of few hours can tell if MTB is present and can also determine resistance.

- The values of LDH are taken in Light's criteria for pleural effusion to determine exudative nature of the fluid
- Adenosine deaminase has 90% sensitivity and 92% specificity for determining the tubercular nature of fluid.
- The question is based on common sense that albumin values in serum and ascitic fluid are evaluated in patients of ascites.

357. Ans. (a) A.T.T

The CXR shows a miliary picture and ATT must be initiated. Since the child is malnourished and is having Miliary TB, his cell mediated immunity is already reduced. Hence steroids would be contraindicated in this case. The antibiotics would be useful in bacterial pneumonia which is ruled out due to radiological picture.

358. Ans. (d) Lung

Ref: Wintrobe's Clinical Hematology, 13th ed. pg. 1583

- It is seen with hyperleucocytosis with WBC count > 10^5/cu. mm. *Leukostasis affects pulmonary and brain circulation.* The presence of dysnea, tachypnea, lethargy and slurred speech is characteristic.
- WBC counts are in excess of 100,000/cu.mm and lead to leukostatic plugging of the capillaries followed by endothelial damage to blood vessels.
- The mortality occurs due to respiratory failure, intracranial hemorrhage and coma.
- The low PO_2 is due to increased consumption of oxygen by leucocytes.
- It is common with acute leukemia subtypes like acute promyelocytic leukemia, acute monocytic leukemia and T cell type of ALL.
- Treatment is leukapheresis

359. Ans. (c) 5th midaxillary space

- The 5th intercostal space in the mid-axillary line is generally used for most situations. This area is commonly known as the "safe triangle", bordered by the anterior border of latissimus dorsi, the lateral border of the pectoralis major, a line superior to the horizontal level of the nipple and an apex below the axilla

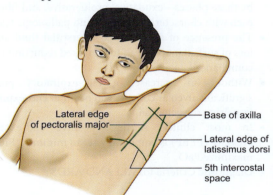

360. Ans. (c) ARDS

Shock Lung/ ARDS is a clinical syndrome caused by diffuse alveolar capillary and epithelial damage. There is usually rapid onset of life-threatening respiratory insufficiency, cyanosis, and severe arterial hypoxemia that is refractory to oxygen therapy and that may progress to multisystem organ failure. The histologic manifestation of ARDS in the lungs is known as *diffuse alveolar damage.*

361. Ans. (a) Staphylococcus aureus

- *S. aureus* is a cause of serious respiratory tract infections in newborns and infants; these infections present as shortness of breath, fever, and respiratory failure.
- Chest X-ray may reveal pneumatoceles (shaggy, thin-walled cavities). Pneumothorax and empyema are recognized complications of this infection.

362. Ans (c) Levofloxacin

Ref: Harrison, 19th ed. pg. 812

Empirical Antibiotic Treatment of Health Care-Associated Pneumonia

Patients without risk factors for MDR pathogens
Ceftriaxone *or*
Moxifloxacin, ciprofloxacin, *or* levofloxacin *or*
Ertapenem

Patients with risk factors for MDR pathogens
- A β-lactam: Ceftazidime or cefepime *or*   Piperacillin/tazobactam, imipenem *plus*   - A second agent active against Gram-negative bacterial pathogens: Gentamicin or tobramycin or amikacin *or*   Ciprofloxacin or levofloxacin *plus*   - An agent active against Gram-positive bacterial pathogens: Linezolid *or* Vancomycin

363. Ans. (d) Fat embolism

- In the clinical setting of fracture of long bone and subsequent respiratory distress and development of petechiae satisfies GURD criteria for diagnosis of fat embolism.

The criteria for diagnosing fat embolism are as follows:

Major criteria
- Symptoms and radiologic evidence of respiratory insufficiency   - Cerebral sequelae unrelated to head injury or other conditions   - Petechial rash

Minor criteria are as follows:
- Tachycardia (heart rate >110 beats/min)   - Pyrexia (temperature >38.5°C)   - Retinal changes of fat or petechiae   - Renal dysfunction

Contd...

FMGE Solutions Screening Examination

- Jaundice
- Acute drop in hemoglobin level
- Sudden thrombocytopenia
- Elevated erythrocyte sedimentation rate
- Fat microglobulinemia

364. Ans. (b) **DU perforation**

- The X-ray shows presence of gas under diaphragm, with clinical findings of rebound tenderness and suggestive of DU perforation.

365. Ans. (d) **Lesion in the brain**

Biot's Breathing: Biot's Breathing is characterized by irregularly irregular breathing with sudden apnea and is seen in CNS lesions and is a sign of increased intracranial pressure.

Kussmaul's Respiration. Kussmaul Breathing is deep rapid respiration in metabolic acidosis and is classically associated with diabetic ketoacidosis

Cheyne-Stokes Respiration. Cheyne-Stokes Respiration is one of increasingly deep respiration followed by a steady diminution of breathing until an apneic episode occurs in neurologic diseases with raised ICP. Obesity may be present. Some patients will show pupillary dilation with rapid breathing and pupillary contraction with apnea.

The differential diagnoses are
- CNS disease
- CHF
- Pneumonia
- Carbon monoxide poisoning
- Medications(eg, morphine).

Apneustic Breathing. Apneustic breathing is seen in severely ill patients with coma. The patient holds his or her breath at the end of inspiration until the Hering-Breuer (carotid body) reflex initiates exhalation. This breathing pattern suggests pontine disease.

366. Ans. (d) **CT with IV contrast**

Ref: Harrison, 19th ed. pg. 1633-64

- A definitive diagnosis of PE depends on visualization of an intraluminal filling defect in more than one projection.
- *Chest CT with contrast has become the main test for diagnosis replacing the older invasive pulmonary angiography.*
- Catheter-based diagnostic testing is used in case of an unsatisfactory chest CT and those patients where catheter-directed thrombolysis or embolectomy is planned.

367. Ans. (a) **Narcotic over-dosage**

- Narcotics cause CNS depression and lead to inability of respiratory centre to respond to increasing carbon dioxide levels.
- Abnormalities of central respiratory drive and reduced central respiratory drive will decrease minute ventilation.

Causes of Reduced Respiratory Drive
- Sedative drugs
- Altered drug metabolism (hepatic/renal failure)
- Iatrogenic drug overdose.
- Head injury, raised intracranial pressure and central nervous system infection
- Severe hypercapnia or hypoxaemia can also depress the respiratory center
- Inadequate ventilation may be caused by reduced respiratory drive, an increase in dead space or an increase in CO_2 production.

368. Ans. (d) **Sulfomethoxazole and trimethoprim**

Ref: Harrison, 19th ed. pg. 492

- Prophylaxis with trimethoprim-sulfamethoxazole prevents many opportunistic infections, including infection with *P. carinii, Toxoplasma gondii,* and community-acquired respiratory, gastrointestinal, and urinary tract pathogens.
- Intolerance of TMP-SMZ is common; desensitization is useful less often in transplant patients than in patients with AIDS.

369. Ans. (a) **Pulmonary hamartoma**

Ref: Harrison, 19th ed. pg. 515-16

- Popcorn calcification is virtually diagnostic on chest radiographs for *pulmonary hamartoma.*
- It characteristically appears as well-defined, solitary pulmonary nodules; they may show varying patterns of calcification, including an irregular popcorn, stippled, or curvilinear pattern, or even a combination of all 3 patterns.

370. Ans. (b) **Alveolar transudate**

Ref: Harrison, 19th ed. pg. 1736-38

- *ARDS is characterised by high protein pulmonary edema and an exudate*. The natural history of ARDS is marked by three phases—exudative, proliferative, and fibrotic—each with characteristic clinical and pathologic features.
- The presence of alveolar and interstitial fluid and the loss of surfactant can lead to a marked reduction of lung compliance.
- Without an increase in end-expiratory pressure, significant alveolar collapse can occur at end-expiration, impairing oxygenation.
- In most clinical settings, positive end-expiratory pressure (PEEP) is empirically set to minimize FIO_2 and maximize PaO_2.
- Diagnostic Criteria for ALI AND ARDS

Oxygenation	Onset	Chest radiograph	Absence of Left Atrial Hypertension
ALI: $PaO_2/FIO_2 \leq 300$ mm Hg	Acute	Bilateral alveolar or interstitial infiltrates	PCWP ≤18 mm Hg or no clinical evidence of increased left atrial pressure
ARDS: $PaO_2/FIO_2 \leq 200$ mm Hg	Acute	Bilateral alveolar or interstitial infiltrates	PCWP ≤18 mm Hg or no clinical evidence of increased left atrial pressure

371. Ans. (b) Lung laceration

- The image shows presence of subcutaneous empysema which is also hinted in line 2 of the question where it mentions crepitus is palpated.
- Chest trauma, a major cause of subcutaneous emphysema, can cause air to enter the skin of the chest wall from the neck or lung.
- Most students mark it as renal shut down which is not the answer because it would not happen within 4 hour of trauma insult.
- Gas gangrene will again take time to develop and would lead to development of crepitus in the injured part.

Causes of subcutaneous emphysema
- Trauma to parts of the respiratory system other than the lungs, such as rupture of a bronchial tube, may also cause subcutaneous emphysema
- May also occur with fractures of the facial bones, neoplasms, during asthma attacks.

When the alveoli of the lung are ruptured, as occurs in pulmonary laceration, air may travel beneath the visceral pleura (the membrane lining the lung), to the hilum of the lung, up to the trachea, to the neck and then to the chest wall.

372. Ans. (d) Increased prostaglandins

Ref: Harrison, 19th ed. pg. 1680

- Aspirin-sensitive asthma is associated with severe rhinosinusitis and recurrent nasal polyposis.
- The complex pathogenesis of aspirin-sensitive asthma involves chronic eosinophilic inflammatory changes, with evidence of increased mast cell activation.
- Aspirin-sensitive asthma is an underdiagnosed condition affecting up to 20% of the adult asthmatic population.
- It is associated with more severe asthma, requires increased use of inhaled and oral corticosteroids, more presentations to hospital and a risk of life- threatening reactions with aspirin.
- The cyclo-oxygenase pathways play a major role in the respiratory reactions that develop after aspirin ingestion.

373. Ans. (c) Low flow oxygen

Ref: Harrison, 19th ed. pg. 1707, 1740

- In COPD, Ventilation/perfusion matching leads to under-ventilated lung which usually has low oxygen content. This leads to localized vasoconstriction limiting blood flow to that lung tissue.
- Supplemental oxygen abolishes this constriction, leading to improved ventilation/perfusion matching.
- High flow oxygen is not tolerated as it leads to crusting, dryness and epistaxis.
- The treatment is guided by PaO_2 which should be maintained at 60 mm Hg or so (SaO_2 of 85-90%). During the period of exercise, sleep or other activities, the flow rate may be increased by another 1–2 L/min.
- While continuous therapy is required for patients who show hypoxaemia at rest, intermittent treatment during specific periods may be used for patients who demonstrate intermittent hypoxaemia

374. Ans. (a) Duration of smoking

Though this is a highly debatable topic most serach results and discussion with faculty and google books (IASLC Textbook of Prevention and Early Detection of Lung Cancer) mention *duration of smoking* to be more important that the number of cigarettes smoked.

375. Ans. (b) Decreased CO_2

Ref: Harrison, 19th ed. pg. 1731-32

- Hyperventilation leads to carbon dioxide washout. It is usually a feature of type 1 respiratory failure.
- *Type 1 respiratory failure is defined as a low level of oxygen in the blood (hypoxemia) without an increased level of carbon dioxide in the blood (hypercapnia), and the $PaCO_2$ may be normal or low.*
- It is typically caused by a ventilation/perfusion (V/Q) mismatch; the volume of air flowing in and out of the lungs is not matched with the flow of blood to the lungs. The basic defect in *Type 1 respiratory failure* is failure of oxygenation characterized by:

P_aO_2	Decreased (<60 mm Hg)
P_aCO_2	Normal or Decreased (<50 mm Hg)
$P_{A-a}O_2$	Increased

376. Ans. (b) Bacterial pneumonia

The image in PA view shows well defined homogenous opacity suggestive of lobar pneumonia.

377. Ans. (a) Right pleural effusion

The image shows presence of Hemi-thorax and tracheal shift to contralateral (left) side. This is suggestive of massive pleural effusion.

FMGE Solutions Screening Examination

378. Ans. (a) Sarcoidosis

Ref: Harrison, 19th ed. pg. 2206

Löfgren syndrome symptoms consist of fever, bilateral hilar lymphadenopathy (BHL), and polyarthralgias

379. Ans. (a) Asbestosis

Ref: Harrison, 19th ed. pg. 1689

- Working with asbestos is the most common risk factor for mesothelioma.
- Indeed, the relationship between asbestos and mesothelioma is so strong that many consider mesothelioma a "signal" or "sentinel" tumor.
- In rare cases, mesothelioma has also been associated with irradiation of the chest or abdomen, intrapleural thorium dioxide (thorotrast) as a contrast medium, and inhalation of other fibrous silicates.

380. Ans. (b) 103 mm Hg

Ref: Harrison, 18th ed. chapter 252

Partial Pressures of blood gases
- Atmosphere: pO_2 = 160 mm Hg, pCO_2 = 0.3 mm Hg
- Alveolar air: **pO_2 = 105 mm Hg,** pCO_2 = 40 mm Hg
- Oxygenated blood: pO_2 = 100 mm Hg, pCO_2 = 40 mm Hg
- Tissues: pO_2 = 40 mm Hg, pCO_2 = 45 mm Hg
- Deoxygenated blood: pO_2 = 40 mm Hg, pCO_2 = 45 mm Hg

> ▶ **Extra Mile**
>
> **O_2 and CO_2 in blood**
> - 1.5% O_2 dissolved in blood
> - 98.5% O_2 carried by hemoglobin (Hb-O_2)
> - Hb can carry up to four molecules of O_2 (four = saturation)
> - PO_2 determines Hb saturation
> - Also pH, temperature and Pco_2 affects Hb-O_2 binding

381. Ans. (d) Long acting beta 2 agonist

Ref: Chapter 254: Harrison, 18th ed.

- LABA improve asthma control and reduce exacerbations when added to ICS, which allows asthma to be controlled at lower doses of corticosteroids.
- LABAs should not be given in the absence of ICS therapy as they do not control the underlying inflammation.
- This observation has led to the widespread use of fixed combination inhalers that contain a corticosteroid and a LABA, which have proved to be highly effective in the control of asthma.

				OCS
			LABA	LABA
		LABA	ICS High dose	ICS High dose
	ICS Low dose	ICS Low dose		
Short –acting B2-agonist as required for symptom relief				
Mild intermittent	Mild persistent	Moderate persistent	Severe persistent	Very severe persistent

382. Ans. (c) Pleural effusion

Ref: Harrison, 18th ed. Chapter 252 and 267

- Severe asthma and pneumonia will require supplemental oxygen so are ruled out.
- Low flow oxygen is mainstay of therapy for Chronic bronchitis.
- Pleural effusion will not be benefitted by supplemental oxygen as lung parenchyma is not involved.

383. Ans. (a) Centri-acinar emphysema

Ref: Harrison, 19th ed. pg. 1701

- Centri-acinar lesions are more common in smokers and severe in the upper lobes, particularly in the apical segments.
- In severe centriacinar emphysema the distal acinus also becomes involved, and so, as noted, the differentiation from panacinar emphysema becomes difficult.

384. Ans. (a) Silicosis

Ref: Chapter 256: Harrison, 18th ed.

Causes of Miliary Mottling
- Miliary tuberculosis
- Fungal infections
- Varicella pneumonia
- Metastases–miliary metastases like thyroid carcinoma, renal cell carcinoma, breast cancer
- Sarcoidosis
- Pneumoconioses
- *Silicosis*
- Coal workers pneumoconiosis
- Pulmonary haemosiderosis
- Hypersensitivity pneumonitis
- Langerhans cell histiocytosis (LCH)
- Pulmonary alveolar proteinosis

385. Ans. (c) Ellis curve

Ellis curve is seen in pleural effusion. It has a S shaped border in axilla where fluid accumulates in pleural cavity. You can see the transverse border of fluid on right lung field in this X ray. Pneumonia does not have a sharp border.

386. Ans. (d) Pneumo-mediastinum

In the area of arrows a *continuous diaphragm sign* is noted. Normally diaphragm is seen below lungs only. This kind of presentation is noted in pneumo-mediastinum.

387. Ans. (c) Systolic Blood pressure is more than 90 mm Hg

Ref: Harrison's, 17th ed. Ch. 251

- CURB 65 also known as the CURB criteria is a clinical prediction rule that has been validated for predicting mortality in Community Acquired Pnemonia.

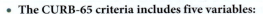

- The CURB-65 criteria includes five variables:
  - Confusion
  - Urea >7 mmol/L
  - Respiratory rate ≥ 30/min
  - **Blood pressure, systolic ≤ 90 mm Hg or diastolic ≤ 60 mm Hg; and**
  - Age ≥65 years
- Each criteria has one point which predicts the mortality in CAP.
  - **Score 0:** 30-day mortality rate is 1.5%- can be treated outside the hospital.
  - **Score 2:** 30-day mortality rate is 9.2%, and patients should be admitted to the hospital.
  - **Score 3:** mortality rates are 22% overall; these patients may require admission to an ICU.

388. Ans. (c) Centriacinar emphysema

Ref: Harrison, 19th ed. pg. 1701

Emphysema: The abnormal permanent enlargement of air spaces distal to the terminal bronchioles, accompanied by the destruction of the walls and without obvious fibrosis. It begins in the respiratory bronchioles and spreads peripherally.

> SMOKING CAUSES intake of TAR which causes ↑ marcrophages in alveolar region. These macrophages secrete enzyme Elastase which causes autodigestion of elastin → leading to ↓ elasticity → Emphysema

Centriacinar emphysema is MOST COMMON FORM.

- Associated with smoking
- Usually seen in apices
- *Causes type-I respiratory failure: 3pO₂, 3pCO₂*
- **MOST RELIABLE radiographic sign: Flattening of the diaphragm**
- **Symptoms:** Persistent cough, Dyspnea, Wheezing, Chest pain, Fever.
- **Upon examination:**
  - Increased RR
  - BARREL SHAPED CHEST (AP diameter > transverse)
  - No cyanosis
  - Pink puffers

> **Extra Mile**
> - Panlobular emphysema: involves entire acinus UNIFORMLY.
> - Paraseptal emphysema: involves only distal acinus *(alveolar ducts and sac). Found near pleura and can result in pneumothorax.*
> - Irregular or cicatricial: can be either of them.

389. Ans. (a) Cyanosis

Ref: Harrison, 19th ed. pg. 1664f

- Emphysema is characterized by damage to respiratory bronchioles **leading to bleb formation**. The air gets trapped in the lungs causing hypoxia. However these patients do not have cyanosis and are called as **PINK PUFFERS.**
- *Cigarette smoking is the most common cause of emphysema* and the type seen is known as centri-acinar emphysema. **These patients develop type 1 respiratory failure** and the resultant hypoxia causes a **barrel shaped chest in** these patients.

390. Ans. (a) Thrombolytic

Ref: Harrison, 19th ed. pg. 1634-35

- Anticoagulation with heparin has long been the standard treatment for normotensive patients with pulmonary embolism. By preventing clot propagation, heparin allows endogenous fibrinolysis to occur, with eventual resolution of thromboemboli. Presumably through this mechanism, heparin therapy has been shown to significantly reduce both the incidence of recurrent pulmonary embolism and patient mortality.
- However in the absence of an absolute contraindication, patients with pulmonary embolism induced hypotension or shock are usually treated with thrombolytic agents. The three thrombolytic agents used in treatment of pulmonary embolism- *streptokinase, urokinase and recombinant tissue-type plasminogen activator(rt-PA).*

391. Ans. (a) Intravenous tissue plasminogen activator

Ref: Harrison, 19th ed. pg. 1634-35

- Massive pulmonary embolism is best managed by thrombolysis using tissue plasminogen activator.
- In case thrombolysis is contraindicated then in these patient fogarthy catheter removal of clot in pulmonary artery would be done.
- In submassive pulmonary embolism heparin is used. Chronic pulmonary embolism leading to pulmonary-hypertension (known as *chronic thromboembolic hypertension*) is treated with a surgical Procedure known as a pulmonary thromboendarterectomy

392. Ans. (a) Allergic Rhinitis Induced Asthama

ARIA stands for Allergic Rhinits Induced Asthma

393. Ans. (a) Streptococcus pneumonia

- Pneumatocoele often occur as a sequela to acute pneumonia, commonly caused by Staphylococcus aureus.
- Pulmonary pneumatoceles are thin-walled, air-filled cysts that develop within the lung parenchyma. They can be

single emphysematous lesions but are more often multiple. **Also occur with other agents, including Streptococcus pneumoniae,** Haemophilus influenzae, Escherichia coli, group A streptococci, Serratia marcescens, Klebsiella pneumoniae, adenovirus, and tuberculosis.". Pneumatocele formation is associated with hyperimmunoglobulin E (IgE) syndrome (Job syndrome).

394. Ans. (d) Bronchocele

- *A bronchocele is a mucous-filled dilated bronchi surrounded by aerated lung.*
- CT chest can identify a bronchocele as a tubular intrapulmonary opacity distinct from vascular shadows
- Their appearance is similar to a "finger in glove"or the shape of the letters V or Y.

395. Ans. (d) Rhinocerebral involvement

Ref: Harrison, 19th ed. pg. 489, 1346

- Rhino-cerebral involvement is seen with mucormycosis in diabetics.
- A rapidly invasive Aspergillus infection in the lungs often causes cough, fever, chest pain, and difficulty breathing. Cavity in lungs in usually caused by A niger. A. fumigatus can be a normal component of sputums

396. Ans. (a) Eosinophiluria

Ref: Harrison, 19th ed. pg. 1346-47

- A.B.P.A allergic brochopulmonary Aspergillosis is hypersensitivity to the antigens on cell wall of aspergillus fumigatus. The clinical profile is an asthmatic patient presenting with passage of browinish plugs in the sputum.
- CXR shows fleeting pulmonary opacities and absolute eosinophil count is increased. Eosinophilia is a feature of asthma anyway but not eosinophiluria
- HRCT shows presence of Central bronchiectasis.
- Treatment of choice for ABPA is steroids.
- **Remember:** Eosinophiluria is a feature of allergic interstitial nephritis.

397. Ans. (b) Cystic fibrosis

Ref: Harrison, 19th ed. pg. 1681, 1686

- Central Bronchiectasis is a classical finding in allergic Bronchopulmonary aspergilloma. It is also documented to be present in cystic fibrosis.
- The cardinal diagnostic tests include an elevated serum level of total IgE (usually >1000 IU/mL), a positive skin-prick test to A. fumigatus extract, or detection of Aspergillus-specific IgE and IgG (precipitating) antibodies.

398. Ans. (a) HRCT scan

Ref: Harrison, 19th ed. pg. 308e-3f, 1694

- The best test to evaluate the destruction and dilatation of large airways which are filled with pus in Bronchiectasis is HRCT
- CT angiography is preferred for pulmonary embolism.
- Pulmonary angiography is done for lung sequestration and is gold standard for pulmonary embolism.

399. Ans. (c) Klebsiella

Ref: Harrison, 19th ed. pg. 1108

- Military mottling or snow storm appearance on CXR is seen in Disseminated TB, Loffler pneumonia, silicosis and chicken pox pneumonia
- Klebsiella causes pneumonia and CXR shows bulging fissure sign due to accumulation of pus in interlobar fissure.

400. Ans. (b) Uveitis

Ref: Harrison, 19th ed. pg. 1112, 1119

- Phlyctenular conjunctivitis occurs as hypersensitivity to tuberculosis bacteria.
- Tubercular lymphadenitis is the most common form of extra-pulmonary TB
- Most common cause of Addison disease in India is tuberculosis though on global scale it is autoimmunity being the leading cause.

401. Ans. (b) Liver

- Congenital transmission usually occurs from a lesion in the placenta through the umbilical vein.
- The tubercle bacilli first reach the fetal liver, where a primary focus with periportal lymph node involvement may occur.
- The bacilli in the lung usually remain dormant until after birth, when oxygenation and pulmonary circulation increase significantly.

402. Ans. (b) Oral corticosteroids

Ref: Harrison, 19th ed. pg. 1676

- Severe persistent asthma is managed with L.A.B.A., inhaled high dose steroids and S.A.B.A. as when required Oral steroids are given in very severe persistent asthma.

403. Ans. (a) Pneumococcus

Ref: Harrison 19th ed. pg. 805

Infection	Causative organism
Lobar pneumonia/Community acquired Pneumonia	Pneumococcus
Nosocomial pneumonia	Staph. aureus

Contd...

Infection	Causative organism
HIV associated pneumonia	P. jiroveci
Meningitis adults (sporadic)	Pneumococcus
Meningitis adults (epidemic)	Neisseria meningitides

404. Ans. (a) Pseudomonas

Ref: Harrison, 19th ed. pg. 1044-45

- *Pseudomonas aeruginosa is a Gram-negative, aerobic, rod-shaped and polar-flagella bacterium with unipolar motility.*
- The coliforms and proteus are gram negative bacteria and only klebsiella is non-flagellated.
- Furthermore, it is an opportunistic pathogen responsible for ventilator-acquired pneumonia (VAP). VAP due to P. aeruginosa is usually multidrug-resistant and associated with severe infection and increased mortality.

405. Ans. (b) TLC ↓

Ref: Harrison, 19th ed. pg. 306e-2f

Parameter	Obstructive	Restrictive
FEV1	Reduced	Reduced
TLC	Normal/increased	Reduced
FVC	Reduced	Reduced
FEV1/FVC RATIO	Reduced	Normal/increased
Residual volume	Increased	Decreased

406. Ans. (a) COPD

Ref: Harrison, 19th ed. pg. 1731-32

Type 2 respiratory failure occurs as a result of alveolar hypoventilation and results in the inability to eliminate carbon dioxide effectively.
- Increased resistive loads e.g., bronchospasm in COPD
- Loads due to reduced lung compliance [e.g., alveolar edema, atelectasis, intrinsic positive end-expiratory pressure).
- Diminished CNS drive to breathe due to drug overdose, brainstem injury, sleep-disordered breathing, and hypothyroidism.
- Reduced strength can be due to impaired neuromuscular transmission (e.g., myasthenia gravis, Gullian-Barré syndrome, amyotrophic lateral sclerosis, phrenic nerve injury).
- Respiratory muscle weakness (e.g., myopathy, electrolyte derangements, fatigue).
- Loads due to reduced chest wall compliance (e.g., pneumothorax, pleural effusion, abdominal distention), and loads due to increased minute ventilation requirements (e.g., pulmonary embolus with increased dead space fraction, sepsis).

407. Ans. (b) Pulmonary embolism

Ref: Harrison, 19th ed. pg. 1631

- The first clinical diagnosis for this case presentation is PE since Venous thromboembolism (VTE), which encompasses deep venous thrombosis (DVT) and pulmonary embolism (PE), is one of the three major cardiovascular causes of death, along with myocardial infarction and stroke.
- *Fracture of femur will lead to immobilization for a long period. Hence PE is all the more likely in this setting.*
- Sudden cardiac death is defined as natural death due to cardiac causes in a person who may or may not have previously recognized heart disease but in whom the time and mode of death are unexpected.

408. Ans. (a) Pulmonary embolism

Ref: Harrison's, 19th ed. pg. 1631

- *PE is the most common preventable cause of death among hospitalized patients. PE and DVT occurring after total hip or knee replacement is currently taken as unacceptable, and steps are taken to prevent it by giving subcutaneous fondaparinux.*
- For patients who have DVT, the most common history is a cramp in the lower calf that persists for several days and becomes more uncomfortable as time progresses. For patients who have PE, the most common history is unexplained breathlessness.

409. Ans. (a) Pulmonary embolism

On chest radiography, the Westermark Sign is a wedge shaped opacity due to pulmonary infarction.

Other Signs in Pulmonary Embolism

- Palla Sign
- Hampton Hump Sign
- IOC – Spirometry
- **Gold Standard IOC** – Pulmonary Angiography

410. Ans. (a) 15 mm Hg

- Pulmonary arterial pressure is about 15 mm Hg, and the pulmonary arterial systolic and diastolic pressures are about 25 and 10 mm Hg, respectively. Pulmonary venous pressure is about 8 mm Hg.

411. Ans. (d) Acts on Alpha 2 Beta 4 Nicotinic receptor

Ref: Harrison, 19th ed. pg. 507, 1705

Average cigarette provides 1 mg of nicotine
- Nicotine's mood-altering effects are different by report: in particular it is both a stimulant and a relaxant. First causing a release of glucose from the liver and epinephrine from the adrenal medulla, it causes stimulation.

FMGE Solutions Screening Examination

- By reducing the appetite and raising the metabolism, some smokers lose weight as a consequence. Nicotinic receptors are known as *alpha 4 beta 2 receptors*.
- At low doses, nicotine potently enhances the actions of norepinephrine and dopamine in the brain, causing a drug effect typical of those of psycho-stimulants.

412. Ans. (a) Non small cell lung Ca

Ref: Harrison, 19th ed. pg. 510-511

- Most common cause of hemoptysis is tuberculosis but at 65 years of age it is more likely a presentation of lung cancer.
- Lung cancers can cause hemoptysis but clubbing is seen with non small cell cancer of the lung only. Remember that *clubbing is absent in small cell cancer of the lung.*

413. Ans. (a) Metastasis to lungs

- Metastatic malignant neoplasms are the most common form of secondary lung tumors. Lung metastases are identified in 30-55% of all cancer patients, though prevalence varies based on the type of primary cancer.
- Chest radiography (CXR) is the initial imaging modality used in the detection of suspected pulmonary metastasis in patients with known malignancies. Chest CT scanning without contrast is more sensitive than CXR
- *The most common radiographic pattern of pulmonary metastasis is the presence of multiple nodules, ranging in size from 3 mm to 15 cm or more.*
- *The nodules are more common in the lung bases (owing to higher blood flow than upper lobes) and in the outer third of the lungs in the subpleural region.*
- They are approximately spherical and of varying sizes. Nodules of same size are believed to originate at the same time, in a single shower of emboli from the primary tumor. Nodules that are smaller than 2 cm are usually round and have smooth margins. Larger nodules are lobulated and have irregular margins; they may become confluent with adjacent nodules, resulting in a conglomerate multinodular mass.

414. Ans. (c) Pulmonary hamartoma

- Pulmonary hamartomas, the most common benign tumors of the lung, are the third most common cause of solitary pulmonary nodules.
- Pulmonary hamartomas are usually asymptomatic and are typically discovered as an incidental coin lesion on a routine chest radiograph.
- On chest X ray pulmonary hamartomas appear as well defined, solitary pulmonary nodules with varying patterns of calcification, including an irregular popcorn, stippled portion. Popcorn calcification is virtually diagnostic.

415. Ans. (b) Hypercapnia

Ref: Harrison, 19th ed. pg. 1736

- ARDS is characterized by *type 1 respiratory failure* which has only hypoxia but the value of CO_2 is normal. ARDS has non cardiogenic pulmonary edema with normal PCWP.
- PCWP (Normal is 8–12 mm Hg) is increased in Cardiogenic pulmonary edema.
- Remember hypercapnia/hypercarbia is a feature of type 2 respiratory failure.

416. Ans. (d) Benzene

Ref: Harrison, 19th ed. pg. 447t, 663

Cigarette smoke product	Effects on human body
Aceta-aldehyde/anabasine	Addictive
Benzene	Carcinogenic + Cardio-toxic + reproductive potential toxicity
Benzopyrine	Carcinogenic
Carbon monoxide	Reproductive potential toxicity
Vinyl chloride	Carcinogenic

417. Ans. (a) Liver cancer

- Smoking DOES NOT cause liver cancer and primary brain cancer.
- Kidney and bladder cancer are associated with smoking.

418. Ans. (a) Pneumothorax

A very surprising question included in medicine as nothing is mentioned about this test in most books.

In cases of spontaneous pneumothorax air leaks into the pleural cavity. This air may be reabsorbed but leaves behind a bronchopleural fistula which on autopsy can be picked by "water test".

This is not a clinical test but done by forensic team post mortem.

Please don't confuse with:
- **Water loading test** is done for SIADH
- **Water deprivation test** is done for diabetes insipidus.

419. Ans. (d) Eosinophilic alveolitis

Ref: Harrison, 19th ed. pg. 1681

Hypersensitivity pneumonitis is seen in conditions like Bagassosis, Farmer's lung. It is a type IV hypersensitivity reaction with normal eosinophil count. The granulomatous involvement of lung explains a reduced DL_{CO}.

420. Ans. (d) Subcutaneous epinephrine

Ref: Harrison, 19th ed. pg. 1680

Medicine

421. Ans. (a) **Hypertension**

    Ref: Harrison, 19th ed. pg. 1724-25

422. Ans. (a) **Dextrocardia**
    - Situs solitus is the normal position, and situs inversus is the mirror image of situs solitus.
    - Cardiac situs is determined by the atrial location.
    - **In situs inversus:**
        - Morphologic right atrium is on the left, and the morphologic left atrium is on the right.
        - Normal pulmonary anatomy is also reversed so that the left lung has 3 lobes and the right lung has 2 lobes.
        - Liver and gallbladder are located on the left
        - Spleen and stomach are located on the right.

423. Ans. (a) **Meniscus sign**

    The CXR shows pleural effusion as both Costophrenic and *Cardiophrenic angles are obliterated in a CXR and also notice the smooth concavity of fluid rising up in a S shape.* This differentiates from pneumonia.

NEPHROLOGY

424. Ans. (b) **Acute renal failure**

    Ref: Harrison 19th ed. P 656
    - The *most serious threat* in adult patients of G6PD is development of *acute renal failure*.
    - In G6PD, acute hemolytic anemia episode occurs due to exposure to fava beans, infections and drugs. *Due to intravascular hemolysis, hemoglobinuria occurs and causes tubular blockage.* The patient passes dark urine and develops jaundice. The peripheral smear shows bite cells and supravital stain reveals *Heinz bodies.*
    - Sequestration crisis is encountered in sickle cell anemia.

425. Ans. (a) **Bicarbonate, uric acid and amino-acids**

Bicarbonate	Urinary bicarbonate loss leads to bicarbatonuria and explains the metabolic acidosis seen in Fanconi's syndrome
Uric acid	Urinary uric acid is derived from tubular secretion, possibly from the S2 segment of the proximal tubule. Overall, 98-100% of filtered urate is reabsorbed; 6-10% is secreted, ultimately appearing in the final urine.
Amino acid	Aminoaciduria is a feature of Fanconi syndrome

426. Ans. (d) **Contrast arteriography**
    - DTPA scan showing decreased uptake on affected side with damaged kidney contributing less than 40% of total kidney function is used for diagnosis of RAS.
    - Doppler ultrasound of the renal arteries produces reliable estimates of renal blood flow velocity and offers the opportunity to track a lesion over time. Positive studies usually are confirmed at angiography, whereas false-negative results occur frequently, particularly in obese patients.
    - Gadolinium-contrast magnetic resonance angiography offers clear images of the proximal renal artery but may miss distal lesions. An advantage is the opportunity to image the renal arteries with an agent that is not nephrotoxic.
    - **Contrast arteriography is the "gold standard" for evaluation and identification of renal artery lesions.**

427. Ans. (c) **Membranous glomerulopathy**

Nephrotic range massive proteinuria	*Intermediate*	Nephritic syndrome haematuria, decreased GFR
FSGS Membranous glomerulopathy Minimal change disease	Membranoproliferative GN Focal proliferative GN IgA nephropathy Idiopathic SLE (Lupus Nephritis) Cryglobulinemia	Diffuse proliferative GN Crescentic GN

428. Ans. (a) **Chronic renal failure**
    - Broad casts are seen in chronic renal failure and occur due to dilated tubules of enlarged nephrons that have undergone compensatory hypertrophy in response to reduced renal mass (i.e. chronic renal failure).

429. Ans. (d) **CRP**
    - The clinical diagnosis is post-streptococcal glomerulonephritis.
    - The antistreptolysin (ASO), antinicotinamide adenine dinucleotidase (anti-NAD), antihyaluronidase (AHase), and anti–DNAse B are commonly positive after pharyngitis and anti–DNAse B and AHase titers are more often positive following skin infections
    - Most patients have marked depression of serum hemolytic component CH50 and serum concentrations of C3
    - The decrease in C3 concentration typically occurs before the increase in ASO titers
    - Urine sediment has red blood cells, red blood cell casts, white blood cells, granular casts, and, rarely, white blood cell casts
    - Dysmorphic red blood cells indicative of glomerular hematuria can usually be detected by performing phase-contrast microscopy.

FMGE Solutions Screening Examination

430. Ans. (a) Interstitial nephritis

- Salt losing nephritis is an interstitial nephritis associated with hyponatremia and hypovolemia.
- Glomerulonephritis follows a skin infection or a pyoderma and presents with hypertension and haematuria with sub-nephrotic proteinuria.
- Lupus nephritis presents with haematuria and hypertension in SLE patients and shows wire loop lesions.
- IgA nephropathy is the most common cause of hematuria and presents after 48 hours of a respiratory tract infection.

431. Ans. (a) GFR

Cockcroft-Gault formula is used for calculation of GFR

Creatinine Clearance (mL/min) =
$$\frac{[140 - \text{age (years)}] \times \text{weight (kg)} \times [0.85 \text{ if female}]}{72 \times \text{serum creatinine}}$$

432. Ans. (c) Norepinephrine

Ref: Harrison, 19th ed. pg. 1761

Septic Shock Management

- Initial management of hypotension should include the administration of IV fluids, typically beginning with 1–2 L of normal saline over 1–2 hours.
- To avoid pulmonary edema, the central venous pressure should be maintained at 2–10 cm H_2O.
- The urine output rate should be kept at >0.5 mg/kg/h by continuing fluid administration; a diuretic such as furosemide may be used if needed.
- In about one-third of patients, hypotension and organ hypoperfusion respond to fluid resuscitation; a reasonable goal is to maintain a mean arterial blood pressure of >65 mm Hg (systolic pressure >90 mm Hg).
- *If these guidelines cannot be met by volume infusion, vasopressor therapy is indicated. Titrated doses of norepinephrine or dopamine should be administered through a central catheter.*

433. Ans. (d) Low complement levels

Ref: Harrison, 19th ed. pg. 1841

- Nephrotic syndrome is kidney disease with proteinuria, hypoalbuminemia, and edema. Nephrotic-range proteinuria is 3 grams per day or more. On a single spot urine collection, it is 2 g of protein per gram of urine creatinine.
- *Persistently low C3 levels are indicative of acute Glomerulonephritis.*
- The most common form of nephrotic syndrome in children, minimal change disease presents with normal C_3 levels. Congenital and hereditary focal glomerulosclerosis may result from mutations of genes that code for podocyte proteins, including nephrin, podocin, or the cation channel 6 protein

434. Ans. (c) ACE inhibitor

Ref: Harrison, 19th ed. pg. 2478-79

- ACE inhibitors may slow the progression of renal disease in CRF.
- ACE inhibitor therapy generally lowers systemic blood pressure, does not alter renal function and decreases proteinuria in patients with CRF.
- The reduction in proteinuria appears to be variable and may depend on pre-treatment glomerular haemodynamics and/or the activity of the renin-angiotensin-aldosterone system.

435. Ans. (a) Diabetic Nephropathy

Ref: Harrison, 18th ed. chapter 279

- Iodinated contrast agents used for cardiovascular and CT imaging are a leading cause of AKI. The risk of AKI, or "contrast nephropathy," is negligible in those with normal renal function but increases markedly in the setting of chronic kidney disease, particularly diabetic nephropathy.
- The most common clinical course of contrast nephropathy is characterized by a rise in SCr beginning 24–48 hours following exposure, peaking within 3–5 days, and resolving within 1 week.
- Contrast nephropathy is thought to occur from a combination of factors
  - Hypoxia in the renal outer medulla due to perturbations in renal microcirculation and occlusion of small vessels
  - Cytotoxic damage to the tubules directly or via the generation of oxygen free radicals, especially since the concentration of the agent within the tubule is markedly increased
  - Management is with N-acetylcysteine and brisk diuresis.

436. Ans. (c) Thiazides

Ref: Harrison, 18th ed. chapter 45

- Diuretics are a particularly common cause due to associated increases in distal tubular Na^+ delivery and distal tubular flow rate in addition to secondary hyperaldosteronism.
- *Thiazides have an effect on plasma K^+ concentration greater than that of loop diuretics despite their lesser natriuretic effect.*

Medicine

- The higher propensity of thiazides to cause hypokalemia may be secondary to thiazide-associated hypocalciuria versus the *hypercalciuria* seen with loop diuretics

---

437. Ans. (b) Chronic renal failure

Ref: Harrison, 19th ed. pg. 1816

ACE inhibitors and ARBs inhibit the angiotensin-induced vasoconstriction of the efferent arterioles of the glomerular microcirculation. This inhibition leads to a reduction in both intra-glomerular filtration pressure and proteinuria.

- Adverse effects from these agents include cough and angioedema with inhibitors, anaphylaxis, and hyperkalemia.
- *The most common cause of chronic renal failure is diabetic nephropathy and is benefitted by above mentioned effects of ACE inhibitors.*
- Choice A bilateral renal artery stenosis leads to hyperkalemia and hence is a contraindication. Choice D is ruled out henceforth.
- Choice C pregnancy, the use of ACE inhibitors has been shown to cause teratogenicity.

---

438. Ans. (b) Decreased insulin

Ref: Harrison, 18th ed. Chapter 344

- Exogenous insulin is normally metabolized by the kidney. However, when there is impairment of kidney function, the half-life of insulin is prolonged because of lower levels of degradation.
- This necessitates *insulin dose reduction.*
- **Also remember:** The clearance of both sulfonylureas and its metabolites is highly dependent on kidney function. In patients with Stage 3-5 CKD, first-generation sulfonylureas should be avoided. Of the second-generation sulfonylureas, glipizide is recommended because its metabolites are not active, and there is a lower potential for development of hypoglycemia.

---

439. Ans. (a) Low sodium diet

Ref: Harrison, 19th ed. pg. 1870-71

- Because calcium and sodium compete for reabsorption in the renal tubules, excess sodium intake and consequent excretion result in loss of calcium in the urine. High-sodium diets are associated with greater calcium excretion in the urine.
- Calcium intake in patients with kidney stones should be normal with adequate water intake.

---

440. Ans. (c) Pericarditis

Ref: Harrison, 19th ed. pg. 1810, 1822

Absolute indication for hemodialysis is uraemic pericarditis followed by uraemic encephalopathy

---

Indications for emergency dialysis is AEIOU

- **A** cidosis, especially if severe (pH < 7.2 and refractory to HCO_3 or unable to give HCO_3 due to volume overload) or symptomatic (arrhythmias).
- **E** lectrolytes, especially potassium with EKG changes. Temporize with Ca, D50, insulin, bicarb, kayexalate.
- **I** ngestions, especially those that cause renal failure such as salicylates or ethylene glycol.
- **O** verload, i.e. volume overload causing pulmonary edema. Temporize with nitrates and mega doses of Lasix (160–200 mg IV) – push slowly to avoid ototoxicity.
- **U** remia, i.e. confusion, pericarditis, seizures, platelet dysfunction with severe bleeding, intractable N/V.

When to start dialysis in CKD?

- Dialysis should be instituted whenever the glomerular filtration rate (GFR) is <15 mL/min and there is one or more of the following: symptoms or signs of uraemia, inability to control hydration status or blood pressure or a progressive deterioration in nutritional status.
- In any case, dialysis should be started before the GFR has fallen to 6 mL/min/1.73m², even if optimal pre-dialysis care has been provided and there are no symptoms.

---

441. Ans. (a) P.S.G.N

Ref: Harrison, 19th ed. pg. 1837

- Acute post-streptococcal glomerulonephritis (PSGN) is the most common type of acute GN. Acute nephritic syndrome is the most serious and potentially devastating form of the various renal syndromes.
- Most often, the patient is a boy, aged 2–14 years, who suddenly develops puffiness of the eyelids and facial edema in the setting of a post-streptococcal infection. The urine is dark and scanty, and the blood pressure may be elevate.
- Rapidly progressive glomerulonephritis (RPGN) is defined as any glomerular disease characterized by extensive crescents (usually >50%) as the principal histologic finding and by a rapid loss of renal function (usually a 50% decline in the glomerular filtration rate [GFR] within 3 mo) as the clinical correlate.

---

442. Ans. (c) CKD is defined as GFR < 30 ml/min/1.73 m² for 4 weeks

Ref: Harrison, 19th ed. pg. 290-91

- CKD is defined as GFR < 60 mL/min/1.73 m² *for 12 weeks/3 months. Hence choice C is wrong.*
- The average rate of decline varies, but it averages about 0.8 mL/min/1.73 m²/year after age of 30 years. The decline accelerates after about age 65 to 70.
- In terms of GFR ranges for specific ages, an average 85-year-old male would be expected to have a glomerular

Explanations

FMGE Solutions Screening Examination

filtration rate around 55–60 mL/min/1.73 m², depending on his GFR at age 30. *Hence choice A is seen.*
- Choice B is correct.

$$C_{CR} = \frac{U_{CR} \times V}{P_{CR}}$$

443. Ans. (d) Malignancy

Ref: Harrison, 18th ed. chapter 283

Cause of Membranous Glomerulopathy

Autoimmune diseases	Infectious diseases	Malignancy
Ankylosing spondylitis	Filariasis	Carcinoma (solid organ)[Q]
Dermatomyositis	Hepatitis B	Leukemia
Hashimoto	Hepatitis C	Lymphoma
MCTD	Leprosy	Melanoma
Rheumatoid arthritis	Malaria	
Sjögren	Syphilis	
SLE		
Scleroderma		
Drugs	***Miscellaneous***	
Captopril[Q]	De novo in renal allografts	
Gold		
Lithium	Kimura disease	
Penicillamine	Sarcoidosis	
Probenecid	Sickle cell disease	

444. Ans. (d) Rhabdomyolysis

Ref: Harrison, 19th ed. pg. 1804-05

- *A urine dipstick test for blood that has positive findings in the absence of red blood cells (RBCS) suggests myoglobinuria.* Myoglobin being a high molecular protein can block kidney tubules leading to acute tubular necrosis.
- In porphyria gross examination of the urine can provide a valuable clue, since urine of porphyria cutanea tarda patients is red to brown in natural light and pink to red in fluorescent light. However since all types of porphyria do not have red color urine, hence it has been kept as second differential diagnosis in this question.
- In hematuria the color of urine is cola color urine.
- In hemolysis state like paroxysmal nocturnal hemoglobinuria the color of urine is brown to black on account of presence of hemoglobinuria.

445. Ans. (b) Acute glomerulonephritis

Ref: Harrison, 18th ed.

Nephritic syndrome	Hematuria, RBC casts Azotemia, oliguria Edema, hypertension
Chronic renal failure	• Azotemia for >3 months • Prolonged symptoms or signs of uremia • Symptoms or signs of renal osteodystrophy • Kidneys reduce in size bilaterally • Broad casts in urinary sediment
Nephrotic syndrome	• Proteinuria > 3.5 g per 1.73 m² per 24 h • Hypoalbuminemia • Edema • Hyperlipidemia

446. Ans. (d) Aminoglycosides

Ref: Harrison, 18th ed. chapter 280

Aminoglycosides lead to development of non-oliguric renal failure.

Common Causes of Chronic Kidney Disease (Decreasing Order of Prevalence)
- Diabetic glomerular disease
- Glomerulonephritis
- Hypertensive nephropathy
- Primary glomerulopathy with hypertension
- *Vascular and ischemic renal disease (Multiple myeloma due to Bence jones proteins and hypercalcemia)*
- Autosomal dominant polycystic kidney disease
- *Other cystic and tubulointerstitial nephropathy(fanconi syndrome)*

447. Ans. (b) Gram positive organisms

Ref: Harrison, 18th edition, chapter 281

- Hemo-dialysis (HD) catheter-related bloodstream infections (CRBSIs) are a major complication of long-term catheter use in HD. *Gram positive organism are seen followed by gram negative organisms.*
- Similarly in peritoneal dialysis, the clinical presentation typically consists of pain and cloudy dialysate, often with fever and other constitutional symptoms. The most common culprit organisms are gram-positive cocci, including *Staphylococcus,* reflecting the origin from the skin. Gram-negative rod infections are less common; fungal and mycobacterial infections can be seen in selected patients, particularly after antibacterial therapy.
- In cases where peritonitis is due to hydrophilic gram negative rods (e.g., *Pseudomonas* sp.) or yeast, antimicrobial therapy is usually not sufficient, and *catheter removal is required to ensure complete eradication of infection.* Non-peritonitis catheter-associated infections (often termed *tunnel infections*) vary widely

448. Ans. (a) IgA nephropathy

Ref: Harrison's, 17th ed. Ch. 277

- IgA nephroathy also known as Bergers disease. IgA antibodies get deposited in mesangial cells and cause dysfunction of mesangial cells and **lead to microscopic/ gross hematuria.**
- It is classically characterized by episodic nature and is one of the most common forms of glomerulonephritis worldwide.
- The two most common presentations of IgA nephropathy are recurrent episodes of macroscopic hematuria during or immediately following an upper respiratory infection in children (Henoch-Schönlein purpura) or asymptomatic microscopic hematuriamost often seen in adults.
- **Minimal change disease** or lipoid nephrosis is the most common nephrotic syndrome in children. Presence of abnormal T-cell release cytokines and cause damage to visceral cell damage i.e., effacement of podocyte which leads to massive proteinuria.
- **In PSGN** the classic presentation is an acute nephritic picture with hematuria, pyuria, red blood cell casts, edema, hypertension, and oliguric renal failure, which may be severe enough to appear as RPGN.

449. Ans. (d) All of the above

Ref: Urologic Emergencies: A Practical Approach, pg. 117-118

- Xantho-granulomatous pyelonephritis (XGP) is the end result of severe, chronic infection of the kidney, seen in ~ 0.6 to 1.4% of renal inflammations.
- *The combination of urinary obstruction, nephrolithiasis, and UTI are important elements in the development of XGP.*
- *Infection is usually secondary to E.coli, or Proteus Mirabilis.*
- Most patients present with recurrent fevers and urosepsis, anemia, and a painful renal mass.
- *Microscopically, there are granulomas and lipid-laden macrophages around the abscess.*

450. Ans. (a) RTA- 1

Ref: Harrison, 19th ed. pg. 332e-7t

- There are three forms of renal tubular acidosis (RTA). Types 1 and 2 may be acquired or primary whereas the **most common form, type 4 RTA,** is usually acquired in association with moderate renal dysfunction and is **characterized by hyperkalemia.**

TYPE-I Distal RTA (dRTA)

- In this type of RTA kidneys are unable to acidify the urine to pH <5.5 in the presence of systemic metabolic acidosis or after acid loading as a result of *impaired hydrogen ion secretion* or bicarbonate reabsorption in the distal nephron.
- **Other features are:** **HYPOKALEMIA,** hypocitraturia, hypercalciuria, nephrocalcinosis, and/or nephrolithiasis. Chronic untreated acidosis may cause rickets or osteomalacia.

TYPE-II Proximal RTA (pRTA)

- It is the result of *impaired bicarbonate reabsorption in* the proximal tubular where the bulk of filtered bicarbonate is recovered. It is most often secondary to various auto-immune, drug-induced, infiltrative, or other tubulopathies or a result of tubular injury from inherited diseases.
- **Clinical features are:** Hyperphosphaturia, hyperuricos-uria, hypercalciuria, nonselective amino aciduria and glycosuria.

451. Ans. (c) Hyperkalemiac acidosis

Ref: Harrison, 19th ed. pg. 1808, 1810

- Acute kidney injury will cause inability to excrete H$^+$ and K$^+$ both leading to hyperkalemic acidosis.
- The acidosis seen is high anion gap metabolic acidosis.

452. Ans. (d) Analgesic nephropathy

Ref: Harrison, 19th ed. pg. 1861

- AKI is a serious complication of snakebites by the viperidae family.
- Pyelonephritis can be hematogenously acquired and cause extensive necrosis of kidney parenchyma.
- Crush injury or Rhabdo-myolysis can result in myoglobinuria causing blockage of kidney tubules and resultant acute tubular necrosis.

Remember: Analgesic nephropathy causes chronic interstitial nephritis and presents with chronic kidney disease.

453. Ans. (a) Present in alkaline urine

Ref: Harrison, 19th ed. pg. 1871

- These struvite stones are also known as triple-phosphate stone.

Two Conditions Must Coexist for the Formation of Struvite Calculi

- Alkaline urine (pH>7.2)
- The presence of ammonia in the urine.

454. Ans. (c) Hypertension

Ref: Harrison, 19th ed. pg. 1841

Essential Features of Diagnosis of Nephrotic Syndrome are:

- Proteinuria >3.5 gms/24 hours period

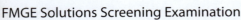

FMGE Solutions Screening Examination

- Hypo-albuminaemia <2.5 gm%
- Edema –peri-orbital edema- pedal edema

Non Essential Features are
- Hyperlidemia- increased cholesterol and increased triglycerides
- Lipiduria
- Loss of protein C /S /AT III in urine leading to hyper-coagulable state.
- **Hypertension as a feature is mainly seen with NEPHRITIC syndrome.** *(Remember Nephritic syndrome has inflammation of kidney blood vessels resulting in vasculitis, reduction in GFR and increase in BP.)*

455. Ans. (c) Nephritic syndrome

Ref: Robbins, 8th ed. / Ch. 14

The presence of red blood cells within the cast is always pathological, and is strongly indicative of glomerular damage, which can occur in
- Glomerulonephritis like P.S.G.N, acute glomerulonephritis, R.P.G.N
- Vasculitis, including Wegener's granulomatosis, systemic lupus erythematosus or Goodpasture's syndrome.
- Renal infarction
- Subacute bacterial endocarditis.
- RBCs may appear normally shaped, swollen by dilute urine (in fact, only cell ghosts and free hemoglobin may remain), or crenated by concentrated urine.
- The presence of dysmorphic RBCs in urine suggests a glomerular disease such as a glomerulonephritis. Dysmorphic RBCs have odd shapes as a consequence of being distorted via passage through the abnormal glomerular structure.

456. Ans. (a) NSAID

Ref: Harrison, 19th ed. pg. 1856

Choices B,C,D lead to acute tubular necrosis and hence by exclusion the answer is A.

Causes of Acute Interstitial Nephritis
- Drugs like beta lactams, quinolones, NSAID,COX-2 inhibitors, phenytoin, valproate and P.P.I
- Infections like streptococcus, staphylococcus
- Connective tissue disorder like SLE, Sjogren
- Light chain nephropathy
- Urate nephropathy

Causes of Chronic Interstitial Nephritis
- V.U.R
- Sickle cell disease
- Hypokalemic nephropathy

457. Ans. (d) Rhabdomyolysis

Ref: Harrison, 19th ed. pg. 1804

- Interstitial nephritis is characterized by tubular damage leading to polyuria.
- Rhabdo-myolysis leads to myo-globinuria and blockage of kidney tubules and subsequent reduction of urine output.

458. Ans. (a) Acute Glomerulonephritis

Ref: Robbins, 8th ed. Chapter 14

- Acute glomerulonephritis is characterized by kidney vasculitis and resultant GFR reduction. This causes high renin hypertension to develop in a patient & lead to edema. The swelling presents first in Peri-orbital area followed by swelling around genitals and then swelling around the feet.
- Acute pyelonephritis is characterized by fever, accelerated heart rate, painful urination, abdominal pain radiating to the back, nausea, and tenderness at the costo-vertebral angle on the affected side
- Chronic glomerulonephritis is bilaterally shrunken kidneys.
- Renal cell carcinoma is characterized by unilaterally enlarged kidneys, painless Haematuria.

459. Ans. (a) Focal segmental glomerulosclerosis

Ref: Robbins, 8th ed. Chapter 14

- HIV nephropathy is associated with development of focal segmental glomerulosclerosis. (Also seen with reflux nephropathy). *It is also the commonest cause of nephrotic syndrome in adults.*

460. Ans. (b) Arteriovenous fistula results in arterialization of vein

Ref: Harrison, 19th ed. pg. 1822-23

- The fistula, graft, or catheter through which blood is obtained for hemodialysis is often referred to as a *dialysis access*.
- A native fistula created by the anastomosis of an artery to a vein (e.g., the Brescia-Cimino fistula, in which the cephalic vein is anastomosed end-to-side to the radial artery) results in arterialization of the vein.
- This facilitates its subsequent use in the placement of large needles (typically 15 Gauge) to access the circulation.
- Fistulas have the highest long-term patency rate of all dialysis access options
- The most important complication of arteriovenous grafts is thrombosis of the graft and graft failure, principally due to intimal hyperplasia at the anastomosis between the graft and recipient vein.

- Many patients undergo placement of an arteriovenous graft (i.e., the interposition of prosthetic material, usually polytetrafluoroethylene, between an artery and a vein) or a tunneled dialysis catheter

461. Ans. (c) Thrice per week

Ref: Harrison, 19th ed. pg. 1823

For the majority of patients with ESRD, between 9 and 12 hours of dialysis are required each week, usually divided into three equal sessions.

Current Targets of Hemodialysis

- Urea reduction ratio (the fractional reduction in blood urea nitrogen per hemodialysis session) of >65–70%.
- Body water–indexed clearance x time product (KT/V) above 1.2 or 1.05.

Remember: Hypotension is the most common acute complication of hemodialysis. Since the introduction of bicarbonate-containing dialysate, dialysis-associated hypotension has become less common. The management of hypotension during dialysis consists of discontinuing ultrafiltration, the administration of 100–250 mL of isotonic saline or 10 mL of 23% saturated hypertonic saline, or administration of salt-poor albumin.

INFECTION

462. Ans. (c) Adequate IVF plus vasopressor

Ref: Harrison, 20th ed. pg. 2050

Saline or balanced crystalloids and nor-epinephrine should be started to obtain a MAP of 65 mm Hg. Vasopressor support is must in patients of septic shock. The preferred vasopressor is nor epinephrine in septic shock and *not* dopamine.

463. Ans. (a) Skin biopsy with fluorescent antibody testing

Ref: Harrison, 20th ed. pg. 1488

- Direct fluorescent antibody testing with rabies virus specific antibodies is highly sensitive and specific for detection of rabies virus antigen in tissues. This test can be easily applied to skin biopsy and brain tissue samples.
- Choice B is ruled out as brain is an immune privileged site, serum antibodies may not develop until late in the disease.
- Choice C is not done . Choice D is an outdated method . Corneal impression is obtained by pressing the surface of sterile glass slide gently but firmly onto the cornea.

464. Ans. (a) C5-C9 deficiency

Ref: Harrison, 20th ed. pg. 1124

The importance of humoral immunity in defence against N. meningitidis infection is best demonstrated by predisposition of persons deficient in terminal component of complement deficiency (C5-C9).

465. Ans. (b) 3

Ref: Harrison, 20th ed. pg. 115

Three consecutive negative blood cultures is mandatory in definition of F.U.O

Definition of fever of unknown origin

- Fever $\geq$ 38.3°C ($\geq$101°F) on at least two occasions
- Illness duration of $\geq$3 weeks
- No known immunocompromised state
- Diagnosis that remains uncertain after a thorough history-taking, physical examination, and the following obligatory investigations: Determination of erythrocyte sedimentation rate (ESR) and C-reactive protein (CRP) level; platelet count; leukocyte count and differential; measurement of levels of hemoglobin, electrolytes, creatinine, total protein, alkaline phosphatase, alanine aminotransferase, aspartate aminotransferase, lactate dehydrogenase, creatine, kinase, ferritin, antinuclear antibodies, and rheumatoid factor, protein electrophoresis; urinalysis; blood cultures ($n = 3$); urine culture; chest X-ray; abdominal ultrasonography; and tuberculin skin test (TST) or interferon γ release assay (IGRA).

466. Ans. (a) Infectious mononucleosis

Ref: Harrison, 20th ed. pg. 1358

- The key word in the question is development of rash after being given ampicillin. Infectious mononucleosis presents as low-grade fever in first 2 weeks of illness. Most common clinical sign is Lymphadenopathy and pharyngitis. Gradually the spleen enlarges. The morbilliform rash on arms and trunk develops both in patients exposed to penicillin derivatives and those who are not exposed to penicillin. *Atypical lymphocytosis is the blood picture with deranged LFT. Most cases are self-limited.*
- Choice B is ruled out as it responds to ampicillin and does not develop after its administration.
- Choice C should have desquamation with mucocutaneous manifestations.
- Choice D does not have a rash and can't be diagnosed on short history of 7 days

FMGE Solutions Screening Examination

467. Ans. (a) No cut off of CD4 count required for initiation of treatment

Ref: www.who.int

The latest guidelines are in favor of initiating ART among all adults living with HIV regardless of WHO clinical stage or at any CD4 cell count.

▶ **Extra Mile**

2014 CDC Case definition for HIV infection among adolescents and adults

Stage	CD4 Count	CD4%	Clinical evidence
Stage 0	Early HIV infection		
Stage 1	≥500 cells/mm³	≥26	No AIDS-defining condition
Stage 2	200-499 cells/mm³	14-25	No AIDS-defining condition
Stage 3	<200 cells/mm³	<14	*or Documentation* of AIDS-defining condition

468. Ans. (d) Lymphocytosis

Ref: Harrison 19th ed. P 1023

Absolute lymphocytosis occurs during *late catarrhal and paroxysmal phases* of pertussis. It correlates with severity of disease.

TABLE: Case definition of pertussis

Acute *coughing illness lasting for >14 days* with at least one characteristic pertussis symptom
- Paroxysmal cough
- Post-tussive vomiting
- Inspiratory whoop

Or

Cough lasting for more than 14 days in an outbreak setting

Contd...

471. Ans. (c) 45–180 days

469. Ans. (b) Ceftriaxone

Ref: Harrison 19th ed. P 1003

- *Ceftriaxone* used as a single IM or IV injection is highly effective in carriage eradication and can be *used for all ages and in pregnancy.*
- Ciprofloxacin or ofloxacin is administered by mouth and is not in recommended in pregnancy. It is given to household contacts.
- Rifampicin is no longer an optimal agent as it fails to eradicated carriage in 15–20% of cases.

470. Ans. (b) Type 3

Ref: Davidson 22nd ed. P 347; Harrison 19th ed. P 1125

- The clinical diagnosis of the patient is *type 2 lepra reaction*. The pathogenesis of type 2 lepra reaction is *type 3 hypersensitivity reaction.*
- Type 2 lepra reaction/Erythema Nodosum Leprosum occur *exclusively in patients with lepromatous end of leprosy* spectrum. The most common clinical features are crops of painful erythematous papules that resolve spontaneously in few days to weeks. Concomitant fever, lymphadenitis, neuritis and anemia may develop.
- Type 1 lepra reaction occurs in half of patients with border line forms of leprosy but *not* in patients with pure lepromatous disease. The type of hypersensitivity reaction is type 4 hypersensitivity.

Ref: Pink Book 2018, CDC Guidelines; Harrison 19th ed. P 2006

TABLE: The ABCs of Hepatitis

	Hepatitis A	Hepatitis B	Hepatitis C
Routes of transmission	Ingestion of fecal matter, even in microscopic amounts, from: • Close person-to-person contact with an infected person • Sexual contact with an infected person • Ingestion of contaminated food or drinks	Contact with infectious blood, semen, and other body fluids primarily through: • Birth to an infected mother • Sexual contact with an infected person • Sharing of contaminated needles, syringes, or other injection drug equipment	Contact with blood of an infected person primarily through: • Sharing of contaminated needles, syringes, or other injection drug equipment Less commonly through: • Sexual contact with an infected person

Contd...

Medicine

	Hepatitis A	Hepatitis B	Hepatitis C
Incubation period	15–50 days (Average: 28 days)	45–160 days (Average: 120 days)	14–180 days (Average: 45 days)
Symptoms of acute infection	Symptoms of all types of viral hepatitis are similar and can include one or more of the following: • Fever • • Fatigue • Loss of appetite • Nausea • Vomiting • Abdominal pain • Gray-colored bowel movements • Joint pain • Jaundice		

472. Ans. (c) Bacterial pneumonia

Ref: Harrison 19th ed. P 1250

- Pulmonary disease is the most frequent complication of HIV infection.
- *The most common manifestation of pulmonary disease is pneumonia.*
- Three of the 10 most common AIDS defining illnesses are recurrent bacterial pneumonia, tuberculosis and *P. jiroveci* pneumonia.
- Encapsulated organisms like *S. pneumoniae* and *H. influenzae* are responsible for most cases of bacterial pneumonia.

473. Ans. (d) Haematocrit

Ref: WHO Handbook for Management of Dengue Fever

- For monitoring patients of severe dengue haematocrit is performed.
- *A rising haematocrit indicates development of dengue shock syndrome*
- *A falling haematocrit indicates bleeding and need for platelet transfusion in case the platelets are less than 10,000/cu.mm.*
- Haematocrit values can be used to monitor fluid resuscitation in patients of dengue.

Dengue without warning signs	Dengue with warning signs		Severe Dengue
Group A **May be sent home**	**Group B** **Referred for in –hospital care**		**Group C** **Require emergency treatment**
Patients who do not have warning signs **AND** Who are able: • To tolerate adequate volume of oral fluids • To pass urine at least once every 6 hours	Patient with any of the following features: • Co-existing conditions such as pregnancy, infancy, old age, diabetes mellitus • Social circumstances such as living alone, living far from hospital	Or Existing warming signs: • Abdominal pain or tenderness • Persistent vomiting • Clinical fluid accumulation • Mucosal bleeding • Lethargy/restlessness • Liver enlargement >2 cm • Laboratory: increase in Hct	Patient with any of the following features • Severe plasma leakage with shock and/ or fluid accumulation with respiratory distress • Severe bleeding • Severe organ impairment
Laboratory tests • Full blood count • Haematocrit	**Laboratory tests** • Full blood Count • Haematocrit		**Laboratory tests** • Full blood count • Haematocrit • Other organ function tests as indicated

474. Ans. (b) Cocksackie

- Hand-foot-and-mouth disease (HFMD) is an acute viral illness that presents as a vesicular eruption in the mouth, but it can also involve the hands, feet, buttocks, and/or genitalia.
- *Coxsackie virus A type 16 (CVA16) is the etiologic agent involved in most cases of HFMD,* but the illness is also associated with coxsackie virus A5, A7, A9, A10, B2, and B5 strains.
- Initially, macular lesions appear on the buccal mucosa, tongue, and/or hard palate. These mucosal lesions rapidly progress to vesicles that erode and become surrounded by an erythematous halo.

475. Ans. (a) Penicillin

For treatment of actinomycosis, the IV administration of 18–24 million units of penicillin daily for 2–6 weeks, followed by oral therapy with penicillin or amoxicillin (total duration, 6–12 months), is recommended guideline for serious infections and bulky disease.

476. Ans. (a) Oseltamivir

- Laboratory testing has found the H1N1 influenza A (swine flu) virus susceptible to the prescription antiviral drugs oseltamivir and zanamivir. Other antiviral agents (e.g. amantadine, rimantadine) are not recommended because of recent resistance to other influenza strains documented over the past several years.

477. Ans. (a) Doxycycline

- *The drug of choice for the treatment of both children and adults with rocky mountain spotted fever is doxycycline, except when the patient is pregnant or allergic to the drug.*
- Because of the severity of RMSF, immediate empirical administration of doxycycline should be strongly considered for any patient with a consistent clinical presentation in the appropriate epidemiologic setting.
- Treatment with chloramphenicol, a less effective drug, is advised only for patients who are pregnant or allergic to doxycycline.
- Beta-lactam antibiotics, erythromycin, and aminoglycosides have no role in the treatment of RMSF, and sulfa-containing drugs are likely to exacerbate this infection. There is little clinical experience with fluoroquinolones, clarithromycin, and azithromycin, which are not recommended.

478. Ans. (b) Azithromycin

Previously healthy and no antibiotics received in past 3 months	Comorbidities or antibiotics received in past 3 months
Macrolide like clarithromycin or azithromycin Doxycycline	Respiratory fluroquinolone like moxifloxacin Beta lactam like Amoxicillin/Clavulanate plus a macrolide

479. Ans. (a) Protein Misfolding

Ref: Harrison, 19th ed. pg. 444e-9

- When a prion enters a healthy organism, it induces existing, properly folded proteins to convert into the misfolded prion form. In this way, the prion acts as a template to guide the misfolding of more proteins into prion form.
- All known mammalian prion diseases are caused by the prion protein, PrP. The endogenous, properly folded form is denoted PrP^C (for *Common* or *Cellular*), whereas the disease-linked, misfolded form is denoted as PrP^{Sc} (for *Scrapie*, after one of the diseases first linked to prions and neurodegeneration.)
- The precise structure of the prion is not known, though they can be formed by combining PrP^C, polyadenylic acid, and lipids in a Protein Misfolding Cyclic Amplification (PMCA) reaction

480. Ans. (c) >25 neutrophils and <10 squamous epithelial cells

Ref: Harrison, 19th ed. pg. 806

- Expectorated sputum is necessarily contaminated by upper respiratory secretions as it passes through the oropharynx and mouth.
- When examining the Gram stain of such a specimen, the examiner should determine whether it is mostly purulent material from the lung or mainly saliva.
- Since squamous epithelial cells line the upper airway but not the tracheo-bronchial tree, their presence indicates that upper airway secretions have contaminated the specimen to some degree.
- *Several criteria have been proposed for determining that a sputum specimen is not excessively contaminated with oropharyngeal flora and is therefore acceptable for culture.*
- *For example:*
  - *Fewer than 10 squamous epithelial cells per field when viewed through a low-power (10x) lens (total magnification 100x) and more than 25 neutrophils per low-power field, or a ratio of neutrophils to epithelial cells greater than 5:1*
- Even if the specimen conforms to those standards, the patient doesn't necessarily have pneumonia.
- That diagnosis depends upon clinical and radiographic information. Patients with viral bronchitis, chronic obstructive lung disease, or tracheal intubation, for example, can have purulent sputum with a predominant organism in the absence of infection of the lung parenchyma.
- In some clearly satisfactory sputum specimens collected from patients with pneumonia due to a single organism (e.g., *Streptococcus pneumoniae*), not only is the infecting organism visible with Gram stain, but often small numbers of other types of bacteria are also present.
- A common mistake is to conclude that the Gram stain shows "mixed flora" and therefore does not help establish a diagnosis.

481. Ans. (a) Nasopharynx

Ref: Harrison's, 19th ed. pg. 997, 999

- *The natural habitat and reservoir for meningococci is the mucosal surfaces of the human nasopharynx and, to a lesser extent, the urogenital tract and anal canal.*
- Approximately 5-10% of adults are asymptomatic nasopharyngeal carriers, but that number increases to as many as 60-80% of members of closed populations (e.g., military recruits in camps).
- The modes of infection include direct contact or respiratory droplets from the nose and throat of infected people.

Medicine

- The incubation period averages 3–4 days (range 1-10 days), which is the period of communicability.
- Bacteria can be found for 2-4 days in the nose and pharynx and for up to 24 hours after starting antibiotics

482. Ans. (b) Serotype B

Ref: Harrison, 19th ed. pg. 1002

- *There are currently three vaccines available in the USA to prevent meningococcal disease, all quadrivalent in nature, targeting serogroups A, C, W-135, and Y.*
- Meningococcal polysaccharide or conjugate vaccines provide no protection against serogroup B disease and MenB vaccines provide no protection against serogroup A, C, W or Y disease. For protection against all 5 serogroups of meningococcus it is necessary to receive both vaccines.
- Only recently vaccine targeting serogroup B has also been created and is *protein* based.

Trade name	Type of vaccine	Serogroups included	Year licensed	Approved ages
Menveo	Conjugate	A, C, W, Y	2010	2 months-55 years
Men Hibrix	Conjugate	C, Y, and Hib	2012	6 weeks-18 months
Trumenba	Protein	B	2014	10-25 years
Bexsero	Protein	B	2015	10-25 years

FLUIDS AND ELECTROLYTES

483. Ans. (d) IV Soda-bicarbonate

Ref: Harrison 19th ed. P 311

- Intravenous bicarbonate has *no role in management of hyperkalemia*. It should not be given in the form of intravenous bolus of undiluted ampoules due to risk of development of hypernatremia. Slow infusion in concomitant metabolic acidosis helps by a *delayed drop* over 4–6 hours.
- Calcium chloride is given to antagonize the effect of potassium on the heart.
- β_2 agonists are useful in case of dangerous hyperkalemia and have additive effect on insulin drip.
- Hemodialysis is the *most effective method* to treat hyperkalemia.

> **Extra Mile**

The most effective drug required to treat dangerous hyperkalemia is *insulin* drip

484. Ans. (b) Diarrhea

Ref: Harrison, 19th ed. P 317

ANION GAP

Increased	Normal	Decreased
KULT	**DR FUSE**	Multiple myeloma
Ketoacidosis	**D**iarrhea	Nephrotic syndrome
Uremia	**R**enal tubular acidosis	
Lactic acidosis	type 1, 2, 4	
Toxins—ethylene	**F**istula	
glycol and methyl	**U**reterosigmoidos-	
alcohol poisoning	tomy	

485. Ans. (a) Renal tubular acidosis

Ref: Harrison 19th ed. P 317

Refer to explanation of above question.

486. Ans. (a) Diarrhea

Ref: Harrison 19th ed. P 2275

- In choice B, extra ADH will lead to gain of water and low plasma osmolality. Same would happen in compulsive water drinking in choice C.
- Cerebral toxoplasmosis leads to SIADH and gain of water.
- Diarrhea will lead to water loss and *hemoconcentration* which can explain increased blood osmolality.

487. Ans. (a) Hypokalemic hypochloremic metabolic alkalosis

Ref: Harrison: 19th ed. P 322

- The repeated vomiting episodes lead to loss of hydrochloric acid. The resultant dehydration triggers activation of RAAS system.
- The elevated aldosterone level lead to excess urinary loss of potassium and hydrogen.
- The resultant manifestation is called hypochloremic hypokalemic metabolic alkalosis.

> **Extra Mile**

- Hypokalemic metabolic acidosis is seen in diarrhea with dehydration.
- Hyperkalemic metabolic acidosis is seen with ureterosigmoidostomy.

488. Ans. (a) Renal tubular acidosis

Normal anion gap (Hyperchloremic Acidosis)	
GI HCO$_3$ –loss	Colostomy
	Diarrhea
	Enteric fistulas
	Ileostomy
	Use of ion-exchange resins
Urologic procedures	Uretero-sigmoidostomy
	Uretero-ileal conduit

Contd...

Explanations

Normal anion gap (Hyperchloremic Acidosis)	
Renal HCO_3 –loss	Tubulo-interstitial disease Renal tubular acidosis, types 1, 2, and 4
Ingestions	$CaCl_2$ Mg sulfate
Parenteral infusion	Arginine lysine Ammonium chloride
Other	Hypoaldosteronism Hyperkalemia Toluene

489. Ans. (a) Starvation

Causes of high anion gap	
Cause	**Examples**
Ketoacidosis	Diabetes Chronic alcoholism undernutrition Fasting
Lactic acidosis (from physiologic processes)	Shock Primary hypoxia due to lung disorders Seizures
Lactic acidosis (from exogenous toxins)	Carbon monoxide Cyanide Iron Isoniazid Toluene
Renal failure	–
Toxins metabolized to acids	Alcohol Methanol Ethylene glycol Paraldehyde Salicylates
Rhabdomyolysis	–

490. Ans. (b) Normal Saline

Ref: Harrison, 19th ed. pg. 1749-50

- *In controlled hemorrhagic shock (CHS),* where the source of bleeding has been occluded, fluid replacement is aimed toward normalization of hemodynamic parameters.
- *In uncontrolled hemorrhagic shock (UCHS),* in which the bleeding has temporarily stopped because of hypotension, vasoconstriction, and clot formation, fluid treatment is aimed at restoration of radial pulse or restoration of sensorium or obtaining a blood pressure of 80 mm Hg by aliquots of 250 mL of lactated Ringer's solution (hypotensive resuscitation).
- *Crystalloid is the first fluid of choice for resuscitation.* Immediately administer 2 L of isotonic sodium chloride solution or lactated Ringer's solution in response to shock from blood loss. Fluid administration should continue until the patient's hemodynamics become stabilized. Because crystalloids quickly leak from the vascular space, each liter of fluid expands the blood volume by 20-30%; therefore, 3 L of fluid needs to be administered to raise the intravascular volume by 1 L.
- Alternatively, colloids restore volume in a 1:1 ratio. Currently available colloids include human albumin, hydroxy-ethyl starch products (mixed in either 0.9% isotonic sodium chloride solution or lactated Ringer's solution), or hypertonic saline-dextran combinations.

491. Ans. (b) Tall T waves in ECG

Ref: Harrison, 19th ed. pg. 307, 310

- *The earliest electrocardiogram (ECG) change associated with hypokalemia is a decrease in the T-wave amplitude.*
- As potassium levels decline further, ST-segment depression and T-wave inversions are seen, while the PR interval can be prolonged along with an increase in the amplitude of the P wave.
- The U wave is described as a positive deflection after the T wave, often best seen in the mid-precordial leads (e.g., V_2 and V_3). When the U wave exceeds the T-wave amplitude, the serum potassium level is <3 mEq/L.
- In severe hypokalemia, T- and U-wave fusion with giant U waves masking the smaller preceding T waves becomes apparent on the ECG.
- A pseudo-prolonged QT interval may be seen, which is actually the QU interval with an absent T wave.

Severe hypokalemia can also cause a variety of tachyarrhythmias, including ventricular tachycardia/fibrillation and rarely atrioventricular block.

492. Ans. (a) Diarrhea

Ref: Harrison, 18th ed. Chapter 45

Diarrhea	Loss of potassium in stool and hypoperfusion of tissues explains the presence of lactic acid leading to metabolic acidosis
Vomiting	Loss of acid in vomiting leads to metabolic alkalosis
Nasogastric suction	Same as above
Conn syndrome	Hyperaldosteronism will promote acid loss leading to metabolic alkalosis.

> **Extra Mile**
>
> **Must know causes of metabolic acidosis = K.U.L.T**
> K = ketoacidosis due to starvation or diabetic complications
> U = uremia
> L = Lactic acidosis
> T = Toxins (methyl alcohol, ethylene glycol)

493. Ans. (b) Biotin deficiency

Ref: Harrison, 18th ed. Chapter 74

Seborrheic dermatitis is seen with following vitamin deficiency
1. Niacin
2. Riboflavin
3. Pyridoxine
4. Biotin

- Niacin deficiency has 3D = diarrhea, dementia and dermatitis (Not in the choices).
- Vitamin A deficiency has night blindness and eye signs and therefore is ruled out
- Riboflavin deficiency is diagnosed by Magenta tongue, angular stomatitis, seborrhea, cheilosis but does not have alopecia and apathy
- In adults, biotin deficiency results in mental changes (depression, hallucinations), paresthesia, anorexia, and nausea. A scaling, *seborrheic,* and erythematous rash may occur around the eyes, nose, and mouth as well as on the extremities.
- In infants, biotin deficiency presents as hypotonia, lethargy, and *apathy.* In addition, infants may develop *alopecia and a characteristic rash* that includes the ears

> **Extra Mile**

Nutrient	Clinical finding
Thiamine	Beriberi: neuropathy, muscle weakness and wasting, cardiomegaly, edema, ophthalmoplegia confabulation
Riboflavin	Magenta tongue, angular stomatitis, seborrhea, cheilosis
Niacin	Pellagra: Pigmented rash of sun-exposed areas, bright red tongue, diarrhea, apathy, memory loss, disorientation
Vitamin B6	Megaloblastic anemia, atrophic glossitic, depression, ↑homocysteine
Vitamin B12	Megaloblastic anemia, loss of vibratory and position sense, abnormal gait, dementia, impotence, loss of bladder and bowel control, ↑ homocysteine, ↑ methylmolonic acid

494. Ans. (c) Renal tubular acidosis

Ref: Harrison's, 17th ed. Chapter 48

- **Anion gap:** The anion gap is the difference between primary measured cations (sodium Na^+ and potassium K^+) and the primary measured anions (chloride Cl^- and bicarbonate HCO_3^-) in serum.

- So we take value of sodium and from it subtract the value of chloride and bicarbonate.
- **Value of Normal anion gap** =10 to 12 mmol/L

AG calculated as follows: AG = Na^+ − (Cl^- + HCO_3^-)

Normal anion gap (Mn: FUSED CAR)	Increased anion gap (Mn: MUDPILES)	Decreased anion gap (Mn: BPH-M)
F- Fistula pancreatic **U-** Ureterosigmoidostomy **S-** Small bowel fistula **E-** Extra chloride **D-** Diarrhea **C-** Carbonic anhydrase Inhibitor *(acetazolamide)* **A-** Adrenal insufficiency **R-** Renal tubular acidosis	**M** - Methanol **U** - Uremia **D** - DKA/AKA/SKA *(diabetic/alcoholic/ starvation)* **P** - Paraldehyde / phenformin **I** - Iron / INH **L** - Lactic acidosis **E** - Ethylene glycol **S** - Salicylates	Bromide intoxication Plasma cell dyscrasia Hypoalbuminemia Monoclonal protein

495. Ans. (d) Renal tubular acidosis

Please refer to above explanation

496. Ans. (b) Diarrhea

Please refer to above explanation

497. Ans. (d) Central pontine myelinosis

Ref: Harrison's, 17th ed. Ch. 334

- Normal serum sodium concentration: 135-145mEq/L. Hypernatremia is defined as a sodium concentration > 145 mEq/L.
- All patients with hypernatremia have hyperosmolality, unlike hyponatremic patients who can have a low, normal, or high serum osmolality.
- Altered mental status is the most common manifestation, ranging from mild confusion and lethargy to deep coma.
- Hyperthermia, delirium, seizures, and coma may be seen with severe hypernatremia (i.e., sodium > 158 mEq/L). Symptoms in the elderly may not be specific; a recent change in consciousness is associated with a poor prognosis.
- The sudden shrinkage of brain cells in acute hypernatremia may lead to *parenchymal or subarachnoid hemorrhages*.
- **Central pontine myelinolysis** *presents most commonly as a complication of treatment of patients with profound, life threatening* **hyponatremia** *(if hypertonic saline is given too rapidly in a patient in whom hyponatremia has been present for >24–48 hours).*

498. Ans. (a) Facial nerve stimulation by tapping over the parotid

Ref: Harrison, 19th ed. pg. 315

Hypocalcemia/Tetany is characterized by irritability of nerves. This can be elicited by tapping over the facial nerve when it is entering into the parotid gland. This will cause twitching of facial musculature. The sign is referred to as Chvostek sign.

499. Ans. (d) Hypertonic fluids

Ref: Harrison, 19th ed. pg. 1779

Hypertonic 3% saline can be used in Raised ICT
- Osmotic therapy (ie, mannitol, hypertonic saline), barbiturate, anesthesia, and neuromuscular blockage, along with concomitant monitoring of intracranial pressure with intracranial pressure monitor is generally required in order to maintain adequate cerebral perfusion pressure of greater than 70 mm Hg.

500. Ans. (b) Heat cramps

Ref: Harrison, 19th ed. pg. 479e-2

Heavy sweating causes heat cramps, especially when the water is replaced without also replacing salt or potassium.

501. Ans. (d) Osteoporosis

Ref: Harrison, 19th ed. pg. 2494-95

- **Osteoporosis** is not due to hypocalcemia but is due to imbalance between the osteoclastic activity and osteoblastic activity
- The IOC for osteoporosis is DEXA scan while the DOC is bisphosphonates along with calcitonin nasal spray.
- Hypocalcemia can cause rickets in children or osteomalacia in adults in which the weakened bone is susceptible to fracture.
- If serum calcium becomes less than 7 mg% then it causes tetany.
- The QT interval in ECG is inversely related to calcium levels in the blood.

502. Ans. (b) Neurogenic

Ref: Harrison, 19th ed. pg. 1750

- In road traffic accident case there can be poly-trauma which can damage the spine as well. The damage to thoracic spine can destroy the sympatho-mimetic outflow to the heart causing bradycardia with hypotension.
- In this question if *tachycardia was given with hypotension, the answer would be hypovolemic shock* secondary to damage to organs like liver and spleen.

503. Ans. (d) Norepinephrine

Ref: Harrison, 19th ed. pg. 444e-3t

Molecule	Half life
Renin	80 minutes
Cortisol	100 minutes
Aldosterone	<20 minutes
Nor epinephrine	2–2.5 minutes
Epinephrine	2–3 minutes

MISCELLANEOUS

504. Ans. (a) Elongation of filiform papillae

Ref: Harrison, 20th ed. pg. 223

Black hairy tongue shows elongation of filiform papillae which become stained by tea, coffee, tobacco or pigmented bacteria. It is seen in elderly smokers, patients on antibiotics, advanced malignancy.

505. Ans. (a) Upper outer

The site is upper outer quadrant to avoid trauma to sciatic nerve.

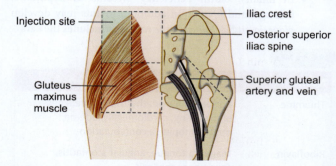

506. Ans. (b) Facial artery

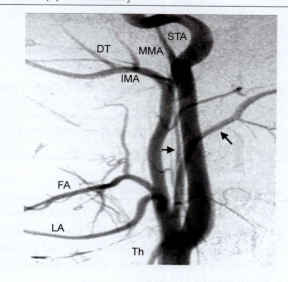

Medicine

- Superior thyroid artery (Th)
- Lingual artery (LA)
- Facial artery (FA)
- Occipital artery (large arrow)
- Ascending pharyngeal artery (small arrow)
- Internal maxillary artery (IMA)
- Middle meningeal artery (MMA)
- Middle deep temporal artery (DT)
- Superficial temporal artery (STA)

507. Ans. (d) Artery puncture

Complications of Jugular Line Insertion

- Arterial puncture. The subclavian artery cannot be compressed; accordingly, the subclavian approach should be avoided in anticoagulated patients.
- Hematoma usually requires monitoring only.
- Hemothorax
- Catheter-related thrombosis may lead to pulmonary embolism.
- An air embolism may be caused by negative intrathoracic pressure, with inspiration by the patient drawing air into an open line hub.
- Dysrhythmia may occur as a consequence of cardiac irritation by the wire or catheter tip. It can usually be terminated by simply withdrawing the line into the superior vena cava. Placing a central venous catheter without a cardiac monitor is unwise.
- Atrial wall puncture can lead to pericardial tamponade.
- Patients who are allergic to antibiotics may experience anaphylaxis upon insertion of an antibiotic-impregnated catheter.
- Chylo-thorax is a possible complication on the left side.

508. Ans. (c) Both

Ref: Harrison, 19th ed. pg. 2107

X-lined severe combined immunodeficiency	Most cases of SCID are due to mutations in the gene encoding the common gamma chain (Yc) a protein that is shared by the receptors for interleukins IL-2, IL-4, IL-7, IL-9, IL-15. *Since the common gamma chain is shared by many interleukin receptors, mutations that result in a non-functional common gamma chain cause widespread defects in interleukin signalling.*
Adenosine deaminase deficiency	The second most common form of SCID after X-SCID is caused by a defective enzyme, adenosine deaminase (ADA), necessary for the breakdown of purines. Lack of ADA causes accumulation of dATP. This metabolite will inhibit the activity of ribonucleotide reductase, the enzyme that reduces ribonucleotides to generate deoxyribonucleotides.

509. Ans. (b) Lymphatics

Ref: Schwartz Surgery, 10th ed. pg. 906

- Buerger's disease, also known as thromboangiitis obliterans, is a progressive non-atherosclerotic segmental inflammatory disease that *most often affects small- and medium-sized arteries, veins, and nerves of the upper and lower extremities.*
- Pathologically, thrombosis occurs in small- to medium sized arteries and veins with associated dense polymorphonuclear leukocyte aggregation, micro-abscesses, and multinucleated giant cells.
- The chronic phase of the disease shows a decrease in the hyper-cellularity and frequent recanalization of the vessel lumen. End-stage lesions demonstrate organized thrombus and blood vessel fibrosis.
- Buerger's disease typically presents in young male smokers, with symptoms beginning prior to age 40. Patients initially present with foot, leg, arm, or hand claudication, which may be mistaken for joint or neuromuscular problems.
- Progression of the disease leads to calf claudication and eventually ischemic rest pain and ulcerations on the toes, feet, or fingers.

510. Ans. (d) Serum amylase

Ref: Harrison 19th ed. Chapter 267

- Acute Physiology and Chronic Health Evaluation II is the most commonly used Severity of illness scoring system in America
- Age, type of ICU admission (after elective surgery vs. nonsurgical or after emergency surgery), a chronic health problem score, and 12 physiologic variables (the most severely abnormal of each in the first 24 h of ICU admission) are used to derive a score.
- The predicted hospital mortality is derived from a formula that takes into account the II score, the need for emergency surgery, and a weighted, disease-specific diagnostic category

VITALS
Rectal temperature, °C
Mean blood pressure, mm Hg
Heart rate
Respiratory rate
Arterial pH
Oxygenation levels
LABS
• Serum sodium
• Serum potassium
• Serum creatinine

Contd...

Explanations

FMGE Solutions Screening Examination

- Hematocrit
- WBC count, 10³/mL
- Glasgow Coma Score

Points Assigned to Age

Points Assigned to Chronic Health

If patient is admitted after elective surgery

If patient is admitted after emergency surgery or for reasons other than after elective surgery

511. Ans. (a) Calf pain

Ref: Harrison 19th ed. pg. 1645-46

- Claudication in the *arch of the foot is an early sign* and is suggestive of, or even specific to, TAO.
- This condition is a manifestation of infrapopliteal vessel occlusive disease.
- As the disease progresses, **typical calf claudication** *and eventually ischemic pain at rest and ischemic ulcerations on the toes, feet, or fingers may develop.*
- Ischemia of the upper limbs is clinically evident in 40–50% of patients, but may be detected in 63% of patients by Allen's test and in 91% of patients by arteriogram of the hand and forearm.

Criteria for diagnosis of TAO

- Onset before age 45
- Current (or recent past) tobacco use
- Distal extremity ischemia (infra-popliteal and/or intra-brachial), such as claudication, rest pain, ischemic ulcers, and gangrene documented with non-invasive testing
- Laboratory tests to exclude autoimmune or connective tissue diseases and diabetes mellitus
- Exclude a proximal source of emboli with echocardiography and arteriography
- Demonstrate consistent Arteriographic findings in the involved and clinically non-involved limbs

512. Ans. (a) External jugular vein

The Peripherally Inserted Central Lines sites are
- Subclavian (preffered)
- Internal jugular vein
- Femoral vein

- In critically ill patients, *barotrauma* (pneumothorax) and puncture of an incompressible artery are probably the most common mechanical complications and can be life-threatening.
- Mechanical complications include
  - Pneumothorax
  - Arterial puncture
  - Catheter malposition can have serious consequences. Positioning of the catheter tip in the cardiac silhouette is associated with an increased risk for cardiac tamponade, and positioning in the subclavian vein with a high risk for thrombus formation in cancer patients.
  - Mediastinal haematoma
  - Hemothorax
  - Injury to adjacent nerves.

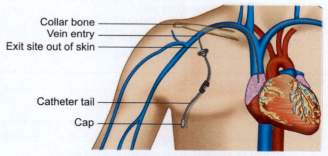

- The recent introduction of more flexible catheters and of the J guide-wire insertion method has decreased the rate of severe mechanical complications.

513. Ans. (a) 35 degrees Celsius

Ref: Harrison, 18th ed. Chapter 19

Accidental hypothermia occurs when there is an unintentional drop in the body's core temperature below 35°C (95°F). At this temperature, many of the compensatory physiologic mechanisms that conserve heat begin to fail. *Primary accidental hypothermia* is a result of the direct exposure of a previously healthy individual to cold. The mortality rate is much higher for patients who develop *secondary hypothermia* as a complication of a serious systemic disorder

514. Ans. (a) Lung cancer

Ref: Table 81.1 Harrison, 18th ed.

The most common cancer in the world is lung cancer, and it is the *most common cause of cancer related death.*

515. Ans. (d) Drug of choice is ciprofloxacin

Ref: Harrison, 19th ed. pg. 1145, 1140

Clinical Features

- Symptoms of leptospirosis include high fever, severe headache, chills, muscle aches, and vomiting, and may include jaundice, red eyes, abdominal pain, diarrhea, and rash.
- Initial presentation may resemble pneumonia. The symptoms in humans appear after a 4–14 day incubation period. More severe manifestations include meningitis, extreme fatigue, hearing loss, respiratory distress, azotemia, and renal interstitial tubular necrosis, which results in renal failure and occasionally liver failure *(the severe form of this disease is known as Weil's disease)*

Investigations

- **Diagnosis**-enzyme-linked immunosorbent assay (ELISA) and polymerase chain reaction (PCR).

Medicine

- Gold standard-The MAT (microscopic agglutination test), a serological test

Treatment

- Doxycycline may be used as a prophylaxis 200–250 mg once a week
- Treatment is a relatively complicated process comprising two main components: suppressing the causative agent and fighting possible complications.
- Effective antibiotics include: Cefotaxime, Doxycycline, Penicillin, Ampicillin, and Amoxicillin.

516. Ans. (b) Fredereich ataxia

Ref: Harrison, 19th ed. pg. 2629-30

Xeroderma pigmentosum	Xeroderma pigmentosum, or XP, is an autosomal recessive genetic disorder of DNA repair in which the ability to repair damage caused by ultraviolet (UV) light is deficient.
Werner syndrome	**Defect is in WRN gene on chromosome 8 which plays an important role in DNA repair and replication.** The clinical presentation is of accelerated ageing. WERNER SYNDROME SHOULD NOT BE CONFUSED WITH WERMER SYNDROME which is multiple endocrine neoplasia type 2A.
Bloom syndrome	**BLM gene on chromosome 15 results in defective DNA repair.** Increased incidence of cancers like leukemia and lymphoma is seen.
Frederi-chataxia	**FRATAXIN gene, disease of trinucleotide repeats.** Friedreich's ataxia is an autosomal recessive inherited disease that causes progressive damage to the nervous system, resulting in symptoms ranging from gait disturbance to dysarthria. HOCM and type 2 diabetes mellitus is associated. **Please DON'T CONFUSE WITH DISEASE OF DEFECTIVE DNA REPAIR ATAXIA TELENGIECTASIA.**

517. Ans. (d) Low output cardiac failure

Ref: Harrison, 19th ed. pg. 426e-1

- Paget disease is a **localized disorder of bone remodeling that typically begins with excessive bone resorption followed by an increase in bone formation.** Therefore, the increase in cardiac output can lead to left ventricular strain and eventually high-output congestive failure.
- Measurement of **serum alkaline phosphatase—in some cases, bone-specific alkaline phosphatase (BSAP)—** can be useful in the diagnosis of Paget disease.
- Most persons with Paget disease are asymptomatic. In these patients, the incidental finding of an elevated serum alkaline phosphatase level or characteristic

radiographic abnormality may lead to detection of the disease. However, when symptoms do occur, **bone pain is the most common complaint.** It may persist or exacerbate during the night.

518. Ans. (d) Malignancy

Ref: Harrison, 19th ed. pg. 501f, 707

- Mycosis Fungoides is a Non-Hogkins lymphoma of T cell variety. It is characterized by skin involvement where a skin biopsy shows findings quizzed in earlier exams by the name of Pautrier's micro-abscess formation.

519. Ans. (a) Lenalidomide

Ref: Harrison, 19th ed. pg. 103e-19

Lenalidomide is used as anticancer agent for multiple myeloma and is also an immun-modulator.

520. Ans. (a) p24 antigen

Ref: Harrison, 19th ed. pg. 1246-47

- Following HIV infection, the sequences of markers to identify infection in their chronologic order of appearance in serum are: viral RNA followed by p24 antigen and lastly anti-HIV antibody.
- ELISA is positive in all babies born to HIV positive mother, due to transplacental transferrin of anti – HIV antibody.
- About 2 weeks after infection, viremia is thought to increase exponentially and then decline to a steady-state level as the humoral and cell-mediated immune responses control HIV replication. This time interval, the serologic "window period," is characterized by seronegativity, occasionally detectable antigenemia, viremia (as measured by RNA), and variable CD4 lymphocyte levels. Detection of specific antibody to HIV signals the end of the window period and labels the individual as seropositive.
- The exact time when HIV RNA, antigen, and antibody can be detected depends on several factors, including the test used, individual host responses, and viral characteristics. Viral RNA can be detected within the first 2 weeks using the highly sensitive RT-PCR method. Antigen, although transient, can appear as early as 2 weeks after infection and lasts 3 to 5 months.

521. Ans. (b) Buerger's disease

Ref: Vascular intervention: A Clinical approach, pg. 219-221

- Buergers disease *(NOT berger disease)* is also known as thrombo angitis obliterans. An inflammatory and obliterative disease of blood vessels of the extremities, mainly lower extremities. *Occurring chiefly in smoker young*

693

Explanations

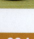

FMGE Solutions Screening Examination

men and leading to ischemia of the tissues and gangrene.
- Involvement of artery vein and nerve, most commonly involved is tibial artery. Intermittent claudication, pain at rest relieved by dangling legs. *Dry gangrene in toes shows shriveled woody induration.*
- **IOC:** duplex USG (ankle brachial index: 0.5 to 0.9)
- **Treatment:** for Claudication pain, reducing the viscosity of blood **pentoxyphylline** is used. For resting pain, lumbar sympathectomy. If gangrene à Amputation done.

522. Ans. (a) Spleen rupture

The image shows CT abdomen with splenic haemorrhage. The abdominal distention is explained by hemoperitoneum. Due to loss of blood, hypovolemic shock ensues and leads to acute tubular necrosis.

523. Ans. (b) MRI scan

The image shows presence of saggital view of abdomen MRI scan. The organs of abdomen and muscle planes are well delineated.

CT scan	MRI
Imaging plane: CT images are acquired only in the axial plane. The axial data set can then be used to reconstruct images in other planes, sagittal and coronal are the most common.	**Imaging plane:** MRI can be acquired in any plane, not just axial
Windows: Images can be "windowed" to bring out different structures, which is a post processing step. For neuroimaging we primarily review images using a "brain window" to look at the parenchyma and ventricular system. We use a bone window to evaluate the osseous structures and air filled cavities including the paranasal sinuses and temporal bone	**Sequences:** In MR, each different type of image is referred to a sequence. The primary MR sequences include T2, T1, T1 with contrast, Diffusion and FLAIR. Each sequence has to be acquired separately, which means that an MRI will take a lot longer to perform than a CT

Contd...

CT scan	MRI
White and black: You will notice that air within the gut is black. The brain parenchyma has a gray appearance and the skull is bright white	**White and black:** You will notice that the same structure may be bright or dark depending on the type of sequence; CSF for example is bright on T2, but dark on T1. The tissue and imaging characteristics are a lot more complicated than CT

Extra Mile

The patient lies on the table along the direction of the magnetic field. All of the protons within the patient's body align with this main magnetic field. The protons are then excited by an RF (Radiofrequency) pulse which elevates the hydrogen atoms to an excited state. These hydrogen atoms then relax to their normal resting state. However the time that it takes for each hydrogen atom to relax depends on their local tissue environment. Hydrogen atoms in water relax at different rates than hydrogen in soft tissue. It is this difference in relaxation times that enables us to generate an MR image

524. Ans. (a) Sapheno-femoral incompetence

Ref: SRB Manual of Surgery, 4th ed. pg. 228

Brodie-Trendelenburg test is used to detect venous incompetence and to differentiate between perforator and Great saphenous incompetence.

525. Ans. (c) Phospholipid precipitates

- The necrotic cell may have a more glassy homogeneous appearance than that of normal cells, mainly as a result of the loss of glycogen particles.
- *Dead cells may ultimately be replaced by large, whorled phospholipid masses called myelin figures.* These phospholipid precipitates are then either phagocytosed by other cells or further degraded into fatty acids; calcification of such fatty acid residues results in the generation of calcium soaps.

ANSWERS TO BOARD REVIEW QUESTIONS

526. Ans. (d) Nevirapine

Ref: http://icmr.nic.in/ijmr/2011/december/1209.pdf

527. Ans. (c) Hemoptysis

Ref: Harrison's 18th ed. ch. : 89

528. Ans. (c) Sweat electrolytes

Ref: Harrison's Medicine 18th ed p 2149-50

529. Ans. (d) Presence of U waves

Ref: See Appendix-54 "ECG CHANGES"

530. Ans. (d) Nifurtimox

Ref: Goodman Gillman 10th ed ch-40, Harrison's 18th ed ch:213

Medicine

531. Ans. (b) Contralateral subthalamus

Ref: Harrison's 18th ed ch:372, Guyton's 11thed p. 709

532. Ans. (a) EEG

Ref: Harrison's 18th ed ch:369

533. Ans. (a) Corpulmonale

534. Ans. (a) Hypercalcemia

535. Ans. (b) Mitral regurgitation

536. Ans. (b) Zonaglomerulosa

537. Ans. (a) Adrenal disease

538. Ans. (b) Stable angina

Duke's criteria is used in infective endocarditis.

539. Ans. (c) Persistent painful erection for >4 hours

540. Ans. (a) Phenformin

541. Ans. (c) Systolic blood pressure is more than 90 mm Hg

542. Ans. (c) Centriacinar emphysema

543. Ans. (a) Rheumatoid nodules

Rheumatoid nodules are a late feature and not considered a diagnostic feature.

544. Ans. (b) Constrictive pericarditis

545. Ans. (d) Carcinoid syndrome

546. Ans. (a) Carbamazepine

547. Ans. (c) Arthritis

548. Ans. (b) Hypotension

549. Ans. (a) RTA-1

550. Ans. (c) Hyperkalemic acidosis

551. Ans. (a) Pigmented

552. Ans. (a) Pyramidal cells

553. Ans. (b) Carcinoma breast

554. Ans. (d) Laryngeal paralysis

555. Ans. (d) Renal tubular acidosis

556. Ans. (a) Obliteration of carotid pulse

557. Ans. (a) Hyponatremia

558. Ans. (c) Polyneuritic leprosy

559. Ans. (a) Inhaled steroids

560. Ans. (c) Calcium

561. Ans. (c) RTA 4

562. Ans. (a) Carotid artery atherosclerosis

Atherosclerosis leads to ischemic stroke which is more common than hemorrhagic stroke.

563. Ans. (a) Ptosis

564. Ans. (a) CAD

565. Ans. (a) Neonatal meningitis

566. Ans. (c) Lacunar stroke

567. Ans. (a) Inflow Right side

568. Ans. (b) Plasma fractionated metanephrine levels

569. Ans. (a) Low dose dexamethasone suppression test

570. Ans. (b) Canagliflozin

571. Ans. (c) Benign rolandic epilepsy

572. Ans. (a) 5 minutes

573. Ans. (c) Lesion in superior temporal gyrus

574. Ans. (b) Vasospasm

575. Ans. (a) Parenchyma

576. Ans. (c) CML

577. Ans. (d) CLL

578. Ans. (c) Marrow hypoplasia

695

Explanations

579. Ans. (b) GH

580. Ans. (b) Iatrogenic steroids

581. Ans. (a) Masked facies

582. Ans. (c) Cortical atrophy

583. Ans. (a) Motor neurone disease

584. Ans. (d) Bladder and bowel involvement

585. Ans. (c) Acromegaly

586. Ans. (a) Automated external defibrillator

Ref: Brunwald 8th ed. ch-33, AHA 2010, guidlines

587. Ans. (a) Parathyroid adenoma

Ref: The Interface of neurology & Internal Medicine by Jose Biller Lippincott publication p-479

588. Ans. (a) Weber syndrome

Ref: Harrison's 17th ed. Chapter 364, Brainstem Disorders by Peter P Urban, Louis R Caplan pg. 205-204

589. Ans. (a) Crohn's disease

Ref: Robbins, 7th ed. pg. 851, Harrison's Internal Medicine 17th ed. Chapter 289

590. Ans. (a) Rectum

Ref: Harrison's, 18th ed. Chapter 295

591. Ans. (d) Liver transplant

Ref: Harrison's, 18th ed. Chapter 279

592. Ans. (c) Peptic ulcer

Ref: Harrison's, 17th ed. Chapter 42-1

593. Ans. (c) Liver

Ref: Textbook of Pulmonary Medicine volume 1 by 2nd ed. D. Behera p-495

594. Ans. (b) Focal segmental glomerulosclerosis

Ref: Harrison's Internal Medicine 17thed ch-182, Human Immunodeficiency Virus Disease: AIDS and Related Disorders

595. Ans. (b) Staphylococcus

Ref: Harrison's 18th ed ch:124, Braunwald's Heart Disease: A Textbook of Cardiovascular Medicine 18th ed. ch-63

596. Ans. (b) Conus medullaris

Ref: Harrison's various references

597. Ans. (c) Mn

Ref: Harrison's 18th ed. ch. 372

598. Ans. (a) Lymphoma

Ref: Harrison's 18th ed. ch. 189

599. Ans. (d) Hypothermia

Ref: Harrison's 18th ed. ch. 368

600. Ans. (c) M3

Ref: Robbin's 8th ed. ch-13

601. Ans. (a) Diagnosis of acute renal failure

Ref: Harrison's 18th ed. ch. 279

602. Ans. (a) Pheochromocytoma

Ref: Harrison's 18th ed. ch. 343

603. Ans. (d) HSP

Ref: Harrison's 18th ed. ch. 326

604. Ans. (a) ASD

Ref: Evidence-Based Cardiology Practice: A 21st Century Approach p-63, Pediatric Cardiology for Practitioners by Myung Kun Park p-26

605. Ans. (d) Atrial fibrillation

Ref: Harrison's 18th ed. ch. 341

606. Ans. (b) Serum ferritin

Ref: Harrison's 18th ed. ch. 103

607. Ans. (a) Vitamin B12 deficiency

Ref: Harrison's 18th ed. ch. 105

608. Ans. (a) EBV

Ref: Harrison's 17th ed. ch. : 105 table 105-4

Medicine

609. Ans. (d) Abdominal fat aspirate

Ref: Harrison's 18th ed. ch. : 112, Amyloidosis: Diagnosis and Treatment by Morie A. Gertz, S. Vincent Rajkumar p-36

610. Ans. (b) Cardiac failure

Ref: Harrison's Internal Medicine 17th ed. ch. 324. Amyloidosis

611. Ans. (a) Ropinirole

Ref: Harrison's, 17th ed. ch. 28

612. Ans. (a) 3rd nerve

Ref: Harrison's, 17th ed. p-1727

613. Ans. (a) Middle Cerebral Artery

Ref: Harrison's 17thed ch-23, http://emedicine.medscape.com/article/323120overview

614. Ans. (b) Putamen

Ref: Harrison's Internal Medicine, 17th ed. ch-364, Cerebrovascular Disease table 364-5

615. Ans. (b) Inferior frontal gyrus

Ref: Gray's Anatomy 39th ed p-415

616. Ans. (c) Superior temporal gyrus

Ref: Gray's Anatomy 39th ed p-415

617. Ans. (b) Hyponatremia

Ref: Harrison's 18th ed. p-347

618. Ans. (c) Steroids

Ref: Harrison's 18th ed. chapter 295

619. Ans. (d) Aortic regurgitation

Ref: Bedside clinics in medicine part 1 by arupkumarkundu p 39

620. Ans. (a) Amyloidosis

Ref: Harrison's 18/e, chapter 238

621. Ans. (d) Acute rheumatic fever

Ref: Harrison 18/e, chapter 322

622. Ans. (a) Sickle cell anemia

Ref: Harrison 18/e, chapter 104

623. Ans. (b) Phytonoyl-CoA α-hydroxylase

Ref: Harrison 18/e, chapter 384

624. Ans. (b) Duloxetine

Ref: Harrison 18/e, chapter 384

625. Ans. (b) Posterior communicating

Ref: Harrison 18/e, chapter 275, Principles and practice of emergency neurology Sid M shah and Kevin M Kelly Textbook of ophthalmology vol. 1 by sunitaagarwal

626. Ans. (a) 75 mg/kg

Ref: Harrison 18/e, chapter 115

627. Ans. (b) Urine output <0.5 ml/kg/h for >12 hours

Ref: Anesthesia for the high-Risk patient edited by Ian McConachie 2/e, p 181, Evidence-Based practice of Critical Care: Expert consult by Clifford S. Deutschman, Patrick J. Neligan 2010 ed table 26-2

628. Ans. (b) Anti-Ro

Ref: Harrison 18/e, table 319-1, Dubois Lupus erythematosus and related syndromes, by Daniel Wallace, bevrahannahshans 8/e, p 326

629. Ans. (a) Atherosclerosis

Ref: Harrison 17/e, chapter 280, CMDT 2009, chapter 22, Brenner and rector's the kidney, 8/e, chapter 43

630. Ans. (a) Liver

Ref: Wintrobe's clinical hematology 12/e, chapter 59, Harrison's Principles of Internal medicine 18/e, chapter 117, 249

631. Ans. (b) Cervical

Ref: Wintrobe's clinical hematology 12/e, chapter 96, Table 96.3, William's hematology 8/e, ch 99

632. Ans. (c) Subclavian artery

Ref: Harrison's Internal Medicine 18/e, Table 326-7, p 2796 and 2798

697

Explanations

FMGE Solutions Screening Examination

633. Ans. (b) Increased TIBC

Ref: Appendix-52 for Types of Anemia

634. Ans. (c) Itraconazole

Ref: Rook 8/e, p 36.74, Harrison's 18/e, ch 206

635. Ans. (b) Beta blocker

Ref: Braunwald's heart disease 9/e, chapter 57, Table 57 G-12

636. Ans. (d) Parenchymal bleed

Ref: Harrison's Internal medicine 18/e, p 3296

637. Ans. (a) Asthma

Ref: Harrison's Internal Medicine 18/e, Figure 252-6, p 2093

638. Ans. (c) Vascular bleeding

Ref: Braunwald's Heart Disease, 9th ed. chapter 20, Table 5

639. Ans. (a) Anti-Sm Antibody

Ref: Harrison's Internal Medicine 18th ed. Chapter 319, Table 319-1, Harrison 17th eds, Table 325-4

640. Ans. (a) Digitalis

Ref: Essentials of medical pharmacology p 498, Harrison's Internal Medicine 18th ed. chapter 227

641. Ans. (a) Pregabalin

Ref: Harrison's Internal Medicine 18th ed. chapter 344, p 2984

642. Ans. (b) Coronary arteriography

Ref: Braunwald's Heart Disease, 9th eds. Chapter 20

643. Ans. (b) Tricuspid regurgitation

Ref: Harrison's Internal Medicine 18th ed. chapter 31

644. Ans. (b) Hematogenous

Ref: Textbook of pulmonary medicine volume 1, 2/e, D. Behara, p 495

645. Ans. (d) Ca2+

Ref: Harrison's Internal medicine 18/e, chapter 387, table 387-10

646. Ans. (c) Spurious polycythemia

Ref: Wintrobe's hematology 12/e, chapter 48, table 48.2, Harrison 18/e, chapter 108

647. Ans. (a) Phrenic nerve

Ref: Cunningham's textbook of anatomy by Daniel john Cunningham p 699, 700, Gray's anatomy 39/e, p 996

648. Ans. (a) Alohol

Ref: Braundwald's Heart Disease Ninth ed. Chapter 64

649. Ans. (b) Hypothermia

650. Ans. (b) Bell's palsy

Ref: Harrison's Internal medicine 18/e, chapter 376, p 3362

651. Ans. (c) Conduction aphasia

Ref: Adams and victor's Principles of neurology 9/e, chapter 23, p 470

652. Ans. (b) Tuberous sclerosis

Ref: Dermatology by Otto Braun falco p 846, Harrison's internal medicine 18/e, chapter 53, p 410

ANSWERS TO IMAGE-BASED QUESTIONS

653. Ans. (c) Pointing index

The image shows presence of point index with lesion of median nerve. The remaining three choices A, C, D are seen in ulnar nerve damage.

654. Ans. (a) Saw tooth appearance

655. Ans. (c) Anterior wall MI

ECG shows presence of ST elevation from V2-V5 diagnostic of anterior wall MI.

656. (a) Sinus tachycardia

Ref: Harrison, 19th ed. pg. 1477

- The ECG shows normal sinus rhythm with heart rate of >100 bpm.
- P waves are normal height and duration. PR interval is 120 msec and QRS duration is 80 msec.
- The findings are diagnostic of sinus tachycardia
- Sinus tachycardia is subdivided into physiological and non-physiological.
- *Inappropriate sinus tachycardia* causes the sinus rate to increase spontaneously at rest or out of proportion to physiological stress or exertion. Affected patients are usually females. Misdiagnosis with anxiety disorder is common.

657. Ans. (c) Mobitz II heart block

Ref: Harrison, 19th ed. pg. 1472

- The ECG shows more P waves than QRS complexes. This suggests a heart block.
- P wave is upright and has a normal morphology. PR interval is 200 msec.
- Dropped beats are present with PR interval remaining the same before the dropped beats.

Comparison of heart blocks

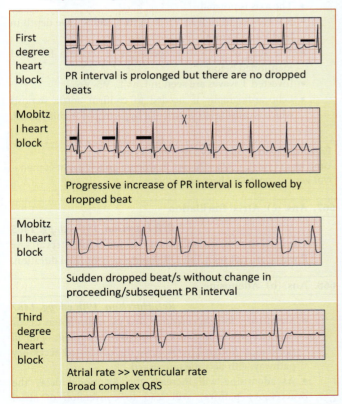

658. Ans. (a) Myocardial ischemia

Ref: Harrison, 19th ed. pg. 1455-56

- The T-wave is upright in all leads except aVR and V1. In the strip provided, notice the predominant T-wave inversion in V1-V4. This is seen in myocardial ischemia.

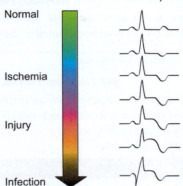

- Diagnosis of myocardial injury needs elevated cardiac biomarkers
- Digoxin leads to ST segment depression
- Digoxin toxicity leads to ventricular bigeminy.

Causes of T-wave inversion:

- Normal in children
- Myocardial ischemia
- Bundle branch block
- Ventricular hypertrophy
- Pulmonary embolism
- Hypertrophic obstructive cardiomyopathy
- Raised intracranial pressure

659. Ans. (a) Hyperacute T-wave

Ref: ACLS Study Guide, 5th ed. pg. 229

The ECG shows presence of large T waves.
They are relatively broad, and are not pointed when compared to Tall tented T waves of hyperkalemia.

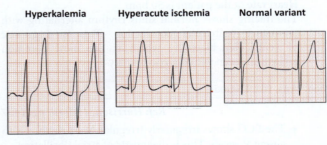

FMGE Solutions Screening Examination

660. Ans. (a) T wave inversion

Ref: Braunwald, 10th ed. pg. 146 and Harrison, 19th ed. pg. 1457

Heart rate is 60 bpm with left axis deviation. *Deep symmetrical T-wave inversion* is noted in the chest leads.

661. Ans. (a) Ventricular bigeminy

Ref: Harrison, 19th ed. Chapter 269e

The ECG strip shows heart rate of approximately 60 bpm. ST segment depression (hockey stick sign) is seen followed by positive deflection of U waves.

Abnormalities of U-wave

Prominent U waves	Inverted U waves
Bradycardia Hypokalemia Hypocalcemia Hypomagnesemia Hypothermia Raised ICP HOCM LVH	Myocardial ischemia HTN Cardiomyopathy

662. Ans. (d) Premature ventricular contractions

Ref: Harrison, 19th ed. pg. 1457

The ECG shows normal sinus rhythm with heart rate of 75 bpm with normal axis.
Raised ST segment in lead V2-V4 and inverted T waves in lead I, aVL, V2-V4 are seen.

663. Ans. (b) Ventricular bigeminy

Ref: Practical Cardiology, 2nd ed. pg. 214

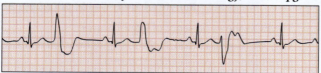

Heart rate of the patient is 50 bpm
The tracing shows normal sinus rhythm alternating with premature ventricular contraction. This is diagnostic of ventricular bigeminy which is the most common arrhythmia seen with digoxin toxicity.

664. Ans. (d) Digoxin

Ref: Harrison, 19th ed. pg. 1457

- The ECG shows irregularly irregular heart rhythm with absent P waves. This is diagnostic of atrial fibrillation.
- Also seen is down-sloping ST segment depression pronounced in V2-V3 and in the rhythm strip.
- This patient of rheumatic heart disease is in atrial fibrillation for which she would have been put on digoxin by her physician.

- The combination of extra-cardiac side effects of digoxin and atrial fibrillation hemodynamic effects would explain the general unwell being of the patient.
- ACE inhibitor can lead to hyperkalemia and diuretics can lead to hypokalemia. However ECG changes of potassium deficit/excess are not seen.

665. Ans. (c) PSVT

Ref: Harrison, 19th ed. pg. 1480-81

- The findings of the ECG are heart rate of 200 bpm. P waves are not visible.
- The axis is normal with narrow qRS complexes.
- This could either be junctional tachycardia or atrio-ventricular nodal re-entrant tachycardia.
- Taking into consideration the age of the patient the incidence of junctional tachycardia can explain the patient experiencing multiple episodes in the past.

666. Ans. (b) Left ventricular hypertrophy

Ref: Harrison, 19th ed. pg. 1454

- The ECG shows normal sinus rhythm with heart rate of 50 bpm
- The axis is normal
- R wave height in lead V5 is 30 mm and S wave depth in lead V1 is 20 mm
- The sum of the two exceeds the set criteria for LVH mentioned below
- Inverted T waves are seen in I, aVL, V5-V6
- Echocardiography is needed to confirm aortic stenosis which is causing left ventricular hypertrophy in this patient.

Voltage criteria for LVH

Precordial leads = SV1 + RV5 or RV6 > 35 mm
Limb leads= RaVL + SV3 > 20 mm in women and >28 mm in men
Not very accurate in obese and athletes

667. Ans. (c) Atrial fibrillation

Ref: Harrison, 19th ed. pg. 1485

The ECG shows a variable heart rate due to RR interval. The P waves are not seen and QRS complex is normal duration.

668. Ans. (b) Adenosine

Ref: Harrison, 19th ed. pg. 1487

- *Serious rhythm degeneration and even death* can occur when *adenosine is inadvertently given to patients of atrial fibrillation/flutter*. This is since the concealed accessory pathway with become unmasked.
- As adenosine will increase the AV nodal delay the accessory pathway will lead to conversion of atrial fibrillation to ventricular fibrillation. This is because the current will now travel preferentially via the accessory pathway.

- In atrial flutter, since the accessory pathway does not have decremental property, the 2:1 conduction will occur at rate of 1:1 leading to rapid clinical decompensation.

669. Ans. (c) Thrombolytic therapy

Ref: Harrison, 19th ed. pg. 1595

- The following ECG shows heart rate of 80 bpm with normal axis. P wave is normal with normal duration QRS seen after each P wave. T waves are hyper-acute in leads V2-V5 with simultaneous presence of ST segment elevation in chest leads V2-V5.
- This is diagnostic of STEMI involving anterior wall and the vessel blocked in left anterior descending artery.
- The symptoms of chest pain and diaphoresis are explained by the ECG findings of the pain.
- Now ideal treatment of STEMI is PCI or thrombolysis.
- Since PCI is not in choices we need to consider thrombolysis for the patient but it is *indicated only within 12 hours of onset of MI*.
- In this question the patient presented late and hence *we will treat with aspirin to prevent future MI episode, Statin to stabilize the vulnerable plaques and morphine to calm the patient and reduce pulmonary edema.*
- E.C.G changes in acute infarction

ECG findings of ischemia	ECG finding of injury	ECG findings of cell death
Tall wide (peaked) T wave T wave inversion	ST elevation (Pardee sign)	• Pathological Q wave

ST Elevation MI Management:
- Nitrates
- Morphine
- Oxygen
- Aspirin
- Start adjunctive treatment
- Beta Blockers (IV)
- Nitroglycerine (IV)
- Heparin (IV)
- Reperfusion therapy is the definitive treatment of choice if patient present <12 hours.
  - Thrombolysis (Streptokinase) Door to needle time < 30 minutes
  - Early primary PCI (Cath lab equipped hospital) Door to balloon time < 90 minutes

670. Ans. (c) Adenosine

Ref: Harrison, 19th ed. pg. 1479

- The ECG is showing heart rate of 200/min.
- Axis is normal.
- Rhythm is regular with absence of P waves.
- Narrow complex QRS (<0.08 sec) is present. P waves buried in the preceding T wave.
- This is seen in paroxysmal supraventricular tachycardia.
- The first line management is adenosine 6 mg intravenously.
- In case the patient is having hemodynamic compromise, electrical cardioversion needs to be done.

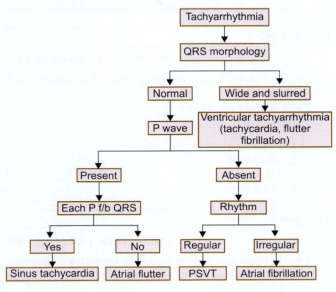

671. Ans. (a) Primary PCI

Ref: Figure 295-4, Harrison, 19th ed. pg. 1604

- The ECG shows heart rate of about 120/min.
- T wave inversion is present from V2-V6
- ST segment elevation >2 mm in noted from V4-V6 exhibiting the traditional Pardee sign
- *STEMI is best managed with primary PCI with first medical contact to device time to be kept <90 minutes*
- If the patient is seen in non PCI capable hospital DIDO time should be less than 30 minutes for thrombolysis.

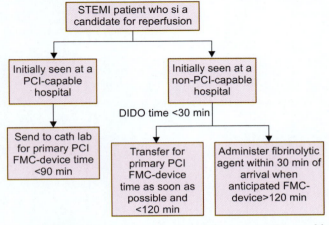

- The patient can be transferred from non PCI capable hospital to PCI capable hospital in case the first medical contact to device time is less than 120 minutes.

- In the question there is no mention of any PCI/ non PCI capable hospital.
- Due to paucity of transport facilities in India, the concept of transfer from non PCI to PCI capable centre with performance of PCI within 120 minutes looks impossible.

672. Ans. (d) 4

Ref: Harrison, 19th ed. pg. 1451

- Corrected QT is defined as QT interval divided by √ R-R interval
- R-R interval in ECG is 4.

Markings in the ECG given:

1. is PR interval
2. is PJ interval
3. is ST segment
4. is RR interval

673. Ans. (c) Phase 2

Ref: Harrison, 19th ed. pg. 1451

- The marked part of the ECG is the isoelectric ST segment which corresponds to the plateau, phase 2 of cardiac action potential
- The rapid upstroke (phase 0) action potential corresponds to onset of QRS.
- Plateau (phase 2) corresponds to isoelectric ST segment.
- Active repolarization (phase 3) corresponds to inscription of T-wave.

674. Ans. (c) Hockey stick sign

Ref: Practical Cardiology, 2nd ed. pg. 125

The image shows rhythm strip exhibiting a variable heart rate with ST segment depression. P-wave is absent with narrow complex. The patient was probably having atrial fibrillation and was started on digoxin which resulted in ST segment depression highlighted below.

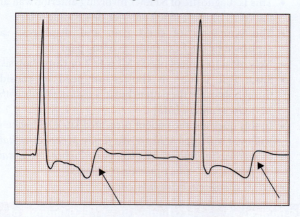

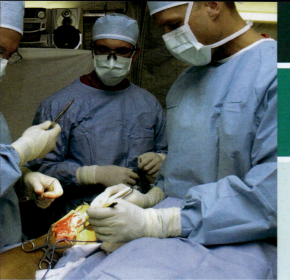

10

Surgery

MOST RECENT QUESTIONS 2019

1. A patient presented to emergency after RTA with multiple rib fractures. He is conscious, speaking single words. On examination, respiratory rate was 40/min and BP was 90/40 mm Hg. What is the immediate next step?
   a. Urgent IV fluid administration
   b. Intubate the patient
   c. Chest –ray
   d. Insert needle in 2nd intercostal space

2. Correct procedure of inserting Nasogastric tube is.
   a. Supine with neck flexed
   b. Supine with neck extended
   c. Sitting with neck flexed
   d. Sitting with neck extended

3. A 7-day old infant presents with bilious vomiting and gross abdominal distention with absent bowel sounds. X ray abdomen shows multiple gas filled loops. Diagnosis is?
   a. Hirschsprung disease
   b. Congenital Hypertrophic pyloric stenosis
   c. Duodenal atresia
   d. Malrotation of gut

4. Meconium ileus is a presentation seen in which of the following diseases?
   a. Mucoviscidosis
   b. Hirschsprung disease
   c. Ileal atresia
   d. Congenital aganglionosis

5. Which is the first investigation to be done in case of Neonate presenting with frothiness in mouth and dyspnoea?
   a. Bronchoscopy with injection of methylene blue
   b. NG Tube insertion and CXR to check position of tube
   c. CT chest
   d. Endoscopy

6. Calculate the GCS of a patient exhibiting eye opening on pain, conscious but confused and cannot tell time and exhibits flexion on painful noxious stimuli to the arm.
   a. 8
   b. 9
   c. 10
   d. 11

7. A 27-year-old woman presents with 26 weeks of gestation with a thyroid lesion which is found to be papillary carcinoma of thyroid. Which is the best treatment for this patient?
   a. Thyroid ablation using radioactive Iodine
   b. Total thyroidectomy
   c. Observation
   d. Hemi-thyroidectomy

8. Which ulcer is likely to develop in a long standing chronic venous ulcer?
   a. Marjolin ulcer
   b. Apthous ulcer
   c. Bazin ulcer
   d. Arterial ulcer

9. Most appropriate management of recurrent keloid is?
   a. Excisional surgery
   b. Intramarginal excision followed by radiation
   c. Cryosurgery
   d. Silicone gel sheeting

10. Seat Belt injury leads to?
    a. Splenic laceration
    b. Splenic contusion
    c. Gut ischemia
    d. Mesenteric adenitis

11. Which complication is seen after Varicose vein stripping procedure?
    a. Neuralgia
    b. Deep vein thrombosis
    c. Acrocyanosis
    d. Telangiectasia

12. Which of the following is not scanned by FAST USG?
    a. Pericardium
    b. Pleural cavity
    c. Spleen
    d. Liver

13. A 40-year-old man is suffering from heaviness in scrotum. A bag of worms feel is observed on scrotal examination and the swelling is seen to reduce in supine position. What is the best treatment?
    a. Suction drainage
    b. Varicocelectomy
    c. Jaboulay procedure
    d. Herniotomy

14. Prophylactic antibiotics to minimise SSI are given_____?
    a. 60 minutes before skin incision
    b. 1-3 hours before skin incision
    c. At time of surgical incision
    d. Night before surgery for peaking of effect

15. Which procedure is done in case of Ranula management?
    a. Incision and drainage   b. Aspiration
    c. Excision   d. Sclerosant injection
16. Which of the following is best for diagnosis of pheochromocytoma?
    a. 24-hour urinary Vaniyll Mandelic acid
    b. 24-hour urinary Fractionated Metanephrine
    c. 24-hour Urinary Hydroxy indole acetic acid
    d. 24-hour Urinary Hydroxy tryptamine
17. Which Instrument is shown below?

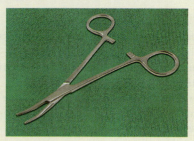

    a. Artery forceps   b. Kocher forceps
    c. Allis forceps   d. Babcock forceps
18. Which instrument is shown below?

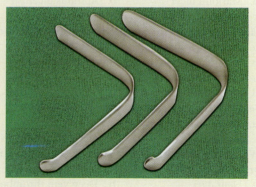

    a. Tongue depressor   b. Doyen retractor
    c. Self-retaining retractor   d. Langenbeck's retractor
19. Comment on the diagnosis?

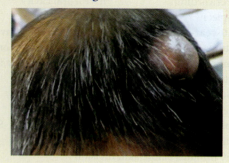

    a. Sebaceous cyst
    b. Implantation dermoid
    c. Angular dermoid
    d. Lipoma
20. Comment on the diagnosis

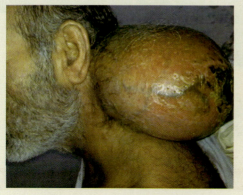

    a. Lipoma   b. Encephalocele
    c. Cystic hygroma   d. Lymphadenopathy
21. What is the location of Killian dehiscence?
    a. Below Superior constrictor
    b. Below Inferior constrictor
    c. Below cricopharyngeal muscle
    d. Below upper 1/3rd of smooth muscle of oesophagus
22. Which organ has highest chances of Graft rejection response?
    a. Cornea   b. Gut
    c. Liver   d. Skin
23. In hypovolemic shock which organ should be assessed for determining under-perfusion?
    a. Kidney   b. Heart
    c. Lung   d. Liver

GASTROINTESTINAL TRACT

24. MC immediate complication of splenectomy?
    (Recent Pattern Question 2018-19)
    a. Haemorrhage
    b. Fistula
    c. Bleeding from gastric mucosa
    d. Pancreatitis
25. Best treatment strategy for Anal cancer?
    (Recent Pattern Question 2018-19)
    a. Chemoradiation   b. Surgery
    c. Radiation   d. Chemotherapy
26. Which is false about Crohn's disease?
    (Recent Pattern Question 2018-19)
    a. No occurrence after surgery
    b. Aphthous ulcer
    c. Skip lesions
    d. Fistula formation
27. Which of the following is not done in Carcinoma oesophagus?   *(Recent Pattern Question 2018-19)*
    a. Biopsy   b. pH-metry
    c. CT chest   d. PET scan

28. A 30-year-old man presents with a four days history of right iliac fossa pain. USG image is shown below. Which is the best management algorithm?

(Recent Pattern Question 2018-19)

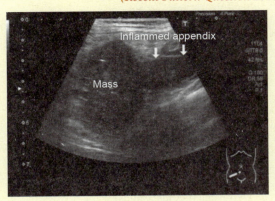

   a. Ochsner-Sherren regimen
   b. Urgent appendicectomy
   c. Extraperitoneal drainage and parenteral antibiotics
   d. Per cutaneous drainage and parenteral antibiotics

29. Comment on the diagnosis of a film shown of a 65-year-old man with acute abdomen.

(Recent Pattern Question 2018-19)

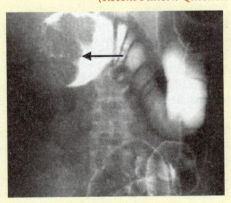

   a. Ileocolic intussusception
   b. Sigmoid volvulus
   c. Toxic megacolon
   d. Colocolic intussusception

30. Surgery is indicated in Ulcerative Colitis in all except?

(Recent Pattern Question 2018-19)

   a. Toxic megacolon
   b. Colonic perforation
   c. Colonic obstruction
   d. Refractory fistula

31. Which is the most common site of the carcinoma of the esophagus? *(Recent Pattern Question 2018)*
   a. Lower 1/3rd
   b. Middle 1/3rd
   c. Upper 1/3rd
   d. GE junction

32. A 9-month-old child presents with excessive cry, right iliac fossa sausage lump and blood in stools. What is the best treatment? *(Recent Pattern Question 2018)*
   a. IVF-antibiotic-NG tube
   b. IVF-antibiotic-air enema
   c. IVF-antibiotics-barium enema
   d. IVF-antibiotics-warm saline enema

33. Metastatic liver disease is found in _____% of patients undergoing surgery for primary colorectal cancer?

(Recent Pattern Question 2018)

   a. 10%
   b. 15%
   c. 33%
   d. 75%

34. Which is the most common cause of hypergastrinemia?
   a. Postvagotomy *(Recent Pattern Question 2018)*
   b. After intake of PPI
   c. Resection of small intestine
   d. Atrophic gastritis

35. What prefix symbol is used to describe the administration of neo-adjuvant treatment given in colorectal cancer?

(Recent Pattern Question 2017)

   a. h
   b. p
   c. y
   d. z

36. A 20-year-old patient presents with RIF pain and fever. USG is shown in image. Diagnosis is?

(Recent Pattern Question 2017)

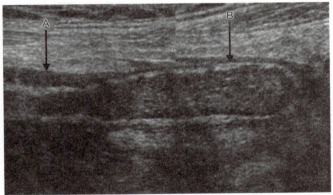

   a. Acute appendicitis
   b. Intussusception
   c. Volvulus
   d. Intestinal obstruction

37. Gastric Outlet Obstruction leads to?

(Recent Pattern Question 2017)

   a. Hypochloremic metabolic alkalosis
   b. Hyperchloremic metabolic acidosis
   c. Hypernatremic metabolic alkalosis
   d. Hyponatremic metabolic acidosis

38. Dysphagia lusoria is due to? *(Recent Pattern Question 2017)*
   a. Aberrant blood vessel
   b. Esophageal diverticulum
   c. Duodenal obstruction
   d. Gastric outlet obstruction

39. Which is the most common site of origin of peritoneal deposits? *(Recent Pattern Question 2016)*
    a. Stomach cancer
    b. Colorectal cancer
    c. Pancreatic cancer
    d. Ovarian cancer

40. What does the arrow in the given CT abdomen show? *(Recent Pattern Question 2016)*

    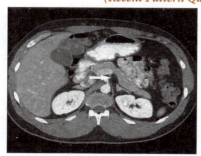

    a. Left adrenal gland
    b. Pancreas
    c. Lesser omentum
    d. Epiploic foramen

41. Which of the following is associated with Gardner syndrome? *(Recent Pattern Question 2016)*
    a. Retinoblastoma
    b. Neuroblastoma
    c. Desmoid tumor
    d. Dermoid cyst

42. Hypertrophic pyloric stenosis presents at *(Recent Pattern Question 2016)*
    a. 3 day
    b. 3 weeks
    c. 3 month
    d. 3 years

43. A 40-year-old chronic alcoholic presents with distended abdomen, hematemesis and fresh blood in stool. On examination huge ascites and distended veins over abdominal wall are noted. Most likely cause of hematemesis is? *(Recent Pattern Question 2016)*
    a. Esophagitis
    b. Esophageal varices
    c. Esophageal cancer
    d. Erosion of gastroduodenal artery

44. A 30-year-old known alcoholic presents to the emergency with massive Upper GIT bleeding. On examination pulse = 110/min and BP = 80/60. First step to be taken is?
    a. Cold saline lavage *(Recent Pattern Question 2016)*
    b. Immediate BT
    c. Transfer for urgent sclerotherapy
    d. Large bore cannula for IVF

45. Which is the rarest position of appendix? *(Recent Pattern Question 2016)*
    a. Retro-caecal
    b. Post-ileal
    c. Post-ileal
    d. Para-caecal

46. Which is the best way to diagnose lower small intestine obstruction? *(Recent Pattern Question 2016)*
    a. Pain abdomen
    b. Multiple air fluid levels
    c. Profuse bilious vomiting
    d. Feculent vomiting

47. What is the location of first constriction of esophagus from the incisor tooth?
    a. 15 cm
    b. 18 cm
    c. 25 cm
    d. 40 cm

48. Which is the best investigation for dysphagia?
    a. Enteroscopy
    b. Barium swallow
    c. Barium enema
    d. Barium meal follow through

49. What is incorrect about Zenker's diverticulum?
    a. Regurgitation of previous day food
    b. Halitosis
    c. Located at killian triangle
    d. Metabolic alkalosis

50. Achalasia Cardia presents with all EXCEPT?
    a. Halitosis
    b. Regurgitation of previous day's food
    c. Dysphagia (liquids >solids)
    d. Corkscrew esophagus

51. Achalasia cardia presents with all EXCEPT:
    a. Increased lower esophagus sphincter tone
    b. Normal peristalsis
    c. Dilatation proximally
    d. Malignancy

52. Dysphagia mainly for liquids is seen with
    a. Achalasia cardia
    b. Zenker diverticulum
    c. Barret esophagus
    d. Diffuse esophageal spasm

53. Lower esophageal sphincter tone is due to
    a. Vasoactive intestinal peptide
    b. Nitrous oxide
    c. Acetylcholine
    d. Pancreatic polypeptide

54. Pseudo-achalasia is seen with
    a. Chagas disease
    b. Scleroderma
    c. Tumor infiltration
    d. Diffuse esophageal spasm

55. Which Metaplasia occurs in lower esophagus in a smoker?
    a. Gastric metaplasia
    b. Goblet cells intestinal metaplasia
    c. Esophageal metaplasia
    d. Intestinal dysplasia

56. Which of the following is more prone to Carcinoma?
    a. Barret esophagus
    b. Boerhaave syndrome
    c. Mallory Weiss tear
    d. Esophageal varices

57. Scoring of esophageal reflux is done by?
    a. Ranson score
    b. Gleason score
    c. Alvarado score
    d. De meester scoring

58. Which is the best investigation for detecting esophageal perforation?
    a. CXR
    b. CT chest
    c. Upper G.I. endoscopy
    d. CT chest with contrast

59. A patient presented to you after assault and penetrating knife injury to abdomen. X-ray shows gas under the diaphragm. Most common organ damaged in this case is:
    a. Spleen
    b. Intestine
    c. Liver
    d. Lung

Surgery

60. Para-esophageal hernia is best diagnosed by:
    a. Chest X-ray   b. Barium study
    c. CT scan   d. Endoscopic ultrasound
61. To differentiate malignancy from benign lesion in GIT. What is the investigation of choice?
    a. USG   b. Biopsy
    c. Endoscopy   d. P.E.T scan
62. Dysphagia lusoria is due to:
    a. Aberrant right subclavian artery
    b. Aberrant left subclavian artery
    c. Aberrant internal carotid artery
    d. Aberrant innominate artery
63. Boerhaave syndrome is
    a. Spontaneous Rupture of esophagus
    b. Traumatic rupture of esophagus
    c. Tear at gastro-esophageal junction
    d. Foreign body esophagus
64. Which is the most important factor for development of appendicitis and its complications?
    a. Bacterial proliferation   b. Age
    c. Increased dietary fiber   d. Bowel lumen obstruction
65. Mc-burney's point is
    a. 1/3rd distance from left anterior superior iliac spine
    b. 2/3rd distance from the anterior superior iliac spine
    c. 1/3rd distance from the umbilicus to ASIS
    d. 1/3rd distance from right anterior superior spine
66. A 25-year-old young male presented with a tender mass in right iliac fossa. On physical examination he has pain and fixed flexed hip. Diagnosis is?
    a. Psoas abscess   b. Appendicitis
    c. Amoeboma   d. Ileocaecal TB
67. Which is the best guide to finding appendix intra operatively?
    a. Locate ileo-ceacal junction
    b. Locate the blind tube of appendix
    c. Locate the anterior taenia of the caecum
    d. Locate the mesenteric supply
68. Identify the structure shown in the given picture

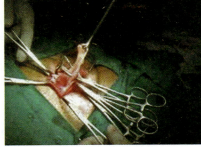

    a. Appendix   b. Meckel diverticulum
    c. Diverticulosis   d. Ligament of Treitz
69. What will be the location of appendix in silent appendix?
    a. Pelvic   b. Preileal
    c. Retro-caecal   d. Pelvic
70. MANTREL score is done for
    a. Acute appendicitis   b. Acute pancreatitis
    c. Acute cholecystitis   d. Acute salpingitis
71. In a child which of the following diseases is misdiagnosed as appendicitis?
    a. Gastroentritis   b. Lymphadenitis
    c. Intussusception   d. All of the above
72. Ochsner sherren regimen is used for management of:
    a. Appendicular mass
    b. Appendicular abscess
    c. Appendicitis
    d. Peritonitis following appendicitis
73. What is true about Carcinoid tumor:
    a. Always benign
    b. Kulchitsky cell tumor
    c. Present with paroxysmal hypertension
    d. Punch biopsy is diagnostic
74. Carcinoid tumor is seen most commonly in?
    a. Ileum   b. Rectum
    c. Appendix   d. Duodenum
75. What is incorrect about peritonitis?
    a. Most common cause is P.U.D
    b. Bile causes more damage than blood in peritoneum
    c. X-ray abdomen shows Gas under diaphragm
    d. Absence of free gas rules out peritonitis
76. Which is the most common organism seen in gastrointestinal perforation peritonitis?
    a. Staph aureus
    b. Pneumococcus
    c. Anaerobic streptococcus
    d. Coagulase-negative staphylococci
77. Non-intestinal peritonitis in females is caused by:
    a. E. coli   b. Klebsiella
    c. Chlamydia   d. Bacteroides
78. Which is the most common tumor of retro-peritoneum?
    a. Stroma   b. Sarcoma
    c. Teratoma   d. Retro-teratoma
79. Which is the most common presentation of retroperitoneal tumor?
    a. Abdominal pain   b. Hydronephrosis
    c. Constipation   d. Abdominal lump
80. Adult patient developing intussusception is due to?
    a. Carcinoid tumor b. Mesenteric insufficiency
    c. Villous adenoma d. Bariatric surgery
81. All are true about intestinal obstruction radio-graphically EXCEPT?
    a. Supine abdominal film is done
    b. More than 2 air fluid levels
    c. Small intestine dilation >3 cm
    d. Pneumatosis intestinalis

FMGE Solutions Screening Examination

82. Best treatment protocol of a Enterogenic cyst?
    a. Enucleation
    b. Resection with intestine part
    c. Aspiration with marsupialization
    d. Observe
83. On removing whole colon (total colectomy) what will be the most common complication?
    a. Anastomotic leak   b. Dys-electrolytemia
    c. Death   d. Fulminant sepsis
84. Which of the following is NOT seen in pyloric stenosis:
    a. Projectile vomiting b. Paradoxical aciduria
    c. Bilious vomiting   d. Metabolic acidosis
85. Congenital pyloric stenosis presents with?
    a. Hypokalemic metabolic acidosis
    b. Hypokalemic metabolic alkalosis
    c. Hyperkalemic metabolic acidosis
    d. Hyperkalemic metabolic alkalosis
86. In Hypertrophic pyloric stenosis, which of the following is seen?
    a. Metabolic acidosis
    b. Metabolic alkalosis
    c. Metabolic alkalosis with paradoxical bicarbonaturia
    d. All of above
87. Which of the following polyp is least likely to turn malignant?
    a. Inflammatory polyp
    b. Familial Adenomatous Polyposis
    c. Hamartomatous polyp
    d. Hyperplastic polyp
88. All are surgical indications in Crohn's disease EXCEPT:
    a. Colonic obstruction b. Refractory fistula
    c. Massive hemorrhage   d. Toxic megacolon
89. A child is passing blood with act of defecation. The probable diagnosis is
    a. Juvenile rectal polyp b. Adenomatous polyposis
    c. Rectal ulcer   d. Post Surgery
90. Earliest complication of ileostomy is:
    a. Obstruction b. Necrosis
    c. Diarrhea   d. Prolapse
91. Post resection of terminal ileum, deficiency of which of the following vitamins is seen along with Steatorrhea?
    a. B12 b. B9
    c. C   d. B6
92. Denver shunt is used in
    a. Ascites   b. Dialysis
    c. Raised ICP d. Headache
93. ROME II criteria is for?
    a. IBS   b. Colonic cancer
    c. Ulcerative colitis d. Colonic hemangioma
94. What is the cause of chronic tropical pancreatitis?
    a. Parasitic infection b. Malnutrition
    c. Idiopathic   d. Genetic

95. Severity of pancreatitis can be best assessed by?
    a. Serial Serum amylase b. Stool trypsin levels
    c. RANSON Score   d. ARDS development
96. Which is not included in APACHE score?
    a. Serum bilirubin b. GCS score
    c. pH of blood   d. Age of patient
97. What is the most common complication after ERCP?
    a. Acute pancreatitis   b. Pseudo-pancreatic cyst
    c. Chronic pancreatitis d. Necrotizing pancreatitis
98. Lisch nodule is seen in?
    a. Neurofibromatosis
    b. Multiple endocrine neoplasia 2A
    c. Turcot syndrome
    d. Familial adenomatous polyposis
99. In case of annular pancreas, what is the surgery of choice?
    a. Duodeno-duodenostomy b. Duodeno-jejunostomy
    c. Pancreato-jejunostomy d. Porto-enterostomy
100. Not a early post-operative complication of splenectomy is?
    a. Thrombocytosis
    b. Splenosis
    c. Sub diaphragmatic abscess
    d. Pulmonary complications
101. Which of the following is a side effect of vagotomy?
    a. Delayed gastric emptying b. Gastric atony
    c. Diarrhea   d. All of the above
102. Pseudo obstruction of intestine is also known as
    a. Hartmann's syndrome b. Ozili's syndrome
    c. Ogilvie's syndrome   d. Mirizzi syndrome
103. What is the most common site of gastric ulcer?
    a. Duodenal cap
    b. Lesser curvature
    c. Second part of duodenum
    d. Greater curvature
104. Posterior perforation of ulcer in Antral canal will lead to fluid deposition in?
    a. Greater Omentum   b. Right Sub-phrenic abscess
    c. Sub-hepatic space d. Lesser sac
105. Purtscher's Retinopathy is due to:
    a. Acute pancreatitis   b. Chronic pancreatitis
    c. Meckel's diverticulum d. Diverticulitis
106. What is the etiology of type-A gastritis?
    a. Hypersensitivity reaction I
    b. Autoimmune
    c. Bacterial
    d. Viral
107. What is the most common location of lymphoma in the G.I.T?
    a. Stomach   b. Ileum
    c. Mesentery d. Colon
108. Sister Mary Joseph nodule is commonly seen with:
    a. Ovarian CA   b. Colon CA
    c. Pancreatic CA d. Stomach CA

109. Krukenburg tumor originates from:
    a. Liver   b. Stomach
    c. Ovary   d. Gallbladder
110. Angiodysplasia is seen in:
    a. Stomach of adult   b. Jejunum of a child
    c. Left side of the colon   d. Right side of the colon
111. Which of the following is *not* a type of mesenteric cyst?
    a. Mesothelial   b. Enterogenous
    c. Chylolymphatic d. Epidermoid
112. What is the most common type of mesenteric cyst?
    a. Simple (mesothelial cyst) b. Chylolymphatic cyst
    c. Enterogenous   d. Dermoid
113. Immunoproliferative lymphoma presents with?
    a. Obstruction   b. Peritonitis
    c. Chronic diarrhea   d. Tenesmus
114. Which of following is used for initial management of rectal prolapse in children?
    a. Digital positioning   b. Transanal surgery
    c. Injection sclerotherapy   d. Resection rectopexy
115. Which is not a cause of acute anal pain?
    a. Thrombosed hemorrhoids
    b. Acute anal fissure
    c. Fistula in ano
    d. Perianal abccess
116. Which of the following is seen in case of fistula-in-ano?
    a. Purulent discharge with bleeding
    b. Serous discharge with bleeding
    c. Painful bleeding with constipation
    d. Painless bleeding with constipation
117. Goodsall's rule in fistula-in-ano is used for distinguishing:
    a. High and low fistula
    b. Anterior and posterior fistula
    c. External and internal fistula
    d. Lateral and medial fistula
118. Which is the most common cancer of anus?
    a. Adenocarcinoma   b. Squamous cell CA
    c. Basal cell CA   d. Melanoma
119. Which is the most common cancer of anus?
    a. Squamous   b. Basaloid
    c. Cuboidal   d. Cloacogenic
120. Anal cancer is associated with
    a. Human papilloma virus b. EBV
    c. HTLV-1   d. Polyoma virus
121. What is the most common site of metastases of carcinoma rectum?
    a. Lung   b. Liver
    c. Brain   d. Vertebra

122. The following image shows

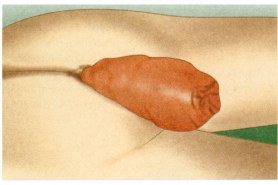

    a. Rectal prolapse   b. Fistula in ano
    c. Perianal abscess   d. Rectal cancer
123. MC complication after hemorrhoidectomy?
    a. Prolapse   b. Urine retention
    c. Fecal incontinence   d. Bleeding
124. What is incorrect about anal canal?
    a. 1/3rd above dentate line and 2/3rd below the dentate line
    b. Extraperitoneal
    c. Anoderm is painful
    d. Keratinization
125. What is true about Ischiorectal fossa boundaries?
    a. Anterior border is formed by inferior fascia of urogenital diaphragm.
    b. Superior border is formed by Gluteus Maximus
    c. Lateral border is formed by Levator Ani
    d. Posterior border is formed by obturator internus muscle.
126. What is the diagnosis?

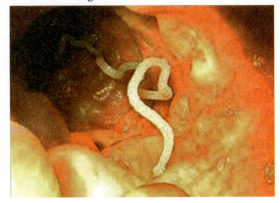

    a. Perforation by Ascariasis
    b. Volvulus by Ascariasis
    c. Ascending cholangitis by Ascariasis
    d. Solitary ascariasis in the bowel

BREAST

127. Dye for Sentinel Lymph node biopsy is injected in which of the following sites? *(Recent Pattern Question 2018-19)*
    a. Axilla
    b. Tail of spence
    c. Nipple
    d. Areola

128. Correct description about Paget's disease of breast?
    (Recent Pattern Question 2018-19)
    a. Eczema of skin of nipple
    b. Eczema of skin of areola
    c. Mastitis carcinomatosis
    d. Atrophic scirrhous carcinoma

129. MC benign breast tumour?
    (Recent Pattern Question 2018-19)
    a. Fibroadenoma
    b. Fibroadenosis
    c. D.C.I.S
    d. Phyllodes tumour

130. Breast triple assessment contains all except?
    (Recent Pattern Question 2018-19)
    a. Clinical examination
    b. Axillary Sampling
    c. USG
    d. FNAC and biopsy

131. Which of the following is not an indication for Fibroadenoma surgery? *(Recent Pattern Question 2018)*
    a. Patient's decision
    b. Size more than 5 cm
    c. Complex type
    d. Recurrence

132. In a breast lump of 4 cm no nodal metastasis is present. Which is the stage of breast cancer?
    (Recent Pattern Question 2018)
    a. Stage I
    b. Stage II
    c. Stage III
    d. Stage IV

133. Peau d'orange appearance in breast cancer is seen with which stage of cancer? *(Recent Pattern Question 2017)*
    a. T4A
    b. T4B
    c. T4C
    d. T4D

134. Breast cancer more than 5 cm is defined as stage_____
    (Recent Pattern Question 2017)
    a. T1
    b. T2
    c. T3
    d. T4

135. What is the diagnosis of the mammography report in a 30 year old woman with breast lump felt on self-examination of breast? *(Recent Pattern Question 2017)*

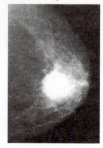

    a. Fibroadenoma
    b. Breast cancer
    c. Fibroadenosis
    d. Brodie's Serocystic disease

136. Which is the most common quadrant for carcinoma Breast? *(Recent Pattern Question 2016)*
    a. Lower outer
    b. Lower inner
    c. Upper outer
    d. Upper inner

137. Which is the most common Familial Breast cancer gene?
    (Recent Pattern Question 2016)
    a. BRCA1
    b. BRCA 2
    c. Li-Fraumeni syndrome
    d. STK 11

138. Skin of nipple and areola drains to which lymph node?
    (Recent Pattern Question 2016)
    a. Anterior axillary
    b. Supra-clavicular
    c. Central
    d. Infra-clavicular

139. A 25-year-old female presents with a breast lump and green discharge from inverted nipples. What is the first differential diagnosis? *(Recent Pattern Question 2016)*
    a. Duct ectasia
    b. Mastitis
    c. Carcinoma
    d. Paget's disease

140. Young female with painless, mobile lump of 4 cm in a breast. What is the diagnosis?
    a. Breast abscess
    b. Breast cyst
    c. Fibroadenoma
    d. Peau d'orange

141. Which breast cancer involves both breasts?
    a. Lobular carcinoma
    b. Mucoid carcinoma
    c. Ductal carcinoma
    d. Ductal carcinoma in situ

142. A biopsy of the opposite breast is considered in which of the following types of breast carcinoma?
    a. Comedo carcinoma
    b. Medullary carcinoma
    c. Mucinous carcinoma
    d. Lobular carcinoma

143. What is correct regarding Peau d'orange in breast carcinoma?
    a. Infiltration of cooper's ligament with cancer cells
    b. Infiltration of skin of breast with cancer cells
    c. Associated with lobular carcinoma of breast
    d. Good prognosis

144. Breast lump in pregnant lady is diagnosed by?
    a. FNAC
    b. Core cut Biopsy
    c. Mammography
    d. MRI

145. Which is the next investigation to be done for painful breast lump in a lactating woman?
    a. Mammography
    b. USG
    c. MRI
    d. FNAC

146. All are true about Paget's disease of breast EXCEPT?
    a. It is often bilateral
    b. Crusting of areola skin
    c. Lumpectomy is performed usually
    d. Paget cells are positive for HER2/neu

147. In breast conservative surgery the healthy margin excised is typically?
    a. 1 cm
    b. 2 cm
    c. 3cm
    d. 4 cm

148. A 35 year pregnant female came to your clinic with lump as shown in the image. What will be the initial screening method?

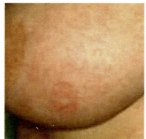

   a. USG b. MRI
   c. Mammogram d. FNAC
149. Breast cancer is called stage 4 when there is?
   a. Involvement of chest wall
   b. Satellite lesion
   c. Ulceration of surface skin
   d. Spread to adrenal gland
150. As per AJCC breast cancer staging T4 is?
   a. Distant metastasis
   b. Satellite lesions
   c. Spread to contralateral axillary lymph nodes
   d. Sentinel lymph node involvement
151. Which is the most important prognostic factor for carcinoma breast?
   a. HER2/Neu b. Histology grade
   c. Tumor staging d. Tumor growth rate
152. What is the probable diagnosis?

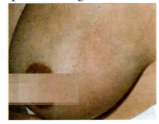

   a. Mastitis b. Mondor disease
   c. Cystosarcoma phyllodes d. Paget disease
153. Sentinel node biopsy is done for all EXCEPT?
   a. Colon carcinoma b. Ocular cancer
   c. Breast cancer d. Malignant melanoma
154. Stage of 3 cm breast cancer involving 4 axillary lymph nodes
   a. Stage I b. Stage II
   c. Stage III d. Stage IV
155. A 28-year-old female presents with infiltrating breast carcinoma with 1 cm hard lump. T1-N0-M0. What is the best treatment?
   a. Radical mastectomy b. Simple mastectomy
   c. Extended radical mastectomy
   d. Super radical mastectomy

THYROID AND SALIVARY GLANDS

156. Sebaceous cyst is not seen in?
   (Recent Pattern Question 2018-19)
   a. Back b. Soles
   c. Scalp d. Scrotum
157. Patient complains of painless swelling over the face with difficulty in swallowing. The appearance of face is shown. The probable diagnosis is?
   (Recent Pattern Question 2018-19)

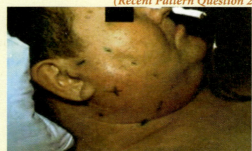

   a. Acute parotitis b. Cancer of parotid gland
   c. Angioedema of face d. Acute Sialpadenitis
158. A 35-year-old lady has presented with a 6-month painless fluctuant, non-transilluminant swelling with a thin watery discharge. Clinical diagnosis is?
   (Recent Pattern Question 2019)

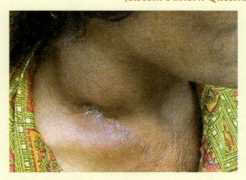

   a. Branchial Cyst b. Secondaries
   c. TB d. Lymphoma
159. Lid lag sign is also known as:
   (Recent Pattern Question 2018)
   a. Stellwag's sign b. Von Graefe's sign
   c. Dalrymple sign d. Mobius sign
160. Which is the most common malignancy of the endocrine system?
   a. Thyroid cancer b. Pancreatic cancer
   c. Pituitary adenoma d. Adrenal malignancy
161. Which of the following is the most useful investigation for thyroid function?
   a. TSH b. T3
   c. T4 d. Thyroglobulin

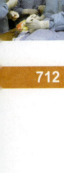

FMGE Solutions Screening Examination

162. Papillary carcinoma of thyroid is spread via?
    a. Lymphatic   b. Hematogenous
    c. Local spread   d. All of the above
163. Which iodine isotope is used for thyroid ablation?
    a. Iodine 131   b. Iodine 123
    c. Iodine 213   d. Iodine 132
164. Which is the most common nerve to be damaged in thyroid surgery?
    a. Recurrent laryngeal nerve
    b. Inferior laryngeal nerve
    c. External branch of superior laryngeal nerve
    d. Internal branch of superior laryngeal nerve
165. Which is the tumor marker for medullary carcinoma of thyroid?
    a. Albumin   b. TSH
    c. Thyroglobulin   d. Calcitonin
166. Which cancer arises from C-cells of thyroid?
    a. Follicular   b. Anaplastic
    c. Papillary   d. Medullary
167. Which thyroid cancer is associated with radiation exposure?
    a. Medullary   b. Papillary
    c. Follicular   d. Anaplastic carcinoma
168. Which thyroid tumor has the best prognosis?
    a. Papillary   b. Follicular
    c. Anaplastic   d. Medullary
169. A male patient with euthyroid state presents with the following condition. What is the diagnosis?

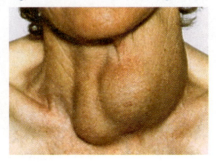

    a. Thyroglossal cyst   b. Multiple nodular goiter
    c. Solitary thyroid nodule d. Toxic nodular goiter
170. FNAC can diagnose all of the following thyroid lesions EXCEPT
    a. Anaplastic carcinoma   b. Papillary carcinoma
    c. Follicular carcinoma   d. Medullary carcinoma
171. Which of the following is not a landmark of facial nerve during superficial parotidectomy?
    a. Tragus
    b. Mastoid process
    c. Posterior belly of digastric muscle
    d. Zygomatic bone

172. Which is the most common parotid gland tumor?
    a. Warthin's tumor
    b. Mucoepidermoid carcinoma
    c. Pleomorphic adenoma
    d. Adenoid cystic carcinoma
173. Nerve invasion is seen in which type of parotid carcinoma?
    a. Muco-epidermoid carcinoma
    b. Adenoid cystic carcinoma
    c. Malignant mixed tumors
    d. Acinic cell carcinoma
174. Warthin's tumor is tumor of which gland?
    a. Parotid gland   b. Submandibular gland
    c. Lingual gland   d. Minor salivary glands
175. Most commonly salivary gland fistula starts from which gland?
    a. Parotid gland   b. Salivary gland
    c. Submandibular glands d. Sublingual glands
176. Salivary gland stone is formed most commonly in:
    a. Submandibular gland b. Mandibular gland
    c. Sublingual gland   d. Parotid gland
177. What is the surgery of choice for pleomorphic adenoma?
    a. Superficial parotidectomy
    b. Total parotidectomy
    c. Radical parotidectomy
    d. Radiotherapy

HERNIA AND HYDROCOELE

178. Bell clapper testis predisposes to?
    (Recent Pattern Question 2018-19)
    a. Torsion testis   b. Varicocele
    c. Cancer of testis   d. Hydrocele
179. In NYHUS classification which of these is called Type 3A hernia?   *(Recent Pattern Question 2018)*
    a. Femoral   b. Direct
    c. Indirect   d. Pantaloons
180. A 40-year-old patient was being operated for direct hernia. During surgery two sacs were seen. The diagnosis is?   *(Recent Pattern Question 2016)*
    a. Pantaloons hernia   b. Richter hernia
    c. Spigelian hernia   d. Littre hernia
181. A 30-year-old obese male patient presents with complete inguinal hernia and on examination doughy consistency is felt with dull note on percussion. This suggests that the contents of the hernia sac contain
    a. Omentum   *(Recent Pattern Question 2016)*
    b. Large intestine
    c. Small intestine
    d. Encysted ascitic fluid

Surgery

182. Deep inguinal ring is a defect in aponeurosis of:
    a. External oblique muscle of abdomen
    b. Internal oblique muscle of abdomen
    c. Transverse abdominis muscle
    d. Transversalis fascia

183. A 3-year-old child presents with red scrotal swelling which shows self resolution by next day morning and is maximum in evening with positive transillumination test. What is the diagnosis?
    a. Scrotal abscess
    b. Congenital hydrocele
    c. Secondary abscess
    d. Infantile hydrocele

184. Hydrocele in a child is managed by:
    a. Herniotomy
    b. Plication of sac
    c. Eversion of sac
    d. Inversion of sac

185. What is not true about hernia in children?
    a. Conservative Management till patient is asymptomatic
    b. Hernia treatment is done with herniotomy
    c. Absorbable mesh is not used
    d. Long standing hernia decreases chances of incarceration

186. The content of Littre's hernia is?
    a. Omentum
    b. Bladder
    c. Meckel's diverticulum
    d. Part of circumference of intestine

187. A 15-year-old male presents with pain in inguinal area and lower abdomen. On examination tenderness over a non-reducible swelling with negative cough impulse is noted. What is the diagnosis?
    a. Strangulated hernia
    b. Testicular torsion
    c. Scrotal abscess
    d. Femoral hernia

188. Femoral hernia presents:
    a. Below and lateral to pubic tubercle
    b. Above and medial to pubic tubercle
    c. Below and medial to pubic tubercle
    d. Above and lateral to pubic tubercle

189. All are true about femoral hernia EXCEPT?
    a. Common in nulliparous women
    b. Lockwood infra-inguinal approach is used
    c. Cough impulse is present
    d. Higher incidence of strangulation than inguinal hernia

190. Which hernia has the highest rate of strangulation?
    a. Direct inguinal hernia
    b. Indirect inguinal hernia
    c. Femoral hernia
    d. Incisional hernia

191. Which of the following hernia presents as emergency?
    a. Direct inguinal hernia
    b. Indirect inguinal hernia
    c. Femoral hernia
    d. Incisional hernia

192. Double sac hernia is known as:
    a. Richter hernia
    b. Cooper's hernia
    c. Littre's hernia
    d. Spigelian hernia

193. A patient has direct inguinal hernia. On operation intra-operative indirect inguinal hernia is seen. What is the diagnosis?
    a. Maydl's hernia
    b. Velpeau hernia
    c. Petit hernia
    d. Saddle bag hernia

194. Meckel's diverticulum forms wall in case of which type of hernia?
    a. Ritcher's hernia
    b. Spigelian hernia
    c. Cooper's hernia
    d. Littre's hernia

195. Spigelian hernia is:
    a. Hernia through petit triangle
    b. Hernia passing through obturator canal
    c. Hernia through linea alba
    d. Hernia at level of arcuate line

196. What is the location of bochdaleck hernia?
    a. Posterolateral
    b. Anteroposterior
    c. Anterolateral
    d. Posteromedial

197. A 25-year-old male presents with fever and red, swollen scrotum. Upon examination testis is felt separate from epididymis because of marked swelling in epididymis. What is the diagnosis?
    a. Testicular torsion
    b. Fournier's gangrene
    c. Epididymo orchitis
    d. Testicular cancer

UROLOGY

198. Which of these is the best for management of a 3cm stone in renal pelvis without evidence of hydronephrosis?
    (Recent Pattern Question 2018-19)
    a. ESWL
    b. PCNL
    c. Antegrade pyeloplasty
    d. Retrograde pyeloplasty

199. Germ cell tumour not seem in males:
    (Recent Pattern Question 2018-19)
    a. Choriocarcinoma
    b. Seminoma
    c. Sertoli cell tumour
    d. Teratoma

200. Cut off for diagnosis of Priapism is?
    (Recent Pattern Question 2018-19)
    a. 1 hours
    b. 2 hours
    c. 3 hours
    d. 4 hours

201. A person could not pass urine after suffering from pelvic fracture. On examination vitals are stable but bladder is not palpable. What is the probable diagnosis?
    (Recent Pattern Question 2018)
    a. Membranous urethra rupture
    b. Bulbar urethra rupture
    c. Recto-urethral injury
    d. Intraperitoneal rupture of bladder

202. The kidney stone whose development is *insensitive* to pH of urine is:
    (Recent Pattern Question 2018)
    a. Calcium oxalate
    b. Triple phosphate
    c. Uric acid
    d. Cystine

FMGE Solutions Screening Examination

203. A 60-year-old smoker male patient presents with painless gross hematuria for 1 day. IVU shows 1.2 cm filling defect at the lower pole of infundibulum. Which is the next best investigation to be done? *(Recent Pattern Question 2018)*
    a. Cystoscopy
    b. Urine cytology
    c. USG abdomen
    d. DMSA scan

204. A 70-year-old man after TURP for BPH develops seizures in postoperative state. What is the diagnosis?
    a. Water intoxication *(Recent Pattern Question 2018)*
    b. Anesthetic over-dosage
    c. Mismatched blood transfusion
    d. Malignant hyperthermia

205. What does the following image show?
    (Recent Pattern Question 2017)

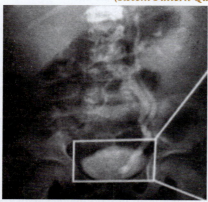

    a. Misplaced Cu-T 380Ag   b. Fecolith
    c. Ureterocele   d. Appendicolith

206. What is the best treatment for metastatic advanced prostate carcinoma? *(Recent Pattern Question 2017)*
    a. T.U.R.P
    b. Androgen ablation
    c. Chemotherapy
    d. Radical prostatectomy

207. Seminoma spreads by? *(Recent Pattern Question 2016)*
    a. Hematogenous route
    b. Direct route
    c. Lymphatics
    d. Directly by spermatic cord

208. In a person if testis cancer is suspected, which test is to be done first? *(Recent Pattern Question 2016)*
    a. Scrotal USG
    b. MRI
    c. FNAC
    d. PET/CT

209. A 28-year-old patient from Bihar presents with on and off pain in right scrotum and then gradual onset swelling develops over the duration of 2 years. Trans illumination test is positive. Top of testis can be reached. The probable diagnosis is? *(Recent Pattern Question 2016)*
    a. Right hydrocele
    b. Right inguinal hernia
    c. Right epididymal cyst
    d. Right encysted hydrocele of cord

210. A 50-year-old patient complains of pain and swelling in right side scrotum for two days. He tells that this swelling has been gradually increasing in size with a dragging sensation for 2 years. On examination there is a large inguinoscrotal irreducible swelling with extreme tenderness and redness. What is the probable diagnosis?
    a. Right hydrocele *(Recent Pattern Question 2016)*
    b. Right strangulated inguinal hernia
    c. Right testicular torsion
    d. Right Pyocele

211. A young boy 18 years of age presents with pain in groin for 2 days. On examination the testis seems high and cremasteric reflex is absent. Elevation of testis worsens the pain. What is the probable diagnosis?
    a. Right testicular torsion *(Recent Pattern Question 2016)*
    b. Right strangulated hernia
    c. Right inguinal hernia
    d. Right epididymo-orchitis

212. Which is the most common type of renal stone?
    a. Calcium oxalate
    b. Triple phosphate
    c. Struvite stone
    d. Urate stone

213. Which renal stone is radiolucent?
    a. Uric acid
    b. Calcium oxalate
    c. Triple phosphate
    d. Calcium phosphate

214. Stag horn calculi associated with proteus infection are:
    a. Uric acid stones
    b. Triple phosphate stones
    c. Calcium oxalate stones
    d. Cystine stones

215. Alkaline urine is seen in:
    a. Uric acid stone
    b. Oxalate stone
    c. Triple phosphate stone
    d. Cystine stone

216. What is the cause of urinary retention?
    a. Vaginal fibroid
    b. Cervical fibroid
    c. Uterine fibroid
    d. Subserosal fibroid

217. What is the most useful investigation for calculus in ureteric colic?
    a. CECT
    b. NCCT
    c. USG
    d. X-ray

218. Transitional cell carcinoma is seen in
    a. Prepuce
    b. Testis
    c. Prostate
    d. Urinary bladder

219. Which is the most common tumor of urinary bladder?
    a. Squamous cell cancer
    b. Carcinosarcoma
    c. Transitional cell cancer
    d. Clear cell cancer

220. What is the most common clinical presentation of bladder cancer?
    a. Painful urinary stasis
    b. Painless urinary stasis
    c. Painful hematuria
    d. Painless hematuria

221. What is the most common clinical subtype of transitional cell carcinoma of bladder?
    a. Local Metastatic
    b. Distant metastasis
    c. Superficial
    d. Deep

222. All are true about transitional cell cancer of urinary tract EXCEPT:
    a. Bladder is a frequent site
    b. Most common risk factor is smoking
    c. Females and males are equally affected
    d. Vitamin A is affective against bladder CA

223. Rupture of urethra above the deep perineal pouch causes urine retention in which region?
    a. Medial aspect of thigh   b. Scrotum
    c. True pelvis only   d. Anterior abdominal wall
224. Which amongst following is the most common cause of UTI?
    a. Instrumentation   b. Urethral diverticulum
    c. Bladder stones   d. Pregnancy
225. Spider leg sign on IVP suggests?
    a. Renal stone   b. Polycystic kidney
    c. Hypernephroma   d. Hydronephrosis
226. Adder head appearance on IVP is seen in
    a. Ureteral duplication   b. Ureterocele
    c. Ureteric hypoplasia   d. Polycystic kidneys
227. Reinke's crystals are seen in?
    a. Leydig cells   b. Sertoli cells
    c. Curschmann spirals   d. Creola bodies
228. Which is the most common testicular tumor?
    a. Seminoma   b. Teratoma
    c. Sertoli cell tumor   d. Chorio-CA
229. Which is the first lymph node involved in lymph node metastasis in testicular tumor?
    a. Inguinal   b. Para aortic
    c. External iliac   d. Internal iliac
230. Which is the most specific marker for prostate cancer?
    a. P.S.A   b. P.A.P
    c. Transrectal USG   d. N.S.E
231. What is incorrect about PSA?
    a. Liquefaction of seminal coagulum
    b. Produced by both normal cells and malignancy
    c. Increased with prostatitis
    d. Persists in blood even after prostatectomy
232. A 70-year-old man with prostate cancer was given radiotherapy. The recurrence of the cancer is monitored biochemically by
    a. Androgens levels
    b. Prostate specific antigen and carcino-embryonic antigen
    c. Prostate specific antigen only
    d. ALP and CEA
233. Three glass urine test with first glass specimen of urine showing threads is diagnostic of
    a. Urethritis   b. Prostatitis
    c. Cystitis   d. Epididymitis
234. Prostate cancer spreads to the vertebral column via?
    a Bateson plexus
    b Inferior hypogastric plexus
    c Superior hypogastric plexus
    d All of above
235. What is the indication for Radical prostatectomy?
    a. Localized prostate cancer, life expectancy < 10 years
    b. Localized prostate cancer, life expectancy > 10 years
    c. Locally advanced prostate cancer, life expectancy < 10 years
    d. Locally advanced disease with extension to lateral pelvic fascia
236. Which of the following is correct about the image given below?

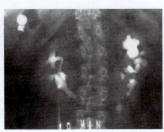

    a. Horse shoe kidney
    b. Undescended left kidney
    c. Congenital absent left kidney
    d. Papillary carcinoma
237. The given picture shows

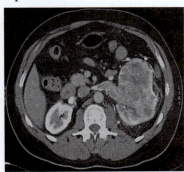

    a. Renal cell cancer   b. Hydronephrosis
    c. Polycystic kidneys   d. Nephrolithiasis
238. What does the given picture show?

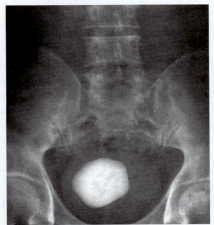

    a. Foreign body   b. Bladder stone
    c. Bladder diverticulum   d. Fecolith

FMGE Solutions Screening Examination

239. What is the probable diagnosis?

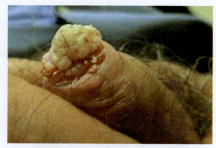

   a. Chancroid b. Carcinoma penis
   c. Chancre d. Bowen disease

240. In carcinoma penis tumor staging, stage III involves:
   a. Shaft of penis
   b. Inguinal lymph node metastasis operable
   c. Inguinal lymph node metastasis inoperable
   d. Confined to prepuce

241. A 5-year-old child pulls penis skin while urinating. Upon examination there is erythema and edema over the prepuce. What is the diagnosis?
   a. Hypospadias b. Urethral Stone
   c. Posterior urethral valve d. Phimosis

242. Chordee is associated with:
   a. Epispadias b. Hypospadias
   c. Phimosis d. Posterior urethral valve

243. The treatment of balanitis xerotica obliterans (BXO) is
   a. Chemotherapy
   b. Circumcision
   c. Radiotherapy
   d. Partial amputation of penis

244. Which is a major cause of death in renal transplant patients?
   a. Uremia b. Malignancy
   c. Rejection d. Infection

HEPATOBILIARY SYSTEM

245. A 6-year-old child is brought with high fever with rigors for 5 days with pain in right hypochondrium. On examination patient is anicteric and tenderness is noted in Right upper quadrant. What is best investigation for this case? *(Recent Pattern Question 2018-19)*
   a. USG
   b. Serology
   c. SGOT/ LFT
   d. Contrast CT scan

246. AFP is a tumour marker for which of the following?
   (Recent Pattern Question 2018-19)
   a. HCC b. RCC
   c. Oncocytoma d. Chordoma

247. Comment on the image shown below.
   (Recent Pattern Question 2018-19)

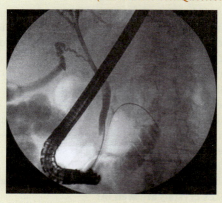

   a. Percutaneous Transhepatic cholangiogram
   b. T tube cholangiogram
   c. E.R.C.P
   d. HIDA scan

248. Which of the following is correct about Zollinger Ellison syndrome? *(Recent Pattern Question 2018)*
   a. Associated with MEN1
   b. Most common site is stomach
   c. Best test for diagnosis is pentagastrin test
   d. Metastasis to adjacent gut

249. Which ligament is compressed in the Pringle maneuver?
   (Recent Pattern Question 2017)
   a. Hepatoduodenal ligament
   b. Gastroduodenal ligament
   c. Gastrohepatic ligament
   d. Lienorenal ligament

250. A patient comes with RUQ pain. The USG image shows?
   (Recent Pattern Question 2017)

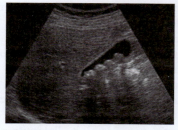

   a. Cholelithiasis b. Cholecystitis
   c. Cholangiocarcinoma d. Porcelain Gallbladder

251. A 28-year-old man from Bihar develops right hypochondriac pain. USG shows 5 × 5 × 4 cm abscess in left lobe of liver. Hydatid serology is negative. What is the treatment?
   a. Anti –Amoebic drugs *(Recent Pattern Question 2016)*
   b. Aspiration + Anti amoebic drugs
   c. Catheter drainage + Anti amoebic drugs
   d. Percutaneous aspiration and infusion of scolicidal agents

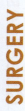

Surgery

252. Aflatoxin leads to? *(Recent Pattern Question 2016)*
    a. Liver cancer
    b. Hepatic adenoma
    c. Bladder cancer
    d. Retinoblastoma
253. What is the ideal management of a hemodynamically unstable patient with suspected liver injury?
    a. Inotropic support *(Recent Pattern Question 2016)*
    b. Exploratory Laparotomy
    c. Rapid transfusion of fresh blood
    d. Rapid infusion of iv crystalloids
254. A 40 year patient is having high grade fever associated with abdominal pain in right upper quadrant, with hepatomegaly and liver dullness on percussion. What is the clinical diagnosis?
    a. Pyogenic liver abscess
    b. Amoebic liver abscess
    c. Hydatid cyst
    d. Neoplastic growth
255. Anchovy sauce pus is seen in?
    a. Amoebic liver abcess
    b. Pyogenic liver abscess
    c. Hydatid cyst
    d. Cold abscess
256. A patient has obstructive jaundice. USG can tell all of the following EXCEPT?
    a. Number of stones in CBD
    b. Peritoneal deposits
    c. Size of liver
    d. Extrahepatic versus intrahepatic causes
257. The organism associated with fish consumption which causes carcinoma gallbladder
    a. Clonorchis sinensis
    b. Gnathostoma
    c. Stronglyoidosiscantonensis
    d. H. diminuta
258. A 30-year-old lady presents with fever and pain in right hypochondrium with presents breath catch up upon palpation. What is the clinical diagnosis?
    a. Acute pancreatitis
    b. Acute cholecystitis
    c. Acute appendicitis
    d. Acute mediastinitis
259. Charcot triad is used for
    a. Acute cholangitis
    b. Acute cholecystitis
    c. Cholelithiasis
    d. Gall bladder CA
260. Murphy sign is seen in:
    a. Acute appendicitis
    b. Acute cholecystitis
    c. Acute pancreatitis
    d. Acute cholangitis
261. Which of the following is *Not* associated with elevation of Right hemi-diaphragm:
    a. Amebic abscess
    b. Pyogenic abscess
    c. Cholecystitis
    d. Sub diaphragmatic abscess
262. Liver biopsy is indicated for diagnosis/evaluation of all EXCEPT?
    a. Autoimmune hepatitis
    b. Storage disorders
    c. Hemangioma
    d. Hepatocellular carcinoma
263. Which is the most common benign liver tumor?
    a. Hemangioma
    b. Hepatocellular carcinoma
    c. Hepatoma
    d. Secondaries
264. Pringle's maneuver is mainly used to control bleeding from
    a. IVC
    b. Hepatic artery
    c. Cystic artery
    d. Hepatic vein
265. What is the true color of cholesterol stone?
    a. Black
    b. Dark yellow
    c. Brown
    d. Pale yellow
266. In Hemolytic anemia which stones are commonly seen?
    a. Pigment stone
    b. Cholesterol stone
    c. Mixed stone
    d. All of above
267. Aspirin protects against all EXCEPT?
    a. MI
    b. Stroke
    c. Colorectal cancer
    d. Liver cancer

HEAD AND NECK

268. All are premalignant conditions of oral cavity except: *(Recent Pattern Question 2018-19)*
    a. Chronic hyperplastic candidiasis
    b. Oral submucosal fibrosis
    c. Oral lichen planus
    d. Leukoplakia
269. Comment on the diagnosis of this 60 year old man. *(Recent Pattern Question 2018-19)*

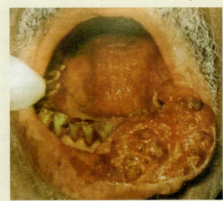

    a. Basal cell Cancer
    b. Plunging Ranula
    c. Epulis
    d. SCC of lip
270. MC subtype of Rodent ulcer is? *(Recent Pattern Question 2018-19)*
    a. Superficial spreading
    b. Acral lentiginous
    c. Nodulocystic
    d. Pigmented
271. Which among the following is the cause of submucosal fibrosis? *(Recent Pattern Question 2018)*
    a. Alcohol
    b. Candidiasis
    c. Betel nut chewing
    d. Pan leaf chewing

272. Which nerve is involved in thoracic outlet syndrome?
 (Recent Pattern Question 2017)
    a. Pain and paraesthesia in axillary nerve distribution
    b. Pain and paraesthesia in median nerve distribution
    c. Pain and paraesthesia in radial nerve distribution
    d. Pain and paraesthesia in ulnar nerve distribution
273. Pott puffy tumor is seen at? (Recent Pattern Question 2017)
    a. Frontal bone   b. Temporal bone
    c. Occipital bone   d. Sphenoid bone
274. Cranio-pharyngioma is a brain tumor arising from?
 (Recent Pattern Question 2016)
    a. Rathke pouch   b. Neurohypophysis
    c. Posterior pituitary d. Median eminence
275. A biker develops a head injury and non-contrast CT scan shows presence of Lentiform hemorrhage. What is the diagnosis? (Recent Pattern Question 2016)
    a. Extradural bleeding
    b. Subdural bleeding
    c. Intraparenchymal bleeding
    d. Intraventricular bleeding
276. Metastasis to neck lymph nodes is from?
    a. Breast cancer   b. Lung cancer
    c. Adrenal carcinoma d. Stomach cancer
277. What is the most common malignant brain tumor?
    a. Astrocytoma   b. Glioblastoma multiforme
    c. Oligodendroglioma d. Ependymoma
278. Stereotactic radiotherapy is used for treatment of?
    a. Brain tumor   b. Lung carcinoma
    c. Cervical cancer   d. Renal carcinoma
279. Which of the following tumors is cured by radiation?
    a. Rhabdomyosarcoma b. Neuroblastoma
    c. Chloroma   d. Seminoma
280. Which is the most common secondary malignancy in retinoblastoma?
    a. Ewing's sarcoma   b. Osteosarcoma
    c. Chondro-sarcoma   d. Rhabdo-myosarcoma
281. All are seen in Trotters' triad EXCEPT:
    a. Unilateral conductive hearing loss
    b. Ipsilateral earache and facial pain
    c. Ipsilateral paralysis of the soft palate
    d. Seen with juvenile nasopharangeal angiofibroma
282. What is true about tongue cancer?
    a. Most common type is adenocarcinoma
    b. Cervical lymph node metastasis is universally present
    c. MC site is on Lateral margin
    d. Slurring of speech is a common complaint
283. What is the most common site of tongue cancer?
    a. Base of tongue
    b. Tip of tongue
    c. Lateral margin of tongue
    d. Posterior attachment of tongue

284. What is your diagnosis?

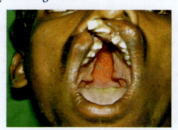

    a. Cleft lip   b. Cleft palate
    c. Cleft lip and palate d. Bifid uvula
285. Secretory sinus in neck, moving upon deglutination:
    a. Branchial sinus   b. Pilonidal cyst
    c. Thyroglossal fistula d. Sublingual dermoid cyst
286. A newborn has a swelling in neck due to soft cystic mass with transillumination test positive. What is the diagnosis?
    a. Potato tumor   b. Branchial cyst
    c. Cystic hygroma   d. Carotid body tumor
287. All of the following are true regarding cystic hygroma EXCEPT
    a. Brilliantly transilluminant
    b. Mostly on posterior neck region
    c. Lined by endothelium
    d. Lined by columnar epithelium

VASCULAR SURGERY

288. Most common complication of below knee stripping of Varicose veins is? (Recent Pattern Question 2018-19)
    a. Haemorrhage   b. Thromboembolism
    c. Neuralgia   d. Infection
289. Which is the most common site of peripheral aneurysm? (Recent Pattern Question 2018)
    a. Femoral artery   b. Radial artery
    c. Popliteal artery d. Brachial artery
290. Intermittent claudication is defined as pain _____?
    a. At rest   (Recent Pattern Question 2018)
    b. On first step of walking
    c. Relieved on standing still
    d. Increase on limb dependency
291. Which of the following is the best management for radiation induced occlusive disease of carotid artery?
    a. Low dose aspirin (Recent Pattern Question 2018)
    b. Carotid angioplasty and stenting
    c. Carotid endarterectomy
    d. Carotid bypass procedure
292. All of the following result after chronic edema to legs EXCEPT?
    a. Marjolin's ulcer b. Thickening of skin
    c. Soft tissue infections d. Varicose veins

Surgery

293. Buerger disease affects which layers of artery?
    a. Tunica media
    b. Tunica adventitia
    c. Tunica intima
    d. All of above
294. All are true about Buerger disease EXCEPT:
    a. Ulnar artery and peroneal arteries involved
    b. Nerve involvement present
    c. Small acral vessels of limb involvement causes hypohidrosis
    d. Phlebitis migrans
295. Patient presents with varicose vein with saphenofemoral incompetence with normal perforators. The best management plan is:
    a. Endovascular striping
    b. Sclero-theraphy
    c. Sapheno-femoral flush ligation
    d. Saphenofemoral flush ligation with stripping
296. Thrombo-angitis obliterans involves?
    a. Arteries
    b. Veins
    c. Nerves
    d. All of above
297. Hoffman Tinel sign is seen in?
    a. Deep vein thrombosis
    b. Nerve regeneration
    c. Pulmonary embolism
    d. Upper motor neuron lesion

GENERAL SURGERY

298. Which of the following is not a hospital acquired infection? *(Recent Pattern Question 2018-19)*
    a. S.S.I
    b. S.T.D
    c. U.T.I
    d. Pneumonia
299. Amount of blood loss in class III circulatory failure/ Haemorrhagic shock? *(Recent Pattern Question 2018-19)*
    a. <15%
    b. 15-30%
    c. 30-40%
    d. >40%
300. Identify the lesion shown.
    (Recent Pattern Question 2018-19)

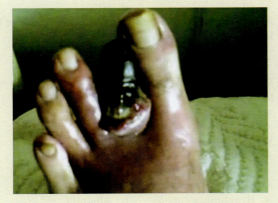

   a. Wet gangrene
   b. Dry gangrene
   c. Frost bite
   d. Ainhum

301. The following patient has presented after chest trauma. On examination crepitus is felt. The clinical diagnosis is? *(Recent Pattern Question 2018-19)*

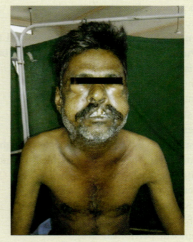

   a. Subcutaneous Emphysema
   b. Gas gangrene
   c. Acute tubular necrosis
   d. SVC syndrome
302. What is the GCS for a brain dead patient?
    (Recent Pattern Question 2018)
    a. 3
    b. 5
    c. 6
    d. 8
303. A 50 kg patient has 40% burn of the body surface area. Calculate the ringer lactate solution to be given for 1st 8 hours of fluid. *(Recent Pattern Question 2018)*
    a. 1 L
    b. 2 L
    c. 4 L
    d. 8 L
304. Which is the best method to administer oxygen in case of burns of airways? *(Recent Pattern Question 2018)*
    a. Elective intubation
    b. Mask
    c. Nasal prongs
    d. Tracheostomy
305. In which of the following conditions is Fogarthy catheter used? *(Recent Pattern Question 2017)*
    a. Acute limb ischemia
    b. Tube thoracotomy with underwater seal
    c. Suprapubic drainage of bladder
    d. Total parenteral nutrition
306. Which of the following needle is used to suture skin?
    a. Cutting needle *(Recent Pattern Question 2017)*
    b. Reverse Cutting needle
    c. Round body needle
    d. Straight needle with eye
307. Shock index is defined as? *(Recent Pattern Question 2017)*
    a. Pulse rate/BP
    b. BP/Pulse rate
    c. CVP/PCWP
    d. PCWP/CVP
308. Which is used to control bleeding?
    (Recent Pattern Question 2017)
    a. Pressure
    b. Packing
    c. Position
    d. All of the above

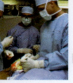

FMGE Solutions Screening Examination

309. What is the preferred fluid used in burns after 24 hours?
    a. Ringer lactate   (Recent Pattern Question 2017)
    b. Colloids
    c. Hypertonic saline
    d. Switch to oral or parenteral nutrition

310. A patient presents with knife stab wound to the Lower neck. Pulse rate is 110/min with BP = 100/70 mmHg. Which is the next step?   (Recent Pattern Question 2017)
    a. Immediate wound exploration
    b. Formal wound exploration in OT in GA
    c. Put stent to prevent pneumothorax
    d. Urgent angiography

311. A patient with abdominal trauma is brought to casualty. On examination the vitals are stable with no evidence of peritonitis. Next best step is? (Recent Pattern Question 2017)
    a. Urgent exploratory laparotomy
    b. CT Abdomen
    c. F.A.S.T
    d. Diagnostic peritoneal lavage

312. Class I haemorrhagic shock is caused by _____ ml loss of blood.   (Recent Pattern Question 2017)
    a. 750   b. 1000
    c. 1500   d. 2000

313. Fogarthy catheter is used in which of the following?
    a. Acute limb ischemia   (Recent Pattern Question 2017)
    b. Suprapubic catheterization of Urinary bladder
    c. Deflating sigmoid volvulus
    d. Coronary stenting

314. A patient underwent inguinal lymph node dissection and drain was placed. On 10th day severe bleeding occurs. What type of bleeding is this?
                                    (Recent Pattern Question 2016)
    a. Reactionary hemorrhage b. Secondary
    c. Primary   d. Tertiary

315. A 25-year-old Patient with abdominal trauma presents with Hypovolemic shock, and is unresponsive to crystalloids. What is the next step?
                                    (Recent Pattern Question 2016)
    a. Albumin   b. Colloids
    c. Blood transfusion   d. Immediate laparoscopy

316. Which is the best parameter to monitor Hypovolemic shock?   (Recent Pattern Question 2016)
    a. Urine output   b. Respiratory rate
    c. Blood pressure   d. Pulse rate

317. A 25-year-old patient presents in emergency with abdominal trauma. Why is FAST done?
                                    (Recent Pattern Question 2016)
    a. Detection of pericardial fluid accumulation
    b. Detection of bowel lacerations
    c. Detection of Mesenteric Tear
    d. Detection of aortic transection

318. Increased cardiac output is seen in which shock?
    a. Septic shock   b. Anaphylaxis
    c. Neurogenic   d. Hemolysis

319. What is given immediately in hemorrhagic shock?
    a. Packed RBC   b. Colloids
    c. Crystalloids   d. Isotonic fluids

320. Plasma expanders are most useful in which shock?
    a. Septic shock   b. Vasovagal shock
    c. Neurogenic shock   d. Cardiogenic shock

321. Neurogenic shock is caused by:
    a. Burns   b. Dehydration
    c. Hemorrhage   d. Anesthesia

322. Which is the preferred fluid in a poly-traumatic patient with shock?
    a. Ringer lactate   b. Normal saline
    c. Dextran   d. Dextrose-normal saline

323. Which is the first fluid of choice in Hypovolemic shock?
    a. Dextran   b. Normal saline
    c. Dextrose normal saline d. Hartmann solution

324. All are criteria for Systemic inflammatory response syndrome in children EXCEPT:
    a. Tachycardia   b. Hypotension
    c. Fever   d. Leukocytosis

325. A new born boy has lumbosacral meningomyelocele and is awaiting surgical repair. The sac is best protected with sterile gauze piece soaked with
    a. Mercurochrome   b. Tincture benzoin
    c. Methylene blue   d. Normal saline

326. In 1 mL of 0.9%, normal saline content of Na is:
    a. 0.1 mEq   b. 0.3 mEq
    c. 0.5 mEq   d. 10 mEq

327. In 1 mL of 3 percent saline what is the quantity of sodium?
    a. 0.5 mEq   b. 1 mEq
    c. 10 mEq   d. 50 mEq

328. In IV fluid what percentage of energy is supplied by glucose when patient is on total parenteral nutrition?
    a. 20   b. 30
    c. 40   d. 50

329. According to "rule of 9". What is the percentage of burn in hand?
    a. 1%   b. 5%
    c. 9%   d. 14%

330. What is the % Body surface area involved in burns of the perineum?
    a. 1%   b. 3%
    c. 5%   d. 9%

331. What is the best solution for burns?
    a. NS 0.9%   b. Ringer's lactate
    c. 25% dextrose   d. Colloid

332. All are given for management of burns EXCEPT?
    a. Hypotonic solutions b. Albumin
    c. 25% dextrose   d. Hartmann solution/ATLS

Surgery

333. What is the first fluid preferred in a burn patient?
   a. Crystalloids
   b. Colloids
   c. Any of above
   d. Both of above

334. All are true about a burn patient EXCEPT:
   a. Hematemesis
   b. For Head and neck burn exposure treatment done
   c. Stridor can be present
   d. Most common infection is by pseudomonas

335. What is the cause of death in 70% burns patient in whom enteral feeding is not given:
   a. Dehydration
   b. Malnutrition
   c. Electrolyte imbalance
   d. Bacterial infection

336. A burn patient is brought to emergency. Upon examination he was found dead. What could be the possible cause?
   a. Sepsis
   b. Hypoxia
   c. Malnutrition
   d. Hypovolemia

337. Which is true about burn?
   a. Above 5% of surface area must be involved to produce shock
   b. Inhaled hot gas will not cause supraglottic airway burn and laryngeal edema.
   c. Early elective intubation is safest
   d. If oral fluids are to be used, salt must be avoided

338. What is correct about 3rd degree burns?
   a. Erythema and painful
   b. Erythema and painless
   c. Painless and cherry red
   d. Painful and cherry red

339. Which virus causes infection in burn patients?
   a. HSV
   b. CMV
   c. EBV
   d. VZV

340. What is the cause of death in early period of burns?
   a. Sepsis
   b. Shock
   c. Dys-electrolytemia
   d. ARDS

341. Burns present as all of the following EXCEPT
   a. Sepsis
   b. Shock
   c. Acute kidney injury
   d. Air embolism

342. Middle area of face fracture (le-fort fracture) is characterized by all EXCEPT
   a. Proptosis
   b. Lengthening of face
   c. Enopthalmos
   d. Ecchymosis

343. In Brown-Sequard syndrome ipsilateral loss will be of?
   a. Pain
   b. Temperature
   c. Tactile discrimination
   d. Proprioception

344. Blow out injury with ptosis occurs due to damage to?
   a. Zygomatic arch
   b. Orbital floor
   c. Sphenoid bone
   d. Palantine and maxillary bones

345. Fournier gangrene is caused by:
   a. Clostridium welchii
   b. Clostridium septicum
   c. Anaerobic Streptococcus
   d. Bacillus subtilis

346. Continuous burrowing ulcer is caused by?
   a. Streptococcus Viridans,
   b. Streptococcus Pyogenes
   c. Staphylococcus aureus
   d. Microaerophilic streptococcus

347. All of the following are released/increased in surgical stress EXCEPT:
   a. ADH
   b. Insulin
   c. ACTH
   d. Cortisol

348. All are true about Keloid EXCEPT:
   a. May be familial
   b. Arises on sternum
   c. Subsides Over Time
   d. Hyperkeratotic

349. Which organ is most commonly affected by blunt trauma to abdomen?
   a. Spleen
   b. Intestine
   c. Liver
   d. Mesentery

350. Wound dehiscence occurs after how many days following surgery?
   a. 2–4 days
   b. Within 2 days
   c. 5–12 days
   d. >2 weeks

351. What does split thickness of skin graft mean?
   a. Is a skin graft including the epidermis and part of the dermis
   b. Is a skin graft including the epidermis and complete dermis
   c. Is a skin graft including part of the epidermis and part of the dermis
   d. Is a skin graft including part of epidermis and whole of the dermis

352. What is a xenograft:
   a. Transplantation of organs from a 1st degree relative
   b. Transplantation of organs from unrelated donor
   c. Transplantation of tissues from self
   d. Transplantation of living tissues/organs from one species to another

353. Fibrosis is seen in all EXCEPT:
   a. Marjolin's ulcers
   b. Buruli ulcer
   c. Venous ulcer
   d. Peptic ulcer

354. Carcinoma developed in a scar is called:
   a. Sarcoma
   b. Adenocarcinoma
   c. Dermoid tumor
   d. Marjolin's ulcer

355. Osteomyelitis first occurs in:
   a. Metaphysis
   b. Epiphysis
   c. Diaphysis
   d. All of above

356. Clean and small wound heals by?
   a. Primary intention
   b. Secondary intention
   c. Tertiary intention
   d. All of above

357. Female patient with injury on her scalp, hair was shaved and sutures were put. On which day sutures should be removed?
   a. 8-10 days
   b. 2 weeks
   c. 3 weeks
   d. 1 month

FMGE Solutions Screening Examination

358. What is incorrect about Laparoscopy?
    a. Smaller incisions
    b. Minimal postoperative pain
    c. Trocar injury in patients with low body mass index
    d. Recovery time is longer
359. A guy driving a car fast suddenly slams on the brakes. He was wearing a seat belt. The organ most likely to be affected is:
    a. Liver
    b. Spleen
    c. Mesentery
    d. Kidney
360. A motor cyclist after multiple trauma is having hypoventilation. What is the cause?
    a. Damage to respiratory centre
    b. Damage to respiratory apparatus
    c. Both
    d. None of the Above
361. What is the best investigation for a hemodynamically stable patient with blunt abdominal trauma?
    a. CECT abdomen
    b. MRI abdomen
    c. Diagnostic Peritoneal lavage
    d. F.A.S.T
362. Painful lockjaw is seen in all of the following EXCEPT?
    a. Tetany
    b. Temporo-mandibular joint abscess
    c. Mandibular abscess
    d. Odontogenic pulp abscess
363. What is the most common site of basal cell carcinoma in lips?
    a. Upper lip
    b. Central 1/3
    c. Lower lip
    d. Commissures
364. Fracture of neck of fibula leads to which nerve injury?
    a. Common peroneal nerve
    b. Obturator nerve
    c. Genitofemoral nerve
    d. Posterior tibial nerve
365. What is the most common Nosocomial infection acquired by a patient undergoing surgery?
    a. S.I.R.S
    b. Surgical site infection
    c. Pneumonia
    d. Catheter based infection
366. Upon aspiration in supine position, food particle goes most commonly to?
    a. Right lower lobe superior basal
    b. Right lower lobe postero basal
    c. Left lower lobe superior basal
    d. Left lower lobe postero basal
367. What is the management of Epidermoid Carcinoma?
    a. 5FU + external beam radiation
    b. Mitomycin + External beam radiation
    c. External beam Radiation
    d. Surgery + Imiquimod
368. In TNM staging, N = ?
    a. Nature of tumor
    b. Number of tumors
    c. Number of lymph nodes
    d. Metastasis

MISCELLANEOUS

369. In TNM staging T indicates. *(Recent Pattern Question 2017)*
    a. Size of tumor
    b. Nodal metastasis
    c. Distant metastasis
    d. Depth of invasion
370. A 65-year-old patient presents with low backache and low grade fever. X-ray spine shows.
    (Recent Pattern Question 2017)

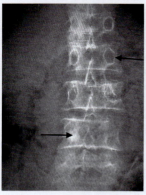

    a. Osteomyelitis
    b. Osteomalacia
    c. Hypoparathyroidism
    d. Metastasis
371. What is correct regarding descent of testes during fetal stage?
    a. Gestational age 1-7 months in abdomen
    b. Gestational age 1-7 months in inguinal canal
    c. Gestational age 7-9 months in scrotum.
    d. Gestational age lies in 7-9 months in abdomen.
372. Which is not a derivative of midgut?
    a. Appendix
    b. Jejenum
    c. Ascending colon
    d. Descending colon
373. All are true about amoebic liver abscess EXCEPT?
    a. Sterile pus
    b. Amoebae reach the right lobe > left lobe
    c. Intercostal tenderness
    d. Hepatocellular jaundice
374. A 30-year-old patient presents with pain in right hypochondrium for 5 days with soft and tender liver and intercostal tenderness. He complains of catch in breath on inspiration and has a non productive cough. On examination the lung fields are clear, patient looks pale and emaciated. What is the probable diagnosis?
    a. Amoebic liver abscess
    b. Pyogenic live abscess
    c. Hydatid cyst
    d. Hepatic adenoma
375. Strawberry Gallbladder is seen in?
    a. Cholesterolosis
    b. Porcelain Gall bladder
    c. Mirizzi syndrome
    d. Wegener's granulomatosis
376. All are features of Saint's triad EXCEPT?
    a. Gall stones
    b. Diverticulitis
    c. Hiatus hernia
    d. Cholesterosis

Surgery

377. **Bent inner tube sign is seen in**
   a. Volvulus
   b. Intussusception
   c. Intestinal obstruction
   d. Gastric antral vascular ectasia

378. **Bird beak sign on barium enema is seen in?**
   a. Achalasia cardia   b. Sigmoid volvulus
   c. Carcinoma esophagus   d. Carcinoma sigmoid colon

379. **All are common causes of ileal obstruction EXCEPT?**
   a. Adhesions   b. Obstructed hernia
   c. Stricture   d. Hirschsprung's disease

380. **What is the most common site of GIST?**
   a. Stomach   b. Liver
   c. Kidney   d. Brain

381. **What is the most common site of lymphoma of GIT?**
   a. Stomach   b. Duodenum
   c. Ileum   d. Colon

382. **The most common cause of intestinal obstruction in infants is?**
   a. Intussusception   b. Congenital bands
   c. Necrotising enterocolitis d. Sigmoid volvulus

383. **The vessel which needs to be ligated in a patient with a bleeding peptic duodenal ulcer is?**
   a. Left gastroepiploic artery
   b. Gastroduodenal artery
   c. Left gastric artery
   d. Superior Pancreatico-duodenal artery

384. **All the following are True regarding FAST-EXCEPT?**
   a. It cannot reliably exclude injury in penetrating trauma
   b. It detects free fluid in the abdomen or pericardium
   c. It is accurate in detecting <50 mL of free blood
   d. It is a focused abdominal sonar for trauma

385. **Wolfe Graft is**
   a. Thin split thickness graft
   b. Medium thickness split thickness skin graft
   c. Full thickness skin graft
   d. Thick split thickness skin graft

386. **Pringle maneuver may be required for treatment of?**
   a. Bleeding Esophageal Varices
   b. Mesenteric Ischemia
   c. Injury to Tail of Pancreas
   d. Live Laceration

387. **Optional timing of administration of prophylactic antibiotic for surgical patients is**
   a. One hour prior to induction of anaesthesia
   b. At the induction of anaesthesia
   c. Any time during the surgical procedure
   d. One hour after induction

388. **What is the raw material used in nylon suture?**
   a. Polyester polymer
   b. Polyamide polymer
   c. Polyethylene terephthalate
   d. Polybutylene terephthalate

389. **All the following statements are true regarding torsion of testis EXCEPT**
   a. Anatomical abnormality is unilateral and contralateral testis should not be fixed
   b. Prompt exploration and twisting & fixation is the only way to save the torted testis
   c. Most common between 10 & 25 years of age
   d. Inversion of testis is the most common predisposing cause

390. **'Fifth vital sign' commonly elicited by anaesthesiologists on surgical patients is:**
   a. FiO_2 b. Pain
   c. Blood pressure   d. Core temperature

391. **The most common cancer of oral cavity is**
   a. Adenocarcinoma
   b. Melanoma
   c. Sarcoma
   d. Squaous cell carcinoma

392. **Barrett's esophagus is diagnosed by**
   a. Squamous metaplasia
   b. Intestinal metaplasia
   c. Squamous dysplasia
   d. Intestinal dysplasia

393. **Boerhaave's syndrome is due to?**
   a. Drug induced esophagus perforation
   b. Corrosive injury
   c. Spontaneous perforation
   d. Gastro-esophageal reflux disease

394. **Which one of the following is not a treatment of Gastroe-sophageal Variceal hemorrhage?**
   a. Sclerotherapy
   b. Sengstaken tube
   c. Trans-jugular intrahepatic Porta-caval shunt
   d. Gastric freezing

395. **"Limey bile" is?**
   a. Present in the CBD
   b. Thin and clear
   c. Like toothpaste emulsion in the gallbladder
   d. Bacteria rich

396. **Major complication of cyst-gastrostomy for pseudo pancreatic cyst is?**
   a. Infection
   b. Obstruction
   c. Fistula   d. Hemorrhage

397. **What is Cullen's sign?**
   a. Bluish discoloration of the flanks
   b. Bluish discoloration in the umbilicus
   c. Migratory thrombophlebitis
   d. Subcutaneous fat necrosis

398. **Which organ is most commonly involved in retroperito-neal fibrosis?**
   a. Aorta   b. Ureter
   c. Inferior vena cava   d. Sympathetic nerve plexus

FMGE Solutions Screening Examination

399. In a case of retro-caecal appendicitis which movement aggravates pain?
a. Flexion
b. Extension
c. Medical rotation
d. Lateral rotation

400. Anal carcinoma is most common carcinoma of type
a. Adeno carcinoma
b. Epidermoid
c. Mixed
d. None of the above

401. After esophagectomy the best substitute as conduit is
a. Stomach
b. Jejunum
c. Right colon
d. Left colon

402. Ranson scoring system is used to predict the severity of
a. Acute pancreatitis
b. Acute Cholecystitis
c. Peritonitis
d. Appendicitis

403. Surgical excision of the liver metastases is well established if the primary is from?
a. Carcinoma lung
b. Colorectal carcinoma
c. Carcinoma breast
d. Melanoma

BOARD REVIEW QUESTIONS

404. The minimum number of polyps necessary for a diagnosis of Familial Adenomatous Polyposis (FAP) is
a. 05
b. 10
c. 50
d. 100

405. Gery turner's sign is seen in
a. Acute appendicitis
b. Acute pancreatitis
c. Acute cholecystitis
d. Acute hepatitis

406. Splenectomy can lead to
a. Leucopenia
b. Thrombocytosis
c. Thrombocytopenia
d. Thrombocytopenia and leucopenia

407. Reversed "3" sign on barium studies is seen in which condition?
a. Ampullary carcinoma
b. Carcinoma stomach
c. Carcinoma head of pancreas
d. Insulinoma

408. The nerve commonly damaged during McBurney's incision is:
a. Subcostal
b. Iliohypogastric
c. 11th thoracic
d. 10th thoracic

409. Most common site of volvulus is:
a. Ileum
b. Appendix
c. Sigmoid colon
d. Caecum

410. Villous adenoma presents as:
a. Hypercalcemia
b. Hypokalemia
c. Hyperphosphaetemia
d. All of the above

411. Sister Mary Joseph nodule is most commonly seen with:
a. Ovarian cancer
b. Stomach cancer
c. Colon cancer
d. Pancreatic cancer

412. Spigelian hernia is:
a. Hernia passing through the obturator canal
b. Hernia passing through the linea alba
c. Hernia through the triangle of petit
d. Hernia occurring at the level of arcuate line

413. Strangulation most commonly occurs in:
a. Femoral hernia
b. Direct inguinal hernia
c. Indirect inguinal hernia
d. Lumbar hernia

414. Multiple strictures in intestine are found in :
a. Radiation enteritis
b. Duodenal ulcer
c. Ulcerative colitis
d. Gastric erosion

415. Colovesical fistula most commonly arises from :
a. Crohn's disease
b. Ulcerative colitis
c. Carcinoma colon
d. Abdomino-perineal resection

416. Sentinel lymph node biopsy is an important part of the management of which of the following conditions?
a. Carcinoma prostate
b. Carcinoma breast
c. Carcinoma lung
d. Carcinoma nasopharynx

417. Most important prognostic indicator for breast Carcinoma is:
a. Age of the patient
b. Lymph node involvement
c. Genetic factors
d. Family history

418. Unilateral breast involvement with scaly skin around the nipple and intermittent bleeding is suggestive of:
a. Galactocoele
b. Paget's disease
c. Eczema
d. Sebaceous cysts

419. Peau d'orange of breast is due to:
a. Obstruction of vein
b. Obstruction of lymphatic ducts,
c. Obstruction of glandular ducts
d. Obstruction of arteries

420. Most common type of breast carcinoma is:
a. Lobular
b. Sarcoma
c. Ductal
d. Granuloma

421. Which type of breast cancer is most likely to be bilateral?
a. Infiltrating duct carcinoma
b. Paget's disease of breast
c. Lobular carcinoma of the breast
d. Medullary carcinoma of the breast

422. Triple examination includes all EXCEPT:
a. Clinical examination
b. Excision biopsy
c. FNAC
d. Mammography

423. Metastasis from follicular carcinoma should be treated by:
a. Radioiodine
b. Surgery
c. Thyroxine
d. Observation

424. Radiation exposure during infancy has been linked to which one of the following carcinoma?
a. Breast
b. Melanoma
c. Thyroid
d. Lung

Surgery

425. **Lateral internal sphincterotomy is useful for:**
   a. Anal fistula
   b. Anal canal strictures
   c. Hemorrhoids
   d. Anal fissure

426. **Erythroplasia of Queyrat occurs in:**
   a. Scrotum
   b. Testes
   c. Penis
   d. Bldder

427. **A 25-year-old man presents with hydrocele on the left side. Associated condition could be a:**
   a. Nephroma
   b. Hepatic malignancy
   c. Testicular tumor
   d. Pepile malignancy

428. **Fournier's gangrene is seen in:**
   a. Scrotum
   b. Shaft of penis
   c. Base of penis
   d. Glans penis

429. **Thimble bladder is seen in:**
   a. Diverticulae
   b. Bladder stones
   c. Schistosomiasis
   d. Tuberculosis

430. **Narrowest part of the urethra is:**
   a. Prostatic urethra
   b. Bulbar urethra
   c. Penile urethra
   d. Membranous urethra

431. **Lord's and Jaboulay's operation is done for:**
   a. Rectal prolapse
   b. Fistula in Ano
   c. Inguinal hernia
   d. Hydrocele

432. **All are causes of bladder cancer EXCEPT:**
   a. Alcohol
   b. Naphthylamine exposure
   c. Cigarette smoking
   d. Schistosoma hematobium

433. **Most common type of hypospadias is:**
   a. Glandular
   b. Penile
   c. Coronal
   d. Perineal

434. **Nissens fundoplication is a first line treatment for?**
   a. GERD
   b. Hitatus hernia
   c. Esophageal atresia
   d. Congenital hypertrophic pyloric stenosis

435. **Concentration of Na (mEq/I) in normal saline is?**
   a. 77
   b. 109
   c. 130
   d. 154

436. **Lipodermatosclerosis is most commonly seen at?**
   a. Anterior aspect of leg
   b. Medial aspect of leg
   c. Anterior aspect of thigh
   d. Posterior aspect of thigh

437. **Greyish discoloration of flank seen in Acute Pancreatitis is referred to as?**
   a. Cullen's sign
   b. Grey Turner sign
   c. Balance's sign
   d. Alvarado's sign

438. **Interstitial cystitis is also known as?**
   a. Eosinophilic cystitis
   b. Radiation cystitis
   c. Hunner's cystitis
   d. Tubercular cystitis

439. **Antibiotic of choice for lymphedema is?**
   a. Penicillin
   b. Amikacin
   c. Metronidazole
   d. Ceftazidime

440. **Most common subtype of thyroid cancer is?**
   a. Medullary carcinoma
   b. Papillary carcinoma
   c. Follicular carcinoma
   d. Anaplastic carcinoma

441. **Maximum & minimum score in Glasgow coma scale is?**
   a. 15 & 0
   b. 14 & 3
   c. 15 & 3
   d. 15 & 1

442. **Alvorado's score is done for?**
   a. Pancreatitis
   b. Appendicitis
   c. Cholecystitis
   d. Cholangitis

443. **Which of the following is not a sign of appendicitis?**
   a. Rovsing's sign
   b. Murphy's sign
   c. Obturator sign
   d. Psoas sign

444. **Most common organism causing appendicitis is?**
   a. Bacteroides
   b. E.coli
   c. Staphylococcus
   d. Streptococcus

445. **Most common site of anorectal abscess is?**
   a. Perianal
   b. Ischiorectal
   c. Pelvirectal
   d. Intersphincteric

446. **Most common site of splenenculi is?**
   a. Omentum
   b. Splenocolic ligament
   c. Gastrocolic ligament
   d. Hilum of spleen

447. **What is the most common presentation of Lobular carcinoma?**
   a. Nipple discharge
   b. Breast mass
   c. Mammographic calcification
   d. Nipple retraction

448. **What is most commonly associated with high risk for carcinoma colon?**
   a. Peutz-Jegher syndrome
   b. Juvenile familial polyposis
   c. Familial adenomatous polyposis
   d. Lynch syndrome

449. **Which is the least common site for spread of melanoma?**
   a. GIT
   b. Lungs
   c. Liver
   d. Renal

450. **Coronary graft is most commonly taken from?**
   a. Femoral vein
   b. Saphenous vein
   c. Axillary vein
   d. Cubical vein

451. **Sentinel lymph node biopsy was first done in?**
   a. Carcinoma breast
   b. Carcinoma colon
   c. Carcinoma penis
   d. Melanoma

452. **Relative humidity in operation theatre should be maintained at?**
   a. 35-45%
   b. 45-55%
   c. 55-65%
   d. 65-75%

453. **In abdominal aortic aneurysm indication of operation is when size of aneurysm is?**
   a. >4 cm
   b. >5.5 cm
   c. >6 cm
   d. 6.6 cm

454. **Bender grading is used for?**
   a. Subarachnoid hemorrhage
   b. Subdural hemorrhage
   c. Extradural hemorrhage
   d. Parenchymal bleed

455. **Murphy's Sign is seen in?**
   a. Acute appendicitis
   b. Acute cholecystitis
   c. Acute Pancreatitis
   d. Ectopic pregnancy

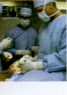

FMGE Solutions Screening Examination

456. Bosniak classification is for?
    a. Renal tuberculosis   b. Renal cysts
    c. RCC   d. VUR
457. Most common cause of nephrolithiasis is?
    a. Hypocitraturia   b. Hyperoxaluria
    c. hyperuricosuria   d. Idiopathic hypercalciuria
458. Which renal stone is radiolucent?
    a. Calcium oxalate   b. Calcium phosphate
    c. Uric acid   d. Struvite
459. Alkalinization of urine helps in dissolution of which type of renal stones?
    a. Calcium oxalate   b. Uric acid
    c. Cystine   d. Struvite
460. Renal stone which is formed due to proteus infection is?
    a. Calcium oxalate   b. Uric acid
    c. Cystine   d. Struvite
461. In tuberculosis of scrotal contents. Which is the first to get affected?
    a. Testis   b. Epididymis
    c. Rete testis   d. Vas deferens
462. Prostatic calculi is made up of?
    a. Calcium carbonate   b. Calcium oxalate
    c. Calcium phosphate   d. Triple phosphate
463. What is the treatment of choice of Warthin tumor?
    a. Radical parotidectomy
    b. Superficial parotidectomy
    c. Superficial parotidectomy with neck dissection
    d. Enucleation
464. Pancreatic pseudocyst is made up of?
    a. Bacteria   b. Pancreatic enzymes
    c. Glucagon   d. Insulin
465. Which is the most common congenital anomaly of pancreas?
    a. Pancreatic divisum   b. Accessory pancreas
    c. Annular pancreas
    d. Developmental pancreatic cysts
466. Best definitive investigation for carcinoma breast is?
    a. Biopsy   b. FNAC
    c. USG   d. Mammography
467. Best investigation for renal calculi is?
    a. X Ray   b. USG
    c. CECT   d. NCCT
468. Saints triad includes all EXCEPT:
    a. Gall stones   b. Cholangitis
    c. Diverticulosis   d. Hiatus hernia
469. Which of the following is used in urinary bladder carcinoma?
    a. 5FU   b. BCG
    c. Cyclophosphamide   d. 6 Mercapto Purine

470. What is the most common site of Esophageal rupture in Rigid Bronchoscopy?
    a. Cervical region   b. Cardiac region
    c. Mid esophagus   d. GE junction
471. Which parotid tumor spreads along nerve sheath?
    a. Pleomorphic adenoma
    b. Mucoepidermoid carcinoma
    c. Adenoid cystic carcinoma
    d. Warthin's tumor
472. Which is the most common carcinoma of minor salivary gland?
    a. Pleomorphic adenoma
    b. Mucoepidermoid carcinoma
    c. Adenoid cystic carcinoma
    d. Warthin's tumor
473. Burn of head region in a child accounts for what percent of burns?
    a. 10%   b. 20%
    c. 30%   d. 40%
474. What is the drug of choice for surgically unresectable renal cell carcinoma?
    a. Sorafenib   b. Sunitinib
    c. Imatinib   d. Cetuximab
475. Heller's operation is done for?
    a. Gastric outlet obstruction
    b. Achalasia cardia
    c. Hiatus hernia   d. Esophageal
476. Pathological nipple discharge is mostly associated with?
    a. Fibroadenoma   b. Duct papilloma
    c. Adenocarcinoma   d. Lobular carcinoma
477. Which is the most common type of hypospadias?
    a. Glandular   b. Penile
    c. Scrotal   d. Perineal
478. What is the best treatment of cystic hygroma?
    a. Radiotherapy   b. Sclerotherapy
    c. Surgical excision   d. Chemotherapy
479. Which is the most common site of aortic dissection is?
    a. Ascending aorta   b. Descending aorta
    c. Arch of aorta   d. Infrarenal portion of aorta
480. In RTA, Injury to aorta causing Aortic rupture is most commonly seen in?
    a. Pedestrian
    b. Motorcyclist
    c. Car driver
    d. Person accompanying car driver
481. Which nerve is involved in parotidectomy?
    a. Trigeminal   b. Mandibular
    c. Auriculotemporal   d. Lingual

Surgery

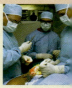

IMAGE-BASED QUESTIONS

482. What does the intraoperative photograph depict?

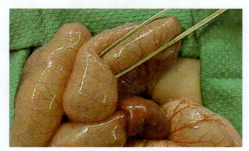

a. Transverse colon   b. Meckel's diverticulum
c. Intussusception   d. Fallopian tube

483. Identify these two surgical instruments.

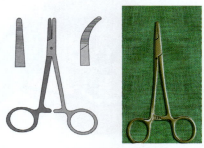

a. Thumb forceps & Sponge Holder
b. Artery Forceps & Needle Holder
c. Sponge Holder & Allis Forceps
d. Needle Holder & Ovum Forceps

484. All are true about the lesion EXCEPT?

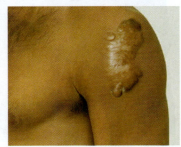

a. Severe itching
b. Claw like process
c. Develops at vaccination sites
d. Collagen bundles are present

485. All are true about the image shown EXCEPT?

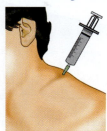

a. Anti-gravity drainage
b. Cold abscess
c. Transillumination test is negative
d. Rubbery consistency of involved lymph nodes

486. All are true about the image shown EXCEPT?

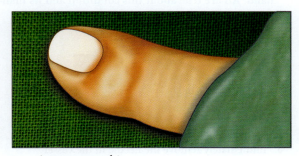

a. Acute paronychia
b. Throbbing pain
c. Ring block with adrenaline used
d. I and D by incising the eponychium

487. Comment on image A and B

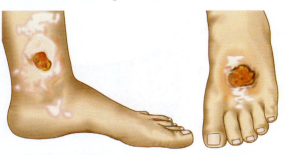

a. A=Venous ulcer and B= ischemic ulcer
b. A=arterial ulcer and B= Venous ulcer
c. A=neuropathic ulcer and B= arterial ulcer
d. A=Venous ulcer and B= neuropathic ulcer

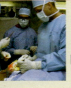

FMGE Solutions Screening Examination

488. Identify the type of ulcer shown

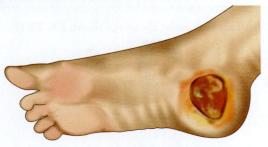

   a. Venous ulcer   b. Arterial ulcer
   c. Neuropathic ulcer d. Bazin's ulcer

489. During induction of anaesthesia, after giving thiopentone injection a patient develops discoloration of hand. All are true about this condition and its management EXCEPT?

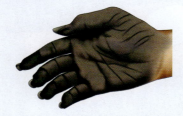

   a. Immediately remove the needle in the vessel
   b. Inject lignocaine
   c. Dilute heparin
   d. Intra-arterial thrombolysis

490. A patient presents with ulcer at the site of previous burn site. All are true about the lesion EXCEPT?

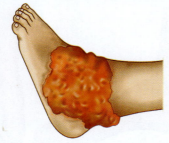

   a. Painless scar   b. Cured by surgery
   c. Lymphatic metastatis d. Marjolin' ulcer

491. What is correct about the diagnosis?

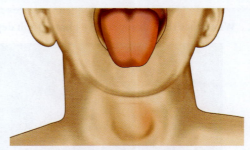

   a. Thyroglossal cyst
   b. Brachial cyst
   c. Cold abscess
   d. Carotid body tumour

492. What is true about the image shown?

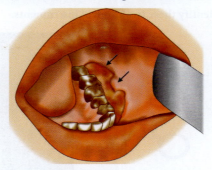

   a. Carcinoma alveolar margin
   b. Leukoplakia
   c. Hyperplastic candidiasis
   d. Fibrous epulis

493. Identify the lesion shown in the figure

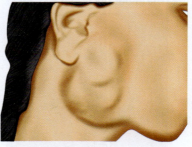

   a. Pleomorphic adenoma
   b. Mumps
   c. Retroauricular lymphadenopathy
   d. Sialadenitis

Surgery

494. All can be seen in this patient EXCEPT

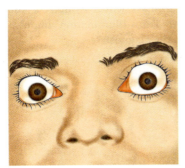

a. Myxedema
b. Dalrymple sign
c. Moist warm hands
d. Constipation

495. All are true about the patient shown in the image EXCEPT?

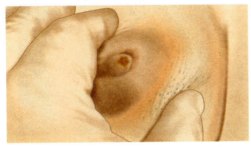

a. Peau d'orange
b. Ulceration of nipple
c. Diagnosis depends on HER2 expression
d. Van Nuys prognostic index

496. A 25-year-old shepherd presents with dragging discomfort in right Hypochondrium and on examination shows presence of enlarged liver 5 cm below costal margins. What is the probable diagnosis?

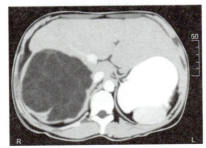

a. Amoebic liver abscess
b. Hydatid cyst
c. Pyogenic liver abscess
d. Hepatic adenoma

497. Which triangle is shown here?

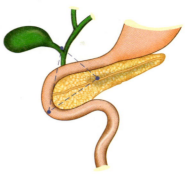

a. Calot's triangle
b. Gastrinoma triangle
c. Hesselbach' triangle
d. Killian's triangle

498. A 65-year-old grandmother presents with feculent nasogastric aspirate. What is the diagnosis?

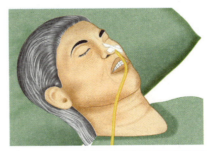

a. Jejunal obstruction
b. Ileal obstruction
c. Diverticulitis
d. Mesenteric ischemia

499. The following disease occurs due to all EXCEPT?

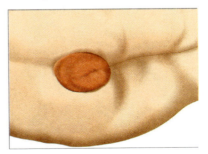

a. Whooping cough
b. Marasmus
c. Obstetric trauma
d. Fistula in ano

FMGE Solutions Screening Examination

500. Which of the following is shown in the image?

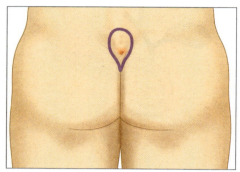

- a. Fistula in ano
- b. Pilonidal sinus
- c. Bowen disease
- d. Hidradenitis suppurativa

501. Identify the structure held with artery forceps?

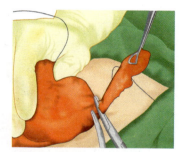

- a. Appendix
- b. Meckel's diverticulum
- c. Zenker's diverticulum
- d. Colostomy procedure

502. Which procedure is shown in the image?

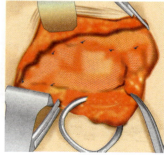

- a. Lichtenstein repair
- b. Bassini herniorrhaphy
- c. Shouldice repair
- d. Lord's procedure

503. A 25-year-old presents with dragging pain and testicular mass which exhibits a cough expansile impulse. Trans-illumination impulse is negative. What is the diagnosis?

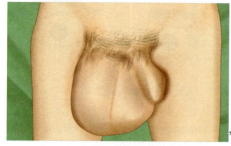

- a. Direct inguinal hernia
- b. Indirect inguinal hernia
- c. Hydrocele
- d. Varicocele

504. All are true about the condition shown EXCEPT:

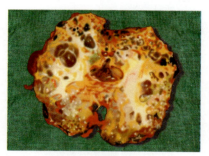

- a. Cysts increase in size with age
- b. Spider leg deformity
- c. Anemia
- d. Low Renin due to pressure atrophy of JG apparatus

505. All are true due to the conditions shown in the figure EXCEPT?

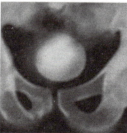

- a. Pain at end of micturition referred to the tip of penis
- b. Holmium laser
- c. Litholapaxy
- d. Painless intermittent hematuria

Surgery

506. The following image shows presence of?

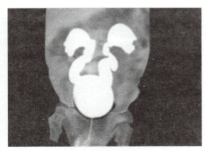

a. Posterior urethral valves
b. Vesico-ureteric reflux
c. Bladder stone
d. Bladder rupture

507. What is incorrect about the image shown?

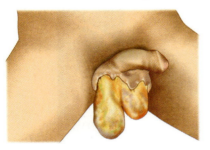

a. Gangrene of scrotum
b. Microaerophilic Hemolytic Streptococci
c. Seen in low socio-economic background
d. Can involve skin of penis

508. The CT chest shows presence of?

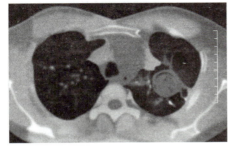

a. Meniscus sign
b. Crescent sign
c. Tree in bud sign
d. Loculated empyema

509. The image shows presence of

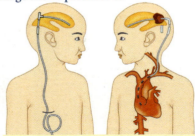

a. A = Ventriculoperitoneal shunt, B = Ventriculo-atrial shunt
b. A = Ventriculo-atrial shunt, B = Ventriculo-peritoneal shunt
c. A = Denver shunt, B = La Veen Shunt
d. A = La Veen Shunt, A = Denver Shunt

510. A 25-year-old patient presents in coma with GCS of 5 and extensor posturing after a bike accident. Which of the following will the best management of the patient?

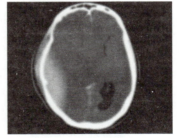

a. Hypertonic saline
b. Thrombolysis
c. Burr hole surgery
d. Hemi-Craniectomy

511. Identify the surgical instrument

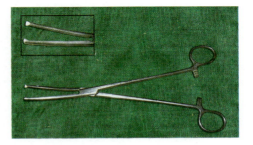

a. Kocher forceps
b. Allis forceps
c. Ovum forceps
d. Artery forceps

512. Identify the instrument shown

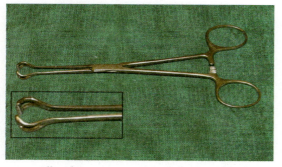

a. Allen forceps b. Mosquito forceps
c. Babcock forceps d. Kocher forceps

515. Identify the image shown

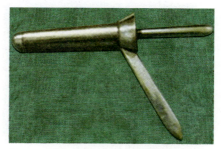

a. Proctoscope b. Sigmoidoscope
c. Anoscope d. Colonoscope

513. Identify the instrument shown

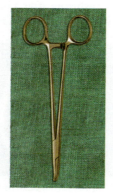

a. Needle holder b. Cheatles forceps
c. Babcock forceps d. Kocher forceps

516. Identify the catheter shown in the figure

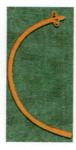

a. Malecot catheter
b. Foley's catheter
c. Red rubber catheter
d. Ryle's tube

514. Identify the image shown

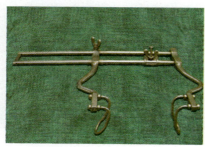

a. Rib Spreader
b. Self-retaining retractor
c. Lister Dilator
d. Male Metallic Catheter

517. Identify the tube shown in the image

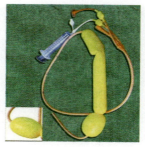

a. Ryle's tube
b. Malecot's Catheter
c. Blakemore Sengstaken Catheter
d. Foley's catheter

Surgery

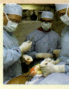

518. What is the clinical diagnosis of the patient?

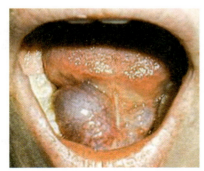

a. Ranula b. Cystic Hygroma
c. Erythroplakia d. Epulis

519. The image shows?

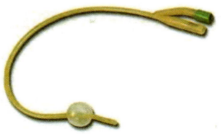

a. Foley's Catheter
b. Swan Ganz catheter
c. Sengstaken Blakemore tube
d. Endotracheal tube

520. Name the retractor

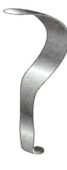

a. Deaver retractor b. Richardson retractor
c. Malleable retractor d. Goulet

Answers to Image-Based Questions are given at the end of explained questions

FMGE Solutions Screening Examination

ANSWERS WITH EXPLANATIONS

MOST RECENT QUESTIONS 2019

1. Ans. (d) Insert needle in 2nd intercostal space

Ref: Harrison 20th ed. pg. 2009

- The clinical diagnosis based on history of rib fractures, respiratory distress and hypotension is pneumothorax. There can be concomitant hemothorax but treatment of obstructive shock caused by pneumothorax is the immediate step.
- This would be done by inserting a wide bore needle in second intercostal space to reduce the impact of obstructive shock and increase systolic blood pressure.

2. Ans. (c) Sitting with neck flexed

Ref: Oxford Handbook of Clinical Medicine, pg. 773

Nasogastric tube should be inserted in a conscious patient in sitting position with slight flexion of the neck.

Procedure for inserting NG tube

- Examine the patient's nostril to check for septal deviation and identify the more patent nostril
- Instil viscous lidocaine into the patient's nostril
- Estimate the length of insertion by measuring the distance from the tip of the nose, around the ear, and down to just below the left costal margin.
- The estimated length falls in between the 2nd and 3rd pre-printed black lines on the tube
- Position the patient sitting upright with the neck partially flexed. Ask the patient to hold a cup of water in his or her hand and put a straw in his or her mouth with instructions to sip water only when asked to.
- Gently insert the NG tube along the floor of the nose, and advance it parallel to the nasal floor (i.e. directly perpendicular to the patient's head, not angled up into the nose) until it reaches the back of the nasopharynx, where resistance will be met (10-20 cm).
- At this time, ask the patient to sip on the water through the straw and start to swallow.
- Notice the flexion in the neck of the patient while the patient is swallowing water through a straw while the NG is advanced forwards.
- Continue to advance the NG tube until the distance of the previously estimated length is reached.

3. Ans. (d) Malrotation of gut

Ref: page 1994: Bailey and love: 26th edition

- Choice A presents with delayed passage of meconium and is ruled out.
- Choice B presents with non-bilious vomiting and is ruled out.
- Choice C presents with bilious vomiting and does not have any abdomen distention. X-Ray abdomen shows double bubble appearance.
- Choice D presents with bilious vomiting and abdominal distention and multiple gas filled loops.

4. Ans. (a) Mucoviscidosis

Ref: Nelson 20th ed. pg. 1802

- Meconium ileus occurs primarily in new-born infants with cystic fibrosis which is also called mucoviscidosis.
- It is an exocrine gland defect of chloride transport that results in abnormally viscous secretions. The distal 20-30cm of ileum is collapsed and filled of pale stool.
- The proximal bowel is dilated and filled with thick meconium that resembles sticky syrup or glue. The peristalsis fails to propel this viscid material forward and becomes impacted in the ileum.

5. Ans. (b) NG Tube insertion and CXR to check position of tube

Ref: Nelson 20th pg. 1783

- The clinical diagnosis of this neonate with frothing and bubbling at the mouth and nose is esophageal atresia.
- The symptoms worsen with episodes of feeding and aspiration of gastric contents if fistula is present
- In setting of early onset respiratory distress, inability to pass a nasogastric or orogastric tube suggests esophageal atresia.
- *Plain X ray will show a coiled feeding tube lying in esophageal pouch and air distended stomach.*
- Choice A bronchoscopy with methylene blue is injected into endotracheal tube and dye is observed in oesophagus during forced inspiration to detect orifice of fistula in TEF.
- Choice C and D are not recommended for diagnosis of esophageal atresia.
- Esophagogram can detect a H type of defect shown.

Types of Tracheo-esophageal Fistula

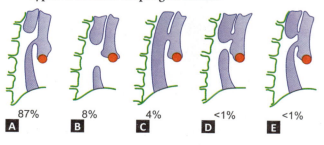

Surgery

6. Ans. (c) 10

Ref: Harrison 20th ed. pg. 3183

Eye opening to pain = 2
Confused= 4
Flexion on painful noxious stimuli to arm= 4
Score = 10

Eye opening (E)		Verbal response (V)	
Spontaneous	4	Oriented	5
To speech	3	Confused	4
To pressure	2	Words	3
None	1	Sounds	2
		None	1
Best motor response (M)			
Obeying commands	6		
Localizing	5		
Normal flexion	4		
Abnormal flexion	3		
Extension	2		
None	1		

7. Ans. (b) Total thyroidectomy

Ref: Bailey and love 26th ed. pg. 766

- Thyroidectomy during pregnancy has not been associated with adverse maternal or neonatal outcomes. There are no indications for termination of pregnancy.
- Whenever possible, the operation should be performed during the second trimester or after delivery.
- *Thyroid cancer, the most common endocrine malignancy, is often detected in young female patients. About 10% of thyroid cancers occurring during the reproductive years are diagnosed during pregnancy or in the early post-partum period.*
- *Patients with large, locally aggressive or metastatic differentiated thyroid cancer require total thyroidectomy with excision of adjacent structures.* Along with this, nodal surgery is done followed by radioiodine ablation with long term TSH suppression.
- Choice A is ruled out since radioactive iodine is not used in pregnancy
- Choice D is ruled out since total thyroidectomy is done for cancer.

8. Ans. (a) Marjolin ulcer

Ref: Bailey and Love 26th ed. pg. 918

- Marjolin's ulcer is a squamous cell cancer that can develop in chronic long standing venous ulcer.

- Failure to heal an ulcer indicates it may have another coexisting cause like malignancy, Rheumatoid arthritis and arterial ulcer.
- Erythema Induratum of Bazin is a tuberculid showing lobular panniculitis. EIB is classified under cutaneous tuberculosis

9. Ans. (b) Intramarginal excision followed by radiation

Ref: SRB, 5th ed. pg. 12

- Excisional surgery alone has been shown to yield a 45-100% recurrence rate and should very rarely be used as a solitary modality, although excision in combination with adjunct measures can be curative.
- Most studies in which excisional surgery was combined with injected steroids reported a recurrence rate of less than 50%.
- *Surgery followed by adjunctive radiotherapy has obtained recurrence rates of 0–8.6%*

10. Ans. (c) Gut ischemia

Ref: Bailey and Love: 26th ed. pg. 882

Mesenteric tears usually occur due to the shearing force applied on the <u>mesentery</u>, which happens while the movable intestines continue moving with the same speed of the car, although the car is decelerated by the act of the brakes (described in physics as the inertia). These tears can be so trivial that a frank intestinal ischemia would not be apparent immediately. The abdominal wall ecchymosis may lead to misdiagnosis as soft tissue injury.

11. Ans. (a) Neuralgia

Ref: Bailey and Love: 26th ed. pg 912

COMPLICATIONS OF STANDARD VARICOSE VEIN SURGERY

- Infection
- Nerve injury. The incidence of saphenous nerve neuralgia is 7% following LSV stripping to the knee. The incidence of sural nerve neuropraxia and common peroneal nerve injury following SSV surgery is fairly high.

12. Ans. (b) Pleural cavity

Ref: Bailey and Love: 26th ed. pg. 109

FAST looks for fluid in following *five* areas

- Perihepatic area and hepatorenal space
- Peri-splenic area
- Left and right Pericolic gutters
- Pelvis
- Pericardium

FMGE Solutions Screening Examination

> **Extra Mile**
>
> **Focused abdominal sonar for trauma**
> - It detects free fluid in the abdomen or pericardium
> - It will not reliably detect less than 100 ml of free blood
> - It does not identify injury to hollow viscus
> - It cannot reliably exclude injury in penetrating trauma
> - It may need pepeating or supplementing with other investigations

13. Ans. (b) Varicocelectomy

Ref: Bailey and Love 26th ed. pg. 1381

The clinical diagnosis of patient is varicocele. The key word is bag of worms feel on scrotal examination. When examined in the erect position, the scrotum on the affected side hangs lower than normal, and on palpation, with the patient standing, the varicose plexus feels like a bag of worms. There may be a cough impulse.

MANAGEMENT
- Operation is not indicated for an asymptomatic varicocele.
- When the discomfort is significant, then embolisation of the gonadal veins is the usual first line intervention.
- If this is not possible, or if the varicocele recurs (as it does in around 20 per cent after embolisation), then *surgical ligation of the testicular veins/* Varicocelectomy is the appropriate treatment.

14. Ans. (a) 60 minutes before skin incision

Ref: Bailey and Love 26th ed. pg. 248

- The timing of antibiotic administration may vary, but the *goal of administering preoperative systemic prophylactic antibiotics is to have the concentration in the tissues at its highest* at the start and during surgery.
- The literature supports at least 30 minutes, but no greater than 60 minutes before the skin incision is the optimal timing for the pre-operative administration of most commonly used antibiotics
- The antibiotic used most commonly is cefazolin
- The antibiotic must be stopped within 48 hours of the surgery.

15. Ans. (c) Excision

Ref: Bailey and Love: 26th ed. pg. 725

- Mucous retention cysts develop in floor of mouth either from obstructed minor salivary glans or from sublingual salivary gland.
- The term ranula applies to mucous extravasation cyst that arises from a sublingual gland producing an appearance of a frog belly.
- It can resolve spontaneously or *requires formal surgical excision of cyst and affected sublingual gland.*
- Incision and drainage results in recurrence.
- Sometimes the cyst may perforate through mylohyoid muscle diaphragm to enter the neck and is called plunging ranula.

16. Ans. (b) 24-hour urinary Fractionated Metanephrine

Ref: Bailey and Love 26th ed. pg. 784

- Catecholamines like nor-epinephrine, epinephrine and dopamine are produced in excess by chromaffin cells of pheochromocytoma.
- The end product of metabolism of these catecholamines is fractionated metanephrine levels.
- Vaniyl mandelic acid levels are used for diagnosis of neuroblastoma.

17. Ans. (a) Artery forceps

Ref: SRB: 5th ed. pg. 1164

The image shows a surgical instrument which has visible transverse serrations in distal blades with a lock in proximal part.

> **Use**
> - To catch bleeding points
> - To open the fascial planes in different surgeries
> - To pass a ligature
> - To hold fascial, peritoneum, aponeurosis
> - To hold sutures
> - To drain an abscess like a sinus forceps

18. Ans. (a) Tongue depressor

Ref: SRB, 5th ed, pg. 1150

The image shows a tongue depressor which can be used for posterior pharyngeal wall visualization to intubation process.

19. Ans. (a) Sebaceous cyst

Ref: SRB: 5th ed, pg. 78

The image shows a sebaceous cyst on the scalp. Other common sites apart from scalp are face and scrotum. It contains a cheesy white material with putty consistency. It is not seen in palms and soles as there are no sebaceous glands.

20. Ans. (a) Lipoma

Ref: SRB: 5th ed, pg. 72

- The image shows a solitary lipoma on dorsum of neck with probably a decubitus ulcer. They are common in males and are common in back, shoulder and upper arm.

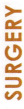

- Choice B is seen in pediatric age group and survival upto adult age group is unlikely. Choice C is seen in posterior triangle of neck
- Choice D is unlikely at occiput.

21. Ans. (b) Below Inferior constrictor

Ref: Bailey and Love: 26th ed. pg. 1018

The Killian's dehiscence is located *below inferior constrictor muscle* and above cricopharyngeal muscle. Laimer's triangle lies below cricophyrageus and above longitudinal muscle of esophagus

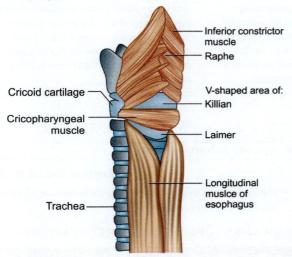

22. Ans. (b) Gut

Ref: Bailey and Love: 26th ed. pg. 1429

Progress in small bowel transplantation has lagged behind others since intestinal transplants stimulate a strong graft rejection response *because small intestine contains large amount of lymphoid tissue.* Moreover, ischemia and rejection increase intestinal permeability and allow translocation of bacteria from the lumen of bowel.

23. Ans. (a) Kidney

Ref: Bailey and Love: 26th ed. pg.18

Urine out-put is a reliable indicator of end organ perfusion. The Brain and heart continue to receive blood supply at the expense of other organs. The Kidney insult in hypovolemic shock indicates decompensation process has started and resuscitative measures are not working.

GASTROINTESTINAL TRACT

24. Ans. (a) Haemorrhage

Ref: Bailey 27th ed. pg. 1186

- Immediate complication is bleeding due to slippage of ligature.
- Gastric dilatation and gastric mucosal damage leading to hematemesis are uncommon complications.
- Fistula can develop due to damage to wall of greater curvature of stomach.
- Damage to tail of pancreas can lead to pancreatitis, localised abscess formation.

25. Ans. (a) Chemoradiation

Ref: SRB 5th ed. pg. 987 and Bailey 26th ed. pg. 1266

- The primary management of anal cancer is by chemoradiotherapy also called Combined Modality Therapy (C.M.T).
- Initially radiotherapy for 3 weeks 3000 rads are given for 3 weeks to the perineum and pelvis.
- The chemotherapy includes a combination of 5FU with mitomycin C or cisplatin.

26. Ans. (a) No occurrence after surgery

Ref: SRB 5th ed. pg. 894

Crohn's disease can recur even after surgical procedures unlike ulcerative colitis where total proctocolectomy cures the disease. Choice B, C and D are characteristic features of Crohn's disease.

TABLE: Difference between Crohn's disease and ulcerative colitis

Crohn's disease	Ulcerative colitis
It affects ileum and often colon but can involve any part of GIT–rectal sparing is common	It affects rectum and colon from distal to proximal
Full thickness–transmural disease	It affects mucosa and submucosa–not deeper
Skin lesions are typical	Skip lesions are not observed
Granulomatous lesion on histology–deep ulcers; pseudopolyps are not found	Not a granulomatous lesion–superficial ulcers, pseudopolyps are present
Stricture and fistula are common	Narrowing can occur but not very common
Anal fissure and perianal abscess are more common	Fissure and perianal disease can occur but not as common as in Crohn's disease
May mimic appendicitis	Will not mimic appendicitis
Bleeding is not common	Bleeding is common
Fever is common	Fever is uncommon
Mass in RIF is common	Mass is not a common feature

Contd...

FMGE Solutions Screening Examination

Crohn's disease	Ulcerative colitis
• Anal pathology very common	• Anal pathology is rare
• Discontinuous segmental asymmetrical colitis	• Continuous mucosal disease–colitis
• Toxic megacolon is rare	• Toxic megacolon is common
• Normal vascular pattern	• Distorted vascular pattern
• Fistula is very common	• Fistula is uncommon
• Recurrence is common after resection	• Total proctocolectomy cures the disease

Ileocolic intussusception	Sigmoid volvulus	Toxic megacolon
The classic meniscus sign can be seen as an abrupt cut off of barium flow at junction of colon and ileum.	The image shows inner tube bent sign diagnostic of sigmoid volvulus. It is called as coffee bean sign and occurs due to anticlockwise rotation of sigmoid colon	Notice the hugely dilated colonic loops suggestive of toxic megacolon. There is **no** meniscus sign/ Claw sign visualised

27. Ans. (b) pH-metry

Ref: SRB 5th ed. pg. 806-807

Biopsy will be done for diagnosis while CT chest will let us know the extent of spread of cancer. PET scan is done to evaluate response to therapy. It will also help to know involvement of lymph nodes which may be involved but are not picked up on a CT scan. *There is no role of pH monitoring in diagnosis or determining prognosis of carcinoma esophagus.*

28. Ans. (a) Ochsner-Sherren regimen

Ref: SRB 5th ed. pg. 946

The image shows an appendicular mass where nature has already contained the infection. If disturbed it will cause fecal fistula. Hence a conservative approach will be followed.

MANAGEMENT PROTOCOL OF APPENDICULAR MASS

- Use conservative Ochsner-Sherren regime
  - IV fluid
  - NGT
  - Analgesics
  - Antibiotics–parenteral
  - Mark the limits of the mass on the abdominal wall using a skin pencil
  - Monitor-vital sign, size of the mass, input/output chart
  - Clinical improvement is expected in 24–48 hours

29. Ans. (d) Colocolic intussusception

Ref: SRB 5th ed. pg. 932

The image shows a barium enema showing a claw sign and haustrations point to etiology of colocolic intussusception. The geriatric age group also point to the presentation of same.

30. Ans. (d) Refractory fistula

Ref: Harrison 20th ed. pg. 2274

Fistula formation is a feature of Crohn's disease. Choices A, B and C will necessitate surgery.

INDICATIONS OF SURGERY IN ULCERATIVE COLITIS

Ulcerative Colitis
Intractable disease
Fulminant disease
Toxic megacolon
Colonic perforation
Massive colonic hemorrhage
Extracolonic disease
Colonic obstruction
Colon cancer prophylaxis
Colon dysplasia or cancer

31. Ans. (b) Middle 1/3rd

Ref: SRB 5th ed. P 805

In spite of the controversy about the topic, the correct answer is middle 1/3rd.

Surgery

Location of cancer esophagus	Incidence
Middle 1/3rd	50%
Lower 1/3rd	33%
Upper 1/3rd	17%

> **Extra Mile**

Esophageal Cancer

- Barrett esophagus predisposes to development of adenocarcinoma.
- Most Common gross presentation is fungating—cauliflower appearance.
- Recent onset dysplasia is the most common presentation; though for dysphagia to develop 2/3rd of lumen should be obliterated.
- Shouldering sign/irregular filling defect is seen on fluoroscopy in barium meal.
- Biopsy is done for histopathological diagnosis and CT chest for staging.

---

32. Ans. (b) IVF-antibiotic-air enema

Ref: Nelson 20th ed. P 2624;
Bailey and Love 26th ed. P 116

- The clinical presentation is of intussusception and needs urgent hydrostatic reduction.
- Three methods are available for reduction of intussusception by hydrostatic pressure
  - Air enema
  - Microbarium sulfate solution
  - Warm saline
- The complications of all of three methods are gut perforation.
- *Gut perforation rate is least with air enema* provided that the pressure is kept below 120 cm of water above the level of buttocks. Hence Bailey mentions this method before others and thus this is the best answer.
- The success rate of radiological hydrostatic reduction under fluoroscopy or ultrasonic guidance is approximately 80–95.

---

33. Ans. (c) 33%

Ref: Bailey and Love 26th ed. P 1164

- Colorectal cancer is the third most common cancer in the world and liver is the most common site of metastasis. The spread occurs via the portal circulation.
- *Metastatic liver disease is found in* **one third** *of patients having surgery for primary colorectal cancer.*
- 50% *will develop* metastasis in case of colorectal carcinoma in due course of time which leads to death.
- Resection and intra-arterial chemotherapy using 5 FU are therapeutic modalities.

---

34. Ans. (d) Atrophic gastritis

Ref: Harrison 19th ed. P 568

In *atrophic gastritis* the parietal cells are damaged and achlorhydria is present. Hence the feedback mechanism results in increased production of gastrin. *It is the most common cause of hypergastrinemia.*

Causes of Hypergastrinemia

- Atrophic gastritis/pernicious anemia
- Rebound after use of PPI
- Zollinger Ellison syndrome
- Menetrier's disease

---

35. Ans. (c) y

Selected Additional Descriptors Encountered in the TNM Classification

m Symbol	The suffix m, in parentheses, is used to indicate the presence of multiple primary tumors at a single site
y Symbol	In those cases in which classification is performed during or following multimodality therapy. The eTNM or pTNM category is identified by a y prefix **This convention should typically be used following neoadjuvant therapies and may be most applicable to induction chemotherapy**
r Symbol	*Recurrent* tumors, when classified after a disease free interval, are identified by the prefix r
R-Classification	The absence of presence of *residual* tumor after treatment is described by the symbol R as follows RX: Presence of residual tumor cannot be assessed R0: No residual tumor R1: Microscopic residual tumor R2: Macroscopic residual tumor

---

36. Ans. (a) Acute appendicitis

The clinical history and USG image is diagnostic of appendicitis. The appendix lumen is dilated >6 mm and wall is hyperechoic.

Sonographic criteria for acute appendicitis	CT criteria for acute appendicitis
Non compressible appendix of size> 6 mm AP diameter Hyperechoic thickened appendix wall > 2 mm: target sign Appendicolith Interruption of submucosal continuity Peri-appendicular fluid	Thickened caecum funnelling contrast into the orifice of appendix called arrow head sign. Thickened meso-appendix Appendicular phlegmon Fecolith

Explanations

FMGE Solutions Screening Examination

37. Ans. (a) Hypochloremic metabolic alkalosis

- The repeated vomiting episode leads to loss of stomach acid and leads to hypochloraemia.
- Due to fluid loss renal blood flow falls which explains the positive stimulus for RAAS system.
- The increase aldosterone leads to urinary loss of hydrogen and potassium.
- Hence GOO leads to *hypochloraemic hypokalemic metabolic alkalosis.*

38. Ans. (a) Aberrant blood vessel

- Dysphagia lusoria is due to aberrant right subclavian artery. *It is also called arteria lusoria, and is one of the most common intrathoracic arterial anomalies.*
- Although mostly asymptomatic, the retroesophageal and retrotracheal course of the lusorian artery might result in-

> - Unspecific thoracic pain
> - Dysphagia
> - Dyspnea
> - Arterio-esophageal fistula with hematemesis
> - Arterio-tracheal fistulae with haemoptysis
> - Aneurysmal formation with risk of rupture

39. Ans. (d) Ovarian cancer

Ref: Grainger & Allison's Diagnostic Radiology 6th ed. pg. 714

Peritoneal seeding is a common mechanism of metastatic dissemination in advanced gynecological malignancy and GIT malignancy

Peritoneal Carcinomatosis

Site of primary	Percentage
Ovarian cancer	71%
Gastric cancer	17%
Colorectal cancer	10%

- Do remember that if only GIT malignancies are mentioned then the answer is Stomach cancer
- The most common seeding site is pouch of Douglas
- More aggressive neoplasms exhibit peritoneal deposits closer to primary tumor.

40. Ans. (b) Pancreas

Remember the marking shown in CT scan Abdomen as this is a favourite question with National Board.

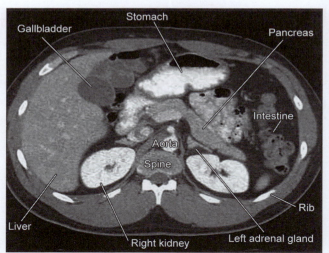

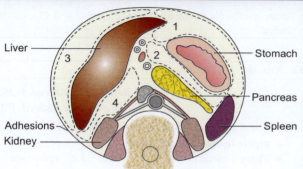

41. Ans. (c) Desmoid tumor

Gardner syndrome is occurrence of familial adenomatous polyposis (FAP) with the extra-colonic manifestations. The polyps in FAP can develop adenocarcinoma colon and hence prophylactic colectomy is performed. Other features seen are

> 1. *Desmoids* or osteomas can cause parietal lumps, obstruction, and bleeding.
> 2. *Dental abnormalities* may develop and may result in jaw pain.
> 3. *Epidermoid cysts* may develop, but they manifest as only cosmetic defects.
> 4. *Gastric polyps* may manifest as epigastric pain or bleeding.
> 5. *Duodenal polyps* may cause pain, bleeding, or jaundice, whereas ileal polyps may cause obstruction.
> 6. *Thyroid carcinoma* (papillary carcinoma) may manifest as a neck mass, hoarseness of voice.

Mnemonic
DAISY **POTS**
Desmoid tumor of abdomen
Polyps
Osteomas
Thyroid cancer
Sebaceous cysts

42. Ans. (b) 3 weeks

Ref: Bailey, 26th ed. pg. 113

- Infantile hypertrophic pyloric stenosis (IHPS) presents with non-bilious projectile vomiting between 2 and 8 weeks of age and is only rarely seen after 13 weeks.
- It is easily distinguished from many other serious causes of vomiting, such as infections because the baby is particularly hungry.
- The non-bilious nature is stressed here to contrast the condition with the bilious vomiting of the potentially life-threatening malrotation and volvulus seen occasionally in neonates.

43. Ans. (b) Esophageal varices

Ref: Bailey, 25th ed. pg. 1043-44

The presence of ascites and dilated veins are suggestive of portal hypertension in a chronic alcoholic. Since patient presents with hematemesis it indicates bleeding esophageal varices for which octreotide infusion should be started with aggressive resuscitation.

44. Ans. (d) Large bore cannula for IVF

Ref: Bailey, 26th ed. pg. 16-17

- The probable clinical diagnosis is portal hypertension with varices
- Volume resuscitation is initiated through *large-bore intravenous lines* with rapid infusion of either isotonic saline (although care must be taken to avoid hyperchloremic acidosis from loss of bicarbonate buffering capacity and replacement with excess chloride) or a balanced salt solution such as Ringer's lactate (being cognizant of the presence of potassium and potential renal dysfunction).

45. Ans. (b) Post-ileal

Ref: Bailey, 26th ed. pg. 1199

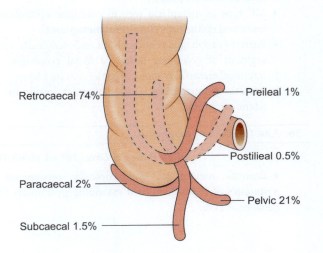

Most common positon of appendix is Retro-caecal 74%
Least common position of appendix is Post-ileal variety

46. Ans. (b) Multiple air fluid levels

Ref: Bailey, 26th ed. pg. 1189

- In intestinal obstruction, fluid levels appear later than gas shadows as it takes time for gas and fluid to separate.
- These are most prominent on an erect film. In adults, two inconstant fluid levels–one at the duodenal cap and the other in the terminal ileum–may be regarded as normal.

47. Ans. (a) 15 cm

Bailey and Love, 26th ed. ch. 62/982

The esophagus has 3 constrictions in its vertical course, as follows:

- **The first constriction is at 15 cm from the upper incisor teeth**, where the esophagus commences at the cricopharyngeal sphincter; this is the narrowest portion of the esophagus and approximately corresponds to the sixth cervical vertebra
- **The second constriction is at 25 cm from the upper incisor teeth,** where it is crossed by the aortic arch and left main bronchus.
- **The third constriction is at 40 cm from the upper incisor teeth,** where it pierces the diaphragm; the lower esophageal sphincter (LES) is situated at this level.

48. Ans. (b) Barium swallow

Ref: Bailey & Love, 26th ed. pg. 989

- Dysphagia is difficulty in swallowing. The cause can be esophageal in origin.
- The motility disorders are best evaluated with esophageal manometry.
  - **Barium swallow:** For esophageal diseases
  - **Barium meal follow through:** Small intestine pathology.
  - **Barium enema:** Colonic and rectal diseases

49. Ans. (d) Metabolic alkalosis

Ref: Bailey & Love, 26th ed. pg. 1018

- In Zenker's diverticulum, the contents of stomach are not lost and therefore metabolic alkalosis cannot occur. *Loss of stomach acid in lieu of reverse peristalsis in chronic vomiting leads to metabolic alkalosis.* When there is excessive pressure within the lower pharynx, the weakest portion of the pharyngeal wall balloons out, forming a diverticulum. Uncoordinated swallowing, impaired relaxation of the cricopharyngeus muscle leads to an increase in pressure within the distal pharynx, so that its wall herniates through the point of least resistance (Killian's triangle).

FMGE Solutions Screening Examination

- Best investigation for Zenker diverticulum is barium swallow and best treatment is surgical resection.

50. Ans. (d) Corkscrew Esophagus

Ref: Bailey & Love, 26th ed. pg. 1014

- Corkscrew esophagus is seen in diffuse esophageal spasm and not in achalasia Cardia.
- **Diffuse esophageal spasm** is a condition in which uncoordinated contractions of the esophagus occur. These spasms do not propel food effectively to the stomach. It can cause dysphagia, regurgitation and chest pain.
- **Esophageal achalasia** is an esophageal motility disorder involving the smooth muscle layer of the esophagus and the lower esophageal sphincter (LES). It is characterized by incomplete LES relaxation, increased LES tone, and lack of peristalsis of esophagus. Diagnosis is reached with esophageal manometry and barium swallow radiographic studies. Permanent relief is brought by Esophageal dilatation and surgical cleaving of the muscle (Heller myotomy).

51. Ans. (b) Normal peristalsis

Ref: Bailey & Love, 26th ed. Ch. 62/1014

- Achalasia is a rare disease caused by loss of inhibitory ganglion cells within the esophageal myenteric plexus
- It leads to a hypertensive lower oesophageal sphincter (LES) which fails to relax on swallowing.
- Long-standing achalasia is characterized by progressive dilatation and sigmoid deformity of the esophagus with hypertrophy of the LES.

Clinical Presentation

- **Progressive dysphagia is the most common presenting symptom. It generally concerns initially liquids and later both liquids and solids from the outset.**
  - **Dysphagia**: Liquids > Solid
- The second most common symptom is the regurgitation of undigested food during or shortly after a meal.

Investigation

- **Screening: Barium study-Bird beak appearance**
- **IOC:** Manometry

Treatment

- **Medical management:**
  - Calcium channel blockers
  - Nitrates
  - Botulinum toxin *(injected into the LES under endoscopic guidance)*

- **Surgical management:**
  - **Harrison states:** *"The only durable therapies for achalasia are **pneumatic dilatation** and **Heller myotomy.**"*
  - **Surgery of choice: Heller's myotomy**

52. Ans. (a) Achalasia Cardia

Please refer to above explanation

53. Ans. (c) Acetylcholine

Ref: Bailey & Love, 26th ed. pg. 988

There are two types of control of LES via the Myenteric plexus:
- Excitatory (cholinergic) ganglionic neurons
- Inhibitory (nitric oxide) ganglionic neurons

Functionally, inhibitory neurons mediate Deglutitive lower esophageal sphincter (LES) relaxation and the sequential propagation of peristalsis.

54. Ans. (c) Tumor infiltration

Ref: Bailey & Love, 26th ed. pg. 1014

- Tumor infiltration, most commonly seen with carcinoma in the gastric fundus or distal esophagus can mimic idiopathic achalasia.
- The resultant "pseudoachalasia" accounts for up to 5% of suspected cases and is more likely with advanced age, abrupt onset of symptoms (<1 year), and weight loss. Hence, endoscopy should be part of the evaluation of achalasia.

55. Ans. (b) Goblet cells intestinal metaplasia

Ref: Sabiston, 19th ed. pg. 1033-36

- Metaplasia of lower esophagus is usually seen in BARRETT'S Esophagus. This condition arises due to severe reflux esophagitis.
- MC type of metaplasia seen in columnar epithelium is intestinal epithelium *(Intestinal metaplasia)*.
- Barrett's esophagus requires both endoscopically visible segment of columnar lining of distal esophagus and *intestinal metaplasia showing goblet cells on biopsy*
- Barret's esophagus is a Premalignant condition for adenocarcinoma

56. Ans. (a) Barrett esophagus

Ref: Bailey & Love, 26th ed. ch 62/1000

- Barrett's metaplasia, endoscopically recognized by tongues of reddish mucosa extending proximally from

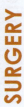

742

the gastroesophageal junction or histopathologically by the finding of specialized columnar metaplasia*(intestinal type with goblet cells),* is associated with at least a 20-fold increased risk for development of **esophageal development of adenocarcinoma.**

57. Ans. (d) De meester scoring

Ranson score	Acute pancreatitis
Gleason score	Prostate cancer
Alvarado score	Acute appendicitis
Di- meester score	GERD

58. Ans. (d) Contrast swallow

Ref: Bailey & Love, 26th ed. pg. 989

- Esophageal perforation causes pleuritic retrosternal pain that can be associated with pneumomediastinum and subcutaneous emphysema.
- Mediastinitis is a major complication of esophageal perforation, and prompt recognition is key to optimizing outcome.
- CT of the chest is most sensitive in detecting mediastinal air, but water soluble contrast (diatrizoate meglumine) will help in determining extravasation.
- *Esophageal perforation is confirmed by a CT with contrast usually Gastrografin followed by thin barium.*
- Treatment includes nasogastric suction and parenteral broad-spectrum antibiotics with prompt surgical drainage and repair in noncontained leaks. Conservative therapy with NPO status and antibiotics without surgery may be appropriate in cases of minor instrumental perforation that are detected early.

59. Ans. (b) Intestine

Ref: Bailey & Love, 26th ed. pg. 973

- Gas under diaphragm sign is seen in case of intestinal perforation. In the above case, patient was stabbed leading to perforation of intestine.
- **MC organ involved in penetrating trauma abdomen**: Intestine.

60. Ans. (b) Barium study

Ref: Bailey & Love, 26th ed. ch. 62/1003

- The symptoms of rolling hernia are mostly due to twisting and distortion of the oesophagus and stomach.
- Dysphagia is common. Chest pain may occur from distension of an obstructed stomach. Classically, the pain is relieved by a loud belch.
- Strangulation, gastric perforation and gangrene can occur.

- The hernia *may be visible* on a plain radiograph of the chest as a gas bubble, often with a fluid level behind the heart.
- *A barium meal is the best method of diagnosis.*
- Symptomatic rolling hernias nearly always require surgical repair as they are potentially dangerous.

61. Ans. (b) Biopsy

Ref: Chapter 91: Harrison, 18th ed.

- Taking multiple biopsies increases the yield. Cytologic examination of tumor brushings complements standard biopsies and should be performed routinely.
- The extent of tumor spread to the mediastinum and para-aortic lymph nodes should be assessed by CT scans of the chest and abdomen and by endoscopic ultrasound.
- Positron emission tomography scanning provides a useful assessment of resectability, offering accurate information regarding spread to mediastinal lymph nodes

62. Ans. (a) Aberrant right subclavian artery

Ref: Bailey & Love, 26th ed. pg. 1022

- During development of aortic arch, if the proximal portion of the right fourth arch disappears instead of distal portion, *the right subclavian artery* will arise as the last branch of aortic arch and is called as aberrant right subclavian artery.
- It then courses behind the esophagus (or rarely in front of esophagus, or even in front of trachea) to supply blood to right arm. This *causes pressure on esophagus and results in dysphagia*. It can sometimes result in upper gastrointestinal tract bleeding

63. Ans. (a) Spontaneous rupture of the esophagus

Ref: Bailey & Love, 26th ed. pg. 992

- Oesophageal rupture in Boerhaave syndrome is thought to be the result of a *sudden rise in internal esophageal pressure produced during vomiting, as a result of neuromuscular incoordination* causing failure of the cricopharyngeus muscle to relax. The syndrome is commonly associated with the consumption of excessive food and/or alcohol as well as eating disorders such as bulimia.
- The *most common anatomical location of the tear in Boerhaave syndrome is at left postero-lateral wall of the lower third of the oesophagus*, 2–3 cm before the stomach
- The most common cause of oesophageal perforation is iatrogenic, which occurs in cervical part of oesophagus.

64. Ans. (d) Bowel lumen obstruction

Ref: Bailey & Love, 26th ed./ch 75 pg. 1201

FMGE Solutions Screening Examination

- Obstruction of the appendix lumen has been widely held to be important, and some form of luminal obstruction, either by a faecolith or a stricture, is found in the majority of cases
- Obstruction of the appendiceal lumen seems to be essential for the development of appendiceal gangrene and perforation.

65. Ans. (d) 1/3 rd distance from the right anterior superior spine

Ref: Bailey & Love, 26th ed. pg. 1203

McBurney's point is the name given to the point over the right side of the abdomen that is *one-third of the distance from the anterior superior iliac spine to the umbilicus*. This point roughly corresponds to the most common location of the base of the appendix where it is attached to the cecum.

66. Ans. (b) Appendicitis

Ref: Bailey & Love, 25th ed. pg. 1208

- The most common symptom of appendicitis is abdominal pain. Typically, symptoms begin as periumbilical or epigastric pain migrating to the right lower quadrant (RLQ) of the abdomen.
- *Patients of appendicitis usually lie down, flex their hips, and draw their knees up to reduce movements* and to avoid worsening their pain. Later, a worsening progressive pain along with vomiting, nausea, and anorexia are described by the patient.
- The duration of symptoms is less than 48 hours in approximately 80% of adults but tends to be longer in elderly persons and in those with perforation.

Clinical Signs in Apppendicitis

- **Rovsing sign** (RLQ pain with palpation of the LLQ): Suggests peritoneal irritation
- **Obturator sign** (RLQ pain with internal and external rotation of the flexed right hip): Suggests the inflamed appendix is located deep in the right hemipelvis
- **Psoas sign** (RLQ pain with extension of the right hip or with flexion of the right hip against resistance): Suggests that an inflamed appendix is located along the course of the right psoas muscle
- **Dunphy sign** (sharp pain in the RLQ elicited by a voluntary cough): Suggests localized peritonitis
- **Markle sign** (pain elicited in a certain area of the abdomen when the standing patient drops from standing on toes to the heels with a jarring landing): Has a sensitivity of 74%

67. Ans. (c) Locate the anterior taenia of the caecum

Ref: Bailey & Love, 26th ed. ch 75/1204

- Three taeniae coli of the caecum, fuse to form the outer longitudinal muscle coat of the appendix.

- During operation, this can be used to find an elusive appendix, as gentle traction on the taeniae coli, particularly the anterior taenia, will lead the operator to the base of the appendix.

68. Ans. (a) Appendix

Ref: Bailey & Love, 26th ed. ch 75/1204

- The base of the appendix can be identified during surgery by following the convergence of the taeniae coli toward the inferior portion of the cecum, forming a continuous muscular layer surrounding the appendix.

The position of the appendicular tip is inconstant and can be situated in the following locations:

- **Retrocecal (65%)** – rigidity is often absent, and even application of deep pressure may fail to elicit tenderness **(Silent appendix)**
- Descending pelvic (31%)
- Transverse and retrocecal (2.5%)
- Ascending, paracecal, and preileal (1%)
- Ascending, paracecal, and postileal (0.4%)

69. Ans. (c) Retro-caecal

Ref: Bailey & Love, 26th ed. Ch 75/1204

70. Ans. (a) Acute appendicitis

Characteristic	Score
M = Migration of pain to the RLQ	1
A = Anorexia	1
N = Nausea and vomiting	1
T = Tenderness in RLQ	2
R = Rebound pain	1
E = Elevated temperature	1
L = Leukocytosis	2
S = Shift of WBCs to the left	1
Total	10

RLQ = right lower quadrant; WBCs = white blood cells

71. Ans. (d) All of the above

Infants	Pre-school Children	School Children
Pyloric Stenosis	Intussusceptions, Meckel's Diverticulitis, Acute Gastroenteritis	The most common mimicker of appendicitis in this population is mesenteric lymphadenitis

Contd...

Adults	Women in their childbearing years	Elderly
Pyelonephritis, Colitis Diverticulitis	(Higher incidence of false-positive diagnoses in this group) Pelvic Inflammatory Disease (PID), Tubo-Ovarian Abscess, Ruptured Ovarian Cyst Or Ovarian Torsion, And Ectopic Pregnancy.	Diverticulitis Bowel Obstruction Malignancies Of The G.I Tract & Reproductive System Perforated Ulcers Cholecystitis

72. Ans. (a) Appendicular mass

Ref: Bailey & Love, 26th ed. pg. 1211

- The appendix that is acutely inflamed may perforate and later wall off from the peritoneal cavity by omentum and adjacent bowel loop to form a tender, palpable right iliac fossa mass. It is a common surgical pathology which occurs in about 2-6% of patients who presented with acute appendicitis.The initial school of thought regards this condition to be managed conservatively, with the famous one being the Ochsner-Sherren regimen. The idea behind this is that, surgery would be hazardous and increase the mortality rate.
- The conservative management of appendicular mass can be summarized by mnemonic "ABCDEF" which is
  - **A:** Analgesic, Antibiotic, antipyretic
  - **B:** Bed rest
  - **C:** Charting (vital sign, size of the mass)
  - **D:** Diet (Keep Nil by Mouth)
  - **E:** Exploratory laparotomy
  - **F:** Fluid maintenance

Three methods are proposed for management of appendicular mass which are:
- Conservative management
- Interval appendectomy
- Early surgical intervention. The selection of methods depends on surgeon preference and patient's condition.

73. Ans. (b) Kulchitsky cell tumor

Ref: Harrison, 18th ed. ch. 350

- Carcinoid tumors arise from argentaffin cells of the crypts of Lieberkühn.
- They are found in distal duodenum to the ascending colon, which are embryologically derived from the midgut.
- *More than **50% of intestinal carcinoids are found in the distal ileum**, with most congregating close to the ileocecal valve.*
- Most intestinal carcinoids are asymptomatic and of low malignant potential, but invasion and metastases may occur, leading to the carcinoid syndrome.

- **Carcinoid tumors are classified as**
  - Typical carcinoid [Kulchitsky cell carcinoma producing 5-HIAA]
  - Atypical carcinoid[producing 5 Hydroxy tryptophan]
- It can be benign or malignant and presents with secretory diarrhea and flushing.
- **Diagnosis** is made by Octreoscan and urinary 5 H.I.A.A (Hydroxy-indole- acetic acid) levels.
- **Drug of choice** is Octreotide.

74. Ans. (a) Ileum

Ref. Harrison, 18th ed. ch 350

Most common site of carcinoid Tumor: Bronchus>ileum >Rectum> appendix

75. Ans. (d) Absence of free gas rules out peritonitis

- The peritoneum, which is a sterile environment, reacts to various pathologic stimuli with a fairly uniform inflammatory response.
- *Primary peritonitis* is most often spontaneous bacterial peritonitis (SBP) caused by chronic liver disease. *Secondary peritonitis* is by far the *most common form of peritonitis* encountered in clinical practice and is most commonly due to PUD. *Tertiary peritonitis* often develops in the absence of the original visceral organ pathology usually in setting of immunocompromised status.
- Chemical (sterile) peritonitis may be caused by irritants such as bile, blood, barium, or other substances or by transmural inflammation of visceral organs (eg, Crohn disease) without bacterial inoculation of the peritoneal cavity. However *bile being alkaline has more irritation than blood.*
- Free air is present in most cases of anterior gastric and duodenal perforation but is much less frequent with perforations of the small bowel and colon and is unusual with appendiceal perforation. Upright films are useful for identifying free air under the diaphragm (most often on the right) as an indication of a perforated viscus.

Remember
- The free gas appears about 1-2 hours after the perforation of bowel
- *Absence of free gas in the peritoneal cavity does not necessarily exclude presence of perforation as it is absent in approximately 25 % cases of perforated duodenal ulcer.*

76. Ans. (c) Anaerobic streptococcus

Ref: Harrison, 19th ed. pg. 972

MICROORGANISMS IN PERITONITIS

Gastrointestinal Sources
- *Escherichia coli*
- *Streptococci(anaerobic)*

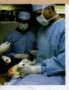

FMGE Solutions Screening Examination

- *Bacteroides*
- *Clostridium*
- *Klebsiella pneumoniae*

Other Sources
- *Chlamydia trachomatis*
- *Neisseria gonorrhoeae*
- *Haemolytic streptococci*
- *Staphylococcus*
- *Streptococcus pneumonia*
- *Mycobacterium tuberculosis* and other spp.
- Fungal infections

77. Ans. (c) Chlamydia

Ref: Harrison, 19th ed. pg. 972

Paths to Peritoneal Infection
- Gastrointestinal perforation, e.g. perforated ulcer, appendix, diverticulum
- Transmural translocation (no perforation), e.g. pancreatitis, ischaemic bowel
- Exogenous contamination, e.g. drains, open surgery, trauma
- *Female genital tract infection, e.g. pelvic inflammatory disease with chylamydia*
- Haematogenous spread (rare), e.g. septicaemia

78. Ans. (b) Sarcoma

Ref: Bailey and Love, 26th ed. ch. 61/985

- One third of malignant tumors that arise in the retroperitoneum are sarcomas, and approximately 15% of soft tissue sarcomas arise in the retroperitoneum.
- Retroperitoneal sarcomas are malignant tumors arising from mesenchymal cells, which are usually located in muscle, fat, and connective tissues. Retroperitoneal sarcomas have varying clinical courses depending on their histologic subtype and grade.

79. Ans. (d) Abdominal lump

Ref: Bailey and Love, 26th ed. ch. 61/985

- Primary retroperitoneal neoplasms are an extremely rare group of tumors (lymphoma is not included in the definition). **The most common type is soft tissue sarcoma (90%).**
- The commonest age range for presentation is around 40–50 years.
- *Sarcomas that arise in the retroperitoneum most commonly present as an abdominal mass, often without other symptoms.*
- Early satiety, gastrointestinal obstruction or bleeding, lower extremity swelling, or pain are among the first symptoms leading to the discovery of a retroperitoneal sarcoma.
- **Investigation:** CT is the most commonly used tool. MRI can be used for further differentiation, but histology is always required. Percutaneous biopsy may be undertaken and for assessment of tumor grade.

80. Ans. (c) Villous adenoma

Ref: Bailey & Love, 26th ed. pg. 1184

ADULT INTUSSCEPTION

- Bowel intussusception in adults is considered a rare condition, accounting for 1%-5% of bowel obstruction.
- Adult cases of intussusception are associated with a lead point which is:
  1. Polyp
  2. Submucosal lipoma
  3. Inflammatory bowel disease
  4. Postoperative adhesions
  5. Meckel's diverticulum
  6. Villous adenoma
  7. Metastatic neoplasms
  8. Iatrogenically, due to the presence of intestinal tubes, jejunostomy feeding tubes or after gastric surgery.

Most common cause of pediatric intussusception is Meckel's diverticulum>polyp.

81. Ans. (d) Pneumatosis intestinalis

Ref: Bailey & Love, 26th ed. pg. 1189

- Plain film radiographs of the abdomen in supine poistion can be helpful in diagnosing small bowel obstruction.
- An upright chest radiograph is best for ruling out free air under the diaphragm.
- Signs of small bowel obstruction include:
  - Bowel dilatation proximal to the site of obstruction, air–fluid levels
  - Paucity of large bowel gas, bowel wall thickening
  - A fixed loop
  - Ground glass appearance signifying intraluminal fluid.
  - Although the cecum may dilate greatly in chronic obstruction without rupturing, perforation should be suspected whenever this portion of the colon is greater than 10 cm in diameter.
- Step ladder pattern of air fluid levels.

82. Ans. (b) Resection with intestine part

Ref: Bailey & Love, 26th ed. pg. 903

- Enterogenous cyst arises from either a diverticulum of the mesentric border of the intestine that has become sequestrated from the intestinal canal during embryonic life or from a duplication of the intestine.
- An enterogenous cyst has a thicker wall than a chylolymphatic cyst and is lined by mucous membrane, sometimes ciliated.
- The content is mucinous and is either colorless or yellowish brown as a result of past haemorrhage. The

Surgery

muscle in the wall of an entric duplication cyst and the bowl with which it is in contact have a common blood supply, *consequently removal of the cyst always entails resection of the related portion of intestine.*

83. Ans. (a) Anastomotic leak

Ref: Bailey & Love, 26th ed. pg. 1150; Advances in Minimally Invasive Surgery, 2nd ed. pg. 250

Anastomotic leak is one of the most dreaded early complications of colorectal surgery. The incidence of anastomotic leak following colectomy is generally reported between 2 and 6%. Anastomotic leaks present in one of three ways.

1. Asymptomatic leak
2. Subtle insidious leak
3. Dramatic early leak

The *asymptomatic leak* is incidentally found during endoscopic or radiographic studies. The incidence of radiographically detected leaks is 4-6 times higher than clinically detected leaks. The *subtle insidious leak* can present peri-operatively with nonspecific signs and symptoms common in the post operative period, and occur 5-14 days following surgery. The *dramatic early leak* can present with any combination of acute abdominal pain, distention, fever, tachycardia, diffuse peritonitis, oliguria, or shock within several days of surgery.

84. Ans. (c) Bilious vomiting

Ref: Sabiston, 19th ed. pg. 1841

- In HPS, hypertrophy of the circular muscle of the pylorus results in constriction and obstruction of the gastric outlet.
- Most commonly clinical presentation is seen between 3-6 weeks of life
- *Clinical features:*
- *Projectile nonbilious vomiting*
- Visible gastric peristalsis may be seen as a wave of contraction from the left upper quadrant to the epigastrium
- The infants usually feed vigorously between episodes of vomiting
- **Typical electrolyte abnormality**: **Hypochloremic, hypokalemic, metabolic alkalosis with paradoxical aciduria.**
- **Remember:** Hypokalemic metabolic acidosis is seen with diarrhea.

Why metabolic alkalosis and paradoxical aciduria?

- Loss of stomach contents will lead to dehydration. This will trigger the R.A.A.S system into an overdrive and lead to release of aldosterone. Since aldosterone leads to potassium and hydrogen loss in the DCT of the kidney,

patient will develop hypokalemic metabolic alkalosis and aciduria (paradoxically)

85. Ans. (b) Hypokalemic metabolic alkalosis

Ref: Bailey & Love, 26th ed. ch 63/1023

86. Ans. (b) Metabolic alkalosis

Please refer to above explanation

87. Ans. (d) Hyperplastic polyp

Ref: Bailey & Love, 26th ed. pg. 1224

Inflammatory polyp	Seen in ulcerative colitis and crohn's disease, and can turn malignant
Familial adenomatous polyposis	- <1% of all colorectal cancers. - Autosomal dominant - > 100 colorectal adenomas, caused by germ-line mutations of the tumor suppressor gene APC
Hamartomatous polyp	They are growths, like tumors found in organs as a result of faulty development. Hamartomatous polyps are seen in Peutz-Jegher Syndrome or Juvenile Polyposis Syndrome.
Hyperplastic polyp	Most common colonic polyps - Quite small - Composed of cells showing dysmaturation and hyperplasia - *No neoplastic potential, but some might have adenomatous changes and should be excised for histopathology.*

88. Ans. (d) Toxic megacolon

Ref: Bailey & Love, 26th ed. pg. 1156

Indications for Surgery in Crohn's Disease

- **Small Intestine**
  - Stricture and obstruction unresponsive to medical therapy
  - *Massive hemorrhage*
  - *Refractory fistula*
  - Abscess
- **Colon and rectum**
- **Intractable disease**
  - Fulminant disease
  - Perianal disease unresponsive to medical therapy
  - Refractory fistula
  - *Colonic obstruction*
  - Cancer prophylaxis
  - Colon dysplasia or cancer

Explanations

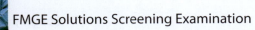

FMGE Solutions Screening Examination

89. Ans. (a) Juvenile rectal polyp

Ref: Bailey & Love, 26th ed. pg. 1224

The most common cause of bleeding per rectum in children is juvenile rectal polyp up to adolescence age. Though in infants and young children (up to 1 yrs) the cause is anal fissure.

90. Ans. (b) Necrosis

Ref: Bailey & Love, 26th ed. pg. 1150

Complications of Ileostomy

Stoma necrosis may occur in the early postoperative period and usually is caused by skeletonizing the distal small bowel and/or creating an overly tight fascial defect.

91. Ans. (a) B12

Ref: Harrison, 18th ed. ch. 294

- Post resection of ileum, vitamin B12 deficiency is seen.
- Steatorrhea is fat malabsorption leading to malodorous stools. Fat malabsorption leads to deficiency of vitamin A, D, E, K.

92. Ans. (a) Ascites

Ref: Bailey & Love, 26th ed. pg. 980

- A peritoneo-venous shunt (also called Denver shunt) is a shunt which drains peritoneal fluid from the peritoneum into veins, usually the internal jugular vein or the superiorvena cava.
- It is sometimes used in patients with refractory ascites.
- It is a long tube with a non-return valve running subcutaneously from the peritoneum to the internal jugular vein in the neck, which flows ascitic fluid to pass directly into the systemic circulation.

93. Ans. (a) IBS

Ref: Bailey & Love, 26th ed. pg. 1179

The Rome criteria is a system developed to classify the functional gastrointestinal disorders (FGIDs), disorders of the digestive system in which symptoms cannot be explained by the presence of structural or tissue abnormality, based on clinical symptoms. *Some examples of FGIDs include irritable bowel syndrome, functional dyspepsia, functional constipation, and functional heart burn.*

94. Ans. (b) Malnutrition

Ref: Bailey & Love, 26th ed. pg. 1134

CHRONIC TROPICAL PANCREATITIS

- Most common cause of chronic pancreatitis is alcohol intake
- *Non alcoholic form of chronic pancreatitis* prevalent in the tropics like Africa, asia and India
- Diabetic stage of the disease referred to as fibrocalculous pancreatic diabetes
- **Etiology:** Malnutrition, cyanogens toxicity (present in insufficiently processed cassava), antioxidant def. and genetic factors
- **Classical triad:** steatorrea, diabetes, abdominal pain
- **Main treatment:** management of diabetes
- **Main cause of death:** complications of diabetes (MC diabetic nephropathy)

95. Ans. (c) RANSON Score

Ref: Bailey & Love, 26th ed. pg. 1128

RANSON CRITERIA

At Admission
- Age in years > 55 years
- White blood cell count > 16000 cells/mm^3
- Blood glucose > 10 mmol/L (> 200 mg/dL)
- Serum AST > 250 IU/L
- Serum LDH > 350 IU/L

Within 48 hours
- Serum calcium < 2.0 mmol/L (< 8.0 mg/dL)
- Hematocrit fall > 10%
- Oxygen (hypoxemia PO$_2$ < 60 mm Hg)
- BUN increased by 1.8 or more mmol/L (5 or more mg/dL) after IV fluid hydration
- Base deficit (negative base excess) > 4 mEq/L
- Sequestration of fluids > 6 L

Alternatively, Pancreatitis severity can be assessed by any of the following:
- APACHE II score ≥ 8
- **CT Scan** - Substantial pancreatic necrosis (at least 30% glandular necrosis according to contrast-enhanced CT)

96. Ans. (a) Serum bilirubin

Ref: Bailey & Love, 26th ed. pg. 1128

APACHE score is: Acute Physiology and Chronic Health Evaluation

The APACHE II point score is calculated from 12 routine physiological measurements:
- Age
- Temperature (rectal)
- Mean arterial pressure
- pH arterial
- Heart rate
- Respiratory rate
- Sodium (serum)
- Potassium (serum)

Surgery

- Creatinine
- Hematocrit
- White blood cell count
- Glasgow Coma Scale

Extra Mile

- Now APACHE III is also available. The APACHE III is used to produce an equation predicting hospital mortality after the first day of ICU treatment.
- **There are 4 components:** Age, Major disease category (reason for ICU admission), Acute (current) physiology, and Prior site of healthcare (e.g. hospital floor, emergency room, etc.).

97. Ans. (a)   Acute pancreatitis

Ref: Schwartz's, 9th ed. pg. 1352

Complications of ERCP

1. *Pancreatitis is the most common ERCP complication.* Transient increase in serum pancreatic enzymes may occur in as many as 75% of patients.
2. Most ERCP-associated *bleeding* is intraluminal, although intra-ductal bleeding can occur.
3. *Post-ERCP cholangitis.*
4. Cardiopulmonary complications
5. Duodenal hematotma
6. Colonic perforation
7. Cardiopulmonary complications

98. Ans. (a) Neurofibromatosis

- **Neurofibromatosis type 1**/von Recklinghausen disease caused by inherited gene, the NF1 gene codes for the protein neurofibromin.
- Patients with neurofibromatosis develop café-au-lait spots, and benign and malignant tumors of the nervous system.
- Benign nervous system involvement include neurofibromas, and the malignant include peripheral nerve sheath tumor.
- *They can also develop distinctive eye lesions called Lisch nodules, which are iris hamartomas*
- The *most common cause of death is CNS tumors.*

Extra Mile

- Turcot syndrome is characterized by intestinal polyposis and CNS tumors: Most commonly glioblastoma or medulloblastoma
- MEN2A sipple consists of parathyroid adenoma, medullary carcinoma thyroid, phaeochromocytoma.

99. Ans. (a)   Duodeno-Duodenostomy

Ref: Bailey & Love, 26th ed. pg. 1194

- Duodenal atresia and stenosis are treated surgically. In patients with duodenal obstruction, a duodenoduodenostomy is the most commonly performed procedure.

- *A duodenojejunostomy is now rarely performed due to its higher risk of long-term complications.*
- Presenting symptoms and signs are the result of high intestinal obstruction. Duodenal atresia is typically characterized by onset of vomiting within hours of birth. While vomitus is most often bilious, it may be non-bilious because 15% of defects occur proximal to the ampulla of Vater.

100. Ans. (b)   Splenosis

Ref: Bailey & Love, 26th ed. pg. 1095-96

Complications of Splenectomy:

- Intraoperative complications:
  - Pancreatic injury
  - Hemorrhage
  - Bowel injury: Colon and stomach
  - Diaphragmatic injuries
- Early post op complications
  - *Pulmonary: Atelectasis, pleural effusion, pneumonitis*
  - *Sub phrenic abscess*
  - Thrombocytopenia and *thrombotic complications*
  - Wound problems
  - Ileus
- Late post op complications:
  - Over whelming post splenectomy infection
  - Splenosis

Splenosis occurs due to seeding of peritoneal cavity with splenic tissue which recruits local blood supply.

101. Ans. (d)   All of the above

Post Vagotomy Complications:

1. **Post vagotomy diarrhea:**
   - About 30% or more of patients suffer from diarrhea after gastric surgery.
2. **Post vagotomy gastric atony:**
   - After vagotomy, gastric emptying is delayed. This is true for both truncal and selective vagotomies but not in the case of highly selective or parietal cell vagotomy.
   - With selective or truncal vagotomy, patients lose antral pump function and therefore have a reduction in their ability to empty solids
3. **Incomplete Vagal Transaction:**
   - It predisposes the patient to the possible development of recurrent ulcer formation. The type of vagotomy performed influences the likelihood of this problem.
   - In highly selective vagotomy, incomplete vagotomy is rarely a problem because of the meticulous dissection required during this procedure.

102. Ans. (c)   Ogilvie's syndrome

Ref: Bailey & Love, 26th ed. pg. 1198

Explanations

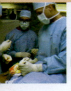

- Pseudo-obstruction of the colon is called as ogilvie's syndrome which is characterized by distention of the colon, with signs and symptoms of colonic obstruction, in the absence of an actual physical cause of the obstruction.
- Mirizzi syndrome is a gallstone becoming impacted in cystic duct or neck of gallbladder causing compression of CBD and resultant obstructive Jaundice.

103. Ans. (b) Lesser curvature

Ref: Bailey & Love, 26th ed. pg. 1034

Most peptic ulcers are caused by *H. pylori* or NSAIDs with lesser curvature being the most common site of gastric ulcer and duodenal cap being the site of duodenal ulcer.

104. Ans. (d) Lesser sac

Ref: Bailey & Love, 26th ed. pg. 1041

Posterior perforation of peptic ulcer leads to escape of contents to enter into lesser sac via foramen of Winslow. Posterior gastric ulcers may erode into the lesser sac behind the stomach. The lesser sac behind the stomach is a potential space and is less effective in sealing off a posteriorly situated gastric ulcer eroding through the wall of the stomach.

105. Ans. (a) Acute pancreatitis

Ref: Bailey & Love, 26th ed. ch. 313

- Purtscher-like retinopathy is seen in:

1. Acute pancreatitis
2. Fat embolization
3. Amniotic fluid embolization
4. Preeclampsia
5. Hemolysis
6. Elevated liver enzymes, and low platelets (HELLP) syndrome; and vasculitic diseases, such as lupus.

- The findings of white lesions in the retina associated with intraretinal and pre-retinal hemorrhages and papillitis are due to lymphatic extravasation from trauma. These lesions are known as Purtscherflecken (larger infarcts of the retinal capillary bed) and cotton-wool spots (small retinal microinfarcts at the level of the nerve fiber layer).
- No proven treatment exists for Purtscher retinopathy that occurs after traumatic injury.

106. Ans. (b) Autoimmune

Ref: Bailey & Love, 26th ed. pg. 1031

- Autoimmune metaplastic atrophic gastritis is an autoimmune disease that attacks parietal cells, resulting in hypochlorhydria and reduced production of intrinsic factor. Consequences include atrophic gastritis, B_{12} malabsorption, and, frequently, pernicious anemia. Risk of gastric adenocarcinoma increases 3-fold. Diagnosis is by endoscopy. Treatment is with B_{12}.
- Type B, or antral-predominant, gastritis is caused by *H. pylori* infection.
- The number of *H. pylori* organisms decreases dramatically with progression to gastric atrophy, and the degree of inflammation correlates with the level of these organisms.
- Early on, with antral-predominant findings, the quantity of *H. pylori* is highest and a dense chronic inflammatory infiltrate of the lamina propria is noted, accompanied by epithelial cell infiltration with Polymorphonuclear leukocytes

107. Ans. (a) Stomach

- Primary **gastric lymphoma** is an uncommon condition, accounting for less than 15% of gastric malignancies and about 2% of all lymphomas. However, the stomach is a very common extranodal site for lymphomas (lymphomas originating somewhere else with metastasis to stomach). It is also the most common source of lymphomas in the gastrointestinal tract.

108. Ans. (d) Stomach CA

Ref: Bailey & Love, 26th ed. ch 63/1050

- Tumor of the stomach may spread via the abdominal cavity to the umbilicus (Sister Joseph's nodule).
- The ovaries may sometimes be the sole site of transcoelomic spread (Krukenberg's tumors).

109. Ans. (b) Stomach

Ref: Bailey & Love, 26th ed. ch 63/1050

110. Ans. (d) Right side of the colon in adults

Ref: Bailey & Love, 26th ed. Ch 69/1171

- *Angiodysplasia is a degenerative lesion of previously healthy blood vessels found most commonly in the cecum and proximal ascending colon.*
- 77% of angiodysplasias are located in the cecum and ascending colon, 15% are located in the jejunum and ileum, and the remainder are distributed throughout the alimentary tract. These lesions typically are non-palpable and small (< 5 mm).
- **Angiodysplasia is the most common vascular abnormality of the GI tract.** After diverticulosis, it is the second leading cause of lower GI bleeding in patients older than 60 years.

111. Ans. (d) Epidermoid

Ref: Schwartz, 9th ed. pg. 1277, Sabiston, 19th ed. pg. 1104-05

Surgery

Types of mesenteric cyst	Features
1. Chylolymphatic cyst	MC age for mesenteric cyst-2nd decade of life
2. Simple (mesothelial cyst)	MC in women
	C/F: painless abdomen swelling>recurrent attack of abdomen pain without vomiting>acute abdomen(torsion,rupture. hrage, infection)
3. Enterogenous	
4. Urogenital remnant	
5. Dermoid	
Diagnosis of mesenteric cyst	CT scan is IOC
Chylolymphatic mesenteric cyst	**Most common type** • Arise from misplaced lymphatic tissue • Located at mesentry of ileum • Thin walled,with clear fluid(pic above) • Unilocular,solitary • Blood supply independent
Treatment of choice	**Chylolymphatic- Enucleation** **Enterogenous- Resection and anastomosis**

112. Ans. (b) Chylolymphatic cyst

Ref: Schwartz, 9th ed./1277, Sabiston 19th ed./1104-05

113. Ans. (c) Chronic diarrhea

- *Immunoproliferative small intestinal disease* (IPSID),is a B cell tumor.
- The presentation includes chronic diarrhea, steatorrhea associated with vomiting and abdominal cramps.
- IPSID presents with intestinal secretions of an abnormal IgA that contains a shortened heavy chain and is devoid of light chains.
- The clinical course is one of exacerbations and remissions, with death due to malnutrition and wasting or the development of a lymphoma.

114. Ans. (a) Digital positioning

Ref: Bailey & Love, 26th ed. pg. 1220

- Patients who present with a prolapsed rectum should undergo manual reduction. Conservative management is appropriate in selected patients. Treatment should be directed to the underlying cause. After treating the underlying cause, conservative management is usually successful.
- The prolapsed bowel may be grasped with lubricated gloved fingers and pushed back in with gentle steady pressure. If the bowel has become edematous, firm

steady pressure for several minutes may be necessary to reduce the swelling and allow for reduction. If the prolapse immediately recurs, it may be reduced again and the buttocks taped together for several hours.

- However, if the prolapse persists after an adequate trial of medical therapy (usually a period of months), surgical intervention may be required. Pain, excoriations, and rectal bleeding are considered indications for surgical treatment.

115. Ans. (c) Fistula in ano

Ref: Bailey & Love, 26th ed. pg. 1259

Causes of Acute Anal Pain

1. Thrombosed hemorrhoids
   - **External hemorrhoids** are located distal to the dentate line and are covered with anoderm. Because the anoderm is richly innervated, thrombosis of an external hemorrhoid **may cause significant pain.**
2. Acute anal fissure
   - Characteristic symptoms include tearing pain with defecation and hematochezia (usually described as blood on the toilet paper)
3. Perianal abccess
   - Severe anal pain is the most common presenting complaint. Walking, coughing, or straining can aggravate the pain.

Fistula in ano presents with

Patients usually complain of intermittent purulent discharge (which may be bloody). Schwartz's 9th ed and oxford textbook of surgery do not mention pain as a feature of fistula in ano

116. Ans. (a) Purulent discharge with bleeding

Ref: Bailey & Love, 26th ed. pg. 1259

- A fistula-in-ano is an abnormal tract with external opening in the perianal area and communicates with the rectum or anal canal by an identifiable internal opening. Fistulas arise as a result of cryptoglandular infection with resultant perirectal abscess.
- The patient may present with recurrent perianal abscesses or with a bloody and purulent discharge.

117. Ans. (b) Anterior and posterior fistula

Ref: Bailey & Love, 26th ed. pg. 1260

- Goodsall's rule used to *indicate the likely position of the internal opening* according to the position of the external opening(s).
- The site of the internal opening may be felt as a point of induration or seen as an enlarged papilla. Whenever possible, it is important to determine by examination the level of the internal opening in relation to the levator mechanism.

Explanations

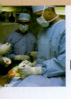

FMGE Solutions Screening Examination

- Goodsall's law indicates that fistulas with an *anterior external opening, drain directly into the anus at the dentate line*, and those with a posterior external opening take a curved course to enter the anal canal in the midline.

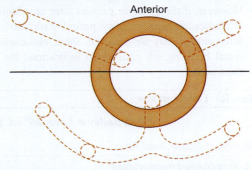

118. Ans. (b) Squamous cell CA

Ref: Sabiston, 19th ed. pg. 1405-06

▌CARCINOMA ANAL CANAL

- Carcinomas arising proximal to the (dentate line) pectinate line are known as **basaloid,** *cuboidal,* or *cloacogenic* tumors; **about one-third of anal cancers have this histologic pattern.**
- Malignancies arising distal to the pectinate line have **squamous histology,** ulcerate more frequently, and **constitute 55% of anal cancer**
  - MC type of CA anal canal: Squamous cell CA > BCC > Melanoma
  - Median age at diagnosis: 60 years
  - MC symptom: Bleeding PR
  - MC site of metastasis: Lung
  - MC site of LN metastasis: Inguinal LNs

Clinical Features of anal Canal CA
- Most patients present with rectal bleeding and pain
- Patients are frequently misdiagnosed as having a benign anorectal condition such as hemorrhoids.
- **Additional symptoms:** Incontinence, change in bowel habits, pelvic pain, and rectovaginal or rectovesical fistulas are ominous.

Diagnosis: IOC for diagnosis of CA anal canal: Proctoscopy with biopsy.

Treatment
- **Nigro regimen:** Chemoradiation is the treatment of choice.
- **Chemotherapy regime:** 5-FU + Mitomycin, Cisplatin
- More than 80% are cured by chemoradiation. If any residual tumor is left behind after chemoradiation, APR is performed.

119. Ans. (a) Squamous

Ref: Bailey & Love, 26th ed. pg. 1267

120. Ans. (a) Human papilloma virus

Ref: Bailey & Love, 26th ed. pg. 1266

- The development of anal cancer is associated with infection by human papilloma virus.
- The infection may lead to:
  - Anal warts (condyloma acuminata)
  - Anal intraepithelial neoplasia
  - Squamous cell carcinoma.
- The risk for anal cancer is increased among homosexual males.
- Anal cancer risk is increased in both men and women with AIDS, because of their immunosuppressed state

121. Ans. (b) Liver

Ref: Bailey & Love, 26th ed. pg. 1226

- Cancers of the colon spread to regional lymph nodes or to the liver through the portal venous circulation.
- *The liver represents the most frequent visceral site of metastasis.*
- Colorectal cancer rarely spreads to the lungs, supraclavicular lymph nodes, bone, or brain without prior spread to the liver.

122. Ans. (a) Rectal prolapse

Ref: Bailey & Love, 26th ed. pg. 1220

- The image shows a rectal prolapse which is a sliding hernia through a defect in the pelvic fascia.

123. Ans. (b) Urine retention

Ref: Bailey & Love, 26th ed. pg. 1256

- Urinary retention is a common complication following hemorrhoidectomy and occurs in 10% to 50% of patients. Many factors are thought to contribute to urinary retention following hemorrhoidectomy, with pain being a major contributor.
- Bleeding is often minor and can be stopped with local pressure.
- Chronic complications include
  - Poor wound healing
  - Abscess
  - Healing
  - Anal stenosis

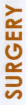

124. **Ans. (a)** 1/3rd above the dentate line and 2/3rd below the dentate line

Ref: Bailey & Love 26th ed./1237

- The anal canal is completely extraperitoneal.
- The length of the (surgical) anal canal is about 4 cm (range, 3–5 cm), with *two thirds of this being above the dentate line and one third below the dentate line (the anatomical anal canal).*
- The epithelium of the (anatomical) anal canal is called anoderm. It is pigmented and keratinised.
- In anatomy texts, the rectum changes to the anal canal at the dentate line. *For surgeons, however, the demarcation between the rectum above and the anal canal below is the anorectal ring.*
- The anorectal ring is situated about 5 cm from anus. At the anorectal angle, the rectum turns backwards to continue as the anal canal

125. **Ans. (a)** Anterior border is formed by inferior fascia of urogenital diaphragm.

Ref: IB Singh Anatomy, 2nd ed./fig. 25.12

ANTERIOR	POSTERIOR	
• Fascia of Colles covering the Transversus perinei superficialis • Inferior fascia of the urogenital diaphragm	• Gluteus maximus • Sacrotuberous ligament	
LATERAL	SUPERIOR	MEDIAL
• Tuberosity of the ischium • Obturator internus muscle • Obturator fascia	• Levator ani **INFERIOR** • Skin	• Levator ani • Sphincter ani externus muscle • Anal fascia

126. **Ans. (d)** Solitary Ascariasis in the bowel

Ref: Bailey & Love, 26th ed. pg. 71

- The image shows a round worm in the bowel.
- While roundworms most commonly reside in the jejunal and ileal lumen, on occasion they may migrate into the duodenum and ampullary orifice.
- While intestinal obstruction is more common in children, adults experience allergic reactions more frequently.

BREAST

127. **Ans. (c)** Nipple

Ref: SRB 5th ed. pg. 543

Sentinel lymph node is localised by pre-operative (within 12 hours) or perioperative injection of isosulfan vital blue or 99m TC radioisotope labelled albumin *near the tumour or into subdermal plexus around the nipple.* Marker will pass into the sentinel node which can be visually detected as blue staining or with hand held gamma camera. It is biopsied with small incision made directly overt it. Frozen section biopsy or touch imprint cytology is done for presence of malignant cells.
Combined approach using Radioisotope Peritumoral injection is done on day of surgery and perioperative injection of patent blue dye in sub-areolar region is used nowadays.

128. **Ans. (c)** Eczema of skin of nipple

Ref: SRB 5th ed. pg. 533

- Paget's disease of the nipple is an intraductal carcinoma of breast. The malignancy spreads within the duct up to the skin of nipple and down into the substance of breast. It mimics eczema of nipple and areola.
- The disease presents as a hard nodule underneath the areola which later ulcerates and causes destruction of nipple. It contains large ovoid clear Paget cells with malignant features.
- Choice C, mastitis carcinomatosis is alternative name for inflammatory carcinoma and is the most aggressive breast cancer.
- Choice D is seen in elderly females and is a slow growing tumour with better prognosis.

129. **Ans. (a)** Fibroadenoma

Ref: SRB 5th ed. pg. 516

The most common benign encapsulated tumour of breast is called as fibroadenoma. It is classified as hyperplasia of single lobule of breast. On mammography is shows a popcorn calcification. Excision is via sub-mammary or circumareolar incision.

130. **Ans. (b)** Axillary sampling

Ref: SRB: 5th ed. pg. 545

Axillary sampling is done after axillary incision and 10-15 nodes are removed for sampling. It is not done now. Triple assessment technique includes choices A, C and D

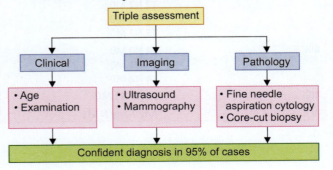

131. Ans. (a) Patient's decision

Ref: SRB 5th ed. P 517

Indications for surgery in Fibroadenoma are:

1. Size >3 cm
2. Multiple
3. Giant type
4. Recurrence
5. Cosmesis
6. Complex type

- *Fibroadenoma which is small (size <3 cm), single lesion and patient's age <30 years can be left alone with regular follow-up with USG at 6 monthly interval.*
- 30% fibroadenomas may disappear or reduce in size over 2–4 years.
- Complex fibroadenoma is a variant of typical fibroadenoma with fibrocystic changes, apocrine metaplasia, cyst formation, sclerosing adenosis. It occurs in old age and occasionally may turn malignant.
- Juvenile fibroadenoma which occurs at young age never turns malignant.

132. Ans. (b) Stage II

Ref: Harrison 19th ed. P 540

- Since size of tumor is 4 cm, it belongs to T2 stage.
- On account of no nodal involvement or distal metastasis the TNM status is T2N0M0. Hence it is stage IIA as per the staging giving below.

Stage Groups

Stage	TNM status
0	Tis N0 M0
IA	T1/T1 mi N0 M0
IB	T0/T1 mi M0
	T1/T1 mi N1 mi M0
IIA	T0 N1 M0
	T1 N1 M0
	T2 N0 M0
IIB	T2 N1 M0
	T3 N0 M0
IIIA	T0 N2 M0
	T1 N2 M0
	T2 N2 M0
	T3 N1 M0
	T3 N2 M0
IIIB	T4 N0 M0
	T4 N1 M0
	T4 N2 M0
IIIC	Any T N3 M0
IV	Any T any N M1

133. Ans. (b) T4B

THE TNM STAGING OF CARCINOMA BREAST (AJCC 7TH EDITION, 2010 PAGE 539: SRB)

T1- Tumor less than 2 cm (20 mm)

T1 mi – Microinvasion 1 mm or less in greatest dimension

T1a – 1–5 mm

T1b – 5–10 mm

T1c – 10–20 mm

T2 – 20–50 mm in greatest dimension

T3 - > 50 mm in greatest dimension

T4 – Any size with direct extension to the chest wall or skin or both.

T4a – Tumor of any size extending into the chest wall, not including only pectoralis muscle invasion/adhesion (Chest wall means ribs, intercostal muscles and serratus anterior but not pectoral muscles).

T4b – *Ulceration or ipsilateral satellite nodules and/or oedema including peaud'orange of the skin which don't meet the criteria for inflammatory carcinoma.*

T4c – T4a and T4b.

T4d – Inflammatory carcinoma

134. Ans. (c) T3

Refer to the explanation of the above question.

135. Ans. (b) Breast cancer

The mammography image shows *mass lesion with surrounding area micro-calcification* diagnostic of a breast cancer. The popcorn lesion will appear as a discrete lesion.

136. Ans. (c) Upper outer

Ref: Bailey, 26th ed. pg. 811

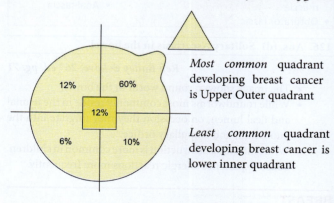

Most common quadrant developing breast cancer is Upper Outer quadrant

Least common quadrant developing breast cancer is lower inner quadrant

137. Ans. (a) BRCA1

Ref: Harsh Mohan Text book of Pathology, 7th ed. pg. 207

Incidence of sporadic, familial and hereditary breast cancer

BRCA1	45%
BRCA2	35%
p 53	1%
STK11	<1%
Sporadic breast cancer	65-75%
Familial breast cancer	20-30%
Hereditary breast cancer	5-10%

138. Ans. (a) Anterior axillary

Ref: Chapter 44: Vishram Singh Anatomy: Volume 1

- Deep lymphatics drain the breast parenchyma and skin of nipple and areola.
- The Nipple and areola drains to the sub-areolar lymphatic plexus of Sappey.
- Most of this drainage occurs to anterior axillary group of lymph nodes.

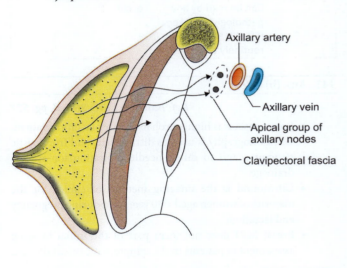

139. Ans. (a) Duct ectasia

Ref: Bailey, 26th ed. pg. 802

Causes of breast discharge

Discharge from the surface
• Paget's disease
• Skin diseases (eczema, psoriasis)
• Rare causes (e.g. chancre)
Discharge from a single duct
• Blood-stained
Intraduct papilloma
Intraduct carcinoma
Duct ectasia

Contd...

Discharge from the surface
• Serous (any color)
Fibrocystic disease
Duct ectasia
Carcinoma
Discharge from more than one duct
• Blood-stained
Carcinoma
Ectasia
Fibrocystic disease
• Black or green
Duct ectasia
• Purulent
Infection
• Serous
Fibrocystic disease
Duct ectasia
Carcinoma
• Milk:
Lactation
Rare causes (hypothyroidism, pituitary tumor)

140. Ans. (c) Fibroadenoma

Ref: Sabiston, 19th ed. pg. 827

- Fibroadenoma aka Breast mouse is the most common benign tumor of breast.
- It is MC seen in young age group females (15-30 yrs)
- Clinically, it is slow growing, painless solitary mass, which is mobile in nature *(that's why known as breast mouse).*
- **IOC:** FNAC
- **Upon mammography:** Popcorn calcification

141. Ans. (a) Lobular carcinoma

Ref: Sabiston, 19th ed. pg. 842, Bailey, 26th ed. pg. 809

LOBULAR CARCINOMA BREAST SALIENT FEATURES

- Mostly Multi-centric and **bilateral**
- Histological hallmark: *Indian file pattern* due to the tendency of tumor cells to invade in linear strand.
- Presenting feature-Breast mass with ill-defined margins
- Cellular feature- cytoplasmic mucoid globule
- *Neighbourhood calcification*-calcification in LCIS typically occurs in adjacent tissues. *It is a unique feature* and adds to diagnosis.

FMGE Solutions Screening Examination

BREAST CANCER- AT A GLANCE

| MC cancer in women (Worldwide) |
| MC cancer in women in urban area (India) |

- MC arise from TDLU (terminal duct lobular unit)
- **MC type-** Invasive ductal
- **MC malignant type-** inflammatory breast CA
- **MC Site-** upper outer quadrant
- MC Site of metastasis is bone (osteolytic) lumbar vertebra>femur>thoracic vertebrae.
- **MC Cause of death-** metastatic disease i.e malignant pleural effusion
- 2nd Most common cause of cancer death in women (*1st is lung in both sexes*)

Evaluation/Diagnosis by triple assessment-
- Clinical
- Imaging (Mammography/USG)
- Histopathology
  - 1st initial Investigation is FNAC
  - **Best/gold standard test-** HPE after biopsy
  - **USG-** for young patient
  - **MRI-** Patient with breast implant condition
  - **PET scan-** For recurrence
  - **Mammography-** For older patient
  - **Mammography:** IOC for micro-calcification

| BIRADS | Breast imaging reporting and data system
0-incomplete assessment
1-Negative
2-Benign
3-Probably benign
4-Suspicious
5-Highly suggestive of malignancy
6-Malignant |

142. Ans (d) Lobular carcinoma

Ref: Bailey & Love, 26th ed. pg. 809

143. Ans. (a) Infiltration of cooper's ligament with cancer cells

Ref: Bailey & Love, 26th ed. pg. 798, 808

- The term implies appearance of dimpled texture of an orange peel. Peau d'orange is caused by *cutaneous lymphatic edema*, which causes swelling.
- The *ligaments of Cooper* are hollow conical projections of fibrous tissue filled with breast tissue; the apices of the cones are attached firmly to the superficial fascia and thereby to the skin overlying the breast. These ligaments account for the dimpling of the skin overlying a carcinoma and can also explain nipple retraction.

144. Ans. (b) Core cut Biopsy

Ref: Sabiston, 10th ed. pg. 830-31

- Since the question asks about diagnosis and NOT screening, the best option will be core-cut biopsy/True-cut biopsy.

- For screening FNAC is preferred.
- **Mammography** is considered as IOC in patients >40 years with breast condition. Since the above given patient is pregnant, mammography will NOT be preferred.
- **USG:** Initial investigation for palpable lesions in women <35 years. But it is Not useful in screening
- **MRI** is indicated in patients with breast implant.

Biopsy Techniques for Breast Lesions

Technique	Advantages	Disadvantages
FNAC	Rapid painless inexpensive No incision prior to selection of local therapy	Does not distinguish invasive from in situ cancer Marker (ER, PR, HER) not routinely available. Requires experienced cytopathologist
True –cut (core-cut) Biopsy	Rapid, relatively painless, inexpensive. No incision Can be read by any pathologist. Markers (ER, PR, HER-2) routinely available	False-negative results, incomplete lesions characterization can occur

145. Ans. (b) USG

Ref: Bailey & Love, 26th ed. pg. 527

- Breast abscess is highly probable in this lactating patient. Ultrasonography is used to distinguish solid from cystic structures and to direct needle aspiration for abscess drainage.
- Ultrasound is the imaging method of choice for the majority of women aged < 40 years and during pregnancy and lactation.
- Breast MRI does not form part of the initial imaging assessment of patients in the symptomatic breast disease.

146. Ans. (a) It is often bilateral

Ref: Bailey & Love, 26th ed. pg. 810

Paget disease of the breast is a malignant condition with appearance of eczema, with skin changes involving the nipple of the breast. *Symptoms usually only affect one breast.* Symptoms may include:

Skin	The first symptom is usually an eczema-like rash. Later, the skin may become flaky or scaly.
Discharge	Straw-colored or bloody.
Sensation	Burning sensation usually occurs in more advanced stages, when serious destruction of the skin often prompts the patient to consult. In more advanced stages, the disease may cause tingling and pain.

Contd...

Nipple changes	May turn inwards
Breast changes	Lump in the breast with redness, oozing and crusting.

- Immunohistochemistry allows definitive diagnosis of mammary PD. Paget cells can be demonstrated by immune - histochemical methods using several antibodies to cell surface and cytoplasmic markers (eg : low-molecular-weight keratins found in simple epithelia, EMA, **HER2/neu,** polyclonal pCEA+).
- Paget's disease of the breast is a type of cancer of the breast. Treatment usually involves a lumpectomy or mastectomy to surgically remove the tumor. Chemotherapy and/or radiotherapy may be necessary, but the specific treatment often depends on the characteristics of the underlying breast cancer.

147. Ans. (a) 1 cm

Ref: Bailey & Love, 26th ed. pg. 813

The amount of breast tissue excised with the lesion may vary with the clinical situation, but is typically 5 mm to 10 mm in all directions. Breast-conserving surgery (BCS): BCS may consist of removal of the tumor with a 1 cm margin of normal tissue (wide local excision) or a more extensive excision of a whole quadrant of the breast (quadrantectomy).

148. Ans. (a) USG

Ref: Scwartz, 10th ed. pg. 527

- The development of a dominant mass during pregnancy or lactation should never be attributed to hormonal changes.
- Breast cysts can be differentiated from solid echogenic abnormalities and will also be used to guide FNAC, core needle biopsy. *In the pregnant lady with breast lump ultrasound will be done initially*, and is a first line investigation modality.
- A dominant mass must be treated with the same concern in a pregnant woman as any other. Breast cancer develops in 1 in every 3000–4000 pregnancies.
- **Differential diagnosis of breast mass in pregnant and lactating patient**
  1. Breast cancer
  2. Fibroadenoma
  3. Lactating adenoma
  4. Galactocele
  5. Fibrocystic changes

149. Ans. (d) Spread to adrenal glands

Ref: Schwartz, 10th ed. pg. 532

- Involvement of chest wall by the cancer, satellite lesions and skin ulceration *constitute stage T4 by TNM staging.*
- Stage 4 of breast cancer can be any T stage, any nodal Stage, but is always M1 stage which is spread to distant organs.
- Do not mix up T_4 with stage 4 as both are fundamentally separate concepts.

150. Ans. (b) Satellite lesions

Ref: Schwartz, 10th ed. pg. 532

To	No evidence of primary tomor
TIS	Carcinoma in situ
T1	Tumor ≤2 cm
T1a	Tumor > 0.1 cm but ≤ 0.5 cm
T1b	Tumor > 0.5 but < 1 cm
T1c	Tumor > 1 cm but ≤2 cm
T2	Tumor > 2 cm but ≤5 cm
T3	Tumor > 5 cm
T4	Extension to chest wall, inflammation, satellite lesions, ulcerations

151. Ans. (c) Tumor staging

Ref: Schwartz, 10th ed. pg. 535

- The most important prognostic variable is tumor staging with *Nodal status>Tumor size>Histological grade*
- The breast cancer markers that are most important in *determining therapy* are estrogen receptor, progesterone receptor and HER-2/neu.
- *Tumor growth rate* correlates with early relapse. S-phase analysis using flow cytometry is the most accurate measure.
- *Histologic classification* of the tumor has also been used as a prognostic factor. Tumors with a poor nuclear grade have a higher risk of recurrence than tumors with a good nuclear grade.
- *Molecular changes in the tumor* are also useful. Tumors that overexpress *erbB2* (HER2/neu) or have a mutated p53 gene have a worse prognosis.

152. Ans. (a) Mastitis

Ref: Bailey & Love, 26th ed. pg. 805, 810

Notice the fullness in lateral quadrant with erythema of overlying skin, diagnostic of Mastitis

Mondor disease	• It involves thrombophlebitis of the superficial veins of the breast and anterior chest wall. • It sometimes occurs in the arm and is known as axillary web syndrome • Patients with this disease often have abrupt onset of superficial pain, with possible swelling and redness of a limited area of their anterior chest wall or breast.
Cystosarcoma phyllodes	• Phyllodes tumors are a fibro-epithelial tumor composed of an epithelial and a cellular stromal component. • They may be considered benign, borderline, or malignant depending on histologic features including stromal cellularity, infiltration at the tumor's edge, and mitotic activity. • All forms of phyllodes tumors are regarded as having malignant potential. They are also known as *serocystic disease of Brodie.*
Paget disease	• Patients with mammary Paget disease (PD) present with a relatively long history of an eczematous skin lesion or persistent dermatitis in the nipple and adjacent areas • *Since in this pic areola is blurred and visible areola appears normal, Paget's is ruled out.*

153. Ans. (b) Ocular cancer

Ref: Bailey & Love, 26th ed. pg. 813

- The **sentinel lymph node** is the **first lymph node** or group of nodes draining a cancer. In case of established cancerous dissemination it is postulated that the sentinel lymph node/s is/are the target organs primarily reached by metastasizing cancer cells from the tumor.
- **The main uses of sentinel lymph node biopsy are in breast cancer and malignant melanoma surgery.** Other cancers which have been investigated with this technique are penile cancer, urinary bladder cancer, prostate cancer, testicular cancer and renal cell cancer.

154. Ans. (c) Stage III A

Since the size of the tumor given is 3 cm, it will be stage T2
Since the number of lymph nodes involved is 4 axillary lymph nodes the stage will be N2
Distant metastasis stage Mo
Stage I and IV are easily ruled out. Stage II has nodal stage 1 (N_1)
Stage III has nodal stage 2 (N_2)

Brief Description of the Terms

Tis : in situ	N0: no regional lymph nodes involved	M0: no metastasis
T0: not evident clinically	N1: ranging from micromeatses to <3 axillary lymph nodes involvement.	M1: presence of metastasis
T1: tumor size 0.1cm-2.0cm	N2: axillary lymph nodes ranging from 3-9 or involvent of intermarry group of lymph nodes	
T2: 2cm – 5cm	N3: >10 axillary lymph-nodes involved or clinically detected inter mammary group of lymph nodes	
T3: >5cm		
T4: Involvement of chest muscle, skin and ulceration.		

155. Ans. (b) Simple mastectomy

Ref: Sabiston, 19th ed. pg. 849-853

- According to staging given in question, this is a case of stage 1 breast CA for which simple mastectomy is preferred.

Types of mastectomy	
Simple or Total mastectomy	Removal of breast tissue, nipple-areola complex, and skin
Extended simple mastectomy	Simple mastectomy + removal of level I axillary LNs.
Modified radical mastectomy	Removes all breast tissue and skin, nipple areola complex, pectoralis major and minor muscles and the level, I, II and III axillary LNs,
Extended radical mastectomy	Radical mastectomy + Removal or internal mammary, LNs
Super radical mastectomy	Radical mastectomy + Removal of internal mammary, mediastinal and supraclavicular LNs

THYROID AND SALIVARY GLANDS

156. Ans. (b) Soles

Ref: SRB: 5th ed. pg. 78

- Sebaceous cyst is a retention cyst which occurs due to blockage of duct of sebaceous gland causing a cystic swelling.

Surgery

- It is commonly seen on scrotum, face and scalp but *not seen in palms and soles as there are no sebaceous glands.*

> **Extra Mile**
>
> *Multiple sebaceous cysts on scrotum is called as strawberry scrotum.*

157. (b) Cancer of parotid gland

Ref: Bailey and Love: 26th ed. pg. 732

The image shows a parotid mass with marking of indelible ink. The painless mass rules out choice A and D while Choice C involves mainly the lips and tongue. The patient is having a parotid tumour and needs an urgent MRI to evaluate the mass followed by FNAC.

158. (c) TB

Ref: Bailey and Love: 25th ed. pg. 700

The image shows a large swelling extending in both anterior and posterior triangle of neck with an orifice of a fistulous tract with some excoriation and inflammation.

Features in favor of TB are:
- Indian patient
- Long standing history
- Location of large abscess overlapping both anterior and posterior triangle of neck
- Non-transilluminant fluctuant swelling.
- Normal overlying skin of abscess

- In contrast Branchial cyst is a *transilluminant fluctuant swelling* in upper or mid 1/3ʳᵈ of sternocleidomastoid containing cholesterol crystals. The site of orifice is lower 1/3ʳᵈ of neck on anterior border of sternocleidomastoid. The internal orifice of branchial fistula is present on posterior faucial pillar behind the tonsil. *The cyst becomes red and infected* before a fistula develops while in this case no evidence of any infection is seen as overlying skin is normal.
- Choice B secondaries is ruled out as they would show a progressive increase and do not have any draining fistula. Same logic is valid for ruling out choice D, Lymphoma.

159. Ans. (b) Von Graefe's sign

Ref: SRB 5th ed. P 470

Lid lag sign or Von Graefe's sign is inability of upper eyelid to keep pace with the eyeball when it looks downwards to follow the examiner's finger.

> **Extra Mile**
>
> Eye signs are common in primary thyrotoxicosis.
> 1. **Lid retraction:** Here upper eyelid is higher than normal; lower eyelid is in normal position. It is due to *sympathetic overactivity* causing spasm of involuntary smooth muscle part of the levator palpebrae superioris (*Muller's muscle*). It is a sign of thyrotoxicosis, not a sign of exophthalmos.
> 2. **Dalrymple's sign:** Upper eyelid retraction, so visibility of upper selera.
> 3. **Stellwag's sign:** Absence of normal blinking—so *staring look*. *First sign to appear.* It is due to widening of palpebral fissure due to lid retraction and also due to contraction of voluntary part of levator palebrae superioris muscle.
> 4. **Joffroy's sign:** Absence of wrinkling on forehead when patient looks up (frowns) with head is bent down/flexed position.
> 5. **Moebius sign:** It is lack of convergence of eyeball. Defective convergence is due to lymphocytic infiltration of inferior oblique and rectus muscles in case of primary thyrotoxicosis. There will be diplopia.
> 6. **Rosenbach's sign:** Tremor of closed eyelids

160. Ans. (a) Thyroid cancer

Ref: Harrison, 18th ed. pg. 341

- Thyroid carcinoma is the most common malignancy of the endocrine system.
- Differentiated tumors, such as papillary thyroid cancer (PTC) or follicular thyroid cancer (FTC), are often curable, and the prognosis is good for patients identified with early-stage disease.
- In contrast, anaplastic thyroid cancer (ATC) is aggressive, responds poorly to treatment, and is associated with a bleak prognosis.

161. Ans. (a) TSH

Ref: Harrison, 19th ed. pg. 341

Best thyroid function test is *TSH as it helps in differentiating between primary and secondary thyrotoxicosis.* The change of TSH values also indicate the improvement in medical condition of the patient. For example after resection of a pituitary adenoma secreting excess of TSH, the values of TSH will come back towards normal.

162. Ans. (a) Lymphatic

Ref: Bailey & Love, 26th ed. pg. 765

- Lymphatic spread is common for papillary carcinoma thyroid whereas follicular carcinoma thyroid spreads

Explanations

FMGE Solutions Screening Examination

via the blood stream. In papillary carcinoma thyroid, total thyroidectomy is performed and approximately 4-6 weeks after surgical thyroid removal, patients must have radioiodine therapy to detect and destroy any metastasis and residual tissue in the thyroid.

163. Ans. (a) Iodine 131

Ref: Bailey & Love, 26th ed. pg. 768

164. Ans. (a) Recurrent laryngeal nerve

Ref: SRB, 5th ed. pg. 493; Bailey & Love, 26th ed. pg. 760

- The recurrent laryngeal nerve is at high risk for injury during thyroid surgery. The damage is transient.
- The recurrent laryngeal nerve innervates all intrinsic muscles of larynx with exception of Cricothyroid muscle. Mechanisms of damage include complete or partial transection, traction, contusion and compromised blood supply. The consequence is true vocal fold paralysis.
- The SLN has 2 divisions: internal and external. The internal branch provides sensory innervation to the larynx. The external branch provides motor function to the crico-thyroid muscle.

165. Ans. (d) Calcitonin

Ref: Bailey and Love, 26th ed. ch. 51/764

- Medullary thyroid cancer is a rare form of thyroid cancer and accounts for 3 to 10% of all thyroid cancers. It grows from specialized thyroid cells called *parafollicular cells*.
- **Parafollicular cells-C-cells**; specialized thyroid cells that secrete calcitonin and play a major role in diagnosis of medullary thyroid cancer.
- Calcitonin is a tumor marker and remember there is no hypocalcemia in medullary carcinoma of thyroid.

166. Ans. (d) Medullary

Ref: Bailey and Love, 26th ed. ch. 5/741

Medullary thyroid cancer grows from specialized thyroid cells called *parafollicular* C-cells which are specialized thyroid cells that secrete calcitonin and play a major role in medullary thyroid cancer.

167. Ans. (b) Papillary

Ref: Bailey & Love, 26th ed. pg. 763-64

- Ionizing radiation can cause genetic mutations leading to malignant transformation.
- This association is much stronger for thyroid cancer than for other malignancies, and radiation is the only well-established environmental risk factor for thyroid malignancy.
- The risk of developing thyroid cancer after exposure to radiation is greater in those exposed during childhood and increases with higher doses of radiation delivered to the thyroid. This is true for exposure to ionizing radiation given for medical purposes and for environmental exposures.
- *The association with radiation is much stronger for papillary than for follicular cancer.*

168. Ans. (a) Papillary

Ref: Bailey & Love, 26th ed. pg. 765-66

THYROID MALIGNANCY

- Papillary carcinoma thyroid (PTC) has excellent prognosis (10yr survival rate >90%)
- **MC type**- Papillary Thyroid CA (PTC)
- Among people exposed to external radiation-PTC
- Lateral abberent thyroid- PTC
- Psammoma bodies-PTC
- Orphan annie nuclei-PTC
- Intranuclear inclusion/pseudo inclusion-PTC
- **Most reliable feature for PTC diagnosis**- nuclear feature i.e. orphan annie nuclei.
- Diagnosis by –FNAC
- **Treatment:** Total or near total thyroidectomy
- Most common thyroid cancer in *iodine sufficient* persons - PTC

169. Ans. (b) Multiple nodular goiter

Ref: Bailey & Love, 26th ed. pg. 749

- Notice the multiple enlarged lobes of this multiple nodular goiter which represents a spectrum of disease ranging from a single hyper-functioning nodule (toxic adenoma) within a multi-nodular thyroid to a gland with multiple areas of hyper function.
- Thyroglossal cyst is ruled out as it is present in midline.
- The answer should not be given as toxic nodular goiter because we cannot comment on thyrotoxicosis status of patient as eye signs etc. are not visible or given and the question also mentions a EUTHYROID status of the patient.

170. Ans. (c) Follicular carcinoma

Ref: Bailey & Love, 24th/785, Schwartz, 8th/1420

- FNAC is unable to distinguish benign follicular lesions from follicular carcinoma. Large follicular tumors (>4 cm) in older men are more likely to be malignant.
- **FNAC is the investigation of choice for solitary thyroid nodules.**

- It cannot distinguish between a follicular Adenoma and a Follicular Carcinoma *as this distinction is dependent not on cytology but on histological criteria such as capsular and vascular invasion.* It therefore cannot be used to diagnose follicular carcinomas.

171. Ans. (d) Zygomatic bone

- **Surgical landmarks to the facial nerve include the tympanomastoid suture line, the tragal pointer, and the posterior belly of the digastric muscle.**
- The tympanomastoid suture line lies between the mastoid and tympanic segments of the temporal bone and is approximately 6-8 mm lateral to the stylomastoid foramen. The main trunk of the nerve can also be found midway between (10 mm posteroinferior to) the cartilaginous tragal pointer of the external auditory canal and the posterior belly of the digastric muscle.

172. Ans. (c) Pleomorphic adenoma

Ref: Bailey & Love, 26th ed. pg. 732

PLEOMORPHIC ADENOMA

- Overall most common tumor of salivary gland
- MC benign salivary gland tumor
- MC tumor of major salivary glands
- MC site is parotid tail (superficial lobe).

Extra Mile

- 2nd MC benign tumor of parotid gland: **Warthin's tumor**
- MC malignant tumor of parotid gland: **Mucoepidermoid CA**
- 2nd MC malignant tumor of parotid gland: **Adenoid cystic CA**

173. Ans. (b) Adenoid cystic carcinoma

Ref: Bailey & Love, 26th ed. pg. 733

- *The adenoid cystic carcinoma is characterized by propensity to spread along nerves.*
- Tumor may be present for more than 10 years and then suddenly infiltrate the adjacent tissues extensively.
- Tumor has affinity for growth along perineural planes.
- Lung metastases are most frequent.

174. Ans. (a) Parotid gland

Ref: Bailey & Love, 26th ed. pg. 733

WARTHIN TUMOR

- *An exclusive tumor of parotid gland*
- Second most common benign parotid tumor (5%)

- Most common *bilateral benign neoplasm of the parotid*
- Marked male as compared to female predominance
- Occurs later in life (sixth and seventh decades)
- Presents as a lymphocytic infiltrate and cystic epithelial proliferation
- May represent heterotopic salivary gland epithelial tissue trapped within intra-parotid lymph nodes
- Incidence of bilaterality and multi-centricity of 10%
- Malignant transformation rare.

175. Ans. (a) Parotid gland

Ref: Schwartz, 10th ed. pg. 600

- MC cause of salivary gland fistula is parotid gland surgery.
- A parotid fistula is a communication through which saliva is discharged.
- Various forms of treatment have been described for parotid gland fistula, including tympanic neurectomy with or without chorda tympani section, radiotherapy and even completion of the parotidectomy.

176. Ans. (a) Submandibular gland

Ref: Bailey and Love, 26th ed. ch. 50/732

- Salivary gland stone (sialolithiasis) is due to duct obstruction, which further lead to calcification.
- This calcification further causes secondary bacterial invasion which leads to **SIALADENITIS**
- **Most common organism associated with sialadenitis: Staph. Aureus and Strep. Viridans**
- **Most common salivary gland associated with sialolithiasis: submandibular gland** *(80 %)* **> Parotid gland (20%)**
- A stone located in the collecting duct or within the gland may be managed by either endoscopic retrieval, lithotripsy or, least likely, surgical removal.
- Sialography is usually required to identify the stone.
- Parotid duct stones are usually radiolucent and rarely visible on plain radiography. They are frequently located at the confluence of the collecting ducts or located in the distal aspect of the parotid duct adjacent to the parotid papilla.

177. Ans. (a) Superficial parotidectomy

Ref: Bailey & Love, 26th ed. pg. 733-34

Treatment of Choice for Pleomorphic Adenoma

- **In parotid gland:** Superficial parotidectomy
- **In other salivary glands:** Excision of the affected gland

> **Extra Mile**
>
> **Indications or radiotherapy in salivary gland tumors**
> - High grade tumors
> - Cervical LN metastasis
> - Large primary lesions
> - Perineural invasion
> - Bone invasion

HERNIA AND HYDROCOELE

178. Ans. (a) Torsion testis

Ref: SRB 5th ed. pg. 1018

- The bell clapper deformity allows the testicle to twist spontaneously on the spermatic cord since the long axis of the testicle is oriented transversely rather than cephalocaudal.
- This congenital abnormality is present in approximately 12% of males and is bilateral in 40% of cases.

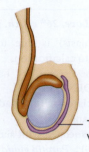

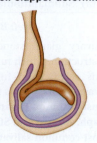

- Torsion occurs as the testicle rotates between 90° and 180°, compromising blood flow to and from the testicle. Complete torsion usually occurs when the testicle twists 360° or more; incomplete or partial torsion occurs with lesser degrees of rotation.

179. Ans. (b) Direct

Ref: SRB 5th ed. p 754

In NYHUS classification, type 3A hernia is direct inguinal hernia.

Type 1: Indirect hernia with normal deep ring
Type 2: Indirect hernia with dilated deep ring
Type 3: Posterior wall defect
3A: Direct hernia
3B: Pantaloon hernia
3C: Femoral hernia
Type 4: Recurrent hernia

180. Ans. (a) Pantaloons hernia

Ref: Bailey, 25th ed. pg. 956

Site of primary	Percentage
Pantaloon hernia	The pantaloons hernia is the simultaneous occurrence of a direct and an indirect hernia. The pantaloons hernia causes two bulges that straddle the inferior epigastric vessels
Ritcher hernia	Richter's hernia is a hernia at any site through which only a portion of the circumference of a bowel wall, usually the jejunum, incarcerates or strangulates. Because the entire lumen is not compromised, symptoms of bowel obstruction can be absent, despite gangrene of the strangulated portion
Spigelian hernia	Spigelian hernia are herniations through the semilunar line, which is the lateral margin of the rectus muscle. At or just below the junction with the semicircular line of Douglas, unlike groin hernias, these hernias lie cephalad to the inferior epigastric vessels. The tight aponeurotic defect predisposes them to incarceration.
Littre hernia	Any groin hernia that contains a Meckel's diverticulum is Littre's hernia. This type of hernia is usually incarcerated or strangulated.

181. Ans. (a) Omentum

Ref: Bed Side Clinics in Surgery: ed. pg. 552: 2014

The clinical finding of doughy feel suggest diagnosis of omentocele.

Comparison of enterocele and omentocele

Omentocele	Enterocele
Doughy feel	Soft elastic feel
Dull note on percussion	Reduction with gurgling sound and resonant percussion note
Absent bowel sounds	Presence of bowel sounds

Other Findings of Hernia

- Expansile impulse on cough
- Reducibility indicates uncomplicated hernia
- Deep ring occlusion test since congenital hernia occurs through the deep ring
- Whether possible to get above the swelling, to differentiate scrotal or inguino-scrotal swelling
- Soft elastic feel with resonant note and audible bowel sounds suggests presence of enterocele.

182. Ans. (d) Transversalis fascia

Ref: Bailey & Love, 26th ed. pg. 955

- Deep inguinal ring is the opening in the *transversalis fascia* through which the ductus deferens and gonadal vessels (or round ligament in the female) enter the inguinal canal.

- Located midway between anterior superior iliac spine and pubic tubercle, it is bounded medially by the lateral umbilical fold (inferior epigastric vessels) and inferiorly by the ilio-pubic tract. Indirect inguinal hernias exit the abdominal cavity through the deep inguinal ring.

183. Ans. (b) Congenital hydrocele

Ref: Bailey & Love, 26th ed. pg. 1382

- Hydrocele is an accumulation of fluid in layers of tunica vaginalis.
- **Vaginal hydrocele:** MC type. Accumulation of fluid within tunica vaginalis layers
- **Infantile hydrocele:** doesn't necessarily appear in infants. The tunica and processus vaginalis are distended to the inguinal ring without any connection with peritoneal cavity.
- **Congenital hydrocele:**
  - It is due to patent processus vaginalis which allows peritoneal fluid to move freely.
  - Size of hydrocele fluctuates usually related to activity
  - **Treatment:** Herniotomy

184. Ans. (a) Herniotomy

Ref: Bailey and Love, 26th ed. ch. 79/1382

- Congenital hydroceles *are treated by herniotomy* if they do not resolve spontaneously
- **Lord's operation** is suitable when the sac is reasonably thin-walled. There is minimal dissection and the risk of haematoma is reduced.
- Eversion of the sac with placement of the testis in a pouch prepared by dissection in the fascial planes of the scrotum is an alternative **(Jaboulay's procedure)**
- Aspiration of the hydrocele fluid is simple, but the fluid always reaccumulates within a week or so. It may be suitable for men who are unfit for scrotal surgery

185. Ans. (a) Conservative Management till patient is asymptomatic

- Most of the pediatric patients with an inguinal hernia have indirect inguinal hernia.
- Inguinal hernias *do not spontaneously heal and must be surgically repaired because of the ever-present risk of incarceration.*
- Only 3 procedures are necessary for the surgical repair of indirect inguinal hernias in children:
  1. High ligation and excision of the patent sac with anatomic closure
  2. High ligation of the sac with plication of the floor of the inguinal canal (the transversalis fascia), and
  3. High ligation of the sac combined with reconstruction of the floor of the canal
- *In patients with a long-standing history of inguinal hernia, the repeated protrusion of abdominal contents through the* inguinal canal enlarges the internal and external rings, reducing the risk of incarceration and strangulation. This makes repair more difficult and recurrence more likely

186. Ans. (c) Meckel's diverticulum

Ref: Bailey & Love, 26th ed. pg. 1170

- When Meckel's diverticulum forms the content of hernia, it is known as Littre's hernia.

187. Ans. (a) Strangulated hernia

Ref: Sabistan, 19th ed. pg. 1127

- Strangulation occurs more often in patients who have a partially reducible or an irreducible hernia
- Indirect inguinal hernias strangulate more commonly, the direct variety not so often because of the wide neck of the sac.
- **MC constricting agent:** Neck of the sac > External inguinal ring in children > Adhesions within the sac.
- **MC contents:** Small intestine > Omentum

Clinical features of strangulated inguinal Hernia

1. Sudden onset inguinal pain
2. Generalized abdomen pain
3. Tense and extremely tender hernia
4. Discoloration of overlying skin with a reddish or bluish tinge
5. There is no expansile cough impulse.

188. Ans. (a) Below and lateral to pubic tubercle

Ref: Bailey and Love, 26th ed, ch. 60/960

- The femoral hernia appears **below and lateral to the pubic tubercle** and lies in the upper leg rather than in the lower abdomen. Inadequate exposure of this area during routine examination leads to failure to detect the hernia.
- The hernia often rapidly becomes irreducible and loses any cough impulse due to the tightness of the neck. It may only be 1–2 cm in size and can easily be mistaken for a lymph node

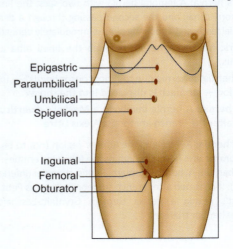

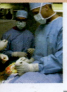

189. Ans. (c) Cough impulse is present

Ref: Bed Side Clinics in Surgery; Makhan Lal Saha, pg. 49

- **Femoral hernias** occur just below the inguinal ligament, when abdominal contents pass through a naturally occurring weakness called the femoral canal. The femoral hernia follows the tract below the inguinal ligament through the femoral canal. The canal lies medial to the femoral vein and lateral to the lacunar (Gimbernat) ligament. *Because femoral hernias protrude through such a small defined space, they frequently become incarcerated or strangulated*
- Femoral hernias are uncommon variety accounting for only 3% of all hernias.
- Femoral hernias mostly develop in women because of the wider bone structure of the female pelvis.
- The *cough impulse is not seen in femoral hernia*. Lockwood infra-inguinal approach is used in repair.

190. Ans. (c) Femoral hernia

Ref: Bailey & Love, 26th ed. Ch. 60/960

- High risk of strangulation is seen with femoral hernia as it has lacunar ligament (Gimbernat's) medially. This is a strong curved ligament with a sharp unyielding edge which impedes reduction of a femoral hernia.
- 50% of cases present as an emergency

191. Ans. (c) Femoral hernia

Please refer to above explanation

192. Ans. (b) Cooper's hernia

Ref: Sabiston, 19th ed. pg. 1126-27

HERNIAS AT A GLANCE

Amyand's hernia: Containing the appendix vermiformis within the hernia sac
Cooper's hernia: A femoral hernia with two sacs, the first being in the femoral canal, and the second passing through a defect in the superficial fascia and appearing almost immediately beneath the skin.
Epigastric hernia: A hernia through the linea alba above the umbilicus.
Hiatus hernia: A hernia due to "short oesophagus" — insufficient elongation — stomach is displaced into the thorax
Littre's hernia: A hernia **involving a Meckel's diverticulum. It** is named after the French anatomist Alexis Littré
Lumbar hernia: A hernia in the lumbar region (not to be confused with a lumbar disc hernia), contains the following entities:
Petit's hernia: A hernia through Petit's triangle (inferior lumbar triangle). It is named after French surgeon Jean Louis Petit.
Grynfeltt's hernia a hernia through Grynfeltt-Lesshaft triangle (superior lumbar triangle).

Maydl's hernia: Two adjacent loops of small intestine are within a hernial sac with a tight neck. The intervening portion of bowel within the abdomen is deprived of its blood supply and eventually becomes necrotic.
Morgagni hernia: A type of hernia where abdominal contents pass into the thorax through a weakness in the diaphragm
Obturator hernia: Hernia through obturator canal.
Pantaloon hernia (Saddle Bag hernia): A **combined direct and indirect hernia**, when the hernial sac protrudes on either side of the inferior epigastric vessels.
Paraumbilical hernia: A type of umbilical hernia occurring in adults
Perineal hernia: A perineal hernia protrudes through the muscles and fascia of the perineal floor. It may be primary but usually is acquired following perineal prostatectomy, abdominoperineal resection of the rectum, or pelvic exenteration.
Richter's hernia: A hernia involving only one sidewall of the bowel, which can result in bowel strangulation leading to perforation through ischaemia without causing bowel obstruction or any of its warning signs.
Sliding hernia: Occurs when an organ drags along part of the peritoneum, or, in other words, the organ is part of the hernia sac. The colon and the urinary bladder are often involved. The term also frequently refers to sliding hernias of the stomach.
Sciatic hernia: This hernia in the greater sciatic foramen most commonly presents as an uncomfortable mass in the gluteal area. Bowel obstruction may also occur. This type of hernia is only a rare cause of sciatic neuralgia.
Velpeau hernia: A hernia in the groin in front of the femoral blood vessels

193. Ans. (d) Saddle bag hernia

Ref: Sabiston, 19th ed. pg. 1126-27

Please refer to above explanation

194. Ans. (d) Littre's hernia

Ref: Sabiston, 19th ed. pg. 1126-27

195. Ans. (d) Hernia at the level of arcuate line

Ref: Bailey and Love, 26th ed. ch. 60/966

Spigelian hernia
- Spigelian hernia herniates through the spigelian fascia, *which is the aponeurotic layer between the rectus abdominis muscle medially, and the semilunar line laterally.*
- **Always occur at or above the arcuate line** because of the lack of posterior rectus sheath. These are inter-parietal hernias, *which penetrate between the muscles of the abdominal wall;* therefore, there is often no notable swelling.

Contd...

Surgery

196. Ans. (a) Posterolateral

Ref: Bailey & Love, 26th ed. pg. 871-72

- Bochdalek's hernia is the most common form of diaphragmatic hernia, occurring in approximately 1 in 2500 births and twice as often in males as in females.
- *Bochdalek's hernia results from failure of normal development of the posterolateral diaphragm during embryogenesis.*
- Separation of the developing thoracic and abdominal cavities occurs during the eighth week of gestation, when the opening between the chest and abdomen (the pleuroperitoneal canal) closes. A congenital diaphragmatic hernia results when the pleuroperitoneal membrane fails to form.
- Most Bochdalek's hernias occur on the left side, allowing protrusion of the abdominal viscera into the chest. The herniated bowel passes through the defect, filling the chest cavity and causing hypoplasia of the left lung and a shift of mediastinal structures to the right side. It is not uncommon for other abnormalities to be associated with Bochdalek's hernia; these may include neural tube defects and cardiovascular abnormalities
- The left-sided Bochdalek hernia occurs in approximately 85% of cases. Left-sided hernias allow herniation of both the small and large bowel and intraabdominal solid organs into the thoracic cavity.
- In right-sided hernias (13% of cases), only the liver and a portion of the large bowel tend to herniate. Bilateral hernias are uncommon and are usually fatal

Remember

- The 3 basic types of congenital diaphragmatic hernia include the posterolateral Bochdalek hernia (occurring at approximately 6 weeks' gestation), the Anterior Morgagni hernia, and the hiatus hernia.

197. Ans. (c) Epididymo orchitis

Ref: Bailey & Love, 26th ed. pg. 1384

ACUTE EPIDIDYMO ORCHITIS

- Inflammation of the epididymis and testis, from an ascending infection from the lower urinary tract.
- *Initially epididymis is involved, after that there is involvement of testis.*
- *Most cases of epididymitis in men younger than 35 years are due to sexually transmitted organisms [C. trachomatis (MC) and N. gonorrhoe]*
- In children and older men this is due to urinary pathogens such as E. coli.
- *Patient presents with fever, swollen, red and tender scrotum.*

- *The epididymis and testis are swollen (Thickened cord with reactive hydrocoele).*
- **Urine analysis** typically demonstrates WBCs and bacteria in the urine or urethral discharge
- **Scrotal USG** showing enlarged epididymis with increased blood flow with reactive hydrocoele.

> **Extra Mile**
>
> - Testicular torsion is commonly seen in pre-pubertal age group (10-25 years). Patients usually presents with sudden agonizing pain.

UROLOGY

198. Ans. (a) PCNL

Ref: SRB 5th ed. pg. 1017

- Kidney stone of size more than 2.5 cm in size is treated with percutaneous nephrolithotomy. In contrast Extracorporeal shock wave lithotripsy is used for stones of size less than 2.5 cm. The piezo-ceramic electromagnetic waves are passed via a water bath and shocks are produced at rate of 2/sec. 1000-4000 shocks are required per stone.
- Pyeloplasty is the surgical reconstruction of the renal pelvis (a part of the kidney) to drain and decompress the kidney. In nearly all cases, the goal of the surgery is to relieve a ureteropelvic junction (UPJ) obstruction.

199. Ans. (c) Sertoli cell tumour

Ref: SRB 5th ed. pg. 1083

Sertoli cell tumour is a sex cord stromal tumour while the remaining choices are germ cell tumours. The prevalence of germ cell tumour is 95%.

Germ cell tumors	Sex cord stromal tumors

- Seminoma
- Spermatocytic seminoma
- Embryonal carcinoma Polyembryoma
- Embryonal carcinoma and teratoma ('teratocarcinoma')
- Teratoma
  Mature
  Immature
  With malignant transformation
- Choriocarcinoma
- Yolk sac tumor
	- Leydig cell tumor
	- Serto cell tumor
	- Granulosa cell tumor
	- Mixed forms

FMGE Solutions Screening Examination

200. Ans. (c) 4 hours

Ref: SRB 5th ed. pg. 1063 and American Urological Association Guidelines

Priapism is a persistent penile erection that continues beyond 4 hours and is unrelated to, sexual stimulation. Typically, only the corpora cavernosa are affected.
Subtypes of priapism include:

- Ischemic (veno-occlusive, low flow) priapism is a nonsexual, persistent erection characterized by little or no cavernous blood flow and abnormal cavernous blood gases (hypoxic, hypercarbic, and acidotic). Ischemic priapism is an emergency.
- Non-ischemic (arterial, high flow) priapism is a nonsexual, persistent erection caused by unregulated cavernous arterial inflow. Typically the penis is neither fully rigid nor painful. Antecedent trauma is the most commonly described etiology.
- Stuttering (intermittent) priapism is a recurrent form of ischemic priapism in which unwanted painful erections occur repeatedly with intervening periods of detumescence.

201. Ans. (a) Membranous urethra rupture

Ref: SRB 5th ed. P 1037 and 1052

- The patient has pelvic fracture which resulted in trauma to membranous and/or prostatic urethra. This is called *posterior urethral rupture.*
- The presentation will be blood at meatus with inability to pass urine.
- There is extravasation of urine to scrotum, perineum and abdominal wall which explains why bladder is empty.
- This extravasation of urine is called extraperitoneal extravasation of urine.
- *Intraperitoneal rupture of bladder* is seen due to kick on abdomen and leads to diffuse abdominal pain, distention and features of peritonitis as urine leaks into peritoneal space. Vitals will reveal presence of shock. X-ray abdomen will show ground glass appearance. Emergency laparotomy is required with bladder repair.

TABLE: Comparison of anterior and posterior urethra rupture

Rupture of anterior urethra	Rupture of posterior urethra
Trauma to *bulbous urethra* due to fall astride projectile object like cycling, manhole cover, gymnasium	Trauma to *membranous and/or prostatic urethra* after pelvic fracture sustained in RTA.

a. Penile urethra
b. Bulbar urethra
c. Membranous urethra
d. Prostatic urethra

a. Penile urethra
b. Bulbar urethra
c. Membranous urethra
d. Prostatic urethra

Contd...

Rupture of anterior urethra	Rupture of posterior urethra
Presentation • Blood at the meatus • Perineal hematoma • *Retention of urine* • Tell patient not to pass urine else extravasation occurs.	*Presentation* • Difficulty in passing urine • Blood at the meatus • Extravasation of urine to scrotum, perineum and abdominal wall and hence bladder is empty.
• PR examination shows normal prostate.	• PR examination shows *floating prostate*.

@Note anterior urethra is undersurface and posterior urethra is dorsal surface.

202. *Ans.* (a) **Calcium oxalate**

Ref: Harrison 19th ed. P 964

- The normal urinary pH is 5.8–6.2.
- Persistent urinary pH less than 5.5 *(acidic urine)* leads to development of uric acid and cystine stones.
- Persistent urinary pH >7.2 *(alkaline urine)* leads to development of struvite stone.
- Urine pH > 7.5 *(alkaline urine)* leads to development of calcium phosphate stone.
- Calcium oxalate stones development is *independent of urinary pH* and is due to idiopathic hypercalciuria.

▶ **Extra Mile**

- Increasing urine pH > 6.2 can dramatically increase uric acid solubility. Hence urinary alkalization is done with potassium citrate. Also give allopurinol.
- For calcium phosphate stones keep pH of urine between 6.2 and 6.5.
- For cystine stones keep pH > 7.0 by urinary alkalization.

203. **Ans.** (a) **Cystoscopy**

Ref: SRB 5th ed. P 1025

- The age of patient, clinical presentation of painless gross hematuria points to etiology as bladder tumor.
- The IVU finding can be explained by the fact that bladder tumor could have *obstructed the ureteric orifice leading to hydronephrosis.*
- Infundibulum in kidney is the area between the calyx and renal pelvis. The filling defect is due to hydronephrosis.
- Cystoscopy must be done for tissue diagnosis of bladder tumor and resection.
- MRI pelvis should be done to check for invasion and pelvic wall extension.
- DMSA scan is done to evaluate for location of scar in pyelonephritis.

204. **Ans.** (a) **Water intoxication**

Ref: Bailey 26th ed. P 1349

- Water intoxication is postoperative complication of TURP.

- The absorption of water into the circulation at the time of transurethral resection can give rise to CCF, hyponatremia and hemolysis. These features can mimic stroke
- Nowadays this is rarely seen due to use of isotonic glycine during irrigation post TURP.

205. Ans. (c) **Ureterocele**

- The image shows a characteristic cobra/adder head appearance of an ureterocele with contrast filling the bladder. The bladder outline is normal.

206. Ans. (b) **Androgen deprivation treatment**

Guidelines for Management of Prostate Cancer

- For advanced disease process, androgen ablation is used. It can be achieved with bilateral capsular orchiectomy or drugs
- Drugs like LHRH agonist and androgen blocking agents like flutamide, bicalutamide are used.
- Radiotherapy is used for bone secondaries. Chemotherapeutic drug used is docetaxel.

Prostate Cancer Treatment Guidelines

Treatmeny by Recurrence Risk

Clinically localized	Therapy
• T3a • Gleason score 8–10 • PSA > 20 ng/mL	• Radiation therapy + Androgen deprivation therapy (2–3 years) • Radial prostatectomy + Pelvic lymph node dissection (in select patients)

Locally advanced	Therapy
T3b–T4 with any Gleason score	• Radiation therapy + Androgen deprivation therapy (2–3 years) • Radiation therapy + Brachytherapy +/– Androgen deprivation therapy (4 to 6 months) • Radical prostatectomy + Pelvic lymph node dissection (in select patients)

Contd...

Locally advanced	Therapy
	• Androgen deprivation therapy (in select patients)
Metastatic	**Therapy**
Any T, N1, M0	• Androgen deprivation therapy • Radiation therapy + Androgen deprivation therapy (2–3 years)
Any T, N, M1	• Androgen deprivation therapy

207. Ans. (c) Lymphatics

Ref: Bailey, 26th ed. pg. 1385

- *Seminomas metastasise mainly via the lymphatics and haematogenous spread is uncommon.*
- The lymphatic drainage of the testes is to the para-aortic lymph nodes near the origin of the gonadal vessels.
- The contralateral para-aortic lymph nodes are sometimes involved by tumor spread, but the inguinal lymph nodes are affected only if the scrotal skin is involved.

There are a number of histological types of non-seminomatous germ cell tumors (NSGCT), which may coexist within a single tumor:

- Embryonal carcinoma. Highly malignant tumors that occasionally invade cord structures.
- Yolk sac tumor. Tumours with this component secrete alpha fetoprotein (AFP)
- Choriocarcinoma. Often produces human chorionic gonadotropin (HCG).This is a highly malignant tumor that metastasizes early via both the lymphatics and the bloodstream
- Teratoma. These tumors contain more than one cell type with components derived from ectoderm, endoderm

208. Ans. (a) Scrotal USG

Ref: Bailey, 26th ed. pg. 1386-87

- *The diagnosis of testicular cancer is confirmed by ultrasound scanning of the testis which is also able to assess the contralateral testis.*
- It is a mandatory test in all suspected cases of testicular tumor.
- Chest X-ray is used to detect Canon Ball metastasis
- CT scan chest and abdomen is used to detect metastasis
- Measure the levels of tumor markers which are raised in around 50 per cent of cases.
- *Rise in AFP* is seen in around 50–70 per cent of NSGCTs
- *Rise in HCG* is seen in 40–60 per cent of NSGCTs and around 30 per cent of seminomas.
- When raised, these markers are used to monitor the response to treatment. The mean serum half-lives of AFP and HCG are 5–7 days and 2–3 days, respectively, and reassessment of the markers following orchidectomy can indicate whether all the tumor tissue has been removed.

209. Ans. (a) Right Hydrocele

Findings in favour of diagnosis of Hydrocele-
- Translucent swelling with positive trans-illumination test
- Possible to 'get above the swelling' on examination of the scrotum
- The swelling usually surrounds the testis and epididymis such that they may become impossible to palpate separately.
- Be wary of an acute hydrocele in a young man since there may be a testicular tumor.
  - *Choice B:* Right inguinal hernia is ruled out as top of testis can be reached
  - *Choice C:* Epididymal cysts are present *bilaterally* and are *present behind the testis* whereas he patient is having a unilateral swelling.
  - *Choice D: Encysted hydrocele of the cord* is a smooth oval swelling near the spermatic cord, which is liable to be mistaken for an inguinal hernia. The swelling moves downwards and becomes less mobile if the testis is pulled gently downwards.
  - Ascites should be considered if the swellings are bilateral.

210. Ans. (d) Right Pyocele

- *The difference in this question from the previous question would be development of an acute on chronic presentation.*
- Scrotal pyoceles are purulent collections within the potential space between the visceral and parietal tunica vaginalis surrounding the testicle.
- The presentation of scrotal pyoceles is subacute onset of pain and swelling, which may mimic other pathology.
- The imaging modality of choice to diagnose a scrotal pyocele is ultrasound.
- Internal echoes within the pyocele fluid collection typically represent cellular debris.
- Other sonographic findings include loculations, septae, and fluid-fluid or air-fluid levels in the tunica vaginalis external to the testicle.
- By contrast, a hydrocele will appear on ultrasound as a simple fluid with an anechoic region that collects anterior and lateral to the testis. If the fluid contains internal echoes on ultrasound, the diagnosis of hematocele (most common in the setting of trauma) or pyocele may be made.
- Fournier's gangrene is the most concerning complication of a scrotal pyocele.

211. Ans. (a) Right Testicular torsion

Ref: Bailey, 26th ed. pg. 1379

- Testicular torsion is most common between 10 and 25 years of age

Clinical Findings

- Sudden agonising pain in the groin and the lower abdomen.
- Feels nauseated and may vomit.
- The testis seems high and the tender twisted cord can be palpated above it.
- The cremasteric reflex is lost.
- Elevation of the testis reduces the pain in epididymo-orchitis and makes it worse in torsion.
- Inversion of the testis is the most common predisposing cause.

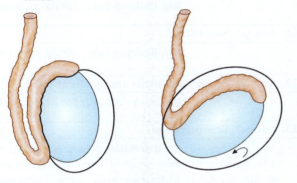

212. Ans. (a) Calcium oxalate

Ref: Bailey and Love, 26th ed. pg. 1292

Types of Renal Stones (Urolithiasis):

1. **Calcium stones (75–85%)**
   - Made of **calcium oxalate**.
2. **Struvite stone/Triple phosphate stone (15% of cases)**
   - Formed mainly after infection by urea splitting bacteria (**Proteus and some staphylococci**) **which cause alkaline urine** lead to precipitation of phosphate crystals.
   - Causes Staghorn calculi, which occupy large position of renal pelvis.
3. **Uric acid stone**
   - Common in patients with hyperuricemia.
   - Cause: Urine of pH less than 5.5 (uric acid is insoluble in acidic urine) à leading to saturation
   - It is radiolucent stone.
4. **Cystine stone**
   - Due to genetic defect in renal absorption of amino acid cysteine à leading to cystinuria.
5. **Xanthine stones due to xanthinuria**

213. Ans. (a) Uric acid

Radiolucent kidney stones mnemonic **L.U.X**
Radio**L**ucent stones are **U**ric acid and **X**anthine stones

214. Ans. (b) Triple phosphate stones

Ref: Bailey & Love, 26th ed. Ch 75/1292

215. Ans. (c) Triple phosphate stone

Ref: Bailey & Love, 26th ed. Ch 75/1292

216. Ans. (c) Uterine fibroid

The complications of fibroid are
- Thrombo-embolism
- Acute torsion of subserosal pedunculated leiomyomata
- *Acute urinary retention by uterine fibroid*
- Renal failure
- Acute pain caused by red degeneration during pregnancy
- Acute vaginal or intra-peritoneal haemorrhage
- Mesenteric vein thrombosis
- Intestinal gangrene

Causes of Urinary Retention and Bladder Outlet Obstruction

ANATOMICAL	
Extrinsic	Pelvic organ prolapse Gynecological e.g. uterine fibroid, tumor Poorly fitting pessary
Urethral	Stricture Meatal stenosis Thrombosed urethral caruncle Diverticulum
Luminal	Stone Bladder/urethral tumor Ureterocoele Foreign body
Impaired detrusor contractility	Senile bladder change Diabetes mellitus Neurological disease
FUNCTIONAL	
Impaired coordination	Primary bladder neck obstruction
Peri-operative	Pain Analgesia or anesthetic e.g. epidural
Infective/inflammatory	UTI Acute vulvovaginitis Vaginal lichen planus/sclerosis Genital herpes
Pharmacological	Opiates Antipsychotics Antidepressants Antimuscarinics

217. Ans. (b) NCCT

Ref: Bailey & Love, 26th ed. pg. 1293

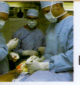

FMGE Solutions Screening Examination

- *Helical computed tomography (CT) scanning without radiocontrast enhancement is now the standard radiologic procedure for diagnosis of nephrolithiasis.*
- The advantages of CT include detection of uric acid stones in addition to the traditional radiopaque stones, no exposure to the risk of radiocontrast agents, and possible diagnosis of other causes of abdominal pain in a patient suspected of having renal colic from stones.
- Ultrasound is not as sensitive as CT in detecting renal or ureteral stones.

218. Ans. (d) Urinary bladder

Ref: Bailey & Love, 26th ed. pg. 1330-35

- Transitional cell epithelium lines → the urinary tract from the renal pelvis to the ureter, urinary bladder, and the proximal two-thirds of the urethra.
- **Transitional cell carcinoma**-Cancers can occur at any point mentioned above:
  - **90% of malignancies develop in the bladder**
  - 8% in the renal pelvis
  - 2% in the ureter or urethra.

Extra Mile

- Bladder cancer is the **fourth (4th)** most common cancer in men and the **thirteenth (1 + 3 = 4)** in women.
- **Among urothelial tumors**-95% are **transitional cell in origin**.
- **Polychronotropism**-urothelial tumors exhibit polychronotropism, which is the tendency to recur over time in new locations in the urothelial tract.
- Most imp risk factor- **Cigarette smoking**
- **Other**-aniline dyes, drugs phenacetin, external beam radiation. Chronic cyclophosphamide, *Schistosoma haematobium* (a parasite-cause both Scc and Tcc)
- Vitamin A - protective.
- 3 clinical subtypes-
  - **Superficial** (75%)
  - Invade muscle (20%)
  - Metastatic (5%)
- Clinical presentation
  1. **Hematuria** (painless)- Most common presentation (80–90% of cases)
  2. Irritative bladder symptoms such as dysuria, urgency, or frequency of urination occur in 20-30% of patients with bladder cancer.
- MC site of lymphatic metastasis: **Pelvic lymph nodes (obturator MC)**
- MC site of hematogenous spread- **LIVER > LUNG**
- **Diagnosis**– diagnosis and initial staging is made **by cystoscopy and TUR.**
  - Newer, voided urine assays (i.e., bladder tumor antigen [BTA-Stat, BTA-TRAK], NMP-22, fibrin/fibrinogen degradation products [FDP]) are being used for the detection and surveillance of urothelial carcinoma.

Contd...

- **Management**-cystoscopy and TUR or biopsy
- Further management depends on stage, grade, size, multiplicity, recurrecnce pattern
- Drugs for intravesical chemo- **Mitomycin, Thiotepa, Epirubicin, BCG (most effective)**

219. Ans. (c) Transitional cell cancer

Ref: Bailey & Love, 26th ed. pg. 1330-35

220. Ans. (d) Painless hematuria

Ref: Bailey & Love, 26th ed. pg. 1330-35

221. Ans. (c) Superficial

Ref: Bailey & Love, 26th ed. pg. 1330-35

222. Ans. (c) Females and males are equally affected

Ref: Bailey & Love, 26th ed. pg. 1330-35

223. Ans. (c) True pelvis only

Ref: Bailey & Love 26th ed. pg. 1361

The prostate has been avulsed from the membranous urethra secondary to fracture of the pelvis. Extravasation occurs above the triangular ligament and is peri-prostatic and perivesical.

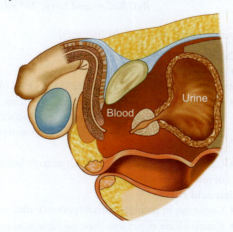

224. Ans. (a) Instrumentation

Ref: Harrison, 18th ed. pg. 288

- Urethral catheterization is the single most important predisposing factor in the development of nosocomial urinary tract infection. Cystoscopy may be followed by a transient bacteremia.
- *The most important risk factor for bacteriuria is the presence of a catheter.* Eighty percent of nosocomial UTIs are related to urethral catheterization, while 5-10% are related to genitourinary manipulation. Catheters inoculate organisms into the bladder and promote

colonization by providing a surface for bacterial adhesion and causing mucosal irritation.

225. Ans. (b) Polycystic kidney

> **Extra Mile**
>
> - **Driven snow appearance** - Pindborg's tumor
> - **Sunray appearance** - Osteogenic Sarcoma, Ewing Sarcoma
> - **Floating Water Lily sign** - Lung Hydatid, Echinococcus
> - **Popcorn calcification** - Pulmonary Hamartoma
> - **Honeycomb appearance** - RA, Scleroderma, Interstitial Lung Disease
> - **Egg shell calcification** - Sarcoidosis, Silicosis, Lymphoma, T.B., Histoplasmosis
> - **Spring water cyst** = Pluero Pericardial cyst
> - **Rib notching** - Neurofibromatosis, Aortic Aneurysm, Taussig-Bing Operation, Aortic obstruction, Coarctation of aorta.
> - **Coeur en Sabot, Flask shape heart** - TOF
> - **Candle wax sign** - Melorheostosis
> - **Football Sign** - Pneumoperitoneum
> - **Thumb Print Sign** - Epiglotis, Ischemic Colitis
> - **Double bubble sign** - Duodenal Atresia
> - **Single bubble sign** - Pyloric stenosis
> - **Soap bubble appearance** - Meconium ileus
> - **Meniscus appearance** - CBD stone on cholangiography
> - **Central dot sign** - Caroli's disease
> - **Chain of lakes appearance** - Chronic pancreatitis
> - **Spongy appearance with central sunburst calcification sign** - serous cyst adenoma
> - **Rim sign in IVP** - Hydronephrosis
> - **Cobra head deformity** - Ureterocele
> - **B/L spider leg sign** - Polycystic Kidney
> - **Golf hole ureter** - T.B.
> - **Flower Vase pattern of pelvis in IVP** - Horse shoe kidney

226. Ans. (b) Ureterocele

> *Ref: Bailey & Love, 26th ed. pg. 1285*

A ureterocele is a congenital saccular dilatation of terminal portion of the ureter. The most common presentation is that of urinary tract infection or uro-sepsis in children. Stasis of urine can lead to calculus formation. Some children may present with palpable mass due to hydro nephrotic kidney .Cyst may prolapse into internal urethral opening causing obstruction to bladder outflow. This condition may remain unrecognized until adult life. Ureterocele is usually discovered on radiological examination or during endoscopy.

227. Ans. (a) Leydig cells

> *Ref: Bailey & Love, 26th ed. pg. 1341*

Rectangular, crystal-like inclusions, composed of protein, with pointed or rounded ends in the interstitial cells of the testis (Leydig cells) and hilus cells in the ovary. *Inside the Leydig cells of human males can be found Reinke's crystals. The purpose of these crystals is uncertain, some believe that they are a by-product of a degenerative process related to aging. They appear to have no contribution to androgen or testosterone production, and they can be used to identify Leydig cells easily when viewing testicular tissue under a microscope.*

228. Ans. (a) Seminoma

> *Ref: Bailey & Love, 26th ed. pg. 1385*

- **Seminoma** is the most common germ cell tumor of the testis or, more rarely, the mediastinum or other extra-gonadal locations. It is a malignant neoplasm and is one of the most treatable and curable cancers, with a survival rate above 95% if discovered in early stages.

229. Ans. (b) Para aortic

> *Ref: Harrison, 19th ed. pg. 589*

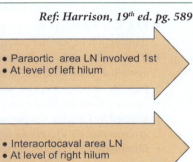

Points to Remember about testicular tumor

- In metastatic disease-Retroperitoneal LN is **Most commonly** involved
- **Metastasis**- Lymphatic >> Blood (m/c lung)
- **exception is Choriocarcinoma where blood metastasis (m/c lung)**>> lymphatic metastasis.
- **Most common testicular tumor- in general** → seminoma
    - Prepubertal adults- Teratoma
    - Infant and children- Yolk sac tumor
- **Most common presentation**- nodule or painless swelling of one gonad
- Most common bilateral testicular tumor- **Malignant lymphoma**
- Most common bilateral primary testicular tumor Seminoma
- FNAC contraindicated
- **Intial IOC**- USG(hypo echoic area within tunica albuginea is suspicious)
- HPE diagnosis by-radical orchiectomy (inguinal approach)
- **Scrotal orchiectomy**- contraindicated
- **Chavesseac maneuver**- soft clamp applied to cord → biopsy from suspicious area → sent for frozen section→ if + ligate cord, do orchiectomy → final HPE

230. Ans. (a) P.S.A (Prostate specific antigen)

Ref: Bailey & Love, 26th ed. pg. 1341

Prostatic acid phosphatase	It is elevated in: • Prostate cancer • Metastatic prostate cancer
Prostate specific antigen	As the PSA level increases, so does the risk of this disease. When the PSA is 1 ng/mL, cancer can be detected in about 8% of men if a biopsy is performed. With a PSA level of 4–10 ng/mL, the likelihood of finding prostate cancer is about 25%
N.S.E (NEURON SPECIFIC ENOLASE)	Neuroblastoma/oat cell cancer

231. Ans. (d) Persists in blood after prostatectomy

Ref: Bailey & Love, 26th ed. pg. 1341

- PSA is a kallikrein-related serine protease that causes liquefaction of seminal coagulum.
- It is produced by both nonmalignant and malignant epithelial cells and, as such, is prostate-specific, not prostate cancer–specific, and serum levels may also increase from prostatitis and BPH. Serum levels are not affected by DRE but the performance of a prostate biopsy can increase PSA levels up to tenfold for 8–10 weeks.
- Elimination of PSA bound to alpha 1-antichymotrypsin is slow (estimated half-life of 1-2 weeks) as it is too large to be cleared by the kidneys. Levels should be undetectable after about six weeks if the prostate has been removed.

232. Ans. (c) Prostate specific antigen only

Ref: Bailey & Love, 26th ed. pg. 1341

- The most common presentation of advanced prostate cancer is a patient with a rising PSA level in whom initial local therapy has failed. Generally, after a radical prostatectomy, the PSA level should be less than 0.2 ng/mL and, after radiation therapy, less than 0.5 ng/mL. Other important prognostic indicators include PSA velocity, time to PSA nadir, time to PSA recurrence, and pattern of PSA recurrence.
- PSA levels for all men with prostate cancer who are having radical treatment should be checked at the earliest 6 weeks following treatment, at least every 6 months for the first 2 years and then at least once a year thereafter.

233. Ans. (b) Prostatitis

Ref Bailey & Love, 25th pg. 1320

The **three-glass urine test** is valuable, if the first glass with the initial voided sample shows **urine containing prostatic threads, prostatic is present**'.

Prostatodynia is diagnosed by presence of perigenital pain in the absence of any objective evidence of prostate inflammation.

234. Ans. (a) Bateson plexus

Ref: Bailey & Love, 26th ed. pg. 527

- The **Bateson venous plexus** is a network of valve-less veins in the human body that connect the deep pelvic veins and thoracic veins to the internal vertebral venous plexuses.
- Because of their location and lack of valves, they are believed to provide a route for the spread of cancer metastases. These metastases commonly arise from cancer of the pelvic organs such as prostate and may spread to the vertebral column.

235. Ans. (b) Localized prostate cancer, life expectancy > 10 years

Ref: Bailey & Love, 26th ed. pg. 1355

- Nerve-sparing RRP is done in patients with clinically localized prostate cancer who have at least a 10-year life expectancy and low comorbidities.
- *Patients with locally advanced disease cannot undergo nerve-sparing RRP; because of the extent of the local tumor burden (especially posteriorly), the nerve-sparing procedure can compromise the adequacy of the operation.*
- The objective of modern RP are to remove the entire cancer with negative surgical margins, minimal blood loss, no serious perioperative complications, and complete recovery of continence and potency.

236. Ans. (a) Horse shoe kidney

Ref: Bailey & Love, 26th ed. pg. 1282

- Since the contrast can be seen on both sides, absent kidney is ruled out. More over the contrast is at normal level, so undescended kidney is unlikely.
- The *horseshoe kidney* consists of two distinct functioning kidneys on each side of the midline, *connected at the lower poles by an isthmus of functioning renal parenchyma or fibrous tissue that crosses the midline of the body*
- The collecting system has a characteristic appearance on intravenous urography because of an incomplete inward rotation of the renal pelvis, which faces anterior. The axis of the collecting system is deviated inward at the lower poles because of the lower pole's connection with the isthmus.

237. Ans. (a) Renal cell cancer

- The large homogenous mass on right shows an enlarged kidney as compared to other side suggestive of malignancy. The hilum of kidney shows renal vein thrombosis.

Surgery

- Due to homogenous mass present unilaterally, polycystic kidney is ruled out. Since no cystic dilatation is present, hydro-nephrosis is ruled out.

238. Ans. (b) Bladder stone

- Notice the densely radio-opaque, single large calculus.
- Fecolith is hardening of feces into lumps of varying size inside the colon, which may appear whenever chronic obstruction of transit occurs, such as in megacolon and chronic constipation but location of this radioopaque shadow in pelvis rules out fecolith

239. Ans. (b) Carcinoma Penis

Ref: Bailey & Love, 26th ed. pg. 1374

- Penile squamous cell carcinoma, the most common penile malignancy, behaves similarly to squamous cell carcinoma in other parts of the skin.This is a slow-growing cancer in its early stages, and because it seldom interferes with voiding or erectile function
- *Bowen's disease* typically presents as a gradually enlarging, well-demarcated erythematous plaque with an irregular border and surface crusting or scaling. *About 60-85% of patients have lesions on the lower leg, usually in previously or presently sun-exposed areas of skin.*

240. Ans. (b) Inguinal lymph node metastasis operable

Ref: Bailey & Love 26th ed. pg. 1373-74

CARCINOMA PENIS

Clinical Features
- Most commonly occur in 6th decade of life
- *Squamous cell carcinoma (80%) is the MC type,* most commonly originates from glans> sulcus > prepuce>shaft.
- Others are transitional cell carcinoma (15%), basal cell carcinoma, malignant melanoma, sarcoma
- **MC symptom**: foul smelling discharge, with little or no pain
- More than 50% patients of CA penis presents with enlarged inguinal lymph nodes.
- **MC and earliest symptom of metastatic CA penis: Priapism**

Jackson (Extent of spread) Staging for CA Penis	
Stage I	Confined to glans or prepuce
Stage II	Extension to shaft
Stage III	Operable inguinal LN metastasis
Stage IV	Inoperable inguinal LN metastasis or local or advanced spread

241. Ans. (d) Phimosis

Ref: Bailey, 26th ed. pg. 1359

PHIMOSIS

- Phimosis is a condition in which the contracted foreskin cannot be retracted over the glans.
- Chronic infection from poor local hygiene is its most common cause.
- Most cases occur in uncircumcised males, although excessive skin left after circumcision can become stenotic and cause phimosis.

Clinical features
- **Difficulty in micturition is the main symptom.**
- Ballooning of prepuce during micturition is suggestive of phimosis.
- *Edema, erythema, and tenderness of the prepuce and the presence of purulent discharge usually cause the patient to seek medical attention.*
- Inability to retract the foreskin is a less common complaint.

HYPOSPADIAS

- Hypospadias results when fusion of urethral folds is incomplete, and urethral meatus opens on the underside of penis or perineum (ventral surface of penis).
- Because fusion of urethral folds is from posterior to anterior, Anterior forms are more common than posterior.
- **Associated pathology:** In addition to ventrally placed ectopic meatus, hypospadias has:
  - **Chordee:** ventral curvature of penis due to contracture of fibrous cord which has replaced the distal urethra and corpus spongiosum.
  - **Hooded prepuce:** Deficient on ventral aspect and excess on dorsal aspect
  - Stenosis of ectopic meatus

EPISPADIAS

- Urethra opens on the dorsum (upper aspect) of the penis in males, in females there is a fissure in the wall of the urethra which opens above the clitoris
- **Females:** Bifid clitoris and separation of the labia. Most are incontinent because of maldevelopment of the urinary sphincters.
- **Males:** Patients with glandular epispadias seldom have urinary incontinence. However, incontinence in penopubic epispadias is 95% and penile epispadias is 75%.

POSTERIOR URETHRAL VALVE

- Exclusively an anomaly of male urethra.
- Symmetrical folds of urothelium extending distally from prostatic urethra to external urinary sphincter.
- Newborns may present with palpable abdominal masses.

- Sometimes, the valves are incomplete and the patient remains without symptoms until adolescence or adulthood.

242. Ans. (b) Hypospadias

Ref: Bailey, 26th ed. pg. 1359

Refer to above explanation

243. Ans. (b) Circumcision

Ref: Bailey & Love, 25th pg. 1371

Balanitis xerotica obliterans (BXO)
- A condition in which the normally pliant **foreskin becomes thickened and will not retract.**
- It is difficult to keep the penis clean and there is a problem with hygiene.
- In later life there is an **increased susceptibility to carcinoma.**
- Treatment is by **circumcision**

244. Ans. (d) Infection

Ref: Cambell's Urology, 8th ed. pg. 346,349

Principal causes of death in renal transplant patients (in decreasing order)
1. Heart disease
2. Infection
3. Stroke

HEPATOBILIARY SYSTEM

245. Ans. (d) Contrast CT scan

Ref: SRB 5th ed. pg. 599, 601

The clinical presentation is suggestive of liver abscess. Since the patient is anicteric, viral hepatitis is a less likely diagnosis. The initial investigation to be performed will be USG which will evaluate the echotexture of liver and give insight into altered echogenicity.

CT scan abdomen with contrast has 95% sensitivity to pick up the abscess, location, size and picks up complications as well.

246. Ans. (a) HCC

Ref: SRB 5th ed. pg. 609

Alpha-fetoprotein is raised to more than 100 IU in Hepatocellular carcinoma. It begins to rise once vascular invasion occurs by the tumour. The fibrolamellar variant of HCC does not show elevated HCC. Other tumour markers for HCC are:
- PIVKA II
- ALP-L3
- DCP (des carboxy prothrombin)

Extra Mile

Tumour marker for fibrolamellar variant of HCC is neurotensin levels and increases in serum vitamin B12 binding protein.

247. Ans. (c) E.R.C.P

Ref: Page 634: SRB, 5th edition

The image shows presence of gastroduodenoscopey at 7'o clock position with a filling defect in CBD. The technique involves cannulation of sphincter of Oddi and dye is injected. It is done under C arm guidance and sedation like midazolam or propofol anaesthesia.

T – Tube cholangiogram	Percutaneous transhepatic cholangiography
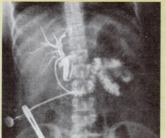	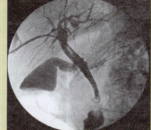
After choledochotomy Kehr's tube is placed in CBD for 14 days and then water-soluble dye is injected into the tube and X-ray is taken. Complete free flow of dye into the duodenum indicates there is no blockage due to residual CBD stones	With help of C arm fluoroscopy *Okuda needle* is passed into dilated biliary duct via the liver parenchyma. It is done to evaluate for high biliary strictures or failure of ERCP.

248. Ans. (a) Associated with MEN1

Ref: Harrison 19th ed. P 569

- Zollinger Ellison syndrome/Gastrinoma is the most common pancreatic tumor seen in multiple endocrine neoplasia type 1.
- The most common site is second part of duodenum and hence choice B is wrong.
- The best test for diagnosis of ZES is secretin study with measurement of fasting gastrin levels and BAO/MAO levels.
- Most common presenting symptom is epigastric pain > diarrhea.
- The most frequent metastasis is *to liver*.

249. Ans. (a) Hepatoduodenal ligament

Pringle maneuver is used to slow bleeding flow during liver surgery. *The Pringle manoeuvre is characterised by clamping of hepatoduodenal ligament.* It is effective as the liver is partially nourished by backflow from the hepatic veins. However intermittent clamping with 15 minutes of clamping and 5 minutes without clamping is less harmful.

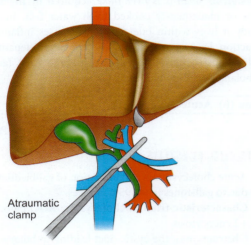

FIGURE: Pringle maneuver. Occlusion of the porta hepatis decreases blood flow to the liver to slow bleeding during liver surgery. It clamps the portal vein and hepatic artery

250. Ans. (a) Cholelithiasis

The USG image shows stones appearing as intraluminal, echogenic, mobile foci that are gravity-dependent and create a clean acoustic shadow. The gravity dependant movement of stone with change of patient position and is called as rolling stone sign.

251. Ans. (b) Aspiration + Anti amoebic drugs

Ref: Bailey, 26th ed. pg. 131

- *The presence of solitary abscess in left lobe points to amoebic liver abscess etiology and needs aspiration and anti- amoebic drugs*
- Liver involvement occurs following invasion of *E histolytica* into mesenteric venules.
- Amebae then enter the portal circulation and travel to the liver where they typically form large abscesses.
- Routine aspiration of liver abscess is not indicated.
- The aspirate is the color of chocolate/ Anchovy sauce due to mixture of blood and liver tissue.
- Choice D is performed for Hydatid cyst.

Indications of aspiration in amoebic liver abscess are
1. Lack of clinical improvement in 24–48 hours
2. Left lobe abscess
3. Thin rim of liver tissue around the abscess

252. Ans. (a) Liver cancer

Ref: Bailey, 26th ed. pg. 131

- Aflatoxin exposure in food is a significant risk factor for Hepatocellular carcinoma.
- Aflatoxins are primarily produced by the food-borne fungi *Aspergillus flavus* and *Aspergillus parasiticus*, which colonize a variety of food commodities, including maize, oilseeds, spices, groundnuts
- Choice B is related to Smoking and aniline dye exposure
- Choice D is related to the earliest detected proto-oncogene Rb.

253. Ans. (c) Rapid transfusion of fresh blood

Ref: Bailey, 26th ed. pg. 16-17 and pg. 109

Choice A	Vasopressor or inotropic therapy is not indicated as first-line treatment of hypovolemic shock.
Choice B	Laparotomy would require General anesthesia which cannot be given in setting of decompensated shock.
Choice C	If blood is being lost, the ideal replacement fluid is blood, although crystalloid therapy may be required while awaiting blood products.
Choice D	While awaiting Blood transfusion crystalloids must be started and is a first line management.

Extra Mile

Role of vasopressors in shock
- Vasopressor agents (phenylephrine, noradrenaline) are indicated in distributive shock states (sepsis, neurogenic shock) where there is peripheral vasodilatation, and a low systemic vascular resistance, leading to hypotension despite a high cardiac output.
- Where the vasodilatation is resistant to catecholamines (e.g. absolute or relative steroid deficiency) vasopressin may be used as an alternative vasopressor.

254. Ans. (b) Amoebic liver abscess

Ref: Sabistan, 19th ed. pg. 1443

AMOEBIC LIVER ABSCESS

- Caused by Entamoeba histolytica whose cysts are acquired through the feco-oral route
- Usually Solitary and more common in **right lobe of liver**.
- It most frequently affects the cecum and ascending colon
- **In colon:** Flask-shaped ulcers (MC site: Cecum and ascending colon)

FMGE Solutions Screening Examination

Clinical Features

- Most common symptoms is abdominal pain
- **Typical clinical picture** (*as seen in the question*): Patient of 20–40 yrs of age, with history of travel to endemic area, presents with fever, chills, anorexia, *right upper quadrant pain*.
- Results from an obligatory colonic infection, a recent history of diarrhea are uncommon.
- USG guided aspiration: Shows anchovy sauce pus

TABLE: Difference between Amoebic liver abscess and Pyogenic liver abscess

Clinical features	Amebic liver abscess	Pyogenic liver abscess
Age (yr)	20–40	>50
Travel in endemic area	Yes	No
Diabetes mellitus	Uncommon	More common
Alcohol use	Common	Common
Jaundice	Uncommon	Common
Elevated bilirubin	Uncommon	Common
Elevated alkaline phosphatase	Common	Common

Extra Mile

- **Most common** symptom of pyogenic abscess: FEVER
- MC sign of pyogenic abscess: RUQ tenderness
- **Most common** symptom of amoebic abscess: **Abdominal pain**
- **Most common** sign of amoebic abscess: **HEPATOMEGALY**
- Hydatid cyst is mostly asymptomatic. If presents with symptom, most common presenting symptom is abdominal pain, vomiting, dyspepsia.

255. Ans. (a) Amoebic liver abcess

Ref: Bailey & Love, 26th ed. pg. 70

256. Ans. (b) Peritoneal deposits

Ref: Bailey & Love, 26th ed. pg. 1100

Advantages of ultrasound in obstructive jaundice

1. Ultrasonography (US) is the least expensive, safest, and most sensitive technique for visualizing the biliary system, particularly the gallbladder
2. Current accuracy is close to 95%. US is the procedure of choice for the initial evaluation of cholestasis and for helping differentiate extrahepatic from intrahepatic causes
3. Visualization of the pancreas, kidney, and blood vessels is also possible.

257. Ans. (a) Clonorchis sinensis

Ref: Bailey & Love, 26th ed. pg. 1115

Clonorchis sinensis is liver fluke acquired by ingestion of raw or inadequately cooked fresh water fish. In human body it lives within bile ducts and causes inflammatory reaction leading to cholangitis, cholangio-hepatitis and biliary obstruction. It is well known to be a risk factor for Cholangio-carcinoma.

258. Ans. (b) Acute cholecystitis

Ref: Sabistan, 19th ed. pg. 1847

ACUTE CHOLECYSTITIS

- Acute cholecystitis is inflammation of gallbladder and is due to gallstones in 90-95% of cases.
- **Characteristic triad of cholecystits:** RUQ pain +Fever + Leucocytosis
- Obstruction of the cystic duct leading to biliary colic is the initial event in acute cholecystitis

Clinical Presentation

1. RUQ pain of much longer duration than biliary colic, is the **MC symptom**
2. **Other common symptoms:** Fever, nausea, and vomiting
3. **Upon Physical examination:** RUQ tenderness and guarding are usually present inferior to the right costal margin.
4. **Murphy's sign:** Inspiratory arrest with deep palpation in the RUQ in acute cholecystitis.
5. **Boas sign:** Hyperesthesia below right scapula in acute cholecystitis

259. Ans. (a) Acute cholangitis

Ref: Sabiston, 19th ed. pg. 1847

- Charcoat triad is seen in case of acute cholangitis.
- **It includes: Pain, Fever, Jaundice**
- Do not mix with triad of cholecystitis

260. Ans. (b) Acute Cholecystitis

Ref: Page 1107, Chapter 67, Bailey and Love, 26th ed.

- In the acute phase of Cholecystitis, the patient may have right upper quadrant tenderness that is exacerbated during inspiration by the examiner's right subcostal palpation (**Murphy's sign).**

261. Ans. (c) Cholecystitis

- Cholecystitis is inflammation of gallbladder wall. Radiological evaluation does not show elevation of right hemidiaphragm in these cases.

Surgery

- Chest radiographs are abnormal in the majority of patients with amebic hepatic abscesses. Findings include **elevation of the right hemi-diaphragm**, right pleural effusion, atelectasis in the region of the base of the right lung, and a right pleural effusion.
- In case of pyogenic liver abscess and subdiaphragmatic abscess also, there is elevation of right hemi-diaphragm.

262. Ans. (c) Hemangioma

Ref: Bailey & Love, 26th ed. pg. 1083

Hemangioma being a *vascular tumor* is diagnosed by imaging techniques and liver biopsy is contraindicated. Cavernous hemangiomas arise from the endothelial cells and consist of multiple, large vascular channels lined by a single layer of endothelial cells and supported by collagenous walls. These tumors are frequently asymptomatic and incidentally discovered at imaging, surgery, or autopsy.

263. Ans. (a) Hemangioma

Ref: Bailey & Love, 26th ed. pg. 1083

- **Hemangiomas:** These are the *most common type of benign liver tumor*. Most of these tumors do not cause symptoms and do not need treatment.
- Hepatic adenomas: These are benign epithelial liver tumors that develop in the liver and are found mainly in women that using estrogens as contraceptives. Symptoms associated with hepatic adenomas are all associated with large lesions which can cause intense abdominal pain.
- Focal nodular hyperplasia (FNH) is the second most common tumor of the liver. This tumor is the result of a congenital arteriovenous malformation hepatocyte response.

264. Ans. (b) Hepatic artery

Ref: Bailey & Love, 26th ed. pg. 1073

- Pringle manoeuvre: Atraumatic clamping of the hilar vessels to control hepatic bleeding from traumatic injuries also known-as the Pringle maneuver.
- This atraumatic clamp is placed at foramen of Winslow, across the hepato-duodenal ligament
- It clamps the portal vein and hepatic artery, and prevents excessive blood loss during parenchymal transection.

265. Ans. (d) Pale yellow

Ref: Bailey & Love, 26th ed. pg. 1106-1107

Morphology of gall stones

Cholesterol stones:
Cholesterol stones arise exclusively in the gallbladder and are composed of cholesterol. *Pure cholesterol stones are pale yellow, round to ovoid, and have a finely granular, hard external surface.* Stones composed largely of cholesterol are radiolucent: Presence of calcium carbonate in stones makes them radiopaque

Mixed stones:
Increasing proportions of calcium carbonate, phosphates, and bilirubin, the stones exhibit discoloration and appear gray-white to black

Pigment gallstones:
- Pigment stones are classified as "black" and "brown." *Black pigment stones* are found in *sterile gallbladder* bile and *brown stones* are found in *infected intrahepatic or extrahepatic ducts*.
- "Black" pigment stones contain oxidized polymers of the calcium salts of unconjugated bilirubin, small amounts of calcium carbonate, calcium phosphate, and mucin glycoprotein.
- "Brown" pigment stones contain pure calcium salts of unconjugated bilirubin, mucin glycoprotein, a substantial cholesterol fraction, and calcium salts of palmitate and stearate.

266. Ans. (a) Pigment stones

Ref: Bailey & Love, 26th ed. pg. 1106-1107

In hemolytic anemia like hereditary spherocytosis, on account of increased extravascular hemolysis, there is production of calcium bilirubinate stones (pigment stones).

267. Ans. (d) Liver cancer

Ref: Harrison, 18th ed. Ch. 91

- Aspirin suppresses cell proliferation by inhibiting prostaglandin synthesis.
- Regular aspirin use reduces the risk of colon adenomas and carcinomas as well as death from large-bowel cancer.

HEAD AND NECK

268. Ans. (c) Oral lichen planus

Ref: SRB 5th ed. pg. 370

Conditions responsible for premalignant lesions of oral cavity

Equivocal risk lesions are
- Oral lichen planus
- Dyskeratosis congenita
- Discoid lupus erythematosus

Medium risk lesions
- Oral submucosal fibrosis
- Syphilitic glossitis
- Sideropenic Glossitis/Plummer Vinson Syndrome

Contd...

FMGE Solutions Screening Examination

High risk Lesions
- Leukoplakia
- Erythroplakia
- Chronic hyperplastic candidiasis

269. Ans. (d) SCC of lip

Ref: SRB 5th ed. pg. 384

The image shows a fungating mass arising from mucosal part of lip. It shows everted edge with induration. The visible staining of teeth indicates that the patient may be using khaini (mixture of tobacco and lime) kept under the lip which is a common cause in Indian patients

The age of patient also favours the diagnosis. It is usually a well differentiated Squamous cell carcinoma.

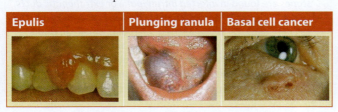

270. Ans. (a) Nodulocystic

Ref: SRB, 5th ed. pg. 290

- The most common subtype of Basal cell cancer is rodent ulcer. It is the most common malignant skin tumour seen on face (Oghren line) and is also called tear cancer. The most common subtype is nodulocystic and noduloulcerative subtype.
- Choices A and B are subtypes of malignant melanoma. Choice D pigmented BCC mimics melanoma.

271. Ans. (c) Betel nut chewing

Ref: Harrison 19th ed. P 369

Causes of Submucosal Fibrosis

1. Prolonged irritation by chilies, tobacco (pan/quid), areca due to arecoline
2. Deficiency of vitamin A and B complex (riboflavin)
3. Localized collagen disorder

- It presents with soreness in mouth which increases during meals. There is trismus and difficulty in protruding the tongue. The entire area turns red and later has stiff fibrotic bands and scarring.
- Common sites are buccal mucosa, faucial pillars and soft palate.
- There is progressive nature of disease even with cessation of causative factors.

272. Ans. (d) Pain and paraesthesia in Ulnar nerve distribution

- Neurologic symptoms occur in 95% of cases of thoracic outlet syndrome. The lower 2 nerve roots of the brachial plexus, C8 and T1, are most commonly (90%) involved, producing pain and paresthesias in the *ulnar nerve* distribution.
- The second most common anatomic pattern involves the upper 3 nerve roots of the brachial plexus, C5, C6, and C7, with symptoms referred to the neck, ear, upper chest, upper back, and outer arm in the radial nerve distribution.

273. Ans. (a) Frontal bone

- *Potts puffy tumor is a misnomer and is an acute osteomyelitis of frontal bone.*
- It has diffuse external swelling of scalp due to subperiosteal pus formation and scalp oedema. It originates in frontal area.
- It presents as a boggy swelling with pitting scalp oedema. X-ray of Skull is done. It is treated with antibiotics and drainage under GA before it spreads to the CNS.
- Once it extends into the cranial cavity, it is managed by neurosurgical decompression using Dandy's Brain Cannula.

Complications
- Osteomyelitis of frontal bone
- Spread of infection of intracranial cavity.
- Cortical venous thrombosis
- Subdural empyema

274. Ans. (a) Rathke pouch

Ref: Harsh Mohan, 7th ed. pg. 787

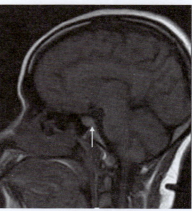

Features of Craniopharyngioma are-
- Slow-growing tumor
- Epithelial-squamous
- Calcified hence visible even on X-ray skull

- Cystic tumor arising from remnants of the craniopharyngeal duct and/or Rathke cleft
- Occupying the (supra)sellar region.

275. Ans. (a) Extradural Bleeding

Ref: Bailey, 26th ed. pg. 316

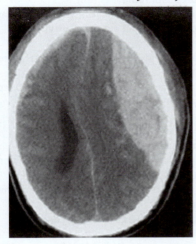

- On CT, extradural haematomas appear as a lentiform (lens shaped or biconvex) hyperdense lesion between skull and brain constrained by the adherence of the dura to the skull.
- Mass effect may be evident, with compression of surrounding brain and midline shift.
- Areas of mixed density suggest active bleeding.

276. Ans. (b) Lung cancer

Ref: Schwartz, 10th ed. pg. 583; Harrison, 18th ed. Ch 99

Metastasis to Cervical lymph Nodes

Squamous cell carcinoma (SCC) is the most common histotype, followed by adenocarcinoma, undifferentiated carcinoma and other malignancies (for example, lymphoma and melanoma)

Common site for metastasis to neck nodes – Head and Neck (M.C.), Lungs (2nd M.C.), esophagus, stomach, ovary, pancreas. Approximately ten percent of patients with abnormal cervical nodes present without obvious primary. *Most common sites for unknown primary:*

1. Nasal Pharynx
2. Pyriform Sinus
3. Tongue Base
4. Tonsillar Crypts
5. Thyroid

The left supraclavicular node is called Virchow's node since it is on the left side of the neck where the lymphatic drainage of most of the body (from the thoracic duct) enters the venous circulation via the left subclavian vein. The metastasis blocks the thoracic duct leading to regurgitation into the surrounding nodes i.e. virchow's node.

Remember

Probable Source of Nodal Metastasis
- **Level 1:** Oral cavity, submandibular gland.
- **Level 2:** Nasal pharynx, oral pharynx, parotid, supraglottic larynx.
- **Level 3:** Oral pharynx, hypopharynx, supraglottic larynx.
- **Level 4:** Subglottic larynx, hypopharynx, esophagus, thyroid.
- **Level 5:** Nasal pharynx, oral pharynx.
- **Level 6 & 7:** Thyroid, larynx, lung.
- **Note:** Bilateral nodes are common with cancers of soft palate, tongue, epiglottis, and nasal pharynx.

277. Ans. (a) Astrocytoma

Ref: Harrison, 18th ed. pg. 379

- MC malignant brain tumor is astrocytoma
- Overall most common brain tumor: Metastasis (Oat cell cancer of lung)

DRAINAGE Sites for Cervical Lymph Nodes

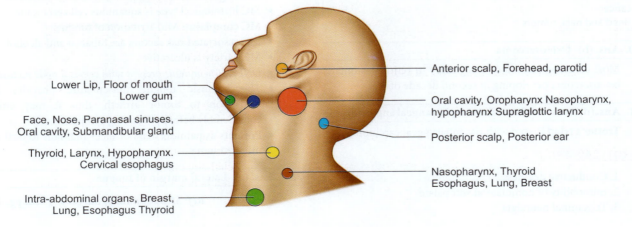

FMGE Solutions Screening Examination

278. Ans. (a) Brain tumor

Ref: Harrison, 18th ed. pg. 379

RADIOSURGERY & STEREOTACTIC RADIOTHERAPY

- Radiosurgery refers to a single treatment with a relatively large dose of radiation by focusing many small beams of radiation from different directions onto a small tumor (up to 3 cm in diameter).
- The CyberKnife is a specially designed imaging-guided system in which a small linear accelerator is moved around the patient by a programmable robotic arm. In addition to treating tumors of the brain, the Cyberknife can be used to treat tumors of the spine and other sites such as the head and neck, prostate, liver, lung, and kidney.

There are two types of Stereotactic Radiation

- Stereotactic radiosurgery (SRS) refers to a single or several stereotactic radiation treatments of the brain or spine.
- Stereotactic body radiation therapy (SBRT) refers to one or several stereotactic radiation treatments with the body, excluding the brain or spine.
- Generally in brain the procedure is referred as stereotactic surgery if it is done in a single session or as **fractionated stereotactic radiotherapy (SRT),** if done in multiple sessions.
- If the therapy is done for other parts of the body then it is generally known as stereotactic radiotherapy

279. Ans. (d) Seminoma

Ref: Bailey & Love, 26th ed. pg. 1385

Radiosensitive tumors	Radioresistant tumors
• Neuroblastoma	• Renal cell cancer
• Seminoma	• Colonic cancer
• Medulloblastoma	• Lung cancer
• Wilm's tumor	• Melanoma
• Early cervical cancer and vaginal cancer	• Sarcoma
• Head and neck tumors	

280. Ans. (b) Osteosarcoma

Most common *secondary malignancy* in retinoblastoma is osteosarcoma developing in second decade of life.

281. Ans. (d) Seen with Juvenile nasopharangeal angiofibroma

Trotter's triad is seen with nasopharyngeal carcinoma

TROTTER'S TRIAD

1. Conductive deafness
2. Immobility of homolateral soft palate
3. Trigeminal neuralgia

Remember Commonly Asked Triads

Extra Mile

Triad of Alports Syndrome
- Sensorineural deafness/Progressive renal failure/Ocular anomalies

Triad of Behcet's Syndrome:
- Recurrent oral ulcers/Genital ulcers/Iridocyclitis [mnemonic: can't see, can't pee, can't eat spicy curry]

Beck's Triad
- Muffled heart sound/Distended neck veins/Hypotension

Gradenigo's Triad
- Sixth cranial n. Palsy/Persistent ear discharge/Deep seated retro orbital pain

Charcot's Triad
- Pain + fever + jaundice

Triad of Hypernephroma
- Pain + hematuria + renal mass Triad of Hypernephroma

Hutchinson's Triad
- Hutchison's teeth/Interstitial keratitis/Nerve deafness

Triad of Kwashiorkar
- Growth retardation/Mental changes/Edema

Saint's Triad
- Gall stones/Diverticulosis/Hiatus hernia

Trotter's Triad
- Conductive deafness/Immobility of homolateral soft palate/Trigeminal neuralgia

Virchow's Triad
- Stasis/Hypercoagulabilty/Vessel injury

Fanconi Syndrome Triad
- Aminoaciduria/Proteinuria/Phosphaturia

282. Ans. (c) MC site is on Lateral margin

Ref: Bailey, & Love, 26th ed. pg. 713-14

TONGUE CANCER

- MC site is middle of lateral border or ventral aspect of the tongue.
- MC histological type is squamous cell carcinoma.
- **MC complaint:** Mid-irritation of tongue.
- MC associated risk factors are tobacco and alcohol.
- MC variety is ulcerative.
- *ONLY 30% patients present with cervical node metastasis.*
- The intrinsic tongue musculature provides little restriction to tumor growth, thus it may enlarge considerably before producing symptoms.
- Presents as painless mass or ulcer that fails to heal after minor trauma.

283. Ans. (c) Lateral margin of tongue

Ref: SRB Manual of Surgery, 4th ed. pg. 1310

Squamous cell cancer of the tongue is the commonest cancer. The location is at the following sites

- Lateral margin -50%
- Posterior 1/3 rd tongue-20%
- Dorsum-6.5%
- Ventral surface-6%
- Tip-10%

284. Ans. (c) Cleft lip and palate

Ref: Bailey & Love, 26th ed. pg. 634

Orofacial clefts (ie, cleft lip [CL], cleft lip and palate [CLP], cleft palate [CP] alone, as well as median, lateral [transversal], oblique facial clefts) are among the most common congenital anomalies. *Approximately 1 case of orofacial cleft occurs in every 500-550 births.*

285. Ans. (c) Thyroglossal fistula

Ref: Dhingra's ENT, 5th ed. pg. 398

- Sublingual dermoid cyst present as midline submental swelling. This cyst is not attached to foramen cecum and hence doesn't move upon tongue protrusion or upon deglutition.
- The **thyroglossal cyst** classically moves upwards with swallowing and notably with tongue protrusion, as it is attached to foramen cecum. It merely indicates attachment to the hyoid bone.

286. Ans. (c) Cystic hygroma

Ref: Bailey & Love, 26th ed. pg. 701

■ CYSTIC HYGROMA/LYMPHANGIOMA

- Cystic hygromas are multiloculated cystic swelling filled with clear lymph lined by endothelial cells
- It results due to sequestration of a portion of the jugular lymph sac from the lymphatic system.
- It is associated with Turner's syndrome
- Most cystic hygromas involve the lymphatic jugular sacs
- **MC site:** Posterior neck region
- **Other common sites:** Axilla, mediastinum, inguinal and retroperitoneal regions
- Approximately 50% of them are present at birth.
- It may show spontaneous regression
- The cysts are filled with clear lymph and **lined by a single layer of endothelium epithelium.**

Clinical Features

- Usually manifests in the neonates or in early infancy (50% present at birth).
- Prone to infection and hemorrhage within the mass.
- Usually present as soft masses that distort the surrounding anatomy, can result in acute airway obstruction.

- Swelling is soft and partially compressible and invariably increases in size when the child coughs or cries.
- **Characteristic features: Brilliantly translucent**

Diagnosis: MRI plays a crucial role in preoperative planning

Treatment: Complete surgical excision is the preferred treatment.

> **Extra Mile**
> - Carotid body tumor aka potato tumor MC presents in 5th decade with firm, rubbery, mobile mass.
> - Branchial cyst most commonly seen in older children or adolescents. However, all branchial remnants are present at the time of birth.

287. Ans. (d) Lined by columnar epithelium

Ref: Bailey & Love, 26th ed. pg. 700-701

VASCULAR SURGERY

288. Ans. (c) Neuralgia

Ref: SRB, 5th ed. pg. 234

Two methods of Venous stripping are:
- Extraluminal collision technique using Myer's stripper
- Invagination technique using Codman stripper

■ COMPLICATIONS OF STRIPPING

- Saphenous neuralgia due to saphenous nerve injury/avulsion
- Numbness or tingling along femoral nerve distribution
- Hematoma
- Infections
- Ulceration
- Recurrence of disease

289. Ans. (c) Popliteal artery

Ref: SRB 5th ed. P 177

- About 70% of peripheral arterial aneurysms are popliteal aneurysm and 20% are iliofemoral aneurysms.
- These aneurysms frequently co-exist with abdominal aortic aneurysms.
- They usually cause limb ischemia and distal embolism.

290. Ans. (c) Relieved on standing still

Ref: Bailey 26th ed. Chapter 53, P 901

Intermittent claudication or vascular claudication is defined as:

FMGE Solutions Screening Examination

- Pain that develops on walking/exercise
- Not seen with the first step (unlike osteoarthritis knees)
- Relieved by standing still (unlike neurogenic claudication)

The distance walked by the patient keeps on progressively reducing.

291. Ans. (b) Carotid angioplasty and stenting

Ref: Schwartz Principles of Surgery, 10th ed. P 903; Harrison 19th ed. p 2571-72

- Radiation induced occlusive carotid artery disease is due to Radiation given to head and neck area. It can lead to development of stroke.
- The best *screening* test is carotid Doppler and measure of carotid intimal thickness is used for diagnosis.
- The gold standard investigation is carotid angiography.
- Carotid angioplasty and stenting is the treatment of choice
- Carotid endarterectomy has higher incidence cranial nerve injury and wound infections which limits its use in these patients.

292. Ans. (d) Varicose veins

Ref: Bailey & Love, 26th ed. pg. 593/903

- Varicose veins are a cause of chronic leg edema and not a result of chronic leg edema.
- Edema is defined as a palpable swelling caused by an increase in interstitial fluid volume. The most likely cause of leg edema in patients over age 50 is venous insufficiency. ***Venous insufficiency affects up to 30% of the population, whereas heart failure affects only approximately 1%.*** The most likely cause of leg edema in women under age 50 is ***idiopathic edema, formerly known as cyclic edema. Pulmonary hypertension and early heart failure can both cause leg edema before they become clinically obvious in other ways.***
- **Marjolin's ulcer** refers to an aggressive ulcerating squamous cell carcinoma presenting in an area of previously traumatized, chronically inflamed, or scarred skin. Histologically, the tumor is a well-differentiated squamous cell carcinoma. This carcinoma is aggressive in nature, spreads locally and is associated with a poor prognosis. Its edge is everted and not always raised.
- The IOC is a wedge biopsy.

293. Ans. (d) All of above

Ref: Bailey & Love, 26th ed. pg. 899-900

- Acute-phase lesions have inflammation involving all coats of the vessel wall, especially of the veins, in association with occlusive thrombosis.

- Intermediate phase is characterized by progressive organization of the occlusive thrombus in the arteries and veins.
- Chronic phase or end-stage lesion is characterized by organization of the occlusive thrombus with extensive recanalization and prominent vascularization of the media.
- In all three phases, the normal architecture of the vessel wall subjacent to the occlusive thrombus and including the internal elastic lamina remains essentially intact.

294. Ans. (c) Small Acral vessels of limb involvement causes hypohidrosis

Ref: Bailey & Love, 26th ed. pg. 899-900

- Arteries affected are plantar and digital vessels of the foot and lower leg. In advanced cases fingers and hands can be involved.
- Sympathetic overactivity can cause excessive sweating and capillary autonomic dysfunction. Raynaud's phenomenon can be a presentation with Buerger disease.
- The visceral and cerebral artery are rarely involved.
- Phlebitis migrans and deep vein thrombosis is attributed to thrombophilia.
- Angiography shows normal proximal vasculature with cork screw collaterals.
- The most frequently affected arteries are anterior (41.4%) or posterior (40.4%) tibial arteries in the lower extremities, and the ulnar artery (11.5%) in the upper extremities.

295. Ans. (d) Saphenofemoral flush ligation with stripping

Ref: Bailey & Love, 26th ed. pg. 903-904

Sapheno-femoral flush ligation if done alone results in development of collaterals and thereby chances of recurrence. The long saphenous vein is not ligated until the T-junction has been confirmed and femoral vein has been exposed. The saphenous trunk is than retrogradely stripped to knee.

296. Ans. (d) All of above

Ref: Bailey & Love, 26th ed. pg. 899-900

- Buerger's disease is an inflammation of the arteries, veins, and nerves in the legs, principally, leading to restricted blood flow. Left untreated, Buerger's disease can lead to gangrene of the affected areas. Buerger's disease is also known as thrombo-angitis obliterans.
- Early symptoms include decrease in the blood supply (arterial ischemia) and superficial (near the skin surface) phlebitis. The main symptom is pain in the affected areas. Inflammation occurs in small and medium-sized arteries and veins near the surface of the limb. The pulse

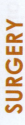

Surgery

in arteries of the feet is weak or undetectable. The lack of blood flow can lead to gangrene. A cold sensitivity in the hands, similar to that seen in Raynaud's disease, can develop.

297. Ans. (b) Nerve regeneration

Ref: Bailey & Love, 26th ed. pg. 471

- **Hoffman Tinel sign** is seen in nerve regeneration and should not be confused with *Homan sign seen in deep vein thrombosis.*
- **Hoffman reflex** is elicited by a reflex test which verifies the presence or absence of lesions in the cortico-spinal tract. It is also known as the **finger flexor reflex**. The test involves tapping the nail or flicking the terminal phalanx

of the middle or ring finger. A positive response is seen with flexion of the terminal phalanx of the thumb.

GENERAL SURGERY

298. Ans. (b) S.T.D

Ref: SRB 5th ed. pg. 36

It is a common sensical question that hospital acquired infections would be surgical site infection. Urinary tract infection and pneumonia. Sexually transmitted infections would be on account of high-risk sexual behaviour prevalent amongst young adults.

299. Ans. (c) 30-40%

Ref: SRB: 5th ed. pg. 120

TABLE: Classification of Hemorrhagic shock

Shock class	Blood loss ml (%)	Heart rate Beats/min	Blood pressure	Respiratory rate Breaths/min	Mental status
I	<750 (15)	<100	Normal	14–20	Slightly anxious
II	750-1500 (15–30)	100–120	Normal	20–30	Mildly anxious
III	1500–2000 (30–40)	120–140	Decreased	30–40	Anxious, confused
IV	>2000 (>40)	>140	Decreased	>35	Confused, lethargic

300. Ans. (a) Wet gangrene

Ref: SRB: 5th ed, pg. 206

The image shows a gangrenous toe of left foot with a vague line of demarcation. The part is putrefied and discoloured. Notice the proximal swelling, erythema and slight ulceration. Usual causes are emboli or trauma.

Feature	Dry gangrene	Wet gangrene	Gas gangrene
Site	Commonly limbs	More common in bowel	Limbs
Mechanism	Arterial occlusion	More commonly venous obstruction	Gases produced by *Clostridium bacteria*
Macroscopy	Organ dry, shrunken, and black	Part moist, soft, swollen, rotten, and dark	Organ red, cold, pale, numb, shriveled up, and auto-amputation
Putrefaction	Limited due to very little blood supply	Marked due to congestion of organ with blood	Marked due to bacteria and infiltration of gases produced by them in tissues
Line of demarcation	Present at the junction between healthy and gangrenous parts	No clear-cut line of demarcation	No clear-cut line of demarcation
Bacteria	Bacteria fail to survive	Numerous present	Major cause
Prognosis	Generally better due to little septicemia	Generally poor due to profound toxemia	Generally poor due to quick spread to the surrounding tissues

Explanations

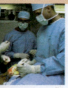

FMGE Solutions Screening Examination

301. Ans. (a) Subcutaneous Emphysema

Ref: Bailey and Love: 26th ed. pg. 933

- The image shows puffiness of face with examination finding of crepitus the diagnosis is subcutaneous emphysema.
- Choice B is ruled out as there is history of any trauma given in the patient
- Choice C is ruled out as no history suggestive of acute kidney injury is given.
- Choice D is ruled out as no facial plethora or dilated collaterals on the chest are seen.

302. Ans. (a) 3

Ref: SRB 5th ed. p 1093

| Eye opening = 1 | Verbal response = 1 | Motor response = 1 |

Hence the total score is 3. GCS is any way not designed to identify brain death but is used to evaluate presence of coma.

Extra Mile
- Mild head injury GCS score: 13–15
- Moderate head injury GCS score: 9–12
- Severe head injury GCS score: 3–8

303. Ans. (c) 4 L

Ref: SRB 5th ed. P 133

Applying the Parkland formula: 4 mL per % of burn per kg body weight

$$4 \times 50 \times 40 = 8000 \text{ mL} = 8 \text{ L}$$

Out of this total 8 L, the first 4 L is given over 8 hours and rest 4 L over the remaining 16 hours.

Extra Mile
In burns patient, Muir and Barclay formula is used to calculate the *colloid* to be given after 24 hours of admission.

304. Ans. (a) Elective intubation

Ref: SRB 5th ed. P 138

- Airway burns are evidenced by singeing of nasal hair and burns on face and neck.
- Hence *elective intubation is recommended with regular performance of pulmonary toilet* to remove the secretions.
- In case routine intubation is not possible, nasopharyngeal intubation should be performed.
- Tracheostomy/cricothyroidotomy can be life-saving especially in case of endotracheal intubation being not possible.
- However tracheostomy performance via burned tissue of neck has *increased complication rate and risk of sepsis as compared to elective intubation*.

305. Ans. (a) Acute limb ischemia

Ref: SRB Surgery: 5th ed. pg. 191

Treatment of Embolism and Thrombosis of Acute Limb Ischaemia

Immediate infusion of 5000-10,000 units of IV heparin and relief of pain are needed first

Surgical

- Embolectomy (surgical exploration and removal of clot) is the choice for embolus. It is done either by interventional balloon 5 French (Fogarty, 1963) embolectomy or open method. It is the standard treatment for arterial embolism. It can be repeated several times until adequate bleeding occurs
- For acute thrombosis causing acute limb ischaemica, open thrombectomy with or without bypass may be the surgical treatment: but it is not the standard treatment for acute thrombosis (standard is thrombolysis, Dotter and co, 1974)

Endovascular therapy

- Intra-arterial thrombolysis using urokinase
- *Percutaneous mechanical thrombectomy*-it is done either by suctioning clot via catheter or dissolution of thrombus by pulverisation and aspiration by high speed motors or fluid jets
- Ultrasound accelerated thrombolysis using catheter based or transdermal using acoustic cavitation to ablate thrombus

Embolectomy

- It is done as early as possible as an emergency, operation.
- Under fluoroscopic guidance. Fogarty catheter (interventional radiology) is passed beyond the embolus and the balloon is inflated. Catheter is withdrawn out gently with embolus. Procedure has to be repeated until embolectomy is completed and good back bleeding occurs. Angiogram is repeated to confirm the free flow
- Postoperatively initially heparin and later oral anticoagulants are used. Procedure is done under general anaesthesia or local anaesthesia.

306. Ans. (a) Cutting needle

- *Cutting needle* is used to suture skin, aponeurosis and tough structures.
- *Reverse cutting needle* is used to suture mucoperiosteum
- *Round body needles* are used in soft structures like peritoneum, muscle, vessel, nerves, tendons, bowel and soft tissues.

Surgical Needles

Types

Based on the edge	
• Round body needle • Cutting needle • Reverse cutting needle	• Taper cut needle • Side-to-side flat—Hagedron needle
Based on curvature	
• Straight needle • Curved needle. Half circle; 5/8 circle, etc.	

Based on Existence of the Eye

- **Atraumatic needle** is eyeless. Here suture material is attached to the needle by swaging. Size of the suture material and that of needle is same and so tissue trauma is less. Needle once used is disposed of (not reusable).
- **Traumatic needle:** It is eyed needle. Needle in the eye area is wider than the body of the needle and so tissue trauma is more. These needles are reusable.

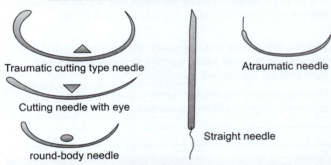

FIGURE: Needles

307. Ans. (a) Pulse rate/BP

Shock index is defined as ratio of pulse rate to blood pressure and value >1 indicates significant blood loss.

Signs of Significant Blood Loss

- Pulse >100/min
- Systolic BP <100 mm Hg
- Diastolic BP drop on sitting or standing >10 mm Hg
- Pallor/sweating

Selective Management of Penetrating Neck Wounds

- Shock index (ratio of Pulse rate to Blood pressure>1)
Tachycardia is not reliable indicator of haemorrhage.

308. Ans. (d) All of the above

Steps to stop blood loss
- **P**ressure
- **P**acking
- **P**osition
- **O**perative **p**rocedures

309. Ans. (b) Colloids

Fluids used in Burns

Fluids used are Ringer lactate, Hartmann fluid, plasma. *Ringer lactate is the fluid of choice.* Blood is transfused in later period (after 48 hours).

First 24 hours only crystalloids should be given (Crystalloids are one which can pass through capillary wall like saline either hypo, iso or hypertonic, dextrose saline, *Ringer lactate*).

Sodium is assessed by formula: 0.52 mmol × kg body weight × % body burns, given at a rate of 4.0 to 4.4 ml/kg hours.

After 24 hours up to 30–48 hours, *colloids* **should be given to compensate plasma loss** (colloids are one which are retained in intravascular compartment). Plasma haemaccel (gelatin), dextrans, hetastarch are used. Usually at a rate of 035–0.5 ml/kg/% burns is used in 24 hours.

310. Ans. (d) Urgent Angiography

- No role exists for probing or local exploration of the neck in the emergency department because this may dislodge a clot and initiate uncontrollable hemorrhage.
- Immediate surgical exploration *is only* done for patients who present with signs and symptoms of shock and continuous haemorrhage from the neck wound.
- **In our case the patient is not in shock. Hence angiography will be done to identify the presence of vascular injury. This is followed by formal neck exploration if required or conservative management is required. Read the protocol mentioned here for better understanding of the topic.**

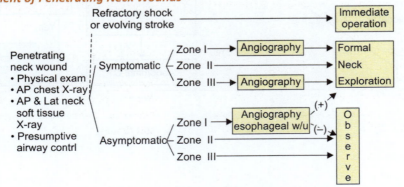

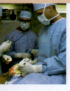

FMGE Solutions Screening Examination

The neck may be divided into 3 zones using anatomic landmarks. Each zone has a group of vital structures that can be injured and may determine the kind of trauma management.

Zones of Penetrating Neck Injury

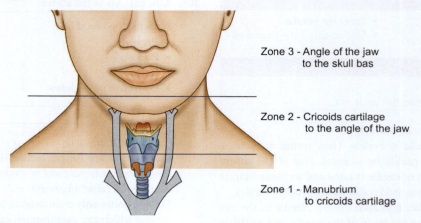

Zone 1	Horizontal area between the clavicle/suprasternal notch and the cricoid cartilage encompassing the thoracic outlet structures	The proximal common carotid, vertebral, and subclavian arteries and the trachea, oesophagus, thoracic duct, and thymus
Zone 2	Area between the cricoid cartilage and the angle of the mandible	Contains the internal and external carotid arteries, jugular veins, pharynx, larynx, esophagus, recurrent laryngeal nerve, spinal cord, trachea, thyroid, and parathyroids
Zone 3	Area that lies between the angle of the mandible and the base of the skull	Distal extracranial carotid and vertebral arteries and the uppermost segments of the jugular veins

311. Ans. (c) F.A.S.T

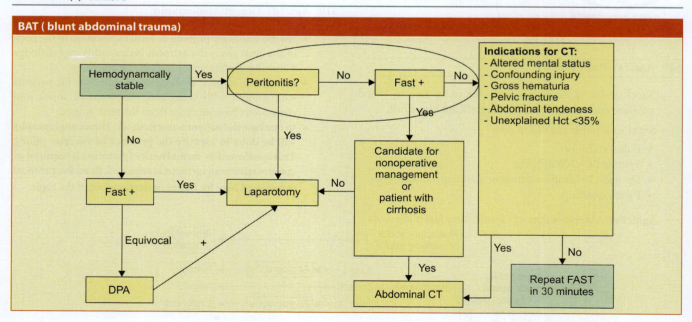

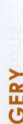

Surgery

312. Ans. (a) 750

CLASSIFICATION OF HAEMORRHAGIC SHOCK (CIRCULATORY FAILURE)

Class	Blood loss	Features
I	Up to 15% (<750 mL)	Normal
II	Blood loss 15–30% (750–1500 mL)	Palor, thirsty, tachycardia
III	Blood loss 30–40% (1500–2000 mL)	Hypotension, tachycardia, oliguria, confusion
IV	Blood loss >40% (>2000 mL)	Rapid pulse, low BP, anuria, unconsciousness, MODS

313. Ans. (a) Acute limb ischemia

Surgical Guidelines for Acute Limb Ischemia

- 5000-10,000 units of heparin
- Relief of pain
- *Embolectomy with 5Fr Fogarthy catheter. The catheter is passed beyond the embolus and balloon is inflated. Catheter is withdrawn gently with the embolus.*
- Surgical exploration and removal of clot if all else fails.

314. Ans. (b) Secondary

Ref: Bailey and Love, 26th ed. pg. 284

Primary hemorrhage	Occurs at the time of surgery or trauma.
Secondary hemorrhage	Secondary haemorrhage is defined as occurring at least 24 hours after surgery, but usually presents several days later, as it is due to postoperative infection.
Reactionary haemorrhage	• Common after first 4–6 hours after surgery. • It may be caused by ▪ Slippage of a ligature ▪ Displacement of blood clot ▪ Cessation of vasospasm, after coughing or increased mobility.

315. Ans. (c) Blood transfusion

Ref: Bailey, 26th ed. pg. 17

Choice A and B	This statement is direct quote from Bailey page 17, 26th edition • *"On balance, there is little evidence to support the administration of colloids, which are more expensive and have worse side-effect profiles."* • Most importantly, the oxygen carrying capacity of crystalloids and colloids is zero.
Choice C	*If blood is being lost, the ideal replacement fluid is blood, although crystalloid therapy may be required while awaiting blood products.*
Choice D	Fluid resuscitation must be done before General anesthesia can be given and surgeon can proceed with immediate laparoscopy.

316. Ans. (a) Urine output

Ref: Bailey, 26th ed. pg. 15

Choice A	As shock progresses, renal compensatory mechanisms fail, renal perfusion falls and urine output dips below 0.5 mL/kg per hour.
Choice C ruled out as	Hypotension is one of the last signs of shock. Children and fit young adults are able to maintain blood pressure until the final stages of shock.
Choice D ruled out	Tachycardia may not always accompany shock. Patients who are on beta-blockers or who have implanted pacemakers are unable to mount a tachycardia

The *minimum* standard for monitoring of the patient in shock is

- Continuous heart rate
- Oxygen saturation monitoring
- Frequent non-invasive blood pressure monitoring
- Hourly urine output measurement.

Since the question is asking for the best parameter, out of the given options urine output is the best answer.

> **Extra Mile**
> - Shock is the most common and therefore the most important cause of death of surgical patients.
> - *Ideal way to manage shock is measure pulmonary capillary wedge pressure> urine output monitoring.*

317. Ans. (a) Detection of Pericardial fluid accumulation

Ref: Bailey, 26th ed. pg. 109

Focused assessment with sonography for trauma (FAST) looks for fluid in the

- Peri-hepatic and hepato-renal space
- Peri-splenic area
- Pelvis
- Pericardium.
  - ▪ It has a role in children but it does not detect solid organ injuries nor replace CT.
  - ▪ Bowel perforation or deep penetrating trauma requires a laparoscopy or laparotomy.
  - ▪ Isolated blunt splenic and/or liver injuries identified on a CT

318. Ans. (a) Septic shock

In Septic shock findings include:

- *Enhanced cardiac output*
- *Peripheral vasodilation*
- *Fever*
- *Leukocytosis*
- *Hyperglycemia*
- *Tachycardia*
- In septic shock, the vasodilatory effects are due in part to the upregulation of the inducible isoform of nitric oxide synthase (iNOS or NOS_2) in the vessel wall.

Explanations

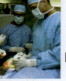

FMGE Solutions Screening Examination

319. Ans. (c) Crystalloids

Ref: Bailey & Love, 26th ed. pg. 16-17

- **Crystalloid is the first fluid of choice for resuscitation.** Immediately administer 2 L of isotonic sodium chloride solution or lactated Ringer's solution in response to shock from blood loss. Fluid administration should continue until the patient's hemodynamics become stabilized. Because crystalloids quickly leak from the vascular space, each liter of fluid expands the blood volume by 20-30%; therefore, 3 L of fluid needs to be administered to raise the intravascular volume by 1 L.
- About the use of RL and NS in hemorrhagic shock, it has been shown that Resuscitation with NS modulates hypercoagulability after trauma and results in increased fluid requirements Administration of RL during resuscitation appears to have no effect on the hypercoagulable state induced by trauma. This hypercoagulable state may reduce bleeding and be protective initially, but may lead to thromboembolic complications later in the course of trauma admission. Due to this reason *RL may be preferred in the trauma (hemorrhagic shock) in the initial phase over NS.*
- As the RL is a little hypotonic solution large volume of RL in patients with head injury may lead to cerebral oedema therefore NS may be preferred over LR in patients of hemorrhagic shock with head injury. (Also remember that head injuries may also precipitate hyponatremia. The most common metabolic abnormality after head injury is SIADH).

320. Ans. (a) Septic shock

Plasma expanders are used to restore circulatory volume in shock, burns, sepsis, hemorrhage, surgery, and other trauma or for prophylaxis of venous thrombosis and thromboembolism.

- *Plasma expanders are most useful when there is faulty distribution* rather than real loss eg- burns, septic/endotoxic shock and trauma. They do not provide oxygen carrying capacity.
- Septic shock is associated with peripheral vasodilatation causing relative hypovolumia
- Antibiotics are the mainstay of treatment of septic shock
- Examples of plasma expanders
  - Dextran 70 & Dextran 40
  - Polyvinyl pyrrolidone
  - Gelatin polymer
  - Albumin
  - Hydroxyl ethyl starch

321. Ans. (d) Anesthesia

Ref: Bailey and Love, 26th ed. ch. 2/15

In high spinal anesthesia, Hypotension occurs due to loss of sympathetic autonomic function and unopposed parasympathetic function. Vasoconstrictor tone is lost and venous pooling occurs. Loss of cardiac accelerator fibres results in bradycardia and patients are unable to increase cardiac output by changes in heart rate.

322. Ans. (b) Normal saline

Ref: Harrison, 18th ed. pg. 270

Normal saline is the preferred fluid for volume expansion in a crashing patient with un-recordable BP. The main point to be noted is that if ringer lactate is infused in these patients, then lactate in the solution will never reach the liver where it is normally converted into bicarbonate. Hence the accumulated lactate will get broken into lactic acid that will worsen the status of patient of poly-trauma who is already acidotic. Dextran would not be indicated as it exhibits anti-thrombotic tendency.

323. Ans. (b) Normal saline

Ref: Harrison, 18th ed. pg. 270

Fluid of choice in Hypovolemic shock is Normal saline.

324. Ans. (b) Hypotension

Ref: Nelson, 18th ed. ch. 176

- Sepsis is defined as SIRS plus evidence of infection like positive blood culture report
- Septic shock is defined as sepsis plus evidence of hypotension for > 1 hour inspite of use of vasoactive agents.

SIRS: 2 out of 4 criteria, 1 of which must be abnormal temperature or abnormal leukocyte count

- Core temperature >38.5°C or <36°C (rectal, bladder, oral, or central catheter)
- Tachycardia: mean heart rate >2 SD above normal for age in absence of external stimuli, chronic drugs or painful stimuli; OR unexplained persistent elevation over 0.5–4 hr; OR in children <1 yr old persistent bradycardia over 0.5 hr (mean heart rate <10th percentile for age in absence of vagal stimuli, β blocker drugs, or congenital heart disease)
- Respiratory rate >2 SD above normal for age or acute need for mechanical ventilation not related to neuromuscular disease or general anesthesia
- Leukocyte count elevated or depressed for age (not secondary to chemotherapy) or >10% immature neutrophils

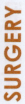

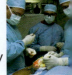

Surgery

325. Ans. (d) Normal saline

Ref: Bailey & Love, 26th ed. pg. 482-83

The first step in the management of a newborn with myelomeningocele is a careful clinical assessment followed by **open defects which should be covered with a saline-moistened non-adherent dressing to prevent injury to and dessication of the neural placode.**

326. Ans. (a) 0.1 mEq

500 mL of 0.9% saline contains about 154 mEq of sodium and chloride per liter. Thus mathematically 1 ml contains 0.15 mEq approximately.

327. Ans. (a) 0.5 mEq

Since 3% NaCl has 513 mEq/L of Na and Cl in 1000 ml, mathematically the answer will be 0.5 mEq.

	Size (mL)	Composition (g/L)	Ionic concentration (mEq/L)		Osmolarity (mOsmol/L)	pH
		Sodium chloride USP (NACL)	Sodium	Chroride		
3% sodium chloride injection, USP	500	30	513	513	1027	50 (4.5 to 7.0)
5% sodium chloride injection, USP	500	50	856	856	1711	5.0 (4.5 to 7.0)

* Normal physiological osmolarity range is approximately 280 to 310 mOsmol/L. Administration of substantially hypertonic solutions (≥ 600 mOsmol/L) may cause vein damage

328. Ans. (d) 50

Ref: Sabiston, 19th ed. pg. 138-39

TPN Formulation	
Without lipid	**With Lipid**
• Calories from amino acids: 20-25% • Calories from dextrose: 75-80%	• Calories from amino acids: 20–25% • Calories from lipids: 20% • Calories from dextrose: 55–60%

329. Ans. (a) 1%

Ref: Sabiston, 9th ed. pg. 523

- This was a confusing question, as most students marked it as 9%, which is true for upper extremity but NOT for hand.
- Bailey in 26th ed. clearly mentions hand as palm and counting it as 1%

Burn size is assessed by Wallace rule of nines (By Alfred Russel Wallace)

- Each upper extremity : 9%
- Head and neck : 9%
- Lower extremities: 18%
- Anterior and posterior aspects of the trunks : 18%
- Perineum and genitalia: 1%

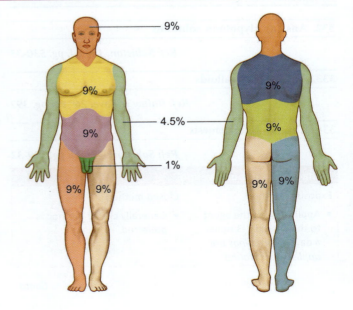

FMGE Solutions Screening Examination

330. Ans. (a) 1%

Ref: Sabiston, 19th ed. pg. 523

Perineum involved in burns is 1% of body surface area.

331. Ans. (b) Ringer's lactate

Ref: Sabiston, 19th ed. pg. 529-30

- **IV fluid resuscitation is immediately required:** In children with burn >10% TBSA and adult with burn >15% TBSA
- Maximum fluid is given in first 8 hours (50%) rest of the fluid will be given in subsequent hours (25% + 25% in next 16 hours).
- **Most commonly used/preferred fluid: Ringer lactate** (Crystalloids). Because it is a relatively isotonic crystalloid solution that is the key component of almost all resuscitative strategies, at least for the first 24-48 hours.
- However, some centers use human albumin, FFP or hypertonic saline.
- RL is preferable to isotonic sodium chloride solution (ie, normal saline [NS]) for large-volume resuscitations because *its lower sodium concentration (130 mEq/L vs 154 mEq/L) and higher pH concentration (6.5 vs 5.0) are closer to physiologic levels.*
- **Hypotonic fluid is not given, as it can lead to hyponatremia and water intoxication.**
- **Maintenance fluid in children:** Dextrose –saline

> **Extra Mile**
> - Hypertonic saline has been effective in treating burn shock as it produces hyperosmolarity and hypernatremia
> - This reduces the shift of intracellular water to the extracellular space

332. Ans. (a) Hypotonic solutions

Ref: Sabiston, 19th ed. pg. 530-33

333. Ans. (a) Crystalloids

Ref: Bailey & Love, 26th ed. pg. 392

334. Ans. (a) Hematemesis

Ref: Sabiston, 19th ed. pg. 529-32

Management of burn wound	
Exposure Method	Closed method
• Application of the agent to the wound 2-3 times a day. *No dressings are applied over wound*	• Generally closed method is preferred

Contd...

Management of burn wound	
• Exposure method is commonly used for face and head	• Occlusive dressing is applied over the agent and changed twice daily
• **Disadvantage:** Increased pain, heat loss Risk of cross-contamination	• **Advantage:** Less pain, less heat loss Less risk of cross-contamination
	• **Disadvantages:** If dressing is not changed twice daily, there is risk of contamination

- *Pseudomonas is the most common infection in burn patients.*
- Due to inhalation of burn particles, stridor can be present.

335. Ans. (a) Dehydration

Ref: Saiston, 19th ed. pg. 534-35

- In this case there is 70% burn and in addition enteral feeding is not given. The most probable cause of death in this case will be dehydration/Hypovolemia.
- MCC of early death in burn patient: **HYPOVOLEMIA**
- MCC of later death in burns: **Septicimia**
- MCC of death in burns: **Septicemia**
- MC CA in burns: **Squamous cell CA**

336. Ans. (d) Hypovolemia

Ref: Sabiston, 19th ed. pg. 534-35

337. Ans. (c) Early elective intubation is safest

Ref: Bailey & Love, 26th ed. pg. 389-90

The shock Reaction after burns
- Burns produce an inflammatory reaction
- This leads to vastly increased vascular permeability
- Water, solutes and proteins move from the intra- to the extravascular space
- The volume of fluid lost is directly proportional to the area of the burn
- *Above 15 per cent of surface area, the loss of fluid produces shock*

Dangers of smoke, hot gas or steam inhalation
- *Inhaled hot gases can cause supraglottic airway burns and laryngeal oedema*
- Inhaled steam can cause subglottic burns and loss of respiratory epithelium
- Inhaled smoke particles can cause chemical alveolitis and respiratory failure
- Inhaled poisons, such as carbon monoxide, can cause metabolic poisoning
- Full-thickness burns to the chest can cause mechanical blockage to rib movement

Initial management of the burned airway
- Early elective intubation is safest
- Delay can make intubation very difficult because of swelling
- Be ready to perform an emergency cricothyroidotomy, if intubation is delayed

Fluids for resuscitation
- In children with burns over 10 per cent TBSA and adults with burns over 15 per cent TBSA, consider the need for intravenous fluid resuscitation
- If oral fluids are to be used, salt must be added
- Fluids needed can be calculated from a standard formula
- The key is to monitor urine output

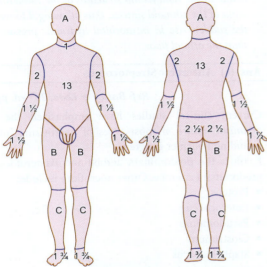

Relative percentage of area affected by growth

Relative percentage of area affected by growth

Age in years	0	1	5	10	15	Adult
A Head	9	8	6	5	4	3
B Head	2	3	4	4	4	4
C leg	2	2	3	3	3	3

338. Ans. (c) Painless and cherry red
Ref: Harrison, 18th ed. ch. 60/390

- **Third-degree burns** appear white, tan, brown, black, or deep cherry red in color.
- The region of third-degree burn is usually painless because of destruction of sensory receptors.
- **Full-thickness burns** are also termed third-degree burns. The epidermis and the dermis are completely destroyed, and deeper tissue may also be involved.

339. Ans. (a) HSV
- **Viral infection in burns:** Burn patients suffer significant immunosuppression during *the first 3 or 4 weeks after hospitalization*. Herpes simplex virus (HSV) infections are commonly seen in immunosuppressed patients and may account for considerable morbidity and some mortality.
- **Bacterial infection in burns:** Burn wound *bacterial infections commonly occur in the first weeks* of hospitalization. **S aureus is the most common pathogen infecting burned** patients, as it is an early colonizer. *K pneumoniae* wound infections occur around the same time as infections by *S aureus* and seem to be more prevalent in the institutions that use systemic perioperative prophylaxis. As would be expected, infections by the nosocomial organisms *P aeruginosa* and *A baumannii* appear later in the course of the hospitalization (after 2 wk of admission).
- **Fungal infection in burns:** Burn wounds are also commonly infected with *fungal pathogens*. These infections are frequent after the use of broad-spectrum antibiotics. *Candida albicans* is the most common fungal infection; nonetheless, a trend towards nosocomially acquired, intrinsically resistant fungal infections (eg, *Candida krusei*) has been reported

340. Ans. (d) Sepsis
Ref: Schwartz, 10th ed. pg. 233

Causes of Death in Burns

Cause	%
ARDS	29%
Brain injury	16%
Shock	8%
Sepsis	**47%**

341. Ans. (d) Air embolism
Ref: Schwartz, 10th ed. pg. 233

The following Complications in burns may occur

- Infections being the most common
- Pneumonia, cellulitis, urinary tract infections
- Anemia secondary to full thickness burns of greater than 10% TBSA is common.
- Electrical burns may lead to compartment syndrome or rhabdomyolysis
- Deep vein thrombosis

Long Term Morbidity with Burns

- The hypermetabolic state result in a decrease in bone density and a loss of muscle mass.
- Keloids may form subsequent to a burn
- Significant psychological trauma
- Social isolation, extreme poverty and child abandonment.

FMGE Solutions Screening Examination

342. Ans. (a) Proptosis

Ref: Bailey & Love, 26th ed. pg. 344

Lefort I	Ecchymosis is present
Lefort II and Lefort III (common)	Gross edema of soft tissue over the middle third of the face, bilateral circumorbital ecchymosis, bilateral sub-conjunctival hemorrhage, epistaxis, CSF rhinorrhoea, dish face deformity, diplopia, enophthalmos, cracked pot sound.
Lefort II	Step deformity at infra-orbital margin, mobile mid face, anesthesia or paresthesia of cheek.
Lefort III	Tenderness and separation at fronto-zygomatic suture, lengthening of face, depression of ocular levels, Enophthalmos, hooding of eyes, tilting of occlusal plane with gagging on one side

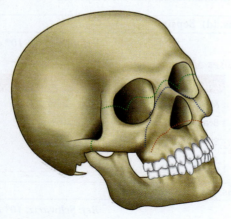

FIGURE: Le-fort fracture

343. Ans. (d) Proprioception

Ref: Harrsion, 18th ed. pg. 377

- Brown sequard consists of ipsilateral weakness (corticospinal tract) and loss of joint position and vibratory sense (posterior column), with contralateral loss of pain and temperature sense (spinothalamic tract) one or two levels below the lesion.
- Segmental signs, such as radicular pain, muscle atrophy, or loss of a deep tendon reflex, are unilateral. Partial forms are more common than the fully developed syndrome.

344. Ans. (b) Orbital floor

- Fracture of the orbital floor is the most common traumatic orbital fracture.
- Eyebrow Ptosis after Blowout Fracture Indicates Impairment of Trigeminal Proprioceptive Evocation That Induces Reflex Contraction of the Frontalis Muscle.
- The force of a blow to the orbit is dissipated by a fracture of the surrounding bone, usually the orbital floor and/or the medial orbital wall. Serious consequences of such injury include diplopia in upgaze where there is significant damage to the orbital floor. In blowout fractures, the medial wall is fractured indirectly.
- Fracture of the medial wall is more common than the floor, since the medial wall is slightly thinner (0.25 mm vs 0.50 mm). *However, it is known that pure blowout fractures most frequently involve the orbital floor. This is due to the honeycomb structure of the numerous bony septa of the ethmoid sinuses, thus allowing it to withstand the sudden rise in intraorbital hydraulic pressure better than the orbital floor*

345. Ans. (c) Anaerobic Streptococcus

Ref: Bailey & Love, 26th ed. pg. 1388

Current clinical studies have emphasized the *multi-organism nature* of most cases of necrotizing infection, including Fournier gangrene.

E.coli is the predominant aerobe and Bacteroides is the predominant anerobe. Other microflora include:

- Proteus
- Enterococcus
- Pseudomonas
- Clostridium
- Staphylococcus
- Streptococcus
- Klebsiella

346. Ans. (d) Microaerophilic streptococcus

Ref: Bailey & Love, 26th ed. pg. 57

- **Chronic undermining burrowing ulcer** (also known as **Meleney gangrene**, or **Meleney's ulcer**) is a cutaneous condition that is a postoperative, progressive bacterial gangrene. Synergistic gangrene is caused by microaerophilic streptococci acting synergistically with aerobic staphylococci, with or without Gram-negative bacilli. It occurs in debilitated patients with other disorders (e.g. diabetes, malnutrition, alcoholism. Infection spreads rapidly along fascial and subcutaneous planes without a severe inflammatory reaction.

347. Ans. (b) Insulin

Ref: Bailey & Love, 26th ed. pg. 4

- The stress response to surgery is characterized by increased secretion of pituitary hormones and

Surgery

activation of the sympathetic nervous system. Release of corticotrophin from the pituitary stimulates cortisol secretion from the adrenal cortex. Arginine vasopressin is secreted from the posterior pituitary and has effects on the kidney. In the pancreas, glucagon is released and insulin secretion may be diminished.

- Logic for ADH increase is that the body is trying to retain water.

Hormones increased	ACTH, GH, AVP, Cortisol, Aldostrone, Small Increase In Glucagon
Hormones decreased	Insulin, Thyroxine (T4) And T3
May increase or decrease	Tsh, Fsh, Lh

348. Ans. (c) Subsides over time

Ref: Bailey & Love, 26th ed. pg. 30

- Keloid formation is a type of scar which, depending on its maturity, is composed mainly of either type III (early) or type I (late) collagen.
- Keloids are firm, lesions or shiny, fibrous nodules, and vary from pink to flesh-colored or red to dark brown in color. A keloid scar is benign and not contagious, but sometimes accompanied by severe itchiness, pain, and changes in texture.
- **They may not improve in appearance over time and can limit mobility if located over a joint.**

349. Ans. (a) Spleen

Ref: Bailey & Love, 26th ed. pg. 1087

- The spleen is the most commonly injured viscus in blunt abdominal trauma and can result from the most trivial of traumas.
- The classical presentation is that of a hemodynamically unstable patient with a history of trauma, with severe abdominal pain and signs of peritonitis.
- The classic physical findings of splenic rupture are left shoulder pain, left upper quadrant pain and tenderness, and Kehr's sign (left shoulder pain from irritation of inferior border of left diaphragm by hematoma).
- Absence of one or more or even all of these signs does not rule out splenic injury. Diagnosis is based on a thorough physical examination and confirmed with the FAST examination

350. Ans. (c) 5-12 days

Ref: Bailey & Love, 26th ed. pg. 279

- Patients maximum at risk for wound dehiscence are those who are/have

- Obese
- Malnourished
- Abdominal distention
- Malignancy
- Multiple trauma to the abdomen
- Infected wounds are also prone to dehiscence.
- **Chronic cough are also at risk.**

Wound separation occurs especially between the fifth and eight postoperative days.

351. Ans. (a) Is a skin graft including the epidermis and part of the dermis

Ref: Bailey & Love, 26th ed. pg. 402

- Skin transplanted from one location to another on the same individual is termed an autograft. If the entire thickness of the dermis is included, the appropriate term is full-thickness skin graft (FTSG).
- *If less than the entire thickness of the dermis is included, this graft is referred to as a split-thickness skin graft (STSG).* STSGs are categorized further as thin (0.005-0.012 in), intermediate (0.012-0.018 in), or thick (0.018-0.030 in), based on the thickness of the harvested graft.

352. Ans. (d) Transplantation of living tissues/organs from one species to another

Ref: Bailey & Love, 26th ed. pg. 833

- **Xenotransplantation** is the transplantation of living cells, tissues or organs from one species to another. Such cells, tissues or organs are called **xenografts** or **xenotransplants**.
- In contrast, the term allotransplantation refers to a same-species transplant. Human xenotransplantation offers a potential treatment for end-stage organ failure, a significant health problem in parts of the industrialized world.

353. Ans. (b) Buruli ulcer

Ref: SRB Manual of Surgery, 23rd ed. pg. 23

- Buruli ulcer is an infectious disease caused by *Mycobacterium ulcerans*. The early stage of infection is characterised by a painless nodule, with non-pyogenic, necrotizing lesions developing in the skin, and occasionally in adjacent bone, as the disease progresses.
- *M. ulcerans* secretes a lipid toxin, mycolactone, which functions as an immune suppressant, necrotising agent and activator of cellular apoptosis in mammalian tissues.
- The disease is primarily an infection of subcutaneous fat, resulting in a focus of necrotic (dead) fat containing

myriads of the mycobacteria in characteristic spherules formed within the dead fat cells. Skin ulceration is a secondary event.
- All other ulcers are associated with significant scarring in the tissues. Scarring in gastric ulcer/duodenal ulcer leads to gastric outlet obstruction.

354. Ans. (d) Marjolin's ulcer

Ref: Bailey & Love, 26th ed. pg. 918

- Marjolin's ulcer is a misnomer. It is a malignant degeneration arising within **a pre-existing cicatrix or scar**
- Most commonly found in the lower extremity→ especially the **heel and plantar foot**.
- Causes:
  - As originally presented by Marjolin, to this day the **leading cause is old burn scars**.
  - The second most common association is malignant degeneration arising within **osteomyelitic fistulae**.
  - Other causes in decreasing order of frequency- secondary to **venous insufficiency** ulcers or pressure ulcers, scarring from lupus, amputation stumps, frostbite, vaccination sites, skin graft donor sites, scars, urinary fistulas, and radiation.
- Marjolin's ulcers are 3 times more likely in **men** than in women.
- Average age of diagnosis is the **fifth decade** of life.
- As a rule, normal healing should be exhibited within the first **2 to 3 weeks**, and ulcers that repeatedly break down, do not respond to treatment and are chronic in nature, are suspicious for malignancy
- Most commonly well-differentiated **squamous cell tumors** found but can be basal cell or melanoma
- **Duration of ulceration** is directly proportional to chance of malignant transformation
- Although there is **no definitive treatment** protocol, therapy generally involves wide local excision with skin grafting or amputation proximal to the lesion depending upon size.
- **Most widely accepted treatment/most definitive option to treat the cancer, and infection/when the bone or joint is involved is amputation.**

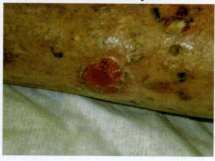

355. Ans. (a) Metaphysis

Ref: Bailey & Love, 26th ed. pg. 541

- **The most common site is the rapidly growing and highly vascular metaphysis of growing bones. The apparent slowing or sludging of blood flow as the vessels make sharp angles at the distal metaphysis predisposes the vessels to thrombosis and the bone itself to localized necrosis and bacterial seeding.**
- Vertebral osteomyelitis at any age is most often a secondary complication of a remote infection with hematogenous seeding.
- Direct or contiguous inoculation osteomyelitis is caused by direct contact of the tissue and bacteria during trauma or surgery.

356. Ans. (a) Primary intention

Ref: Bailey & Love, 26th ed. pg. 25

HEALING BY PRIMARY INTENTION

- It involves epidermis and dermis without total penetration of dermis healing by process of epithelialization when wound edges are brought together so that they are adjacent to each other (re-approximated).
- This minimizes scarring
- Most surgical wounds heal by primary intention healing
- Wound closure is performed with sutures (stitches), staples, or adhesive tape
- **Examples:** well-repaired lacerations, well reduced bone fractures, healing after flap surgery

357. Ans. (a) 8-10 days

Ref: Sabiston, 18th ed. pg. 2134

Scalp suture should be removed on 6th to 8th day. Given these options, 8-10 days is the best choice.

TABLE: Day of suture removal from different body areas

Body area	Suture removal on
Scalp	6 – 8 days
Face	3 – 5 days
Chest, Abdomen	8 – 10 days
Ear	10 – 14 days
Extremities, back	12 – 14 days

358. Ans. (d) Recovery time is longer

- Laparoscopy is a technique in which operations in the abdomen are performed through small incisions (usually 0.5–1.5 cm) as opposed to the larger incisions needed in laparotomy.
- Rather than a minimum 20 cm incision as in traditional (open) cholecystectomy, four incisions of 0.5–1.0 cm

Surgery

will be sufficient to perform a laparoscopic removal of a gallbladder.

- Since the gallbladder is similar to a small balloon that stores and releases bile, it can usually be removed from the abdomen by suctioning out the bile and then removing the deflated gallbladder through the 1 cm incision at the patient's navel.
- *Post operative stay in hospital is short.*
- The risk of Trocar injuries is increased in patients who have a low body mass index or have a history of prior abdominal surgery.
- Vascular injuries can result in hemorrhage that may be life threatening. Injuries to the bowel can cause a delayed peritonitis. It is very important that these injuries be recognized as early as possible.

---

359. Ans. (c) Mesentery

Ref: Bailey & Love, 26th ed. pg. 982

- Seat belt syndrome is characterized by tear of mesentery on sudden deceleration while the patient is using a seat belt.
- **In the absence of seat belt being worn by the car passenger, the chest of the victim would slam into the steering wheel resulting in hemo-pericardium and a resultant high mortality.**

---

360. Ans. (a) Damage to respiratory centre

Ref: Bailey & Love, 26th ed. pg. 310

The Cushings triad is the triad of bradycardia, hypertension, and respiratory irregularity that often occupies a herniation event clinically. It is likely due to brainstem compression.

---

361. Ans. (a) CECT

Ref: Bailey & Love, 26th ed. pg. 208

Since the patient is in shock with history of blunt abdomen trauma, the first investigation to be done should be FAST. The main role of ultrasound includes the assessment of intraperitoneal fluid and haemopericardium In the presence of free intraperitoneal fluid and an unstable patient, the ultrasound allows the trauma surgeon to explore the abdomen as a cause of blood loss.

In the presence of fluid and a haemodynamically stable individual, further assessment by way of CT shall be performed. Occasionally, a second ultrasound scan may show free fluid in the presence of an initially negative FAST scan.

---

362. Ans. (a) Tetany

Ref: Harrison, 18th ed. pg. 352

- Painful lock jaw is related to inflammation of anatomical structures of jaw and surrounding structures. Tetanus is

characterized by release of tetano-spasmin toxin which causes painful muscle spasm and lockjaw.

- However in the question the choice A is Tetany/ Hypocalcemia where either Chvostek sign and Carpo-pedal spasm is seen.

---

363. Ans. (c) Lower lip

Ref: Bailey & Love, 26th ed. pg. 710

- Lip cancer is the most common malignant lesion of the oral cavity, constituting 25-30% of all oral cavity cancer cases and is the second most common malignancy of the head and neck overall (after cutaneous malignancy). Unlike other sub-sites of the oral cavity, sun exposure is a well established risk factor for development of lip cancer.
- 95% of carcinoma of lip arise on lower lip and 15% rise in central one-third and commissures. The lymph nodes involved are submental and submandibular groups.

---

364. Ans. (a) Common peroneal nerve

- Common peroneal nerve originates from the dorsal branches of the fourth and fifth lumbar and the first and second sacral nerves. It descends obliquely along the lateral side of the popliteal fossa to the head of the fibula, close to the medial margin of the biceps femoris muscle. **Where the common peroneal nerve winds round the head of the fibula, it is palpable and vulnerable to injury.**

Remember

- Tarsal tunnel syndrome- Posterior tibial nerve
- MeralgiaParasthetica- Lateral cutaneous nerve of thigh
- Claw hand-ulnar nerve
- Mononeuritis multiplex is most commonly caused by Polyarteritis Nodosa.(If asked for India Ans. as leprosy).

---

365. Ans. (b) Surgical site infection

Ref: Bailey & Love, 26th ed. pg. 136/140

- Surgical site infections (SSIs) have been reported to be one of the most common causes of nosocomial infections; accounting for 20% to 25% of all nosocomial infections worldwide. SSIs have been responsible for the increasing cost; morbidity and mortality related to surgical operations and continue to be a major problem worldwide.
- Globally, surgical site infection rates have been reported to range from 2.5% to 41.9%. *Nosocomial infections can be defined as those occurring within 48 hours of hospital admission, 3 days of discharge or 30 days of an operation.*

---

366. Ans. (a) Right lower lobe superior basal

Ref: Complete Review of Medicine by Deepak Marwah, 1st ed.

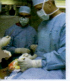

FMGE Solutions Screening Examination

- *In supine position and with the patient on back superior segment of RLL is the most dependent segment.*
- In right lateral decubitus position the axillary subsegments of anterior and posterior segments of RUL are the dependant site for aspiration. Abscess is located in the middle of lateral CXR corresponding to RUL bronchus take off.
- When the patient is on abdomen, aspiration does not occur, thus it is extremely unlikely for any anterior segments, middle lobe and lingula to be the site for aspiration lung abscess.
- **The superior segments of Right Lower Lobe and axillary subsegments of anterior and posterior segments of RUL are common sites for aspiration and will account for 85% of all Lung abscesses.**

367. Ans. (d) Surgery + Imiquimod

Ref: Schwartz, 10th ed pg. 647;
Bailey & Love, 26th ed. pg. 463

- Most cancers of the anus, cervix, head and neck, and vagina are epidermoid carcinomas and also called squamous cell carcinoma.
- Treatment modalities for SCC include cautery and ablation, cryotherapy, drug therapy including imiquimod, surgical excision, Moh's microsurgery, and radiation therapy.
- Topical fluorouracil is FDA-approved treatment for superficial Basal Cell Carcinoma.

368. Ans. (c) Number of lymph nodes

MISCELLANEOUS

369. Ans. (a) Size of tumor

TNM is based on 3 components:

Letter	Stands for	Description
T	Tumour	Indicates the size of the primary tumor and the degree of spread into nearby tissues (local invasion)
N	Lymph nodes	Indicates whether or not the cancer has spread to nearby lymph nodes, the size of the nodes that contain cancer and how many lymph nodes contain cancer
M	Metastasis	Indicates whether or not cancer has spread (metastasized) to distant organs

Additional letters or numbers are placed after T, N and M to provide more specific details:

- X means the tumor or lymph nodes cannot be assessed or evaluated.
- T followed by a number (0–4) describes the size of tumor and how much nearby tissue it has invaded.
- N followed by a number (0–3) describes the degree of spread to the lymph nodes.
- M followed by the number 0 or 1 describes whether or not cancer has spread to other parts of the body.
- Lowercase letters (a, b or c) are used to subdivide the tumor, lymph nodes or metastasis categories to make them more specific.

370. Ans. (d) Metastasis

The X-Ray spine AP shows multiple lytic lesions suggestive of malignancy metastasizing to the vertebra. The most probable origin is from the prostate which is the leading cancer is males.

Also notice the combination of osteolytic and osteosclerotic secondaries.

371. Ans. (a) Gestational age 1-7 months in abdomen

Ref: Human Embryology, 10th ed. pg. 311

- *The testes remain high in the abdomen until the 7th month of gestation, when they move from the abdomen through the inguinal canals into the two sides of the scrotum.*
- In first phase, movement across the abdomen to the entrance of the inguinal canal appears controlled by anti-müllerian hormone (AMH)
- In second phase, in which the testes move through the inguinal canal into the scrotum, is dependent on androgens (most importantly testosterone).
- In many infants with inguinal testes, further descent of the testes into the scrotum occurs in the first 6 months of life. This is attributed to the postnatal surge of gonadotropins and testosterone that normally occurs between the first and fourth months of life.

372. Ans. (d) Descending colon

Ref: High Yield Embryology, 5th ed. pg. 294

373. Ans. (d) Hepatocellular jaundice

Ref: Manipal Manual of Surgery, 4th ed. pg. 520

- The anchovy sauce pus of ameobic liver abscess is sterile and is produced due to broken RBCs and damaged hepatocytes.
- Due to right branch of portal vein being more in line with portal vein the organism will have higher chances of seeding in the right lobe than the left lobe.
- Most patients will be male and alcoholic from lower socio-economic background and will present with severe right hypochondrium pain and symptoms of pleurisy and right shoulder pain.
- On examination intercostal tenderness is seen
- Bed side USG is the investigation of choice.

- Jaundice is not seen usually or if seen is of obstructive type.

374. Ans. (a) Ameobic liver abscess

Ref: Manipal Manual of Surgery, 4th ed. pg. 521

Refer to the above explanation

Hydatid cyst	Usually clinically silent *Enlarged liver with smooth surface and is non tender.*
Pyogenic liver abscess	Multiple abscess leading to spiky fever and enlarged liver.
Hepatic adenoma	Presents in young women on OCP and is solitary. Liver enlargement may or may not be seen.

375. Ans. (a) Cholesterolosis

Ref: Bailey & Love, 26th ed pg. 1108

- The submucous aggregation of cholesterol crystals in mucosa of gallbladder lends it appearance to be called strawberry gallbladder.
- Porcelain gallbladder exhibits calcification and is a risk factor for malignancy of gallbladder.

Extra Mile

Strawberry Tongue	Kawasaki Disease
Strawberry nose	Rhinosporidosis
Strawberry vagina	Bacterial vaginosis
Strawberry gingiva	Wegener granulomatosis

376. Ans. (d) Cholesterosis

Ref: Manipal Manual of Surgery, 4th ed. pg. 584

377. Ans. (a) Volvulus

Ref: Manipal Manual of Surgery, 4th ed. pg. 739

- In sigmoid volvulus, the X-ray abdomen erect shows hugely dilated sigmoid loop called bent inner tube sign.
- Acute sigmoid volvulus presents as intestinal obstruction and starts after straining at stool. *It occurs in anticlockwise direction and after one and a half turns, the entire loop becomes gangrenous.*
- The percussion note on the abdomen shall be tympanitic note.

378. Ans. (b) Sigmoid Volvulus

Ref: Manipal Manual of Surgery, 4th ed. pg. 738

- In sigmoid volvulus the loop of bowel twists to result in tympanitic note all over the abdomen. Hypovolemic shock develops within 6-8 hours and per rectum shows rectum to be empty.
- On performing a *contrast enema*, when the barium enters the rectum, it tapers into sigmoid colon called as *Bird Beak sign*.
- Bird beak sign on barium swallow occurs with achalasia cardia.

379. Ans. (d) Hirschsprung's Disease

Ref: Manipal Manual of Surgery, 4th ed. pg. 731

Common causes of ileal obstruction	Common causes of colonic obstruction
- Adhesions - Obstructed hernia - Stricture - Intussusception - Ileocaecal TB - Bands	- Fecal impaction - Carcinoma colon - Hirschsprung's disease - Anorectal malformations

380. Ans. (a) Stomach

Ref: Bailey and Love 26th ed. pg. 1160

- GIST is a mesenchymal tumor with increased size and high levels of c-kit (CD117)
- *GIST tumors are found most commonly in the stomach*
- Occur most commonly in the 50-70-year age group.
- Presents with pain, nausea, hematemesis or melena.
- Surgery is the most effective way of removing GISTs, as they are radio-resistant.
- Imatinib Mesylate is the best drug

381. Ans. (a) Stomach

Ref: Advances in Oncology, Vol. 3/137

The most common extra-nodal site of lymphoma is GIT with the most common site being the stomach followed by small intestine and ileo-caecal region.

382. Ans. (a) Intussusception

Ref: Schwartz 10th ed. pg. 1237

The intraoperative picture shows presence of intussusception.

- Most common lead point causing intussusception in children = Meckel's Diverticulum
- Most common type of intussusception in children= Ileo-colic (Post Rota virus diarrhea)
- Most common lead point causing intussusception in Adults= Polyp (Villous Adenoma)

FMGE Solutions Screening Examination

- Most common type of intussusception in adults = Colo-colic
- Most common small bowel tumor in children causing intussusception = lymphoma

383. Ans. (b) Gastroduodenal artery

Ref: Bailey and Love, 26th ed. pg. 1023

- Perforations involving the gastroduodenal artery complex occur as a sequel to transmural ulceration of the posterior duodenal wall.
- The gastroduodenal artery, is a branch of the hepatic artery, passes behind the first part of the duodenum, and is responsible for bleeding in duodenal ulcer.

384. Ans. (c) It is accurate in detecting <50 mL of free blood

Ref: Bailey and Love, 26th ed. pg. 359

- FAST does not reliably detect less than 100ml of free blood. Hence choice **C is False**.
- It does not identify injury to hollow viscus. It cannot reliably exclude injury in penetrating trauma.

Focused assessment with sonography for trauma (FAST) should include views of
- Hepato-renal recess (Morison pouch)
- Peri-splenic view
- Sub-xiphoid pericardial window
- Supra-pubic window (Douglas pouch).

If an extended FAST (E-FAST) examination is performed, views of
- The bilateral hemithoraces and
- The upper anterior chest wall, should also be obtained.

385. Ans. (c) Full thickness skin graft

Ref: Bailey and Love, 26th ed. pg. 404

If the entire thickness of the dermis is included, the appropriate term is full-thickness skin graft (FTSG). If less than the entire thickness of the dermis is included, this graft is referred to as a split-thickness skin graft (STSG).

STSGs are categorized further as

- Thin (0.005-0.012 in)
- Intermediate (0.012-0.018 in)
- Thick (0.018-0.030 in)
- Split-thickness skin grafts (of varying thickness). These are sometimes called Thiersch grafts. They are used to cover all sizes of wound, are of limited durability and will contract. They may be used to provide valuable temporary wound closure before better cosmetic secondary correction after rehabilitation.
- *Full-thickness skin grafts (Wolfe grafts):* Used for smaller areas of skin replacement where good elastic skin that will not contract is required (such as fingers, eyelids, facial parts).
- *Composite skin grafts (usually skin and fat, or skin and cartilage).* Often taken from the ear margin and useful forrebuilding missing elements of nose, eyelids and fingertips

386. Ans. (d) Liver Laceration

Ref: Bailey and Love 26th ed. pg. 1073

- Pringle manoeuvre is used for control of bleeding in liver trauma
- This technique enables surgeons to *halt hemorrhage and find the source of bleeding*, allowing time for repair of the vessel. In the setting of hepatic resection of benign and malignant lesions, this maneuver *can be used to assist with control of bleeding*.
- It involves vascular inflow occlusion by placing an atraumatic clamp across the foramen of Winslow.

387. Ans. (b) At the induction of anaesthesia

Ref: Bailey and Love 26th ed. pg. 1109

- Prophylaxis is uniformly recommended for all clean-contaminated, contaminated and dirty procedures.
- Timing of antibiotic administration is critical to efficacy. The first dose should always be given before the procedure, preferably within 30 minutes before incision.
- Re-administration at one to two half-lives of the antibiotic is recommended for the duration of the procedure.
- In general, postoperative administration is not recommended.
- There is a delay before host defences can become mobilised after a breach in an epithelial surface, whether caused by trauma or surgery. The acute inflammatory, humoral and cellular defences take up to 4 hours to be mobilised. This is called the 'decisive period', and it is the time when the invading bacteria may become established in the tissues.
- Cefazolin provides adequate coverage for most other types of procedures.

388. Ans. (b) Polyamide polymer

Ref: Bailey and Love, 26th ed. pg. 37

Surgery

TABLE: Non-absorbable suture materials

Suture	Types	Raw Material
Silk	Braided or twisted multi-filament Dyed or undyed Coated (with wax or silicones) or uncoated	Natural protein Raw silk from silk-worm
Linen	Twisted	Long staple flax fibres
Nylon	Monofilament or multifilament	An alloy of Iron, nickel and chromium
Polyester	Monofilament or braided multifilament	Polyamide polymer
Polybut-ester	Monofilament Dyed or undyed	Polybutylene terephthalate and polytetramethylene ether glycol
Polypro-pylene	Monofilament Dyed or undyed	Polybutylene terephthalate and polytetramethylene Polymer of propylene

389. Ans. (a) Anatomical abnormality is unilateral and contralateral testis should not be fixed

Ref: Bailey and Love, 26th ed. pg. 1379

Anatomical abnormality is unilateral and contralateral testis should not be fixed	The other testis should also be fixed because the anatomical predisposition is likely to be bilateral. An infarcted testis should be removed and prosthetic device deployed.
Prompt exploration and twisting & fixation is the only way to save the torted testis	Patient presents with sudden agonising pain in the groin and the lower abdomen. The patient feels nauseated and may vomit. If the testis is viable when the cord is untwisted it should be prevented from twisting again by fixation with non-absorbable sutures between the tunica vaginalis and the tunica albuginea.
Most common between 10 & 25 years of age	Testicular torsion is most common between 10 and 25 years of age, although a few cases occur in infancy.
Inversion of testis is the most common predisposing cause	Inversion of the testis is the most common predisposing cause. The testis is rotated so that it lies transversely or upside down.

390. Ans. (b) Pain

Ref: Handbook of Clinical Anesthesia, 3rd ed. pg. 783

Pain should be recorded as the fifth vital sign along with blood pressure, heart rate, respiratory rate and temperature.

391. Ans. (d) Squamous cell carcinoma

Ref: Devita, 9th ed. pg. 729

- Most common site oral Cancer: Carcinoma Tongue > Carcinoma Lip
- Most common histological type: Squamous Cell Cancer
- Most common site of oral Cancer in India: Cancer of Buccal Mucosa
- Max Risk of L.N. Metastasis: Carcinoma Tongue
- Min Risk of L.N Metastasis: Carcinoma lip > hard palate
- Most common age: 50-60 years

392. Ans. (b) Intestinal metaplasia

Ref: Sabiston, 19th ed. pg. 1033

- Barrett's esophagus is characterized by metaplasia of esophageal squamous epithelium into columnar in distal esophagus.
- For diagnosis of Barrett's esophagus it requires both endoscopically visible segment of columnar lining of distal esophagus and intestinal metaplasia showing goblet cells on biopsy.
- Barrett's esophagus is the single most important risk factor for adenocarcinoma of esophagus.
- Adenocarcinoma develops at the squamo-columnar junction or within 2 cm from the junction.

393. Ans. (c) Spontaneous Perforation

Ref: Sabiston, 19th ed/1043, SRB manual of Surgery/1287

- Boerhaave's syndrome is spontaneous perforation of esophagus, occurring usually due to severe barotrauma when a person vomits against a closed glottis.
- Most common location of perforation is left posterolateral side of the distal esophagus.
- Tear is full thickness penetrating complete through all the layers of esophageal wall with spillage of contents into the mediastinum. (In Mallory Weiss tear it is partial thickness, extends through the mucosa and submucosa, but not through the muscular layer.)
- **Clinical finding – *Mackler's triad***
  - Vomiting
  - Thoracic pain
  - Cervical subcutaneous emphysema

394. Ans. (d) Gastric freezing

Ref: Harrison, 18th ed. pg. 2598

- Endoscopy followed by endoscopic variceal ligation should be performed.

- Balloon tamponade with Sengstaken Blakemore tube or Minnesota tube can be used in patients who cannot get endoscopic therapy immediately or who need stabilization prior to endoscopic therapy.
- Some endoscopists will use variceal injection therapy (sclerotherapy) as initial therapy, particularly when bleeding is vigorous.
- Shunt therapy (Transjugular intrahepatic portacaval shunt) has been shown to control refractory bleeding.

Pharmacologic Therapy for Variceal Hemorrhage

- Vasopressin, most potent vasoconstrictor, use is limited by side effects.
- Somatostatin and octreotide
- Octreotide is the preferred pharmacological agent

395. Ans. (c) Like toothpaste emulsion in the gallbladder

Ref: Harrison, 18th ed. pg. 2622

- It is a complication of chronic cholecystitis.
- Calcium salts in the lumen of the gallbladder in sufficient concentration may produce calcium precipitation and diffuse, hazy opacification of bile or a layering effect on plain abdominal radiography.
- This so called **limey bile or milk of calcium bile**, is usually clinically innocuous but cholecystectomy is recommended, especially when it occurs in a hydropic gallbladder.
- In the entity called porcelain gallbladder, calcium salt deposition within the wall of a chronically inflamed gallbladder may be detected on the plain abdominal film.

396. Ans. (d) Hemorrhage

Ref: CSDT, 11th ed. pg. 638

- Serious post-op hemorrhage from cyst occurs from cystogastrostomy.
- Most common cause of pseudopancreatic cyst is pancreatitis.
- It may resolve spontaneously, so it is followed with serial ultrasonic studies.

Indications of Surgical Intervention

- Age of cyst more than 6 weeks without resolution
- Size of cyst greater than 6 cm
- Evidence of secondary infection
- Development of any other complications

Surgical Methods

- Internal drainage – most preferred surgical management
- There are three options:
    - Cysto-Jejunostomy
    - Cysto-gastrostomy
    - Cysto-Duodenostomy
- Excision of pseudocyst
- External drainage

397. Ans. (b) Bluish discoloration in the umbilicus

Ref: Sabiston, 19th ed. pg. 1524

Signs indicative of retroperitoneal bleeding in severe pancreatitis

Flank ecchymosis	Grey turner sign
Periumbilical ecchymosis	Cullen's sign
Inguinal ecchymosis	Fox sign

Radiological Signs of Acute Pancreatitis
- Renal halo sign
- Gasless abdomen
- Ground glass appearance
- Colon cut off sign
- Sentinel loop

Radiological Signs of Chronic Pancreatitis
- Chain of lakes appearance
- String of pearl appearance
- Beaded appearance

398. Ans. (b) Ureter

Ref: Campbell, 10th ed. pg. 1108-1112

- Ureters are involved most commonly.
- MC site is lower third.
- Obstructive uropathy is the **earliest and most common specific** symptom.
- 70% cases are primary or idiopathic (Ormond's disease)
- **Investigation of choice** is CT scan.
    - In patients with renal compromise, MRI is the investigation of choice.

399. Ans. (b) Extension

Ref: Sabiston, 19th ed. pg. 1280

Blumberg's sign	Rebound tenderness at Mc Burney's point
Cope's psoas test	Pain on hyperextension of right hip Suggestive of retro-caecal appendix.
Dunphy's sign	Pain on coughing
Rovsing's sign	Pain in the right lower quadrant during palpation of the left quadrant
Obturator sign	Pain on internal rotation of the hip Suggestive of pelvic appendix

400. Ans. (b) Epidermoid

Ref: Maingot's, 10th ed. pg. 1505

- Epidermoid carcinoma of the anus includes squamous cell carcinoma, cloacogenic carcinoma, transitional carcinoma and basaloid carcinoma. The clinical behavior and natural history of these tumors is similar.
- Mainly 3 types of malignant neoplasm are seen in anal canal –
  - Squamous cell carcinoma (most common)
  - Basal cell carcinoma (2nd most common)
  - Melanoma
- Most common rectal and colon carcinoma is adenocarcinoma.

401. Ans. (a) Stomach

402. Ans. (a) Acute pancreatitis

403. Ans. (b) Colorectal carcinoma

ANSWERS TO BOARD REVIEW QUESTIONS

404. Ans. (d) 100
405. Ans. (b) Acute pancreatitis
406. Ans. (b) Thrombocytosis
407. Ans. (c) Carcinoma head of pancreas
408. Ans. (b) Iliohypogastric
409. Ans. (c) Sigmoid colon
410. Ans. (b) Hypokalemia
411. Ans. (b) Stomach cancer
412. Ans. (d) Hernia occurring at the level of arcuate line
413. Ans. (a) Femoral hernia
414. Ans. (a) Radiation enteritis
415. Ans. (a) Crohn's disease
416. Ans. (b) Carcinoma breast
417. Ans. (b) Lymph node involvement
418. Ans. (b) Paget's disease
419. Ans. (b) Obstruction of lymphatic ducts
420. Ans. (c) Ductal
421. Ans. (c) Lobular carcinoma of the breast
422. Ans. (b) Excision biopsy
423. Ans. (a) Radioiodine
424. Ans. (c) Thyroid
425. Ans. (b) Anal canal strictures
426. Ans. (c) Penis
427. Ans. (a) Nephroma
428. Ans. (a) Scrotum
429. Ans. (d) Tuberculosis
430. Ans. (d) Membranous urethra
431. Ans. (d) Hydrocele
432. Ans. (a) Alcohol
433. Ans. (a) Glandular
434. Ans (b) Hitatus hernia

Ref: Bailey & Love, 25th ed. pg. 1021, Sabiston, 18th ed ch-42

435. Ans. (d) 154

Ref: Essentials of General Surgery edited by Richard M. Bell, Merril T. Dayton p-51 4th ed

436. Ans. (b) Medial aspect of leg

Ref: Sabiston, 18th ed. ch-68

437. Ans. (b) Grey Turner sign

Ref: Bailey & Love 25th ed p 967 & 1140, Schwartz's 8th ed. ch-34, Sabiston Textbook of Surgery 18th ed ch-55

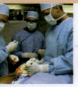

FMGE Solutions Screening Examination

438. Ans. (c) Hunner's cystitis

Ref: Smith Urology 17th ed/576

439. Ans. (a) Penicillin

Ref: Mastery of Vascular and Endovascular Surgery edited by Gerald B. Zelenock, Thomas S. Huber, Louis M. Messina, Alan B. Lumsden, Gregory L. Monet/-567

440. Ans. (b) Papillary carcinoma

Ref: Sabiston 18th ed ch-36, Schwartz 9th ch-38

441. Ans. (c) 15 & 3

Ref: Schwartz 9th ed table 42-2, Sabiston 18th ed table 20-2

442. Ans. (b) Appendicitis

Ref: Schwartz 9th ed ch-30 table 30-2, Bailey & Love 25th ed/1211

443. Ans. (b) Murphy's sign

Ref: Sabiston 19th ed ch-49

444. Ans. (a) Bacteroides

Ref: Sabiston 18th ed ch-49

445. Ans. (a) Perianal

Ref: Pfenninger and Fowler's Procedures for Primary Care: Expert Consult 3rd ed by John L. Pfenninger, Grant C. Fowle Ch-107, The ASCRS Textbook of Colon and Rectal Surgery 2nd ed/220

446. Ans. (d) Hilum of spleen

Ref: Essentials of General Surgery/427

447. Ans. (b) Breast mass

Ref: With text

448. Ans. (c) Familial Adenomatous polyposis

Ref: Sabiston Textbook of Surgery 18th ed Table 50-4

449. Ans. (d) Renal

Ref: DeVita, Hellman, and Rosenberg's Cancer: Principles & Practice of Vol I/1931

450. Ans. (b) Saphenous vein

Ref: Introductory Guide to Cardiac Catheterization- Arman T. Askari, Medhi H. Shishehbor, Ronnier J. Aviles/59

451. Ans. (c) Carcinoma penis

Ref: Mastery of surgery 5th ed volume 2 p-1531, Schwartz 9th ed various chapter

452. Ans. (c) 55-65

Ref: Bailey & Love 26th ed. page 248, 25th ed page 210

453. Ans. (b) >5.5 cm

Ref: Rutherford: Vascular Surgery, 6th ed page 1408-122, Harrison 18th ed chapter 248

454. Ans. (b) Subdural hemorrhage

Ref: Schwartz 9th ed Chapter 42

455. Ans. (b) Acute cholecystitis

Ref: Bailey and love 25th edition page 967 & 1140, Schwartz's 8th edition chapter 34, Sabiston Textbook of Surgery, 18th ed chapter 55

456. Ans. (b) Renal cysts

Ref: Smith urology page 511

457. Ans. (d) Idiopathic hypercalciuria

Ref: Robbin's 8th ed Table 20-12, Sabiston Textbook of Surgery, 18th ed chapter 77,

458. Ans. (c) Uric acid

Ref: Robbin's 8th ed Table 20-12, Sabiston Textbook of Surgery, 18th ed chapter 77,

459. Ans. (b) Uric acid

Ref: :Robbin's 8th ed Table 20-12, Sabiston Textbook of Surgery, 18th ed chapter 77,

460. Ans. (d) Struvite

Ref: :Robbin's 8th ed Table 20-12, Sabiston Textbook of Surgery, 18th ed chapter 77,

461. Ans. (b) Epididymis

Ref: Smith urology page 219, Textbook of Pathology By V. Krishna/347

462. Ans. (c) Calcium phosphate

Ref: Smith Urology 17th ed page 273, Schwartz 9th ed chapter 40

Surgery

463. Ans. (b) Superficial parotidectomy

Ref: sabiston Textbook of Surgery, 18th ed chapter 33

464. Ans. (b) Pancreatic enzymes

Ref: Schwartz 9thed chapter 33

465. Ans. (a) Pancreatic Divisum

Ref: Schwartz 9th ed chapter 33, Sabiston 18th ed chapter 55, Robbin's pathology 8th ed chapter 19

466. Ans. (a) Biopsy

Ref: Bailey & Love 25th ed./289, 290

467. Ans. (d) NCCT

Ref: Smith Urology 17th ed/79, 81

468. Ans. (b) Cholangitis

Ref: Srb's Manual of surgery 4th ed p-1287, The ASCRS Textbook of Colon and Rectal Surgery: Second Edition-edited by David E. Beck, Patricia L. Roberts, Theodore J. Saclarides, Anatomy J. Senagore, Michael J. Stamos, Steven D. Wexner 2nd ed p-383

469. Amns. (b) BCG

Ref: Sabiston Textbook of surgery 18th ed Table 77-6

470. Ans. (a) Cervical region

Ref: Bailey & Love 25th ed p 1014-1015, Sabiston 18th ed ch-41

471. Ans. (c) Adenoid cystic carcinoma

Ref: Sabiston Textbook of surgery 18th ed ch-33

472. Ans. (c) Adenoid cystic carcinoma

Ref: Bailey & Love 25th ed p 752, Schwartz's 9th ed ch-18

473. Ans. (b) 20%

Ref: Schwartz's 9th ed ch-8 table 8-2, Bailey & Love 25th ed p 382, Practical plastic surgery by Zol B. Kryger, Mark Sisco p-155

474. Ans. (b) Sunitinib

Ref: Sabiston Textbook of surgery 18th ed ch-77, NCCN Guidelines Version 1.2013

475. Ans. (b) Achalasia cardia

Ref: CSDT 11th ed p.478, Bailey & Love 24th ed p 1019, Maingot's 10th ed/847

476. Ans. (b) Duct papilloma

Ref: Bailey & Love 24th ed p 828, Schwartz 9th ed ch-17

477. Ans. (a) Glandular

Ref: Bailey & Love 24th ed p 1389

478. Ans. (c) Surgical excision

Ref: Schwartz 9th ed ch-39

479. Ans. (a) Ascending aorta

Ref: Harrison's 17th ed ch:242

480. Ans. (c) Car driver

Ref: Bailey & Love 25th ed p 343, Critical care Medicine: The Essentials By John J. Marini, Arthur P. Wheeler/635

481. Ans. (c) Auriculotemporal

Ref: Dhingra's ENT 4th ed/220

Explanations

ANSWERS TO IMAGE-BASED QUESTIONS

482. Ans. (c) Intussusception

Ref: Page 1234, Schwartz 10th edition

The intraoperative picture shows presence of intussusception.
- Most common lead point causing intussusception in children= Meckel's Diverticulum
- Most common type of intussusception in children= Ileocolic (Post Rota virus diarrhea)
- Most common lead point causing intussusception in Adults= Polyp (Villous Adenoma)
- Most common type of intussusception in adults= Colo-colic
- Most common small bowel tumor in children causing intussusception = lymphoma

483. Ans. (b) Artery Forceps & Needle Holder

Thumb forceps

Sponge holder

Artery forceps

Needle holder

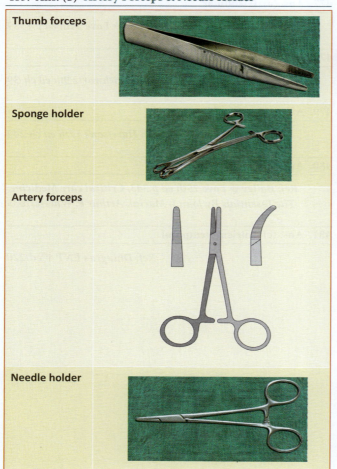

Contd...

Allis forceps

Ovum forceps

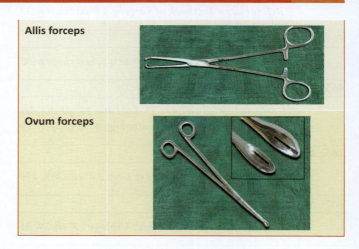

484. Ans. (d) Collagen bundles are present

The picture shows presence of keloid, which is called so as it extends to normal tissues with its claw like processes.

Hypertrophic scar	Keloid
Itching not present or mild	Severe itching and worsens after 1 year
Never crosses boundaries of original incision	Extends to normal tissues and has claw like lesions
Occurs at original site of incision and has minimal vascularity	Occurs at vaccination sites, injection and incision sites and piercing sites.
Occurs due to hypertrophy of mature fibroblasts with minimal blood vessels	*Immature fibroblasts with immature blood vessels and exhibits high tendency to recur and collagen bundles are absent.*

485. Ans. (d) Rubbery consistency of involved lymph nodes

The image shows anti gravity drainage of a cold abscess being done. The upper deep cervical lymph nodes are usually involved. On palpation matting of lymph nodes is characterstic feature while the rubbery consistency of lymph nodes is seen in hodgkins lymphoma.

Cold Abscess Features are
- No local rise of temperature
- No redness
- Transillumination test is negative
- On sternocleidomastoid contraction test, it becomes less prominent indicating it is deep to deep fascia.

Surgery

486. Ans. (c) Ring block with adrenaline used

- The image shows presence of commonest hand infection which is acute paronychia. It occurs due to trimming of nail or ingrown toe nail. The infection starts in subcuticular area and spreads all around as eponychium is adherent to nail base.
- *Use of digital block and I and D is done by incising the eponychium. Adrenaline is not used for infiltration in the finger, penis and ear lobule.*

487. Ans. (a) Venous ulcer; (b) Arterial ulcer

- Image A shows presence of ulcer on lateral aspect of leg with granulation tissue present
- Image B shows presence of ulcer on dorsal aspect of foot with wet gangrene visible.
- Neuropathic ulcer in diabetes can occur on the heel or pressure point in the sole of the foot

Characteristics of Arterial and Venous Ulcer

Venous ulcer	Ischemic ulcer
Occur at medial or lateral aspect of leg	Dorsum of foot Typical arterial ulcers occur on tips of toes
Single and oval	Irregular
Superficial and does not penetrate deep fascia	Deep ulcer and penetrates the deep Fascia
Pigmentation present	Pigmentation present

488. Ans. (c) Neuropathic ulcer

Venous ulcer	Occurs above medial or lateral malleolus with granulation tissue and surrounding pigmentation
Arterial ulcer	Occurs on toes with poor peripheral pulses
Neuropathic ulcer	Occurs on heel
Bazin's ulcer	Occurs in obese young females in ankle region with abnormal amount of subcutaneous fat. Lesions begin as erythematous purplish nodules which rupture producing non healing ulcer

489. Ans. (a) Immediately remove the needle in the vessel

This is a case of inadvertent intra-arterial injection of thiopentone into one of the high division of brachial artery resulting in blanching and severe pain in the hand. Steps to be followed are

- *Do not remove* the needle
- Inject 5 ml of 1% lignocaine or 2 % papaverine

- Intra-arterial dilute heparin
- Intra-arterial streptokinase
- Brachial plexus block to reduce sympathetic activity induced spasm of blood vessels

490. Ans. (c) Lymphatic metastasis

- The image shows presence of marjolin's ulcer which grows very slowly and develops at the site of previous burn site or varicose ulcer, snake bite scar or osteomyelitis scar.
- It is painless scar and doesnot exhibit metastasis. It is cured by surgery and radiotherapy is not useful.

491. Ans. (a) Thyroglossal Cyst

- The image shows presence of midline swelling which is moving with movement of the tongue. The most common site is sub-hyoid cyst. It is a cystic fluctuant trans-illumination negative swelling and moves as it is attached to hyoid bone.
- Branchial cyst arises from the vestigial remnants of 2nd branchial arch and is located in the anterior triangle of the neck partly under cover of the upper 1/3rd of the anterior border of sterno-mastoid. The swelling on aspiration contains cholesterol crystals
- Cold abscess occurs in anterior triangle of the neck and does not move with tongue movement.
- Carotid body tumor is called chemodectoma and occurs at the upper part of anterior triangle of the neck, at the level of hyoid bone beneath the anterior edge of the sternomastoid muscle. It is firm to hard and is called classical potato tumor.

492. Ans. (a) Carcinoma alveolar margin

- The image shows presence of staining of teeth, with an exophytic lesion with everted margins suggestive of diagnosis of a malignancy.
- Leukoplakia is a white patch in the mouth that cannot be scraped off.
- Hyperplastic candida involves the commissures of the mouth with candida invasion and shows no response to drugs, surgery and laser.
- Fibrous epulis is a fibroma arising from periodontal membrane and is slow growing without any ulceration.

493. Ans. (a) Pleomorphic adenoma

- The image shows a nodular growth at location of parotid gland and also notice the ear lobule of the patient is elevated with obliterated retromandibular groove.
- In mumps bilateral parotid enlargement is seen and does not have a bosselated appearance.

- Sialadenitis occurs due to stones and is more common in submandibular gland (80% of stones occur in submandibular gland). Even if parotid is involved bosselated or nodular appearance is suggestive of a tumor.

494. Ans. (d) **Constipation**

- The image shows presence of upper sclera above the limbus visible in the patient suggestive of diagnosis of thyrotoxicosis. Contraction of the Muller's muscle due to sympathomimetic overdrive results in lid spasm
- Pretibial myxedema is a feature in Grave's Disease, and patient has tachycardia with excessive sweating leading to moist warm hands.
- *Constipation is a feature of hypothyroidism*

495. Ans. (c) **Diagnosis depends on HER2**

- 25% of all breast cancers overexpress HER-2 which is a transmembrane tyrosine kinase receptor. These patients should be given Trastuzumab. HER-2/neu is a *prognostic and not a diagnostic marker.*
- Modified Van Nuys prognostic index includes size of tumor, margins, pathology grade and age in years.
- 5 year disease free survival for VPIN 4-6 =100%
- The image shows nipple ulceration and infiltration of skin by the tumor called as peau'd orange. Remember puckering or dimpling of skin is seen due to infiltration of ligaments of cooper.

496. Ans. (b) **Hydatid cyst**

- The image shows a CT scan of the liver with classical Cart wheel appearance, suggestive of multiple hydatid cysts. The calcified cysts are left alone as they are dead cysts.
- Medical treatment with Albendazole for 21 days is given and surgery is done in case of symptomatic cysts or asymptomatic patient with cyst> 5cm or a non-calcified infected cyst.

497. Ans. (b) **Gastrinoma triangle**

The image shows gastrinoma triangle where ZES gastrinoma is located. The boundaries are from the *confluence* of cystic duct and Common hepatic duct, *confluence* of second and third part of duodenum and *junction* of neck and body of pancreas.

Hesselbach triangle

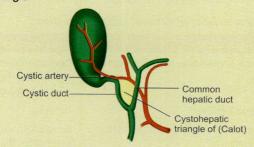

Triangular area on the inferior aspect of the anterior abdominal wall within the groin. Its boundaries are:
- Base is the inguinal ligament
- Lateral border is formed by the inferior epigastric vessels
- Medial border is the lateral edge of the rectus sheath.

Calot's triangle

- Triangle formed by cystic duct, common hepatic duct and base of liver and contains the cystic artery.

Killian triangle
- Site for Zenker Diverticulum

498. Ans. (b) **Ileal obstruction**

- Vomiting of feculent contents indicates terminal ileal obstruction. It does not contain fecal matter but contains terminal ileal contents which undergo bacterial degradation and fermentation resulting in smell of fecal matter.
- Jejunal obstruction results in bilious vomiting while diverticulitis produces hematochezia.
- Mesenteric ischemia will lead to abdominal angina.

499. Ans. (d) **Fistula in ano**

- The image shows presence of rectal prolapse and occurs due to habitual constipation undeveloped sacral curve, whooping cough, marasmus and torn perineum in obstetric trauma

Surgery

500. Ans. (b) Pilonidal sinus

- The image shows a presence of external sinus opening just above the anal verge in midline over the coccyx. This is diagnostic of pilonidal sinus.
- Methylene blue shall be injected to demonstrate the branches of the sinus followed by excision
- Fistula of ano is located around the anal orifice and is due to infection of the anal glands.
- It is squamous cell carcinoma in situ of the anus, and is the precursor to the invasive squamous cell carcinoma. It is associated with HPV type 16 and 18.
- Hidradenitis suppurativa is recurrent suppuration of apocrine glands in the skin, resulting in multiple abscesses which rupture causing *multiple sinuses*.

501. Ans. (a) Appendix

- *The structure shown is closer to caecumis appendix whereas Meckel's Diverticulum is seen about 60 cm from the ileo-caecal junction.*
- *Intra-operatively, appendix can be identified by tracing Taenia Coli which converges onto the base of the appendix.*

502. Ans. (a) Lichtenstein repair

- The image shows polypropylene mesh which is used in hernia repair called as *Lichtenstein repair*.
- Bassini repair is a herniotomy with approximation of posterior wall of inguinal canal; by suturing the conjoined tendon above to the inguinal ligament below by using interrupted non absorbable suture material such as nylon.
- Shouldice method is method of tensionless repair in three layers where in the above image only a mesh can be seen.
- Lord's procedure is ruled out as it is done for hydrocele.

503. Ans. (b) Indirect inguinal hernia

- Direct inguinal hernia pushes through the posterior wall and hence it is *unusual for it to descend into the scrotum*. It is common in elderly whereas the patient is only 25 years of age.
- Expansile impulse on coughing is diagnostic of hernia and indirect hernia can occur in any age group and is mainly unilateral.
- Trans-illumination test is positive in vaginal hydrocele and impulse on coughing is absent.

504. Ans. (d) Low Renin due to pressure atrophy of JG apparatus

- The picture shows autosomal dominant polycystic kidneys in which there is progressive enlargement of cysts with new ones developing with age. The IVU shows a spider leg deformity of the calyces.

- The damage to the kidney results in decrease in amount of erythropoietin leading to normocytic normochromic anemia.
- The damage to the kidney results in development of reduction in GFR and positive feedback to R.A.A.S system results in increase in renin levels as well as high Blood pressure.

505. Ans. (d) Painless intermittent hematuria

- The image shows presence of large vesical calculus. The stone is more common in males and shows pain aggravated by jumping or jolting and is referred to tip of penis at the end of urination.
- Laser lithotripsy (Holmium Laser) can break most large stones and ultrasound lithotripsy is very safe but only for small stones.
- In litholaplaxy, the stone is grasped firmly and broken while the small fragments are evacuated by using a evacuator

506. Ans. (b) Vesico-ureteric reflux

- The image shows presence of Vesico-ureteric Reflux with dye from the bladder refluxing into the tortuous dilated ureters. This is seen with stage V of V.U.R.
- The investigation of choice is MCU: Micturating Cystourethrography

507. Ans. (a) Gangrene of testis

- The diagnosis is Fournier gangrene characterised by extensive gangrene of scrotal skin. The sloughed skin exposes the testicles. In some cases the gangrene can involve the skin of penis, anterior abdominal wall.
- *The testis is not involved as it has a thick tunica albuginea.*

508. Ans. (b) Crescent sign

- The CT scan shows an air crescent sign with rim of air surrounding the aspergilloma or fungus ball caused by aspergillus species. The fungus settles in the cavity which is pre-existing and grows into a ball.
- Meniscus sign is seen in pleural effusion while tree in bud appearance is seen in pneumocystis carinii infection and tuberculosis.
- Loculated empyema would in the periphery of lung.

509. Ans. (a) A = Ventriculoperitoneal shunt, B = Ventriculo-atrial shunt

La Veen and Denver shunts are used in portal Hypertension and start from peritoneal cavity and hence choice C and D are ruled out.

510. Ans. (c) Burr Hole surgery

The image shows presence of extra-dural haemorrhage due to presence of biconvex lenticular opacity. Due to risk of

FMGE Solutions Screening Examination

brain herniation leading to death best management will be burr hole surgery.

511. Ans. (a) Kocher forceps
- The forceps has serrations with a sharp tooth at the tip which differentiates it from artery forceps. It is used to hold tough structures like aponeurosis, fascia.
- Allis forceps has a ratchet and has triangular expansion at the tip where serrations are present.

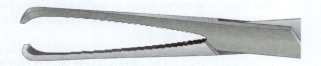

512. Ans. (c) Babcock forceps
The instrument shows expansion with fenestrations at the operating end but does not have teeth. It is used to hold intestines during anastomosis.

513. Ans. (a) Needle holder
The needle holder has two small blades with serrations and is used to hold curved needles which are used to suture the parts.

514. Ans. (b) Self-retaining catheter
The image shows presence of strong heavy instrument used to spread the laparotomy wound and is called as self-retaining retractor.

515. Ans. (a) Proctoscope
The image shows a proctoscope with outer sheath and inner blunt part called as obturator. It is used to diagnose hemorrhoids, carcinoma rectum or rectal ulcers.

516. Ans. (a) Malecot catheter
The image shows a red rubber catheter with a flower shaped ending to ensure that it is a self-retaining catheter. This is used to drain an amoebic liver abscess

517. Ans. (c) Blackmore sengastaken catheter
It is a double balloon and triple lumen tube used for control of bleeding esophageal varices.

518. Ans. (a) Ranula
Ranula is a pseudocyst that is associated with mucus extravasation into the surrounding soft tissues. These lesions occur as the result of trauma or obstruction to the salivary gland excretory duct and spillage of mucin into the surrounding soft tissues.

519. Ans. (a) Foley catheter

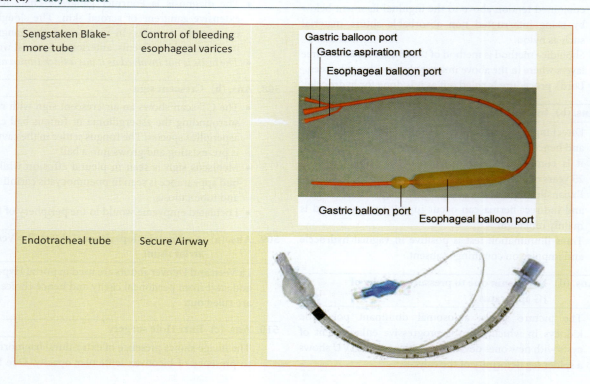

| Sengstaken Blakemore tube | Control of bleeding esophageal varices |
| Endotracheal tube | Secure Airway |

520. Ans. (a) Deaver retractor

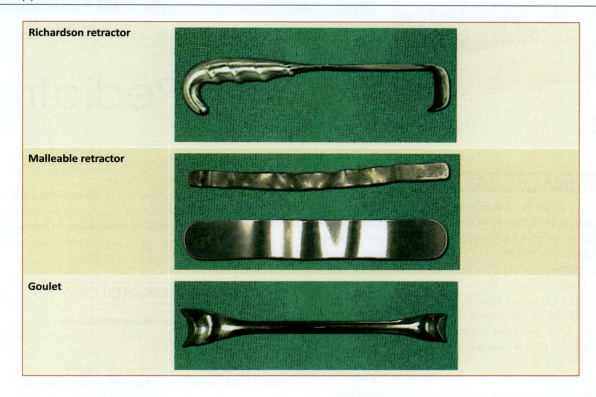

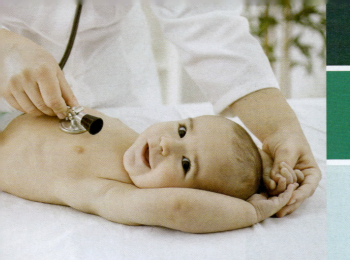

11

Pediatrics

MOST RECENT QUESTIONS 2019

1. A 3-year-old child with weight of 12 kg is having loose motions. He is thirsty, drinks eagerly, tears are absent and skin pinch goes back slowly. What is the best treatment plan for this child?
   a. 1200 ml RL over 12 hours
   b. 600ml RL over 6 hours
   c. ORS 100 ml per episode of loose stool
   d. ORS 50 ml per episode of loose stool

2. Wide open posterior fontanelle with large tongue with rough dry skin is seen in?
   a. Pellagra m
   b. Down syndrome
   c. Hypothyroidism
   d. Nutritional rickets

3. Chronic malnutrition in child is best evaluated by?
   a. Weight for height
   b. Weight for age
   c. Height for age
   d. Ponderal index

4. Neonatal jaundice becomes detectable at serum bilirubin exceeding?
   a. 2 mg%
   b. 3 mg%
   c. 4 mg%
   d. 5 mg%

5. Severity of cyanosis in Fallot's physiology is best decided by?
   a. V.S.D
   b. Overriding of aorta
   c. Concentric RVH
   d. Subpulmonic stenosis

6. Infant is admitted with respiratory distress and prolonged expiration with Rhonchi in chest are heard. CXR shows hyperinflation. What is the diagnosis?
   a. Pneumonia
   b. Croup
   c. Asthma
   d. Bronchiolitis

7. Which of these is used in treatment of bronchiolitis?
   a. Ribavarin
   b. Amantadine
   c. Racemic epinephrine
   d. Corticosteroids

8. 6th day disease is?
   a. Erythema Infectiosum
   b. Exanthema subitum
   c. Erythema marginatum
   d. Erythema nodosum

9. Protein in Cow's milk in comparison to human milk is?
   a. Double
   b. Triple
   c. Quadruple
   d. Same

NEONATOLOGY

10. Maximum heat loss in neonate is from:
    (Recent Pattern Question 2018-19)
    a. Head
    b. Skin
    c. Respiration
    d. Trunk

11. All are features of congenital syphilis except?
    (Recent Pattern Question 2018-19)
    a. Gumma
    b. Saddle nose
    c. Osteochondritis
    d. Charcot joints

12. Which is the best marker for NTD?
    a. αFP *(Recent Pattern Question 2018)*
    b. hCG
    c. Pseudocholinesterase
    d. Inhibin-A

13. The pupil of a newborn is:
    a. Dilated *(Recent Pattern Question 2018)*
    b. Mid-dilated
    c. Constricted
    d. Normal

14. Gynecomastia in neonate is seen due to:
    (Recent Pattern Question 2018)
    a. Mother intake of estrogen
    b. Mother intake of progesterone
    c. GnRH
    d. Gonadotropins

15. Which is the most common cause of neonatal sepsis in India? *(Recent Pattern Question 2018)*
    a. *Klebsiella pneumoniae*
    b. *Mycoplasma pneumoniae*
    c. Group B Streptococcus
    d. Listeria monocytogenes

16. A term child is brought with complaints of having jaundice on day 3 of life. How much should be the minimum level to cause jaundice?
    (Recent Pattern Question 2017)
    a. 5 mg%
    b. 10 mg%
    c. 15 mg%
    d. 20 mg%
17. A term baby is apneic and has a heart rate 90/min. Bag and mask ventilation was given for 30 seconds. Subsequently the Heart rate is still less than 100 bpm. What is the next step? *(Recent Pattern Question 2017)*
    a. Reduce oxygen supply
    b. Check chest movement
    c. Give supplemental oxygen
    d. Give chest compression
18. What is the diagnosis of the child shown in the image, whose mother is having Bronchial asthma?
    (Recent Pattern Question 2016)

    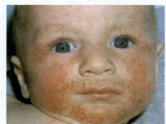

    a. Atopic dermatitis   b. Contact dermatitis
    c. Seborrheic dermatitis d. Irritant dermatitis
19. Apgar score system contains all of the following criteria EXCEPT:
    a. Respiratory rate   b. Color
    c. Motor activity   d. Heart rate
20. For accurate measurement of axillary temperature in newborn, thermometer is kept for?
    a. 1 min   b. 2 min
    c. 3 min   d. 5 min
21. Anterior fontanelle corresponds to all structures EXCEPT:
    a. Frontal bones   b. Coronal suture
    c. Lambdoid suture   d. Saggital suture
22. What is the most common cause of Jaundice in term newborns requiring treatment?
    a. Rh incompatibility   b. ABO incompatibility
    c. Physiological jaundice d. Sepsis
23. In neonatal sepsis, acute phase reactant is:
    a. WBC   b. Alpha anti trypsin
    c. IL-6   d. CRP
24. True about Cephal-hematoma:
    a. Jaundice is prolonged due to cephal-hematoma
    b. Crosses the suture line
    c. Appears on occiput in first few hours of life
    d. Due to rupture of bridging arteries
25. Hutchinson teeth are seen in:
    a. Early congenital spirochete infection
    b. Late congenital syphilis
    c. Rickets
    d. Scurvy
26. Congenital Rubella Syndrome has all of the following EXCEPT:
    a. Sensorineural deafness b. Cataract
    c. Cardiac Defects   d. Hydrocephalus
27. A 28-year-old woman gave birth to a small for age newborn at 38 weeks of pregnancy. On examination, the newborn was found to have rhinitis, distended abdomen; wrinkled skin, and palmoplantar blisters. The woman had an earlier history of abortion and stillbirth. The most likely diagnosis is:
    a. Neonatal pemphigus   b. Scabies
    c. Congenital syphilis d. Congenital HIV infection
28. Physiological jaundice in a full term new born usually resolves by:
    a. One week   b. Two weeks
    c. Three weeks   d. Four weeks
29. The time usually taken for air to reach the descending colon after birth in a normal infant is:
    a. 1–2 hrs   b. 3–4 hrs
    c. 5–6 hrs   d. 8–9 hrs
30. In neonatal resuscitation which is correct?
    a. Put cold water on back   b. Slap on back
    c. Tickle the sole   d. Suspend head down
31. Drug of choice for acute lead encephalopathy
    a. Succimer
    b. d-penicillamine
    c. EDTA
    d. Zinc acetate
32. Key features of kangaroo mother care are all the following EXCEPT?
    a. Skin to skin contact between mother and baby
    b. Exclusive breast feeding
    c. Initiated in a facility and continued at home
    d. Done for babies with cyanosis
33. Nipple confusion means?
    a. Baby fed with a bottle finding it difficult and confusing to suckle at breast
    b. Baby not able to suckle with bottle
    c. Baby not able to feed with spoon
    d. Baby not able to feed with paladi
34. Bag and mask ventilation is contraindicated in newborn resuscitation with clinical suspicion of?
    a. Diaphragmatic hernia
    b. Intracranial hemorrhage
    c. Meconium ileus
    d. Pneumothorax

FMGE Solutions Screening Examination

35. A mother complains that baby is more comfortable and breathes better when held against shoulder. What important clinical problem do you suspect?
    a. Nose block
    b. Psychological anxiety or insecurity
    c. Aerophagy with abdominal fullness
    d. Orthopnea
36. The following component of human milk is not protective against GIT infections?
    a. Lysozyme   b. Lactoferrin
    c. Bifidus factor d. β_2 transferrin
37. Increased oxygen delivery during prematurity causes all the following EXCEPT:
    a. Vasoconstriction   b. Vasodilation
    c. Vaso obliteration d. Neovascularisation
38. Expressed breast milk can be stored at room temperature for how many hours?
    a. 4   b. 8
    c. 16 d. 24
39. Pathological jaundice criteria includes all EXCEPT:
    a. 24 hours later but within 72 hours
    b. More than 14 days persistence
    c. >2 mg/dL conjugated bilirubin
    d. Clay colored stool
40. Growing fetus derives energy from?
    a. Amino acid
    b. Carbohydrate
    c. Lipid
    d. Minerals
41. The ratio of chest compression to breathing in neonatal life support is?
    a. 3:1   b. 4:1
    c. 5:1   d. 6:1
42. Which type of cerebral palsy is most commonly seen as a sequel of bilirubin encephalopathy?
    a. Spastic quadriparesis
    b. Spastic diplegia
    c. Atonic cerebral palsy
    d. Extra pyramidal cerebral palsy
43. Hemorrhagic disease of the newborn is attributed to the deficiency of?
    a. Vitamin A   b. Vitamin E
    c. Vitamin K   d. Vitamin C
44. In neonate which is the indication for chest compressions?
    a. Irregular breathing with heart rate 80 after 30 seconds
    b. Regular breathing with heart rate 80 after 30 seconds
    c. AMBU Bag ventilation for 30 seconds with heart rate of 50
    d. Regular breathing with Cyanosis

MILESTONES IN CHILDREN

45. What is the cut off level of imbecile?
    (Recent Pattern Question 2018)
    a. 0–20   b. 20–49
    c. 50–69   d. >70
46. A baby with tripod position, bi dextrous approach, recognises strangers and can spell out mono syllable by what age:
    a. 7 months   b. 12 months
    c. 9 months   d. 10 months
47. Beyond what age, absence of social smile is regarded as abnormal:
    a. 12 weeks   b. 14 weeks
    c. 16 weeks   d. 18 weeks
48. Moro's reflex disappears by which age?
    a. 3 month   b. 6 months
    c. 9 months   d. 12 months
49. Most common cause of neonatal mortality in India?
    a. Prematurity
    b. Congenital malformation
    c. Pneumonia
    d. Metabolic (hypoglycemia)
50. A baby placed in the prone position is able to lift the head and upper chest on extended arms by?
    a. 1 month   b. 3 months
    c. 6 months   d. 9 months

BREASTFEEDING

51. Best management for formula fed child with severe Cow milk protein allergy?   *(Recent Pattern Question 2016)*
    a. Soya milk
    b. Hydrolysed formula feed
    c. Amino acid based formula
    d. Total Parenteral nutrition
52. All of the following are signs of good attachment during breast feeding EXCEPT:
    a. Baby's mouth is wide open
    b. Baby's lower lip is inverted
    c. Upper areola is more visible than lower
    d. Baby's chin touching the breast
53. All of the following are signs of good attachment during breast feeding EXCEPT:
    a. Baby's mouth is wide open
    b. Baby's lower lip is everted
    c. Lower areola is more visible than upper
    d. Baby's chin touching the breast
54. Recommendation for exclusive breast feeding is up to:
    a. 3 months   b. 4 months
    c. 5 months   d. 6 months

Pediatrics

55. Breast milk contains all EXCEPT?
   a. Lacta globulin
   b. Lactoalbumin
   c. Whey protein
   d. Avidin

56. "Good attachment" of infant to mother's breast during breast feeding includes all of the following EXCEPT:
   a. Chin of the infant touches mother's breast
   b. Upper part of areola is visible more than the lower part
   c. Lower lip of infant is inverted
   d. Mouth of infant is wide open

57. Which amino acid, present in human milk in large amount helps in brain development?
   a. Alanine
   b. Tyrosine
   c. Lysine
   d. Taurine

GROWTH AND DEVELOPMENT

58. Swallowing reflex appears at?
   (Recent Pattern Question 2017)
   a. 6 week
   b. 16 weeks
   c. 18 weeks
   d. 22 weeks

59. Undescended testis is a feature of?
   (Recent Pattern Question 2016)
   a. Prematurity
   b. Post term
   c. Term child
   d. Term small for date

60. How many teeth are present in a 3 year child?
   a. 8 teeth
   b. 12 teeth
   c. 18 teeth
   d. 20 teeth

61. False regarding the testicular development during fetal stage:
   a. Develop in abdomen
   b. Gubernaculum plays decisive role
   c. 7 months into scrotum
   d. Scrotum empty at 7 months

62. All of the following are common problems of pre-school children EXCEPT:
   a. Temper tantrums
   b. Sleep problems
   c. Truancy
   d. Pica

63. Early sign of puberty in male is enlargement of testes. In females it is determined by:
   a. Pubarche
   b. Menarche
   c. Thelarche
   d. Menstruation

64. Nocturnal Enuresis is occurrence of involuntary voiding at night in a child more than
   a. 2 ½ years
   b. 3 ½ years
   c. 4 years
   d. 5 years

65. An infant is considered anemic at Hemoglobin less than gm%?
   a. 8
   b. 9
   c. 10
   d. 12

66. A 3-year-old Child who has diurnal enuresis and soiling of clothes. Treatment required?
   a. Urethroplasty
   b. Put catheter for 7 days
   c. Circumcision at 10 years
   d. Behaviour modification

67. Rickets in India is most commonly caused by?
   a. Malnutrition
   b. Lack of sun exposure
   c. Lactose intolerance
   d. Genetics

68. Age at which child can tell gender?
   a. 2 years
   b. 3 years
   c. 4 years
   d. 5 years

69. Concerning attention deficit hyperactivity disorder which is true?
   a. Impulsive behavior is a feature
   b. Higher incidence in tic disorders
   c. May respond to treatment with stimulants such as amphetamine
   d. All the above

70. X-ray of choice for age detection in 6 months old child is?
   a. Skull
   b. Hand
   c. Knee
   d. Shoulder

71. Most common location of supernumerary teeth is?
   a. Between incisors
   b. Between canines
   c. Between molars
   d. Between premolars

72. Birth weight doubles by?
   a. 3 months
   b. 5 months
   c. 9 months
   d. 12 months

73. Birth length doubles by what age?
   a. 1 year
   b. 2 years
   c. 3 years
   d. 4 years

74. At what age do first permanent teeth appear?
   a. 5 years
   b. 6 years
   c. 7 years
   d. 8 years

75. Vocabulary of a 2 year old child is?
   a. 20 words
   b. 50 words
   c. 100 words
   d. 200 words

76. A child draws Triangle at what age?
   a. 3 years
   b. 4 years
   c. 5 years
   d. 7 years

77. A 18 month baby can do which of the following?
   a. Hide & seek game
   b. Write Alphabet
   c. Say short sentence
   d. Walk short distance

78. Which of the following is called as red flag sign in child development, if not attained?
   a. Vocalization at 2 months
   b. Walking at 12 months
   c. Single word at 12 months
   d. Social smile at 3 months

79. To diagnose anemia in age group 6 month to 6 years, level of hemoglobin should be?
    a. Hb 10g/dL b. Hb 11g/dL
    c. Hb 12g/dL d. Hb 13g/dL
80. By what age can a child tell his/her own gender?
    a. 1.5–2 years b. 2.5–3 years
    c. 3.5–4 years d. 4.5–5 years
81. Which of the following-is the first sign of sexual maturity in boys?
    a. Increase in height b. Appearance of facial hair
    c. Change in voice d. Increase in testicular size
82. At what age (in years) does-a child attain a height of 100 cms?
    a. 2 b. 3
    c. 4 d. 5

PROTEIN ENERGY MALNUTRITION

83. Which is the most specific clinical feature for diagnosis for Kwashiorkor? *(Recent Pattern Question 2018)*
    a. Fatty liver b. Easy pluckable hair
    c. Low serum albumin d. Edema
84. Adaptive starvation with increased metabolism:
    (Recent Pattern Question 2018)
    a. Bulimia b. Kwashiorkor
    c. Marasmus d. Cachexia
85. Which of the following defects will lead to this presentation? *(Recent Pattern Question 2017)*

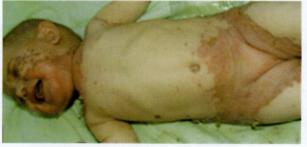

    a. ABCD1 b. SLC39A4
    c. ATP7B d. ATP7A
86. Chronic malnutrition is measured by:
    a. Weight/height b. Height/age
    c. Weight/age d. Mid arm circumference
87. Which is the best parameter for acute severe malnutrition:
    a. Weight/height b. Height/age
    c. Weight/age d. Mid arm circumference
88. BMI is measured in children by:
    a. Wt.kg/Ht.m^2 b. Wt.kg/Ht.cm^2
    c. Wt.gm/Ht.cm^2 d. Wt.gm/Ht.m^2
89. Very low birth weight child weighs:
    a. 1000 gm b. < 1500 gm
    c. < 2500 gm d. < 750 gm

90. Extremely low birth weight baby is defined as?
    a. <1000 gms b. <1500 gms
    c. <2500 gms d. <2800 gms
91. What is the mid upper arm circumference – cut off value for malnutrition of a child:
    a. 12.5 cm b. 10.5 cm
    c. 14.5 cm d. 9.5 cm
92. Ponderal index in malnourished babies is?
    a. <1 b. <2
    c. <4 d. <6
93. A 4-year-old boy, with swollen bleeding gums, petechiae and dry eyes. Diagnosis:
    a. Rickets b. Marasmus
    c. Scurvy d. Dehydration
94. Flag hair sign is seen in
    a. Kwashiorkor b. Marasmus
    c. Scurvy d. Pellagra
95. All are seen in Marasmus EXCEPT:
    a. Muscle wasting b. Hepatomegaly
    c. Low insulin d. Muscle wasting
96. All are seen in Kwashiorkor EXCEPT
    a. Increase appetite b. Flag sign on hair
    c. Hepatomegaly d. Apathy
97. Nutritional rickets is treated by a single dose of Vitamin D of
    a. 5,000 mcg b. 10,000 mcg
    c. 15,000 mcg d. 20,000 mcg
98. All are seen in nutritional Rickets EXCEPT?
    a. Pseudoparalysis
    b. Delayed dentition
    c. Widening of the wrist joint
    d. Double medial malleolus
99. The metabolic defect in hereditary fructose intolerance is due to deficiency of enzyme:
    a. Fructokinase b. Aldolase-B
    c. Xylitol dehydrogenase d. Phosphofructokinase
100. Chronic malnutrition diagnosis is based upon?
    a. Decreased weight for age
    b. MAC< 11.5 cm
    c. <3.5 gm% serum protein
    d. Decreased height for age
101. All are seen in marasmus EXCEPT?
    a. Hunger b. Wasting
    c. Loose folds skin d. Apathy

PEDIATRIC NEUROLOGY

102. Medulloblastoma is: *(Recent Pattern Question 2018)*
    a. Malignant tumor in adults
    b. Malignant tumor in children
    c. Benign brain tumor
    d. Malignant cerebellar tumor in adults

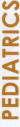

Pediatrics

103. Elevated amniotic fluid acetylcholinesterase is used for diagnosis of? *(Recent Pattern Question 2017)*
   a. Neonatal myasthenia gravis
   b. Spinal dysraphism
   c. Hydrops fetalis
   d. Neonatal heart block

104. Which of the following is a neural tube marker?
   (Recent Pattern Question 2017)
   a. Pseudo-cholinesterase   b. Acetylcholinesterase
   c. Transketolase   d. Beta 2 transferrin

105. NTD with maximum viability is?
   (Recent Pattern Question 2017)
   a. Spina bifida occulta   b. Anencephaly
   c. Myelomeningocele   d. Meningocele

106. SSPE is caused by? *(Recent Pattern Question 2017)*
   a. Rubella   b. Rubeola
   c. Varicella   d. Variola

107. A 1-year-old baby brought by the mother complaining of a cystic mass on back and inability to move both legs ever since birth. Possible diagnosis?
   a. Pilonidal cyst   b. Meningocoele
   c. Meningomyelocoele   d. Sacrococcygeal teratoma

108. All are true regarding congenital hydrocephalus EXCEPT:
   a. Stenosis of aqueduct can contribute
   b. Mostly Hereditary in nature
   c. Can be seen together with Spina bifida
   d. Broad forehead and wide open anterior fontannel

109. Continuous prophylactic anticonvulsant therapy is not needed in a child with febrile convulsion with?
   a. Developmental delay
   b. Family history of epilepsy
   c. Typical simple Febrile fits
   d. Persistent neurological deficit

110. In a child diagnosed with H. influenza meningitis, what investigation must be done before discharging him from the hospital?
   a. BERA   b. MRI
   c. CT scan   d. X-ray skull

111. Most common cause of meningo-encephalitis in children is?
   a. HSV   b. Measles
   c. Adenovirus   d. Enterovirus

112. Treatment of Rolandic epilepsy is?
   a. Phenytoin   b. Lamotrigine
   c. Carbamezapine   d. ACTH

113. All of the following are manifestations of hypervitaminosis A EXCEPT?
   a. Loss of hair
   b. Generalized exfoliation
   c. Decreased Intracranial pressure
   d. Muscle pains

GENETICS

114. Trisomy of Down's syndrome is:
   a. 21   b. 22
   c. 18   d. 13

115. Which is correct about estriol level in Down syndrome?
   a. No change   b. Low
   c. Elevated   d. Double-triple

116. Trisomy 18 is? *(Recent Pattern Question 2016)*
   a. Down syndrome   b. Edward syndrome
   c. Patau syndrome   d. Turner syndrome

117. Anti-mongoloid facies, Short stature, undescended testis, and pulmonic stenosis are seen in?
   (Recent Pattern Question 2016)
   a. Noonan syndrome   b. Down syndrome
   c. Klinefelter syndrome   d. Angelman syndrome

118. Recent marker for Down syndrome:
   a. HCG   b. Alpha feto protein
   c. Inhibin   d. Estriol

119. All are seen in Down's syndrome EXCEPT:
   a. Low IQ   b. Brachycephaly
   c. Umbilical hernia   d. Hypothyroidism

120. For Prenatal diagnosis of Down's syndrome, all are true EXCEPT?
   a. Reduced femur and humerus length
   b. Nuchal fold thickness >2.5 mm
   c. Increased umbilical blood flow
   d. Ventricular septal defect may be present

121. Neural tube defects marker
   a. Estriol
   b. Beta hCG
   c. Alpha feto-protein
   d. Acetylcholine esterase

122. The earliest congenital anomaly identified by ultrasound is:
   a. Hydrocephalus
   b. Encephalocele
   c. Spina bifida
   d. Anencephaly

PEDIATRIC CARDIOLOGY

123. Most common cardiac anomaly associated with Noonan syndrome: *(Recent Pattern Question 2018-19)*
   a. Pulmonic stenosis   b. Coarctation of aorta
   c. VSD   d. TAPVR

124. Continuous murmur is heard in?
   (Recent Pattern Question 2018-19)
   a. Patent ductus arteriosus b. VSD
   c. ASD   d. Tetralogy of Fallot

FMGE Solutions Screening Examination

125. All of the following statements are true regarding TOF, EXCEPT: *(Recent Pattern Question 2018)*
 a. Right ventricular hypertrophy
 b. ASD
 c. Overriding of aorta
 d. Subpulmonic stenosis

126. The innocent murmur is best heard in children at:
 a. Pulmonic area *(Recent Pattern Question 2018)*
 b. Aortic area
 c. Left lower sternal border
 d. Apex

127. A 2-week-old child presents with cyanosis. Which of the following heart disease will have highest chances of 1 year survival? *(Recent Pattern Question 2017)*
 a. T.O.F
 b. T.G.A
 c. T.A.P.V.C
 d. Tricuspid Atresia

128. Which of the following is a feature of Tetralogy of fallot?
 a. Pan-systolic murmur *(Recent Pattern Question 2017)*
 b. Congestive heart failure
 c. Pulmonic stenosis
 d. Normal Cardiothoracic ratio

129. Structure with functional closure immediately after birth? *(Recent Pattern Question 2017)*
 a. Foramen Ovale
 b. Ductus venosus
 c. Ductus arteriosus
 d. Umbilical artery

130. Most common heart defect in children?
 (Recent Pattern Question 2016)
 a. Muscular V.S.D   b. Membranous VSD
 c. Ostium Secondum   d. Ostium Primum

131. Which of the following is an acyanotic heart disease:
 a. TOF   b. TGA
 c. PDA   d. COA

132. All are seen in Kawasaki disease EXCEPT:
 a. Mitral regurgitation
 b. Ischemic heart disease
 c. Myocarditis
 d. Pericardial tamponade

133. Which of the following is synonymous with Muco-cutaneous lymph node syndrome?
 a. Scarlet fever
 b. Kawasaki disease
 c. Behcet's syndrome
 d. Tuberculosis

134. In septum primum type of ASD over burden occurs in which chamber?
 a. RV   b. LV
 c. RA   d. LA

GASTROINTESTINAL TRACT

135. A 1-month-old baby presents with lethargy, non-bilious vomiting, excessive crying and F.T.T. The diagnosis is?
 a. Ileal atresia   *(Recent Pattern Question 2017)*
 b. Duodenal atresia
 c. Hypertrophic pyloric stenosis
 d. Trachea-esophageal fistula

136. What is the dose of zinc given to 4 month old child in diarrhoea? *(Recent Pattern Question 2016)*
 a. 5 mg   b. 10 mg
 c. 15 mg   d. 20 mg

137. In pediatrics, differential for Acute appendicitis are all EXCEPT:
 a. Gastroenteritis   b. Volvulus
 c. Trauma   d. Torsion

138. Useful in acute diarrhea:
 a. Zinc   b. Magnesium
 c. Calcium   d. Potassium

139. IOC for congenital hypertrophic pyloric stenosis:
 a. X-ray   b. CT San
 c. MRI   d. Ultrasound

140. Which drug consumption by pregnant lady can lead to baby developing hypertrophic pyloric stenosis?
 a. Vancomycin
 b. Nifedipine
 c. Erythromycin
 d. Phenyl propalamine

141. Double bubble appearance is seen in?
 a. Jejunal atresia
 b. Duodenal atresia
 c. Obstructive jaundice
 d. Pyloric atresia

142. What is the most-likely diagnosis of a 26-day-old infant presenting with recurrent nonbilious vomiting with constipation and loss of weight?
 a. Esophageal atresia
 b. Annular pancreas
 c. Ileal atresia
 d. Pyloric stenosis

143. All are seen in lactose intolerance EXCEPT?
 a. Benedict test positive in urine
 b. Alkaline urine
 c. Acidic stool
 d. Lactase enzyme deficiency

144. All are seen in lactose intolerance EXCEPT?
 a. Benedict test positive in urine
 b. Non Reducing sugar in urine
 c. Acidic stool
 d. Lactase enzyme deficiency

145. A child presents with bilious vomitting on day 2 of life and the mother gives history of polyhydramnios. The radiological imaging is shown. What's your probable diagnosis?

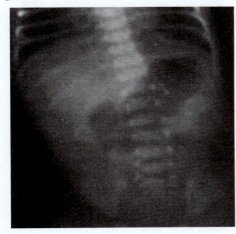

   a. Duodenal atresia
   b. Hypertrophic pyloric stenosis
   c. Ileal atresia
   d. Congenital Mega-colon

146. In Hypertrophic pyloric stenosis which electrolyte should be replenished first?
   a. Na⁺
   b. K⁺
   c. Cl⁻
   d. HCO³⁻

147. A 5-year-child came with dehydration. Plan A was proposed for treatment of dehydration. How much ORS should be given per loose stool?
   a. 0–50 mL
   b. 50–100 mL
   c. 100–200 mL
   d. 200–300 mL

FLUID & ELECTROLYTE BALANCE

148. 24 hour normal fluid requirement for a one year old child weighing 8 kg is
   a. 700 mL
   b. 800 mL
   c. 900 mL
   d. 1000 mL

149. The sodium concentration of low osmolarity ORS is:
   a. 45 mmol/L
   b. 60 mmol/L
   c. 75 mmol/L
   d. 90 mmol/L

150. A 2-year-old female child was brought to a PHC with a history of cough and fever for 4 days with inability to drink for last 12 hours. On examination, the child was having weight of 5 kg and respiratory rate of 45 per minute with fever. The child will be classified according to IMNCI as suffering from:
   a. Very severe pneumonia
   b. Severe pneumonia
   c. Pneumonia
   d. No pneumonia

151. Calculate the Fluid requirement for severe dehydration in a one year old child weighing 8 kg:
   a. 600 mL
   b. 800 mL
   c. 900 mL
   d. 1000 mL

152. What serum level of albumin is considered as mild degree of malnutrition:
   a. 4.0 g/dL
   b. 3.5 g/dL
   c. 3.0 g/dL
   d. 2.5 g/dL

153. Severe dehydration is seen in 2-year-old child. IV fluid to be given:
   a. 30 mL in 60 min
   b. 30 mL in 30 min
   c. 70 mL in 360 min
   d. 70 mL in 180 min

154. Intraosseous line is placed in which bone in children?
   a. Femur
   b. Tibia
   c. ASIS
   d. Iliac crest

155. Low Osmolar ORS composition is?
   a. Na 90 + 311 mOsm
   b. Na 75 + 245 mOsm
   c. Na 60 + 245 mOsm
   d. Na 60 + 240 mOsm

VACCINES

156. What is the upper limit of initiation of first dose of Rotavirus vaccine? *(Recent Pattern Question 2017)*
   a. 6 weeks
   b. 10 weeks
   c. 12 weeks
   d. 15 weeks

157. Which of the following vaccine can be given to AIDS positive child?
   a. DPT
   b. BCG
   c. Measles
   d. OPV

158. Which among the following is vaccine for cholera?
   a. PPV 23
   b. Dukoral
   c. Ty 21 a vaccine
   d. JE-MB Nakayama

159. Osteomyelitis is side effect of which vaccine?
   a. Hepatitis B vaccine
   b. BCG
   c. Measles vaccine
   d. IPV

KIDNEY

160. Mutation in NPHS 1 gene causes which disease?
   a. Alport syndrome
   b. Congenital Finnish type nephrotic syndrome
   c. Focal segmental glomerulonephritis
   d. Nail patella syndrome

161. Child presents with Pathological fracture, Renal stone and Psychiatric symptoms. Most probable diagnosis is?
   a. Renal tubular acidosis
   b. Hyperparathyroidism
   c. Polycystic kidney disease
   d. CRF

162. Henoch Schonlein purpura commonly involves which age group?
   a. 4–8 years
   b. 10–15 years
   c. 15–20 years
   d. > 25 years

FMGE Solutions Screening Examination

RESPIRATORY SYSTEM

163. Which of the following clinical presentation is correct for a child with pneumonia?
 (Recent Pattern Question 2018)
 a. <50/min RR, with age of 2 months
 b. >40/min RR, for 2–12 months
 c. >40/min RR, for 12–60 months
 d. <60/min RR, for 0–2 months

164. Most common cause of common cold in children is?
 a. RSV
 b. Rhinovirus
 c. Influenza
 d. Allergic

INBORN ERRORS OF METABOLISM

165. A normal born child presents with mental retardation, blond hair and convulsions at 1 year of age. Most probable diagnosis is?
 a. Albuminuria
 b. Phenylketonuria
 c. Gaucher's disease
 d. Tyrosinemia

ENDOCRINOLOGY

166. Nelson syndrome is seen in?
 a. Adrenalectomy
 b. Hypopituitarism
 c. Deficiency of beta cells
 d. Deficiency of growth hormone

MISCELLANEOUS

167. Hand foot mouth disease is usually caused by:
 (Recent Pattern Question 2018)
 a. Coxsackie A   b. Adenovirus
 c. Rotavirus   d. Hepatitis B virus

168. Which of the following is the cause of development of acute scrotum in a 2-year-old child?
 (Recent Pattern Question 2017)
 a. Torsion of appendix of testis
 b. Epididymitis
 c. Testicular trauma
 d. Idiopathic swelling of scrotum

169. An 8 month baby presents with fever, cough and confluent rash on hairline, face, neck and body. Which of the following is a causative organism?
 (Recent Pattern Question 2017)
 a. Varicella   b. Variola
 c. Rubella   d. Rubeola

170. Slapped cheeks appearance is seen in?
 (Recent Pattern Question 2016)

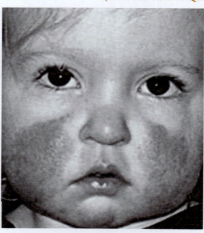

 a. Erythema infectiosum   b. Measles
 c. Chicken pox   d. Erythema nodosum

171. Post streptococcal glomerulonephritis in children is diagnosed by
 a. Heavy proteinuria, high cholesterol, high ASO titre
 b. Heavy proteinuria, hematuria, low ASO titre
 c. Mild proteinuria, high hematuria, high ASO titre
 d. Mild proteinuria, high cholesterol, normal ASO titre

172. Acrodermatitis enterohepatica is due to:
 a. Pustular psoriasis   b. Zinc toxicity
 c. Zinc deficiency   d. Collodion baby

173. What is the dose of isoniazid in infants:
 a. 5 mg/kg   b. 10 mg/kg
 c. 15 mg/kg   d. 20 mg/kg

174. Precocious puberty and patchy skin pigmentation is known as:
 a. Albright's syndrome
 b. Litter Siwe disease
 c. Asherman's syndrome
 d. Morquio's syndrome

175. All are seen at Congenital rubella syndrome EXCEPT?
 a. SN hearing loss
 b. Cataract
 c. Headlight in fog appearance
 d. PDA

176. The following is helpful in a child with severe falciparum malaria with high parasitemia?
 a. IV corticosteroids
 b. Exchange transfusion
 c. Hyperbaric oxygen
 d. IVIG

177. Most common age for pediatric TB is?
 a. < 1 year   b. 1–4 years
 c. 5–8 years   d. 8–14 years

Pediatrics

178. **In mechanical ventilation of a newborn with ARDS, the end tidal volume is kept at?**
   a. 5 mL/kg
   b. 7 mL/kg
   c. 10 mL/kg
   d. 15 mL/kg

179. **Regarding Wilson's disease, the true statement is:**
   a. Hemolytic anemia
   b. Autosomal dominant inheritance
   c. Decreased urinary copper excretion
   d. Normal hepatic copper level

180. **Which of the following is the most common symptom of Henoch-Schonlein Purpura?**
   a. Abdominal pain
   b. Joint pain
   c. Decreased urine output
   d. Rashes

181. **Which of the following cannot be done by a four year old child?**
   a. Count 10 pennies
   b. Hop on one foot
   c. Copy a bridge
   d. Identity the longer of two lines

182. **What is the most common cause of congenital hypothyroidism?**
   a. Maternal antibiotics
   b. Dyshormonogenesis
   c. Thyroid dysgenesis
   d. Maternal medications

183. **The most common type of congenital oesophageal atresia is?**
   a. Proximal end blind, distal end communicating with trachea
   b. Distal end blind, proximal end communicating with trachea
   c. Proximal and distal ends open and communicating with trachea
   d. Both ends blind

184. **Which one of the following infections is characterized by an increased TLC with absolute lymphocytosis?**
   a. Diphtheria
   b. Measles
   c. MI
   d. Pneumonia

185. **All of the following methods are used for the diagnosis of HIV infection in a 2 month old child EXCEPT:**
   a. DNA PCR
   b. Viral culture
   c. HIV ELISA
   d. p 24 antigen assay

186. **Sub-periosteal hemorrhage in the long bones is usually seen in?**
   a. Osteogenesis imperfecta
   b. Scurvy
   c. Rickets
   d. Hemophilia

187. **Acrodermatitis Enterohepatica occurs due to deficiency of?**
   a. Ascorbic acid
   b. Vitamin B12
   c. Zinc
   d. Riboflavin

BOARD REVIEW QUESTIONS

188. **Most common cause of respiratory distress in newborn baby after caesarean section?**
   a. Hyaline membrane disease
   b. Meconium aspiration syndrome
   c. Transient Tachypnea of new-born
   d. Primary pulmonary hypertension

189. **Incorrect about breast milk is?**
   a. 65 kcal /100 mL
   b. High lactaglobulin
   c. Contains IgA
   d. Deficient in vitamin K

190. **Air Broncho gram in CXR of a neonate is diagnostic of**
   a. Hyaline membrane disease
   b. Meconium aspiration syndrome
   c. Transient Tachypnea of new-born
   d. Primary pulmonary hypertension

191. **Phototherapy works by?**
   a. Photo-oxidation
   b. Structural isomerization
   c. Configuration isomerization
   d. Photo-dissolution

192. **Breastfeeding is contraindicated in**
   a. Cleft palate
   b. HIV positive mother
   c. Unilateral breast abscess
   d. Inverted nipple

193. **All are true about a baby born to a mother with gestational diabetes mellitus, EXCEPT?**
   a. Congenital malformations
   b. Polycyathemia
   c. Jaundice
   d. Hyperinsulinemia

194. **DPT is contraindicated in**
   a. Epilepsy
   b. Mental retardation
   c. Cerebral palsy
   d. Fever after last shot

195. **Persistent diarrhoea is defined as diarrhoea lasting more than?**
   a. 7 days
   b. 14 days
   c. 21 days
   d. 28 days

196. **Feature of Wilson disease is**
   a. Decreased serum copper
   b. Decreased urinary copper
   c. Decreased hepatic copper
   d. Increased ceruloplasmin

197. **Neonate with cyanosis on day 0?**
   a. Tricuspid atresia
   b. TGA
   c. TAPVC
   d. VSD

198. **Upper segment: lower segment ratio becomes 1:1 at**
   a. Birth
   b. 3 years
   c. 6 years
   d. 10 years

FMGE Solutions Screening Examination

199. Kanawati index is
     a. Mid arm circumference/head circumference
     b. Head circumference/weight
     c. Weight/head circumference
     d. Weight/length^3
200. Hutchinson teeth are seen in:
     a. Early congenital spirochete infection
     b. Late congenital syphilis
     c. Rickets   d. Scurvy
201. All are seen in Kwashiorkor EXCEPT:
     a. Increase appetite   b. Flag sign on hair
     c. Hepatomegaly   d. Apathy
202. Short stature is defined as less than _____
     a. 3rd centile   b. 10 centile
     c. 25 centile   d. 50 centile
203. Child can lift head, greater part of chest while supporting weight on extended arms at
     a. 2 months   b. 4 months
     c. 6 months   d. 8 months
204. Hopping is seen at
     a. 2 years   b. 3 years
     c. 4 years   d. 5 years
205. Child helps in household chores, dresses and undresses at
     a. 2 years   b. 3 years
     c. 4 years   d. 5 years
206. Apgar score system contain all of the following criteria EXCEPT:
     a. Respiratory rate   b. Color
     c. Motor activity   d. Heart rate
207. A baby with tripod position, bi dexterous approach, recognizes strangers and can spell out mono syllable by what age?
     a. 7 months   b. 12 months
     c. 9 months   d. 10 months
208. Most common type of seizures in neonate is?
     a. Subtle   b. Absence
     c. GTCS   d. Myoclonic seizure
209. Most common brain tumour in children
     a. Medulloblastoma   b. Cerebellar astrocytoma
     c. Germinoma   d. Pinealoma
210. Most common type of cerebral palsy?
     a. Spastic   b. Athetoid
     c. Mixed   d. Dystonic
211. All of the following are signs of good attachment during breast feeding EXCEPT:
     a. Baby's mouth is wide open
     b. Baby's lower lip is everted
     c. Lower areola is more visible than upper
     d. Baby's chin touching the breast
212. How many teeth are present in 3 year child:
     a. 8 teeth   b. 12 teeth
     c. 18 teeth   d. 20 teeth

213. What is the most common cause of Jaundice in term newborns requiring treatment?
     a. Rh incompatibility   b. ABO incompatibility
     c. Physiological jaundice d. Sepsis
214. Chronic malnutrition is measured by
     a. Weight/height   b. Height/age
     c. Weight/age   d. Mid arm circumference
215. Very low birth weight child weights
     a. 1000 g   b. <1500 g
     c. <2500 g   d. <750 g
216. Extremely low birth weight
     a. <1000   b. <1500
     c. <2500   d. <2800
217. Malnutrition of a child mid upper arm circumference – cut off value is
     a. 12.5 cm   b. 10.5 cm
     c. 14.5 cm   d. 9.5 cm
218. Ponderal index in malnourished babies is:
     a. <1   b. <2
     c. <4   d. <6
219. Flag hair sign is seen in
     a. Kwashiorkor   b. Marasmus
     c. Scurvy   d. Pellagra
220. Harrison groove is seen in
     a. Rickets
     b. Scurvy
     c. Vitamin D resistant rickets
     d. Chondrocalcinosis
221. Keshan disease is due to deficiency of?
     a. Selenium   b. Chromium
     c. Zinc   d. Iodine
222. Asymmetric tonic neck reflex disappears at
     a. 3 month   b. 6 month
     c. 9 month   d. 12 months
223. Drug of choice for lipoid nephrosis
     a. Statin   b. Steroid
     c. Cyclophosphamide d. High protein diet
224. Lymphoma in children is predominantly seen at what age?
     a. < 4 years   b. < 14 years
     c. > 14 years   d. < 1 year
225. Infective endocarditis is least common in?
     a. Severe MR   b. Severe AR
     c. Small VSD   d. Small ASD
226. Alpha-1- antitrypsin deficiency presents as?
     a. Emphysema   b. Bronchitectasis
     c. Empyema   d. Bronchogenic carcinoma
227. Percentage of dose given as basal insulin in bolus-basal regimen in children is?
     a. 0–25%   b. 25–50%
     c. 50–75%   d. None of these

Pediatrics

228. Most common birth defect in north India is?
   a. CTEV
   b. Neural tube defects (Spina bifida)
   c. Down's syndrome
   d. Hemoglobinophathies

229. In children renal failure in terms of urine output is defined as?
   a. Less than 0.3 mL/kg/hr
   b. Less than 0.5 mL/kg/hr
   c. Less than 0.8 mL/kg/hr
   d. Less than 1 mL/kg/hr

230. Average gain of height in first year is?
   a. 25 cm
   b. 50 cm
   c. 75 cm
   d. 100 cm

231. Treatment of breath holding spells is?
   a. Pyridoxine
   b. Zinc
   c. Iron
   d. Molybdenum

232. Conjugated bilirubin is increased in?
   a. Rotor Syndrome
   b. Gilbert's syndrome
   c. CrigglerNajjar syndrome 1
   d. CrigglerNajjar syndrome 2

233. At what age do first permanent teeth appear?
   a. 5 years
   b. 6 years
   c. 7 years
   d. 8 years

234. Most common cardiac anomaly in Turner's Syndrome is?
   a. Coarctation of aorta
   b. Bicuspid aortic value
   c. Ventricular septal defect
   d. Atrial septal defect

235. Adolescence starts at the age of?
   a. 7 years
   b. 10 years
   c. 14 years
   d. 17 years

236. Child draws triangle at what age?
   a. 3 years
   b. 5 years
   c. 6 years
   d. 7 years

237. Which of the following has no role in diagnosis of childhood TB?
   a. ELISA
   b. Mantoux
   c. CXR
   d. FNAC

238. A child 4-month-old has 10 episodes of vomiting and 2–3 episodes of loose stools and crying since the last 24 hours, best line of management will be?
   a. Intravenous fluids
   b. ORS
   c. Intravenous fluids then ORS
   d. Hospitalise and treat

239. True about Wilson's disease is?
   a. Increased serum ceruloplasmin
   b. Decreased liver copper
   c. Increased urinary copper excretion
   d. Decreased urine copper excretion

240. Most common enzyme deficiency leading to childhood hypertension is?
   a. 17-Alpha hydroxylase
   b. 21-Beta hydroxylase
   c. 11-Beta hydroxylase
   d. 3-Beta hydroxy steroid dehydrogenase

241. Blood volume in preterm neonate is?
   a. 90 mL/kg
   b. 80 mL/kg
   c. 70 mL/kg
   d. 60 mL/kg

242. Preterm neonate target oxygen saturation is?
   a. 85–95%
   b. >95%
   c. 70–95%
   d. <80%

FMGE Solutions Screening Examination

ANSWERS WITH EXPLANATIONS

MOST RECENT QUESTIONS 2019

1. Ans. (c) ORS 100 ml per episode of loose stool

Ref: OP Ghai, 8th ed. pg. 294

- The diagnosis of this child who is thirsty and drinks eagerly with absent tears is some dehydration. Hence ORS is to be given to this child for correction of dehydration at rate of 75 ml/Kg over the next 4–6 hours plus ongoing losses.
- For ongoing losses in children over 2 years, 100 ml per episode of loose stool should be given extra over the correction mentioned in first point.
- Choice A and B are ruled out as intravenous correction is done for severe dehydration.

Age	Amount of ORS to be given after each loose stool
<24 months	50–100 ml per episode
2–10 years	100 ml-200 ml per episode
>10 years	Ad Lib

2. Ans. (c) Hypothyroidism

Ref: Nelson 20th ed. pg. 2269

- Choice A Pellagra manifests as edema, erythema, and burning of sun-exposed skin on the face, neck, and dorsal aspects of the hands, forearms, and feet.
- Choice B presents as protuberant tongue with brachycephaly and early closure of fontanelles.
- Choice D presents as wide open anterior fontanelle.
- Choice C Congenital Hypothyroidism presents with patent posterior fontanelle with myxedema leading to large tongue and coarse dry skin. The leading cause of congenital hypothyroidism is thyroid dysgenesis.

3. Ans. (c) Height for age

Ref: Nelson 20th ed. pg. 298

- Height for age is a measure of linear growth and a deficit represents cumulative effect of adverse events in first 1000 days from conception. It results in chronic malnutrition and stunting. Conversely a low weight for height or wasting indicates acute malnutrition.
- Weight for age is most commonly used index of nutritional status although is does not differentiate between wasting and stunting.

4. Ans. (d) 5mg%

Ref: Nelson 20th ed. pg. 871

Jaundice in neonates becomes apparent in cephalocaudal progression starting from face and progressing to abdomen and feet. Dermal pressure reveals anatomic progression. Jaundice on face starts at 5 mg/dl.

5. Ans. (d) Subpulmonic stenosis

Ref: Nelson 20th ed. pg. 2212

The major determinant of cyanosis in TOF is subpulmonic stenosis which will decide the amount of blood entering into lungs.

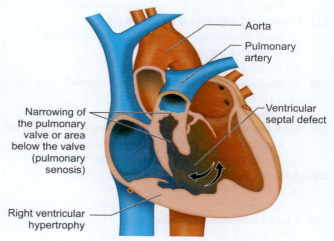

6. Ans. (d) Bronchiolitis

Ref: Nelson 20th ed. pg. 245

- The characteristic feature of bronchiolitis is prolonged expiration due to airway inflammation. It is caused by Respiratory syncytial virus.
- Choice A has presence of Bronchial breathing and crepitations and is ruled out.
- Choice B manifests as hoarseness, a seal-like barking cough, inspiratory stridor, and a variable degree of respiratory distress.
- Choice C has episodic attacks on exposure to allergens.

7. Ans. (a) Ribavarin

Ref: Nelson 20th ed. pg. 1608

Bronchiolitis caused by respiratory syncytial virus is managed with aerosol of Ribavarin. It causes only modest improvement. Hence, humified oxygen is the main stay of treatment. Latest approach is to use palivizumab for prophylaxis in high risk infants.

Pediatrics

Virus	Clinical syndrome	Antiviral agent of choice	Alternative antiviral agents
Influenza A	Treatment	Oseltamivir (> 1yr old)	Rimantadine Amantadine
	Prophylaxis	Oseltamivir (> 1yr old)	Amantadine Rimantadine Zanamivir (> 7 yr old)
Influenza B	Treatment	Oseltamivir	Zanamivir (> 7 yr old)
Respiratory syncytial virus	Bronchiolitis or pneumonia in high-risk host	Oseltamivir Ribavirin aerosol	

8. Ans. (b) Exanthema subitum

Ref: Nelson 20th ed. pg. 1594

- Human herpes-6A, Herpes-6B and HHV7 causes Roseola infantum or exanthema subitum and is called sixth disease.
- The most common cause is primary infection with human herpesvirus 6B.
- The classic presentation of roseola infantum is a 9- to 12-month-old infant who acutely develops a high fever and often a febrile seizure. After 3 days, a rapid defervescence occurs, and a morbilliform rash appears.

> **Extra Mile**

Number	Other names for the disease	Etiology (ies)
First disease	Rubeola, measles, hard measles, 14-day measles, morbilli	Measles virus
Second disease	Scarlet fever, scarlatina	*Streptococcus pyogenes*
Third disease	Rubella, German measles, 3-day measles	Rubella virus
Fourth disease	Filatov-Duke's disease, staphylococcal scalded skin syndrome, Ritter's disease	Some say the disease does not exist. Other believe it is due to *Staphylococcus aureus* strains that make epidermolytic (exfoliative) toxin
Fifth disease	Erythema infectiosum	Erythrovirus (Parvovirus) B19
Sixth disease	Exanthem subitum, roseola infantum, "Sudden Rash", rose rash of infants, 3-day fever	Human herpes virus 6B or human herpes virus 7

9. Ans. (b) Triple

Ref: Nelson 20th ed. pg. 417

Compositions of human colostrum, mature breast milk, and cow's milk (g/L)			
Compositions	**Human colostrum**	**Human breast milk**	**Cow's milk**
Total protein	23	11	31
Immunoglobulins	19	0.1	1
Fat	30	45	38
Lactose	57	71	47
Calcium	0.5	0.3	1.4
Phosphorus	0.16	0.14	0.90
Sodium	0.50	0.15	0.41

FMGE Solutions Screening Examination

NEONATOLOGY

10. Ans. (a) Head

Ref: Op Ghai, 8th ed. pg. 143

Maximum heat loss in neonates occurs from the scalp.

11. Ans. (d) Charcot joints

Ref: Nelson 20th ed. pg. 2050-51

- Congenital syphilis can lead to development of rare hypersensitivity phenomenon like soft tissue gumma.
- Depression of nasal route as a result of syphilitic rhinitis destroying the adjacent bone and cartilage leads to saddle nose.
- Osteochondritis is painful and results in inability to move the involved extremity and is called as pseudo-paralysis of parrot.
- Seen in late congenital syphilis clutton joints are unilateral or bilateral painless joint swelling (usually involving knees) from synovitis with sterile synovial fluid. Spontaneous remission occurs after several weeks.
- Charcot joints are seen in Tabes dorsalis in adult patient of syphilis.

12. Ans. (a) αFP

Ref: Nelson 20th ed. P 2802

- Failure of closure of the neural tube allows excretion of fetal substances (α-fetoprotein [αFP], acetylcholinesterase) into the amniotic fluid, serving as biochemical markers for a NTD.
- Prenatal screening of maternal serum for αFP in the 16th-18th week of gestation is an effective method for identifying pregnancies at risk for fetuses with NTDs in utero.

> **Extra Mile**
> - Inhibin-A is a part of quadruple test for Down syndrome screening.
> - Inhibin-B has negative feedback on FSH.
> - It is used as tumor marker for granulosa cell tumor.

13. Ans. (c) Constricted

Ref: Advanced Pediatric Assessment, By Ellen M. Chiocca; p 320

- Pupil size is measured against a standardized size gauge; the normal range in infants and children is 2–6 mm
- Infants normally have miotic (constricted) pupils. Children normally have larger pupils than infants or adults.

14. Ans. (a) Mother intake of estrogen

Ref: OP Ghai 8th ed. P 135

- Transient breast enlargement in the newborn has been reported in 20% to 30% of newborn babies. It is usually the result of the transplacental transfer of maternal and placental estrogens.
- Engorged breasts should not be squeezed or massaged as it could lead to soreness and infection.

15. Ans. (a) *Klebsiella pneumoniae*

Ref: AIIMS Newborn Protocols

- Data from National Neonatal Perinatal Database 2000 suggests that *Klebsiella pneumoniae* and *Staphylococcus aureus* are the most common causes of neonatal sepsis in India.
- Worldwide, the most common cause is Group B *Streptococcus*
- Neonatal sepsis is the second most common cause of neonatal mortality contributing to 23% of all neonatal deaths.

16. Ans. (a) 5 mg%

Ref: Nelson, 20th ed. pg. 1928

Since the neonate developed Jaundice on day 3 of life it indicates physiological jaundice. It appears when total serum bilirubin exceeds 5 mg% and progresses in cephalo-caudal direction.

Dermal pressure may reveal the anatomic progression of
1. Face = 5 mg/dL
2. Mid-abdomen = 15 mg/dL
3. Soles = 20 mg/dL

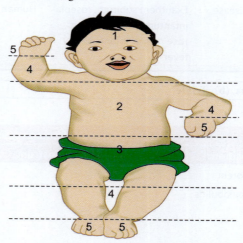

Numbers here indicate progression of Jaundice

- The yellow color usually results from the accumulation of *unconjugated, nonpolar, lipid-soluble bilirubin pigment in the skin.*
- This unconjugated bilirubin is an end product of heme-protein catabolism from a series of enzymatic reactions by heme-oxygenase and biliverdin reductase and non-enzymatic reducing agents in the reticuloendothelial cells

17. Ans. (b) Check chest movement

Ref: 2016 Update on Neonatal Resuscitation by AAP

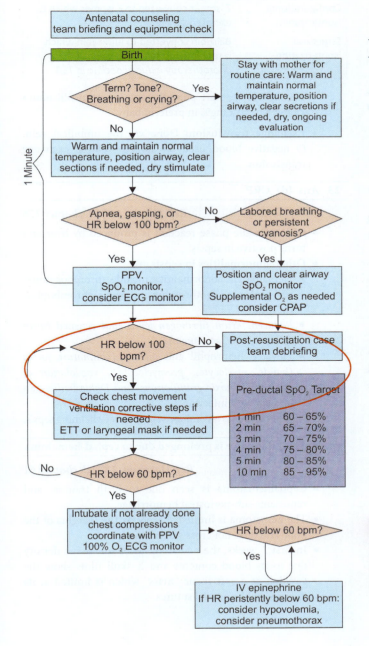

- Since 30 seconds of PPV has already been administered and heart rate is still less than 100/min, check chest movement to take ventilation corrective steps.
- It could be that the face mask used is not of appropriate size or proper seal was not obtained leading to impaired ventilation.
- If the heart rate stabilizes to 100/min and spontaneous respiration is established then continue supplemental oxygen and post resuscitation care should be established.
- It is a must for you to know neonatal resuscitation. So please write down the algorithm and read it one day before the examination. For adult resuscitation protocol refer to the medicine section.

18. Ans. (a) Atopic dermatitis

Ref: Nelson, 20th ed. pg. 1096

- The most common chronic relapsing skin disease seen in infancy and childhood is atopic dermatitis.
- Affects 10–20% of children worldwide
- Frequently occurs in families with asthma, allergic rhinitis, and food allergy.
- "Atopic march." is a term used to define infants with Atopic Dermatitis is predisposed to developing allergic rhinitis and/or asthma later in childhood.

Major Clinical Features of Atopic Dermatitis

Pruritus
Facial and extensor eczema in infants and children
Flexural eczema in adolescents
Chronic or relapsing **dermatitis**
Personal or family history of **atopic** disease

19. Ans. (a) Respiratory rate

Ref: OP Ghai, 8th ed. pg. 126

- **Apgar score:** A numerical expression of condition of new born infant, usually determined at 1 minute and 5 minute after birth.
- Can be remembered as APGAR (Appearance, Pulse rate, Grimace, Activity, RESPIRATORY EFFORT)
- Remember, its NOT respiratory rate you count in APGAR scoring, rather its respiratory effort.

	Score 0	Score 1	Score 2
Appearance	Blue or pale all over	Blue at extremities	Pink all over
Pulse rate	Absent	<100	>100

Contd...

FMGE Solutions Screening Examination

	Score 0	Score 1	Score 2
(Grimace) Reflex irritability	No response	Grimace	Cry or pull away when stimulated
Activity	None	Some flexion	Flexed arms and legs that resist extension
Respiratory effort	Absent	Weak, irregular, gasping	Strong, lusty cry

Total score	: 10
No distress	: 7–10
Mild distress	: 4–6
Severe distress	: 0–3

20. Ans. (c) 3 min

Ref: OP Ghai, 8th ed. pg. 144

HOW TO TAKE ARMPIT (AXILLARY) TEMPERATURES in new born

- Place the tip of the thermometer in a dry armpit.
- Close the armpit by holding the elbow against the **chest for 3 minutes**.
- Remove the thermometer after you hear the signal (usually a series of beeps) and read the temperature on the screen.
- A child has a fever if the armpit temperature is over 99°F (37.2°C). If you're not sure if it is correct, check it by taking a rectal temperature.

21. Ans. (c) Lambdoid suture

Ref: OP Ghai, 8th ed. pg. 41

- Well you can look at the diagram for the logic and memorize the diagram as it will help you in anatomy also.

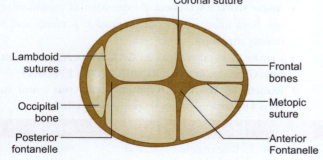

- Lambdoid suture corresponds with posterior fontanelle.

22. Ans. (a) Rh incompatibility

Ref: OP Ghai, 8th ed. pg. 175

- Most common cause of pathological jaundice in children is Rh incompatitbility.
- **Characteristics of pathological jaundice**
  - Appears within first 24 hours of birth
  - Peak values exceed >15 mg%
  - Rate of rise of Serum bilirubin >5 mg/dL/day

Management
Principles of Phototherapy

Configurational isomerization	Z isomer converted to E isomer which is excreted slowly
Structural isomerization	Bilirubin converted to lumirubin which is rapidly excreted and *responsible for phototherapy induced decline in TSB*

- **Phototherapy:** Start phototherapy if serum bilirubin> 15 mg% or >12 mg% in preterm baby.
- **Exchange transfusion:** Done via the umbilical vein. O negative blood used for double volume exchange transfusion.

23. Ans. (d) CRP

Ref: Nelson, 18th ed. chapter 176

- CRP, an acute phase reactant is produced by liver and turns positive in sepsis.
- **Other abnormalities in sepsis are:**
  - Hematologic abnormalities include thrombocytopenia, prolonged prothrombin and partial thromboplastin times,
  - *Reduced serum fibrinogen levels and elevated fibrin split products, and anemia.*
  - Elevated neutrophil and *increased immature forms (bands, myelocytes, promyelocytes), vacuolation of neutrophils, toxic granulations, and Döhle bodies* can be seen with infection.
  - Neutropenia is an ominous sign of overwhelming sepsis.

24. Ans. (a) Jaundice is prolonged due to cephal-hematoma

Ref: Harrison, 18th ed. chapter 61

- Cephalhematoma is seen due to birth trauma, and represents sub-periosteal hemorrhage.
- The hematoma is limited sharply by the margins of the bone and does not cross suture lines.
- In first 2 weeks, the hematoma is of soft tissue density due to its blood contents and X skull films show the swelling as a soft tissue "mass" which is limited at its margins by the cranial sutures.

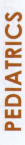

25. Ans. (b) Late congenital syphilis

Ref: OP Ghai, 8th ed. pg. 273

It is a common pattern of presentation for congenital syphilis, and consists of three phenomena *aka Hutchinson triad*:
- Interstitial keratitis
- Hutchinson incisors
- Eighth nerve deafness.

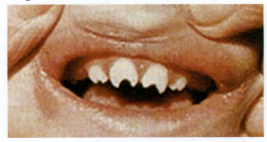

26. Ans. (d) Hydrocephalus

Ref: OP Ghai, 8th ed. pg. 272

The classic Triad for Congenital Rubella Syndrome is:

1. Sensorineural deafness (58% of patients)
2. Eye abnormalities—especially retinopathy, cataract and microphthalmia (43% of patients)
3. Congenital heart disease—especially patent ductus arteriosus (50% of patients)

*"Salt-and-pepper" retinopathy is the most common ocular manifestation of congenital rubella.

Other Manifestations of CRS may Include:

- Spleen, liver or bone marrow problems
- Mental retardation
- Microcephaly^Q
- Eye defects
- Low birth weight
- Thrombocytopenic purpura (presents as a characteristic blueberry muffin rash)^Q
- Hepatomegaly
- Micrognathia

27. Ans. (c) Congenital syphilis

Ref: OP Ghai, 8th ed. pg. 182, 273

Early manifestations of congenital infection vary and involve multiple organ systems.

- About 60% of infants born with congenital syphilis are asymptomatic at birth.
- Symptoms develop within the first 2 months of life. In symptomatic infants, the *most common physical finding, seen in 100% of cases, is hepatomegaly.*
- The other common findings are skeletal abnormalities, rash, and generalized lymphadenopathy.
- Radiographic abnormalities, periostitis or osteitis, involve multiple bones. Sometimes, the lesion is painful and an infant will favor an extremity (pseudopalsy).
- The rash is maculopapular and may involve palms and soles. In contrast to acquired syphilis, a vesicular rash and bullae may develop. These lesions are also highly contagious.
- Mucosal involvement may present as rhinitis ("*snuffles*"). Nasal secretions are highly contagious.
- Hematological abnormalities include anemia and thrombocytopenia.

Late-onset congenital syphilis (diagnosed >2 y)
Manifestations include neurosyphilis and involvement of the teeth, bones, eyes, and the eighth cranial nerve, as follows:

1. Bone involvement - Saber shins^Q, saddle nose
2. Teeth involvement - Notched, peg-shaped incisors (Hutchinson teeth)^Q
3. Pigmentary involvement - Linear scars (rhagades)^Q at the corners of the mouth
4. Interstitial keratitis - Presents in the first or second decade of life
5. Sensory-neural hearing loss (eighth cranial nerve deafness)
6. Classic Hutchinson triad^Q - (1) defective incisors, (2) interstitial keratitis, (3) eighth cranial nerve deafness.

28. Ans. (b) Two weeks

Ref: OP Ghai, 8th ed. pg. 172

- Physiological jaundice is seen in most infants due to elevation of un-conjugated bilirubin concentration during their first week.
- **Term infants** - Jaundice lasts for about 10 days with peak of serum bilirubin up to 15 mg/dL by 3 days of age.
- **Preterm infants** - Jaundice lasts for about two weeks, with a rapid rise of serum bilirubin up to 12 mg/dL.

Mechanisms involved in physiological jaundice are mainly:

- Relatively low activity of the enzyme glucuronosyl transferase^Q
- Shorter life span of fetal red blood cells^Q, being approximately 80 to 100 days in a full term infant, compared to 100 to 120 days in adults.
- Relatively low conversion of bilirubin to urobilinogen by the intestinal flora^Q, resulting in relatively high absorption of bilirubin back into the circulation.

FMGE Solutions Screening Examination

29. Ans. (d) 8-9 hrs
- There is no gas in the abdomen of a new born baby. It takes 8 hours for the air to reach the descending colon and performing the X-ray shall be useful.
- Invertogram in neonates with suspected ano-rectal malformations should be done after 24 hours of life.

30. Ans. (c) Tickle the sole

Ref: Chapter 100: Delivery Room Emergencies: Nelson 18th edn.

Immediately after birth, an infant in need of resuscitation should be placed under a radiant heater and dried (to avoid hypothermia), *positioned head down and slightly extended, the airway cleared by suctioning, and gentle tactile stimulation provided (slapping the foot, rubbing the back)*. Simultaneously, the infant's color, heart rate, and respiratory effort should be assessed

31. Ans. (a) Succimer

Ref: Nelson 20th edn. pg. 3433

Children with blood lead levels >45 µg/dL require 2, 3 Dimercaptosuccinic acid/succimer.

32. Ans. (d) Done for babies with cyanosis

Ref: OP Ghai, 8th ed. pg. 148

- **Kangaroo care** is a technique practiced on newborn, usually preterm, infants wherein the infant is held, skin-to-skin, with an adult.
- The kangaroo position provides ready access to nourishment.
- The parent's stable body temperature helps to regulate the neonate's temperature more smoothly than an incubator, and allows for readily accessible breastfeeding.
- Babies who are eligible for kangaroo care include pre-term infants, weighing less than 1,500 grams, and breathing independently.
- Cardiopulmonary monitoring, oximetry, supplemental oxygen or nasal (continuous positive airway pressure) ventilation, intravenous infusion, and monitor leads do not prevent kangaroo care.
- Babies who are in kangaroo care tend to be less prone to apnea and bradycardia and have stabilization of oxygen needs.

33. Ans. (a) Baby fed with a bottle finding it difficult and confusing to suckle at breast

Ref: OP Ghai, 8th ed. pg. 153

- A problem that may beset a bottlefed baby in which it forgets how to nurse on mother' nipple

- Breastfeeding requires far more vigorous mouth and tongue motions and greater muscle coordination than bottlefeeding.
- On bottle nipples or even pacifiers, a newborn can forget how to nurse properly.
- This confusion can lead to diminished or discontinued nursing. Nipple confusion is usually not a concern after the early weeks, once the baby is nursing well.

34. Ans. (a) Diaphragmatic hernia

Ref: OP Ghai, 8th ed. pg. 129

- In diaphragmatic hernia: Bag and mask will lead to over-distention of the stomach which is already lying in chest cavity. This *will worsen the mediastinal shift and compress the ipsilateral lung further leading to worsening of the patient.*
- Bag and mask ventilation is also not to be done in meconium aspiration syndrome. In choice C, it is written meconium ileus.

35. Ans. (d) Orthopnea

Ref: OP Ghai, 8th ed. pg. 397-98

- Breathing difficulty in children when lying down is a condition in which a child has trouble catching his or her breath or breathing normally when lying down.

Breathing difficulty in children when lying down (pediatric orthopnea) includes:
- Airway obstruction e.g., foreign object
- Chronic obstructive pulmonary disease
- Cystic fibrosis
- Corpulmonale
- Heart failure

Baby feels better when held against shoulders.

36. Ans. (d) β_2 transferrin

- Macrophages in human milk may synthesize complement, lysozyme, and lactoferrin. Breast milk contains lactoferrin, an iron-binding whey protein that is normally saturated with iron and has an inhibitory effect on the growth of *Escherichia coli* in the intestine.
- Further, the lower pH of the stool of breast-fed infants is thought to contribute to the favorable intestinal flora of these infants compared with formula fed infants (more bifidobacteria and lactobacilli; fewer *Escherichia coli*), and this helps protect against infections caused by some species of *E. coli*.

37. Ans. (b) Vasodilation

Ref: Nelson's, 18th ed. Ch: 97.2

Supplemental O_2 helps in vasoconstriction and ductal closure. Both functional and anatomical closure of ductus arteriosus is attributed to increasing O_2 levels. Increased O_2

Pediatrics

is also responsible for neovascularization and development of retinopathy of prematurity.

Oxygen causes tissue injury through the formation of reactive oxygen intermediates and peroxidation of membrane lipids.

---

38. Ans. (b) 8

Ref: OP Ghai, 8th ed. pg. 155

Expressed breast milk can be stored in:
- Room temperature-for 8 hours
- Refrigerator-for 24 hours
- Deep freezer-for 3 months

---

39. Ans. (a) 24 hours later but within 72 hours

Ref: OP Ghai, 8th ed. pg. 172

Presence of any of the following signs denotes that the jaundice is pathological
- Clinical jaundice detected before 24 hours of age
- Rise in serum bilirubin by more than 5 mg/ dL/day
- Serum bilirubin more than 15 mg/dL
- Clinical jaundice persisting beyond 14 days of life
- Clay/white colored stool and/or dark urine staining the clothes yellow.
- Direct bilirubin >2 mg/dL at any time.

Characteristics of Physiological Jaundice
- First appears between 24–72 hours of age
- Maximum intensity seen on 4–5 th day in term and 7th day in preterm neonates.
- Does not exceed 15 mg/dL.
- Clinically undetectable after 14 days.
- No treatment is required but baby should be observed closely for signs of worsening jaundice.

---

40. Ans. (b) Carbohydrate

Ref: OP Ghai, 8th ed. pg. 8–9

- In order to supply the fetus with energy, the pregnant woman increases her hepatic glucose production by 16–30%. The transfer of glucose from the maternal circulation to the fetus takes place by facilitated diffusion involving glucose transporter 1. (GLUT1)
- A considerable part of the trans-placentally transferred glucose is used by the fetal brain. Although enzyme systems that are necessary for glucose production (gluconeogenesis) develop early, the fetus only produces its own glucose under extreme condition such as during maternal starvation.

---

41. Ans. (a) 3:1

Ref: Ghai, 7th ed. pg. 691–2

- Ratio of chest compressions to rescue breaths in neonates is 3:1. In pediatric resuscitation with single rescuer, the ratio is 30:2.
- In resuscitation in adults the ratio is again 30:2 with a single/two rescuers.

Sternum should be compressed to depress approximately *one third to one half of the anteroposterior diameter* of the chest. Chest compression should be delivered providing *equal time in compression and relaxation phases.*

---

42. Ans. (d) Extra pyramidal cerebral palsy

Ref: Ghai, 7th ed. pg. 559-560

Extrapyramidal cerebral palsy is caused by **bilirubin encephalopathy.** It is also associated with deafness.

Clinical Manifestations Include:
- Dyskinesia such as athetosis, choreiform movements, dystonia, tremors and rigidity
- *Early indicator is inability to reach for and grasp a dangling ring by the age of 6 months.*

Types of Cerebral palsy

Spastic cerebral Palsy: Most common type of cerebral palsy. It is of the following subtypes:
Spastic Quadriparesis: More in **term babies**   Spastic Diplegia: More in **preterm babies;** associated with periventricular leukomalacia   Spastic Hemiplegia: recognized after 4-6 months of age
Hypotonic (atonic) cerebral palsy
Extrapyramidal cerebral palsy/athetoid cerebral palsy: Kernicterus

---

43. Ans. (c) Vitamin K

- Vitamin K is produced by our gut flora. The gut of a New-born baby is sterile and hence no vitamin K is being produced.
- Moreover vitamin K is negligible in breast milk. *In lieu of these factors all babies are susceptible to development of Hemorrhagic disease of New-born.*
- To prevent this from happening therefore, as standard operating procedure in all hospitals injection vitamin K_1 1 mg intramuscular is given to prevent hemorrhagic disease of new born.
- In our country where a large number of children are born via home deliveries, no vitamin K would be given to the child and therefore the *child may be brought to the hospital on day 5 with umbilical stump bleeding.*
- For management: the child should be given injection vitamin K 1mg intravenously. If bleeding is still present then FFP needs to be administered.

Explanations

FMGE Solutions Screening Examination

> **Extra Mile**
> - Type of vitamin K used for treatment of H.D.N= vitamin K$_1$
> - Umbilical stump bleeding in child on day 1 of life= factor 13 deficiency
> - Umbilical stump bleeding in child on day 5 of life= H.D.N
> - Male baby with excessive circumcision bleeding= Hemophilia A
> - Vaginal bleeding in a girl child on day 5 of life= No intervention required (occurs due to transplacental transfer of hormones)

44. Ans. (c) AMBU Bag Ventilation for 30 seconds with heart rate of 50

Ref: Nelson, 18th ed. Chapter 100,

- *If the heart rate does not improve after 30 sec with bag and mask (or endotracheal) ventilation and remains below 100/min, ventilation is continued and chest compression should be initiated over the lower third of the sternum* at a rate of 120/min. The ratio of compressions to ventilation is 3:1.
- If the heart rate remains <60 despite effective compressions and ventilation, administration of epinephrine should be considered.
- AAP guidelines are given below.

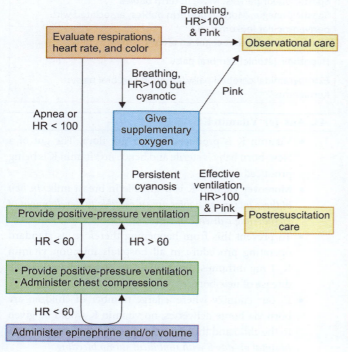

MILESTONES IN CHILDREN

45. Ans. (b) 20–49

Ref: Nelson 20th ed. P 217

IQ range	Classification
140 and over	Genius or near genius
120–140	Very superior intelligence
110–120	Superior intelligence
90–110	Normal or average intelligence
80–90	Dullness
70–80	Borderline deficiency
50–69	Moron
20–49	Imbecile
Below 20	Idiot

TABLE: Identification of cause in children with severe intellectual disability

Cause	Examples	Percent of total
Chromosomal disorder	Trisomies 21, 18, 13 Klinefelter syndrome	~20
Genetic syndrome	Fragile X syndrome Prader-Willi syndrome Rett syndrome	~20
Nonsyndromic autosomal mutations	Variations in copy number, *denovo* mutations in *SYNGAP 1*, *GRIK2*, *TUSC3*	~10
Developmental brain abnormality	Hydrocephalus ± meningomyelocele, lissencephaly	~8
Inborn erros of metabolism or neurodegenerative disorder	PKU, Tay-Sachs	~7
Congenital infections	HIV, toxoplasmosis, rubella, CMV, syphilis, herpes simplex	~3
Perinatal causes	HIE, meningitis, IVH, PVL, fetal alcohol syndrome	4
Postnatal causes	Trauma (abuse), meningitis, hypothyrodism	~4
Unkown	Cerebral palsy	~20

46. Ans. (a) 7 months

Ref: OP Ghai, 8th ed. pg. 49

- Lets evaluate data step wise to arrive at answer.
  1. Baby can sit in tripod position by 5th month.
  2. Bi dextrous approach by 5th month.
  3. Monosyllables by 6th month.
  4. Stranger anxiety by 7th month.

47. Ans. (a) 12 weeks

Ref: OP Ghai, 8th ed. pg. 52

There are Two Types of Smiles for Babies
- The *spontaneous* or almost reflexive smile that can occur early in the newborn period.
- The *social smile* that occurs in response to something, like when you talk or sing to baby
- The social smile is a developmental milestone that infants reach when they are one to two months old.
- Not having a social smile by three months of age is a red flag for child to be evaluated by an expert.

48. Ans. (b) 6 months

Ref: OP Ghai, 8th ed. pg. 142

- **Moro reflex persists until 6 months.** It is sometimes referred to as the startle reflex.
- The Moro reflex is present at birth, peaks in the first month of life, and *completely disappears around 6 months of age.*
- It is likely to occur if the infant's head suddenly shifts position, the temperature changes abruptly, or they are startled by a sudden noise.
- **The legs and head extend while the arms jerk up and out with the palms up and thumbs flexed. Shortly afterward the arms are brought together and the hands clench into fists, and the infant cries loudly.**
- *Bilateral absence* of the reflex may be linked to damage to the infant's central nervous system, while a *unilateral absence* could mean an injury due to birth trauma (e.g., a fractured clavicle or injury to the brachial plexus). Erb's palsy or some other form of paralysis is also sometimes present in such cases.

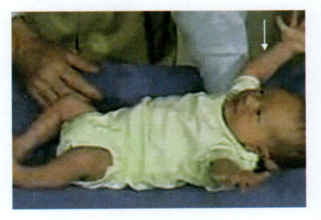

49. Ans. (a) Prematurity

Ref: OP Ghai, 8th ed. pg. 124

- Most common cause of neonatal mortality in India is prematurity (obviously lack of hospital care).
- Metabolic causes like hypoglycemia infant of diabetic mother, can be asked in questions.

50. Ans. (c) 6 Months

Ref: OP Ghai, 8th ed. pg. 154

- Head lag disappears by 3 months
- Head control is achieved by 4 months
- A child in prone position at 3 months can lift chin off the bed, but it takes a while for the shoulder muscles to develop sufficient strength so as to lift the chest and head off the bed. This activity would be possible by 6 months
- Wave bye-bye by 9 months
- Stand without support at 12 months
- Run by 18 months

BREASTFEEDING

51. Ans. (c) Amino acid based formula

Ref: Nelson, 20th ed. pg. 288-89

- Most common cause associated with food intolerance during infancy: **Cow's milk proteins > Soyabean milk**
- Nearly, 50% of children affected by cow's milk protein intolerance develop soy protein intolerance as well if they are fed with soy based formulas.
- Therefore soy-based formulas should not be used for the treatment of cow's milk protein intolerance

Management of Cow Milk Protein Allergy

Exclusively breast fed child	Formula fed child
Maternal exclusion diet avoiding food containing Cow Milk Protein and hen's eggs is advised, since these are excreted in breast milk.	Elimination diet and avoid egg protein The elimination diet should be continued for a minimum of 2 weeks, and up to 4 weeks in cases of atopic dermatitis or allergic colitis.
If *no improvement* start Extensively hydrolyzed formula feed (eHF)	If no improvement, start *amino acid based formula*

- Use complete milk protein hydrolysates in infants who cannot be breastfed. Occasionally, children may develop intolerance toward complete hydrolysated formulas. In these cases, use amino acid–based formulas, which are now widely available and are balanced in trace elements and vitamins.

FMGE Solutions Screening Examination

52. Ans. (b) Baby's lower lip is inverted

Correct Positioning During Breast feeding

1. The *mother should be seated comfortably* in an upright position, so that her breasts fall naturally and she has good support for her back, arms and feet
2. The *infant should be supported* behind the shoulders and facing the mother, with his or her body flexed around the mother's body. The position must be a comfortable drinking position for the infant
3. The chin should be tucked well into the breast, and the infant's *mouth should be wide open*, with the bottom lip curled *back. More areola will be evident above* the *infant's top lip than below the bottom lip*
4. After an initial short burst of sucking, the rhythm will be slow and even, with deep jaw movements that should not cause the mother any discomfort – pauses are a normal part of the feed and they become more frequent as the feed continues

- If the cheeks are being sucked in or there is audible 'clicking', the infant is not attached correctly
- The infant should stop feeding of his or her own accord by coming off the breast spontaneously

53. Ans. (c) Lower areola is more visible than upper

Ref: OP Ghai, 8th ed. pg. 154

Please refer to above explanation.

54. Ans. (d) 6 months

Ref: OP Ghai, 8th ed. pg. 150

- Exclusive breast feeding is up to 6 months and should be continued uptil 2 years.
- Prelacteal feeds like water, honey, and so called health tonics are contraindicated in children less than 6 months of age.

55. Ans. (d) Avidin

Ref: Nelson, 18th ed. Chapter 42

- Human milk contains a variety of cells, including macrophages, T cells, stem cells, and lymphocytes.
- In early lactation, the breastfed infant may consume as many as 10^{10} maternal leukocytes per day.
- About 80% of the cells in early milk are breast milk macrophages, which originate as peripheral blood monocytes that exit the bloodstream and migrate into milk through the mammary epithelium.
- The proteins of human milk are divided into the whey and casein fractions or complexes, with each comprising of a remarkable array of specific proteins and peptides.

- The most abundant proteins are casein, α-lactalbumin, lactoferrin, secretory immunoglobulin IgA, lysozyme, and serum albumin.

56. Ans. (c) Lower lip of infant is inverted

Ref: OP Ghai, 8th ed. pg. 154

- The basic concept is that when the child suckles the breast the lower lip should be EVERTED.

57. Ans. (d) Taurine

Clinical studies have elucidated various mechanisms by which taurine promotes brain development, the main effect being on neurotransmitter production.

In previous year same question was asked with different choices and you need to remember that DHA- Docosa Hexanoic Acid plays an important role in brain myelination in infants. Infact studies have shown that IQ of breast fed baby is higher than that of cow milk fed baby with DHA making all the difference.

GROWTH AND DEVELOPMENT

58. Ans. (b) 16 weeks

Ref: Rudolph Paediatrics, 22nd ed. pg. 183

Must know time line for fetal development

Appearance of fetal pole shadow (USG)	5–6 weeks fertilization
Heart beat (USG)	6–7 weeks
Erythropoiesis	
In liver	6 weeks
In bone marrow	16 weeks
Development of lymphocytes	
In thymus	9 weeks
In lymph nodes	10 weeks
Breathing movement	11–12 weeks
Swallowing reflex	16 weeks
Appearance of meconium	20 weeks
Secretion of urine	End of first trimester

59. Ans. (a) Prematurity

- Prenatal ultrasonography shows no testicular descent before 28 weeks' gestation, other than transabdominal movement to the internal inguinal ring.

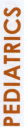

Pediatrics

- Transinguinal migration, thought to be under hormonal control, occurs at 28–40 weeks' gestation, usually resulting in a scrotal testis by the end of a full term of gestation

TABLE: New ballard scoring for determining prematurity

	−1	0	1	2	3	4
Skin	Sticky friable transparent	Gelatinuos red, translucent	Smooth pink, visible veins	Superficial peeling &/or rash. Few veins	Cracking pale areas rare veins	Parchment deep cracking no vessels
Plantar surface	Heel-toe 40-50 mm: −1 < 40 mm: − 2	> 50 mm no crease	Faint red marks	Anterior transverse crease only	Creases ant. 2/3	Creases over entire sole
Breast	Imperceptible	Barely perceptible	Flat areola no bud	Stippled areola 1–2 mm bud	Raised areola 3–4 mm bud	Full areola 5-10 mm bud
Eye/Ear	Lids fused loosely;−1 tightly;−2	Lids open pinna flat stays folded	Slightly Curved pinna; soft; slow recoil	Well-curved pinna; soft but ready recoil	Formed & firm instant recoil	Thick cartilage ear stiff
Genitals Male	Scrotum flat, smooth	Scrotum empty faint rugae	Testes in upper canal	Testes descending few rugae	Tests down good rugae	Testes pendulous deep rugae
Genitals Female	Clitoris prominent labia flat	Prominent clitoris small labia minora	Prominent clitoris enlarging minora	Major & minora equally prominent	Majora large minora small	Majora cover clitoris & minora

60. Ans. (d) 20 teeth

- All 20 teeth (10 in the upper jaw and 10 in the lower jaw) have come in by the time the child is 2 ½ to 3 years old. The complete set of primary teeth is in the mouth from the age of 2 ½ to 3 years of age to 6 to 7 years of age.
  - Basic rule of thumb is that approximately 4 teeth will erupt for every 6 months of life.
  - Lower teeth erupt before upper teeth with teeth in both jaws usually erupting in pairs.
  - Primary teeth are whiter and smaller in color than the permanent teeth that will follow.
  - By the time a child is 2 to 3 years of age, all primary 20 teeth should have erupted.
- Shortly after age 4, the jaw and facial bones of the child begin to grow, creating spaces between the primary teeth.
- Between the ages of 6 and 12, a mixture of both primary teeth and permanent teeth reside in the mouth.

61. Ans. (c) 7 months into scrotum

Ref: OP Ghai, 8th ed. pg. 540

From the 3rd month of pregnancy and its end the testes migrate from the lumbar area to the future scrotum.

This transfer is secondary to

- Combination of growth processes and hormonal influences.

- Gubernaculum testis also plays a decisive role in this phenomenon.

Scrotum is empty at 7 months. The testis descents into inguinal canal at 7 months.

62. Ans. (c) Truancy

- *Pre-school children are classified as children between 2 to 5 years. The usual problems seen are:*

  1. **Temper tantrums** Control is a central issue.
     Tantrums normally appear toward the end of the 1st yr of life and peak in prevalence between 2 and 4 yr of age. Tantrums lasting more than 15 min or regularly occurring more than 3 times/day may reflect underlying medical, emotional, or social problems
  2. Sleep problems
  3. Pica involves repeated or chronic ingestion of non-nutritive substances, which may include plaster, charcoal, clay, wool, ashes, paint, and earth.

- **Truancy is seen in school going children. Truancy and run-away behavior are never** developmentally appropriate. Approximately ½ of school refusal incidents result from child and adolescent behavioral problems; the other ½ of incidents are related to mood and anxiety symptoms. **Often, truancy represents disorganization within the home, developing personality problems, or both.**

FMGE Solutions Screening Examination

63. Ans. (c) Thelarche

Ref: Nelson, 18th ed. Adolescence: chapter 12

IN GIRLS

- The first visible sign of puberty and the hallmark of SMR2 (Sexual maturity rating) is the **appearance of breast buds,** between 8 and 12 yr of age.
- Menses typically begins 2–2½ yr later, during SMR3–4 (median age, 12 yr), around the peak height velocity.

IN BOYS

- *The first visible sign of puberty and the hallmark of SMR2 is testicular enlargement, beginning as early as 9½ yr.* This is followed by penile growth during SMR3. Peak growth occurs when testis volumes reach approximately 9–10 cm³ during SMR4.
- Under the influence of LH and testosterone, the seminiferous tubules, epididymis, seminal vesicles, and prostate enlarge. The left testis normally is lower than the right. Erections are common, and nocturnal emissions may occur. The voice deepens, and linear growth is accelerated.

Also remember: Precocious puberty is defined as the onset of secondary sexual characteristics before 8 year of age in girls and 9 year in boys.

64. Ans. (d) 5 yrs

- OP ghai states enuresis as urinary incontinence beyond the age of 4 years for daytime and 6 years for night-time enuresis.
- It is said to be present if it occurs twice per week for 3 consecutive months.
- *Most of children attain complete bladder control by age of 5 years*
- The prevalence of enuresis is 7% in boys and 3% in girls at age of 5 years and keeps on decreasing for every subsequent year.
- Treatment of choice for nocturnal enuresis is alarm devices with desmopressin nasal spray.

65. Ans. (d) 12 g%

Ref: Nelson, 18th ed. Table 447-1

TABLE: Hematologic values during infancy and childhood

Age	Hemoglobin (G/DL)	
	Mean	Range
Cord blood	16.8	13.7–20.1
2 week	16.5	13.0–20.0
3 month	12.0	9.5–14.5

Contd...

	Hemoglobin (G/DL)	
6 mo-6 year	12.0	10.5–14
7–12 year Adult	13.0	11.0–16.0
Female	14	12.0–16.0
Male	16	14.0–18.0

66. Ans. (d) Behavior modification

Ref: Nelson, 18th ed. Chapter 573

- In children with overactive bladder, urge incontinence, and dysfunctional voiding, voiding at predetermined times aids in retraining the child to exercise voluntary bladder control.
- *Behavioral modification has remained the mainstay of treatment for daytime wetting. These measures focus on relearning and training the normal responses from the bladder and urethra.*
- Bladder irritants such as caffeine should be eliminated from the diet.
- The child voids on waking, and subsequently at least every 2 h, during waking hours. As urgency improves, the interval between voids can be extended. In children with infrequent voiding, in whom an elevated PVR volume is encountered, double voiding will both increase functional bladder capacity and decrease the risk of infection.

67. Ans. (a) Malnutrition

Ref: Nelson, 18th ed. Chapter 45

- **Rickets,** a disease of growing bone, occurs in children due to malnutrition in India. It occurs before fusion of the epiphyses, and is due to un-mineralized matrix at the growth plates.
- Earliest presentation is craniotabes and presentation after 6 months of age is widening of Bilateral wrist joints.

68. Ans. (b) 3 years

Ref: Nelson, 18th ed. Chapter 9

Milestones at 3 years of age
1. Can tell age gender and recall story
2. Rides tricycle
3. Stands momentarily on one foot
4. Makes tower of 10 cubes; imitates construction of "bridge" of 3 cubess
5. Copies circle
6. Imitates cross
7. Plays simple games (in "parallel" with other children)
8. Helps in dressing (unbuttons clothing and puts on shoes)
9. Washes hands

Pediatrics

69. Ans. (d) All of the above

Ref: OP Ghai, 8th ed. pg. 59

- Attention deficit hyperactivity disorder in the (ICD-10) is a psychiatric disorder of the neurodevelopmental type in which there are significant problems of attention, hyperactivity, or acting impulsively that are not appropriate for age.
- *Symptoms must begin by age six to twelve years and persist for more than six months for a diagnosis to be made.* In school-aged individuals inattention symptoms often result in poor school performance

Symptoms

1. Inattention
2. Hyperactivity (restlessness in adults)
3. Disruptive behavior, and
4. Impulsivity, are common in ADHD
   - Academic difficulties are frequent as are problems with relationships. Based on the presenting symptoms ADHD can be divided into three subtypes predominantly inattentive, predominantly hyperactive-impulsive, or combined.

An individual with hyperactivity may have some or all or the following symptoms:

- Fidget and squirm in their seats.
- Talk nonstop.
- Dash around, touching or playing with anything and everything in sight.
- Have trouble sitting sill during dinner, school, doing homework, and story time.
- Be constantly in motion.
- Have difficulty doing quiet tasks or activities.

70. Ans. (d) Shoulder

Ref: Ghai, 8th ed. pg. 6

Skeletal age determination	
Age	X-ray
Newborn	Knee
Infant between 3-9 months	Shoulder
1–13 years	Single film of Hand & Wrist
12–14 years	Elbow & hip

71. Ans. (a) Between incisors

Ref: Shafer's Textbook of Oral Pathology, 6th ed. pg. 46

- Supernumerary tooth or hyperdontia refers to presence of an extra tooth. It can be one or more than one.
- It develops from third tooth bud arising from the dental lamina near the permanent tooth bud or possibly by splitting of permanent tooth bud itself.

- *The most common location is anteriorly between the maxillary incisors*

72. Ans. (b) 5 months

Ref: O.P Ghai, 8th ed. pg. 4

Birth weight doubles at 5 months, triples in an year and is four times at 2 years and becomes 5 times at 3 years.
Note: Newborns lose 10% of body weight in first ten days due to loss of extracellular water, after which they gain 25–30 g/day for first 3 months of life.

73. Ans. (d) 4 years

Ref: O.P Ghai, 8th ed. pg. 5

Time	Length
At birth	50 cm
3 months	60 cm
9 months	75 cm
2 years	90 cm
41/2 years	100 cm

Indian children gain 5 cm height every year until 10 years of age.

74. Ans. (b) 6 years

Ref: Nelson, 18th ed. Ch 8

75. Ans. (c) 100 words

Ref: Nelson's, 18th ed. ch: 32.2

76. Ans. (c) 5 years

Ref: Nelson's, 18th ed ch: 9

77. Ans. (d) Walk short distance

Ref: Nelson, 18th ed. chapter 10

Hide and seek game Do not confuse with peak a boo	Not mentioned but by my experience >3 years
Write alphabet	6 years
Say short sentence	2 years
Walk short distance	18 months

78. Ans. (d) Social smile at 3 months

79. Ans. (c) Hb = 12 g/dL

Ref: OP Ghai, 8th ed /298

Hemoglobin levels below 12 g/dL in children from 6 months to 6 years and below 13 g/dL in older children is suggestive of anemia.

FMGE Solutions Screening Examination

80. Ans. (b)   2.5–3 years

Ref: OP Ghai, 8th ed. pg. 52 Table 3.3

By the age of three years a child can tell his/her age and gender. They can recall experiences for example - a child ate my lunch in the play school

Extra Mile
- Child can draw a circle by the age of = 3 years
- Autism diagnosis in children can be made by age of = 3 years
- ADHD diagnosis in children by the age of = 6 years
- Nocturnal enuresis cut off age = 6 years

81. Ans. (d)   Increase in testicular size

Please refer explanation of question 40

82. Ans. (c)   4 years

Ref: OP Ghai 8th ed./13

- Length of Indian baby at birth = 50 cm
- Length at 1 year = 75 cm
- Length at 4½ years = 100 cm
- Subsequently 5–6 cm/year
- Pubertal growth spurt = 6–8 cm/year

PROTEIN ENERGY MALNUTRITION

83. Ans. (d)   Edema

Ref: OP Ghai 8th ed. P 99

- Kwashiorkor usually affects children aged 1–4 years.
- The main sign is *pitting edema*, usually starting in the legs and feet and spreading, in more advanced cases, to the hands and face.
- Because of edema, children with Kwashiorkor may look healthy because of which their parents view them as well fed.

84. Ans. (c)   Marasmus

Ref: Nelson 20th ed. P 2802

- Individuals with *marasmus* appear cachectic and wasted due to long-term deficits of all nutrients, especially energy and protein.
- In marasmus, the normal *adaptive* response to uncomplicated *starvation* is to utilize body energy stores while preserving lean body mass, leading to a wasted appearance.

85. Ans. (b)   SLC39A4

Ref: Nelson, 20th ed. pg. 3238-3239

- The image shows rash at peri-oral area, groin and spreading to involve the inguinal folds and genitals. This is seen in acro-dermatitis entero-hepatica and occurs due defect in the gene *SLC39A4*.
- The SLC39A4 gene encodes a transmembrane protein that is part of the zinc/iron-regulated transporter–like protein (ZIP) family *required for zinc uptake.*
- This protein is expressed in the enterocytes in the duodenum and jejunum and the patient will have a *decreased ability to absorb zinc from dietary sources.*

86. Ans. (b)   Height/age

Ref: Nelson's Pediatrics, 18th ed. Ch 43

The nutritional indices commonly calculated for young children are:

- **Weight for height** – an index used to measure wasting or acute malnutrition; (WHAM)
- **Height for age** – an index used to measure stunting or chronic malnutrition; (HA-CM)
- **Weight for age** – an index used to measure underweight (or wasting and stunting combined). (WASW)
- **Mid arm circumference** is a specific indicator of wasting or acute malnutrition.

Remember:
- Weight reflects only present health status of the child, whereas height indicates events in the past also
- Most sensitive measure of physical growth- WEIGHT
- Single best parameter for assessment of physical growth- WEIGHT

87. Ans. (a)   Weight/height

Please refer to above explanation.

88. Ans. (a)   Wt.kg/Ht.m²

Ref: Nelson, 18th ed. chapter 44

Also note that the way we diagnose obesity in children is different from adults

BMI percentile for age	Weight status
<5th percentile	Underweight
5th–84th percentile	Normal weight
85th–94th percentile	At risk for overweight
≥95th percentile	Overweight

The obesity guidelines for adults are

BMI (kg/m²)	Weight status
<18.5	Underweight
18.5–24.9	Normal weight

Contd...

Pediatrics

BMI (kg/m²)	Weight status
25–29.9	Obesity
30–39.9	Obese
40–49.9	Morbid obesity
≥50	Super morbid obesity

89. Ans. (b) <1500 g

Ref: OP Ghai, 8th ed. pg. 125

- Normal birth weight - 2800 g- 3000 g
- Low birth weight (LBW) - <2500 g
- Very low birth weight (VLBW) - <1500 g
- Extremely low birth weight (ELBW) - <1000 g.

90. Ans. (a) <1000 g

Ref: OP Ghai, 8th ed. pg. 125

Refer to above explanation

91. Ans. (a) 12.5 cm

Ref: OP Ghai, 8th ed. pg. 97

- Mid arm circumference is measured by a Field instrument → Shakir's tape
- Among age group: 1–5 yrs
- <12.5 cm shows severe malnutrition

92. Ans. (b) <2

Ref: Rudolph Pediatrics, 22th ed. pg. 191

Ponderal index = Weight in grams/ (Length of baby in cm)³ multiplied by 100

- Value is less than 2 = Asymetrical IUGR
- Value is normal in Symmetrical IUGR
- Asymmetrical IUGR is more common. In asymmetrical IUGR, there is restriction of weight followed by length. The head continues to grow at normal or near-normal rates (head sparing). This is a protective mechanism that may have evolved to promote brain development. This type of IUGR is most commonly caused by extrinsic factors that affect the fetus at later gestational ages.
- Symmetrical IUGR is less common and is more worrisome. This type of IUGR usually begins early in gestation. Since most neurons are developed by the 18th week of gestation, the fetus with symmetrical IUGR is more likely to have permanent neurological sequelae.

93. Ans. (c) Scurvy

Ref: OP Ghai, 8th ed. pg. 120

Features of Scurvy:
- Frog leg appearance[Q]

- Bone pain
- Myalgias may occur because of reduced carnitine production.
- Skin changes with roughness, easy bruising and petechiae, gum swelling & bleeding, loosening of teeth, poor wound healing.

94. Ans. (a) Kwashiorkor

Ref: Nelson's Pedia, 19th ed. Ch 670

KWASHIORKOR

Disease occurs due to decreased protein and caloric intake.

Clinical Features are:

- **Hypoalbuminemia:** Which leads to pedal edema. This pedal oedema can mask weight loss.
- **Hepatomegaly:** Hallmark feature of kwashiorkor
- **Skin:** Sun-exposed skin is relatively spared, as are the feet and dorsal aspects of the hands;
- **Hair and Nail:** Nails are thin and soft, and hair is sparse, thin, and depigmented, sometimes displaying a **flag sign** of alternating light and dark bands that reflect alternating periods of adequate and inadequate nutrition.
- Apathy[Q]
- Lack of appetite[Q]
  - **Pellagra** presents with edema, erythema, and *burning of sun-exposed skin on the face, neck, and dorsal aspects of the hands, forearms, and feet.*
  - **Scurvy** presents initially with follicular hyperkeratosis and *coiling of hair.* Perifollicular erythema and hemorrhage, swollen, erythematous gums; stomatitis; Subperiosteal hematomas lead to frog leg appearance (Pseudo-paralysis)

95. Ans. (b) Hepatomegaly

Ref: OP Ghai, 8th ed. pg. 99

- **Marasmus** is characterized by failure to gain weight and irritability, followed by weight loss and listlessness until emaciation results. *The skin loses turgor and becomes wrinkled and loose as subcutaneous fat disappears. Loss of fat* from the sucking pads of the cheeks often occurs late in the course of the disease. The infant's face gives *wizened old man's look.*
- *The abdomen may be distended or flat,* with the intestinal pattern readily visible. There is muscle atrophy and resultant hypotonia.
- **Kwashiorkor** is characterized by development of pedal edema which can mask weight loss. Dietary protein deficiency leads to brain damage and apathy, and/or irritability. *When advanced, there is lack of growth, lack*

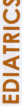

of stamina, loss of muscle tissue, increased susceptibility to infections, vomiting, diarrhea, anorexia, flabby subcutaneous tissues, and edema.. It is often present in internal organs before it is recognized in the face and limbs.
- Hepatomegaly due to fatty liver is seen with flag sign on hair and skin showing flaky paint dermatosis.

96. Ans: (a) Increase appetite

Ref: OP Ghai, 8th ed. pg. 99

- Kwashiorkor is protein and calorie deficiency and hence the serum albumin of the child is very low. This causes the child to develop pedal edema and generalized anasarca later.
- Since the child is not eating proteins, essential amino acids like phenylalanine is deficient and therefore the child forms less of melanin. *This results in hair of the child being reddish in color. This color change of hair strand is seen as FLAG sign.*
- The children with kwashiorkor have a FATTY liver and thereby a hepatomegaly.
- Apathy means lack of interest in surroundings and therefore this child is not interested in playing with the mother or toys. This occurs due to brain damage secondary to chronic protein deprivation.
- **Note:** *Increased appetite can be seen in patients with Marasmus.*

97. Ans. (c) 15,000 mcg

Ref: OP Ghai, 8th ed. pg. 113

- 1mcg of vitamin D = 400 I.U.
- For treatment of rickets, cholecalciferol can be given in a single-day dose of 15,000 mcg (600,000 U), which is usually divided into 4 or 6 oral doses. An intramuscular injection is also available.
- An alternative regimen is to give 125–250 mcg (5000-10,000 U) daily for 2–3 months until healing is well established and the alkaline phosphatase concentration is approaching the reference range.

98. Ans. (a) Pseudoparalysis

Ref: OP Ghai, 8th ed. pg. 113

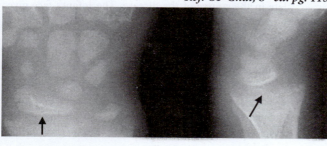

- Note the distal end of radius on the left and ulna on right. Even without experience you can notice that distal end has fraying. Mentally visualize a paint brush. The distal end of bone is widened (SPLAYED).
- **Rickets due to deficiency of calcium and vitamin D will have delayed dentition which is defined as (ZERO TEETH AT >13 months of age.**
- The widening of wrist joint is seen usually beyond 6 months of age when the child starts crawling and creeping and weight of body fall on distal radius.
- Double medial malleolus
- Bowing of legs (GENU VARUM) and knock knees (GENU VALGUM) is seen.
- Pigeon chest with rachitic rosary *(non tender).*

99. Ans. (b) Aldolase-B

Ref: OP Ghai, 8th ed. pg. 696

- Hereditary fructose intolerance, or the presence of fructose in the blood (fructosemia), is caused by a deficiency of aldolase B, the second enzyme involved in the metabolism of fructose. This enzyme deficiency results in an accumulation of fructose-1-phosphate, which inhibits the production of glucose and results in diminished regeneration of adenosine triphosphate. Clinically, patients with hereditary fructose intolerance are much more severely affected than those with essential fructosuria, with elevated uric acid, growth abnormalities and can result in coma if untreated.

Remember and Don't Confuse with:
- *Essential fructosuria caused by a deficiency of the enzyme hepatic fructokinase* is a clinically benign condition characterized by the incomplete metabolism of fructose in the liver, leading to its excretion in urine.

100. Ans. (d) Decreased height for age

Ref: Nelson, 18th ed. Chapter 14

- Height for age is used for chronic malnutrition which leads to Stunting. The term "stunting" is used to describe a condition in which children fail to gain sufficient height, given their age.
- In acute malnutrition the best parameter used is weight for height.

101. Ans. (d) Apathy

Ref: Nelson, 18th ed. Chapter 43

- **Marasmus** is characterized by weight loss and listlessness until emaciation results :MONKEY FACIES
- The skin loses turgor and becomes wrinkled and loose as subcutaneous fat disappears from buttocks leading to BAGGY PANTS appearance.

Pediatrics

- Loss of fat from the sucking pads of the cheeks often occurs late in the course of the disease; thus, the infant's face may retain a relatively normal appearance compared with the rest of the body.
- *These children are irritable and have a voracious appetite. Apathy is a feature of kwashiorkor.*
- The abdomen has muscle wasting leading to pot belly with the intestinal pattern readily visible.

PEDIATRIC NEUROLOGY

102. Ans. (b) Malignant tumor in children

Ref: OP Ghai 8th ed. P 571

Medulloblastoma

- These are midline cerebellar tumors and occur in infancy.
- They are fast growing and malignant.
- Craniospinal spread along neuraxis is common and death occurs early.

103. Ans. (b) Spinal dysraphism

Ref: Nelson, 20th ed. pg. 2802-2803

- Elevated amniotic fluid acetylcholinesterase is used for diagnosis of neural tube defects which are also called spinal dysraphism.
- *Tests for antenatal diagnosis of spina bifida occulta.*
  - Antenatal USG showing Frog sign
  - Amniotic fluid acetylcholinesterase

104. Ans. (b) Acetylcholinesterase

Ref: Nelson, 20th ed. pg. 2802-2803

Refer to the explanation of the question above.

105. Ans. (a) Spina bifida occulta

Ref: Nelson, 20th ed. pg. 2802-2803

- Most common neural tube defect is Spina bifida occulta.
- Most severe neural tube defect is Cranioraschisis totalis
- Best prognosis and maximum viability (survival chances) is seen with Spina bifida occulta
- If spina bifida occulta is not in choices then answer is Meningocele.

106. Ans. (b) Rubeola

Ref: Rudolph Paediatrics, pg. 2186

This disease is a complication of measles virus called rubeola. Features of SSPE

- Slowly progressive disease characterized by seizures and progressive deterioration of cognitive and motor functions, with death occurring 5–15 years after measles virus infection.

- SSPE most often develops in persons infected with measles virus at <2 years of age.
- Investigation of choice is antibody to measles virus in CSF
- EEG shows sharp wave complexes called as Rademacher's complex.
- DOC is inosine prabonex.

107. Ans. (c) Meningomyelocele

Ref: Nelson's, 18th ed. Ch 592

- **Myelomeningocele** is a type of spina bifida in which the spinal canal does not close before birth.
- A **meningocele** is formed when the meninges herniate through a defect in the posterior vertebral arches. The spinal cord is usually normal and assumes a normal position in the spinal canal.
- In Meningocele, just the membranes extend through, *while in Myelomeningocele, the spinal cord also pushes through the hole within the sac that the meninges makes by extending through the opening.*

108. Ans. (b) Mostly Hereditary in nature

Ref: Nelson's, 18th ed. Ch 592.11

- Hydrocephalus is not a specific disease; rather, it represents a diverse group of conditions that result from impaired circulation and absorption of CSF
- Congenital hydrocephalus implies hydrocephalus is present at birth. Most common cause of congenital hydrocephalus is aqueductal stenosis.

Other Causes of Congenital Hydrocephalus can be

- Dandy Walker syndrome
- Arnold chiari malformation
- Toxoplasmosis
- CMV

Clinical Manifestation

1. An accelerated rate of enlargement of the head is the most prominent sign.
2. *The anterior fontanelle is wide open and bulging, and the scalp veins are dilated.*
3. *The forehead is broad*, and the eyes may deviate downward because of impingement of the dilated suprapineal recess on the tectum, producing the *setting-sun eye sign.*

109. Ans. (c) Typical Simple Febrile fits

Ref: OP Ghai, 8th ed. pg. 556-57

Typical febrile seizures are the most common type of seizures in children. For management intermittent prophylaxis with oral diazepam is required. For atypical febrile seizures continuous prophylaxis is recommended.

FMGE Solutions Screening Examination

110. Ans. (a) BERA

Ref: OP Ghai, 8th ed. pg. 619; Oski's Pediatrics

Due to high incidence of deafness post H. influenzae meningitis, BERA should be done.

111. Ans. (d) Enterovirus

- **Meningo-encephalitis is caused by:**
  - Enterovirus (Commonest cause)
  - Coxsackie virus, echo virus – spread is mainly by mouth to mouth transmission
  - Flavi-Virus – West Nile virus, Japanese B Encephalitis
  - Herpes virus
  - Measles and mumps

112. Ans. (c) Carbamezapine

Ref: Nelson's, 18th ed. ch: 593.3

Rolandic epilepsy or Benign Epilepsy of Childhood with Centro-temporal Spike is one of the epilepsy syndromes of childhood with a good prognosis.

- It occurs in children aged 2–14 years and EEG shows centro-temporal spikes
- The disorder occurs in children with positive family history of epilepsy. The seizures usually manifest as
  - Partial seizures with somatosensory symptoms are often confined to the face.
  - Oropharyngeal symptoms include tonic contractions, guttural noises, dysphagia, and excessive salivation
- Consciousness may or may not be impaired, and the partial seizure may proceed to secondary generalization
- Carbamazepine is the preferred drug, which is continued for at least 2 years or until 14–16 year of age

113. Ans. (c) Decreased Intracranial pressure

Ref: OP Ghai, 8th ed. pg. 111-112

- Manifestations of **acute toxicity** include muscle and bone tenderness, especially over the long bones of the upper and lower extremities, as well as neurologic manifestations with signs of increased intracranial pressure (eg, children may have bulging fontanelles).
- Manifestations of **chronic toxicity** include the following: Alopecia/xeroderma with itchy skin/Skin erythema/Skin desquamation/itching/Brittle nails/Exanthema/Cheilitis/Petechiae/Premature epiphysial closure in children/Hepato-splenomegaly/Peripheral neuritis/Benign intracranial hypertension.

> **Extra Mile**
> - Pseudotumor cerebri/benign intracranial hypertension = vitamin A toxicity
> - Earliest sign of vitamin A deficiency = Conjunctival xerosis
> - Treatment of vitamin A deficiency = vitamin A orally 2 LAC IU on day 0,1 and day 14.

GENETICS

114. Ans. (a) 21

Ref: O.P Ghai 8th Ed. P 420

- Down syndrome is the most common chromosomal disorder, occurring with a frequency of 1:800 to 1:1000 newborns.
- Chromosome number 21 is present in triplicate, the origin of the extra chromosome 21 being maternal (due to maternal meiotic non disjunction).

115. Ans. (b) Low

Ref: Rudolph Paediatrics, 22nd ed. pg. 1415

Aneuploidies	AFP	Estriol	hCG	Inhibin A
Down's syndrome	Low	Low	High	High
Turner's syndrome	Decreased	Decreased	Very high	Very high
Edward's syndrome	Unchanged	Low	Very low	Unchanged
Patau's syndrome	Increased	Normal	Normal	Normal

116. Ans. (b) Edward syndrome

Ref: Nelson, 20th ed. pg. 611

Syndrome	Description
Down syndrome	Trisomy 21
Edward syndrome	Trisomy 18
Patau syndrome	Trisomy 13 *Patau syndrome is the least common and most severe of the viable autosomal trisomies. Median survival is fewer than 3 days.*
Turner syndrome	45 XO

117. Ans. (a) Noonan syndrome

Ref: Nelson, 20th ed. pg. 2747-48

NOONAN SYNDROME

- The term is applicable to males and females with normal karyotypes who have certain phenotypic features that occur also in females with Turner syndrome.
- Inheritance pattern is *Autosomal dominant* with variable expression.

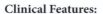

Pediatrics

Clinical Features:
1. Hypertelorism, epicanthus, *downward slanted palpebral fissures known as antimongoloid facies.*
2. Short stature, webbing of the neck
3. Pectus carinatum or pectus excavatum
4. Cubitus valgus
5. The cardiac defect is most often *pulmonary valvular stenosis*, hypertrophic cardiomyopathy, or atrial septal defect.

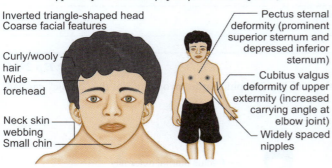

118. Ans. (c) Inhibin

Ref: Nelson, 18th ed. pg. Ch. 95

- Triple test can screen trisomy 21. (Diagnostic sensitivity 70%)
- In addition to Down syndrome, the triple and quadruple tests screen for fetal trisomy 18 also known as Edward's syndrome, open neural tube defects, and may also detect an increased risk of Turner syndrome, trisomy 16 mosaicism, fetal death, Smith-Lemli-Opitz syndrome, and steroid sulfatase deficiency

> **Extra Mile**
>
> **Quadruple test incorporates the above parameters and Inhibin A**
> - High LEVELS are seen in Trisomy 21.
> - Low levels are seen in Trisomy 18.
> - Variable levels in Trisomy 13 (Patau syndrome)

Triple test parameters	Alpha feto protein	Unconjugated Estriol	Beta HCG
Down syndrome	Low	Low	High
Edward syndrome	Low	Low	Low
Neural tube defects Omphalocele, multiple gestation	High	Not applicable	Not applicable

119. Ans. (c) Umbilical hernia

Ref: OP Ghai, 8th ed. pg. 638

- Brachycephaly implies small skull, due to premature fusion of the coronal suture. Therefore the brain is not able to grow and results in mental retardation.
- Overall the most common cause of mental retardation is idiopathic > Down syndrome.
- Thyroid abnormalities in form of either thyroid agenesis or autoimmune thyroditis are seen in Down syndrome.
- Eye findings of down syndrome have also been asked and should be remembered as *(MEBB)*
  1. Mongoloid slant of eyes
  2. Epicanthal folds
  3. Blue dot cataract
  4. Brushfield spots in the iris

Clinical features of Down syndrome
- Flattened facies and low set ears
- Mental retardation
- Single transverse palmar crease and atypical finger prints
- Clinodactyly
- Hypotonia
- Brachycephaly
- Congenital heart disease (ASD): Endocardial cushion defect
- Macroglossia
- Epicanthix fold
- Strabismus
- Brushfield spots (Iris)

120. Ans. (c) Increased Umbilical blood flow

Ref: OP Ghai, 8th ed. pg. 639

- Best way for prenatal diagnosis of Down syndrome is Chorionic villus sampling. However antenatal ultrasound features are:
  - Reduced length of femur and humerus
  - Nuchal fold translucency >2.5 mm
  - Congenital heart disease like ASD, VSD.

121. Ans. (d) Acetylcholine esterase

Ref: OP Ghai, 8th ed. pg. 575-76

- NTD *(anencephaly, open spina bifida or meningomyelocele, and encephalocele)* are a heterogeneous group of congenital malformations resulting from a failure of fusion of the neural tube.
- When a NTD is suspected based upon maternal serum alpha-fetoprotein (AFP) screening results or diagnosed via ultrasound, analysis of AFP and acetylcholinesterase (AChE) in amniotic fluid are useful diagnostic tools.

FMGE Solutions Screening Examination

- AChE is primarily active in the central nervous system with small amounts of enzyme found in erythrocytes, skeletal muscle, and fetal serum.
- *Normal amniotic fluid does not contain AChE, unless contributed by the fetus as a result of an open NTD.*

122. Ans. (d) Anencephaly

Ref: Nelson, 18th ed. pg. Ch. 592.6

- Anencephaly is absence of cranial vault posteriorly with brain and meninges exposed. This condition can be detected by antenatal USG as early as 11–12 weeks. The USG sign is called as *frog eye sign*.

PEDIATRIC CARDIOLOGY

123. Ans. (a) Pulmonic stenosis

Ref: Nelson 21st/E p 2995

Pulmonary stenosis, with or without dysplastic pulmonary valve and hypertrophic cardiomyopathy, are the "classic" cardiac defects reported in Noonan syndrome.

Features of Noonan Syndrome

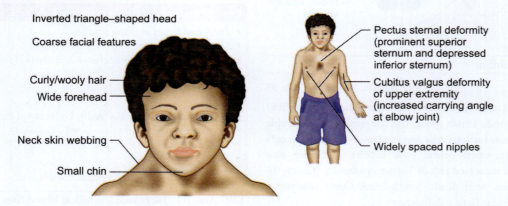

124. Ans. (a) Patent ductus arteriosus

Ref: Op ghai 8th ed page 417

- Continuous murmur is heard in PDA due to huge pressure difference between aorta and pulmonary artery. It is heard both in systole and diastole and peaks at S2.
  Causes of Continuous Murmurs
  1. Patent ductus arteriosus
  2. Coronary arteriovenous
  3. Ruptured sinus of Valsalva aneurysm
  4. Aortic-pulmonary window
  5. Anomalous left coronary artery origin from pulmonary artery
  6. Coarctation of aorta
  7. Pulmonary artery atresia
  8. Truncus arteriosus
  9. Pulmonary artery stenosis
  10. Systemic arteriovenous fistula
  11. Pulmonary arteriovenous fistula
  12. Mammary souffle
  13. Venous hum

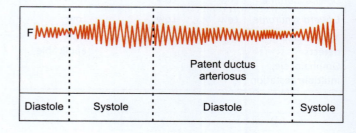

125. Ans. (b) **ASD**

Ref: OP Ghai 8th ed. P 420

Classic Tetrad of TOF
1. Severe right ventricle outflow obstruction due to sub-pulmonic stenosis
2. Large VSD
3. Over-Riding of aorta
4. Right ventricular hypertrophy.

> **Extra Mile**
> - Major determinant of central cyanosis in TOF is sub-pulmonic stenosis.
> - IOC for TOF is T.T.E
> - DOC for TOF is Alprostadil
> - Palliative surgery for TOF is Blalock Taussig shunt.

126. Ans. (c) **Left lower sternal border**

Ref: Nelson 20th ed. P 2169

- Many murmurs in children are *not associated* with significant hemodynamic abnormalities. They are called "innocent" murmurs.
- The most common innocent murmur is a medium-pitched, vibratory or "musical," relatively short *systolic ejection murmur*, which is heard best along the left lower and midsternal border and has no significant radiation to the apex, base or back.

127. Ans. (a) **TOF**

Ref: Nelson 20th ed. pg. 2212-2213

- Tetralogy of Fallot is the most common cyanotic heart disease and will have the maximum viability out of the structural defects given in the choices. *After successful total correction, patients are generally asymptomatic and are able to lead unrestricted lives.*
- TGA will present with cyanosis on day 0 and will result in death due to mixing of two circulations unless atrial septostomy is done followed by switch operation. Without treatment, the prognosis is poor; most patients succumb in the 1st year of life because of heart failure, hypoxemia, and pulmonary hypertension.
- Tricuspid atresia with pulmonic atresia will lead to cyanosis on day 0 and has bad prognosis.
- TAPVC will cause overloading of right side of heart with obstructive flow in infra-cardiac variety. It again has a bad prognosis.

128. Ans. (d) **Normal Cardiothoracic ratio**

Ref: Nelson 20th ed. pg. 2212-2213

Tetralogy of Fallot has
1. Sub-pulmonic stenosis (Ejection Systolic murmur)
2. VSD (Right to Left Shunting)
3. Concentric right ventricular hypertrophy
4. Over- riding aorta

Due to right ventricular hypertrophy the chances of RVF is unlikely. On CXR boot shaped heart is seen with normal CT ratio.

> **Extra Mile**
> - Most common cause of cyanosis with normal sized heart is TOF.
> - Most common cause of cyanosis with left sided enlargement of heart is tricuspid atresia.

129. Ans. (a) **Foramen Ovale**

Ref: Langman Embryology, pg. 47

Key Functional Changes after Birth

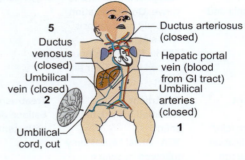

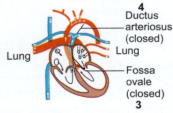

1. & 2 Umbilical cord clamped (Closure of Umbilical arteries and vein)
3. Foramen ovale closed
4. Ductus arteriosus closed
5. Ductus venosus closed

130. Ans. (b) **Membranous VSD**

Ref: Nelson, 20th ed. pg. 2194-95

VSD is the most common cardiac malformation and accounts for 25% of congenital heart disease. Defects may occur in any portion of the ventricular septum, but most are of the membranous type.

FMGE Solutions Screening Examination

Types of VSD
- Membranous
- Muscular VSD or Swiss cheese type multiple defects
- Supra-cristal VSD

Types of ASD
- Ostium secondum (most common type)
- Ostium primum (associated with Down Syndrome)
- Sinus venous variety (associated with Partial anomalous venous connection)

131. Ans. (c) PDA

Ref: Nelson, 18th ed. Chapter 426

Acyanotic heart disease	Cyanotic heart disease	Obstructive heart disease
PDA VSD ASD	TOF Tricuspid atresia Transposition of great arteries	Coarctation of aorta
Presents with recurrent pneumonia and congestive heart failure	Presents with cyanosis. Tet spells and failure to thrive. On examination the child has cyanosis with single S2. CXR in TOF shows Boot shaped heart/ Coer en sabot	Presents with hypertension
Treatment PDA = Indomethacin/ surgical ligation VSD = Dacron patch ASD = Occlusion device	Treatment Modified Blalock taussig shunt TGA= Atrial Septostomy followed by switch operation	Treatment Balloon dilation with stenting

132. Ans. (d) Pericardial tamponade

Ref: Nelson, 18th ed./ Ch. 165

Cardiac Manifestations of Kawasaki Disease
- Coronary artery aneurysms develop in up to 25% of untreated patients in the 2nd-3rd wk of illness and are best detected by two-dimensional echocardiography.
- Myocarditis, manifested as tachycardia out of proportion to fever occurs in at least 50% of patients
- Valvular regurgitation: Mitral and Aortic regurgitation have been associated with Kawasaki disease in both early and chronic phase of the disease.
- Pericarditis with a small pericardial effusion is common during the acute illness.
- Giant coronary artery aneurysms (>8 mm internal diameter) pose greatest risk for rupture, thrombosis or stenosis, and myocardial infarction.

133. Ans. (b) Kawasaki Disease

Ref: OP Ghai, 8th ed. pg. 631

134. Ans. (d) LA

Ref: OP Ghai, 8th ed. pg. 413

- Ostium primum ASDs commonly present with a cleft in the anterior leaflet of the mitral valve. This is sometimes termed a partial AV canal defect or a partial AV septal defect.
- Due to cleft in mitral valve, the LV decompresses into LA leading to overloading of left atrium. In contrast in O. Secundum ASD it is right atrium and right ventricular that develop overloading.

GASTROINTESTINAL TRACT

135. Ans. (c) Hypertrophic pyloric stenosis

Ref: Nelson, 20th ed. pg. 1787

Ileal atresia	Presents as bilious vomiting and triple bubble sign on X-ray Abdomen.
Duodenal atresia	Presents as bilious vomiting and double bubble appearance on X-Ray abdomen
Hypertrophic pyloric stenosis	The presentation is after 2 weeks of life in usually a first born boy baby. The child presents with non-bilious vomiting.
Trachea-esophageal fistula	Presents with choking after feeds with failure to thrive. Drooling of saliva in neonates indicates esophageal atresia.

136. Ans. (b) 10 mg

Ref: Nelson, 20th ed. pg. 1872-73

Zinc supplementation is given at a dose of 2RDA per day (20 mg per day for >6 months and 10 mg per day for younger than 6 months) for 14 days is effective in reducing severity of diarrhea as well as duration of episode.

137. Ans. (c) Trauma

Ref: Nelson's Pedia, 18th ed. Ch. 340

- The list of illnesses that can mimic acute appendicitis includes: 1. Gastroenteritis; 2. Mesenteric adenitis; 3. Meckel diverticulitis; 4. Inflammatory bowel disease; 5. Pneumonia; 6. Cholecystitis; 7. Urinary tract infection; 8. Infectious enteritis; 9. Testicular torsion.

138. Ans. (a) Zinc

Ref: OP Ghai, 8th ed. pg. 121

- The World Health Organization (WHO) and UNICEF *recommend daily 20 mg zinc supplements for 10–14*

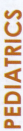

Pediatrics

days for children with acute diarrhea, and 10 mg per day for infants under six months old, to curtail the severity of the episode and prevent further occurrences in the ensuing -two to three months, thereby decreasing the morbidity considerably.

- One out of every five children who die of diarrhea worldwide is an Indian. Daily around 1,000 children die of diarrhea in India, which means 41 children lose their lives every hour.

139. Ans: (d) Ultrasound

Ref: Nelson, 18th ed. pg. Ch. 326.1

ULTRASONOGRAPHY

- *The criterion standard imaging technique for diagnosing HPS*
- *Muscle wall thickness 3 mm* or greater and *pyloric channel length 14 mm* or greater *are considered abnormal* in infants younger than 30 days.

BARIUM UPPER GI STUDY

- Effective when Ultrasonography is not diagnostic.
- Should demonstrate an elongated pylorus with antral indentation from the hypertrophied muscle.
- May show the "double track" sign when thin tracks of barium are compressed between thickened pyloric mucosa or the "shoulder" sign when barium collects in the dilated pre-pyloric antrum.
- Serum electrolytes should be measured to document adequacy of fluid resuscitation and correction of electrolyte imbalances before surgical repair.
- The definitive treatment of pyloric stenosis is with surgical pyloromyotomy known as Ramstedt's procedure
- It is done by simple incision of about 3-4 cm which leads to relaxation of pyloric muscles and hence gastric outlet opens up.

The classic biochemical abnormality seen in case of HPS is hypochloremic, hypokalemic metabolic alkalosis with paradoxical aciduria.

140. Ans. (c) Erythromycin

- Exposure to erythromycin between 3 and 13 days of life is associated with an eightfold risk of infantile hypertrophic pyloric stenosis (IHPS) developing shortly thereafter, according to the results of a retrospective cohort study published in the July, 2015 issue of the Archives of Pediatric and Adolescent Medicine.

> **Extra Mile**

Perinatal drug exposure	Teratogenic effect
Lithium	Ebstein anomaly
Vitamin D3	William syndrome (supravalvular aortic stenosis)
Thalidomide	Phocomelia
Erythromycin	Infantile hypertrophic pyloric stenosis
Carbimazole/ methimazole	Aplastic cutis congenital
Warfarin	Nasal hypoplasia and phalangeal defects
Steroids	Cleft lip and palate

141. Ans. (b) Duodenal atresia

Ref: Nelson, 18th ed. pg. Ch. 327.1

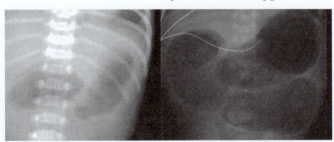

Look at the two X-rays. The left one shows double bubble appearance of duodenal atresia and the right one shows triple bubble sign of jejuno-ileal atresia.

142. Ans. (d) Pyloric stenosis

Ref: Nelson, 18th ed. pg. Ch. 326.1

- All babies REGURGITATE curdled milk. So the mother is instructed to always put the baby to shoulder after breast feeding the child as this shall help the child burp and expel the swallowed air.
- However if a male infant, first born, 2-3 weeks old is brought to your clinic with recurrent vomiting which is non-bilious and associated with failure to gain weight, then suspect-HYPERTROHPIC PYLORIC STENOSIS
- A lump may be palpable to gentle examination in the epigastrium with finding of visible peristalsis. The investigation of choice shall be USG abdomen. Surgery to be done shall be a pyloromyotomy (Ramstedt operation).

FMGE Solutions Screening Examination

> **Extra Mile**
> - **Hypokalemic hypochloremic metabolic alkalosis** is seen in = Hypertrophic pyloric stenosis
> - **Hyperkalemic hyperchloremic metabolic acidosis** is seen in = Uretero-sigmoidostomy
> - MC cause of hematochezia in a preterm neonate = Necrotizing Enterocolitis
> - MC cause of hematochezia in children= Rectal Prolapse> Meckel's Diverticulum
> - Double bubble sign= duodenal atresia
> - Inverto-gram(Special X-ray of the baby in inverted position) isused for = Ano-rectal malformations

143. Ans. (b) Alkaline urine

Ref: Lippincott's, 4th ed. pg. 85

LACTOSE INTOLERANCE/ LACTASE DEFICIENCY

The classic example of osmotic diarrhea is lactose intolerance due to lactase enzyme deficiency. *The colonic bacteria ferment the non-absorbed lactose to short-chain organic acids, generating an osmotic load and causing water to be secreted into the lumen.*
- Lactose is by far the most commonly Mal-absorbed carbohydrate.
- Secondary lactose intolerance follows small bowel mucosal damage (celiac disease, rotavirus infection) and is usually transient, improving with mucosal healing.
- Lactase deficiency can be diagnosed by hydrogen breath test or by measurement of mucosal lactase concentration with small bowel biopsy
- *Confirmatory diagnosis is made by stool acidity test, undigested lactose creates lactic acid that can be detected in stool sample.*
- Undigested lactose may get absorbed and eliminated in urine (Lactoseuria), hence acidic urine.
- In lactose intolerance reducing substance will be positive by Benedict's test in urine.
- Diagnostic testing is not mandatory and often simple dietary changes that produce symptom relief. Eliminate lactose from the diet result in symptom relief
- *Treatment* of lactase deficiency *consists of a milk-free diet.*

144. Ans. (b) Non reducing sugar in urine

Ref: Lippincott's, 4th ed. pg. 85

Refer to above explanation.

145. Ans. (a) Doudenal Atresia

Ref: Bailey and love 24th ed., /1199,

- The hallmark of duodenal obstruction is **bilious vomiting** without abdominal distention, which is usually noted on the 1st day of life.

- A history of **polyhydramnios** is present in half the pregnancies and is caused by a failure of absorption of amniotic fluid in the distal intestine.
- The diagnosis is suggested by the presence of a "**double-bubble sign**" on plain abdominal radiographs. *The appearance is caused by a distended and gas-filled stomach and proximal duodenum*

146. Ans. (b) K+

Ref: Sabiston, 18th ed. /Ch .71

- Hypertrophic pyloric stenosis presents with *hypokalemic, hypochloremic metabolic alkalosis with paradoxical aciduria.*
- Treatment includes replacement of the volume deficit with isotonic saline and then potassium replacement once adequate urine output is achieved.
- For most infants, administration of fluid containing 5% dextrose and 0.45% saline with **2 to 4 mEq/kg of added potassium at a rate of approximately 150 to 175 mL/kg for 24 hours** will correct the underlying deficit. After resuscitation, a Fredet-Ramstedt pyloromyotomy is performed
- Fluid resuscitation with correction of electrolyte abnormalities and metabolic alkalosis is essential before induction of general anesthesia for operation.

147. Ans. (c) 100–200 mL

Ref: OP Ghai, 6th ed. pg. 273

PLAN A

Home Based Treatment of Dehydration

Age	Amount of ORS to give after each loose stool or other culturally appropriate ORT fluids	Amount of ORS to provide for use at home
< 2 years	50–100 mL	500 mL/day
2–10 years	100–200 mL	1000 mL/day
>10 years	As much as desired	2000 mL/day

FLUID & ELECTROLYTE BALANCE

148. Ans. (b) 800 mL

Ref: OP Ghai, 8th ed. pg. 73, 293

The fluid requirement of children less than 10 kg is *100 mL per kg of body weight.* The preffered fluid shall be N/5 in 5% dextrose with added potassium for daily requirements.

Pediatrics

149. Ans. (c) 75 mmol/L

Ingredient	g/L	Mmol/L
Sodium chloride	2.6g	75
Anhydrous glucose	13.6	75
Potassium chloride	1.5	20
Trisodium citrate	2.9	10

The low osmolality ORS has osmolality of 245 mOsm.

150. Ans. (a) Very severe pneumonia

Ref: OP Ghai, 8th ed. pg. 294

- The clinical presentation of severely malnourished child with fast breathing will be classified as very severe pneumonia
- Integrated management of childhood illness encompasses a holistic approach towards a sick child where criteria based diagnosis is made and treatment initiated as per the protocol.
- The primary criteria for diagnosis of pneumonia are based on respiratory rate and the age of child

Age of child	Pneumonia diagnosed if respiratory rate is
Less than 2 months	>60 breaths/min
2–12 months	>50 breaths/min
>1–5 yrs	>40 breaths/min

The disease is Classified as Very Severe if any of the Following is Present

- Cyanosis
- Inability to drink or breast feed
- Seizures/encephalopathy
- *PEM grade 4*

The disease is Classified as Severe Pneumonia in presence of

- Chest in-drawing
- Sub-costal and or intercostals recessions
- Use of accessory muscles of respiration like nasal flaring/sterno-mastoid prominent

151. Ans. (b) 800 mL

Ref: Harrison 18th ed., Chapter 54: Deficit therapy

- For correction of severe dehydration, the fluid requirement the formula = 100 mL/Kg
- The total fluid required in 8 kg child would be therefore 800 mL
- The initial fluid here would be given at a rate of 30 mL/kg = 240 mL given over 1 hour.
- The remainder fluid here would be given at a rate of 70 ml/kg = 560 mL over 5 hours.

152. Ans. (b) 3.5 g/dL

All the following criteria must be met for diagnosis of mild malnutrition

- Patient is 20% below usual weight or significant history of weight loss documented
- Serum albumin < 3.4 g/dL

153. Ans. (b) 30 mL in 30 min

Ref: Nelson's Pediatrics, 18th ed. Ch. 54

MILD DEHYDRATION

- **In infant:** <5% of body weight is dehydrated
- **In older child or adult:** <3% of body weight is dehydrated.
- Normal or increased pulse; decreased urine output; thirsty; normal physical findings

MODERATE DEHYDRATION

- **In infant:** 5–10% of body weight is dehydrated
- **In older child or adult:** 3–6% of body weight is dehydrated.
- Tachycardia; *little or no urine output;* irritable/lethargic; *sunken eyes and fontanel;* decreased tears; dry mucous membranes; mild delay in elasticity (skin turgor); *delayed capillary refill (>1.5 sec).*

SEVERE DEHYDRATION

- **In infant:** >10% of body weight is dehydrated
- **In older child or adult:** >6% of body weight is dehydrated.
- Rapid and weak or absent peripheral pulses; decreased blood pressure; *no urine output; very sunken eyes and fontanel; no tears*; parched mucous membranes; delayed elasticity *(poor skin turgor);* **very delayed capillary refill (>3 sec)**; cold and mottled; limp, depressed consciousness.
- *For a child > 1 yr - 30 mL/kg is given in 1/2 hour and 70 mL/kg is given in 2½ hour (total over 3 hours).*

FMGE Solutions Screening Examination

Treatment for Severe Dehydration

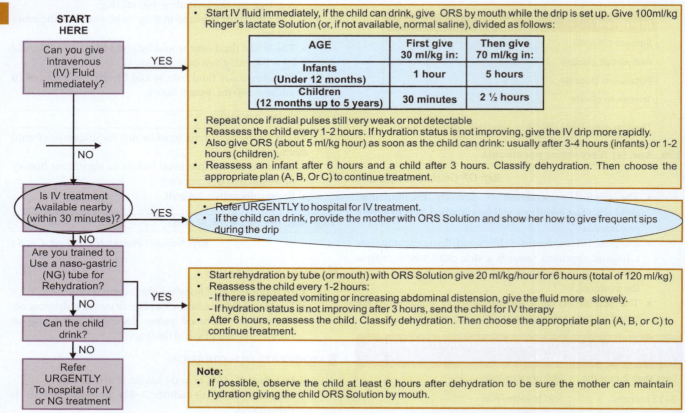

154. Ans. (b) Tibia

Ref: Nelson's, 18" ed./ ch. 66

- If venous access is not available in an arrest situation within 1 min, an intraosseous line should be placed in the anterior tibia (with care taken to avoid traversing the epiphyseal plate)
- The needle should penetrate the anterior layer of compact bone, with its tip advanced into the spongy interior of the bone.
- Intraosseous needles are special rigid, large-bore needles that resemble those used for marrow aspiration. Current recommendations urge the use of intraosseous cannulation in patients for whom intravenous access proves difficult or unattainable, even in older children.
- Once the patient has received initial drug and fluid therapy through the IO line, every effort should be made to obtain more conventional central venous access and remove the IO line as soon as possible.
- Alternative sites for intraosseous (IO) insertion include **the distal tibia, distal femur, sternum, and humerus**

Complications of IO Infusion

1. Extravasation of fluid is the most common complication and occurs when a needle is misplaced
2. Compartment syndrome is a risk with IO insertion.
3. Extravasation of hypertonic or caustic medications, such as sodium bicarbonate, dopamine, or calcium chloride, can result in necrosis of the muscle.
4. Infection and osteomyelitis are relatively rare complications and occur most commonly if aseptic technique is not followed during insertion.
5. Other possible complications include local hematoma, pain, fracture and growth plate injuries (with incorrect placement), and fat microemboli and compartment syndrome

155. Ans. (b) Na 75 mEq + 245 mOsm

Ref: OP Ghai, 8th ed. pg. 294

The concentration of sodium in low osmolality ORS is 75 mEq. The osmolality is 245 mOsm.

Pediatrics

849

Extra Mile

- WHO recommends a special ORS formulation, known as **ReSoMal**, for management of diarrhoea in **severely malnourished children** that contains a lower amount of sodium (45mmol/L) and higher amount of potassium (40 mmol/L) than the standard WHO-ORS.

VACCINES

156. (d) 15 weeks

Ref: IAP 2016 Guidelines

ROTAVIRUS (RV) VACCINES

Routine Vaccination

- Minimum age: 6 weeks for all available brands (RV-1) [Rotarix], RV-5 [RotaTeq] and RV-116E [Rotavac])
- Only two doses of RV-1 are recommended
- RV1 should preferably be employed in 10 and 14 week schedule.
- If any dose in series was RV-5 or RV-116E or vaccine product is unknown for any dose in the series, a total of 3 doses of RV vaccine should be administered.

Catch-up vaccination

- **The maximum age for the first dose in the series is 14 weeks, 6 days**
- Vaccination *should not be initiated for infants aged 15 weeks, 0 days or older*
- The maximum age for the final dose in the series is 8 months, 0 days

157. Ans. (a) DPT

Ref: OP Ghai, 8th ed. pg. 193

- Since all live vaccines are contraindicated in immune-compromised patients hence only DPT can be given. *Please note that the question mentions an AIDS positive patient and "not a child born to HIV positive mother".*
- If a child is born to HIV positive mother, the child may or may-not be acquire HIV infection from the mother. Hence WHO recommends BCG should be given to a baby born to HIV positive lady. *Textbook clearly mentions that if baby has documented AIDS then live vaccines are contraindicated. In such cases I.P.V. can be given in place of O.P.V.*

158. Ans. (b) Dukoral

*Ref: Nelson, 18th ed chapter 173, http://wwwnc.cdc/gov/
eid/article/17/11 11-0822 article*

- Dukoral is indicated for active immunization against disease caused by *Vibrio cholerae*s ero group O1 in adults and children from 2 years of age who will be visiting endemic/epidemic areas
- The standard primary course of vaccination with Dukoral against cholera consists of 2 doses for adults and children from 6 years of age. Children 2 to below 6 years of age should receive 3 doses. Doses are to be administered at intervals of at least one week. If more than 6 weeks have elapsed between doses, the primary immunization course should be re-started.
- Immunization should be completed at least 1 week prior to potential exposure to *V. cholerae* O1.

159. Ans. (b) BCG

Ref: OP Ghai, 8th ed. pg. 191

BCG

- Although BCG vaccination often causes local reactions, serious or long-term complications are rare. *Reactions that can be expected after vaccination include moderate axillary or cervical lymphadenopathy and induration and subsequent pustule formation at the injection site*; these reactions can persist for as long as 3 months after vaccination.
- Most serious complication of BCG vaccination is disseminated BCG infection.
- The most frequent disseminated infection is BCG osteomyelitis

KIDNEY

160. Ans. (b) Congenital Finnish type nephrotic syndrome

Ref: Nelson, 18th ed./ Table 527.1

- Congenital nephrotic syndrome is one of the Finnish heritage diseases and rare form of nephrotic syndrome.
- It occurs predominantly in families of Finnish origin and manifests shortly after birth
- The condition is caused by a defect in the protein nephrin, which is found in the kidney.
- Gene responsible is NPHS 1.

161. Ans. (b) Hyperparathyroidism

Renal Tubular acidosis	RTA 1 can present with Nephrocalcinosis and renal rickets but pathological fractures and psychiatric symptoms are not seen
Hyperparathy-roidism	The increased bone resorption explains pathological fracture. Hypercalcemia leads to deposition of calcium in the kidney parenchyma. Psychiatric symptoms are seen in hyperparathyroidism.

Contd...

Explanations

FMGE Solutions Screening Examination

Polycystic kidneys	Presents with CRF with cystic kidneys
CRF	Can have pathological fracture due to Osteitis Cystica Fibrosa due to secondary Hyperparathyroidism.

162. Ans. (a) 4-8 years

Henoch schonlein purpura is the most common type of vasculitis in children and presents at 4–8 years of age. IgA is incriminated in pathogenesis of HSP. The commonest presentation is extensor purpura.

RESPIRATORY SYSTEM

163. Ans. (c) >40/min RR, for 12–60 months

Ref: OP Ghai 8th ed. P 381

As per WHO clinical classification of acute lower respiratory infection, pneumonia is defined as:

Increased respiratory rate:	
<2 months old	>60 per minute
2–12 months old	>50 per minute
12–60 months old	>40 per minute

164. Ans. (b) Rhinovirus

Ref: Harrison, 18th ed. chapter 186, Nelson, 18th ed. chapter 376

The most common pathogens associated with the common cold are the rhinoviruses.
In contrast bronchiolitis is caused by RSV.

Pathogens Associated with the Common Cold

Association	Pathogen	Relative Frequency
Agents primarily associated with colds	Rhinoviruses Coronaviruses	Frequent Occasional
Agents primarily associated with other clinical syndromes that also cause common cold symptoms	Respiratory syncytial viruses *(MC cause of bronchiolitis)*	Occasional
	Influenza viruses	Occasional
	Parainfluenza viruses	Uncommon
	Adenoviruses	Uncommon
	Enteroviruses	Uncommon

INBORN ERRORS OF METABOLISM

165. Ans. (b) Phenylketonuria

Ref: Nelson, 18th ed. chapter 85.1, Harrison's 17th ed. Ch 358

Clinical Manifestations of Classic Phenylketonuria

- The affected infant is normal at birth.
- Mental retardation may develop gradually and may not be evident for the 1st few months.
- Vomiting, sometimes severe enough to be misdiagnosed as pyloric stenosis, may be an early symptom.
- Older untreated children become hyperactive, with purposeless movements, rhythmic rocking, and Athetosis.
- Infants are lighter in their complexion than unaffected siblings with blonde hair.
- These children have an unpleasant odor of Phenyl-acetic acid, which has been described as musty or mousey.
- Most infants are hypertonic with hyperactive deep tendon reflexes.
- Microcephaly, prominent maxilla with widely spaced teeth, enamel hypoplasia, and growth retardation are other common findings in untreated children.

ENDOCRINOLOGY

166. Ans. (a) Adrenalectomy

Ref: Nelson, 18th ed. / Ch. 578

Nelson syndrome is seen post adrenalectomy. The rise of ACTH post-operatively leads to hyper pigmentation of palm, sole creases.

MISCELLANEOUS

167. Ans. (a) Coxsackie A

Ref: OP Ghai 8th ed. P 219

- Hand-foot-mouth disease is a common viral illness primarily affecting children below 5 years of age.
- The most common causes of hand foot mouth disease are Coxsackie virus A16 and enterovirus 71.

168. Ans. (a) Torsion of appendix of testis

Ref: Nelson, 20th ed. pg. 2595-96

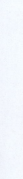

Pediatrics

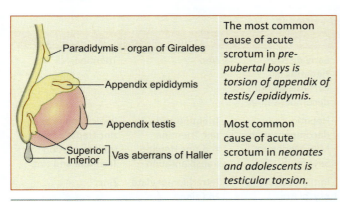

	The most common cause of acute scrotum in *pre-pubertal boys is torsion of appendix of testis/ epididymis.*
	Most common cause of acute scrotum in *neonates and adolescents is testicular torsion.*

Drug	Pediatric dose in mg/kg	Side effect	MAX adult dose
INH	*15 mg /kg thrice weekly, under RNCTP 20-30 mg twice weekly dosages*	Peripheral neuritis	300 mg
Rifampicin	15 mg/kg	Hepatitis	600 mg
Pyrazinamide	30–35	Gout	2000 mg
Ethambutol	20–25	Optic neuritis	1500 mg

Please note that the values for INH and rifampicin under the revised programme are equal.

169. Ans. (d) Rubeola

Ref: Nelson, 20th ed. pg. 1544

- The clinical presentation given is of measles (Aka Rubeola) and is characterised by rash on face, neck and spreading to rest of the body.
- Chicken pox rash appears on extremities and is maculo-papulo-vesicular. The rash is red but has vesicles which are not given in the clinical presentation above.
- Rubella presents as measles but has posterior cervical lymphadenopathy.
- Variola is the small pox virus and the vaccine for small pox is made from a virus called *vaccinia*.

170. Ans. (a) Erythema infectiosum

- Erythema infectiosum (also known as fifth disease) is usually a benign childhood condition characterized by a *classic slapped-cheek appearance* and lacy exanthem.
- It results from infection with human parvovirus (PV) B19, an erythrovirus

171. Ans. (c) Mild proteinuria, high hematuria, high ASO titre

Ref: OP Ghai, 8th ed. pg. 474-75

- Glomerulo-nephritis is characterized by inflammation of glomerulus leading to hematuria with sub-nephrotic proteinuria. The inflammation follows a skin infection or a sore throat and therefore requires serological evidence in form of elevated ASO titer or anti DNA-ase-B.

172. Ans. (c) Zinc deficiency

Ref: Pediatric Dermatology, 3rd ed. pg. 1137

- Zinc toxicity can cause zinc shakes especially after inhalation of zinc following welding of galvanized metals.
- Zinc deficiency is known as acrodermatitis enterohepatica

173. Ans. (c) 15 mg/kg

Ref: OP Ghai, 8th ed. pg. Table 10.9

174. Ans. (a) Albright's syndrome

Ref: Nelson, 18th ed. Ch. 563

McCune Albright syndrome is suspected when two of the three following features are present:

1. Endocrine hyperfunction such as precocious puberty
2. Polyostotic fibrous dysplasia
3. Unilateral Cafe-au-lait spots

175. Ans. (c) Headlight in Fog appearance

Ref: Nelson, 18th ed.,: Table 244-1

Headlight in fog appearance is seen in Toxoplasmosis

Cardiovascular	PDA Pulmonary artery stenosis VSD (ASD is not seen)
Central nervous system	Parenchymal necrosis Vasculitis with calcification Chronic meningitis
Eye	Microphthalmia Cataract Iritis Ciliary body necrosis Glaucoma Salt and Pepper Retinopathy[Q]
Ear	Cochlear damage Endothelial necrosis

176. Ans. (b) Exchange transfusion

Ref: OP Ghai 8th ed./176

- *Supportive therapy is very important in falciparum malaria and includes red blood cell transfusion(s) to maintain the hematocrit above 20%, exchange transfusion in life-threatening P. falciparum malaria with parasitemia>5%.*
- Supplemental oxygen and ventilatory support is required for pulmonary edema or cerebral malaria.

FMGE Solutions Screening Examination

- Careful intravenous rehydration for severe malaria, intravenous glucose for hypoglycemia, anticonvulsants for cerebral malaria with seizures and dialysis for renal failure. *Corticosteroids are no longer recommended for cerebral malaria.*

177. Ans. (b) 1–4 years

Ref: Park, 22nd ed pg. 178

178. Ans. (a) 5 mL/kg

Ref: Nelson's, 18th ed. ch: 101.4

- During mechanical ventilation of newborns, it has been found out that large tidal volumes can lead to lung injury; therefore small tidal volumes are recommended.
- In a healthy newborn tidal volume of 5–8 mL/kg may be used, however in a newborn with ARDS, a tidal volume of 4–6 mL/kg is recommended.
- PEEP levels of 4-6 cm H_2O are usually safe and effective

179. Ans. (a) Hemolytic anemia

Ref: OP Ghai, 8th ed. pg. 320

- Hemolytic anemia is a feature of Wilson's disease. Hemolytic anemia occurs because large amounts of copper derived from hepatocellular necrosis are released into the bloodstream.
- Wilson disease is an *autosomal recessive* trait caused by mutations in the *ATP7B gene in chromosome 13*
- ATP7B protein deficiency impairs biliary copper excretion, resulting in copper toxicity affecting the liver and brain
- Hepatic features: may present as hepatitis, cirrhosis or as hepatic decompensation
- Most common Neurological feature in Wilson is dysarthria followed by dystonia

Investigations

1. Serum Ceruloplasmin is decreased. Serum ceruloplasmin should not be used for definitive diagnosis, because they are normal in up to 10% of affected patients.
2. 24-hour urine copper excretion – increased: Screening test
3. Hepatic copper content – Increased
4. Liver biopsy:
    - Gold standard test for Wilson's disease
    - Liver copper >**200 microgram/gram** dry weight of liver is suggestive of Wilson's disease.
    - Copper stain — Rhodamine stain

Treatment

Disease status	First choice	Second choice
Early disease Hepatitis or cirrhosis without decompensation	Zinc	Trientine
Hepatic decompensation: Mild Moderate Severe	Trientine and zinc Trientine and zinc Hepatic transplantation	Penicillamine and zinc Hepatic transplantation Trientine and zinc
Initial neurologic/psychiatric	Tetrathiomolydate and zinc	Zinc
Maintenance	Zinc	Trientine
Pediatric	Zinc	Trientine
Pregnant	Zinc	Trientine

Prognostic index of Nazer is used to asses severity of Wilson's disease

- Parameters: Bilirubin, AST, Prothrombin time

180. Ans. (d) Rashes

Ref: OP Ghai, 8th ed. pg. 632-633

HENOCH-SCHONLEIN PURPURA

- Most common cause of non-thrombocytopenic purpura in children
- **Age group:** 4–7 years. However, the disease may also be seen in infants and adults. Males > Females.
- Etiology is unknown, but typically follows an upper respiratory tract infection and is associated with increased IagA levels.

Clinical Features

1. In pediatric patients, *palpable extensor purpura is seen in virtually all patients.*
2. Damage to cutaneous vessels also results in local angioedema, which may precede the palpable purpura.
3. Polyarthralgias
4. GI involvement is characterized by colicky abdominal pain usually associated with nausea, vomiting, diarrhea or constipation and is frequently associated with passage of blood and mucus per rectum.

Renal involvement is characterized by mild glomerulo-nephritis leading to proteinuria and microscopic hematuria.

181. Ans. (a) Count 10 pennies

Ref: Nelson Textbook of Pediatrics, table 9.1

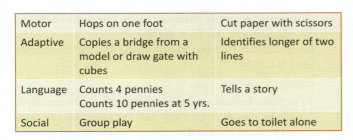
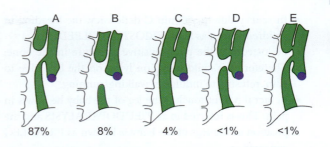

Motor	Hops on one foot	Cut paper with scissors
Adaptive	Copies a bridge from a model or draw gate with cubes	Identifies longer of two lines
Language	Counts 4 pennies Counts 10 pennies at 5 yrs.	Tells a story
Social	Group play	Goes to toilet alone

182. Ans. (c) Thyroid dysgenesis

Ref: OP Ghai, 8th ed. pg. 516

- Most cases of congenital hypothyroidism are not hereditary and result from thyroid dysgenesis.
- Some cases may be familial, usually caused by one of the inborn errors of thyroid hormone synthesis, and may be associated with Goiter.
- In many cases, the deficiency of thyroid hormone is severe, and symptoms develop in the early weeks of life. In others, lesser degrees of deficiency occur, and manifestations may be delayed for months.
- The prevalence of congenital hypothyroidism based on nationwide programs for neonatal screening is 1/4,000 infants worldwide

183. Ans. (a) Proximal end blind, distal end communicating with trachea

Ref: Nelson chapter 316, Congenital Anomalies of Esophagus

- Esophageal atresia (EA) is the most frequent congenital anomaly of the esophagus, affecting ≈1/4,000 neonates. Of these, >90% have an associated tracheoesophageal fistula (TEF).
- In the *most common form of EA*, the upper esophagus ends in a blind pouch and the TEF is connected to the distal esophagus.
- The inability to pass a nasogastric or orogastric tube in the newborn is suggestive of esophageal atresia.

TEF can be detected by

1. *Plain radiography* in the evaluation of respiratory distress may reveal a coiled feeding tube in the esophageal pouch and/or an air-distended stomach.
2. Pure EA may present as an *airless, scaphoid abdomen*.
3. *Esophagogram* with contrast medium injected under pressure may demonstrate the defect.
4. The orifice may be detected at *bronchoscopy* or when methylene blue dye injected into the endotracheal tube during endoscopy is observed in the esophagus during forced inspiration

184. Ans. (b) Measles

Ref: T Singh, 2nd pg. 148-9

Lymphocytosis is defined as *more than 45% lymphocytes* in the peripheral blood. Examples include:
1. TB, brucellosis, syphilis
2. CLL, NHL with spillover
3. Infectious mononucleosis
4. Mumps, **measles**, chicken pox
5. Toxoplasmosis
6. Viral infections

Diphtheria, MI and pneumonia cause neutrophilia.

185. Ans. (c) HIV ELISA

Ref: OP Ghai, 8th ed. pg. 234

The question tests your elementary knowledge of the fact that IgG class of antibody present in the body of the infected mother can be passively transmitted to the baby. These antibodies are detected by ELISA test and will test positive in every baby born to HIV positive lady. This does not mean that the baby has mother's infection but only acquired antibodies.

The transmission of infection from mother to child is best detected by DNA PCR. We can determine the viral load in the baby through the same test. Viral culture would tell you regarding viral load and changes after HAART. The p 24 antigen was done routinely till DNA PCR was available.

> **Extra Mile**
>
> - Peri-natal transmission rate for HIV = 30%
> - Best drug to reduce Perinatal transmission rate for HIV= nevirapine single dose to mother and baby
> - By how much % does the Perinatal transmission rate for HIV reduce after nevirapine = 50% reduction.
> - BCG is indicated in baby born to HIV lady but if the question asks whether BCG/live vaccine should be given to a child with AIDS then the answer is NO.

186. Ans. (b) Scurvy

Ref: OP Ghai, 8th ed. pg. 120

FMGE Solutions Screening Examination

- In scurvy due to vitamin C deficiency, the bleeding in children is seen as SUBPERIOSTEAL BLEEDING.
- Periosteum is the pain sensitive structure in the bone. Therefore the child keeps on lying on the bed, due to pain, refusing to indulge in walking/running.
- In fact if parent touches the leg of the baby he howls in pain. This is referred to as PSEUDOPARALYSIS and the position of the legs of the baby is known as FROG LEG appearance.
- The usual clinical history given shall be a 1 year old child from poor family, exclusively breastfed at 1 year of age, no complimentary feeds given is brought to the hospital with complaints on irritability and cannot bear weight on standing. Always get an X-ray knee joint (unlike X-ray WRIST joint in rickets)

> **Extra Mile**
> - X-ray knee in scurvy shows damage at = Metaphyseal end as compared to epiphyseal end in rickets.
> - X-ray knee in scurvy shows findings as = Pelkan spur, Wimberger Ring and white line of Frankel
> - Wimberger line is seen in syphilis

187. Ans. (c) Zinc

Ref: OP Ghai, 8th ed. pg. 121

Autosomal recessive disorder caused by an inability to absorb sufficient zinc from the diet.
Genetic defect is in the intestinal zinc specific transporter gene SLC39A4.

Clinical Manifestations
1. Vesiculo-bullous, eczematous, dry, scaly, or psoriasiform skin lesions symmetrically distributed in the *peri-oral*, and *perineal areas* and on the *cheeks*, knees, and elbows.
2. The hair often has a peculiar reddish tint
3. Ocular manifestations include photophobia, conjunctivitis, blepharitis, and corneal dystrophy
4. Chronic diarrhea, stomatitis, glossitis, nail dystrophy, growth retardation
5. Delayed wound healing
6. Lymphocyte function and free radical scavenging are impaired.

> **Extra Mile**
> - DOC acrodermatitis enterohepatica = ZINC therapy rapidly abolishes the manifestations of the disease.
> - Radiological findings of rickets = Cupping, Fraying, Splaying on distal end of radius.
> - Dose of vitamin D for rickets= 6 lac IU intramuscular single dose or 60,000IU orally X10 days.
> - Keshan disease = Selenium deficiency

ANSWERS TO BOARD REVIEW QUESTIONS

188. Ans. (c) Transient Tachypnea of new-born
189. Ans. (b) High lactaglobulin
190. Ans. (a) Hyaline membrane disease
191. Ans. (b) Structural isomerization
192. Ans. (a) Cleft palate
193. Ans. (a) Congenital malformations
194. Ans. (a) Epilepsy
195. Ans. (b) 14 days
196. Ans. (a) Decreased serum copper
197. Ans. (b) TGA

198. Ans. (d) 10 years
199. Ans. (a) Mid arm circumference/head circumference
200. Ans. (b) Late congenital syphilis
201. Ans. (a) Increase appetite
202. Ans. (a) 3rd centile
203. Ans. (c) 6 months
204. Ans. (c) 4 years
205. Ans. (d) 5 years
206. Ans. (a) Respiratory rate
207. Ans. (a) 7 months

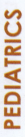

Pediatrics

208. Ans. (a) Subtle

209. Ans. (b) Cerebellar astrocytoma

210. Ans. (a) Spastic

211. Ans. (c) Lower areola is more visible than upper

212. Ans. (d) 20 teeth

213. Ans. (a) Rh incompatibility

214. Ans. (b) Height /age

215. Ans. (b) <1500 gm

216. Ans. (a) <1000 gm

217. Ans. (a) 12.5 cm

218. Ans. (b) <2

219. Ans. (a) Kwashiorkor

220. Ans. (a) Rickets

221. Ans. (a) Selenium

222. Ans. (b) 6 month

223. Ans. (b) Steroid

224. Ans. (c) > 14 years

Ref: Nelson, 19th ed. pg. 1739

225. Ans. (d) Small ASD

Ref: OP Ghai, 7th ed. pg. 390

226. Ans. (a) Emphysema

Ref: Robbins 8thEdn /684, 685, Harrison 18thed chapter 309, Nelson Textbook of Pediatrics, 18thed chapter 390

227. Ans. (b) 25–50%

Ref: Nelson, 18th ed. Ch 590

228. Ans. (b) Neural tube defects (Spina bifida)

229. Ans. (a) Less than 0.3 ml/kg/hr

Ref: Principles of Pediatric and Neonatal Emergencies By Krishan Chugh, 3rded /158

230. Ans. (a) 25 cm

Ref: Nelson's 18th ed. Ch 14, Essence of Paediatrics Prof. MR Khan 4thed /59

231. Ans. (c) Iron

Ref: Pediatrics by Lucy M. Osborn Pg 758, Nelson's 18th ed. Ch 594

232. Ans. (a) Rotor Syndrome

Ref: Harrison's, 17th ed. Ch Table 43-1

233. Ans. (b) 6 years

Ref: Nelson, 18th ed. Ch 8

234. Ans. (b) Bicuspid aortic value

Ref: Nelson's, 18th ed. Ch 587

235. Ans. (b) 10 years

Ref: Nelson's, 18th ed. ch: 12

236. Ans. (b) 5 years

237. Ans. (a) ELISA

Ref: O.P Ghai, 6th ed. pg. 235

238. Ans. (b) ORS

Ref: OP Ghai, 6th ed pg. 273

239. Ans. (c) Increased urinary copper excretion

Ref: Harrison's, 18th ed. chapter 360

240. Ans. (c) 11-Beta Hydroxylase

Ref: Nelson's, 18th ed. ch: 445

241. Ans. (a) 90 ml/kg

Ref: Maternal, Fetal, and Neonatal Physiology By Susan Tucker Blackburn 4th ed. pg. 235,

242. Ans. (a) 85–95%

Ref: Assisted Ventilation of the Neonate, pg. 136

Explanations

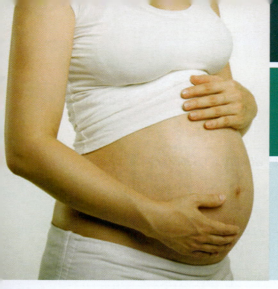

12

Obstetrics and Gynecology

OBSTETRICS

MOST RECENT QUESTIONS 2019

1. A 16-year-old girl presented with primary amenorrhea with orderly appearance of secondary sexual characteristics like breast and pubic hair. What is the next best step for this patient:
   a. Reassure
   b. USG
   c. HSG
   d. Hormonal study

2. A 19-year-old primigravida, presents with 8 weeks amenorrhea, light bleeding and pain. USG reveals intra uterine pregnancy. What is preferred management in this case?
   a. Estrogen plus Progesterone therapy
   b. D and C
   c. Bed rest and Progesterone
   d. Beta hCG

3. A 35 year female presented with complaints of infertility. She has previous history of PID. Preliminary investigations like USG showed normal organs and hormone levels were also normal. What is the next best investigation?
   a. Repeat USG
   b. Hysterosalpingography
   c. Endometrial biopsy
   d. Urine culture and sensitivity

4. Couvelaire uterus is seen in:
   a. Placenta previa
   b. Vasa previa
   c. Abruptio placenta
   d. Placenta percreta

5. Risk of endometrial cancer is least in:
   a. Nullipara
   b. Obesity
   c. Late menopause
   d. Multigravida

6. A grand multipara is a women who has given birth to ___ births:
   a. >2
   b. >3
   c. >4
   d. >5

7. A 26 weeks pregnant female presented with HTN for the first time. There is no proteinuria. Diagnosis of such condition
   a. Chronic hypertension
   b. Eclampsia
   c. Gestational Hypertension
   d. Preeclampsia

8. Minimum sperm count for normal semen analysis according to WHO:
   a. 2 million/mL
   b. 5 million/mL
   c. 10 million/mL
   d. 20 million/mL

9. Endometrial biopsy for infertility test in women should be done at:
   a. Ovulatory phase
   b. Menstrual phase
   c. Anytime during cycle
   d. Premenstrual period

10. In this normal menstrual cycle graph, the mark 'X' graph is due to:

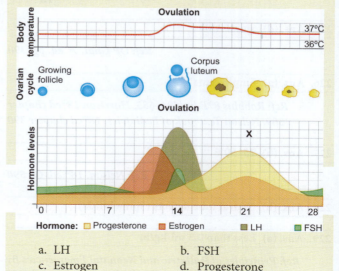

   a. LH
   b. FSH
   c. Estrogen
   d. Progesterone

Obstetrics and Gynecology

11. A patient who was using CuT for contraception, presented with a 20 weeks pregnancy. The IUCD is placed at fundus, tail visible at OS and she wants to continue the pregnancy. What is your next step in this patient:
    a. Leave IUD in-situ, continue pregnancy
    b. Do medical termination of Pregnancy
    c. Remove IUCD and continue pregnancy
    d. Remove IUCD and do MTP

12. Which of the following can be a cause of Oligohydramnios?
    a. Multiparity   b. Twins
    c. Renal agenesis   d. Macrosomia

ANATOMY AND PHYSIOLOGY

13. Beta hCG is secreted by:
    (Recent Pattern Question 2018-19)
    a. Yolk sac   b. Placenta
    c. Syncytiotrophoblast d. Umbilical cord

14. At 24 weeks the fundus height reaches to:
    (Recent Pattern Question 2018)
    a. Symphysis pubis to umbilicus
    b. Symphysis pubis to mid of umbilicus
    c. Between umbilicus to xiphisternum
    d. At xiphisternum

15. Constipation in pregnancy is due to:
    (Recent Pattern Question 2017)
    a. Uterus enlargement b. Estrogen effect
    c. Progesterone effect d. Excessive micturition

16. During pregnancy urine frequency increases in which trimester? *(Recent Pattern Question 2017)*
    a. T1   b. T2
    c. T3   d. Puerperium

17. Change in BMR(%) during pregnancy:
    (Recent Pattern Question 2017)
    a. Rise by 25%   b. Fall by 25%
    c. Rise by 50%   d. Fall by 50%

18. Which is the largest diameter of fetal head?
    (Recent Pattern Question 2017)
    a. Mentovertical   b. Occipitofrontal
    c. Submentobregmatic d. Suboccipitofrontal

19. Placenta develops completely by—age of gestation:
    (Recent Pattern Question 2016)
    a. 3 weeks   b. 4 weeks
    c. 6 weeks   d. 12 weeks

20. Vessel which disappears in placenta:
    (Recent Pattern Question 2016)
    a. Left umbilical artery b. Left umbilical vein
    c. Right umbilical vein   d. Right umbilical artery

21. Blood is carried from placenta to inferior vena cava through: *(Recent Pattern Question 2016)*
    a. Ductus arteriosus b. Ductus venosus
    c. Right umbilical vein d. Left umbilical vein

22. Which of the following decreases during pregnancy
    (Recent Pattern Question 2016)
    a. Systemic venous resistance
    b. CO
    c. HR
    d. Plasma volume

23. Normal pH of vagina *(Recent Pattern Question 2016)*
    a. 2–2.5   b. 3.5–4.5
    c. 4.5–5.5   d. 5.0–6.5

24. Nulliparous cervix: body uterus ratio
    (Recent Pattern Question 2016)
    a. 50–50   b. 60–40
    c. 30–70   d. 70–30

25. In a normal menstrual cycle, lowest amount of estrogen and progesterone is seen at:
    (Recent Pattern Question 2016)
    a. Follicular phase   b. Ovulation
    c. At beginning of menses d. Secretory phase

26. True support of uterus:
    a. Broad ligament   b. Round ligament
    c. Cardinal ligament d. Uterosacral ligament

27. Which gland opens on posterolateral margin of vaginal opening:
    a. Skene gland   b. Cooper gland
    c. Bartholin's gland d. Bulbourethral gland

28. Which is the smallest transverse diameter of fetal head:
    a. Biparietal   b. Bitemporal
    c. Bimastoid   d. Super subparietal

29. Longest diameter of fetal skull is:
    a. Occipitofrontal   b. Submentobregmatic
    c. Suboccipitofrontal d. Mentovertical

30. Shortest diameter of pelvic outlet:
    a. Anteroposterior   b. Intertuberous
    c. Oblique   d. Interspinous

31. Largest diameter of pelvic inlet:
    a. Transverse   b. True conjugate
    c. Oblique   d. Bituberous

32. What is the least diameter of pelvic inlet?
    (Recent Pattern Question 2017)
    a. Sacrococcygeal   b. Pubococcygeal
    c. Transverse   d. Sacrocotyloid

33. Prominent iliac spine is seen in which type of pelvis:
    a. Gynaecoid   b. Platypelloid
    c. Android   d. Anthropoid

34. Which of the following is not increased during pregnancy:
    a. Plasma volume   b. RBC count
    c. Platelet count   d. Hemoglobin

35. In pregnancy which clotting factor will be decreased:
    a. Factor II   b. Factor V
    c. Factor VII   d. Factor XI

FMGE Solutions Screening Examination

36. Most common cause of secondary amenorrhea
    a. Turner syndrome   b. Pregnancy
    c. Mullerian agenesis   d. Kallmann syndrome
37. When is the best time to do breast self-exam?
    a. 3 days after menstruation
    b. 3 days before menstruation
    c. During menstruation
    d. During ovulation
38. When is the time for ovulation:
    a. 14 days after menstruation
    b. Along with LH surge
    c. 1 week before menstruation
    d. 2 weeks before next menstruation
39. Oxygenated blood from placenta goes to fetal heart via:
    a. Ductus arteriosus   b. Ductus venosus
    c. Foramen ovale   d. Umbilical artery
40. Which of the following closes before birth:
    a. Ductus arteriosus   b. Ductus venosus
    c. Cardinal vein   d. Umbilical vein
41. Uterus is at the level of umbilicus at which age of gestation:
    a. 12 weeks   b. 22 weeks
    c. 20 weeks   d. 24 weeks
42. Oxytocin will not do the following action:
    a. Milk production
    b. Milk let down
    c. Contraction of myo-epithelial cells
    d. Vascular contraction

EMBRYOLOGY

43. After 28 weeks AOG major amount of amniotic fluid is secreted from: *(Recent Pattern Question 2018-19)*
    a. Fetal skin   b. Fetal urine
    c. Placental cell membrane d. Plasma
44. In a general population, the screening of Down syndrome is done by: *(Recent Pattern Question 2018)*
    a. USG
    b. Serum biomarkers
    c. Chorionic villus sampling
    d. Amniocentesis
45. Which of the following is best done for intrapartum fetal monitoring? *(Recent Pattern Question 2018)*
    a. Fetal echocardiography
    b. Fetal scalp pH
    c. Continuous electrical fetal monitoring
    d. Physical examination
46. Amniocentesis is best done by:
    (Recent Pattern Question 2018)
    a. 10–11 weeks   b. 12–13 weeks
    c. 15–18 weeks   d. 20–35 weeks
47. Size of graffican follicle at the time of ovulation:
    a. 10 mm   b. 15 mm
    c. 20 mm   d. 25 mm

48. Which of the following is not related with fertilization:
    a. Sperm crosses corona radiata
    b. Implantation after 6 days
    c. Zona pellucida facilitation by hyaluronidase
    d. Zona reaction attracts the sperms
49. What is the function of zona pellucida?
    (Recent Pattern Question 2017)
    a. Prevent wrong implantation of embryo
    b. Formation of blastocyst
    c. Prevention of multiple sperm entry
    d. Prevent wrong attachment of sperm
50. Which of the following is a true statement:
    a. Placenta is formed at morula stage
    b. Implantation starts on 10th day
    c. During initial weeks corpus luteum survival is due to LH
    d. Fertilization takes place in ampula
51. Implantation occurs after fertilization:
    a. 5–6 days   b. 7–8 days
    c. 8–10 days   d. 10–12 days
52. Gestational sac can be visualized via USG by:
    a. 4 weeks   b. 5 weeks
    c. 8 weeks   d. 10 weeks
53. Corpus luteum formation occurs on _____ of menstrual cycle:
    a. 15th day   b. 22nd day
    c. 1st day   d. 28th day
54. Doubling of Beta hCG levels is seen in:
    a. 24 hours   b. 48 hours
    c. 72 hours   d. 96 hours
55. Placental blood supply is established on:
    (Recent Pattern Question 2016)
    a. 2nd week   b. 3rd week
    c. 5th week   d. 8th week
56. Labia minora is homologous to which organ in males?
    (Recent Pattern Question 2017)
    a. Glans penis   b. Scrotum
    c. Corpus cavernosa   d. Penile urethra
57. Inferior 1/3rd of vagina is derived from:
    (Recent Pattern Question 2017)
    a. Metanephric bud   b. Urogenital sinus
    c. Mullerian duct   d. Genital fold
58. When is the embryo termed as fetus?
    a. End of 7th week *(Recent Pattern Question 2017)*
    b. After 10 weeks from LMP
    c. End of 8th week after LMP
    d. From end of 2nd trimester
59. Fertilization most commonly occurs at:
    (Recent Pattern Question 2017)
    a. Ampulla   b. Interstitium
    c. Isthmus   d. Uterine cavity
60. When does Haematopoiesis shift to liver from yolk sac:
    a. 10 weeks   b. 12 weeks
    c. 16 weeks   d. 20 weeks

Obstetrics and Gynecology

61. **Maximum number of oogonia:**
    a. 6 million
    b. 4 million
    c. 5 million
    d. 7 million

62. **1st polar body is released at the time of:**
    a. Birth
    b. Puberty
    c. Menstruation
    d. Fertilization

63. **What is released at the time of ovulation:**
    a. 1st polar body
    b. Primary oocyte
    c. Female pronucleus
    d. 2nd polar body

64. **Ovulation occurs after the extrusion of:**
    a. Primary oocyte
    b. Female pronucleus
    c. 1st polar body
    d. 2nd polar body

65. **Maternal side of placenta is derived from which layer:**
    a. Decidua basalis
    b. Zona capsularis
    c. Zona parietalis
    d. Inner cell mass

66. **True about fetal surface of placenta:**
    a. Derived from decidua basalis
    b. It has spongy and rough surface
    c. It has umbilical cord attachment site
    d. It has cotyledons

LABOR AND DELIVERY

67. **During childbirth all of the following can cause prolapse EXCEPT:** *(Recent Pattern Question 2018-19)*
    a. Precipitated labour
    b. Prolonged 2nd stage
    c. Premature bearing down
    d. 3rd degree perineal tear

68. **A 32-year-old pregnant female presented with 34-week pregnancy with complaints of pain in the abdomen, and decreased fetal movements. Upon examination, BP = 90/60, FHR = 100, upon per vaginum examination there is blood seen and cervix is closed. What is the preferred management?** *(Recent Pattern Question 2018-19)*
    a. Tocolytics
    b. Induce labour
    c. Immediate LSCS
    d. Wait and watch

69. **Uterus relaxation in order to delay the labor is caused by:** *(Recent Pattern Question 2018)*
    a. Ritodrine
    b. Tolterodine
    c. Oxytocin
    d. Labetalol

70. **Which of the following the presenting part in the fetus in left occiput anterior (LOA) position:** *(Recent Pattern Question 2018)*
    a. Suboccipito-bregmatic
    b. Submentoverical
    c. Brow
    d. Vertex

71. ***Pacemaker* of uterine contraction is located at:**
    a. Fundus
    b. Anterior wall
    c. Posterior wall
    d. Tubal ostia

72. **1/5 head is palpable suprapubic. True statement regarding this is:** *(Recent Pattern Question 2016)*
    a. Brow presentation
    b. 1/5 of head at pelvic brim
    c. Fetal head is engaged
    d. 1/5th of the head below ischial spine

73. **According to the rule of 5th, when is the fetal head engagement:**
    a. 1/5th of the fetal head palpable
    b. 2/5th of the fetal head palpable
    c. 3/5th of the fetal head palpable
    d. 4/5th of the fetal head palpable

74. **Moulding of fetal head** *(Recent Pattern Question 2016)*
    a. Disappears in few weeks
    b. Can damage brain
    c. No alteration in shape of head
    d. Complicates the delivery

75. **During the 3rd stage of labor, what is the pressure in the uterus:**
    a. 30–40 mm Hg
    b. 100–120 mm Hg
    c. 80–100 mm Hg
    d. 40–60 mm Hg

76. **Pressure inside uterus during early phase of active labor:**
    a. 50 mm Hg
    b. 100 mm Hg
    c. 150 mm Hg
    d. 200 mm Hg

77. **Force developed from uterine contraction:**
    a. 7 kg
    b. 14 kg
    c. 21 kg
    d. 25 kg

78. **Duration of 2nd stage of labor in primigravida:**
    a. 30 minutes
    b. 2 hours
    c. 15 minutes
    d. 4 hours

79. **To monitor fetal heart rate in a normal delivery partogram, it should be repeated every:**
    a. 30 minutes
    b. 1 hours
    c. 2 hours
    d. 90 minutes

80. **While doing partogram, pelvic examination is done at:**
    a. 30 minutes
    b. 1 hours
    c. 2 hours
    d. 4 hours

81. **Peak of prostaglandins occurs in what stage:**
    a. 1st stage of labor
    b. 2nd stage of labor
    c. 3rd stage of labor
    d. Before 1st stage of labor

82. **Amniotic fluid at term:**
    a. 1000–1200 mL
    b. 800–1000 mL
    c. 1200–1500 mL
    d. 700–800 mL

83. **Amniotic fluid is maximum at:**
    a. 22–26 weeks
    b. 34–36 weeks
    c. 38–40 weeks
    d. 40–42 weeks

84. **Bishop score includes all EXCEPT:**
    a. Cervical consistency
    b. Dilatation of cervix
    c. Position of cervix
    d. Cervical length

85. **Most common fractured bone during birth is:**
    a. Humerus
    b. Scapula
    c. Clavicle
    d. Radius

86. **Cord compression leads to:**
    a. Late deceleration
    b. Early deceleration
    c. Variable deceleration
    d. Acceleration

87. **Late deceleration is due to:**
    a. Head compression
    b. Cord compression
    c. Uteroplacental insufficiency
    d. All of the above

Questions

FMGE Solutions Screening Examination

88. Identify the progress of partogram:

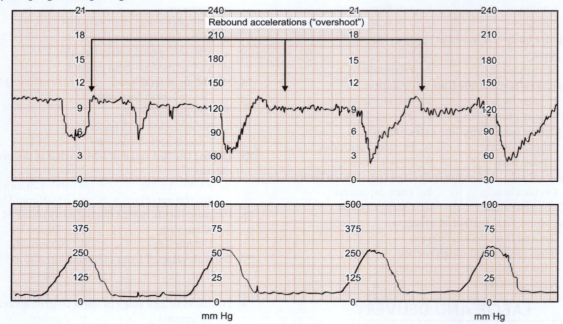

   a. Early deceleration
   b. Variable deceleration
   c. Late deceleration
   d. Normal partogram

89. As compared to mediolateral episiotomy, median episiotomy has complications because of:
   a. Poor repair
   b. Cosmetic problem
   c. Extension to rectum
   d. More blood loss

90. Arrest disorder is defined as the cessation of cervical dilatation in active phase of labor of more than:
   a. 1 hour
   b. 1.2 hours
   c. 1.5 hours
   d. 2 hours

ANTEPARTUM AND POSTPARTUM PERIOD

91. EDD calculated by: *(Recent Pattern Question 2018-19)*
   a. Young's rule
   b. Naegele's formula
   c. Cardiff formula
   d. Hadlock formula

92. True sign of placental separation are all EXCEPT:
   (Recent Pattern Question 2018)
   a. Gush of blood
   b. Raised fundal height
   c. Lengthening of cord
   d. Discoid uterus

93. Which is correct about iron status in pregnancy?
   (Recent Pattern Question 2016)
   a. Serum iron is increased
   b. TIBC increased
   c. Serum ferritin increased
   d. Serum iron: TIBC ratio increased

94. Lactiferous duct of breast contraction is due to
   (Recent Pattern Question 2016)
   a. Progesterone
   b. Estrogen
   c. Oxytocin
   d. Prolactin

95. First investigation to be done for screening the presence of fetus:
   a. TVS
   b. TAS
   c. MRI
   d. Doppler

96. Placental circulation is established by:
   a. 15 days
   b. 16 days
   c. 21 days
   d. 25 days

97. A 35 year primigravida visited your clinic. USG given below: What is the diagnosis?

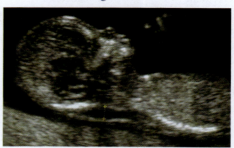

   a. Anencephaly
   b. Holoprocencephaly
   c. Nuchal translucency
   d. Hydrocephaly

Obstetrics and Gynecology

98. Iron and folic acid supplement during pregnancy:
   a. 500 mg iron + 100 mcg folic acid
   b. 100 mg iron + 500 mcg folic acid
   c. 100 mg iron + 100 mcg folic acid
   d. 20 mg iron + 100 mcg folic acid

99. Test which identifies fetal well being by detecting fetal heart rate acceleration and fetal movement:
   a. Bio-Physical profile
   b. Stress test
   c. Non-stress test
   d. Contraction stress test

100. Biophysical profile scoring includes all EXCEPT:
   a. FHR deceleration
   b. Fetal breathing
   c. Fetal movement
   d. Amniotic fluid

101. Length of lower uterine segment at term:
   a. 5 cm
   b. 10–12 cm
   c. 15 cm
   d. 20 cm

102. Hegar sign is seen earliest at:
   a. 6 weeks
   b. 10 weeks
   c. 14 weeks
   d. 15 weeks

103. Jacquemier's sign of pregnancy occurs in which week:
   a. 6th week
   b. 8th week
   c. 10th week
   d. 12th week

104. Obstetric care will mostly affect:
   a. Infant mortality rate
   b. Early neonatal mortality rate
   c. late neonatal mortality rate
   d. Perinatal mortality rate

105. LMP of patient is 30 June 2015, EDD is__:
   a. 7 March, 2016
   b. 7 April, 2016
   c. 30 March, 2016
   d. 30 April, 2016

106. Lochia lasts for:
   a. 5 days
   b. 2 weeks
   c. 3 weeks
   d. 4 weeks

107. The most common site of puerperal infection is:
   a. Placental site
   b. Cervical laceration
   c. Episiotomy wound
   d. Vaginal laceration

108. Following are signs of placental separation EXCEPT:
   a. Uterus rises in abdomen
   b. Uterus becomes discoid
   c. Lengthening of cord
   d. Fresh gush of blood from the vagina

109. Which of the following is a sign of placental separation in stage III of labor:
   a. Gushing of blood
   b. Discoid uterus
   c. Filling of placenta in vagina
   d. Increase in blood pressure

110. The signs and symptoms of placental separation include all of the following EXCEPT:
   a. Raised fundal height
   b. Fundus of uterus below umbilicus
   c. Gush of Vaginal bleeding
   d. Lengthening of cord

111. Common cause of 3rd day Puerperal fever:
   a. Breast Engorgement
   b. UTI
   c. Puerperal sepsis
   d. Pulmonary

112. What is the most common cause of maternal mortality in India?
   a. Haemorrhage
   b. Obstructed Labor
   c. Cardiac arrest
   d. Anemia

113. Most common indirect cause of maternal mortality:
   a. Sepsis
   b. Hemorrhage
   c. Obstructed labor
   d. Anemia

114. Which of the following is the cause of amenorrhoea in a lactating mother:
   a. Increased release of LH
   b. Increased GnRH secretion
   c. Hyperestrogenic state
   d. Increased prolactin level

115. Weight of uterus immediately after delivery:
   a. 60 g
   b. 500 g
   c. 1000 g
   d. 800 g

116. Heart rate returns to normal after delivery:
   a. Immediately
   b. 4 weeks
   c. 4 hours after
   d. 6 weeks

117. Cardiac output return to normal how many days after delivery:
   a. 1 hour
   b. 4 hours
   c. 2 weeks
   d. 4 weeks

118. The uterus becomes pelvic organ how many days after normal delivery:
   a. 5–7 days
   b. 12–14 days
   c. 16–18 days
   d. 20–22 days

119. Blood loss of fetal origin:
   a. Placenta previa
   b. Vasa previa
   c. Abruption Placenta
   d. Circumvallate placenta

120. A pregnant patient after delivery presented with hemorrhage. Immediate hysterectomy is done in:
   a. Pre-eclampsia
   b. Rupture of uterus
   c. Atonic uterus
   d. Inversion of uterus

121. During delivery there is a perineal tear involving the anal sphincter but anal mucosa is not involved. Which is the degree of tear?
   a. I
   b. II
   c. III
   d. IV

ABORTION AND THIRD TRIMESTER BLEEDING

122. A G4P2 lady presented with history of two abortions at 16 weeks and 20 weeks AOG. Which of the following could be the most suspected cause for this abortions?
   (Recent Pattern Question 2018-19)
   a. Chromosomal abnormality
   b. Cervical incompetence
   c. Placenta previa
   d. Thyroid abnormality

123. Most common cause of miscarriage in 1st trimester abortions: *(Recent Pattern Question 2018)*
    a. Trisomy
    b. Monosomy X
    c. Triploidy
    d. Tetraploidy
124. Most common cause of bleeding in early pregnancy *(Recent Pattern Question 2016)*
    a. Spontaneous abortion
    b. Missed abortion
    c. Ectopic pregnancy
    d. Abruption placenta
125. Most common cause of 1st trimester abortions:
    a. Trisomy
    b. Monosomy X
    c. Triploidy
    d. Tetraploidy
126. Commonest cause of first trimester miscarriage is:
    a. Syphilis
    b. Cervical incompetence
    c. Chromosomal abnormalities
    d. Rhesus isoimmunisation
127. In Inevitable abortion:
    a. Uterus size larger than to AOG, cervix open
    b. Uterus size equal to AOG, cervix close
    c. Uterus size smaller than to AOG, cervix open
    d. Uterus size smaller than to AOG, cervix close
128. Treatment of choice of inevitable abortion less than 10 week:
    a. Dilatation and evacuation
    b. Suction and evacuation
    c. Medical management
    d. Complete hysterectomy
129. For MTP which of the following drug dosage is used:
    a. 200 mg mifepristone + 400 mg misoprostol
    b. 200 mg misoprostol + 400 mg mifepristone
    c. 200 mg mifepristone + 400 mcg misoprostol
    d. 400 mcg mifepristone + 200 mg misoprostol
130. Which one of following is the legal drug used for MTP in India?
    a. Misoprostol + Methotrexate
    b. Mitoprostane + Methotrexate
    c. Mifepristone 200 mg + Misoprostol 400 mcg oral
    d. None
131. Which of the following is not used in MTP?
    a. Misoprostol
    b. Mifepristone
    c. Misoprostol + Tamoxifen
    d. Mifepristone + Misoprostol
132. Dangerously low lying placenta is:
    a. Type I anterior
    b. Type II anterior
    c. Type I posterior
    d. Type II posterior
133. McAfee and Johnson regimen is used for:
    a. Eclampsia
    b. Placenta previa
    c. Placental abruption
    d. Placenta accrete
134. Patient with 37 week AOG, centrally located placenta previa presented with bleeding per vaginum. Management:
    a. Caesarean section
    b. Abortion
    c. Vaccum delivery
    d. Forceps delivery
135. Umbilical cord attached to the margin of placenta:
    a. Circumvallate placenta
    b. Battledore placenta
    c. Velamentous insertion
    d. Vasa previa
136. Nitabuch's membrane is absent in:
    a. Placenta accreta
    b. Vasa previa
    c. Abruption placenta
    d. Placenta previa
137. Absence of Nitabuch's membrane leads to in all EXCEPT:
    a. Placenta previa
    b. Placenta accreta
    c. Placenta increta
    d. Placenta percreta
138. Recurrence of hydatiform mole is assessed by:
    a. AFP level
    b. β-hCG level
    c. LDH level
    d. Estrogen level
139. Complete mole contains
    a. 46 YY
    b. 46 XY
    c. 46 XXY
    d. 69 XXX
140. In gestational trophoblastic disease, metastases most commonly occurs to:
    a. Brain
    b. Liver
    c. Lungs
    d. Bone
141. Theca lutein cyst are seen in
    a. Complete mole
    b. Partial mole
    c. Tubal ectopic
    d. Missed abortion
142. In a patient who underwent post molar evacuation by dilatation and curettage. Which of the following test used to define successful removal of H. Mole:
    a. Beta hCG
    b. Per speculum
    c. Progesterone
    d. USG
143. The risk of uterine rupture after previous lower transverse uterine incision at Caesarean Section is:
    a. 1%
    b. 3%
    c. 5%
    d. 7%

TWIN PREGNANCY

144. If a zygote divides 2–3 days after fertilization, which of the following type of twining is seen: *(Recent Pattern Question 2018-19)*
    a. Monochorionic, Monoamniotic
    b. Monochorionic, Diamniotic
    c. Diamniotic, Dichorionic
    d. Dichorionic, Monoamniotic
145. Division of zygote took place on 5th day after fertilization. What is the type of twinning?
    a. Monochorionic, monoamniotic
    b. Monochorionic, diamniotic
    c. Dichorionic, diamniotic
    d. Dichorionic, monoamniotic
146. Most common type of twin gestation is:
    a. Monochorionic monoamniotic
    b. Diamniotic, monochorionic
    c. Conjoined twins
    d. Dichorionic monoamniotic

Obstetrics and Gynecology

147. Best position of twins for normal vaginal delivery:
a. A non-vertex, B vertex
b. A vertex, B non-vertex
c. A vertex, B vertex
d. A non-vertex, B non-vertex

148. Twin pregnancy is earliest detected at:
a. 10 weeks
b. 12 weeks
c. 6 weeks
d. 8 weeks

149. Twin pregnancy is least associated with:
a. Multigravida
b. Genetic
c. Young female
d. Patient receiving fertilization treatment

ECTOPIC PREGNANCY

150. In a patient with ectopic tubal pregnancy which is the earliest to rupture? *(Recent Pattern Question 2018-19)*
a. Interstitial
b. Isthmus
c. Ampulla
d. Infundibulum

151. Most common site of ectopic pregnancy:
(Recent Pattern Question 2017)
a. Ampulla
b. Interstitium
c. Isthmus
d. Fimbrae

152. Which is the most dangerous site for Ectopic pregnancy:
(Recent Pattern Question 2017)
a. Isthmus
b. Ampulla
c. Interstitial
d. Fimbrae

153. A 29-year-old female presented with 7 weeks of pregnancy. She has complaint of vaginal spotting. USG shows empty uterus. Best treatment:
(Recent Pattern Question 2017)
a. If sac >3.5 cm do medical management
b. Laparoscopy with salpingostomy
c. Laparotomy with salpingectomy
d. Laparatomy

154. Ectopic pregnancy with adnexal mass <2.5 cm. Treatment:
a. Medical management *(Recent Pattern Question 2017)*
b. Surgical management
c. Laparoscopy
d. Laparoscopy with salpingectomy

155. Most common complaints of ectopic pregnancy
(Recent Pattern Question 2016)
a. Pain
b. Vaginal bleeding
c. Infection
d. Amenorrhea

156. Pain is more common than bleeding in
(Recent Pattern Question 2016)
a. Ectopic pregnancy
b. Complete mole
c. Incomplete abortion
d. Missed abortion

157. Suspected ectopic pregnancy is best diagnosed by
(Recent Pattern Question 2016)
a. MRI
b. TVS
c. X-ray abdomen supine
d. HSG

158. Drug used for ectopic pregnancy
(Recent Pattern Question 2016)
a. Mifepristone + misoprostol
b. Misoprostol 200 mg
c. Methotrexate 50 mg IM
d. Progesterone

159. Triad of ectopic pregnancy are all EXCEPT:
a. Vomiting
b. Bleeding
c. Abdominal pain
d. Amenorrhea

160. All are true about ectopic pregnancy EXCEPT
a. Most common cause is Progestasert
b. Can be diagnosed by hCG level
c. A negative pregnancy test excludes the diagnosis
d. Methotrexate is used as medical management

161. Most sensitive diagnostic test for ectopic pregnancy:
a. Transvaginal USG
b. Serial monitoring of beta hCG
c. Culdocentesis
d. MRI

162. Criteria for medical termination of ectopic pregnancy:
a. Beta hCG < 5000
b. Mass of >3.5 cm
c. Present fetal heart beat
d. 6 week pregnancy

MALPRESENTATION, DIFFICULT DELIVERY AND INSTRUMENTATION

163. The pressure used for gynecological laparoscopy:
(Recent Pattern Question 2018)
a. 10–15 mm Hg
b. 15–20 mm Hg
c. 20–30 mm Hg
d. 30–50 mm Hg

164. Upon hysteroscopy which of the following cannot be seen? *(Recent Pattern Question 2018)*
a. OS
b. Cervix
c. Endometrium
d. Uterus surface

165. True about frank breech:
(Recent Pattern Question 2018)
a. Mostly associated with congenital anomaly
b. Footling presentation
c. ECV done after 34 weeks
d. Has hip extended and knee flexed

166. Which is the most prominent part in transverse lie?
(Recent Pattern Question 2016)
a. Acromion
b. Sternum
c. Buttock
d. Mentum

167. In face presentation what is the presenting denominator? *(Recent Pattern Question 2016)*
a. Cheek
b. Mentum
c. Forehead
d. Lips

168. Breech presentation with footling. Management is:
a. Vaginal delivery
b. Ceasarean section
c. Forceps delivery
d. Internal podalic version

Questions

863

169. Which of the following is most common compound presentation:
    a. Head with foot
    b. Head with hand
    c. Hand, head and foot
    d. Both hand and foot
170. In Brow presentation, head of the fetus:
    a. Complete hyperextension
    b. Partial extension
    c. Complete flexion
    d. Moderate flexion
171. What is the presentation of the given image:

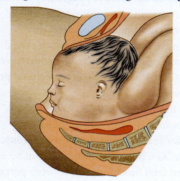

    a. Face presentation
    b. Transverse lie
    c. Brow presentation
    d. Vertex
172. Fetus in transverse position. Which of the following is true:

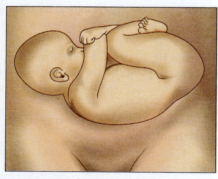

    a. Polyhydramnios is a cause
    b. It can be caused by abruptio placenta
    c. It results to hand prolapsed in all cases
    d. Shoulder dystocia is a major threat
173. Treatment of choice of acute hydramnios with fetal distress in pregnancy:
    a. Amniocentesis
    b. Cordocentesis
    c. Indomethacin
    d. Termination
174. Which of the following is a contraindication for trial of vaginal delivery in VBAC:
    a. Breech presentation
    b. Previous CS of more than 2
    c. Presence of anesthesiologist
    d. Informed consent
175. All are contraindications of Internal cephalic version EXCEPT:
    a. Shoulder presentation of first fetus
    b. Face presentation
    c. Transverse lie of second fetus in a twin pregnancy
    d. Breech presentation of 2nd fetus in a twin.
176. External cephalic version is done in all EXCEPT:
    a. Primigravida
    b. Flexed breech
    c. Anemia
    d. PIH
177. Following are contraindications to External Cephalic Version EXCEPT:
    a. Contracted pelvis
    b. Antepartum hemorrhage
    c. Multiple pregnancy
    d. Hydramnios
178. Low forceps are applied when:
    a. Scalp is visible at the introitus
    b. Fetal head is at pelvic floor
    c. Fetus is at station + 2
    d. Fetal head is engaged

DISEASES DURING PREGNANCY

179. Feature of hydrops fetalis in a fetus can be due to:
    (Recent Pattern Question 2018-19)
    a. Ebstein barr virus
    b. Human papilloma virus
    c. Parvovirus B19
    d. Influenza virus
180. Cut off point for 50 gram glucose challenge test at 1 hour mg%: *(Recent Pattern Question 2018-19)*
    a. 100
    b. 140
    c. 180
    d. 200
181. Chromosome pattern in complete mole:
    (Recent Pattern Question 2018-19)
    a. 46 XY both maternal origin
    b. 46 XX both maternal origin
    c. 46 XX both paternal origin
    d. 46 YY both paternal origin
182. Agent used for status eclampticus?
    (Recent Pattern Question 2017)
    a. Hydralazine
    b. Thiopentone sodium
    c. Valproate
    d. Magnesium sulfate
183. In an eclamptic patient with raised ICT, which drug should be given: *(Recent Pattern Question 2017)*
    a. Mannitol
    b. Furosemide
    c. Labetalol
    d. Hydralazine
184. Maximum risk of pre-eclampsia is due to
    (Recent Pattern Question 2016)
    a. CRF
    b. Heart disease
    c. Anemia
    d. Liver disease
185. Drugs not useful in emergency in pregnancy:
    a. Nifedipine
    b. Labetalol
    c. Ritodrine
    d. Phenobarbitone

Obstetrics and Gynecology

186. **In pregnancy with hypertension which drug is given:**
    a. Propranolol
    b. Acebutalol
    c. Metoprolol
    d. Labetalol

187. **Which of the following anti-hypertensive is contraindicated in pregnancy:**
    a. Beta blockers
    b. ACE inhibitors
    c. Methyldopa
    d. Ca channel blockers

188. **Drug contraindicated in pregnancy:**
    a. Angiotensin receptor blockers
    b. Beta blockers
    c. Calcium channel blockers
    d. Methyl dopa

189. **Antenatal mother with epilepsy on phenytoin therapy must be given:**
    a. Folic acid supplementation
    b. Vitamin B_{12} supplementation
    c. Vitamin B_6 supplementation
    d. Vitamin A supplementation

190. **A 42 years primigravida presents at 28 weeks period of gestation and has left upper breast mass. Choose the best investigation modality:**
    a. Mammography
    b. CT scan
    c. MRI
    d. High Resonance ultrasound

191. **Best marker in intrahepatic cholestasis of pregnant women:**
    a. Bile acid
    b. Bilirubin
    c. Alkaline phosphatase
    d. SGPT

192. **All of the following can cause DIC in women EXCEPT:**
    a. Amniotic fluid embolism
    b. Sepsis
    c. Placenta previa
    d. HELLP

193. **All are true about HELLP syndrome EXCEPT:**
    a. Increased LDH
    b. Low platelet
    c. Increased live enzymes
    d. Hyponatremia

194. **DOC for candidiasis in pregnancy**
    a. Metronidazole 500 mg
    b. Tinidazole 500 mg
    c. Fluconazole 150 mg
    d. Metronidazole 1 g

195. **A pregnant women with BP 150/100 mm Hg, proteinuria after 20 weeks. Diagnosis?**
    a. Pre-eclampsia
    b. Pregnancy induced hypertension
    c. Renal hypertension
    d. Eclampsia

196. **All can be done in pre-eclampsia EXCEPT:**
    a. Diuretics
    b. Anti hypertensives
    c. $MgSO_4$
    d. Admission and wait

197. **For controlling eclamptic patient with convulsion, which of the following will be used:**
    a. Mannitol
    b. Furosemide
    c. Hydralazine
    d. $MgSO_4$

198. **A patient presented with a pregnancy of 32 weeks with antepartum haemorrhage. Patient with hypertension. Management at this point of time:**
    a. Caesarean section
    b. Observation on OPD basis
    c. Hospitalization and observation
    d. Induce labor

199. **A pregnant lady with PIH is having bleeding per vagina. The decision to continue pregnancy is based on:**
    a. Presence of fetal cardiac activity
    b. Availability of blood
    c. Blood pressure
    d. Adequate medical facilities

200. **In a diabetic mother, most common fetal complication will be:**
    a. Neural tube defect
    b. Congenital sacral agenesis
    c. Congenital heart disease
    d. Hydrocephalus

201. **DOC for hyperthyroidism in pregnancy:**
    a. Propylthiouracil
    b. Methimazole
    c. I-131
    d. Thyroxine

FETAL GROWTH AND DEVELOPMENT

202. **Best parameter to find out age of gestation in first trimester:** *(Recent Pattern Question 2018)*
    a. Dates of menstrual period
    b. CRL
    c. Femur length
    d. Weight of the fetus

203. **Breathing movement of fetus on USG is first detected at:** *(Recent Pattern Question 2017)*
    a. 11 weeks
    b. 20 weeks
    c. 24 weeks
    d. 26 weeks

204. **During intrauterine life fetal waste is excreted by?** *(Recent Pattern Question 2017)*
    a. Straight into mother's blood by simple diffusion
    b. Diffusion into amniotic fluid
    c. Ultrafiltration
    d. Leakage

205. **Fetal haemoglobin is maximum secreted by** *(Recent Pattern Question 2016)*
    a. Liver
    b. Yolk sac
    c. Spleen
    d. Bone marrow

206. **Deoxygenated blood from the fetus to the mother is carried via:**
    a. Umbilical artery
    b. Umbilical veins
    c. Pulmonary artery
    d. Pulmonary vein

207. **Cardiac activity in fetus can be asessed via transabdominal scan by:**
    a. 6–7 weeks
    b. 8–9 weeks
    c. 9–11 weeks
    d. 12–14 weeks

FMGE Solutions Screening Examination

208. Crown rump length at 12 weeks:
    a. 7 cm   b. 10 cm
    c. 12 cm   d. 25 cm
209. At 12 weeks pregnancy "CRL" is:
    a. 60 mm   b. 100 mm
    c. 120 mm   d. 250 mm
210. Radiotherapy is most harmful in which week of gestation:
    a. 4–16 weeks   b. 18–23 weeks
    c. 28–32 weeks   d. 36–38 weeks
211. In folate + vitamin B12 combined deficiency which of the following is/are mainly seen?
    a. Neural tube defects   b. Megaloblastic anemia
    c. Abruptio placentae   d. Placenta previa

INTRAUTERINE FETAL DEATH

212. Intrauterine death is least likely caused by:
    a. Rh-incompatibility   b. Obstructed labor
    c. Low birth weight   d. Placental insufficiency
213. Which of the following sign is seen in intrauterine fetal demise:
    a. Von Braun-Fernwald's sign
    b. Roberts sign   c. Goodell's sign
    d. Osiander sign
214. Which of the following is most likely cause of intrapartum death?
    a. Cord prolapsed   b. Abruptio placentae
    c. Hyaline membrane disease
    d. Eclampsia

215. Methotrexate is indicated mainly in:
    a. Pre-eclampsia   b. IUD
    c. Prematurity   d. Ectopic pregnancy

MISCELLANEOUS

216. Which of the following statement is Not true about placenta:
    a. Weight of full term placenta is 508 and volume is 497 ml
    b. At 17th week weight of placenta is equal to weight of fetus
    c. It has 4 to 6 lobes
    d. Total of lobes remain the same throughout the gestation
217. Level of which hormone are increased during post menopausal women:
    a. Estrogen   b. Progestron
    c. FSH   d. Cortison
218. Drug contraindicated in pregnancy:
    a. Oral penicillin   b. Cephalosporin 1st generation
    c. Chloramphenicol   d. Erythromycin
219. Antibody to cross placenta
    a. IgA   b. Ig G
    c. Ig E   d. Ig M
220. Earliest sex-determination is done at:
    a. 1 month   b. 2 months
    c. 3 months   d. 4 months
221. The dose of anti-D immunoglobulin to be given to non-immune Rh D negative women after delivery is:
    a. 50 µg   b. 150 µg
    c. 300 µg   d. 450 µg

GYNECOLOGY

ANATOMY, MENARCHE AND MENOPAUSE

222. A 58-year-old lady with menopause and hot flushes presents to the physician. Which is correct?
    (Recent Pattern Question 2018-19)
    a. Increased FSH, increased estrogen
    b. Decreased FSH, decreased estrogen
    c. Decreased FSH, increased estrogen
    d. Increased FSH, decreased estrogen
223. A girl is said to have primary amenorrhea in absence of secondary sexual characters by what age:
    (Recent Pattern Question 2018)
    a. 12   b. 13
    c. 14   d. 16
224. Which of the following is the most common cause of secondary amenorrhea? *(Recent Pattern Question 2018)*
    a. Pelvic irradiation   b. Diabetes
    c. Kallmann syndrome   d. Imperforate hymen

225. Marker of ovarian reserve in a premenopausal female:
    (Recent Pattern Question 2018)
    a. Antral follicle size   b. Raised LH/FSH ratio
    c. Decreased inhibin A
    d. Anti-mullerian hormone
226. According to American fertility society classification system, unicornuate uterus is classified under this class:
    a. Class I   b. Class II
    c. Class III   d. Class IV
227. Thelarche definition: *(Recent Pattern Question 2017)*
    a. Growth of pubic and axillary hair
    b. Growth of breast
    c. Increase in height
    d. Onset of menstruation
228. The hormone which increases on thelarche:
    (Recent Pattern Question 2017)
    a. GnRH   b. Estrogen
    c. Progesterone   d. GH

Obstetrics and Gynecology

229. Average age of menopause:
(Recent Pattern Question 2017)
a. 40　　　　　　　b. 45
c. 55　　　　　　　d. 60

230. Precocious puberty in females is defined as:
(Recent Pattern Question 2016)
a. Occurrence of menarche before age of 8 years
b. Occurrence of menarche before age of 12 years
c. Appearance of secondary sexual characteristics before 8 years
d. Appearance of secondary sexual characteristics before 10 years

231. Follicles in ovary are decreasing with age, the first change is: *(Recent Pattern Question 2016)*
a. Increase FSH　　　b. Increase LH
c. Increase inhibin　　d. Increase estradiol

232. Menstrual blood stored in vagina in:
a. Pyometra　　　　　b. Hematometra
c. Hematocolpos　　　d. Hematosalphinx

INFECTION

233. Which is correct about presentation of *C. trachomatis* infection? *(Recent Pattern Question 2018-19)*
a. Pruritic Vaginitis
b. Leads to Infertility
c. Uveitis
d. Inclusion body pneumonitis

234. Which of the following infections can commonly lead to infertility: *(Recent Pattern Question 2018-19)*
a. Chlamydia　　　　b. Trichomoniasis
c. Candidiasis　　　　d. Bacterial vaginosis

235. A 32-year-old female presented with acute history of profuse mucoid vaginal discharge, abdominal pain and deep dyspareunia. Per speculum examination reveal erosion of cervix and a reddened area around cervix external os. Which of the following treatment option is preferred for this patient:
(Recent Pattern Question 2018-19)
a. Laser therapy　　　b. Conization operation
c. Cryosurgery　　　　d. Policresulen

236. Common mode of transmission in pyogenic TB salpingitis: *(Recent Pattern Question 2018)*
a. Hematogenous　　　b. Lymphatic
c. Direct invasion　　　d. Sexually transmitted

237. A 25-year-old lady who presents with curdy white discharge from vagina is likely to be suffering from:
(Recent Pattern Question 2018)
a. Gonococcal vulvovaginitis
b. Candida vaginitis
c. Trichomoniasis
d. Chlamydia trachomatis

238. Temperature in puerperal pyrexia:
(Recent Pattern Question 2018)
a. 98.4°F　　　　　　b. 99°F
c. 100.4°F　　　　　　d. 104°F

239. Which of the following organism is common cause of tubal blockage?
a. Chlamydia　　　　　b. Herpes simplex
c. Candida　　　　　　d. HPV

240. A 29-year-old female presents with PID, what is the indication to hospitalize?
(Recent Pattern Question 2017)
a. Pregnancy　　　　　b. Cervical discharge
c. TB　　　　　　　　d. Acute mild PID

241. Most common presentation in fallopian tube TB:
(Recent Pattern Question 2017)
a. Infertility　　　　　b. Pain
c. Abdominal cramps　d. Bleeding

242. Recurrent vulvo-vaginitis is defined as:
(Recent Pattern Question 2016)
a. >2 infection in a year　b. >3 infection in a year
c. >4 infection in a year　d. >5 infection in a year

243. Clue cells are seen in: *(Recent Pattern Question 2016)*
a. Bacterial vaginosis　　b. Cystitis
c. Candida albicans　　　d. Trichomoniasis

244. 10% KOH is used for diagnosing:
(Recent Pattern Question 2016)
a. Candida　　　　　　b. Trichomonas
c. Mycoplasma　　　　d. Gardenella vaginalis

245. Fishy odor in whiff test is seen in:
(Recent Pattern Question 2016)
a. Giardia　　　　　　b. Bacterial vaginosis
c. Trichomoniasis　　　d. Candidiasis

246. Trichomoniasisis is caused by:
a. Bacteria　　　　　　b. Virus
c. Protozoa　　　　　　d. Chlamydia

247. All of the following statement are true about Bacterial vaginosis EXCEPT:
a. Cause by gardenella vaginalis
b. Fishy odor upon whiff test
c. Infection seen when vaginal pH is <4.5
d. It is not an STD

248. Clue cells are seen in:
a. Bacterial vaginosis　　b. Candidiasis
c. Trichomoniasis　　　d. Gonoccocal

249. Whiff test done for:
a. Gonococcal infections　b. Gardenella
c. Trichomoniasis　　　d. Candiasis

250. In patients with asymptomatic carrier of Chlamydia, organisms resides most commonly in:
a. Vagina　　　　　　b. Urethra
c. Ectocervix　　　　　d. Endocervix

FMGE Solutions Screening Examination

251. First symptom of fallopian tube TB:
    a. Pain   b. Bleeding
    c. Watery discharge   d. Uterine prolapse
252. Clubbing of fimbrial end of Fallopian tube is seen upon HSG. What could be the possible pathology:
    a. Tuberculosis   b. Gonococcal
    c. Hydrosalpinx   d. Mullerian anomaly
253. A young female was worked up for examined for her infertility by hysterosalpingography reveals 'Bead — like' fallopian tube and clubbing of ampulla. Which of the following is the most likely cause?
    a. Gonococcus   b. Mycoplasma
    c. Chlamydia
    d. Mycobacterium tuberculosis
254. PID can be due to:
    a. IUCD insertion   b. Oral contraceptive
    c. Condom   d. Hypertension
255. A 40-year-old woman presents with PID. Best investigation to be done:
    a. USG   b. CT
    c. MRI   d. Laproscopy

CERVICAL CANCER

256. Cervical cancer is mostly caused by:
    (Recent Pattern Question 2018-19)
    a. HPV 6   b. HPV 16
    c. HPV 31   d. HPV 56
257. Most common type of cervical cancer:
    a. Squamous cell CA   b. Small cell CA
    c. Adeno CA   d. Adenoma
258. All of the following statements are true regarding etiology of cervical cancer EXCEPT:
    a. Both active and passive cigarette smoking increases the risk of cervical cancer
    b. Oral contraceptives decreases the risk of cervical cancer
    c. Abstinence from sexual activity and barrier protection decrease cervical cancer risk
    d. Low education increases cervical cancer risk
259. Most common cause of CA cervix:
    a. HPV 6 and 18   b. HPV 16 and 18
    c. HPV 6   d. HPV 6 and 11
260. Most commonly associated human papilloma virus with Cancer Cervix is?
    a. HPV 16   b. HPV 24
    c. HPV 32   d. HPV 36
261. Secondary level prevention of CA cervix:
    a. Vaccination   b. Pap smear
    c. Colposcopy   d. Spectroscopy
262. Screening test for cervical cancer is:
    a. Biopsy   b. Papaniculaou smear
    c. Visual inspection d. Colposcopy
263. Cancer cervix screening according to WHO guidelines:
    a. Women between the ages of 21 and 29 should have a Pap test every 3 years
    b. Women between the ages of 30 and 65 should have both a Pap test and an HPV test every 5 years
    c. Women over age 65 who have had regular screenings with normal results should NOT be screened for cervical cancer
    d. All of the above

ENDOMETRIAL AND FALLOPIAN TUBE CANCER

264. Effect of tamoxifen: *(Recent Pattern Question 2018)*
    a. Increased risk of endometrial carcinoma
    b. Decreased risk of ovarian CA
    c. Causes cardiotoxicity
    d. Increased risk of osteoporosis
265. In endometriosis which of the following is not given?
    (Recent Pattern Question 2018)
    a. Gonadotropin analogue
    b. Aromatase inhibitor
    c. Mifepristone
    d. Estradiol
266. Radiological test for staging of endometrial carcinoma is best done with: *(Recent Pattern Question 2018)*
    a. MRI
    b. Sonosalpingography
    c. PET-CT
    d. Doppler USG
267. Most common presentation of adenomyosis?
    (Recent Pattern Question 2017)
    a. Dyspareunia   b. Infertility
    c. Dysmenorrhea   d. Hypomenorrhea
268. _____% women with postmenopausal bleeding found to have endometrial cancer:
    a. 20   b. 30
    c. 40   d. 50
269. This type of endometrial hyperplasia leads to increased risk of endometrial cancer:
    a. Simple   b. Proliferative
    c. Atypical   d. Secretive
270. Best prognostic for endometrial pathology
    a. Transvaginal ultrasound   b. Biopsy
    c. Hysteroscopy   d. Fractional curettage
271. What would be the appropriate treatment of stage-I endometrial cancer:
    a. Conservative management
    b. Chemo therapy followed by radio therapy
    c. Simple hysterectomy
    d. Bilateral salpingo oophorectomy

Obstetrics and Gynecology

272. **Earliest presentation of fallopian tube cancer:**
   a. Painless watery discharge
   b. Painless vaginal bleeding
   c. Painful watery discharge
   d. Painful vaginal bleeding

273. **Tumor erodes serosa/adnexa of uterus in this stage of endometrial CA:**
   a. Ib   b. II
   c. IIIa   d. IIIb

OVARIAN CANCER

274. **Call exner bodies are seen in:**
   (Recent Pattern Question 2017)
   a. Granulosa cell tumor   b. Yolk cell tumor
   c. Teratoma   d. Krukenberg tumor

275. **Theca lutein cysts are common in**
   (Recent Pattern Question 2016)
   a. Vagina   b. Uterus
   c. Ovary   d. Cervix

276. **All of the following are germ cell tumor EXCEPT:**
   a. Dysgerminoma   b. Choriocarcinoma
   c. Clear cell tumor   d. Teratoma

277. **Most common germ cell ovarian tumor:**
   a. Dysgerminoma   b. Teratoma
   c. Endodermal sinus tumor d. Clear cell tumor

278. **Most common malignant germ cell ovarian tumor:**
   a. Yolk sac tumors
   b. Dysgerminoma
   c. Dermoid cyst
   d. Brenners

279. **Most frequent epithelial tumors of ovary:**
   a. Papillary serous cystadenoma
   b. Brenners
   c. Endometrioid
   d. Mucinous cyst adenoma

280. **Most common malignant ovarian tumor?**
   a. Clear cell tumor
   b. Serous cyst adenocarcinoma
   c. Mucinous cyst adenocarcinoma
   d. Granulosa cell tumor

281. **All of the following statements are true about choriocarcinoma EXCEPT:**
   a. Can present with epigastric pain
   b. Ovary is the primary site
   c. Lungs are common site of metastasis
   d. Snow storm appearance upon CXR

282. **Syncitiotrophoblast is seen in:**
   a. Partial mole
   b. Complete mole
   c. Choriocarcinoma
   d. Placental site of trophoplastoma

283. **Treatment of choice in choriocarcinoma is**
   a. Chemotherapy
   b. External beam radiotherapy
   c. Hysterectomy
   d. Intracavitary brachytherapy

284. **Tumor marker of CA ovary for follow up**
   a. CEA   b. PSA
   c. CA 125   d. BETA hCG

VULVAR AND VAGINAL CANCER

285. **In a patient with Vulval ulcer. Which of the following will lead to malignancy?**
   a. HSV1   b. HSV2
   c. STD   d. HPV

286. **Vulval cancer spreads to urethra at what stage?**
   a. Stage I A   b. Stage I B
   c. Stage II   d. Stage III A

287. **Urethra is involved in which stage of Vulvar neoplasia?**
   a. Stage I   b. Stage II
   c. Stage III   d. Stage IV

288. **A Vulvar cancer of 3 cm, no lymph node involved. Treatment:**
   a. Simple partial vulvectomy with lymphadenectomy
   b. Simple partial vulvectomy without lymphadenectomy
   c. Wide local excision with lymphadenectomy
   d. Radical vulvectomy

289. **Treatment for vulval cancer stage 1**
   a. Complete radical Vulvectomy
   b. Partial vulvectomy
   c. Total vulvectomy and bilateral groin lymph node resection
   d. CT or RT followed by resection of residual tumor

290. **Infertility occurs due to carcinoma of all EXCEPT:**
   a. Endometrial carcinoma b. Ovarian carcinoma
   c. Vaginal carcinoma   d. Cervix CA

DYSFUNCTIONAL UTERINE BLEEDING (DUB) AND DYSMENORRHEA

291. **True about endometriosis:**
   (Recent Pattern Question 2018-19)
   a. Presence of endometrial gland in deep myometrium
   b. Presence of endometrium at ectopic locations
   c. Treated with hysterectomy
   d. Not associated with infertility

292. **A 29-year-old female presented with infertility. There is history of abdominal pain, dyspareunia, dysmenorrhea, menorrhagia. Most likely cause:**
   (Recent Pattern Question 2018-19)
   a. Adenomyomatosis   b. Endometriosis
   c. Myomas   d. Cervicitis

FMGE Solutions Screening Examination

293. In a 25-year-old lady with primary dysmenorrhea, which of the following statement is true?
     (Recent Pattern Question 2018)
     a. No clinical significant pelvic pathology is found
     b. Menorrhagia and dyspareunia
     c. More commonly seen after 3rd decade
     d. Biochemical parameters are always normal

294. Most common cause of dysfunctional uterine bleeding:
     a. PID   b. Endometriosis
     c. Dermoid cyst d. Anovulatory

295. Which of the following is an acyclical bleeding:
     a. Menorrhagia   b. Polymenorrhoea
     c. Metrorrhagia d. Oligomenorrhoea

296. A 15-year-old girl presented with dysmenorrhea in every menstrual period. Menarche occurs at 13 years of age. Since then she experiences this very severe pain at right side associated with nausea and vomiting. She can't attend the school during menses from past year for which she consulted and started to take NSAIDs. Initially it is effective but after some time it is ineffective. What is next line of management?
     a. Pelvic and abdomen USG
     b. Oral contraceptive pills
     c. Dilatation and curretage
     d. High dose of non-specific steroid

297. Drug of choice in case of Puberty menorrhagia:
     a. Progesterone   b. OCP
     c. IUCD   d. Endometrial curretage

FIBROID

298. During caesarean section which fibroid is the easiest to remove: *(Recent Pattern Question 2018-19)*
     a. Pedunculated   b. Interstitial
     c. Cervical   d. Intramural

299. Which of the following is *not* associated with pain in submucosal fibroids? *(Recent Pattern Question 2018)*
     a. Torsion   b. Large size
     c. Sarcomatous change   d. Red degeneration

300. Most common type of uterine tumor is:
     (Recent Pattern Question 2018)
     a. Leiomyoma   b. Endometrial cancer
     c. Adenomyoma   d. Leiomyosarcoma

301. Retention of urine is caused by which type of fibroid:
     (Recent Pattern Question 2017)
     a. Subserosal   b. Cervical
     c. Intramural   d. Submucosal

302. Hysteroscopical excision can be done for all EXCEPT:
     a. Uterine fundus fibroid   b. Submucous fibroid
     c. Subserous fibroid   d. Endometrial polyp

303. Laproscopic surgery is most applicable to which types of fibroid:
     a. Subserous fibroid   b. Uterine fundus fibroid
     c. Submucous fibroid   d. Endometrial polyp

304. A pregnant female with 16 week AOG presented with bleeding. Upon USG Fibroid detected. Management:
     a. Conservative management
     b. Laparoscopic myomectomy
     c. Curettage
     d. Hysterectomy

305. Drug indicated in uterine fibroid:
     a. Danazol   b. GnRH analogue
     c. Mifepristone   d. All of the above

CHROMOSOMAL ANOMALIES

306. In Turner syndrome all are seen EXCEPT:
     a. Webbed neck
     b. Tall stature
     c. Widening of long bones of leg
     d. XO inheritance

307. Which of the following is true about Turner syndrome?
     a. 45 X Chromosome   b. Primary Amenorrhea
     c. Coarctation of acrta d. All of the above

308. Turner syndrome is
     a. 45 XO   b. 47 XXY
     c. Trisomy 13   d. Trisomy 18

309. Turner syndrome presents with which heart defect?
     a. PDA   b. TOF
     c. Coaractation of aorta d. Mitral stenosis

310. In Down's syndrome, 2nd trimester quadruple test includes all EXCEPT:
     a. Alpha fetoprotein
     b. hCG
     c. Inhibin A
     d. PAPP

311. Young female comes in with primary amenorrhea with normal breast, normal pubic hair. USG reveals absent uterus and cervix with short vaginal pouch and normal ovaries. Diagnosis:
     a. Klinefelter syndrome
     b. Mullerian agenesis
     c. Gonadal dysgenesis
     d. XYY

312. Female pseudohermaphroditism, all are true EXCEPT:
     a. Mullerian inhibiting substance is not produced
     b. Karyotype 46 XX
     c. Ovaries and uterus are absent
     d. Fused posterior labia with prominent clitoral hypertrophy

Obstetrics and Gynecology

TROPHOBLASTIC TUMORS

313. **Most common site of metastasis of choriocarcinoma**
     (Recent Pattern Question 2016)
     a. Lung   b. Liver
     c. GIT   d. Ovaries

314. **After evacuation of molar pregnancy, monitoring is done with** *(Recent Pattern Question 2016)*
     a. Serial TVS   b. Serial serum β hCG level
     c. Speculum examination   d. LDH level

315. **Which of the following is not trophoblast related:**
     a. Choriocarcinoma
     b. H. mole
     c. Placental Site tropboblast tumor
     d. Chorioangioma

INFERTILITY AND CONTRACEPTION

316. **28-year-old lady (G_2P_1) who does not want to conceive after abortion, which is the preferred mode of contraception:** *(Recent Pattern Question 2018-19)*
     a. OCP   b. IUD
     c. Barrier   d. Implant

317. **After a normal delivery OCP is to be started after___:**
     (Recent Pattern Question 2018-19)
     a. 2 weeks   b. 6 weeks
     c. 12 weeks   d. 3 months

318. **In a couple, initial work-up done for infertility:**
     (Recent Pattern Question 2018-19)
     a. Semen analysis, CXR, Montoux
     b. Semen analysis, Tubal patency test, Ovulation test
     c. Ovulation, tubal patency, Montoux test
     d. Testicular biopsy, USG, sperm penetration test

319. **Absolute contraindication of OCP's are all EXCEPT:**
     (Recent Pattern Question 2018)
     a. Smoking   b. Age <35 years
     c. Lactation   d. Breast cancer

320. **OCP can lead to:** *(Recent Pattern Question 2018)*
     a. Hepatic adenoma   b. Thyroid adenoma
     c. Fibroadenoma   d. Myoma

321. **Which of the following is the preferred mode of contraception recommended during lactation?**
     (Recent Pattern Question 2018)
     a. IUCD   b. DMPA
     c. Progesterone only pills   d. OCP

322. **Which of the following is the first line drug for follicle induction in infertility?** *(Recent Pattern Question 2018)*
     a. Clomiphene citrate   b. GnRH agonist
     c. OCP   d. hCG therapy

323. **Which of these is true about RU_486 given for abortion?**
     a. Used till 11th week   *(Recent Pattern Question 2017)*
     b. Teratogenic effect
     c. Used for emergency contraception
     d. Protects from ectopic pregnancy

324. **Most common complication of IUD insertion**
     (Recent Pattern Question 2016)
     a. Pain   b. Vaginal bleeding
     c. Expulsion   d. Infection

325. **Unexplained infertility is diagnosed in:**
     a. 1% of infertile couples   b. 5% of infertile couples
     c. 10% of infertile couples   d. 2S% of infertile couples

326. **Testicular biopsy is best indicated in diagnostic workup of patient with:**
     a. Azoospermia   b. Oligospermia
     c. Necrospemnia   d. Pyospermia

327. **A couple after four days of having sex, contraceptive recommended:**
     a. Oral contraceptive pills
     b. CuT 380
     c. Yuzpe method
     d. Low dose POP with norgesterol

328. **Failure rate of Pomeroy's technique of sterilization is:**
     a. 0.1% to 0.3%   b. 0.3% to 1%
     c. 1.0% to 1.5%   d. 1.6% to 2.0%

329. **Contraceptive effect of CuT-380A lasts for how many years?**
     a. 5   b. 10
     c. 15   d. 20

330. **Levo-norgesterol all statement are true EXCEPT:**
     a. Used in combined OCP with estrogen
     b. Composition in combined OCP is 0.15 mg
     c. Should be given for 21 days
     d. They are lipid friendly

331. **True about pearl index:**
     a. Population study
     b. Family planning
     c. Contraceptive methods
     d. Contraceptive failure

332. **All are benefits of OCPs EXCEPT:**
     a. Improve menstrual abnormality
     b. Protect against unwanted pregnancy
     c. Protect from breast cancer
     d. Protect from endometrial cancer

333. **Non-contraceptive benefit of combined oral contraceptive pills include all EXCEPT:**
     a. Protection against endometrial cancer
     b. Protection against cervical cancer
     c. Relief of dysmenorrhoea
     d. Relief of menorrhagia

871

Questions

334. Mechanism of action of combined OCP:
    a. Prevent implantation of ovum
    b. Prevent fertilization
    c. Prevent release of ovum from ovary
    d. Reduce sperm motility

POLYCYSTIC OVARIAN SYNDROME (PCOS)/STEIN LEVANTHAL SYNDROME

335. MC cause of hirsutism:
    (Recent Pattern Question 2018-19)
    a. Drug induced   b. PCOS
    c. Endometriosis   d. Adenomyosis
336. The number of ovarian follicles are increased in:
    (Recent Pattern Question 2018)
    a. Turner syndrome   b. Klinefelter syndrome
    c. PCOD   d. Primary amenorrhea
337. Most common cause of hirsutism in females is:
    a. Metropathica heamorrhagica
    b. PCOD
    c. Endometriosis
    d. PID
338. Patient with history of amenorrhea and hirsutism. USG of uterus given below. Diagnosis:

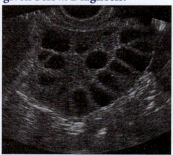

    a. PCOS   b. Endometriosis
    c. Adenomomatosis   d. Choriocarcinoma

339. Primary treatment for hirsutism in PCOD:
    a. Minoxidil
    b. Progesterone
    c. GnRH analogue
    d. Combined OCP

PROLAPSE

340. True about Pessary used in prolapse:
    (Recent Pattern Question 2018-19)
    a. Filling type pessary used
    b. Not preferred in pregnancy
    c. Needs to be changed every 3 months
    d. Never used with Gel to insert
341. Conservative treatment for pelvic organ prolapse:
    (Recent Pattern Question 2018-19)
    a. Perineorrhaphy
    b. Shirodkar procedure
    c. Pessary
    d. Le Fort repair

MISCELLANEOUS

342. A patient presented to you Post hysterectomy with osteoporosis and in need of HRT. What will be the choice of HRT for such patient:
    a. Progestin
    b. Estrogen
    c. Estrogen and progestin both
    d. Testoesterone
343. Best gas used for creating pneumoperitoneum at laparoscopy is
    a. N_2
    b. O_2
    c. CO_2
    d. N_2O

BOARD REVIEW QUESTIONS

344. The ratio of fetal weight and placental weight at term is?
    a. 4:1   b. 5:1
    c. 6:1   d. 7:1
345. Velocity of sperms in female genital tract is?
    a. 0–1 mm/min   b. 1–2 mm/min
    c. 4–5 mm/min   d. 5–6 mm/min
346. True about circumvallate placenta is?
    a. Fetal plate smaller than basal plate
    b. Basal plate smaller than fetal plate
    c. Has accessory lobes
    d. Is membranous

347. Vaccine preventable cancer is?
    a. Endometrial cancer   b. Breast cancer
    c. Cancer cervix   d. Ovarian cancer
348. Subpubic angle in Gynaecoid pelvis is?
    a. 75°   b. 80°
    c. 100°   d. 120°
349. Investigation for bacterial vaginosis is?
    a. Pap smear
    b. Gram stain
    c. Culture
    d. Microscopy

Obstetrics and Gynecology

350. **Vaccum cup is placed?**
   a. Anterior to anterior fontanelle
   b. Posterior to posterior fontanelle
   c. Anterior to posterior fontanelle
   d. Posterior to anterior fontanelle

351. **Intrauterine contraceptive device with an effective life of 10 years is?**
   a. Cu T 380 A
   b. Mirena
   c. Cu T 200
   d. Progestasert

352. **Mirena releases _____ microgram of LNG/day?**
   a. 20
   b. 55
   c. 65
   d. 380

353. **Today vaginal sponge failure rate is:**
   a. 5%
   b. 9%
   c. 16%
   d. 20%

354. **Which of the following causes OCP failure?**
   a. Carbamazepine
   b. Rifampicin
   c. NSAIDS
   d. Ethambutol

355. **Maximum transmission of rubella occurs in:**
   a. 1st trimester
   b. 2nd trimester
   c. 3rd trimester
   d. Labor

356. **Narrowest part of fallopian tube is?**
   a. Infundibulum
   b. Ampulla
   c. Cornual
   d. Interstitium

357. **Glucose challenge test is done with _____ grams of glucose and is seen at _____ hours?**
   a. 75 g and 2 hours
   b. 100 g and 2 hours
   c. 50 g and 1 hour
   d. 75 g and 1 hour

358. **Earliest sign in Sheehan syndrome is?**
   a. Hypomenorrhea
   b. Amenorrhea
   c. Lack of lactation
   d. Cold intolerance

359. **Drug of choice in pregnant women with Secondary Syphilis is?**
   a. Doxycycline
   b. Benzathine Penicillin
   c. Ceftriaxone
   d. Cotrimoxazole

360. **Calcium requirement in pregnancy is?**
   a. 1 g
   b. 1.2 g
   c. 1.5 g
   d. 2 g

361. **Father of obstetrics ultrasound is?**
   a. John Wild
   b. Ian Donald
   c. Mc Donald
   d. Mc Roberts

362. **Number of follicles in female newborn is?**
   a. 1 million
   b. 2 million
   c. 3 million
   d. 4 million

363. **Normal development of a female with absent uterus and vagina indicates?**
   a. Turner's syndrome
   b. Testicular feminizing syndrome
   c. Mullerian agenesis
   d. Gonadal dygenesis

364. **Most common type of conjoined twin is:**
   a. Throracopagus
   b. Craniopagus
   c. Pyopagus
   d. Ischiopagus

365. **Medical management of unruptured tubal pregnancy**
   a. Methrotrexate
   b. Oxytocin
   c. Progesterone
   d. All of above

366. **Biggest fetal skull diameter is**
   a. Biparietal
   b. Bitemporal
   c. Mento vertical
   d. Submentobregmatic

367. **Dusky hue of vestibule and anterior vaginal wall is**
   a. Chadwick sign
   b. Osiander sign
   c. Goodel sign
   d. Hegar sign

368. **Most common Type of female pelvis**
   a. Gynaecoid
   b. Anthropoid
   c. Android
   d. Platy pelloid

369. **Most common cause of Breech presentation**
   a. Prematurity
   b. Twins
   c. Android pelvis
   d. Previous LSCS

370. **A pregnant women with BP 150/100 mmHg, proteinuria after 20 weeks. Diagnosis?**
   a. Pre-eclampsia
   b. Pregnancy induced hypertension
   c. Renal hypertension
   d. Eclampsia

371. **If zygote divides after 8 days it will lead to twin:**
   a. Dichorionic, diamniotic
   b. Monochorionic diamniotic
   c. Monochorionic monoamniotic
   d. Conjoined twins

372. **Incidence of uterine rupture in previous LSCS**
   a. 1%
   b. 0.1%
   c. 5%
   d. 10%

373. **Smallest transverse diameter of fetal head:**
   a. Biparietal
   b. Bitemporal
   c. Bimastoid
   d. Mentovertical

374. **Minimum pressure of uterine contraction to cause pain:**
   a. 10 mm Hg
   b. 15 mm Hg
   c. 30 mm Hg
   d. 45 mm Hg

375. **Piskacek's sign is seen at?**
   a. 6 weeks
   b. 8 weeks
   c. 12 weeks
   d. 16 weeks

376. **Page/Sher classification is used for;**
   a. Placenta previa
   b. Abruption placenta
   c. Eclampsia
   d. None

377. **True abut bacterial vaginosis, is all EXCEPT**
   a. Whiff's test positive
   b. Itchy/pruritus
   c. Clue cells
   d. Grey white discharge

378. **Distention of fallopian tube on ampullary end is seen in**
   a. Hydrosalpinx
   b. Pyosalpinx
   c. Salpingitisisthmicanodosa
   d. Chronic interstitial salpingitis

FMGE Solutions Screening Examination

379. Most common site of genital TB
    a. Fallopian tube   b. Uterus
    c. Cervix   d. Ovary
380. Tadpole cells are seen in?
    a. Invasive carcinoma
    b. Koilocytosis
    c. Carcinoma in situ
    d. Mild dyskaryosis
381. Best test for gonorrhea
    a. Nucleic acid amplification
    b. Gram stain
    c. Culture in Thayer martin media
    d. Elisa
382. Fitz hugh Curtis syndrome is seen with?
    a. Chancroid
    b. L.G.V
    c. Chlamydia
    d. Donovanosis
383. In spinnbarkeit:
    a. Mucus can withstand stretching up to 5 cm
    b. Mucus can withstand stretching up to 10 cm
    c. Mucus can withstand stretching up to 15 cm
    d. Mucus can withstand stretching up to 20 cm
384. Most common type of cervical cancer:
    a. Squamous Cell Ca   b. Small Cell Ca
    c. Adeno Ca   d. Adenoma
385. Best prognostic for endometrial pathology
    a. Transvaginal Ultrasound   b. Biopsy
    c. Hysteroscopy   d. Fractional Curettage
386. Earliest Presentation of Fallopian Tube Cancer:
    a. Painless watery discharge   b. Painless vaginal bleeding
    c. Painful watery discharge   d. Painful vaginal bleeding
387. Most common malignant germ cell ovarian tumor:
    a. Yolk Sac Tumors   b. Dysgerminoma
    c. Dermoid Cyst   d. Brenners
388. Tumor Marker of CA Ovary for follow up
    a. CEA   b. PSA
    c. CA 125   d. BETA hCG
389. Most common cause of dysfunctional uterine bleeding:
    a. PID   b. Endometriosis
    c. Dermoid Cyst   d. Anovulatory
390. Turner syndrome presents with which ....defect?
    a. PDA   b. TOF
    c. Coaractation of aorta   d. Mitral stenosis
391. In down's syndrome, 2nd trimester quadruple test includes all EXCEPT:
    a. Alpha Fetoprotein   b. hCG
    c. Inhibin A   d. PAPP
392. Testicular biopsy is best indicated in diagnostic workup of patient with:
    a. Azoospermia   b. Oligospermia
    c. Necrospemnia   d. Pyospermia
393. A couple presents after four days of having sex, contraceptive recommended.
    a. Oral Contraceptive Pills
    b. CuT 380
    c. Yuzpe Method
    d. Low dose pop with norgesterol
394. Most Common Cause of Hirsutism in Females is:
    a. Metropathica Heamorrhagica
    b. POCD
    c. Endometriosis
    d. PID
395. Ashermann syndrome is:
    a. Adhesion in uterus post curettage
    b. Adhesion in uterus, post salpingectomy
    c. Adhesion in uterus, post salpingitis
    d. All of above
396. All are emergency contraceptives EXCEPT
    a. Copper I.U.D   b. Mifepristone
    c. Levonorgenstrel   d. Norplant
397. Essure is:
    a. Male contraception
    b. Transcervical sterilization
    c. Combined injectable contraceptive
    d. Transdermal patch
398. True about Female condom is all EXCEPT:
    a. Single use
    b. Inner ring smaller than outer ring
    c. Protect against P.I.D
    d. Beneficial in immunological infertility
399. Main support of uterus is:
    a. Cardinal ligament   b. Broad ligament
    c. Uterocervical ligament   d. Pubocervical ligament
400. Presentation when the engaging diameter is Mento-vertical is:
    a. Brow   b. Face
    c. Vertex   d. Breech
401. WHO modified partogram charting starts at cervical dilatation of:
    a. 2 cm   b. 3 cm
    c. 4 cm   d. 5 cm
402. HIV transmission is maximum during?
    a. Labor   b. Early pregnancy
    c. Late pregnancy   d. Post delivery
403. Cause of acidic pH of vagina is due to:
    a. Doderlein Bacilli   b. Gardnerella
    c. Mobilincus   d. Glycogen
404. Most common cause of obstructed Labor in India is:
    a. Android pelvis
    b. Gynecoid pelvis
    c. Platypelloid pelvis
    d. Anthropoid pelvis

Obstetrics and Gynecology

405. At what age the product of conception is called as "Embryo"?
   a. 72 hours
   b. 1 week
   c. 3 weeks
   d. 8 weeks

406. Not seen in endometriosis is:
   a. Vaginal discharge
   b. Dyspareunia
   c. Pelvic pain
   d. Dysmennorrea

407. Amniocentesis is done at what intrauterine age:
   a. 10–12 weeks
   b. 12–20 weeks
   c. 20–25 weeks
   d. 25–30 weeks

408. Sign seen in USG in monochorionic diamniotic twins is?
   a. Lambda sign
   b. Twin peak sign
   c. T sign
   d. Membrane thickness >2 mm

409. In dizygotic twin there is:
   a. Always same sex
   b. Always different sex
   c. Seprate chorion and amnion
   d. None

410. Cervix effacement suggestive of onset of Labor is:
   a. 25 mm
   b. 30 mm
   c. 35 mm
   d. 15 mm

411. Most common genital infection in pregnancy is:
   a. Candida
   b. Trichomonas
   c. Chlamydia
   d. Gonorrhea

412. Uteroplacental circulation is established after fertilization:
   a. 1 weeks
   b. 2 weeks
   c. 3 weeks
   d. 4 weeks

413. Fetus most radiosensitive at:
   a. 8–15 weeks
   b. 10–15 weeks
   c. 15–20 weeks
   d. >20 weeks

414. Investigation of choice in post-menopausal bleeding is:
   a. Fractional curettage
   b. D and C
   c. Colposcopy guided endometrial biopsy
   d. PAP smear

415. Amsel criteria for the diagnosis of bacerial vaginosis does not include:
   a. Plenty of lactobacilli
   b. pH > 4.5
   c. Whiff's test positive
   d. Clue cells

416. Billing's method of contraception is a:
   a. Hormonal method
   b. Barrier method
   c. Behavioral method
   d. None

417. Drug of choice for chemotherapy of cervical cancer is:
   a. Cisplatin
   b. Vincristine
   c. Cyclophosphamide
   d. Etoposide

418. Blood volume returns to normal pre pregnant levels, how many weeks after pregnancy?
   a. 1 week
   b. 3 weeks
   c. 4 weeks
   d. 6 weeks

419. Most common cause of rupture uterus in India is:
   a. VBAC
   b. Obstructed Labor
   c. Precipitate Labor
   d. Multiparity

420. A pregnant woman is on anticoagulant therapy is shifted to heparin at:
   a. 28 weeks
   b. 32 weeks
   c. 36 weeks
   d. At the onset of labor

421. Which of the following is known as pregnancy tumor?
   a. Fundal fibroid with pregnancy
   b. Ovarian tumor with pregnancy
   c. Cervical fibroid with pregnancy
   d. Pyogenic granuloma

422. Puerperal sepsis/infection occurs up to:
   a. 1 week
   b. 2 weeks
   c. 3 weeks
   d. 4 weeks

423. Le Forts operation is done in:
   a. Young patient with utero-vaginal prolapse
   b. Elderly patient with utero-vaginal prolapse
   c. Multiparous with utero-vaginal prolapsed
   d. Pregnant patient with utero-vaginal prolapsed

424. In a case of pre-eclampsia Doppler USG will show?
   a. Reversed blood flow in ductusvenosus at 22 weeks
   b. Absent blood flow in umbilical artery at 22 weeks
   c. Diastolic notch in umbilical artery at 22 weeks
   d. Increase peak systolic flow velocity in middle cerebral artery

425. First sign of magnesium sulphate toxicity is:
   a. Loss of deep tendon reflexes
   b. Respiratory depression
   c. Cardiac arrest
   d. Decrease urinary output

426. Treatment of choice of Perimenopausal adenomyosis is:
   a. OCPS
   b. GnRH agonists
   c. LNG IUS
   d. Hysterectomy

427. Clue cells are seen in:
   a. Bacterial vaginosis
   b. Herpes virus
   c. Syphilis
   d. Toxoplasmosis

428. Preterm baby is born before:
   a. 28 weeks
   b. 32 weeks
   c. 34 weeks
   d. 37 weeks

429. Most common cardiovascular condition leading to maternal death in pregnancy is:
   a. ASD
   b. Mitral stenosis
   c. Aortic stenosis
   d. Pulmonary hypertension

430. First symptom of vulval hematoma is:
    a. Pain
    b. Itching
    c. Retention of urine
    d. Swelling of vulva
431. PAP smear invented by:
    a. John papanicolaou
    b. George papanicolaou
    c. Vladimir papanicolaou
    d. Ben papanicolaou
432. Most common site of ectopic pregnancy is ampulla because:
    a. Fertilisation takes place here
    b. It is the widest part
    c. It has very thick mucosal layer
    d. It has less propulsive activity
433. Incidence of breech presentation at term is:
    a. 1%
    b. 3%
    c. 7
    d. 10%
434. Genital tuberculosis most common disseminates by:
    a. Lymphatic
    b. Hematogenous
    c. Local spread
    d. None
435. Which contraceptive should be used after molar pregnancy:
    a. Barrier
    b. Hormonal contraceptives
    c. IUCD
    d. Natural method
436. Drug of choice for eclampsia is:
    a. Magnesium sulphate
    b. Clonazepam
    c. Antihypertensives
    d. Beta blockers
437. Amniotic fluid volume in polyhydramnios is more than:
    a. 500 mL
    b. 1000 mL
    c. 1500 mL
    d. 2000 mL
438. Prepuberty ratio of corpus of uterus and cervix is:
    a. 1:2
    b. 1:1
    c. 2:1
    d. 3:1
439. Serous carcinoma of endometrium is associated with which mutation:
    a. p53
    b. PTEN
    c. k ras
    d. p16k
440. Surfactant appears in amniotic fluid at:
    a. 20 weeks
    b. 24 weeks
    c. 28 weeks
    d. 30 weeks
441. Single best parameter to assess fetal well being is:
    a. Femur length
    b. Head circumference
    c. Abdominal circumference
    d. Amniotic fluid volume
442. RDA of iodine in pregnancy is:
    a. 200 mcg/day
    b. 220 mcg/day
    c. 240 mcg/day
    d. 260 mcg/day
443. Size of ovarian follicle at ovulation is:
    a. 0.5–1 cm
    b. 1–1.5 cm
    c. 1.5–2 cm
    d. 2–2.5 cm
444. Partial mole is:
    a. Haploid
    b. Diploid
    c. Triplod
    d. Polyploid
445. Heart disease with worst prognosis in pregnancy is:
    a. Aortic Stenosis
    b. Pulmonary Hypertension
    c. Uncorrected fallot
    d. Marfan s syndrome with normal aorta
446. Usual causative organism of endocervicitis is:
    a. Herpes simplex virus
    b. Chlamydia
    c. Trichomoniasis
    d. Candida
447. First maneuver to be done incase of shoulder dystocia is:
    a. McRoberts
    b. Wood's corkscrew
    c. Lovset
    d. Zavanelli
448. A 33-year-old female presents with history of 6 months amenorrhea. Biochemical investigations showed increased FSH and decreased Estradiol. Diagnosis is:
    a. PCOD
    b. Hyperprolactinemia
    c. Premature menopause
    d. Ectopic pregnancy
449. What is seen in a menopausal women (2018)
    a. Inc FSH and LH
    b. Dec FSH and LH
    c. Inc FSH and Dec LH
    d. Dec FSH and Inc estrogen
450. Postmenopausal cardiac problem is due to: (2018)
    a. Increase in FSH
    b. Decrease in estrogen
    c. Increase in progesterone
    d. Increase in androgen
451. Contraindication of CuT insertion are all EXCEPT: (2018)
    a. PID
    b. Ectopic pregnancy
    c. Multiparity
    d. Suspected pregnancy
452. Mittelschmerz pain is noted during: (2018)
    a. Ovulation
    b. Menstruation
    c. Delivery
    d. Copulation

Obstetrics and Gynecology

IMAGE-BASED QUESTIONS

453. A 35-year-old lady presents with vaginal discharge. Smears from vaginal discharge show presence of:

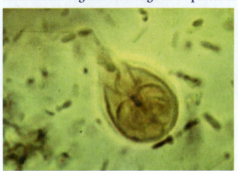

a. Trichomonas
b. Entamoeba histiolytica
c. Toxoplasma
d. Giardia

454. Identify the instrument shown below:

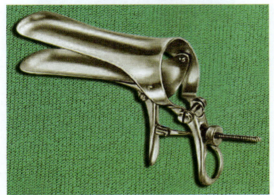

a. Sims speculum
b. Cusco speculum
c. EB curette
d. Deaver's retractor

455. Identify the instruments shown in the figure:

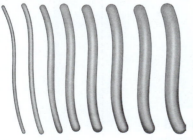

a. Uterine sound
b. Hegar dilator
c. Sims self retaining speculum
d. Interlocking nails

456. The vaginal smear shows presence of:

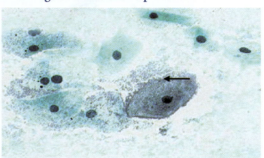

a. Bacterial vaginosis
b. Candidiasis
c. Human papilloma virus
d. Trichomonas vaginalis

457. Least common site of ectopic pregnancy:

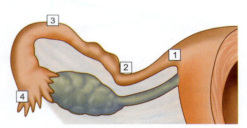

a. Interstitial part
b. Isthmus
c. Ampulla
d. Fimbrial end

458. The HSG report shows:

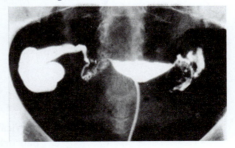

a. Hydrosalpinx
b. Uterus didelphys
c. Adenomyosis
d. Endometriosis

459. The following instrument is called as:

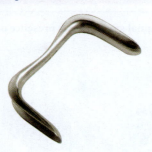

a. Cusco's speculum
b. Vulsellum
c. Sims speculum
d. Vaginal sling

461. The image shows:

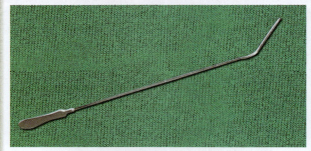

a. Uterine sound
b. Vere's needle
c. Hegar dilator
d. Curette

460. Which instrument is shown below:

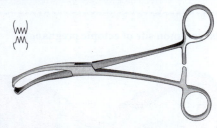

a. Cusco's speculum
b. Vulsellum
c. Sims speculum
d. Vaginal sling

462. The image shows:

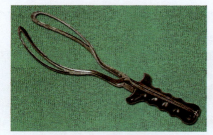

a. Outlet forceps
b. Keilland forceps
c. Piper forceps
d. Artery forceps

463. Identify the image and its use:

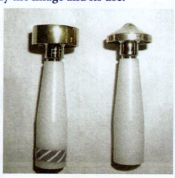

a. Cervical dilator   b. Uterine sound
c. Babcock   d. Cryotherapy probe

Answers to Image-Based Questions are given at the end of explained questions

Obstetrics and Gynecology

ANSWERS WITH EXPLANATIONS
OBSTETRICS
MOST RECENT QUESTIONS 2019

1. Ans. (b) USG

Ref: Shaw's Gynecology 16th ed. P 329

- In a patient with primary amenorrhea and secondary sexual characteristics, we need to rule out conditions like androgen insensitivity syndrome and MRKH syndrome. But before that checking the presence or absence of uterus with help of ultrasonography decides the further steps like karyotyping or hormonal studies.
- *Please refer the flowchart below*

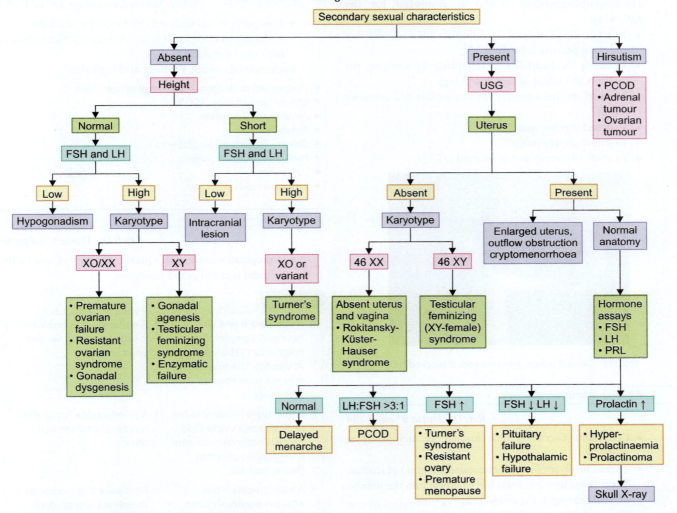

FLOW CHART: Investigations in amenorrhea

2. Ans. (c) Bed rest and Progesterone

Ref: DC Dutta 9th ed. P 153-54

- The patient is a case of threatened abortion, which can present with brisk bleeding.
- This bleeding usually stops spontaneously upon bed rest.
- **Definition of Threatened abortion:** "a clinical entity where the process of miscarriage has started but has not progressed to a state from which recovery is impossible"

FMGE Solutions Screening Examination

- **Treatment:**
  - Bed rest and sternuous activity restriction
  - Treatment with progesterone induces immunomodulation to shift the Th1 (proinflammatory response) to Th2 (anti-inflammatory response)
- **Note:** Use of hCG is not preferred.

3. Ans. (b) **Hysterosalpingography**

    Ref: Shaw's Gynecology 16th ed. P 111-12

- Pelvic inflammatory disease can cause tubal blockage, which can cause infertility.
- Therefore HSG is done to rule out PID induced tubal blockage

Hysterosalpingography (HSG) is employed for the following:

- To study the patency of the fallopian tubes in infertility and postoperative tuboplasty.
- To assess the feasibility of tuboplasty by studying the location and extent of tubal pathology.
- To study uterine anomaly such as septate and cornuate uterus.
- To detect uterine synechiae.
- To detect uterine polyp.
- To study incompetence of internal OS.

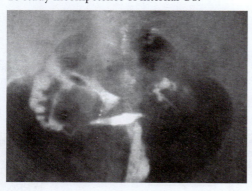

FIGURE: Genital tuberculosis—beaded blocked tubes

4. Ans. (c) **Abruptio placenta**

    Ref: DC Dutta 9th ed. P 238

- Couvelaire Uterus is also known as uteroplacental apoplexy.
- It leads to severe form of concealed abruptio placentae. There is massive intravasation of blood into the uterine musculature up to the serous coat.
- The condition can only be diagnosed on laparotomy.
- Upon naked eye examination of such uterus, it is dark port wine color which may be patchy or diffuse.
- **Note:** Presence of couvelaire uterus is not an indication per se for hysterectomy.

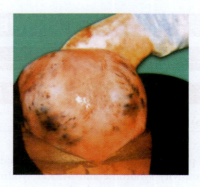

5. Ans. (d) **Multigravida**

    Ref: Shaw's Gynecology 16th ed P 508

- Low parity is an increased risk factor for development of endometrial CA. Out of given choices, multigravida is at least risk of endometrial CA

Endometrial cancer: Etiology and high risk

- Unopposed oestrogen or high level of oestrogen
- Chronic anovulation, PCOD
- Familial predisposition
- Tamoxifen
- Obesity, hypertension, diabetes
- Feminizing ovarian tumour
- Low parity
- Late menopause

6. Ans. (c) **>4**

    Ref: DC Dutta 9th ed pg 86

- A pregnant woman with a previous history of four births or more is called grand multipara.

Extra Mile

A nullipara is one who has never completed a pregnancy to the stage of viability. She may or may not have aborted previously.	**A nulligravida** is one who is not now and never has been pregnant
A primipara is one who has delivered one viable child. Parity is not increased even if the fetuses are many (twins, triplets)	**A primigravida** is one who is pregnant for the first time
A multigravida is one who has previously been pregnant. She may have aborted or have delivered a viable baby	**Multipara** is one who has completed two or more pregnancies to the stage of viability or more
A parturient is a women in labor	**A puerpera** is a woman who has just given birth

Obstetrics and Gynecology

7. Ans. (c) Gestational Hypertension

Ref: DC Dutta 9th ed P 207

TABLE: Classification of hypertension in pregnancy (National high blood pressure education program 2000 and ACOG-2013)

Disorder	Definiton	Disorder	Definition
Hypertension	BP ≥140/90 mm Hg measured two times with at least 6-hour interval	Chronic hypertension with superImposed preeclampsia and eclampsia	The common causes of chronic hypertension: • Essential hypertension • Chronic renal disease (renovascular) • Coarctation of aorta • Endocrine disorders (diabetes mellitus, pheochromocytoma, thyrotoxicosis) • Connective tissue diseases (Lupus erythematosus) The criteria for diagnosis of superimposed preeclampsia: • New onset of proteinuria >0.5 g/24 hours specimen • Aggravation of hypertension • Development of HELLP syndrome • Development of headache scotoma, epigastric pain
Proteinuria	Urinary excretion of >0.3 g protein/24 hours specimen or 0.1 g/L		
Gestational hypertension	BP >140/90 mm hg for the first time in pregnancy after 20 weeks, without proteinuria		
Preeclampsia	Gestational hypertension with proteinuria		
Eclampsia	Women with preeclampsia complicated with grand mal seizures and/or coma		
HELLP syndrome	• Hemolysis (H) • Elevated liver enzymes (EL) • Low platelet count (LP)		
Chronic hypertension	Known hypertension before pregnancy or hypertension diagnosed first time before 20 weeks of pregnancy		
Superimposed preeclampsia or eclampsia	Occurrence of new onset of proteinuria in women with chronic hypertension		

8. Ans. (d) 20 million/mL

Ref: Shaw's Gynecology 16th ed. P 243-44

TABLE: Latest WHO recommendations of normal semen analysis reference values

- Volume: 1.5–5.0 mL
- pH: >7.2
- Viscosity: <3 (scale 0–4)
- Sperm concentration: >20 million/mL
- Total sperm number: >40 million/ejaculate
- Percent motility: >50%
- Forward progression: >2 (scale 0–4)
- Normal morphology: >50% normal
- Round cells: <5 million/mL
- Sperm agglutination: <2 (scale 0–3)

Source: WHO guidelines

9. Ans. (d) Premenstrual period

Ref: Shaw Gynecology 16th ed. P 255

ENDOMETRIAL BIOPSY

- Although endometrial biopsy has been widely replaced for serial ultrasound monitoring, if ever needed, it is preferably done 1 or 2 days before the onset of menstruation.
- The material removed should be fixed immediately in formalin saline and submitted to histological scrutiny.
- Secretory changes prove that the cycle has been ovulatory.

FMGE Solutions Screening Examination

10. Ans. (d) Progesterone

- The shown graph in question marked with X is due to progesterone effect in luteal phase.
- Follow the image for better understanding:

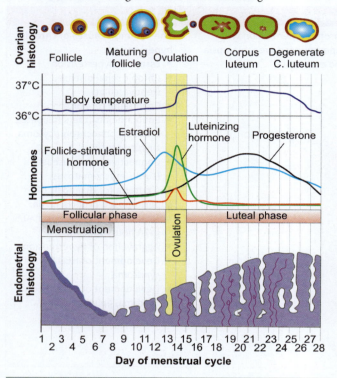

11. Ans. (c) Remove IUCD and continue pregnancy

Ref: Shaw's Gynaecology 16th ed. pg. 271, 272

- In patients with in-situ IUCD, pregnancy occurs in 1–3 per 100 women years.
- If this happens, it is important to do ultrasound and rule out ectopic pregnancy.
- The uterine pregnancy can cause severe infection. It is therefore mandatory to remove the IUCD if the tail is visible through the os.
- While doing so, the risk of abortion should be explained to the woman. If the thread of the IUCD is not seen, termination of pregnancy is offered, not because IUCD has any teratogenic effect but because the risk of uterine infection is considerable. Alternatively, the pregnancy is continued after counselling and explaining the risk.

12. Ans. (c) Renal agenesis

Ref: DC Dutta 9th ed. pg. 203, 204

- Oligohydramnios is an extremely rare condition **where the liquor amnii is deficient in amount to the extent of** less than 200 mL at term.
- **Sonographically, it is defined** when the maximum vertical pocket of liquor is less than <2 cm or when amniotic fluid index (AFI) is less than 5 cm (less than 5 percentile).
- Absence of any measurable pocket of amniotic fluid is defined as Anhydramnios. AFI between 5 and 8 is termed as borderline AFI or borderline Oligohydramnios.
- Internal organ malfunction like renal agenesis can cause this problem.

Causes:

Fetal cause	Maternal cause

• Renal cause (MCC)
  ▪ Renal agenesis
  ▪ Polycystic kidney
  ▪ Urethral obstruction
• Fetal growth restriction
• Premature rupture of membranes
• Post-term pregnancy
• Fetal death
• Drugs exposure like: PG inhibitor, ACE inhibitor
	• Hypertension
	• Uteroplacental insufficiency
	• Dehydration
	• Idiopathic

ANATOMY AND PHYSIOLOGY

13. Ans. (c) Syncytiotrophoblast

Ref: DC Dutta 9th ed. P 53-54

- From placenta, syncytiotrophoblast is the principal site of protein and steroid hormone synthesis.
- **hCG:**
  - A glycoprotein hormone
  - MW: 36000–40,000 dalton
  - Has 2 subunits: α and β
  - α: Hormone non-specific (92 Amino acid). **Biochemically similar to LH, FSH and TSH.**
  - β: Hormone specific (145 Amino acid). Unique for hCG.
- **Functions:**
  - Rescue and maintenance of corpus luteum till 6 weeks of pregnancy
  - Stimulate leydig cell of male fetus (to produce testosterone)
  - Immunosuppressive activity
  - Stimulate both adrenal and placental steroidogenesis
  - Promote secretion of relaxin from the corpus luteum.

Obstetrics and Gynecology

> **Extra Mile**
> - hCG disappears from circulation within 2 weeks following delivery
> - **hPL (Human Placental Lactogen)** aka human chorionic somato-mammotropin; Similar to GH and prolactin.
>   - First detected during the 3rd week of gestation. Its plasma concentration rises proportionatally to placental mass
>   - **Func:** Causes maternal lipolysis and promote transfer of glucose and amino acid to the fetus.
> - **Pregnancy specific β-1 Glycoprotein (PS β-1G):** Produced by trophoblast cell. Detected in maternal serum 18–20 days after ovulation. Potent immunosuppressor → prevent rejection of conceptus.

14. Ans. (a) Symphysis pubis to umbilicus

Ref: DC Dutta Obstetrics 8th ed. P 78

DC Dutta states: During progression of pregnancy the height of uterus is:
- Midway between the symphysis pubis and umbilicus at 16th week
- At the level of umbilicus at 24th week and
- At the junction of the lower third and upper two-thirds of the distance between the umbilicus and ensiform cartilage at 28th week.

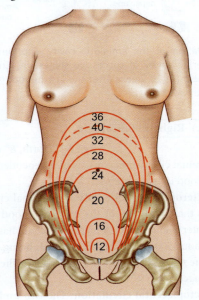

The level of fundus uteri at different weeks.
Note: *The change of uterine shape*

15. Ans. (c) Progesterone effect

Ref: DC Dutta 8th ed. P 114

Dutta states: *"Constipation is a quite common ailment during pregnancy. Atonicity of the gut due to the **effect of progesterone**, diminished physical activity and pressure of the gravid uterus on the pelvic colon"*

> **Extra Mile**
> **Reasons of other ailments during pregnancy**
> - **Leg cramps** during pregnancy may be due to deficiency of diffusible serum calcium or elevation of serum phosphorus.
> - **Backache:** Physiological changes that contribute to backache are: joint ligament laxity (relaxin, estrogen), weight gain, hyperlordosis and anterior tilt of the pelvis. It is a common problem (50%) in pregnancy.

16. Ans. (a) T1

Ref: DC Dutta, 8th ed. pg. 53

- **Dutta states:** *"Increased frequency of micturition is noticed at 6–8 weeks of pregnancy which subsides after 12 weeks"*.
- Urine frequency increases initially in first trimester. Normally, uterus is anteverted in position and is exaggerated up to 8 weeks.
- This enlarged uterus may lie on the bladder rendering it incapable of filling, clinically evident by increased frequency of micturition. Afterwards, it becomes erect, the long axis of the uterus conforms more or less to the axis of the inlet.

17. Ans. (a) Rise by 25%

Ref: DC Dutta, 8th ed. pg. 70

- During pregnancy glomerular filtration rate increases, which causes increased renal clearance of iodine.
- **Maternal serum iodine levels fall** due to increased renal loss and also due to transplacental shift to the fetus. These cause hyperplasia of the gland.
- **Therefore** iodine intake during pregnancy should be increased from 100 μg/day to 200 μg/day (as recommended by WHO).
- **There is rise in the basal metabolic rate**, which **begins at about the third month**, reaches a value of **+25% during the last trimester**.
- This increase in BMR is probably due to increase in net oxygen consumption of mother and fetus.

18. Ans. (a) Mentovertical

Ref: DC Dutta, 8th ed. pg. 96

- **Largest fetal head diameter is Mentovertical.**

FMGE Solutions Screening Examination

TABLE: Important diameters of the skull

Diameters	Measurement in cm (Inches)	Attitude of the Head	Presentation
Suboccipitobregmatic—extends from the nape of the neck to the center of the bregma	9.5 cm (3 ¾")	Complete flexion	Vertex
Suboccipito-frontal—extends from the nape of the neck to the anterior end of the anterior fontanel or center of the sinciput	10 cm (4")	Incomplete flexion	Vertex
Occipitofrontal—extends from the occipital eminence to the root of the nose (Glabella)	11.5 cm (4 ½")	Marked deflexion	Vertex
Mentovertical—extends from the midpoint of the chin to the highest point on the sagittal suture	14 cm (5 ½")	Partial extension	Brow
Submentovertical—extends from junction of floor of the mouth and neck to the highest point on the sagittal suture	11.5 cm (4 ½")	Incomplete extension	Face
Submentobregmatic—extends from junction of floor of the mouth and neck to the center of the bregma	9.5 cm (3 ¾")	Complete extension	Face

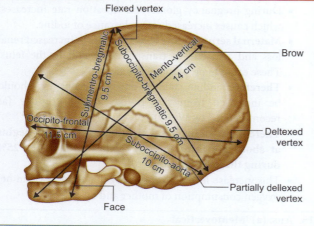

19. Ans. (d) 12 weeks

Ref: DC Dutta, 8th ed. pg. 32-33

- The placenta is developed from two sources:
  - **Fetal component:** The principal component *(which develops from the chorion frondosum)*
  - **Maternal component** consists of decidua basalis. *(Only the decidua basalis and the blood in the intervillous space are of maternal origin.)*
- **At 3rd–4th week:** Lacunar spaces become confluent with one another and form a multilocular receptacle lined by syncytium and filled with maternal blood. This space becomes the future intervillous space.
- **At 6th week:** Decidua capsularis becomes thinner and both the villi and the lacunar spaces in the embryonic area get obliterated, converting the chorion into chorion laeve.
- Because of this there is compensatory growth and proliferation of the **decidua basalis** and enormous and exuberant division and subdivision of the chorionic villi in the embryonic pole (**chorion frondosum**).
- **These two, i.e., chorion frondosum and the decidua basalis form the discrete placenta. It begins at 6th week and is completed by 12th week**

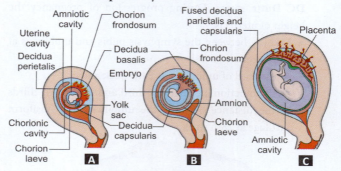

FIGURE: Relation of the amniotic cavity, chorionic cavity and uterine cavity of successive stages; (A) End of the 8th week; (B) 10 weeks after the last period; (C) End of the 12th week

20. Ans. (c) Right umbilical vein

Ref: DC Dutta, 8th ed. pg. 37-38

- Placental circulation consists of independent circulation of blood in two systems:
  - **Uteroplacental circulation** (maternal circulation): It is the circulation of the maternal blood through the intervillous space. A mature placenta has a volume of about 500 mL of blood; **350 mL being occupied in the villi system** and **150 mL lying in the intervillous space**[Q].
  - **Fetoplacental circulation:** The **two umbilical arteries** carry the impure blood from the fetus. The fetal blood flow through the placenta is about 400 mL/min.
  - **Note:** Of the two umbilical veins, **the right one disappears by the 4th month**, **leaving behind left umbilical vein**, which carries oxygenated blood from the placenta to the fetus.

Obstetrics and Gynecology

- Umbilical artery carry deoxygenated blood from fetus to mother

Extra Mile

TABLE: Summary of intervillous hemodynamics (V. Imp)

Volume of blood in mature placenta	500 mL
Volume of blood in intervillous space	150 mL
Blood flow in intervillous space	500–600 mL/min
Pressure in intervillous space: • During uterine contraction • During uterine relaxation	30–50 mm Hg
Pressure in the supplying uterine artery	70–80 mm Hg
Pressure in the draining uterine vein	8 mm Hg

TABLE: Summary of fetal hemodynamics (V. Imp)

Fetal blood flow through the placenta	400 mL/min	
Pressure in the umbilical artery	60 mm Hg	
Pressure in the umbilical vein	10 mm Hg	
Fetal capillary pressure in villi	20–40 mm Hg	
	Umbilical artery	**Umbilical vein**
O$_2$ saturation	50–60%	70–80%
PO$_2$	20–25 mm Hg	30–40 mm Hg

21. Ans. (b) Ductus venosus

Ref: DC Dutta, 8th ed. pg. 49

- **The umbilical vein carrying the oxygenated blood (80% saturated) from the placenta**, enters the fetus at the umbilicus and runs along the free margin of the falciform ligament of the liver. In the liver, it gives off branches to the left lobe of the liver and receives the deoxygenated blood from the portal vein.
- The greater portion of the oxygenated blood, mixed with some portal venous blood, short circuits the liver through the **ductus venosus** to enter the inferior vena cava (IVC) and thence to right atrium of the heart.

TABLE: Hormonal Levels in Different Phases of Menstrual Cycle

22. Ans. (a) Systemic venous resistance

Ref: DC Dutta, 8th ed. pg. 60

Changes during pregnancy:
- Increased in cardiac output
- Increase in HR
- Increase in plasma volume
- **Decrease in SVR** by (−21%) due to smooth muscle relaxing effect of progesterone, NO, prostaglandins or ANP.
- In spite of the large increase in cardiac output, the **maternal BP (BP = CO × SVR) is decreased** due to decrease in SVR. **There is overall decrease in diastolic blood pressure (BP) and mean arterial pressure (MAP) by 5–10 mm Hg**

23. Ans. (c) 4.5–5.5

pH of vagina: Normally it is acidic due to duoderlins bacilli, estrogen. Acidic pH prevents uterus from infection *(since age group is not mentioned, we will be considering the adult in reproductive age group)*
- **Normal pH throughout reproductive life is 4–4.5**
- pH during pregnancy: Less than 4 (becomes more acidic)
- pH at birth: 5.5–6.0
- pH during pre-pubertal age, menstruation and Menopause is similar: 6.5–7.5

24. Ans. (c) 30–70

Ref: DC Dutta, 8th ed. pg. 7 - 8

Cervix: Corpus ratio *(since age group is not mentioned, we will be considering the adult in reproductive age group)*
- **At birth**- 1:1
- **Before puberty**- 2:1
- **After puberty**- 1:2
- **Reproductive life**- 1:3
- **Menopause**- 1:1

25. Ans. (a) Follicular phase

Ref: Shaws, 16th ed. pg. 47

- In follicular phase estradiol level is 100/200 pg/mL and progesterone level is 1 ng/mL, which is least amount together in the menstrual cycle phases.
- *Compare the levels from table*

	NORMAL			
Hormone	**Follicular phase**	**Ovulation**	**Luteal phase**	**Menstrual phase**
FSH	5–15 mIU/mL	12–30	2–9	3–15 mIU/mL
LH	6–14 mIU/mL	25–100	2–13	3–12 mIU/mL
E$_2$	100/200 pg/mL	300–500 pg/mL	100–200	–
Progesterone	1 ng/mL	–	15 ng/mL	–

Contd...

FMGE Solutions Screening Examination

	NORMAL				
Hormone	Follicular phase	Ovulation	Luteal phase	Menstrual phase
17 ketosteroid	Normal	5–10 mg/daily	–	>25 mg in adrenal hyperplasia
Testosterone	Normal	0.2 –0.8 ng/mL	–	>2 ng/mL in ovarian tumors
Androstenedione	Normal	1.3–1.5 ng/mL	–	–
DHEA	Normal	<5 mcg/mL	–	>5 mcg in adrenal hyperplasia
Cortisol	–	<5 mcg/dL	–	–
DHEAS	800 ng/mL	–	–	Adrenal hyperplasia, tumor

26. Ans. (c) Cardinal ligament

Ref: DC Dutta, 8th ed. pg. 7

- Cardinal ligament is also known as Mackenrodt's ligament.
- It is considered as true support of uterus.
- Normal position of uterus is: Anteversion and Anteflexion
- **Function of cardinal ligament:**
  - Lateral stabilization of cervix at the level of ischial spine
  - Primary vascular conduits of the uterus and vagina
- Other ligaments like round and broad ligament act as a guyrope with a steadying effect on the uterus. *They have no role in preventing descent of uterus.*

27. Ans. (c) Bartholin's gland

Ref: Gray's Basic Anatomy/248

- The orifice of urethra and vagina are associated with opening of glands.
- The ducts of para-urethral glands (**skene's gland**) opens into the vestibule, one on each side of the lateral margin of urethra.
- The ducts of greater vestibular gland (**Bartholin's gland**) open adjacent to the **postero-lateral margin of the vaginal opening** in the crease between the vaginal orifice and remanants of hymen.
- Bartholin gland the female homologues of the bulbourethral glands in men.

> **Extra Mile**
> - When bartholin's gland is blocked, a fluid filled cyst named bartholin's cyst develops.
> - TOC for bartholin's cyst: **Marsuplization.**

28. Ans. (c) Bimastoid

Ref: DC Dutta, 8th ed. pg. 94-97

TRANVERSE DIAMETERS OF FETAL HEAD

- Biparietal: 9.5 cm
- Bitemporal: 8 cm
- Bimastoid: 7.5 cm; smallest transverse diameter
- Super subparietal: 8.5 cm

29. Ans. (d) Mentovertical

Ref: DC Dutta, 8th ed. pg. 94-97

DIAMETERS OF SKULL

- The anteroposterior diameters of the head which may engage are:

Diameters	Measurment (In cm)	Presentation
Suboccipitobregmatic	9.5 cm	Vertex
Suboccipitofrontal	10 cm	Vertex
Occipitofrontal	11.5 cm	Vertex
Mentovertical: extend from mid-point of chin to the highest point on the saggital suture	14 cm	Brow
Submentovertical	11.5 cm	Face
Submentobregmatic	9.5 cm	Face

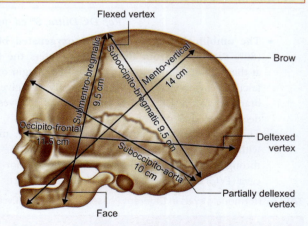

- The transverse diameters which are concerned in the mechanism of labor are
  - **Biparietal diameter** – 9.5 cm: extends between two parietal eminences.
  - **Super-subparietal** – 8.5 cm
  - **Bitemporal diameter**: 8 cm
  - **Bimastoid diameter** – 7.5 cm

Obstetrics and Gynecology

30. Ans. (b) **Intertuberous**

Ref: *DC Dutta, 8th ed. pg. 94-97; William's 23rd ed. Chapter 2, Maternal Pelvic Anatomy*

- Most of the students answer interspinous for this question. Obviously interspinous is having the least diameter (10cm), but it belongs to mid pelvis.
- The question is asking about the shortest diameter of **pelvic outlet**, which is intertuberous *(diameter between ischial tuberosity)* diameter ~ **11 cm**.

PLANES AND DIAMETERS OF THE PELVIS

The pelvis is described as having four imaginary planes:
- The plane of the **pelvic inlet**—the superior strait
- The plane of the **mid pelvis**—the least pelvic dimensions
- The plane of the **pelvic outlet**—the inferior strait
- The plane of greatest pelvic dimension—of no obstetrical significance.

TABLE: Summarized data of maternal Pelvis planes and diameters *(all the numerical datas are derived from standard reference i.e. william's 23rd ed.)*

Plane	Diameter	Measured Between	Size
Pelvic Inlet	Transverse	Greatest distance between the linea terminalis on either side	~ 13 cm
	A-P diameter aka **true conjugate**	Extends from the upper-most margin of the symphysis pubis to the sacral promontory	11cm
	Oblique diameter	Extends from one of the sacroiliac synchondroses to the iliopectineal eminence on the opposite side.	12 cm
Mid Pelvis Measured at level of ischial spine	Interspinous diameter	Between the ischial spines	10 cm
	Anteroposterior	At the level of ischial spine	11.5 cm
Pelvic outlet Makes 2 traingles with common base	Antero-posterior	Coccyx to symphysis pupis	11.5 cm
	Transverse	Between ischial tuberosities	11 cm
	Posterior saggital	Sacro-Coccygeal angle to the midline imaginary line at base	11.5/2 cm

Contd...

FMGE Solutions Screening Examination

Plane	Diameter	Measured Between	Size
Other important pelvic diameters	Obstetrical conjugate	Shortest distance between the sacral promontory and the symphysis pubis	10 cm. obstetrical conjugate is estimated indirectly by subtracting 1.5 to 2 cm from the diagonal conjugate
	Diagonal conjugate	From the lower margin of the symphysis to the sacral promontory	11.5-12 cm

31. Ans. (a) Transverse

Ref: DC Dutta, 8th ed. pg. 99-104

- If such questions are asked regardless of pelvic plain, then **transverse diameter of pelvic inlet has largest diameter (13 cm).** If it is not in option, next best option is oblique diameter (12 cm)
- Smallest diameter regardless of pelvic plain- **Bispinous (10 cm)**
- For more details, please refer to above explanation.

32. Ans. (d) Sacrocotyloid

Ref: DC Dutta, 8th ed. pg. 101

- **Sacrocotyloid—9.5 cm (3¾")**: It is the distance between the midpoint of the sacral promontory to iliopubic eminence (Fig.).
- It represents the space occupied by the biparietal diameter of the head while negotiating the brim in flat pelvis.
- **Other diameter of pelvic inlet:**
  - Anteroposterior: 11 cm
  - Transverse: 13 cm
  - Oblique: 12 cm

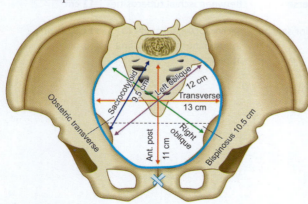

FIGURE: Different diameters of the inlet of obstetrical significance. Bispinous diameter is also demonstrated

33. Ans. (c) Android

Ref: DC Dutta 8th ed. pg. 99-104

- Prominent ischial spine is seen in case of android type of pelvis.
- Pelvis type most favorable for delivery: **Gynecoid**
- MC type of pelvis in females: **Gynecoid**
- Heart shaped pelvis: **Android**
- Flat pelvis: **Platypelloid**

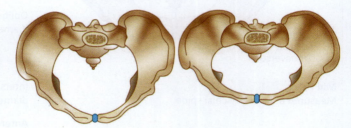

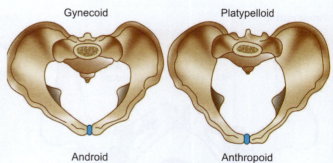

FIGURE: Types of pelvis

- Pelvis MC associated with face and brow presentation: **Platypelloid**
- Pelvis MC associated with occipitoposterior presentation: **Android**
- Pelvis MC associated with face to pubis delivery: **Anthropoid**

Obstetrics and Gynecology

34. Ans. (c) Platelet count

Ref: DC Dutta, 8th ed. pg. 58-59

- During pregnancy, physiological demand increases as the pregnancy advances.
- Plasma volume, RBC count and Hb count increased, but platelet count decreased (*Idiopathic dilutional thrombocytopenia*).
- Following hematological parameters are altered:

Parameters	Alterations
Hb	Increased by: 20%
RBC	Increased by: 20-30%
Blood volume	Increased by: 30-40%
Plasma volume	Increased by: 40-50%
Packed cell volume	Decreased
Platelet count	Decreased (dilutional thrombocytopenia)

- Maximum plasma volume is seen at **36** week AOG: **50%**
- Maximum cardiac output: Immediately post partum (highest cardiac output).
- BP fall post partum because of relaxation of all blood vessels.

35. Ans. (d) Factor XI

Ref: DC Dutta, 8th ed. pg. 58; William's Obstetrics 23rd ed. pg. 121-122

- Pregnancy is a hypercoagulable state. All clotting factors are increased during pregnancy except **factor XI and XIII which decreases** (11 and 13).
- Note: Clotting time and bleeding time remains unaffected during pregnancy.

36. Ans. (b) Pregnancy

Ref: Dutta's Obstetrics, 7th ed. pg. 431-438

- Amenorrhea is the absence of menstrual bleeding. It is a normal feature in prepubertal, pregnant, and postmenopausal females.
- **Primary amenorrhea** is defined as the absence of menses by age 16 in the presence of normal developmental and secondary sexual characteristics or by age 14 if secondary sexual characteristics have failed to develop
- **Secondary amenorrhea** refers to the absence of menses for 6 months or more in a women with previously regular menstrual cycles.

Causes

- Primary amenorrhea may result from congenital reproductive tract abnormalities or endocrine disorders that delay the onset of puberty.
  - Ex: HPA dysfunction, Kallman's syndrome, CNS tumors, turner syndrome, mullerian agenesis etc.

- The most common cause of secondary amenorrhea is pregnancy.
- Other causes of secondary amenorrhea can be: Tubercular Endometritis, PCOS, Cushing's disease, Sheehan's syndrome, Uterine synechiae secondary to vigorous curettage.

37. Ans. (a) 3 days after menstruation

Ref: DC Dutta, 8th ed. pg. 56, 7th ed. pg. 540

- **Breast self-examination** (BSE) is a screening method used in an attempt to detect early breast cancer. The method involves the woman herself looking at and feeling each breast for possible lumps, distortions or swelling.
- **For premenopausal women**, the most commonly recommended time is **just after the end of menstruation**, because the breasts are least likely to be swollen and tender at this time.
- According to given options, 3 days after menstruation is the best choice for BSE.
- For postmenopausal or have irregular cycles might do a self-exam once a month regardless of their menstrual cycle.

38. Ans. (d) 2 weeks before next menstruation

Ref: DC Dutta, 8th ed. pg. 22, 7th ed. pg. 19

- Ovulation is a process whereby a secondary oocyte is released from the ovary following rupture of a mature Graafian follicle and becomes available for conception.
- *In relation to the menstrual period, the event occurs about 14 days prior to the expected period.*

39. Ans. (b) Ductus venosus

Ref: DC Dutta, 8th ed. pg. 36; William's Obstetrics 23rd ed. Ch: 4

- Ductus venosus carries oxygenated blood from placenta and drains into IVC.
- Ductus arteriosus is a connection between aorta and pulmonary arteries, thereby bypassing lung. Persistence of ductus arteriosus leads to a congenital heart condition called Patent Ductus Arteriosus.
- Foramen ovale is connection between right atrium and left atrium.
- Umbilical artery carries deoxygenated blood from fetus to mother.

40. Ans. (c) Cardinal vein

Ref: DC Dutta, 8th ed. pg. 50

- The cardinal veins form as the basis for the intraembryonic venous part of the circulatory system. Various venous systems appear in various stages of the embryo-

FMGE Solutions Screening Examination

genesis and partially disappear again. Very early in the development two paired systems appear:
- The **superior cardinal veins** bring the blood from the head region via the left and right common cardinal vein
- The **inferior cardinal veins** drain the blood from the lower half of the body into the two common cardinal veins
- From here, the blood is emptied into the **sinus venosus** and into the atrium via the **sinus horns**.

Rest of structures given in option closes AFTER birth, with following sequence:
U- Umbilical vein
F- Foramen ovale
A- Ductus Arteriosus
V- Ductus Venosus

41. Ans. (d) 24 weeks

Ref: DC Dutta, 8th ed. pg. 54, 78; 7th ed pg. 69

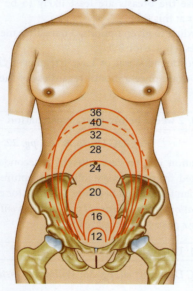

Dutta in 8th ed. States
The height of uterus is midway between symphysis pubis and umbilicus at 16 week and at the level of umbilicus at 24th week.

TABLE: Gestational age and fundal height

Gestational age	Fundal height landmark
12 weeks	Pubic Symphysis
24 weeks	Umbilicus
36 weeks	Xiphoid Process of Sternum
37–40 weeks	Regression of fundal height between 36-32 cm

42. Ans. (a) Milk production

Ref: DC Dutta, 8th ed. pg. 136, 574

Milk production is by Prolactin.

EMBRYOLOGY

43. 24. Ans. (b) Fetal urine

Ref: DC Dutta 9th ed. P 34

- The exact origin of amniotic fluid is not well understood. It is believed that it is mainly due to mixed maternal and fetal origin.
  - **Early stages:** Skin and placenta
  - **12–14 weeks AOG:** Lung and kidney
  - **20 weeks AOG:** Kidney
- The water in the amniotic fluid is completely changed and **replaced in every 3 hours**

Production	Removal
• **Transudation** of maternal serum across the placental membranes • **Transudation** from fetal circulation across the umbilical cord or placental membranes • **Secretion** from amniotic epithelium • **Transudation** for fetal plasma through the highly permeable **fetal skin** before it is keratinized at 20th week • **Fetal urine:** Daily output at term is about 400-1,200 ml • **Fetal lung** that enters the amniotic cavity add to its volume	• **Fetus swallows** about 500-1000 mL of liquor every day • **Intramembranous absorption** of water and solutes (200–500 mL/day) from the amniotic compartment to fetal circulation through the fetal surface of the placenta.

- Volume of amniotic fluid according to AOG:
  - At 12 weeks: 50 mL
  - At 20 weeks: 400 mL
  - At 36–38 weeks: 1 Litre (peak)
  - At **term: 600–800 mL**
  - 43 week: 200 mL

> **Extra Mile**

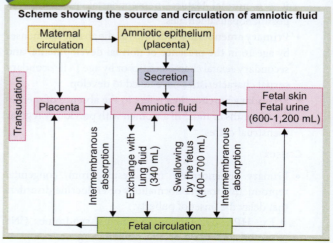

Scheme showing the source and circulation of amniotic fluid

Obstetrics and Gynecology

44. Ans. (a) USG
Ref: DC Dutta Obstetrics 8th ed. P 41

- In general population the investigation modality to screen Down syndrome is USG, which is readily available.
- **Nuchal translucency**—Increased fetal nuchal skin thickness (in the first trimester) >3 mm by TVS is a strong marker for chromosomal anomalies (trisomy 21, 18, 13, triploidy and Turner's syndrome).
- **For confirmation** fetal karyotyping is done.
- **Earliest investigation which can confirm the diagnosis is chorionic villi sampling, which can be done transcervically** between 10 weeks and 13 weeks and **transabdominally** from 10 weeks to term.

TABLE: Prenatal diagnosis: CVS, amniocentesis and cordocentesis

	Chorionic villus sampling	Amniocentesis	Cordocentesis
Time	• Transcervical 10–13 weeks • Transabdominal 10 weeks to term	After 15 weeks (early 12–14 weeks)	18–20 weeks
Materials for study	Trophoblast cells	• Fetal fibroblasts • Fluid for biochemical study	• Fetal white blood cells (others—infection and biochemical study)
Karyotype result	• Direct preparation: 24–48 hours • Culture: 10–14 days	• Culture: 3–4 weeks	• Culture: 24–48 hours
Fetal loss	0.5–1%	0.5%	1–2%
Accuracy	Accurate; may need amniocentesis for confirmation	Highly accurate	Highly accurate
Termination of pregnancy when indicated	1st trimester—safe	2nd trimester—risky	2nd trimester—risky
Maternal effects following termination of pregnancy	Very little	More traumatic; physically and psychologically	Same as amniocentesis

Extra Mile

TABLE: Ultrasound markers of chromosomal abnormalities (General sonography)

Observation	Chromosomal abnormality
Head • Choroid plexus cyst • Strawberry skull • Hydrocephalus • Holoprosencephaly	Trisomy 18, 13 triploidy
Face • Cleft lip/palate • Micrognathia • Low set ears	Trisomy 13, 18, Meckel-Gruber syndrome Triploidy
Nuchal translucency >3 mm	Trisomy 21, 18, 13, Turner syndrome
Cardiac defects	Trisomy 13, 18, 21
Renal anomalies • Horseshoe kidney • Bilateral dilatation of renal pelvis • Cystic dysplasia	Trisomy 13, 18, 21 Triploidy
Hands/feet • *Flexed overlapping fingers* • Rockerbottoms/club foot • Polydactyly • Wide gap between 1st and 2nd toes • Clinodactyly • Short femur	 Trisomy 18 Trisomy 13 Trisomy 21
GI system • Echogenic bowel • Omphalocele • Duodenal atresia	Trisomy 13, 18 Trisomy 21
General • Early IUGR • Hydrops	Trisomy 13, 18, 21 Triploidy, 45XO

FMGE Solutions Screening Examination

45. Ans. (c) Continuous electrical fetal monitoring

Ref: DC Dutta Obstetrics 8th ed. P 693-94

- Continuous electronic fetal monitoring is done by using ultrasound Doppler effect. The transducers are placed on the maternal abdomen, one over the fundus and the other at a site where the fetal heart sound is best audible.
- Frequency of uterine contractions and uterine pressure are recorded simultaneously by tocodynamometer.
- **Book states:** *"Intermittent auscultation is an effective method. Fetuses with abnormal FHR pattern on auscultation should have EFM."*
- *"EFM is most reliable when FHR pattern is reassuring and when there is fetal acidosis."*

Advantages of EFM over clinical monitoring:
- Accurate monitoring of uterine contractions.
- Significant improvement of perinatal mortality.
- Can detect hypoxia early and can explain the mechanism of hypoxia and its specific treatment.
- Improvement of intrapartum fetal death by threefold.
- It is an important record for medicolegal purpose.

46. Ans. (c) 15–18 weeks

Ref: DC Dutta Obstetrics 8th ed. P 741

- Amniocentesis is the deliberate puncture of the amniotic fluid sac per abdomen for diagnostic and therapeutic purposes.
- **It is best done in early months at around 15–20 weeks. For diagnosis** of chromosomal and genetic disorders like:
  - Sex-linked disorders
  - Karyotyping
  - Inborn errors of metabolism
  - Neural tube defects.

47. Ans. (c) 20 mm

Ref: DC Dutta 8th ed./22; Shaw's 15th ed. /Harrison 19/e

- Preovulatory graffian follicle is **18–20 mm**
- Rate of growth of follicle **2–3 mm/day**
- Growth and size of follicle measured by **TVS**, started on 10th day of cycle (in case of infertility), done alternate day.
- Just prior to ovulation its size of follicle is **18–20 mm**, and endometrium is **trilaminar** in appearance.
- When the egg enters the fallopian tube, it is surrounded by a cumulus of granulosa cells (cumulus oophorus) and intimately surrounded by a clear zona pellucida.
- In most mammals, including humans, the egg is released from the ovary in the metaphase II stage.

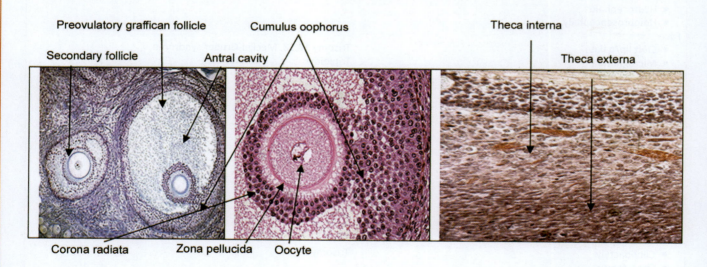

Obstetrics and Gynecology

Stages of Development of Ovum

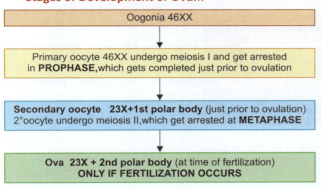

48. Ans. (d) Zona reaction attracts the sperms

Ref: DC Dutta, 8th ed. pg. 23, 7th ed. pg. 21

Once an ovum is fertilized, zona reaction takes place.
- **Zona reaction**-Once sperm penetrates zona pellucida, the ovum become impermeable to other sperms, this prevents polyspermy. *Therefore zona reaction DOESN'T ATTRACT sperm.*
- When more than one sperm manages to enter the ovum (dispermy = 2; triploidy = 3), the fetus nearly always aborts
- 1st Cell division then occurs (20 hour) → gives rise to two-cell embryo

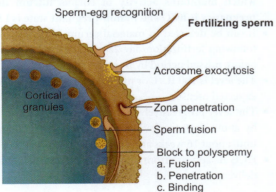

Complete Steps of Fertilization

- **Capacitation** - A period of conditioning that occurs in the **female reproductive tract.**
- **Chemotaxis** -sperm are **attracted to an egg** through the process known as chemotaxis
- Binding of **progesterone** + surface receptor on the sperm → increase in intracellular calcium ion concentration → which increases **sperm motility** (chemokinesis).
- **Acrosome reaction** *(perforations form in the acrosome)* **occurs in ampulla**

- Zonapellucida is a glycoprotein layer surrounding the membrane of oocytes (see image).
- Once sperm reaches ova, there is release of hyluronidase → **penetration of corona radiata** and cumulus cells by sperm.
- Glycoproteins on the outer surface of the sperm then bind with glycoproteins on the zonapellucida of the ovum.

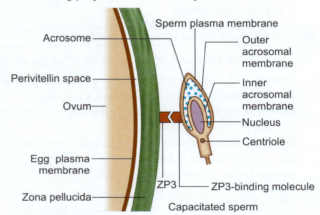

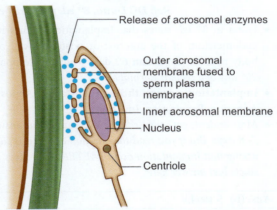

- Release of acrosin occurs → Acrosin digests the zonapellucida and membrane of the oocyte
- After this Sperm enters the cytoplasm → intracytoplasmic structures, the coronal granules, arrange themselves in an orderly fashion (around the outermost portion of the cytoplasm just beneath the cytoplasmic membrane). Swelling of sperm head then occurs, giving rise to male pronucleus.
- Doing this the egg completes its **second meiotic division,** casting off the **second polar body to a position beneath the zonapellucida.**

49. Ans. (c) Prevention of multiple sperm entry

Ref: DC Dutta, 8th ed. pg. 24

- Zona pellucida is a glycoprotein layer surrounding the membrane of oocytes.

- Once sperms reach ova, there is release of hyluronidase → **penetration of corona radiata** and cumulus cells by sperm.
- Glycoproteins on the outer surface of the sperm then bind with glycoproteins on the zona pellucida of the ovum.
- **Zona reaction:** Once sperm penetrates zona pellucida, the ovum become impermeable to other sperms, this prevents polyspermy.

50. Ans. (d) Fertilization takes place in ampula

Ref: DC Dutta, 8th ed. pg. 32-36, 7th ed. pg. 21-22

Option A-Placenta is formed by trophoblast which 1st appear at blastocyst stage, hence option A is wrong.
Option B-Implantation starts on 6th day and completes by 10th day
Option C-During initial weeks corpus leuteum surviaval is due to HCG, not due to LH.
Option D-site of fertilization is ampulla.

51. Ans. (a) 5-6 days

Ref: DC Dutta, 8th ed. pg. 25, 8th ed. 25

- Dutta in 8th ed. states that Implantation occurs in the endometrium of the anterior or posterior wall of the body near the fundus **on 6th day**, which corresponds to 20th day of a regular normal cycle.
- **Implantation occurs through 4 stages**: Apposition, Adhesion, Penetration, Invasion.
- Most students got confused here and marked the answer as 7- 8 days. But if you read the question again, it is cleverly asking that implantation occurs AFTER. 5 – 6 days is the single best answer here.

52. Ans. (b) 5 weeks

Ref: DC Dutta, 8th ed. pg. 734, 7th ed. pg. 68

- 1st radiological investigation for diagnosis of pregnancy is visualisation of gestational sac by TVS.
- **4 ½ weeks**- TVS
- **5 weeks** - by both TVS & TAS

*TVS: Transvaginal scan
*TAS: Transabdominal scan

53. Ans. (a) 15th day

Ref: DC Dutta, 8th ed. pg. 22; Williams Obstetrics 23rd ed. Ch: 3

- Following ovulation (14th day) the remaining follicular cells left by the ovulated follicle differentiate into the corpus luteum (meaning *yellow body.*).
- Corpus luteum secrets progesterone, which causes secretory changes in endometrium.

MENSTRUAL PHASES

Cycle Day	1-5	6-14	15-28
Ovarian phase	Early follicle	Follicular	Luteal
Endometrial phase	Menstrual	Proliferative	Secretory
Estrogen/Progesterone	Low levels	Estrogen	Progesterone

54. Ans. (b) 48 hours

Ref: DC Dutta, 8th ed. pg. 23, 8th ed. pg. 66, 7th ed. pg. 58-59

hCG

- hCG is a glycoprotein which is synthesized by syncytiotrophoblast of the placenta.
- The half-life of hCG is 36 hours.
- In early pregnancy the doubling time of hCG is 1.4–2 days.
- It has 2 subunits:
  - α-biologically similar in LH, FSH and TSH. (i.e. nonspecific)
  - β-subunit-unique to HCG. (i.e. specific)
- Structurally it is similar to- FSH, LH, TSH but functionally it is similar to LH (i.e. luteotropic), i.e. helps in maintaining corpus luteum. So, the **main hormone which maintains activity of corpus luteum during pregnancy is hCG** and in **non-pregnant state is LH**.
- It can be detected in material serum as early as 8 days following fertilization/day 22 of menstrual cycle/5 days before missed period by immuno assay.°
- The level is 100 IU/L or mIU/mL around the time of the expected menses.
- The level progressively rise and reach maximum levels by about 8-10 weeks/70days/1st trimester. It then falls until about 16 weeks and remains at low level up to term.
- HCG disappears from circulation by 2 weeks following delivery.

Action

- Sustains the corpus luteum and thereby maintains the hormonal support to the pregnancy in early weeks.
- Stimulates the leydig cells of the male fetus to produce testosterone and thereby induces development of the male external genitalia

55. Ans. (b) 3rd week

Ref: DC Dutta, 8th ed. pg. 32

- **After interstitial implantation is completed on day 11th**, the blastocyst is surrounded on all sides by lacunar spaces around cords of syncytial cells, called trabeculae.

Obstetrics and Gynecology

- **On 13th day** stem villi develops from the trabeculae which connect the chorionic plate with the basal plate.
- **On 13th, 16th and 21st day** Primary, secondary and tertiary villi are successively developed respectively from the stem villi.
- **Arterio-capillary-venous system in the mesenchymal core of each villus is completed on 21st day (week 3).**

> **Extra Mile**

TABLE: Important events following fertillization

'0' hour	Fertilization (day-15 from LMP)
30 hours	Two-cell stage (blastomeres)
40–50 hours	Four-cell stage
72 hours	Twelve-cell stage
96 hours	16 cell stage. Morula enters the urterine cavity
5th day	Blastocyst
4–5th day	Zone pellucida disappears
5–6th day	Blastocyst attachment to endometrial surface
6–7th day	Differentiation of cyto and syncytiotrophoblastic layers

10th day	Synthesis of hCG by syncytiotrophoblast
9–10th day	Lacunar network forms
10–11th day	• Trophoblasts invade endometrial sinusoids establishing uteroplacental circulation • Interstitial implantation completed with entire decidual coverage
13th day	Primary villi
16th day	Secondary villi
21st day	Tertiary villi
21st–22nd day	Fetal heart. Fetoplacental circulation

56. Ans. (d) Penile urethra

Ref: Shaw, 16th ed. pg. 1

TABLE: Embroyological structure and its derivative in female and male counterparts

Embroyological structure	Female derivative	Male derivative
Genital swelling	Labia majora	Scrotum
Genital fold	Labia minora	Penile urethra
Genital ridge	Ovary	Testis
Genital tubercle	Clitoris	Penis

57. Ans. (b) Urogenital sinus

Ref: Shaw, 16th ed. pg. 124

- Vagina is embroyologically derived from:
  - **Upper 2/3rd:** Mesoderm of Mullerian duct
  - **Lower 1/3rd:** Sinovaginal bulb of endodermal sinus

58. Ans. (b) After 10 weeks from LMP

Ref: DC Dutta, 8th ed. pg. 46

The chronology in the fetal period is expressed in terms of menstrual age and not in embryonic age

Three periods are distinguished in the prenatal development of the fetus.

- **Ovular period or germinal period**—lasts for first 2 weeks following ovulation.
- **Embryonic period:** From 3rd week to 10 weeks following ovulation (8 weeks post conception).
- **Fetal period:** Begins 10 week after ovulation (after 8th week following conception) and ends in delivery.

59. Ans. (a) Ampulla

Ref: DC Dutta, 8th ed. pg. 23

- Fertilization is the process of fusion of the spermatozoon with the mature ovum.
- Almost always, fertilization occurs in the ampullary part of the fallopian tube.

60. Ans. (a) 10 weeks

Ref: DC Dutta, 8th ed. pg. 19, 7th ed. pg. 42

- **Fetal Blood:** Haematopoiesis is demonstrated in the embryonic phase first in the yolk sac by 14th day.
- By 10th week, the liver becomes the major site.
- Gradually, the red cells production sites extend to the spleen and bone marrow and near term, the bone marrow becomes the major site of red cell production.

61. Ans. (d) 7 million

Ref: DC Dutta, 8th ed. pg. 19

- The gonads begin to differentiate. During the 4th or 5th week of development.
- If there is absence of the Y chromosome, the gonads will differentiate into ovaries. As the ovaries differentiate, ingrowths called cortical cords develop where the primordial germ cells collect.
- The primordial germ cells grow and begin to differentiate into oogonia during the 6th to 8th week of female (XX) embryonic development.
- Oogonia then proliferate via mitosis during the 9th to 22nd week of embryonic development.
- By the 8th week of development,there can be up to 600,000 oogonia and **up to 7,000,000 by the 5th month of development.**

62. Ans. (b) Puberty

Ref: DC Dutta, 8th ed./19-20, 8th ed./ 21, 7th ed./17 & 19

- **Oogenesis:** The process involved in the development of a mature ovum is called Oogenesis.
- At 20th week AOG, the number of oogonia reaches at its maximum number, about 7 million.
- While the majority of the oogonia continue to divide, some enter into the prophase of the first meiotic division and are called primary oocytes.
- At birth, total number of oocyte is about 2 million.
- *The primary oocytes do not finish the first meiotic division until puberty is reached.*
- *Now, first meiotic division of primary oocyte takes place at puberty, which give rise to secondary oocyte and first polar body.*
- These two are of unequal size, the *secondary oocyte* contains nearly all the cytoplasm and haploid number of chromosomes (23, X), but the *polar body* contains scanty cytoplasm and half of the chromosomes (23, X).
- Ovulation takes place soon after the formation of the secondary oocyte.
- **2nd meiotic division of secondary oocyte takes place only after fertilization of ova by the sperm.**
- This results in the formation of two unequal daughter cells, each possessing 23 chromosomes (23, X): larger one is the mature ovum and the smaller one is the second polar body containing the equal number of chromosomes.
- The first polar body may also undergo the second meiotic division.
- In the absence of fertilization, the secondary oocyte does not complete the second meiotic division and degenerates as it is.
- *Refer to the flowchart below (must remember it. There's question in almost every exam from this topic)*

Scheme showing gametogenesis

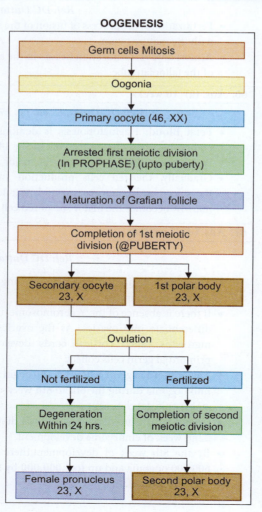

Obstetrics and Gynecology

> **Extra Mile**
> - 1ST polar body released: At time of puberty/ovulation
> - 2nd polar body released: At time of fertilization
> - 1st site of fetal hematopoiesis: Yolk sac.

63. Ans. (a) 1st polar body

Ref: DC Dutta, 8th ed. pg. 19-20; Shaws, 15th ed. pg. 74

PROCESS OF FERTILIZATION

- Certain changes are necessary before the primary oocyte can mature for fertilization. **Oogonia that enter the prophase of the first meiotic division are known as primary oocytes.** Those oogonia which do not begin the first meiotic division and those not surrounded by granulosa layer atrophy.
- At puberty, under the LH surge, primary oocyte completes the first meiotic division and gives rise to secondary oocyte, containing most of the cytoplasm, 23X chromosomes, and a small polar body.
- This secondary oocyte completes its second meiotic division only after fertilization, and gives out second polar body.
- Thus, the first stage of maturation of the oocyte occurs within the graafian follicle, but the second division occurs only after the fertilization in the fallopian tube.
- Please refer to above explanation and flowchart also for detailed explanation.

64. Ans. (c) 1st polar body

Ref: DC Dutta, 8th ed. pg. 21-22, 8th ed. pg. 21, 7th ed. pg. 17,19

65. Ans. (a) Decidua basalis

Ref: DC Dutta, 8th ed. pg. 32

SAILENT FEATURE OF PLACENTA

- Weight-500 g
- Ratio of weight of placenta: Weight of fetus = 1: 6
- Human placenta is discoidal (disc shape) and deciduate (shed off during delivery), hemochoroidal (in contact with maternal blood)
- **Derived forms decidua basalis**
- Placental circulation established at 21-22nd day (same time heart is formed, hence fetal circulation is established.)

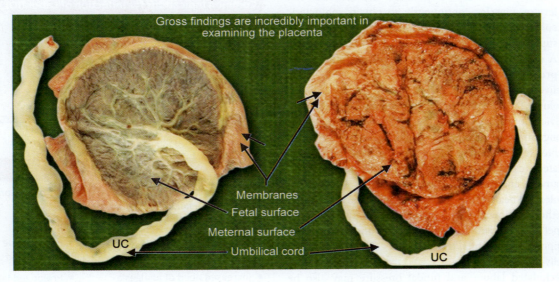

66. Ans. (c) It has umbilical cord attachment site

Ref: DC Dutta, 8th ed. pg. 34-35, 7th ed. pg. 29

Maternal surface of placenta covered by remnant of the deciduas basalis (compact and spongy layer)

Fetal surface	Maternal surface
• Smooth, glistening	• Rough, spongy
• Covered by amnion (above) and chorion (below)	• Covered by remnant of deciduas basalis
• Umbilical cord is attached	• Has 15-20 lobes/cotyledons
• 4/5 of placenta is fetal origin	• 1/5 is maternal origin
• Develops from chorionic sac (chorion frondosum)	• Derived from endometrium (functional layer - Decidua basalis)

LABOR AND DELIVERY

67. And. (d) 3rd degree perineal tear

Ref: DC Dutta 9th ed. P 349-50

- Prolapse is protrusion of the vaginal walls at the vaginal orifice during straining.
- In severe cases, the cervix, uterus and whole of the vaginal wall may be pushed down to the level of the vulva or sometimes it may extrude from the vagina
- MC seen in postmenopausal and multiparous women.
- **Causes of prolapse:**
- **Most important cause:** Atonicity and asthenia that follow menopause.
- Birth injury (overstretching causes atonicity).
    - Book states: *"A perineal tear is less harmful than the excessive stretching of the pelvic floor muscles and ligaments that occurs during childbirth"*
    - Patient with complete perineal tear exercises her levator muscles continuously to obtain sphincteric control over rectum. This tones up all ligamentary support in pelvis in addition to pelvic floor muscles.
    - A complete perineal tear therefore **not followed by prolapse**
- Delivery done by untrained dais/midwives
- Prolong 2nd stage of labour (cause undue stretching of pelvic floor muscles)
- Congenital weakness of pelvic floor muscles
- Ventouse extraction of the fetus before the cervix is fully dilated (causes overstretching of both Mackenrodt's ligaments and the uterosacral ligaments)
- Prolonged bearing down in the second stage and Credè's method of downward vigorous push on the uterus to expel the placenta (it may weaken the ligamentary supports of the genital tract).
- Delivery of a big baby
- Precipitated labour and fundal pressure may also be responsible for prolapse
- Rapid succession of pregnancies
- Raised intra-abdominal pressure due to chronic bronchitis

- Surgical procedures: Abdominoperineal excision of the rectum and radical vulvectomy.

Extra Mile

- Use of forceps is protective against prolapse
- **Classification of Prolapse**
    - **Anterior vaginal wall**
        - Upper two-third Cystocele
        - Lower one-third Urethrocele } Cystourethrocele
    - **Posterior vaginal wall:**
        - Upper 1/3rd: Enterocele (pouch of Douglas hernia)
        - Lower 2/3rd: Rectocele

68. Ans. (c) Immediate LSCS

Ref: DC Dutta 8th ed. P 267

- In this case fetal distress and maternal condition does not warrant tocolytic or wait and watch policy. Therefore immediate CS should be performed.

INDICATIONS OF CESAREAN SECTION

- **When an urgent termination is indicated and the cervix is unfavorable** (unripe and closed).
- **Severe preeclampsia** with a tendency of prolonged induction—delivery interval.
- **Associated complicating factors,** such as elderly primigravidae, contracted pelvis, malpresentation, etc.

Extra Mile

Common Indications for Induction of Labor (IOL)
- Postmaturity
- Pre-eclampsia/eclampsia
- Intrauterine fetal death
- Premature rupture of the membranes
- Congenital malformation of the fetus
- Antepartum hemorrhage
- Chronic hydramnios

TABLE: Dangers of indication of labor

Maternal	Fetal
• Psychological upset when there is induction failure and cesarean section is done	• Iatrogenic prematurity
• Tendency of prolonged labor due to abnormal uterine action	• Hypoxia due to uterine dysfunction
• Increased need of analgesia during labor	• Prolonged labor
• Increased operative interference	• Operative interference
• Increase morbidity	

Obstetrics and Gynecology

69. Ans. (a) Ritodrine

Ref: DC Dutta 8th ed. P 583

- **Preterm labor and delivery** can be delayed by drugs in order to improve the perinatal outcome. These agents are known as tocolytic agents.
- The commonly used drugs are:
  - **Betamimetics:** Ritodrine, Isoxuprine. Causes relaxation of uterus.
  - **Prostaglandin synthetase inhibitors/COX inhibitor:** Indomethacin, sulindac.
  - **Magnesium sulfate:** Act as **competitive inhibitor** of calcium ion.
  - **Calcium channel blockers:** Nifedipine, nicardipine.
  - **Oxytocin receptor antagonists:** Atosiban. Used as IV infusion.
  - **Nitric oxide donors:** Glyceryl trinitrate (used as patches).
  - Progesterone.

70. Ans. (d) Vertex

Ref: DC Dutta 8th ed. P 87

- **Anterior, posterior, right or left position is referred in relation to the maternal pelvis**, with the mother in erect position.
- **Vertex occupying the left anterior quadrant of the pelvis is the most common one** and is called left occipitoanterior (LOA). This is the first vertex position.

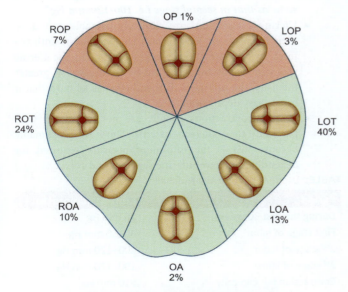

The position and relative frequency of the vertex at the onset of labor

TABLE: Pelvic diameter and presenting part

Diameters	Measurment (in cm)	Presentation
Suboccipitobregmatic	9.5 cm	Vertex
Suboccipitofrontal	10 cm	Vertex
Occipitofrontal	11.5 cm	Vertex
Mentovertical: Extend from midpoint of chin to the highest point on the sagittal suture	14 cm	Brow
Submentovertical	11.5 cm	Face
Submentobregmatic	9.5 cm	Face

71. Ans. (d) Tubal ostia

Ref: William's Obstetrics, 23rd ed. Ch: 18

- The normal contractile wave of labor originates near the uterine end of one of the fallopian tubes (tubal ostia). Thus, these areas act as "pacemakers"

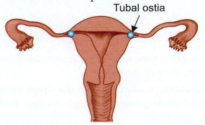

- The right pacemaker usually predominates over the left and starts most contractile waves.
- Contractions spread from the pacemaker area throughout the uterus at 2 cm/sec, depolarizing the whole organ within 15 seconds. This depolarization wave propagates downward toward the cervix.
- Intensity is greatest in the fundus, and it diminishes in the lower uterus.

72. Ans. (c) Fetal head is engaged

Ref: DC Dutta, 8th ed. pg. 153

- Since the type of pelvis may vary from one woman to another (gynaecoid, android, anthropoid and platypelloid), the only effective measure of fetal head descent that reflects engagement is the suprapubic assessment of how much of the fetal skull remains palpable.
- The amount of fetal head felt suprapubically in finger breadth is assessed by placing the radial margin of the index finger above the symphysis pubis successively until the groove of the neck is reached.
- Progressive descent of the head can be usefully assessed abdominally by estimating the number of "fifths" of the head above the pelvic brim
- **Dutta states:** *"when the fetal head is **one-fifth above** (pelvic brim), only the sinciput can be felt abdominally and nought-fifths represents a head entirely in the pelvis with no poles felt abdominally"*

73. Ans. (a) 1/5th of the fetal head palpable

Ref: DC Dutta, 8th ed. pg. 153, 7th ed. pg. 131

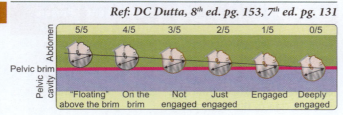

74. Ans. (b) Can damage brain

Ref: DC Dutta, 8th ed. pg. 97

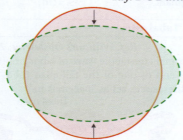

FIGURE: Diagrammatic representation showing the principle of moulding of the head

- **Moulding is alteration of the shape of the fore-coming head while passing through the resistant birth passage during labor.**
- There is very **little alteration** in size of the head.
- Normally, an alteration of **4 mm in skull diameter** commonly occurs.
- It doesn't complicate the delivery, instead it enables the head to **pass more easily,** through the birth canal.
- *Mechanism:* There is compression of the engaging diameter of the head with corresponding elongation of the diameter at right angle to it (Fig.)
- During the process, the parietal bones tend to overlap the adjacent bones, viz.
    - Posteriorly with occipital bone behind
    - Anteriorly, with frontal bones and the
    - At sides, with temporal bones
- **Molding disappears within few hours after birth.**

GRADING

- **Grade-1**—The bones touching but not overlapping
- **Grade-2**— Overlapping but easily separated and
- **Grade-3**—Fixed overlapping *(most severe form)*

Importance:

- **Slight molding is inevitable and beneficial.** It enables the head to **pass more easily,** through the birth canal.
- Extreme molding can result in severe intracranial disturbance in the form of **tearing of tentorium cerebelli or subdural haemorrhage.**
- Can tell the presenting part while delivery.

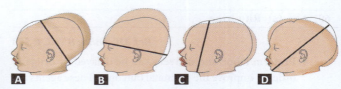

FIGURE: Types of molding in cephalic presentations (shown by dotted line): (A) Vertex presentation with well flexed head; (B) Vertex presentation with deflexed head (sugar loaf head); (C) Face presentation; (D) Brow presentation

75. Ans. (b) 100–120 mm Hg

Ref: William's Obstetrics, 23rd ed. Ch.18 intrapartum Assessment (Internal Uterine Pressure Monitoring)

- A fluid-filled plastic catheter with its distal tip located above the presenting part is used to measure amnionic fluid pressure between and during contractions.
- Clinical labor usually commences when uterine activity reaches values between *80 and 120 Montevideo units*. This translates into approximately three contractions of 40 mm Hg every 10 minutes *(40 × 3 = 120)*.
- **During the first 30 weeks**, uterine activity is comparatively quiescent. Contractions are seldom greater than 20 mm Hg.
- **During first-stage labor**, uterine contractions increase progressively in intensity from approximately *25 mm Hg at* commencement of labor to **50 mm Hg at the end.**
- **DC Dutta states:** "intrauterine pressure is raised to 40-50 mm Hg during 1st stage and about 100-120 mm Hg in second stage of labor during contractions. In spite of diminished pain in 3rd stage, the pressure is probably the same as that in second stage i.e. 100-120 mm Hg"
- Uterine contractions are clinically palpable only after their intensity exceeds 10 mm Hg. Moreover, until the intensity of contractions reaches 40 mm Hg, the uterine wall can readily be depressed by the finger. At greater intensity, the uterine wall then becomes so hard that it resists easy depression.
- Uterine contractions usually are not associated with pain until their intensity *exceeds 15 mm Hg,* presumably because this is the minimum pressure required for distending the lower uterine segment and cervix.

TABLE: Uterine Pressure in a Nutshell

Period	Contraction pressure
During the first 30 weeks	20 mm Hg
First stage of labor	40–50 mm Hg
2nd stage of labor	100–120 mm Hg
3rd stage of labor	100–120 mm Hg
Contraction felt clinically	>10 mm Hg
Contraction associated with pain	15 mm Hg
Pressure required for distending lower uterine segment	15 mm Hg

Obstetrics and Gynecology

76. Ans. (a) 50 mm Hg

Ref: William's Obstetrics, 23rd ed. pg. ch 18

- According to the given options, 50 mmHg is best answer that can be chosen.
- *Please refer to above explanation.*

77. Ans. (a) 7 kg

- *No definite literature or data was found on this question. However we tried to come out with this answer with little bit of physics.*
- Please convert the mm H_2O pressure to kg per mm square it will be almost around 6.79755. Close to 7 kg
- The volume of amniotic fluid controls the pressure inside the uterus. As the volume of amniotic fluid decreases, the pressure inside the uterus increases. While the pressure inside the uterus increases, the amount of force exerted on the fetus increases as well. This can be demonstrated by the following formula:

$$P \text{ (pressure)} = F \text{ (force)}/A \text{(area)}$$

(Pressure can be in the unit of a Pascal or Newton/meter². Standard pressure is 1 atm (atmosphere) or 1.01×10^5 Pa (Pascals). Normal intrauterine pressure is considered any measurement 20 mm over water pressure.)

78. Ans. (b) 2 hours

Ref: DC Dutta, 8th ed. pg. 153

Stages of Labor	Duration	
	Primipara	**Multipara**
Stage I: From uterine contraction to full cervical dilatation (10 cm)	12 hours	6 hours
Stage II: Full dilatation to delivery of baby	*2 hours*	30 mins
Stage III: Delivery of baby to placental delivery	15 mins	15 mins
Satge IV: 1 hour post partum to rule out PPH and vulvar hematoma.	1 hour	1 hour

79. Ans. (a) 30 minutes

Ref: William's 23rd ed. Chapter 17, Normal Labor and Delivery; Preadmission and Admission Electronic Fetal Heart Rate Monitoring

- American Academy of Pediatrics and American College of Obstetricians and Gynecologists (2007) recommend that during the first stage of labor, in the absence of any abnormalities, the fetal heart rate should be checked immediately after a contraction at least every 30 minutes and then every 15 minutes during the second stage.

- *If continuous electronic monitoring is used, the tracing is evaluated at least every 30 minutes* during the first stage and at least every 15 minutes during second-stage labor.
- For women with pregnancies at risk, fetal heart auscultation is performed at least every 15 minutes during the first stage of labor and every 5 minutes during the second stage.
- *Given the above options, every 30 minutes monitoring is the best choice.*

80. Ans. (d) 4 hours

Ref: Williams, 23rd ed. Ch: 17

- On admission, the cervical dilatation should be plotted on the partogram, provided the diagnosis of Labor has been made.
- A partogram was designed by the World Health Organization (WHO) for use in developing countries
- The partograph is similar for nulliparas and multiparas.
- Labor is divided into a latent phase (8 hrs), and an active phase. The active phase starts at 3 cm dilatation, and progress should be no slower than 1 cm/hr.
- An alert line is drawn at 1 cm/h once the active phase of Labor has been reached, and an action line is then drawn parallel and to the right of this.
- Pelvic examination is done at 4 hours.

81. Ans. (c) 3rd stage of labor

Ref: High risk pregnancy 4th ed. by James et. al, ch 75- Normal third stage of Labor

There are four stages of labor

- **The first stage** is from the onset of true labor to complete dilation of the cervix.
- **The second stage** is from complete dilation of the cervix to the birth of the baby.
- **The third stage** is from the birth of the baby to delivery of the placenta.
- **The fourth stage** is from delivery of the placenta to stabilization of the patient's condition, usually at about 6 hours postpartum.

■ PROSTAGLANDINS

- Prostaglandin F (PGF), $PGF_{2\alpha}$, and oxytocin are the biochemical agents primarily involved in the third stage of labor.
- During the first and second stages of labor, only $PGF_{2\alpha}$ and oxytocin are significantly raised in maternal plasma compared with pre-labor concentrations.
- *At 5 minutes after birth, maternal PGF and $PGF_{2\alpha}$ concentrations peak at about twice the levels found at*

the commencement of the second stage. A rapid increase in prostaglandin concentrations is also found in umbilical cord venous blood, suggesting that this postpartum prostaglandin surge originates in the placenta.
- After placental separation, the concentrations decrease but at rates slower than the metabolic clearance of prostaglandin, indicating that its production continues in the decidua and myometrium.
- Plasma oxytocin also drops to prelabor levels within 30 minutes of delivery, unless sustained by exogenous infusion.

Extra Mile

Hormones	Peak level at:
Oxytocin	At birth
Prolactin	Levels decrease during labor but then rise steeply at the end of labor and **peak with birth**

82. Ans. (b) 800–1000 mL

Ref: Wiliams Obstetrics, 24th ed. pg. 250

NORMAL AMNIOTIC FLUID VOLUME

- Amniotic fluid volume increases as the age of gestation increases:
  - 10 weeks: 30 mL
  - 16 weeks: 200 mL
  - 3rd trimester: 800 mL
- Amniotic fluid is maximum at 28–36 week age of gestation (1000 mL).
- This fluid is approximately 98-percent water. A full-term fetus contains roughly 2800 mL of water, and the placenta another 400 mL, such that the term uterus holds nearly 4 liters of water.
- Fetal urine production begins between 8 and 11 weeks, but it does not become a major component of amniotic fluid until the second trimester.

TABLE: In order to attempt any question related to this topic we have summarized this table of the amount of amniotic fluid, fetal weight according to gestational age **(william's OB 23rd ed. Ch 21).**

Weeks' Gestation	Fetus wt (g)	Amniotic fluid (mL)	Placenta (g)
16 weeks	100	200	100
28 weeks	1000	1000	200
36 weeks	2500	900–1000	400
40 weeks	3300	800	500

Note: If question formed as amniotic fluid is maximum at then single best answer will be 36 weeks.

- This latter observation explains why fetuses with lethal renal abnormalities may not manifest severe oligohydramnios until after 18 weeks.
- *Fetal urination is the primary amnionic fluid source by the second half of pregnancy*.
- By term, fetal urine production may exceed 1 liter per day—such that the entire amnionic fluid volume is recirculated on a daily basis. Fetal urine osmolality is significantly hypotonic to that of maternal and fetal plasma and similar to that of amnionic fluid.

83. Ans. (b) 34–36 weeks

Ref: Wiliams Obstetrics, 24th ed.,/250

Please refer to above explanation

84. Ans. (d) Cervical length

Ref: Dutta's Obstetrics 7th ed. 523

- **Bishop score is used to predict** success rate of the induction of the labor
- **Bishop score includes:** (**Note:** it doesn't include length of cervix)
- Dilation of the cervix.
- Position of the cervix.
- The presenting part of the fetus
- Consistency of the cervix

85. Ans. (c) Clavicle

Ref: "Clavicle fracture in labor: risk factors and associated morbidities". J Perinatol (Dec '01)

- *Clavicle fractures are the most frequently encountered birth injury (0.5%).*
- *Brachial plexus is also injured during child birth due to its stretch. The brachial plexus is stretched when the head is pulled in one direction and the arm in the opposite.*
- *Femur fractures also occur in as the leg is awkwardly twisted during delivery. These are rare injuries that are much less common than clavicle fractures.*

86. Ans. (c) Variable deceleration

Ref: Dutta's Obstetrics, 7th ed. pg. 612

- Deceleration is transient decrease in FHR below the baseline by 15 bpm or more and lasting for more than or equal to 15 secs.
- Three basic type of deceleration are observed:
  - **Early Deceleration:** Due to head compression
  - **Late deceleration:** Uteroplacental insufficiency and fetal hypoxia
  - *Variable deceleration: Cord compression (MC type)*

87. Ans. (c) Uteroplacental insufficiency

Ref: Dutta's Obstetrics, 7th ed. pg. 612

Please refer to above explanation

88. Ans. (b) Variable deceleration

The given partogram shows variable deceleration. Now compare the different partograms

FETAL MONITOR PATTERNS

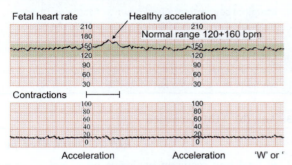

REASSURING PATTERN

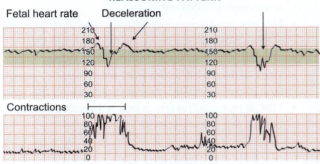

VARIABLE DECELERATIONS

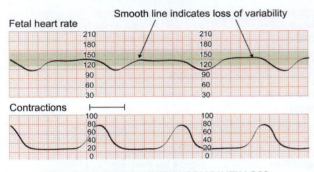

LATE DECELERATION WITH VARIABILITY LOSS

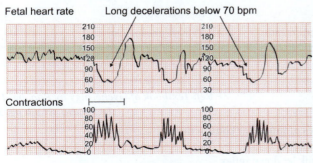

SEVERE VARIABLE DECELERATIONS

89. Ans. (c) Extension to rectum

Ref: DC Dutta, 8th ed. pg. 649-50, 5th ed. pg. 606

- **Episiotomy:** is defined as a surgical incision of the perineum made to increase the diameter of the vulval outlet during child-birth (and not the whole birth canal).
- **Types of episiotomy:** (Only the median or mediolateral episiotomy are done commonly).
- Medio-lateral
  - Median
  - Lateral
  - 'J' shaped

Median	Mediolateral
• Muscles are not cut	• Muscles are cut
• Blood loss is less	• Blood loss is more
• Repair is easy	• Repair is difficult
• Healing is superior	• Healing is less superior
• Dyspareunia is rare	• Dyspareunia is more
• Extension, if occurs, may involve rectum	• Relative safety from rectal involvement from extension
• Incision cannot be extended	• Incision can be extended

90. Ans. (d) 2 hours

Ref: Dutta 8th ed. pg. 154-156

- **Secondary arrest** is defined when the **active phase of labor (cervical dilatation)** commences normally but stops or **slows significantly for 2 hours** or more prior to the full dilatation of the cervix.
- It is commonly **due to malposition or cephalopelvic disproportion.**

'Cessation of active phase of dilatation by more than 2 hours is defined as arrest': Danforth.

ANTEPARTUM AND POSTPARTUM PERIOD

91. Ans. (b) Naegele's formula

Ref: DC Dutta 9th ed. P 88

- Calculation of the expected date of delivery is done according to **Naegele's formula**
- 1st day of LMP + 9 months + 7 days

Extra Mile

- **Cardiff "count 10" formula:** fetal movement count. If <10 kicks in 12 hours on two successive days → Fetal compromise.
- **Hadlock formula and Shepard formula:** For fetal weight estimation according to gestational age using fetal biometric data (BPD, Head circumference, Abdominal circumference and femur length)
- **Johnsons formula:** Also for fetal weight estimation.
  - Height of uterus above symphysis pubis minus 12
- **Crichton's Fifth formula:** Assessment of progressive descent of fetal head.

FMGE Solutions Screening Examination

- Count 3 calendar month back from 1st day of LMP +7 days
- For IVF pregnancy, date of LMP is 14 days prior to date to embryo transfer
- Based on formula labor starts on expected date in 4%. Its prediction range is about 50% with 7 days on either side of EDD.

92. Ans. (d) Discoid uterus

Ref: DC Dutta Obstetrics 8th ed. P 143-44

- The 3rd stage of labor comprises of placental separation, its descent into lower segment and its expulsion.
- After the birth of the baby, the uterus measures about 20 cm (8″) vertically and 10 cm (4″) anteroposteriorly and the shape become discoid (before separation).

Signs Before and After Placental Separation

- **Before separation:** Uterus becomes *discoid in shape*, firm in feel and nonballottable.
    - Fundal height reaches slightly below the umbilicus
- **After separation:**
    - Uterus becomes globular firm and ballotable
    - *The fundal height is slightly raised*
    - Sudden gush of vaginal bleeding upon separation
    - Permanent lengthening of the cord.

> **Extra Mile**
>
> - **The separation is facilitated partly** by uterine contraction and mostly by weight of the placenta as it descends down from the active part.
> - There are two types of separation of placenta:
>   i. **Marginal separation:** Also known as Mathews-Duncan separation and starts from the margin. It is the most common type.
>   ii. **Central separation:** Also known as **Schultze** separation. Starts at center, blood accumulates retroplacentally until whole of the placenta gets detached.

93. Ans. (b) TIBC increased

Ref: DC Dutta, 8th ed. pg. 304

- Total iron requirement during pregnancy is estimated approximately 1,000 mg
- This iron need is not squarely distributed throughout the pregnancy but mostly limited to the third trimester.
- Pregnancy is an inevitable iron deficiency state.
- There is **decreased** serum iron, serum ferritin (storage form of iron) and reduced serum iron: Serum TIBC ratio.
- TIBC is increased (as serum iron is decreased).

> **Extra Mile**
>
> **TABLE:** Normal blood values in non-pregnant and pregnant state
>
> | Blood values | Non-pregnant | Second half pregnancy |
> |---|---|---|
> | Hemoglobin (Hb) | 14.8 gm/100 mL | 11–14 gm/100 mL |
> | Red blood cells (RBC) | 5 million/cu mm (mm^3) | 4–4.5 million/mm^3 |
> | Packed cell volume (PCV) (Hematocrit) | 39–42% | 32–36% |
> | Mean corpuscular hemoglobin (MCH) | 27–32 micromicron (picogram-pg) | 26–31 pg |
> | Mean corpuscular volume (MCV) | 75–100 cubic micron (μ^3) | 75–95 μ^3 |
> | Mean corpuscular hemoglobin concentration (MCHC) | 32–36% | 30–35% |
> | Serum iron | 60–120 µg/100 mL | Slightly lowered (65–75 µg/100) |
> | Total iron blinding capacity (TIBC) | 300–350 µg/100 mL | Increaed (300–400 µg/100 mL) |
> | Saturation percentage (Ratio-serum Iron: TIBC) | 30% | Less than 16% |
> | Serum ferritin | 20–30 µg/L (mean) | 15 mg/L (mean) |

94. Ans. (c) Oxytocin

Ref: Textbook of Gyenecolgy by Rao, pg. 17; DC Dutta, 8th ed. pg. 17

- **Oxytocin** primarily results in stimulation of **two specific types of muscular contraction:**
    - Uterine muscular contraction during parturition
    - Breast lactiferous duct myoepithelial contraction during milk let down reflex.

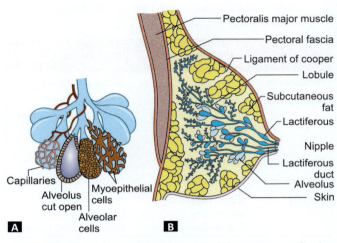

FIGURE: (A) Structure of the basic unit of the mammary gland; (B) Structure of adult female breast

A Brief on Breast Functional Anatomy

- **The areola** is central, pigmented portion of breast with a diameter of about 2.5 cm.
- Accessory glands located around the periphery of the areola are **Montgomery glands** *(they can secrete milk)*.
- **The nipple** ccommodates **about 15–20 lactiferous ducts** and their openings.
- Each milk duct (**lactiferous duct**) dilates to form lactiferous sinus at about 5–10 mm away from its opening in the nipple. Lactiferous sinus acts as reservoir of milk.
- The lining epithelium of the duct near the opening is stratified squamous. Each alveolus is lined by columnar epithelium where milk secretion occurs.
- **Myoepithelial cells are the** network of branching longitudinal striated cells which surround the alveoli and the smaller ducts. There is a dense network of capillaries surrounding the alveoli. These are situated between the basement membrane and epithelial lining.
- **Contraction of these cells (in response to oxytocin) squeezes the alveoli and ejects the milk into the larger duct.**

95. Ans. (b) TAS

Ref: DC Dutta, 8th ed. pg. 733

- For screening transabdominal sonography is the best modality. However if question framed as "best investigation" or "earliest detection" then the answer will be transvaginal sonography.

96. Ans. (c) 21 days

Ref: DC Dutta, 8th ed. pg. 32

- Placental circulation is established by 21 days
- Fetal circulation is established by 21 days

> **Extra Mile**
> - Weight of placenta at term: **500 gm**
> - Functional unit of placenta: **Lobule**
> - Surface area of placenta at term: 12m^2
> - Placenta takes over function of corpus luteum at 8 weeks (8–10 weeks)

97. Ans. (c) Nuchal translucency

Ref: DC Dutta, 8th ed. pg. 735

- **Nuchal translucency** is a fluid behind the neck of the fetus. It is an anechoic space visible and seen in all fetuses between 11–14 weeks of age
- **The most common cause of increased nuchal translucency (>3 mm) is aneuploidy** where TURNER syndrome is the most common cause followed second by Down syndrome.
- The reason why it is seen in 11–14 weeks is because at that time fetal lymphatics are developing and peripheral resistance is high and gradually disappears.
- **Remember**: Cystic hygroma which is seen in Turner syndrome is high incidence is due to defective development of lymphatics.

98. Ans. (b) 100 mg iron + 500 mcg folic acid

Ref: DC Dutta, 8th ed. pg. 241

- **Adult** iron + folic acid tablet given in pregnancy: 1 tab/day × 100 days
- **Kids** iron + folic acid tablet given: 1 tab/day x 100 days per year- 0 to 5 years of age.

Iron and Folic Acid Tablet Content

	Iron	Folic acid
Adult tab	100 mg	500 mcg
Kids tab (1/5th)	20 mg	100 mcg

99. Ans. (c) Non-stress test

Ref: DC Dutta, 8th ed. pg. 122

NON-STRESS TEST (NST)

- In NST, continuous electronic monitoring of fetal heart rate with fetal movements are noted.
- There is an observed association of FHR acceleration with fetal movements, which when present, indicates a healthy fetus.
- It can reliably be used as a screening test.
- The FHR accelerations associated with fetal movements is basically *reflex mediated*.
- *It should be noted that the test is valuable to identify the fetal wellness rather than illness.*

Interpretation
- **Reactive (Reassuring)** – two or more accelerations of more than 15 beats per minute which lasts for 15 seconds or more in a 20 minute observation.
- **Non-reactive (Non-reassuring)** – Absence of any fetal reactivity.

Contraction stress test (CST) is based to observe the response of the fetus at risk for utero placental insufficiency in relation to uterine contractions.

100. Ans. (a) FHR deceleration

Ref: Dutta's Obstetrics, 7th ed. pg. 109

Biophysical Profile Scoring (Manning – 1992)				
Observation for 30 minutes Normal score: 2 Abnormal: 0			BPP score	Interpretation
Parameters	**Minimal normal criteria**	**Score**		
Non stress Test (NST)	Reactive pattern	2	8–10	No fetal asphyxia
Breathing movements	≥1 episode lasting > 30 sec	2	6	Suspect Chronic asphyxia
Gross body movement	≥3 discrete body/ limb movements	2	4	Suspect Chronic asphyxia
Fetal muscle tone	≥1 episode of extension (limb or trunk) with return of flexion	2	0–2	Strongly suspect asphyxia
Amniotic fluid	≥1 pocket measuring 2 cm in two perpendicular planes	2		

101. Ans. (b) 10–12 cm

MATERNAL CHANGES DURING PREGNANCY

- Both ovaries are enlarged due to increased vascularity
- Uterus weight increases from 50 gm in non-pregnant state to 1000 gm at term.
- Capacity, shape and blood flow of uterus increases during pregnancy
- Formation of lower uterine segment: After 12 weeks, the isthmus (0.5 cm) starts to expand gradually to form the lower uterine segment **which measures 10 cm in length at term** (7.5-10 cm according to Dutta).
- The vagina becomes soft, warm, and moist with increased secretion and violet in color (Chadwick's sign) due to increased vascularity.

Difference between upper uterine segment and lower uterine segment

	Upper uterine segment	Lower uterine segment
Peritoneum	Firmly-attached	Loosely-attached
Myometrium	3 layers; outer longitudinal, middle oblique and inner circular	2 layers; outer longitudinal and inner circular
Decidua	Well-developed	Poorly-developed
Membranes	Firmly-attached	Loosely-attached
Activity	Active, contracts, retracts and becomes thicker during labor	Passive, dilates, stretches and becomes thinner during Labor

102. Ans. (a) 6 weeks

Ref: DC Dutta 8th ed. pg. 74-75

The pelvic changes during pregnancy are divers and appear different at different periods:

Signs	At AOG
Palmer's sign: Regular and rhythmic uterine contraction	4-8 weeks
Vaginal sign: Softened vaginal wall with copious mucoid discharge	6th week
Goodell's sign: Cervix feels soft and congested	6th week
Hegar's sign: Uterus is enlarged and soft; cervix empty.	6-10 weeks
Osiander sign: Increased pulsation at lateral fornices	8th week
Chadwick's sign or Jacquemier's sign: Dusky hue of the vestibule and anterior vaginal wall (due to local vascular congestion)	8th week
Piskacek's sign: Asymmetrical enlargement of the uterus if there is lateral implantation	8th week

103. Ans. (b) 8th week

Please refer to above explanation.

104. Ans. (d) Perinatal mortality rate

Ref: DC Dutta 8th ed./687

- **Perinatal period** is from 28th week age of gestation to 7th day of newborn life.
- Perinatal mortality rate includes late fetal deaths and early neonatal deaths.
- A better obstetric care will be able to diagnose any fetal stress which will result in early intervention, which will certainly helps in delivering a healthy baby.
- Therefore an obstetric will mostly affect Perinatal mortality rate.

Obstetrics and Gynecology

105. Ans. (b) 7 April, 2016

> *Ref: DC. Dutta's Textbook of Obstetrics, 8th ed. pg. 83-108*

- Calculation of the expected date of delivery is done according to **naegele's formula**
- 1st day of LMP +9 months + 7 days
- Count 3 calender month back from 1st day of LMP +7 days
- Here LMP= 30th June

EDD

30th June 2015
+7 day +9 month
7th April, 2016

106. Ans. (c) 3 weeks

> *Ref: DC Dutta, 7th ed. pg. 146*

LOCHIA

- It is the vaginal discharge for the first fortnight during puerperium.
- It has 3 phases, which may extend upto 3 weeks.
  - Lochia rubra: 1–4 days; red in color
  - Lochia serosa: 5–9 days; the color is yellowish or pink or pale brownish
  - Lochia alba: 10–15 days; pale white color
- Duration of the Lochia alba beyond 3 weeks suggests local genital lesion

107. Ans. (a) Placental site

> *Ref: Dutta's Obstetrics, 7th ed. pg. 433*

PUERPERAL SEPSIS

- An infection of the genital tract which occurs as a complication of delivery is termed puerperal sepsis.
- Sources of infection may be endogenous where organisms are present in the genital tract before delivery.

Mode of Infection

- Puerperal sepsis is generally a wound infection.
- Placental site being a raw surface in the endometrium is the most common site for infection.
- Other causes of puerperal sepsis may be laceration of the genital tract or may be CS section wound infection by organisms like anaerobic strep, E. Coli, staph etc.
- *Anaerobic streptococcus is the most common cause of Puerperal sepsis.*
- The primary sites of infections are: Uterus, Perineum, Vagina, Cervix.

108. Ans. (b) Uterus becomes discoid

> *Ref: DC Dutta, 7th ed. pg. 131-312*

Clinical Course of Third Stage of Labor

- Third stage includes separation, descent and expulsion of the placenta with its membrane.

Signs before and after placental separation

- **Before Separation:** uterus becomes *discoid in shape*, firm in feel and non-ballottable.
  - Fundal height reaches slightly below the umbilicus
- **After Separation:**
  - Uterus becomes globular firm and ballotable
  - *The fundal height is slightly raised*
  - Sudden gush of vaginal bleeding upon separation.
  - Permanent lengthening of the cord.

109. Ans. (a) Gushing of blood

> *Ref: D.C Dutta, 7th ed. pg. 131-312*

Please refer to above explanation.

110. Ans. (b) Fundus of the uterus below umbilicus

> *Ref: D.C Dutta, 7th ed. pg. 131-312*

111. Ans. (c) Puerperal sepsis

> *Ref: D.C Dutta, 7th ed. pg. 432, 433, 435*

PUERPERAL PYREXIA (FEVER)

- A rise of temperature reaching 100.4°F (39°C) or more on 2 separate occasions at 24 hours apart (excluding first 24 hours) within first 10 days following delivery is called *puerperal pyrexia.*
- **Causes of pyrexia are:** Peurperal sepsis, Urinary tract infection, Mastitis, Infection of caesarean section wound, Pulmonary infection, Septic pelvic thrombophlebitis etc.

PUERPERAL SEPSIS

- An infection of the genital tract which occurs as a complication of delivery is termed puerperal sepsis.
- Sources of infection may be endogenous where organisms are present in the genital tract before delivery.
- *Anaerobic streptococcus is the most common cause of Puerperal sepsis.*
- The primary sites of infections are: Perineum, Vagina, Cervix, Uterus
- *Remember: A case of puerperal pyrexia is considered to be due to genital unless proved otherwise.*

112. Ans. (a) Haemorrhage

> *Ref: Dutta's Obstetrics, 7th ed. pg. 411*

- Most common Indirect cause of maternal mortality in India: Anemia

Explanations

907

- Most common cause of maternal mortality in India: Post partum hemorrhage (PPH)
- Most common direct cause of MMR: PPH

Direct maternal mortality	Indirect maternal mortality
It results from obstetric complication of pregnant state (pregnancy, labor and puerperium) from interventions or incorrect treatment.	It results from previous existing disease or disease that develops during pregnancy.
Ex: PPH, Obstructed labor, Sepsis	Anemia, HTN, gestational DM, Epilepsy

113. Ans. (d) Anemia

Please refer to above explanation.

114. Ans. (d) Increased prolactin level

Ref: DC Dutta, 8th ed. pg. 171, 614; 6th pg. 148
Breast feeding increases the levels of prolactin which lead to the following consequences:
- Reduced ovarian response to FSH leading to **hypo-estrogenic state**
- Suppression of LH release thereby **preventing LH surge and inhibiting ovulation**
- **Reduces GnRH secretion**

115. Ans. (c) 1000 g

Ref: Dutta's Obstetrics, 7th ed. pg. 144.
- Immediately following delivery, the uterus becomes firm and retracts with alternate hardening and softening.
- Immediately postpartum the uterus weighs about 1000 g and measures about 20 × 17 × 7.5 cm.
- **6 weeks post partum**, its measurement is almost similar to that of non-pregnant state and **weighs about 60 g**.

116. Ans. (b) 4 weeks

Ref: DC Dutta, 8th ed. pg. 53-54
- Heart rate returns to pre-pregnant value at around 4 weeks postpartum

117. Ans. (d) 4 weeks

Ref: Dutta's Obstetrics, 7th ed. pg. 53
- The cardiac output (CO) starts to increase from 5th week of pregnancy, reaches its peak **40-50% at about 30-40 weeks.**
- CO is lowest in the sitting or supine position and highest in the right or left lateral or knee chest position.
- It increases further during labor (+50%) and immediately following delivery (+70%) over the pre-labor values.
- Within 1–2 hours following birth, the cardiac output is estimated to be about 500 ml/min and Hr ~ 120–140/min
- **CO returns to pre labor values one hour after delivery.**
- *It returns to the pre-pregnancy level in 4 weeks time.*

118. Ans. (b) 12–14 days

Ref: Dutta's Obstetrics, 7th ed. pg. 144-145
- Uterus becomes pelvic organ in about 2 weeks after normal delivery.
- The rate of involution of uterus after delivery is 1.25 cm or half inch/day.
- **It regains its pre-pregnancy size at the end of 6 weeks.**

> **Extra Mile**
> - During pregnancy, uterus remains pelvic organ till 2 week of pregnancy. Thereon, it starts to ascend in abdomen.

119. Ans. (b) Vasa previa

Ref: Dutta's Obstetrics, 7th ed. pg. 259

VASA PREVIA

- In a vilamentous insertion of cord, the leash of blood vessels may traverse through membranes overlying the internal OS, in front of the presenting part. This condition is called Vasa previa.
- Rupture of the membranes involves the overlying vessels and leads to vaginal bleeding.
- This vaginal bleeding is, thus, entirely from fetal blood and may result in fetal exsanguination and even death.

120. Ans. (b) Rupture of uterus

Ref: William's, 23rd ed. Ch 35
- *Postpartum hemorrhage has been defined as the loss of 500 mL of blood or more after completion of the third stage of labor.*
- According to the given case scenario, ruptured uterus is the only indication to do immediate hysterectomy.
- Other given options like pre-eclampsia, atonic uterus or involution of uterus may present with post delivery hemorrhage, but they are not an indication for immediate hysterectomy and managed conservatively first.
- **Pre-eclampsia:** Because of the poorly contractile nature of the lower uterine segment, there may be uncontrollable hemorrhage following placental removal. When bleeding is not controlled by conservative means, other methods like oversewing the implantation site, bilateral internal iliac artery ligation or uninterrupted chromic sutures is the next best choice *(William's 23rd)*. If such conservative methods fail, and bleeding is brisk, then hysterectomy is necessary.
- **Uterine atony** is the most common cause of obstetrical hemorrhage. Managed initially with oxytocin, ergot

Obstetrics and Gynecology

derivatives, Prostaglandin analogues (PGF2α). If no effect with conservative management then hysterectomy is the choice.

- **Note:** For women whose placenta previa is implanted anteriorly in the site of a prior hysterotomy incision, there is an increased likelihood of associated placenta accreta and need for hysterectomy.
- **Inversion of the uterus** most often associated with immediate life-threatening hemorrhage. The recently inverted uterus with placenta already separated from it may often be replaced simply by pushing up on the fundus with the palm of the hand and fingers in the direction of the long axis of the vagina followed by fluid infusion and blood transfusion. If no relief then reduction via laparotomy is performed.

---

121. Ans. (c) III

Ref: DC Dutta, 7th ed. pg. 422-23

PERINEAL TEARS

1st degree	Is a laceration of the vaginal mucosa and the perineal skin but not the underlying fascia and muscle.
2nd degree	Involves the vaginal mucosa perineal skin and the fascia and muscles of the perineal body.
3rd degree	Involves the vaginal mucosa skin and perineal body and the anal sphincter is also disrupted
4th degree	In addition the rectal mucosa is also torn.

ABORTION AND THIRD TRIMESTER BLEEDING

---

122. Ans. (b) Cervical incompetence

Ref: DC Dutta 9th ed. P 161

- The patient in the given case is of 2nd trimester abortion. Cervical incompetence is the most common cause that can be suspected for this patient

TABLE: Common causes of miscarriage

1st trimester	2nd trimester
• Genetic factors (50%) • Endocrine disorders like thyroid abnormalities, diabetes • Immunological disorder • Infections • Unexplained	• Anatomical abnormalities ▪ Cervical incompetence ▪ Mullerian fusion defect-bicornuate/sepatate uterus ▪ Uterine synechiae ▪ Uterine fibroid • Maternal medical illness • Unexplained

Cervical Incompetence/Insufficiency

- Causes of cervical incompetence can be:
  - ▪ Congenital uterine abnormalities
  - ▪ **Acquired:** More common.
    - ♦ History of D&C or D and E operation
    - ♦ Cervix amputation
    - ♦ Vaginal operative delivery through undilated cervix
    - ♦ Multiple gestations
- Patient usually present with history of mid-trimester, painless cervical dilatation and escape of liquor amnii followed by painless expulsion of the product of conceptus.
- Passage of 6–8 number hegar dilator without resistance and pain is highly suggestive

Treatment:

- *Cerclage operation:* Two types of operation are in current use during pregnancy
  - ▪ **Shirodkar**
  - ▪ **McDonald**
- **Principle:** It reinforces the weak cervix by a nonabsorbable tape, placed around the cervix at the level of internal os.
- **Time of operation:** Around 14 weeks of pregnancy or at least 2 weeks earlier than the previous miscarriage, as early as the 10th week.
- *Removal of stitch*: **The stitch should be removed at 37th week** or earlier if labor pain starts (preferably in OT).

> **Extra Mile**

TABLE: Types of miscarriage and the diagnostic features

Type	Symptoms	Uterine Size	Cervix (Ext. Os)	Ultrasonography
Threatened	• Vaginal bleeding present • Pelvic pain	Corresponds to gestational age	Closed	• Fetus alive • Retroplacental hemonhage+
Inevitable	• Vaginal bleeding present • Pelvic pain	Same or smaller	Open with palpable conceptus	• Fetus often dead Retroplacental hemorrhage+
Incomplete	Vaginal bleeding (may be heavy)	Smaller	Open	Products of conception partly retained

Contd...

FMGE Solutions Screening Examination

Extra Mile

Type	Symptoms	Uterine Size	Cervix (Ext. Os)	Ultrasonography
Complete	Vaginal bleeding—trace or absent	Smaller	Closed	Uterine cavity empty
Missed	Vaginal bleeding—trace, brownish in color	Smaller	Closed	Blighted ovum or fetus without cardiac activity
Septic	Vaginal discharge: purulent, foul smelling with features of sepsis	Variable, may be larger	Open	Products of conception retained, presence of foreign body (±), free fluid in the peritoneal cavity/POD

123. Ans. (a) Trisomy

Ref: Williams 24th ed. P 370

- Approximately 50% of miscarriages during first trimester are anembryonic. The other 50% are embryonic miscarriages.
  - **Anembryonic:** With no identifiable embryonic elements.
  - **Embryonic:** Display a developmental abnormality of the zygote, embryo, fetus, or at times, the placenta.
- Of 50% embryonic miscarriages, 25% of all abortion are aneuploid abortions (*abnormal chromosome number*). The remaining cases are euploid (*abnormal chromosome development*) abortions.

Chromosomal aneuploidy	Incidence %
Trisomy	22–32
Monosomy X (45,X)	5–20
Triploidy	6–8
Tetraploidy	2–4
Structural anomaly	2

Note: *Most common cause of first trimester bleeding: Abortion*

124. Ans. (a) Spontaneous abortion

Ref: DC Dutta, 8th ed. pg. 185-86

- **Spontaneous abortion** is the expulsion or extraction from its mother of an embryo or fetus weighing 500 g or less when it is not capable of independent survival
- **Incidence:**
  - About 75% miscarriages occur before the 16th week and of these **about 80% occur before the 12th week of pregnancy.**

Common Causes of Miscarriage
- *First trimester:*
  - **Genetic factors (50%)- MCC.**
  - Endocrine disorders (LPD, thyroid abnormalities, diabetes).
  - Immunological disorders (autoimmune and alloimmune).
  - Infection.
  - Unexplained.
- *Second trimester:*
  - Anatomic abnormalities—
    - Cervical incompetence (congenital or acquired).
    - Mullerian fusion defects (bicornuate uterus, septate uterus).
    - Uterine synechiae
    - Uterine fibroid.
  - Maternal medical illness
  - Unexplained
- **Third trimester**: Most common cause of bleeding is: Abruptio placenta > placenta previa

125. Ans. (a) Trisomy

Ref: Williams 24th ed. pg. 370

- Approximately 50% of miscarriages during first trimester are anembryonic. The other 50% are embryonic miscarriages.
  - **Anembryonic:** With no identifiable embryonic elements.
  - **Embryonic:** Display a developmental abnormality of the zygote, embryo, fetus, or at times, the placenta.
- Of 50% embryonic miscarriages, 25% of all abortion are aneuploid abortions (*abnormal chromosome number*). The remaining cases are euploid (*abnormal chromosome development*) abortions.

Chromosomal aneuploidy	Incidence %
Trisomy	22-32
Monosomy x (45, X)	5-20
Triploidy	6-8
Tetraploidy	2-4
Structural anomaly	2

Note: *Most common cause of first trimester bleeding: Abortion*

Obstetrics and Gynecology

126. Ans. (c) Chromosomal abnormalities

Ref: Dutta, 6th ed. pg. 160

With respect to first trimester abortions, 75% of the abortions take place before 16th week and out of these, about 75% occur before the 8th week of pregnancy.
- **Chromosomal abnormality in the conceptus is the commonest cause of miscarriage.**
- **Autosomal trisomy** particularly **Trisomy 16** is the commonest cause for spontaneous abortion.

127. Ans. (c) Uterus size small to AOG, cervix open

Ref: Dutta's Obstetrics, 7th ed. pg. 163

- In Inevitable abortion, condition is progressed to a stage from where continuation of pregnancy is not possible.
- Patient usually presents with bleeding per vaginum with **size of uterus smaller than age of gestation and open cervix.**
- **USG finding:** Dead fetus

Extra Mile

Abortion	Size of uterus	Cervix OS	USG finding
Threatened	Equal to AOG	Closed	Fetus alive
Missed	Smaller than AOG	Closed	Dead fetus
Incomplete	Smaller than AOG	Open	Retained products of conception
Complete	Smaller than AOG	Closed	Uterine Cavity empty

128. Ans. (a) Dilatation and evacuation

Ref: D.C Dutta, 7th ed. pg. 161-162

INEVITABLE MISCARRIAGE

- It is the clinical type of abortion where the changes have progressed to a state from where continuation of pregnancy is impossible.
- **Clinical feature:**
  - Increased vaginal bleeding
  - Aggravation of pain in the lower abdomen
  - Dilated internal OS
- **Treatment**
  - Before 12 weeks
    - *Dilatation and evacuation* followed by curettage using analgesia or under general anaesthesia
    - Alternative, suction evacuation followed by curettage is also done.
  - **After 12 weeks:** Product of conception is evacuated by Oxytocin drip which increases uterine contraction.

129. Ans. (c) 200 mg mifepristone + 400 mcg misoprostol

Ref: D.C Dutta, 7th ed. pg. 173-174

Following are the indications for termination under the MTP Act:
- **To save the life of the mother (Therapeutic or medical termination):** Ex: Grade 3–4 cardiac disease, malignant HTN, CGN, cervical or breast malignancies etc.
- **Social indications:** To prevent grave injury to the physical and mental health of the pregnant woman.
- **Humanitarian ground:** Pregnancy because of rape or incest.
- **Eugenic:** Substantial risk of the child being born with serious physical and mental abnormalities so as to be handicapped in life.

Remember
- Termination is permitted up to 20 weeks of pregnancy. When the pregnancy exceeds 12 weeks, opinion of two medical practitioners is required

Medical Methods of First Trimester Abortion
- 200 mg of mifepristone orally is given on day 1. On day 3, misoprostol (PGE$_1$) 400 µg orally or 800 µg vaginally is given for the MTP.

130. Ans. (c) Mifepristone 200 mg + Misoprostol 400 mcg oral

Ref: Dutta's Obstetrics, 7th ed. pg. 173

Medical methods of first trimester abortion
- 200 mg of mifepristone orally is given on day 1.
- On day 3, misoprostol (PGE$_1$) 400 µg orally or 800 µg vaginally is given for the MTP.

131. Ans. (c) Misoprostol + Tamoxifen

Ref: Dutta's Obstetrics, 7th ed. pg. 173

- *200 mg of mifepristone orally is given on day 1. On day 3, misoprostol (PGE$_1$) 400 µg orally or 800 µg vaginally is given for the MTP.*
- Tamoxifen is an estrogen antagonist, which is basically used in breast cancer.

132. Ans. (d) Type II posterior

Ref: DC Dutta 8th ed./283-84; William's 23rd ed. Ch. 35.

PLACENTA PREVIA

Placenta previa is used to describe a placenta that is implanted over or very near the internal cervical os. There are several possibilities:
- **Total placenta previa**—the internal os is covered completely by placenta
- **Partial placenta previa**—the internal os is partially covered by placenta

FMGE Solutions Screening Examination

- **Marginal placenta previa**—the edge of the placenta is at the margin of the internal os
- **Low-lying placenta**—the placenta is implanted in the lower uterine segment such that the placental edge does not reach the internal os, but is in close proximity to it.
  - *Low lying placenta type II is posteriorly located and is considered dangerous because it* can be compressed by the presenting part and this will cause severe fetal asphyxia and sometimes fetal death.
- **Vasa previa**—the fetal vessels course through membranes and present at the cervical os

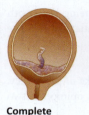 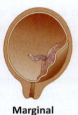 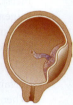

Complete   Partial   Marginal   Low Lying

133. Ans. (b) Placenta previa

Ref: DC Dutta, 8th ed./290, Williams 22nd ed./ 822-823

- **MacAfee and Johnson Regimen** is a Conservative Management in Placenta Previa: This consists of complete bed rest, tocolysis, and close observation of patient.
- Steroids are generally given to enhance lung maturity.
- **To undertake this regimen (to wait and watch) all three criteria should be fulfilled:**
  - Mother should be hemodynamically stable
  - There should be no fetal distress
  - Pregnancy less than 36 weeks of gestation.
- If any of the criteria is not met then the patient should be delivered by LSCS.

> **Extra Mile**
> - Classification of abruption placentae: page/sher's/classification
> - **Zuspan regimen** for the treatment of eclampsia using Magnesium sulphate (zuspan aka sibai)
> Other regimens using MgSO$_4$ for treatment of eclampsia are
> Pritchard's regimen (intramuscular)
> Sibai regimen (intravenous)
> - Most appropriate treatment of eclampsia: MgSO$_4$

134. Ans. (a) Caesarean section

Ref: DC Dutta, 8th ed. pg. 290-92; William's, 23rd ed. Chapter 35.

- Placenta previa-placenta located at LUS.
- One of the most common cause of APH.
- In case of centrally located placenta previa –mode of delivery is always CS.

Management of placenta previa depends on its type- 4 types

Indication for termination(by vaginal/CS)	Indication for conservative management
• POG-37 weeks or beyond • Pt continuously bleeding • Fetal distress • Hemodynamically unstable mother • Pt is active Labor • IUD • Congenital malformation of baby which are incompatible with life	Done in patient who do not obey previous 7 rule
Termination by vaginal delivery or CS (depending on type of PP)	Ma caffe's protocol for conservative management • Bed rest • Monitor vitals-mother and baby • Blood transfusion(if needed)
Type 1 (low lying)-vaginal delivery Type 2 (marginal)-vaginal if placenta anterior, CS-if posterior Type 3 (incomplete/partial)- always CS Type 4(complete/central)- always CS	If POG <34 weeks- give betamethasone 12 mg IM 2 dose, 24 hrs apart, for lung maturity.

Mark CS as management option for placenta previa if any of following points give in Question
- Mother unstable
- Fetal distress
- Major degree of PP-type 3 (incomplete/partial), type 4 (complete/central)

135. Ans. (b) Battledore placenta

Ref: William's Obstetrics, 23rd ed. Ch: 27

- Normally, the cord usually is inserted at or near the center of the fetal surface of the placenta.
- Cord insertion at the placental margin is sometimes referred to as a **Battledore placenta**. It is found in about 7% of term placentas.
- **Velamentous insertion:** This type of insertion is of considerable clinical importance. The umbilical vessels spread within the membranes at a distance from the pla-

Obstetrics and Gynecology

cental margin, which they reach surrounded only by a fold of amnion. As a result, vessels are vulnerable to compression, which may lead to fetal anoxia. Incidence: 1%

136. Ans. (a) Placenta accreta

Ref: Williams Obstetrics, 23rd ed. Ch 35.

- The nitabuch *layer* is a zone of fibrinoid degeneration in which invading trophoblasts meet the decidua. *If the decidua is defective, as in placenta accreta, the Nitabuch layer is usually absent.*

> **Extra Mile**
>
> - **Placenta accreta** indicates that villi are attached to the myometrium.
> - **Placenta increta,** villi actually invade the myometrium.
> - **Placenta percreta** defines villi that penetrate through the myometrium and to or through the serosa.

137. Ans. (a) Placenta previa

Ref: Williams Obstetrics, 23rd ed. Ch 35.

Absence of nitabuch membrane can lead to placenta accreta, increta or percreta.

138. Ans. (b) β-hCG level

Ref: DC Dutta, 8th ed. pg. 227

Hydatiform moles are abnormal pregnancies characterized histologically by aberrant changes within the placenta. Specifically, the chorionic villi in these placentas show varying degrees of trophoblastic proliferation and edema of the villous stroma. **They are of two types: Partial and complete.**

Complete mole	Partial mole
• A molar pregnancy with some normal and some swollen villi plus fetal, cord, and/or amniotic membrane elements.	• A molar pregnancy with swelling of all placental villi.
• *Fetal tissue absent.*	• *Fetal tissues are present.*
• **Karyotype:** 46, XX or 46, XY	• **Karyotype:** 69, XXX or 69, XXY
• **Villous edema:** diffuse	• **Villous edema:** focal
• **Typical clinical presentation:** Molar gestation	• **Typical clinical presentation:** Missed abortion
• **Postmolar malignant sequelae-** 15-20%	• **Postmolar malignant sequelae-** 2-4%

Investigation

- Diagnosing in first-trimester is now common because of the routine use of serum β-hCG measurements *(as they produce excess β-hCG due to trophoblastic proliferation)* and transvaginal sonography.

- Although β-hCG levels are helpful, *the diagnosis of molar pregnancy more frequently is found sonographically* because of the identifiable diffuse swelling and enlargement of the chorionic villi.
- **Appearance on USG:** Snow storm appearnce

Treatment

- Suction curettage is the preferred method of evacuation regardless of uterine size in patients who wish to remain fertile.

POSTMOLAR SURVEILLANCE

- Gestational trophoblastic neoplasia (GTN) develops after approximately 15-20 % of complete moles and 2-4% in partial moles.
- **Postmolar surveillance with serial quantitative serum β-hCG levels is the standard.**

> **Extra Mile**
>
> - GTD INCLUDES: H.Mole, Invasive mole, ChorioCA, PSTT (Placental Site Trophoblastic Tumor)
> - **MC site of metastasis of GTD: Lungs**

139. Ans. (b) 46 XY

Ref: DC Dutta, 8th ed. pg. 230

Please refer to above explanation.

140. Ans. (c) Lungs

Please refer to above question.

141. Ans. (a) Complete mole

Ref: DC Dutta, 8th ed. pg. 226-30

THECA LUTEIN CYST

- **Theca lutein cysts yellow colored cyst seen in H. mole due to high circulating levels of hCG.**
- Size: microscopic to 10 cms size.
- **Theca lutein cyst are also seen in case of:**
  - Fetal hydrops
  - Placental hypertrophy
  - Multifetal pregnancy

142. Ans. (a) Beta hCG

MONITORING

- After suction Evacuation: We send **weekly serum β-hCG.** Till they Become Normal.

Avg. time for hCG to Came Back to Normal

- After a complete Mole – 9 weeks
- After a partial Mole – 7 weeks
- After a Molar – 9 weeks
- Once hCG is Normal
- We send hCG values Monthly × 6 months

Explanations

913

FMGE Solutions Screening Examination

143. Ans. (a) 1%

Ref: William's Obstetrics 23/table 26-3

Types of prior uterine incisions and risk of uterine rupture

Prior incison	Rupture rate (percentage)
1. Classical	4-9%
2. T-shaped	4-9%
3. Low-vertical	1-7%
4. Low-transverse	0.2-1.5%

TWIN PREGNANCY

144. Ans. (c) Diamniotic, Dichorionic

Ref: DC Dutta 9th ed. P 189

TABLE: Division of zygote and types of twinning

Division of Zygote on/after	Types of Twining
Within 72 hours/3 days	Dichorionic, Diamniotic
Between 4 and 8 days	Monochorionic, Diamniotic
Between 8 and 12 days	Monochorionic, Monoamniotic
>12 days	Siamese, Conjoined Twins

145. Ans. (b) Monochorionic, Diamniotic

Ref: Dutta, 8th ed. pg. 233

TABLE: Division of zygote and types of Twinning

Division of Zygote on/ after	Types of Twining
Within 72 hours/3 days	Dichorionic, Diamniotic
Between 4 – 8 days	Monochorionic, Diamniotic
Between 8 – 12 days	Monochorionic, Monoamniotic
>12 days	Siamese, Conjoined Twins

Extra Mile

- Most common type of twinning is dizygotic twins: 69%
- Monozygotic twins in: 31%
- **MC TYPE OF TWIN GESTATION:** Diamniotic Monochorionic (70–75%)
- **Least common type of twin gestation:** Conjoined twins (<1%)
- **Hellin rule** is associated with multiple **pregnancy** as per which chance of twins is a1 in 80 pregnancies, triplets 1 in 80² and so on. It can result in complications
- **Prematurity** is the **commonest fetal complication**
- **Post partum hemorrhage** is the commonest **maternal complication.**
- **Twin to twin transfusion syndrome is seen in:** MC-DA

146. Ans. (b) Diamniotic, monochoronic

Ref: Dutta, 8th ed. pg. 233

147. Ans. (c) A vertex, B vertex

Ref: Dutta, 7th ed. pg. 202-203

- Vertex twin i.e. both baby in vertex presentation has best prognosis.

Presentations

- Both vertex (Most common) 60%
- Vertex (1st) – Breech (2nd) 20%
- Breech (1st)- Vertex (2nd) 10%
- Both Breech 8-10%

Mode of Delivery in twin presentation

- **Vertex Twin:** Mode of Delivery is Vaginal i.e. $(V_x$-$V_x)$
- **1st Breech & 2nd vertex** *C.S
  - Interlocking most commonly seen with this presentation
  - After coming head of 1st twin gets locked with forecoming Head of 2nd Twin
- **1st Twin** Vertex and 2nd Any: Vaginal Delivery
- **1st Twin** Transverse: C.S

148. Ans. (a) 10 weeks

Ref: D.C Dutta, 8th ed. 237

Dutta 8th ed states: "sonography in multifetal pregnancy is done for confirmation of diagnosis as early as **10th week AOG".** It also helps in assessing:

- Viability of fetuses
- Chorionicity *(Lambda or twin peak sign)*
- Pregnancy dating
- Fetal growth monitoring
- Fetal anomalies
- Placental localization
- Amniotic fluid volume

Extra Mile

- Chorionicity of placenta is best diagnosed at 10–13th week AOG by USG
- **Lambda or Twin peak sign:** Indicates dichorionic placenta. In dichorionic twins there is thick septum between the two gestational sacs. It is best identified at the base of membrane where a triangular projection is seen.

149. Ans. (c) Young female

Ref: Dutta, 7th ed. pg. 202

Twin pregnancy associated with increased maternal age.

The incidence of Dizygotic twins increases with:

- Increasing maternal age

Obstetrics and Gynecology

- Increasing parity
- Family history of twinning
- Ovulation induction with clomiphene citrate or gonadotrophins.

ECTOPIC PREGNANCY

150. Ans. (b) Isthmus

Ref: DC Dutta 9th ed. P 170

- Most common site of ectopic pregnancy is Ampullary part of the fallopian tube
- **Least common variety of ectopic tubal pregnancy: Interstitial**

- MC site of tubal rupture in ectopic pregnancy: Isthmus (narrow part of tube and less distensible).
- Isthmic rupture usually occurs in:
  - **Isthmic part:** 6–8 weeks (earliest to rupture)
  - **Ampullary part:** 8–12 weeks
  - **Interstitial part:** Up to 4 months

151. Ans. (a) Ampulla

Ref: DC Dutta, 8th ed. pg. 207

- An ectopic pregnancy is one in which the fertilized ovum is implanted and develops outside the normal endometrial cavity.
- Most common site of ectopic pregnancy is fallopian tube, Ampullary part.

Sites of Implantation

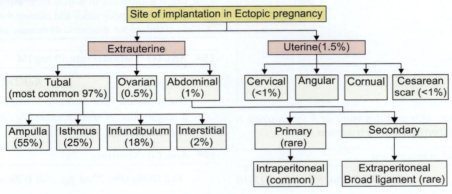

152. Ans. (c) Interstitial

Ref: DC Dutta 8th ed. pg. 214

- **Interstitial ectopic pregnancy is the rarest variety of tubal pregnancy.** Because of the thick and vascular musculature of the uterine wall with greater distensibility, the fetus grows dissecting the muscle fibers for a longer period **(12-14 weeks)** before termination occurs.

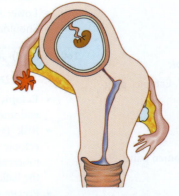

FIGURE: Interstitial pregnancy

- The usual termination is rupture. It is **associated with massive intraperitoneal hemorrhage** due to its combined vascularization by the uterine and ovarian arteries.

FMGE Solutions Screening Examination

153. Ans. (b) Laparoscopy with salpingostomy

Ref: DC Dutta, 8th ed. pg. 217-18

- The USG finding of empty uterus indicates this case as ectopic pregnancy.

Table: Management of unruptured ectopic pregnancy can be done by:

Medical management: methotrexate 50 mg/m² IM	Expectant management	Surgical management
• Serum hCG level should be <3000 IU/L • Gestational sac size <3.5 cm • Hemodynamically stable patient • Tubal diameter should be less than 4 cm without any fetal cardiac activity • There should be no intra-abdominal hemorrhage	• If sac size <3 cm • HCG < 1000 IU/L and subsequent levels are falling	• Laparoscopy is preferred over laparotomy • Salpingostomy is preferred over salpingectomy

Note: *If patient presents with unstable vitals or if laparoscopy is contraindicated, then laparotomy is advised.*

154. Ans. (a) Medical management

Ref: DC Dutta, 8th ed. pg. 217-18

155. Ans. (a) Pain

Ref: Dutta Obs, 7th ed. pg. 182; William Obs, 22nd ed. pg. 258

- An ectopic pregnancy is one in which the fertilized ovum is implanted and develops outside the normal endometrial cavity.
- **Classic Triad of Ectopic Pregnancy**
  - **Pain (100%)**
  - **Amenorrhea (75%)**
  - **Bleeding per vaginum (70%)**

Note: *Triad is present only in 50% case of ectopic*

- **Most common/Consistent** finding of Ectopic pregnancy: **Pain**

Symptoms

- Nausea and Vomiting
- Lower Abdominal pain/generalized Abdomen pain
- Shoulder tip pain (25%)
- Syncopal attacks (10%)

156. Ans. (a) Ectopic pregnancy

Ref: Dutta Obs, 7th ed. pg. 182; William Obs, 22nd ed. pg. 258

157. Ans. (b) TVS

Ref: DC Dutta, 8th ed. pg. 213

- Investigation of choice in a case of ectopic pregnancy/suspected case of ectopic pregnancy is Transvaginal scan.
- Findings raising suspicion of ectopic on TVS:
  - **Empty uterine cavity: most important**
  - Finding of complex adnexal mass
  - Fluid (echogenic) in the pouch of Douglas.
  - Adnexal mass clearly separated from the ovary.
  - Rarely cardiac motion may be seen in an unruptured tubal ectopic pregnancy.

Extra Mile

- **Estimation of β-hCG:** Urine pregnancy test—ELISA is sensitive to 10-50 mIU/mL and is positive in 95% of ectopic pregnancies. A single estimation of β-hCG level either in the serum or in urine confirms pregnancy but cannot determine its location.
- **Gold standard for diagnosis of ectopic pregnancy:** Laproscopy

158. Ans. (c) Methotrexate 50 mg IM

Ref: DC Dutta, 8th ed. pg. 216

Dutta states: *"For systemic therapy of ectopic pregnancy, a single dose of methotrexate (MTX) 50 mg/M² is given intramuscularly."*

159. Ans. (a) Vomiting

Ref: Dutta Obs, 7th ed. pg. 182; William Obs, 22nd ed. pg. 258

CLASSIC TRIAD OF ECTOPIC

- **Pain+ Amenorrhea+ Bleeding per vaginum**
  Triad is present only in 50% case of ectopic
- **M.C/Consistent** finding of Ectopic →**pain**

Symptoms

- Nausea & Vomiting
- Lower Abdom. pain/generalized Abdom pain
- Shoulder tip pain Syncopal attacks

160. Ans. (c) A negative pregnancy test excludes the diagnosis

Ref: DC Dutta 8th ed./212, Williams Obst. 21st ed./ 892

- **Ectopic pregnancy:** Pregnancy that occurs outside the endometrial lining of uterus.
- Risk factors for ectopic pregnancy include previous ectopic pregnancies and conditions like tubal surgery, tubercular infection that disrupt the normal anatomy of the Fallopian tubes.
- Previous salpingitis/tubal disease is the most common cause of ectopic pregnancy.
- Among contraceptives, use of progestasert is the most common cause of ectopic pregnancy.

Obstetrics and Gynecology

- The major health risk of ectopic pregnancy is rupture leading to internal bleeding.
- It can be diagnosed by Beta HCG level. It doesn't rise as fast as it rises in uterine pregnancy.
- *It can also be diagnosed by pregnancy test, but a negative pregnancy test doesn't rule out the diagnosis of ectopic pregnancy.*
- On transvaginal scan presence of an adnexal mass and the absence of an intrauterine pregnancy increases the likelihood of an ectopic pregnancy.
- *Methotrexate is considered as drug of choice for ectopic pregnancy.*

161. Ans. (a) Transvaginal USG

Ref: DC Dutta, 8ᵗʰ ed. pg. 212, Williams Obst, 21ˢᵗ ed. pg. 892

Diagnosis of Ectopic Pregnancy

- Most definite diagnosis of pregnancy is by demonstrating intrauterine sac.
- An absence of the intrauterine sac in a patient who is complaining of pain, bleeding and positive pregnancy test raise the suspicion of ectopic pregnancy.
- By doing **transvaginal USG, ectopic pregnancy can be ruled out.** If the USG demonstrates live intrauterine fetus then ectopic pregnancy is very unlikely.
- On the other hand, if the uterus is empty, an ectopic pregnancy can be diagnosed based on the visualization of an adnexal mass separate from the ovaries.
- **Beta-hCG** also helps in diagnosis of pregnancy. It is positive in virtually 100% of ectopic pregnancies.
- A positive test only confirms pregnancy and does not indicate whether it is intrauterine or extrauterine (ectopic).
- *In normal pregnancy beta-HCG should double up every 2 days but in ectopic pregnancy the rate of increase of beta HCG is slow.*

CULDOCENTESIS

- Culdocentesis is the transvaginal passage of a needle into the posterior cul-de-sac in order to determine whether free blood is present in the abdomen.
- This procedure will reveal non-clotted blood if intra-abdominal bleeding has occurred.
- Clotted bloods signify ruptured ectopic pregnancy.
- If culdocentesis is positive, laparoscopy or laparotomy should be performed immediately.

162. Ans. (a) Beta hCG < 5000

Ref: DC Dutta, 8ᵗʰ ed. pg. 209

CRITERIA FOR MEDICAL MANAGEMENT OF ECTOPIC PREGNANCY USING METHOTREXATE

Absolute Rquirements

- Hemodynamic stability
- No evidence of acute intra-abdominal bleeding
- Reliable commitment to comply with required
- Follow-up care

Preferable Requirements

- Absent or mild pain
- Serum beta hCG level less than 10, 000 IU/L *(best results seen with hCG < 2000 IU/L)*
- Absent embryonic heart activity
- Ectopic gestational mass less than <3.5 cm in diameter.

MALPRESENTATION, DIFFICULT DELIVERY AND INSTRUMENTATION

163. Ans. (a) 10–15 mm Hg

Ref: Shaw's Gyencology 16ᵗʰ ed. P 93-94

- Laparoscope is a rigid telescope varying in diameter between 4 mm and 10 mm and it is 30 cm long.
- CO_2 machine to create pneumoperitoneum is specially designed for laparoscopy. About 100 mL/min is instilled into the peritoneal cavity, maintaining intraperitoneal pressure **below 15 mm** Hg.
- About 1000 mL is required for adequate pneumoperitoneum.

164. Ans. (d) Uterus surface

Ref: Shaw's Gyenecology 16ᵗʰ ed. P 103-104

- Hysteroscopy is a diagnostic and therapeutic modality for the intrauterine pathology.
- It can visualize the OS, cervix, endometrium and their associated pathologies like fibroids, endometrial polyps, endometrial TB, adhesion of septum, *in situ* placed or misplaced IUCD.
- It cannot visualize the outer surface of uterus.
- For the procedure the uterine cavity is distended with CO_2 at the rate of 70 mL/min and pressure less than 100 mm Hg, or with saline, dextrose, hyskon or glycine 1.5%.
- **Types of hysteroscopes:**
  - **Microhysteroscope:** Provides magnification of 30–150 times.
  - **Contact hysteroscope:** A diagnostic tool without distending medium.

Contraindications of Hysteroscopy

- During menstruation, view is obscured and infection rate increases.
- Genital tract infection.

FMGE Solutions Screening Examination

- Pregnancy.
- **Scarred uterus and enlarged uterus more than 12 weeks** size form relative contraindications.
- **Cervical stenosis** can cause cervical tear and uterine perforation.
- **Cardiopulmonary disorders:** Due to risk of fluid overload or anesthesia risk.

165. Ans. (c) ECV done after 34 weeks

Ref: DC Dutta 8th ed. P 435

- Breech is the most common malpresentation, with reduced incidence as the age of gestation progresses *(20% at 28th week and drops to 5% at 34th week and to 3–4% at term)*.
- Thus in 3 out of 4, **spontaneous correction into vertex presentation occurs by 34th week.**
- So external cephalic version (ECV) **should not be done before 34 weeks**.
- They are **not** associated with any specific congenital anomaly.
- There are two varieties of breech presentation (*see* Fig.):
  - Complete
  - Incomplete

Complete (Flexed Breech)
- Thighs are flexed at hips and legs at knees.
- **Presenting part:** Two buttocks, external genitalia and two feet.
- **It is commonly present in multiparae (10%).**

Incomplete: Three varieties are possible:
- **Breech with extended legs (Frank breech):** In this condition, **thighs are flexed on the trunk and legs are extended at the knee joints** (*see* **Fig. A**). The presenting part consists of the two buttocks and external genitalia only.
  - **It is commonly present in primigravidae,** about 70% (due to tight abdominal wall and good uterine tone).

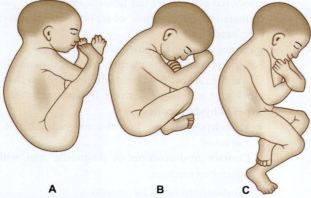

FIGURE: Varieties of breech presentation—(A) Breech with extended legs (Frank breech); (B) Flexed breech (Complete breech); (C) Footling presentation

- **Footling presentation (25%):** Both thighs and legs are partially extended bringing the legs to present at brim.
- **Knee presentation:** Thighs are extended but the knees are flexed, bringing the knees down to present at the brim. Footling and knee presentation are not so common.

166. Ans. (a) Acromion

Ref: DC Dutta, 8th ed. pg. 454

- When the long axis of the fetus lies perpendicularly to the maternal spine or centralized uterine axis, it is called transverse lie.
- In transverse lie, acromion is the presenting part/most prominent part upon vaginal examination.

Extra Mile

Presentation	Presenting part
Face	Mentum
Shoulder	Acromion
Breech	Sacrum
Cephalic	Vertex

167. Ans. (b) Mentum

Ref: DC Dutta, 8th ed. pg. 449

- Face is a rare variety of cephalic presentation where the **presenting part** is the face.
- **There is complete extension of the head** so that the occiput is in contact with the back. **The denominator is mentum.**
- Face presentation results most likely from complete extension of deflexed head of a vertex presentation.

Note: *Most common fetal cause of face presentation is anencephaly.*

168. Ans. (b) Ceasarean section

Ref: DC Dutta 8th ed./441-42, Williams 22/e/571

- **Because Breech presentation with footling has very high incidence of cord prolapse, delivery by caesarean section is recommended in these patients.**
- Indication of C.S in breech are:
- Big baby (Wt> 3.5 kg.)
- Hyperextension of head (stargazing fetus)
- **Footling presentation (risk of cord prolapse)**
- Suspected pelvic contraction
- Severe IUGR

169. Ans. (b) Head with hand

Ref: DC Dutta, 7th ed. pg. 397

COMPOUND PRESENTATION

When a cephalic presentation is complicated by the presence of:
- A hand or a foot or both alongside the head or
- Presence of one or both hands by the side of the breech, it is called compound presentation.
- ***The commonest one being the head with hand***
- *Rarest one being the presence of head, hand and a foot.*
- The incidence is about 1 in 600.

Causes of Compound Presentation
- Prematurity (commonest),
- Contracted pelvis
- Pelvic tumors
- Multiple pregnancy
- Macerated fetus
- High head with premature or early rupture of the membranes.

170. Ans. (b) Partial extension

Ref: William's Obstetrics, 23rd ed. Ch 17

- In cephalic presentation, the fetal head may assume a position between these extremes:
  - **Vertex presentation:** Head is flexed sharply so that the chin is in contact with the thorax. The occipital fontanel is the presenting part, and this presentation is referred to as a *vertex* or *occiput presentation*.
  - **Sinciput/Military presentation:** Partially flexed head in some cases, with the anterior (large) fontanel, or bregma, as presenting.
  - **Brow presentation:** head is partially extended (see Fig).
  - These two presentations (sinciput and brow) are usually transient. As labor progresses, sinciput and brow presentations almost always convert into vertex or face presentations by neck flexion or extension, respectively.
  - **Face presentation:** Much less commonly, the fetal neck may be sharply extended so that the occiput and back come in contact, and the face is foremost in the birth canal, giving it the *face presentation*.

171. Ans. (a) Face presentation

Ref: DC Dutta 8th ed./449, Dutta's Obstetrics P 392

CEPHALIC PRESENTATIONS

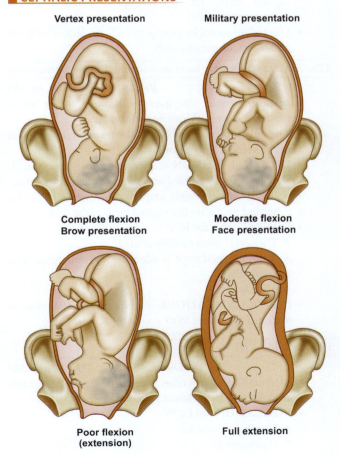

ABNORMAL PRESENTATIONS

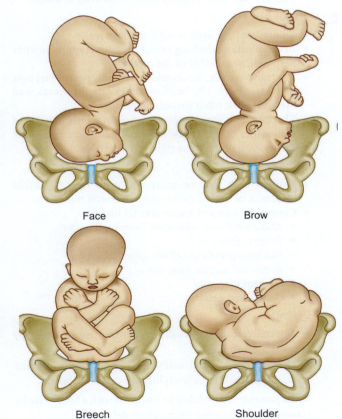

FACE PRESENTATION

- Seen in 0.5% of cases.
- With this presentation, the head is hyperextended so that the occiput is in contact with the fetal back, and the chin (mentum) is presenting.
- The fetal face may present with the chin (mentum) anteriorly or posteriorly, relative to the maternal symphysis pubis

Etiology

- Causes of face presentations are numerous and include conditions that favor extension or prevent head flexion:
  - Preterm infants
  - Anencephalic fetuses naturally present by the face
  - In contracted pelvis or large fetuses
  - High parity is a predisposing factor to face presentation

172. Ans. (a) Polyhydramnios is a cause

Ref: William's Obstetrics 23rd ed. Ch 20, Abnormal Labor

- *For this question, most of the students usually go for 'D' shoulder dystocia is a threat for this condition. But remember one thing that shoulder dystocia usually results in longitudianal lie, where head of the baby is born and rest of the body below neck is stuck. It occurs can be secondary to contracted pelvis, macrosomic baby etc.*
- This is a clear case of transverse lie (as seen in image).

TRANSVERSE LIE

- Transverse lie is seen in 0.3% of the cases.
- In this position, the long axis of the fetus is approximately perpendicular to that of the mother.
- In a transverse lie, the shoulder is usually positioned over the pelvic inlet. The head occupies one iliac fossa, and the breech the other *(as seen in question)*.
- This creates a *shoulder presentation* in which the side of the mother on which the acromion rests determines the designation of the lie as right or left acromial.

Etiology

- Women with four or more deliveries have a 10-fold incidence of transverse lie compared with nulliparas.
- **Common causes of transverse lie include:**
  - Abdominal wall relaxation from high parity
  - Preterm fetus
  - *Placenta previa (NOT abruption placentae)*
  - Abnormal uterine anatomy
  - *Hydramnios, and*
  - Contracted pelvis.

Diagnosis

- A transverse lie is usually recognized easily, often by inspection alone.
- The abdomen is unusually wide, whereas the uterine fundus extends to only slightly above the umbilicus

Management: Active labor in a woman with a transverse lie is usually an indication for cesarean delivery.

173. Ans. (a) Amniocentesis

Ref: DC Dutta, 8th ed. pg. 248-50

174. Ans. (b) Previous CS of more than 2

Ref: Dutta's Obstetrics, 7th ed. pg. 330

Recommendations of American college of obstetricions & Gynecologists (ACOG) for vaginal birth after cesarian delivery (VBAC):

Indications

- *No more than 1 previous lower segment transverse scar*
- Availability of anesthesia and personnel for emergency cesarean delivery.
- Clinically adequate pelvis
- No history of previous uterine rupture or other uterine scars.
- Availability of physician throughout active labor.

Contraindications

- *Prior classical or T-shaped uterine incision.*
- *Previous 2 or more LSCS*
- History of uterine rupture.
- Medical or obstetrical complications that preclude vaginal birth. Ex: pre-eclampsia, placenta previa, malpresentation etc.
- Limited resources for emergency CS. Ex: lack of surgeon, anesthesia, or nursing staff.

175. Ans. (c) Transverse lie of second fetus in a twin pregnancy

Ref: DC Dutta, 7th ed. pg. 585

- *In other words, this question actually asking about condition where ICV can be performed.*
- **The only indication of ICV is the transverse lie in case of the second baby of twins.**
- **INTERNAL VERSION**: is always a podalic version and is almost always completed with the extraction of the fetus.
  - It is most commonly employed for the delivery of a second twin after the vaginal birth of the first.
- **CONDITIONS for ICV**
  - The cervix must be fully dilated
  - Amniotic fluid must be adequate for intrauterine fetal manipulation
  - Alive fetus.
- **CONTRAINDICATIONS**: *it must not be attempted in neglected obstructed labor even if the baby is living.*

176. Ans. (d) PIH

Ref: DC Dutta, 7th ed. pg. 379-380 and 583

- External Cephalic version is done to bring the favorable cephalic pole in the lower pole of the uterus.
- **INDICATIONS of ECV:**
  - Breech presentation
  - Transverse lie

Obstetrics and Gynecology

- **Benefits of ECV:**
  - Reduces maternal morbidity due to caesarean or vaginal breech delivery
  - Reduces the incidence of breech presentation at term.
  - Reduces the number of caesarean delivery
  - The success rate of external version is about 60%
- **CONTRAIDICATIONS OF ECV**
  - Multiple pregnancy
  - Previous caesarean delivery
  - Antepartum hemorrhage
  - Fetal causes like hyperextension of the head, dead or large fetus (> 3.5kg).
  - Ruptured membranes
  - Known congenital malformation of the uterus
  - Contracted pelvis
  - *Obstetric complications like Severe pre-eclampsia, obesity, Elderly primigravida, Bad obstetric History (BOH).*

Note: Breech with extended legs is not a contraindication for external version.

177. Ans. (d) Hydramnois

Ref: DC Dutta, 7th ed. pg. 379-380 and 583

- It's asking here about condition where ECV can be performed.
- Hydramnios always helps in bringing the favorable cephalic pole in the lower pole of the uterus.
- *Please refer to the previous Explanation.*

178. Ans. (c) Fetus is at station + 2

Ref: DC Dutta, 7th ed. pg. 573

TABLE: Classification for operative vaginal (forceps /ventouse) delivery (ACOG-2000)

Procedure	Criteria
Outlet	Scalp is visible at the introitus without separating the labia. Fetal skull at the level of the pelvic floor or on the perineum. Saggittal suture is in direct AP diameter or in the right or left occiput anterior or posterior position.
Low	Leading point of the fetal skull (station) is at +2 cm or more but has not yet reached the pelvic floor. Rotation is <45 degree Rotation is >45 degree
Mid	Fetal head is engaged. Head is 1/5 palpable per abdomen but presenting part is above +2 cm station.
High	Head is not engaged. *This type is not included in classification*

DISEASES DURING PREGNANCY

179. Ans. (c) Parvovirus B19

Ref: DC Dutta 9th ed. P 200, 313

- Hydrops fetalis is the most serious form of Rh hemolytic disease
- Hemolysis produces → severe anemia → Damage to liver → leading to hypoproteinemia → Causing generalized edema/Hydrops fetalis, ascites and hydrothorax.
- Hydrops fetalis is due to:
  - Rh immunization
  - Non-immune hydrops
  - Cardiothoracic anomalies
  - Fetal cirrhosis and
  - Fetal infections with TORCH and Parvovirus B19 infection.
- Incidence is 13 times higher is Rh +ve males
- **USG:** Budha position (with halo around head due to edematous scalp)
- To counter the adversity of hypoxia due to hemolysis there is **Hyperplasia of placental tissue** as well.
- Cause of fetal death: **Cardiac failure**

180. Ans. (b) 140

Ref: DC Dutta 9th ed. P 263

- As a screening method for high risk pregnant patients, 50 gram oral glucose challenge test is done regardless of meal or time of the day.
- Done between 24 and 28 weeks of pregnancy
- A plasma glucose value of 140 mg% at 1 hour is considered as a cut-off point

Extra Mile

TABLE: Criteria for diagnosis of GDM with 100 gm oral glucose (O'sullivan and Mahan modified by Carpenter and Coustan) and national diabetes data group

GTT: Venous Plasma (mg/dL)		
Time	**Carpenter & Coustan**	**NDDG**
Fasting	95	105
1 hour	180	190
2 hours	155	165
3 hours	140	145
GDM is diagnosed when any two values are met or elevated		

TABLE: Criteria for diagnosis of impaired glucose tolerance and diabetes with 75 gm oral glucose (american diabetes association)

Time	Normal Tolerance	Impaired Glucose Tolerance	Diabetes
Fasting	<100	≥100 and <126	≥126
2 hours post: glucose	<140	≥140 and < 200	≥200

181. Ans. (c) 46 XX both paternal origin

Ref: DC Dutta 9th ed. P 181

- Complete mole commonly has 46XX karyotype (in 85%), the molar chromosome are derived entirely from the father.
  - Less commonly the chromosomal pattern may be 46Xy or 45X
- An empty ovum is fertilized by a haploid sperm, which duplicates its own chromosome after meiosis → Phenomenon called **Androgenesis**.
- Complete mole shows paternal: maternal ratio of 2:0, whereas partial mole shows 2:1 ratio.

TABLE: Important features of complete and partial moles

Features	Complete Mole	Partial Mole
Embryo/Fetus	Absent	Present
Hydropic degeneration of villi	Pronounced and diffused	Variable and focal
Trophoblast hyperplasia	Diffuse	Focal
Uterine size	More than the date (30-60%)	Less than the date
Theca lutein cysts	Common (25-50%)	Uncommon
Karyotype	46, KX (85%), Paternal in origin	Triploid (90%), diploid (10%)
β-hCG	High (>50,000)	Slight elevation (<50,000)
Classic clinical symptoms	Common	Rare
Risk of persistent GTN	20%	<5%
Immunostaining (p57^{KF2})	Negative	Positive

182. Ans. (b) Thiopentone sodium

Ref: DC Dutta, 8th ed. pg. 270

- During pregnancy when fits are multiple, recurring at varying intervals **in quick succession, it is called status eclampticus**.

Treatment of status eclampticus
- **Thiopentone sodium 0.5 g** dissolved in 20 mL of 5% dextrose is given intravenously very slowly.
- **If the procedure fails**, use of complete anesthesia, muscle relaxant and assisted ventilation may be employed.
- **In unresponsive cases**, cesarean section in ideal surroundings may be a lifesaving attempt.

183. Ans. (a) Mannitol

Ref: DC Dutta, 8th ed. pg. 275

- A deeply unconscious patient with raised intracranial pressure needs steroid and/or diuretic therapy.
- DOC for eclampsia: $MgSO_4$.

184. Ans. (b) Heart disease

Ref: DC Dutta, 8th ed. pg. 256

- **Pre-eclampsia** is a multisystem disorder of unknown etiology characterized by development of hypertension to the extent of **140/90 mm Hg** or more with proteinuria after the 20th week in a previously normotensive and non-proteinuric woman.
- The incidence in primigravidae is about 10% and in multigravidae 5%.

Etiopathogenesis of Pre-eclampsia

- **Hypertension:** The underlying basic pathology is **endothelial dysfunction** and intense **vasospasm**, affecting almost all the vessels, particularly those of uterus, kidney, placental bed and brain. The basic underlying pathology remains as **endothelial dysfunction** and **vasospasm**.

Risk Factors for Pre-eclampsia

- Primigravida: Young or elderly (first time exposure to chorionic villi)
- Family history: Hypertension, preeclampsia
- Placental abnormalities:
  - Hyperplacentosis: Excessive exposure to chorionic villi-(molar pregnancy twins, diabetes
  - Placental Ischemia)
- Obesity: BMI > 35 kg/m², insulin resistacne
- Pre-existing vascular disease
- New paternity
- Thrombophilias [antiphospholipid syndrome, protein C, S deficiency, Factor V leiden

185. Ans. (a) Nifedipine

Ref: KDT, 6th ed. pg. 323

- Nifedipine is a calcium channel blocker which is used as an alternative drug for premature labor.
- Influx of calcium ions play an important role in uterine contractions. CCB's reduce tone of myometrium and oppose contractions.
- These drugs especially Nifedipine can postpone labor only if started early enough.
- In emergency situation, Ritodrine (β2 selective agonist) is considered as the drug of choice to suppress preterm labor.

> **Extra Mile**
> - Drug of choice for hypertension in pregnancy: LABETALOL
> - Drug of choice for epilepsy in pregnancy- LAMOTRIGINE

186. Ans. (d) **Labetalol**

Ref: Dutta Obs, 7th ed. 228, William Obs, 22nd ed. pg. 728

187. Ans. (b) **ACE inhibitors**

Ref: KDT, 6th ed. 553; Williams, 24th ed, pg. 1025

- ACE's are the drugs which inhibit the conversion of angiotensin-I to angiotensin-II. They can cause severe fetal malformations when given in the second and third trimesters.
- **These include:** Hypocalvaria and renal dysfunction and are also teratogenic and because of this, they are not recommended during pregnancy
- *Angiotensin-receptor blockers act in a similar manner.* But, instead of blocking the production of angiotensin-II, they inhibit binding to its receptor. *They are presumed to have the same fetal effects as ACE inhibitors and thus are also contraindicated.*

Antihypertensive to be avoided during pregnancy	Antihypertensive safer during pregnancy
- ACE inhibitors (Ex- captopril, enelapril etc.) - Angiotensin antagonist (losartan, telmesartan) - Thiazide diuretics (Ex- hydrochlorthiazide) - Furosemide - Propanolol - Nitroprusside	- Hydralazine - Methyldopa - Atenolol - Metoprolol - *Labetalol- DOC* - Nifedipine - Prazosin and Clonidine

Drugs and their respective risk
- **Diuretics:** Tend to reduce blood volume; increase risk of placental infarcts, fetal wastage, stillbirth.
- **ACE inhibitors, AT1 antagonists:** growth retardation and fetal damage risk.
- **Propanolol:** Causes low birth weight, neonatal hypoglycemia and bradycardia.
- **Nitroprusside:** Contraindicated in eclampsia.

188. Ans. (a) **Angiotensin receptor blockers**

Ref: KDT 6th ed. pg. 553

Please refer to above explanation.

189. Ans. (a) **Folic acid supplementation**

Ref: DC Dutta, 8th ed. pg. 585

- Use of anti- epileptic drugs like phenytoin, valproate and even phenobarbitone has been shown in pregnancy to contribute to acquire folic acid deficiency.

- If a lady is deficient in folic acid at the time of her pregnancy, then the baby most likely will born with neural tube defect.
- Traditionally we study that folic acid should be taken peri-conceptionally 2 months before and 3 months later to pregnant status at dose of 400 micrograms.
- However with the use of anti-epileptics drugs like phenytoin, valproate etc. the dose of folic acid needs to be supplemented at a dose of 4 mg once per day.

190. Ans. (c) **MRI**

Ref: William's Gyne, chapter 12- Breast Diseases; Breast CA screening

MAGNETIC RESONANCE IMAGING

- This screening option has recently been evaluated among genetically high-risk women. It is particularly attractive in this group of women, who develop breast cancer at a rate of 2 percent per year between the ages of **25 and 50,** a time during which mammography sensitivity is reduced by dense breast tissue.
- *In general, MR imaging shows higher sensitivity and specificity than mammography.*
- *In the case given, patient is a 42 year primigravida, which in-itself is at high risk of developing congenital anomaly. By giving tests like mammography, condition can be worsened. Hence MRI is considered as the best modality of screening. Also it has higher sensitivity and specificity than other given tests.*

SCREENING MAMMOGRAPHY

- Considered as screening IOC.
- This radiographic test is currently the best available and most thoroughly validated breast cancer screening test available.
- At this time, it is generally accepted that for women aged 50 to 69 years, screening mammography reduces breast cancer mortality.

Screening Sonography: This modality identifies mammographically occult breast cancer in less than 1 percent of women.

191. Ans. (a) **Bile acid**

Ref: William's 23rd ed. Ch 50, Hepatic GB and pancreatic disorders; Intrahepatic cholestasis of Pregnancy

INTRAHEPATIC CHOLESTASIS OF PREGNANCY

- This disorder also has been referred to as recurrent jaundice of pregnancy, cholestatic hepatosis, and icterus gravidarum.
- It is characterized clinically by pruritus, icterus, or both.

FMGE Solutions Screening Examination

Pathogenesis

- The cause of obstetrical cholestasis is unknown, but it probably occurs in genetically susceptible women.
- Whatever the inciting cause(s), bile acids are cleared incompletely and accumulate in plasma. *Of note, total bile acid concentration may already be elevated 10- to 100-fold in normal pregnancy.*
- Even *before* bile acid levels increase, associated dyslipidemia is apparent
- Total cholesterol levels are significantly higher compared with those of normal pregnancy, and *low-density lipoprotein (LDL) cholesterol levels become elevated earliest.*
- **Hyperbilirubinemia** results from retention of conjugated pigment, but total plasma concentrations rarely exceed 4 to 5 mg/dL.
- **Alkaline phosphatase** is usually elevated even more so than in normal pregnancy.
- **Serum transaminase** levels are normal to moderately elevated but seldom exceed 250 U/L
- Liver biopsy shows mild cholestasis with bile plugs in the hepatocytes and canaliculi of the centrilobular regions, but without inflammation or necrosis.

Note: *These changes disappear after delivery but often recur in subsequent pregnancies or with estrogen-containing contraceptives.*

192. Ans. (c) Placenta previa

Ref: Willaims, 24th ed. pg. 827

- Disseminated intravascular coagulation (DIC) aka consumptive coagulopathy is a pathologic disruption of the finely-balanced process of hemostasis.
- Massive activation of the clotting cascade results in widespread thrombosis, *which leads to depletion of platelets and coagulation factors and excessive thrombolysis,* because all the clotting factors and platelets are consumed in intravascular coagulation. The end result is multiorgan failure and hemorrhage.
- **Placental Abruption:** is the most common cause of severe consumptive coagulopathy in obstetrics
- **Causes of DIC in pregnancy:**
  - Placental abruption (NOT placenta previa): most common cause.
  - Amnionic-fluid embolism.
  - Sepsis
  - Thrombotic microangiopathies
  - Acute kidney injury
  - Pre- eclampsia and
  - HELLP (Hemolysis, Elevated liver enzyme levels, low Platelet count) syndromes.

193. Ans. (d) Hyponatremia

Ref: DC Dutta's Textbook of Obstetrics, 7th ed. pg. 222

HELLP syndrome is rare complication of pre-eclamsia (10-15%), but can also develop without maternal hypertension.
- H-Hemolysis (bilirubin >1.2 mg/dl)
- EL-Elevated Liver enzyme (ASL and ALT >70 IU/L), **LDH >600 IU/L**, Bilirubin (>1.2mg/dl)
- LP-Low Platelets (1, 00, 000/mm³)

194. Ans. (c) Fluconazole 150 mg

Ref: Shaws, 15th ed. pg. 352

CANDIDAL (MONILIAL) VAGINITIS

- It is a fungal infection caused by yeast-like microorganisms called Candida or Monilia.
- The commonest species causing human disease is Candida albicans

Clinical Features

- Vulval itching is the most common symptom, accompanied by vaginal irritation, dysuria, or both
- Thick curdy or flaky vaginal discharge.

Diagnosis

- Essentially based on clinical findings. But the diagnosis can be confirmed on microscopic examination of a smear of the vaginal discharge treated with 10% KOH solution.
- Pap smear shows **thick red-stained hyphae and dark red spores.**

Treatment

- **A single dose of fluconazole 150 mg has been found to be very effective.**
- Ideally, both partners should be treated and the underlying predisposing factor corrected to give long-term relief.
- Recurrent infection requires fluconazole orally 150 mg every 72 hours for 3 doses.

195. Ans. (a) Pre-eclampsia

Ref: William's Obstetrics 23rd ed. Ch 34.

GESTATIONAL HYPERTENSION CRITERIA

- Systolic BP >140 or diastolic BP >90 mm Hg for first time during pregnancy
- No proteinuria
- BP returns to normal before 12 weeks postpartum
- Final diagnosis made only postpartum
- May have other signs or symptoms of preeclampsia, for example, epigastric discomfort or thrombocytopenia.

PREECLAMPSIA

- BP >140/90 mm Hg **after 20 weeks'** gestation
- Proteinuria >300 mg/24 hours or >1+ dipstick

Eclampsia: Symptoms of pre-eclampsia + seizures *that cannot be attributed to other causes in a woman with preeclampsia.*

196. Ans. (a) Diuretics

Ref: KDT, 6th ed. pg. 553

- Diuretics are contraindicated in preeclampsia as they are teratogenic.

Antihypertensives in Pregnancy

Safe	Contraindicated
Labetalol-DOC	ACE inhibitors
Calcium Channel blockers	
Hydralazine	Diuretics
Alpha methyldopa	Reserpine
Sodium nitroprusside+/−	Loratidine

197. Ans. (d) MgSO$_4$

Ref: DC Dutta, 8th ed. pg. 271, Dutta Obs, 6th ed. pg. 235

Medical Management

- *Seizure treatment*
  - The drug of choice for the control and prevention of convulsions is Pritchard's regimen i.e. magnesium sulphate.

Extra Mile

- DOC in eclampsia – MgSO$_4$
- 2nd DOC in eclampsia is hydralazine.

198. Ans. (c) Hospitalization and observation

Ref: DC Dutta, 8th ed. pg. 264-65

- Given these options, the best choice is hospitalization and do the observation under supervision conservatively.
- As the AOG is premature, CS or induction of labor can complicate the baby's outcome.

199. Ans. (a) Presence of fetal cardiac activity

Ref: DC Dutta, 8th ed. pg. 264

Please follow the flowchart given

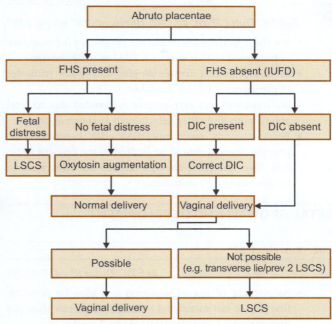

200. Ans. (c) Congenital heart disease

Ref: Danforth's Obstetrics and Gynecology, 10th ed. pg. 249-250

- In **infant of diabetic mother**, maternal hyperglycemia causes fetal hyperglycemia. In response of that, there is fetal β cell hyperplasia, which secretes enough insulin to counteract excess insulin coming from mother. This excess glucose causes glycogen and fat deposition leading to fetal macrosomia **(20-25%)**.
- Soon after birth, when the cord is clamped and cut, there is cessation of glucose supply from mother while there is still higher insulin production in neonate, leading to à Hypoglycemia **(25–40%)**.
- **Danforth's OBG states** *"Most frequent type of malformation involves central nervous system, cardiovascular system, gastrointestinal, genitourinary, and skeletal anomalies, with **cardiovascular system being the most common**"*
- This ventricular wall and septal hypertrophy is thought to be due to glucose toxicity (from mother) and hyperinsulinemic state of the fetus.
- **Other fetal complications:**
  - Neonatal hyperbilirubinemia: 20–25%
  - Myocardial and septal hypertrophy: 10%
  - Congenital sacral agenesis: ~1%

201. Ans. (a) Propylthiouracil

Ref: DC Dutta 7th ed. pg. 287; Harrison's 19th ed. pg. 2297

- For the hyperthyroidism during pregnancy the mainstay of treatment in 1st trimester is PTU or methimazole.
- Methimazole is preferable avoided during first trimester of pregnancy if PTU is available.
- Methimazole and carbimazole is avoided due to fetal aplasia cutis and other defects such as choanal atresia.
- Because of its rare association with hepatotoxicity, propylthiouracil should be limited to the first trimester and then maternal therapy should be converted to methimazole (or carbimazole).

FETAL GROWTH AND DEVELOPMENT

202. Ans. (b) CRL

Ref: DC Dutta 8th ed. P 81, 84

- Assessment of age of gestation can also be done by first day of last menstrual period. It is greater than the postconception (fertilization) age by 2 weeks.
- The length is more reliable criterion than the weight to calculate the age of the fetus.
- In the **first trimester**, CRL (mm) + 6.5 = gestational age in weeks.
- **Best fetal parameter to find out AOG in 1st trimester:** CRL (Crown rump length). Variation ± 5 days.
- **Best fetal parameter to find out AOG in 2nd trimester:** BPD (Biparietal diameter). Most accurate when done between 12 and 20 weeks.
- **Best fetal parameter to find out AOG in 3rd trimester:** Femur length. Less reliable, variation ± 16 days.

203. Ans. (a) 11 weeks

Ref: DC Dutta, 8th ed. pg. 48

Dutta states: *"Breathing movements are identified by 11 weeks but are irregular until 20th week. Their frequency varies from 30–70 per minute and is dependent on the maternal blood sugar concentration."*

204. Ans. (a) Straight into mother's blood by simple diffusion

Ref: DC Dutta, 8th ed. pg. 41

Mechanisms involved in the transfer of substances across the placenta are:

- **Respiratory function:** Although the fetal respiratory movements are observed as early as 11 weeks, there is no gaseous exchange. Intake of oxygen and output of carbon dioxide take place by **simple diffusion** across the fetal membrane.
- **Excretory function:** Waste products from the fetus such as urea, uric acid, and creatinine are excreted in the maternal blood **by simple diffusion.**
- **Nutritive function:**
  - **Glucose,** the principal source of energy is transferred to the fetus **by facilitated diffusion.**
  - **Amino acids** are transferred by active transport
  - **Lipids, triglycerides and fatty acids** are transferred from mother and synthesized in fetus as well.
  - **Water and electrolytes** such as sodium, potassium and chloride cross through the fetal membrane by simple diffusion, whereas calcium, phosphorus and iron cross **by active transport.**
  - **Hormones:** Insulin, steroids from the adrenals, thyroid, chorionic gonadotropin or placental lactogen cross the placenta at a very slow rate.

Extra Mile

- Neither parathormone nor calcitonin cross the placenta.

205. Ans. (a) Liver

Ref: DC Dutta, 8th ed. pg. 47; PubMed

- Hematopoiesis is **first started in the yolk sac** by 14th day.
- **By 10th week,** the **liver becomes the major site.** The great enlargement of the early fetal liver is due to its erythropoietic function. Gradually, the red cell production sites extend to the spleen and bone marrow
- Near term, the bone marrow becomes the major site of red cell production.
- During the first half, the hemoglobin is of fetal type (α-2, γ-2) but from 24 weeks onwards, adult type of hemoglobin (α-2, β-2) **appears and at term about 75–80% of the total hemoglobin is of fetal type** (HbF).

206. Ans. (a) Umbilical artery

Ref: DC Dutta, 8th ed. pg. 36

- Deoxygenated blood from fetus to mother is carried via umbilical artery.
- Oxygenated blood is via umbilical vein.

207. Ans. (a) 6–7 weeks

Ref: DC Dutta, 8th ed. pg. 734

- Cardiac activity be assessed at the earliest by trans-vaginal scan by 5 weeks
- Cardiac activity be assessed by trans-abdominal scan by 6 weeks
- Fetal heart sound can be assessed by Doppler- 10 weeks
- Fetal heart sound can be assessed by stethoscope-18 weeks

Obstetrics and Gynecology

208. Ans. (a) 7 cm

Ref: DC Dutta 7th ed./ 41; William's Obstetrics 22nd ed./ 91

- To determine the length of the fetus, the measurement is commonly taken from the vertex to the coccyx (crown-rump length) in earlier weeks of gestation.
  - By the end of the 12th week of pregnancy, when the uterus usually is just palpable above thesymphysis pubis, the crown-rump length of the fetus is *6 to 7 cm.*
  - **At 16th week, CRL:** 12 cm and the weight is about 110 gm.
  - **At 28th week, CRL:** 25 cm and the weight is about 1100 gm.
  - **At 32nd week, CRL:** 28 cm and the weight is about 1800 gm.
  - **At 36th weeks, CRL:** 32 cm and the weight is about 2500 gm.
- From the end of 20th week onwards, the measurement is taken from the vertex to the heel (crown –heel length).

Extra Mile

- Best fetal parameter to find out AOG in 1st trimester: CRL (Crown Rump length)
- Best fetal parameter to find out AOG in 2nd trimester: BPD (Biparietal diameter)
- Best fetal parameter to find out AOG in 3rd trimester: Femur Length.

209. Ans. (a) 60 mm

Ref: DC Dutta 7th ed./41; William's Obstetrics 22nd ed. pg. 91

- By the end of the 12th week of pregnancy, when the uterus usually is just palpable above the symphysis pubis, the crown-rump length of the fetus is *6 to 7 cm i.e. 60 to 70 mm.*
- *Please refer to above explanation for more details.*

210. Ans. (a) 4-16 weeks

Ref: Dutta's Obstetrics, 7th ed. pg. 647

RADIATION HAZARDS

1. **Teratogenecity:** Diagnostic range of radiation exposure (<5 Rads) is not associated with any congenital malformation.
2. **Oncogenecity:** Dividing cells particularly in **first trimester** are more sensitive to injury from radiation. Diagnostic radiation with fetal exposure is associated with an increased risk of malignancy.
3. **Genetic damage and intrauterine death**

NOTE: **radiation during early stage of pregnancy can damage the embroyo. This risk can be minimized by using the "10 day rule". This rule states that:** *"No women should be exposed to X-Ray for a non-urgent indication outside 10 days from her last period during reproductive period"*

211. Ans. (b) Megaloblastic anemia

Ref: Dutta's Obstetrics, 7th ed. pg. 268-69

- This is a bit confusing question though. But if we read the question carefully it is asking the outcome of combined vit B12 and folate deficiency, which is Megaloblastic anemia according to the question.
- Neural tube defect is due to deficiency of folic acid (Vit B9).
- Abruption placentae can be secondary to Vit B12 deficiency.

INTRAUTERINE FETAL DEATH

212. Ans. (b) Obstructed labor

Ref: D.C Dutta, 7th ed. pg. 322-323

INTERAUTERINE FETAL DEATH (IUD)

- All fetal deaths weighing 500 gram or more occurring during pregnancy (antepartum death) or during labor (intrapartum).
- It is least likely caused by maternal factors like prolonged or obstructed labor, or due to uterine rupture.
- IUFD most commonly caused by fetal factors like Rh incompatibility, chromosomal abnormalities etc.

Causes of IUD

MATERNAL: 5-10%	FETAL: 25-40%
• Hypertensive disorder in pregnancy	• Chromosomal abnormalities
• Diabetes in pregnancy	• *Rh-incompatibility*
• Anti-phospholipid syndrome	• Non immune hydrops
• Thrombophilias	• *Growth restriction*
• *Abnormal labor: Prolonged or obstructed labor, ruptured uterus*	
• Post term pregnancy	
• Lupus Erythematosus	
PLACENTAL: 20-35%	**IATROGENIC**
• Antepartum haemorrhage	• External cephalic version
• Cord accident	• Drugs
• TTTS	
• *Placental insufficiency*	**IDIOPATHIC: 25-35%**

213. Ans. (b) Robert's sign

Ref: Dutta's Obstetrics, 7th ed. pg. 324

- **Robert's sign** refers to the presence of a gas shadow within the heart or the greater vessels, in cases of fetal death.
  - It is a rare sign caused by postmortem blood degeneration, usually seen 1–2 days after death

FMGE Solutions Screening Examination

- **Spalding sign:** Overlapping of skull bone. *Also a sign of fetal demise.*
- **Goodell's sign:** Softening of the vaginal part of the cervix during the first trimester
- **Von Braun-Fernwald's sign:** Softening of the uterine fundus at the site of implantation at 4–5 weeks gestation.
- **Osiander sign:** Increased pulsation at lateral fornices of vagina seen at ~8th week of pregnancy.

> **Extra Mile**
> **Robert Pelvis:** aka transversely contracted pelvis. Ala of both the sides are absent and sacrum is fused with innominate bones.

214. Ans. (a) Cord prolapsed

Ref: Dutta's Obstetrics, 7th ed. pg. 398

- Most common cause of intrapartum fetal death is cord prolapsed. Overall perinatal mortality is 15-50%.
- In other cases like abruption, Eclampsia, there are chances that we can terminate the pregnancy via emergency CS. But once there is cord prolapsed, there is sudden hypoxia to fetus leading to death.

215. Ans. (d) Ectopic pregnancy

Ref: DC Dutta, 8th ed. pg. 204, 216, 228, 486,588

- DOC for ectopic pregnancy → Methotrexate

MISCELLANEOUS

216. Ans. (c) It has 4 to 6 lobes

Ref: William's obstetrics, 23rd ed. Implantation, Embryogenesis and Placental development

PLACENTAL GROWTH

- *In the first trimester, placental growth is more rapid than that of the fetus.*
- By approximately 17th weeks period of gestation, placental and fetal weights are approximately equal.
- By term, placental weight is approximately one sixth of fetal weight.

- The average placenta at term is 185 mm in diameter and 23 mm in thickness, **with a volume of 497 mL and a weight of 508 g.** These measurements vary widely.
- From the maternal surface, the number of slightly elevated convex areas, *called lobes, varies from 10 to 38.*
- Lobes are incompletely separated by grooves of variable depth that overlie *placental septa,* which arise from folding of the basal plate.
- Although grossly visible lobes are commonly referred to as cotyledons.
- *The total number of placental lobes remains the same throughout gestation,* and individual lobes continue to grow—although less actively in the final weeks.

217. Ans. (c) FSH

Ref: D.C Dutta, 6th ed. pg. 56

- There is a significant fall in the level of serum estradiol from 50–300 pg/ml before menopause to 10-20 pg/ml after menopause
- This decrease the negative feedback effect on hypothalamopituitary axis resulting in increase in FSH.
- The increase in FSH is also due to diminished inhibin.

218. Ans. (c) Chloramphenicol

Ref: DC Dutta, 8th ed. pg. 587-89

- Chloramphenicol causes grey baby syndrome due to bone marrow suppression.
- **Antibiotics which are safe in pregnancy-**
  - Cephalosporin
  - Penicillin
  - Erythromycin or macrolide group

219. Ans. (b) IgG

Ref: Robbin's, 9th ed. pg. 198-199

220. Ans. (c) 3 months

Ref: DC Dutta, 8th ed. pg. 735

221. Ans. (c) 300 µg

Ref: DC Dutta, 8th ed. pg. 387, 721

GYNECOLOGY

ANATOMY, MENARCHE AND MENOPAUSE

222. (d) Increased FSH, decreased estrogen

Ref: Shaw, 16th ed. pg. 66 – 67

- Menopause is a retrospective diagnosis as it takes 12 months of amenorrhoea to confirm that menopause has set in.

- Menopause normally occurs between the ages of **45 and 50 years,** the **average age being 47 years.**
- At the time of menopause there is cessation of ovarian activity and a fall in the oestrogen and inhibin levels → cause a rebound increase in the secretion of FSH and LH by the anterior pituitary gland.
- The FSH level may rise as much as 50-fold and LH 3–4 folds.

Obstetrics and Gynecology

- There is 50% reduction in androgen production and 66% reduction in oestrogen at menopause
  - There is a significant fall in the level of serum estradiol from 50–300 pg/ml before menopause to 10-20 pg/ml after menopause

> **Extra Mile**

Prediction of approaching menopause:
- A fall in the level of inhibin B (not inhibin A) causes a rise in follicle-stimulating hormone (FSH) level.
- A **fall in the level of anti-müllerian hormone** suggests low ovarian reserve and low antral follicular count.
- Rise of FSH level more than normal luteinizing hormone (LH) level.

223. Ans. (c) 14

Ref: DC Dutta 7th ed. P 371

- The normal upper limit of menarche is 15 years.
- According to recent recommendation, primary amenorrhea is defined as:
  - Absence of menses by 14 years of age in absence of sexual characters.
  - Absence of menses by 16 years of age regardless of presence of secondary sexual characteristics.

224. Ans. (a) Pelvic irradiation

Ref: DC Dutta 7th ed. P 376

- Secondary amenorrhea is defined as: *"absence of menstruation for 6 months or more in a women in whom normal menstruation has been established"*
- **Book states:** *"Amenorrhea in a woman with reproductive age should be considered as pregnancy unless proved otherwise"*. Therefore, pregnancy is considered as most common cause of amenorrhea in a woman of reproductive age.
- **Note:** Amenorrhea is physiological before puberty, during pregnancy and lactation and following menopause.
- **The most common cause of secondary amenorrhea** (pathological) is hypothalamic dysfunction. Pelvic irradiation is one of the causes of hypothalamic dysfunction.
  - Kallmann syndrome and imperforate hymen are usually associated with primary amenorrhea.
  - Diabetes and hypothyroidism is the systemic cause of secondary amenorrhea.
- **MCC of cryptomenorrhea** is imperforate hymen.
- **MCC of primary amenorrhea** is gonadal failure, abnormal chromosomal pattern, developmental defect of genital tract and disturbed action of HPO axis.

225. Ans. (d) Anti-mullerian hormone

Ref: Shaw's Gynecology 16th ed, P 65-66, 260

929

Test for ovarian reserve is indicated in:
- Women >35 years of age, smokers, presence of only one ovary and unexplained infertility.
- It involves standard day 3 FSH estimation, along with administration of 100 mg CC from day 5 to day 9, repeat FSH on day 10. FSH values must be the same as on day 3 of the cycle.

Prediction of approaching menopause:
- A fall in the level of inhibin B (not inhibin A) causes a rise in follicle-stimulating hormone (FSH) level.
- A **fall in the level of anti-müllerian hormone** suggests low ovarian reserve and low antral follicular count.
- Rise of FSH level more than normal luteinizing hormone (LH) level.

Anti-müllerian Hormone (AMH)
- AMH is a peptide secreted by the sertoli cells in the testis and granulosa cells in the ovary.
- During intrauterine life AMH inhibits the development of **müllerian** system in males. Absence of AMH results in hermaphrodite.
- In the female it helps in the follicular development and oocyte maturation.
  - Normal value is 2–6.8 ng/mL
  - **Poor ovarian reserve:** 1 ng/mL
  - **PCOD and hyperstimulation syndrome:** 0.10 ng/mL
- Estimation of serum AMH is used in the study of ovarian reserve in an infertile woman and a woman with secondary amenorrhea.
- Its level is related to precocious and delayed puberty, infertility and premature menopause.
- Its level is related and reflects the number of growing follicles.

226. Ans. (b) Class II

Ref: Shaw's 16th ed. P 118

American fertility society classification system classified müllerian malformations into 6 classes:
- **Class I (agenesis, hypoplasia).** Uterus is absent in total agenesis. Partial agenesis is identified as unicornuate uterus. In hypoplasia, the endometrial cavity is small with reduced intercornual distance of less than 2 cm.
- **Class II (unicornuate uterus)** appears **banana-shaped** without the rounded fundus and triangular-shaped uterine cavity. If present, rudimentary horn presents as a soft tissue mass with similar myometrial echogenicity. Obstruction in the rudimentary horn is recognized as haematometra on one side.
- **Class III (uterus didelphys).** The two horns are widely separated, but vaginal septum is difficult to identify.

Explanations

- **Class IV (bicornuate uterus)** shows two uterine cavities, with concave fundus, with fundal cleft greater than 1 cm, and this differentiates between the bicornuate and the septate uterus. The intercornual distance is more than 4 cm.
- **Class V (septate uterus)** shows a convex or flattened fundus. The intercornual distance is normal (<4 cm) and each cavity is small.
- **Class VI (arcuate uterus)** with no fundus is of no clinical importance.

227. Ans. (b) Growth of breast

Ref: Shaw, 16th ed. pg. 56

Thelarche

- The first sign of puberty is the development of the breasts. Breast budding usually appears between the ages of 9–11 years.
- It is indicative of the competency of the hypothalamic–pituitary–ovarian axis.

228. Ans. (a) GnRH

Ref: Shaw, 16th ed. pg. 56

Endocrine mechanisms underlying puberty: These have been highlighted in the following:

- **Early in puberty**, the sensitivity of the gonadostat to the negative effects of low estradiol (E2) gradually decreases.
- **Late in puberty**, maturation of positive E2 feedback initiates the LH surge.
- Basal levels of pituitary gonadotropins **increase throughout puberty** due to enhanced hypothalamic GnRH pulse amplitude rather than frequency.

229. Ans. (b) 45

Ref: Shaw, 16th ed. pg. 66

- Menopause is defined as the time of cessation of ovarian function resulting in permanent amenorrhoea.
- Menopause is a retrospective diagnosis as it takes 12 months of amenorrhoea to confirm that menopause has set in.
- Menopause normally occurs between the ages of **45 and 50 years,** the **average age being 47 years.**

> **Extra Mile**
>
> - **Climacteric** is the phase of waning ovarian activity, and may begin 2–3 years before menopause and continue for 2–5 years after it. The climacteric is thus a phase of adjustment between the active and inactive ovarian function.
> - Menopause setting **before the age of 40** is known as **premature menopause.**
> - Menopausal age is NOT related to menarche, race, socioeconomic status, number of pregnancies and lactation, or taking of oral contraceptives.

230. Ans. (c) Appearance of Secondary sexual...

Ref: Shaw's, 16th ed. pg. 59

- **Precocious puberty:** This is defined as the appearance of any of the **secondary sexual characteristics before the age of 8 years** or the **occurrence of menarche before the age of 10** years
- Precocious puberty in females is pubertal changes before the age of 8 years.
- In males it is onset of puberty before the age of 9 years

231. Ans. (a) Increase FSH

Ref: Yen and Jaffe's Reproductive Endocrinology, pg. 155

- FSH levels increase with age, before increases in LH or decrease in estradiol and a number of studies have demonstrated an inverse relationship between increase in FSH and decreasing inhibin B in association with reproductive aging."
- **Ref states:** *"Reproductive aging is associated with decline in fertility that **begins in third decade**, which accelerates after age 35. A gradual decrease in pool of ovarian follicles which first accelerates around the same age would appear to underlie this decline in fertility. **It is also at age 35 that an increase in FSH is first seen."***

> **Extra Mile**
>
> - The first evidence of primordial follicle appears at about 20 weeks of fetal life. The fetal ovary contains **7 million primordial follicles** but most degenerate, and **the newborn contains only 2 million follicles.**
> - At birth, about 2 million follicles seen are reduced **to 400,000 at puberty;**
> - Only 400 follicles are available during the childbearing period for fertilization.

232. Ans. (c) Hematocolpos

Ref: Shaws, 15th ed. pg. 96-98

- **Hematocolpos** is a medical condition in which the vagina fills with menstrual blood. It is often caused by the combination of menstruation with an imperforate hymen.
- **Hematometra:** A related disorder is, where the uterus is filled with menstrual blood.
- **Pyometra:** a type of uterine infection. Disease of the dogs, but has been also noted in humans.
- **Hematosalphinx:** bleeding and collection of blood in fallopian tube. MCC is tubal (ectopic) pregnancy.

Obstetrics and Gynecology

INFECTION

233. Ans. (b) Leads to Infertility

Ref: Harrison 20th ed. Page 1319 - 1321

- The chlamydia species are classified mainly into 4 species:
  - *C. trachomatis*
  - *C. pneumonia*
  - *C. psittaci* (separated into 3 species: C. psittaci, C. felis, C. abortus)
  - *C. pecorum* (the last species being found in ruminants)

Infections associated with Chlamydia trachomatis

- **Trachoma:** C. trachomatis (serotype A, B, Ba and C)- can cause ocular infection trachoma and adult inclusion conjunctivitis.
- **Oculogenital infections (serotype D – K)**
  - Transmitted during sexual contact or from mother to baby during childbirth. Associated with:
    - ♦ **Female:** Cervicitis, salpingitis, acute urethral syndrome, endometritis, ectopic pregnancy, infertility, pelvic pain and PID.

* Untreated PID and High levels of antibody to human heat-shock protein have been associated with tubal factor infertility and ectopic pregnancy.
- ♦ **Males:** Urethritis, proctitis, and epididymitis
- ♦ **Infants:** Conjunctivitis (inclusion body conjunctivitis) and pneumonia
- **LGV (L1, L2, L3)**
  - Characterized by acute lymphadenitis with bubo formation and/or acute hemorrhagic proctitis.

> **Extra Mile**

- *C. pneumoniae* is a common cause of human respiratory diseases, such as pneumonia and bronchitis
- It mainly causes atypical pneumonia as seen with mycoplasma pneumonia
- The clinical spectrum of *C. pneumoniae* infection includes acute pharyngitis, sinusitis, bronchitis, and pneumonitis, primarily in young adults

234. Ans. (a) Chlamydia

Ref: Harrison 20th ed. Page 1319 - 1321

Refer to above explanation

> **Extra Mile**

TABLE: Contraindications of gastric lavage

	Symptoms signs	Examination findings	pH	Wet mount
Normal	White floccular or curdy, odorless	Discharge present in dependent portions of vagina	3.8–4.5	Normal
Bacterial vaginosis	Increased white thin discharge, increased odor	Thin whitish gray homogenous discharge sometimes frothy	>4.5 basic	Clue cells >20% shift in flora, amine odor after KOH smear
Candidiasis	Increased white thick discharge, pruritus, dysuria, burning	Thick curdy discharge, vaginal erythema	<4.5 Acidic	Hyphae or spores
Trichomonas	Increased yellow frothy discharge, increased odor, pruritus, dysuria	Yellow frothy discharge with or without vaginal or cervical erythema	>45 Basic	Motile trichomonads Increased white cells

235. Ans. (c) Cryosurgery

Ref: Shaw's Gynecology 16th ed. 173-74

- The patient in this case is a case of cervicitis.
- **Acute cervicitis:** More commonly secondary to STD (chlamydia trachomatis, gonorrhoea), septic abortion and puerperal sepsis.
- **Chronic cervicitis:** More common than acute variant. Usually due to traumatic childbirth, D&C or a sequel of STD.

- **Clinical features:**
  - Profuse mucoid vaginal discharge, which can be blood stained
  - Postcoital bleeding
  - Antepartum haemorrhage
  - Low backache, abdominal pain and dyspareunia
- **Upon examination:**
  - Cervical erosion
  - Erosion takes the form of a reddened area around the external os, with its inner margin continuous with

Explanations

the endocervical lining and with a well-defined outer margin.
- In chronic cases cervix is fibrosed, bulky with nabothian follicles around the area of erosion
• **Treatment:**
- **Diathermy cauterization:** Tissues of cervix are coagulated and columnar epithelium is destroyed. It also destroys all infection lying in the depths of the racemose glands and in due course healthy epithelium grows down from the upper part of the cervical canal to cover the raw area.
  ♦ Require opening of cervical os and anaesthesia
- **Cryosurgery:** More preferred nowadays. Safer than cautery as it is painless and avoids accidental burn in vagina. Doesn't require anaesthesia
  ♦ The refrigerants used in cryosurgery are carbon dioxide (–78°C), Freon (–81°C), nitrous oxide (–88°C) and nitrogen (–186°C).
  ♦ **Disadvantage:** extensive tissue destruction → hypokalemia
- **Laser therapy:** Highly preferred in chronic cervicitis.
  ♦ Fast healing and accurate/precise excision or burning of tissue
- **Conization operation:** Preferred if above methods are ineffective or if there is extensive area involved.
- **Policresulen:** One gram of Policresulen contains 360 mg of protein. It coagulates necrotic, pathologically altered tissue without destroying the healthy tissue.
  ♦ Contraindicated during pregnancy

236. Ans. (a) Hematogenous

Ref: Shaw's Gyencology 16th ed. P 188

- The general distribution of involvement of reproductive organs in cases of genital TB are as follows:
  - **Fallopian tube:** 90–100%
  - **Endometrium:** 50–60%
  - **Ovaries:** 20–30%
  - **Cervix:** 5–15%
  - **Vulva and vagina:** <1%
- The tubal mucosa is the most favorable nidus for **bloodborne** spread of the disease resulting in endosalpingitis—usually bilateral.
- It is the earliest lesion with a propensity for transluminal spread to the ovary and endometrium.
- Hence, fallopian tubes play the central role in the initiation and dissemination of pelvic tuberculosis.
- **Radiological appearance:** Tobacco pouch appearance.

237. Ans. (b) Candida vaginitis

Ref: Shaw's 16th ed. P 164

- Candidiasis is a fungal infection caused by yeast-like microorganisms called *Candida* or *Monilia*.
- The most common species causing human disease is *Candida albicans*. It can be sexually transmitted.

Risk Factors
- These include promiscuity, immunosuppression, HIV, pregnancy, steroid therapy, following long-term broad-spectrum antibiotic therapy, oral contraception pills, diabetes mellitus, poor personal hygiene and obesity.

Clinical Features
- **Pruritus vulva is the cardinal symptom:** It is often accompanied by vaginal irritation, dysuria, or both, and **passage of thick curdy or flaky discharge.**
- Speculum examination reveals vaginal wall congestion with **curdy discharge** often visible at the vulval mucocutaneous junction and in the posterior fornix.

Diagnosis
- Microscopic examination 10% KOH mount
- Culture on **Sabouraud agar or Nickerson's medium** helps to identify *Candida*.
- Pap smear shows thick red-stained hyphae and dark red spores.

Treatment
- **DOC:** Fluconazole 150 mg single dose. Both partners should be treated.
- Local intravaginal application of antifungal agents such as imidazole, miconazole, clotrimazole, butoconazole or terconazole vaginal pessaries or creams used for 3–6 days is very effective.

> **Extra Mile**
> - **Trichomoniasis** present with typical discharge, which is profuse, thin, creamy or slightly green in color, irritating and frothy. Itchy tender, angry looking vaginal walls and strawberry vagina.
> - **Chlamydia infection** (a STD) is usually asymptomatic but may develop vaginal discharge, dysuria and **increased frequency** of micturition, and at times cervicitis. Sometimes, chlamydia may cause Reiter's syndrome with arthritis, skin lesions, conjunctivitis and genital infection.
> - **Gonococcal vulvovaginitis** presents with urinary frequency and dysuria, dyspareunia, rectal discomfort, vaginal discharge. Vulvovaginal/perineal infection often results in inflammation, discharge, irritation causing pruritus and dysuria.

238. Ans. (c) 100.4°F

Ref: DC Dutta 8th ed. P 500

- Puerperal pyrexia is defined as a rise of temperature reaching **100.4°F (38°C)** or more (measured orally) on two separate occasions at 24 hours apart (excluding first 24 hours) within first 10 days following delivery.

Obstetrics and Gynecology

Causes of Puerperal Pyrexta
• Puerperal sepsis
• **Urinary tracht infections:** Cystitis, pyelonephritis
• Mastitis, breast abscess
• **Wound infections:** CS or episiotomy
• **Pulmonary infections:** Atelectasis, pneumonia
• Septic pelvic thrombophlebitis
• A recrudescence of malaria or pulmonary tuberculosis
• **Others:** Pharyngitis, gastroenteritis

239. Ans. (a) Chlamydia

Ref: Shaw's Gynecology 16th ed. P 181

- Pelvic inflammatory disease is a leading cause of tubal obstruction and the most common associated organism is chlamydia.
  - **Shaw's states:** *"Chlamydial infection causes more damage to the mucosa and the wall of the tube than gonorrhoea, leading to fibrosis and tubal blockage"*
  - **Other causes** of tubal obstruction can be: Gornorrheal infeaction, tuberculosis of uterus and fallopian tube, postoperative

240. Ans. (a) Pregnancy

Ref: Shaw, 16th ed. pg. 177-78, 183

- Pelvic inflammatory disease (PID) implies inflammation of the upper genital tract involving the fallopian tubes as well as the ovaries.
- The most common cause of PID is *sexually transmitted diseases* (STD).
- Gonococcal and chlamydial infections are most common, the incidence of the two varying in different communities. **Chlamydia being the commonest.**

Indications for hospitalization in PID

- The mild cases of acute PID are treated at home with antibiotics.
- Moderate and severe cases of PID need hospitalization.
- Those who need the diagnosis to be confirmed also require to be admitted for investigations.
- Those who need intravenous therapy need admission.

241. Ans. (a) Infertility

Ref: Shaw, 16th ed. pg. 188

- Most common site of genital TB is fallopian tube: 90–100%

Other sites:

- Endometrium: 50–60%
- Ovaries: 20–30%
- Cervix: 5–15%
- Vulva and vagina: 1%

Clinical feature:

- **Infertility:** This is an important presenting symptom. In fact, in 35–60% cases it may be the only complaint for which the patient seeks medical attention.

- **Menstrual irregularity:** This has been observed in 10–40% of cases. The menstrual disturbances reported include menorrhagia, menometrorrhagia, intermenstrual bleeding, oligomenorrhoea, hypomenorrhoea, amenorrhoea and even postmenopausal bleeding.

Chronic pelvic pain:

- Vaginal discharge
- Abdominal mass
- Fistula
- Ectopic pregnancy

242. Ans. (b) >3 infection in a year

Ref: Katz Comprehensive Gyenecology, 5th ed. Ch 22

Katz states: *"Recurrent vulvo-vaginits (bacterial vaginosis/vulvovaginal candidiasis) is defined as three or more documented episodes in one year"*

243. Ans. (a) Bacterial vaginosis

Ref: Shaws, 15th ed. pg. 309

Gardnerella (Bacterial) Vaginosis

- **Bacterial vaginosis** is termed vaginosis rather than vaginitis, because it is associated with alteration in the normal vaginal flora rather than due to any specific infection.
- Bacterial vaginosis is a vaginal infection casued by **Gardenella vaginalis.**
- Bacterial vaginosis is diagnosed on the basis of the following findings:
  - Vaginal secretions are gray and thinly coat the vaginal walls.
  - The pH of these secretions is *higher than 4.5* (usually 4.7 to 5.7).
  - Microscopy of the vaginal secretions reveals an *increased number of clue cells, and leukocytes are conspicuously absent.*
  - The addition of **10% KOH to the vaginal secretions (the "whiff" test)** releases a fishy, amine-like odor.
- This infection can cause PID, chorioamnionitis, premature rupture of membrane (PROM) and preterm Labor.

Treatment: Metronidazole 500 mg BD × 1 week is effective

244. Ans. (d) Gardenella vaginalis

Ref: Shaws's, 15th ed. pg. 309

245. Ans. (b) Bacterial vaginosis

Ref: Shaws, 15th ed. pg. 309

246. Ans. (c) Protozoa

Ref: Shaws, 15th ed. pg. 308-310

Explanations

TRICHOMONIASIS

- Most common in clinical practice. Patients complain of pruritus.
- Vulvae harbour this organism. Infection is sexually transmissible, it can be acquired.
- It is not uncommon during pregnancy and is often associated with gonococcal infection.
- **The Trichomonas is a protozoan,** actively motile and is anaerobic. *Trichomonas vaginalis, is the type found in the vagina.*

Symptoms

- 20% remain asymptomatic. 70% show profuse, thin, creamy or slightly green in color, irritating and frothy discharge.
- The vaginal walls are tender, angry looking and the discharge causes pruritus and inflammation of the vulva.
- There are often multiple small punctate strawberry spots *(strawberry vagina).*
- Urinary symptoms, such as dysuria and frequency, and a low-grade urethritis, Abdominal pain, low backache and dyspareunia may also be complained of if pelvic infection occurs.

Diagnosis

- The culture is 98% reliable. Trichomonas may also be diagnosed on a smear stained for cytology.

Treatment

- Metronidazole 200 mg oral TDS × 1 week both the partners
- The recent modality of treatment is to shorten the duration of therapy by giving 2 g metronidazole for 1 day only.

247. Ans. (c) Infection seen when vaginal pH is < 4.5

Ref: Shaws, 15th ed. pg. 308-310

- *After reading this question, usually we get this tendency to mark option D, which says bacterial vaginosis is NOT a STD, but this statement is true.*
- Bacterial vaginosis is a vaginal infection casued by Gardenella vaginalis (NOT a STD).
- **Bacterial vaginosis is diagnosed on the basis of the following findings:**
  - Vaginal secretions are gray and thinly coat the vaginal walls.
  - The pH of these secretions **is *higher than 4.5*** (usually 4.7 to 5.7).
  - Microscopy of the vaginal secretions reveals an **increased number of clue cells, and leukocytes are conspicuously absent.**
  - The addition of KOH to the vaginal secretions *(the "whiff" test)* releases a fishy, amine-like odor.

> **Extra Mile**
>
> - Most common vaginal infections during pregnancy is candidiasis
> - Bacterial vaginosis (BV) is the most common vaginal infection in women of childbearing age
> - Genital human papillomavirus the most common sexually transmitted infection.

248. Ans. (a) Bacterial vaginosis

Ref: Shaws, 15th ed. pg. 309

249. Ans. (b) Gardenella

Ref: Shaws, 15th ed. pg. 131-132

- Whiff test or amine test is done for gardenella (bacterial) vaginosis.
- It is performed by adding a small amount of potassium hydroxide (KOH) to a microscopic slide containing the vaginal discharge. *A characteristic fishy odor is considered a positive whiff test* and is suggestive of bacterial vaginosis.

250. Ans. (b) Urethra

Ref: Shaws, 15th ed. pg. 350

CHLAMYDIA

- Chlamydial infection is common in young, sexually active women. The incubation period is 6-14 days. It is sexually transmitted by vaginal and rectal intercourse.
- Chlamydia trachomatis is a small gram-negative bacteria, an obligate intracellular parasite that appears as intra cytoplasmic inclusion body, and is of two varieties, one that causes lympho granuloma venereum (LGV) and the other of non-LGV, which causes non-specific lower genital tract infection.
- Often, the infection is asymptomatic but may develop vaginal discharge, dysuria and frequency of micturition, and at times cervicitis.
- *In asymptomatic cases, Chlamydia resides most commonly in urethra.*
- Sometimes, chlamydia may cause Reiter's syndrome with arthritis, conjunctivitis and genital infection associated with skin lesions. *(can't see, can't pee & can't walk)*

The cervix is the first site of infection. Ascending upwards causes salpingitis and infertility

Diagnosis

- The use of fluorescein-conjugated monoclonal antibody in immunofluorescence tests on smears prepared from urethral and cervical secretion allows a direct diagnosis of the infection to be made.

Obstetrics and Gynecology

Note:

- Cervical ectopy with bleeding on touch and mucopurulent discharge is seen when the cervix is infected.
- Chlamydial infection and gonococcal infection often coexist and both attack the columnar epithelium of the genital tract and urethra. ***Urine can be cultured in suspected chlamydial infection.***

Treatment

- Tetracycline 500 mg and clindamycin 500 mg 6 hourly × 2 weeks is effective.

---

251. Ans. (a) Pain

> *Ref: Katz: Comprehensive Gynecology, 5th ed. Ch 23,*
> *Tuberculosis William's gynecology, ch 18*

- Pelvic TB are uncommon, but when occurs, it involves **fallopian tube in most of the cases.**
- Without pasteurization of milk, bovine tuberculosis produces primary infections in the human gastrointestinal tract. This leads to Subsequent lymphatic or hematogenous dissemination results in pelvic tuberculosis.
- **The clinical presentations of this chronic infection are:**
  - ***Mild to moderate chronic abdominal and pelvic pain occur (in 35% patients)***
  - Infertility and abnormal uterine bleeding.
  - Often times, the advanced cases presents with ascites while some women may be asymptomatic.
  - The remaining patients have bilateral adnexal masses and mild adnexal tenderness, with an inability to manipulate the adnexa because of scarring and fixation.

---

252. Ans. (c) Hydrosalpinx

> *Ref: Williams Gynecology, ch. 9, Pelvic mass; Fallopian*
> *Tube pathology*

HYDROSALPINX

- Results secondary to chronic PID.
- ***Grossly, the fine fimbria and tubal ostia are obliterated and replaced by a smooth, clubbed end.*** The ballooned, thin walls of the elongated tube are whitish and translucent, and the tube is typically distended with a clear serous fluid.
- Depending on the degree and location of the ipsilateral ovary, the hydrosalpinx may be adhered to it.
- Hydrosalpinx may be found in asymptomatic women during pelvic examination or incidentally during sonography or HSG done for other indications. Some women note infertility or chronic pelvic pain.

Treatment

- For women not wishing to preserve fertility, laparoscopic treatment may include lysis of adhesions and salpingectomy.
- In women who desire fertility, surgical intervention depends on the degree of tubal damage.

> **Extra Mile**

- **HYSTEROSALPINGOGRAPHY:** To study the patency of the fallopian tubes in infertility and postoperative tuboplasty and also employed to study uterine anomalies.
- *If in the question, clubbing of ampullary end is asked, the answer would be tuberculosis.*

---

253. Ans. (d) Mycobacterium tuberculosis

> *Ref: Shaws 15th ed. /158-159; DC Dutta 8th ed./ 158-159*

TB is also an important cause of **infertility**. Other salient features about TB are as follows:

- Most common presentation of genital TB is infertility.
- HSG is contraindicated in case of genital TB
- Best time to do HSG is **within 10 days** of LMP.
- Vaginal epithelium is resistant to TB.
- MC mode of spread of genital TB is **hematogenous**.
- TB salpingitis belong to stage V of PID.
- Conception rate even after treatment of genital TB is quite low.

---

254. Ans. (a) IUCD insertion

> *Ref: William's Gyenecology ch 3*

- IUCD acts by causing local inflammation at endometrial site. It increases the risk of PID in female.
- Oral contraceptives decreases the risk of PID.

TABLE: Pelvic Inflammatory Disease Risk Factors

Douching
Single status
Substance abuse
Multiple sexual partners
Lower socioeconomic status
Recent new sexual partner (s)
Younger age (10 to 19 years)
Other sexually transmitted infections
Sexual partner with urethritis or gonorrhea
Previous diagnosis of pelvic inflammatory disease
Not using mechanical and/or chemical contraceptive barriers
Endocervical testing positive for *N. Gonorrhoeae* or *C. Trachomatis*

---

255. Ans. (d) Laproscopy

> *Ref: Shaws, 15th ed. pg. 451, DC Dutta, 8th ed. pg. 451*

- Laproscopy is helpful in confirming the diagnosis as well as to know extent of disease.
- It is the current criterion standard for the diagnosis of PID. No single laboratory test is highly specific or sensitive for the disease.

FMGE Solutions Screening Examination

- Other investigations are-
  - ESR
  - Hemogram

CERVICAL CANVER

256. Ans. (b) HPV 16

Ref: Shaw's Gynecology 16th ed. P 485

- Women with STD, HIV infection, herpes simplex virus 2 infection, human papilloma virus (HPV) infection **(16, 18, 31, 33)** or condylomata have a high predisposition to cancer.
- Out of these HPV is now considered the most important cause.
- Most commonly caused by **HPV 16 and 18**

Other causes/risk factors for cervical cancer:
- Coitus before the age of 18 years
- Multiple sexual partners
- Delivery of the first baby before the age of 20 years
- Multiparity
- Poor personal hygiene
- Poor socioeconomic status
- Smoking and alcohol abuse
- COC and progestogens use over 8-year periods
- Exposure to diethylstilbestrol

Extra Mile

- Average age for cervical CA: 35–45 years
- **Gardasil** is a quadrivalent vaccine against HPV 16, 18, 31, 38 to be given to adolescents at 0, 2 and 6 months intramuscularly in the deltoid muscle.
- **Cervarix** is bivalent against HPV 16, 18 to be given (0.5 mL) at 0, 1 and 6 months. Immunity is expected to last 10 years.

257. Ans. (a) Squamous cell CA

Ref: Shaws, 15th ed. pg. 964

- The two most common histologic subtypes of cervical cancer are squamous cell and adenocarcinoma.
- Of these, *squamous cell tumors predominate, comprise 85 percent* of all cervical cancers, and arise from the ectocervix
- Adenocarcinomas comprise **10 to 15 percent** of cervical cancers and arise from the endocervical mucus-producing glandular cells.

258. Ans. (b) Oral contraceptives decreases the risk of cervical cancer

Ref: Williams Gynecology chapter 29-30

For this question, most of the students claimed option "D" but according to william's "Lower educational attainment, older age, obesity, smoking, and neighborhood poverty are independently related to lower rates of cervical cancer screening, which contribute to increased risk of cervical cancer".

- **Use of combined oral contraceptives doesn't decrease the risk,** *but it increases the risk.* COC users and women who are within 9 years of use have a significantly higher risk of developing both squamous cell and adenocarcinoma of the cervix *(william's gyne).*
- In women who are positive for cervical HPV DNA and who use COCs, risks of cervical carcinoma increase by up to fourfold compared with women who are HPV-positive and never users of COCs.
- *Both active and passive cigarette smoking increases the risk of cervical cancer.*
- An increased number of sexual partners and early age of first intercourse have been shown to increase cervical cancer risks.
- *Abstinence from sexual activity and barrier protection during sexual intercourse have been demonstrated to decrease cervical cancer incidence.*

TABLE: Risk Factors for Cervical Neoplasia

Behavioral risk factors	Demographic risk factors	Medical risk factors
• Infrequent or absent cancer screening Pap tests • Early coitarche • Multiple sexual partners • Male partner who has had multiple sexual partners • Tobacco smoking • Dietary deficiencies	• Ethnicity (Latin American countries, U.S. minorities) • Low socioeconomic status • Age	• Cervical high-risk human papillomavirus infection • Parity • Immuno-suppression

TABLE: Summarized staging of Cervical CA

Stage I	Tumor confined to the cervix
Stage IA	Microinvasion (preclinical)
Stage IB	All other cases confined to the cervix
Stage IIA	Tumor spread to the upper two thirds of the vagina
Stage IIB	Tumor spread to paracervical tissue but not to the pelvic walls
Stage IIIA	Tumor spread to the lower third of the vagina
Stage IIIB	Tumor spread to the pelvic wall or obstruction of either ureter by tumor
Stage IV	Tumor spread to the mucosa of the bladder or rectum or outside the pelvis

Obstetrics and Gynecology

259. Ans. (b) HPV 16 and 18

Ref: Shaws, 15ᵗʰ ed. pg. 952

- Women with STD, HIV infection, herpes simplex virus 2 infection, human papilloma virus (HPV) infection (**16, 18, 31, 33**) or condylomata have a high predisposition to cancer.
- Of these, HPV is now considered the most important cause, *most commonly cause by **HPV 16 and 18***
- Most HPV infection 16, 18 are symptomless in young women and clear within 2 years.
- Persistent infection is the cause of cancer of the cervix in 70-90% cases.

260. Ans. (a) HPV 16

Ref: Shaws, 15ᵗʰ ed. pg. 952

- HPV 16 and 18 are most commonly associated with cervical cancer.
- HPV 31, 33, 35, 51 are also associated with cervical cancer, but are relatively less commonly.

261. Ans. (b) Pap smear

Ref: Shaws, 15ᵗʰ ed. pg. 957; International Journal of Obstetrics and Gynecology 2006

Cervix cancer is the second most common cause of female specific cancer after breast cancer

- **Primary prevention** of a disease requires warding it off before the pathogenic process can occur. In the case of cervical cancer, this would require that infection of the will be cervix prevented. It could be achieved either by complete abstinence from sexual activity or *with a vaccine.*
- **Secondary prevention** stops the progression of disease once it has already started. *A good example of secondary prevention is cytologic screening to detect cervical cancer precursors, followed by treatment to prevent progression to cancer.*

Diagnosis

- Diagnosis of cervical dysplasia is mainly based on cytological screening of the population and by signs and symptoms:
  - Many are asymptomatic.
  - Some complain of postcoital bleeding or discharge.
  - On inspection, the cervix often appears normal, or there may be cervicitis or an erosion which bleeds on touch.
  - Some present with postmenopausal bleeding.
- Routine cytological screening or Pap smear Should be done to all women above the age of 21 years who are sexually active for at least 3 years. In all women with abnormal Pap tests showing mild dysplasias, it is important to treat any accompanying inflammatory

pathology and repeat the Pap test. If it persists to be abnormal, consider **colposcopic** examination and selective biopsies.

262. Ans. (b) Papaniculaou smear

Ref: Shaw's Gynae, 15ᵗʰ ed. pg. 403

- Pap smear is taken from cervix, with Arye spatula, rotated 360° to pick up cells from squamo-columnar junction. Vaginal smear for hormonal evaluation is taken from lateral fornix
- The objective of screening is to reduce the incidence and mortality from cervical cancer
- Pap smear test has been effective reducing the incidence of cervical cancer by 80% and the mortality by 70%.
- *Please refer to above explanation also.*

263. Ans. (d) All of the above

Ref: Shaws, 15ᵗʰ ed. pg. 403

The latest recommendations for cervical CA screening are:

- All women should begin cervical cancer screening at age 21 years.
- *Women between the ages of 21 and 29 should have a Pap test every 3 years.* They should not be tested for HPV unless it is needed after an abnormal Pap test result.
- *Women between the ages of 30 and 65 should have both a Pap test and an HPV test every 5 years.* This is the preferred approach, but it is also acceptable to have a Pap test alone every 3 years.
- *Women over age 65 who have had regular screenings with normal results should not be screened for cervical cancer.* Women who have been diagnosed with cervical pre-cancer should continue to be screened.
- Women who have had their uterus and cervix removed in a hysterectomy and have no history of cervical cancer or pre-cancer should not be screened.
- Women who have had the HPV vaccine should still follow the screening recommendations for their age group.
- Women who are at high risk for cervical cancer may need to be screened more often. Women at high risk might include those with HIV infection, organ transplant, or exposure to the drug DES. They should talk with their doctor or nurse.

ENDOMETRIAL AND FALLOPIAN TUBE CANCER

264. Ans. (a) Increased risk of endometrial carcinoma

Ref: Shaw's Gynecology 16ᵗʰ ed. P 554

- Tamoxifen is a selective estrogen receptor modulator, given for breast CA treatment.

FMGE Solutions Screening Examination

- Tamoxifen given to women with breast cancer increases the risk of endometrial hyperplasia and cancer to two- to three-folds. It also increases the risk of ovarian CA.
- Raloxifene has no adverse effect on the endometrium.
- Tamoxifen is effective in primary and secondary prevention of breast cancer.
- It **prevents spread to the other breast and recurrence by 50% and mortality by 25%.**
- It is also bone (decrease risk of osteoporosis) and cardioprotective.
- Side effects (two-fold increase) are hot flushes, vaginal dryness (anti-E2 action), endometrial hyperplasia, polyp, endometrial carcinoma and sarcoma. Other side effects are: DVT, retinopathy, ischemic heart disease.

Extra Mile

Risk Factors for Endometrial Cancer
- Endogenous estrogen dependent
- Nulliparity, low parity
- Polycystic ovary syndrome (PCOS)
- Early menarche, late menopause
- Functioning ovarian tumors
- Obesity, hypertension, diabetes, hyperlipidemia
- Exogenous estrogen
- Unopposed estrogen therapy
- Tamoxifen therapy
- Hered.ary

265. Ans. (d) Estradiol

Ref: Shaw's Gynecology 16th ed. P 409

- Endometriosis is ectopic benign endometrial tissues outside the cavity of the uterus, which responds to ovarian hormones.
- Usual sites of ectopic endometrial tissue is pelvic endometriosis (pelvic peritoneum, pouch of douglas, uterosacral ligament), rectovaginal endometriosis, ovary, appendix, pelvic lymph nodes, or at the scar site known as scar endometriosis.
- Symptoms can range from simple abdominal pain, dysmenorrhea, dyspareunia to infertility.

Treatment
- Endometriosis is estrogen dependent. Hormones act on the receptors in the endometriotic tissue and cause their atrophy and shrinkage.
- The purpose of administration of various hormones or drugs is to act as antiestrogens.
  - Continuous administration of gonadotropin analogue is useful in precocious puberty to down regulate and suppress pituitary gonadotropins. It causes atrophy of the endometriotic tissue in 90% cases. Drugs are: Goserelin, buserelin, nafarelin, cetrorelix, leuprolide.
  - Aromatase inhibitors available are letrozole (2.5 mg), anastrozole (1–2 mg) and rofecoxib (12.5 mg) daily

  for 6 months. It has antiestrogenic activity inhibiting conversion of androgen to estrogen.
  - **Combined OCP:** Intermittently or continuously, oral contraceptives may alleviate the disease. Not used much due to side effects.
  - **Oral progestogens:** They exert an antioestrogenic effect and their continuous administration causes decidualization and endometrial atrophy. Drugs commonly in use are: Norethisterone 5.0–20.0 mg daily, or dydrogesterone 10–30 mg daily. *This hormone does not prevent ovulation and is suitable for a woman trying to conceive.*
  - Mifepristone has some beneficial influence on shrinkage of fibroids and endometriosis (10–25 mg daily for 3 months).
  - Raloxifene, 60 mg daily used in endometriosis, do not cause endometrial hyperplasia.
- *Note:* Estradiol being the estrogen agonist will aggravate the symptoms. Hence should not be given.

266. Ans. (c) PET-CT

Ref: Shaw's 16th ed. 510

Radiological Tests in Endometrial CA
- **PET–CT reveals metabolic activity in the tissue and is a gold standard for staging.**
- *CT* has a predictable rate of 85% in studying the extent of spread of the lesion. Hypodensity in the myometrium suggests myometrial infiltration.
- *MRI* is superior to CT in detecting myometrial involvement and nodal enlargement with 90% detection rate and without radiation hazard.
- *Sonosalpingography* is very useful in detecting endometrial polyps which could be malignant.
- *Ultrasound* is useful in studying the endometrial thickness, irregular line, detecting polyps and associated ovarian tumor or ovarian metastasis.

267. Ans. (c) Dysmenorrhea

Ref: Shaw, 16th ed. pg. 420

Adenomyosis
- This condition is also termed as uterine endometriosis. It is observed frequently in elderly women aged more than 40.
- The disease often coexists with uterine fibromyomas, pelvic endometriosis (15%) and endometrial carcinoma.

Clinical presentation
- Some are asymptomatic, others present with **menorrhagia** and progressively increasing dysmenorrhoea.
- **Other symptoms:** Pelvic discomfort, backache and dyspareunia
- **Clinical examination** reveals a painful symmetrical enlargement of the uterus that rarely exceeds that of a 3-month pregnancy and is often mistaken for a myoma.

- A myoma is rarely painful. Therefore, a **painful, symmetrical enlargement of the uterus should suggest the diagnosis of adenomyosis.**
- **Shaw states:** *"If a patient gives a history of menorrhagia with accompanying dysmenorrhoea, one should always consider the possibility of adenomyosis"*

Investigation:
- MRI is superior to ultrasound.

Treatment
- Since most women are elderly and past the age of childbearing, **total hysterectomy** is the treatment.

268. Ans. (c) 40

Ref: Shaws, 15th ed. pg. 151

POSTMENOPAUSAL BLEEDING

- Postmenopausal bleeding and abnormal premenopausal and perimenopausal bleeding the primary symptoms of endometrial carcinoma.
- Normally a 1-year period of amenorrhea after the age of 40 is considered as menopause. However, vaginal bleeding occurring anytime after 6 months of amenorrhoea in a menopausal age should be considered as postmenopausal bleeding and investigated.
- Even without amenorrhoea or irregular bleeding, if a woman over the age of 52 years continues to menstruate, she needs investigations to rule out endometrial hyperplasia and malignancy of the genital tract.
- *Thirty to fifty percent of postmenopausal bleeding is attributed to malignancy of the genital tract, the most common being endometrial cancer, cervical cancer and ovarian tumors.*
- Common benign conditions are endometrial hyperplasia and polypi.

269. Ans. (c) Atypical

Ref: Shaw's Gynaecology, 15th ed. pg. 724

ENDOMETRIAL HYPERPLASIA

This occurs in:
- Anovulatory cycles with unopposed oestrogen acting on the endometrium
- Metropathia haemorrhagica
- Obese women
- Polycystic ovarian disease
- a woman on tamoxifen
- feminizing ovarian tumors
- Hyperplasia may be simple hyperplasia, glandular or atypical hyperplasia.
- Simple hyperplasia is at a risk of endometrial cancer in 2% and glandular hyperplasia in 4-10%. *Atypical hyperplasia, however, has the tendency to develop carcinoma in as much as 60-70%.*

Extra Mile
- 80% cases of simple hyperplasia respond to progestogens, response of atypical hyperplasia is only 50%, but with the risk of malignancy.
- For this reason, atypical endometrial hyperplasia should be treated by hysterectomy and not merely by ablative technique.

270. Ans. (b) Biopsy

Ref: Dutta's Obstetrics, 7th ed. pg. 341 and 345

Diagnosis of Endometrial Carcinoma

- Postmenopausal bleeding is considered to be due to endometrial carcinoma unless proven otherwise.
- **Endometrial biopsy:** Histology is the definitive diagnosis
- Papanicolaou smear not a reliable test for endometrial CA. It is Positive only in 30 per cent cases of endometrial cancer.
- **Ultrasound and color Doppler (TVS):** Findings suggestive of endometrial carcinoma are:
  - Endometrial thickness ≥ 4 mm
  - Hyperechoic endometrium with irregular outline.
  - Increased vascularity
  - Intrauterine fluid
- **Hysteroscopy:** helps in direct visualization of endometrium and to take target biopsy.
- **Fractional curettage:** is not only the definite method of diagnosis but can detect the extent of growth.

Prognosis

- Tumors showing poor prognosis are:
  - Poorly undifferentiated
  - Greater myometrial penetration
  - Lymphovascular space invasion
- Aneuploid tumors: worst prognosis

TABLE: Most of the prognostic factors given below in the table can be evidenced by endometrial biopsy

Prognostic factors in endometrial carcinoma
- Age at diagnosis: Older the patient poorer the prognosis.
- Stage of the disease
- **Histologic type:**
  - Typical adenocarcinomas- better prognosis;
  - Papillary serous, clear cell carcinoma-poor prognosis.
- Histologic differentiation.
- Histologic grade: Grade 3 tumors have 5 times more risk of recurrence and low 5 year survival rate.
- Myometrial penetration.
- Lymphovascular space invasion.
- Lymph node metastasis.

FMGE Solutions Screening Examination

271. Ans. (c) Simple hysterectomy

Ref: William's Gyne. Ch 33

Surgical treatment options for patients with endometrial cancer:
- Simple Hysterectomy
- BSO (Bilateral salpingo oophorectomy)
- Radical hysterectomy
- Vaginal hysterectomy

- Almost three quarters of patients are stage I at diagnosis.
- *In general, an extrafascial ("simple") hysterectomy is sufficient*, but radical hysterectomy may be preferable for women with clinically obvious cervical extension of endometrial cancer.
- **Contraindications of primary surgery include:** a desire to preserve fertility, massive obesity, high operative risk, and clinically unresectable disease.
- Vaginal hysterectomy with or without BSO is another option for those women who cannot undergo systematic surgical staging because of comorbidities.

> **Extra Mile**
>
> *"Just so you don't miss any further question on endometrial CA staging, following table has been summarized"*

TABLE: FIGO staging for endometrial CA

I A	Tumor confined to the uterus, no or < ½ myometrial invasion
I B	Tumor confined to the uterus, > ½ myometrial invasion
II	Cervical stromal invasion, but not beyond uterus
III A	Tumor invades serosa or adnexa
III B	Vaginal and/or parametrial involvement
III	Metastasis to pelvic and paraaortic lymph nodes
III C1	Pelvic node involvement
III C2	Para-aortic involvement
IV-A	Tumor invasion bladder and/or bowel mucosa
IV-B	Distant metastases including abdominal metastases and/or inguinal lymph nodes

Note:
- Paclitaxel (*Taxol*), doxorubicin (*Adriamycin*) and cis-platin (TAP) **chemotherapy** is the adjuvant treatment of choice for advanced endometrial cancer.
- In practice, **cytotoxic chemotherapy frequently is combined with radiotherapy** in patients with advanced endometrial cancer.
- **Primary radiation therapy** usually is considered only in rare instances when a patient is an exceptionally poor surgical candidate.

272. Ans. (a) Painless watery discharge

Ref: Shaws, 15th ed. pg. 999

FALLOPIAN TUBE CANCERS

- Primary cancer of the fallopian tubes is uncommon and account for only 0.3%.
- The tumor is often an adenocarcinoma though chorio-carcinoma may develop in a tubal ectopic pregnancy or in a tubal mole.
- The tumor is highly malignant and spreads rapidly through lymphatics to the pelvic organs..

FIGO classification does not exist, Erez classification is as follows:
- **Stage I:** The tumor is limited to the mucosa and muscle.
- **Stage IIA:** The serosa is breached but the tumor has not spread to other organs.
- **Stage IIB:** The tumor invades the pelvic organs.
- **Stage III:** Metastasis outside the pelvis but within the abdominal cavity.
- **Stage IV:** Extra-abdominal metastasis is present.

Clinical features
- The tumor occurs in menopausal women, most of them of them are nulliparous.
- *The early symptom is painless watery discharge per vagina*, which may at times be amber-colored. Sooner or later, postmenopausal bleeding develops.
- A lump may be too small to be felt on clinical examination.
- *Pain is a late symptom.*

273. Ans. (c) IIIa

Ref: Refer to staging Shaws, 15th ed. pg. 421

OVARIAN CANCER

274. Ans. (a) Granulosa cell tumor

Ref: Shaw 16th ed. P 442

- Granulosa call tumor is an estrogen secreting tumor, characterized histopathologically by **Call exner body.**

> **Extra Mile**

Ovarian tumor	HPE characteristics
Serous cystadenoma	Psamomma bodies
Clear cell tumor	Hobnail cell
Yolk sac tumor	Schiller duval bodies
Granulosa cell tumor	Call exner bodies
Krukenberg tumor	Signet ring cell

Obstetrics and Gynecology

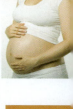

275. Ans. (c) Ovary

Ref: Shaws, 16th ed. pg. 430

Lutein Cysts of the Ovary

Two types of lutein cysts are recognized:
- Granulosa lutein cysts found within the corpus luteum.
- Theca lutein cysts associated with trophoblastic disease and chorionic gonadotropin therapy.

Corpus Luteum (Granulosa Lutein) Cysts

- Corpus luteum cysts are functional, non-neoplastic enlargements of the ovary.
- **Clinical presentation:** local pain, tenderness or delayed menstruation. These cysts are often palpable clinically.
- Ultrasound reveals **spider-web-like structure** with or without a clot.

Theca Lutein Cysts

- **Theca lutein cysts (TLC)**, also known as **hyperreactio luteinalis (HL)**, are a type of **functional ovarian cyst**. They are typically multiple and **seen bilaterally** and filled with straw-colored fluid.
- It is commonly associated with hydatidiform moles, choriocarcinoma and gonadotropin (hCG) or clomiphene therapy.
- The cysts spontaneously regress after elimination of the mole, therapeutic curettage, treatment of choriocarcinoma or discontinuation of gonadotropin therapy.

276. Ans. (c) Clear cell tumor

Classification of ovarian tumor

Epithelial tumor (80%)	Germ cell tumor	Sex cord tumor
• Clear cell tumor • Brenner's tumor • Serous tumor *(MC)* • Endometrioid tumor • Mucinous tumor	• Choriocarcinoma • Dysgerminoma • Endodermal sinus tumor • Polyembroyoma • Teratoma *(MC)*	• Theca cell tumor • Granulosa cell tumor • Androblastoma • Gynandroblastoma • Arrhenoblastoma
Mn: CBSE-M	Mn: C- DEPT:	Mn: The GAGA

277. Ans. (b) Teratoma

Ref: Williams Gynae, 1st ed. Ch 36

- Germ cell tumors arise from the ovary's germinal elements and comprise a third of all ovarian neoplasms.
- The **mature cystic teratoma**, also called **dermoid cyst, is by far the most common subtype.** This accounts for 95% of all germ cell tumors and is **clinically benign.**
- In contrast, **malignant germ cell** tumors comprise fewer than 5 percent of malignant ovarian cancers in Western countries and include *dysgerminoma, yolk sac tumor, immature teratoma,* and other less common types.

Extra Mile

- Overall, MC ovarian tumor: **Epithelial cell tumor**
- Overall, MC benign tumor of the ovary: **Dermoid cyst**
- MC benign epithelial tumor of the ovary: **Serous cystadenoma**
- MC malignant ovarian tumor: **Serous cystadenocarcinoma**
- **MC germ cell tumor: Mature Teratoma (Dermoid Cyst)**
- Most common ovarian tumor associated with pregnancy: **Dermoid Cyst**
- Most common ovarian tumor which undergo torsion: **Dermoid cyst**
- MC malignant germ cell tumor: **Dysgerminoma**
- Ovarian tumor mostly in young age: **Dysgerminoma**
- Ovarian tumor metastasized to contralateral tumor: **Granulosa cell tumor**

278. Ans. (b) Dysgerminoma

Ref: Shaws, 15th ed. pg. 933

Please refer to above explanation.

YOLK SAC TUMORS

- Yolk sac tumors account for 20% of all malignant ovarian germ cell tumors
- *Microscopically Schiller-Duval bodies* are pathognomonic when present.

279. Ans. (a) Papillary serous cystadenoma

Ref: William's Gynecology, Ch 35; Epithelial tumors of ovary

TABLE: Epithelial Ovarian Tumor Cell Types
(Katz: Comprehensive Gynecology, 5th ed.)

Ovarian Cancers	Approximate Frequency (%)
Serous	35–40
Mucinous	6–10
Endometrioid	15–25
Clear cell (mesonephroid)	5–10
Brenner	Rare

SEROUS TUMORS

- Serous tumors are the most frequent ovarian epithelial tumors. **The malignant forms account for 40% or more of ovarian cancers.**
- During frozen section evaluation, *psammoma bodies are essentially pathognomonic* of an ovarian-type serous carcinoma

MUCINOUS ADENOCARCINOMAS

- About 5 to 10 percent of true epithelial ovarian cancers are mucinous adenocarcinomas

- These cells resemble cells of the endocervix or may mimic intestinal cells, which can pose a problem in the differential diagnosis of tumors that appear to originate from the ovary or intestine.

ENDOMETRIOID ADENOCARCINOMAS

- About 15 to 25 percent of epithelial ovarian cancers are endometrioid adenocarcinomas, *the second most common histologic type.*

CLEAR CELL TUMORS

- Comprising 5 to 10 percent of epithelial ovarian cancers, *clear cell adenocarcinomas are the most frequently associated with pelvic endometriosis.*
- Microscopically **hobnail cells** are characteristic finding. These are cells with abundant glycogen and nuclei of the cells protrude into the glandular lumen.

BRENNER TUMOR

- These tumors constitute only 2% to 3% of all ovarian tumors.
- Brenner tumors consist of cells that resemble the transitional epithelium of the bladder and Walthard nests of the ovary.

280. Ans. (b) Serous cyst adenocarcinoma

Ref: Shaws, 15th ed. pg. 422

- Most common ovarian tumor: Serous Cystadenoma (50%)
- *Malignant form of serous cystadenoma is serous cystadenocarcinoma.*
- Largest ovarian tumor: Mucinous cystadenoma
- Clear cell tumor is a malignant ovarian tumor of epithelial origin, characterized histopathologically by **Hobnail Cell.**
- Granulosa call tumor is an estrogen secreting tumor, characterized histopathologically by **Call exner body.**

Extra Mile

Ovarian tumor	HPE characteristics
Serous cystadenoma	Psamomma bodies
Clear cell tumor	Hobnail cell
Yolk sac tumor	Schiller duval bodies
Granulosa cell tumor	Call exner bodies
Krukenberg tumor	Signet ring cell

281. Ans. (b) Ovary is the primary site

Ref: Shaws, 15th ed. pg. 424

- **Choriocarcinoma** is a highly malignant tumor arising from the chorionic epithelium.

- About 3-5 per cent of all patients with molar pregnancies develop choriocarcinoma.
- The primary site is usually anywhere in the uterus *(secondary involvement).*
- *Rarely, it starts in the tube or ovary.*
- The lesion is usually localized nodular type.
- **Spread:** The common sites of metastases are lungs (80%), Anterior vaginal wall (30%), brain (10%), liver (10%).

Symptoms

- Irregular vaginal bleeding, at times brisk
- Continued amenorrhoea.
- **Lung:** Cough, breathlessness, haemoptysis.
- **Cerebral:** Headache, convulsion, paralysis or coma.
- **Liver:** epigastric pain, jaundice.
- **Chest X-ray:** Shows 'cannon ball' shadow or 'snow storm' appearance due to numerous tumor emboli.

282. Ans. (c) Choriocarcinoma

Ref: Shaws, 15th ed. pg. 424

CHORIOCARCINOMA

- Generally, choriocarcinoma is a part of a mixed germ cell tumor. Its origin as a teratoma can be confirmed in prepubertal girls, when the possibility of its gestational origin can be definitely excluded. The tumors are very vascular.
- *Histologically the tumor shows a dimorphic population of syncytiotrophoblasts and cyto-trophoblasts.* It secretes large quantities of human chorionic gonadotropin (hCG) hormone, which forms an ideal tumor marker in the diagnosis and management of the tumor. The tumor is highly malignant, and metastasizes by bloodstream to the lungs, brain, bones and other organs.

283. Ans. (a) Chemotherapy

Ref: Shaws, 15th ed. pg. 124-125

- The treatment of choice of choriocarcinoma is mainly chemotherapy both for local and distal metastasis.
- The drug of choice for the same is **methotrexate.** It is given orally 5 mg five times a day for 5 days.
- Side effects of Methotrexate are ulcerative stomatitis, gastric hemorrhage, skin reaction, alopecia, bone marrow suppression, Liver and Kidney damage.

284. Ans. (c) CA 125

Ref: Shaws, 15th ed. pg. 422-928

- Tissue markers such as CA-125 and NB/70k are useful mainly in the follow-up of certain tumors.
- **CA-125** is a glycoprotein and surface cell antigen which is secreted by the malignant epithelial tumors.

Obstetrics and Gynecology

- Level of CA-125 more than 35 U/ml suggests malignant and residual tumor, and indicates the need of chemotherapy.
- CA-125 is also raised in abdominal tuberculosis and endometriosis.
- CEA (carcinoembryonic antigen) more than 5 mg/l is seen in mucinous ovarian tumor.
- **NOTE:** CA-125 is raised in only 50% cases in Stage I and 90% in Stage II ovarian cancer.

VULVAR AND VAGINAL CANCER

285. Ans. (d) HPV

Ref: William's Gyenecology Ch 31

HPV (16, 18) most comman cause of vulvar carcinoma.

- HPV infects the female →vulva, vagina, and cervix
- Male → urethra, penis, and scrotum.
- Both genders → Perianal, anal, and oropharyngeal area.

Salient Features of Vulvar Cancer

MC site- labia majora and minora
MC symptom pruritus.
MC type- SCC, epidermoid type (same for vaginal CA)
MC implicated factor- HPV 16, 18.

Premalignant lesion of vulva	
• VIN (MC) vulvar intraepithelial lesion • /ts ds • Condyloma accuminata	• Lichen sclerosis • Erythroplasia of querat • Bowen disease (type of VIN)

MC mode of spread- lymphatic 1st LN- Superficial inguinal LN 2nd LN- Deep inguinal LN

286. Ans. (c) Stage II

Ref: Shaws 15 ed. p-941

Carcinoma of the Vulva (FIGO staging 2008)

Stage I	Tumor confined to the vulva
I a	Lesions ≤ 2 cm is size, confined to the vulva or perineum and with stromal invasion ≤1 mm, no nodal metastasis
I b	Lesions >2 cm in size or with stromal invasion >1.0 mm, confined to the vulva or perineum, with negative nodes
Stage II	**Tumor of any size with extension to adjacent perineal structures (1/3rd lower urethra, 1/3rd lower vagina, anus) with negative nodes**
Stages III	Tumor of any size with or without extension to adjacent perineal structures (one-third lower urethra, one-third lower vagina, anus) with positive inguino-femoral lymph nodes

Contd...

IIIA	• With lymph node metastasis (≥5 mm) or • 1-2 lymph node metastasis(es) (<5 mm)
IIIB	• With two or more lymph node metastases (≥5 mm) or • 3 or more lymph node metastases (<5 mm)
Stage IV A	Tumor involving any of the following: • Upper urethral and/or vaginal mucosa, bladder mucosa, rectal mucosa, or fixed to pelvic bone, or • Fixed or ulcerated inguino-femoral lymph nodes.
Stage IV	Distant metastasis including pelvic lymph nodes

Note: *According to old FIGO staging (1995) for vulvar CA (as mentioned in William's), only in stage III there is invlovement of adjacent organs like lower urethra and/or the vagina or the anus. So don't be confused, and mark answers according to latest staging as mentioned above.*

287. Ans. (b) Stage II

Ref: William's Gyenecology, Ch 31

288. Ans. (b) Simple partial vulvectomy without lymphadenectomy

Ref: William's Gyenecology Ch: 31

FIGO Staging of Vulvar cancer	Treatment
Stage I: Tumor confined to the vulva, Negative nodes	**Microinvasive surgery:** Simple/wide local excision. No Lymphadenectomy required
IA: size < 2cm; stromal invasion < 1mm	
IB: size > 2cm; stromal invasion > 1mm	
Stage II: Tumor of any size, with spread to lower urethra, lower vagina or anus with negative nodes	**Radical vulvectomy or Modified radical vulvectomy + inguinofemoral lymphadenectomy**
Stage III: II + Regional lymph node metastasis (inguinal, femoral)	
Stage IVA: Tumor invades upper urethra, upper vagina, bladder mucosa, rectal mucosa + Nodes	**RT + Surgery**
Stage IVB: Vulvar cancer with distant metastasis including pelvic lymph nodes	**Stage IVB: Palliative therapy**

Extra Mile

- **Radical Vulvectomy:** An operation that removes the entire vulva, including subcutaneous and fatty tissue, the labia minora and majora, perineal skin, and clitoris, to treat cancer.
- **Skinning Vulvectomy:** An operation that removes the skin of the vulva, including the labia majora and minora, the clitoris, and perineal skin.

FMGE Solutions Screening Examination

289. Ans. (b) Partial vulvectomy

Ref: Shaws, 15th ed. pg. 943; William's Gynecology Ch 31, Invasive CA of Vulva

Please refer to above explanation.

290. Ans. (c) Vaginal carcinoma

- Primary vaginal carcinoma is rare and comprises only 1 to 2 percent of all gynecologic malignancies.
- The most common histologic type of primary vaginal cancer is squamous cell carcinoma, followed by adenocarcinoma.
- Vaginal carcinoma has no direct role in infertility.

Causes of Infertility

Infertitlity factors	%
Male factor	30% (most common cause)
Ovarian/anovulation factors	25%
Tubal/uterine factors	25%
Cervical factors	10%
Unexplained	10%

DYSFUNCTIONAL UTERINE BLEEDING (DUB) AND DYSMENORRHEA

291. Ans. (b) Presence of endometrium at ectopic locations

Ref: Shaw's Gynecology 16th ed. P 409-410

- Endometriosis is the occurrence of ectopic benign endometrial tissues outside the cavity of the uterus.
- The ectopic endometrial tissue responds to ovarian hormones.
- **Note:** PID closely mimics endometriosis

Endometriosis	Adenomyosis
• It is also a cause of DUB • Presence of endometrium outside uterus • **MC site:** Ovary **Rarest site:** CNS • It presents as chocolate cyst of ovary • Present with menorrhagia, pain, Infertility. • **MC symptom:** Congestive dysmenorrhea • **Gold standard Inv:** Laparoscopy (diagnostic + therapeutic)	• Also a cause of DUB • Presence of endometrial gland in myometrium • Seen in patients around 40 years • Present with menorrhagia, dysmenorrhea and pain but *no Infertility* • Uterus is tender and enlarged: 12-14 week size • Diagnosed with Histopathology • **Treatment of choice:** Hysterectomy

292. Ans. (b) Endometriosis

Ref: Shaw's Gynecology 16th ed. P 409-410
Refer to above explanation

293. Ans. (a) No clinical significant pelvic pathology is found

Ref: Shaw's Gynecology 16th ed. P 471

- Dysmenorrhea means cramping abdominal pain accompanying menstruation. It can be of 2 types:
- **Primary dysmenorrhea:**
  - These are not associated with any identifiable pelvic pathology.
  - Pathogenesis of pain is attributed to a biochemical derangement.
  - It affects more than 50% postpubescent women in the age group of 18–25 years with ovulatory cycles.
- **Secondary dysmenorrhea:**
  - These are associated with the presence of organic identifiable pelvic pathology, i.e. fibroids, adenomyosis, pelvic inflammatory disease (PID) and endometriosis.
  - Unilateral dysmenorrhea occurs in a rudimentary horn of a bicornuate uterus.
  - It is also seen in some women wearing intrauterine contraceptive device (IUCD) and in cases of cervical stenosis.

TABLE: Differentiating features of primary and secondary dysmenorrhea

Differentiating features	Primary	Secondary
Onset	Within 2 years of menarche	20–30 years, maybe pre- and postmenstrual
Description	Cramping–hypogastrium, back, inner things	Variable dull ache
Symptomatology	Nausea, vomiting, diarrhea, headache, fatigue	Dyspareunia, infertility, menstrual disorders
Pelvic findings	Normal	Variable, depending on cause
Etiology	Excessive myometrial contraction, ischemia, excessive prostaglandin production	Endometriosis, PID, adenomyosis, fibroids, pelvic vein congestion
Management	Reassurance, analgesics, NSAIDs, antispasmodics, OC pillls, in rare cases, surgery–Cotte's operation or laparoscopic uterosacral nerve ablation (LUNA)	Treatment directed to the cause

Obstetrics and Gynecology

294. Ans. (d) Anovulatory

Ref: Shaws, 15th ed. pg. 301-307

- Dysfunctional uterine bleeding is irregular, abnormal uterine bleeding that is not caused by a tumor, infection or **pregnancy.**
- Dysfunctional uterine bleeding is a disorder that occurs most frequently in women at the beginning and end of their reproductive lives.
- It is of 2 types:
- **Ovulatory:** after adolescent years and before perimenopausal years.
- **Anovulatory:** postmenarcheal, premenopausal.
- Half of the cases occur in women over 45 years of age and about one fifth occur in women under age 20.
- Dysfunctional uterine bleeding is diagnosed when other causes of uterine bleeding have been eliminated.
- Failure of the ovary to release an egg *(anovulatory)* during the menstrual cycle occurs in about 70% of women with DUB. This is probably related to a hormonal imbalance.

Extra Mile

- **Normal menstruation duration:** 28 +/- 7 days, mean of 4 days duration, not more than 7 days
- **Menorrhagia or hypermenorrhea:** prolonged (>7 days) or excessive (>80 ml) bleeding at regular intervals
- **Metrorrhagia:** bleeding in irregular but frequent intervals, variable amount
- **Menometrorrhagia:** Prolonged bleeding at irregular intervals
- **Polymenorrhea:** bleeding in regular intervals < 21 days
- **Oligomenorrhea:** Regular intervals > 35 days

Endometriosis	Adenomyosis
It is also a cause of DUB.	Also a cause of DUB
Presence of endometrium outside uterus.	Presence of endometrial gland in myometrium
MC site: ovary Rarest site: CNS	Seen in patients around 40 years.
In ovary, it present at chocolate cyst ovary.	Present with menorrhagia, dysmenorrhea and pain BUT no Inftertility.
Present with menorrhagia, pain, Infertility.	Uterus is tender and enlarged: 12- 14 week size.
MC symptom: Congestive Dysmenorrhea.	Diagnosed with Histopathology.
Gold standard Inv: Laparoscopy (diagnostic + therapeutic)	Treatment of choice: Hysterectomy

295. Ans. (c) Metrorrhagia

Ref: Shaw, 15th pg. 283

296. Ans. (a) Pelvic and abdomen USG

Ref: William's Gynecology 1st ed. Ch 11

- **Dysmenorrhea** is Cyclic pain with menstruation and accompanies most menses. This pain is classically described as cramping and is often accompanied by low backache, nausea and vomiting, headache, or diarrhea.
  - **Primary dysmenorrhea** describes cyclic menstrual pain without an identifiable associated pathology.
  - **Secondary dysmenorrhea** is cyclic menstrual pain which may frequently complicates endometriosis, leiomyomas, PID, adenomyosis, endometrial polyps, and menstrual outlet obstruction.
- The above given case is a patient of chronic pelvic pain secondary to dysmenorrhea.
- First line drug/DOC in dysmenorrhea is: NSAIDs
- If NSAIDs doesn't relieve the symptom, further work-up must be performed to rule out other pathologies.
- The next best choice for this patient is Pelvic and abdominal ultrasonography.

297. Ans. (a) Progesterone

Ref: Shaws, 15th ed. pg. 303-304

- Puberty menorrhagia is anovulatory. Therefore our first line or **DOC in puberty menorhhagia is cyclical progestin therapy.**

FIBROID

298. Ans. (a) Pedunculated

Ref: Shaw's Gynecology 16th ed. P 410-402

- Myomectomy is the most common surgical procedure done for fibroids during caesarean section
  - *Myomectomy* refers to the removal of fibroids, leaving the uterus behind
- Pedunculated myomas can easily be removed and hemostasis can be secured at the same time without endangering mother's life.
- **Vaginal myomectomy:**
  - Indicated in submucous fibroid
  - In Cervical fibroids and pedunculated fibroid polypus
  - If more than 50% submucous fibroids project into the cavity
- **Hysteroscopic myomectomy**
  - Hysteroscopic myomectomy has become possible for **submucous fibroids** not removable by the simple vaginal route.
  - The fibroid is excised either by cautery, laser or resectoscope. It is best done under laparoscopic guidance to avoid uterine perforation.

FMGE Solutions Screening Examination

> **Extra Mile**
> - Anterior and posterior fibroids lodged in the pouch of Douglas cause increase in frequency and retention of urine
> - Broad ligament fibroids can cause hydroureter and hydronephrosis

299. Ans. (b) Large size

Ref: Shaw's 16th ed. P 397

- In torsion very severe abdominal pain is experienced.
- **Book states:** "*Acute pain is seen when a fibroid is complicated by torsion, hemorrhage and red degeneration.*"
- Pain in a rapidly growing fibroid in an elderly woman may be due to sarcoma.
- Sarcomatous change in a myoma is extremely rare and is usually associated with intramural and submucous tumors which have a higher potential for sarcomatous change than subserous tumors.
  - It is more commonly seen in a postmenopausal woman when it is observed that the tumor grows suddenly, **causing pain** and postmenopausal bleeding.
- **A large fibroid** may be observed as an abdominal tumor which grows slowly or not at all over a long period. A rapid growth only occurs during pregnancy, due to oral contraceptive hormones and malignancy. *As many as 50% women are asymptomatic.* These fibroids are detected during gynecological check-up or ultrasound done for unrelated symptoms.

> **Extra Mile**
>
> **Table: Clinical symptomatology and complications associated with uterine fibromyomas**
> - Menstrual disturbances—menorrhagia, polymenorrhagia, intermenstrual bleeding, continuous bleeding, postmenopausal bleeding
> - Infertility
> - Pain—spasmodic dysmenorrhea, backache, abdominal pain
> - Lump in the abdomen or mass protruding at the introitus
> - Pressure symptoms on adjacent viscera—bladder, ureters, rectum
> - Pergnancy losses, postpartum hemorrhage, uterine inversion
> - Vaginal discharge

300. Ans. (a) Leiomyoma

Ref: Shaw's 16th ed. P 507

- Most common benign tumor of uterus is leiomyoma (fibroid).
- Most common malignant tumor of uterus is endometrial carcinoma.
- **Overall most common uterine tumor:** Leiomyoma.

Endometrial CA

- Endometrial cancer is 20–25% of all genital cancers in the developed countries (*in developing countries cervical CA still predominates due to poor screening*).
- The peak incidence of endometrial cancer is 55–70 years, 20–25% occur in perimenopausal women and only 5% develop in women below the age of 45 years.
- Seventy-five percent of the tumors are localized in the uterus when diagnosed and surgery is the cornerstone in its management.
- There are two varieties of endometrial cancer:
  - **Type I are estrogen-dependent** and account for 90% growths. The source of estrogen may be endogenous or exogenous. They are well-differentiated with good prognosis.
  - **Type II are estrogen-independent** and develop in atrophic endometrium. They are mostly undifferentiated with poor prognosis. P_3 mutations are recognized in type II tumors.

301. Ans. (b) Cervical

Ref: Shaw's, 16th ed. pg. 392

- The distribution of myoma/Fibroid in the body of the uterus is broadly classified as follows (Figure):
- Intramural (interstitial) 75%
- Submucous 15%
- Subserous 10%
- The majority of myomas arise in the uterus. Tumors can therefore be classified as uterine and extrauterine.
- The uterine growth is further divided into those that arise from the body and those that arise from the cervix.

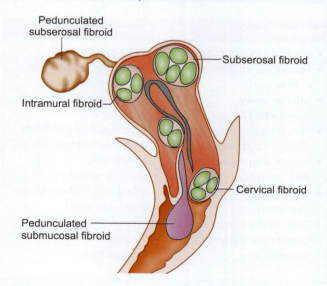

FIGURE: Varieties of submucous fibroid. Various anatomical sites of fibromyomas

Obstetrics and Gynecology

Cervical Fibroid
- Cervical fibroid is a single fibroid encountered in 1% of all fibroids. It may develop as a central, anterior, posterior fibroid or grow laterally in the broad ligament.

Symptoms
- A cervical fibroid exerts pressure on the bladder, ureter and in rare cases on the rectum. A woman may feel a lump in the lower abdomen. **During pregnancy, it can cause retention of urine**. Obstructed Labor occurs if the cervical fibroid lies below the presenting part.

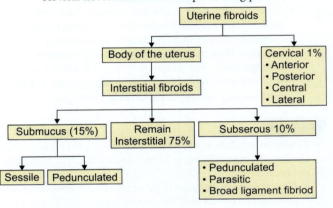

302. Ans. (c) Subserous fibroid

Ref: Shaws, 15th ed. pg. 359

- Uterine fibroids are noncancerous growths of the uterus that often appear during childbearing years. It is aka leiomyomas
- They aren't associated with an increased risk of uterine cancer and almost never develop into cancer.

Types
- **Intramural fibroids** are located within the wall of the uterus and are the **most common type.**
- **Subserosal fibroids** are located underneath the mucosal (peritoneal) surface of the uterus and can become very large. They can also grow out in a papillary manner to become pedunculated fibroids.
  - Therefore hysteroscopical excision is not possible.
  - It can be resected lapascopically or by open laparotomy.
- **Submucosal fibroids** are located in the muscle beneath the endometrium of the uterus and distort the uterine cavity; even small lesions in this location may lead to bleeding and infertility
- **Cervical fibroids** are located in the wall of the cervix (neck of the uterus)

303. Ans. (a) Subserous fibroid

Ref: Shaws, 15th ed. pg. 359
Please refer to above explanation.

304. Ans. (a) Conservative management

Ref: Shaws, 15th ed. pg. 364;
William Obstetrics 23rd ed. Ch 40

- Uterine leiomyomas (*fibroids*) are common benign smooth muscle tumors. Their incidence during pregnancy is probably about 2 percent and depends on population characteristics and the frequency of routine sonography.
- **Treatment of symptomatic myomas consists of analgesia and observation.** Most often, signs and symptoms abate within a few days, but inflammation may stimulate labor.
- Surgery is **rarely** necessary during pregnancy.

305. Ans. (d) All of the above

Ref: Shaws, 15th ed. pg. 359; Williams Gynecology Ch: 9

- Leiomyomas are benign smooth muscle neoplasms that typically originate from the myometrium. They are often referred to as uterine myomas, and are incorrectly called **fibroids** because the considerable amount of collagen contained in many of them creates a fibrous consistency.
- Drugs used to decrease the size of the fibroid:
  - GnRH analogue (Buserelin, Nafarelin, Goserelin, Triptorelin, Leuprorelin acetate)
  - GnRH antagonist: Cetrirelix, Ganirelix
  - Mifepristone (anti-progesterone)
  - Danazol

CHROMOSOMAL ANOMALIES

306. Ans. (b) Tall stature

Ref: Shaws, 15th ed. /110-111; Harrison 19/e 635;
William's Gynecology, Ch 16

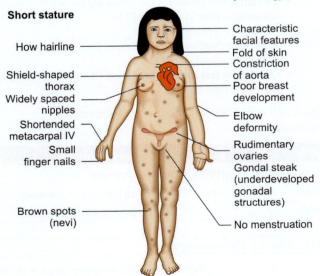

FMGE Solutions Screening Examination

In turner syndrome
- Deletion of genetic material from an X chromosome accounts for about two thirds of gonadal dysgenesis which leads to a condition called turner syndrome (XO).
- A 45, X karyotype is found in about half of these patients, most of whom have associated somatic defects including **short stature, webbed neck,** low hairline, shield-shaped chest, widening of long bones, STREAK GONADS, renal anomalies (Horse-shoe kidney) and cardiovascular defects (COA).
- Other features of turners syndrome is summarized in the image given.

307. Ans. (d)   All of the above

Ref: Shaws, 15th ed. /110-111, Harrison, 19th ed. pg. 635; DC Dutta, 6th ed. pg. 422-423

Please refer to above explanation.

308. Ans. (a)   45 XO

Ref: Shaws 15th ed. /110-111; Harrison 19/e 635; William's Gynecology Ch 16

309. Ans. (c)   Coaractation of aorta

Ref: Shaws, 15th ed. pg. 111, DC Dutta, 6th ed. pg. 422-423

- Cardiac anomaly seen with turner syndrome is *coaractation of aorta.*
- Single most common cause of increased mortality in children with Turner's syndrome: **Cardiovascular abnormalities (COA)**
- Single most important cause of primary amenorrhea: *Turner's syndrome.*

310. Ans. (d)   PAPP

- The triple test measures the following three levels in the maternal serum: *(sensitivity 71%)*
  - Alpha-fetoprotein (AFP)
  - Human chorionic gonadotropin (hCG)
  - Unconjugated estriol (UE3)
- **Quadruple test include:** triple test + Inhibin A: *increases sensitivity upto 80%*

The levels may indicate increased risk for certain conditions:

AFP	UE3	hCG	Associated conditions
Low	Low	High	Down's syndrome
Low	Low	Low	Trisomy 18 (Edward's syndrome)
High	-	-	NTD, omphalocoele, gastrochisis

311. Ans. (b)   Mullerian agenesis

Ref: William's Gynecology chapter 19-20

MULLERIAN AGENESIS

- Congenital absence of both uterus and vagina is referred as *müllerian aplasia, müllerian agenesis,* or *Mayer-Rokitansky-Küster-Hauser syndrome.*
- In classic müllerian *agenesis*, patients have a **shallow vaginal pouch**, only measuring up to 1.5 inches deep. *In addition, the uterus, cervix, and upper part of the vagina are absent.*
- Typically, a portion of the distal fallopian tubes are present. *In addition, normal ovaries are present*, given their separate embryonic origin.
- Most patients with müllerian *agenesis* have only small rudimentary müllerian bulbs without endometrial activity.
- Surgical excision of symptomatic rudimentary bulbs is required. With müllerian *agenesis*, traditional conception is impossible, but pregnancy may be achieved using sophisticated technology involving oocyte retrieval, fertilization, and implantation into a surrogate.

Extra Mile

- **Klinefelter syndrome, 47, XXY,** is a common sex chromosome abnormality associated with maternal age and occurs in 1/1000 live male births.
  - **Clinical features** include tall gynecoid stature, gynecomastia (with an increased risk for breast cancer), and testicular atrophy and low IQ.
- **Gonadal dysgenesis:** is the most common cause of primary amenorrhea. It is most frequently due to a chromosomal disorder or deletion of all or part of an X chromosome.

In order to figure out all the MCQs based on absence or presence or breast/uterus, following table is summarized: *(Katz: Comprehensive Gynecology, 5th ed.)*

Absent breast development; uterus present
- 45, X (Turner's syndrome)
- 46, X, abnormal X (e.g., short- or long-arm deletion)
- Mosaicism (e.g., X/XX, X/XX, XXX)
- 46, XX or 46, XY pure gonadal dysgenesis
- Kallman syndrome
- 17α-hydroxylase deficiency with 46, XX
- Pituitary failure
- Hypothalamus failure

Present breast development; uterus absent
- Androgen resistance (*testicular feminization*)
- Congenital absence of uterus (*utero-vaginal agenesis*)

Absent breast development; uterus absent
- 17, 20-desmolase deficiency
- Agonadism
- 17α-hydroxylase deficiency with 46, XY karyotype

Breast development; uterus present
- Hypothalamic etiology
- Pituitary etiology
- Ovarian etiology
- Uterine etiology

Obstetrics and Gynecology

312. Ans. (c) Ovaries and uterus are absent

Ref: Shaws 15th ed. /101

FEMALE PSEUDOHERMAPHRODITISM

- Results from excessive androgen exposure of an embryo or fetus
- Müllerian-inhibiting substance is not produced.
- The karyotype is 46, XX and ovaries are present.
- Because müllerian-inhibiting substance is not produced, the ovaries and female internal ductal structures such as the *uterus, cervix, and upper vagina are present*
- Clitoral hypertrophy will be more pronounced along with fused posterior labia.
- These patients are fertile

Male Pseudohermaphroditism
- Insufficient androgen exposure of a fetus destined to be a male leads to male pseudohermaphroditism.
- The karyotype is 46, XY and testes are present.
- The uterus is generally absent as a result of normal embryonic MIS production.
- These patients are most often sterile from abnormal spermatogenesis and have a smaller or inadequate phallus for sexual function.

TROPHOBLASTIC TUMORS

313. Ans. (a) Lung

Ref: Katz Comprehensive Gyenecology, 5th ed. Ch 35

- **Choriocarcinoma** is a highly malignant tumor arising from the chorionic epithelium.
- *About 3-5% of all patients with molar pregnancies develop choriocarcinoma.*
  - The primary site is usually anywhere in the uterus (secondary involvement).
  - Rarely, it starts in the tube or ovary.
  - The lesion is usually localized nodular type.
  - **Spread:** The common sites of metastases are **lungs (80%),** Anterior vaginal wall (30%), brain (10%), liver (10%)

Symptoms

- Irregular vaginal bleeding, at times brisk
- Continued amenorrhoea
- **Lung:** Cough, breathlessness, haemoptysis
- **Cerebral:** Headache, convulsion, paralysis or coma
- **Liver:** *Epigastric pain, jaundice*
- **Chest X-ray:** Shows **'cannon ball'** shadow or **'snow storm'** appearance due to numerous tumor emboli.

314. Ans. (b) Serial serum β hCG level

Ref: Katz Comprehensive Gyenecology, 5th ed. Ch 35

Postmolar Surveillance

- Gestational trophoblastic neoplasia (GTN) develops after approximately 15–20% of complete moles and 2–4% in partial moles.
- **Postmolar surveillance with serial quantitative serum β-hCG levels** is the standard.

315. Ans. (d) Chorioangioma

- **Chorioangioma** *the most common tumor of the placenta*
- It is a benign vascular tumor of placental origin, and is usually found incidentally.
- They are thought to arise as a malformation of the primitive angioblastic tissue of the placenta.
- *The angiomas are perfused by the fetal circulation. Therefore when they are large, they may represent a significant impediment to fetal cardiac activity.*
- These angiomas may also sequester platelets and can in turn give a fetal thrombocytopenia
- They can also cause increase in levels of maternal serum alpha-fetoprotein (MSAFP) and may prompt sonographic evaluation.

TABLE: Modified WHO Classification of Gestational Trophoblastic Disease

Molar lesions	Nonmolar lesions

• Hydatidiform mole
  ▪ Complete
  ▪ Partial
• Invasive mole
	• Choriocarcinoma
	• Placental site trophoblastic tumor
	• Epithelioid trophoblastic tumor

- **Choriocarcinoma:** A morphologic term applied to a highly malignant type of trophoblastic neoplasia in which both the cytotrophoblast and syncytiotrophoblast grow in a malignant fashion.
  - Chorionic villi are absent. These tumors tend to be hemorrhagic and necrotic
- **H. Mole:** A placental abnormality involving swollen placental villi and trophoblastic hyperplasia with loss of fetal blood vessels. There are two types: partial and complete.
  - **Partial:** A molar pregnancy with swelling of all placental villi partial. *Fetal tissues are present.*
  - **Complete:** A molar pregnancy with only villi, cord, and/or amniotic membrane elements.
- **Placental-Site Trophoblastic Tumor** A rare type of GTD arising in the uterus that secretes human placental lactogen and human chorionic gonadotrophin (hCG).
- **Note:** Persistent abnormal bleeding following normal pregnancy, abortion, or ectopic pregnancy should lead

to a consideration of the diagnosis of GTD. *The finding of pulmonary nodules on chest radiograph after normal pregnancy suggests GTD.*

INFERTILITY AND CONTRACEPTION

316. Ans. (b) IUD

Ref: DC Dutta 9th ed. P 498

- The best contraceptive method postplacental and postabortion is IUD
- IUD is the most effective reversible contraceptive methods.
- IUD is generally contraindicated in unmotivated persons, but since in this case the patient herself doesn't wish to conceive in near future, IUD is preferred.

Advantages of IUD:
- Ease of insertion
- Prevent uterine synechiae
- Longer action and inexpensive
- Contraceptive effect is reversible by simply removal of IUD
- Free of systemic metabolic side effects as seen with pills
- No need for continuous motivation (as seen with pills or barrier method). Only a single act of motivation is required.

Ideal IUD Candidate:
- In monogamous relationship
- Has borne at least one child
- No history of PID
- Has normal menstrual period
- Willing to check the IUD tail
- Has access to follow up and treatment

Timing of Insertion
- During menstruation or within 10 days of beginning of a menstrual period (diameter of cervical canal is greater)
- Can be done during the **first week after the delivery** before she leaves hospital *(immediate postpartum insertion).*
  - Special care required during first week as it has greater risk of perforation
- **Loop insertion:** Convenient time for loop insertion is 6–8 weeks after delivery *(postpuerperal insertion)*
- Can also be taken up immediately after first trimester abortion
  - IUD insertion after second trimester is NOT recommended → Increased risk of infection

317. Ans. (b) 6 weeks

Ref: DC Dutta 9th ed. P 623; Shaw's Gynecology 16th ed. P 273

- Within 6 weeks postpartum OCP's are contraindicated if the mother is lactating. In a lactating mother OCP can be started after 6 weeks (42 days) after delivery.
  - In the early phase of post-partum there is increased coagulability, which can be worsened due to estrogen containing hormonal contraceptives. Moreover lactation can also be affected.
- **The book states:** *"In a nonlactating woman, OC can be started after 3 weeks of delivery, but can be given soon after an abortion, MTP or an ectopic pregnancy"*
- **Note:** Contraceptive of choice during lactation: Mini-pill (aka Lactation pill)

Extra Mile

TABLE: Contraindications of combined oral contraceptives (WHO/FRM/FPP-2001)

Absolute			Relative
(A) Circulatory diseases (past or present) Thromboembolic disorder (current or past) • Arterial or venous thrombosis • Severe hypertension, stroke • Valvular heart disease, ischemic heart disease, angina • Diabetes with vascular complications • Focal migraine • Severe hypercholesterolemia • Smokers over age 35 years	**(B) Diseases of the liver** • Active liver disease • Liver adenoma, carcinoma • Liver tumors	**(C) Others** • Pregnancy • Undiagnosed genital tract bleeding • Estrogen-dependent neoplasm; e.g. breast cancer • Breast-feeding (within 6 weeks postpartum) • Major surgery or prolonged immobilization	• Age >40 years • Smoker or <35 years history of jaundice • Diabetes • Gallbladder disease • Hyperlipidemia • Postbreast cancer • Breastfeeding (postpartum 6 weeks to 6 months) • Sickle cell disease • CIN

318. Ans. (b) Semen analysis, Tubal patency test, Ovulation test

Ref: Shaw's Gynecology 16th ed. P 240-42

- Infertility implies apparent failure of a couple to conceive, while sterility indicates absolute inability to conceive, for one or more reasons.
- If a couple fails to achieve pregnancy after 1 year of 'unprotected' and regular intercourse, it is an indication to investigate the couple.

PATHOLOGY OF INFERTILITY

- 1/3rd cases: male is directly responsible
- 1/3rd cases: both partners are at fault
- 1/3rd cases female is directly responsible

Faults in the Male. The factors involved include:
- Disorders of spermatogenesis—50% (Ex: Hypothalamic disorder, Kallmann syndrome, orchitis etc.)
- Obstruction of the efferent ducts—30%
- Disorders of sperm motility—15% (Kartagener syndrome)
- Sexual dysfunction- Unexplained—15% (premature ejaculation, impotence, hypospadias)

Initial work-up in an infertile couple is:
- History and physical examination
- Ovulation assessment
- Hysterosalpingogram (to check tubal patency)
- Semen analysis

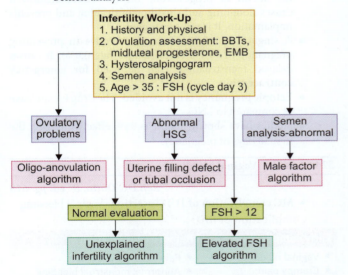

Note: *Please refer to textbook for the complete discussion of all the algorithm*

Extra Mile

Semen analysis
- It is the most important part of the male investigation.
- The best specimen is one obtained by masturbation in the vicinity of the laboratory (condom specimen is discouraged)
- Specimen best collected after a 3–5 days of abstinence.

WHO 2010 Semen Analysis
- Total volume, 2 mL (1.5 mL)
- PH—7.2–7.8
- Viscosity-3 (scale 0–4)
- Sperm concentration 20 million/mL or more (15 million/mL)
- Sperm count, >40 million/per ejaculate or more. Ten motile sperms per high field are considered normal.
- Motility >50% or more with progressive motility
- Morphology. 14% strict criteria (4%)
- Viability >75% or more (50%)
- White blood cells <1 million/mL
- Round cells <5 million/mL
- Sperm agglutination <2
- Pus cells: Absent
- **Postcoital test** (*Sims' or Huhner's test, PCT*): Postcoital (2 hs), cervical mucus collected study the sperm antibody in cervical mucus
- **Miller–Kurzrok test:** To study the penetration of sperms under the microscope.
  - Penetration less than 3 cm at 30 minutes is abnormal
- **Testicular biopsy:** Indicated in azoospermia to distinguish between testicular failure and obstruction in the vas deferens.
- **FSH level:** A high FSH level denotes primary gonadal failure

319. Ans. (b) Age <35 years

Ref: Shaw's Gyenology 16th ed. P 275

OCP Pills are contraindicated in:
- Cardiac disease, hypertension, smoker >35 years.
- **Diabetes:** Because carbohydrate tolerance may be reduced
- **History of thrombosis, myocardial infarct, sickle cell anemia, severe migraine:** OCP increases the risk of thrombosis and therefore it can worsen these pathologies.
- **Chronic liver diseases such as cholestatic jaundice of pregnancy, cirrhosis of liver, adenoma, porphyrias:** Adenomas have been reported and though they are benign, rupture of a hepatoma can be fatal.
- **Breast cancer:** OCP is proved to increase the risk of breast cancer in a high-risk woman. The progestogen component of OCP has a high potential for breast cancer.
- **Gallbladder disease:** Gallbladder function may be adversely affected.
- Gross obesity.
- Patient on enzyme-inducing drugs like rifampicin, and antiepileptic except sodium valproate.
- 4–6 weeks prior to planned surgery.
- **Lactating woman:** As lactation is suppressed with combined pills.
- **Monilial vaginitis:** As oral pills are associated with monilial vaginitis

FMGE Solutions Screening Examination

Book states: *The woman can take OC for several years up to the age of 35, and thereafter until 45 years if she is healthy, slim and nonsmoker.*

320. Ans. (a) Hepatic adenoma

Ref: Shaw's Gynecology 16th ed. P 274

Book states: "Liver adenomas have been reported and though they are benign, rupture of a hepatoma can be fatal. Because the hormones are metabolized in the liver, chronic liver diseases and recent jaundice contraindicate the use of OCP".

- OCP has no adverse effect on thyroid.
- It has shown to increase the risk of malignant breast CA if started in young, nulliparous females.
- No adverse effect is noted on uterine fibroids, and it is oestrogen singly that increases their size.
- It has shown to increase the risk of monilial vaginitis and endocervical CA and pituitary adenoma.

321. Ans. (c) Progesterone only pills

Ref: Shaw's Gynecology 16th ed. P 275

- **Minipill/Progestogen-only pill (POP).** The low-dose POP *(norethisterone 350 mcg, norgestrel 75 mcg or LNG 30 mcg)* have been introduced to avoid the side effects of estrogen in the combined pills.
- Given as once daily dosing, to be started within 5–7 days of menstruation and taken at the same time every day *(with a leeway of 3 hours either early or late)*.
- Contraceptive agent of choice during lactation is POP.

TABLE: Advantages and disadvantages of POP

Advantages	Disadvantages
They are recommended to: • Lactating women • Women over 35 years • Those with focal migraine • Those intolerant to estrogen or estrogen contraindicated • Diabetic, hypertensive woman, sickle cell anemia • Faster return of fertility than COC users because ovulation is not suppressed in all cases (suppressed in 40%)	• Strict daily compliance • Irregular bleeding • Amenorrhea • Depression • Headache • Weight gain • More failure rate than COCP (2–3/100 women years) • Ectopic pregnancy

Contraindications of COCP
- Previous ectopic pregnancy
- Ovarian cyst, breast and genital cancers
- Abnormal vaginal bleeding
- Active liver and arterial disease
- Porphyria
- Liver tumor
  - Because of osteopenia, it is contraindicated in adolescents and young women.

322. Ans. (a) Clomiphene citrate

Ref: Shaw's 16th ed. P 258

- Anovulation is a common problem encountered in infertility.
- **Clomiphene citrate (CC).**
  - Ovulation should be induced with CC, with a dose of 50 mg/day starting from day 2 to day 6 of the cycle for 5 days.
  - Ovulation is monitored by serial ultrasound monitoring of the follicular size, and occurrence of ovulation.
  - If the response to 50 mg CC is not satisfactory, the dose of CC should be increased to 100 mg/day from day 2 to day 6.
- If clomiphene therapy fails following 6–8 cycles, FSH and hCG therapy is recommended.
- In hypothalamic disorder, GnRH is given to stimulate the pituitary FSH and LH and the folliculogenesis monitored.

323. Ans. (c) Used for emergency contraception

Ref: Shaw, 16th ed. pg. 279

RU 486 (Mifepristone)

- RU 486 is a steroid with an affinity for progesterone receptors. It does not prevent fertilization but by blocking the action of progesterone on the endometrium, it causes sloughing and shedding of decidua and prevents implantation. It is **not teratogenic.**
- A single dose of 25–50 mg is effective in preventing pregnancy in 99.1% cases (failure rate 0.9%). It causes delayed menstruation. Can be **used for emergency contraception.**
- **Ectopic pregnancy is not avoided.** The drug is expensive as compared to LNG.
- Studies have shown than it is 95% effective during the first 50 days of pregnancy.

324. Ans. (b) Vaginal bleeding

Ref: DC Dutta, 8th ed. pg. 618

- MC complication of IUD insertion: Vaginal bleeding

Complication of IUD:

Early complication	Remote complication
• Vaginal bleed • Crampy pain • Syncopal attack • Partial or complete perforation	• Pain • Abnormal menstrual bleeding • PID • Spontaneous expulsion • Perforation

325. Ans. (c) 10% of infertile couples

Ref: Shaw, 15th pg. 202, 209

Definition of infertility: Inability to conceive even after 1 year of unprotected sexual intercourse.

Relative Prevalence of Cause of Infertility

Obstetrics and Gynecology

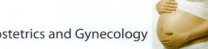

- Male Factor 25–40%
- Female Factor 40–55 %
- Both 10%
- Unexplained 10%
  - **Disorders of the spermatogenesis** are the most common cause of **male infertility**.
  - **Ovarian causes** are the most common cause of **female infertility**.

Extra Mile

- WHO cut off limit for sperm count is 20 million/ml.
- Post coital test (Sim's or Huhner's test) is done for cervical factor of infertility
- Effective sperm count is 50 million/ml.
- Testicular biopsy can differentiate obstructive lesion at vas deferens from testicular failure.
- Most treatable form of infertility is anovulation.
- **Best investigation** for tubal patency is **laproscopic chromotubation**.
- Clomiphene citrate is the ovulation induction agent of choice
- **Ferning of cervical mucus** occurs due to **estrogen**.
- Bromocriptine is used to treat hyperprolactinemia.
- Ovarian hyperstimulation syndrome is most commonly the side effect of human menopausal gonadotropin injections used for ovulation induction.

326. Ans. (a) Azoospermia

Ref: Shaws, 15th ed. pg. 203

- Azoospermia is defined as complete absence of sperm from the ejaculate.
- It is present in about 1% of all men and in approximately 15% of infertile men.
- Azoospermia is different from aspermia, in that aspermia is the complete absence of seminal fluid emission upon ejaculation.
- In order to distinguish between obstructive and non-obstructive causes of azoospermia, **diagnostic testicular biopsy is indicated for patients with normal testicular size, at least one palpable vas deferens and a normal serum follicle-stimulating hormone level**.
- *Testicular biopsy is indicated in azoospermic men* with a normal-sized testis and normal findings on hormonal studies to rule out ductal obstruction.

Relative indications for testicular biopsy

- Ruling out partial obstruction in patients with severe oligospermia
- Evaluating patients with hypogonadotropism to select those likely responsive to treatment.
- Respond to gonadotropin replacement retrieving spermatozoa in azoospermic patients undergoing IVF or ICSI.

Extra Mile

- **Aspermia:** Absence of semen
- **Azoospermia:** Absence of sperm
- **Hypospermia:** Low semen volume
- **Oligozoospermia:** Low sperm count
- **Asthenozoospermia:** Poor sperm motility
- **Teratozoospermia:** Sperm carry more morphological defects than usual
- **Necrozoospermia:** All sperm in the ejaculate are dead

327. Ans. (b) CuT 380

Ref: Shaws, 15th ed. pg. 549

COPPER-T IUCD

- Can be Inserted within 5 days of intercourse
- **MOA:** prevents implantation of a fertilized ovum.
- **Advantages:**
  - It can be inserted as late as 5 days after the unprotected intercourse.
  - cheap.
  - **Failure rate is EXCEPTIONALLY low which is 0.1%.**
  - It is long lasting, can remain as ongoing contraceptive method for 3 to 5 years.

Contraceptive	Failure rate	Method/time of administration
CuT	0.1%	Inserted within 5 days of UNPROTECTED sex
Levonorgestrel (LNG)	1.1%.	One tablet should be taken within 72 hours of unprotected sex and another 12 hours later.
Combined pill	3.2 per 100 woman years	Taken within 72 hours of intercourse followed by 2 tablets taken 12 hours later **(Yuzpe and Lancee method)**
RU 486 (mifepristone)	Failure rate 0.9%	Single dose of 10 mg
Ethinyloestradiol	failure rate 0 to 1.5%	1 mg daily for 5 days, starting within 72 hours of unprotected sex **(Haspels and Andriesse method)**

328. Ans. (a) 0.1% to 0.3%

Ref: Shaw 15th ed. pg. 240

The most popular technique of tubal ligation is Pomeroy **technique (a type of minilaprotomy;** abdominal incision should be less than 5 cm). The failure rate is **only 0.4%. Catgut suture** is being used for this method of sterilization.

329. Ans. (b) 10 years

Ref: Shaw, 15th ed. pg. 227-8

FMGE Solutions Screening Examination

Name of device	Effective period
• CuT 380A	10 years
• Nova T-Silver	5 years
• Multiload 375	5 years
• Multiload 250	3 years

330. Ans. (d) They are lipid friendly

Ref: D.C Dutta, 7th ed. pg. 543-545

- Levonorgesterol is a progestin which is used in combined OCP with estrogen.
- The combined oral steroidal contraceptives is the most effective reversible method of contraception.
- The commonly used progestins are either levonogestrel or norethisterone or desogestrel.
- *Lipid friendly, third generation progestins are namely desogestrel, gestodene, norgestimate.*
- The oestrongens are principally confined to either ethinyl-oestradiol or menstronal.
- **Composition in OCP:** Levonorgestrel 0.15 + Ethinyl oestradiol 30
- It should normally be started on day one of the cycle.
- One tablet is to be taken daily preferably at bed time for consecutive 21 days. It is continued for 21 days and then has a seven days break.
- *Thus a simple regime of "3 weeks ON and 1 week off" is to be followed.*

331. Ans. (d) Contraceptive failure

Ref: Park's PSM, 21st ed. pg. 472

- Pearl index is used to measure the contraceptive efficacy/contraceptive failure.
- It is defined as the number of failures per 100 women-years (HWY) of exposure.

$$PI = \frac{\text{Total accidental pregnancies}}{\text{Total months of exposure}} \times 1200$$

- Another method used to measure contraceptive failure/efficacy is *life table analysis.*
- Life table analysis: calculates failure rates for each month of use.

332. Ans. (c) Protect from breast cancer

Ref: D.C Dutta, 8th ed. pg. 625

BENEFITS OF COMBINED ORAL CONTRACEPTIVES (COCS)

- **Contraceptive benefits:**
  - Protection against unwanted pregnancy *(failure rate- 0.1 per 100 women year)*
  - Convenient to use
  - Not intercourse related
  - Reversibility
  - Improving maternal and child health care

- **Non-contraceptive benefits:**
  - Improvement of menstrual abnormalities
  - Reduction of dysmenorrhea (40%)
  - Reduction of menorrhagia (50%)
  - Reduction of premenstrual tension syndrome (PM)
  - Prevention of malignancies like Endometrial cancer (50%), Epithelial ovarian cancer 50%, Colorectal cancer (40%).
- It increases risk of breast CA, cervical CA

333. Ans. (b) Protection against cervical cancer

Ref: D.C Dutta, 7th ed. pg. 547

334. Ans. (c) Prevent release of ovum from ovary

Ref: DC Dutta, 8th ed. pg. 622

- Combined OCP is in combination with estrogen and progesterone. It acts by inhibiting ovulation.

POLYCYSTIC OVARIAN SYNDROME (PCOS)/STEIN LEVANTHAL SYNDROME

335. Ans. (b) PCOS

Ref: Shaw's Gynecology 16th ed. P 145-46

- MCC of hirsutism is: PCOS
- *Polycystic ovarian syndrome accounts for 70 to 80% of cases of hirsutism*, with idiopathic hirsutism being the second most frequent cause.
- In a female, hirsutism is defined as the presence of coarse, dark, terminal hairs distributed in a male pattern.
- Hirsutism in PCOS is secondary to hyperandrogenism.

Latest Definition of PCOS *(To include two out of three of the following)*

- Oligomenorrhea or anovulation
- Clinical and/or biochemical signs of **hyperandrogenism**
- Polycystic ovaries (with the exclusion of related disorders)

Signs and Symptoms/Consequences

- Patients with PCOS, complaints stem from varied endocrine effects and may include:
  - Menstrual irregularities, infertility, manifestations of androgen excess, or other endocrine dysfunction.

Short-term consequences	Long-term consequences
• Irregular menses	• Diabetes mellitus
• Hirsutism/acne androgenic alopecia	• Cardiovascular disease
• Infertility	• Endometrial cancer
• Obesity	
• Metabolic disturbances	
• Abnormal lipid levels/ glucose intolerance	

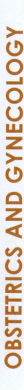

Obstetrics and Gynecology

336. Ans. (c) PCOD

Ref: Shaw's Gynecology 16th ed. P 145-46

PCOD

In PCOD, upon USG:
- There are enlarged ovaries (increased size and stroma).
- Ovarian volume will be more than 10 mm^3.
- It shows 12 or more small follicles each of 2–9 mm in size placed peripherally.

Note: *In PCOD, there is hyperandrogenism. Androgen suppresses the growth of the dominant follicle and prevents apoptosis of smaller follicles which are normally destined to disappear in the late follicular phase. Hence there are increased numbers of follicles.*

Turner's Syndrome
- In Turner syndrome, either the short arm of X chromosome is deleted or the nucleus possesses only 45 chromosomes, i.e. 22 pairs of autosomes plus a sex chromosome XO.
- Sometimes, it is also referred as ovarian agenesis or gonadal dysgenesis because of presence of undifferentiated stromal cells with absence of sex cells, known as **streak gonads**.
- The **ovaries in Turner syndrome do not contain graafian follicles, so estrogen is not produced.**
- **In primary amenorrhea**, there is failure of HPO axis causing absence of ovarian follicles.
- In Klinefelter syndrome, there are masculine gonads.

337. Ans. (b) PCOD

Ref: Shaws, 15th ed. pg. 274; William's Gyne, Ch 17 PCOD

Please refer to above explanation for more details

> **Extra Mile**
> - **Ferriman-Gallwey Scoring System:** To quantify the degree of hirsutism
> - **Most common areas affected with excess hair growth in women with PCOS include:** the upper lip, chin, sideburns, chest, and linea alba of the lower abdomen.
> - Hirsutism should be distinguished from **hypertrichosis**, which is a generalized increase in lanugo, that is, the soft, lightly pigmented hair associated with some medications and malignancies.

338. Ans. (a) PCOS

Ref: Shaws, 15th ed. pg. 115-116

- **GARLAND/NECKLACE pattern on USG:** PCOS
- **Comet tail appearance:** Adenomyomatois
- **Snowstorm appearance:** Choriocarcinoma

339. Ans. (d) Combined OCP

Ref: Williams Gynecology Ch 17

- Polycystic ovarian syndrome is also called Androgen insensitivity syndrome, where there is excess of androgen in female patient.
- Elevated androgen levels play a major role in determining the type and distribution of hair. Within a hair follicle, testosterone is converted by the enzyme 5a-reductase to dihydrotestosterone (DHT).
- Although both testosterone and DHT convert short, soft vellus hair to coarse terminal hair, **DHT is markedly more effective than testosterone.** Conversion is irreversible, and only hairs in androgen-sensitive areas are changed in this manner to terminal hairs. As a result the most common areas affected with excess hair growth in women with PCOS include the upper lip, chin, sideburns, chest, and linea alba of the lower abdomen.
- A first-line treatment for menstrual irregularities is combination oral contraceptive pills (COCs), which will induce regular menstrual cycles. In addition, COCs reduce androgen levels, Thereby, decreasing the severity of hirsutism.
- Specifically, COCs suppress gonadotropin release, which results in decreased ovarian androgen production. Moreover, the estrogen component increases SHBG levels. The progestin component antagonizes the endometrial proliferative effect of estrogen, thus reducing risks of endometrial hyperplasia due to unopposed estrogen.

PROLAPSE

340. Ans. (c) Needs to be changed every 3 months

Ref: Shaw's Gynecology 16th ed. P 356; DC Dutta 9th ed. P 293

- Ring pessary is used for prolapse
- The ring pessary is made of soft plastic polyvinyl chloride material and is available in different sizes.
- It is inserted using gel
- Pregnant woman with prolapse needs a ring pessary in the first trimester of pregnancy
  - Uterus grows abdominally, the prolapse gets reduced, and the pessary can then be removed.
- **Current indications for use of pessary are:**
  - A young woman planning a pregnancy
  - During early pregnancy
  - Puerperium
  - Temporary use while clearing infection and decubitus ulcer
  - A woman unfit for surgery
  - In case a woman refuses for surgery

341. Ans. (c) Pessary

Ref: Shaw's Gynecology 16th ed. P 359-60

- Pessary is the conservative treatment for prolapse.
- All other choices are surgical repair

FMGE Solutions Screening Examination

TABLE: Management of genital prolapse

Nulliparous	Abdominal sling operations
Pregnancy Postnatal	Ring pessary up to 16 weeks • Ring pessary and pelvic floor exercises for 3-6 months • Surgery if required thereafter
Young woman <40 years	Conservative vaginal surgery (fertility sparing surgery) • Cystocele, rectocele repair • Manchester repair • Sling operation
Woman beyond 40 years and multipara	Vaginal hysterectomy and pelvic floor repair

Extra Mile

Surgeries of prolapse
- **Anterior colporrhaphy:** To repair cystocoele and cystourethrocele
- **Posterior colporrhaphy:** to repair rectocoele and deficient perineum
- **Fothergill's Repair (Manchester Operation):** Anterior colporrhaphy with amputation of cervix
  - Preserves menstrual and childbearing functions
- **Shirodkar's Procedure:** Anterior colporrhaphy and attachment of Mackenrodt ligaments to the cervix on each side is exposed
  - The cervix is not amputated and subsequent pregnancy complications avoided
- **Le Fort's Repair:** reserved for the very elderly menopausal patient with an advanced prolapse.
- **Sling operation:** best for nulliparous prolapse
  - Abdominal sling operation
  - Khanna sling operation
  - Abdominal wall cervicopexy

MISCELLANEOUS

342. Ans. (b) Estrogen

Ref: Shaws, 15th ed. pg. 66-67

- HRT stands for Hormone Replacement Therapy
- Estrogen plays a key role throughout the body. It affects the brain, the bones, the skin, the heart, the blood vessels, and more. While estrogen levels lower gradually during natural menopause, they plummet with surgical menopause (hysterectomy).
- Hormone therapy after surgery—either with estrogen and progestin or with estrogen alone—is a way to counteract the supply of estrogen lost due to hysterectomy.
- *Women who have both the uterus and ovaries removed usually just get estrogen replacement therapy (ERT) alone.*
- *Combination therapy with both estrogen and progestin is considered in patients who have underwent oophorectomy (removal of ovaries). That's because estrogen alone can increase the risk of cancer in the uterus. Adding progestin removes this risk.*
- HRT using a combination of estrogen and progestin *can also be* used after a hysterectomy if widespread *endometriosis* is found at the time of surgery.
- **Note:** testoesterone replacement is considered in patients who do not respond to estrogen alone. Some doctors recommend testosterone replacement along with estrogen replacement because testosterone helps in energy levels, mood and libido.

Factors in favor of taking HRT include:
- Family history of osteoporosis
- High risk category related to osteoporosis
- Family history of heart disease
- High risk category related to heart disease
- Severe climateric symptoms
- Post hysterectomy

343. Ans. (c) CO_2

Ref: Shaws, 15th ed. pg. 492

Pnenumoperitoneum in created with CO_2 or nitrous oxide. CO_2 is preferred because nitrous oxide can cause explosion in the presence of volatile anaesthetic drug.

ANSWERS TO BOARD REVIEW QUESTIONS

344. Ans. (c) 6:1

Ref: COGT 10th ed ch-8, William's 23rd ed ch-3 p-54

345. Ans. (b) 1–2 mm/min

Ref: Ganong's 22nd ed p-427, Guyton 11th edn p-999

346. Ans. (a) Fetal plate smaller than basal plate

Ref: William's obs ch-27 p.578

347. Ans. (c) Cancer cervix

Ref: Novak's Gyne 15th ed ch-19.P 581

348. Ans. (c) 100°

Ref: Appendix-103 for "Caldwell-Moloy Classification Of Types Of Pelvis"

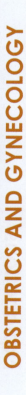

Obstetrics and Gynecology

349. Ans. (d) Microscopy

Ref: Novak's 14th ed p 544

350. Ans. (c) Anterior to posterior fontanelle

351. Ans. (a) Cu T 380 A

Ref: Novak's 14th ed ch: 10

352. Ans. (a) 20

Ref: Novak's 14th ed ch 10

353. Ans. (b) 9%

Ref: Appendix-115 for "METHODS OF CONTRACEPTION"

354. Ans. (b) Rifampicin

Ref: KDT 7th ed p-317

355. Ans. (a) 1st trimester

Ref: William's obstetrics 23rd ed p-145

356. Ans. (d) Interstitium

Ref: Williams 23ed p. 28, Textbook of Obstetrics byPadubidri p.11, Novak's 14th ed ch: 5

357. Ans. (c) 50 g and 1 hour

Ref: Williams Obst. 23rd ed Ch: 52

358. Ans. (c) Lack of lactation

Ref: The pituitary: 3rded by ShlomoMelm ed p. 403

359. Ans. (b) Benzathine Penicillin

Ref: Danforth's Obstetrics and Gynecology, 10th ed p 613

360. Ans. (a) 1 g

Ref: Park 20th ed p-552, Williams 23rd ed ch: 8 p.203

361. Ans. (b) Ian Donald

Ref: Williams obs. Ed 23 ch: 16 p. 349

362. Ans. (a) 1 million

Ref: Novak's 14th ed. ch: 7 p. 177, Gray's Anatomy 39th ed p-1392

363. Ans. (c) Mullerian agenesis

Ref: Shaw's 13th ed p-87

364. Ans. (a) Throracopagus

365. Ans. (a) Methrotrexate

366. Ans. (c) Mento vertical

367. Ans. (a) Chadwick sign

368. Ans. (a) Gynaecoid

369. Ans. (a) Prematurity

370. Ans. (a) Preeclampsia

371. Ans. (c) Monochorionic monoamniotic

372. Ans. (b) 0.1%

373. Ans. (c) Bimastoid

374. Ans. (b) 15 mm Hg

375. Ans. (b) 8 weeks

376. Ans. (b) Abruption placenta

377. Ans. (b) Itchy/pruritus

378. Ans. (a) Hydrosalpinx

379. Ans. (a) Fallopian tube

380. Ans. (a) Invasive carcinoma

381. Ans. (a) Nucleic acid amplification

382. Ans. (c) Chlamydia

383. Ans. (b) Mucus can withstand stretching up to 10 cm

384. Ans. (a) Squamous Cell Ca

385. Ans. (b) Biopsy

386. Ans. (a) Painless watery discharge

387. Ans. (b) Dysgerminoma

Explanations

388. Ans. (c) CA 125
389. Ans. (d) Anovulatory
390. Ans. (c) Coaractation of aorta
391. Ans. (d) PAPP
392. Ans. (a) Azoospermia
393. Ans. (b) CuT 380
394. Ans. (b) POCD
395. Ans. (a) Adhesion in uterus post curettage
396. Ans. (d) Norplant
397. Ans. (b) Transcervical sterilization
398. Ans. (a) Single use
399. Ans. (a) Cardinal ligament
400. Ans. (a) Brow

Ref: Dutta 6th ed p-393

401. Ans. (c) 4 cm

Ref: Dutta 6th ed p-528, Midwifery Education Modules By WHO, World Health Organization P: 55

402. Ans. (a) Labor

Ref: Dutta 6th ed p-300

403. Ans. (a) Doderlein Bacilli

Ref: Shaw 13th ed p. 125, Novak's Gynecology 12thed p-192, Jeffcoate 7ed p-27

404. Ans. (a) Android pelvis

Ref: Dutta 6th ed p-347, William's 22nd ed ch-2, Danforth's 10th ed p-474

405. Ans. (c) 3 weeks

Ref: Dutta 6th ed p-24

406. Ans. (a) Vaginal discharge

Ref: Duttagynaecology 4th ed p-287

407. Ans. (b) 12–20 weeks

Ref: Current OB/Gyn 10th edn ch-13

408. Ans. (c) T sign

Ref: William's 23rd ed p-864, Danforth 10th ed p-243, Obstetric Ultrasound by Trish Chudleigh 3rd ed p-48

409. Ans. (c) Seprate chorion and amnion

Ref: William's 23rd ed p-864, Danforth 10th ed p-243, Obstetric Ultrasound by Trish Chudleigh 3rd ed p-48

410. Ans. (d) 15 mm

Ref: Manual Of Obstretics 3rd ed by Daftary p-250, Textbook of Basic Nursing by Caroline Bunker Rosdahl, Mary T. Kowalski 9thed p-906

411. Ans. (a) Candida

Ref: Dutta obs. 64th ed. p-306, Shiela'sBTextbook of Gynaecology, p-205, Danforth's Obstetrics and Gynecology, 10th ed p-609

412. Ans. (b) 2 weeks

Ref: With text

413. Ans. (a) 8-15 weeks

Ref: Radiation Injury Prevention and Mitigation in Human by Kedar N. Prasad p-62

414. Ans. (a) Fractional curettage

Ref: Novak's Gynecology 13thedn p-453, Dutta 4thed p-331, TeLinde 9thed p-1379

415. Ans. (a) Plenty of lactobacilli

Ref: Shaw 13th ed p-129, Novak's Gynecology 12thedn p-192, CGDT 9thed p-654

416. Ans. (c) Behavioral method

Ref: William's 23rd ed ch-32

417. Ans. (a) Cisplatin

Ref: Berek& Novak's Gynecology, 14th ed p-1431

418. Ans. (a) 1 week

Ref: Williams Obstetrics 23rd ed ch-30 p-649; Ch: 5 p-115

419. Ans. (b) Obstructed Labor

Ref: Williams obstetrics 23rd ed ch: 35 p-784, Duttas obstetrics 7th ed ch: 28 p-426

420. Ans. (c) 36 weeks

Ref: Williams Obstetrics 23rd ed p-964

Obstetrics and Gynecology

421. Ans. (d) Pyogenic granuloma

Ref: Williams Obstetrics 22nd ed ch:56

422. Ans. (b) 2 weeks

Ref: Williams Obstetrics 22nd ed ch: 20; Current Diagnosis & Treatment Obstetrics & Gynecology, Tenth Ed.ion ch: 32

423. Ans. (b) Elderly patient with utero-vaginal prolapse

Ref: Practical Gynacecolgy and Obstetrics by V. Padubidri p-47, Danforth's 10thed p-867, Current OB/GYN ch-44 Pelvic Organ Prolapse

424. Ans. (c) Diastolic notch in umbilical artery at 22 weeks

Ref: Obstetric Ultrasound by Trish Chudleigh, BaskyThilaganathan 3rd ed p-228-232, Williams 23rd ed p-364, Dutta 6thed p-464

425. Ans. (a) Loss of deep tendon reflexes

Ref: William's 23 ed e. p-738

426. Ans. (d) Hysterectomy

Ref: Novak's Gynaecology 14th ed p-521, Dutta 6th ed. p-295

427. Ans. (a) Bacterial vaginsis

Ref: Shaw 13th ed p-129, Novak's Gynecology 12th ed. p-192

428. Ans. (d) 37 weeks

Ref: William's obstetrics 23rd ed ch-36, American journal of Obs and gynaec, Nov. 2013 no. 529

429. Ans. (d) Pulmonary hypertension

Ref: Dutta 6th ed. p-279

430. Ans. (a) Pain

Ref: William's Obstetrics 23rd e. ch-35 p-783

431. Ans. (b) George papanicolaou

Ref: Cervical Cancer: Current and Emerging Trends in Detection and Treatment

432. Ans. (a) Fertilization takes place here

Ref: With text

433. Ans. (b) 3%

Ref: Dutta 6th ed. p-374

434. Ans. (b) Hematogenous

Ref: A comprehensive Textbook of Obstetrics and Gynecology By Sadhana Gupta 1st ed. p-215

435. Ans. (b) Hormonal contraceptives

Ref: William's 22nd ed ch-11

436. Ans. (a) Magnesium sulfate

Ref: William's 22nd ed ch-34, Current Diagnosis & Treatment Obstetrics & Gynecology 10th ed Table 19-2, Table 19-4, Danforth 10th ed p-264

437. Ans. (d) 2000 mL

Ref: John Hopkin's Manual For Gynaecology& Obstetrics p-110

438. Ans. (a) 1:2

Ref: Shaw 13thed p-9, Keith L Moore 7th ed p-394

439. Ans. (a) p53

Ref: Robbin's 8th ed p-1034

440. Ans. (c) 28 weeks

Ref: Nelson 18th ed Ch-101

441. Ans. (c) Abdominal circumference

Ref: Dutta 6th ed p-464

442. Ans. (a) 200 mcg/day

Ref: Appendix-127 for "Indian Reference, Recommended Dietary Allowance"

443. Ans. (c) 1.5–2 cm

Ref: William's 22nd ed ch-3, Guyton 12th ed p-990

444. Ans. (c) Triplod

Ref: Danforths obstetrics and Gynecology 10th ed. p-10374, Dutta 6th ed. p-200

445. Ans. (b) Pulmonary hypertension

Ref: Dutta 6th ed. p-279

446. Ans. (b) Chlamydia

Ref: Harrison's 17th ed. Ch: 124

447. Ans. (a) McRoberts

Ref: William's obstetrics 23nd ed. Ch-483

448. Ans. (c) Premature menopause

Ref: William's 22nd ed. Ch-16

449. Ans. (a) Inc FSH and LH

Ref: Shaw's 16th ed. P 66

- Menopause normally occurs between the ages of 45 and 50 years, the average age being 47 years.
- Menopause setting before the age of 40 is known as premature menopause.
- At menopause ovarian activity declines. Cessation of ovarian activity and a fall in the oestrogen and inhibin levels cause a rebound increase in the secretion of FSH and LH by the anterior pituitary gland. The FSH level may rise as much as 50-fold and LH 3–4 fold.
- There is 50% reduction in androgen production and 66% reduction in oestrogen at menopause

450. Ans. (b) Decrease in estrogen

Ref: Shaw's 16th ed. P 66-67

- **Oestrogen is cardioprotective by maintaining:**
  - High level of high density lipoprotein (HDL)
  - Lowering the low density lipoprotein (LDL) and triglycerides.
- Oestrogen deficiency therefore can cause atherosclerosis, ischaemic heart disease and myocardial infarction.
- Oestrogen prevents atherosclerosis through its antioxidant property.

> **Extra Mile**
> - Oestrogen level of over 40 pg/mL exerts bone and cardiotrophic effect.
> - Level below 20 pg/mL may predispose to osteoporosis and ischaemic heart disease
> - Post menopausal Alzheimer's disease is also related to decreased level of estrogen

451. Ans. (c) Multiparity

Ref: Shaw's Gynecology 13th ed. P 270

- **Copper T (CuT) is a copper containing IUCD with** copper wire of **surface area 200 to 250 mm** is wrapped round the vertical stem of a polypropylene frame.
- Available CuT devices are: CuT 200, Copper 7, Multiload Copper 250, CuT 380, CuT 220 and Nova-T.
- These copper devices are more expensive than inert devices andexert a better contraceptive effect, with fewer side effects.
- It is preferred in multiparous women.

Contraindications of IUCD

- Suspected pregnancy
- Pelvic inflammatory disease (PID), lower genital tract infection
- Presence of fibroids—because of misfit
- Menorrhagia and dysmenorrhoea, if Copper T is used
- Severe anaemia
- Diabetic women who are not well controlled—because of slight increase in pelvic infection
- Heart disease—risk of infection
- Previous ectopic pregnancy
- Scarred uterus
- Preferably avoid its use in unmarried and nulliparous patients because of the risk of PID and subsequent tubal infertility
- LNG IUCD in breast cancer
- Abnormally shaped uterus, septate uterus

> **Extra Mile**
> - Mirena (32 x 32 mm) contains 52 mg LNG, eluting 20 mcg daily. It can be retained for 5 years,
> - Failure rate of mirena: 0.1–0.4 per 100 woman years.

452. Ans. (a) Ovulation

- **Mittelschmerz pain** (intermenstrual pain) is one sided lower abdominal pain associated with ovulation, which occurs during mid cycle or 14 days before the next menstrual cycle.
- It usually lasts a few minutes to few hours.

ANSWERS TO IMAGE-BASED QUESTIONS

453. Ans. (a) Trichomonas

The image shows presence of anaerobic flagellated protozoan parasite, which causes vaginitis in women with development of greenish malodorous discharge.

454. Ans. (b) Cusco speculum

455. Ans. (b) Hegar dilator

456. Ans. (a) Bacterial vaginosis

The image shows *presence of clue cells* which are vaginal epithelial cells, coated with bacteria. The patient presents with whitish vaginal discharge with a fishy odor.

457. Ans. (a) Interstitial part

The image shows a fallopian tube with ovary seen close to the fimbrial end of the tube. The chances of ectopic pregnancy is highest in ampulla (choice c), and least in interstitial part (Choice a).

458. Ans. (a) Hydrosalpinx

459. Ans. (c) Sims speculum

460. Ans. (b) Vulsellum

461. Ans. (a) Uterine sound

462. Ans. (a) Outlet forceps

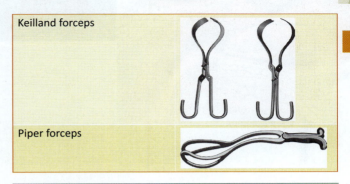

Keilland forceps

Piper forceps

463. Ans. (d) Cryotherapy probe

The shown image is cryotherapy probe.
Used in cervical cancer

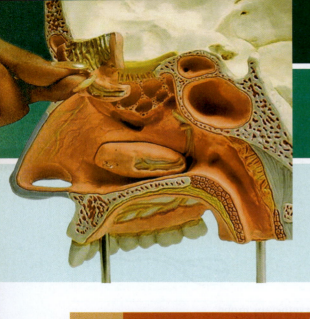

13

ENT

EAR AND ITS DISEASES

MOST RECENT QUESTIONS 2019

1. Narrowest part of airway in infant:
   a. Glottis
   b. Subglottis
   c. Supraglottis
   d. Epiglottis
2. A 15 year boy presents with recurrent episodes of epistaxis, unilateral obstruction of nostril. Most likely cause:
   a. Nasal polyp
   b. Angiofibroma
   c. Nasopharyngeal CA
   d. Pharyngitis
3. Abductor of vocal cord:
   a. Posterior cricoarytenoid muscle
   b. Interarytenoid muscle
   c. Cricothyroid muscle
   d. Thyroarytenoid muscle
4. In ranula management which of the following step is correct?
   a. Excision of ranula and sublingual gland duct
   b. Excision of only the cystic swelling
   c. In large ranula marsuplization not preferred
   d. In small ranula marsuplization is preferred
5. High tracheostomy is done in which condition?
   a. Laryngeal carcinoma
   b. Laryngeal stenosis
   c. Respiratory obstruction
   d. Foreign body
6. A patient presented with profound sensorineural deafness, not responding to hearing aids, with intact auditory nerve function. Which of the following procedure is preferred in this patient?
   a. BAHA
   b. Cochlear implant
   c. Brainstem implant
   d. Tympanoplasty
7. A patient presented with nasopharyngeal CA with bilateral LN, epistaxis and hearing loss. What is the most common cause of deafness in this patient:
   a. Nerve deafness
   b. Ossicular damage
   c. Serous otitis media
   d. Auditory canal obstruction

8. Nasal mass with extension from maxillary sinus is most likely a case of:
   a. Antrochoanal polyp
   b. Ethmoid polyp
   c. Glomus tumor
   d. Rhinoscleroma

ANATOMY OF AURICLE AND EXTERNAL AUDITARY CANAL & EMBRYOLOGY

9. Which of the following is the derivative of first pharyngeal arch: *(Recent Pattern Question 2018-19)*
   a. Stapedius muscle
   b. Anterior belly of digastric muscle
   c. Posterior belly of digastric muscle
   d. Hyoid bone
10. What is the Ossicles-lever ratio?
    (Recent Pattern Question 2018)
    a. 1.3:1
    b. 1.8:1
    c. 21:1
    d. 14:1
11. Endolymph is secreted by: *(Recent Pattern Question 2018)*
    a. Basilar membrane
    b. Reissner's membrane
    c. Stria vascularis
    d. Tectorial membrane
12. Surgical landmark for mastoid antrum:
    (Recent Pattern Question 2017)
    a. Korner septum
    b. MacEwen's triangle
    c. Fallopian triangle
    d. Antral triangle
13. Which muscle arises from 4th phyrangeal arch:
    (Recent Pattern Question 2016)
    a. Cricothyroid
    b. Cricoarytenoid
    c. Posterior cricoarytenoid
    d. Thyroarytenoid
14. Ear lobule is made of:
    a. Skin only
    b. Cartilage
    c. Skin with fat
    d. Fibrous tissue
15. All of the following nerves supply auricle of ear EXCEPT?
    a. Greater auricular nerve
    b. Lesser petrosal nerve
    c. Auriculotemporal nerve
    d. Lesser Occipital nerve

ENT

963

16. **All of the following nerves supply the medial aspect of auricle EXCEPT:**
   a. Greater auricular nerve   b. Lesser occipital nerve
   c. Facial nerve   d. Auriculotemporal nerve

17. **Major portion of auricle is supplied by:**
   a. Greater auricular nerve
   b. Lesser occipital nerve
   c. Facial nerve
   d. Auriculotemporal nerve

18. **Arnold nerve is a branch of:**
   a. Vagus nerve   b. Hypoglossal nerve
   c. Glossopharyngeal nerve   d. Trigeminal nerve

19. **Jacobson's nerve is a branch of:**
   a. Vagus nerve   b. Hypoglossal nerve
   c. Glossopharyngeal nerve   d. Trigeminal nerve

20. **Which of these is not a derivative of 3rd pharyngeal/ branchial arch:**
   a. Lesser cornu   b. Greater cornu
   c. Stylopharyngeus   d. Lower hyoid

21. **Greater cornu of hyoid is derived from which branchial arch:**
   a. I   b. II
   c. III   d. IV

22. **Which of the following intrinsic laryngeal muscles is not derived from branchial arch VI:**
   a. Cricoarytenoid muscle   b. Interarytenoid muscle
   c. Thyroarytenoid muscle   d. Cricothyroid muscle

23. **Thyroid cartilage is derived from which branchial arch:**
   a. II and III   b. III and IV
   c. IV and V   d. IV and VI

24. **Stapes is derived from which branchial arch:**
   a. I   b. II
   c. III   d. IV

25. **All are derived from branchial arch EXCEPT?**
   a. Ultimobranchial body   b. Stapes
   c. Laryngeal cartilage   d. Mandible

26. **All are true about external auditory meatus EXCEPT:**
   a. It extends from the bottom of concha to tympanic membrane & measures 24 cms in length
   b. Fissure of santorini in cartilaginous part can transmit infection to the parotid or superficial mastoid infection.
   c. Foramen of Huschke may present from Antero-inferior part of bony canal
   d. Outer 1/3rd is bony and inner 2/3rd is cartilaginous

27. **Length of cartilaginous part of external auditory canal:**
   a. 1.5 cm   b. 2.4 cm
   c. 8 cm   d. <1 cm

28. **Foramen of Huschke is a congenital pathology located between:**
   a. Bony part of EAC and submandibular gland
   b. Cartilaginous part of EAC and submandibular gland
   c. Bony part of EAC and parotid gland
   d. Cartilaginous part of EAC and parotid gland

29. **All are true about external ear EXCEPT:**
   a. Auricle is made up of frame work of single yellow elastic cartilage covered with skin
   b. Area between tragus and crus of helix without cartilage is incisura terminalis
   c. Cartilage from the tragus can be used in reconstructive surgery of nose
   d. Composite grafts of cartilage & skin from pinna cannot be used for correction of defects of nasal ala

30. **What is the length of external auditory canal?**
   a. 2.5 cm   b. 1.5 cm
   c. 1 cm   d. 2 cm

31. **Ceruminous glands are seen in which part of external auditory canal:**
   a. 2/3 outer and 1/3 inner b. 1/3 outer and 2/3 inner
   c. 1/3rd outer   d. 2/3rd inner

32. **Retromolar trigone is located at:**
   a. Posterior part of mandible
   b. Ascending ramus of mandible
   c. Submandibular area
   d. Digastric muscle

ANATOMY OF MIDDLE EAR & INNER EAR

33. **Which is the peripheral receptor of hearing?**
   (Recent Pattern Question 2017)
   a. Organ of corti   b. Ampulla
   c. Utricle   d. Semicircular canal

34. **The semi-circular canal is responsible for:**
   (Recent Pattern Question 2017)
   a. Hearing   b. Balance
   c. Cough reflex   d. Sneezing reflex

35. **Promontory is seen in which wall of middle ear?**
   (Recent Pattern Question 2017)
   a. Anterior   b. Medial
   c. Posterior   d. Lateral

36. **Eustachean tube opens in:** *(Recent Pattern Question 2017)*
   a. Nasopharynx   b. Oropharynx
   c. Trachea   d. Laryngopharynx

37. **Stria vascularis is present in:** *(Recent Pattern Question 2016)*
   a. Cochlea   b. Saccule
   c. Utricle   d. Semi-circular canals

38. **Autoconia is seen in:** *(Recent Pattern Question 2016)*
   a. Utricle
   b. Superior semicircular canal
   c. Lateral semicircular canal
   d. Cochlea

39. **Least blood supply goes to:** *(Recent Pattern Question 2016)*
   a. Handle of malleus
   b. Body of incus
   c. Long process of incus
   d. Stapes

Questions

FMGE Solutions Screening Examination

40. Corda tympani is seen on which wall of middle ear:
    a. Anterior wall
    b. Medial wall
    c. Posterior wall
    d. Lateral wall
41. Anterior wall of middle ear is also known as:
    a. Outer wall
    b. Mastoid wall
    c. Carotid wall
    d. Jugular wall
42. Which of the following is not a content of medial wall of middle ear?
    a. Oval window
    b. Round window
    c. Processus cochleariformis
    d. Aditus ad antrum
43. Tegmen tympani separates middle ear from:
    a. Anterior cranial fossa
    b. Posterior cranial fossa
    c. Middle cranial fossa
    d. Superior cranial fossa
44. Otosclerosis is seen which wall of middle ear:
    a. Anterior
    b. Posterior
    c. Lateral
    d. Medial
45. Tensor typmani is inserted in:
    a. Tympanic membrane
    b. Malleus
    c. Incus
    d. Stapes
46. Fallopian canal contains which cranial nerve?
    a. 5
    b. 6
    c. 7
    d. 8
47. Length of internal acoustic meatus:
    a. 5 mm
    b. 1 cm
    c. 2 cm
    d. 3 cm
48. Shortest length of middle ear:
    a. 2 mm
    b. 4 mm
    c. 6 mm
    d. 1 cm
49. Bill's bar divides:
    a. Facial nerve and cochlear nerve
    b. Facial nerve and superior vestibular cochlear nerve
    c. Facial and inferior vestibule cochlear nerve
    d. Superior and inferior vestibule cochlear nerve
50. Cochlea main function is:
    a. Balancing
    b. Hearing
    c. Otolith organ
    d. Olfaction
51. All are required for balancing EXCEPT:
    a. Visual system
    b. Olfactory system
    c. Proprioception
    d. Vestibule and cochlea
52. Cupula is seen in:
    a. Saccule
    b. Utricle
    c. Semicircular canal
    d. Cochlea
53. Stria vascularis are seen in:
    a. Vestibule
    b. Utricle
    c. Cochlea
    d. Middle ear

TESTS OF AUDITORY SYSTEM

54. Why is cold water not used in syringing?
    (Recent Pattern Question 2018-19)
    a. Cold water leads to wax impaction
    b. Cold water leads to foreign body impaction
    c. Can cause tympanic membrane rupture
    d. Can cause vertigo
55. In audiometry a notch is seen at 4000 Hz. This is most likely due to: *(Recent Pattern Question 2018-19)*
    a. Otosclerosis
    b. Meniere's disease
    c. Noise induced hearing loss
    d. Age related hearing loss
56. Maximum tolerable noise according to Government of India guidelines: *(Recent Pattern Question 2018)*
    a. 85 dB, 8 hrs/day for 5 days per week
    b. 90 dB in 8 hrs/day for 5 days per week
    c. 95 dB, 8 hrs/day for 5 days per week
    d. 115 dB, 8 hrs/day for 6 days per week
57. The graph for otosclerosis in tympanometry is:
    (Recent Pattern Question 2017)
    a. Ad
    b. As
    c. A
    d. B
58. Which test is used for screening for neonatal deafness?
    (Recent Pattern Question 2017)
    a. Tuning fork test
    b. ABR
    c. Impedance audiometry
    d. Tympanometry
59. Otoacoustic emission comes from:
    (Recent Pattern Question 2017)
    a. Utricle
    b. Cochlea
    c. Saccule
    d. Semicircular canal
60. Tone decay is seen in: *(Recent Pattern Question 2017)*
    a. Otosclerosis
    b. Glue ear
    c. Ossicular disruption
    d. Acoustic neuroma
61. Gelle test is done for: *(Recent Pattern Question 2016)*
    a. Otosclerosis
    b. Senile deafness
    c. Traumatic deafness
    d. Congenital deafness
62. Negative Rinne test indicates:
    (Recent Pattern Question 2016)
    a. Meniere's disease
    b. CSOM
    c. BPPV
    d. Sensorineural hearing loss
63. Pure tone audiometry symbol 'X' is used for
    (Recent Pattern Question 2016)
    a. Right ear, air conduction
    b. Right ear, bone conduction
    c. Left ear, air conduction
    d. Left ear, bone conduction
64. Most common frequency of tuning fork used in ENT:
    a. 256 Hz
    b. 512 Hz
    c. 1024 Hz
    d. 2048 Hz

ENT

965

65. Which of the following is the best tuning fork to do Rinne's and Weber's tests?
   a. 128 Hz
   b. 256 Hz
   c. 512 Hz
   d. 1024 Hz

66. All of the following are tuning fork test EXCEPT:
   a. Gelle test
   b. Rinne test
   c. Schwabach's test
   d. Pure tone audiometry

67. Otoacoustic emissions are derived from:
   a. Tympanic membrane
   b. Ossicles
   c. Cochlea
   d. Vestibule

68. Sensorineural deafness in neonates is best diagnosed by:
   a. ABR
   b. Audiometry
   c. Tympanometry
   d. Electrocochleography

69. Caloric test is done for assessing:
   a. Vestibular function
   b. Auditory function
   c. Tactile function
   d. Ocular function

70. Calorie test with warm and cold water stimulates which of the following structures?
   a. Saccule
   b. Lateral semicircular canal
   c. Superior semicircular canal
   d. Posterior semicircular canal

71. Vestibular function is tested by:
   a. Fistula test
   b. Acoustic reflex
   c. Galvanic stimulation
   d. Impedance Audiometry

DISEASES OF EAR, TREATMENT AND REHABILITATION

72. Mainstay of treatment of Glue ear:
   (Recent Pattern Question 2018-19)
   a. Antibiotics
   b. Nasal decongestants + Antibiotics
   c. Myringectomy + Gromet insertion
   d. Myringotomy + Gromet insertion

73. The drug whose side effect is cochleotoxicity:
   (Recent Pattern Question 2018)
   a. Kanamycin
   b. Streptomycin
   c. Gentamycin
   d. Minocycline

74. Most common cause of facial nerve palsy:
   (Recent Pattern Question 2018)
   a. Idiopathic Bell's palsy
   b. Herpes zoster oticus
   c. Mastoid surgery
   d. Chronic suppurative otitis media

75. Flamingo pink appearance of tympanic membrane is seen in:
   (Recent Pattern Question 2018)
   a. Glomus tumor
   b. Otosclerosis
   c. Acoustic neuroma
   d. Cholesteatoma

76. Ear pain, tinnitus and vertigo along with feeling of blocked ear is a feature of: *(Recent Pattern Question 2018)*
   a. Gradenigo's syndrome
   b. Cantrell disease
   c. Costen syndrome
   d. Lermoyez syndrome

77. A patient presents with symptoms of facial nerve palsy and bulla on tympanic membrane and meatus. Possible diagnosis: *(Recent Pattern Question 2017)*
   a. Bells' palsy
   b. Ramsay hunt syndrome
   c. Herpes oticus
   d. Melkersson syndrome

78. Granulomatous lesion in tympanic membrane and middle ear lateral wall is seen in: *(Recent Pattern Question 2016)*
   a. CSOM
   b. Bullous myringitis
   c. Chronic myringitis
   d. Herpes zoster otiticus

79. Ventilation tube is put in the ear in cases of:
   (Recent Pattern Question 2016)
   a. Otoscleorsis
   b. Labryinthitis
   c. Serous otitis media
   d. CSOM

80. Impaction of wax is treated by:
   a. Syringing
   (Recent Pattern Question 2016)
   b. Softening followed by syringing
   c. Instrumentation
   d. Suction

81. In tympanic membrane perforation, graft is taken from temporalis muscle fascia. What type of graft this:
   (Recent Pattern Question 2016)
   a. Autograft
   b. Allograft
   c. Xenograft
   d. Isograft

82. Normal hearing range:
   a. 20–20,000 Hz
   b. 30–30,000 Hz
   c. 200–2000 Hz
   d. 300–3000 Hz

83. According to WHO moderate hearing loss is defined at:
   a. 30–40 dB
   b. 41–60 dB
   c. 56–70 dB
   d. 71–90 dB

84. Noise induced hearing loss is seen maximum at:
   a. 1–2 khz
   b. 3–4 khz
   c. 5–6 khz
   d. 7–10 khz

85. Myringitis bullosa is commonly caused by:
   a. Bacteria
   b. Virus
   c. Fungi
   d. Protozoa

86. Bullous myringitis is caused by:
   a. Virus
   b. Bacteria
   c. Fungus
   d. Autoimmune

87. Acute otitis media is most commonly caused by:
   a. Streptococcus pneumoniae
   b. Hemophilus influenzae
   c. Staphylococcus aureus
   d. Klebsiella pneumoniae

88. Which of the following is resorbed in otitis media development:
   a. Pus
   b. Blood
   c. Air
   d. All of the above

Questions

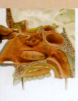

89. According to TOS classification of chronic otitis media in which stage is the retraction pocket adherent to the handle of malleus and full extent of the retraction pocket can be clearly seen.
    a. Stage 1
    b. Stage 2
    c. Stage 3
    d. Stage 4
90. All are extracranial complications of chronic otitis media EXCEPT:
    a. Ossicular damage
    b. Petrositis
    c. Gradenigo syndrome
    d. Lateral sinus thrombophlebitis
91. Most common intracranial manifestation of late chronic otitis media:
    a. Brain abscess
    b. Cerebellar abscess
    c. Lateral sinus thrombophlebitis
    d. Labyrinthine fistula
92. Most common extracranial complication of CSOM:
    a. Meningitis
    b. Ossicle damage
    c. Mastoiditis
    d. Labyrinthine fistula
93. Most common type of hearing loss in TB otitis media
    a. Conductive hearing loss
    b. SNHL
    c. Presbycusis
    d. Hyperacusis
94. Which one of the following is classical sign of tubercular otitis media?
    a. Marginal perforation of tympanic membrane
    b. Multiple perforation of pars tensa
    c. Large central perforation of tympanic membrane
    d. Attic perforation
95. Which of the following ear ossicle is 1st to get affected in otitis media?
    a. Long process of incus
    b. Stapes
    c. Handle of malleus
    d. Body of malleus
96. Gardenigo's syndrome involves which cranial nerve:
    a. CN IV, V
    b. CN V, VI
    c. CN VII, VIII
    d. CN IX, X
97. Which is not a component of Gardenigo's syndrome:
    a. Deafness
    b. Ear discharge
    c. Retroorbital pain
    d. Double vision
98. Which is a causative organism for malignant otitis externa:
    a. Virus
    b. Bacteria
    c. Fungi
    d. Protozoa
99. Malignant otitis externa affects which cranial nerve:
    a. 7th
    b. 8th
    c. 9th
    d. 10th
100. Ramsay hunt syndrome is due to:
    a. Herpes zoster virus
    b. Herpes simplex virus
    c. Varicella zoster
    d. Pseudomonas
101. What will be the probable site of lesion causing slowly progressive facial palsy?
    a. Skull
    b. Parotid
    c. Geniculate ganglion
    d. Middle ear
102. Schwartz's sign is seen in:
    a. Otosclerosis
    b. Meniere's disease
    c. Retrocochlear lesion
    d. None
103. Carhart's notch dips at:
    a. 2 Hz
    b. 200 Hz
    c. 2000 Hz
    d. 2000 MHz
104. Which of the following is earliest and consistent symptom of glomus tumor?
    a. Hoarseness
    b. Tinnitus
    c. Otorrhea
    d. Dysphagia
105. Hennebert sign is seen in:
    a. Otosclerosis
    b. Vestibular neuritis
    c. Menier's disease
    d. Rotatory nystagmus
106. Hearing defect in menier's disease:
    a. Hyperacusis
    b. Hypoacusis
    c. Diplacusis
    d. Paracusia Willi
107. In case of BPPV, which semicircular canal is affected:
    a. Lateral semicircular canal
    b. Posterior semicircular canal
    c. Anterior semicircular canal
    d. Superior semicircular canal
108. Referred pain in the ear is commonly from:
    a. Mandibular cancer
    b. Carcinoma of tongue
    c. Laryngeal cancer
    d. Maxillary carcinoma
109. Trotter's triad consists of all of the following EXCEPT:
    a. Palatal paralysis
    b. Trigeminal Neuralgia
    c. Sensorineural deafness
    d. Conduction deafness
110. Which of the following is most prominent symptom of acoustic neuroma?
    a. Ataxic gait
    b. Diplopia
    c. Sensorineural hearing loss
    d. Parasthesia
111. Which one of the following is not a feature of adenoid hypertrophy?
    a. Dull expression
    b. Open mouth
    c. Pinched up nose
    d. Crowding of lower tooth
112. Adenoidectomy is contraindicated in:
    a. Glue ear
    b. Recurrent rhinosinusitis
    c. Mouth breathing
    d. Cleft palate
113. All of the following are the indications of adenoidectomy EXCEPT?
    a. Obstructive sleep apnea
    b. Allergic rhinitis
    c. Recurrent glue ear
    d. Prior to orthodontic treatment
114. Adenoidectomy with Grommet insertion is treatment of choice for:
    a. Serous otitis media in adults
    b. Serous otitis media in children
    c. Adenoiditis in children
    d. Otitis interna in children

ENT

115. A 5-year-old child presents to your clinic with complaint of recurrent respiratory tract infection. Mother complains about this recurrent infection, mouth breathing and decreased hearing. Treatment of choice for this condition is:
   a. Myringoplasty
   b. Adenoidectomy
   c. Grommet insertion
   d. Myringotomy

116. Graft used for tympanoplasty:
   a. Antral fascia
   b. Temporalis fascia
   c. Preauricular fascia
   d. Postauricular fascia

117. Electrode of cochlear implant is passed via:
   a. Round window
   b. Oval window
   c. Lateral semicircular canal
   d. Around the auditory nerve

NOSE AND PARANASAL SINUSES

118. Most common symptom of Nasopharyngeal cancer:
   (Recent Pattern Question 2018-19)
   a. Airway Obstruction
   b. Conductive hearing loss
   c. Neck swelling
   d. Epistaxis

119. Continuous watery discharge from nose after trauma is most likely a feature of: *(Recent Pattern Question 2018-19)*
   a. CSF otorrhea
   b. Common colds
   c. CSF Rhinorrrhea
   d. Anterior epistaxis

120. After a head trauma a patient is unable to smell coffee and asafoetida but can smell ammonia. Which of the following statements is true about the patient
   (Recent Pattern Question 2018-19)
   a. Ammonia is used for testing olfactory nerve
   b. The Olfaction system is not damaged
   c. Ammonia irritates trigeminal nerve
   d. All of the above

121. A male trauma patient admitted was to hospital with watery discharge from nose. On investigation it showed damage in cribriform plate. What is the possible diagnosis? *(Recent Pattern Question 2018)*
   a. CSF rhinorrhea
   b. Vasomotor rhinitis
   c. Allergic rhinitis
   d. Atrophic rhinitis

122. Young operation is done in:
   (Recent Pattern Question 2018)
   a. Otosclerosis
   b. Atrophic rhinitis
   c. Viral rhinitis
   d. Rhinitis sicca

123. Direct branch of internal carotid artery in Kiesselbach's plexus: *(Recent Pattern Question 2018)*
   a. Sphenopalatine artery
   b. Anterior ethmoidal artery
   c. Superior labial artery
   d. Greater palatine artery

124. Samter's triad includes: *(Recent Pattern Question 2017)*
   a. Allergy, asthma, nasal polyp
   b. Allergy, asthma aspirin intolerance
   c. Aspirin sensitivity, asthma, nasal polyp
   d. Allergy, polyp, bronchiectasis

125. Which of the followng is best to prevent rhinitis medicamentosa? *(Recent Pattern Question 2017)*
   a. Give oral drug to relieve symptoms
   b. Nasal drop withdrawal
   c. Antihistaminic
   d. Shift to nasal steroids

126. Which is the most common cancer of paranasal sinus?
   (Recent Pattern Question 2017)
   a. Squamous cell CA
   b. Basal cell CA
   c. Adenoid cystic CA
   d. Melanoma

127. Sphenoid sinus opens into:
   a. Superior meatus
   b. Middle meatus
   c. Inferior meatus
   d. Supreme meatus

128. Location of the nasolacrimal duct:
   a. Inferior meatus
   b. Superior meatus
   c. Sphenoethmoidal recess
   d. Middle meatus

129. Nasolacrimal duct opens into:
   a. Mouth opposite to 2nd molar
   b. Middle meatus of the nose
   c. Superior meatus of the nose
   d. Inferior meatus of the nose

130. Antrochoanal polyp opens in which meatus:
   a. Middle meatus
   b. Superior meatus
   c. Inferior meatus
   d. Sphenoethmoidal recess

131. What is the likely source of infection for Pus from sphenoethmoidal recess?
   a. Sphenoid sinus
   b. Ethmoidal sinus
   c. Maxillary sinus
   d. Frontal sinus

132. Which sinus opens in inferior meatus:
   a. Maxillary sinus
   b. Frontal sinus
   c. Anterior ethmoidal sinus
   d. None

133. Kiesselbach's plexus does not involve:
   a. Superior labial artery
   b. Anterior ethmoidal artery
   c. Greater palatine artery
   d. Posterior ethmoidal artery

134. Which of the following vessel of Little's area is not a branch of external carotid artery?
   a. Sphenopalatine artery
   b. Greater palatine artery
   c. Anterior ethmoidal artery
   d. Superior labial artery

135. Which of the following is not an etiologically derived cause for epistaxis:
   a. Nose picking
   b. Intra nasal tumours
   c. Vascular disorders or blood dyscrasias
   d. Hereditary hemorrhagic telangiectasia

Questions

FMGE Solutions Screening Examination

136. **Esthesioneuroblastoma arises from:**
    a. Olfactory epithelium   b. Ethmoid sinus
    c. Maxillary sinus   d. Sphenoid sinus
137. **All of the following paranasal sinuses are present at birth EXCEPT:**
    a. Maxillary sinus   b. Ethmoid sinus
    c. Sphenoid sinus   d. None
138. **Sinus absent at the birth:**
    a. Maxillary sinus   b. Ethmoidal sinus
    c. Frontal sinus   d. Temporal sinus
139. **Radiological evidence of frontal sinus can be seen at:**
    a. 2 years   b. 4 years
    c. 6 years   d. 8 years
140. **Sphenoid sinus reaches adult size at:**
    a. 5 years   b. 10 years
    c. 15 years   d. 28 years
141. **Ethmoid sinus reaches adult size at:**
    a. 5 years   b. 8 years
    c. 10 years   d. 12 years
142. **Largest sinus:**
    a. Frontal sinus   b. Maxillary sinus
    c. Ethmoidal sinus   d. Aphenoid sinus
143. **Caldwell luc's operation is done for:**
    a. Frontal sinusitis   b. Maxillay sinusitis
    c. Ethmoid sinusitis   d. Sphenoid sinusitis
144. **Young's operation is done for:**
    a. Atrophic rhinitis   b. Vasomotor rhinitis
    c. Antro-choanal polyp   d. Allergic rhinitis
145. **Which one of the following is a cause of nasal obstruction in Atrophic Rhinitis:**
    a. Secretions   b. Deviated nasal septum
    c. Polyp   d. Crusting
146. **Which of the following is the most common presentation of nasopharyngeal carcinoma:**
    a. Epistaxis   b. Lymphadenopathy
    c. Nasal obstruction   d. Apnea
147. **Miculicz and Russel body upon biopsy is seen in:**
    a. Rhinophyma   b. Rhinoscleroma
    c. Rhinosporidiosis   d. Rhinolith
148. **Rhinophyma is associated with which of the following:**
    a. Hypertrophy of sebaceous gland
    b. Infection of hair follicles
    c. Congenital deformity of the nose
    d. Hypertrophy of sweat gland
149. **Cause of rhinosporidiosis:**
    a. Bacterial   b. Viral
    c. Fungal   d. Protozoa
150. **A patient presents to you with big nasal cavity, thick crust formation and woody hard external nose. What is the probable diagnosis?**
    a. Vasomotor rhinitis   b. Rhinoscleroma
    c. Rhinosporidiosis   d. Atrophic rhinitis

151. **Woody induration of rhinoscleroma is initially seen at which stage:**
    a. Catarrhal stage   b. Strophic stage
    c. Granulomatous stage   d. Cicatricial stage
152. **Rhinoscleroma is caused by:**
    a. Virus   b. Bacteria
    c. Fungus   d. Anaerobes
153. **Most common fractured bone on face:**
    a. Nasoethmoid bone   b. Zygomatic bone
    c. Nasal bone   d. Mandible
154. **Chevallet fracture of nasal septum is:**
    a. Horizontal fracture   b. Vertical fracture
    c. Comminuted fracture   d. Serpentine fracture
155. **Impact of force in case of jarjavay septal fracture is from:**
    a. Above   b. Below
    c. Front   d. Behind
156. **Most common site of fracture of mandible is:**
    a. Neck of condyle   b. Angle of mandible
    c. Symphysis   d. Ramus

THROAT/PHARYNX

157. **A patient presented with 3 days history of fever, throat pain, difficulty in deglutition with deviation of uvula. Most likely diagnosis:** *(Recent Pattern Question 2018-19)*
    a. Quinsy   b. Pre-tracheal abscess
    c. Retopharyngeal abscess   d. Epiglottitis
158. **Hypoglossal nerve supplies all of these muscle EXCEPT:** *(Recent Pattern Question 2018-19)*
    a. Palatoglossus   b. Styloglossus
    c. Genioglossus   d. Hyoglossus
159. **Picket fence fever is seen in:** *(Recent Pattern Question 2018-19)*
    a. Lateral sinus thrombophlebitis
    b. Quincy
    c. Laryngitis sicca
    d. Croup
160. **Which of the following is NOT a premalignant lesion/condition:** *(Recent Pattern Question 2018-19)*
    a. Chronic hypertrophic candidiasis
    b. Oral submucosal fibrosis
    c. Lichen planus
    d. Aphthous ulcer
161. **The treatment of nasopharyngeal carcinoma:** *(Recent Pattern Question 2018)*
    a. Chemoradiation   b. Surgery
    c. Chemotherapy   d. Radiation
162. **All of the following is seen when superior laryngeal nerve is damaged EXCEPT:** *(Recent Pattern Question 2018)*
    a. Aspiration   b. Stridor
    c. Bowed vocal cords   d. Loss of pitch

ENT

163. **Recurrent laryngeal nerve supplies all EXCEPT:**
(Recent Pattern Question 2018)
a. Cricothyroid
b. Cricoarytenoid
c. Aryepiglottic
d. Interarytenoid

164. **Most common site for laryngeal web is:**
a. Supraglottic
b. Subglottic
c. Glottis level
d. Epiglottis level

165. **A 15-year-old boy presented with history of fever since 2 days, unable to swallow the food with muffled voice. On examination it is noted that right tonsil is shifted to midline. What is the diagnosis?**
a. Quincy *(Recent Pattern Question 2018)*
b. Acute tonsillitis
c. Parapharyngeal abscess
d. Acute retropharyngeal abscess

166. **Juvenile recurrent laryngeal papillomatosis is caused by:**
(Recent Pattern Question 2018)
a. EBV
b. HSV
c. HPV
d. VZV

167. **A 60-year-old man presents with right sided ear pain and dysphagia. Diagnosis:** *(Recent Pattern Question 2017)*
a. Achalasia cardia
b. Lower esophageal carcinoma
c. Carcinoma of pyriform sinus
d. Postcricoid carcinoma

168. **Passavant's ridge is formed by:**
(Recent Pattern Question 2017)
a. Palatopharyngeus
b. Cricopharyngeus
c. Genioglossus
d. Stylopharyngeus

169. **Omega shaped glottis is seen in:**
(Recent Pattern Question 2017)
a. Laryngeal TB
b. Laryngomalacia
c. Tracheal stenosis
d. Laryngeal malignancy

170. **Peritonsillar abscess management:**
a. Drainage *(Recent Pattern Question 2017)*
b. Analgesic plus antibiotic
c. Analgesic with antibiotic and drainage
d. Wait and watch

171. **Elective tracheostomy is done in:**
(Recent Pattern Question 2017)
a. Deep burn of chest wall
b. Radiation burn of face
c. Burn of head and neck
d. Acid burn on ingestion

172. **High tracheostomy is done in:**
(Recent Pattern Question 2017)
a. Carcinoma larynx
b. Laryngomalacia
c. Thyroid surgery
d. Diptheria infection

173. **A singer presents with sore throat, GERD and vocal nodule. Medical treatment:**
a. Direct laryngoscopy *(Recent Pattern Question 2017)*
b. PPI
c. Microscopic laryngeal surgery
d. Speech therapy plus PPI

174. **Narrowest part of glottis in pediatric age group:**
(Recent Pattern Question 2017)
a. Lower part of thyroid cartilage
b. Upper part of thyroid cartilage
c. Glottis
d. Epiglottis

175. **Head and neck tumour stage III according to TNM classification involves:** *(Recent Pattern Question 2016)*
a. Unilateral mobile lymph nodes <3 cm
b. Unilateral mobile lymph node >3 cm
c. Bilateral mobile lymph nodes <6 cm
d. Bilateral mobile lymph nodes >6 cm

176. **Abductor of vocal cords:** *(Recent Pattern Question 2016)*
a. Cricothyroid
b. Posterior cricothyroid
c. Posterior cricoarytenoid
d. Interarytenoid

177. **Mouse nibbled vocal cord is seen in:**
(Recent Pattern Question 2016)
a. Laryngeal CA
b. Laryngeal TB
c. Laryngeal papilloma
d. Vocal cord palsy

178. **Hot potato voice is seen in** *(Recent Pattern Question 2016)*
a. Acute epiglottis
b. Antrochonal polyp
c. Peri-tonsillar abscess
d. Carcinoma larynx

179. **Narrowest part of airway in a child:**
(Recent Pattern Question 2016)
a. Glottis
b. Supraglottis
c. Subglottis
d. Epiglottis

180. **Nasopharyngeal angiofibroma is most commonly seen in:**
a. Elderly males
b. Females
c. Young males
d. Infants

181. **A 13-year-old child presents with 3 year history of gradual swelling of maxilla with medial displacement of turbinates with mild proptosis. What is the most likely diagnosis:**
a. Olfactory neuroblastoma
b. Angiofibroma
c. Carcinoma of maxilla
d. Fibrous dysplasia

182. **Crypts are seen in:**
a. Tonsils
b. Adenoids
c. Lymph nodes
d. Parotids

183. **Mallampati score is done for assessing:**
a. Size of the airway
b. Oral cavity of patient for intubation
c. Mobility of neck
d. Size of Ryle's tube

184. **Which of the following muscle is not supplied by recurrent laryngeal nerve:**
a. Cricothyroid
b. Lateral cricoarytenoid
c. Thyroarytenoid
d. Posterior cricoarytenoid

185. **Which one of the following is an abductor of vocal cords:**
a. Posterior cricoarytenoid
b. Transverse arytenoids
c. Cricothyroid
d. Aryepiglotticus

186. **Recurrent laryngeal nerve supplies all EXCEPT:**
a. Cricothyroid
b. Thyroaretenoid
c. Lateral cricoaretenoid
d. Posterior cricoaretenoid

Questions

FMGE Solutions Screening Examination

187. Warthins tumor is seen in:
    a. Submandibular gland   b. Parotid gland
    c. Sublingual gland   d. All of the above
188. Glossopharyngeal nerve supplies:
    a. Glossopharyngeus muscle
    b. Stylopharyngeus muscle
    c. Anterior 2/3 of the tongue
    d. All of the above
189. Omega shaped epiglottis is seen in:
    a. Epiglottitis   b. Laryngomalacia
    c. Epiglottis CA   d. Tuberculosis
190. Thumb sign is seen in:
    a. Acute laryngitis
    b. Acute epiglottitis
    c. Acute laryngo trachea bronchitis
    d. Acute tonsillitis
191. Bezold's abscess is in relation to:
    a. Digastric muscle
    b. Sternocleidomastoid muscle
    c. Behind the mastoid
    d. Submandibular region
192. Which of the following sites represents the location of Bezold abscess?
    a. Diagastric triangle
    b. Sternocleidomastoid muscle
    c. Infra temporal region
    d. Sub mandibular region
193. All are complication of tonsillitis EXCEPT:
    a. Otitis media
    b. Abscess
    c. Malignant change
    d. Subacute bacterial endocarditis
194. Which of the following cyst doesn't move upon deglutition:
    a. Ranula   b. Thyroglossal cyst
    c. Sublingual dermoid cyst   d. Thymic cyst
195. In the early stage of which of the following carcinoma, no lymphatics involved:
    a. Glottic CA   b. Infraglottic CA
    c. Supraglottic CA   d. Hypopharyngeal CA
196. Radiation therapy is mostly useful for:
    a. Glottis CA   b. Epiglottis CA
    c. Sub-glottis CA   d. Supraglottis CA
197. Hot potato voice is seen in all EXCEPT:
    a. Quinsy   b. Carcinoma thyroid
    c. Carcinoma tonsil   d. Streptococcus pharyngitis
198. Transillumination test is positive in:
    a. Branchial cyst   b. Thymic cyst
    c. Ranula   d. Thyroglossal duct cyst
199. Male patient with female like voice. This condition is called:
    a. Puberphonia   b. Androphonia
    c. Rhinolalia aperta   d. Rhinolalia clausa
200. Female patient with male like voice. Type of thyroplasty done:
    a. I   b. II
    c. III   d. IV
201. In a patient with vocal cord paralysis, the surgeon is afraid of aspiration. Thyroplasty done in order to prevent aspiration:
    a. Type I   b. Type II
    c. Type III   d. Type IV
202. Most common complication of tracheostomy:
    a. Hemorrhage
    b. Tracheal stenosis
    c. Recurrent laryngeal nerve damage
    d. Infection

BOARD REVIEW QUESTIONS

203. Dysphagia lusoria is caused by:
    a. Abdominal aorta   b. Thoracic aorta
    c. Aberrant right subclavian artery
    d. None of the above
204. Glomus jugulare are seen in:
    a. Hypotympanum   b. Promontory
    c. Epitympanum   d. None of these
205. Endolymphatic sac decompression is treatment for:
    a. Meniere's disease   b. Facial nerve injury
    c. Ostosclerosis   d. Otitis media
206. A pregnant lady comes to ENT OPD with hearing loss, tinnitus and soft spoken voice. Most probable diagnosis is:
    a. Otosclerosis   b. Meniere's disease
    c. Retrocochlear hearing loss
    d. Malingering
207. A patient on ATT develops tinnitus and hearing loss due to:
    a. Isoniazis   b. Pyrazinamide
    c. Streptomycin   d. Rifampicin
208. Most superior sinus in the face is?
    a. Frontal sinus   b. Ethmoid sinus
    c. Maxillary sinus   d. Sphenoid sinus
209. Most common fractured bone in the face is:
    a. Nasal   b. Malar
    c. Zygomatic   d. Temporal
210. Where is electrode kept in cochlear implant:
    a. Round window   b. Oval window
    c. Scala vestibule   d. Scala tympani
211. Otosclerosis shows which kind of tympanogram?
    a. Low compliance   b. High compliance
    c. Normal compliance   d. No effect on compliance

ENT

212. **Bony nasal septal perforation is seen in:**
   a. Tuberculosis
   b. Syphilis
   c. Leprosy
   d. Rhinosporidiosis

213. **Foramen of huschke is present in:**
   a. Bony part of external auditory canal
   b. Cartilaginous part of external auditory canal
   c. Middle ear, anterior wall
   d. Middle ear, posterior wall

214. **"Dilator tubae" muscle is a portion of:**
   a. Tensor tympani
   b. Levator veli palatini
   c. Tensor veli palatini
   d. Salpingopharyngeus

215. **Ostmann's pad of fat is related to:**
   a. Ear lobule
   b. Opening of eustachian tube
   c. Closing of eustachian tube
   d. Mastoid process

216. **Which of the following test for Eustachean tube function utilizes negative pressure?**
   a. Catheterization
   b. Valsalva test
   c. Politzer test
   d. Toynbee's test

217. **Van der hoeve syndrome is related with:**
   a. Glomus tumor
   b. Facial nerve paralysis
   c. Otosclerosis
   d. Cholesteatoma

218. **Most common tumor of ear:**
   a. Squamous cell CA
   b. Basal cell CA
   c. Glomus tumor
   d. Acoustic neuroma

219. **A female patient is having male like voice. Thyroplasty of choice:**
   a. Type 1
   b. Type 2
   c. Type 3
   d. Type 4

220. **In the early stage of which of the following carcinoma, no lymphatics are involved:**
   a. Glottic CA
   b. Infraglottic CA
   c. Supraglottic CA
   d. Hypopharyngeal CA

221. **Otalgia in tonsillitis. Nerve involved:**
   a. Glossopharyngeal nerve
   b. Trigeminal nerve
   c. Facial nerve
   d. Vagus nerve

222. **Which is most effective in glue ear:**
   a. Antibiotics
   b. Nasal Decongestants
   c. Steroids
   d. Tympanoplasty

223. **Malignant otitis externa is a:**
   a. Autoimmune condition
   b. Pre-malignant condition
   c. Malignant condition
   d. Infective condition

224. **Brown sign is seen in:**
   a. Glomus tumor
   b. Meniere's disease
   c. Acoustic neuroma
   d. Otoscelrosis

225. **Toynbee's muscle is:**
   a. Stapedius
   b. Tensor tympani
   c. Scalenusminimus
   d. Levatorani

226. **Rhinosporidiosis is caused by:**
   a. Protozoal infection
   b. Viral infection
   c. Bacterial infection
   d. Fungal infection

227. **First branch of the facial nerve is:**
   a. Greater petrosal nerve
   b. Lesser petrosal nerve
   c. Chorda-tympani nerve
   d. Nerve to the stapedius

228. **The pressure difference that can cause atmosphere and middle ear barotraumas is:**
   a. 60 mm Hg
   b. 60-70 mm Hg
   c. 70-80 mm Hg
   d. >90 mm Hg

229. **Common age for otosclerosis is:**
   a. 5-10 years
   b. 10-20 years
   c. 20-30 years
   d. 30-45 years

230. **Earliest symptom of glomus tumor is:**
   a. Pulsatile tinnitus
   b. Deafness
   c. Headache
   d. Vertigo

231. **Stapedius muscle is supplied by:**
   a. 5th nerve
   b. 6th nerve
   c. 7th nerve
   d. 8th nerve

232. **'Trench mouth' is:**
   a. Sub mucosal fibrosis
   b. Tumor at uveal angle
   c. Ulcerative lesion of the tonsil
   d. Retention cyst of the tonsil

233. **A diabetic patient presents with black necrotic mass filling the nasal cavity. Most likely fungal infection is:**
   a. Rhinosporidiosis
   b. Aspergillosis
   c. Mucormycosis
   d. Candidiasis

234. **Nasal perforation in bony part is seen in:**
   a. Syphilis
   b. Tuberculosis
   c. Wegner's granuloma
   d. Allergic rhinitis

235. **Carhart's notch is seen in:**
   a. Otosclerosis
   b. Acoustic neuroma
   c. Meniere's disease
   d. CSOM

236. **Only abductor of the vocal cord is:**
   a. Lateral cricoarytenoid
   b. Posterior cricoarytenoid
   c. Cricothyroid
   d. Thyroarytenoid

237. **The most common location of vocal nodules is:**
   a. Junction of the ant: 1/3 and posterior 2/3
   b. Junction of the ant: 2/3 and posterior 1/3
   c. Junction of the posterior ¼ and ant: 2/3
   d. Anterior commisure

238. **Caldwell luc operation is done in:**
   a. Maxillary sinusitis
   b. Ethmoidal sinusitis
   c. Sphenoidal sinusitis
   d. Frontal sinusitis

239. **'Steeple sign' on AP radiograph is seen in:**
   a. Laryngotracheobronchitis
   b. Epiglottitis
   c. Retrobulbar abscess
   d. Laryngeal diphtheria

240. **Mastoid tip is involved in:**
   a. Bezold abscess
   b. Luc's abscess
   c. Citelli's abscess
   d. Parapharyngeal abscess

FMGE Solutions Screening Examination

241. Most common organism causing CSOM:
   a. Moraxella catarrhalis
   b. Hemophilus influenzae
   c. Streptococcus pneumoniae
   d. Pseudomonas
242. Recurrent polyp are seen in:
   a. Antrochoanal polyp   b. Ethmoidal polyp
   c. Nasal polyp   d. Hypertrophic turbinate
243. Acute tonsillitis is caused commonly by:
   a. Parainfluenza virus
   b. Beta-hemolytic streptococcus
   c. Staphylococcus aureus   d. Moraxella
244. A 17-year-male presented with swelling in the cheek with recurrent epistaxis. Most likely diagnosis:
   a. Angiofibroma   b. Carcinoma nasopharynx
   c. Rhabdomyosarcoma   d. Ethmyoid polyp
245. Oro-antral fistula is seen most commonly in:
   a. Dental extraction   b. Carcinoma maxilla
   c. Mucocele of the maxilla   d. Fracture of the maxilla
246. Most common intracranial complication of CSOM:
   a. Lateral sinus thrombosis   b. Meningitis
   c. Temporal lobe abscess   d. Orbital cellulitis
247. Mikulicz cell is seen in:
   a. Rhinoscleroma   b. Rhinosporidiosis
   c. Aspergillosis   d. TB
248. Reactionary hemorrhage occurs within:
   a. 24 hours   b. 48 hours
   c. 72 hours   d. 5 days
249. Bill's bar divides:
   a. Facial nerve and cochlear nerve
   b. Facial nerve and superior vestibular nerve
   c. Facial and inferior vestibule cochlear nerve
   d. Superior and inferior vestibule cochlear nerve
250. Most common type of hearing loss in TB otitis media:
   a. Conductive hearing loss   b. SNHL
   c. Presbycusis   d. Hyperacusis
251. Antrochoanal polyp opens in which meatus:
   a. Middle meatus   b. Superior meatus
   c. Inferior meatus   d. Sphenoethmoidal recess
252. Young's operation is done for:
   a. Atrophic rhinitis   b. Vasomotor rhinitis
   c. Antro-choanal polyp   d. Allergic rhinitis
253. Degree of Eustachian tube from horizontal line is:
   a. 35°   b. 45°
   c. 55°   d. 65°
254. Space of Tucker is seen in:
   a. Larynx   b. Oesophagus
   c. Femoral canal
   d. Laparoscopic approach to hernia
255. Which of the following syndrome is associated with Anosmia?
   a. Kallmann's syndrome   b. Turner's syndrome
   c. Down's syndrome   d. Klinefelter's syndrome

256. Bryce's sign is seen in:
   a. Laryngocele   b. Post cricoid carcinoma
   c. Angiofibroma   d. Chronic tonsillitis
257. Isthmus of thyroid corresponds to which tracheal rings?
   a. 1-3   b. 2-4
   c. 4-6   d. 6-8
258. A patient presents with diplopia, fever and ear discharge. The most probable diagnosis is:
   a. CSOM   b. Meningitis
   c. Lateral sinus thrombosis   d. Petrositis
259. Ground glass appearance of maxillary sinus is seen in:
   a. Maxillary sinusitis   b. Maxillary carcinoma
   c. Maxillary polyp   d. Maxillary fibrous dysplasia
260. Mucocele is commenest in which among the following sinuses?
   a. Frontal   b. Maxillary
   c. Ethmoid   d. Sphenoid
261. Schuller's view and law's view is for:
   a. Sphenoid sinus
   b. Mastoid air cells
   c. Foramen ovale and spinosum
   d. Carotid conal
262. Most common nerve damage in maxillary fracture:
   a. Supraorbital nerve   b. Infraorbital nerve
   c. Facial nerve   d. Lingual nerve
263. SADE's classification is used for:
   a. Cholesteatoma   b. Pars Flaccida
   c. Pars Tensa   d. ASOM
264. Who described Meniere's disease first?
   a. Arthur Toynbee   b. Valsalva
   c. Prosper Meniere   d. MacEwan
265. Cochlear aqueduct connects:
   a. Middle ear to subarachnoid space
   b. Inner ear to middle ear
   c. Inner ear to subarachnoid space
   d. Inner ear to nasal cavity
266. Mouse nibbled appearance of vocal cord is seen in:
   a. Vocal cord palsy   b. Vocal nodules
   c. Larynx Ca   d. TB larynx
267. Gutzmann pressure test is done for:
   a. Laryngomalacia   b. Puberphonia
   c. Laryngeal polyps   d. Vocal cord palsy
268. Inability to vocalise is:
   a. Aphonia   b. Mutism
   c. Alogia   d. Dysarthria
269. Otolith organs are concerned with function of:
   a. Vestibular reflex   b. Position sense
   c. Linear acceleration   d. Angular acceleration
270. Frequency range in normal human hearing is:
   a. 20-4000 Hz   b. 20-8000 Hz
   c. 20-10000 Hz   d. 20-20000 Hz

ENT

271. As per Factory Act in India maximum audible tolerance is:
    a. 90 dB for 6 hours   b. 90 dB for 8 hours
    c. 85 dB for 6 hours   d. 85 dB for 8 hours
272. Imaging study of choice for para nasal sinuses is:
    a. USG   b. CT scan
    c. X-ray PNS   d. FDG PET scan
273. Semicircular canal perceives:
    a. Linear acceleration b. Angular acceleration
    c. Both   d. None
274. Most common site of carcinoma of paranasal sinus is:
    a. Frontal   b. Ethmoid
    c. Maxillary   d. Sphenoid
275. Most common cause of acute otitis media in children is:
    a. Staphylococcus aureus b. Streptococcus pneumonia
    c. Haemophilus influenzae d. Moraxella catarrhalis
276. Treatment of choice of nasopharyngeal carcinoma is:
    a. Surgery   b. Chemotherapy
    c. Radiotherapy   d. Medical management
277. Location of adenoids on pharyngeal wall is:
    a. Superiorly   b. Laterally
    c. Inferiorly   d. Posteriorly
278. Otosclerosis presents with:
    a. Conductive deafness
    b. Sensorineural deafness
    c. Mixed hearing loss
    d. Fluctuating hearing loss
279. Most common part affected in otosclerosis is:
    a. Anterior part of foot plate of stapes
    b. Posterior part of foot plate of stapes
    c. Middle part of foot plate of stapes
    d. Annular ligament of stapes
280. Rhinitis sicca is characterised by:
    a. Drying of anterior 1/3rd of the nasal cavity
    b. Drying of middle 1/3rd of the nasal cavity
    c. Drying of the posterior 1/3rd of the nasal cavity
    d. Drying of the nasal septum
281. Vidian neurectomy is done in:
    a. Allergic rhinitis   b. Vasomotor rhinitis
    c. Atrophic rhinitis   d. Rhinitis medicamentosa
282. Crooked nose is due to:
    a. Deviated Ala
    b. Deviated septum
    c. Hump in nasal septum
    d. Deviated dorsum and septum
283. Intrinsic laryngeal muscle having life saving action, leading to passage of air through glottis: *(2018)*
    a. Lateral cricoarytenoid   b. Posterior cricoarytenoid
    c. Cricothyroid   d. Interarytenoid
284. CSOM patient with hectic picket fence fever, rigor and tenderness around mastoid. This is typical sign of: (ENT)
    a. Meningitis   *(2018)*
    b. Petrositis
    c. Abscess
    d. Lateral sinus thrombophlebitis
285. Most common site of laryngeal web: *(2018)*
    a. Anterior laryngeal wall b. Posterior laryngeal wall
    c. Supraglottis   d. Subglottis
286. Most common organism causing fungal infection of ear:
    a. Candida albicans   b. Aspergillus Niger *(2018)*
    c. Mucormycosis   d. Aspergillus fumigatus
287. Most common cause of SNHL: *(2018)*
    a. Noise induced   b. Mennier's disease
    c. Labyrinthitis   d. Presbycusis

FMGE Solutions Screening Examination

IMAGE-BASED QUESTIONS

288. A 21-year-old college student presents with hot potato voice and trismus. Throat examination was done. Clinical diagnosis is:

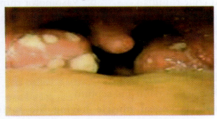

a. Quinsy
b. Epiglottitis
c. Infectious mononucleosis
d. Chronic tonsillitis

289. The shown image is section taken from:

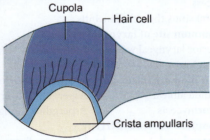

a. Cochlea
b. Vestibule
c. Semicircular canal
d. Bill's bar

290. Diagnosis based on your otoscopic finding:

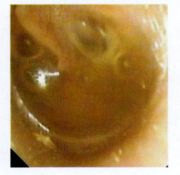

a. Acute otitis media   b. Chronic otitis media
c. Serous otitis media d. Serous otitis externa

291. Diagnosis based on your otoscopic finding:

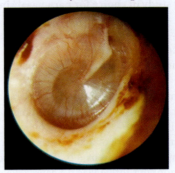

a. Acute otitis media   b. Chronic otitis media
c. Serous otitis media d. Serous otitis externa

292. A 14-year-male from Chhattisgharh presented with swelling of nose which is increasing gradually from last 3-4 months. Upon examination, nose has woody touch. Possible diagnosis:

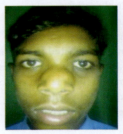

a. Rhinoscleroma   b. Rhinophyma
c. Rhinosporidiosis d. Rhinohyperplasia

293. Diagnosis:

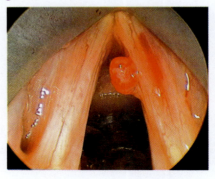

a. Vocal cord nodule   b. Vocal cord polyp
c. Vocal cord granuloma d. Papilloma

294. This patient was prepared for surgery. Your senior resident did this marking before proceeding the incision. What is the name of this:

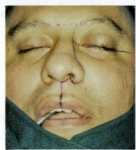

a. Ohngren's line
b. Weber fergusson incision
c. Lederman incision
d. Frontal sinosotomy

296. The given image is used for:

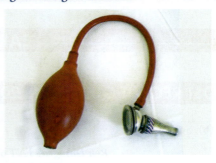

a. Cleaning the external auditory canal
b. Visualizing the whole external ear
c. Packing ear canal or nasal cavity
d. Checking the mobility of tympanic membrane

295. A 13-year-old patient presented with history of recurrent epistaxis. Upon general evaluation you noted the swelling of cheek. Most likely diagnosis:

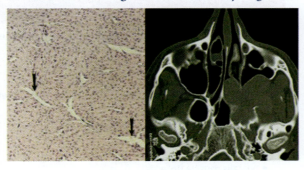

a. Rhinoscleroma
b. Angiofibroma
c. Antral polyp
d. Ethmoidal polyp

297. The below given sign is seen in:

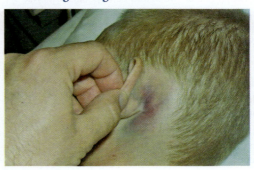

a. Otosclerosis
b. Cholesteatoma
c. Lateral sinus thrombophlebitis
d. Laryngeal pathology

298. Spot diagnosis:

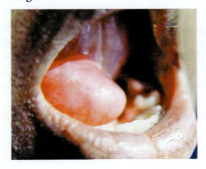

a. Tongue tie
b. Potato tumor
c. Ranula
d. Thyroglossal cyst

Answers to Image-Based Questions are given at the end of explained questions

ANSWERS WITH EXPLANATIONS

EAR AND ITS DISEASES

MOST RECENT QUESTIONS 2019

1. Ans. (b) Subglottis

Ref: Dhingra's ENT 6th ed. P 285

- Book states: "infants larynx is small and conical. The diameter of cricoid cartilage is smaller than the size of glottis, making subglottis the narrowest part."
- Note: in adults the dimensions of glottis–subglottis is same and larynx is cylindrical. However glottis is considered as the narrowest part of adult larynx

TABLE: Difference between adult and pediatric larynx

	Adult larynx	Pediatric larynx
Location	C3–C6	High in neck At rest: C3 or C4 While swallowing: C1 or C2
Cartilage	Soft	Softer
Thyroid cartilage	Elevated at thyroid angle	Flat
Shape	Cylindrical	Conical
Length of vocal cord	Female: 15–19 mm Male: 17–23 mm	Female: 6 mm Male: 8 mm

Note: In contrary to what book says, there are recent studies that says that the narrowest portion of child larynx is same as adult i.e. glottis.
- However many anatomist are still not agreeing to this.
- We are therefore referring here the textbook to answer this question.

2. Ans. (b) Angiofibroma

Ref: Dhingra's ENT 6th ed. P 246–47

- Angiofibroma is a benign vascular tumor of nasopharyngeal area.
- It is the most common pharyngeal tumor of adolescent male, mostly in second decade of life.
- This tumor is thought to be testosterone dependent
- MC site: Sphenopalatine foramen

CLINICAL FEATURE

- MC clinical feature: Recurrent epistaxis
- Progressive nasal obstruction and denasal speech
- Otitis media with effusion and conductive hearing loss
- Hollman miller sign/Antral sign: Cheek swelling- Pathognomonic feature
- Frog eye sign: Proptosis

IOC: CECT

Treatment: Surgical excision

3. Ans. (a) Posterior cricoarytenoid muscle

Ref: Dhingra's ENT 6th ed. P 283

- The only abductors of vocal cord is posterior cricoarytenoid muscle

MUSCLES OF LARYNX

Intrinsic muscles of Larynx: Attaches laryngeal cartilage with each other

Muscles acting on vocal cord	Muscles acting on Laryngeal inlet
• **Abductors:** Posterior cricoarytenoid • **Adductors** ▪ Lateral cricoarytenoid ▪ Interarytenoid ▪ Thyroarytenoid (external part) • **Tensors:** ▪ Cricothyroid ▪ Vocalis muscle (internal part of thyroarytenoid)	• **Opener of laryngeal inlet** ▪ Thyroepiglottic muscle (part of thyroarytenoid) • **Closers of laryngeal inlet** ▪ Interarytenoid ▪ Aryepiglottic muscle

Extrinsic muscles of vocal cord: Connects larynx with neighbouring structure
- **Elevators of larynx:**
  - **Primary elevator:** Stylopharyngeus, Salpingopharyngeus, Palatopharyngeus and Thyrohyoid
  - **Secondary elevator:** Mylohyoid (main), Digastric muscle, Stylohyoid and Geniohyoid
- **Depressors:**
  - Sternohyoid, Sternothyroid and Omohyoid

4. Ans. (a) Excision of ranula and sublingual gland duct

Ref: Dhingra's ENT 6th ed. P 224

- Ranula is cystic translucent lesion at the floor of mouth on one side of frenulum.
- It pushes the tongue upwards
- Arises due to obstruction of sublingual salivary gland duct.
- Sometimes when it extends into the neck → Known as plunging ranula

TREATMENT
- If small: Complete surgical excision of cyst and its duct
- If large: Marsupialization preferred

5. Ans. (a) Laryngeal carcinoma

Ref: Dhingra's ENT 6th ed. P 316-17

Types of Tracheostomy
- **Emergency tracheostomy:** Done in emergency/urgent setting. Vertical midline incision made in 2nd and 3rd tracheal rings
- **Elective/Routine tracheostomy/Tranquil:** Planned procedure. Transverse incision
- **Permanent tracheostomy:** May be required in bilateral abductor paralysis or laryngeal stenosis

Tracheostomy is also classified on the basis of site:
- **High tracheostomy:** Done above level of isthmus. Damages first tracheal ring
  - Complication: Perichondritis
  - Only indication: Laryngeal CA *(total laryngectomy is anyway required)*
- **Mid tracheostomy:** Preferred type. Done through 2nd or 3rd tracheal ring. Divides thyroid isthmus
- **Low tracheostomy:** Done below the level of isthmus. A difficult one, not generally recommended.

6. Ans. (b) Cochlear implant

Ref: Dhingra's ENT 6th ed. P 125

- In the above patient of profound SNHL, cochlear implant is preferred.
- Indication of cochlear implant:
  - Bilateral Severe/profound SNHL
  - Intact auditory nerve system
- Implant has external and internal component (image). Electrode array is placed in scala tympani of cochlea.

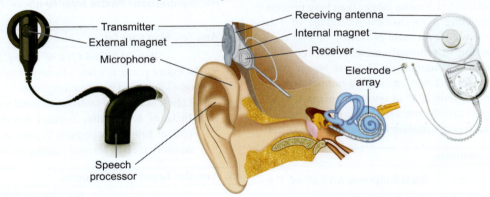

Illustration of cochlear implant components. The external parts are shown on the left, the internal components of the implant on the right. The scheme in the middle shows the position of the cochlear implant components *in situ*

7. Ans. (c) Serous otitis media

Ref: Dhingra's ENT 6th ed. P 250-51

- In a patient with nasopharyngeal CA, most common clinical presentation is cervical lymphadenopathy.
- Upon superior invasion it can invade floor of skull invading several cranial nerve
- First cranial nerve to be involved: CN 6
- An anterior growth can cause eustachean tube obstruction → serous otitis media/glue ear
- **Clinical feature:** Trotter's triad
  - Soft palate palsy (due to CN 10 invasion)
  - Deep facial pain (due to CN 5 invasion)
  - Conductive hearing loss (due to eustachean tube obstruction)
- **Note:** in adult patient with unilateral glue ear, nasopharyngeal CA should be ruled out first.

8. Ans. (a) Antrochoanal polyp

- The mentioned case is very much suggestive of antrochoanal polyp.
- These are the single polyp originated from maxillary sinus and protrudes into nasal cavity.

ANATOMY OF AURICLE AND EXTERNAL AUDITARY CANAL & EMBRYOLOGY

9. Ans. (b) Anterior belly of digastric muscle

Ref: Diseases of ENT, by Dhingra, 6th ed. Pg. 285

TABLE: Derivatives of branchial/pharyngeal arches

1st Branchial arch	2nd Branchial arch	3rd Branchial arch	4th Branchial arch	6th Branchial arch
• Malleus and Incus • Maxilla • Mandible • Muscle of mastication • Anterior belly of digastric muscle • Tensor tympani muscle • Sphenomandibular ligament	• Stapes (except foot plate) • Upper half of body of hyoid • Lesser cornu of hyoid • Muscle of facial expression • Posterior belly of digastric muscle • Stylohyoid ligament	• Lower part of body of hyoid • Greater cornu of hyoid • Stylopharyngeus muscle • Common carotid artery	• Upper thyroid cartilage • Cricothyroid muscle • Extrinsic laryngeal and pharyngeal muscle	• Lower half of thyroid cartilage • Arytenoid cartilage • All intrinsic laryngeal muscle except cricothyroid
Nerve: Mandibular branch of CN 5th	**Facial Nerve**	**Glossopharyngeal nerve**	**Vagus + Superior Laryngeal nerve**	**Vagus + Recurrent laryngeal nerve**

Note: Laryngeal cartilage like cricoid, coneiform, corniculate are formal due to fusion of Branchial arch 4 and 6.
- Epiglottic cartilage derived from hypobranchial eminence.

10. Ans. (a) 1.3 : 1

Ref: Dhingra's ENT 6th ed. P 15

- Handle of malleus is 1.3 times longer than long process of incus, providing a mechanical advantage of 1.3, giving the **ossicular-lever ratio of 1.3:1**
- **Hydraulic action of tympanic membrane:** The total area of tympanic membrane is 21 times bigger than footplate of stapes (3.2 mm), giving it a ratio of **21:1**
- As we know that only 2/3rd of tympanic membrane is effective, it gives an effective aerial ratio of 14:1
- Therefore **total transformation ratio** is: 14 × 1.3 = **18.2:1**

11. Ans. (c) Stria vascularis

Ref: Dhingrwa's ENT 6th ed. P 9

- **Cochlea is divided into 3 compartments:** Scala tympani, scala media and scala vestibuli by the two membranes **basilar membrane and Reissner's membrane.**
- Another membrane, i.e. stria vascularis is present on the wall of scala tympani and secretes endolymph.

12. Ans. (b) MacEwen's triangle

Ref: Dhingra's ENT, 6th ed. pg. 5

- Mastoid antrum is the largest air cell of mastoid. Its depth is ~15 mm from skin due to the thick plate of bone over it.
- Antrum is marked externally on the surface of mastoid by **Suprameatal triangle/MacEwen's triangle.**

▶ **Extra Mile**

- Development of mastoid is from squamous and petrous bone. Persistence of petrosquamous suture is known as **Korner's septum.**

13. Ans. (a) Cricothyroid muscle

Ref: Diseases of ENT, by Dhingra, 6th ed. pg. 285
For explanations Please refer to above Table.

14. Ans. (c) Skin with fat

Ref: Dhingra's ENT, 6th ed. pg. 2, 5th ed. pg. 3-4
- The entire pinna is made of one yellow elastic cartilage except lobule and incisura terminalis.
  - Lobule is made of fat tissue covered with skin.
  - **Incisura terminalis:** Located between tragus and crus of helix. Can be used to gain access in external auditory meatus without cutting the cartilage.

15. Ans: (b) Lesser petrosal nerve

Ref: Dhingra's ENT, 6th ed. pg. 4

■ **NERVE SUPPLY OF AURICLE/PINNA**

Lateral Surface

- **Greater Auricular nerve**
- **Vagus (Arnold's nerve) + Facial Nerve:** Supplies concha
- **Auriculotemporal nerve**

Medial Surface

- **Lesser occipital nerve:** Supplies upper 1/3rd
- **Greater auricular nerve: Supplies lower 2/3rd**
- **Vagus (Arnold's nerve) + Facial nerve:** Supplies conchal protrusion medially (see Image)

---

16. Ans. (d) Auriculotemporal nerve

Ref: Dhingra's ENT, 6th ed. pg. 4

- Auriculotemporal nerve supplies only on the lateral aspect of auricle.

---

17. Ans. (a) Greater auricular nerve

Ref: Dhingra's ENT 6th ed. pg. 4

- Greater auricular nerve has major contribution of auricle. It supplies major portion on lateral aspect as well as on the medial aspect.

---

18. Ans. (a) Vagus nerve

Ref: Dhingra's ENT, 6th ed. pg. 4

- **Arnold's nerve** is the auricular branch (also known as the mastoid branch) of the vagus nerve (CN X).
- It originates from the superior ganglion of the vagus nerve
- Arnold's nerve along with facial nerve innervates concha of auricle and the external acoustic meatus *(posterior and inferior wall).*

---

19. Ans. (c) Glossopharyngeal nerve

Ref: Dhingra's ENT, 6th ed. pg. 4

- Jacobson's nerve is a branch of glossopharyngeal nerve (CN- IX) in middle ear.
- It supplies medial aspect of tympanic membrane.

---

20. Ans. (a) Lesser cornu

Ref: Inderbir Singh's Embroyology, 7th ed. pg. 119-120

---

21. Ans. (c) III

Ref: Inderbir Singh's Embroyology, 7th ed. pg. 119-120

- Lower part of hyoid and greater cornu of hyoid is derived from branchial arch III.
- Upper part of hyoid and lesser cornu of hyoid is derived from branchial arch II

---

22. Ans. (d) Cricothyroid muscle

Ref: Inderbir Singh's Embroyology, 7th ed. pg. 119-120

- All intrinsic laryngeal muscles is derived from branchial arch VI EXCEPT cricothyroid muscle.
- Cricothyroid muscle is derived from branchial arch IV.

---

23. Ans. (d) IV and VI

Ref: Inderbir Singh's Embroyology, 7th ed. pg. 119-120

- Thyroid cartilage is derived from branchial arch IV and VI.
  - Upper part: Branchial arch IV
  - Lower part: Branchial arch VI

---

24. Ans. (b) II

Ref: Inderbir Singh's Embroyology, 7th ed. pg. 119-120

- Ear ossicles are derived from branchial arch I and II
- Malleus and incus: BA-I
- Stapes: BA-II

---

25. Ans. (a) Ultimobranchial body

Ref: Inderbir Singh's Embroyology, 7th ed. pg. 119-120

- In humans, the ultimobranchial body is an embryological structure that gives rise to the calcitonin-producing cells—**also called parafollicular cells or C cells**—of the thyroid gland.
- In humans, this body is a derivative of the ventral recess of the **fourth pharyngeal pouch.**
- **Stapes:** from 2nd Branchial arch
- **Laryngeal cartilage:** from 6th branchial arch
- **Mandible:** from 1st branchial arch

---

26. Ans. (d) Outer 1/3rd is bony and inner 2/3rd is cartilaginous

Ref: Dhingra's ENT, 6th ed. pg. 4-5

- In External auditory canal /meatus: **outer 1/3rd is cartilaginous, inner 2/3rd is bony**. Length is 8 mm and 16 mm respectively.
- EAC extends from bottom of concha to tympanic membrane having a total length of 24 mm.
- **Congenital pathologies associated with EAC:**
  - **Fissure of santorini:** From anterior wall of cartilaginous part of EAC to parotid gland
  - **Foramen of Huschke:** From anteroinferior wall of bony part of EAC to parotid gland
- **Note:** Any infection in parotid gland can spread to EAC or vice versa through these congenital pathologies.

---

27. Ans. (d) <1 cm

Ref: Dhingra's ENT, 6th ed. pg. 4-5

- **Total Length of EAC:** 24 mm (2.4 cm)
  - **Outer 1/3rd is cartilaginous: 8 mm (0.8 cm)**
  - Inner 2/3rd is bony: 16 mm (1.6 cm)

---

28. Ans. (c) Bony part of EAC and parotid gland

Ref: Dhingra's ENT, 6th ed. pg. 2

- **Congenital pathologies associated with EAC:**
  - **Fissure of santorini:** From anterior wall of cartilaginous part of EAC to parotid gland
  - **Foramen of Huschke:** From anteroinferior wall of bony part of EAC to parotid gland

29. Ans. (d) Composite grafts of cartilage & skin from pinna are not used for correction of defects of nasal ala

Ref: Dhingra's ENT, 6th ed. pg. 2

- **Composite grafts of cartilage & skin from pinna are used sometimes for correction of defects of nasal ala.**
- All other statements mentioned above are true.

> Extra Mile
> - CARTILAGE from the tragus, perichondrium from the tragus or concha and fat from lobule are frequently used for reconstructive surgery of middle ear.
> - Tragal cartilage can be used to correct the depressed nasal bridge
> - Incisura terminalis is area between tragus and crus of helix. It is devoid of cartilage.

30. Ans. (a) 2.5 cm

Ref: Dhingra's ENT, 5th ed. pg. 4

- Length of external auditory canal- 24 mm (2.4 cm)
- Shape: S-shaped
- Outer 1/3rd cartilaginous part (8 mm)
- Inner 2/3rd: Bony part (16 mm)

31. Ans. (c) 1/3rd outer

Ref: Dhingra's ENT, 5th ed. / 4

- Outer 1/3rd of EAC is cartilaginous. It has hair follicles and ceruminous glands which secretes sebum.

32. Ans. (b) Ascending ramus of mandible

Ref: Dhingra's ENT, 5th ed./227

- Retromolar trigone is a triangular area of mucosa covering **anterior surface of the ascending ramus of mandible.**
- Base of retromolar trigone is posterior to the last molar while its apex is adjacent to the tuberosity of maxilla.

ANATOMY OF MIDDLE EAR & INNER EAR

33. Ans. (a) Organ of corti

Ref: Dhingra's ENT, 6th ed. pg. 9, 10

- Organ of corti is sensory organ of hearing.

34. Ans. (b) Balance

Ref: Dhingra's ENT, 6th ed. pg. 9, 17

- There are 3 semicircular canals; the posterior, lateral and superior. They all lie in planes at right angles to each other.
- It is responsible for *balancing angular acceleration*.
- Macula, present in utricle and saccule is responsible for balancing linear acceleration.

35. Ans. (b) Medial

The most prominent portion of the medial wall of the middle ear cavity is the promontory. The projection is raised by underlying basal turn of cochlea. It has number of grooves containing tympanic plexus of nerves.

36. Ans. (a) Nasopharynx

- ET opens on lateral wall of nasopharynx.
- Bounded by ridge–Torus Tubarius

37. Ans. (a) Cochlea

Ref: Dhingra's ENT, 5th ed. pg. 12

- Upon taking the section of cochlea, we see 3 compartments and 3 membranes:
  - **Scala vestibuli:** Contains perilymph
  - **Scala media:** Contains endolymph
  - **Scala tympani:** Contains perilymph

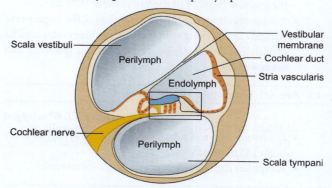

- **Three membranes are:**
  - **Reissner's membrane:** Separates scala vestibule from scala media.
  - **Basilar membrane:** Separates scala tympani from scala media. Also supports organ of corti.
  - **Stria vascularis:** On the wall of scala media. Converts perilymph into endolymph.

38. Ans. (a) Utricle

Ref: P.L. Dhingra's ENT, 6th ed. pg. 16

- Sensory organ of utricle and saccule: Macula

Structure of Macula
- Made of 2 parts:
  - A **sensory neuroepithelium** made of type 1 and type 2 hair cells
  - An **otolith membrane**. This membrane is made up of a gelatinous mass and on top, there is crystal of calcium carbonate called **otoconia or otolith.**

ENT

> **Extra Mile**
>
> - Sensory organ of linear motion/acceleration: Macula (In utricle and saccule)
> - Sensory organ of angular motion/acceleration: Crista ampularis (in Semicircular canal, ampulated portion)

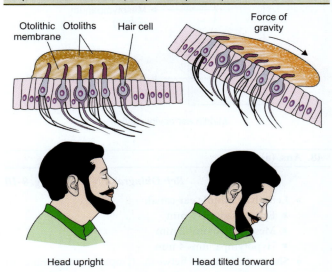

39. Ans. (c) Long process of incus

Ref: PubMed

40. Ans. (c) Posterior wall

Ref: Dhingra's ENT, 6th ed. pg. 4-5

- Chorda tympani is a branch of facial nerve which is located on posterior wall of middle ear.
- **Middle wall is box shaped cavity having 6 walls.**
- Corda tympani is a branch of facial nerve which is located on posterior wall of middle ear. It has sensory and secretomotor branches and supplies:
  - Anterior 2/3rd of tongue
  - Sublingual gland
  - Submandibular gland

> **Extra Mile**
>
> **TABLE:** Middle ear walls and their contents
>
> | Wall | Made of significance |
> |------|---------------------|
> | • Superior wall/roof | Made of tegmen tympani, a very thin plate of bone. **Separates middle ear from middle cranial fossa** |
> | • Inferior wall/floor | Aka **Jugular wall**. It is formed by tympanic plate of temporal bone. Below the floor lies inferior jugular vein |
> | • Lateral wall | Aka **outer wall**. Formed by tympanic membrane |
> | • Anterior wall | Aka **carotid wall**. Separates middle ear from Internal carotid artery. |
>
> *Contd...*
>
> | Wall | Made of significance |
> |------|---------------------|
> | | **Contents of anterior wall:** Opening of eustachean tubve 2 Drains on lateral wall of nasopharynx Canal of tensor tympani- Gives origin to tensor tympani muscle |
> | • Medial wall | Aka **labyrinth wall**. Separates middle ear from inner ear. **Contents:** • **Promontory:** Due to basal coil of cochlea • **Oval window:** Covered by foot plate of stapes • **Round window:** Covered by secondary tympanic membrane • **Processus cochleariformis:** Hook like structure, anterior to oval window. Tensor tympani muscle takes a turn here before inserting to neck of malleus • **Fistula ante-fenestrum:** MC site for ostosclerosis • **Fallopian canal/Facial canal:** Facial nerve runs here in horizontal direction. |
> | • Posterior wall | Aka **mastoid wall**. Separates middle ear from mastoid cavity. **Contents:** • **Pyramid:** Bony protrusion. Origin of stapedius muscle from tip of pyramid • **Aditus ad-antrum:** Doorway to antrum of mastoid. Located on postero-superior wall. • **Facial nerve in facial canal** in vertical direction. **Gives rise to chorda tympani** • **Facial recess**-Landmark for intact canal wall surgery |

41. Ans. (c) Carotid wall

Ref: Dhingra's ENT, 6th ed. pg. 5

Anterior wall is also known as carotid wall. Separates middle ear from Internal carotid artery. Contents of anterior wall:

- **Opening of eustachean tube:** Drains on lateral wall of nasopharynx
- **Canal of tensor tympani:** Gives origin to tensor tympani muscle.

42. Ans. (d) Aditus ad antrum

Ref: Dhingra's ENT, 6th ed. pg. 5-6

- Aditus ad antrum is located on posterior wall. It is a doorway to antrum of mastoid.
- Antrum is largest mastoid air cell.

43. Ans. (c) Middle cranial fossa

Ref: Dhingra's ENT, 6th ed. pg. 5

FMGE Solutions Screening Examination

- Roof of middle ear is formed by tegmen tympani, a very thin plate of bone.
- It separates middle ear from middle cranial fossa.

44. Ans. (d) Medial

Ref: Dhingra's ENT, 6th ed. pg. 5

- MC site for ostosclerosis: **Fistula ante-fenestrum**
- **Location of fissula ante-fenestram:** Medial wall of middle ear

45. Ans. (b) Malleus

Ref: Dhingra's ENT, 5th ed. pg. 12

There are two important muscles of middle ear:

Muscle	Origin	Insertion	Nerve supply
Tensor tympani	Canal of tensor tympani (anterior wall)	Neck of malleus	Mandibular branch of CN- V
Stapedius	Tip of pyramid (posterior wall)	Neck of stapes	CN- VII

46. Ans. (c) 7

Ref: Dhingra's ENT, 5th ed. pg. 6

- Fallopian canal is also known as facial canal present on the walls of middle ear.
- **Direction:**
  - Entry from media wall. Facial nerve runs in horizontal direction
  - Exits on posterior wall. Facial nerve here runs in vertical direction.
  - Exits via stylomastoid foramen.

47. Ans. (b) 1 cm

Ref: Dhingra's ENT, 6th ed. pg. 9-10

- The opening to the internal acoustic meatus is located inside the cranial cavity, near the center of the posterior surface of the petrous part of the temporal bone.
- The size varies considerably; its margins are smooth and rounded. **The canal is short (about 1 cm)** and runs laterally into the bone.
- Length of external acoustic canal: **24 mm.**
- **Length of middle ear canal:**
  - Epitympanum- 6 mm
  - Mesotympanum- 2 mm
  - Hypotympanum- 4 mm
- **Shortest** distance between tympanic membrane to promontory: 2 mm.

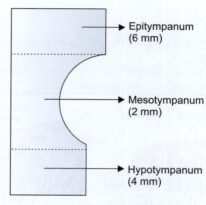

Middle ear cavity section

48. Ans. (a) 2 mm

Ref: Dhingra's ENT, 6th ed. pg. 9-10

- **Length of middle ear canal:**
  - Epitympanum- 6 mm
  - Mesotympanum- 2 mm
  - Hypotympanum- 4 mm
- **Shortest** distance between tympanic membrane to promontory: 2 mm.

49. Ans. (b) Facial nerve and superior vestibular cochlear nerve

Ref: Dhingra's ENT, 6th ed. pg. 90-91

- Bill's bar divides the superior compartment of the internal acoustic meatus into an anterior and posterior compartment.
- *Anterior to Bill's bar, are the facial nerve (in the anterior superior quadrant) and nervus intermedius, **and posterior to it is the superior division of the vestibular nerve (in the posterosuperior quadrant).***

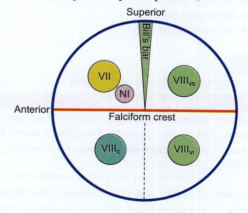

50. Ans. (b) Hearing

Ref: Dhingra's ENT, 5th ed. pg. 11

- The main function of cochlea is hearing via the hair cells present on basilar membrane
- **Sensory organ of hearing:** Organ of Corti
- **Otolith organ:** Utricle and Saccule

51. Ans. (b) Olfactory system

Ref: Dhingra's ENT, 5th ed. pg. 22

- **Requirements for balancing:**
  - Vision
  - Vestibule and cochlea
  - Proprioception
  - Cerebellum

52. Ans. (c) Semicircular canal

Ref: Dhingra's ENT, 5th ed. pg. 20

- Sensory organ of angular motion is crista ampularis which is located in semicircular canal.
- Structure of crista ampularis is a crest like mound of connective tissue on which lie the sensory epithelial cells. These sensory hair cells project into the cupula.
- **Cupula is a gelatinous mass** of polysachharides and contains canals into which project the cilia of sensory cells.

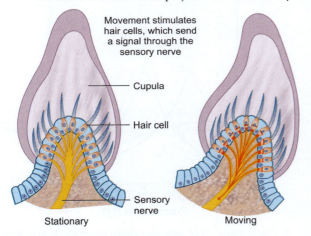

53. Ans. (c) Cochlea

Ref: Dhingra's ENT, 5th ed. pg. 12

- Upon taking the section of cochlea, we see 3 compartments and 3 membranes:
  - Scala vestibuli: Contains perilymph
  - Scala media: Contains endolymph
  - Scala tympani: Contains perilymph
- 3 membranes are:
  - **Reissner's membrane:** Separates scala vestibule from scala media.
  - **Basilar membrane:** Separates scala tympani from scala media. Also supports organ of corti.
  - **Stria vascularis:** On the wall of scala media. Converts perilymph into endolymph.

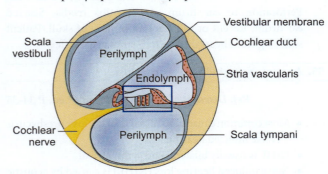

TESTS OF AUDITORY SYSTEM

54. Ans. (d) Can cause Vertigo

Ref: Diseases of ENT by Dhingra 6th ed. P 53-54

- **External ear syringing** is done to clean/remove wax from external auditory canal.
- **Indications:**
  - Removal of wax
  - Dried fungal debris
  - Epithelial debris
  - Blunt foreign bodies
- **Direction of flow:** Postero-superior wall
- **Water** that is used is normal room temperature water (pre-boiled and cooled to room temperature)
- If too cold or too warm water used → It can stimulate labyrinth as in caloric testing and can cause vertigo.

REQUIREMENTS AND PROCEDURE OF SYRINGING

Requirements: Aural syringe 50 or 100 cc capacity, a kidney tray and warm saline at body temperature (Not to produce caloric reaction and vertigo)

Procedure: Patient sits before the operator with the ear to be syringed facing him. The nozzle of the syringe is detached and the syringe is filled with water/saline. The nozzle is then tightly reapplied and air pushed out of the syringe in vertical position. Light is thrown on to the patients ear by means of head mirror/light. The kidney tray is held below the ear. The pinna of the patient is pulled **upwards, backwards and outwards** with one hand of the operator to straighten out the meatus and by means of the syringe, the jet of the fluid is ordinarily directed towards the postero-superior wall of the meatus. The force used should be moderate and canal washed of wax. The meatus should be inspected after each

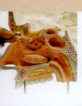

FMGE Solutions Screening Examination

syringing to see the TM so that operator does not go on syringing unnecessarily. After syringing, the meatus should be dried with cotton wool on carrier.

Contraindications: Generalized & Localized otitis externa, Perforation of ear drum, Acute otitis media, Scarred ear drum, Recent or old fracture of base of skull, Patient suffering from heart disease for fear of vagal reflex.

55. Ans. (c) Noise induced hearing loss

Ref: Diseases of ENT by Dhingra 6th ed. P 34-35

- Most common cause of acquired hearing loss: presbycusis > Noise induced hearing loss
- NIHL is usually bilateral and symmetrical
- Noise induced hearing loss (NIHL) is caused by acoustic trauma which is characterized by specific pattern of audiogram finding.
- NIHL can damage hair cells, starting in the basal turn of cochlea. Outer hair cells are affected first followed by inner hair cells.
- NIHL usually affect a person's hearing sensitivity in the higher frequencies like 3000 Hz, 4000 Hz or 6000 Hz.
- Upon audiogram a notch is seen especially at 4000 Hz.
- Tinnitus is the first symptom without any hearing impairment.

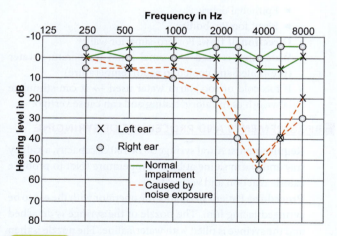

Extra Mile

- **Carhart Notch:** A sudden dip/notch at 2000 Hz. Seen in otosclerosis
- **Acoustic trauma:** Sudden, permanent, SNHL due to single exposure to an intense sound (130–140 dB) for < 0.2 sec.

56. Ans. (b) 90 dB in 8 hrs/days for 5 days per week

Ref: Dhingra's ENT 6th ed. P 35

Book states: *"a noise of 90 dB, 8 hours a day for 5 days per week is the maximum safe limit as recommended by the ministry of labour, GOI."*

TABLE: Permissible exposure in cases of continuous noise or a number of short-term exposure (Ministry of Labor, GOI): Factory Act 1948

Noise level (dBA)	Permitted daily exposure (hour)
• 90	8
• 92	6
• 95	4
• 97	3
• 102	1 ½
• 105	1
• 110	½
• 115	¼

Note: 5 dB rule of time intensity states that "any rise of 5 dB noise level will reduce the permitted noise exposure time to half".

57. Ans. (b) As

Ref: Dhingra's ENT, 6th ed. pg. 25

Types of tympanogram graphs and their interpretation:
- A: Normal
- As: Otosclerosis (reduced compliance at ambient pressure)

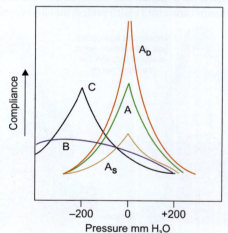

- Ad: Disruption of ossicular chain (increased compliance at ambience pressure)
- B: Glue ear/Fluid in middle ear (**Flat or dome shaped**)
- C: Eustachean tube obstruction (Maximum compliance at pressure more than −200 mm H_2O; Negative pressure in middle ear)—**negative tympanogram**

58. Ans. (b) ABR

Ref: Dhingra's ENT, 6th ed. pg. 27

ABR is auditory brainstem response. It is used for:
- Screening infants hearing
- To determine threshold of hearing in infant and in uncooperative patient.

- To diagnose brainstem pathology. E.g. multiple sclerosis.
- For intraoperative monitoring of CN.
- In acoustic neuroma surgery
- **OAE** is also used for screening of hearing in neonates.

59. Ans. (b) Cochlea

Ref: Dhingra's ENT, 6th ed. pg. 27

Otoacoustic emission test will determine cochlear, hair cell function. It is used for—
- Screening neonates exposed to aminoglycoside antibiotics.
- Differentiating sensory and neural components of sensori-hearing loss.
- Test for feign (maligned) hearing loss.
- To differentiate cochlear vs retrocochlear hearing loss

Note: *Sedation does not interfere with OAE test.*

60. Ans. (d) Acoustic neuroma

Ref: Dhingra's ENT 6th ed. pg. 450

- **Tone decay** also known as auditory fatigue, is a change in auditory threshold when a continuous tone is presented to the ear.
- It is seen in **acoustic neuroma** and other retrocochlear lesion.

61. Ans. (a) Otosclerosis

Ref: Diseases of ENT, by Dhingra, 6th ed. pg. 22-23

- Gelle's test is a Tuning fork test which can be performed using tuning fork of different frequencies such as: 128, 256, 512, 1024, 2048, 4096 Hz.
- MC used/ideal for routine clinical practice is of **512 Hz.**
- **Tests done with tuning fork:**
  - Rinne's test
  - Weber's test
  - Absolute bone conduction (ABC) test
  - Bing test
  - Gelle's test
  - Lewis test

> **POINTS TO KNOW ABOUT GELLE'S TEST**
>
> - Gelle's test is a bone conduction test and examines effect of increased air pressure in ear canal (*using siegel's speculum*) on hearing.
> - This test is performed by placing a vibrating tuning fork on mastoid, while changes in air pressure in the ear canal are brought about by siegel's speculum.
> - In normal individuals, increased air pressure in ear canal, pushes tympanic membrane inwards which raises intralabyrynthine pressure → immobility of basilar membrane → decreased hearing **(POSITIVE TEST).**
> - In patients with fixed ossicular chain (otosclerosis) or disconnected ossicular chain, there is no change in hearing **(NEGATIVE TEST).**
> - **Note:** *Earlier it was a popular test for otosclerosis. Now it is superceded by tympanometry.*

62. Ans. (b) CSOM

Ref: Diseases of ENT, by Dhingra, 6th ed. pg. 22

TABLE: Tests done with help of tuning fork and their interpretation

> - Rinne's is a tuning fork test, which is done to test the air conduction and bone conduction.
> - It is done by placing the tuning fork on mastoid (Bone conduction) followed by bringing it in front of ear canal (air conduction).
> - In normal individual and in SNHL sound is still heard when tuning fork is brought in front of ear canal (**AC > BC → Positive Rinne**)
> - In patients with conductive hearing loss, sound transmitted via bone conduction (mastoid) is more as compared to air conduction (**BC > AC → Negative Rinne**).
> - All the given conditions in options causes sensorinueral hearing loss, except the CSOM, which causes conductive hearing loss.

63. Ans. (c) Left ear, air conduction

Ref: Diseases of ENT, by Dhingra, 6th ed. pg. 30

Symbols and Lines used in Audiogram
- Broken line for bone conduction (Mn: B–B)
- Continuous line for air conduction
- Red line for right ear (Mn: R–R)
- Blue line for left ear

TABLE: Symbols used in Audiogram charting

Test modality	Right ear	Left ear
AC unmasked	O	X
AC masked	△	□
BC unmasked	<	>
BC masked	[	]

64. Ans. (b) 512 Hz

Ref: Dhingra's ENT, 5th ed. pg. 26

- Tuning fork test can be performed using tuning fork of different frequencies such as: 128, 256, 512, 1024, 2048, 4096 Hz.
- MC used/ideal for routine clinical practice is of 512 Hz.
- Tuning fork of lower frequencies produce sense of bone vibration while those of higher frequencies have a shorter decay time and are thus not routinely preferred.
- Tuning fork of
- **Tests done with tuning fork:**
  - Rinne's test
  - Weber's test
  - Absolute bone conduction (ABC) test
  - Bing test
  - Gelle's test
  - Lewis test

FMGE Solutions Screening Examination

65. Ans. (c) 512 Hz

Ref: Dhingra's ENT, 6th ed. pg. 22, 5th ed. pg. 26

66. Ans. (d) Pure tone audiometry

Tests done with help of tuning fork and their interpretation:

Test	Normal	CHL	SNHL
RINNE	AC > BC	BC > AC	AC > BC
WEBER	NO Lateralization	Lateralization deaf side	Lateralization normal side
ABC	Equal	Equal	Reduced
Schwabach's	Equal	Increased	Reduced

67. Ans. (c) Cochlea

Ref: Dhingra's ENT 5th ed. / 32

- Otoacoustic emission (OAE) are low intensity sounds **produced by outer hair cells of a normal cochlea.**
- These sounds produced by outer hair cells travels in a reverse direction: Outer hair cells 2 basilar membrane 2 perilymph 2 oval window 2 ossicles 2 tympanic membrane 2 ear canal.
- When outer hair cells are damaged, OAE are absent. Hence it helps to know the function of cochlea.

68. Ans. (a) ABR

Ref: Dhingra's ENT, 5th ed. pg. 31-32

- **ABR** is considered as best test for screening of hearing in neonates
- **ABR is** auditory brainstem response. Can be used as screening procedure and threshold of hearing in infants. Mainly used to diagnose retrocochlear pathology. Ex: Acoustic Neuroma.
- **Tympanometry** is considered as IOC for otosclerosis.
- **Electrocochleography:** Used to find out threshold of hearing in young infants and children. It is also the most sensitive test for Meniere's disease.

69. Ans. (a) Vestibular function

Ref: Dhingra's ENT, 5th ed. pg. 48

- Caloric test is used to assess vestibular function. The basis of this test is to induce nystagmus by thermal stimulation of the vestibular system.
- Done by taking water of 2 temperatures, cold (30°C) and hot (44°C).
- **Position of the test:** Supine then lift head at 30° forward or patient sitting with bending backwards 60°.
- **This position is used in order to make lateral/horizontal SCC in vertical position.**
- Cold water elicits nystagmus in opposite eye and warm water elicit nystagmus in same eye (Mn: COWS).
- **Interpretation:**
  - **Normal: Time** taken from start of irrigation to end point of Nystagmus is taken and it is **80 seconds —120 seconds.**
  - **Canal paresis:** Duration of Nystagmus shortened i.e. <80 sec.
- Indicates depressed function of ipsilateral Labyrinth, vestibular nerve and vestibular nuclei.
- **It is seen in:**
  - Meniere's disease
  - Acoustic neuroma
  - Vestibular neuritis
  - Vestibular nerve section
  - Postural vertigo

70. Ans. (b) Lateral semicircular canal

Ref: Dhingra's ENT, 6th ed. pg. 43

71. Ans. (a) Fistula test

Ref: Dhingra's ENT, 6th ed. pg. 41

FISTULA TEST

- The aim of this test is to induce nystagmus by increasing pressure in labyrinth which is performed by applying pressure at tragus.
- **If there is fistula between middle ear and inner ear, this increased pressure leads to stimulation of labyrinth which results in nystagmus and vertigo.**
- In normal population the test is negative because the pressure changes in the external auditory canal cannot be transmitted to the labyrinth.
- **Fistula test is positive in the following cases:**
  - When there is erosion of lateral/horizontal semicircular canal as in cholesteatoma
  - After fenestration operation- **type V tympanoplasty** *(a surgically created window in the horizontal canal)*
  - Post stapedectomy fistula *(Abnormal opening in the oval window post-stapedectomy)*
  - After rupture of round window membrane
  - **A positive fistula also implies that the labyrinth is still functioning.**
- **It is absent when labyrinth is dead.**
- A false negative fistula test is also seen when cholesteatoma covers the site of fistula and doesn't allow pressure changes to be transmitted to the labyrinth.
- A false positive fistula test is seen in case of menier's disease aka endolymphatic hydrops.

ENT

987

Extra Mile

- **Impedance audiometry** is done in order to determine the status of the tympanic membrane and middle ear via tympanometry.
  - The other purpose of this test is to evaluate acoustic reflex pathways, which include cranial nerves VII and VIII and the auditory brainstem.
- **Galvanic vestibular stimulation** is the process of sending specific electric messages to a nerve in the ear that maintains balance.

DISEASES OF EAR, TREATMENT AND REHABILITATION

72. Ans. (d) Myringotomy + Gromet insertion

Ref: Diseases of ENT by Dhingra 6th ed. P 65

- Main cause of otitis media is Eustachean tube obstruction/dysfunction. Can occur due to chronic rhinitis, chronic sinusitis
  - In child: MC due to adenoid hypertrophy
  - Adult: Raise suspicion of nasopharyngeal carcinoma
- **Upon examination:**
  - Severely retracted tympanic membrane
  - Dull/pale tympanic membrane
  - Presence of fluid level with air bubbles
- **Initial management:**
  - Nasal decongestant
  - Anti-allergic measures
  - Antibiotics (in cases of URTI)
  - Valsalva manuever/Politzerisation- for middle ear aeration
- Mainstay of treatment of glue ear is **myringotomy with grommet insertion** with or without adenoidectomy.
- Indications of surgery in glue ear:
  - Chronic effusion >3 months
  - CHL 40 dB
  - Suspicion of malignancy
- **Preferred site:** Postero-inferior quadrant of tympanic membrane

Extra Mile

- If aspirate is thick/glue like → two incisions are made: Antero-superior and antero-inferior quadrant known as "Beer can principle"

73. Ans. (a) Kanamycin

Ref: Goodman & Gillman 13th ed. P 1044-45

- All aminoglycosides have the potential to produce reversible and irreversible vestibular, cochlear, and renal toxicity and neuromuscular blockade.

- Aminoglycoside-induced ototoxicity may result in irreversible, bilateral, high-frequency hearing loss or vestibular hypofunction.
- A high-pitched tinnitus often is **the first symptom** of cochlear toxicity.
- Drugs like amikacin, neomycin and kanamycin are specifically cochleotoxic > vestibulotoxic.
- Gentamicin, streptomycin is vestibular > cochleotoxic
- Tobramycin: Cochlear = Vestibular toxicity

74. Ans. (a) Idiopathic Bell's palsy

Ref: Dhingra's ENT 6th ed. P 95

- Facial nerve palsy can be central or peripheral.
- Peripheral lesion can involve nerve in its intracranial, intratemporal or extratemporal part. Peripheral lesions are more common and 2/3rd of them are idiopathic variety.
- **MCC:** 60–75% of the facial paralysis is due to **bell's palsy.** It is defined as idiopathic, peripheral facial paralysis or paresis of acute onset.
  - **Causes:** Viral infection (HSV, HZV or EBV), vascular ischemia, hereditary (~10% of patients have positive family history), autoimmune disorder.

75. Ans. (b) Otosclerosis

Ref: Dhingra's ENT 6th ed. P 87

- Otosclerosis is a sclerotic bone disease having two stages:
  - **Otospongiotic stage** also known as active stage
  - **Otosclerotic stage** also known as passive stage
- It is most commonly seen in females, in the age group of 20–30 years and the condition worsens during pregnancy.
- **Clinical features/Symptoms:**
  - Progressive conductive hearing loss
  - Tinnitus
  - Vertigo
  - **Paracusis willis:** Patient hears better in noisy environment (as a normal person raises voice in noisy environment)
- **Signs**
  - **Schwartz sign:** Reddish hue/flamingo pink coloration seen on the promontory through tympanic membrane.
  - Pure tone audiometry shows loss of air conduction more for lower frequencies. At 2000 Hz, there is sudden dip/notch formation known as **Carhart Notch**
- **IOC: Tympanometry (finding will be "As")**
- **Treatment: Stapedectomy/Stapedotomy** with a placement of prosthesis is treatment of choice.

76. Ans. (c) Costen syndrome

Ref: Dhingra's ENT 6th ed. P 447

- **Costen syndrome:**

Explanations

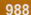

- It is an abnormality of temporomandibular joint, and is characterized by otalgia, feeling of blocked ear, tinnitus and often vertigo as well.
- Pain in Costen syndrome also radiates to frontal, parietal and occipital region.
- **Gradenigo's syndrome:** It is a severe form of petrositis (complication of otitis media) and involves CN V and VI. It consists of:
  - Ear discharge
  - Diplopia (due to CN VI involvement)
  - Retro-orbital pain (due to CN V involvement)

77. Ans. (b) Ramsay hunt syndrome

Ref: Dhingra's ENT, 6th ed. pg. 55, 96

- **Herpes zoster oticus** is a condition which is characterized by the appearance of vesicles on tympanic membrane, deep meatus, retroauricular sulcus and concha.
- If herpes zoster oticus involves facial nerve, this condition is called **Ramsay Hunt syndrome.** Patient may present in symptoms of facial nerve paralysis along with facial anesthesia, giddiness and hearing impairment due to involvement of 5th and 8th cranial nerve.
- **Treatment:** Acyclovir + Steroids

> **Extra Mile**
>
> - **Bell's palsy** is usually idiopathic. However it can be infective or hereditary in origin as well. It is always diagnosis of exclusion.
> - **Myringitis bullosa** is a painful condition characterized by formation of haemorrhagic blebs on the tympanic membrane and deep meatus. Involvement of facial nerve is very less likey.
> - **Melkersson syndrome** is an idiopathic condition present with triad of recurrent facial nerve paralysis, lip swelling and fissured tongue.

78. Ans. (c) Chronic myringitis

Ref: Diseases of ENT, by Dhingra, 6th ed. pg. 55

- **Myringitis granulosa**
  - It is a non-specific granulation on the outer/lateral surface of tympanic membrane.
  - It may be associated with external ear infection, impacted wax or long-standing foreign body.

79. Ans. (c) Serous otitis media

Ref: Dhingra, 5th ed. pg. 71-72

- Serous otitis media is also known as Glue ear.
- It is an insidious condition characterized by accumulation of non-purulent effusion in the middle ear cleft.
- One of common causes of serous otitis media (Glue ear) in children is blockage of Eustachian tube secondary to adenoid hyperplasia.

- Therefore, the treatment aims at removal of adenoid (adenoidectomy) and drainage of middle ear by grommet/Ventillation tube.
  - **Grommet** is a small tube inserted in tympanic membrane to drain the middle ear.
- Serous otitis media in adults should arouse suspicion of nasopharyngeal carcinoma and hence the treatment aims at removal of carcinoma.
- Adenoiditis is an acute condition and requires treatment conservatively.

80. Ans. (b) Softening followed by syringing

Ref: PL Dhingra's ENT, 6th ed. pg. 53

Dhingra states: *"If the wax is too hard and impacted to be removed by syringing or instruments, it should be softened by drops of 5% sodium bicarbonate in equal parts of glycerine and water instilled 2–3 times a day for a few days."*

Note:

- Hydrogen peroxide, liquid paraffin or olive oil may also achieve same result.
- Commercial drops like 2% paradichlorobenzene (ceruminolytic agent) can also be used to soften the wax.

> **Extra Mile**
>
> - If a fly or any crawling insect enters the ear canal, no attempt should be made to catch them alive. First they should be killed by instilling oil, spirit or chloroform, then suctioned out.

81. Ans. (a) Autograft

Ref: PubMed

- **Autograft:** Transplantation of tissue to the same person, from whom the tissue is harvested.
- **Isograft:** Transplantation of organ or a tissue from a donor to a genetically identical recipient like the twins
- **Allograft:** Transplant of an organ or tissue between two genetically non-identical members of same species
- **Xenograft:** Transplant of organ or tissues from one species to another.

> **Extra Mile**
>
> - Tympanoplasty is repairing of tympanic membrane in cases of ruptured tympanic membrane either due to infection or trauma.
> - Temporalis fascia is used for tympanoplasty. It has **very low basal metabolic rate**, hence very high rate of survival.

82. Ans. (a) 20–20,000 Hz

Ref: Dhingra's ENT, 6th ed. pg. 14-15

- Normal hearing capacity is from 20 Hz to 20,000 Hz.
- Function of hearing is by cochlea, which has 2 ends broadly. Apex and Base. Apex is for low frequency sound (20 Hz) and Base is for high frequency sound (20,000 Hz).

ENT

83. Ans. (b) 41–60 dB

Ref: Dhingra's ENT, 6th ed. pg. 38

WHO classification for hearing loss:

0–25 dB	Normal hearing
26–40 dB	Mild hearing loss
41–60 dB	Moderate hearing loss
61–80 dB	**Severe hearing loss**
>80 dB	Profound hearing loss

84. Ans. (c) 5–6 khz

*Ref: Noise-Induced Hearing Loss: Scientific Advances;
edited by Colleen G. Le Prell, Donald Henderson,
Richard R. Fay, Arthur Poppe*

- When the ear is exposed to excessive sound levels or loud sounds over time, the overstimulation of the hair cells on basilar membrane leads to heavy production of reactive oxygen species, leading to oxidative cell death.
- Damage ranges from exhaustion of the "hair" (hearing) cells in the ear to loss of those cells.
- NIHL usually occurs initially at high **frequencies (3, 4, or 6 kHz),** and then spreads to the low frequencies (0.5, 1, or 2 kHz)".

85. Ans. (b) Virus

Ref: Dhingra, 5th ed. pg. 62

- **Myringitis bullosa**
  - It is a painful condition characterized by formation of haemorrhagic belbs on the tympanic membrane and deep meatus.
  - **It is most commonly caused by virus-Adenovirus**
  - However it can also be caused by mycoplasma Pneumonia
- **Another similar disease entity is:**
  - **Myringitis granulosa**
    - ◆ It is non-specific granulations on the outer surface of tympanic membrane.
    - ◆ It may be associated with external ear infection, impacted wax or long-standing foreign body.

86. Ans. (a) Virus

Ref: Dhingra, 5th ed. pg. 62

Please refer to above explanation

87. Ans. (a) Streptococcus pneumoniae

Ref: Dhingra's ENT, 6th ed. pg. 62

- Acute otitis media is most commonly caused by Streptococcus Pneumonia. However it can also be caused by H. influenzae and Moraxella catarrhalis.

> **Extra Mile**

Common Infections and their most Common Causative Agents:

Infection	MC organism
Perichondritis	Pseudomonas
Malignant otitis externa	Pseudomonas
Localized otitis externa	Staphylococcus aureus
Acute suppurative otitis media	Strep pneumoniae
Chronic otitis Media	Pseudomonas

88. Ans. (c) Air

Ref: Dhingra's ENT, 5th ed. pg. 69-70

Otitis media is acute inflammation of middle ear by pyogenic organism secondary to:
- Eustachian tube blockage (MCC)
- Tympanic membrane perforation

Stages of Otitis Media Development

- **Stage of tubal occlusion:** Edema and hyperemia of nasopharyngeal end of eustachian tube blocks the tube leading to absorption of air and negative intratympanic pressure and retraction of TM with handle of malleus.
- **Stage of pre-suppuration:** Prolonged suppuration leads to growth of pyogenic organism causing appearance of inflammatory exudates, characterized by **cart-wheel appearance of TM**
- **Stage of suppuration:** Marked formation of pus in middle ear and to some extent in mastoid air cells, characterized by red and bulging tympanic membranes with loss of landmarks. X-rays shows clouding of air cells.
- **Stage of resolution:** Rupture of TM with release of pus and subsidence of symptoms, characterized by a small perforation in antero-inferior quadrant of pars-tensa.
- **Stage of complication:** If resolution doesn't take place, disease spreads, causing mastoiditis, facial paralysis, petrositis, meningitis etc.

89. Ans. (b) Stage 2

Ref: Dhingra's ENT, 6th ed. pg. 67-69

■ PARS FLACCIDA RETRACTION

- This classification described by Toss is fairly simple to apply, the only difficulty being the difficulty in making a distinction between stages 3 and 4. Hence for practical purposes these two stages are grouped together.
- Pars flaccida retractions have a vital role to play in the pathophysiology of cholesteatoma. Tos et al classified pars flaccida retraction in to four stages:

- **Stage I:** Pars flaccida is dimpled and is more retracted than normal. It is not adherent to the malleus.

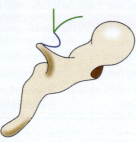

- **Stage II:** *In this stage the retraction pocket is adherent to the handle of malleus. The full extent of the retraction pocket can be clearly seen.*

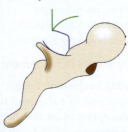

- **Stage III:** In this stage part of the retraction pocket may be hidden. There may also be associated erosion of the outer attic wall (scutum).

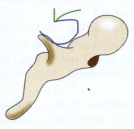

- **Stage IV:** In this stage there is definite erosion of the outer attic wall. The extent of the retraction pocket cannot be clearly seen as most of it are hidden from the view.

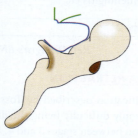

90. Ans. (d) Lateral sinus thrombophlebitis

Ref: Dhingra's ENT, 5th ed. pg. 94 and 84-86

- Lateral sinus thrombophlebitis is an inflammation of inner wall of lateral venous sinus with formation of thrombus.
- It occurs as a complication of acute coalescent mastoiditis, masked mastoiditis or chronic suppurative otitis media.

Intra cranial	Extra cranial
• Meningitis- **MC**	• Ossicular damage
• Lateral sinus thrombophlebitis	• Mastoiditis **(MC)**
• Sub dural abscess	• Gardenigo's syndrome

Intra cranial	Extra cranial
• Extra dural abscess	• Labyrinthine fistula/ Labyrinthitis
• Otitis hydrocephalus	• Petrositis
• Cerebral abscess (2ⁿᵈ MC)	• Facial nerve palsy
• Mn: Men Like S-Ex On Call	• Mn: OMG Lady Love Peters Face

91. Ans. (a) Brain abscess

Ref: Dhingra's ENT, 5th ed. pg. 84-86, 94

- MC Intracranial complication of CSOM Meningitis > Cerebral Abscess

Please refer to above explanation

92. Ans. (c) Mastoiditis

Ref: Dhingra's ENT 5th ed./ 84-86, 94

- Overall, MC complication of csom → Mastoiditis
- MC extracranial complication → Mastoiditis.

93. Ans. (a) Conductive hearing loss

Ref: Dhingra's ENT, 5th ed. pg. 83

Clinical features of Tubercular otitis media:
- **Painless foul smelling ear discharge:** Very characteristic finding.
- **Perforation:** Multiple perforations usually 2–3 on pars tensa is classical sign of disease.
- **Hearing loss:** There is a severe hearing loss, out of proportion to symptoms. **Mostly conductive**, it may be SNHL if labyrinth is involved.
- Facial paralysis
- In the presence of secondary pyogenic infection, tubercular otitis media may be indistinguishable from chronic suppurative otitis media. Culture of ear discharge for tubercle bacilli, histopathological examination of granulations and other evidence of tuberculosis in the body help to confirm the diagnosis.

ENT

Treatment

- **Systemic antitubercular therapy** as being carried for primary focus.
- **Local treatment** in the form of aural toilet and control of secondary pyogenic infection. Mastoid surgery is indicated for complications. Healing is delayed in tuberculous cases. Wound break-down and fistula formation are common.

---

94. Ans. (b) Multiple perforation of pars tensa

Ref: Dhingra's ENT, 5th ed. pg. 83

Please refer to above explanation

---

95. Ans. (a) Long process of incus

Ref: Dhingra's ENT, 5th ed. pg. 78 & 81

■ OSSICULAR NECROSIS IN OTITIS MEDIA

Dhingra States

- In case of tubo-tympanic CSOM *"ossicular chain is usually intact and mobile but may show some degree of necrosis, **particularly of the long process of incus"***
- In case of atticoantral type CSOM *"ossicular necrosis is common in atticoantral type of CSOM. **Destruction may be limited to the long process of incus** or may also involves stapes superstructure, handle of malleus or the entire ossicular chain"*

---

96. Ans. (b) CN V, VI

Ref: Dhingra's ENT, 6th ed. pg. 447

- Petrositis is inflammation of petrous bone.
- Gardenigo's syndrome results due to severe petrositis, which is a complication of CSOM (Chronic Suppurative Otitis Media).
- Two cranial nerves are involved in case of Gardenigo's syndrome: CN V and CN VI.
- **It is characterized by 3 D's:**
  - Discharge
  - Diplopia
  - Deep pain/retro-orbital pain
- Remember, there is NO Deafness in case of Gardenigo's syndrome.

---

97. Ans. (a) Deafness

Ref: Dhingra's ENT, 6th ed. pg. 447

---

98. Ans. (b) Bacteria

Ref: Dhingra's ENT, 5th ed. pg. 57-58

- Malignant otitis externa is caused by pseudomonas infection in elderly, diabetics & patients on the immune-compromised drugs.
- Early manifestation resembles diffuse otitis externa. Patients have severe pain and appearance of granulation in meatus.

Infectious Etiology of Ear Canal

Bacterial	Fungal	Viral
• Localized otitis externa • Diffuse otitis externa • Malignant otitis externa	• Otomycosis	• Herpes zoster oticus • Otitis externa hemorrhagica

---

99. Ans. (a) 7th

Ref: Dhingra's ENT, 6th ed. pg. 52-53

- Malignant otitis externa is an inflammatory condition caused by pseudomonas infection usually in elderly diabetic & those on immune-compromised drugs.
- Facial nerve paralysis is common.

---

100. Ans. (a) Herpes zoster virus

Ref: P.L. Dhingra, 5th ed. pg. 107

- In some cases of herpes zoster oticus, there is facial paralysis along with vesicular rash in the external auditory canal and pinna. This condition is called Ramsay Hunt Syndrome.
- **Treatment:** Acyclovir + Steroids

---

101. Ans. (c) Geniculate ganglion

Ref: Dhingra's ENT, 5th ed. pg. 102, 109

Course of Facial Nerve

- Motor fibres take origin from the nucleus of VIIth nerve. It leaves the brainstem at pontomedullary junction, travels through posterior cranial fossa and enters the internal acoustic meatus.
- Origin of facial nerve in inner ear is from geniculate ganglion. If there is a lesion at geniculate ganglion it can cause slow progressive facial palsy

Branches of Facial Nerve

- **Greater superficial petrosal nerve:** Arises from geniculate ganglion and carries secretomotor fibres to lacrimal gland and glands of nasal mucosa
- Nerve to stapedius
- Chorda tympani: Sensory to anterior 2/3rd of tongue and secretomotor fibres to sublingual and submandibular gland.
- Communicating branch

Explanations

- Posterior auricular nerve
- Muscular branch: To stylohyoid and posterior belly of digastric
- Peripheral branches.

102. Ans. (a) Otosclerosis

Ref: Dhingra, 5th Ed. pg. 461, 98-99

- **Schwartz sign** is a pink reflex, seen through intact tympanic membrane, in the area of oval window. It indicates active otosclerosis usually during pregnancy.
- Otosclerosis is an abnormal bone growth in the middle ear that causes conductive hearing loss.

Symptoms
- Hearing loss (CHL)
- **Paracusis willi**: An otosclerotic patient hears better in noisy surrounding.
- Tinnitus
- Vertigo
- Speech

Signs
- **Schwartz's sign**: A reddish hue seen on the promontory through the tympanic membrane. This is indicative of active focus with increased vascularity.
- Pure tone audiometry shows loss of air conduction, more for lower frequencies
- **Carhart's notch**: there is a sudden dip at 2000 Hz in bone conduction curve.

Extra Mile
- Don't get confused between schwartz sign and Schwartz surgery.
- Schwartz surgey is a simple mastoidectomy or cortical mastoidectomy in case of mastoiditis.

103. Ans. (c) 2000 Hz

- **Carhart Notch** is an audiogram finding and is an important feature in patients with Otosclerosis.
- There is a sudden dip (notch) at 2000 Hz in bone conduction curve.
- Carhart's notch disappears after stapedectomy.

104. Ans. (b) Tinnitus

Ref: Dhingra, 5th ed. pg. 120-121

- **GLOMUS TUMOR** is the most common benign neoplasm of middle ear and is so-named because of its origin from the glomus bodies.
- The tumor is often seen in the middle age (40–50 years)
- Females are affected five times more than males.
- There are two types of glomus tumor:
  - **Glomus jugulare** arise from the dome of jugular bulb. Invade the hypotympanum and jugular foramen.
    - They may compress jugular vein or invade its lumen
  - **Glomus tympanicum** arise from the promontory of the middle ear and cause aural symptoms and sometimes with facial paralysis.

Clinical Features
- **Earliest symptoms are tinnitus** and hearing loss.
  - Tinnitus is pulsatile and of swishing character.
  - Hearing loss is conductive and slowly progressive.
- Otoscopy shows a red reflex through intact tympanic membrane.
- **"Rising sun"** appearance is seen when tumor arises from the floor of middle ear.
- In addition to hearing loss and tinnitus, there is history of profuse bleeding from the ear either spontaneously or on attempts to clean it
- Dizzines or vertigo and facial paralysis may appear
- Ear ache is less common
- Otorrhea may occur due to secondary infection and the condition may simulate chronic suppurative otitis media with polyp.
- IXth to XIIth cranial nerves may be paralyzed
- There is dysphagia and hoarseness with unilateral paralysis of the soft palate, pharynx and vocal cord with weakness of the trapezius and sternomastoid muscles.
- **Rule of 10's** Remember that 10% of the tumors are familial, 10% multicentric and up to 10% functional, i.e. they secrete catecholamines.

105. Ans. (c) Meniere's disease

Ref: Dhingra's ENT, 6th ed. pg. 448

Meniere's disease aka Endolymphatic Hydrops is a condition which is characterized by triad of:
- Episodic Vertigo
- Sensorineural Hearing loss
- Tinnitus

Meniere's disease has some special features:
- **Hennebert's sign:** False positive fistula sign
- **Tulio's phenomenon:** Vertigo in noisy environment
- Diplacusis

106. Ans. (c) Diplacusis

Ref: PL Dhingra, 5th ed. pg. 112

WHY DIPLACUSIS IN MENIERE'S DISEASE?

- In the abnormal ear, neurons respond to a broader range of stimulus frequencies. But due to CNS preconditioning, the brain interprets any activity in a particular neuron as resulting from a stimulus of its normal characteristic frequency. Thus a single stimulus simultaneously processed by the normal and abnormal cochlea will be perceived as two different stimuli by the CNS, thus leading to diplacusis.

107. Ans. (b) Posterior semicircular canal

Ref: Dhingra's ENT, 6th ed. pg. 45-46

- BPPV is Benign Paroxysmal Positional Vertigo
- It occurs **due to an otolith in posterior semicircular canal,** which can result either due to head trauma, infection or drugs.
- This condition can be diagnosed by typical history and Dix- Hallpike Manoeuvre.
- This condition can be treated by Epley's Maneuver, where repositioning of otolith is done from posterior semicircular canal to Utricle.

108. Ans. (b) Carcinoma of tongue

Ref: Dhingra, 5th ed. pg. 240

- Referred pain in the ear is most likely due to carcinoma of tongue.
- Due to common nerve supply of the tongue (lingual nerve) and ear (auriculo temporal) from the mandibular division of the trigeminal nerve, a referred pain of tongue CA presents with ipsilateral ear pain.

CARCINOMA OF TONGUE

- Carcinoma involving anterior 2/3rd of tongue is commonly seen in men in the age group of 50-70 years.
- It may also develop on a pre-existing leukoplakia, long standing dental ulcer or syphilitic glossitis
- Most common type of tongue CA: Squamous cell type
- **Site: Most common site is middle of the lateral border** or the ventral aspect of the tongue

Clinical Presentation

- A submucous nodule with induration of the surrounding tissue.
- An exophytic lesion like a papilloma
- A non-healing ulcer with rolled edges, grayish white shaggy base and induration.

Symptomatology

- Early lesions are painless and remain asymptomatic for a long time
- Pain in the tongue locally at the site of ulcer
- **Pain in the ipsilateral ear:** Due to common nerve supply of the tongue (lingual nerve) and ear (auriculo temporal) from the mandibular division of the trigeminal nerve
- A lump in the mouth
- Enlarged lymph node mass in the neck
- Dysphagia, difficulty to protrude the tongue, slurred speech and bleeding from the mouth are late features.

109. Ans. (c) Sensorineural deafness

Ref: Dhingra's ENT, 6th ed. pg. 446-47

- Trotter's triad is seen in case of nasopharyngeal carcinoma. **It is also called Sinus of Morgagni Syndrome. Trotter's triad includes:**
  - Ipsilateral soft palate palsy (Due to CNX)
  - Conductive hearing loss (Due to ET obstruction)
  - Trigeminal neuralgia (Due to CN V).

110. Ans. (c) Sensorineural hearing loss

Ref: Dhingra's ENT, 5th ed. pg. 124

ACOUSTIC NEUROMA

- Acoustic neuroma is also known as vestibular schwannoma, neurilemmoma or eighth nerve tumor.
- It arises from superior division of vestibular nerve.
- The tumor arises from the Schwann cells of the vestibular, but rarely from the cochlear division of 8th nerve within the internal auditory canal.

Clinical Features

- **Age and sex:** Mostly seen in age group of 40-60 years. Both sexes are equally affected.
- **Cochleovestibular symptoms**
  - They are the earliest symptoms.
  - Most commonly manifests by Progressive unilateral sensorineural hearing loss, often accompanied by tinnitus.
  - Vestibular symptoms are imbalance or unsteadiness.
- **Cranial nerve involvement**
  - **Cranial nerve 5th is the earliest nerve to be involved** (after 8th)causing loss of corneal reflex
  - **MC clinical finding of acoustic** neuroma-loss of corneal reflex
  - CN 7th involvement: although rare, it causes numbness or paraesthesia of face
  - **Hitzelberger sign**: Hypoaesthesia around posterior auricular area (due to CN 7th involvement)
  - In CN 8th Sensory fibres are affected early.
  - **9th and 10th nerves:** There is dysphagia and hoarseness due to palatal, pharyngeal and laryngeal paralysis.
- **Brainstem involvement**
  - There is ataxia, weakness and numbness of the arms and legs with exaggerated tendon reflexes.
- **Cerebellar involvement**
  - Revealed by finger-nose test, knee-heel test, dysdiadochokinesia, ataxic gait, inability to walk along a straight line with tendency to fall to the affected side.
- **Raised intracranial tension**
- This is also a late feature.
- There is headache, nausea, vomiting, diplopia and papilloedema with blurring of vision.

111. Ans. (d) Crowding of lower tooth

Ref: Dhingra's ENT, 6th ed. pg. 243-44

- Enlargement of adenoid tonsils due to infection can lead to adenoid hypertrophy.

Clinical Features of Adenoid Hypertrophy

- Signs and symptoms of adenoid hypertrophy doesn't depend on the absolute size of the adenoid mass but are relative to the available space in the nasopharynx.
- This hypertrophy may cause nasal, aural or general symptoms.

A. Nasal Symptoms

- **Commonest symptom of adenoid hypertrophy: Nasal obstruction.**
- **Nasal discharge:** It is partly due to choanal obstruction, as the normal nasal secretions cannot drain into nasopharynx and partly due to associated chronic rhinitis. The child often has a wet bubbly nose.
- **Sinusitis:** Adenoid hypertrophy can lead to persistent nasal discharge and infection which can cause Chronic maxillary sinusitis. Reverse is also true that a primary maxillary sinusitis may lead to infected and enlarged adenoids.
- **Epistaxis:** When adenoids are acutely inflamed, epistaxis can occur with nose blowing.
- **Voice change:** Decreased nasality in voice *(Rhinolalia Clausa).*

B. Aural Symptoms

- **Tubal obstruction.** Adenoid mass blocks the eustachian tube leading to retracted tympanic membrane which causes conductive hearing loss.
- Persistence can cause Chronic suppurative otitis media which may fail to resolve due to presence of infected adenoids.
- **Serous otitis media:** The waxing and waning size of adenoids causes intermittent eustachian tube obstruction with fluctuating hearing loss.

C. General Symptoms

- **Adenoid facies:** Mouth breathing and Chronic nasal obstruction can lead to characteristic facial appearance called **adenoid facies.**
  - *In adenoid facies, the child has an elongated face with dull expression, open mouth,* **prominent crowded upper teeth***, and hitched up upper-lip,* **pinched-in nose appearance** *due to disuse atrophy of alae nasi.*
- **Highly arched hard palate** as the moulding action of the tongue on palate is lost. *This high arched hard palate can cause deviated nasal septum.*
- **Pulmonary hypertension:** Long-standing nasal obstruction due to adenoid hypertrophy can cause pulmonary hypertension and cor-pulmonale.

112. Ans. (d) Cleft palate

Ref: Dhingra, 5th ed. pg. 442

- **Adenoids**, also known as **pharyngeal tonsil**, or **nasopharyngeal tonsil**, are located at the back of the throat, above the tonsils, and are small lumps of tissue.
- They form part of the immune system of babies and young children.
- In case of their hyperplasia, there are several difficulties faced by patients like rhinousinusitis, mouth breathing, snoring etc.
- Adenoidectomy is surgical removal of adenoids to overcome those problems.

Indications and Contraindications of Adenoidectomy

Indications	Contraindications
• Adenoid hypertrophy causing snoring	• Cleft palate or submucous palate
• Mouth breathing sleep apnea syndrome or speech abnoramlities, i.e. (rhinolalia clausa)	• Removal of adenoids causes velopharyngeal insufficiency in such cases
• Recurrent rhinosinusitis	• Haemorrhagic diathesis
• Chronic secretory otitis media associated with adenoid hyperplasia	• Acute infection of upper respiratory tract.
• Recurrent ear discharge in benign CSOM associated with adenoiditis/adenoid hyperplasia	• Bleeding disorders
	• Allergic rhinitis
	• Polio epidemic
• Dental malocclusion	

113. Ans. (b) Allergic rhinitis

Ref: Dhingra's ENT, 6th ed. pg. 431-432

114. Ans. (b) Serous otitis media in children

Ref: Dhingra, 5th ed pg. 71-72

- Serous otitis media is also known as Glue ear.
- It is an insidious condition characterized by accumulation of non-purulent effusion in the middle ear cleft.
- One of common causes of serous otitis media (Glue ear) in children is blockage of Eustachian tube secondary to adenoid hyperplasia.
- Therefore, the treatment aims at removal of adenoid (adenoidectomy) and drainage of middle ear by grommet.
  - Grommet is a small tube inserted in tympanic membrane to drain the middle ear.

ENT

995

- Serous otitis media in adults should arouse suspicion of nasopharyngeal carcinoma and hence the treatment aims at removal of carcinoma
- Adenoiditis is an acute condition and requires treatment conservatively.

115. Ans. (b) Adenoidectomy

Ref: Dhingra's ENT, 6th ed. pg. 431-32

Please refer to the previous question for explanation.

116. Ans. (b) Temporalis fascia

Ref: Dhingra's ENT, 6th ed. pg. 29-30, 400

- Tympanoplasty is repairing of tympanic membrane in cases of ruptured tympanic membrane either due to infection or trauma.
- Temporalis fascia is used for tympanoplasty. It has very low basal metabolic rate, hence very high rate of survival of graft.

117. Ans. (a) Round window

Ref: Dhinga's ENT, 5th ed. pg. 138

- Cochlear implant is an electronic device that can provide useful hearing and improved communication abilities for a person with profound sensorineural hearing loss.
- **Cochlear implant consists of 2 components:**
  - **External component:** Include external speech processor and a transmitter. Speech processor may be body worn or behind the ear type.
  - **Internal component:** It is surgically implanted and comprises the receiver/stimulator package with an electrode array. Electrode array is **passed via round window** and is *inserted into the cochlea (scala tympani) deeper in skull.*

NOSE AND PARANASAL SINUSES

118. Ans. (c) Neck swelling

Ref: Diseases of ENT by Dhingra 6th ed. P 250-251

Nasopharyngeal cancer
- Commonly seen in chinese, elderly population (30 – 50/100,000 population)
- **MC site:** Fossa of Rosenmuller
- The tumor from fossa of Rosenmuller can grow in any direction.
  - Anterior: Can block Eustachean tube → CHL
  - Inferior: Can cause difficulty in deglutition
  - Superior: Can involve several cranial nerve if skull base is involved

- All cranial nerves can be affected (First CN involved: CN-VI)
- Frequently involved CN are V, VI, IX and X
- Involvement of nerve supplying ocular muscles are also seen

- **Symptoms:**
  - Neck mass: Due to cervical lymphadenopathy- most common clinical picture that patient present with
  - Trotter's triad: CHL, soft palate palsy, deep facial pain
  - Diplopia, nasal dysfunction, headache, etc.
- **WHO classification-on basis of histopathology**

Type I (25%)	Squamous cell carcinoma
Type II (12%)	Non-keratinising carcinoma • Without lymphoid stroma • With lymphoid stroma
Type III (63%)	Undifferentiated carcinoma • Without lymphoid stroma • With lymphoid stroma

- **Treatment:**
  - Radiotherapy is definitive treatment (it is most radiosensitive tumor of head and neck).

119. Ans. (c) CSF Rhinorrrhea

Ref: Dhingra's ENT 6th ed. P 305

- It is a case of CSF rhinorrhea due to cribriform plate fracture.
- Cribriform plate, which is a thin plate of bone, forms the roof of nose. In patients with trauma, there is clear watery nasal discharge with or without blood tinged.
- **Causes of CSF rhinorrhea:**
  - Trauma: Most common cause
  - Surgical: During FESS, transphenoidal surgery
  - Neoplasm invading the skull base
  - Infection and mucoceole of sinuses eroding bone and dura
  - Congenital: Meningocoele, meningoencephalocoele and glioma with skull base defect
- **Symptoms:**
  - Clear watery nasal discharge which cannot be sniffed back
  - Reservoir sign: When rising in morning CSF collected in sinuses on bending head.
  - Handkerchief sign: Handkerchief stiffens if it is due to nasal discharge due to its mucus content.
- **Investigation:**
  - Beta 2 transferrin: Most sensitive and specific.
  - HRCT: IOC
  - MRI: To locate site of leak and if any associated CNS pathology.
- **Treatment:**
  - Conservative treatment along with prophylactic antibiotics.

Explanations

FMGE Solutions Screening Examination

996

- Surgical repair if there is no relief from conservative management.

120. Ans. (c) Ammonia irritates trigeminal nerve

Ref: Physical Medicine and Rehabilitation, 4th ed. P 12

- The patient here is presenting with history of trauma, which can cause damage to olfactory nerve → leading to anosmia.
  - MC cranial nerve damaged in head trauma: Olfactory nerve
- Remember, for olfaction system two separate nerves are responsible:
  - CN I: Responsible for perception associated with quality of odour
  - CN V: Produces sensation of irritation or pungency
- Odour sensation from olfactory nerve usually do not produce physiological response. But sensation from trigeminal nerve can produce response such as runny nose, red eyes, sneezing when an irritant like ammonia/vinegar is detected.

121. Ans. (a) CSF rhinorrhea

Ref: Dhingra's ENT 6th ed. P 305

- It is a case of CSF rhinorrhea due to cribriform plate fracture.
- Cribriform plate, which is a thin plate of bone, forms the roof of nose. In patients with trauma, there is clear watery nasal discharge with or without blood tinged.
- **Symptom:**
  - Watery nasal discharge which cannot be sniffed back.
- **Investigation:**
  - **Beta 2 transferrin:** Most sensitive and specific.
  - **HRCT:** IOC.
  - **MRI:** To locate site of leak and if any associated CNS pathology.
- **Treatment:**
  - Conservative treatment along with prophylactic antibiotics
  - Surgical repair if there is no relief from conservative management.

122. Ans. (b) Atrophic rhinitis

Ref: Dhingra's ENT 6th ed. P 154

- Atrophic rhinitis is the chronic inflammation of nose characterized by atrophy of nasal mucosa and turbinate bone. This makes the nasal cavity roomy and filled with foul smelling nasal crust.
- **Pathology:** Ciliated columnar epithelium is lost and is replaced with stratified squamous type of epithelium.
- **Treatment:**
  - Alkaline nasal douching using Na^+ bicarbonate, Na^+ biborate and NaCl.

- Followed by local application of 25% glycerin → it inhibits the growth of proteolytic organisms.
- Antibiotics (streptomycin 1 g/day × 10 days)
- Surgery:
  - **Young's operation:** Complete closure of both nostrils by nasal flaps.
  - **Modified Young's operation:** Keep the nostrils partially open ~3 mm. Its efficacy is similar to Young's operation.
  - **Lautenslager operation:** Medicalization of lateral wall of nose
  - **Wittmack's operation:** It is the transposition of the parotid duct into the maxillary sinus for moistening the nasal cavity.
  - Submucosal Teflon paste injection.

123. Ans. (b) Anterior ethmoidal artery

Ref: Dhingra's ENT 6th ed. P 177

- Kiesselbach's plexus is the arterial plexus present at the anteroinferior part of septum just above the vestibule and the area is also known as Little's area.
- **Arteries of the plexus are:**
  - Sphenopalatine artery (branch of maxillary artery → Br. of external carotid artery)
  - Greater palatine artery (branch of maxillary artery → Br. of external carotid artery)
  - Superior labial artery (branch of facial artery → Br. of External carotid artery)
  - Anterior ethmoidal artery (branch of ophthalmic artery → Br. of internal carotid artery)

124. Ans. (c) Aspirin sensitivity, asthma, nasal polyp

Ref: Dhingra's ENT, 6th ed. pg. 240

- **Samter's triad** consists of nasal polyp, bronchial asthma and aspirin sensitivity.

125. **Ans. (b) Nasal drop withdrawal**

    Ref: Dhingra's ENT, 6th ed. pg. 170

    - Topical nasal decongestants can sometimes cause rebound phenomenon if used for long time, the condition is known as **rhinitis medicamentosa.**
    - **It is treated by:**
        - **Withdrawal of nasal drops**
        - Short course of systemic steroid therapy
        - Surgical reduction of turbinates in some cases if hypertrophied.

126. **Ans. (a) Squamous cell CA**

    Ref: Dhingra's ENT, 6th ed. pg. 205-206

    - Paranasal sinus CA most commonly affects males of age above 50 years.
    - **Most common paranasal sinus CA is squamous cell CA.** Rest are adenocarcinoma, adenoid cystic CA, melanomas and various other sarcomas.
    - Most common sinus associated with CA: **Maxillary sinus.**
    - Most common sinus CA among workers of furniture/wood industry: **Adenocarcinoma**

127. **Ans. (d) Supreme meatus**

    Ref: Dhingra's ENT, 6th ed. pg. 187-88

    - On the lateral wall of the nose are three turbinates and four meatuses.
    - **The inferior turbinate is the longest turbinate**
    - The supreme meatus is also called sphenoethmoidal recess

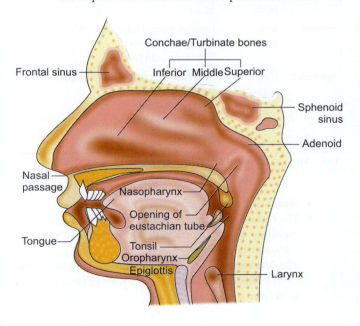

Ostia Opening in Meatuses

Meatus	Ostia
• Supreme meatus/Sphenoethmoidal recess	Sphenoid sinus ostia
• Superior meatus	Posterior ethmoidal sinus ostia
• Middle meatus	Has three ostias • Maxillary sinus • Frontal sinus • Anterior ethmoidal sinus
• Inferior meatus	**Has no Ostia.** It has Nasolacrimal duct opening

Remember: Direction of nasolacrimal duct is *downwards, backwards and outward.*

128. **Ans. (a) Inferior meatus**

    Ref: Dhingra's ENT, 6th ed. pg. 187-88

    - **Late**ral wall of the nose **contains inferior meatus** which has no ostia, **instead it has naso-lacrimal duct.** The nasolacrimal duct (sometimes called the tear duct) carries tears from the lacrimal sac into nasal cavity.
    - Inferior nasal meatus is partially covered by a mucosal fold called **valve of Hasner** or *plica lacrimalis*).

129. **Ans. (d) Inferior meatus of the nose**

    Ref: Dhingra's ENT, 6th ed. pg. 187-88

    Refer to above explanation

130. **Ans. (a) Middle meatus**

    Ref: Dhingra's ENT, 6th ed. pg. 173-75

    - ANTROCHOANAL POLYP most commonly seen in children. They are unilateral, usually arises from the mucosa of maxillary antrum near its accessory ostium, comes out of it & grows in the chonaa & nasal cavity.
    - Maxillary sinus opens into the middle meatus.

131. **Ans. (a) Sphenoid sinus**

    Ref: Dhingra's ENT, 6th ed. pg. 138

    - Spheno ethmoidal recess is situated above the superior turbinate. Sphenoid sinus opens into it.
    - Sphenoid sinus. It has an anterior part & posterior part.
        - **Anterior part:** Roof related to the olfactory tract, optic chiasma, frontal lobe while the lateral wall is related to optic nerve, internal carotid artery & maxillary nerve.
        - **Posterior part:** Roof is related to the pituitary gland in the sella turcica while each lateral wall is related to cavernous sinus, internal carotid artery and CN 3rd and all division of 5th nerve.

132. **Ans. (d) None**

    Ref: Dhingra's ENT, 6th ed. pg. 138-40

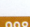

FMGE Solutions Screening Examination

- Please read the question carefully! The question is about the sinus opening.
- In inferior meatus there is no opening of any sinuses. *It has opening for nasolacrimal duct.*

133. Ans. (d) Posterior ethmoidal artery

Ref: Dhingra's ENT, 6th ed. pg. 147, Dhingra 4th ed. pg. 140

- Kiesselbach's area, aka Kiesselbach's plexus and Little's area, is an area on the nasal septum located on the antero-inferior part of the septum.
- In this area four arteries anastomose to form a vascular plexus called Kiesselbach's plexus.
- **The arteries are**
  1. Sphenopalatine artery (from the maxillary artery): **Main artery of plexus**
  2. Greater palatine artery (from the maxillary artery)
  3. Anterior ethmoidal artery (from the ophthalmic artery)
  4. Septal branch of the superior labial artery (from the facial artery)

> **Extra Mile**
> - Only artery of Kisselbach's plexus which is a branch of internal carotid artery: Anterior ethmoidal artery. The other three are branches of external carotid artery.
> - Most common site of epistaxis: Kisselbach's area/Little's area
> - **Artery of epistaxis: Sphenopalatine artery**
> - **Posterior epistaxis is from:** Woodruf's plexus (very difficult to control)
> - **Woodruf's Plexus:** Situated in the posterior part of meatus. Formed when sphenopalatine artery anastomosis with postpharyngeal artery.

134. Ans. (c) Anterior ethmoidal artery

Ref: Dhingra's ENT, 6th ed. pg. 147-48

- Anterior and posterior Ethmoid artery is a branch of ophthalmic artery, which is derived from internal carotid artery.
- It is only anterior ethmoidal artery (of internal carotid) which contributes to little's area.
- **Branches from external carotid artery** *(indirectly)* **contributing to little's area:** Sphenopalatine artery, Greater palatine artery and superior labial artery.

135. Ans. (d) Hereditary hemorrhagic telangiectasia

Ref: Dhingra's ENT, 6th ed. pg. 176-77

ETIOLOGY OF EPISTAXIS

- One of the most common local causes is trauma, due to nose picking or fractures.
- Some of the other local causes include nasal sprays, inflammatory reactions, anatomical deformities (i.e. septal deviation, septal spurs), foreign bodies, intranasal tumors, chemical irritants, and nasal prongs for oxygen. Systemic causes include hypertension, vascular disorders, blood dyscrasias, hematologic malignancies, allergies, malnutrition, alcohol, drugs, and infection.
- Hereditary Hemorrhagic Telangiectasia is a rare cause causing bleeding. This is also known as **Osler-Weber-Rendu disease** and an **autosomal dominant** disease.

> **Extra Mile**
> - MCC of epistaxis overall: Trauma
> - MCC of epistaxis in adult: Trauma
> - MCC of epistaxis in elderly: Hypertension
> - MCC of epistaxis in child: Digital trauma from nose picking.

136. Ans. (a) Olfactory epithelium

Ref: Dhingra's ENT, 6th ed. pg. 204

- **Esthesioneuroblastoma** usually arise from the olfactory epthelium. It's a rare tumor of any age group.
- **Presentation of tumor:** cherry red, polypoidal spots mass in upper third of nasal cavity. It is a vascular tumor that bleeds profusely on biopsy.

137. Ans. (c) Sphenoid sinus

Ref: Dhingra, 5th ed. pg. 203

TABLE: Development and growth of paranasal sinuses

Sinuses	Status at birth	Growth	First radiologic evidence
Maxillary	Present at birth	Rapid growth from birth to 3 years and from 7-12 years. Adult size-15 yrs	4-5 months after birth
Ethmoid	Present at birth	Reach Adult size by 12 years	1 years
Frontal	Not present	Invades frontal bone at the age of 4 years. Size increases until teens	6 years
Sphenoid	Not present	Reaches sella turcica by the age of 7 years. **Reaches full size between 15 years to adult age**	4 years

138. Ans. (c) Frontal sinus

Ref: Dhingra, 5th ed. pg. 203

- *Please refer to above table*
- The first sinus that starts to develop in human embryo is maxillary sinus. It starts to develop around 10 weeks of intra-uterine life.
- *The last sinus to develop in human embryo is frontal sinus. This sinus is absent at the time of birth & starts to develop postnatally.*

ENT

- Frontal sinus can be visualized radiologically at 6 yrs of age.

139. Ans. (c) 6 years

Ref: Dhingra, 5th ed. pg. 203

140. Ans. (c) 15 years

Ref: Dhingra, 5th ed. pg. 203

141. Ans. (d) 12 years

Ref: Dhingra, 5th ed. pg. 203

142. Ans. (b) Maxillary sinus

Ref: Dhingra, 5th ed. pg. 203-204

- Maxillary sinus is largest sinus with volume of around 15 cc.

143. Ans. (b) Maxillay sinusitis

Ref: Dhingra's ENT, 6th ed. pg. 411-12

- **Most common sinus involved in sinusitis: Maxillary sinus** (aka Antrum of Highmoore)
- Treatment of acute cases is by antibiotics and symptomatic.
- Chronic cases and recurrent cases are treated by surgery. Usually performed surgeries are:
- Antral wash
- **Caldwell-Luc operation**
- FESS (Functional Endoscopic Sinus Surgery)- Most preferred currently. Best surgical option

Caldwell Luc operation Indications:	Technique
- In case of chronic maxillary sinusitis - Dental cyst or Oro-antral fistula - Fracture of maxilla or blow out fracture of orbit - Antrochoanal polyp	- Horizontal Incision below gingivolabial sulcus - Elevation of flap à Opening of Antrum à Removal of deseased antral mucosa/polyp - Making of naso-antral window - Packing the antrum à Closure of wound

144. Ans. (a) Atrophic rhinitis

Ref: Dhingra, 5th ed. pg. 170

ATROPHIC RHINITIS (OZAENA)

- **Etiology** (Remember Mnemonic HERNIA)
  - **H**ereditary factors
  - **E**ndocrinal disturbance: Disease usually starts at puberty, involves females more than males.
  - **R**acial factors: White and yellow races are more susceptible than equatorial African natives.

- **N**utritional deficiency. Disease may be due to deficiency of vitamin A, D or iron
- **I**nfective.
  - **Kelbsiella ozaenae: Most common cause**
  - Diphtheroids, P. vulgaris, Esch. coli, staphylococci and Streptococci

Clinical Features

- Foul smell from the nose
- **Merciful anosmia**
- **Nasal obstruction:** *Due to large crusts filing the nose*
- Epistaxis: May occur when the crusts are removed

Treatment

Medical: Nasal irrigation and removal of crusts by Alakaline Douche- **Best Treatment**

- **Alakaline nasal douche** is prepared from (**in ratio of 1:1:2):**
  - Sodium bicarbonate
  - Sodium biborate
  - Sodium chloride

Surgical

- **Young's operation:** Both the nostrils are closed completely just within the nasal vestibule by raising flaps. They are opened after 6 months.
- **Modified young operation:** To avoid the discomfort of bilateral nasal obstruction, modified Young's operation aims to partially close the nostrils.

145. Ans. (d) Crusting

Ref: Dhingra, 5th ed. pg. 170

Please refer to above explanation

146. Ans. (b) Lymphadenopathy

Ref: Dhingra's ENT, 6th ed. pg. 446-47

NASOPHARYNGEAL CARCINOMA

- Nasopharyngeal carcinoma is caused by **Ebstein Barr virus (EBV).**
- It is seen most commonly in Chinese population or South East Asian peoples.
- Most common site of nasopharyngeal carcinoma: **Fossa of Rosenmuller.**
  - This is a pyramidal shaped fossa on the lateral wall of nasopharynx.
- The most common type of nasopharyngeal carcinoma is undifferentiated carcinoma of nasopharyngeal type.

Clinical Presentation

- The most common presentation is cervical lymphadenopathy.

Explanations

FMGE Solutions Screening Examination

- Other important presentations are
  - Nasal obstruction
  - Nasal bleeding
  - Unilateral glue ear in adult leading to conductive hearing loss.
  - Cranial nerve palsies. *All the nerves from 3rd to 12th may be involved.*
- **Trotter's triad** seen in case of nasopharyngeal carcinoma. It is also called Sinus of Morgagni Syndrome.
  - Ipsilateral soft palate palsy
  - Conductive hearing loss
  - Trigeminal neuralgia.

147. Ans. (b) Rhinoscleroma

Ref: Dhingra's ENT, 5th ed. pg. 172

RHINOSCLEROMA

- Caused by gram negative coccobacillus- Klebsiella Rhinoscleromatis.
- **It passess through 3 stages:** Catarrhal, Granulomatous and Cicatricial.
- It causes woody infiltration of upper lip, so it is also known as Woody Nose.
- Upon biopsy characteristic cells seen are: Miculicz's cell and Russel Bodies.
- Tx: Streptomycin (1 g/day) and tetracycline (2 g/day) are given together for 4-6 weeks.

RHINOPHYMA

- It is due to hypertrophy of sebaceous glands of nasal tip.
- Associated with Acne Rosacea.
- Nose becomes big and ugly, hence also known as Potato Nose.

RHINOLITH

- It is old, calcified foreign body in nose.
- Present with foul smelling, one sided yellowish nasal discharge.

RHINOSPORIDIOSIS

- Caused by Rhinosporidiosis Seeberi
- *Present as strawberry/mulberry polyp in the nose.*
- It has very higher tendency to bleed. Hence also known as Bleeding Polyp.

148. Ans. (a) Hypertrophy of sebaceous gland

Ref: PL Dhingra, 5th ed. pg. 159, 461

RHINOPHYMA/POTATO NOSE/RUM NOSE/COPPER'S NOSE/TOPPER'S NOSE/BRANDY NOSE

- Benign tumor due to **hypertrophy of sebaceous glands of tip of nose.**
- Seen in cases of long-standing **acne rosacea.**
- Precipitated by: Spicy food, Heat, Alcohol
- **Treatment: Laser (CO_2) Excision with skin grafting and Avoidance of alcohol.**

149. Ans. (d) Protozoa

Ref: Dhingra's ENT, 6th ed. pg. 158-59

- Currently rhinosporidiosis is considered as a protozoal infection caused by **RHINOSPORIDIOSIS SEEBERI.** It is most commonly seen in the coastal parts of the world, most commonly in India, Pakistan and Sri Lanka. In india most commonly reported from the coastal part Tamil Nadu.
- It most commonly infects nose and nasopharynx. Other sites: Lip, Palate, conjunctiva, brochi, skin, vulva, vagina.
- It presents as polypoid mass which bleeds easily on touch, hence also known as Bleeding polyp.
- According to very recent papers, it is classified as **aquatic protist**

Treatment
- **Medical:** Dapsone
- **Surgical:** Complete excision of mass with diathermy knife and cauterization of base

150. Ans. (b) Rhinoscleroma

Ref: Dhingra's ENT, 6th ed. pg. 156-57, 5th ed. pg. 172

RHINOSCLEROMA

- It is a chronic granulomatous disease caused by gram negative coccobacillus-**Klebsiella Rhinoscleromatis.**
- It has 3 stages:
  - **Catarrhal or atrophic stage:** characterized by foul smelling purulent nasal discharge and crusting *(causing obstruction). This stage resembles atrophic rhinitis.*
  - **Granulomatous stage:** In this stage there are painless and non-ulcerative granulomatous nodules in nasal mucosa. *There is also subdermal infiltration of lower part of external nose and upper lip giving a 'woody' feel.*
  - **Cicatricial stage:** The last stage which causes adverse conditions like stenosis of nares, distortion of upper lip, adhesions in the nose, nasopharynx and

ENT

oropharynx. There may be subglottic stenosis with respiratory distress.
- Rhinoscleroma causes woody infiltration of nose, so it is also known as **Woody Nose.**
- Characteristic cells upon biopsy are: **Miculicz's cell and Russel Bodies.**
- **Treatment:** Streptomycin (1g/day) and tetracycline (2g/day) are given together for 4-6 weeks.

151. Ans. (c) Granulomatous stage

Ref: Dhingra's ENT, 6th ed. pg. 156-57, 5th ed. pg. 172

152. Ans. (b) Bacteria

Ref: Dhingra's ENT, 6th ed. pg. 156-57
Please refer to above explanation for more details.

153. Ans. (c) Nasal bone

Ref: Dhingra's ENT, 6th ed. pg. 147-148

- **Facial trauma,** also called **maxillofacial trauma,** is any physical trauma to the face.
- Commonly injured facial bones include the nasal bone, maxilla, and the mandible. The mandible may be fractured at its symphysis, body, angle, ramus, and condyle.
- *Nasal fracture is the most common facial fracture, and the third most common fracture of the skeleton overall.*
- Facial fractures occur for a variety of reasons related to sports participation: Contact between players (eg, a head, fist, elbow); contact with equipment (eg, balls, pucks, handle bars); or contact with the environment, obstacles, or a playing surface (e.g., wrestling mat, gymnastic equipment, goalposts, trees).
- Facial fractures may be associated with head and cervical spine injuries and it requires a significant amount of force.

154. Ans. (b) Vertical fracture

Ref: Dhingra's ENT, 6th ed. pg. 147-48

- There are two main types of fracture of septum namely: Chevallet and Jarjavay fracture

TABLE: Fracture of nasal septum

Fracture	Injury type	Impact of force
Chevallet fracture	Vertically	From below
Jarjavay fracture	Horizontally	From front

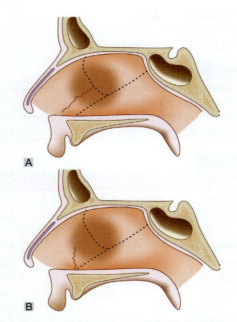

FIGURE: Fracture showing (A) Jarjaway type (B) Chevallet type

155. Ans. (c) Front

Ref: Dhingra's ENT, 6th ed. pg. 147-48

156. Ans. (a) Neck of condyle

Ref: Dhingra's ENT, 6th ed. pg. 185

- Neck of condyle is the most common site of fracture of mandible followed by angle of mandible.

THROAT/PHARYNX

157. Ans. (a) Quinsy

Ref: Diseases of ENT by Dhingra 6th ed. P 265

- **Quinsy is** peritonsillar abscess where crypta magna gets infected and sealed off leading to intratonsillar abscess which then burst through tonsillar capsule leading to collection of pus in peritonsillar tissues → Peritonsillar abscess.
- **MC organism:** *Streptococcus pyogenes, Staph aureus*
- **Symptoms:** Severe throat pain, odynophagia (refusal to eat), halitosis, hot potato voice, ipsilateral earache
- **Upon examination:** Congested tonsil with edematous pillar, contralateral deviation of uvula

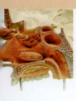

FMGE Solutions Screening Examination

- **Treatment:**
  - IV antibiotics and fluid
  - Surgical drainage by incision

> **Extra Mile**
> - **Infection in pretracheal space** can lead to is dangerous and can compress major vessels, lower airways and upper digestive tract. Infection in this space is secondary to thyroiditis or perforation of anterior cervical esophagus.
> - **Retropharyngeal abscess** patient can present with dysphagia, difficulty in breathing, stridor, croupy cough and torticollis (neck become stiff). Upon examination- bulge in the posterior pharyngeal wall usually seen on one side of midline.

> **Extra Mile**
>
> | | Croup | Epiglottitis | Bacterial tracheitis | Retro-pharyngeal abscess |
> |---|---|---|---|---|
> | Peak age | 1-2 years | 2-7 years | 1-6 years | 1-5 years |
> | Onset | Gradual (days) | Sudden (hours) | Gradual (days) with progressive worsening | Gradual (days) with progressive worsening |
> | Prodromal URTI | Yes | Minimal, short | Yes | Yes |
> | Fever | Low grade | High grade | Variable severity | High grade |
> | Cough | Barking | Minimal, muffled | Barking, croup-like | Minimal |
> | Stridor | Harsh | Soft, may become inaudible | Harsh | Variable (20-71% cases) |
> | Discriminating features | Well child; worsens at night | Drooling: leans forward in 'tripod' posture | Painful swallow; poor response to croup treatment | Painful swallow; neck stiffness or torticollis |
>
> URTI = Upper Respiratory Tract Infection

158. Ans. (a) Palatoglossus

- The hypoglossal nerve (CN- XII) runs inferior to the tongue and innervates tongue muscles.
- All the intrinsic and extrinsic muscles of tongue (genioglossus, styloglossus, hyoglossus) is supplied by CN-XII except palatoglossus.
- Palatoglossus is supplied by CN- X

> **Extra Mile**
>
> **Sensory supply of tongue**
> - **Anterior 2/3rd:**
>   - General sensation: Lingual nerve
>   - Special sensation: Chorda tympani (branch of CN- VII)
> - **Posterior 1/3rd:**
>   - General and special sensation: Glossopharyngeal nerve
> - **Base of tongue:**
>   - General and special sensation: Internal laryngeal nerve

159. Ans. (a) Lateral sinus thrombophlebitis

Ref: Diseases of ENT by Dhingra 6th ed. P 84-85

- Lateral sinus thrombophlebitis is an intracranial complication of CSOM.
- The patient usually present with intermittent high grade fever termed as hectic picket fence fever associated with rigor, chills, headache.

Other clinical features:
- Anemia
- Thrombocytopenia
- Papilledema
- **Griesinger sign:** Edema over posterior part of mastoid, due to thrombosis of mastoid emissary veins.
- **Tobey- Ayer test:** If internal jugular vein compressed on healthy side, there is rise in CSF pressure.
- **Crowe- Beck test:** Pressure applied on the jugular vein of healthy side produces engorgement of retinal veins and supraorbital veins (because of thrombosed opposite side).

160. Ans. (d) Aphthous ulcer

Ref: Diseases of ENT by Dhingra 6th ed. P218

- **Apthous ulcer** can be due to autoimmune process, nutritional deficiency of Vitamin B12, folic acid and iron, infection, stress or food allergy.
- **Site:** mucosa of inner surface of lips and buccal mucosa, tongue, floor of mouth, soft palate
- **Spares** mucosa of hard palate and gingiva.
- **Occur in 2 forms:**
  - Minor form: 2–10 mm; multiple in number with central necrotic area and a red halo; heals without any scar in 2 weeks.
  - Major form: 2–4 cm; heals with a scar

- **Treatment:**
  - Topical application of steroids
  - Cauterization with 10% silver nitrate
  - In severe cases: 250 mg of tetracycline dissolved in 50 ml water → given as mouth rinse then to be swallowed (4 times/day)
  - Lignocaine viscous: For local pain

Extra Mile

- Erosive form of **lichen planus** can be a premalignant lesion. There is painful erosion of buccal mucosa, gigiva or lateral tongue surrounded by a keratotic periphery.
  - Malignant potential: 0.4 to 3.7%
- **Chronic hypertrophic candidiasis** aka candidial leukoplakia.
  - MC site: anterior buccal mucosa just behind angle of mouth
  - It appears as white patch that cannot be wiped off
- **Oral submucal fibrosis** mostly associated with betel-nut chewing. Alcohol further increases the risk by 2 fold.
  - It is a premalignant condition. Malignant transformation is seen in 3 – 7.6% of cases
  - Leukoplakia and squamous cell CA is associated with submucous fibrosis, possible due to common etiological factors involved

TABLE: Some premalignant lesion and conditions

Premalignant lesions	Premalignant conditions
• Erythroplakia (aggressive)	• Oral submucous fibrosis
• Leukoplakia	• Oral lichen planus
• Candidiasis	• Actinic keratosis
• Carcinoma in situ	• Syphilis
• Leukokeratosis nicotina palatinae	• Discoid lupus erythematosus
	• Sideropenic dysphagia

161. Ans. (a) Chemoradiation

Ref: Dhingra's ENT 6th ed. P 252

- Nasopharyngeal carcinoma is the most common malignant carcinoma (CA) of nasopharyngeal area and is most commonly seen in Chinese population.

TREATMENT OF NASOPHARYNGEAL CA:

- **Stage I and II:** Radiotherapy is the treatment of choice.
- **Stage III and IV:** Radiotherapy + chemotherapy.
- **Book states:** "Stage III and IV CA can be cured by radiotherapy alone, but cure rate is doubled when chemotherapy is combined with radiotherapy".
- Cisplatin or cisplatin + 5FU is used for chemotherapy.

MUST KNOW QUESTIONS ABOUT NASOPHARYNGEAL CA:

- **Most common site for nasopharyngeal CA:** Fossa of Rosenmüller
- Most common type of nasopharyngeal carcinoma is Type III (63%).

- **Trotter's triad** is associated with nasopharyngeal CA includes: Conductive hearing loss, soft palate palsy and deep facial pain.
- First cranial nerve (CN) to be affected is: CN VI (Abducens nerve).
- Nasopharyngeal CA can involve multiple cranial nerves like II, III, IV, V, VI, IX, X, XI, XII.
- Involvement of CN IX, X, XI causes *jugular foramen syndrome*.

162. Ans. (a) Aspiration

Ref: Dhingra's ENT 6th ed. P 326

- External branch of superior laryngeal nerve supplies cricothyroid and is mainly responsible for pitch of the voice.
- If it is injured, it causes bowing and inferior placement of vocal cord with consequent loss of pitch.

163. Ans. (a) Cricothyroid

Ref: Dhingra's ENT 6th ed. P 284, 298

- All the muscles of larynx are supplied by either recurrent laryngeal nerve or superior laryngeal nerve.
- External branch of **superior laryngeal nerve supplies cricothyroid muscle** and is mainly responsible for pitch of the voice. Rest all the muscles are supplied by recurrent laryngeal nerve (RLN).
- Right RLN arises from the vagus at the level of subclavian artery, hooks around it and then ascends between the trachea and esophagus.
- Left recurrent laryngeal nerve arises from vagus and hooks around arch of aorta, loose around it and then ascends into the neck in tracheoesophageal groove.
- The left RLN has much longer course and is more prone to injury and paralysis as compared to right side.

164. Ans. (c) Glottis level

Ref: Dhingra's ENT 6th ed. P 295

- Laryngeal web is due to incomplete recanalization of larynx.
- Most common site of this web is between the vocal cords (at the glottis level) and has a concave posterior margin.
- **Clinical features:**
  - Airway obstruction
  - Weak cry
  - Aphonia (dating from birth)
- **Treatment:**
  - **If thin webs:** Cut with a knife or CO_2 laser
  - **Thick web:** Excision via laryngofissure and placement of a silicon keel and subsequent dilatation.

FIGURE: Laryngeal web

165. Ans. (a) Quincy

Ref: Dhingra's ENT 6th ed. P 265

QUINCY

- It is collection of pus in the peritonsillar space, which lies between the tonsillar capsule and superior constrictor muscle.
- It usually follows acute tonsillitis, though it may arise de novo as well.
- **MCC:** *Streptococcus pyogenes, Staphylococcus aureus.*
- **Symptoms:**
  - Acute onset high grade fever
  - Severe throat pain, usually unilateral
  - Marked odynophagia; patients are even unable to swallow their own saliva
  - **Muffled voice,** often **called hot potato voice**
  - Foul breath due to sepsis in oral cavity
  - Trismus and ipsilateral earache.
- **Signs:**
  - Swollen/enlarged tonsil
  - Swollen uvula and pushed to opposite side
  - Soft palate and anterior pillar bulging
  - Cervical lymphadenopathy.
- **Treatment:**
  - IV fluids + antibiotics + analgesics + oral hygiene
  - Surgery:
    - Incision and drainage
    - Interval tonsillectomy (I/D → then tonsillectomy after 4–6 weeks).

> **Extra Mile**
> - **Parapharyngeal and acute retropharyngeal abscess** is usually seen in children below 3 years. Symptoms can be dysphagia, stridor, bulge in posterior pharyngeal wall.

166. Ans. (c) HPV

Ref: Dhingra's ENT 6th ed. P 305

- Juvenile papillomatosis also known as respiratory papillomatosis is the most common benign neoplasm of larynx in the children.
- It is most commonly caused by **HPV type 6 and 11.**
- Affected children acquire this infection at birth itself from the mothers who had vaginal HPV virus infection.
- Papilloma's mostly affects supraglottic and glottic region of larynx but can also involve subglottis, trachea and bronchi.
- **Symptoms:** Hoarseness, aphonia, respiratory difficulty, stridor.
- **Treatment:** CO_2 laser surgery.

167. Ans. (c) Carcinoma of pyriform sinus

Ref: Dhingra's ENT, 6th ed. pg. 273

Pyriform Sinus Carcinoma

- It is the most common hypopharyngeal cancer
- Mostly affect males above 40 years of age. The growth is asymptomatic for long time due to large size of the pyriform sinus.
- It can spread locally or via lymphatic spread.
- Most common and first lymph node involved: Cervical lymph node.

Clinical feature:

- Patient usually describes it as "something sticking in throat and pricking sensation" while swallowing. It is also the **earliest symptom**.
- **First sign: Mass of lymph nodes** high up in the neck
- Referred otalgia, pain on swallowing and increasing dysphagia are other symptoms which may follow.

IOC: Endoscopic biopsy
Treatment:
- If no nodal involvement: Radiotherapy
- If nodal involvement: Surgery

> **Extra Mile**
> **Postcricoid carcinoma** arises from postcricoid region and most commonly affects females in early 20's–30's. Its most common presenting symptom is progressive dysphagia.

168. Ans. (a) Palatopharyngeus

Ref: Dhingra's ENT, 6th ed. pg. 240

- **Passavant ridge** is a mucosal ridge raised by fibres of palatopharyngeus.
- It encircles the posterior and lateral walls of nasopharyngeal isthmus

ENT

- **Advantage of ridge:** Soft palate while contraction makes a firm contact with this ridge to cut off Nasopharynx from the oropharynx during speech or deglutition.

169. Ans. (b) Laryngomalacia

Ref: Dhingra's ENT, 6th ed. pg. 295

TABLE: Different shape of glottis and conditions

Finding	Condition
Key hole shaped glottis	Phonasthenia
Omega shaped glottis	Laryngomalacia
Thumb sign	Acute epiglottitis
Steeple sign	Croup/Laryngotracheobronchitis
Turban shaped glottis	Laryngeal TB

170. Ans. (c) Analgesic with antibiotic and drainage

Ref: Dhingra's ENT, 6th ed. pg. 264-65

Treatment of Peritonsillar Abscess (Quinsy)

- IV fluids to cover dehydration
- Antibiotics to cover both aerobic and anerobic organisms
- Analgesics to relieve pain
- Oral hygiene
- Incision and drainage of abscess
- Interval tonsillectomy: Tonsils are removed 4–6 weeks following attack of quinsy.

171. Ans. (c) Burn of head and neck

Ref: Dhingra's ENT, 6th ed. pg. 316

- Burn of face and neck can lead to airway edema and will require a planned tracheostomy. Elective tracheostomy can be therapeutic to relieve respiratory obstruction, remove tracheobronchial secretions. Prophylactic tracheostomy is done to guard against anticipated respiratory obstruction or aspiration of blood.
- **Elective tracheostomy** also known as routine tracheostomy is a planned, unhurried procedure. It is done when all surgical facilities are available, endotracheal tube can be put and local or general anesthesia can be given.

172. Ans. (a) Carcinoma larynx

Ref: Dhingra's ENT, 6th ed. pg. 316

- Tracheostomy can be divided into: High, Mid or Low
  - **High tracheostomy** is done above the level of thyroid isthmus. It violates the 1st ring of trachea. Only indication for high tracheostomy is CA larynx, because in such cases total larynx would ultimately be removed and in a lower down area, a fresh tracheostome is made.
  - **Mid tracheostomy** is the preferred one. Done through 2nd or 3rd ring by dividing or retracting isthmus upwards.
- **Low tracheostomy** is done below the level of isthmus. Diptheria is a common indication.

173. Ans. (d) Speech therapy plus PPI

Ref: Dhingra's ENT, 6th ed. pg. 303

- The given condition is a case of singer's nodule also known as screamer's nodule.
- It is medically treated with **speech/voice therapy** and PPI should be added to relieve GERD, which might be an aggravating factor for the patient.
- For large nodules or long standing nodules, surgery (Microscopic laryngeal surgery) may be required.

174. Ans. (a) Lower part of thyroid cartilage

Ref: Dhingra's ENT, 6th ed. pg. 285

- Infants larynx is small and conical. The diameter of cricoid cartilage is smaller than size of glottis, making **subglottis the narrowest part.**
- Cricoid cartilage is located at the lower part of thyroid cartilage, hence it is the best answer of choice given these options.

TABLE: Difference between pediatric and adult larynx

	Infant	Adult
Anatomical level of glottis	C2-C3	C3-C6
Shape	Conical	Tubular
Narrowest at	Subglottis	Glottis
Functional difference	Can swallow and breath at same time (due to high positioning)	Can not swallow and breath at the same time
Cartilage	Softer	Soft

175. Ans. (d) Bilateral mobile lymph nodes >6 cm

Ref: Diseases of ENT, by Dhingra, 6th ed. pg. 308

FMGE Solutions Screening Examination

TABLE: Tumor staging

Tumor	Node	Metastasis
T1- One focal area involved T2- 2-3 area involved T3- Pre-epiglottic, Para-Glottic, Paralysis of VC, Posterior cricoid space T4- Trachea, Tongue base muscle Thyroid muscle	N0- No LN involved N1- <3 cm, single, 1/L N2a: 3–6 cm single, 1/L N2b: 3–6 cm multiple, 1/L N$_2$C: 3–6, multiple, B/L N$_3$: >6 cm	M0: no mets M1: + Mets Mx: Can not be assessed

176. Ans. (c) Posterior cricoarytenoid

Ref: P.L. Dhingra, 6th ed. pg. 283-84

Movement	Muscles	Nerve supply
Abduction of vocal cords	Posterior cricoarytenoids only	Recurrent laryngeal nerve
Adduction of the vocal cords	• Lateral cricoarytenoids • Interarytenoids • Thyroarytenoids (external part)	Recurrent laryngeal nerve
Tensor of vocal cords	• Cricothyroid • Vocalis (internal part, part of Thyroarytenoid)	Superior laryngeal nerve
Relaxor of vocal cord	Thyroarytenoid	Recurrent laryngeal nerve
Elevation of larynx	Thyrohyoid, mylohyoid	
Depression of larynx	Sternothyroid, sternohyoid	

177. Ans. (b) Laryngeal TB

Ref: Diseases of ENT, by Dhingra, 6th ed. pg. 293

- Laryngeal TB is always secondary. It is primary most commonly from lungs.
- Most commonly involved part: Posterior wall
- First part to get affected in case of laryngeal TB: **Interarytenoid fold**
- **Important Features:**
  - **Turban epiglottis**—due to pseudo edema
  - **Mouse nibbled appearance:** Due to ulceration of vocal cord
- **Cobble stone appearance**

178. Ans. (c) Peri-tonsillar abscess

Ref: Dhingra's ENT, 5th ed. pg. 279

- Hot potato voice is muffled and thick speech.
- MCC of hot potato voice is **Quincy (peritonsillar abscess)**, which is an extremely painful condition.
- However it can also be seen in conditions like CA tonsil and streptococcus pharyngitis.

179. Ans. (c) Subglottis

Ref: Diseases of ENT, by Dhingra, 6th ed. pg. 285

TABLE: Difference between infant and adult larynx

Features	Infant/Child	Adult
Anatomical level	C2–C3	C3–C6
Shape	Conical	Tubular
Narrowest at	Subglottis	Glottis
Important feature	Can swallow and breath at the same time	Can not swallow and breath at the same time
Cartilage	Softer	Soft

▶ **Extra Mile**

TABLE: Difference between male and female larynx

Features	Male	Female
Length	44 mm	36 mm
AP diameter	43 mm	41 mm
Transverse diameter	36 mm	26 mm

180. Ans. (c) Young males

Ref: Dhingra's ENT, 5th ed. pg. 261

"Nasopharyngeal angiofibroma is seen almost exclusively in ADOLESCENT **males in the age group of 10-20 years.**"

ABOUT NASOPHARYNGEAL ANGIOFIBROMA

- It is a vascular tumor with lots of fibrous tissue without muscular coat. Hence it causes severe bleeding because of inability to contract.
- **Most common benign tumour** of nasopharynx.
- Arises from the posterior part of nasal cavity close to superior margin of **sphenopalatine foramen.**
- **Frog face deformity**—if tumor Extends to orbit and causes proptosis
- **Antral/Holman-Millar sign**—Anterior bowing of posterior wall of maxillary sinus is pathognomonic.
- Investigation of choice is **C.E.C.T.** scan
- Treatment of choice is **surgical excision.**

181. Ans. (b) Angiofibroma

Ref: Dhingra's ENT, 5th ed. pg. 261

ENT

182. Ans. (a) Tonsils

Ref: Dhingra's ENT, 6th ed. pg. 257-58

- Crypts are inward folding of the mucosa which are found in tonsils and they increase the surface area.
- Crypts are also seen in small intestine.

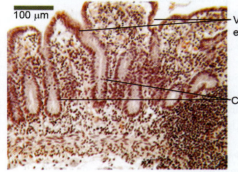

183. Ans. (b) Oral cavity of patient for intubation

- Mallampati score, also known as Mallampati classification is used to assess the oral cavity of patient to predict the ease of intubation.
- It is assessed by looking at the anatomy of the oral cavity; specifically, it is based on the visibility of the base of soft palate, uvula, fauces, and pillars.
- A high Mallampati score (class 3 or 4) is associated with more difficult intubation as well as a higher incidence of sleep apnea.

MODIFIED MALLAMPATI SCORING

- Class I: Soft palate, uvula, fauces, pillars visible.
- Class II: Soft palate, uvula, fauces visible.
- Class III: Soft palate, base of uvula visible.
- Class IV: Only hard palate visible

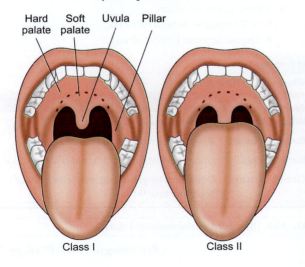

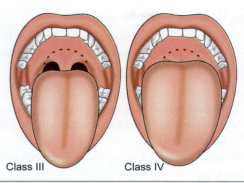

184. Ans. (a) Cricothyroid

Ref: P.L. Dhingra, 5th ed. pg. 317; BD Chaurasia Vol: 3 pg. 242, 244

- All intrinsic muscles of the larynx are supplied by the recurrent laryngeal nerve except cricothyroid which is supplied by external branch of superior laryngeal nerve.
- Recurrent laryngeal nerve supplies posterior cricoarytenoid, lateral cricoarytenoid, transverse and oblique arytenoids, aryepiglotticus, thyroarytenoid, thyroepiglotticus muscle.

185. Ans. (a) Posterior cricoarytenoid

Ref: P.L. Dhingra, 5th ed. pg. 317

Please refer to above explanation

186. Ans. (a) Cricothyroid

Ref: P.L. Dhingra, 5th ed. pg. 317

Please refer to above explanation

187. Ans. (b) Parotid gland

Ref: Dhingra's ENT, 5th ed. pg. 248

WARTHINS TUMOR

- Warthins tumor is also known as Adenolymphoma
- It is a benign, mixed type tumor of salivary gland.
- It occurs exclusively in parotid gland.
- It is the 2nd most common benign tumor of parotid gland.
- Most common benign & overall tumor of parotid gland is pleomorphic adenoma

Extra Mile

- Most common salivary gland tumors occurs in Parotid Gland (85% benign): **Pleomorphic adenoma**.
- Overall, **mucoepidermoid carcinoma** is the most common malignant tumor of the parotid gland or any salivary gland. It can be divided into low-grade and high-grade tumors.
- Second most common tumor of parotid gland is **Warthin's tumor**
- Most common malignant tumor of parotid gland is **mucoepidermoid carcinoma**
- Parotid tumor which spreads by perineural invasion is Adenoid cystic carcinoma.

FMGE Solutions Screening Examination

188. Ans. (b) Stylopharyngeus muscle

- Cranial nerve IX (glossopharyngeal nerve) is a mixed nerve that carries afferent sensory and efferent motor information.

Functions
- **Branchial motor:** Supplies the stylopharyngeus muscle
- **Visceral motor:** provides parasympathetic innervation to the parotid gland
- **Visceral sensory:** Carries visceral sensory information from the carotid sinus and carotid body.
- **General sensory**: Provides general sensory information from the skin of the external ear internal surface of the tympanic membrane, upper pharynx and the posterior one-third of the tongue.
- **Special sensory:** Provides taste sensation from the posterior one-third of the tongue including circumvallate papillae.

189. Ans. (b) Laryngomalacia

Ref: Dhingra's ENT, 6th ed. pg. 295

LARYNGOMALACIA

- The most common congenital disease of larynx is Laryngomalacia.
- Laryngeal cartilages are extremely soft and flabby in a child with laryngomalacia.
- **Most common clinical presentation of laryngomalacia: Stridor**
- The stridor is mainly inspiratory and increases during supine position but decreases during prone position.
- Laryngomalacia may involve all the cartilages but epiglottis and aryepiglottic folds are mainly involved.
- **IOC:** Direct laryngoscopy.
- The finding is Omega shaped epiglottis (long and tubular epiglottis with curled up tip).

Extra Mile

TABLE: Different shape of glottis and conditions

Glottis shape	Condition
• Key hole shaped	Phonasthenia
• Omega shaped	Laryngomalacia
• Thumb sign	Acute epiglottitis
• Steeple sign	Croup/Laryngotracheobronchitis
• Turban shaped	Laryngeal TB

190. Ans. (b) Acute epiglottis

Ref: Dhingra's ENT, 6th ed. pg. 289, 4th ed. pg. 267

	Acute epiglottitis	**Acute laryngo-tracheo-bronchitis (or croup)**
Causative organism	• Strep. pneumoniae > Haemophilus influenza type B	Para influenza virus type I and II
Age	2–7 years	3 months to 3 years
Pathology	Supraglottic larynx	Subglottic area
Prodromal symptoms	Absent	Present
Onset	Sudden	Slow
Fever	High	Low grade or no fever
Patient's look	Toxic	Non-toxic
Cough	Usually absent	Present, (Barking seal-like)
Stridor	Present and may be marked	Present
Odynophagia	Present, with drooling of secretions	Usually absent
Radiology	*Thumb sign on lateral view*	*Steeple sign on AP view of neck*
Treatment	Humidified oxygen, third generation cephalosporin or amoxicillin	Humidified O$_2$ tent, steroids

Note: According to recent papers Strep. pneumoniae is MCC of acute epiglottitis

191. Ans. (b) Sternocleidomastoid muscle

Ref. PL Dhingra, 5th pg. 87

- **Mastoid tip is in relation to two muscles:**
  - Sternocleidomastoid muscle
  - Digastric muscle (posterior belly)
- If there is abscess from:
  - **SCM muscle**: Bezold's abscess
  - **Digastric area**: Citelli's abscess.

Extra Mile

Different MASTOID Abscess

Abscess	Location
Wild's abscess	Subperiosteal mastoid abscess
Bezold's abscess	Deep to Sternomastoid muscle
Luc's abscess	Under periosteum of the roof of bony canal
Citelli's abscess	Digastric triangle (along posterior belly of digastric muscle)

192. Ans. (b) Sternocleidomastoid muscle

Ref: Dhingra's ENT, 6th ed. pg. 78

Please refer to above explanation

ENT

193. Ans. (c) Malignant change

Ref: Dhingra's ENT, 5ᵗʰ ed. pg. 272-273

- Acute tonsillitis often affects school-going children, but it can also affect adults.

Cause:
- **MCC:** Group A Beta Hemolytic streptococcus
- Acute infections of tonsil may involve these components and are thus classified as:
    - **Acute catarrhal or superficial tonsillitis:** generalized pharyngitis and is mostly seen in viral infections.
    - **Acute follicular tonsillitis:** Infection spreads into the crypts which become filled with purulent material.
    - **Acute parenchymatous tonsillitis:** Uniformly enlarged and red tonsil.
    - **Acute membranous tonsillitis:** It is a stage ahead of acute follicular tonsillitis. In this, exudation from the crypts coalesces to form a membrane on the surface of tonsil.

Symptoms
- Sore throat, Difficulty in swallowing, Fever, Eearache, odynophagia, dysphagia
- **Constitutional symptoms**
    - Headache, general body aches, malaise and constipation.

Treatment
- Patient is put to bed and encouraged to take plenty of fluids.
- Analgesics
- Antimicrobial therapy (DOC: Penicillin)

Complications
- Chronic tonsillitis with recurrent acute attacks. This due to incomplete resolution of acute infection.
- *Peritonsillar abscess.*
- *Parapharyngeal abscess.*
- Cervical abscess due to suppuration of jugulodigastric lymph nodes.
- *Acute otitis media.*
- Rheumatic fever.
- Acute glomerulonephritis.
- *Subacute bacterial endocarditis.*

Note: *Malignancy is never a complication of tonsilittis.*

194. Ans. (c) Sublingual dermoid cyst

Ref: Dhingra's ENT, 5ᵗʰ ed. pg. 398

- Sublingual dermoid cyst present as midline submental swelling. This cyst is not attached to foramen cecum and hence does not move upon tongue protrusion or upon deglutition.
- The thyroglossal cyst classically moves upwards with swallowing and notably with tongue protrusion, as it is attached to foramen cecum. It merely indicates attachment to the hyoid bone.

195. Ans. (a) Glottic CA

Ref: Dhingra's ENT, 5ᵗʰ ed. pg. 327

- Most common laryngeal malignancies are squamous cell CA (90-95%).
- It can be any of these three sites:

Supraglottis	2ⁿᵈ MC site. Nodal metastasis occur early. MC to middle jugular nodes
	Symptom: Throat pain, Dysphagia, referred pain to ear > Hoarseness
Glottis	**MC site.** Local spread present. *Nodal metastasis is always absent as glottis has no (or very few) lymphatics.*
	Symptoms: Hoarseness > Stridor > laryngeal obstruction
Subglottis	3ʳᵈ MC site. Lymph nodes involved are: Prelaryngeal, Pretracheal, Paratracheal and Lower jugular nodes.
	Symptoms: Stridor > Hoarseness

196. Ans. (b) Epiglottis CA

Ref: Dhingra's ENT, 5ᵗʰ ed. pg. 329

- Treatment of laryngeal CA depends upon site of lesion, extent of lesion, presence or absence of nodal metastasis.
- **It consists of:**
    - Radiotherapy
    - Surgery (conservative laryngeal surgery, total laryngectomy)
    - Combined therapy
- **Radiotherapy:** Reserved for early lesions which neither impair cord mobility nor invade the cartilage or cervical nodes.
- **Superficial exophytic lesions, especially of the tip of epiglottis, and aryepiglottic folds give 70-90% cure rate.**
- RT doesn't give good results in lesions with fixed cords, subglottic extension, cartilage invasion and nodal metastasis.
- **Note:** *Early stages of all these cancers, gives good prognosis with radiotherapy. But once cord mobility is impaired, surgery is the next best choice.*

197. Ans. (b) Carcinoma thyroid

Ref: Dhingra's ENT, 5ᵗʰ ed. pg. 279

- Hot potato voice is muffled and thick speech.
- MCC of hot potato voice is Quincy (peritonsillar abscess), which is an extremely painful condition.
- However it can also be seen in conditions like CA tonsil and streptococcus pharyngitis.

198. Ans. (c) Ranula

Ref: Dhingra's ENT, 5th ed. pg. 237-38, 400

- **Ranula** is a cystic **transilluminant** swelling seen in the floor of mouth on one side of frenulum. It arises due to obstruction of sublingual salivary gland duct.
    - **Treatment:** complete surgical excision if small, or marsupialization if large.
- **Thymic cyst** can be cystic or solid. Present as a neck mass anterior and deep to middle third of SCM muscle.
- **Branchial cyst** is non-transilluminant, round, fluctuant, non-tender mass present in upper part of neck anterior to SCM muscle.
- **Thyroglossal duct cyst** is cystic midline swelling in the course of thyroid duct.

199. Ans. (a) Puberphonia

Ref: Dhingra's ENT, 6th ed. pg. 314-15

- **Androphonia:** Female patient with male like voice. Cause can be psychological or organic
- **Puberphonia:** Male patient with female like voice. Cause can be psychological or organic
- **Rhinolalia aperta:** Hypernasality in voice. **Cause can be:** cleft palate, Post adenoidectomy, oroantral fistula etc.
- **Rhinolalia clausa:** Hyponasality in voice. Caused due to any pathology causing nasal obstruction.

200. Ans. (d) IV

There are 4 types of thyroplasty done, depending on the pathology
- **Type I:** Medialization (Done for Abducted Vocal Cord)
- **Type II:** Lateralization (Done for Adducted Vocal Cord)
- **Type III:** Relaxation, shortening *(in order to lower down the pitch)*
- **Type IV:** Tensioning, Lengthening *(in order to increase the pitch)*

201. Ans. (a) Type I

- Type I thyroplasty is medialization. It is done in patient with lateralized vocal cord to prevent complications like aspiration.

202. Ans. (a) Hemorrhage

Ref: Dhingra's ENT, 6th ed. pg. 319

- Most common complication of tracheostomy: Hemorrhage > Tracheal stenosis
- MC damaged structure while tracheostomy: Isthmus of thyroid

ANSWERS TO BOARD REVIEW QUESTIONS

203. Ans. (c) Aberrant right subclavian artery
Ref: Srb's Manual of Surgery by Sriram Bhat pg. 720

204. Ans. (a) Hypotympanum
Ref: Dhingra, 4th ed. pg. 107

205. Ans. (a) Meniere's disease
Ref: Dhingra, 4th ed. pg. 416

206. Ans. (a) Otosclerosis
Ref: Dhingra, 4th ed. pg. 86

207. Ans. (c) Streptomycin
Ref: Dhingra, 4th ed. pg. 39
- It is ototoxic and nephrotoxic.

208. Ans. (a) Frontal sinus
Ref: Gray's Basic Anatomy, 40th ed pg. 562

209. Ans. (a) Nasal
Ref: Clinical anatomy by Regions, 8e by Richard S. Snell pg. 679

210. Ans. (d) Scala tympani
Ref: ochlear Implants: Principles and practice edited by John K Niparko pg. 45

211. Ans. (a) Low compliance
Ref: Appendix-48 for "Types of Tympanogram

212. Ans. (b) Syphilis
Ref: Dhingra, 5th ed. pg. 166

213. Ans. (a) Bony part of external auditory canal

214. Ans. (c) Tensor veli palatini

215. Ans. (c) Closing of eustachean tube

ENT

216. Ans. (d) Toynbee's test

217. Ans. (c) Otosclerosis

218. Ans. (a) Squamous cell CA

219. Ans. (d) Type 4

220. Ans. (a) Glottic CA

221. Ans. (a) Glossopharyngeal nerve

222. Ans. (b) Nasal decongestants

223. Ans. (d) Infective condition

224. Ans. (a) Glomus tumor

225. Ans. (b) Tensor tympani

226. Ans. (a) Protozoal infection

227. Ans. (a) Greater petrosal nerve

228. Ans. (d) >90 mm Hg

229. Ans. (c) 20-30 years

230. Ans. (a) Pulsatile tinnitus

231. Ans. (c) 7th nerve

232. Ans. (c) Ulcerative lesion of the tonsil

233. Ans. (c) Mucormycosis

234. Ans. (a) Syphilis

235. Ans. (a) Otosclerosis

236. Ans. (b) Posterior cricoarytenoid

237. Ans. (a) Junction of the ant: 1/3 and posterior 2/3

238. Ans. (a) Maxillary sinusitis

239. Ans. (a) Laryngotracheobronchitis

240. Ans. (a) Bezold abscess

241. Ans. (d) Pseudomonas

242. Ans. (b) Ethmoidal polyp

243. Ans. (b) Beta-hemolytic streptococcus

244. Ans. (a) Angiofibroma

245. Ans. (a) Dental extraction

246. Ans. (b) Meningitis

247. Ans. (a) Rhinoscleroma

248. Ans. (a) 24 hours

249. Ans. (b) Facial nerve and superior vestibular nerve

250. Ans. (a) Conductive hearing loss

251. Ans. (a) Middle meatus

252. Ans. (a) Atrophic rhinitis

253. Ans. (b) 45°

Ref: Gray's Anatomy 40th edCh: 36, Head & Neck Surgery: Otolaryngology Byron J. Bailey, Jonas T. Johnson, Shawn D Newlands 4th ed. pg. 1254

254. Ans. (a) Larynx

Ref: http://www.ncbi.nlm.nih.gov/m/pubmed/8793218

255. Ans. (a) Kallmann's syndrome

Ref: Differential Diagnosis in Otolaryngology: Head and Neck surgery edited by Michael Stewart, Samuel Selesnick

256. Ans. (a) Laryngocele

Ref: Essential Otolaryngology: Head and Neck Surgery, 10th ed. p-254

257. Ans. (b) 2-4

Ref: Dhingra's, 4th ed. pg. 292

258. Ans. (d) Petrositis

Ref: Dhingra's 4thed p-400 Handbook of Neurosurgery Mark S. Greenberg 7thed p-836

259. Ans. (d) Maxillary fibrous dysplasia

Ref: Ballenger's Otorhinolaryngology: Head & Neck Surge: by James Byron Snow, Phillip A. Wackym, John Jacob Ballenge centennial ed p-506

Explanations

260. Ans. (a) Frontal

> Ref: *Dhingra's 4th ed p-188, Sutton 7th ed p-1552*

261. Ans. (b) Mastoid air cells

> Ref: *Dhingra's 4th ed p-383*

262. Ans. (b) Infraorbital nerve

> Ref: *Peterson's Principles of Oral and Maxillofacial surgery, Volume 1 p-442*

263. Ans. (c) Pars Tensa

> Ref: *Scott & Brown's Otolaryngology 7th ed p-947*

264. Ans. (c) Prosper meniere

> Ref: *Scott & Brown's Otolaryngology, Head and Neck Surgery 7th ed p-3695*

265. Ans. (c) Inner ear to subarachnoid space

266. Ans. (d) TB larynx

> Ref: *Dhingra, 4th ed. pg. 270*

267. Ans. (b) Puberphonia

> Ref: *Dhingra, 4th ed. pg. 289*

268. Ans. (a) Aphonia

> Ref: *Kaplan 10th ed ch-8, Oxford Handbook of Psychiatry edited by David Semple, Roger Smyth*

269. Ans. (c) Linear acceleration

> Ref: *Dhingra, 4th ed. pg. 17*

270. Ans. (d) 20-20000 Hz

> Ref: *Dhingra, 4th ed. pg. 16, 21*

271. Ans. (b) 90 db for 8 hours

> Ref: *Dhingra's 3rd ed p-46, http://www.who.int/occupational_health/publications/noise4.pdf*

272. Ans. (b) CT scan

> Ref: *Scott-Brown's Otorhinolaryngology: Head and Neck Surgery 7th ed. pg.1086*

273. Ans. (b) Angular acceleration

> Ref: *Dhingra's ENT, 4th ed. pg. 18*

274. Ans. (c) Maxillary

> Ref: *Dhingra's, 4th ed. pg. 195*

275. Ans. (b) Streptococcus pneumonia

> Ref: *Dhingra's, 4th ed. pg. 61*

276. Ans. (c) Radiotherapy

> Ref: *Nasopharyngeal Carcinoma By Andrew Van Hasselt, Alan G. Gibb 2nd ed p-4, Dhingra's 4th ed. pg. 235*

277. Ans. (d) Posteriorly

> Ref: *Dhingra's 4th ed. pg. 221, 224, 228*

278. Ans. (a) Conductive deafness

> Ref: *Dhingra's, 4th ed. pg. 86, 400*

279. Ans. (a) Anterior part of foot plate of stapes

> Ref: *Scott-Brown's Otorhinolaryngology: Head and Neck Surgery 7thed edited Vol-1 p-3456, Diseases of Ear, Nose and Throat By Mohan Bansal 1st ed 2013 / 152*

280. Ans. (a) Drying of anterior 1/3rd of the nasal cavity

> Ref: *Dhingra's, 4th ed. pg. 148*

281. Ans. (b) Vasomotor rhinitis

> Ref: *Dhingra's, 4th ed. pg. 160*

282. Ans. (d) Deviated dorsum and septum

> Ref: *Dhingra's, 5th ed. p-158, Sss-Otorhinolaryngology and Head & Neck Surgery by George 2010 ed. pg. 139*

283. Ans. (b) Posterior cricoarytenoid

- Posterior cricoarytenoid muscle is the only abductor of vocal cord, leading to air passage to lungs. Therefore it is said that this muscle is having life saving action.
- Other intrinsic laryngeal muscles like lateral cricoarytenoid, cricothyroid, interarytenoid having adduction action, which is helpful in voice production.

284. Ans. (d) Lateral sinus thrombophlebitis

- Lateral sinus thrombophlebitis is an intracranial complication of CSOM.
- The patient usually present with intermittent high grade fever termed as hectic picket fence fever associated with rigor, chills and headace.
- Other clinical features:
  - Anemia

ENT

- Papilledema
- **Griesinger sign:** Edema over posterior part of mastoid, due to thrombosis of mastoid emissary veins.
- **Tobey- Ayer test:** If internal jugular vein compressed on healthy side, there is rise in CSF pressure.
- **Crowe- Beck test:** pressure applied on the jugular vein of healthy side produces engorgement of retinal veins and supraorbital veins (because of thrombosed opposite side).

285. Ans. (a) Anterior laryngeal wall

Ref: Kendig's Disorders of the Respiratory Tract in Children E-Book, P 305

- Laryngeal web is a rare congenital anomaly, which result from failure of recanalization of laryngotracheal tube during 3rd month of gestation.
- Most common site of these webs are anterior commissure.
- **Cohen's classification** subdivides laryngeal web into four types:

- **Type I:** Anterior web, involving 35% of glottis or less
- **Type II:** Anterior web involving 35-50% of glottis
- **Type III:** Anterior web involving 50 – 70% of glottis
- **Type IV:** Anterior web involving 75 – 90% of glottis
- Most common presentation: **Hoarseness**

286. Ans. (b) Aspergillus Niger

- Most common organism causing fungal infection of ear (Otomycosis) is: Aspergillus Niger.
- Common organism causing otomycosis: Aspergillus Niger > Aspergillus fumigatus > Candida

287. Ans. (d) Presbycusis

- Overall, most common cause of SNHL: Prebycusis
- Hallmark of prebycusis is bilateral, high frequency SNHL.
- Noise induced hearing loss is the second most common cause of SNHL among adults
- Most common infectious cause of congenital SNHL: CMV infection

ANSWERS TO IMAGE-BASED QUESTIONS

288. Ans. (a) Quinsy

- The image shows a deviated uvula indicating a Peritonsillar abscess and clinical history of hot potato voice confirms the diagnosis of quinsy

289. Ans. (c) Semicircular canal

290. Ans. (c) Serous otitis media

- During otoscopy, fluid level with air bubble is very suggestive of Glue ear/serous otitis media.

291. Ans. (a) Acute otitis media

- Upon otoscopy, red congested tympanic membrane with fluid level is suggestive of acute suppurative otitis media.
- The shown image shows cart wheel appearance which is due to dilatation of vessels of tympanic membrane due to inflammation.

292. Ans. (a) Rhinoscleroma

- Woody nose is seen in granulomatous stage of rhinoscleroma.

293. Ans. (b) Vocal cord polyp

- The shown image is vocal cord polyp.
- Site: Junction of anterior 1/3rd and posterior 2/3rd

- Most common site is junction of anterior 1/3rd and posterior 2/3rd

294. Ans. (b) Weber fergusson incision

- The shown incision line is weber fergusson incision.
- It is done for maxillectomy in maxillary sinus carcinoma.

295. Ans. (b) Angiofibroma

- The shown case and radiological image is diagnostic of Juvenile nasopharyngeal carcinoma.
- The shown HPE image shows endothelial lining which is also a finding of angiofibroma.

296. Ans. (d) Checking the mobility of tympanic membrane

The shown image is of **siegel speculum** which is used for checking the mobility of tympanic membrane.

297. Ans. (c) Lateral sinus thrombophlebitis

- The shown sign is known as **Griesinger sign**, which is mastoid emissary vein thrombosis seen in case of lateral sinus thrombophlebitis.

298. Ans. (c) Ranula

- The shown image is ranula. It is retention cyst of sublingual gland.

Explanations

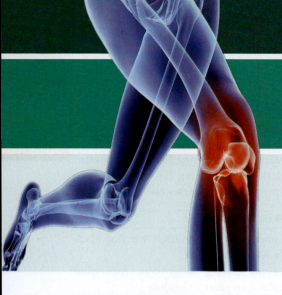

14

Orthopedics

MOST RECENT QUESTIONS 2019

1. A 6-year-old child is suspected with supracondylar fracture of right hand, complaining of pain and swelling. X-ray of right elbow was not significant. What is the next best step in this case?
   a. Compare with X-ray of left hand
   b. Closed reduction and slab
   c. Closed reduction with K wire fixation
   d. Casting
2. A patient presented with following serum parameters: Normal serum ALP, normal PTH level and increased Ca+ and PO_4. Most likely cause:
   a. Vitamin D increase
   b. Hyperparathyroidism
   c. Osteoporosis
   d. Osteomalacia
3. Three point bony relationship has diagnostic value in:
   a. Elbow fracture
   b. Monteggia fracture
   c. Galeazzi fracture
   d. Colles' fracture
4. Management of olecranon fracture as seen in the image:

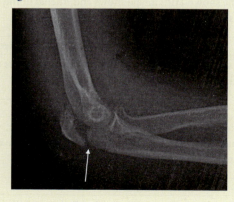

   a. Above elbow plaster slab
   b. Below elbow plaster slab
   c. Close reduction with Tension band wiring
   d. Open reduction with Tension band wiring

GENERAL ORTHOPEDICS AND FRACTURES

5. A lady presented in emergency with history of trauma to neck region. Identify the shown fracture in image:
   (Recent Pattern Question 2018-19)

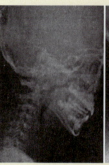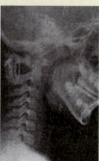

   a. Atlanto-axial dislocation
   b. Jefferson fracture
   c. Hangman fracture
   d. Clay-shoveler fracture
6. Jefferson fracture is: *(Recent Pattern Question 2017)*
   a. C2 fracture   b. C1 fracture
   c. Fracture of talus   d. Atlanto-axial dislocation
7. Hangman fracture is: *(Recent Pattern Question 2017)*
   a. C1 ring fracture
   b. C2 odontoid process fracture
   c. C2 pars interarticularis fracture
   d. C7 fracture
8. A male patient presents after trauma with popliteal vessel injury and fracture of 0.5 cm × 0.5 cm. What is the Anderson Gustillo classification?
   (Recent Pattern Question 2017)
   a. 1   b. 2
   c. 3A   d. 3C
9. What is the treatment of Anderson Gustillo classification grade 3B? *(Recent Pattern Question 2017)*
   a. Intramedullary nailing   b. Intramedullary wiring
   c. Close reduction   d. K wire

Orthopedics

10. Connection of Haversian canal are by
    (Recent Pattern Question 2016)
    a. Canaliculi   b. Volkmann canal
    c. Osteon   d. Central canal

11. Stress fracture occurs most commonly in:
    a. Metatarsals   b. Metacarpals
    c. Calcaneum   d. Talus

12. Runners fracture occurs in which bone
    a. Fibula   b. Metatarsals
    c. Tibia   d. Calcaneum

13. Fracture and dislocation of lateral clavicle. Best treatment is:
    a. Figure of 8 splint b. Open reduction
    c. Normal sling   d. Surgical repair

14. Avascular necrosis can be a possible sequelae of fracture of all of the following bones, EXCEPT:
    a. Femur neck   b. Scaphoid
    c. Talus   d. Calcaneum

15. Mason's classification is used for:
    a. Clavicle fracture   b. Colle's fracture
    c. Radial head fracture d. Monteggia fracture

16. Which of the following fracture most likely leads to malunion:
    a. Clavicle fracture
    b. Femur neck fracture
    c. Scaphoid fracture
    d. Ulna fracture

UPPER LIMB

17. A Tennis player presents with a history of spontaneous shoulder dislocation, labrum injury. Now he states that he can himself correct the dislocation. This condition most likely is: *(Recent Pattern Question 2018-19)*
    a. Recurrent anterior shoulder dislocation
    b. Recurrent posterior shoulder dislocation
    c. Reverse hill sach's lesion
    d. Inferior shoulder dislocation

18. Herberden's arthropathy affects:
    (Recent Pattern Question 2018)
    a. Lumbar spine
    b. Sacroiliac joint
    c. Distal interphalangeal joint
    d. Knee joint

19. Muscle in 2nd compartment of wrist:
    (Recent Pattern Question 2018)
    a. Extensor pollicis brevis
    b. Extensor carpi radialis brevis and longus
    c. Abductor pollicis longus
    d. Extensor pollicis longus

20. A patient received an electric shock and fell down. He cannot do external rotation of shoulder and cannot move arm. What is the diagnosis?
    (Recent Pattern Question 2018)
    a. Anterior dislocation   b. Posterior dislocation
    c. Clavicle fracture   d. Luxation erecta

21. Terrible triad of elbow is: *(Recent Pattern Question 2017)*
    a. Humerus fracture with medial epicondyle fracture
    b. Shaft fracture with dislocation and ulnar fracture
    c. Elbow dislocation with shaft fracture
    d. Elbow dislocation with radial head and coronoid fracture

22. What is true about supracondylar fracture?
    (Recent Pattern Question 2017)
    a. Mostly seen in elderly population
    b. Females are mostly affected
    c. Most common type is extension type
    d. Can cause non union

23. Nerve involved in shaft of humerus fracture
    (Recent Pattern Question 2016)
    a. Median   b. Anterior interossues
    c. Posterior interosseus d. Radial

24. Nerve involved in carpal tunnel syndrome
    (Recent Pattern Question 2016)
    a. Ulnar nerve   b. Radial nerve
    c. Median nerve   d. Medial nerve

25. Which of the following is static stabilizer of shoulder joint:
    a. Supraspinatus   b. Infraspinatus
    c. Negative pressure in glenoid cavity
    d. Subscapularis

26. Supraspinatus injury leads to which of the following:
    a. Frozen shoulder   b. Winging of scapula
    c. Cannot abduct   d. Cannot adduct

27. In Anterior dislocation of shoulder which nerve is commonly affected:
    a. Axillary nerve   b. Radial nerve
    c. Ulnar nerve   d. Median nerve

28. In a man lifting up suitcase, posterior dislocation of glenohumeral joint is prevented by:
    a. Deltoid   b. Latissimus dorsi
    c. Coracobrachialis   d. Short head of biceps

29. Which of the following test of shoulder dislocation is verified by just looking at the axillary fat folds:
    a. Dugas test   b. Callway test
    c. Hamilton ruler test d. Bryants's test

30. Hill Sach's lesion is seen in:
    a. Hip joint dislocation   b. Elbow dislocation
    c. Shoulder Dislocation   d. Jaw dislocation

31. Colle's fracture which of the following tendons likely to rupture:
    a. Flexor pollicis longus b. Flexor policis brevis
    c. Extensor policis longus d. Extensor policis brevis

32. Kienbock disease is avascular necrosis of:
    a. Scaphoid   b. Trapezoid
    c. Trapezium   d. Lunate
33. Monteggia fracture is:
    a. Fracture of distal radius with dislocation of head of ulna
    b. Fracture of the proximal third of the ulna with dislocation of the head of the radius.
    c. Fracture of distal third of ulna with dislocation of head of radius
    d. Fracture of proximal one third of radius with dislocation of head of radius
34. Injury in radial groove of humerus will lead to:
    a. Wrist drop   b. Chauffeur's fracture
    c. Skier's thumb   d. Mallet finger
35. Content of anatomical snuff box
    a. Radial artery   b. Ulnar artery
    c. Median nerve   d. Superficial artery
36. Which of the following does not indicate ulnar nerve injury:
    a. Clawing of medial 2 digits
    b. Froment sign is present
    c. Abductor Pollicis longus palsy
    d. Loss of sensory supply of medial little finger and medial half of ring finger
37. First sign of volkman's ischemia is:
    a. Pulselessness   b. Pallor
    c. Paralysis   d. Pain
38. A pregnant woman aged 30 years, after trauma feeling tingling pain and numbness at the tips of thumb, index finger and middle finger, on examination doctor presses between the wrist joint for 30 seconds and the patient develops more pain at the tips of the middle, index finger and thumb. What is the diagnosis
    a. Carpal tunnel syndrome   b. Cubital tunnel syndrome
    c. Tarsal tunnel syndrome   d. Pronator syndrome
39. Finkelstein test is done for:
    a. Compound palmar ganglia
    b. Carpal tunnel syndrome
    c. De-quervain tenosynovitis
    d. Tennis elbow
40. Dupuytren's contracture is associated with all EXCEPT:
    a. Usually not painful
    b. Involves the ring and little finger
    c. Table top test is negative
    d. Clostridial collagenase for resolution
41. Gun stock deformity is seen in:
    a. Supracondylar fracture of humerus
    b. Lateral condyle fracture
    c. Radial head fracture
    d. Ulnar head fracture

42. A 20-year-old male presents with anterior shoulder dislocation. This injury is usually caused as a combination of which of the following?
    a. Abduction and external rotation
    b. Abduction and internal rotation
    c. Adduction and external rotation
    d. Adduction and internal rotation
43. A 24-year-old sustained the fracture shown in the X-ray below. The nerve most likely to be injured is:

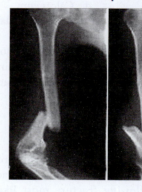

    a. Ulnar nerve
    b. Median nerve
    c. Radial nerve
    d. Musculocutaneous nerve
44. Eponym for fracture shown in below X-ray is:

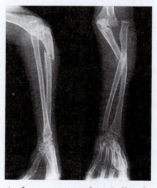

    a. Monteggia fracture   b. Colles fracture
    c. Galezzei fracture   d. Smith fracture

LOWER LIMB

45. The triad of triple arthrodesis includes all EXCEPT:
    (Recent Pattern Question 2018)
    a. Calcaneocuboid joint   b. Talonavicular joint
    c. Tibiotalar joint   d. Subtalar joint
46. Lauge-Hansen classification belongs to:
    (Recent Pattern Question 2018)
    a. Femur fracture   b. Elbow fracture
    c. Ankle fracture   d. Shoulder fracture

47. Triple deformity is seen in all of the following conditions EXCEPT: *(Recent Pattern Question 2017)*
    a. Knee TB
    b. Reactive arthritis
    c. Iliotibial contracture
    d. Poliomyelitis
48. Triple deformity of knee includes all EXCEPT:
    a. Knee flexion
    b. Posterior subluxation of femur
    c. Lateral rotation of tibia
    d. Posterior subluxation of tibia
49. A patient with fracture of femur shaft develops petechiae, respiratory distress and decreased sPO₂, 5 days after injury. Possible diagnosis is *(Recent Pattern Question 2016)*
    a. Hypostatic pneumonia
    b. Haemolytic anemia
    c. Crush syndrome
    d. Fat embolism
50. Anterior cruciate ligaments prevent:
    a. Anterior dislocation of ulna
    b. Posterior dislocation of ulna
    c. Anterior dislocation of tibia
    d. Posterior dislocation of tibia
51. Which nerve is injured in fracture of fibula:
    a. Posterior tibial nerve
    b. Anterior tibial nerve
    c. Common peroneal nerve
    d. Deep peroneal nerve
52. Bumper fracture is?
    a. Fracture of fibula
    b. Fracture of distal tibia
    c. Fracture of medial tibial plateau
    d. Fracture of lateral tibial plateau
53. Main extensor of knee:
    a. Gastrocnemius
    b. Quadriceps femoris
    c. Hamstrings
    d. Peroneal muscles
54. Q angle is increased in
    a. Patellar subluxation
    b. Genu varum
    c. Femoral ante-flexion
    d. Medial positioning tibial tuberosity
55. Gallow's traction is used for fracture of:
    a. Neck of femur
    b. Shaft of femur
    c. Shaft of tibia
    d. Tibial plafond
56. The ligaments connecting the menisci to the tibia are known as:
    a. Coronary
    b. Arcuate
    c. Transverse
    d. Oblique
57. In patient with femoral head fracture associated with femur neck fracture. What is the grading according to pipkin classification:
    a. Grade I
    b. Grade II
    c. Grade III
    d. Grade IV
58. Spot diagnosis:

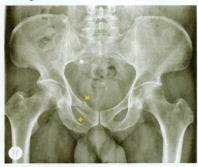

    a. Malgaigne fracture
    b. Straddle fracture
    c. Pubic rami with penile fracture
    d. Sacroiliac joint dislocation only

PELVIS AND HIP

59. A 79-year-old lady presents with history of fall. There is right sided intertrochanteric fracture of hip evidenced by the given X-ray. Best management for this patient is: *(Recent Pattern Question 2018-19)*

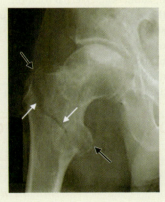

    a. Bipolar Hemiarthoplasty
    b. Intramedullary nail
    c. Hip-Spica
    d. Internal fixation
60. A 30-year-old male fell from a tree. Thereafter he complains of pain and is unable to move his legs *(image given)*. Next management *(Recent Pattern Question 2016)*

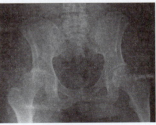
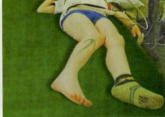

    a. Open reduction
    b. Urgent Closed reduction
    c. Traction
    d. Observation

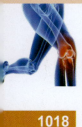

FMGE Solutions Screening Examination

61. Patient came into emergency department with flexion, adduction and internal rotation of hip. Diagnosis?
    a. Anterior dislocation of hip
    b. Posterior dislocation of hip
    c. Femur neck fracture
    d. Femur head fracture

62. Posterior dislocation of hip results in:
    a. Abduction, internal rotation, extension
    b. Adduction, internal rotation, extension
    c. Adduction, internal rotation, flexion
    d. Abduction, external rotation, flexion

63. 82-year-old female with necrotic head of femur and bilateral osteoarthritis. What is the next step of management:
    a. Uncemented total hip replacement
    b. Cemented total hip replacement
    c. Hemi-arthroplasty
    d. Observation

64. In anterior dislocation of hip, attitude of limb is:
    a. Flexion, abduction, internal rotation
    b. Flexion, abduction, external rotation
    c. Flexion, adduction, internal rotation
    d. Flexion, adduction, external rotation

65. What is the position of leg in tubercular arthritis in synovitis stage:
    a. Flexion, adduction, Internal rotation
    b. Flexion, abduction, Internal rotation
    c. Flexion, abduction, External rotation
    d. Extension, abduction internal rotation

INFECTION & TUBERCULOSIS OF BONE AND JOINTS

66. The spina ventosa is seen in:
    (Recent Pattern Question 2018)
    a. Carpals
    b. Phalanges
    c. Dorsal spine
    d. Shoulder joint

67. Most common type of lesion in Pott's spine:
    (Recent Pattern Question 2018)
    a. Central
    b. Anterior
    c. Paradiscal
    d. Appendiceal

68. A 4-year-old child presented with limping and fever and has the given X-ray. Most likely diagnosis:
    a. Osteomyelitis   *(Recent Pattern Question 2017)*
    b. Osteosarcoma
    c. Enchondroma
    d. Aneurysmal bone cyst

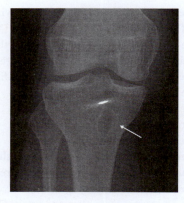

69. Most common organism causing osteomyelitis:
    a. Staph Aureus   b. Strep pneumonia
    c. H. Influenza   d. E. coli

70. Most common site for osteomyelitis:
    a. Epiphysis   b. Metaphysis
    c. Diaphysis   d. Sub-chondral growth plate

71. Earliest X-ray finding in osteomyelitis:
    a. Involucrum   b. Sequestrum
    c. Cloacae   d. Periosteal reaction

72. Felon means infection of:
    a. Epinychium   b. Terminal pulp space
    c. Deep palmar abscess d. Subcuticular space

73. Spina ventosa is:
    a. Tubercular dactylitis   b. TB of spine
    c. TB of vertebral pedicles d. Extra-axial

74. Triple deformity of knee includes all EXCEPT:
    a. Posterior subluxation of tibia
    b. Medial rotation of tibia
    c. Lateral rotation of tibia
    d. Flexion

75. Triple deformity in tubercular arthritis of the knee is:
    a. Flexion, posterior subluxation and external rotation
    b. Flexion, posterior subluxation and internal rotation
    c. Extension, anterior subluxation and external rotation
    d. Extension, anterior subluxation and internal rotation

76. Most common area involved in tubercular spine is:
    a. Paradiscal area   b. Central type
    c. Anterior involvement d. Appendicle involvement

77. True about bony ankylosis:
    a. Painful condition
    b. Tubercular arthritis is most common cause
    c. Septic arthritis leads to bony ankylosis
    d. Spine tuberculosis is the leading cause

78. The most common sequelae of tuberculous spondylitis is:
    a. Fibrous ankylosis   b. Bony Ankylosis
    c. Pathological dislocation d. Chronic osteomyelitis

79. Kanavel sign includes all EXCEPT:
    a. Tenderness   b. Flexion
    c. Pain upon passive flexion d. Uniform swelling

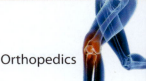

Orthopedics

BONE ONCOLOGY AND JOINT DISORDERS

80. Most common site of Adamantinoma:
    (Recent Pattern Question 2018-19)
    a. Radius   b. Humerus
    c. Tibia   d. Femur

81. Sunray appearance in osteosarcoma is due to:
    a. Bone destruction *(Recent Pattern Question 2018)*
    b. Periosteal reaction
    c. Vascular calcification
    d. Bone hypertrophy

82. A child with pain in lower limb presented with this X-ray. Which is the probable diagnosis?
    (Recent Pattern Question 2017)

    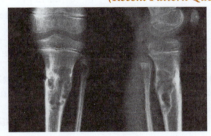

    a. Osteosarcoma
    b. Osteoid osteoma
    c. Ewing's sarcoma
    d. Osteofibrous dysplasia

83. Which of the following is an epiphyseal tumor?
    (Recent Pattern Question 2017)
    a. Osteoid osteoma
    b. Adamantinoma
    c. Osteosarcoma
    d. Chrondroblastoma

84. An intramedullary tumor occurring in the lower metaphysis of the tibia in a 15-year-old male is most likely to be:
    a. Ewing's sarcoma
    b. Giant cell tumor
    c. Chondrosarcoma
    d. Osteosarcoma

85. Sun burst appearance usually seen in:
    a. Osteosarcoma
    b. Osteopetrosis
    c. Osteomyelitis
    d. Osteoradionecrosis

86. Aspirin is useful in which type of bone tumor:
    a. Osteonecrosis   b. Osteopetrosis
    c. Osteoid osteoma   d. Ewing sarcoma

87. Most common presenting age of Ewing's sarcoma is:
    a. First decade   b. Second decade
    c. Third decade   d. Fourth decade

88. X-ray wrist showing soap bubble appearance in epiphyseal region. Diagnosis:

    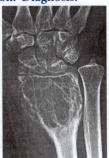

    a. Giant cell tumor   b. Osteosarcoma
    c. Osteochondroma   d. Osteoid osteoma

JOINT DISORDERS

89. Which is the most common joint involved in *thalassemia*?
    (Recent Pattern Question 2017)
    a. Hip   b. Knee
    c. Shoulder   d. Ankle

90. Which of the following condition present as arthritis with conjunctivitis? *(Recent Pattern Question 2017)*
    a. Reiter's syndrome   b. Kaplan syndrome
    c. Pneumoconiosis   d. Aspergillosis

91. Joint *not* involved in Rheumatoid Arthritis:
    a. DIP   b. PIP
    c. MC   d. Wrist

92. Which of the following is seen in Boutonniere's deformity:
    a. Extension of PIP and DIP
    b. Flexion of PIP and DIP
    c. Flexion contracture of PIP and extension of DIP
    d. Flexion of DIP and extension of PIP

93. All are seen in Rheumatoid arthritis EXCEPT:
    a. Boutonniere's deformity b. Heberden nodes
    c. Involvement of PIP   d. Swan neck deformity

94. A 35-year-old female presented with MCP and PIP pain. Diagnosis:
    a. Rheumatoid arthritis   b. Rheumatic fever
    c. Gouty arthritis   d. Psoariatic arthritis

95. Diagnosis of the picture given:

    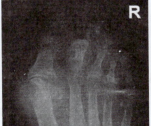 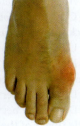

    a. Osteoarthritis   b. Gouty arthritis
    c. Rheumatoid arthritis   d. Pseudogout

FMGE Solutions Screening Examination

96. Drug of choice for acute gouty arthritis:
    a. Indomethacine   b. Allopurinol
    c. Colchicine   d. Aspirin
97. Correct meaning of Poncet disease:
    a. TB with Rheumatoid arthritis
    b. TB of short bones
    c. TB with polyarthritis
    d. TB of shoulder

VERTEBRA & NEUROMUSCULAR DISEASE

98. Cubital tunnel syndrome involves which nerve?
    a. Radial nerve   *(Recent Pattern Question 2017)*
    b. Ulnar nerve
    c. Anterior interosseous nerve
    d. Median nerve
99. In the lumbar spine, 90% of the disc herniations occur at which of the following level:
    a. L1-L2   b. L2-L3
    c. L3-L4   d. L4-L5
100. Injury to cervical nerve C5, C6 causes:
     a. Erb's paralysis   b. Klumpke paralysis
     c. Horner syndrome   d. Central cord syndrome
101. Sciatic nerve damage most commonly due to:
     a. Degenerative   b. Iatrogenic
     c. Traumatic   d. Vascular
102. Condition in which there is anterior or posterior displacement of a vertebra in relation to the vertebrae below:
     a. Spondylosis   b. Spondylitis
     c. Spondylolisthesis   d. Spondylolysis
103. Motor march is seen in:
     a. Neurapraxia   b. Axonotmesis
     c. Neurotmesis   d. None of these
104. Card test/book test is done for which nerve injury:
     a. Radial nerve   b. Ulnar nerve
     c. Median nerve   d. Tibial nerve
105. Froment's sign is a feature of:
     a. Radial nerve palsy   b. Ulnar nerve palsy
     c. Median nerve palsy   d. Tibial nerve palsy
106. Ulnar nerve paralysis causes:
     a. Ape thumb deformity b. Wrist drop
     c. Claw finger deformity d. Meralgia perasthetica
107. Cockup splint is used in paralysis of:
     a. Ulnar nerve   b. Radial nerve
     c. Median nerve   d. Sciatic nerve
108. Neuropraxia is a condition characterized by:
     a. Division of nerve sheath b. Division of axons
     c. Division of nerve fibres d. Physiological block
109. Little finger of the hand corresponds to:
     a. C6 dermatome   b. C7 dermatome
     c. C8 dermatome   d. T1 dermatome

110. Pain due to postamputation neuroma is best treated by:
     a. Infrared therapy   b. Interference therapy
     c. Ultrasound therapy d. Stump bandaging
111. The picture given below shows a hand following a nerve injury. Identify the nerve:

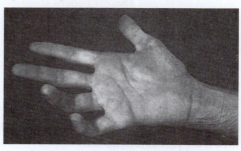

     a. Median nerve   b. Ulnar nerve
     c. Radial nerve   d. Musculocutaneous nerve

PEDIATRIC ORTHOPEDICS

112. A 5-year-old child presents with limping and limb shortening. Based on the following finding seen on X-ray, this is most likely a case of:
     (Recent Pattern Question 2018-19)

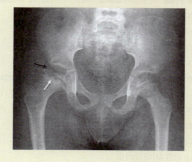

     a. DDH   b. Hip dislocation
     c. Perthes disease d. Stage I TB hip joint
113. True about Blount disease:
     (Recent Pattern Question 2018-19)
     a. Dysplasia of proximal epiphysis
     b. Metaplasia of distal epiphysis
     c. Dysplasia of diaphysis
     d. Metaplasia of diaphysis
114. Most common joint dislocation in pediatric population:
     (Recent Pattern Question 2017)
     a. Wrist   b. Sternoclavicular
     c. Elbow   d. Hip
115. Trethovan sign is used for diagnosis of:
     a. Talar fracture *(Recent Pattern Question 2017)*
     b. Congenital hip dysplasia
     c. Clavicle fracture
     d. Slipped capital femoral epiphysis

Orthopedics

116. Investigation for screening congenital dislocation of hip in an infant is:
    a. X-ray b. USG
    c. CT scan d. MRI
117. Barlow test is used for testing:
    a. Talar fracture
    b. Slipped capital femoral epiphysis
    c. Congenital dislocation of hip
    d. Rickets
118. Which ligament is involved in Pes-planus:
    a. Spring ligament
    b. Deep transverse ligament
    c. Long & short plantar ligament
    d. Deltoid ligament
119. Clutton's joint is seen in:
    a. Early congenital syphilis b. Late congenital syphilis
    c. Tertiary syphilis d. All of the above
120. Vertical talus is associated with:
    a. Congenital flat foot b. Ankle dislocation
    c. Talus fracture d. Pes cavus

METABOLIC BONE DISORDERS

121. Marble Schonberg disease is:
    (Recent Pattern Question 2018-19)
    a. Osteomalacia b. Osteosclerosis
    c. Osteopetrosis d. Osteoporosis
122. A patient presented finger deformity and pain in knee and fingers. In which of the following condition there is involvement of DIP, PIP, CMC (carpometacarpal joint) and sparing of wrist: *(Recent Pattern Question 2018-19)*
    a. Psoriatic arthritis b. Rheumatoid Arthritis
    c. Pseudogout d. Osteoarthritis
123. Which of the following is the management for postmenopausal women with osteoporosis:
    (Recent Pattern Question 2018)
    a. Raloxifene b. Tamoxifen
    c. Bisphosphonates d. Calcitonin
124. X-ray Wrist and hand of a child is given below. There is prominent cupping and widening of growth plate. What is the diagnosis: *(Recent Pattern Question 2017)*

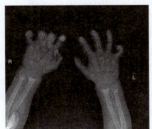

    a. Fluorosis b. Plumbism
    c. Vitamin C deficiency d. Vitamin D deficiency

125. A case of young patient presents to you with knee pain, irritability and gum bleeding. Upon X-ray of leg, cortex is significantly thin with a white line at the metaphysis. What could be possible cause:

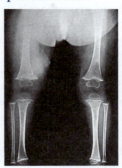

    a. Fluorosis b. Rickets
    c. Scurvy d. Caffey's disease
126. A 1-year-old breast fed child with excessive crying and gum bleeding and the below shown X-ray is a feature of:

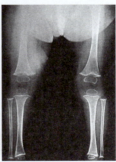

    a. Rickets b. Scurvy
    c. Kwashiorkor d. Marasmus
127. A 7-year-old boy presented with double medial malleolus. X-Ray was performed. What is the treatment?

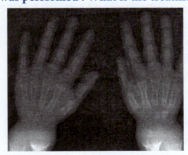

    a. Vitamin B b. Vitamin C
    c. Vitamin D d. Vitamin E
128. A child from a small village of Bihar has long bone pain, is weak and lethargic and on examination he has bow legs. The X-ray reports shows increase in bone density, osteophytes and dismorphic joint space. Possible diagnosis:
    a. Fluorosis b. Rickets
    c. Scurvy d. Caffey's disease

FMGE Solutions Screening Examination

129. Osteopetrosis results due to defective
    a. Osteoblasts   b. Osteoclasts
    c. Bone collagen
    d. Phosphate deposition in trabecular bone
130. "Bone within bone" appearance is classically seen in
    a. Osteomalacia   b. Osteopetrosis
    c. Renal osteodystrophy   d. Vitamin C deficiency
131. Stoss therapy is used for:
    a. Scurvy   b. Vit D deficiency Rickets
    c. Vit D Resistant rickets   d. Paget's disease
132. All of the following are true about osteomalacia EXCEPT:
    a. Vitamin D deficiency   b. Proximal myopathy
    c. Raised serum calcium
    d. Bone biopsy shows increased demineralized bone matrix
133. Looser's zones are seen in:
    a. Osteoporosis   b. Osteomalacia
    c. Osteosarcoma   d. TB spine
134. Multiple fractures in a child without healing are seen in which condition:
    a. Battered baby syndrome   b. Hypoparathyroidism
    c. Resistant rickets   d. Osteogensis Imperfecta
135. Gower's sign is seen in:
    a. Gullian barre syndrome
    b. Duchenne muscular dystrophy
    c. Congenital myopathy
    d. All of the above
136. Short 4th and 5th metacarpal is seen in:
    a. Pseudohypoparathyroidism
    b. Hyperparathyroidism
    c. Hyperthyroidism   d. Hypothyroidism
137. Sub-periosteal bone absorption is best seen in
    a. Radius   b. Metacarpals
    c. Phalanges   d. Ulna
138. Most common cause of bone disease especially in women in India:
    a. Steroid-induced osteoporosis
    b. Nutritional deficiency
    c. Paget's disease   d. Sarcoidosis
139. The following X-ray is diagnostic of which of the following condition:

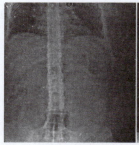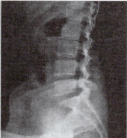

    a. Rheumatoid arthritis   b. Ankylosing spondylitis
    c. Hyperparathyroidism   d. Pagets disease

BOARD REVIEW QUESTIONS

140. Most common cause of Sciatic nerve damage?
    a. Iatrogenic   b. Traumatic
    c. Vascular   d. Degenerative
141. All are seen in Rheumatoid arthritis EXCEPT?
    a. Heberden nodules   b. Involvement of PIP
    c. Swan neck deformity   d. Boutonniere deformity
142. Which ligament is involved in Pesplanus?
    a. Spring ligament
    b. Deep transverse ligament
    c. Long & short plantar ligament
    d. Deltoid ligament
143. Clutton's joint is seen in?
    a. Early congenital syphilis   b. Late congenital syphilis
    c. Tertiary syphilis   d. All of the above
144. Runners fracture occurs in which bone?
    a. Fibula   b. Femur
    c. Tibia   d. All of the above
145. Most common presenting age of Ewings sarcoma is?
    a. First decade   b. Second decade
    c. Third decade   d. Fourth decade
146. True about osteosarcoma:
    a. Very radio sensitive tumor
    b. Sunburst appearance exclusively found here
    c. Most commonly seen in diaphyseal area
    d. Tissue biopsy is investigation of choice
147. Broadie's abscess, false statement:
    a. Can be seen in Chronic osteomyelitis
    b. Can be seen in Subacute osteomyelitis
    c. Can be seen in Acute osteomyelitis
    d. Organism is staph aureus
148. Bony ankylosis is noticed in case of
    a. TB arthritis   b. Pyogenic arthritis
    c. Rheumatoid arthritis   d. None
149. Kanavel's sign is seen in:
    a. Tenosynovitis   b. Trigger finger
    c. Dupuytrens contracture   d. Carpal tunnel syndrome
150. Triple deformity of knee includes all EXCEPT:
    a. Posterior subluxation of tibia
    b. Medial rotation of tibia
    c. Lateral rotation of tibia
    d. Flexion

Orthopedics

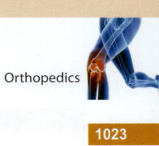

151. MC malignant bone tumor is:
    a. Osteosarcoma   b. Osteoclastoma
    c. Secondaries   d. Multiple myeloma
152. Most common bone tumor in hand:
    a. Exostosis   b. Giant cell tumor
    c. Enchondroma   d. Synovial sarcoma
153. Hill Sach's lesion is seen in:
    a. Hip joint dislocation   b. Elbow dislocation
    c. Shoulder dislocation   d. Jaw dislocation
154. What is uncommon in Colle's fracture:
    a. Non-union   b. Mal-union
    c. Rupture of EPL tendon   d. Dinner fork deformity
155. Fallen leaf sign is seen in?
    a. Aneurysmal bone cyst   b. Simple bone cyst
    c. Osteosarcoma   d. Osteoclastoma
156. Most common site of tuberculosis of spine is?
    a. Thoracolumbar   b. Sacral
    c. Cervical   d. Lumbosacral
157. Nerve involved in foot drop is?
    a. Deep peroneal   b. Common peroneal
    c. Anterior tibial   d. Posterior tibial
158. Fairbank's Triangle is seen in?
    a. Tibia vara   b. Genu valgum
    c. Hip fracture   d. Coxa vara
159. Terry Thomas sign is seen in?
    a. Keinbock's disease   b. Carpal instability
    c. Calcaneal disorders   d. Hip trauma
160. Classical sign of scaphoid fracture is?
    a. Pain with limited range of motion
    b. Pain in snuffbox
    c. Scaphoid ring sign
    d. Swelling of wrist
161. Most common part of spine affected by Rheumatoid arthritis is?
    a. Lumbar spine   b. Thoracic spine
    c. Cervical spine   d. Sacrum
162. Fracture of distal tibial epiphysis with anterolateral displacement is called as?
    a. Pott's fracture   b. Cotton's fracture
    c. Triplane fracture d. Tillaux fracture
163. Postitive trendelenburg's sign is seen in paralysis of?
    a. Gluteus maximus   b. Gluteus medius
    c. Calf muscles   d. Hamstrings
164. Most common primary malignancy of bone is?
    a. Multiple myeloma b. Osteoid osteoma
    c. Osteosarcoma   d. PNET
165. Axillary nerve damage is caused by damage to?
    a. Shaft of humerus b. Surgical neck humerus
    c. Medial epicondyle d. Lateral epicondyle
166. Osgood schlatters disease involves?
    a. Tibial tuberosity
    b. Femoral condyle
    c. Lateral malleolus
    d. Medial malleolus
167. Jones operation is done for?
    a. CTEV   b. Hallux valgus correction
    c. Cavus deformity of foot   d. Claw hallux
168. C6–C7 cervical spine fracture is seen in?
    a. Chance fracture   b. Clay shoveller's fracture
    c. Hangman's fracture   d. Jefferson fracture
169. Bone cement setting time is?
    a. 30 seconds   b. 1–2 min
    c. 8–10 min   d. >30 min
170. A 65-year-old male has been diagnosed with osteoarthritis, feature or deformity seen is?
    a. Swan neck deformity   b. Boutonniere deformity
    c. Heberden's nodes   d. Opera glass deformity
171. Most common deformity seen in osteoarthritis is?
    a. Genu valgum   b. Genu varum
    c. Genu recurvatum   d. Triple knee deformity
172. Hawkin sign denotes?
    a. Retained vascularity   b. Non union
    c. Decrease vascularity   d. Avascular necrosis
173. Phalen test is done for?
    a. De quervain's tenosynovitis
    b. Carpal tunnel syndrome
    c. Rotator cuff injury
    d. Tennis elbow
174. Finkelstein test is used for diagnosis of?
    a. Thoracic outlet syndrome
    b. Carpal tunnel syndrome
    c. Tarsal tunnel syndrome
    d. De quervain tenosynovitis
175. Keller's operation is done for?
    a. Hallax valgus   b. Hallux varus
    c. Genu varus   d. CTEV
176. Charlie chaplin gait is seen in?
    a. Congenital coxavara   b. Tibial torsion
    c. Genu valgus   d. CDH
177. Joint spared in osteoarthritis: (2018)
    a. DIP   b. PIP
    c. Knee   d. Ankle
178. Most common joint involved in OA: (2018)
    a. Knee   b. Elbow
    c. Shoulder   d. Hip
179. Keinbock disease involves: (2018)
    a. Capitate   b. Lunate
    c. Talus   d. Trapezoid

IMAGE-BASED QUESTIONS

180. Diagnosis is:

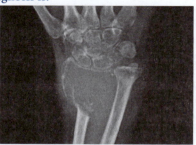

a. Unicameral bone cyst
b. Aneurysmal bone cyst
c. Giant cell tumor
d. Osteosarcoma

181. Diagnosis is:

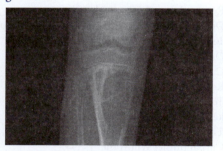

a. Unicameral bone cyst
b. Aneurysmal bone cyst
c. Giant Cell tumor
d. Osteosarcoma

182. Spot diagnosis for foot deformity?

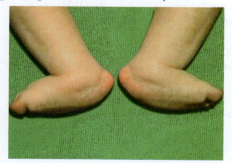

a. CTEV   b. Congenital vertical talus
c. Rocker bottom foot   d. Pes Cavus

183. 18-year-old Male has history of trauma. X-ray is shown below. The diagnosis is?

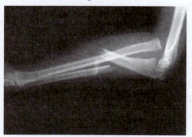

a. Supra-Condylar Fracture
b. Colle's Fracture
c. Galeazzi fracture
d. Monteggia fracture

184. Identify the periosteal reaction:

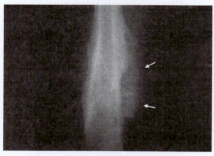

a. Onion peel appearance
b. Codman's Triangle
c. Sun Burst appearance
d. Onion ring appearance

185. The image shows presence of?

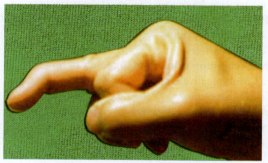

a. Swan neck deformity   b. Boutonnierre Deformity
c. Mallet finger   d. Duputyren's Contracture

186. The image shows ?

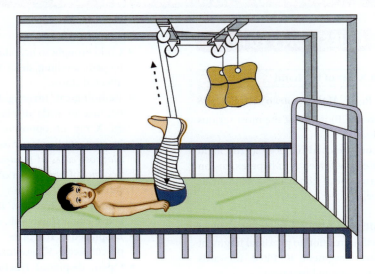

    a. Gallow's Traction
    b. 90-90 traction
    c. Russel traction
    d. Agnes hunt traction

Answers to Image-Based Questions are given at the end of explained questions

FMGE Solutions Screening Examination

ANSWERS WITH EXPLANATIONS

MOST RECENT QUESTIONS 2019

1. Ans. (a) Compare with X-ray of left hand

Ref: J. Maheshwari 6th ed. P 97–98

- Supracondylar fracture (SCF) is one of the most serious fracture in childhood.
- **Mechanism:** Fall on outstretched hand → as the hand strikes the ground → elbow forced into hyperextension → fracture of humerus above condyles → Known as supracondylar fracture.
- **Types of SCF:**
  - **Extension type (MC type):** Distal fragment is tilted backwards (extended) in relation to proximal fragment
  - **Flexion type:** Distal fragment is tilted forwards (flexed) in relation to proximal fragment.

- **Diagnosis:**
  - Child brought to hospital with history of fall, followed by pain, swelling, deformity and inability to move the affected elbow.
  - **Radiological investigation:** Commonly diagnosed because of wide displacement. A comparison with an X-ray of opposite shoulder might be helpful in suspected cases *(this is done in some difficult to diagnose cases of minimally displaced fracture due to presence of ossification centres around the elbow)*
- **Treatment:**
  - **Undisplaced fracture:** Require immobilisation in an above-elbow plaster slab, with elbow in 90 degree flexion.
  - **Displaced fracture:** Closed reduction and percutaneous K wire fixation
  - **Open, displaced fracture:** Open reduction and K wire fixation.

2. Ans. (a) Vitamin D increase

Ref: J. Maheshwari 6th ed. P 308, 313

TABLE: Actions of PTH, Vit D, and FGF23 on Gut, Bone, and Kidney

	PTH	**Vitamin D**	**FGF23**
Intestine	↑CA and P absorption (by ↑1,25 [OH]$_2$ D production)	↑Ca and phosphate absorption by 1,25 (OH)$_2$D	↓Ca and P absorption by ↓1,25 (OH)$_2$ production
Kidney	↓Ca excretion, ↑P excretion	↓Ca and P excretion by 25(OH)D and 1,25(OH)$_2$D[1]	↑P excretion
Bone	↑Ca and P resorption high doses. Low doses may increase bone formation	↑Ca and P resorption by 1,25(OH)$_2$D; ↑bone formation by 1,25(OH)$_2$D and 24,25(OH)$_2$D	↓mineralization due to hypophosphatemia
Net effect on serum levels	↑Serum Ca, ↓Serum P	↑Serum Ca and P	↓Serum P

Note:
- In hyperparathyroidism serum ALP, Ca+ is high and PO$_4$ is low.
- In osteoporosis all serum parameters are normal.
- Osteomalacia is due to dietary deficiency of Vitamin D causing decreased Serum Ca+ and PO$_4$.

3. Ans. (a) Elbow fracture

Ref: J. Maheshwari 6th ed. P 107

- Three point bony relation is made with medial malleolus, lateral malleolus and olecranon process
- This three point relationship comes in a horizontal line if elbow is extended.
- In olecranon fracture this three point bony relation is disrupted
- In supracondylar fracture, three point bony relation is maintained

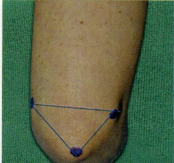

Flexion
- Medial epicondyle
- Lateral epicondyle
- Olecranon

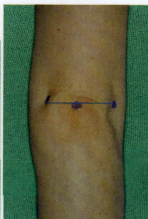

Extension

ORTHOPEDICS

Orthopedics

4. Ans. (d) Open reduction with Tension band wiring

Ref: J. Maheshwari 6th ed. P 105-106

- Olecranon fracture is commonly seen in adults due to direct injury after a fall onto the point of elbow.
- It can be of three types:

Fracture type	Treatment
Type I: Crack without displacement of fragments	Immobilize the elbow with an above elbow plaster slab in 30 degree of flexion
Type II: Clean break with separation of fragments	Open reduction and internal fixation using the technique of tension-band wiring. It is NOT possible to keep the fragments together in the plaster alone because of constant pull exerted by triceps
Type III: Comminuted fracture	**If not separated:** Treated in a plaster slab **If fragments are separated:** Tension band wiring or excision of fragments may be required.

GENERAL ORTHOPEDICS AND FRACTURES

5. Ans. (a) Atlanto-axial dislocation

Ref: Essential Orthopaedics, Maheshwari & Mhaskar, 6th ed. P 3

- The shown image is a case of atlanto-axial dislocation
- Atlantoaxial dislocation commonly present with fracture, as compared to pure dislocation of C1 (Atlas) and C2 (Axis)
- Pure dislocation commonly associated with neurological deficit
- MC dislocation in atlanto-axial dislocation: Anterior
- **Treatment:**
  - Skull traction followed by immobilisation using **Minerva jacket.**

Extra Mile

- **Hangman fracture:** Fracture through pedicle and lamina of C2 vertebra, with subluxation of C2 over C3. This type of fracture seen in hanging.
- **Jefferson fracture:** Fracture of C1 vertebra
- **Clay-shoveler fracture:** Avulsion fracture of spinous process of one or more of the lower cervical or upper thoracic vertebra. Name is given as it is caused by muscular action in shovelling by labourers.

6. Ans. (b) C1 fracture

Ref: Apley's System of Orthopaedics, 9th ed. pg. 813

- **Jefferson's fracture:** Sudden severe load on the top of the head may cause a 'bursting' force which fractures the ring of the atlas.
- There is no encroachment on the neural canal and, usually, **no neurological damage**.

7. Ans. (c) C2 pars interarticularis fracture

Ref: Apley's System of Orthopaedics, 9th ed. pg. 814

- In the true judicial 'hangman's fracture' there are bilateral fractures of the pars interarticularis of C2 and the C2/3 disc is torn.
- The mechanism is extension with distraction.

8. Ans. (d) 3C

Ref: Apley's System of Orthopaedics, 9th ed. pg. 706

- If there is arterial injury that needs to be repaired, regardless of the amount of other soft tissue damage, it is considered as grade IIIC.

Grade	Characteristics of fracture
I	Open fracture with a wound < 1 cm
II	Open fracture with a wound > 1 cm without extensive soft-tissue damage
III	Open fracture with extensive soft-tissue damage
IIIa	3 with adequate soft-tissue coverage
IIIb	3 with soft tissue loss and periosteal stripping and bone exposure
IIIc	3 with arterial injury needing repair

9. Ans. (a) Intramedullary nailing

Ref: Anderson JT, Gustilo RB. Orthopedics clinics of North America, 1980; 11:569

- For open fractures like 3B intramedullary nails are preferred over K wires.
- With the evolution of available nails like antibiotic impregnated nails, intramedullary nailing is now performed even in 3B fractures.
- Although there was initial phobia for the use of intramedullary nails, their usage has become widespread not only in grade 1 and 2 but even in grade 3 injuries.

10. Ans. (b) Volkmann canal

Ref: Wheater's Functional Histology: A Text and Colour Atlas pg. 192

- Basic structural unit of lamellar bone is osteon. These osteons consist of concentric bone layers called lamella.
- Lamella sorrounds a long passageway/central canal, known as **Haversion canal** aka longitudinal canal (*a neurovascular canal*).

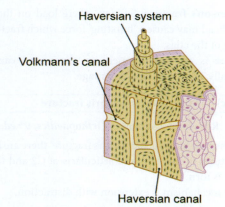

- These haversion canals are joined by a transverse canal known as **Volkmann canal** (see image). The neurovascular bundles connects the endosteum from periosteum via this volkmann canal.

11. Ans. (a) Metatarsals

Ref: Essential Orthopedics Maheshwari, 5th ed. pg. 167

- Stress fractures often develop from overuse, such as from high-impact sports like distance running or basketball.
- Most stress fractures occur in the weight-bearing bones of the foot and lower leg. Studies show that athletes participating in tennis, track and field, gymnastics, dance, and basketball are at high risk for stress fractures.
- It most commonly occurs in metatarsals.
- It is seen due to imbalance between load and resistance on the bone.
- **2 Types of stress fracture:**
  - **FATIGUE #:** Increased load, Normal resistance of bone
  - **INSUFFICIENCY #:** Normal load, Decreased resistance of bone
- **Examples of stress fracture:**
  - **Lower extremity:** March #- 2nd MT > 3rd MT
  - **Upper extremity:** Olecranon #
  - **Note:** MC site of stress # → lower 3rd tibia > 2nd MT

12. Ans. (a) Fibula

Ref: Apley's Orthopedics, 9th edn. pg. 724

The most common site of runner's fracture is distal shaft of fibula.

13. Ans. (d) Surgical repair

Ref: Maheshwari, 5th ed. pg. 88; Disorders of shoulder: Diagnosis and management, volume 1/ 961

- Since best treatment for *lateral third fracture* and dislocation of clavicle is asked, the best choice here will surgical repair.

References State
- "Distal third of fracture of clavicle accounts for 15% of all clavicle fracture. Non-displaced fractures of the distal clavicle are splinted and treated symptomatically with ice, analgesics and sling."
- Dislocated fractures of the distal third requires surgical intervention because of the rupture of coracoclavicular ligament.
- If displaced fracture is treated conservatively, it may cause non-union

Extra Mile
- CLASSIFICATION used for clavicular fracture → Craig's, Campbell Allman, Robinson's

14. Ans. (d) Calcaneum:

Ref: Maheshwari 5th ed. pg. 50, 2nd pg. 41; Adams 9th/62

Common sites of avascular necrosis	Causes
Head of femur	• Fracture neck femur • Posterior dislocation of hip
Proximal pole of scaphoid	Fracture through waist of scaphoid
Body of Talus	Fracture through neck of talus
Lunate	Dislocation

15. Ans. (c) Radial head fracture

Fracture classification

Classification	Used for
• Mason's	• Head of radius fracture
• Campbell	• Clavicle fracture
• Neer	• Proximal humerus
• Bado	• Monteggia fracture
• Melon's	• Colle's fracture
• Garden's/Pauwels	• Neck of femur
• Pipkin	• Head of femur
• Judet	• Acetabulum #
• Tiles	• Pelvic fracture

16. Ans. (a) Clavicle fracture

- Malunion and non-union is always a worrisome complication associated with fractures.
- **Malunion** is when the fracture heals in a deformed position or with limb shortening. It can be due to improper or inadequate reduction. **It can be seen in following fractures:**
  - Intertrochantric fracture
  - Humerus supracondylar fracture

Orthopedics

- ♦ *Clavicle fracture*
- ♦ *Colle's fracture*
- **Nonunion** is when the bone doesn't heal properly leaving the limb with pain and disability. It can be due to poor blood supply, infection.
- Femur neck #, Scaphoid #

UPPER LIMB

17. Ans. (a) Recurrent anterior shoulder dislocation

Ref: Essential Orthopaedics, Maheshwari & Mhaskar, 6th ed. P 89-90

- **Most common joint dislocation in body:** Shoulder dislocation
- **MC type of shoulder dislocation:** Anterior
- **Shoulder instability:** Head of the humerus is NOT stable in the glenoid. It can present with:
  - **Loose shoulder/minor shoulder instability:** Patient present with pain in shoulder upon using it. Pain occurs as a result of stretching of capsule, as the head moves out, without actual dislocation
  - **Frank dislocation:** Patient presents with abnormal movement of the head of humerus → partial movement → gets spontaneously reduced or dislocated
- **Mechanism of injury:**
  - **MC:** Fall on outstretched hand with the shoulder abducted and externally rotated.
  - Direct force (as seen in tennis player) pushing humerus head from glenoid cavity.
- **Classification of anterior shoulder dislocation:**
  - **Preglenoid:** Head of humerus lies in front of glenoid
  - **Subcoracoid:** MC type; head lies below the coracoid process
  - **Subclavicular:** Head lies below the clavicle

> **Extra Mile**
> - **Posterior shoulder dislocation** is associated with epileptiform convulsion or as a consequence of electric shock.
> - **Luxatio Erecta -** inferior dislocation. Rare type of shoulder dislocation. Head comes to lie in the subglenoid position.
> - **Hill–Sachs lesion**, also **Hill-Sachs fracture**, is a cortical depression in the **posterolateral** head of the humerus bone. It is seen in anterior shoulder dislocation.
> - **Reverse Hill Sach's lesion** is due to posterior shoulder dislocation. Micro avulsion is seen on **antero-medial** aspect of humeral head.
> - **Bankart lesion** is avulsion of anterior glenoid labrum.

18. Ans. (c) Distal interphalangeal joint

Ref: Colour Atlas of Clinical Pharmacology by N Bellamy, pg. 60

- *Heberden's arthropathy/node* is a form of joint pathology seen in osteoarthritis and involves distal interphalangeal joint.
- Another similar pathological involvement of proximal interphalangeal joint in osteoarthritis is known as *Bouchard's nodes*.

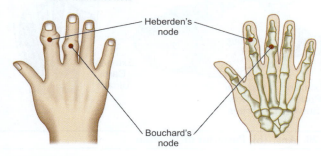

> **Extra Mile**

TABLE: Joint involvement in several conditions

	Osteoarthritis	Rheumatoid arthritis	Psoriatic arthritis
Joint involved	PIP DIP and 1st carpometacarpal joint (1st CMC) Knee	• PIP • MCP • Wrist	• DIP • PIP and any other joints
Joint spared	MCP and wrist	DIP	Any

19. Ans. (b) Extensor carpi radialis brevis and longus

Ref: Hand and Wrist edited by James R. Doyle. P 94

- Second compartment of the wrist **contains two muscles namely: Extensor carpi radialis longus and extensor carpi radialis brevis.**
- On the other hand 1st dorsal compartment of hand contains muscles like abductor pollicis longus and extensor pollicis brevis.

Extensor compartment of the wrist

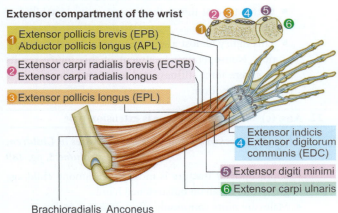

FMGE Solutions Screening Examination

Anatomy - Compartments

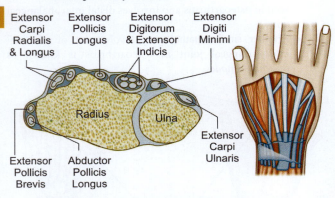

20. Ans. (b) Posterior dislocation

Ref. The Shoulder volume 1, Charles A Rockwood, P 151

- Electrical injury is a rare cause of posterior shoulder dislocation. Injury mechanism in electrical injury is similar to epileptic seizures, where the shoulder is forced to internal rotation, flexion and adduction.
- Posterior dislocation is seen in 2–4% patients.
- It is usually seen after electric shock, epileptic seizure, extreme trauma known as triple E syndrome.

21. Ans. (d) Elbow dislocation with radial head and coronoid fracture

Ref: Mastering Orthopedic techniques: Intra-articular Fractures by Rajesh Malhotra, pg. 149

Terrible triad of elbow includes/aka terrible triad of Hotchkiss

- Elbow dislocation
- Radial head fracture
- Coronoid fracture
  - It is called terrible because after this fracture, the joint becomes extremely unstable and fracture segments are usually quite small and hence difficult to repair.
  - In this type of injury there is recurrent instability of elbow joint.
  - This injury almost always requires surgical intervention. Non-operative treatment of this injury results in severe joint stiffness and a non-functional elbow range of motion.

22. Ans. (c) Most common type is extension type

Ref: Rockwood and Wilkins' Fractures in Children, Volume 3, pg. 489

- Supracondylar fracture is mostly seen among child age group due to fall on outstretched hand.
- Males are more commonly affected than females

- Well known complications of supracondylar fracture are:
  - Anterior interosseous nerve damage
  - Malunion of union → can cause **gun stock deformity.**
- There are two types of supracondylar fracture, based on location of its distal fragment:
  - **Extension type (MC type 75–80%):** Distal fragment displaced in posterior aspect
  - **Flexion type:** Distal fragment displaced in volar aspect.

23. Ans. (d) Radial

TABLE: Shoulders pathology and nerve involved:

Fracture	Nerve involved
Anterior shoulder dislocation	Axillary Nerve
Surgical neck humerus #	Axillary Nerve
Humerus shaft #	Radial Nerve
Supracondylar #	Anterior Interosseous Nerve > Median Nerve
Cubitus valgus	Tardy ulnar nerve palsy
Medial condyle humerus #	Ulnar Nerve

24. Ans. (c) Median nerve

TABLE: Entrapment syndromes

Entrapment syndrome	Nerve involved
Carpal tunnel syndrome aka Pronator syndrome	• Median nerve (at wrist) Median nerve (proximally compressed beneath – ligament of struthers, bicipital aponeurosis or origins of pronator teres or flexor digitorum superficialis)
Cubital tunnel syndrome/ Guyon's canal syndrome	• Ulnar nerve (between two heads of flexor carpi ulnaris or arcade of struthers) • Ulnar nerve (at wrist)
Tarsal tunnel syndrome	Posterior tibial nerve (behind & below medial malleolus)
Thoracic outlet syndrome	Lower trunk of brachial plexus, (C8 & T1) & subclavian vessels (between clavicle & first rib)
Meralgia paresthetica	Lateral cutaneous nerve of thigh
Morton's metatarsalgia	Interdigital nerve compression (usually of 3rd, 4th toe)

25. Ans. (c) Negative pressure in glenoid cavity

Ref: Maheshwari, 5th ed. pg. 87

- Shoulder joint is the most mobile joint of the body. Being the most mobile, it is also stable at its position. This can be due to following factors.

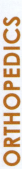

Orthopedics

TABLE: Static stabilizer vs dynamic stabilizer of shoulder joint

Static stabilizer	Dynamic stabilizer (SITS)
• Glenoid labrum • Glenohum ligament • Negative pressure in glenoid cavity	• Supraspinatus • Infraspinatus • Teres minor • Subscapularis

▶ **Extra Mile**

- **SITS** muscle is also known as rotator cuff muscle.
- **SIT** (Supraspinatus, Infraspinatus, Teres minor) inserts on greater trochanter *(Mn: SIT on GT)*
- **Subscapularis** inserts on lesser trochanter.
- Tendon passes in intertubercular groove-Long head of biceps brachii

26. Ans. (c) Cannot abduct

Ref: Apley's System of Orthopaedics & Fractures, 8th ed. pg. 281-82

In case of supraspinatus injury, abduction is restricted.

Function of Rotator Cuff Muscle

- **Supraspinatus:** Assists deltoid in *abduction of arm* by fixing head of humerus against the glenoid cavity.
- **Infraspinatus & Teres minor:** *Laterally (externally) rotates arm* & stabilizes the shoulder joint.
- **Subscapularis:** Internal rotation

27. Ans. (a) Axillary nerve

Ref: Maheshwari, 5th ed. pg. 91

- The shoulder is the most frequently dislocated joint. It moves almost without restriction but pays the price of stability. The shoulder's integrity is maintained by the gleno-humeral joint capsule, the cartilaginous glenoid labrum (which extends the shallow glenoid fossa), and muscles of the rotator cuff.
- *Anterior dislocations occur in as many as 98% of cases. Anterior displacement of the humeral head is the most common dislocation seen by emergency physicians.*
- An inferior shoulder dislocation is the least common form of shoulder dislocation. The condition is also called luxatio erecta because the arm appears to be permanently held upward or behind the head, in fixed abduction. It is caused by a hyper-abduction of the arm that forces the humeral head against the acromion.

28. Ans. (c) Coracobrachialis

Ref: Maheshwari, 5th ed. pg. 88

- Glenohumeral joint is *the most important joint of shoulder complex.*
- It is a *synovial ball and socket* articulation between the head of the humerus and glenoid cavity of scapula.

- Movements at this joint includes *flexion, extension, abduction, adduction, medial rotation, lateral rotation and circumduction.*
- Posterior dislocation of glenohumeral (shoulder) joint would be prevented by the muscle which originate posteriorly and inserted anteriorly.
  - **For example: Corachobrachialis muscle** originate from **Coracoid process of scapula** and inserted at Medial aspect of shaft of humerus.
- The net vector of pull of this muscle would be anteriorly, opposing the posterior dislocation of shoulder joint.

Origin & Insertions of Muscles Around Shoulder Joint:

Muscle	Origin	Insertion
Deltoid	Ant. Fibres- Lateral 1/3rd of anterior border of clavicle Middle Fibres- Lateral border of acromion Posterior Fibres-Lower lip of crest of spine	Deltoid Tuberosity of humerus
Coracobra-chialis	Coracoid process of scapula	Medial aspect of shaft of humerus
Latissimus dorsi	Posterior 1/3rd of iliac crest, lumbar fascia, spine of lower 6 thoracic vertebrae, lower 4 ribs inferior angle of scapula	Floor of bicipital groove
Biceps	**Long head:** Supra glenoid tubercle of scapula **Short head:** Coracoids process of scapula	Tuberosity of radius

The classical clinical feature of posterior dislocation of shoulder is- *arm is held in medial rotation and is locked in that position,* and an examiner can not externally rotate it.

29. Ans. (d) Bryant's test

Ref: Practical Orthopedics, 2th ed. pg. 479

Tests for Shoulder Dislocation can be Memorized by Simple Mnemonic: B.D.C.H.

- **Bryants test:** Look at the axillary fat fold on the dislocated side. It is displaced inferiorly if compared to normal side.
- **Dugas test:** Instruct the patient to put the hand on opposite shoulder, then bring the elbow close to chest. Inability to perform it, means positive test.
- **Callaways test:** Check for the circumference of dislocated shoulder and compare it with normal side. Circumference on dislocated side will be more than that of normal side.
- **Hamilton ruler test:** If a ruler is placed on upper arm, its two ends can easily touch the acromion and lateral condyle in a straight line. In normal person it will not be possible due to humeral head prominence.

FMGE Solutions Screening Examination

30. Ans. (c) Shoulder Dislocation

Ref: Maheshwari, 5th ed. pg. 90

- A **Hill–Sachs lesion**, also **Hill-Sachs fracture**, is a cortical depression in the **postero-lateral** head of the humerus bone.
- It is seen in anterior shoulder dislocation due to forceful impaction of the humeral head against the antero-inferior glenoid rim.

> **Extra Mile**
> - **Reverse Hill Sach's lesion** is due to posterior shoulder dislocation. Micro avulsion is seen on **antero-medial** aspect of humeral head.
> - **Bankart lesion** is avulsion of anterior glenoid labrum.

31. Ans. (c) Extensor policis longus

Ref: Apley's, 9th ed. pg. 772-74

- Colle's fracture is a fracture of distal radius at corticocancellous junction with dorsal displacement of distal segment.
- **Mechanism of injury:** Fall on outstretched hand with wrist in hyperextension.

Complication of Colle's

- **Joint stiffness-most common**
- Malunion- 2nd most common
- Sudeck's osteodystrophy
- **Rupture of extensor pollicis longus tendon:** Less common complication, usually seen after 4th week of injury.

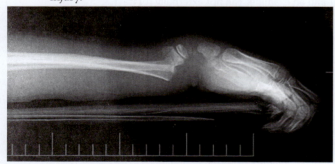

32. Ans. (d) Lunate

Ref: Maheshwari, 5th ed. pg. 318

- It is breakdown of the lunate bone, a carpal bone in the wrist that articulates with the radius in the forearm.
- *Specifically, Kienbock's disease is another name for avascular necrosis with fragmentation and collapse of the lunate.*

- This has classically been attributed to arterial disruption, but may also occur after events that produce venous congestion with elevated inter-osseous pressure.

33. Ans. (b) Fracture of the proximal third of the ulna with dislocation of the head of the radius.

Ref: Maheshwari, 5th ed. pg. 110

- **Monteggia fracture:** Fracture of the proximal third of the ulna with dislocation of proximal radio-ulnar joint.
- **Posterior interosseous nerve** is damaged in case of monteggia fracture dislocation.
- **Cause of monteggia fracture:** Fall on an outstretched hand with the forearm in excessive pronation (hyper-pronation injury).

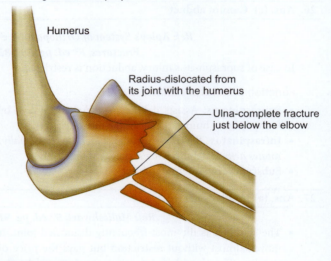

> **Extra Mile**
> - **Galeazzi Fracture:** *Fracture of the distal third of radius and dislocation of the distal radio – ulnar joint.*
> - Isolated ulnar shaft fractures are most commonly seen in defence against blunt trauma (e.g. nightstick injury). Such an isolated ulnar shaft fracture is not a Monteggia fracture. It is called a **'nightstick fracture'**.

34. Ans. (a) Wrist drop

Ref: Maheshwari, 5th ed. pg. 117

- **Wrist drop:** Due to injury to radial nerve
- **Skier's thumb:** Sprain or rupture of ULNAR collateral ligament. It is due to forceful radial and palmar hyperabduction of thumb, because of snow skiing accidents.
- **Chauffeur's fracture:** Fracture of radial styloid process
- **Mallet finger:** It is flexion deformity of the **distal inter-phalangeal joint**, due to avulsion of extensor tendon of distal phalanx.

Orthopedics

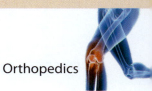

35. Ans. (c) Radial artery

Contents of Anatomical Snuff Box
- **Radial artery:** Only content which runs in groove *(all others are either floor or roof)*
- Tendon of abductor pollicis longus
- Tendon of extensor pollicis brevis
- Scaphoid bone-Floor

> **Extra Mile**
> - Superficial cutaneous branch of radial nerve
> - Partial tear of supraspinatus: Painful arc syndrome.
> - **Winging of scapula:** Long thoracic nerve palsy
> - **Frozen shoulder:** Also known as *Adhesive Capsulitis*. In frozen shoulder, all range of motion is restricted. Associated with DM, hyperthyroidism, dupuytren's disease, cardiac disease etc.

36. Ans. (c) Abductor Pollicis longus palsy

Ref: Maheshwari, 5th ed. pg. 65,67

- *The abductor pollicis longus muscle is innervated by the posterior interosseous nerve, which is a continuation of the deep branch of the radial nerve after it passes through the supinator muscle.*
- *Froment's sign* tests for palsy of the **ulnar nerve, specifically, the action of adductor pollicis.** To perform the test, a patient is asked to hold an object, usually a flat object such as a piece of paper, between their thumb and index finger (pinch grip). The examiner then attempts to pull the object out of the subject's hands. A normal individual will be able to maintain a hold on the object without difficulty.
- However, with ulnar nerve palsy, the patient will experience difficulty maintaining a hold and will compensate by flexing the FPL (Flexor Pollicis Longus) of the thumb to maintain grip pressure causing a pinching effect.
- Injury of the ulnar nerve at different levels causes varying motor and sensory deficits.

37. Ans. (d) Pain

Ref: Maheshwari, 5th ed. pg. 102

Clinical Features of Volkman's Ischemic Contracture (VIC)
- Pain out of proportion to physical examination findings.
- **Pain on passive stretching: 1st sign**
- Pressure increased
- Pallor/may also be pink
- Pulselessness
- Paresthesia
- Paralysis

(Pulselessness is a late sign and is unreliable for diagnosis of compartment syndrome)

> **Extra Mile**
> - Nerve involved in VIC: Anterior Interosseous Nerve > Median nerve

38. Ans. (a) Carpal tunnel syndrome

Ref: Maheshwari, 5th ed. pg. 303

Entrapment syndrome	Nerve involved
Carpal tunnel syndrome aka Pronator syndrome	Median nerve (at wrist) Median nerve (proximally compressed beneath–ligament of struthers, bicipital aponeurosis or origins of pronator teres or flexor digitorum superficialis
Cubital tunnel syndrome/ Guyon's canal syndrome	Ulnar nerve (between two heads of flexor carpi ulnaris or arcade of struthers) Ulnar nerve (at wrist)
Tarsal tunnel syndrome	Posterior tibial nerve (behind & below medial malleolus)
Thoracic outlet syndrome	Lower trunk of brachial plexus, (C8 & T1) & subclavian vessels (between clavicle & first rib)
Meralgia parasthetica	Lateral cutaneous nerve of thigh
Morton's metatarsalgia	Interdigital nerve compression (usually of 3rd, 4th toe)

39. Ans. (c) De-quervain tenosynovitis

Ref: Maheshwari, 5th ed. pg. 303

- Finkelstein's test is one way to determine if there is tenosynovitis in the abductor pollicis longus and extensor pollicis brevis tendons of the wrist. These two tendons belong to the first dorsal compartment.
  - **Finkelstein's test** is used to diagnose De-Quervain's tenosynovitis in people who have wrist pain.
  - To perform the test, the examining physician grasps the thumb and the hand is ulnar deviated sharply. If sharp pain occurs along the distal radius it is indicative of tenosynovitis.

40. Ans. (c) Table top test is negative

Ref: Maheshwari, 5th ed. pg. 302

- Dupuytren's contracture is a condition in which the fascia or tissue lining underneath the skin on the palm and fingers becomes thickened and scarred. As a result, the tissue lining shortens and may cause puckering of the skin or limit the ability to straighten the finger joints.
- It is usually an unpainful condition and is usually seen in northeastern European population.

- **Cause:** Idiopathic
- **Most commonly affects** Ring finger > little finger. Thumb is rarely involved
- **Most common joint involved:** Metacarpophalangeal joint > PIP joint
- Table top test involves placing palm on the table, which in presence of contracture would turn out to be impossible. *Table top test is positive in case of Duputren's contracture.*
- No definite treatment but Clostridial collagenase injections have shown excellent results and are becoming the preferred method of treatment for this condition.

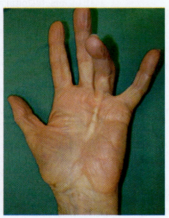

Extra Mile
- **Dupuytren disease is** another disease entity. It doesn't only affect the palms of the hands but it can also involve the back of their finger joints giving a nodule like appearance called "Garrod pads", "knuckle pads", or "dorsal Dupuytren nodules"
- Dupuytren disease can cause lumps in the arch of the feet **(Ledderhose disease)**. In severe cases, it can also involve wrist joint.

41. Ans. (a) Supracondylar fracture of humerus

Ref: Maheshwari, 5th ed. pg. 102; Essential Orthopedics by J. Maheshwari, pg. 98

- Most common complication of supracondylar fracture is malunion, which further can lead to cubitus varus deformity. This is because of the reason that fracture unites with the distal fragment tilted medially and in internal rotation.
- This cubitus varus is usually termed as gun stock deformity.
- Most common nerve damaged in supracondylar fracture: **Anterior Interosseous Nerve.**

Extra Mile
A pressure >30 mm Hg → can cause compartment syndrome

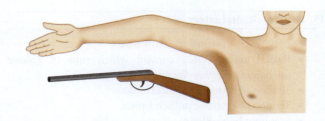

42. Ans. (a) Abduction and external rotation

Ref: Maheshwari's 'Essential Orthopaedics'; 3rd ed. p-74
- A fall on the outstretched hand with the shoulder abducted and externally rotated is the common mechanism of injury of anterior shoulder dislocation.
- Occasionally, it may result from a direct force pushing the humerus head out of the glenoid cavity.
- A posterior dislocation may result from a direct blow on the front of the shoulder, driving the head backwards.
- More often, however, the posterior dislocation is a consequence of an electric shock or an epileptiform convulsion.

Pathology (in recurrent cases)
- Bankart's lesion is stripping off (or an avulsion of) fibrocartilage labrum from anterior glenoid and neck of scapula.
- Hill Sachs lesion is compression fracture of postero lateral humeral head due to impression (friction) of glenoid rim which occur during repeated dislocation.

Tests for Anterior Shoulder Dislocation
- **Dugas' test:** Inability to touch the opposite shoulder.
- Hamilton ruler test:
  - Because of the flattening of the shoulder, it is possible to place a ruler on the lateral side of the arm.
  - This touches the acromion and the lateral condyle of the humerus simultaneously.
- **Callway's test:** The vertical circumference of the axilla is increased compared to the normal side.

Management:
- Commonly used reduction techniques are Stimson's gravity method, Hippocratic method and Kocher's method.
- Force direction in other dislocations of shoulder
- Posterior dislocation—Indirect force producing marked internal rotation and adduction.
- So the arm is flexed and internally rotated.

Extra Mile

| Positions of leg in hip dislocation ||
Dislocation of hip	Position of limb
Anterior	Flexion, Abduction, External Rotation
Posterior	Flexion, Adduction, Internal Rotation
Fracture neck of femur	Flexion, Adduction, External Rotation

Orthopedics

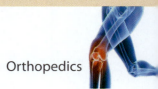

43. Ans. (c) Radial nerve

Holstien Lewis Fracture

- The radiograph shows a fracture shaft of humerus.
- The nerve most likely to get damaged is radial nerve, as this nerve is very close to the shaft of humerus.
- **Holstein Lewis fracture:** Entrapment of radial nerve between fragments in the oblique fracture of distal third of humerus.
- Radial nerve, which is fixed to proximal fragment by lateral intermuscular septum, is trapped between fragments when closed reduction is attempted.

44. Ans. (a) Monteggia fracture

- The radiograph shows a fracture of proximal part of ulna and dislocation of head of radius (disruption of upper radioulnar joint).
- This is called Monteggia fracture dislocation.
- Treatment of Monteggia Fracture
  Acute fractures:
  - **In children:** Closed reduction and Plaster cast
  - **In adults:** ORIF with plate. Radial head reduces spontaneously.
- Old, malunited fractures: ORIF with plate for ulna fracture and radial head excision.

LOWER LIMB

45. Ans. (c) Tibiotalar joint

Ref: Atlas Foot and Ankle Surgery, 2nd ed. P 272

- **Triple arthrodesis** is a surgical procedure done in order to relieve pain in the rear part of the foot, improve stability of the foot, and in some cases correct deformity of the foot, by fusing of the three main joints of the hindfoot:
  - The subtalar joint
  - Calcaneocuboid joint and
  - Talonavicular joint.

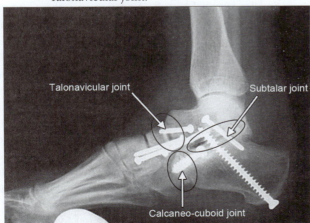

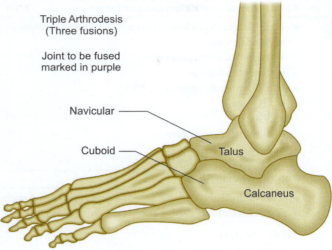

- It is commonly carried out on patients with joint degeneration resulting from arthritis or a severe flat foot deformity.

46. Ans. (c) Ankle fracture

Ref. Rockwood and Green's Fractures in Adults, Volume 1 by Charles A Rockwood, P 1980

- Lauge-Hansen classification is a system of categorizing ankle fractures based on the foot position and the force applied.

> **Extra Mile**

Some fracture classification nomenclature

- **Femur fracture:** Winquist classification
- **Femur neck fracture:** Pauwel and Garden classification
- **Elbow fracture:** Mayo classification
- **Lateral condyle fracture:** Milch classification
- **Proximal humerus fracture:** Neer classification

47. Ans. (b) Reactive arthritis

Ref: Textbook of Orthopedics by Kotwal, pg. 98

- Triple deformity of knee can result due to spasm and contracture of biceps femoris and tensor fascia lata. It consists of:
  - Flexion at knee
  - Postero-lateral subluxation at tibia
  - Lateral rotation and abduction of the leg
- It is seen in following conditions *(remembered as TRIP)*:
  - TB knee
  - Rheumatoid arthritis
  - Iliotibial contracture
  - Polio

48. Ans. (b) Posterior subluxation of femur

- Triple deformity of knee is seen in TB knee. It includes:
  - Knee flexion
  - Posterior subluxation tibia
  - Lateral roatation
- Triple deformity seen in: (TRIP)
  - TB knee
  - RA
  - Iliotibial contracture
  - Polio

49. Ans. (d) Fat embolism

- A **fat embolism** is often caused by physical trauma such as **fracture of long bone,** soft tissue trauma and burns.

Clinical Feature

- Tachycardia, tachypnea, increased temeperature, **hypoxemia (decreased sPO$_2$)**, hypercapnea, thrombocytopenia.
- **Pathognomonic sign: Petechial rash** on the upper anterior portion of the body, including the chest, neck, upper arm, axilla, shoulder, oral mucosa and conjunctivae.

TABLE: Factors favoring fat embolism

Traumatic	Nontraumatic
• Fracture of long bones eg. Femur • Reaming • Mobility of fracture	• Diabetes • Fatty liver • Pancreatitis • Sickle cell anemia • Decompression sickness • Extensive burns • Inflammation of bone & soft tissue • Oil or fat introduced to body

Extra Mile

- **Crush injury** is compression of extremities or other parts of the body that causes muscle swelling and/or neurological disturbances in the affected areas of the body, while crush *syndrome* is localized crush injury with systemic manifestations. It is Characterized by major shock and renal failure after a crushing injury to skeletal muscle.
- **Hypostatic pneumonia** is usually seen in elderly and debilitating patients. It results from infection developing in the dependent portions of the lungs due to decreased ventilation of those areas, with resulting failure to drain bronchial secretions.

50. Ans. (c) Anterior Dislocation of tibia

Ref: Maheshwari, 5th ed. pg. 148-149

- The anterior cruciate ligament (ACL) stretches from the lateral condyle of femur to the anterior intercondylar area.

- *The ACL is critically important because it prevents the tibia from being pushed too far anterior relative to the femur.* It is often torn during twisting or bending of the knee.

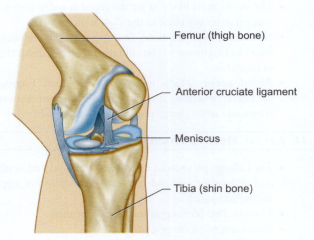

- *ACL is considered as the major stabilizer of the knee. Therefore, ACL Tears are the most common knee injuries.*
- If there is ACL tear, reconstruction is most commonly done by autograft, meaning the tissue used for the repair is from the patient's body.
- **The two most common sources for tissue are** the patellar tendon and hamstrings tendon
- **The posterior cruciate ligament (PCL)** stretches from medial condyle of femur to the posterior intercondylar area.
- This ligament prevents posterior displacement of the tibia relative to the femur.

51. Ans. (c) Common peroneal nerve

Ref: Maheshwari, 5th ed. pg. 158

- Smaller terminal branch of sciatic nerve, the common peroneal nerve arises in the lower third of thigh. It runs downward through the popliteal fossa (lateral side) closely following the medial border of biceps femoris muscle. It leaves the fossa by crossing superficially the lateral head of the gastrocnemius muscle. It then passes behind the head of the fibula, winds laterally around the neck of the bone, pierces the peroneus longus muscle, and divides into two terminal branches superficial and deep peroneal nerve.
- *The common peroneal nerve is extremely vulnerable to injury by direct trauma and fractures of fibula as it winds around the neck of fibula.*
- Injury to common peroneal nerve causes **foot drop**.

Orthopedics

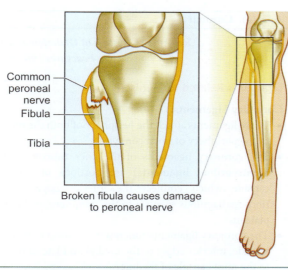

52. Ans. (d) Fracture of lateral tibial plateau

Ref: BRS: Gross Anatomy, 7th ed. pg. 83

- **Bumper fracture** is a fracture of the *lateral tibial plateau* caused by a forced valgus applied to the knee usually by the impact bumper of a moving car on the lateral side of the knee while the foot is planted on the ground.
- This causes the lateral part of the distal femur and the lateral tibial plateau to come into contact, compressing the tibial plateau and causing the tibia to fracture.

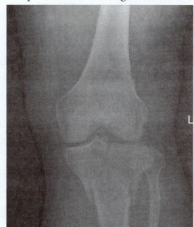

53. Ans. (b) Quadriceps femoris

Ref: Maheshwari, 5th ed. pg. 145

- Quadriceps is a large muscle group that includes the four prevailing muscles on the front of the thigh. It is the great extensor muscle of the knee. It is subdivided into four separate portions or 'heads', which have received distinctive names:
    - **Rectus femoris** occupies the middle of the thigh, covering most of the other three quadriceps muscles.

It originates on the ilium. It is named from its straight course.
- The other three lie deep to rectus femoris and originate from the body of the femur, which they cover from the trochanters to the condyles:
    - **Vastus lateralis** is on the *lateral side* of the femur (i.e on the outer side of the thigh).
    - **Vastus medialis** is on the *medial side* of the femur (i.e. on the inner part thigh).
    - **Vastus intermedius** lies between vastus lateralis and vastus medialis on the *front* of the femur (i.e. on the top or front of the thigh), but deep to the rectus femoris. Typically, it cannot be seen without dissection of the rectus femoris.
- *Quadriceps femoris is the main and only extensor of knee.*
    - It produces locking action as a result of medial rotation of the femur during the last stage of extension.
    - To reverse this lock popliteus muscle comes into action and does so by the lateral rotation of femur
- **Remember: Lock is: Quadriceps femoris muscle and, Key is popliteus muscle.**

54. Ans. (a) Patellar subluxation

Ref: Practical Orthopedics, 2th ed. pg. 511

Q angle is the angle formed by a line drawn from the ASIS to central patella and a second line drawn from central patella to tibial tubercle.

- An increased Q-angle is a risk factor for patellar subluxation
- Normally Q angle is 14 degree for males and 17 degree for females

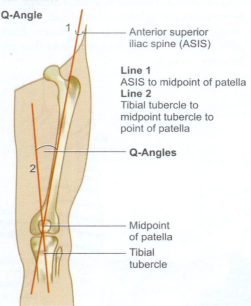

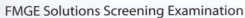

FMGE Solutions Screening Examination

- Q angle is increased in:
  - Genu valgum
  - *Increased femoral anteversion*
  - External tibial torsion
  - Laterally positioned tibial tuberosity
  - Tight lateral retinaculum

55. Ans. (b) **Shaft of femur**

Ref: Apley's 'System of Orthopaedics and Fractures'; 9/e, p-861

Gallow's Traction
- This is used in infants and children with femoral shaft fractures.
- **Indications of Gallow's traction**
  - Child must weigh less than 12 kg
  - Femoral fractures
  - Skin must be intact
- Both the fractured and the well femur are placed in skin traction and the infant is suspended by these from a special frame.
- Vascular compromise is the biggest danger.
- Check the circulation twice daily.
- The buttocks should be just off the bed.

Bryant's or Gallow's Traction
- Do not use for children older than 18 months, best for infant under 1 year.
- Weight limit of child: 16–18 kg.
- Lie child supine with the hips flexed 90°, the legs being pulled directly upwards.
- Apply only enough weight or elevate the infant just enough to allow you to slip your hand under the nappy.
- Gallows traction has been associated with vascular problems, including severe compartment syndrome.
- This is due to the elevated position of the legs, straightness of the knees and tightness of bandages.
- Avoid complications, apply the traction carefully, use adhesive skin traction, allow some knee flexion and don't bandage too tight.

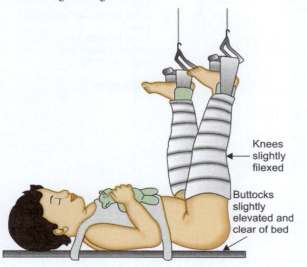

56. Ans. (a) **Coronary**

Ref Apley's 'System of Orthopaedics and Fractures'; 9/e, p-583

Ligaments Related to Menisci

Coronary Ligaments:
- These ligaments attach the periphery of both the menisci to the periphery of tibial condyles.
- The coronary ligaments of the knee (also known as **meniscotibial ligaments**) are portions of the joint capsule which connect the inferior edges of the fibrocartilaginous menisci to the periphery of the tibial plateaus.
- The coronary ligaments function to connect parts of the outside, inferior edges of the medial and lateral menisci to the joint capsule of the knee.

Meniscofemoral Ligaments:
- These ligaments attach the posterior part of lateral meniscus to the femur.
- These are of two types:
  - Anterior meniscofemoral ligament (Ligament of Humphrey): Runs anterior to PCL.
  - Posterior meniscofemoral ligament (Ligament of Wrisberg): Runs posterior to PCL.

Transverse Ligament:
It attaches the anterior edges of medial and lateral meniscus to each other.
- **Option 'B': Arcuate**
  Arcuate ligament is the ligament between the posterolateral femoral condyle to the fibular head. It covers the popliteus tendon.
- **Option 'D': Oblique**
  Oblique popliteal ligament is the ligament from semi-membranous to lateral femoral condyle and it is derived from semimembranous.

57. Ans. (c) **Grade III**

Pipkin classification for femur head fracture (#)
- I-femoral head # caudal to fovea
- II-femoral head # cephalad to fovea
- III-femoral head # associated with femoral neck #
- IV-any of the above with acetabular #

58. Ans. (a) **Malgaigne fracture**

- **Straddle #-** B/L Pubic rami
- **Malgaigne#** I/L Pubis with ilium near sacroiliac joint. The image shows malgaigne's fracture
- Classification for pelvic bone fracture → Tiles classification

Orthopedics

PELVIS AND HIP

59. Ans. (d) Internal fixation

Ref: Essential Orthopaedics, Maheshwari & Mhaskar, 6th ed. P 138

- In elderly population the intertrochanteric fracture is usually sustained by a sideway fall or a blow over the greater trochanter.
- In young population it occurs due to violent trauma usually due to road traffic accident.
- In the fracture the distal fragment rides up so that the femoral neck-shaft angle is reduced (coxa-vara). In most cases the fracture is comminuted and displaced.

TREATMENT:

- Most of these fractures unite by themselves if femoral neck-shaft angle is maintained. Done by conservative means like traction (require bed rest of 3-4 months).
  - **MC used traction:** Russei's traction
- In elderly population internal fixation is preferred.
  - Prolong bed rest in elderly can cause further complications like pneumonia, bed sores etc.

> **Extra Mile**
> - **Hemiarthroplasty:** Used for femoral neck fracture
> - **Hip spica:** used for femoral shaft fracture (age >2 to 16 years)
> - **Gallows traction:** Used for femoral shaft fracture (birth to 2 years)

TABLE: Differences between fracture neck of the femur and intertrochanteric fracture

	Fracture neck femur	Intertrochanteric fracture
Age	After 50 years	After 60 years
Sex	F > M	M > F
Injury	Trivial	Significant
Ability to walk	May walk in impacted fracture	Not possible
Pain	Mild	Severe
Swelling	Nil	Severe
Ecchymosis	Nil	Present
Tenderness	In Scarpa's triangle	On the greater trochanter
Ext. rotation deformity	Less than 45°	More than 45°
Shortening	Less than 1 inch	More than 1 inch
Treatment	Int. fixation always	Can be managed in traction
Complications	Non-union	Malunion

60. Ans. (b) Urgent Closed reduction

- The shown image is case of posterior hip dislocation
- Posterior hip dislocation is usually reduced under general anesthesia as soon as possible (within the 7 day of injury).
- Most commonly this reduction is done by **closed reduction.**
- **Indication of surgical reduction:**
  - In case of failed closed reduction.
  - If associated with acetabular fracture, making hip unstable
  - Intra-articular loose fragment
- **Complications of posterior hip dislocation:**
  - Avascular necrosis of femoral head
  - Sciatic nerve injury
  - Osteoarthritis
  - Femoral head damage

61. Ans. (b) Posterior dislocation of hip

Ref: Maheshwari, 5th ed. pg. 130

POSTERIOR DISLOCATION OF HIP

- It is most common type of hip dislocation in adults and children.
- Usually this occurs in a road accident when someone seated in car is thrown forwards, striking the knee against the dashboard *(dashboard injury)*
- It is the position (direction) of hip at the time of injury that decides the pattern of injury.

Pattern of injury	Position of Hip at the time of injury
Pure posterior dislocation	Flexion, adduction, internal rotation
Posterior fracture dislocation	Less flexion, less adduction (neutral or slight abduction), internal rotation
Anterior dislocation	Hyper abduction + Extension

Classification Schemes for Posterior Hip Dislocations

Thompson & Epstein	
Type I	Dislocations without or with minor fracture
Type II	Dislocation with a single large fracture of posterior acetabular rim
Type III	Dislocation with comminution of posterior acetabular rim
Type IV	Dislocation with fracture of acetabular floor
Type V	Dislocation with fracture of femoral head

1039

Explanations

FMGE Solutions Screening Examination

Stewart and Miford	
Type I	Dislocation without fracture
Type II	Dislocation with posterior rim fracture (one or more fragments), but the hip is stable after reduction
Type III	Dislocation with fracture of rim producing gross instability
Type IV	Dislocation with fracture head or neck of femur

Type V Thompson & Epstein is Subdivided by Pipkin into Four Types (Pipkin Classification)
I. Femoral head fracture caudal to fovea centralis
II. Femoral head fracture cephalad to the fovea
III. Femoral head fracture associated with femoral neck fracture
IV. Type I, II, or III associated acetabular fracture

Note: *Thomson & Epstein, and Stewart & Milford are posterior dislocation injuries of hip and Pipkin's fracture is fracture of femoral head (& / or neck) in posterior dislocation injuries.*

62. Ans. (c) Adduction, internal rotation, flexion

Ref: Maheshwari, 5th ed. pg. 130

- Posterior dislocations comprise approximately 80-90% of hip dislocations caused by Motor Vehicle Crash.
- In posterior hip dislocations, the femoral head goes posteriorly causing the femur to get adducted and internally rotated.
- **Posterior dislocation:** The hip is Flexed, ADducted and Internally Rotated (Mn: FADIR)
- **Anterior dislocation:** The hip is minimally Flexed, markedly ABducted, and Externally Rotated *(Mn: FABER).*

63. Ans. (b) Cemented total hip replacement

Ref: Maheshwari, 5th ed. pg. 138

TOTAL HIP REPLACEMENT

- Total Hip replacement may be preferable in patients with *acetabular damage (osteoarthritis, rheumatoid arthritis, AVN),* metastatic disease or Paget's disease.
- Originally the *primary indication* for THR was the *alleviation of incapacitating* pain in patients **older than 65** years of age who could not be relieved, sufficiently by non surgical means & for whom the only surgical alternative was resection of hip joint (Girdle stone resection arthroplasty). Secondary importance is improved function of hip.
- Therefore it is mostly used for hip arthritis *(rheumatoid, ankylosing, osteoarthritis),* **avascular necrosis of femoral head,** non-union of femoral head and, or neck.

64. Ans. (b) Flexion, abduction, external rotation

Ref: Maheshwari, 5th ed. pg. 130

65. Ans. (c) Flexion abduction External rotation

Ref: Maheshwari, 5th ed. pg. 196

- The tuberculosis of hip mainly progresses through three stages.
  - **Stage of Synovitis (FABER - AL)**
  - Stage of Arthritis (FADIR - AS)
  - Stage of Erosion (FADIR - TS)
- The mnemonics indicate the orientation and appearance of the lower limb during those stages of TB
  - **FABER – AL:** stands for Flexion, ABduction, External Rotation and Apparent Lengthening.
  - **FADIR – AS:** stands for flexion, adduction, internal rotation and apparent shortening.
  - **FADIR – TS:** stands for flexion, adduction, internal rotation and true shortening.

Staging	Clinical findings	Radiologic features
Ist stage of synovitis	Flexion, abduction, external rotation, appearent lengthening	Haziness, rarefaction
IInd stage of early arthritis	Flexion, adduction, internal rotation, apparent shortening	Rarefaction, osteopenia, bony lesion in femoral head, acetabulum or both. No reduction in joint space
IIIrd stage of arthritis	Flexion, adduction, internal rotation, shorting	All of the above and destruction of articular surface, reduction in joint space
IVth stage of advanced arthritis	Flexion, adduction, internal rotation with gross shortening	Complete destruction, no joint space, wandering acetabulum

Source: Babhulkar and Pande, Clin Ortho Rel Res 2002

INFECTION & TUBERCULOSIS OF BONE AND JOINTS

66. Ans. (b) Phalanges

Ref: Textbook of Orthopedics by John Ebnezar, Rakesh John P 554

- Spina ventosa is a rare skeletal tuberculosis of short tubular bones like phalanges, metacarpals, metatarsals.
- This condition is uncommon after the age of 5 years. It is also known as tuberculosis dactylitis.
- In this condition hand is more frequently involved than foot.

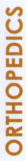

- Due to abundant blood flow through the large nutrient artery, almost in the middle of the bone, the first inoculum of infection, lodged in the center of marrow cavity, leads to spindle shaped expansion of bone called *spina ventosa*.

> **Extra Mile**
> - Caries sicca: TB shoulder
> - Poncet disease- TB associated with polyarthritis
> - Pott's disease

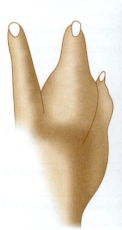
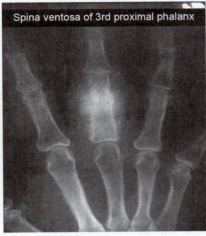

Spina ventosa of 3rd proximal phalanx

67. Ans. (c) Paradiscal

Ref. Tuberculosis of the Skeletal system, SM Tuli, P 223

- There are 4 patterns of vertebral involvement in Pott's spine:
  I. Paradiscal (due to arterial spread)
  II. Central (due to venous spread)
  III. Anterior (due to subperisteal spread)
  IV. Appendiceal and articular type (occur in isolation involving pedicles, laminae, transverse process and spinous process or in conjunction with typical paradiscal variant).

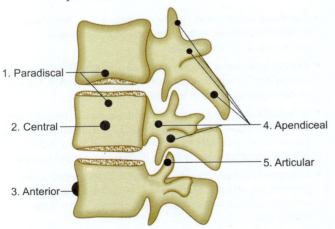

- Paradiscal is the most common type of lesion in Pott's spine.
- It spreads through arterial supply, causing reduced disc space and loss of vertebral margins.

68. Ans. (a) Osteomyelitis

Ref: Apley's System of Orthopaedics, 9th ed. pg. 36

- The given image is a case of Brodie's abscess showing sclerotic margin which can be manifested sometimes in subacute osteomyelitis.

> **Extra Mile**
> - Most common bone involved in acute osteomyelitis: Lower end of femur
> - Most common bone involved in subacute and chronic osteomyelitis: Upper end of tibia
> - Most common organism for osteomyelitis: Staphylococcus aureus

69. Ans. (a) Staph Aureus

Ref: Maheshwari, 5th ed. pg. 168

Note that responsible pathogens may be isolated in only 35-40% of infections. Bacterial causes of acute hematogenous and direct osteomyelitis include the following:

- Most common organism causing acute osteomyelitis: Staph. Aureus
- MCC of osteomyelitis in **sickle cell anemia patient: SALMONELLA**
- MCC of osteomyelitis in **IV drug abuser: PSEUDOMONAS**
- MC organism causing osteomyelitis in **open foot injury: PSEUDOMONAS**
- MC organism causing osteomyelitis in **HIV patient: Staph. Aureus**
- MC organism causing osteomyelitis in case of **animal bite: Pasteurella Multiocida**
- MC organism causing osteomyelitis in case of **human bite: Eikenella Corrodens**

70. Ans. (b) Metaphysis

Ref: Maheshwari, 5th ed. pg. 168

- Hematogenous osteomyelitis is an infection caused by bacterial seeding from the blood.
- Acute hematogenous osteomyelitis is characterized by an acute infection of the bone caused by the seeding of the bacteria within the bone from a remote source. This condition primarily occurs in children.
- The most common site is the rapidly growing and highly vascular metaphysis of growing bones. The apparent slowing or sludging of blood flow as the vessels make sharp angles at the distal metaphysis predisposes the vessels to thrombosis and the bone itself to localized necrosis and bacterial seeding.

FMGE Solutions Screening Examination

> **Extra Mile**
> - MC site of OM in child: Lower end of femur
> - MC site of OM in adults: Thoraco-Lumbar vertebra (Thoracic > Lumbar)
> - MC site of OM in infants: Hip

71. Ans. (d) Periosteal reaction

Ref: Maheshwari, 8th ed. pg. 169; Harrison's, 18th ed. Ch 126

- **Earliest X-ray change:** Loss of soft tissue plane which is seen after 24 hours. In case of osteomyelitis X-Ray is normal during first 24 hours.
- 2nd X-ray change seen is periosteal reaction, which is usually seen 7–10 days after infection.
- **Periosteal reaction can be of 3 types:**
  - **No reaction:** seen in case of TB
  - **Narrow zone of activity:** Benign condition (Ex: in infection like osteomyelitis)
  - **Wide zone of activity:** Malignant condition (Ex: Codman's triangle in osteosarcoma)

72. Ans. (b) Terminal pulp space

Ref: Maheshwari, 5th ed. pg. 206

- Felons/Whitlow are closed-space infections of the fingertip pulp. Infection occurring within these compartments can lead to abscess formation, edema, and rapid development of increased pressure in a closed space. This increased pressure may compromise blood flow and lead to necrosis of the skin and pulp.
- **Clinical feature:** Felons are characterized by marked throbbing pain, tension, and edema of the fingertip pulp.
- **Causes:** Staphylococcus aureus, is the most common cause.
- **Management:** The felon should be incised in the area of maximum tenderness. The incision should not cross the distal interphalangeal (DIP) joint to prevent formation of a flexion contracture at the DIP flexion crease. Probing is not carried out proximally to avoid extension of infection into the flexor tendon sheath.
- **Complication of felon:** Osteomyelitis > Tenosynovitis

73. Ans (a) Tubercular dactylitis

Ref: Maheshwari, 5th ed. pg. 203

- **Spina ventosa** ("wind-filled sail") refers to the end-stage radiographic appearance of tuberculosis dactylitis. Cystic expansion of the short tubular bones with bone destruction.
- Tuberculous dactylitis is the painless tuberculous involvement of the fingers and toes and is more common in children. It begins with fusiform soft-tissue swelling with or without periostitis.

> **Extra Mile**
> - **MC site bone TB:** Spine > Hip > Knee
> - MC site in spine is *Thoracolumbar (paradiscal)*
> - **Earliest symptom:** BACK PAIN
> - **Triad of TB joint:** *Decreased joint space + articular damage + Juxta-articular osteoporosis*
> - **Spina ventosa-** TB of short bones
> - **Caries sicca:** TB shoulder
> - **Poncet disease:** TB associated with polyarthritis

74. Ans. (b) Medial rotation of tibia

Ref: Practical Orthopedics, 2th ed. pg. 173

- Tuberculosis of the knee is classical cause of triple deformity. It includes:
  - Flexion
  - Lateral (external) rotation of tibia
  - Posterior subluxation of tibia
- Better treatment results are seen with ATT and arthrodesis
- This condition can also be seen in Rheumatoid arthritis.

75. Ans. (a) Flexion, posterior subluxation and external rotation

Ref: Practical Orthopedics, 2th ed. pg. 173

76. Ans. (a) Paradiscal Area

Ref: Maheshwari, 8th ed. pg. 185

- **Most common site of skeletal tuberculosis:** TB Spine (50% of cases)
- **Most common site in spine:** Thoraco Lumbar vertebra followed by cervical vertebra (Thoracic vertebra > Lumbar)
- The spinal TB is always secondary to a primary lesion (ex: in lungs) and occurs due to hematogenous spread.
- **IOC for TB spine:** MRI

Clinically there are four types of Pott's Spine

> - **Paradiscal lesion (most common)** begins in the metaphysis, erodes the cartilage and destroys the disc, resulting in narrowing of the disc space.
> - **Central type** begins in the midsection of the body which further gets softened under gravity and muscle action, leading to compression, collapse and bony deformation.
> - **Anterior lesions** lead to cortical bone destruction beneath the anterior longitudinal ligament. Spread of the infection is in the subperiosteal and sub ligamentous planes resulting in the loss of periosteal blood supply to the body with resultant collapse.
> - **In appendicle type**, the infection settles in the pedicles, the laminae, the articular processes or the spinous processes and causes initial ballooning of the structure followed by destruction.

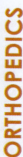

Orthopedics

77. Ans. (c) Septic arthritis leads to bony ankylosis

Ref: Maheshwari, 5th ed. pg. 182

TABLE: Bony Ankylosis vs Fibrous Ankylosis

Bony	Fibrous
• Painless • MCC: Septic arthritis > TB spine	• Painful • MCC: Tubercular arthritis of hip and knee

78. Ans. (b) Bony ankylosis

Ref: Maheshwari, 5th ed. pg. 189

- Tuberculous spondylitis is most commonly localized in the thoracic portion of the spine.
- The infection coming from primary site (ie: lungs) then spreads from two adjacent vertebrae into the adjoining intervertebral disc space. If only one vertebra is affected, the disc is normal, but if two are involved, the disc, which is avascular, cannot receive nutrients and collapses. The disc tissue dies and is broken down by caseation, leading to vertebral narrowing and eventually to vertebral collapse (Bony ankylosis) and spinal damage.
- From the choices given in the question, the most logical answer is bony ankylosis.
- Actual late complications of Tubercular spondylitis is: Vertebral collapse resulting in kyphosis, Spinal cord compression, sinus formation, paraplegia.
- **Most common cause of bony ankylosis: Septic arthritis > TB spine**

79. Ans. (c) Pain upon passive flexion

Kanavel sign is seen in tenosynovitis… infl of tendon sheath of flexor aspect of hand. It includes 4 components:
- Tenderness
- Uniform swelling
- Flexed finger
- *Pain upon passive extension*

BONE ONCOLOGY AND JOINT DISORDERS

80. Ans. (c) Tibia

Ref: Campbell Orthopaedics, 12th ed. P 922; Essential Orthopaedics, Maheshwari & Mhaskar, 6th ed. P 237

- Adamantinoma is an uncommon tumor (<1%) of long bones containing epithelial—like islands of cells
- **MC site of adamantinoma:** Tibia (85%) > Mandible
  - In mandible, it is termed as ameloblastoma
  - Can involve ipsilateral fibula
- **MC age group:** 10–35 years
- **MC symptom:** Pain
- **On X-ray:** Honey coomb like appearance/Sharply demarcated radiolucent lesions
- **Treatment:** Wide surgical resection

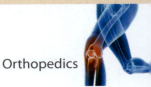

TABLE: Most common sites of primary bone tumors

Tumor	Site
Chondroblastoma	Epiphyseal (most common tumor in this region before puberty)
Osteoclastoma	Epiphyseal (most common tumor in this region after puberty)
Chondrosarcoma, osteochondroma, bone cyst, enchondroma, osteosarcoma, osteoclastoma	Metaphyseal
Ewing's tumor, lymphoma, multiple myeloma, adamantinoma, osteoid osteoma	Diaphyseal

TABLE: Most common sites of individual bone tumors

Tumor	Site
Solitary bone cyst	Upper end of humerus
Aneurysmal bone cyst	Lower limb metaphysis
Osteochondroma	Distal femur
Osteoid osteoma	Femur
Osteoblastoma	Vertebrae
Osteoma	Skull, facial bones
Enchondroma	Short bones of hand
Chordoma	Sacrum
Adamantinoma	Tibial
Ameloblastoma	Mandible
Osteoclastoma	Lower end femur
Fibrous dysplasia	Polyostotic–craniofacial Monostotic–upper femur
Multiple myeloma	Lumbar vertebrae
Osteosarcoma	Lower end femur
Ewing's sarcoma	Femur
Chondrosarcoma	Pelvis
Secondary tumors	Dorsal vertebrae

81. Ans. (b) Periosteal reaction

Ref: Fundamentals of Orthopedics, by Mukul Mohindra, Jitesh Kumar Jain P 500

- Sunray appearance in osteosarcoma is due to periosteal reaction, causing calcification along Sharpey's fiber.

IMPORTANT X-RAY SIGNS

- **Fibrous dysplasia:** Ground glass appearance, Rind sign (sclerotic margin around tumor), Shephard crook deformity (collapse of medial part of femoral neck so that proximal femur becomes hook shaped, seen in Paget's disease and Osteogenesis imperfecta also)
- **Simple bone cyst:** Fallen leaf sign (can be seen in ABC but less often).

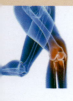

- **Hemangiome:** Corduroy appearance (Jail house sign), Polka dot pattern.
- **Osteoid osteoma:** Nidus <1.5 cm and osteoblastoma >1.5 cm.
- **Giant cell tumor:** Soap bubble appearance.
- **Osteosarcoma:** Codman's triangle, Sunray appearance (due to calcification along sharpey's fibers).
- **Chondrosarcoma:** Popcorn like calcification.
- **Ewing's sarcoma:** Onion peel appearance (intense periosteal reaction in layers), Codman's triangle.
- **Eosinophilic granuloma:** Punched out lytic lesions in skull with double contours.
- **Multiple myeloma:** Punched out lesions without a reactive/sclerotic surrounding zone.

82. Ans. (d) Osteofibrous dysplasia

- In the given image, the lesion is in tibial shaft. Given these choices, osteofibrous dysplasia is the single best answer.
- **Apley's states:** *"tumors in the tibial shaft is fairly rare. A condition that particularly affects the tibial shaft is osteofibrous dysplasia, a tumor that almost always occurs on the tibia, predominantly in shaft area"*
- **Note:** This condition is a very close differential diagnosis of malignant adamantinoma

83. Ans. (d) Chrondroblastoma

Ref: Apley's System of Orthopaedics, 9th ed. pg. 198

CHONDROBLASTOMA
- This benign tumor of immature cartilage cells is one of the few lesions to **appear primarily in the epiphysis**, usually of the **proximal humerus**, **femur or tibia**.
- The presenting symptom is a constant ache in the joint; the tender spot is actually in the adjacent bone.
- X-ray shows a rounded, well-demarcated radiolucent area in the epiphysis with no hint of central calcification.

84. Ans. (d) Osteosarcoma

Ref: Maheshwari, 5th ed. pg. 239

Osteosarcoma is a malignant bone tumor, which most commonly originates from metaphyseal region and is common in second decade.

TABLE: Tumors according to their origin site in long bone

Epiphysis (Mn: ECG)	Metaphysis (Mn: ME-BOO)	Diaphysis (DEMO–A)

• Chondroblastoma- before physeal closure
• Giant cell tumor- after physeal closure
	• Enchondroma (short bones)
	• Bone cyst (MC in upper humerus)
	  ▪ UBC, ABC
	  ▪ Osteochondroma (EXOSTOSIS)
	  ▪ Osteosarcoma
		• Ewing's sarcoma
		• Multiple myeloma
		• Osteoid osteoma
		• Adamantioma

UBC = Unicameral bone cyst
ABC = Aneurysmal bone cyst

85. Ans. (a) Osteosarcoma

Ref: Maheshwari, 5th ed. pg. 239

- Osteosarcoma is an aggressive malignant neoplasm arising from primitive transformed cells of mesenchymal origin (and thus a sarcoma) that exhibit osteoblastic differentiation and produce malignant osteoid.
- Sun Ray Appearance It is the most common radiological finding of primary bone cancer.
- If the lesion grows rapidly but steadily, the periosteum will not have enough time to lay down thin shell of bone, and in such cases, the tiny fibers that connect the periosteum to the bone *(Sharpey's fibers)* become stretched out perpendicular to the bone.
- **When these fibers ossify, they produce a pattern sometimes called "sunburst" periosteal reaction.**

86. Ans. (c) Osteoid osteoma

Ref: Maheshwari, 5th ed. pg. 235

- Osteoid osteoma is a benign bone tumor characterized by pain which is relieved by non-steroidal anti-inflammatory drugs (NSAIDs), such as aspirin.
- To clarify the mechanism of the pain, five osteoid osteomas were studied immune-histochemically using polyclonal antibodies against prostaglandin E2 (PGE2), S-100 protein and protein gene product.

87. Ans. (b) Second decade

Ref: Maheshwari, 5th ed. pg. 243

"Ewing's sarcoma is generally a lesion of children and adolescents, occurring most commonly (80% to 94%) in the first 2 decades, with a peak incidence in the second decade"

EWING'S SARCOMA
- Highly malignant, undifferentiated peripheral primitive neuro ectodermal tumor (PNET)
- Most common site is diaphysis of femur
- Common in 10–20 year old male
- Histopathology shows round cells containing glycogen and reticulin; PAS positive and diastase digestible
- 80–95% tumors possess translocation; t(11, 22)
- X-ray reveals laminated periosteal new bone formation also known as *"Onion peel appearance"*

Extra Mile

TABLE Bone tumors and their Incidence age wise

Tumor	Seen at age
Unicameral bone cyst	1st decade
Aneurysmal bone cyst	2nd decade
Giant cell tumor	2nd to 4th decade

88. Ans. (a) Giant cell tumor

Ref: Maheshwari 5th ed. pg. 237; Orthopedic Pathology by Vincent J Vigorita pg. 294

- GCT is an epiphyseal tumor
- GCT usually involves subarticular region distal radius and distal femur, the proximal tibia being most common site.
- If there is a soap bubble appearance in diaphyseal region, it is adamantioma.

Extra Mile

- **Sun burst appearance:** Osteosarcoma
- **Nidu/Seed in cortex:** Osteioid osteoma
- **Onion skin appearance:** Ewing's sarcoma
- **Exostosis (cartilage cap):** Osteochondroma

JOINT DISORDERS

89. Ans. (b) Knee

- Most common joint involved in thalassemia is Knee joint.
- Most common orthopaedic symptom in thalassemia is leg pain.

Extra Mile

- Most common joint involved in haemophilia: Knee > Elbow > Ankle > Shoulder > Hip

90. Ans. (a) Reiter's syndrome

Ref: Apley's System of Orthopaedics, 9th ed. pg. 70

REITER'S SYNDROME

- It is a clinical **triad** of **urethritis, arthritis and conjunctivitis** occurring some weeks after either dysentery of genitourinary infection. It is now recognized that this is one of the classic forms of reactive arthritis, i.e. an aseptic inflammatory arthritis associated with non-specific infection

Cause

- First-degree relatives and a close association with HLA-B27 point to a genetic predisposition.
- Gut pathogens include Shigella flexneri, Salmonella, Campylobacter species and Yersinia enterocolitica. Lymphogranuloma venereum and Chlamydia trachomatis have been implicated as sexually transmitted infections.

Clinical Features

- The acute phase of the disease is marked by an asymmetrical inflammatory arthritis of the lower limb joints–usually as well. The joint may be acutely painful, hot and swollen with a tense effusion, suggesting gout or infection.
- The chronic phase is more characteristic of a spondyloarthropathy.

91. Ans. (a) DIP

Ref: Maheshwari, 5th ed. pg. 287

- Rheumatoid arthritis characteristically causes swelling of small joints in the hand like the PIP, MCP and the wrist joint bilaterally.
- Isolated DIP joint involvement is seen in psoriatic arthropathy.
- DIP joint involvement is also seen with osteoarthritis but the involvement is with pain at the base of thumb. Knee joint is the commonest large joint involved in these patients.

92. Ans. (c) Flexion contracture of PIP and extension of DIP

Ref: Maheshwari, 5th ed. pg. 288

- **Boutonniere deformity** is a deformed position of the fingers or toes, in which the joint nearest the knuckle (PIP) is permanently bent toward the palm while the farthest joint (DIP) is bent back away *(PIP flexion with DIP hyperextension)*.
- It is commonly caused by injury or by an inflammatory condition like rheumatoid arthritis.

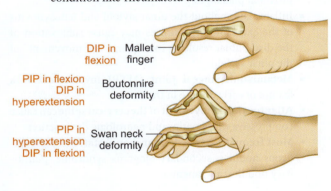

Extra Mile

- **'Z-deformity'** i.e. radial deviation of the wrist with ulnar deviation of the digits, often with palmar subluxation of proximal phalanges.
- **'Swan – neck deformity'** i.e. hyperextension of PIP joints with compensatory flexion of the distal interphalangeal joints.
- **Wind –** sweep deformities of toes i.e. valgus deformities of toes in one foot and varus in other, *(as wind sweeps all the structure in one direction).*

93. Ans. (b) Heberdens nodes

Ref: Harrison, 18th ed./ch. 332

- *"Heberden's nodes are hard or bony swellings that develop in the distal interphalangeal joints (DIP) in a case of osteoarthritis"*

Clinical Features of Rheumatoid Arthritis

- The presenting symptoms of RA typically result from inflammation of the joints, tendons, and bursae.
- Early morning joint stiffness lasting more than 1 hour and easing with physical activity.
- The earliest involved joints are typically the small joints of the hands and feet. The initial pattern of joint involvement may be monoarticular, oligoarticular (<4 joints), or polyarticular (>5 joints), usually in a symmetric distribution.
- *Wrists, metacarpophalangeal (MCP) and proximal interphalangeal (PIP) joints stand out as the most frequently involved joints.*
- **Frequent hallmark of RA:** Flexor tendon tenosynovitis.

Deformities

- Ulnar deviation of the hand.
- *Swan-neck deformity:* Hyperextension of the PIP joint with flexion of the DIP
- *Boutonniere deformity:* Flexion of the PIP joint with hyperextension of the DIP joint
- *Z deformity:* Radial deviation of wrist with ulnar deviation of digits, often with palmar subluxation proximal phalanges.
- Inflammation about the ulnar styloid and tenosynovitis of the extensor carpi ulnaris may cause subluxation of the distal ulna, resulting in a "piano-key movement" of the ulnar styloid
- **Metatarsophalangeal joint (MTP)** involvement is a feature of early disease in the feet
- **Atlantoaxial involvement of the cervical spine** can cause compressive myelopathy and neurologic dysfunction
- **Most frequent extraarticular manifestations:** Subcutaneous nodules, secondary Sjogren's syndrome, pulmonary nodules, and anemia.

---

94. Ans. (a) Rheumatoid Arthritis

Ref: Harrison's, 18th ed. Ch. 321

Clinical Features of RA

- Incidence of RA increases between 25 and 55 years of age.
- **Gender:** Female > Male
- Early morning joint stiffness lasting more than 1 hour and easing with physical activity.
- The earliest involved joints are typically the small joints of the hands and feet.
- The wrists, metacarpophalangeal (MCP), and proximal interphalangeal (PIP) joints stand out as the most frequently involved joints. Distal interphalangeal (DIP) joint involvement may occur in RA, but it usually is a manifestation of coexistent osteoarthritis.

---

95. Ans. (b) Gouty arthritis

Ref: Harrison's, 18th ed. Ch 332, 333

TABLE: Pathology and Common Joint Involved

Pathology	Common joint involved
Gout	1st MTP; GREAT TOE
OA	DIP, PIP- sparing MCP, wrist, elbow, ankle (DIP > KNEE)
RA	Involving PIP, MCP joint
Psoriasis	DIP
Pseudogout	Knee

---

96. Ans. (a) Indomethacin

Ref: Harrison's, 18th ed. Ch 333

- **MC site of gout:** Meta-tarsophalangeal joint of great toe.
- In gout there is deposition of uric acid in the joint.
- **Intake of Alcohol, Diuretics and aspirin are precipitating factors of gout.**

Treatment:

- NSAIDs given in full anti-inflammatory doses are effective in ~ 90% of patients.
- The most effective drugs are NSAIDS *(except aspirin)* with a short half-life and include **indomethacin 25–50 mg TID**; naproxen, ibuprofen and diclofenac.
- **Colchicine** given orally is a traditional and effective treatment if used early in an attack. It causes GI disturbance thereby reducing the compliance.
- Ultimate control of gout requires correction of the basic underlying defect: The hyperuricemia. Uricosuric drugs like **Allopurinol and Febuxostat** both are xanthine oxidase inhibitors. *These drugs are never preferred during acute attacks and whenever given, they should always be covered by NSAIDS.*
- **DOC for chronic gout: Allopurinol.**

---

97. Ans. (c) TB with polyarthritis

- **Spina ventosa-TB** of short bones
- **Caries sicca-TB** shoulder
- **Poncet disease-TB with polyarthritis**
- **Pott's-TB spine**

VERTEBRA & NEUROMUSCULAR DISEASE

98. Ans. (b) Ulnar nerve

Ref: Apley's System of Orthopaedics, 9th ed. pg. 290

- The ulnar nerve is easily felt behind the medial epicondyle of the humerus (the 'funny bone'). It can be trapped or compressed within the cubital tunnel (by bone abnormalities, ganglia or hypertrophied synovium).

Orthopedics

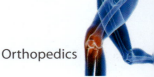

- Sometimes it is stretched by a cubitus valgus deformity or simply by holding the elbow flexed for long.

Extra Mile

TABLE: Neuropathy and Nerve involved

Carpal tunnel syndrome	Median nerve
Cubital tunnel syndrome	Ulnar nerve
Guyon canal syndrome	Ulnar nerve
Meralgia paresthetica	Lateral cutaneous nerve of thigh
Cheralgia paresthetica	Superficial radial nerve

99. Ans. (d) L4-L5

Ref: Maheshwari, 5th ed. pg. 253

- **Most common site of spinal disc herniation: Lumbar region (95% in L4-L5 or L5-S1).**
- **The second most common site is the cervical region (C5-C6, C6-C7).**
- Thoracic region accounts for only **0.15% to 4.0%** of cases.
- Herniations usually occur posterolaterally, where the annulus fibrosis is relatively thin and is not reinforced by the posterior or anterior longitudinal ligament.
- In the cervical spinal cord, a symptomatic posterolateral herniation between two vertebrae will impinge on the nerve which exits the spinal canal between those two vertebrae on that side. For example, a right posterolateral herniation of the disc between vertebrae C5 and C6 will impinge on the right C6 spinal nerve.

100. Ans. (a) Erb's paralysis

Ref: Apley's Orthopedics, 9th ed. pg. 279-80

Erb's paralysis	- Erb's palsy or Erb–Duchenne palsy is a paralysis of the arm caused by injury to the upper group of the arm's main nerves, specifically the severing of the upper trunk C5–C6 nerves. **Position of hand in Erb's paralysis:** Adducted, Internally rotated, and pronated
Klumpke's paralysis	Klumpke's Palsy involves the eighth cervical vertebra and the first thoracic vertebra (C8 and T1). **Position of hand:** Elbow flexed, arm supinated There may be unilateral horner syndrome
Horner syndrome	Seen with Pancoast tumor and presents with Ptosis, Miosis, enopthalmos, anhydrosis, loss of ciliospinal reflex.
Central cord syndrome	Seen most often after a hyperextension injury in an individual with long-standing cervical spondylosis. It presents with features of corticospinal pathway.

101. Ans. (b) Iatrogenic

Ref: Maheshwari, 5th ed. pg. 264

- The most common pathological mechanisms for sciatic nerve injury are compression, traction or direct injury by mechanical disruption as is seen in intragluteal muscle injection, or called as Sciatic neuritis.
- **Division of the main sciatic nerve is rare except in gunshot wounds or operative (iatrogenic) accidents.**
- The sciatic nerve is the nerve most commonly injured during total hip replacement.
- Sciatic nerve is the most common nerve injured by intramuscular injections, especially in children.

102. Ans. (c) Spondylolisthesis

Ref: Maheshwari, 5th ed. pg. 283-284

Spondylosis	Degenerative osteoarthritis of the joints between the center of the spinal vertebrae and/or neural foramina
Spondylitis	Spondylitis is an inflammation of the vertebra. It is a form of spondylopathy. In many cases spondylitis involves one or more vertebral joints as well, which itself is called spondylarthritis
Spondylolisthesis	Spondylolisthesis is the anterior or posterior displacement of a vertebra or the vertebral column in relation to the vertebrae below
Spondylolysis	Defect of a vertebra. More specifically it is defined as a defect in the pars interarticularis of the vertebral arch

103. Ans. (b) Axonotemesis

Ref: Maheshwari, 5th ed. pg. 63

104. Ans. (b) Ulnar nerve

Ref: Clinical assessment & examination in Orthopedics pg. 67

Tests for ulnar nerve

• Card test	Palmar interossei are Adductors (PAD) tested by asking the patient to hold a card between the extended fingers and assess resistance against pulling
• Egawa test	Dorsal interossei are Abductors (DAB) supplied by the ulnar nerve. It is tested by asking the patient to place the palm on table and move the middle finger both ways, i.e. towards index finger and ring finger. In Dorsal interossei palsy patient will be unable to abduct the middle finger
• Book test/ Froment's sign	To test adductor pollicis ask the patient to grasp a book or card between extended thumb and index finger. An ulnar nerve palsy patient tries to grasp the book by flexing the inter-phalangeal joint of thumb.

1047

Explanations

FMGE Solutions Screening Examination

> **Extra Mile**
> - OSCHNER CLASP TEST and PEN TEST is used to check for MEDIAN NERVE PALSY.

105. Ans. (b) Ulnar nerve palsy

Ref: Maheshwari, 5th ed. pg. 64

Please refer to above explanation

106. Ans. (c) Claw finger deformity

Ref: Maheshwari, 5th ed. pg. 64

- In ulnar nerve palsy especially in long standing cases, the hand assumes the characteristic **"claw" deformity.** It is also known as partial claw hand deformity.
- Complete claw hand deformity is due to palsy of ulnar and median nerve both.

Condition	Features
Median Nerve Palsy / Labourer Nerve Palsy	• Pointing index • Pen test • Ape thumb deformity • Carpal tunnel syndrome
Ulnar Nerve Palsy / Musician nerve palsy	• Book test (froment sign) • Card test • Egawa's test • Claw finger deformity
Radial Nerve Palsy	• Wrist drop • Thumb drop • Finger drop
Lateral cutaneous nerve of thigh (entrapped)	• Meralgia paraesthetica
Erb's palsy	**Policeman tip deformity (Porter's tip deformity)**

107. Ans. (b) Radial nerve

Ref: Maheshwari, 5th ed. pg. 25 Table 4.1

Cockup splint is used in cases of radial nerve injury.

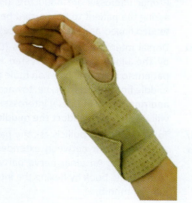

TABLE: Different splint and their Uses

Splint	Used In
Knuckle bender splint	Ulnar nerve
Aeroplane splint	Brachial plexus injury
Dennis brown splint	CTEV
Bohler Brown splint	Fracture femur (anywhere from neck to supracondylar region)
Turn buckle splint	VIC (Volkmann ischemic contracture)

108. Ans. (d) Physiological block

Ref: Apley's, 8th ed. pg. 231

TABLE: Patterns of nerve injury

Neuropraxia	Axonotmesis	Neurotmesis
• Reversible physiological nerve conduction block • It is seen in crutch palsy, **tourniquet palsy,** and saturday night palsy	• There is *loss of conduction* because *of axonal interruption* but the nerve is in continuity and the neural tubes are intact • Seen in closed *fractures* and dislocations	• There is complete division of nerve with complete loss of conduction (i.e. epineurium, perineurium, endoneurium, & axon all have lost their continuity) • Seen in open *wounds*

109. Ans. (c) C8 dermatome

Ref: Apley's system of Orthopaedics & Fractures, 9/e, pp- 229, 272

Clinically Important Dermatomes

Upper Extremity
- C6- Thumb
- C7 - Middle finger
- C8 - Little finger
- T1 - Inner forearm
- T2 - Upper inner arm

Lower Extremity
- L3-Knee
- L4 - Medial malleolus
- L5 - Dorsum of foot
- L5 - Toes 1–3
- SI - Toes 4 and 5; lateral malleolus

Others
- C2 and C3 - Posterior head and neck
- T4 - Nipple
- T10 - Umbilicus

Orthopedics

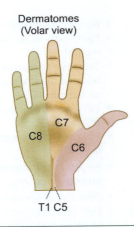

Dermatomes (Volar view)

- Clawing of figers is caused by Lumbrical muscle paralysis. It is also called as Intrinsic Minus Deformity or **Duchenne's sign**.
- Lumbricals of little finger and ring figer are supplied by Ulnar nerve.
- Lumbricals of Index finger and Middle finger are supplied by Median nerve.
- The ulnar nerve palsy causes partial claw hand involving little and ring fingers; **Ulnar nerve and Median Nerve combined injury causes Total claw hand involving all four fingers**
- Knuckle bender splint is used to correct the claw hand deformity.

110. Ans. (c) Ultrasound therapy

Ref: De Lisa's 'Physical Medicine and Rehabilitation: Principles and Practice'; 5/e, Vol II, p-1304

Treatment of Post-amputation Neuroma and Scar Pain

- Repeated injection of a local anaesthetic has proven to be an extremely useful technique.
- This should be followed by appropriate **physical therapy to the scar, usually ultrasound** followed by stretching or deep massage of the scar.
- This type of treatment has provided permanent or prolonged pain relief for longer than 6 months in many patients.
- When the local anaesthetics, with or without steroids, do not provide prolonged relief, other methods should be considered.
- Cryoanalgesia using a cryoprobe and freezing the neuroma for 1 minute at 20°C has been used with good success.
- The advantage of a cryoprobe lies in the fact that it is a physical method of blocking the nerve without further neuroma or neuritis.
- Neurolytic agents such as phenol or alcohol have been used to relieve neuroma and scar pain.
- However, incomplete block with these agents can resul: In neuritis, producing severe pain.
- These neurolytic techniques should be used only after repeated injections of local anaesthetics produce consistent pain relief proportional to the duration or action of the local anaesthetic agent.
- Although surgical revision of the scar is often considered, it is not very successful when the scar cannot be stretched out and there is significant nerve entrapment.

111. Ans. (b) Ulnar nerve

Ulnar Claw Hand

- The deformity in the picture is Partial Claw Hand, i.e. Hyperextension of MCP joints and Hyperflxion of interphalangeal joints of ring and little fingers.

PEDIATRIC ORTHOPEDICS

112. Ans. (c) Perthes disease

Ref: Essential Orthopaedics, Maheshwari & Mhaskar, 6th ed. P 318

PERTHES DISEASE

- Also known as Coxa plana or Pseudocoxalgia
- It is an osteochondritis of the epiphysis of the femoral head
- The femoral head here becomes avascular → Avascular necrosis of femoral head
- **MC age group:** 5–10 years
- **The disease progress through 3 stages:**
  - Stage of synovitis
  - Stage of trabecular necrosis
  - Stage of healing
- **Clinical picture:**
  - Pain in hip, radiating to knee
  - Limping or hip stiffness
- **Upon examination:**
  - Limb shortening
  - Limitation of abduction and internal rotation
- **X-ray:**
  - Sclerosis of femoral head epiphysis *(as seen in image of this patient)*
  - Hip joint space is increased
- **Treatment:**
  - Head containment (by plaster, splint or surgical)—Head is kept inside the acetabulum while revascularisation takes place

OTHER OPTIONS

- There is no history of trauma, so hip dislocation is unlikely
- DDH usually seen in infant, and the clinical presentation also doesn't correlate with DDH
- In Stage 1 hip there is apparent limb lengthening

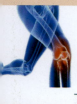

FMGE Solutions Screening Examination

113. Ans. (a) Dysplasia of proximal epiphysis

Ref: Essential Orthopaedics, Maheshwari & Mhaskar, 6th ed. P 320

BLOUNT'S DISEASE

- Disease caused by abnormality of proximal posteromedial tibial epiphysis
- Classically seen in African-American obese male child (first 3 years) and in west Indies
- Presents as pathologic tibia vara (bowed legs)

TABLE: Some other developmental abnormalities of orthopaedic interest

• Olliers disease (multiple enchondromas) • Dyschondroplasia	• Not familial • Masses of cartilage in the metaphysis remain unossified • Defective ossification
Melorheostosis	• Candle bone disease
Osteopathia striata	• Striped bones disease
Osteopoikilosis	• Spotted bones disease
Morquio disease	• Familial (autosomal recessive) disease • Gives rise to dwarfism affecting both, limbs and trunk • Mental development normal • Corneal opacity sometimes present • X-ray – typical 'tonguing' of lumbar vertebrae • Keratan sulfhate in urine
Hunter's disease	• Familial x-linked disease • Defect is the excretion of large amount of Keratan sulfhate in urine • Dwarf with dorso lumbar kyphosis, knock knees, flat feet • Mental deficiency may occur • No corneal opacity
Hurler's disease (Gargoylism)	• Familial (autosomal recessive) disease • Give rise to dwarfism of both, limbs and trunk • Defect is an error in development of fibroblasts • There is excretion of dermatan sulfate and hepartan sulfate in urine • Typical facial appearance • Mental development abnormal • Corneal opacity present • X-ray typical 'beak ' in 2nd lumbar vertebra
Engelmann's disease	• Familial (autosomal recessive) disease • Symmetrical, fusiform enlargement and sclerosis of shafts of the long bones in children. Femur affected commonly. • Epiphysis is spared

Contd...

Caffey's disease (infantile cortical hyperostosis)	• Nonfamilial disease • Starts early in life (before the 5th month) • There is a formation of sub-periosteal bone on the shafts of long bones, and on the mandible • Self-limiting course, resolves by 3 years of age • Tibia more common than ulna in familial form
Albright's syndrome	• Polyostotic fibrous dysplasia and precocious puberty
Arthrogryposis multiplex congenita (AMC)	• Defective development of muscles • Stiff, deformed joints • Multiple joint dislocations with 'shapeless extremities' • May present as clubfoot
Myositis ossificans progressiva	• Ectopic ossification, often beginning in trunk • Short big toe
Multiple epiphyseal dysplasia	• Least rare type • Affects all the epiphyses, resulting in stunted growth, deformities (varum, valgum etc.) • Epiphysis looks ill defined, irregular on X-rays
Spondylo-epiphyseal dysplasia	• Spine is also involved in addition to limb epiphyses
Metaphyseal dysplasia (Pyle's disease)	• Autosomal recessive • A modelling defect results in 'Erlenmeyer flask' deformity of the distal femur and proximal tibia
Blount's disease	• The growth of the medial-half of the proximal tibial epiphysis is retarded, resulting in severe tibia vara deformity in childhood, common in West Indies
Cleidocranil dysostosis	• Faulty development of membranous bones • Clavicles are absent • Skull sutures remain open • Coxa vara • Wide foramen magnum
Nail patella syndrome	• Familial disorder • Hypoplastic nails and absence of patella
Marfans syndrome (Arachnodactyly)	• Spider fingers • Associated atrial regurgitation • Ocular lens dislocation
Apert syndrome	• Tower shaped head

114. Ans. (c) Elbow

- Most common joint dislocation in pediatric population: **Elbow joint**
- Most common joint dislocation in adult population: **Humerus Joint**

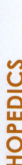

Orthopedics

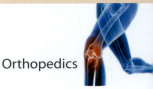

115. **Ans. (d) Slipped capital femoral epiphysis**
    - The usual presentation of SCFE is an overweight child who has poorly localized groin, thigh or knee pain.
    - Usual age of presentation is 11–14 years. M>F
    - Upon examination leg is shortened and externally rotated.
    - Upon radiological investigation:
        - **Trethovan's sign:** A line drawn along the superior border of the femoral neck on the AP view should pass through the femoral head. In SCFE, the line passes superior to the head rather than through the head.

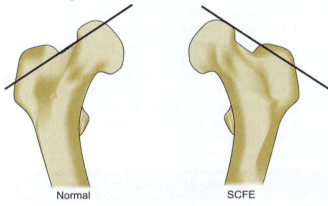

Normal   SCFE

116. **Ans. (b) USG**

Ref: Maheshwari, 5th ed. pg. 222

TABLE: Investigations of congenital dislocation of Hip

USG	• Post natal diagnosis within the first year is best made by an ultrasound • Allows assessment even in first two months when plain radiographs can be normal • Considered as screening test of choice in case of CDH

X-Ray	Plain films may be normal in first 2–3 months, however subtle changes begin to appear at 6 weeks
	• Reliable depiction of DDH made after 4–6 months
	• Most useful in period between 2–8 months
	• Classical findings: (putti's triad)
	  1. Absent or small proximal femoral capital epiphyses
	  2. Lateral displacement of femur
	  3. Shallow acetabulum with an increased inclination of acetabular roof > 30 degrees
	• Disruption of shenton's line
	• Head lies in outer and upper quadrant

CT	Used for pre-surgical planning
MRI	Considered as IOC/Best investigation for diagnosis of CDH

117. **Ans. (c) Congenital dislocation of hip**
    - Physical examination used for testing congenital dislocation of hip (CDH)- done together
        - ♦ **Barlow test:** Hip is dislocated by Adduction
        - ♦ **Ortolani test:** relocation done by Abduction

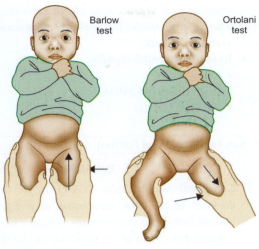

118. **Ans: (a) Spring ligament**

Ref: Maheshwari, 5th ed. pg. 210

- *"Pesplanus or a flat foot is a disorder of laxity of medial longitudinal arch which is maintained by the spring ligament and plantar aponeurosis"*
- The term pesplanus denotes an excessively flat foot. There is no precise degree of flatness that defines pesplanus, but it may be either physiological or pathological.
- In physiological pesplanus, the feet are flexible and rarely problematic. In marked contrast, pathological pesplanus is often associated with stiffness and pain.
- The windlass (or 'Jack's great toe') test involves passively dorsiflexing the hallux at the metatarsophalangeal joint. This tightens the plantar aponeurosis and, in flexible pesplanus, results in accentuation of the medial longitudinal arch.
- In pathological pesplanus, no accentuation of the arch is seen. This test can also be carried out by asking the individual to stand on tiptoe and viewing the hind foot from behind. In flexible flat feet, the calcaneus swings into a varus position; in pathological pesplanus it does not.

119. **Ans. (b) Late congenital syphilis**

Ref: Maheshwari, 5th ed. pg. 178

- **The clinical manifestations of congenital syphilis include:**
    - **Early manifestations:** Infection appear within the first 2 years of life (often at 2–10 weeks of age)
    - **Late manifestations,** are noninfectious and appear after 2 years
- Late congenital syphilis (untreated after 2 years of age) is subclinical in 60% of cases; the clinical spectrum in the remainder of cases may include interstitial keratitis (which

occurs at 5–25 years of age), eighth-nerve deafness, and recurrent arthropathy. Bilateral knee **effusions are known as clutton's joints.**
- **Triad of congenital syphilis:**
  - Keratitis
  - Heart defect (MC: PDA)
  - Deafness (SNHL)

120. Ans. (a) Congenital flat foot

Ref: Maheshwari, 5th ed. pg. 326

- Congenital vertical talus (CVT) is an uncommon disorder of the foot, manifested as a rigid rocker-bottom flatfoot. Its characteristic radiographic feature is a dorsal dislocation of the navicular on the talus. If left untreated, CVT results in a painful and rigid flatfoot with weak push-off power. CVT has been referred to in the literature by several synonyms, including congenital convex pes valgus.
- **Presentation:**
- Presents as a rigid flatfoot with **a rocker-bottom appearance** of the foot.
- The forefoot is abducted and dorsiflexed.
- **Treatment:** Serial casting should be the initial treatment, although prior to the Dobbs article, it was usually thought to be unsuccessful. A single-stage surgical correction is another option and can be accomplished via either the **Cincinnati approach** or the dorsal approach.

METABOLIC BONE DISORDERS

121. Ans. (c) Osteopetrosis

Ref: Essential Orthopaedics, Maheshwari & Mhaskar, 6th ed. P 317

OSTEOPETROSIS

- Also known as Marble bone disease or Albers-Schonberg disease
- It is characterized by dense but brittle bones also known as marble bones which occur due to reduced bone resorption and diffuse symmetrical skeletal sclerosis due to impaired formation or function of osteoclast.
- **X-ray appearances**
  - Bone within Bone appearance
  - Erlenmeyer flask deformity of long bone disease ends (flask shaped metaphysis)
  - Rugger jersey spine
  - Increased bone density

It can occur in two forms:

Autosomal dominant	Congenital Autosomal recessive
• Less severe	More severe form
• Has tendency to fracture	In child it is associated with severe anemia, jaw osteomyelitis and cranial nerve palsies
• Better survival	Poor survival

122. Ans. (d) Osteoarthritis

Ref: Harrison's 19th ed. P 2226

- Osteoarthritis (OA) is the most common type of arthritis.
- Commonly affected joints include the cervical and lumbosacral spine, hip, knee, and first metatarsal phalangeal joint (MTP).
- In the hands, the distal and proximal interphalangeal joints and the base of the thumb are often affected.
- Joints Spared: Wrist, elbow, and ankle
- Deformity can be due to bouchard nodes (PIP) and heberden nodes (DIP)

TABLE: Joint involvement in several conditions

	Osteoarthritis	Rheumatoid arthritis	Psoriatic arthritis
Joint involved	PIP DIP and 1st carpometacarpal joint (1st CMC)	• PIP • MCP • Wrist	• DIP • PIP and any other joints
Joint spared	MCP and wrist	DIP	Any

123. Ans. (c) Bisphosphonates

Ref. Postmenopausal Osteoporosis, Hormones & Other therapies by Andrea R Genazzari, P 289-90

- Bisphosphonates act by inhibiting osteoclast mediated bone resorption. Currently the 3rd generation bisphosphonate is commonly used.
- Zoledronate is the most potent and is also considered as *drug of choice for treatment and prophylaxis of osteoporosis.*
- It is also used for treatment of hypercalcemia associated with malignancy and for treatment of Paget's disease.
- Bisphosphonates have poor oral absorption. Therefore given empty stomach, around 30 minutes before meal with a glass of water. They are known to cause esophagitis, so patients are asked to remain upright after drug intake.

TABLE: Classification of bisphosphonates

1st generation	2nd generation	3rd generation
• Etidronate • Clodronate • Medronate	• Alendronate • Pamidronate	• Zoledronate (2–5 mg/year) • Risedronate (150 mg/month)

Orthopedics

1053

124. Ans. (d) Vitamin D deficiency

Ref: Apley's System of Orthopaedics, 9th ed. pg. 135-36

- The given image and the information on cupping and widening points towards rickets.
- Rickets and osteomalacia are different expressions of the same disease: inadequate mineralization of bone.
- The inadequacy may be due to defects anywhere along the metabolic pathway for vitamin D: Nutritional lack, underexposure to sunlight, intestinal malabsorption, decreased 25-hydroxylation (liver disease, anticonvulsants) and reduced 1α-hydroxylation (renal disease).

Clinical Features of Rickets

- The infant with rickets may present with **tetany** or convulsions. Later the parents may notice that there is a **failure to thrive**, listlessness and **muscular flaccidity**. Early bone changes are deformity of the skull **(craniotabes)** and thickening of the knees, ankles and wrists from physeal overgrowth. Enlargement of the costochondral junctions (**'rickety rosary'**) and lateral indentation of the chest **(Harrison's sulcus)** may also appear.
- Distal tibial bowing has been attributed to sitting or lying **cross-legged**.
- In active rickets there is thickening and **widening of the growth plate**, **cupping of the metaphysis** and, sometimes, bowing of the diaphysis. The metaphysis may remain abnormally wide even after healing has occurred.

125. Ans. (c) Scurvy

Ref: Maheshwari, 5th ed. pg. 315

Scurvy causes failure of collagen synthesis and osteoid formation. It clinically presents with:
- Irritability
- Gum bleeding
- Pseudoparalysis (due to subperiosteal haemorrhage)
- Anemia and beading of costochondral junction.

Radiological features are: Frenkel's line (dense line between metaphysic and physis/epiphysis), ring sign, *thin cortex,* scurvy line (band of rarefaction on the diaphyseal side) and metaphyseal osteopenia, cleft and fractures.

Pathology: Deficiency causes failure of collagen synthesis or primitive collagen formation, throughout the body, including in blood vessels, predisposing to haemorrhage.

> **Extra Mile**

Rickets	Scurvy
• **Metaphysis:** *indistinct, frayed, splaying, and cupping of margin.* Patchy sclerosis in case of intermittent dietary deficiency	• **Metaphysis:** Frankel's white line, Trummerfeld, lucent zone, Pelkan spur due to fracture.
• Widened epiphysis with hazed cortical margin	• Wimberger's sign (small epiphysis surrounded by sclerotic rim)
• Generalized reduction in bone density	• Subperiosteal hemorrhage with periosteal elevation
• Looser's zone (less common)	• Ground glass appearance of bone with pencil thin cortex.
• Severe cases show Genu valgum, bow legs, thoracic kyphosis, pigeon chest, *ricketic rosary,* skull bossing, cox vera.	

126. Ans. (b) Scurvy

Please refer to above explanation

127. Ans. (c) Vitamin D

Ref: Maheshwari, 5th ed. pg. 311

- Double malleoli is sign of rickets which is seen due to deficiency of vitamin D.

Please refer to above explanation

128. Ans. (a) Fluorosis

Ref: Maheshwari, 5th ed. pg. 314

- Hint in the question is child from a village of Bihar with Genu varum/bow legged, long bone pain and X-Rays showing increased bone density, this characteristically focuses towards Fluorosis.

GENU VALGUM (KNOCK KNEE)

- It is *abnormal approximation of knees* with abnormally *divergent ankles.* It can be estimated by measuring the distance between the medial malleolis, when the knees are touching with the patella facing forwards; it is usually *<5 cm.* Valgus alignment of lower extremities is normal in child between *2–8 years* of age (Known as *physiological valgus* & is maximum between 2–4 years). The commonest cause of genu valgum (knock knee) is *idiopathic > rickets.*

Explanations

FMGE Solutions Screening Examination

GENU VARUM (BOW LEGS)

- Knee are abnormally divergent and ankles approximated. B/L bow legs can be estimated by measuring the distance between the medial malleoli when heels are touching; it should be <6 cm. Normal children show maximum varus at 6 months to 1 year of age. The *causes of genu varum are similar to genu val gum* except that the defective growth is on the medial side.

FLUOROSIS

- Fluorine in very low concentration- *1 part per million (ppm)* or less is used to reduce the incidence of dental caries. At slightly higher levels *(2–4 ppm)* it may produce *mottling of teeth*.
- In some parts of India and Africa, where fluorine concentration in the drinking water may be above *10 ppm*- chronic fluorine intoxication (flurosis) is endemic and results in skeletal anomalies.
- **Characterstic pathological feature** is *subperiosteal new bone accretion and osteosclerosis (increased bone density)*, most marked in vertebrae, ribs, pelvis, forearm and leg bones, together with *hyperostosis at the bony attachments of ligaments, tendons and fascia*.
- Despite the apparent thickening and density of skeleton, tensile strength is reduced and the bones fracture more easily.
- First clinical manifestation is usually a stress fracture, **back pain, bone pain, joint stiffness** and neurological defects (due to hyperostosis encroaching vertebral canal).
- **Characterstic X-ray features** are *osteosclerosis, osteophytosis and ossification of ligamentous and fascial attachments*. It can be radiologically mistaken for other osteosclerotic conditions as *Paget's disease, osteopetrosis, renal osteodystrophy, idiopathic skeletal hyperostosis* etc.
- **Note:** *Fluorine stimulates osteoblastic activity; fluoroapatite crystals* are laid down in bone and these are usually *resistant to osteoclastic resorption*. This leads to *calcium retention* impaired mineralization and *secondary hyperparathyroidism*.

> **Extra Mile**
>
> - **Infantile cortical hyperostosis (Caffeys Disease)** is a *self limiting disorder* characterized by *soft tissue swelling, rapid subperiosteal new bone formation, cortical thickening of under lying bones,* fever and irritability. Classically, the onset of disease *occurs before 5th month* of life with *resolution by 3 years of age*.
> - In sporadic cases, *mandible is the most common site of involvement presenting as jaw tumor* or swelling i.e. is firm, tender without heat or redness.

129. Ans. (b) Osteoclasts

Ref: Robbin's Pathology, 8th pg. 1212

"**Osteopetrosis** also known as **marble bone disease** and **Alber's Schon-berg disease** is characterized by reduced bone resorption and diffuse symmetrical skeletal sclerosis due to impaired formation or function of **osteoclasts**."

Disease	Cause
Osteogenesis imperfecta	Deficiency in synthesis of type 1 collagen
Osteopetrosis	Osteoclasts dysfunction
Osteoporosis	Loss of bone mass
Paget disease (Osteitis Deformans)	Both osteoclast and osteoblast dysfunction
Rickets and osteomalacia	Vitamin D deficiency
Scurvy	Vitamin C deficiency

130. Ans. (b) Osteopetrosis

Ref: Sutton, 7th pg. 1339, 1355, 1365

Disease	Radiological feature
Osteoporosis	• **Cod fish vertebrae** • Pencilling-in-vertebrae (loss of density of vertebral body with radiodense end plates)
Osteomalacia	• **Looser's zone/Pseudo fracture** is the Hallmark feature (B/L radiolucent band of uncalcified osteoid due to pressure of pulsating artery) • **Cod Fish** (marked biconcave) vertebrae • Pencilling in vertebrae
Osteopetrosis/ Marble Bone disease/Alberg Schowenberg disease	• **Bone within Bone appearance** • Erlenmeyer flask deformity of long bone disease ends (flask shaped metaphysis) • **Rugger jersey spine** • Increased density of bones

131. Ans. (b) Vit D deficiency Rickets

Ref: Maheshwari 5th ed. pg. 317, 311; http://www.indianpediatrics.net/july 2013/july-669-675.htm

- Different methods of treating vitamin D deficiency have been advocated, ranging from small doses for a few months to a single mega dose *(high dose)*, an approach referred to as *stoss therapy*.
- Vitamin D deficiency rickets occurs secondary to vitamin D deficiency which can take place secondary to many factors:

Orthopedics

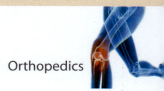

Decreased vitamin D synthesis	Due to chronic liver disease
Decreased nutritional intake of vitamin	In strict vegetarian diet
Age and physiology related	Elderly, obese and institutionalized patients
Decreased maternal vitamin D stores	Exclusive breast feeding
Malabsorption	Celiac disease, pancreatic insufficiency (cystic fibrosis), biliary obstruction (biliary atresia)
Increased degradation of 25 (OH) D_3	Due to intake of drugs such as rifampicin, isoniazid, anticonvulsants, glucocorticoids

Recommended Treatment Regimen
- **Common recommendations include** vitamin D 1000-5000 units/day for several weeks or single IM injection of 6 lakh units (Stoss therapy) or 50,000 U of vitamin D_2 weekly for 8 weeks.
- Another advantage of Stoss therapy is that vitamin D is efficiently stored in adipose tissue and muscle and is continuously converted into active form.
- Stoss therapy regimens with large oral or parenteral dose of vitamin D_3 has been shown to cause increased and sustained higher levels of 25 (OH) D_3 levels, especially the regimen with **6 lakh IU.**

Note: Vitamin D stimulates renal and GI absorption of calcium.

PAGET'S DISEASE
- It is characterized by *excessive disorganized bone turnover,* that encompasses *excessive osteoclastic activity initially followed by disorganized excessive new bone formation.*
- **Treatment of choice for paget's disease: Calcitonin.**

132. Ans. (c) Raised serum calcium

Ref: Maheswari's, 5th pg. 310, 311

"In **osteomalacia** the **serum calcium level is low**, the phosphates are low, and alkaline phosphatase is high."

PATHOPHYSIOLOGY OF OSTEOMALACIA

Lack of sunlight exposure, nutritional deficiency of **vitamin D,** malabsorption syndrome, partial gastrectomy
↓
Failure of absorption of **calcium and phosphorous (Decreased serum calcium and phosphorous)**
↓
Decreased turnover of calcium and phosphorus in bone matrix
↓
Demineralization of bone and bony substance replaced by soft osteoid tissue
↓
Bone pains, muscular weakness (myopathy), spontaneous fractures

Note: Osteoid matrix is secreted at normal rate but the mineralization is decreased (i.e. decrease in mineral apposition rate). This leads to increased osteoid maturation time.

Radiological Features
- **Looser's Zone (pseudo fracture)**- Are radiolucent zones at sites of stress.
- **Triradiate pelvis** in female.

133. Ans (b) Osteomalacia

Ref: Maheshwari, 5th ed. pg. 312

- **Cortical infarctions** are wide transverse lucencies traversing bone usually at right angles to the involved cortex and are *associated most frequently with osteomalacia* and rickets. They are pseudofractures and considered a type of insufficiency fracture.
- Typically, the fractures have sclerotic irregular margins, and are often symmetrical.

Causes of Looser's Zone
- Osteomalacia
- Renal osteodystrophy
- Fibrous dysplasia
- Hyperthyroidism
- Paget's disease of bone
- X linked hypophosphataemia
- Osteogenesis Imperfecta

134. Ans. (d) Osteogenesis Imperfecta

Ref: Maheshwari, 5th ed. pg. 316

- In case of Osteogenesis Imperfecta patients are born with defective connective tissue, or without the ability to make it.
- This condition usually arises because of a **deficiency of type I collagen.**
- Deficiency of type I collagen arises from an amino acid substitution of glycine to bulkier amino acids in the collagen triple helix structure.
- The replaced larger amino acid side-chains create steric hindrance that creates a bulge in the collagen complex, which in turn influences both the molecular nano-mechanics and the interaction between molecules, which are both compromised.

FMGE Solutions Screening Examination

Radiological Findings in Limbs in Osteogenesis Imperfecta

- Thin and under tabulated gracile bones which are normal in length or shortened
- **Thickened or deformed bones (due to multiple fractures)**
- **Banana fracture:** pathological fractures tend to be oriented transversely within long bones
- Shaft fractures and metaphyseal abnormalities with florid or exuberant callus formation that can mimic an osteosarcoma.

> **Extra Mile**
> - Battered baby syndrome in this question is ruled out since fractures are seen in it in various stages of healing.
> - Hypo-parathyroidism can present with short stature and features of rickets like delayed dentition.

135. Ans. (b) Duchenne muscular dystrophy

Ref: Harrison, 19th ed. pg. 462e-5

- *Gowers' sign is classically seen in Duchenne muscular dystrophy* but also presents itself in centro nuclear myopathy, myotonic dystrophy and various other conditions associated with proximal muscle weakness.
- This causes the patient to get up in a peculiar fashion taking support of his body or a nearby object.

136. Ans. (a) Pseudohypoparathyroidism

Ref: Harrison 19th ed. pg. 2485

Differential Diagnosis of Short 4th and 5th Metacarpal

- Post traumatic
- Ishemic diseases like sickle cell anemia
- Pseudohypoparathyroidism
- Pseudo-pseudo hypoparathyroidism
- Turner's syndrome

137. Ans. (c) Phalanges

Ref Sutton 7th ed. pg. 1339, 1362

Hallmark or characteristic feature of hyperparathyroidism is- subperiosteal erosion of bone, particularly aspect of middle pharynx of middle and index finger.

> **Extra Mile**
> - Other sites of subperiosteal resorption include the phalangeal tufts; medial aspect of the proximal ends of the tibia, humerus and femur; superior and inferior margins of the ribs; and lamina dura.

138. Ans. (b) Nutritional deficiency (most probably)

- **Nutritional bone disease** is defined as a **syndrome of bone disease and deformities** in which the bone is affected as a tissue, primarily as a consequence to deficiencies of vitamin D and calcium; or imbalances of the nutrients which are critically important for the growth and development of the bone; its mineralization and maintenance of calcium homeostasis and the structural integrity and health of the skeleton.
- Vitamin D deficiency is widespread in both genders in India.

139. Ans. (b) Ankylosing spondylitis

Radiological features of Ankylosing Spondylitis
- Sacroiliitis is a pre-requisite for diagnosis. The SI joints may show erosion, sclerosis at early stage and ankylosis in late stages.
- Spine: Squaring of vertebral bodies
- Syndesmophyte formation
- Bamboo spine' appearance

ANSWERS TO BOARD REVIEW QUESTIONS

140. Ans. (a) Iatrogenic

Ref: Apley's Concise system of Orthopaedics and Fractures 3rd p 118

141. Ans. (a) Heberden nodules

Ref: Harrison's 18th ed. ch. : 321

142. Ans. (a) Spring ligament

Ref: Gray's Anatomy 40th ed. ch. : 84, 39th ed p 1512, Keith L Moore 4th ed p 400

143. Ans. (b) Late congenital syphilis

Ref: Harrison's 18th ed. ch. : 169

144. Ans. (a) Fibula

Ref: Rockwood 7th ed. ch. : 19

145. Ans. (b) Second decade

Ref: Apley's system of orthopaedics 8th edn p 190, Turek's orthopaedics 6th ed p 307

Orthopedics

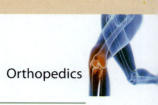

146. Ans. (d) Tissue biopsy is investigation of choice
- Sunburst appearance can also be found in other bone malignancy

147. Ans. (c) Can be seen in Acute osteomyelitis
- MCC of brodies = Subacute OM >> chronic OM.

148. Ans. (b) Pyogenic arthritis

149. Ans. (a) Tenosynovitis

150. Ans. (b) Medial rotation of tibia

151. Ans. (c) Secondaries

152. Ans. (c) Enchondroma

153. Ans. (c) Shoulder dislocation

154. Ans. (a) Non-union

155. Ans. (b) Simple bone cyst

Ref: Essentials in Bone and Soft-Tissue Pathology-By Jasvir S. Khurana, Edward F. McCarthy Paul J. Zhang p-70

156. Ans. (a) Thoracolumbar

Ref: Apley 387-389, Schwartz's Principles of Surgery 9th ed ch-29 M Tuli 3rded p-192

157. Ans. (b) Common peroneal

Ref: Gray's Anatomy 39th ed Grant's Atlas of Anatomy, 12th ed p-428

158. Ans. (d) Coxa vara

Ref: Textbook of orthopaedics and Trauma by GS Kulkarni p -3635

159. Ans. (b) Carpal instability

Ref: Essential Orthopaedics p-307

160. Ans. (b) Pain in snuffbox

Ref: Rockwood and Green's Fractures in Adults by Robert W. Bucholz p 791

161. Ans. (c) Cervical spine

Ref: Orthopedic surgery essentials-Spine by Christopher M. Bono, Steven R. Garfin p-188

162. Ans. (d) Tillaux fracture

Ref: Rockwood and wilkins' fractures in children p 991

163. Ans. (b) Gluteus medius

Ref: Keith L. Moore 4/e, p 348/354

164. Ans. (a) Multiple myeloma

Ref: Apley's 8/e, p 191

165. Ans. (b) Surgical neck humerus

Ref: Grant's atlas of anatomy, 12/e, p 524

166. Ans. (a) Tibial tuberosity

Ref: Apley's system of Orthopaedics and fractures edited by Louis Solomon, Dividwarwick, Selvadurainayagam 9/e, p 575-576, 887

167. Ans. (d) Claw hallux

Ref: Textbook of Orthopaedics and trauma G. S. Kulkarni 2/e, p 575, Essential orthopaedicsmaheshwari 4/e, p 341

168. Ans. (b) Clay shoveller's fracture

Ref: Essntial Orthopaedics by J. Maheshwar 4/e, p 265

169. Ans. (c) 8–10 min

Ref: Essential orthopaedics by J. Maheshwari 4/e, p 338

170. Ans. (c) Heberden's nodes

171. Ans. (b) Genu varum

Ref: Apley's orthopaedics 9/e, p 572

172. Ans. (a) Retained vascularity

Ref: Rockwood and wilkins' Fractures in children p 1020, Lovell and winter's pediatric orthopaedics vol-1, 6/e, p 1512

173. Ans. (b) Carpal tunnel syndrome

Ref: Appendix-135 for "Tests used in orthopedics

174. Ans. (d) De quervain tenosynovitis

Ref: Appendix-135 for "Tests used in orthopedics

175. Ans. (a) Hallax valgus

Ref: Essential orthopaedics J. Maheshwari 4/e, p 341, Srb's Manual of surgery by bhat 4/e, p 173

FMGE Solutions Screening Examination

176. Ans. (b) **Tibial torsion**

Ref: Segen's Medical dictionary

177. Ans. (d) **Ankle**

Ref: Skeletal radiology: Bare bones, P 225

- In hand osteoarthritis primarily affects PIP, DIP and basal joint of thumb (1st carpometacarpal joint).
- Isolated involvement of basal joint of thumb is diagnostic of primary osteoarthritis (Specific joint involved).
- Other joints involved are: 1st metatarsophalangeal joint, hips and knees, cervical and lumbar spine.
  - Lumbar spine is the most frequent spinal location for osteoarthritis
- **Joints which are spared in osteoarthritis:**
  - Metacarpophalangeal joint (MCP)
  - Wrist
  - Elbow
  - Shoulder
  - Ankle

178. Ans. (a) **Knee**

- Among the given options knee is the more commonly affected joint in osteoarthritis.
- Knee joint is also the most common lower limb joint affected in osteoarthritis.

179. Ans. (b) **Lunate**

Ref: Textbook of Orthopedics by Kotwal; P 124-125

- Keinbock disease is avascular necrosis of lunate bone.

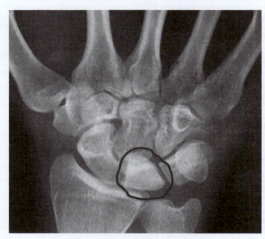

Other avascular necrosis of bones are:
- **Kohler disease:** AVN of Navicular
- **Freiberg disease:** 2nd MT head
- **Islene disease:** 5th MT base
- **Perthes disease:** Avascular necrosis of Head of Femur
- **Scheuermann's disease:** vertebral epiphysis avascular necrosis

ANSWERS TO IMAGE-BASED QUESTIONS

180. Ans. (c) **Giant cell tumor**

The image shows X-ray of wrist joint with presence of Soap Bubble appearance.
Soap bubble appear once is seen in Adamantinoma (MC site of Adamantinoma: Tibia > mandible)

"Soap Bubble appearance as a term" is to be remembered also for:
- Hydronephrosis
- Osteoclastoma (Giant cell tumor)
- Meconium ileus

181. Ans. (b) **Aneurysmal bone cyst**

- The image shows X-ray of the knee joint with presence of multiple lytic lesions suggestive of aneurysmal bone cyst.
- Unicameral bone Cyst is more common in upper humerus.

182. Ans. (c) **Rocker bottom foot**

The image shows convexity at the sole of the foot sole. In CTEV the bilateral feet and toes point inwards facing each other.

183. Ans. (d) **Monteggia fracture**

- The image shows X-ray of the Elbow joint with fracture of upper ulna diagnostic of Monteggia Fracture.
- Galeazzi fracture is an isolated fracture of the junction of the distal third and middle third of the radius with associated subluxation or dislocation of the distal radio-ulnar joint

184. Ans. (c) **Sunburst appearance**

- The image shows a sun burst appearance lesion which grows rapidly but steadily, and the periosteum will not have enough time to lay down thin shell of bone.
- Therefore in such cases, the tiny fibers that connect the periosteum to the bone (Sharpey's fibers) become stretched out perpendicular to the bone. When these fibers ossify, they produce a pattern sometimes called "sunburst" periosteal reaction.
- It is usually seen in osteosarcoma, but can also be seen in other bone malignancies.

Orthopedics

185. Ans. (c) **Mallet finger**

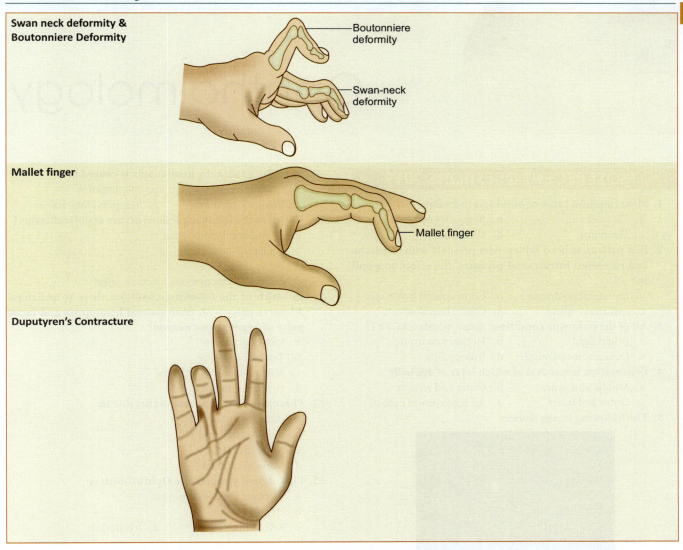

186. Ans. (a) **Gallow's Traction**

Gallow's traction	Fracture shaft of femur in children <2 years
90–90 traction	Fracture shaft femur in children
Russel traction	Conventional skin traction
Agnes hunt traction	Hip deformity

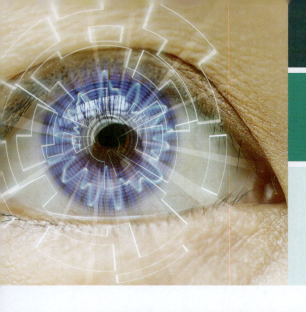

15

Ophthalmology

MOST RECENT QUESTIONS 2019

1. Most common cause of blindness in India:
    a. Cataract
    b. Refractive error
    c. Trachoma
    d. Glaucoma
2. In a patient of head injury, who presents with headache and increased intracranial pressure, the effect on pupil is:
    a. Ipsilateral mydriasis
    b. Contralateral mydriasis
    c. Ipsilateral miosis
    d. Contralateral miosis
3. All of the following conditions cause miosis EXCEPT:
    a. Bright light
    b. Horner syndrome
    c. Oculomotor paralysis
    d. Iridocyclitis
4. Evisceration is removal of which layer of eye ball?
    a. Middle and inner
    b. Outer and middle
    c. Outer and inner
    d. All the layers of eyeball
5. The following image shows:

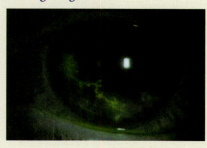

    a. Bacterial keratitis
    b. Fungal keratitis
    c. Viral keratitis
    d. Syphilitic keratitis
6. Drug contraindicated in keratitis
    a. Tear drops
    b. Steroids
    c. Cycloplegics
    d. Timolol
7. Which of the following is seen retinitis pigmentosa?
    a. Arteriolar attenuation
    b. Neovascularization
    c. Retinal artery thrombosis
    d. Papilledema
8. Not used for color vision testing:
    a. Holmgren wool test
    b. Ishihara chart
    c. FM 100 Hue test
    d. Ames test
9. Superior quadrantic hemianopia is caused by:
    a. Craniopharyngioma
    b. Meningioma
    c. Pituitary adenoma
    d. Temporal lobe lesion
10. Which of the following lesions occurs at optic chiasma?
    a. Bitemporal hemianopia
    b. Unilateral blindness
    c. Pie in floor
    d. Bilateral homonymous macular defect
11. In which of the following condition there is ipsilateral 3rd nerve palsy with contralateral hemiplegia and facial palsy of upper motor neuron?
    a. Weber syndrome
    b. Terson syndrome
    c. Millard-Gubler syndrome
    d. Foville's syndrome
12. Phacomorphic glaucoma occurs due to:
    a. Intumescent cataract
    b. Morgagnian cataract
    c. Nuclear cataract
    d. Cortical cataract
13. First sign of sympathetic Ophthalmitis is:
    a. Circumcorneal congestion
    b. Hypopyon
    c. Retrolental flare
    d. Iris nodule

ANATOMY, PHYSIOLOGY AND EXAMINATION OF EYE

14. Corneal endothelium is derived from?
    (Recent Pattern Question 2018-19)
    a. Neuroectoderm
    b. Neural crest
    c. Mesoderm
    d. Surface ectoderm
15. True about retinoscopy:
    (Recent Pattern Question 2018-19)
    a. In Hypermetropia the red glow moves in opposite direction
    b. In high myopia, the red glow moves in same direction
    c. In emmetropia the red glow moves in opposite direction
    d. Done from 1 meter distance from patient

Ophthalmology

16. A child presents with night blindness, delayed dark adaptation. Which investigation to be done further to confirm the diagnosis? *(Recent Pattern Question 2018-19)*
    a. Dark adaptometry
    b. ERG
    c. EOG
    d. Retinoscopy

17. Newborn is hypermetropic by?
    (Recent Pattern Question 2018)
    a. +2 to +3 D
    b. +1 to +2 D
    c. +3 to +4 D
    d. +2 to +4 D

18. Structure with highest refractive index:
    (Recent Pattern Question 2018)
    a. Cornea
    b. Lens
    c. Aqueous humor
    d. Vitreous humor

19. Which is True about PHPV?
    (Recent Pattern Question 2018)
    a. Visual prognosis is good
    b. Generally unilateral
    c. Associated with microphthalmia
    d. Associated with exophthalmos

20. Maximum visual field is seen in?
    (Recent Pattern Question 2016)
    a. Temporal
    b. Nasal
    c. Inferior
    d. Superior

21. Normal intraocular pressure _____ mm Hg?
    (Recent Pattern Question 2016)
    a. 5–10
    b. 10–20
    c. 20–25
    d. 25–30

22. Axial length of orbit:
    a. 2.5 mm
    b. 2.5 cm
    c. 2 mm
    d. 2 cm

23. The junction between the retina and ciliary body is called:
    a. Pars plana
    b. Pars plicata
    c. Ora serrata
    d. Equator

24. All of the following ocular muscles are supplied by CN III EXCEPT:
    a. Superior rectus
    b. Superior oblique
    c. Inferior rectus
    d. Medial rectus

25. All of the following statement are true about oculomotor nerve EXCEPT:
    a. Supplies extrinsic ocular muscles
    b. Its nucleus is located in lower midbrain
    c. Its nucleus is located in upper midbrain
    d. Palsy may lead to ptosis

26. All are glands of eyelids EXCEPT:
    a. Glands of zeis
    b. Lacrimal gland
    c. Meibomian gland
    d. Glands of moll

27. Person is not able look down. Which extra ocular muscle is affected:
    a. Superior oblique
    b. Inferior oblique
    c. Superior rectus
    d. Lateral rectus

28. The secondary actions of superior rectos muscle are:
    a. Adduction and intorsion
    b. Abduction and intorsion
    c. Adduction and extorsion
    d. Abduction and extorsion

29. Person is not able look down. Which extra ocular muscle is affected:
    a. Inferior oblique
    b. Inferior rectus
    c. Superior rectus
    d. Lateral rectus

30. In lateral rectus palsy of the right side, the face of the patient is turned to which of the following sides?
    a. Upwards
    b. Downwards
    c. Towards the right side
    d. Towards the left side

31. Synergistic muscle of right inferior oblique:
    a. Right superior oblique
    b. Left superior rectus
    c. Left inferior rectus
    d. Right superior rectus

32. The oculomotor and trochlear nerve passes through:
    a. The superior orbital fissure
    b. The inferior orbital fissure
    c. The optic canal
    d. None of the above

33. Maddox rod test is used for:
    a. Strabismus
    b. Refractive error
    c. Retinal hemorrhage
    d. Color blindness

34. By pinhole visual acuity is neutralized till:
    a. 1 D
    b. 2 D
    c. 3 D
    d. 4 D

35. Which component of the eye has maximum refractive index:
    a. Anterior surface of the lens
    b. Posterior surface of the lens
    c. Centre of the lens
    d. Cornea

36. Power of cornea is?
    a. 41 D
    b. 40 D
    c. 45 D
    d. 47 D

37. Shallow anterior chamber is seen in?
    a. Myopia
    b. Phacomorphic glaucoma
    c. Phacolytic glaucoma
    d. Aphakia

38. Accommodation is maximum in:
    a. Children
    b. Young male
    c. Elderly
    d. None

39. Surface ectoderm forms:
    a. Lens of eye
    b. Retina
    c. Iris
    d. Corneal stroma

40. Lens develops from.
    a. Neuroectoderm
    b. Surface ectoderm
    c. Mesoderm
    d. Neural crest

41. Outer epithelium of cornea is derived from?
    a. Mesoderm
    b. Endoderm
    c. Surface ectoderm
    d. Neural ectoderm

42. Which of the following has maximum field of vision:
    a. Superior
    b. Inferior
    c. Temporal
    d. Nasal

FMGE Solutions Screening Examination

43. Neuroretinal rim is broadest in which area:
    a. Temporal area
    b. Inferior
    c. Superior
    d. Supero temporal
44. Which of the following is better diagnosed with distant direct ophthalmoscopy:
    a. Retinal hemorrhage
    b. Subluxation of lens
    c. Ciliary body injury
    d. Opacity in the refractive media
45. Macular edema is seen with:
    a. Indirect ophthalmoscopy
    b. Direct ophthalmoscopy
    c. Slit lamp + 90 D
    d. Distant direct ophthalmoscopy
46. Hirschberg test measures?
    a. Strabismus
    b. Glaucoma
    c. Cataract
    d. Refractive error
47. Muscle first affected in thyroid ophthalmopathy is:
    a. Medial rectus
    b. Lateral rectus
    c. Inferior rectus
    d. Superior rectus
48. True about Color blindness:
    a. Males are more prone
    b. Males and females equally affected
    c. Autosomal dominant
    d. Males are carrier

CORNEA, CONJUNCTIVA AND SCLERA

49. True about pterygium: *(Recent Pattern Question 2018-19)*
    a. Inflammation of cornea
    b. Fatty deposition over sclera
    c. Conjunctiva invasion making a flap over cornea
    d. Dead epithelial debris accumulation
50. Cause of acute hemorrhagic conjunctivitis:
    (Recent Pattern Question 2018)
    a. Coronavirus
    b. Adenovirus
    c. Enterovirus
    d. Herpes virus
51. Klebsiella pneumoniae causes:
    (Recent Pattern Question 2018)
    a. Stye
    b. Keratitis
    c. Chalazion
    d. Entropion
52. True about dendritic ulcer:
    (Recent Pattern Question 2018)
    a. Corneal sensation decreased
    b. Increased corneal thickness
    c. Descemetocele
    d. Hypopyon
53. Which is therapeutic indication of keratoplasty?
    (Recent Pattern Question 2018)
    a. Optic nerve atrophy
    b. Keratoconus
    c. Myopia
    d. Hypermetropia

54. Swimming pool conjunctivitis is caused due to?
    (Recent Pattern Question 2017)
    a. Streptococcus
    b. Staph aureus
    c. Chylamydia
    d. Hemophilus
55. To prevent disease transmission from a conjunctivitis patient, which is the most effective way:
    (Recent Pattern Question 2017)
    a. Rinse eye
    b. Wearing black sunglasses
    c. Antibiotics
    d. Clean hand
56. Stocker line is seen in? *(Recent Pattern Question 2017)*
    a. Pingencula
    b. Pterygium
    c. Keratitis bacterial
    d. Keratitis viral
57. Most common cause of bacterial corneal ulcer:
    (Recent Pattern Question 2017)
    a. Pseudomonas
    b. Acanthamoeba
    c. Pneumococcus
    d. Staphylococcus
58. Salmon patch is seen in? *(Recent Pattern Question 2017)*
    a. Mooren's ulcer
    b. Viral keratits
    c. Interstitial keratitis
    d. Allergic keratitis
59. Munson sign is seen in? *(Recent Pattern Question 2017)*
    a. Corneal degeneration
    b. Keratoconus
    c. Mooren ulcer
    d. Pinguecula
60. Angular conjunctivitis is most commonly caused by:
    (Recent Pattern Question 2017)
    a. Moraxella
    b. H. influenzae
    c. Strep. Pneumoniae
    d. Staph. Aureus
61. In case of Neurotropic keratitis which nerve is involved:
    (Recent Pattern Question 2016)
    a. Trigeminal nerve
    b. Oculomotor
    c. Facial
    d. Trochlear
62. Colored halos in conjunctivitis are due to excess:
    (Recent Pattern Question 2016)
    a. Lacrimation
    b. Edema
    c. Flakes of mucus
    d. Dryness
63. Angular conjunctivitis is caused by:
    (Recent Pattern Question 2016)
    a. Moraxella
    b. Streptococcus
    c. Gonococcus
    d. Corynebacterium
64. Fleischer ring is seen in: *(Recent Pattern Question 2016)*
    a. Wilson's disease
    b. Keratoconus
    c. Fungal infection
    d. Protozoal keratitis
65. True about bowman's membrane:
    a. True elastic membrane
    b. Most regenerative layer
    c. Prevents infection more than descemet's membrane
    d. Cellular layer
66. Keratometer is used to assess:
    a. Thickness of cornea
    b. Refractive power
    c. Astigmatism
    d. Curvature of cornea
67. Thickness of cornea is best detected by:
    a. Keratometry
    b. Pachymetry
    c. Placido disc
    d. Tonometry

Ophthalmology

68. All are seen in Keratoconus EXCEPT:
   a. Progressive vision loss due to increasing myopia and irregular astigmatism
   b. Keyser Fleischer Ring
   c. Scissoring reflex in retinoscopy
   d. Munson sign Positive

69. Recurrent corneal erosion are seen in:
   a. Corneal dystrophy   b. Keratoconus
   c. Keratoglobus   d. Corneal degeneration

70. Recurrent corneal erosion are seen in:
   a. Corneal degeneration   b. Keratitis
   c. Corneal dystrophy   d. Keratoconus

71. Which of the following drug has corneal staining property:
   a. Thioridazine   b. Isoniazid
   c. Quinines   d. Acetazolamide

72. In case of xeropthalmia secondary to Vitamin A deficiency, what does X2 indicate according to WHO:
   a. Conjunctival xerosis   b. Bitot's spot
   c. Corneal xerosis   d. Corneal ulcer

73. Which of the following does not occur due to vitamin A intoxication:
   a. Xerophthalmia   b. Pseudotumor cerebri
   c. Dry skin   d. Vomiting

74. First sign of papilledema:
   a. Hyperemia of disc margin
   b. Abolition of cups
   c. Blurring of disc
   d. Soft exudates

75. Treatment of mooren's ulcer is?
   a. Topical steroids   b. Corneal graft
   c. Immunosuppressives   d. All of the above

76. Kayer fleischer ring affects:
   a. Conjunctiva   b. Epithelium layer
   c. Bowman's layer   d. Descemets membrane

77. Giant dendritic ulceration on cornea is seen in case of:
   a. Fungal infection   b. Chlamydial infection
   c. HSV infection   d. Pneumococcal infection

78. Which one of the following drugs is contraindicated in treatment of dendritic corneal ulcer:
   a. Atropine   b. Cefazolin
   c. Acyclovir   d. Dexamethasone

79. Herpes Simplex Virus infection with disc shaped ulceration is seen in:
   a. Epithelial keratitis   b. Stromal keratitis
   c. Syphilitic keratitis   d. Interstitial keratitis

80. Nummular keratitis is seen in:
   a. Bacterial keratitis   b. Herpes zoster keratitis
   c. Acanthamoeba keratitis d. Fungal keratitis

81. Interstitial keratitis is seen in:
   a. Trachoma   b. Bacterial conjunctivitis
   c. Fungal conjunctivitis   d. Syphilis

82. Which of the following is used in Acanthamoebic keratitis treatment:
   a. Topical corticosteroids
   b. Propamidine isothionate
   c. Acetazolamide
   d. Artificial tear

83. Acanthamoebic keratitis is associated with which of the following:
   a. Lacrimal gland inflammation
   b. Inturning of eyelids
   c. Wearing of soft contact lenses
   d. Dry eye

84. Giant Papillary Conjunctivitis is caused by:
   a. Contact Lens wear
   b. Ocular Prosthesis
   c. Protruding corneal sutures
   d. All of the above

85. Giant papillary conjunctivitis can be secondary to:
   a. Trachoma
   b. Contact lens
   c. Phlyctenular conjunctivitis
   d. Vernal kerato conjunctivitis

86. Which of the following is seen in chronic contact lens wearer:
   a. Inclusion conjuntivitis
   b. Giant papillary conjunctivitis
   c. Vernal keratoconjuntivitis
   d. Follicular conjunctivitis

87. Complication in a patient with Long term use of contact lens is most commonly caused by?
   a. Aspergillus   b. Acanthameoba
   c. Pneumococcus   d. Pseudomonas

88. In which of the following corneal ulcers signs are more than symptoms:
   a. Fungal corneal ulcer
   b. Bacterial corneal ulcer
   c. Viral corneal ulcer
   d. Herpetic corneal ulcer

89. Satellite lesion on cornea are seen in:
   a. Viral ulcer
   b. Bacterial ulcer
   c. Fungal ulcer
   d. Herpetic ulcer

90. Treatment of choice of trachoma:
   a. Azithromycin   b. Tetracycline
   c. Erythromycin   d. Penicillin

91. Location of Arlt's line:
   a. Sclera
   b. Lens
   c. Lower palpebral conjunctiva
   d. Upper palpebral conjunctiva

FMGE Solutions Screening Examination

92. **Herbert pits are seen in trachoma at:**
    a. Limbus
    b. Lid margin
    c. Palpebral conjunctiva
    d. Bulbar conjunctiva
93. **Swimming pool conjunctivitis is caused by:**
    a. Pneumococcus
    b. Adeno virus
    c. Pox virus
    d. Staph Aureus
94. **Cobble stoning of conjunctiva is seen in:**
    a. Vernal keratoconjunctivitis
    b. Simple allergic conjunctivitis
    c. Gaint papillary conjuntivitis
    d. Acute hemorrhagic conjunctivitis
95. **Spring catarrh is treated with which of the following drugs:**
    a. Olopatadine drops
    b. Normal saline eye drops
    c. Ciprofloxacin
    d. Carboxymethylcellulose (CMC) eye drops
96. **Chlymadia trachomatic A-C will cause which of the following?**
    a. Opthalmia Neonatorum
    b. Vernal Kerato conjunctivitis
    c. Paratrachoma
    d. Trachoma
97. **Ropy discharge is seen in:**
    a. Conjunctival conjunctivitis
    b. Bacterial conjunctivitis
    c. Fungal conjunctivitis
    d. Veneral conjunctivitis
98. **Fat like nodules on bilateral nasal side of conjunctiva is seen in?**
    a. Pterygium
    b. Pinguecula
    c. Chalazion
    d. Hordeolum
99. **Intercalary staphyloma:**
    a. Sloughing corneal ulcer
    b. Degenerative high myopia
    c. Bulge in limbal area lined by root of iris
    d. Penetrating injuries
100. **Ciliary staphyloma is a complication of:**
    a. Episcleritis
    b. Degenerative myopia
    c. Perforated corneal ulcer
    d. Scleritis
101. **Posterior staphyloma is seen in:**
    a. High hypermetropia
    b. Astigmatism
    c. Emmetropia
    d. Degenerative myopia
102. **Scleritis is commonly seen with:**
    a. Reiter's syndrome
    b. Rheumatoid arthritis
    c. Ankylosing spondylitis
    d. Wegner's syndrome
103. **Keratoconjunctivitis sicca is due to:**
    a. Mucin deficiency
    b. Lipid deficiency
    c. Aqueous deficiency
    d. Impaired eyelid function

RETINA AND UVEAL TRACT

104. **Sarcoidosis is associated with:**
    (Recent Pattern Question 2018-19)
    a. Cataract
    b. Ectopia lentis
    c. Anterior uveitis
    d. Keratitis
105. **Cattle track appearance is seen in:**
    (Recent Pattern Question 2018)
    a. Central retinal vein occlusion
    b. Central retinal artery occlusion
    c. Central serous retinopathy
    d. Diabetic retinopathy
106. **What is the size of optic disc?**
    (Recent Pattern Question 2018)
    a. 0.5 mm
    b. 1.5 mm
    c. 2 mm
    d. 2.5 mm
107. **In uveitis, site of keratic precipitate is:**
    (Recent Pattern Question 2018)
    a. Corneal stroma
    b. Corneal endothelium
    c. Lens anterior part
    d. Lens posterior part
108. **How many years does it take to develop retinopathy in case of uncontrolled diabetes mellitus type I?**
    (Recent Pattern Question 2018)
    a. 1–5
    b. 6–10
    c. 11–15
    d. 16–20
109. **Which of the following is used for immediate management of acute uveitis?** *(Recent Pattern Question 2017)*
    a. Cycloplegics
    b. Steroids
    c. Antimicrobials
    d. Eye patching
110. **Granular keratic precipitates are seen in:**
    (Recent Pattern Question 2017)
    a. Nongranulomatous uveitis
    b. Granulomatous uveitis
    c. Syphilitic uveitis
    d. Infective uveitis
111. **Mutton fat KP is seen in:** *(Recent Pattern Question 2017)*
    a. Granulomatous uveitis
    b. Non-granulomatous uveitis
    c. Traumatic uveitis
    d. Acute anterior uveitis
112. **Which of the following condition presents with Uveitis with arthritis:** *(Recent Pattern Question 2017)*
    a. Kaplan syndrome
    b. Pneumoconiosis
    c. Reiter syndrome
    d. Aspergillosis
113. **Retinopathy of prematurity is due to?**
    (Recent Pattern Question 2017)
    a. Hypoxia
    b. Hyperoxia
    c. Hypercapnea
    d. Apnea
114. **Koeppe nodules are seen in**
    (Recent Pattern Question 2016)
    a. Iris stroma
    b. Periphery of pupil
    c. Papilla
    d. Cornea

Ophthalmology

115. Retinal detachment occurs between which layers of retina?
     a. Sensory and nuclear layer
     b. Inner nuclear layer and outer nuclear layer
     c. Sensory and pigmentary layer
     d. Outer plexiform and inner plexiform layer
116. Which of the following is true about inverse Retinitis pigmentosa?
     a. X linked
     b. Bony spicule in fovea
     c. Bony spicule in para fovea
     d. Progressive Choroid degeneration
117. All of the following are features of retinitis pigmentosa EXCEPT:
     a. Bone spicule pigmentation in retina
     b. Waxy pallor of disc
     c. Central scotoma
     d. Ring scotoma
118. A diabetic patient taking Insulin for the past 10 years complains of gradual painless loss of vision. Most likely cause of his condition is:
     a. Total rhegmatogenous retinal detachment.
     b. Cataract
     c. Tractional retinal detachment not involving the macula
     d. Vitreous haemorrhage.
119. Early stage non proliferative diabetic retinopathy is present as:
     a. Microaneurysms   b. Dot and Blot hemorrhages
     c. Hard exudates   d. Soft exudates
120. Classical sign of neovascular glaucoma is:
     a. Retinal neovascularization
     b. Disc neovascularization
     c. Ciliary body neovascularization
     d. Iris neovascularization
121. All are anti-VEGF EXCEPT:
     a. Pegaptanib   b. 5FU
     c. Bevacizumab   d. Ranibizumab
122. Sudden painless loss of vision is due to:
     a. Iridocyclitis   b. Chorioretinitis
     c. Vitreous hemorrhage   d. Diabetic retinopathy
123. In a diabetic patient sudden severe painless loss of vision is due to?
     a. Vitreous Haemorrhage
     b. Tractional Retinal Detachment
     c. Diabetic retinopathy
     d. Neovascularization
124. The most common cause of vitreous hemorrhage in a young normal male is:
     a. Diabetes
     b. Anemia
     c. Hypertensive retinopathy
     d. Trauma
125. A hypertensive pregnant patient presented to you with sudden painless loss of vision what could be the possible cause?
     a. Tractional retinal detachment
     b. Exudative retinal detachment
     c. Vitreous hemorrhage
     d. Rhegmatogenous retinal detachment
126. Malignant melanoma of the choroid will produce:
     a. Exudative retinal detachment
     b. Traction retinal detachment
     c. Retinal dialysis
     d. Rhegmatogenous retinal detachment
127. All of the following are predisposing factors for rhegmatogenous retinal detachment EXCEPT:
     a. Myopia   b. Diabetic retinopathy
     c. Trauma   d. Aphakia
128. Cherry red spot NOT seen in?
     a. Trauma   b. Tay Sach's
     c. CRAO   d. CRVO
129. The only condition amongst the following associated with cystoid macular edema is?
     a. Overuse of ocular analgesics
     b. Glaucoma
     c. Central retinal vein occlusion
     d. Topical steroid therapy
130. Candle Wax retinopathy seen in?
     a. Sarcoidosis   b. Amyloid
     c. Diabetic retinopathy d. Hypertensive retinopathy
131. Snow banking is typically seen in:
     a. Pars planitis   b. Endophthalmitis
     c. Coat's disease   d. Eale's disease
132. Duration of cycloplegic by atropine in an adult:
     a. 6 hours   b. 2–3 days
     c. 7–10 days   d. 1–2 days
133. Drug contraindicated in uveitis is:
     a. Pilocarpine   b. Acetazolamide
     c. Atropine   d. Steroids
134. All of the following drugs are used for acute iridocyclitis EXCEPT:
     a. Atropine eye ointment   b. Steroid eye drops
     c. Pilocarpine eye drops   d. Timolol eye drops
135. Most common complication of acute anterior uveitis:
     a. Secondary glaucoma   b. Cataract
     c. Retinal detachment   d. Macular oedema

EYELID AND LACRIMAL APPARATUS

136. In Dacryocystorhinostomy (DCR), lacrimal gland opens into: *(Recent Pattern Question 2018-19)*
     a. Inferior meatus   b. Middle meatus
     c. Supreme meatus   d. Superior meatus

137. **Site of internal hordeolum:**
    (Recent Pattern Question 2018)
    a. Zeiss gland   b. Meibomian gland
    c. Moll gland   d. Conjunctiva

138. **Adhesion of margin of two eyelids:**
    a. Symblepharon   b. Lagophthalmos
    c. Ankyloblepharon   d. Blepharophimosis

139. **Treatment of choice for the chronic dacrocystitis?**
    a. Syringing
    b. Dacrocystectomy
    c. Conjunctivo-dacryocystorhinostomy
    d. Dacrocystorhinostomy

140. **In case of Ptosis which cranial nerve will be completely paralyzed?**
    a. 3rd CN palsy   b. 4th CN palsy
    c. 5th CN palsy   d. 6th CN palsy

LENS/CATARACT

141. **For Laser iridotomy which laser is used?**
    (Recent Pattern Question 2018-19)
    a. Double argon laser b. ND:YAG laser
    c. Excimer laser   d. CO_2 laser

142. **Rossette cataract is seen after:**
    (Recent Pattern Question 2018-19)
    a. Blunt trauma to eye
    b. Penetrating injury to eye
    c. Copper foreign body in eye
    d. Infection

143. **Ectopia lentis is seen in:**
    (Recent Pattern Question 2018-19)
    a. Homocystinuria   b. Refsum's disease
    c. Wilson's disease   d. Sarcoidosis

144. **Laser used in after cataract surgery:**
    (Recent Pattern Question 2017)
    a. Nd:YAG   b. Argon
    c. CO_2 d. Excimer

145. **Rosette cataract is caused due to:**
    (Recent Pattern Question 2017)
    a. Blunt trauma   b. Diabetes
    c. Myotonic dystrophy d. Wilsons disease

146. **Second sight is a feature of** *(Recent Pattern Question 2016)*
    a. Congenital cataract b. Cortical cataract
    c. Nuclear cataract
    d. Posterior subscapular cataract

147. **A 65-year-old patient presented with gradual painless reduction in vision 1 year after vitrectomy. Possible cause**
    a. Secondary glaucoma *(Recent Pattern Question 2016)*
    b. Anterior uveitis
    c. Lens protein leakage
    d. Posterior-subscapular cataract due to long term use of steroids

148. **Most common cause of blindness in world is:**
    a. Cataract   b. Refractive errors
    c. Trachoma   d. Glaucoma

149. **Which laser is used for Posterior capsular cataract:**
    a. Krypton   b. ND-YAG
    c. Argon   d. Diode laser

150. **Ideal site for intraocular lens implantation:**
    a. Behind the lens capsule b. Anterior to the pupil
    c. Behind the cornea d. In the lens capsule

151. **All of the following are Clinical features of complicated cataract EXCEPT:**
    a. Polychromatic lustre
    b. Axial spread of opacity
    c. Opacity along sutures
    d. Posterior subcapsular opacity

152. **Complicated cataract caused by all EXCEPT:**
    a. Subluxation of lens b. Retinal detachment
    c. Vitreous movement   d. Anterior Uveitis

153. **Rossete cataract is seen in?**
    a. Trauma   b. Diabetes
    c. Galactosemia   d. Wilson's disease

154. **Vossius ring is seen at:**
    a. Iris
    b. Cornea
    c. Anterior capsule of the lens
    d. Posterior capsule of the lens

155. **The type of immature cataract which causes severe loss of vision is:**
    a. Posterior subcapsular cataract
    b. Capsular cataract
    c. Cortical cataract
    d. Nuclear sclerosis

156. **Rainbow cataract is due to:**
    a. Phenylketonuria   b. Galactosemia
    c. Diabetes mellitus d. Secondary cataract

157. **All of the following systemic diseases may be associated with cataract EXCEPT:**
    a. Phenylketonuria   b. Galactosemia
    c. Diabetes mellitus d. Wilson's disease

158. **Anterior lenticonus is found in:**
    a. Lowe's syndrome   b. William's syndrome
    c. Down's syndrome   d. Alport's syndrome

159. **In Marfan's syndrome which of the following will be seen in eyes:**
    a. Inferonasal subluxation of lens
    b. Superotemporal subluxation of lens
    c. Corneal edema
    d. Increased IOP

160. **Location of lens in Marfan's syndrome is:**
    a. Inferior and nasally b. Superior and temporally
    c. Forward subluxated   d. Upward displacement

161. Jack in a box is seen in:
    a. Pseudophakia   b. Aphakia
    c. Squint   d. Cataract
162. Side effect of oral steroid:
    a. Glaucoma
    b. Cataract
    c. Basement membrane thickening
    d. Blepharoconjunctivitis
163. Iridodonesis is seen with?
    a. Iridocyclitis   b. Subluxation of lens
    c. Mature cataract d. Intumescent cataract

GLAUCOMA

164. Which of the following is the carbonic anhydrase inhibitor used in glaucoma?
    (Recent Pattern Question 2018)
    a. Timolol   b. Mannitol
    c. Latanoprost   d. Dorzolamide
165. Vertically fixed mid-dilated pupil seen in:
    a. Cataract   b. Open angle glaucoma
    c. Angle closure glaucoma d. Uveitis
166. In case of Angle closure glaucoma, what is the shape of pupil:
    a. Vertically dilated b. Horizontally dilated
    c. Fully constricted   d. Irregular constricted fixed
167. A 50-year-old female, presented with redness, painful, sudden loss of vision. She also claims about seeing colored haloes. Diagnosis:
    a. Angular conjunctivitis
    b. Retinal detachment
    c. Acute congestive glaucoma
    d. Keratitis
168. Primary open angle glaucoma is best treated by:
    a. Peripheral Iridectomy b. Latanoprost
    c. Trabeculoplasty   d. Laser Iridotomy
169. Clinically earliest visual field defect in primary open angle glaucoma:
    a. Seidel scotoma   b. Arcuate scotoma
    c. Parcentral scotoma d. Nasal spur
170. MOA of acetazolamide used in glaucoma:
    a. Increase aqueous production
    b. Increase uveo-scleral outflow
    c. Increase trabecular outflow
    d. Decrease aqueous production
171. The first line of treatment of advanced open angle glaucoma is:
    a. Epinephrine   b. Latanoprost
    c. Pilocarpine   d. Acetazolamide
172. Safest anti-glaucoma drug in children:
    a. Acetazolamide   b. Latanoprost
    c. Timolol   d. Dorzolamide

173. Which of the following drug is contraindicated in a glaucoma patient suffering from bronchial asthma:
    a. Timolol maleate   b. Latanoprost
    c. Betaxolol   d. Brimonidine
174. A patient of 18 year, presents with swollen, watery eyes. Examination confirms glaucoma. Which of the following is the best step that provides earliest relief:
    a. Gonioscopy   b. Medical management
    c. Surgical management d. Ophthalmoscopy
175. Treatment for the given case (bilateral big blue eyes in image due to increased IOP)

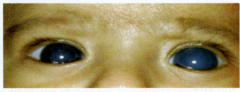

    a. Goniotomy   b. Trabeculotomy
    c. Trabeculectomy   d. Laser iridotomy
176. Treatment of angle closure glaucoma.
    a. Peripheral Iredectomy b. Trabeculectomy
    c. Trabeculoplasty   d. Laser Iridotomy
177. Laser iridotomy is useful in:
    a. Angle closure glaucoma b. Neovascular glaucoma
    c. Open angle glaucoma   d. Secondary glaucoma
178. In acute congestive glaucoma, best prophylaxis for the other eye is:
    a. Laser Iridotomy
    b. Topical steroids
    c. Trabeculectomy
    d. Surgical peripheral Iridectomy
179. Treatment of choice for the other eye in open angle glaucoma is:
    a. Peripheral iridectomy b. Laser trabeculoplasty
    c. Laser iridotoomy   d. Trabeculectomy
180. Colored haloes least seen in:
    a. Cataract   b. Open angle glucoma
    c. Angle closure glaucoma d. Purulent conjunctivitis
181. A man present with frequent change of presbyopic lens. Diagnosis:
    a. Open angle glaucoma b. Angle closure glaucoma
    c. Cataract   d. Astigmatism
182. Krukenberg spindles are seen at?
    a. Cornea anterior surface b. Cornea posterior surface
    c. Lens posterior surface   d. Lens anterior surface

REFRACTIVE ERROR

183. A newborn is hypermetropic by:
    (Recent Pattern Question 2018-19)
    a. +2.5 D   b. 5 D
    c. 10 D   d. 1 D

FMGE Solutions Screening Examination

184. Obstacle in manifest squint-concomitant type is:
    (Recent Pattern Question 2018-19)
    a. Motor obstacle   b. Sensory obstacle
    c. Central obstacle   d. All of the above

185. Crowding phenomenon is seen in:
    (Recent Pattern Question 2018)
    a. Hypermetropia   b. Amblyopia
    c. Strabismus   d. Retinitis pigmentosa

186. What is the best treatment of Amblyopia?
    a. Occlusion   *(Recent Pattern Question 2018)*
    b. Atropine penalization
    c. Correction of refractive error
    d. Surgery

187. Which is true statement for a patient with paralytic squint?   *(Recent Pattern Question 2017)*
    a. Head tilt opposite to rectus muscle paralysis
    b. Head tilt towards the rectus muscle paralysis
    c. Amblyopia
    d. Decreased visual acuity

188. Least common cause of blindness:
    a. Cataract   *(Recent Pattern Question 2016)*
    b. Corneal opacity
    c. Refractive error
    d. Glaucoma

189. Convex lenses are used for:
    a. Myopia   *(Recent Pattern Question 2016)*
    b. Hypermetropia
    c. Astigmatism
    d. Myopic astigmatism

190. In convergent squint what is the angle of deviation?
    (Recent Pattern Question 2016)
    a. 10°   b. 15°
    c. 20°   d. 30°

191. In case of Myopia, the following is seen:
    a. Large optic disc   b. Small optic disc
    c. Normal eye   d. None of above

192. Excessive accommodation causes:
    a. Pseudomyopia
    b. Pseudohypermetropia
    c. Astigmatism
    d. Presbyopia

193. Treatment of anisometropia:
    a. Glasses   b. Contact lens
    c. Trabeculectomy   d. Trabeculoplasty

194. Lens used in Astigmatism:
    a. Convex lens
    b. Cylindrical
    c. Concave lens
    d. Contact lens

195. Worth 4 dot test is done for:
    a. Color deficiency   b. Strabismus
    c. Binocular vision   d. Squint

196. Different refractive power between two eyes is known as?
    a. Combined astigmatism   b. Aniseikonia
    c. Anisometropia   d. Ametropia

197. Cylindrical lens is used for:
    a. Presbyopia   b. High myopia
    c. Hypermetropia   d. Astigmatism

OCULAR INJURY AND MALIGNANCY

198. A patient with a history of fall on symmetrical surface, presents with enophthalmos, diplopia on upward gaze and loss of sensitivity over cheek. True statement about this is: *(Recent Pattern Question 2018-19)*
    i. Strongly suspecting orbital floor fracture
    ii. It is a blow-out fracture
    iii. Zygomatic bone is most likely injured
    iv. Frontal bone fracture
    a. Only i and ii are correct
    b. II, III and IV are correct
    c. I, II, and III are correct
    d. All are correct

199. Blow out fracture can be due to:
    a. Tennis ball injury   *(Recent Pattern Question 2018-19)*
    b. Chisel and hammer injury
    c. Sudden fall
    d. Punch at the chin from below

200. Most common malignant orbital tumour in children:
    (Recent Pattern Question 2017)
    a. Rhabdomyosarcoma   b. Retinoblastoma
    c. Lipoma   d. Neuroblastoma

201. Tear drop sign is seen in fracture of?
    (Recent Pattern Question 2017)
    a. Orbital roof   b. Orbital floor
    c. Orbital lateral wall   d. Orbital medial wall

202. Which gene is associated with Knudson two hit hypothesis?   *(Recent Pattern Question 2017)*
    a. RB gene   b. PTEN
    c. P16   d. P53

203. A patient presents with ocular trauma and blood in anterior chamber. Which is the best treatment?
    (Recent Pattern Question 2017)
    a. Eye patch   b. Hospital admission
    c. Steroid   d. Conservative

204. Corneal curvature is measured by:
    (Recent Pattern Question 2017)
    a. Perimetry   b. Gonioscopy
    c. Pachymetry   d. Keratometry

205. Which of the following is an etiology of axial proptosis?
    (Recent Pattern Question 2017)
    a. Lacrimal gland tumour   b. Optic nerve glioma
    c. Orbital floor fracture   d. Forehead tumour

Ophthalmology

206. Most common primary intraocular tumor in children?
   a. Retinoblastoma   *(Recent Pattern Question 2016)*
   b. Malignant melanoma of choroid
   c. Malignant melanoma of ciliary body
   d. Rhabdomyosarcoma

207. Unilateral oculomotor nerve paralysis leads to?
        (Recent Pattern Question 2016)
   a. Loss of accommodation
   b. Argyll Robertson pupil
   c. Eyeball turned up and out
   d. Diplopia

208. Ciliary muscle damage leads to:
        (Recent Pattern Question 2016)
   a. Angle closure glaucoma
   b. Loss of accommodation
   c. ARP
   d. Diplopia

209. Tolosa Hunt syndrome involves:
   a. Orbital floor   *(Recent Pattern Question 2016)*
   b. Orbital apex
   c. Orbital roof
   d. Orbital space

210. Which one is seen after penetrating injury in ciliary body?
   a. Iridocyclitis
   b. Sympathetic ophthalmitis
   c. Endophthalmitis
   d. Corneal ulceration

211. Sympathetic ophthalmitis usually results due to:
   a. Glaucoma
   b. Trachoma
   c. Penetrating injury to Ciliary body
   d. Uveitis

212. Most common foreign body to cause penetrating injury to ciliary body:
   a. Ball   b. Hammer and chisel
   c. Gun bullet   d. Vegetative material

213. Most common cause of subconjunctival hemorrhage:
   a. Hypertension   b. Trauma
   c. Pertussis   d. Diabetes

214. Pupillary reaction to light is still normal in lesion/injury to:
   a. Optic nerve
   b. Optic disc
   c. Optic tract
   d. Optic chiasm

215. Blow out fracture of orbit is characterized by all EXCEPT:
   a. Orbital floor and medial wall involvement are common
   b. Tear drop sign on X-ray
   c. Diplopia
   d. Exophthalmos

216. Lisch Nodules on Iris is a feature of:
   a. Amyloidosis   b. Neurofibromatosis
   c. Tuberous Sclerosis   d. None of these

217. Most common malignant eyelid tumor:
   a. Squamous cell carcinoma b. Basal carcinoma
   c. Sebaceous carcinoma   d. Malignant melanoma

218. Most common epithelial tumor of lacrimal gland:
   a. Choroid melanoma   b. Pleomorphic adenoma
   c. Basal cell CA   d. Rhabdomyosarcoma

219. Commonest site of distant metastasis of retinoblastoma is:
   a. Liver   b. Brain
   c. Lungs   d. Long bones

220. A child with retinoblastoma will have this:
   a. Esotropia   b. Exotropia
   c. Hypotropia   d. Heterotropia

NEURO-OPHTHALMOLOGY

221. Bilateral temporal hemianopia is due to:
        (Recent Pattern Question 2016)
   a. Bilateral optic nerve damage
   b. Pituitary adenoma
   c. Unilateral optic tract damage
   d. Bilateral optic tract damage

222. Colour blindness in ethambutol toxicity:
   a. Red blue   b. Red green
   c. Blue   d. Red green blue

223. What will be the treatment of ptosis due to Horner syndrome:
   a. Unilateral sling operation
   b. Bilateral sling operation
   c. Cut levator palpebrae superioris 15 mm
   d. Fasanella servat operation

224. Which of the following muscle is affected in increased cranial pressure:
   a. Inferior oblique   b. Lateral rectus
   c. Middle rectus   d. Superior oblique

225. Lesion in occipital lobe will cause?
   a. Binasal hemianopia
   b. Bitemporal hemianopia
   c. Homonymous superior quadrantonopia
   d. Homonymous hemianopia with macular sparing

226. Lesion of optic tract causes?
   a. Binasal hemianopia
   b. Bitemporal hemianopia
   c. Homonymous superior quadrantonopia
   d. Homonymous hemianopia

227. Right homonymous hemianopia is caused by lesion of:
   a. Right optic nerve
   b. Right optic radiation
   c. Left optic tract
   d. Right geniculate body

FMGE Solutions Screening Examination

228. The characteristic field defect seen in pituitary tumors is
    a. Homonymous hemianopia
    b. Complete vision loss
    c. Binasal hemianopia
    d. Bitemporal hemianopia
229. Isolated third nerve palsy with pupillary sparing is seen in which of the following conditions:
    a. Aneurysmal rupture
    b. Trauma
    c. Diabetes
    d. Raised ICT
230. Which amongst the following is associated with Altitudinal visual field defect:
    a. Optic neuritis
    b. AION (Anterior lschemic Optic Neuropathy)
    c. Intracranial tumor
    d. Papillitis
231. All are true about Adie's pupil EXCEPT:
    a. Seen due to inflammation of ciliary ganglion secondary to post viral illness
    b. Pupil is super sensitive to pilocarpine
    c. Bilateral constricted and irregular pupil
    d. Adie's pupil shows no response to light

BOARD REVIEW QUESTIONS

232. Volume of eye ball is?
    a. 30 ml   b. 6.5 ml
    c. 20 ml   d. 10 ml
233. Oral dose of Vitamin A given to child with Xeropthalmia is?
    a. 10,000 IU per dose   b. 100,000 IU per dose
    c. 20,000 IU per dose   d. 200,000 IU per dose
234. Hirschberg test is used for?
    a. Ptosis   b. Keratitis
    c. Corneal curvature   d. Strabismus
235. Papillodema is seen in?
    a. Optic neuritis   b. Optic nerve glioma
    c. CRVO   d. CRAO
236. Vitamin B12 deficiency causes?
    a. Scotoma   b. Hemianopia
    c. Myopia   d. Quadrantanopia
237. Most common cause of optic atrophy in children is:
    a. Retinopathy of prematurity
    b. Optic nerve glioma
    c. Dwarfism
    d. Hydrocephalus
238. Hemorrhagic conjunctivitis is caused by?
    a. Enterovirus 70   b. Coxsackie virus
    c. Enterovirus 72   d. Calcivirus
239. Most common cause of vitreous hemorrhage in adults?
    a. Hypertension   b. Eale's disease
    c. Diabetes   d. HIV
240. Schwalbe's line is?
    a. The posterior limit of Descemet's membrane of cornea
    b. The posterior limit of Bowman's membrane of cornea
    c. The anterior limit of Descemet's membrane of cornea
    d. The posterior limit of Bowman's membrane of cornea
241. Optic nerve is which order neuron in visual pathway?
    a. First   b. Third
    c. Second   d. Fourth
242. What is the definition of blindness according to WHO?
    a. 1/60   b. 3/60
    c. 6/60   d. 6/18
243. Candle wax droppings on fundus examination are seen in:
    a. Sarcoidosis
    b. Undulant fever
    c. Anterior uveitis
    d. Juvenile rheumatoid arthritis
244. Earliest manifestation of sympathetic opthalmitis in uninjured eye?
    a. Esotropia
    b. Loss of accommodation
    c. Epiphora
    d. Circum-corneal congestion
245. Aqueous humour is produced by:
    a. Pars plana   b. Pars plicata
    c. Pars intermedialis   d. Iris
246. Vitamin present in aqueous humour is?
    a. Vitamin A   b. Vitamin B
    c. Vitamin C   d. Vitamin D
247. Swinging flashlight test is done for?
    a. Optic neuritis   b. Papilledema
    c. Papillitis   d. Perception of light
248. Most common type of cataract?
    a. Nuclear   b. Cortical
    c. Posterior subscapular   d. Anterior subscapular
249. Most common cause of angle closure glaucoma?
    a. Hyperopia   b. Myopia
    c. Pupillary block   d. Space occupying tumour
250. Latanoprost acts by?
    a. Increase uveo-scleral outflow
    b. Decrease aqueous production
    c. Decrease aqueous resistance
    d. Decrease aqueous consistency
251. Placido disc is used for measuring?
    a. Corneal thickness
    b. Corneal surface
    c. Corneal staining
    d. Corneal curvature

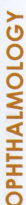

Ophthalmology

252. Most common type of hypermetropia is:
- a. Simple
- b. Pathological
- c. Functional
- d. Physiological

253. Marcus gunn sign seen in:
- a. Optic neuritis
- b. Hypertensive retinopathy
- c. Anterior ischemic optic neuropathy
- d. Tobacco amblyopia

254. Metamorphopsia is seen in:
- a. Scleritis
- b. Optic nerve inflammation
- c. Iridocyclitis
- d. Choroiditis

255. All are true about rods and cones EXCEPT?
- a. Cones for photopic vision
- b. Form sense at fovea
- c. Purkinje shift is all colours seen as grey in bright light
- d. Rhodopsin is the visual pigment

256. Preferred treatment of Ophthalamia neonatorum?
- a. Crede's method
- b. Ceftriaxone
- c. Azithromycin
- d. Neomycin

257. Night blindness can occur due to all EXCEPT?
- a. Retinitis pigmentosa
- b. Post LASIK
- c. Central cataract
- d. Vitamin A deficiency

258. Not a feature of alport syndrome?
- a. Sensorineural Hearing loss
- b. Posterior lenticonus
- c. Hematuria
- d. COL4 gene defect

259. What is true about Eale's disease?
- a. Painful loss of vision
- b. Young females commonly affected
- c. Seen after reactivation with Syphillis
- d. ATT with Steroids given

260. Fundus showing splashed tomato appearance is seen in:
- a. CRVO
- b. CRAO
- c. Cystoid macular edema
- d. Hypertensive retinopathy

261. All are true about ROP EXCEPT?
- a. Prematurity
- b. Direct ophthalmoscopic screening done at 32 weeks post conceptional age
- c. Earliest sign is dilatation of veins
- d. Seen with FiO_2 > 50%

262. Best test for Best disease?
- a. EOG
- b. ENG
- c. EMG
- d. ECG

263. Treatment of tractional retinal detachment?
- a. Par plana vitrectomy
- b. Scleral buckling
- c. Pan-retinal photocoagulation
- d. All of the above

264. Blue sclera is seen in?
- a. Buphthalmos
- b. Osteogenesis imperfecta
- c. Ehler danlos syndrome
- d. All of the above

265. Laser iridotomy is useful in:
- a. Angle closure glaucoma
- b. Neovascular glaucoma
- c. Open angle glaucoma
- d. Secondary glaucoma

266. Shaffer sign is seen in:
- a. Retinitis pigmentosa
- b. Retinal detachment
- c. Vitreous haemorrhage
- d. Scotoma

267. Secondary malignancy in retinoblastoma:
- a. Chondroma
- b. Osteosarcoma
- c. AML
- d. Malignant melanoma

268. Rollable intraocular lens is made of?
- a. PMMA
- b. Acrylate
- c. Hyaluronic acid
- d. Hydrogel

269. Salt and pepper fundus is seen in:
- a. Congenital rubella
- b. Congenital syphilis
- c. Leber amaurosis
- d. Congenital herpes

270. Most serious complication of cataract surgery:
- a. Hyphema
- b. Malignant glaucoma
- c. Vitreous loss
- d. Cystoid macular edema

271. Roth spots are seen in:
- a. Infective endocarditis
- b. Libman sacks endocarditis
- c. Hypertension retinopathy
- d. NBTE

272. Sudden increase in sugar in diabetics leads to:
- a. Myopia
- b. Presbyopia
- c. Hypermetropia
- d. Anisometropia

273. Child attains 6/6 vision of the age of:
- a. 3 years
- b. 6 years
- c. 7 years
- d. 14 years

274. Tear production in child begins at:
- a. 4 weeks
- b. 4 months
- c. 6 months
- d. 9 months

275. Retinal astrocytoma is seen in:
- a. Tuberous sclerosis
- b. Retinitis pigmentosa
- c. Choroid melanoma
- d. All of the above

276. All are used for distant vision EXCEPT?
- a. Landolt C chart
- b. Snellen chart
- c. E chart
- d. Jaeger chart

277. Bevacizumab is used in:
- a. Central serous retinopathy
- b. Phylectenular conjunctivitis
- c. Diabetic retinopathy
- d. CRVO

278. Which of these is not a feature of Horner syndrome in children:
- a. Ptosis
- b. Heterochromia iridis
- c. Exopthalmos
- d. Anhidrosis

279. All are useful in treatment of keratomalacia EXCEPT?
- a. Injection vitamin A
- b. Vitamin C drops
- c. Amniotic membrane transplant
- d. Eye patching

FMGE Solutions Screening Examination

280. **Dua's layer is present between:**
   a. Between deep stroma and descemet membrane
   b. Deep stroma and bowman membrane
   c. Bowman and descemet membrane
   d. Superficial stroma and bowman membrane

281. **Optic tract lesion leads to:**
   a. Homonymous hemianopia
   b. Homonymous hemianopia with macular sparing
   c. Pie in the sky
   d. Pie in floor

282. **Organism leading to angular conjunctivitis:**
   a. Corynebacterium diphtheria
   b. Moraxella axenfeld
   c. Mobiluncus
   d. Staph aureus

283. **Acute hemorrhagic conjunctivitis is caused by:**
   a. Enterovirus 70   b. HSV1
   c. Chylamydia   d. Moraxella

284. **All are true about trachoma EXCEPT?**
   a. Spread via houseflies   b. Sago grain follicles
   c. Pannus   d. White ropy discharge

285. **Horner tranta spots are seen at:**
   a. Limbus   b. Palpebral conjunctiva
   c. Bulbar conjunctiva d. Puncta

286. **Most common cause of corneal ulcer:**
   a. Staphylococcus aureus
   b. Coagulase negative staphylococcus
   c. Pneumococcus
   d. H. influenza

287. **Most common cause of viral corneal ulcer:**
   a. Herpes zoster   b. Herpes simplex
   c. Adenovirus   d. Enterovirus

288. **Fleischer ring is seen in:**
   a. Wilson disease   b. Keratoconus
   c. Menke disease   d. Hemosiderosis

289. **Corneal ulceration can be seen due to damage to which nerve:**
   a. Fifth   b. Sixth
   c. Seventh   d. Ninth

290. **Tubular vision is seen in:**
   a. Retinitis pigmentosa
   b. Bread crumb cataract
   c. Balint syndrome
   d. Central serous retinopathy

291. **Champagne cork appearance of optic disc is seen in:**
   a. Papilledema   b. Papillitis
   c. Optic atrophy   d. Optic neuritis

292. **Unilateral papilledema with contralateral optic atrophy is a feature of:**
   a. Foster Kennedy syndrome   b. ICSOL
   c. Retinitis pigmentosa   d. CRVO

293. **Correct action of superior rectus:**
   a. Elevation and intortion
   b. Depression and intortion
   c. Elevation and extortion
   d. Depression and extortion

294. **Maddox rod is used for:**
   a. Latent squint in near vision
   b. Latent squint in distant vision
   c. Manifest squint in distant vision
   d. Manifest squint in near vision

295. **Stye is:**
   a. Inflammation of gland of zeis
   b. Inflammation of meibomian glands
   c. Inflammation of tarsal cyst
   d. Inflammation of tenon capsule

296. **Loss of eye lashes is known as:**
   a. Tylosis   b. Madarosis
   c. Entropion   d. Trichiasis

297. **Madarosis is seen in:**
   a. Leprosy   b. Angular conjunctivitis
   c. Style   d. Sarcoidosis

298. **Kerato conjunctivitis sicca is seen in:**
   a. Sjogren syndrome   b. Sarcoidosis
   c. Mikulicz syndrome d. HIV

299. **Cobble stone appearance of conjunctiva is seen in:**
   a. Trachoma   b. Vernal conjunctivitis
   c. Opthalmia neonatorum d. Bacterial conjunctivitis

300. **Which component of eye has highest refractive index:**
   a. Cornea   b. Lens cortex
   c. Vitreous humour d. Aqueous humour

301. **Amaurotic cat eye reflex is seen in:**
   a. Cridu chat syndrome   b. Retinoblastoma
   c. Trachoma   d. Retinitis pigmentosa

302. **X3A in WHO staging of vitamin A deficiency is:**
   a. Keratomalacia   b. Corneal ulcer
   c. Conjunctival xerosis d. Xeropthalmia

303. **Most common cause of visual loss in an AIDS patient is:**
   a. Ocular Kaposi sarcoma b. CMV retinitis
   c. HIV retinitis   d. Toxoplasma

304. **Scleritis is most commonly associated with?**
   a. Ankylosing spondylitis b. Rheumatoid arthritis
   c. Giant cell arteritis   d. Ehler danlos syndrome

305. **Altitudinal field defects are seen in:**
   a. Anterior ischemic optic neuritis
   b. Papilledema
   c. Papillitis
   d. Rieter syndrome

306. **Intraocular calcification is seen with:**
   a. Retinoblastoma
   b. Retrolental fibroplasia
   c. Persistent hyperplastic vitreous
   d. Chloroma

Ophthalmology

307. Investigation of choice for retinal detachment is:
- a. Indirect ophthalmoscopy
- b. Direct ophthalmoscopy
- c. Retinoscopy
- d. Slit lamp

308. Foster fuch spots are seen in:
- a. Opthalmia neonatorum
- b. Sympathetic opthalmatis
- c. Myopia
- d. Presbyopia

309. Mutton fat keratic precipitates are seen in:
- a. Granuloma uveitis
- b. Non granulomatous uveitis
- c. Choroiditis
- d. Posterior staphyloma

310. Hudson stahli line is seen in limbus due to:
- a. Iron deposition
- b. Melanin deposition
- c. Copper deposition
- d. Heavy metal deposition

311. All are features of hypercholesterolemia EXCEPT:
- a. Lipemia retinalis
- b. Tendon xanthoma
- c. Arcus senilis
- d. Hollenhurst fundus plaques

312. Size of optic disc is?
- a. 0.5 mm
- b. 1.5 mm
- c. 5.5 mm
- d. 10.5 mm

313. Most common etiology of Phlyctenular conjunctivitis is?
- a. Bacterial
- b. Fungal
- c. Protozoal
- d. Tuberculous

314. Krukenberg's spindles are seen in?
- a. Pigmentary glaucoma
- b. Sympathetic opthalmitis
- c. Chalazion
- d. Retinitis pigmentosa

315. Macular edema is seen in?
- a. Diabetes mellitus
- b. Age related macular degeneration
- c. Papilloedema
- d. CRAO

316. Photoretinitis is caused by?
- a. Solar eclipse
- b. Welder's flash
- c. Arc lamp
- d. Lightening

317. Shafer's sign is seen in?
- a. Retinal detachment
- b. Vitreous break
- c. Glaucoma
- d. Iritis

318. Where does squamous cell carcinoma of conjunctiva originate from?
- a. Limbus
- b. Fornix
- c. Nasal conjunctiva
- d. Temporal conjunctiva

319. Cupuliform cataract arises from?
- a. Posterior capsule
- b. Anterior capsule
- c. Posterior cortex
- d. Anterior cortex

320. Most common intraocular malignancy in adults is?
- a. Melanoma of choroid
- b. Melanoma of uvea
- c. Retinoblastoma
- d. Rhabdomyosarcoma

321. Which of the following do not penetrate cornea?
- a. Gonococci
- b. Neisseria meningitis
- c. Pseudomonas
- d. Corynebacterium diphtheria

322. Angle kappa is formed between which axis?
- a. Anatomical and visual axis
- b. Anatomical and horizontal axis
- c. Between two visual axes
- d. Visual axis and vertical axis

323. How is posterior chamber examined in mature cataract?
- a. Laser interferometry
- b. Optical coherence tomography
- c. B scan
- d. A scan

324. Diagnosis of CMV retinitis is primarily by?
- a. Fundoscopy
- b. Retinal biopsy
- c. CMV DNA
- d. ELISA

325. Snow banking is seen in:
- a. Anterior uveitis
- b. Posterior uveitis
- c. Intermediate uveitis
- d. None of these

326. Which is not a differential diagnosis of blue sclera?
- a. Homocystinuria
- b. Ehlers-Danlos syndrome
- c. Neurofibromatosis
- d. Marfan's syndrome

1073

Questions

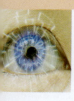

FMGE Solutions Screening Examination

327. Physiological blue sclera is seen in?
    a. Elderly
    b. Pregnancy
    c. Premature newborn
    d. None of these

328. Most common ocular feature in rheumatoid arthritis is?
    a. Uveitis
    b. Ectopia lentis
    c. Keratoconjunctivitis sicca
    d. Episcleritis

329. Pseudoproptosis is seen in?
    a. High myopia
    b. Thyrotoxicosis
    c. Orbital proptosis
    d. Deep orbital tumour

330. Most common complication of corneal transplant is?
    a. Lenticonus
    b. Melting of cornea
    c. Neovascularisation
    d. Post transplant astigmatism

331. Rhodopsin gene is seen in which chromosome?
    a. Chromosome 3
    b. Chromosome 7
    c. Chromosome 10
    d. X Chromosome

332. Corneal ulcer leads to?
    a. Anterior staphyloma
    b. Posterior staphyloma
    c. Lenticomus
    d. Keratoconus

333. Which of the following is the most common cause of anterior uveitis?
    a. Idiopathic
    b. HLA-B27
    c. Sarcoidosis
    d. Tuberculosis

334. Chronic use of systemic steroids most commonly leads to which ocular complication?
    a. Cataract
    b. Glaucoma
    c. Uveitis
    d. Conjuctival and lid papilomatis

335. Muscles responsible for accommodation are innervated by nerves passing through?
    a. Devilotschaw nucleus
    b. Edinger-westphal nucleus
    c. Nucleus coeruleus
    d. Dorsal nucleus

336. Normal flora of the eye constitutes?
    a. E. coli
    b. B. proteus
    c. C. gonococci
    d. Diptheroids

337. Transparency of cornea is mainly due to which layer?
    a. Endothelium
    b. Descemet's membrane
    c. Bowman's membrane
    d. None of these

338. Most common cause of retinal detachment is?
    a. Myopia
    b. Hypermetropia
    c. Tractional
    d. Exudates

339. Muddy appearance of iris is seen in?
    a. Glaucoma
    b. Iridocyclitis
    c. Persistent papillary membrane
    d. Iris cyst

340. Glaukomflecken is a feature of?
    a. Acute angle-closure glaucoma
    b. Pigmentary glaucoma
    c. Primary open angel glaucoma
    d. Congenital glaucoma

341. Most common muscle involved in Graves ophthalmopathy is?
    a. Medial rectus
    b. Lateral rectus
    c. Inferior rectus
    d. Superior rectus

342. Posterior capsular cataract is treated by which laser?
    a. Argon laser
    b. CO_2 laser
    c. Excimer
    d. Nd:YAG

343. Tarsal muscles are supplied by?
    a. Ophthalmic nerve
    b. Nasociliary nerve
    c. Sympathetic nerves
    d. Oculomotor nerve

344. Lens is derived from?
    a. Endoderm
    b. Surface ectoderm
    c. Lambert Eaton syndrome
    d. Hyperthyroidism

345. Optic cup develops into?
    a. Lens
    b. Retina
    c. Cornea
    d. Sclera

346. Corneal endothelial counting is done by?
    a. Tachymetry
    b. Pachymetry
    c. Specular microscope
    d. Perimetry

347. Normal corneal endothelial count is?
    a. 500/mm^2
    b. 2500/mm^2
    c. 4500/mm^2
    d. 6500/mm^2

348. According to WHO best definition of blindness is:
    a. <3/60
    b. <6/60
    c. <6/6
    d. <3/6
    (2018)

Ophthalmology

IMAGE-BASED QUESTIONS

349. Which eye abnormality is shown?

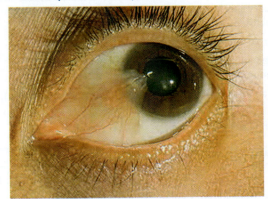

   a. Pinguecula   b. Pterygium
   c. Keratomalacia   d. Entropion

351. What is the following fundus finding shown below?

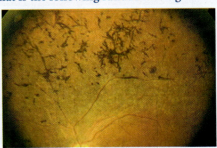

   a. Retinitis Pigmentosa
   b. Age related macular degeneration
   c. Papilledema
   d. Papillitis

350. The image shows?

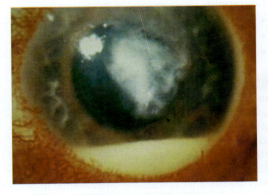

   a. Hypopyon   b. Hyphaema
   c. Stye   d. Chalazion

352. The fundus finding shows presence of?

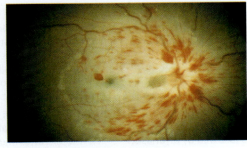

   a. Splashed tomato appearance
   b. Dot blot haemorrhages
   c. Cottage cheese and tomato appearance
   d. Cattle trucking appearance

Answers to Image-Based Questions are given at the end of explained questions

FMGE Solutions Screening Examination

ANSWERS WITH EXPLANATIONS

MOST RECENT QUESTIONS 2019

1. Ans. (a) Cataract

Ref: A K Khurana 6th ed. P 477

- Globally, MCC of blindness is cataract, affecting 17.6 million (39%), followed by glaucoma which affects 4.5 million (10%) population.
- MCC of blindness in India: Cataract
- MCC of blindness in developed countries: Age Related Macular Degeneration (50% of all blindness in developed countries)
- MCC of blindness in developing countries: Cataract
- MC preventable cause of blindness worldwide: Trachoma

2. Ans. (a) Ipsilateral mydriasis

Ref: A K Khurana 6th ed. P 335

Ocular signs in head injury can be seen due to concussion injury or base of skull bone fracture

Concussion Injury: Associated with subdural hemorrhage and unconsciousness, and produces following ocular signs:	Fractured skull base • **Cranial nerve palsies:** Commonly associated with fractured base of skull. MC being ipsilateral facial paralysis of lower motor neuron type.
• **Hutchinson pupil:** Characterized by ipsilateral miosis followed by mydriasis, with no light reflex due to raised ICP. • **Papilloedema:** If occurs within 48 hours of trauma → indicates extra or intracerebral hemorrhage. If occurs after a week of head injury, it is usually due to cerebral edema	• **Optic nerve injury:** Can cause optic nerve atrophy 2-4 weeks after injury • Subconjunctival Hemorrhage • **Pupillary signs:** Inconsistent sign. Pupil size is usually dilated on the affected side.

3. Ans. (c) Oculomotor paralysis

Ref: A K Khurana 6th edit pg 504

TABLE: Condition causing miosis and mydriasis

Causes of Miosis	Causes of Mydriasis
• Parasympathomimetic drugs	• Topical sympathomimetic drug (Phenylephrine)
• Systemic morphine	• Topical parasympatholytics (Atropine)

Contd...

Causes of Miosis	Causes of Mydriasis
• Iridocyclitis (irregular, non-reactive pupil)	• Acute congestive glaucoma; Absolute glaucoma
• Horner's syndrome	• Optic atrophy
• Head injury (pontine hemorrhage)	• Retinal detachment
• As an effect of strong light	• CN 3 (oculomotor nerve) palsy
• During sleep	• Belladonna poisoning

4. Ans. (a) Middle and inner

Ref: A K Khurana 6th ed. P 173

- Eyeball has 3 layers: Sclera, Choroid and Retina
- Evisceration is removal of content of eyeball leaving behind the sclera (the outer layer).
- Frill evisceration is preferred over simple evisceration, where about 3 mm frill of the sclera is left round the optic nerve.

Indications:
- Panophthalmitis
- Expulsive choroidal hemorrhage
- Bleeding anterior staphyloma

> **Extra Mile**
>
> - **Enucleation** is excision of eyeball.
> - In adults performed under local anaesthetics and in children under general anaesthetics
> - **Indications:**
>   ▪ Retinoblastoma and Malignant melanoma
>   ▪ Painful blind eye
>   ▪ MC indication for enucleation: Eye donation from cadaver

5. Ans. (c) Viral keratitis

Ref: A K Khurana 6th ed. P 108-109

- The image shows dendritic ulcer, which is typical lesion for viral keratitis.
- **Signs:**
  ▪ **Punctate epithelial keratitis:** Fine or coarse punctate lesion
  ▪ **Dendritic ulcer:** Typical lesion for recurrent epithelial keratitis. Ulcer in irregular, zigzag, branching shape. Floor of ulcer stains with fluorescein, and the margin is stained with rose Bengal dye.
  ▪ **Geographical ulcer:** Branches of dendritic ulcer coalesce to form geographical ulcer.

Ophthalmology

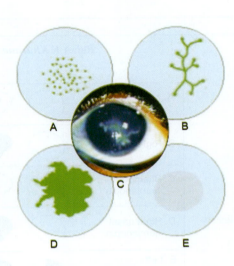

Figure: A. Punctate keratitis; B. Dendritic ulcer; C & D. Geographical Ulcer; E. Disciform keratitis

- **NOTE:** FM-100 Hue test is the most sensitive test for color vision testing

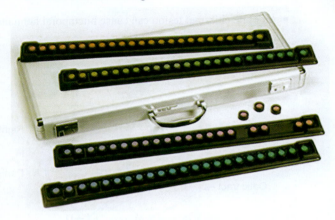

Figure: FM 100 Hue

6. Ans. (b) Steroids

Ref: A K Khurana 6th ed. P 64, 75

- Using steroids in active inflammation can cause flare-up of bacterial infection and corneal ulcer may develop.

7. Ans. (a) Arteriolar attenuation

Ref: A K Khurana 6th ed. P 288

Fundal changes in retinitis pigmentosa:
- Retinal pigmentary changes: Perivascular, jet black spots resembling bony corpuscles in shape
- Retinal arterioles are attenuated (narrowed), may become thread like in later stages
- Thinning and atrophy of retinal pigment epithelium
- Pale, waxy optic disc

Clinical features of RP:
- Night blindness: characteristic earliest feature
- Delayed dark adaptation
- Tubular vision (preserved central vision, lost after many years)

RP is inherited as:
- AR: most common (intermediate severity)
- AD: least severe
- X-Linked: least common (Most severe)

8. Ans. (d) Ames test

Ref: A K Khurana 6th ed. P 330-331

- Ames test is utilized to determine the mutagenic activity of chemicals by observing they can cause mutation in test bacteria or not.
- All other test in choices are utilized in color vision testing.

9. Ans. (d) Temporal lobe lesion

Ref: A K Khurana 6th edit pg 314

- Superior quadrantic hemianopia is also termed as *"pie in the sky"*.
- It is produced when inferior fibres are involved in temporal lobe lesions. Inferior most fibres of optic radiation form the so called Meyer's loop.
- Remember, inferior fibres of optic radiations contain fibres from ipsilateral lower temporal retina and contralateral lower nasal retina.
- Inferior quadrantic hemianopia is *"pie on the floor"*. It is produced when superior fibres are involved in parietal lobe lesions
- Other choices like pituitary adenoma (MCC), craniopharyngioma and meningioma are the causes of chiasmal lesions, which causes bitemporal hemianopia.

Lesion of parietal lobe (Pie on floor)
Inferior quadrantic hemianopia

Lesion of temporal lobe (Pie on sky)
Superior quadrantic hemianopia

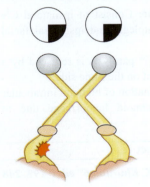
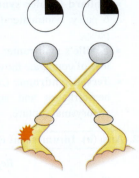

FMGE Solutions Screening Examination

10. Ans. (a) Bitemporal hemianopia

Ref: A K Khurana 6th ed. P 312

- An optic chiasmal lesion can cause bitemporal hemianopia.

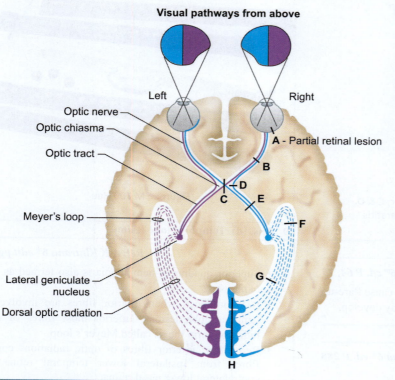

11. Ans. (a) Weber syndrome

Ref: A K Khurana 6th ed. P 334

- **Weber syndrome:** Characterized by ipsilateral CN 3 palsy, contralateral hemiplegia and facial palsy of upper motor neuron type.
- **Benedict's syndrome:** Characterized by ipsilateral CN 3 palsy associated with tremors and jerky movements of the contralateral side due to involvement of the red nucleus.
- **Millard-Gubler syndrome:** Consist of ipsilateral CN 6 palsy, contralateral hemiplegia and ipsilateral facial palsy.
- **Foville's syndrome:** CN 6th paralysis is replaced by a loss of conjugate movement on the same side.
- **Terson syndrome:** Combination of bilateral intraocular hemorrhages and subarachnoid hemorrhage due to aneurysmal rupture.

12. Ans. (a) Intumescent cataract

Ref: A.K. Khurana 6th ed. P 193, 248

- Phacomorphic glaucoma is most common lens induced glaucoma (secondary ACG).
- It is caused due to intumescent/swollen, cataractous lens.
- The swollen lens pushes the iris forward resulting in secondary ACG.

13. Ans. (c) Retrolental flare

Ref: A K Khurana 6th ed. P 437

- Sympathetic ophthalmitis is bilateral granulomatous panuveitis. It occurs as a result of penetrating ocular trauma (exciting eye), which can involve the contralateral eye (sympathizing eye) due to uveal pigment allergen released from the injured eye.
- **Symptom:**
  - Photophobia and transient indistinctness of near object
- **Signs:**
  - **First sign:** Presence of retrolental flare and cells or the presence of few keratic precipitates at the back of cornea.
  - Mild ciliary congestion
  - Edematous disc
- **Treatment:**
  - **Best prophylactic therapy:** Early excision of injured eye

Ophthalmology

- **If there is hope of saving injured eye:** Repair the wound + topical and systemic steroid and antibiotics along with atropine
- If no relief or photophobia, KP and lacrimation persist after 2 weeks of treatment → excise the injured eye immediately

ANATOMY, PHYSIOLOGY AND EXAMINATION OF EYE

14. Ans. (b) Neural crest

Ref: Comprehensive Ophthalmology by A.K Khurana 6th ed. P 12-13

- Corneal epithelium is derived from surface ectoderm, while corneal endothelium is derived from neural crest.

TABLE: Embryology of eye

Surface ectoderm	Neuroectoderm	Neural crest	Mesoderm
• Tarsal plate • Epithelium of cornea & conjunctiva • Lens • Lacrimal gland	• Retina • Optic nerve • Smooth muscle of iris • Epithelium of iris and ciliary muscle, retina • Secondary vitreous	• Trabecular meshwork • Ciliary muscles • Endothelium of cornea • Stroma of cornea • **Sclera EXCEPT temporal part**	• Extraocular muscles • Primary vitreous • **Temporal sclera** • Blood Vessels
Mn: TÉLL	ROSES	To MESS	Extra Pulm. TB

15. Ans. (d) Done from 1 meter distance from patient

Ref: Comprehensive Ophthalmology by A.K Khurana 6th ed. P 5771

- Retinoscopy aka skiascopy or shadow test is done to check the error of refraction by method of neutralization.
- Patient is made to sit at a distance of 1 meter from examiner → a light is thrown into patient's eye → through a hole in retinoscope mirror, the examiner observes the red reflex in the pupillary area of patient.
- Examiner Look for movement of red reflex/orange streak/bar of light.
  - **If NO movement:** Myopia = –1 D
  - **If opposite movement:** Myopia > –1
  - **Same side movement:** Myopia < – 1; Emmetropia = 0; Hypermetropia: +1

16. Ans. (b) ERG

Ref: Comprehensive Ophthalmology by A.K Khurana 6th ed. P 287

- Dark adaptation is ability of the eye to adapt itself to decreasing illumination. The time taken to see in dim illumination is dark adaptation time.
- Rods are more sensitive to low light (scotopic vision) while cones are for bright light.
- **Delayed dark adaptation:** Occur due to disease of rods. Ex: Deficiency of vitamin A, retinitis pigmentosa.

RETINITIS PIGMENTOSA

- Degenerative disease of the rods
- MC affects males in childhood and progress slowly
- Inherited as:
  - AR- in 25% cases; intermediate severity
  - AD- in 25% cases; least severe
  - X-linked- least common (10%); most severe
- **Clinical feature:**
  - Night blindness
  - Delayed dark adaptation
  - Tubular vision
  - **Triad:** Arterioles constriction, Bony spicule pigmentation, Waxy pallor of disc
- **IOC:** Electroretinogram (B wave affected before A wave)
- **Treatment:** Vitamin A 15000 IU orally qd, slow down progression.

17. Ans. (a) +2 to +3 D

Ref: Comprehensive Ophthalmology by Khurana; 6/ed. P 9

EYE AT BIRTH

- AP diameter is 16.5 mm, adult size is attained by 7 to 8 years (24 mm).
- Corneal diameter 10 mm, adult size attained by 2 years.
- Lens spherical.
- Lacrimal gland underdeveloped, tears not secreted.
- Orbit is more divergent.
- Visual acuity 6/60.
- Myelination of optic nerve has reached lamina cribrosa.

18. Ans. (b) Lens

Ref: Comprehensive Ophthalmology by Khurana 4/ed. P 4

- Among the given choices, lens has the highest refractive index of about 1.38 to 1.40

Refractive index of different ocular structure

Structure	Refractive index
• Lens	1.38 – 1.40
• Cornea	1.376
• Aqueous humor	1.336
• Vitreous humor	1.336

19. Ans. (c) Associated with microphthalmia

Ref: Ocular Pathology; E-book, P 664

- The primary vitreous used information of the eye during fetal development remains in the eye upon birth and is hazy and scarred.
- The persistence of primary vitreous even after birth is said to be persistent hyperplastic primary vitreous (PHPV).
- **Symptoms are:** Leukocoria, strabismus, nystagmus and blurred vision, blindness.
- It is seen almost always unilateral (~90% of the cases)
- It is associated with:
  - Small eye (typically occurs in a microphthalmic eye)
  - Retinal detachment
  - Vitreous hemorrhage
- If diagnosed at an early stage it may be possible to aspirate the lens followed by excision of the retrolental membrane and vitrectomy.
- Visual prognosis is poor.

20. Ans. (a) Temporal

Extent of normal visual field (in degrees)

- Superior: 50°
- Nasal: 60°
- Inferior: 70°
- Temporal: 90–100°

21. Ans. (b) 10–20

Ref: A.K Khurana's Ophthalmology, 6th ed. pg. 223

- Normal IOP refers to pressure exerted by intraocular fluids on coats of eyeball.
- Normal IOP varies **between 10 to 21 mm Hg** (mean 16.5 +/– 2.5 mm Hg).
- This pressure is essentially maintained by a dynamic equilibrium between the formation and outflow of aqueous humor.
- Normal aqueous production rate: 2.3 μl/L
- Normal aqueous outflow rate: 0.22/min/mm Hg

22. Ans. (b) 2.5 cm

Ref: A.K. Khurana, 6th ed. pg. 3

- Axial length of orbit is 24 mm i.e. 2.4 cm
- Volume of orbit: 6 ml
- Depth of anterior chamber: 3 mm
- Eyeball Made of 3 layers:
  - Sclera: Outer
  - Choroid: Middle *(vascular layer; a dangerous layer)*
  - Retina: Inner
- Cornea forms **anterior 1/6th** of eyeball and sclera forms **posterior 5/6th** of eyeball

23. Ans. (c) Ora serrata

Ref: A.K. Khurana, 6th ed. pg. 264

The ciliary body extends backward as far as the ora serrata, at which point the retina proper begins abruptly. The transition from the ciliary body to the choroid, on the other hand is gradual, although this line is conveniently accepted as the limit the two structures. The ora serrata thus circles the globe, but is slightly more anterior on the nasal than on the temporal side.

24. Ans. (b) Superior oblique

Ref: A.K. Khurana, 6th ed. pg. 5-6, 337

EXTRA-OCULAR MUSCLES

- The extraocular muscles control the movement of the eye.
- **Levator Palpabrae Superioris (LPS):** Muscle which elevates the palpabrae upwards resulting in opening the eye.
- When LPS gets tired, muller's muscle and frontalis muscle helps in elevation of eyelid.
- **Eyeball muscles (6):**
  - **4 Recti muscles:** Superior (SR), inferior (IR), lateral (LR) and medial rectus (MR)]
  - **2 Oblique muscles:** Superior oblique and inferior oblique
- The muscles supplied by the occulomotor nerve (**CN III**) are: superior, inferior and medial rectus and inferior oblique, sphincter papillae and ciliary muscle.
- Lateral rectus is supplied by abducens (VI)
- Trochlear nerve (CN IV) supplies superior oblique muscle.
- *Mnemonic:* LR6, SO4, O3; which means lateral rectus is supplied by sixth nerve, superior oblique by fourth nerve and all other by EOM by third cranial nerve.

25. Ans. (b) Its nucleus is located in lower midbrain

Ref: A.K. Khurana, 6th ed. pg. 7-8

- Location of **CN III** (occulomotor nerve) nucleus is **upper midbrain**
- Location of **CN IV** (trochlear nerve) nucleus is in the **lower mid-brain.**

TABLE: CN, their Respective Nucleus Location and their Function

Cranial Nerve	Nucleus Location	Function
Oculomotor III	Upper midbrain	Eyeball movements: extrinsic ocular muscles
Trochlear IV	Lower midbrain	Eyeball movements: extrinsic ocular muscles
Abducens VI	Pons	Eyeball movements: extrinsic ocular muscles
Hypoglossal XII	Medulla	Tongue muscles and movements

Ophthalmology

26. Ans. (b) Lacrimal gland

Ref: A.K. Khurana, 6th ed. pg. 386

GLANDS OF EYELIDS

- **Meibomian glands**: Also known as tarsal glands present in the stroma of tarsal plate and are arranged vertically.
  - They are modified sebaceous glands. Their ducts open at the lid margin. Their secretion constitutes the oily layer of tear film.
- **Glands of Zeis**: These are also sebaceous glands which open into the follicles of eyelashes.
- **Glands of Moll**: These are modified sweat glands situated near the hair follicle. They open into the hair follicles or into the ducts of Zeis glands.
- **Accessory lacrimal glands of Wolfring.** These are present near the upper border of the tarsal plate.

Note: *Lacrimal gland is one of the gland of lacrimal apparatus. It is NOT among the eyelid glands.*

27. Ans. (a) Superior oblique

Ref: A.K. Khurana, 6th ed. pg. 337-39

- The function of superior oblique is quite contrary to its name. Its action is depression of eyeball, which helps to see down.
- Its yoke muscle is inferior rectus, which also has the similar function as superior oblique. If superior oblique is affected patient will develop difficulty in looking down
- There are 9 Gaze:
  - Primary : Straight
  - Secondary: Up, down, left, right
  - Tertiary : Up left, Up, right, Down left, Down right
- **ACTIONS OF EOM**

Muscle	Function		
	Primary	Secondary	Tertiary
Lateral rectus	Abduction	–	–
Medial Rectus	Adduction	–	–
Inferior Rectus	Depression	Extortion	Adduction
Superior rectus	Elevation	Intortion	Adduction
Inferior Oblique	Extortion	Elevation	Abduction
Superior oblique	Intortion	Depression	Abduction

- **Mnemonics:** *SinRad (all superior muscles causes Intortion; all rectus muscles causes Adduction EXCEPT Lateral rectus)*

28. Ans. (a) Adduction and intorsion

Ref: A.K. Khurana, 6th ed. pg. 339

29. Ans. (b) Inferior rectus

Ref: A.K. Khurana, 6th ed. pg. 337-39

- The function of inferior rectus is depression of eyeball, which helps to see down.
- Its yoke muscle is superior oblique, which also has the similar function as inferior rectus.

30. Ans. (c) Towards the right side

Ref: A.K. Khurana, 6th ed. pg. 337-39

- *VIth nerve palsy leads to loss of abduction/lateral gaze leading to **abnormal head posture towards the side** of affected muscle*
- *There is Presence of **convergent squint also.***

> **Extra Mile**

IVth nerve palsy
- Diplopia on looking down
- Inability to look inferomedially

31. Ans. (d) Right superior rectus

Ref: A.K. Khurana, 6th ed. pg. 339

- **Synergistic muscle** is two muscles *functioning as same, in the same eye.* Function of superior rectus is to elevate the eye, which is same with inferior oblique.
  - Right inferior oblique and right superior rectus elevate the right eye
- Yoke muscle on the contrary, is two extraocular muscles from two eyes having same function.
  - **Ex:** Yoke muscle of right inferior oblique is left superior rectus.

32. Ans. (a) The superior orbital fissure

Ref: A.K. Khurana, 6th ed. pg. 337, BDC, 4th ed. Vol III, pg. 25-6

TABLE: Structures passing through superior orbital fissure

Superior orbital fissure		
Medial /lower part	**Middle part (through tendinous ring)**	**Lateral/ Upper part**
• Inferior Opthalmic vein	• Nasociliary nerve	• Superior Opthalmic vein
• Sympathetic nerves around internal carotid artery	• Occulomotor nerve	• Lacrimal nerve
	• Abducent nerve	• Frontal nerve
Mn: Inferior sympathy	***Mnemonic –"NOA"***	• Trochlear nerve
		Mn – "Superior LFT"

Explanations

1081

FMGE Solutions Screening Examination

Examination of a Case of Heterophoria
- Testing for vision and refractive error.
- Cover-uncover test.
- Prism cover test
- **Maddox rod test:** Patient is asked to fix on a point light in the centre of Maddox tangent scale at a distance of 6 meters.
- A Maddox rod is placed in front of one eye with axis of the rod parallel to the axis of deviation.
- The Maddox rod converts the point light image into a line. Thus, the patient will see a point light with one eye and a red line with the other.
- Due to dissimilar images of the two eyes, fusion is broken and heterophoria becomes apparent.
- **Maddox wing test:** Also used to measure phoria of near distance.

Extra Mile
Structures passing through Inferior orbital fissure
- Zygomatic branch of maxillary nerve
- Infraorbital nerve & vessels
- Rami of Pterygoid ganglion
- Communicating vein b/w inferior ophthalmic & pterygoid plexus of veins.

Mn-"ZIPC"

33. Ans. (a) Strabismus

Ref: A.K. Khurana, 6th ed. pg. 346

- **Strabismus:** A misalignment of the visual axes of the two eyes is called squint or strabismus.
- **It is classified as:**
  - Pseudostrabismus (apparent squint)
  - Heterophoria (latent squint)
  - Heterotropia (manifest squint)

HETEROPHORIA

- Hterophoria also known as 'Latent strabismus'
- It is a condition in which the tendency of the eyes to deviate is kept latent by fusion.

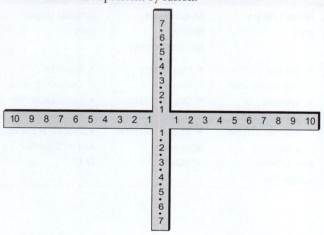

34. Ans. (c) 3 D

Ref: A.K. Khurana, 6th ed. pg. 578

- By pinhole test visual acuity can be neutralized till 3 D. It can't accommodate more than that.
- It is a test to distinguish a refractive error from organic disease.
- A refractive error may, be corrected with glasses, whereas organic disease may signal the development of preventable blindness. If visual acuity is improved after pin hole test, the defect is refractive; if not, it is organic.
  - **Pinhole improves vision:** Refractive error, peripheral cataract
  - **Pinhole worsen vision:** Macular diseases, central lens opacities
  - **Vision static with pinhole:** Amblyopia

35. Ans. (c) Centre of the lens

Ref: A.K. Khurana 6th ed. /179; Parson's 20/e p-52-53

REFRACTIVE INDEX OF DIFFERENT MEDIUM
- Highest refractive index is of *center of lens* (1.406)
- Anterior and posterior lens cortex forming anterior & posterior lens surface (1.386)
- Cornea (1.376)
- Aqueous and vitreous humor (1.336)
- Air (1)

36. Ans. (c) 45 D

Ref: A.K. Khurana, 6th ed. pg. 95

POWER
- Lens= +16D
- Cornea= +44D
- Total= +60D

Ophthalmology

37. Ans. (b) Phacomorphic glaucoma

Ref: A.K. Khurana, 6th ed. pg. 3, 192-93

- **Deep anterior chamber is seen in**: Young, males and myopes
- **Shallow anterior chamber is seen in**: Women, Elderly, and Children (WEC)

> **Extra Mile**

Phacomorphic Glaucoma
- Phacomorphic glaucoma is angle closure glaucoma caused by mature cataract *making the anterior chamber shallow.*

Phacolytic glauoma
- Phacolytic glaucoma is open angle glaucoma caused by hypermature cataract in which the *anterior chamber is deep* by leaking lens material which blocks the trabecular meshwork.
- Treatment is cataract surgery

Myopia
- Myopia or 'Short sight' is a refractive error that most commonly presents as indistinct distant vision in which the light rays are focused in front of retina. As the maximum distance of clear vision is reduced the far point comes nearer. Following are types of myopia-
    - Axial Myopia
    - Curvature Myopia
    - Index Myopia
- **Axial Myopia-** eyeball larger than normal causes myopia. Every 1 mm increase in axial length has 3D increase in 1 mm = 3D
- **Curvature Myopia-** axial length normal. Cornea is curved as in keratoconus. 1 mm of curvature = 6D. So they are very high myopes.
- **Index Myopia-** corneal curvature normal. Refractive Index increases. More the difference → more the bending between two media.

Myopics are typically called short sighted, so all myopics wear concave lenses. Minification 1D = 2%

Aphakia: Aphakia means absence of crystalline lens from eye.

38. Ans. (a) Children

Ref: A.K. Khurana 6th ed. /45-49; Khurana's 4th Ed./ 39-41

ACCOMODATION

- Mechanism by which we can focus the diverging rays coming from a near object on the retina in an attempt to see clearly is called accommodation.
- During this there occurs increase in the power of crystalline lens due to increase in the curvature of its surface.

Mechanism of Accommodation
- When the eye is at rest (unaccomodated), the ciliary ring is large and keeps the zonules tense.
- Because of zonular tension the lens is kept compressed (flat) by the capsule.
- Ciliary muscles and zonules have inverse relation in function.
- Ciliary ring is shortened due to contraction of the ciliary muscle which releases zonular tension on the lens capsule. This allows the elastic capsule to act unrestrained to deform the lens substance. The lens then alters its shape to become more convex (conoidal).
- The lens assumes conoidal shape due to configuration of the anterior lens capsule which is thinner at the centre and thicker at the periphery
- **Note:** *The crystalline protein of lens and contraction of ciliary muscle is finest in child as compared to adult and elderly. Hence children have maximum accommodation.*

39. Ans. (a) Lens of eye

Ref: A.K. Khurana 6th ed. /12

TABLE: Embryology of eye

Surface ectoderm	Neuroectoderm	Neural crest	Mesoderm
• Tarsal plate • Epithelium of cornea & conjunctiva • Lens • Lacrimal gland	• Retina • Optic nerve • Smooth muscle of iris • Epithelium of iris and ciliary muscle, retina • Secondary vitreous	• Trabecular meshwork • Ciliary muscles • Endothelium of cornea • Stroma of cornea • **Sclera EXCEPT temporal part**	• Extraocular muscles • Primary vitreous • **Temporal sclera** • Blood Vessels
Mn: TELL	ROSES	To MESS	Extra Pulm. TB

40. Ans. (b) Surface ectoderm

Ref: A.K. Khurana, 6th ed. pg. 12

41. Ans. (c) Surface ectoderm

Ref: A.K. Khurana, 6th ed. pg. 12

Please refer to above explanation

Explanations

42. Ans. (c) Temporal

Ref: A.K. Khurana, 6th ed. pg. 505, Khurana, 4th ed. pg. 481

Extent of Normal Visual Field:
- Superior: 50
- Inferior: 70
- Nasal: 60
- Temporal: 90-100

43. Ans. (b) Inferior

Ref: A.K. Khurana, 6th ed. pg. 265-66

- Neuroretinal rim is the tissue outside the cup and contains the retinal nerve axons as they enter the nerve head.
- It is broadest in lower segment of the disc, then above followed by nasally and temporally.
- There is greater axonal mass and vascularity in the infero-temporal region.
- In case of primary open angle glaucoma, there is progressive loss of retinal ganglion cells, leading to enlargement of the cup, particularly in lower and upper poles of disc, leading to vertically oval cup.

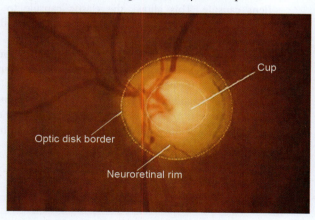

44. Ans. (d) Opacity in the refractive media

Ref: A.K. Khurana, 6th ed. pg. 586

DISTANT DIRECT OPHTHALMOSCOPY

- Used to get a preliminary idea about the status of the ocular media and fundus
- This should be done routinely before doing a direct ophthalmoscopy
- **Equipment needed** - self illuminated ophthalmoscope or plane mirror with a hole in centre
- **Procedure**
  - Should be performed in a semi dark room
  - The ophthalmoscope should be kept at a distance of 20-25 cm from the patient's eye
  - Normally a red reflex is seen at the pupillary area
- **Uses**
  - Opacities in the ocular media are seen as dark spots in the red glow at the pupillar area
  - The plane of the opacities can be assessed by asking the patient to move the eye from side to side while the examiner is observing the pupillary glow (based on parallax principle)
    - Opacities in front of the pupil move in the direction of eye movement
    - Opacities in the pupillary plane do not move
    - Opacities behind the pupillary plane move opposite the direction of eye movement
- To differentiate between a mole on the iris and a hole in the iris
  - In oblique illumination, both appear dark
  - In distant direct ophtalmoscopy
    - Mole–appears dark
    - Hole–red glow is seen
- To detect a retinal detachment or fundal mass
  - Both of them are visible as a grayish reflex
  - It is not possible to differentiate them in distant direct ophthalmoscopy
- The image in Indirect Ophthalmoscopy is inverted both vertically as well as laterally, which means: *What appears as right upper quadrant is actually in the left lower quadrant.*

> **Extra Mile**

Direct ophthalmoscope	Indirect Ophthalmoscope
Virtual, Erect and Magnified 15 times: "VEM"	Real, Inverted and 4-5 times Magnified: "RIM"
Mneomonic: "DEV" i.e. Direct = Erect + Virtual	Mnemonic: "IIR" i.e. Indirect = Inverted + Real

45. Ans. (b) Direct ophthalmoscopy

Ref: A.K. Khurana, 6th ed. pg. 586; Khurana 4th ed. pg. 565

- **Direct ophthalmoscopy:** Disc and macula
- **Indirect ophthalmoscopy:** Whole retina, vitrous (*choice of test in retinal detachment*)
- **Distant direct ophthalmoscopy-** for any opacity, cataract, detachment
- **Retinoscopy:** For calculating refractive error

46. Ans. (a) Strabismus

Ref: A.K. Khurana, 6th ed. pg. 344-58

Classification of Squints (Strabismus)

LATENT SQUINT/HETROPHORIA

- A condition in which the tendency of eyes to deviate is kept latent by fusion. Therefore when the influence of fusion is removed the visual axis of one eye axis of one eye deviates away (Orthophoria is a condition of perfect alignment of two eyes)

Ophthalmology

- Types Esophoria is a tendency to converge
  - Exophoria is a tendency to diverge
  - Hyperphoria is a tendency to deviate upwards
  - Hypophoria is a tendency to deviate downwards
  - Cyclophoria is a tendency to rotate around A–P axis
- Evaluation
  - Refraction
  - Uncover test (tells about present & type of hetrophoria)
  - Maddox rod test (amount of hetrophoria in degrees)
  - **Maddox wing test** (amount of phoria for near distance i.e. 33 cm)
- Treatment:
  - Refraction
  - Occlusion therapy (in presence of amblyopia)
  - Orthoptic exercise
  - Operative correction
  - Prism correction for remaining error.

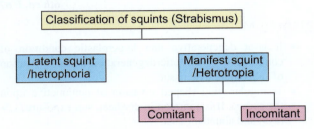

MANIFEST SQUINT (HETEROTROPIA)	
Comitant	**Incomitant**
• Amount of deviation in squinting eye remains constant (unaltered) in all directions of gaze & there is no limitation of ocular movements.	• Manifest squint in which amount of deviation varies in different directions of gaze.

• Types
  ■ **Alternating squint:** when one eye fixes, the other eye deviates & either of the eyes can adopt fixation alternately & freely
  ■ Esotropia (Convergent squint)
  ■ Exotropia (Divergent squint)
  ■ Hypertropia (Vertical squint)
	• Types
	  ■ Paralytic squint
	  ■ "A" & "V" pattern hetrotrophias
	  ■ Special ocular motality defects
	  ■ **Clinical presentation:** is diplopia, confusion, nausea, vertigo & ocular deviation with restriction of eye movements, compensatory head posture & false projection & orientation, loss of stereoposis, normal visual acuity & no amblyopia.

• Evaluation
  ■ Refraction, visual acuity, ocular motality
  ■ Direct cover test (confirms the presence of manifest squint)
  ■ Alternate cover test (reveal whether the squint is U/L or alternate and to differentiate concomitant squint from paralytic squint).
  ■ Estimation of angle of deviation.
  ■ **Hirschberg corneal reflex test:** Roughly the angle of squint is 15° and 45° when the corneal light reflex falls on the border of pupil & limbus respectively. The premise is that every millimeter of deviation from centre of pupil is equal to 7° (15Δ)
	• Evaluation
	  ■ All tests of comitant squint
	  ■ Diplopia carting
	  ■ **Hess screen test**
	  ■ Forced duction test
	• Treatment of cause, diplopia (by occlusion), surgery (if no recovery in 6 months).

47. Ans. (c) Inferior rectus

Ref: A.K. Khurana, 6th ed. pg. 414

- In thyroid eye ophthalmopathy, the ocular motility defects due to restrictive myopathy *(in order of frequency)* are:
  - Elevation (due to fibrosis of inferior rectus)
  - Depression (due to fibrosis of superior rectus)
  - Abduction (due to fibrosis of medial rectus)
  - Adduction (due to fibrosis of lateral rectus).

Mnemonic - "I M Shy Lad"

48. Ans. (a) Males are more prone

Ref: A.K. Khurana, 6th ed. pg. 329

- Color blindness is an **X-Linked recessive condition**. Females are always carrier and males are always affected. Hence males are more affected than females.
- Most common type of color blindness: Deutranopia (Green color blindness)

FMGE Solutions Screening Examination

CORNEA, CONJUNCTIVA AND SCLERA

49. Ans. (c) Conjunctiva invasion making a flap over cornea

Ref: Comprehensive Ophthalmology by A.K Khurana 6th ed. P 87

PTERYGIUM

- It is a degenerative and hyperplastic condition of conjunctiva → elastotic degeneration and proliferation of subconjunctival tissue
- Triangular/wing shaped invasion of conjunctiva upon the cornea. It is common in dry heat, sun exposure (UV rays) and abundant dust.
- Iron deposition in the corneal epithelium at the advancing head of the pterygium is called **Stocker line.**
- It usually asymptomatic.
- **MC site:** Nasal side
   - **Primary double pterygium:** Involvement of both nasal and temporal side
- The corneal epithelium, bowman's layer and superficial stroma are destroyed
- **Treatment:** Surgical excision.
   - The commonest problem after excision is recurrence which is reduced by postoperative use of mitomycin-C/ thiotepa or by doing surgical excision with free conjunctival graft from same/ other eye.

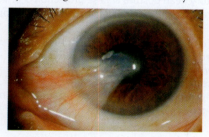

Extra Mile

TABLE: Differences between pterygium and pseudopterygium

	Pterygium	Pseudopterygium
Etiology	Degenerative process	Inflammatory process
Age	Usually occurs in elder persons	Can occur at any age
Site	Always situate in the palpebral aperture	Can occur at any site
Stages	Either progressive, regressive or stationary	Always stationary
Probe test	Probe cannot be passed underneath	A probe can be passed under the neck

50. Ans. (c) Enterovirus

Ref: Comprehensive Ophthalmology by Khurana 6/ed. P 23

- **Acute hemorrhagic conjunctivitis:** It is also called Apollo conjunctivitis.
- It is caused by picornavirus (enterovirus type 70).

51. Ans. (b) Keratitis

Ref: Yanoff Duker Ophthalmology; P 220

- Bacteria which cause purulent keratitis after epithelial injury are pseudomonas, *Staphylococcus aureus, Pneumococcus, Moraxella, Streptococcus epidermidis, E. coli, Proteus, Klebsiella*.
- **Clinical feature of keratitis:** Pain, lacrimation, photophobia, red eye, blurred vision.

52. Ans. (a) Corneal sensation decreased

Ref: Comprehensive Ophthalmology by Khurana 6/ed. P 27

- Dendritic ulcer is seen in viral keratitis which is most commonly caused by HSV. It can involve any layer of cornea but when only corneal epithelium is involved it is known as dendritic ulcer.
- Recurrent ocular herpes present as geographic ulcer, superficial punctate keratitis.
- When stroma is involved it presents as disciform keratitis and diffuse stromal necrotic keratitis.
- The characteristic hypopyon corneal ulcer is caused by pneumococcus (ulcus serpens) and pseudomonas.
- In recurrent epithelial keratitis, there is decreased corneal sensation

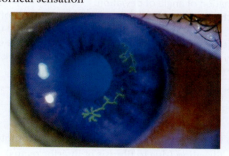

53. Ans (b) Keratoconus

Ref: Yanoff Duker; 4/ed. P 254

- Keratoconus is degenerative disease of cornea, where it becomes conical. It is best treated by keratoplasty.
- Keratoplasty is corneal grafting or in more simple term, corneal transplantation.

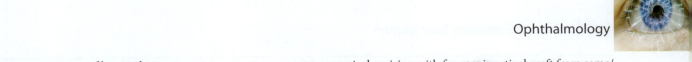

Ophthalmology

- There are two types of keratoplasty:
  - **Penetrating keratoplasty (PK)** also known as full thickness keratoplasty
  - **Lamellar keratoplasty (LK)** also known as partial thickness keratoplasty. It has highest success rate as compared to PK.
- **Indication for keratoplasty:**
  - Corneal scar
  - Non-healing ulcer
  - Chemical injuries
  - Keratoconus
  - Pseudophakic bullous keratopathy

54. Ans. (c) Chylamydia

Ref: Khurana, 6th ed. pg. 73

- **Adenovirus** is considered as the **most common** cause of swimming pool conjunctivitis. Chlorine is unable to eliminate the virus, hence it can often present as an outbreak. But it was not given in choice.
- **However, it can also be caused by chlamydia trachomatis serotypes D to K** and the condition is said to be adult inclusion conjunctivitis.

Adult inclusion conjunctivitis.

- Caused by **chlamydia trachomatis serotypes D to K.**
- **Usually** affects sexually active males and primary source of infection is urethritis in males and cervicitis in females.
- **Transmission: Either** via contaminated fingers or more commonly through contaminated water of swimming pool. Therefore it is also said to be swimming pool conjunctivitis.

55. Ans. (d) Clean hand

Ref: Khurana, 64

- Frequent handwashing is the most effective way to reduce the risk of transmission to the close contacts.
- **Other measures can be:** avoid sharing towels, handkerchief and pillows.

56. Ans. (b) Pterygium

Ref: Khurana, 88

Pterygium

- Triangular invasion of conjunctiva upon the cornea. It is common in dry heat, sun exposure and abundant dust.
- Iron deposition in the corneal epithelium at the advancing head of the pterygium is called **STOCKER LINE.** Usually asymptomatic.
- **Treatment:** Surgical excision. The commonest problem after excision is recurrence which is reduced by post-operative use of mitomycin C/thiotepa or by doing surgical excision with free conjunctival graft from same/ other eye.

57. Ans. (d) Staphylococcus

Ref: Khurana, 99

- The common cause of corneal ulcer in India is Streptococcus Pneumoniae (causes central corneal ulcer) whereas the **commonest cause overall is staphylococcus aureus** (causes peripheral corneal ulcer).
- The bacterial ulcer can present with the formation of a hypopyon (sterile).
- The characteristic hypopyon corneal ulcer is due to pneumococcus and is called ulcus serpens.
- **Treatment:** topical gentamicin/ tobramycin and cephalozin with cycloplegics(atropine ointment or drops) and analgesics.

58. Ans. (c) Interstitial keratitis

Ref: Khurana, 121

- Inflammation of corneal stroma without primary involvement of epithelium or endothelium is called interstitial keratitis.
- It can have many causes like: Congential syphilis, TB, Cogan's syndrome, acquired syphilis, malaria, sarcoidosis, leprosy.

Syphilitic interstitial keratitis

- It is associated more frequently with congenital syphilis and manifestation develops between 5-15 years of age.

Clinical features:

- Can present with Hutchinson triad i.e. interstitial keratitis, Hutchinson teeth and vestibular deafness.
- **Clinically it can present with 3 stages:**
  - **Initial progressive stage:** Lasts for 2 weeks. Begins with edema of endothelium and deeper stroma secondary to anterior uveitis.
  - **Florid stage:** Lasts for 2 months there is development of radial bundle of brush like vessels on cornea. Since these vessels are covered by hazy cornea, they look dull reddish pink which is called **salmon patch appearance.**
  - **Regression stage:** May last for 1–2 years. The acute inflammation resolves with progressive appearance of vascular invasion. Resolution of the lesion leaves behind some opacities and **ghost vessels.**

Treatment:

- **Local:** Topical corticosteroid drops e.g: dexamethasone 0.1%, Atropine ointment 1% 2–3 times a day, Dark goggles or keratoplasty in case of dense corneal opacity.
- **Systemic:** Penicillin, systemic steroid.

FMGE Solutions Screening Examination

59. Ans. (b) Keratoconus

Ref: Khurana, 131

- **Munsen's sign:** Localized bulging of lower lid when patient looks down. Seen in late stages of keratoconus.

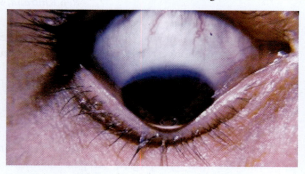

60. Ans. (a) Moraxella

Ref: A.K Khurana's Ophthalmology, 6th ed. pg. 66

Conjunctivitis type	MC organism/comments
• Acute mucopurulent	• Staphylococcus • It is MC type of bacterial conjunctivitis • (+) Halo
• Acute Purulent Conjunctivitis	• Gonococcus
• Membranous Conjunctivitis	• C. Diphtheria • Bleeds on separation
• Pseudomembranous Conjunctivitis	• Adeno/Staph/Strep • Separates easily
• Angular Conjunctivitis	• **Moraxella Axenfeld-** MCC
• Epidemic Keratoconjunctivitis/Madras eye	• Adenovirus: MCC

• Acute hemorrhagic/Apollo Conjunctivitis	• PicoRNA virus
	  ▪ Enterovirus 70: MCC
	  ▪ Echovirus
	  ▪ Coxsackie virus

61. Ans. (a) Trigeminal nerve

Ref: A.K Khurana's Ophthalmology, 6th ed. pg. 108-109

- Neurotropic keratitis is a corneal degenerative disease characterized by a reduction or absence of corneal sensitivity.
- In this condition, corneal innervation by **trigeminal nerve** is impaired.
- Most common ocular conditions associated with NK are herpes keratitis (zoster and simplex),
- **Other causes can be:** Topical anesthetic abuse, chemical and physical burns, contact lens abuse, topical drug toxicity, irradiation to eye or adnexa and corneal surgery.

62. Ans. (c) Flakes of mucus

Ref: A.K Khurana's Ophthalmology, 6th ed. pg. 63

- Any condition which causes fluid accumulation on cornea, can cause colored haloes.
- **Differential diagnosis of color haloes:**
  ▪ ACG
  ▪ Cataract
  ▪ Mucopurulent conjunctivitis: Due to prismatic effect of mucus present on cornea

> **Extra Mile**
> - Acute bacterial conjunctivitis is aka as acute mucopurulent conjunctivitis.
> - **Causes:** Staph Aureus, Koch-weeks bacillus, Pneumococcus and streptococcus

63. Ans. (a) Moraxella

Ref: A.K Khurana's Ophthalmology, 6th ed. P 66

64. Ans. (b) Keratoconus

Ref: A.K Khurana's Ophthalmology, 6th ed. pg. 132

- **Fleischer rings** are pigmented rings in the peripheral cornea, resulting from iron deposition in basal epithelial cells, in the form of hemosiderin.
- Fleischer rings are indicative of keratoconus, a degenerative corneal condition that causes the cornea to thin and change to a conic shape.
- Signs of keratoconus:
  ▪ **Munsen Sign:** V-Shaped protrusion of cornea on down gaze
  ▪ **Vogt's Striae:** Break in descemet's membrane
  ▪ **Fleischer ring:** Iron deposition at back of cornea
  ▪ Scissoring of reflex upon retinoscopy

> **Extra Mile**
> - **Kayser-Fleischer rings** are due to copper deposition, seen in case of Wilsons disease
> - **Immune ring of pessary:** In case of fungal keratitis
> - **Ring shaped ulcer: Protozoal keratitis**

65. Ans. (c) Prevents infection more than descemet's membrane

Ref: A.K Khurana 6th ed. pg. 96, Khurana, 4th ed. pg. 80.89

- Bowman's layer of cornea is acellular mass of condensed collagen fibrils
- **Thickness:** 12 μm
- It is NOT a true elastic membrane but simply a condensed superficial stroma
- Once destroyed, never regenerates

- It shows considerable resistance to *infection (descemet membrane maintains integrity of eyeball)*

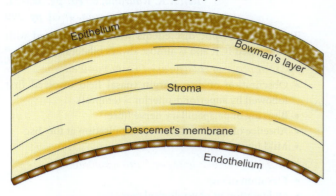

66. Ans. (d) Curvature of cornea

Ref: A.K. Khurana, 6th ed. pg. 575

Few Instruments Which are Used for Ocular Examination

Measurement parameter	Instruments/for:
• Corneal thickness	Pachymeta
• Corneal curvature	Keratometer
• Angle of anterior chamber	Gonioscope
• Corneal surface	Placido disc
• Corneal endothelium	Specular microscope
• Direct ophthalmoscope • Rememberd as: "DEV"	Routine fundus examination. *"Image formed is Erect and Virtual and magnified, 15 times"*
• Indirect ophthalmoscope	For assessment of retinal detachment and other peripheral retinal lesions. *The image is real, inverted and magnified 5 times.*
• Perimetry	Optic nerve function

67. Ans. (b) Pachymetry

Ref: A.K. Khurana, 6th ed. pg. 95-96; Khurana, 4th ed. pg. 89

- Corneal thickness is measured by the method known as pachymetry. Normal corneal thickness is around (0.52 mm – 0.7 mm) 500–700 µm.

Extra Mile

- PLACIDO DISC- for corneal surface
- Keratometry- Corneal curvature
- Tonometry- for IOP

68. Ans. (b) Keyser Fleischer Ring

Ref: A.K. Khurana 6th ed. pg. 131; Khurana, 4th ed./ 141

- Fleischer's ring is seen in keratoconus and not KF rings.
- KF ring is seen in Wilsons disease (Chalcosis)

KERATOCONUS

- Keratoconus (conical cornea) is a non-inflammatory bilateral (85%) ecstatic condition of cornea in its axial part.

Clinical Feature

- Patient presents with a defective vision due to progressive myopia and irregular astigmatism, which does not improve fully despite correction with glasses.
- Slit lamp examination may show thinning and ectasia of central cornea, *opacity at the apex and* **Fleischer's ring at the base of cone**, folds in Descemet's and bowman's membranes.
- **Vogt lines:** Very fine, vertical, deep stromal striae which disappear with external pressure on the globe are peculiar feature.
- On retinoscopy a yawning reflex *(scissor reflex)*
- **Munsen's sign:** Localized bulging of lower lid when patient looks down is positive in late stages.

69. Ans. (a) Corneal dystrophy

Ref: A.K. Khurana, 6th ed. pg. 124-31;
Corneal dystrophies are inherited disorders in which the cells have some inborn defect due to which pathological changes may occur with time leading to hazy cornea.

- Corneal dystrophies are classified according to anatomical site involved: Anterior dystrophy, Stromal dystrophies, Posterior dystrophies.
- Among anterior dystrophies, **epithelial basement membrane dystrophy aka Cogan's microcystic dystrophy is the most common.**
- These lesions involve corneal epithelium and present as bilateral dot-like microcystic or linear finger print opacities. In 10% of cases there is recurrent corneal erosion and majority of cases remains asymptomatic.
- It is characterized by the failure of the cornea's outermost layer of epithelial cells to attach to the underlying basement membrane (Bowman's layer).
- The condition is excruciatingly painful because the loss of these cells results in the exposure of sensitive corneal nerves.
- **Cause:** There is often a history of previous corneal injury (corneal abrasion or ulcer).

- It may also be due to corneal dystrophy or corneal disease.
- **Treatment-** Patching with plain ointment for 1-2 days.

70. Ans. (c) Corneal dystrophy

Ref: A.K. Khurana, 6th ed. pg. 124-31

Please refer to above explanation

71. Ans. (a) Thioridazine

Ref: A.K. Khurana, 6th ed. pg. 502

- Thioridazine is an antipsychotic agent.
- Its ocular side effect (corneal staining) limits its use.
- **Note:** ATT drug **Ethambutol** also causes corneal staining.

72. Ans. (c) Corneal xerosis

Ref: A.K. Khurana, 6th ed. pg. 468

- **Xeropthalmia:** all the ocular manifestation of Vitamin A deficiency.
- **First clinical sign of Vitamin A deficiency:** *Conjunctival Xerosis*
- **First clinical symptom of vitamin A deficiency:** *Night blindness*

WHO Classification of Xeropthalmia

CLASS	SIGNS
X1A	Conjunctival xerosis
X1B	Conjunctival xerosis with bitot's spot
X2	Corneal xerosis
X3A	Corneal xerosis with ulceration
X3B	Keratomalacia

73. Ans. (a) Xerophthalmia

Ref: Harrison's, 19th ed. pg. 96e-6

- MC ocular manifestation of vitamin A deficiency is xerophthalmia. This condition includes milder stages of night blindness and conjunctival xerosis (dryness) with bitot's spot.

Other Features of Vitamin A Deficiency:

- Diarrhea, Dysentry, measles, malaria or respiratory. These condition can pose risk to life if associated with vitamin A deficiency.

Features of Vitamin A toxicity:

- **Acute:** Increased ICP leading to bulging fontanels, vertigo, diplopia, seizure and exfoliative dermatitis.
- **Chronic:** dry skin, Chielosis, glossitis, alopecia, bone demineralization, hyperlipidemia, hypercalcemia, amenorrhea and features of pseudotumor cerebri with increased ICP and papilledema.

74. Ans. (c) Blurring of disc

Ref: A.K. Khurana, 6th ed. pg. 323-24, Khurana, 4th ed. pg. 299

Papilledema: Optic disc edema which is associated with the increased ICP, and is almost always bilateral.

Ophthalmoscopic Features of Early Papilledema:

- Obscuration of disc margin (nasal field involved first followed by superior > inferior > tempral).
- Blurring of peripapillary nerve fibre
- Absence of spontaneous venous pulsation at the disc
- Mild hyperemia

Features of Fully developed/Late papilledema

- Elevation of cup
- Obliteration of physiological cup
- Marked hypermia of disc
- Multiple soft exudates
- Tortuous and engorged veins
- Separation of nerve-fibre layer by edema.

75. Ans. (d) All of the above

Ref: A.K. Khurana, 6th ed. pg. 116, 4th ed. pg. 109-110

■ **MOOREN'S ULCER**

- Mooren's Ulcer/chronic serpiginous or rodent ulcer is a severe inflammatory peripheral ulcerative keratitis.
- **Treatment:**
  - Topical corticosteroids
  - Immunosuppressives with systemic steroids, e.g. cyclosporine
  - Soft contact lens
  - Lamellar or full thickness corneal grafting.

76. Ans. (d) Descemets membrane

Ref: A.K. Khurana, 6th ed. pg. 434

- **Chalcosis:** Refers to the specific changes produced by accumulation of copper in the eye.
- **Clinical feature:**
  - **Kayser-fleischer ring:** It is a golden brown ring which occurs due to deposition of copper in the peripheral parts of the *Descemet's membrane of the cornea.*
  - **Sunflower cataract:** Produced by deposition of copper on the posterior capsule of the lens.
  - **Retina:** It may show deposition of golden plaques at the posterior pole which reflect the light with a metallic sheen.

77. Ans. (c) HSV infection

Ref: A.K. Khurana, 6th ed. pg. 108

- Viral keratitis causes corneal ulceration. It is caused most commonly **by Herpes simplex, Herpes Zoster and Adenoviruses.**

Ophthalmology

- Dendritic & geographical corneal ulcers are seen in herpes simplex ocular disease.
- Dendritic ulcer (branching ulcer with knobbed ends), resembles no other condition, and is *pathognomic of herpes simplex ocular infection*.
- The use of **steroids** in dendritic ulcer hastens the formation of geographical ulcer so it is **contraindicated**.

78. Ans. (d) Dexamethasone

Ref: A.K. Khurana, 6th ed. pg. 108-109

- **Dendritic ulcer** is an irregular linear branching ulcer with knobbed ends and reduced corneal sensations seen in epithelial keratitis
- It is caused by herpes simplex infection.
- Steroids cause progression of dendritic ulcer, into **geographical ulcer** so, they are **contraindicated**.
- The treatment is done with **3% acyclovir ointment** and mechanical debridement. Other antibiotics may be required if there is a secondary infection.

79. Ans. (b) Stromal keratitis

Ref: A.K. Khurana, 6th ed. pg. 108-109

STROMAL KERATITIS

- It manifests as disciform keratitis (*disc shape ulcer with a surrounding Wessley immune ring formed due to delayed hypersensitivity to **HSV antigen***) or **diffuse stromal necrotic keratitis** (due to active viral invasion and tissue destruction).
- **Treatment:** Steroid drops with acyclovir 3%

> **Extra Mile**
>
> **Epithelial keratitis**
> - Caused by herpes simplex virus. It manifests as dendritic ulcer (irregular, linear, branching ulcer with knobbed ends and reduced corneal sensation) or geographical ulcer (large " amoeboid ulcer"). Steroids cause progression of dendritic ulcer into geographical ulcer, so, they are contradicated.
> - Treatment: 3% acyclovir ointment and mechanical debridement.

80. Ans. (b) Herpes zoster keratitis

Ref: A.K. Khurana, 6th ed. pg. 108-109

81. Ans. (d) Syphilis

Ref: A.K. Khurana, 6th ed. pg. 120-121

- Keratitis means corneal inflammation
- **Interstitial Keratitis** basically means corneal scarring due to chronic inflammation of the corneal stroma. Interstitial means space between cells i.e. corneal stroma which lies between the epithelium and the endothelium.
- It is most commonly seen in infection like syphillis

SYPHILITIC KERATITIS

- It is seen more frequently with congenital syphilis than acquired syphilis. It may present as part of Hutchinson's traid of:
  - **Interstitial keratitis**
  - Hutchinson teeth
  - Vestibular deafness

82. Ans. (b) Propomidine isothionate

Ref: A.K. Khurana, 6th ed. pg. 112

ACANTHAMOEBA KERATITIS

- Acanthamoeba is a free lying amoeba found in soil, fresh water, well water, sea water, sewage and air.
- **Mode of infection**- direct corneal contact with any material or water contaminated with the organism. **For eg:**
  - *Contact lens wearers using home-made saline from contaiminated tap water is the commonest situation recognized for acanthamoeba infection.*
  - Other situations may be: mild trauma associated with contaminated vegetable matter, salt water diving, wind blown contaminant and hot tub use.
  - Opportunistic infection
- **Symptoms**. Very severe pain (out of proportion to the degree of inflammation), watering, photophobia, blepharospasm and blurred vision.
- **Treatment:** Specific medical treatment includes:
  - *0.1 % propamidine isothionate (brolene) drops;*
  - Neomycin drops
  - Polyhexamethylene biguanide (0.01% - 0.02% solution)
  - Chlorhexidine

83. Ans. (c) Wearing of soft contact lenses

Ref: A.K. Khurana, 6th ed. pg. 112

84. Ans. (d) All of the above

Ref: A.K. Khurana, 6th ed. pg. 82-83

GIANT PAPILLARY CONJUNCTIVITIS

- It is the inflammation of conjunctiva with formation of very large sized papillae.
- **Cause:** It is a localized allergic response to a physically rough or deposited surface (*contact lens, prosthesis, left out nylon sutures*).
- **Symptoms:** Itching, stringy discharge and reduced wearing time of contact lens or prosthetic shell.
- **Treatment:** The offending cause should be removed.
  - Disodium cromoglycate is known to relieve the symptoms and enhance the rate of resolution.

Explanations

FMGE Solutions Screening Examination

85. Ans. (b) Contact lens

Please refer to previous explanation.

86. Ans. (b) Gaint papillary conjunctivitis

Ref: A.K. Khurana, 6th ed. pg. 82-83

Please refer to above explanation

> **Extra Mile**
>
> **Inclusion Conjuntivitis**
> - Caused by Chlamydia trachomatis D–K within 5–14 days of birth. Clinical features include mucoid/mucopurulent discharge, redness in conjunctiva, swollen lids and pain in eyeballs.
>
> **Follicular conjunctivitis**
> - It is characterized by redness in conjunctiva, formation of follicles and discharge from the eyes. It is of following types:
>   - **Epidemic keratoconjunctivitis:** Adenovirus 8, 19; can cause "acute pseudomembranous conjunctivitis" in severe infection.
>   - **Pharyngo-conjunctival fever:** Caused by adenovirus.
>   - **Herpetic conjunctivitis:** Caused by HSV1 (more commonly) and HSV 2 (less commonly)

87. Ans. (d) Pseudomonas

Ref: A.K. Khurana, 6th ed. pg. 98

PSEUDOMONAS
- Pseudomonas is the commonest organism affecting long term use of contact lens followed by acanthameoba. SIGNS suggesting the former infection: presence of ring shaped ulcer, lack of vascularization, pain out of proportion, pseudodendritis.

PNEUMOCOCCUS
- The commonest cause of corneal ulcer in India is Streptococcus Pneumonia (causes central corneal ulcer) whereas the commonest cause in the world is staphylococcus aureus (causes peripheral corneal ulcer).
- The bacterial ulcer can present with the formation of a hypopyon (sterile).
- The characteristic hypopyon corneal ulcer is due to pneumococcus and is called **ulcus serpens**.
- **Treatment:** Topical gentamicin/tobramycin and cephalozin with cycloplegics (atropine ointment or drops) and analgesics.

88. Ans. (a) Fungal corneal ulcer

Ref: A.K. Khurana 6th ed./106, Khurana 4th ed./100

- Fungal corneal ulcer aka fungal keratitis is most commonly caused by **Aspergillus fusarium**. Patient in this condition presents with history of trauma with vegetative matter.
- Symptoms shown by patients here are milder than signs. Signs are dry looking, greyish white corneal ulcers with feather finger like extensions (due to hypae)

Signs of Fungal Keratitis:
- **Satellite nodule** (satellite lesion present around ulcer)
- **Large organized hypopion** (non-sterile)
- **Immune ring of pessary**

Predisposing factors- topical steroids, organic matter. Worst prognosis.

Treatment: 5% natamycin or .2%fluconazole for 6-8 weeks.

89. Ans. (c) Fungal ulcer

Ref: A.K. Khurana, 6th ed. pg. 106, Khurana, 4th ed. pg. 100

Please refer to above explanation

90. Ans. (a) Azithromycin

Ref: A.K. Khurana, 6th ed. pg. 65-66

- Trachoma is caused by C. Trachomatis.
- I.P.- 5-12 days
- SAFE strategy used for control of trachoma
  - S: Surgery
  - A: Antibiotic
  - F: Face wash
  - E: Environment
- DOC for Trachoma: Azithromycin > tetracycline

91. Ans. (d) Upper palpebral conjunctiva

Ref: A.K. Khurana, 6th ed. pg. 69

- Conjuctival scarring seen in **trachoma** as irregular stellate shaped scars over sulcus subtarsalis is called Arlt's line.
- It is seen in upper palpebral conjunctiva.

92. Ans. (a) Limbus

Ref: A.K. Khurana, 6th ed. pg. 69-70; Parson's 21st ed. pg. 173

- Herbert pits are oval or circular scar which is left after healing of Herbert pit in the limbus area.

Other Signs of Trachoma:
- Conjunctival scarring (Arlt's line)
- **Sago grain** follicles/Bulbar follicles (*pathognomonic*)

93. Ans. (b) Adeno virus

Ref: AK Khurana, 6th ed. pg. 73-74

- Adenovirus is considered as most common cause of swimming pool conjunctivitis.
- Chlorine is unable to eliminate the virus, hence it can often present as an outbreak.

Disease	Causative agent
Swimming pool conjunctivitis	Adenovirus
Swimming pool granuloma	Mycobacterium marinum
Swimmer's itch	Schistosoma mansoni S. japonicum

Ophthalmology

94. Ans. (a) Vernal keratoconjunctivitis

Ref: A.K. Khurana, 6th ed. pg. 79

CONJUNCTIVITIS

- The inflammation of the conjunctiva is characterized by redness associated with watery or mucopurulent discharge.

VERNAL KERATO-CONJUNCTIVITIS OR SPRING CATARRH

- It is a recurrent, bilateral, interstitial, self limiting, allergic inflammation of the conjunctiva seen in children usually in summer months.
- **Etiology:** It is considered a hypersensitivity reaction to some exogenous allergen such as grass pollen etc.
- **Clinical features:** Characterized by marked burning and itching sensation which is usually in tolerable.
  - Lacrimation.
  - Stringly (**ropy**) discharge.
  - Usually upper tarsal conjunctiva of both eyes are involved.
  - Lesion are characterized as **"cobble-stone"** or "pavement stone" fashion.
  - **Horner Tranta's spots:** Presence of discrete whitish raised dots along the limbus.
- **Treatment**
  - Mast Cell Stabilizers (Olopatadine)
  - Sodium Chromoglycate

Simple allergic conjunctivitis: Non specific allergic rhinitis associated with hay fever or seasonal/perennial allergic conjunctivitis.

GIANT PAPILLARY CONJUNCTIVITIS

- Conjunctivitis with formation of large sized papillae in upper tarsal conjunctiva due to localized allergy
- Against contact lens /nylon sutures/prosthesis.
- **Treatment:** Removal of offending agent
  - Mast Cell Stabilizers
- **Acute hemorrhagic conjunctivitis:** It is also called Apollo conjunctivitis. It is caused by picornavirus (enterovirus type 70).

> **Extra Mile**

Discharge	Etiological Agent
• Purulent/ mucopurulent	• Bacterial conjunctivitis
• Watery	• Viral conjunctivitis
• Ropy	• Allergic conjunctivitis
• Mucopurulent	• Chlamydial conjuntivitis

95. Ans. (a) Olopatadine drops

Ref: A.K. Khurana, 6th ed. pg. 79-80

Please refer to above explanation

96. Ans. (d) Trachoma

Ref: A.K. Khurana, 6th ed. pg. 61, 65

Trachoma: is a chronic keratoconjunctivitis, primarily affecting the superficial epithelium of conjunctiva and cornea simultaneously.

- It is one of the leading causes of preventable blindness in the world.

Etiology

- **Causative organism:** Caused by Chlamydia trachomatis.
- The organism is epitheliotropic and produces intra-cytoplasmic inclusion bodies called H.P. bodies.
- There are 11 identified serotypes of Chlamydia: A, B, Ba, C, D, E, F, G, H, J and K
- *Serotypes A, B, Ba and C are associated with hyperendemic (blinding) trachoma*
- *Serotypes D-K are associated with paratrachoma.*

OPHTHALMIA NEONATORUM

- Bilateral inflammation of the conjunctiva occurring in an infant, less than 30 days old.

Source and Mode of Infection

- **Before birth:** Very rare; through infected amniotic fluid in case of ruptured membranes.
- **During Birth:** Most common mode of infection; from infected birth canal when the child is born with face presentation or with forceps.
- **After birth:** Infection during first bath of newborn or from infected clothes or hands.

Causative Agents

- **Chemical conjunctivitis:** Silver nitrate or antibiotics used for prophylaxis.
- **Gonococcal infection**
- **Neonatal inclusion conjuncitivitis** *caused by serotypes D to K of Chlamydia trachomatis* is the commonest cause of ophthalmia neonatorum.

97. Ans. (d) Veneral conjunctivitis

Ref: A.K. Khurana, 6th ed. pg. 79-80

Please refer to above explanation

98. Ans. (b) Pinguecula

Ref: A.K. Khurana, 6th ed. pg. 86

PINGUECULA

- Conjunctival fatty degeneration near limbus. It is bilateral condition, **affects more commonly nasal side** followed by involvement of the temporal side. No treatment required.
- Totally benign.

FMGE Solutions Screening Examination

PTERYGIUM
- Triangular invasion of conjunctiva upon the cornea. It is commoner in dry heat, sun exposure and abundant dust. Iron deposition in the corneal epithelium at the advancing head of the pterygium is called STOCKER LINE. Usually asymptomatic.
- **Treatment:** Surgical excision. The commonest problem after excision is recurrence which is reduced by postoperative use of mitomycin C/thiotepa or by doing surgical excision with free conjunctival graft from same/other eye.

CHALAZION
- Chronic granulomatous inflammation of Meibomian Gland. No pain.
- **Treatment:** Incision and drainage

HORDEOLUM
- **External hordeolum/ STYE**- Staphlococcus infection of Zeiss gland.
    - **Treatment**
        - Topical antibiotics.
        - Hot fomentation.
- **Internal hordeolum**-Acute Staphlococcus infection of Meibomian gland. Extremely painful.
    - **Treatment :** Incision and Drainage.

99. Ans. (c) Bulge in limbal area lined by root of iris

Ref: A.K. Khurana, 6th ed. pg. 144

- **Intercalary staphyloma** is a localized ectasia of limbal tissue lined by the root of iris.
- **Cause:** perforating injury of the peripheral cornea or perforation of marginal corneal ulcer.

> **Extra Mile**
> - **Anterior staphyloma:** Formation of pseudo cornea after perforation of a large sloughing corneal ulcer.
> - **Ciliary staphyloma:** Incarceration of ciliary body and is **arises due to complication of scleritis.**
> - **Equatorial staphyloma:** The ectasia of the sclera of equatorial region with incarceration of the choroid is known as equatorial staphyloma.
> - **Posterior staphyloma** is an ectasia of the sclera at the posterior pole which is lined by the choroid.

100. Ans. (d) Scleritis

Ref: A.K. Khurana, 6th ed. pg. 144

101. Ans. (d) Degenerative myopia

Ref: A.K. Khurana, 6th ed. pg. 144
- Posterior staphyloma is seen in conditions like pathological myopia, posterior scleritis and perforating injuries.

Important Features Associated with Myopia
- **Simple/developmental myopia is the commonest type of myopia.**
- Foster fucks flecks is the choroidal haemorrhage in the macular region.
- Lacquer cracks are breaks in the bruchs membrane
- **Retinal detachment** is the **most serious complication** of myopia.

102. Ans. (b) Rheumatoid arthritis

Ref: A.K. Khurana, 6th ed. pg. 141, Khurana, 4th ed. pg. 129
- Scleritis is chronic inflammation of the sclera. Most commonly seen in elderly females (40-70 years).
- Scleritis is associated with autoimmune collagen disorders, **most commonly with rheumatoid arthritis.**
- Other causes can be PAN, SLE, ankylosis spondylitis, Wegener's granulomatosis, thyrotoxicosis, TB, syphillis.

103. Ans. (c) Aqueous deficiency

Ref: A.K. Khurana, 6th ed. pg. 389

Tear Film Consists of 3 Layers:
- **Lipid layer**-Outermost layer. Secreted by Meibomian, Zeiss and Moll gland
- **Aqueous layer**-intermediate layer. Forms bulk of tear. Secreted by lacrimal gland
- **Mucous/Mucin layer:** Innermost layer. Secreted by conjunctival goblet cells

KERATOCONJUNCTIVITIS SICCA
- It is the disease entity most commonly seen due to aqueous tear deficiency.
- Causes can be: Sjogren syndrome, hyposecretion, congenital alacrimia. Decreased secretion or lack of secretion from other tear glands also contribute to this condition.
- **Symptoms of keratoconjunctivitis sicca:** Foreign body sensation, photophobia. Test is done by wetting of a filter paper (Schirmer strip test)

> **Extra Mile**
> **Mucin layer deficiency** can lead to xerophthalmia, conjunctival scarring. Can be seen in SJS, chemical burns, trachoma.

RETINA AND UVEAL TRACT

104. Ans. (c) Anterior uveitis

Ref: Comprehensive Ophthalmology by A.K Khurana 6th ed. P 167

UVEITIS IN SARCOIDOSIS

- Sarcoidosis is one of the chronic granulomatous disease that can cause non-infective uveitis
- **MC age group:** 20–50 years; F > M
- **Associated feature:** Bilateral hilar lymphadenopathy, pulmonary infiltration, skin and ocular lesions
- 20–50% of sarcoidosis patients present with ocular lesions like:
- **Sarcoid uveitis:** Can cause anterior, posterior or intermediate panuveitis
  - **Anterior uveitis:** Large mutton fat KP, busaca nodule, anterior chamber cells and flare
  - **Intermediate uveitis:** Characterized by snow balls and snow banking
  - **Posterior uveitis:** Present with cystoid macular edema, periphlebitis reinae with sheathing, appearing as candle wax dripping, peripheral multifocal chorioretinitis characterised by small, punched out atrophic spots *(it is highly suggestive of sarcoidosis)*.
- **Uveoparotid fever:** Aka Heerfordt's syndrome:
  - Characterized by bilateral granulomatous paniuveitis with painful enlargement of parotid gland, rash, fever and cranial nerve palsies.

DIAGNOSIS:

- Abnormal Chest X-ray (in 90% cases)
- Kveim test: +ve
- Serum ACE level

Treatment: Steroids

105. Ans. (b) Central retinal artery occlusion

Ref: Walsh and Hoyt; Vol. 3, P 3370

- **Central retinal artery occlusion (CRAO):** Presents with sudden painless loss of vision. Causes are:
  - **Artery occlusion by the Emboli:** It is most common cause.
  - **Other causes:** Giant cell arteritis, SLE, scleroderma.
  - Fundus appears milky white because of retinal edema. There is cherry red spot. Due to embolus the blood column within the retina is segmented and is known as cattle tracking.
- **Central retinal vein occlusion (CRVO):** Its incidence is more common than CRAO. Causes are:
  - Hypertension, diabetes mellitus, atherosclerosis.
  - **Upon examination:** Tortuous and engorged veins, disc edema, soft exudate and evidence of rubeosis iridis (new vessel on iris)
- **Central serous retinopathy (CSR):** It is due to accumulation of transparent fluid at the posterior pole specially macula causing a circumscribed area of retinal detachment in the macular region. Causes are:
  - Raised aldosterone level usually among type A personalities
  - Cushing syndrome, idiopathic. Fluorescein angiography shows ink blot pattern and smoke stack pattern.
- **Diabetic retinopathy:** It is of 2 types:
  - **Nonproliferative diabetic retinopathy (NPDR):** Findings/changes in NPDR are:
    - **Microaneurysm:** Earliest change
    - Retinal hemorrhage
    - Hard and soft exudates.
  - **Proliferative diabetic retinopathy (PDR):** Findings/changes in PDR are:
    - **Neovascularization:** Hallmark
    - Vitreous hemorrhage, and
    - Retinal detachment.

106. Ans. (b) 1.5 mm

Ref: Comprehensive Ophthalmology by Khurana 6/ed. P 6

- The average optic disc is 1500 microns (or 1.5 millimeters) in size where optic nerve enters into the back of the eye.
  - Small optic disc is said when vertical diameter of optic disc is <1.5 mm
  - Large disc is said when size of vertical diameter is >2.2 mm.
- Length of optic nerve is 47–50 mm and has 4 parts:
  - **Intraocular:** 1 mm
  - **Intraorbital:** 30 mm
  - **Intracanalicular:** 6–9 mm
  - **Intracranial:** 10 mm

107. Ans. (b) Corneal endothelium

Ref: Comprehensive Ophthalmology by Khurana 6/ed. P 34

- Keratic precipitate (KP) is deposition of protein on the corneal endothelium in patients with anterior uveitis.
- This KP is deposited in a triangular fashion, known as Arlt's triangle.
- In some chronic granulomatous diseases like sarcoidosis, leprosy, TB, there is deposition of special KP's known as mutton fat KP.

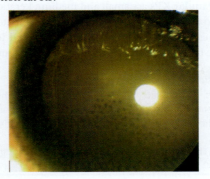

FMGE Solutions Screening Examination

108. Ans. (a) 1–5

Ref: Harrison 19th ed. P 2424

- **Poor sugar control** (glycosylated hemoglobin > 7%) leads to development of diabetic retinopathy within 5 years in type 1 diabetes mellitus and over 15–20 years in type 2 diabetes mellitus.
- Diabetics have *25 times* higher chances of blindness as compared to nondiabetics.

Extra Mile

- Most common cause of *visual loss* in a diabetic is macular edema.
- Best method to *detect visual loss* is FFA or optical coherence tomography.
- Most common cause of blindness in diabetic is retinal detachment.
- Diabetic retinopathy and nephropathy progress over same duration and *always co-exist*.
- Best *predictor for development of retinopathy* is duration of diabetes.

109. Ans. (a) Cycloplegics

Ref: Khurana, 6th ed. pg. 159-60

- **DOC for acute anterior uveitis:** Topical glucocorticoids
- **1st line agent for immediate management of acute uveitis:** Cycloplegics
- **Khurana states:** *"Cycloplegics are very useful and most effective during acute phase of iridocyclitis"*
- Commonly used drug is 1% atropine sulphate eye ointment or drops to be instilled 2-3 times a day.
- **Mechanism of action:**
  - Relieves spasm of iris sphincter and ciliary body, which gives immediate relief and comfort from pain.
  - Prevents synechiae formation and breaks them as well.
  - Decreases hyperemia which reduces exudation.
  - Increases blood supply to anterior uvea by relieving pressure on anterior ciliary artery, which adds to more absorption of toxin.

110. Ans. (a) Nongranulomatous uveitis

Ref: Khurana, 6th ed. pg. 154

- **Granular KPs** are small and medium keratic precipitate, and are pathognomonic of non-granulomatous uveitis.
- These are small, dirty white KP arranged irregularly at the back of cornea and are usually numerous.

Extra Mile

- **Fine KP:** Aka stellate KP. They usually cover whole corneal endothelium and form endothelial dusting. They are seen in: Fuch's heterochromic iridocyclitis, Herpetic iritis and CMV retinitis.
- **Old KP:** They are irregular in shape and this is a sign of healed uveitis.

111. Ans. (a) Granulomatous uveitis

Ref: Khurana, 6th ed. pg. 154

- **Mutton fat keratic precipitates** are typically seen in granulomatous uveitis. These are composed of epithelioid cells and macrophages.
- These are large, thick, fluffy, lardaceous KP having waxy or greasy appearance. They are usually 10-15 in number

112. Ans. (c) Reiter syndrome

Ref: Khurana, 6th ed. pg. 168

- **Reiter syndrome** is characterized by triad of: Urethritis, arthritis and conjunctivitis with or without iridocyclitis.
- It mostly affects males who are positive for HLA B27.

113. Ans. (b) Hyperoxia

Ref: Khurana, 6th ed. pg. 283

- Retinopathy of prematurity (ROP), *(earlier known as retrolental fibroplasia)* is a bilateral proliferative retinopathy occurring in premature infants with low birth weight who often have been exposed to high concentration of oxygen.
- **Risk factors:**
  - Low gestation age <32 weeks
  - Low birth weight <1500 gm
  - Supplemental oxygen therapy
  - Vitamin E deficiency in mothers, respiratory distress syndrome, asphyxia, shock etc.

114. Ans. (b) Periphery of pupil

Ref: A.K Khurana's Ophthalmology, 6th ed. pg. 153

- Granulamotous uveitis is characterized by infiltration with lymphocytes, plasma cells and mobilization and proliferation of large mononuclear cells → collectively known as iris nodule
- Iris nodule is a feature of granulomatous uveitis.
- If formed near pupillary border: **Koeppe's nodule**
- If formed near collarette: **Busaca nodule**
- If deposited at the back of cornea: Keratic precipitates

115. Ans. (c) Sensory and pigmentary layer

Ref: A.K. Khurana, 6th ed. pg. 299

- Retina has 10 layers.
- Inner 9 layers are known as neurosensory layer and outer one layer is known as pigmentary layer.
- *Retinal detachment is defined as separation of neurosensory layer of retina from pigmentary retinal layer.*

116. Ans. (a) X linked

Ref: A.K. Khurana, 6th ed. pg. 287

INVERSE RETINITIS PIGMENTOSA

- Inverse RP is a degeneration of the nerve cells in the macula, which is located in the center of the retina.

Ophthalmology

Inverse or central RP is characterized by a bilateral and often symmetrical loss of cone function in the presence of a reduced rod function. Individuals with macular degeneration secondary to a central vision loss experience difficulty reading, recognizing faces, shapes and contours of objects or things.

- This is a general term for a disparate group of rod-cone dystrophies characterized by progressive **night blindness,** visual field constriction with a **ring scotoma/ tubular vision**, **loss of acuity**, **waxy pallow optic disc,** and an abnormal electroretinogram (ERG).
- It occurs sporadically or in an autosomal recessive, dominant, or **X-linked pattern.**
- **MC inheritance pattern: Autosomal Recessive**
- Irregular black **deposits of clumped pigment in the peripheral retina,** called *bone spicules* because of their vague resemblance to the spicules of cancellous bone, give the disease its name.
- **No definite treatment. However, Vitamin A can slow down the progression.**

117. Ans. (c) Central scotoma

Ref: A.K. Khurana, 6th ed. pg. 233, 287-88

Central scotoma is a feature of open angle glaucoma.

All other choices are considered as triad of retinitis pigmentosa (Bony spicule on retina, waxy pallor disc, Ring scotoma)

Visual field abnormalities in glaucoma are initially observed on kinetic perimetry are as follows

- **Relative paracentral scotoma:** These are areas where smaller or dimmer targets are not visualized by the patient, but larger or brighter targets are appreciated.
- **Bjerrum's Scotoma:** Extension of the blind spot in the shape of an arc in the central bjerrum's area.
- **Siedel scotoma:** One that appears to start at the poles of the blind spot and arches over the macular area, without reaching the horizontal meridian nasally.
- **Arcuate scotoma:** Also appear to start at the superior or inferior poles of the blind spot and arch over the macular area, widening as they curve down or up to end as a horizontal line nasally, which never crosses the horizontal divide of the visual field.
- **Double arcuate or ring scotoma:** Advanced glaucomatous field defects - only central and temporal islands of vision are left when two arcuate scotomas expand to involve the peripheral visual field
- **Nasal step:** The appearance of a horizontal shelf in the nasal visual field is caused by an asymmetry in the nerve fiber loss at the two poles.
- **End-stage or near-total field defect** with only a residual temporal island of vision, occurs at the last stage, sparing of blind spot.

118. Ans. (c) Tractional retinal detachment not involving the macula

Ref: A.K. Khurana, 6th ed. pg. 276-77

- Diabetic retinopathy leads to tractional retinal detachment, which presents with slowly progressive loss of vision.
- There is no photopsia or floaters unless macula is involved because the vitreo-retinal traction develops very slowly.

119. Ans. (a) Microaneurysms

Ref: A.K. Khurana, 6th ed. pg. 276-77

DIABETIC RETINOPATHY

- The retinal change seen in diabetes are called as diabetic retinopathy. In diabetes, there is pericytes necrosis. Normally ratio 1 pericytes: 1 endothelial cell. But in diabetic retinopathy 1 pericyte: 3 endothelial cell. The vessels wall is weakened and leakage occurs. Classification–
  - Non proliferative diabetic retinopathy
  - Proliferative diabetic retinopathy

Non proliferative diabetic retinopathy (NPDR)	Proliferative diabetic retinopathy (POR)
• **Microaneurysms-** early manifestation • Dot and Blot hemorrhages • Hard exudates • Soft exudates	• Neovascularization of the disc • Neovascularization of anywhere else from the disc • Neovascularization of iris-RUBIOSSIS IRIDIS

120. Ans. (d) Iris neovascularization

Ref: A.K. Khurana, 6th ed. pg. 250-51

- Neovascular glaucoma results from the formation of a neovacular membane involving the anterior chamber secondary to diffuse retinal hypoxia. There is release of factors like vascular endothelial growth factor (VEGF) from the vitreous which causes formation of abnormal new blood vessels over the iris. The fibrovascular membrane then progressively closes the angle of the anterior chamber.
- It is usually associated with **neovascularisation of the iris (rubeosis iridis).**

121. Ans. (b) 5FU

Ref: A.K. Khurana, 6th ed. pg. 251-52

- Anti-VEGF are class of drugs which are used for treatment of diabetic retinopathy with neovascularization (proliferative diabetic retinopathy-PDR).
- Available anti-VEGF are: Ranibizumab, Bevacizumab, Pegaptanib.

Note: *TOC for PDR- Laser photocoagulation*

122. Ans. (c) Vitreous hemorrhage

Ref: A.K. Khurana, 6th ed. pg. 260-61

- Vitreous haemorrhage usually occurs from the retinal vessels and may present as pre-retinal or an intragel haemorrhage.

CAUSES

Causes of Vitreous Haemorrhage are as Follows:
- **Spontaneous** vitreous haemorrhage from retinal breaks especially those associated with PVD.
- **Trauma to eye:** Blunt or perforating
- **Inflammatory diseases** such as chorioretinitis and periphlebitis
- **Vascular disorders** e.g., hypertensive retinopathy, and centreal retinal vein occlusion.
- **Metabolic diseases** as diabetic retinopathy.
- **Blood dyscrasias** eg: Retinopathy of anaemia, leukaemias, polycythemias sickle-cell
- **Neoplasms**

Clinical Features
- **Symptoms**: Sudden development of floaters occurs when the vitreous haemorrhage is small.
  - In massive vitreous haemorrhage, sudden painless loss of vision.
- **Signs**
  - Distant direct ophthalmoscopy reveals black shadows against the red glow in small haemorrhages and no red glow in a large haemorrhage.
  - Direct and indirect ophthalmoscopy may show presence of blood in the vitreious cavity.
  - Ultrasonography with b-scan is particularly helpful in diagnosing vitreous haemorrhage.

123. Ans. (a) Vitreous haemorrhage

Ref: A.K. Khurana, 6th ed. pg. 260-61

Causes of Painless and Painful Loss of Vision

Sudden painless loss of vision	Sudden painful loss of vision
• Vascular occlusion (CRAO, CRVO) • *Retinal detachment* • **Vitreous hemorrhage** • Ischemic optic neuropathy	• Acute iridocyclitis • Chemical injuries • Mechanical injuries • Acute congestive glaucoma • Optic neuritis
Gradual painless loss of vision	**Gradual painful loss of vision**
• Progressive pterygeum involving the pupil • Corneal degeneration • Corneal dystrophy • Developmental cataracts • Senile cataracts • Optic atrophy • Chorioretinal degeneration • Age- related macular degeneration • *Diabetic retinopathy* • Refractive errors • Papilloedema and Papillitis	• Chronic iridocyclitis • Corneal ulceration • Chronic simple glaucoma

124. Ans. (d) Trauma

Ref: A.K. Khurana, 6th ed. pg. 260-61

- Vitreous hemorrhage is defined as the presence of extravasated blood within the space outlined by the zonular fibers and posterior lens capsule anteriorly, the nonpigmented epithelium of the ciliary body laterally, and the internal limiting membrane of the retina (lamina limitans interna) posteriorly and posterolaterally.
- **The 3 most common causes of vitreous hemorrhage are proliferative diabetic retinopathy,** posterior vitreous detachment (PVD) with or without retinal tears, and ocular trauma (eg, shaken baby syndrome).
  - Any cause of peripheral neovascularization may result in vitreous hemorrhage, **but trauma is the leading cause of vitreous hemorrhage in young people**.

The most common cause found in adults is diabetic retinopathy
MCC of recurrent vitrous hemorrhage in young adult: Eale's disease

125. Ans. (b) Exudative retinal detachment

Ref: A.K. Khurana, 6th ed. pg. 273

Please refer to above table.

RETINAL DETACHMENT

- Retinal detachment is the separation of neurosensory retina from the retinal pigmentary epithelium by subretinal fluid. Depending on the mechanism of subretinal fluid accumulation retinal detachment are of following types:
  - Exudative retinal detachment
  - Tractional retinal detachment
  - Rhegmatogenous retinal detachment

Exudative retinal detachment: Lesions of retinal pigment epithelium. **Commonest causes are:**
- **Malignant melanoma of choroid**
- *Followed by pregnancy induce hypertension, 140/90 after 20th week of gestation.*
- Malignant hypertension 200/120 end stage hypertension.

TRACTIONAL RETINAL DETACHMENT

- Caused by mechanical traction (progressive contraction) of fibrovascular membranes over large areas of vitreoretinal adhesion. *Characterized by slow painless loss of vision* (only retinal detachment that is slow). Causes are:
  - *Most common cause is diabetes mellitus*
  - Retinopathy of pregnancy
  - Sickle cell anemia

RHEGMATOGENOUS RETINAL DETACHMENT

- Characterized by the presence of retinal break held open by vitreo retinal traction that allows accumulation of liquefied vitreous (syneresis) under neurosensory retina, separating it from retinal pigment epithelium.

Ophthalmology

1099

- The predisposing conditions of **rhegmatogenous retinal detachment** are **Myopia**, previous intraocular surgery such as **aphakia** or pseudophakia, a family history of retinal detachment, **trauma** and inflammation.

VITREOUS HEMORRHAGE

- Vitreous hemorrhage is not a (clinical) feature of retinal detachment. *Characterised by sudden painless loss of vision; floaters, no flashing of light.* **Causes are:**
  - **Diabetic retinopathy: most common cause**
  - In young patient most common cause is Trauma and Eale's disease.

---

126. Ans. (a) Exudative retinal detachment

> *Ref: A.K. Khurana, 6th ed. pg. 273, 299*

---

127. Ans. (b) Diabetic retinopathy

> *Ref: A.K. Khurana, 6th ed. pg. 273, 299; Parson's Ophthalmology 20/312*

---

128. Ans. (d) CRVO

> *Ref: A.K. Khurana, 6th ed. pg. 269, 431*

Cherry Red Spot of Retina is seen in—

- CRAO
- Trauma (Blunt trauma, Berlin's edema)
- Neimann pick disease
- Gaucher's disease
- Tay – Sach's disease
- Sand hoff's disease

Mnemonic: Cherry Tree Never Grow Tall in Sand.

---

129. Ans. (c) Central retinal vein occlusion

> *Ref: A.K. Khurana, 6th ed. pg. 214, 271, 294*

CYSTOID MACULAR EDEMA (CME)

- Collection of fluid in the **outer plexiform (Henle's layer) a nuclear layer** of the retina is called CME.
- It is associated with Central Retinal Vein Occlusion/ post operative complication of cataract extraction and penetrating keratoplasty/ diabetic retinopathy/ Retinitis pigmentosa
- Minimal to moderate loss of vision is seen.
- It is **best examined with slit lamp/+90D** lens
- Ophthalmoscopy shows **"honeycomb appearance"** of macula.
- Fundus fluorescein angiography shows **"flowerpetal appearance".**
- Treatment of underlying primary cause and drugs (topical steroids triamcinofone/ topical NSAIDs like flurbiprofen) is beneficial.

Extra Mile

- **100 day glaucoma'** is seen with CRVO
- **CATTLE TRUCK** appearance seen with CRAO
- IRVIN GASS SYNDROME is seen with post cataract CME

---

130. Ans. (a) Sarcoidosis

SARCOIDOSIS

- Sarcoidosis is a granulomatous disease of unknown etiology.
- It occurs most frequently in young adults (20 to 40 years), has a predilection for women.
- Around 20% patients with sarcoidosis has ocular involvement.
- **The most prevalent ocular sign** is unilateral, anterior, granulomatous uveitis.
- The common clinical ocular findings associated with sarcoid uveitis include:
  - Decreased or hazy vision, pain, photophobia, lacrimation, conjunctival injection, cells and flare in the anterior chamber, granulomatous iritis with large *"mutton fat"* keratic precipitates scattered over the back surface of the corneal endothelium, iritis spill over leading to anterior vitritis, true vitritis with white exudative debris in the region of the ora serrata (snowball or snowbank retinopathy) with retinal vasculitis *(candle wax drippings)* and phlebitis (venous sheathing).

AMYLOIDOSIS

- **Orbit/adnexal:** Include ptosis, keratoconjunctivitis sicca, proptosis, ocular motility disturbances, palpable mass lesions and pupillary abnormalities. Pain uncommonly accompanies orbital amyloidosis, and its presence should prompt the examiner to consider alternative diagnosis.
- **Conjunctiva:** Ptosis, a visible or palpable mass, and recurrent subconjunctival hemorrhage are commonly reported symptoms.
- **Anterior chamber/iris:** A "scalloped" configuration of the iris margin may signify amyloid deposition in the iris stroma or, alternatively, disruption of the parasympathetic innervation of the iris sphincter. Anterior chamber involvement appears as whitish, flocculent debris in the aqueous, on the lens capsule or on the iris surface.
- **Lens:** Pseudopodia lentis, punctate dots on the posterior capsule resembling ameboid foot processes, are considered pathognomonic of vitreoretinal amyloidosis in patients with heredofamilial disease.
- **Vitreous/retina:** Vitreoretinal amyloidosis manifests as **"lacy," "cobweb-like," "sheet-like" or "stringy"** veils of gray or yellowish-white material in the vitreous. Symptoms include floaters, blurry vision or glare, or patients may be asymptomatic.

Explanations

FMGE Solutions Screening Examination

- **Diagnosis:** Congo red staining demonstrating apple-green birefringence when viewed through crossed polarimetric filters remains the gold standard for establishing the diagnosis of amyloidosis.
- **Treatment:** Surgical excision or debulking remains the treatment of choice.

131. Ans. (a) Pars planitis

Ref: A.K. Khurana, 6th ed. pg. 150-51

INTERMEDIATE UVEITIS (PARS PLANITIS)

- It denotes inflammation of pars plana part of ciliary body and most peripheral part of the retina.
- **Etiology:** It is an idiopathic disease usually affecting both eyes (80 percent) of children and young adults.

Clinical Features

- **Symptoms:** Most of the patients present with history of floaters.
- **Signs:** The eye is usually quiet.
  - Slit-lamp examination may show: mild aqueous flare, and fine KPs at the back of cornea.
  - Fundus examination with indirect ophthalmoscope reveals the whitish exudates in the inferior quadrant present near the ora serrata.
  - These typical exudates are referred as *snow ball opacities*. These may coalesce to form a grey white plaque called *snow banking*.

Extra Mile

TABLE: Comparison of Anterior, Intermediate and Posterior Uveitis

	Anterior	Intermediate	Posterior
Aka	Iridocyclitis	Pars Planitis	Chorioretinitis
Cause	Idiopathic	Idiopathic	Toxoplasmosis
Clin. Feature	Sudden painless loss of vision	Floaters	Sudden painless loss of vision
Cells	WBC's **Keratic precipitate**	**Snowballs/ snowbanks**	**Headlight in fog appearance**
Treatment	Topical steroids-DOC Cycloplegics	Inj: Triamcinilone	Antimicrobials Systemic steroids

132. Ans. (c) 7–10 days

Ref: A.K. Khurana, 6th ed. pg. 573, Khurana, 4th ed. pg. 146

TABLE: Cycloplegics and its duration of action

Drug	Duration of Effect (days)
Atropine	7–10
Scopolamine	3–7

Contd...

Drug	Duration of Effect (days)
Homatropine	1–3
Cyclopentolate	1
Tropicamide	days (6 hrs)

133. Ans. (a) Pilocarpine

Ref: A.K. Khurana, 6th ed. pg. 159-50, Khurana's, 4th ed. pg. 146, 47

- **DOC for acute anterior uveitis:** Topical glucocorticoids
- **1st line agent:** Cycloplegics
- In case of uveitis, there is spasm of ciliary muscle and constriction of pupil (miosis). Pilocarpine is a parasympathomimetic agent, which causes further spasm of ciliary muscles and miosis.
- **Note:** *In case of anterior uveitis, there is irregular constriction of pupil called, festooned pupil.*

134. Ans. (c) Pilocarpine eye drops

Ref: A.K. Khurana, 6th ed. pg. 159-60

135. Ans. (a) Secondary glaucoma

Ref: A.K. Khurana, 6th ed. pg. 157

Complications of Anterior Uveitis:

- *Secondary glaucoma (most common)*
- Band shaped keratopathy: More common in children with JRA
- Anterior & posterior synechiae
- Seclusio occlusio pupillae
- *Complicated cataract*
- Pseudoglioma due to vitreous exudation
- *Cystoid macular oedema* is common cause of visual impairment
- Pthisis & atrophic bulbi
- Tractional retinal detachment

Extra Mile

- Retinal detachment is a rare and late complication of anterior uveitis
- It is more common in pars-planitis and posterior uveitis).

EYELID AND LACRIMAL APPARATUS

136. Ans. (b) Middle meatus

Ref: Comprehensive Ophthalmology by A.K Khurana 6th ed. P 396

- **Dacryocystorhinostomy** (DCR) is a surgical procedure of choice in patients with dacryocystitis (inflammation of lacrimal sac)

Ophthalmology

- It is done by creating a new drainage of tear into nose, which opens in middle meatus.
  - **Remember:** Normally nasolacrimal duct opens into inferior meatus.
- The medial wall of lacrimal sac is anastomosed with middle meatus of nose → overcoming the obstruction at the junction of lacrimal sac and nasolacrimal duct.
- Performed in patients below 60 years.

Extra Mile

- **Dacryocystectomy (DCT):** used only when DCR is contraindicated or when the patient is too young (<4 years) or too old (>60 years) or in cases of chronic granulomatous disease induced obstruction like syphilis, TB, leprosy.
- **Conjunctivodacryocystorhinostomy (CDCR):** Done in presence of blocked canaliculi

137. Ans. (b) Meibomian gland

Ref: Yanoff Duker; 4/ed. P 1431

GLANDS OF EYE AND ITS ASSOCIATED PATHOLOGY

Gland	Associated pathology
Meibomian gland	**Internal hordeolum:** Staphylococcal infection of meibomian gland. Painful condition. Treated with I/D and antibiotics support **Chalazion:** Chronic granulomatous disease occurred due to blocked meibomian gland. Non painful condition. Treated with incision and curettage.
Zeis gland	**External hordeolum/Stye:** Staphylococcal infection of Zeis gland. Treated with topical antibiotics.

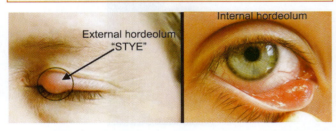

138. Ans. (c) Ankyloblepharon

Ref: A.K. Khurana, 6th ed. pg. 377

- **Symblepharon:** Lids become adherent with the eyeball as a result of adhesions between the palpebral and bulbar conjunctiva.
- **Ankyloblepharon:** Adhesions between margins of the upper and lower lids.
  - It may occur as a congenital anomaly or may result after healing of chemical burns, thermal burns, ulcers and traumatic wounds of the lid margins.

- **Blepharophimosis:** In this condition the extent of the palpebral fissure is decreased. It appears contracted at the outer canthus.
- **Lagophthalmos:** This condition is characterized by inability to voluntarily close the eyelids

139. Ans. (d) Dacrocystorhinostomy

Ref: A.K. Khurana, 6th ed. pg. 395-96

Dacrocystits is inflammation of the lacrimal sac

CHRONIC DACROCYSTITIS

- Chronic dacryocystitis is more common than the acute dacrocystitis.
- **Cause:** Vicious cycle of stasis and mild infection of long duration.
- **Factors responsible for stasis of tears in lacrimal sac:**
  - **Anatomical factors:** Narrow bony canal
  - **Foreign bodies** in the sac may block opening of NLD.
  - **Excessive lacrimation**
  - **Mild grade inflammation:** May block the NLD
  - **Obstruction of lower end of the NLD** by nasal diseses such as polyps, hypertrophied inferior concha, severe deviated nasal septum.
- **Source of infection:** It may get infected from the conjunctiva, nasal cavity (retrograde spread), or paranasal sinuses by: Staphylococci, pneumococci, streptococci and pseudomonas pyocyanea.
- **Clinical Feature**
  - **Stage of chronic catarrhal dacryocystitis:** Characterised by mild inflammation of the lacrimal sac associated with blockage of NLD.
  - **Stage of lacrimal mucocoele:** Characterized by constant epiphora associated with a swelling just below the inner canthus.
  - **Stage of chronic suppurative dacryocystitis:** Characterized by epiphora, associated recurrent conjunctivitis and swelling at the inner canthus with mild erythema.
  - **Stage of chronic fibrotic sac:** Repeated infections may result in a small fibrotic sac due to thickening of mucosa, which is associated with epiphora and discharge.
- **Treatment**
  - **Conservative treatment** by repeated lacrimal syringing.
  - *Dacryocystorhinostomy (DCR). It is considered as surgery of choice as it re-establishes the lacrimal drainage.*
  - **Dacryocystectomy (DCT).** It should be performed only when DCR is contraindicated.
  - **Conjunctivodacryocystorhinostomy (CDCR).** It is performed in the presence of blocked canaliculi.

FMGE Solutions Screening Examination

140. Ans. (a) 3rd CN palsy

Ref: A.K. Khurana, 6th ed. pg. 379

- Ptosis is drooping of eyelid.
- Eyelid is comprised of 4 muscles:

TABLE: Muscles, their innervation and function

Muscle	CN innervation	Function
LPS	III	Opens the eyelid
Muller's muscle	III	Opens eyelid when LPS tired
Frontalis	VII	Closes the eyelid
Orbicularis oculi	VII	Closes the eyelid

- CN III palsy leads to drooping of eyelid (Ptosis).
- CN VII palsy may also cause ptosis.

> **Extra Mile**
> - All the extraocular muscles are supplied by CN III except lateral rectus and superior oblique.
> - Lateral rectus supplied by- CN VI
> - Superior oblique supplied by- CN IV

Remember: LR6, SO4; all other by CN III

LENS/CATARACT

141. Ans. (b) ND:YAG laser

Ref: Comprehensive Ophthalmology by A.K Khurana 6th ed. P 462

- Lasers for glaucoma:
  - Laser iridotomy for ACG (uses ND:YAG laser)
  - Argon laser trabeculoplasty for OAG
  - Laser goniopunctures for developmental glaucoma
  - Pan retinal photocoagulation: For prophylactic/treatment of neovascular glaucoma
  - **Cyclophotocoagulation:** For absolute glaucoma or near absolute glaucoma
- Nd:YAG laser typically emits light with wavelength of **1064 nm** in the infrared
- Uses of Nd:YAG laser:
  - Correct posterior capsular opacification
  - Peripheral laser iridotomy in ACG
  - Double frequency ND:YAG (wavelength: 532 nm) used for pan-retinal photocoagulation.

> **Extra Mile**
> - **Excimer lasers** are used for photoablation—these lasers act by tissue remodelling. Used for:
>   - Photorefractive keratectomy (PRK)
>   - LASIK surgery
>   - Phototherapeutic keratectomy (PTK) for corneal diseases such as band shaped keratopathy.

TABLE: Lasers used in ophthalmology

Type of laser	Wave length (nm)	Atomic environment used	Effects produced
• Argon	514	Argon gas	Photocoagulation
• Krypton	647	Krypton gas	Photocoagulation
• Diode	840	Diode crystal	Photocoagulation
• Diode Pumped frequency doubled Nd:YAG	532	Diode and Nd:YAG crystals	Photocoagulation
• Nd: YAG	1064	A liquid dry or a solid compound of yttrium-aluminium garnet and neodymium	Photodisruption
• Excimer	193	Helium and fluorine gas	Photoablation
• Femtosecond	1053	Neodymium-glass	Photodisruption

142. Ans. (a) Blunt trauma to eye

Ref: Comprehensive Ophthalmology by A.K Khurana 6th ed. P 430

BLUNT TRAUMA TO LENS CAN PRODUCE

- **Vossius ring:** Circular ring of brown pigment at the anterior capsule. Occurs due to striking of pupillary margin against lens capsule.
- **Concussion cataract:** Mainly due to imbibition of aqueous on the lens fibres. It can assume following shapes:

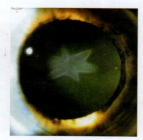

- **Discrete sub epithelial opacity:** Most commonly occurred
- **Early rosette cataract (Punctate):** Most typical form. Appears as feathery lines of opacities along the star shaped suture lines, in posterior cortex
- **Late rosette cataract:** Develops 1-2 years after injury in the posterior cortex
- Traumatic zonular cataract
- Diffuse concussion cataract

Ophthalmology

143. Ans. (a) Homocystinuria

Ref: Comprehensive Ophthalmology by A.K Khurana 6th ed. P 216

Systemic conditions associated with ectopia lentis:
- **Marfan syndrome:** MCC of hereditary ectopia lentis. AD condition. Lens displaced supero-temporally (bilaterally symmetrical)
- **Homocystinuria:** 2nd MCC of of hereditary ectopia lentis. AR condition. Lens subluxated inferior and nasally.
- **Weil Marchesani syndrome:** AR condition. Associated with mental retardation, short stature and stubby fingers. Lens subluxated anteriorly.
- **Sulphite oxidase deficiency:** AR condition. Ectopia lentis is universal ocular feature
- Hyperlysinnemia

> **Extra Mile**
> - **Simple ectopia lentis:** Superior displacement of lens
> - **Sunset syndrome:** Inferior subluxation of IOL
> - **Sunrise syndrome:** Superior subluxation of IOL
> - **Lost lens syndrome:** Complete dislocation of IOL into vitreous cavity.

144. Ans. (a) Nd:YAG
- ND-YAG (Neodymium- Yttrium-Aluminium-Garnet) laser is used for posterior capsulotomy in after cataract surgery.

145. Ans. (a) Blunt trauma
- Rosette cataract is seen in concussion injuries which appears as feathery line of opacities along the star shaped suture lines.
- In rosette cataract there is circular ring of brown pigment of pupillary margin seen on anterior capsule of lens.

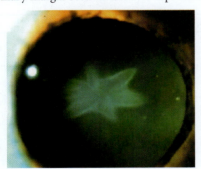

146. Ans. (c) Nuclear cataract

Ref: A.K Khurana's Ophthalmology, 6th ed. pg. 191
- Nuclear cataract can cause nuclear sclerosis, which causes deterioration of distant vision (due to progressive index myopia). These patients may be able to read without presbyopic glasses. This improvement in near vision is referred to as *"second sight"*

147. Ans. (d) Posterior-subscapular cataract due to long term use of steroids

Ref: A.K Khurana's Ophthalmology, 6th ed. pg. 194-95

148. Ans. (a) Cataract

Ref: A.K. Khurana, 6th ed. pg. 180-81, Khurana 4th ed. pg. 171, 175
- **MCC of blindness in world & India:** Cataract
- Cataract most commonly seen in females
- **2nd MCC of blindness-** Glaucoma
- **MC infective cause of blindness-** Trachoma
- **MCC of ocular morbidity-** Refractive error

149. Ans. (b) ND-YAG

Ref: A.K. Khurana, 6th ed. pg. 187-89
- ND-YAG (Neodymium- Yttrium-Aluminium-Garnet) laser is used for posterior capsulotomy in after cataract.
- Diode, Argon and Krypton laser is used for retinal photocoagulation.

150. Ans. (d) In the lens capsule

Ref: A.K. Khurana, 6th ed. pg. 186, 195-96

INTRAOCULAR LENS IMPLANTATION
- Presently, intraocular lens (IOL) implantation is the method of choice for correcting aphakia.

Types of Intraocular Lenses
- **Anterior chamber IOL:** These lenses lie in front of the iris and are supported in the angle of anterior chamber.
- ACIOL can be inserted after ICCE or ECCE *(Intra/Extra Capsular Ccataract Extraction)*.
- **Iris –supported lenses:** These lenses are fixed on the iris with the help of sutures or claws.
- **Posterior Chamber lenses:** PCIOL implanted behind the iris. They may be supported by the ciliary sulcus or capsular bag.
- **At present** the trend is *"In the Bag"* fixation.

> **Extra Mile**
>
> **Cataract Surgeries and their Main Indications**
>
> | Cataract | Surgery |
> |---|---|
> | Immature cataract | Phacoemulsification |
> | Mature/hyper mature cataract | ECCE |
> | Subluxated | ICCE |

151. Ans: (c) Opacity along sutures

Ref: A.K. Khurana, 6th ed. pg. 194-95

- **Complicated cataract**: Cataract secondary to some intraocular disease which may be:
  - **Anterior** *cortical* in anterior segmental lesion as glaucoma, acute iritis, or,
  - **Posterior cortical** in posterior segmental lesion as uveitis, RD, pigmentary retinal dystrophy.
- The second type of complicated cataract presents with posterior cortical bread crumb appearance/ polychromatic lusture or rainbow cataract.
- *Bread crumbs appearance* is Pathognomonic of posterior cataract.
- *Opacity usually commence in posterior cortex and spread axially and NOT along sutures.*
- Vision is much impaired even in early stage, owing to the position of the opacity near the nodal point of the eye.

152. Ans. (c) Vitreous movement

Ref: A.K. Khurana, 6th ed. pg. 194-95

- **Complicated cataract occurs secondary intraocular disease e.g.**
  - Inflammatory conditions as uveitis.
  - Degenerative conditions as retinitis pigmentosa, high myopia etc.
  - Intraocular tumors
  - Retinal detachment, Glaucoma etc.

Extra Mile

TABLE: Types of cataract and their causes

Type of cataract	Cause
Snow flake/snow storm cataract	Diabetes mellitus/Down's syndrome
Sunflower/Petals of flower cataract	Wilson's disease Chalcosis (mild reaction to copper) Penetrating trauma (with retention to copper)
Blue dot cortical cataract	Atopic dermatitis Myotonic dystrophy
Vossius ring/Rosette shaped cataract	Blunt trauma
Christmas tree cataract	Myotonic dystrophy
Oil drop cataract Dust like lenticular opacity	Galactosemia
Breadcrumb appearance Polychromatic lusture Rainbow cataract	Complicated cataract/Secondary cataract
Morgagnian cataract	Hypermature senile cataract

153. Ans. (a) Trauma

Ref: A.K. Khurana, 6th ed. pg. 429, Khurana, 4th ed. pg. 405

154. Ans. (c) Anterior capsule of the lens

Ref: A.K. Khurana, 6th ed. pg. 429, Parsons' Diseases of the Eye, 20th ed. pg. 367

- **Blunt trauma** to eye leads to formation of **vossius ring on anterior surface of lens**
- It is a faint or stippled opacity seen on the anterior capsule of the lens due to multitudes of brown amorphous granules of pigment lying on the capsule
- Produced by the impress of the iris on the lens as a result of a force that drives cornea and iris backwards.
- It is about the same diameter as the *contracted pupil.*

155. Ans. (a) Posterior subcapsular cataract

Ref: Levin's ophthalmology, 232

"**Posterior sub capsular cataracts** typically account for less than 10% of age related cataracts. They arise from epithelial cells that fail to differentiate properly into fiber cells. These cells migrate or are carried by their neighbors to the posterior pole of lens where they swell and form a plaque that scatters light. Because these plaques are in the **optic axis** they **significantly degrade vision** even when quite small.

156. Ans. (d) Secondary cataract

Ref: A.K. Khurana, 6th ed. pg. 214

157. Ans. (a) Phenylketonuria

Ref: A.K. Khurana, 6th ed. pg. 181-215

158. Ans. (d) Alport's syndrome

Ref: A.K. Khurana, 6th ed. pg. 218-219

- Anterior lenticonus is seen *in Alport's syndrome* (90%)
- It is a disorder of basement membrane and is characterized by:
  - *Familial haemorrhagic nephritis*
  - *Sensory-neural deafness* and
  - *Ocular features like anterior lenticonus,* cataract, retinal flecks and posterior polymorphous corneal dystrophy.

159. Ans. (b) Superotemporal subluxation of lens

Ref: Khurana, 4th ed. pg. 202

- Marfan's syndrome is an **autosomal dominant** condition.
- Subluxation of lens is a common finding, which is seen in upward and temporal area, bilaterally symmetrical.

- Other abnormalities includes: Spider finger, long extremities, high arched palate and dissecting aortic aneurysm with normal IQ.

> **Extra Mile**
>
> **Suluxation of lens also seen in-**
> - **Homocystinuria:** Autosomal Recessive condition; Downward and nasally displaced lens.
> - **Weil marchesani syndrome:** Forward subluxation and spheroaphakia
> - **Sulphite oxidase deficiency:** Ectopia lentis is universal ocular feature
> - **Ehler's danlos syndrome**
> - **Hyperlysinemia**
> - **Stickler syndrome**

160. Ans. (b) Superior and temporally

Ref: A.K. Khurana, 6th ed. pg. 215

Please refer to above condition

161. Ans. (b) Aphakia

Ref: A.K. Khurana, 6th ed. pg. 37, 187

- Jack in a box phenomenon is seen after cataract surgery where the lens of the patient is removed. This causes disproportion in power of the eye. To correct aphakia, patients are prescribed with glasses.
- To correct the refractive error in aphakia about 10 dioptre of convex lenses are required for distance vision and about 13 dioptre for near vision. Such high power lenses are associated with numerous physical and optical problems. The most important of these problems are:
  - Magnification
  - Roving Ring Scotoma
  - **Jack-in-the-box Phenomenon**

162. Ans. (b) Cataract

- Side of oral/systemic steroid: **Cataract**
- Side effect of topical steroid: **Glaucoma**
  - Mn: *GTCS (Glaucoma-topical; Cataract- Systemic)*
- Blepharoconjuncivitis is Side effect of **Timolol**

163. Ans. (b) Subluxation of lens

Ref: A.K. Khurana, 6th ed. pg. 215, 500; Khurana, 4th ed. pg. 203-204, 473

- Iridodonesis is tremulousness of iris.
- It is observed when its posterior support is lost as in aphakia and subluxation of lens.

GLAUCOMA

164. Ans. (d) Dorzolamide

Ref: Katzung Pharmacology; 11/ed. P 89

- **Timolol:** Beta blocker. Decreases aqueous secretion from ciliary epithelium. DOC for POAG in India.
  - Overall, DOC for OAG is latanoprost.

- **Mannitol:** A hyperosmotic agent. Reduces vitreous volume and deepens anterior chamber.
- **Prostaglandin analogue: Latanoprost, Bimatoprost:** Increases uveoscleral aqueous outflow. Considered as DOC for OAG.
- **Carbonic anhydrase inhibitor:** Acetazolamide, dorzolamide, brinzolamide. Acts by decreasing aqueous secretion.

165. Ans. (c) Angle closure glaucoma

Ref: A.K. Khurana, 6th ed. pg. 239-40

- In case of angle closure glaucoma, pupil is mid-dilated, vertically fixed. At this position of pupil, iris and lens are at maximum approximation which precipitate the condition and patient presents with sudden painful loss of vision.
- Open angle glaucoma is due to blockage of trabecular meshwork. Patient gives a history of slow painless loss of vision.
- Uveitis is inflammation of uveal component. Pupil here called festooned pupil *(anterior uveitis)*.

166. Ans. (a) Vertically dilated

Ref: A.K. Khurana, 6th ed. / 239-40, Khurana 4th ed./ 225

- In case of angle closure glaucoma, pupil is mid dilated, vertically fixed.
- Irregularly constricted fixed pupil is seen in anterior uveitis *(known as festooned pupil)*.

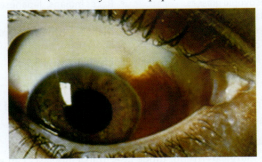

167. Ans. (c) Acute congestive glaucoma

Ref: A.K. Khurana, 6th ed. pg. 239-41

- Acute congestive glaucoma usually presents with sudden painful loss of vision associated with colored haloes. ACG more commonly seen in middle to elderly females.
- D/dx of color haloes:
  - ACG
  - Cataract
  - Mucopurulent conjunctivitis (Not in angular)
- RD presents with sudden painless loss of vision associated with flashes of light.

FMGE Solutions Screening Examination

168. Ans. (b) Latanoprost

Ref: A.K. Khurana, 6th ed. pg. 228-30

GLAUCOMA

- It is a group of conditions characterized by progressive optic neuropathy with characterstic optic disc appearance and irreversible visual field defects.
- It is caused due to retinal ganglion cell death by increase in intraocular pressure (IOP) (usually) or other factors (excitotoxicity/optic nerve spasm)

Classical Triad
- Increase IOP (>21)
- Visual Field decrease
- Optic disk/ Nerve changes (damage)

Atleast 2 conditions is required for diagnosis

PRIMARY OPEN ANGLE GLAUCOMA

- It is also known as chronic simple glaucoma of adult onset and is characterized by the-
  - Slowly progressive raised IOP
  - Optic disc cupping
  - Specific visual field defects

Clinical Features and Risk Factors for OAG

Clinical features	Risk factors
• Frequent change in presbyopic glasses. • Delayed dark adaption. • Painless • No corneal edema • No loss of vision • No coloured halos	• Age • Race- Indians, Japanese. • Myopes • Diabetes, hypertension, hyperthyroidism • Mustard oil intake

Treatment: POAG is best treated by PG analogue Latanoprost (DOC)

Surgery: Trabeculectomy
- Surgical–Argon/ diode laser trabeculoplasty can also be done.

Extra Mile
- **Peripheral Iridectomy:** Surgical treatment done in primary angle closure glaucoma. *Treatment of choice for acute congestive glaucoma.*
- **Laser Iridotomy:** Treatment of choice for angle closure glaucoma.

169. Ans. (c) Parcentral scotoma

Ref: A.K. Khurana, 6th ed. pg. 233, 238

Visual field defects in glaucoma
1. Isopter contraction: *Earliest*
2. Baring of blind spot
3. Isolated paracentral scotoma (earliest chinically significant)
4. Seidel scotoma
5. Bjerrum or arcuate scotoma
6. Roenne's central nasal step
7. Double arcuate scotoma leads to tubular vision
8. Temporal island of vision is also lost with no light perception

170. Ans. (d) Decrease aqueous production

Ref: A.K. Khurana, 6th ed. pg. 451-52

- **ACETAZOLAMIDE** is a carbonic anhydrase inhibitor which acts in OAG by decreasing aqueous production.
- **Carbonic anhydrase derivatives are:** Acetazolamide, **Dorzolamide,** Brinzolamide
- Dorzolamide is mildest carbonic anhydrase inhibitor, hence considered as DOC for glaucoma in children.
- Alpha-2 agonist (Brimonidine, Apraclonidine) also act by decreasing aqueous production.
- **Class of drugs which act by increasing outflow:**
  - ↑ **Trabecular outflow:** Pilocarpine, Epinephrine
  - ↑**Uveoscleral outflow:** PG Analogue (Latanoprost)

Extra Mile

TREATMENT OF Glaucoma
- **First line DOC for ACG:** Mannitol
- **TOC for ACG:** Laser iridotomy
- **DOC for OAG:** PG analogue (Latanoprost)
- **Most powerful anti glaucoma drug:** Latanoprost
- **DOC for OAG in India-** Timolol
- **Safest anti-glaucoma for children-** Dorzolamide

171. Ans. (b) Latanoprost

Ref: A.K. Khurana, 6th ed. pg. 453

172. Ans. (d) Dorzolamide

Ref: A.K. Khurana, 6th ed. pg. 452-454

173. Ans. (a) Timolol maleate

Ref: A.K. Khurana, 6th ed. pg. 236-37

- Although timolol is considered as DOC for OAG in India, it is contraindicated in glaucoma patients suffering from bronchial asthma.
- Timolol is a non selective Beta blocker which might aggravate the asthma of the patient.
- For such patient Betaxolol is next best choice.

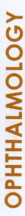

174. Ans. (c) Surgical management

Ref: A.K. Khurana, 6th ed. pg. 225-227

- Once the patient presents with symptoms of primary developmental glaucoma like photophobia, blepharospasm, lacrimation, eye rubbing, the next procedure is to do careful examination in which following things done: IOP measurement, ophthalmoscopy and gonioscopic examination of the angle of anterior chamber.
- The next best step once examination confirms glaucoma is to undergo surgical management (goniotomy) in order to decrease the IOP.

175. Ans. (b) Trabeculotomy

Ref: A.K. Khurana, 6th ed. pg. 225-227,

- Manifestation of congenital glaucoma below age of 3 years is termed as buphthalmos *(as given in case)*. This condition occur due to developmental anomaly of the angle of anterior chamber.
- **Treatment:**
  - **Goniotomy** is preferred treatment, where barkaan's goniotomy knife is used to make an incision in the angle under gonioscopic control.
  - **Trabeculotomy** is preferred when corneal clouding prevents visualization by gonioscopy. *(as seen in given case)*
  - **Combined trabeculotomy and trabeculectomy** is preferred treatment nowadays with better result.

176. Ans. (d) Laser iridotomy

Ref: A.K. Khurana, 6th ed. pg. 247

- **Laser Iridotomy:** Treatment of choice for angle closure glaucoma.
- **Peripheral Iredectomy:** Surgical treatment done in primary angle closure glaucoma. Treatment of choice for acute congestive glaucoma.
- **Trabeculectomy:** It is a filtration surgery done in primary open angle glaucoma.
- **Trabeculoplasty:** Primary open angle glaucoma is also treated by Trabeculoplasty.

177. Ans. (a) Angle closure glaucoma

Ref: A.K. Khurana, 6th ed. pg. 247

178. Ans. (a) Laser Iridotomy

Ref: A.K. Khurana, 6th ed. pg. 247-48

- Please refer to above explanation
- Treatment of choice for primary angle closure glucoma (*fellow eye*, latent stage, *subacute or intermittent stage, chronic stage*) is *laser iridotomy*
- Peripheral surgical iridectomy can also be used.
- In acute congestive stage of PACG drug of choice is Pilocarpine, till the time laser iridotomy can be performed.

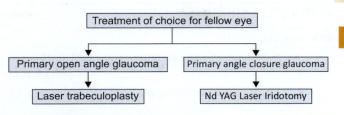

179. Ans. (b) Laser trabeculoplasty

Please refer to above explanation

180. Ans. (b) Open angle glucoma

- In case of OAG colored haloes are very late feature.
- Coloured halos are most commonly seen in **primary angle closure glaucoma, cataract & acute purulent conjunctivitis.** These are differentiated by:
  - **Emsley-Fincham's test:** a stenopaeic slit is passed across the pupil.
    - In case of Primary angle closure glaucoma: Haloes remain intact
    - In case of Immature cataract: Haloes broken into segments.
  - **Conjunctivitis:** Haloes eliminated after irrigating the discharge.
- Therefore given these options, our best choice will be OAG.

181. Ans. (a) Open angle glaucoma

Ref: A.K. Khurana, 6th ed. pg. 229

Frequent change of presbyopic lens is a typical characteristic feature of open angle glaucoma.

> **Extra Mile**
>
> FREQUENT CHANGE OF GLASSES in young:
> - If power also increases → PATHOLOGICAL Ex: OAG
> - If NO increment in power → KERATOCONUS

182. Ans. (b) Cornea posterior surface

Ref: A.K. Khurana, 6th ed. pg. 250; Khurana, 4th ed. pg. 234

- Krukenberg spindles are pigmentary granules which are seen on posterior surface of cornea in shape of spindles in **cases of secondary open angle glaucoma** (pigmentory glaucoma). It can be seen on iris.
- This condition is most commonly seen in young males and myopics.

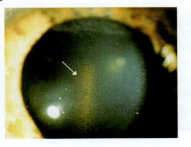

FMGE Solutions Screening Examination

REFRACTIVE ERROR

183. Ans. (a) +2.5 D

Ref: Comprehensive Ophthalmology by A.K Khurana 6th ed. P 13

- A newborn is hypermetropic by +2 to +3 D (average: 2.5 D)

EYE AT BIRTH

- **AP diameter:** 16.5 mm (adult size 24 mm by 7–8 years)
- **Corneal diameter:** 10 mm (adult size 11.7 mm 2 years)
- NB hypermetropic by 2–3 D
- Fixation starts at 1 month. Completed by 6 months
- **Retina:** Fully developed except macular area
  - Macula fully developed by 4–6 months
  - Fusional reflex and accomodation well developed by 4–6 months
  - 3D depth perception/stereopsis - 6 years
- **Lacrimal gland:** Underdeveloped (tears not secreted)
- **Anterior chamber:** Shallow and angle is narrow
- Orbit is more divergent (50°) as compared to adults (45°)

184. Ans. (d) All of the above

Ref: Comprehensive Ophthalmology by A.K Khurana 6th ed. P 347-348

- **Manifest squint is of two types:** Concomitant squint and Incon-comitant squint.
- Concomitant squint:
  - Due abnormality/obstacle in binocular vision development, namely sensory, motor and central

TABLE: Obstacle in central vision development

Sensory obstacle	Motor obstacle	Central obstacle
• Refractive error • Corneal and lenticular opacity • Macular disease • Incorrect spectacle use • Optic atrophy	• Congenital abnormality of shape and size of orbit • Abnormalities of extraocular muscles (faulty innervation & insertion) • Abnormalities of accommodation and convergence	• Deficient development of fusion • Abnormality of cortical control of ocular movement (as seen in mental trauma, hyperexcitability of CNS)

185. Ans. (b) Amblyopia

Ref: Handbook of Pediatric Strabismus and Amblyopia edited by Kenneth W. Wright, Peter H. Spiegel, P 116

The visual deficit associated with amblyopia has certain unique characteristics, including the crowding phenomenon, the neutral density filter effect, and eccentric fixation. The crowding phenomenon relates to the fact that patients with amblyopia have better visual acuity reading single optotype than reading multiple optotypes in a row (linear optotypes). Often, patients with amblyopia will perform 1 or 2 Snellen lines better when presented with single optotypes versus linear optotypes. This crowding phenomenon may have something to do with the relatively large receptive field associated with amblyopia. Crowding bars are often used around a single optotype to provide a more sensitive test for amblyopia.

186. Ans. (a) Occlusion

Ref: Comprehensive Ophthalmology by Khurana; 6/ed. P 63

- Amblyopia refers to a reversible decrease of vision, and is also referred as to lazy eye.
- Treatment of amblyopia should be started as early as possible, younger the child better is the prognosis.
- Occlusion therapy is the mainstay of therapy in which healthy eye is occluded to force the fixation of amblyopic eye.
- Before occlusion any opacity in the media should be removed and any refractive error should be corrected.
- However atropine penalization can also be done in better eye. Atropine causes cycloplegia and hence blurring of vision, which also forces the fixation of amblyopic eye.

187. Ans. (b) Head tilt towards the rectus muscle paralysis

Ref: Khurana, 6th ed. pg. 354

Paralytic squint
- Refers to ocular deviation resulting from complete or incomplete paralysis of one or more extraocular muscles.
- **Causes may be:** Neurogenic, myogenic or at the level of neuromuscular junction.

Clinical features:

Symptoms	Signs
• Diplopia: It is the main symptom and is more marked in the field of action of paralyzed muscle • Confusion • Nausea and vertigo • Ocular deviation	• **Primary deviation:** Deviation of the affected eye and is away from the action of paralyzed muscle. Eg: if medial rectus palsy, the eye is diverged. • **Secondary deviation:** Deviation of normal eye • **Ocular movement restriction:** Occurs in direction of action of paralyzed muscle • **Compensatory head posture:** In the direction of action of paralyzed muscle. It is adopted to avoid diplopia and confusion.

Note: In case of paralytic squint, visual acuity is normal and there is no amblyopia as in most cases paralytic squint develops in adults when visual acuity has already developed.

188. Ans (c) Refractive error

Ref: A.K Khurana's Ophthalmology, 6th ed. pg. 34-36; Harrison's, 19th ed. pg. 195

- Most common cause of blindness in the world: Cataract
- Second Most common cause of blindness in world: Glaucoma> ARMD
- Most common infective cause of blindness: Trachoma
- Most common cause of ocular morbidity: Refractive error
- Given these choices, refractive error is the least common cause of blindness. **Harrison states:** "*Refractive errors usually develop slowly and **remain stable** after adolescence, except in unusual circumstances. For example, the acute onset of diabetes mellitus can produce sudden myopia because of lens edema induced by hyperglycemia.*"
- Corneal opacities like Nebula, Macula and Leucoma also contribute significantly to blindness.

189. Ans. (b) Hypermetropia

Ref: A.K Khurana's Ophthalmology, 6th ed. pg. 36

- Convex lens (plus lens) is used for treatment of hypermetropia.

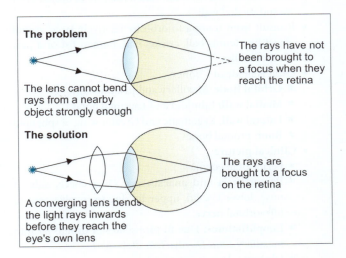

Extra Mile

- Lens used in myopia: Concave lens (Minus lens)
- Lens used in presbyopia: Convex lens

190. Ans. (d) 30°

Ref: A.K Khurana's Ophthalmology, 6th ed. pg. 348

Concomitant squint is of three types:
- Convergent squint (esotropia)
- Divergent squint (exotropia)
- Vertical squint (hypertropia)

CONVERGENT SQUINT (ESOTROPIA)

- It denotes inward deviation of one eye. It is the most common type of squint in children

TYPES

- **Infantile esotropia**
    - **Clinical features:**
        - **Age:** Onset at 1–2 month, but can occur at any time in first 6 months of life
        - **Angle of deviation:** Usually constant and fairly large (>30°)
        - Amblyopia in 25–40% of cases
        - Fixation pattern: Binocular vision does not develop and there is alternate fixation in primary gaze and cross fixation in lateral gaze.
    - TOC: Surgery
    - Time for surgery: Between first 6 months to 2 years (preferable before 1 year of age).
- **Accommodative esotropia:** Develops at around 2–3 years of age. Associated with high hypermetropia (+4 to +7 D)
- **Acquired non-accomodative esotropia**
- **Sensory esotropia**
- **Consecutive esotropia**

191. Ans. (a) Large optic disc

Ref: A.K. Khurana, 6th ed. pg. 38

MYOPIA

- Also known as short sightedness.
- It is a type of refractive error in which parallel rays of light coming from infinity are focused in front of retina when accommodation is at rest.
- Myopic patients have short eyeballs.

Fundus Examination of Myopia

- *Optic disc appears large and pale* and at its temporal edge a characteristic myopic crescent is present
- Degenerative changes in retina and choroid are common in progressive myopia
- Posterior staphyloma at posterior pole may be apparent due to ectasia of sclera.
- Degenerative changes in vitreous include: liquefaction, vitrous opacities, and posterior vitreous detachment (PVD).

192. Ans. (a) Pseudomyopia

Ref: A.K. Khurana, 6th ed. pg. 47

"Accommodation refers to a process whereby a change in position as well **as increased curvature of the crystalline lens** increases the conjugation power of the eye i.e. its ability to **converge an image to focus on retina.**

From the above paragraph it can be concluded that more is the accommodation, more is the curvature of lens and the ray will converge more and hence image will be formed in front of retina i.e. pseudomyopia.

193. Ans. (b) Contact lens

Ref: A.K. Khurana, 6th ed.

- Anisometropic patients cannot wear glasses as it causes diplopic vision so contact lens are prescribed.
- Glasses can only tolerate and correct upto 4D.
- **Trabeculectomy:** It is a filtration surgery done in primary angle closure glaucoma.
- **Trabeculoplasty:** Primary open angle glaucoma is treated by Trabeculoplasty.

194. Ans. (b) Cylindrical

Ref: A.K. Khurana, 6th ed. pg. 42-423

- Astigmatism is a common eye condition that's easily corrected by eyeglasses, contact lenses, or surgery.
- It is caused by an eye that is not completely round. It is a type of refractive error.
- **Cause:** Astigmatism is a natural and commonly occurring cause of blurred or distorted vision. The exact cause in not known.
- **Symptom:** Blurring of vision which can be associated with fatigue and eyestrain.
- **Cylindrical lens** is used for the management of astigmatism.

> **Extra Mile**
> - Myopics are said to be short sighted. Concave lenses are used in myopics
> - Convex lens are used in hypermetropics.

195. Ans. (c) Binocular vision

Ref: A.K. Khurana, 6th ed. pg. 342

- **Worth four dot test (WFDT)** is a test for binocular vision using red-green color dissociation.
- It is a dissociation test which can be used with both distance and near fixation and differentiate between binocular single vision, abnormal retinal correspondence and suppression.
- **Note:** Result of WFDT can only be interpreted if the presence or absence of manifest squint is known at the time of testing.

196. Ans. (c) Ansiometropia

Ref: A.K. Khurana, 6th ed. pg. 44-45, Khurana, 4th ed. pg. 38

- **Isometropia:** Two eye with equal refraction
- **Anisometropia:** Two eye with unequal refraction of power >2.5D
- **Aniseikoinia:** Difference in size/shape of image of >5% on visual cortex by retina.

197. Ans. (d) Astigmatism

Ref: A.K. Khurana, 6th ed. /42-43, Harrison's 19th ed./ 195

- Astigmatism is a type of refractive error which arises due to irregular curvature of cornea.
- Correction of astigmatism is done by using cylindrical lens.

OCULAR INJURY AND MALIGNANCY

198. Ans. (a) Only i and ii are correct

Ref: Comprehensive Ophthalmology by A.K Khurana 6th ed. P 422-23

- Blow out fracture is comminuted fracture of orbital floor >> and medial wall.
- It result from trauma to orbit by relatively large, round object like tennis ball, cricket ball, human fist or a part of automobile.
- Orbit is made of 7 bones:
  - **Orbital floor:** Maxillary and palatine bone
  - **Medial wall:** Ethmoid and Lacrimal bone
  - **Lateral wall:** Zygomatic and Greater wing of sphenoid
  - **Roof:** Frontal bone
- Clinical picture:
  - Perioribtial edema
  - **Paraesthesia and anaesthesia:** Over cheek, side of nose, lower eye-lid, upper lip due to involvement of infraorbital nerve.
  - **Enophthalmos:** Due to protrusion of orbital fat into maxillary *sinus (X-ray: Tear drop sign).*
  - **Diplopia:** Due to extraocular nerve entrapment
- **Treatment:**
  - Avoid nose blowing
  - Systemic antibiotics (as prophylaxis) and analgesics
  - Cold compress (decreases swelling by vasoconstriction)
  - Surgical repair of plate (10–14 days after injury)

199. Ans. (a) Tennis ball injury

Ref: Comprehensive Ophthalmology by A.K Khurana 6th ed. P 422-23

Refer to above explanation

Ophthalmology

200. Ans. (a) Rhabdomyosarcoma

Common Malignancies of Eye

- *Retinoblastoma is most common secondary intraorbital tumor of children*
- *Squamous cell CA is most common secondary orbital tumor of adult*
- **Rhabdomyosarcoma** *is most common primary malignant orbital tumor of children* and most common soft tissue malignancy of childhood.
- Lymphoma is the most common primary malignant orbital tumor of adult
- **Choroid melanoma** *is most common intraocular malignancy in adult*
- **Capillary haemangioma** is most common tumor of orbital & periorbital areas in children.
- **Cavernous haemangioma** is most common benign orbital tumor in adults.
- **Pleomorphic adenoma** (benign mixed tumor) is most common epithelial tumor of lacrimal gland.
- **Neuroblastoma** is *most common cause of orbital metastasis in children*
- **Breast** (> Bronchus > Prostate > Skin melanoma) is the most common cause of orbital metastasis in adult.
  - CA Breast (Female)
  - CA Breast (Male)
- **Choroid** is the most common site for metastasis (90%) followed by iris & ciliary body. *Metastatic tumors to choroid are more common than primary malignancies.*

201. Ans. (b) Orbital floor

- Orbital floor is made of maxillary and palatine bone. In case of orbital floor fracture, content of orbit protrudes into maxillary sinus which on radiological image is seen as tear drop.

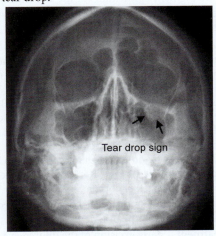
Tear drop sign

202. Ans. (a) RB gene

Ref: Khurana, 6th ed. pg. 303

- Retinoblastoma (RB) gene has been identified as 14 band on long arm of chromosome 13 (13q14) and is a cancer suppressor or antioncogenic gene. Deletion or inactivation of both the normal alleles of this protective gene by two mutation **(Knudson two hit hypothesis)** results in occurrence of retinoblastoma.

203. Ans. (d) Conservative

Ref: Khurana, 6th ed. pg. 429

- It is a case of traumatic hyphaema (blood in anterior chamber).
- **Khurana states:** *"Conservative treatment is aimed at prevention of rise in IOP and occurrence of secondary haemorrhage. A small hyphaema usually clears up with conservative treatment, however a large non resolving hyphaema should be drained to avoid blood staining of cornea"*
- If hyphaema is associated with rise in IOP, it can be lowered by acetazolamide and hyperosmotic agents.

204. Ans. (d) Keratometry

INSTRUMENTS USED FOR OCULAR EXAMINATION

Measurement parameter	Instruments for:
• Corneal thickness	Pachymeter
• Corneal curvature	Keratometer
• Angle of anterior chamber	Gonioscope
• Corneal surface	Placido disc
• Corneal endothelium	Specular microscope
• Direct ophthalmoscope (Remembered as: "DEV")	Routine fundus examination. "Image formed is **Erect** and **Virtual** and magnified, 15 times"
• Indirect ophthalmoscope	For assessment of retinal detachment and other peripheral retinal lesions. *The image is real, inverted and magnified 5 times.*
• Perimetry	Optic nerve function

205. Ans. (b) Optic nerve glioma

Ref: Khurana, 6th ed. pg. 419

Optic nerve glioma

- It is a slow growing tumor arising from the astrocytes, usually occurs in 1st decade of life in a child between 4-8 years of age.
- It may present either as a solitary tumor or as a part of von Recklinghausen neurofibromatosis.

Clinical features:
- It is characterized by gradual vision loss associated with a gradual, **painless unilateral axial proptosis.**
- **Fundus exam shows:** Optic atrophy or papilloedema and venous engorgement.

Treatment: observation, followed by surgical excision.

206. Ans. (a) Retinoblastoma

Ref: A.K Khurana's Ophthalmology, 6th ed. pg. 303

COMMON MALIGNANCIES OF EYE

- *Retinoblastoma* is most common intraocular (not orbital) malignancy in children (1 in 15000 to 20,000 live births)
- *Retinoblastoma* is confined to infancy and very young children usually seen between 1 and 2 years of age.
- Occurs bilaterally in 25-30% cases

207. Ans. (a) Loss of accommodation

Ref: A.K Khurana's Ophthalmology, 6th ed. pg. 355

FUNCTION OF OCULOMOTOR NERVE (CN.III)

- The third cranial nerve controls the movement of four of the six eye muscles. These muscles move the eye inward, up and down, and they rotate the eye. The third cranial nerve also controls constriction of the pupil, the positioning of the upper eyelid, and the ability of the eye to focus.
- With unilateral third nerve palsy, diplopia is masked due to development of ptosis.
- Other findings:
  1. Ptosis: Due to paralysis of LPS muscle
  2. Deviation: Eyeball is turned *downward and outward*
  3. Restricted ocular movements in all direction except outward.
  4. Fixed and dilated pupil: Due to paralysis of sphincter pupillae muscles.
  5. **Accommodation is completely lost** due to paralysis of ciliary muscle.

208. Ans. (b) Loss of accommodation

Ref: A.K Khurana's Ophthalmology, 6th ed. pg. 147-48

FUNCTION OF CILIARY BODY

- Formation of aqueous humor (*by pars plicata*)
- Ciliary muscles helps in accommodation (*its damage leads to loss of accomodation*)

209. Ans. (b) Orbital apex

Ref: A.K Khurana's Ophthalmology, 6th ed. pg. 413

- Tolosa hunt syndrome refers to idiopathic non-specific granulomatous inflammation involving the superior orbital fissure and/or orbital apex and/or cavernous sinus

- **Clinical presentation:**
  - Depending on the involvement of orbital, it can present as either orbital apex syndrome or as superior orbital fissure syndrome.
    - **Superior orbital fissure syndrome:** Symptoms depend on involvement of structure passing through the superior orbital fissure.
      - ★ CN V #: Retroorbital pain, loss of sensation in ophthalmic division of CN V.
      - ★ CN III, IV, VI #: Ipsilateral ophthalmoplegia
      - ★ CN III #: Ptosis
  - **Orbital apex syndrome:** Symptoms are due to involvement of structure present at orbital apex. Optic nerve involvement causing early vision loss and afferent pupil defect plus symptoms of superior orbital fissure syndrome.

210. Ans. (b) Sympathetic ophthalmitis

Ref: A.K Khurana, 6th ed. pg. 163, 437

- Sympathetic ophthalmitis is a serious bilateral granulomatous panuveitis which usually occurs due to penetrating trauma to ciliary body.
- The injured eye is called exciting eye.
- Fellow eye which also develops uvieitis is called sympathizing eye.

Features
- Always follows a penetrating wound.
- More common in children than in adults.
- It doesn't occur when actual suppuration develops in the injured eye

Pathologies
- Uveal pigment acts as allergen and excites plastic uveitis in the sound eye.
- Dalen-Fuchs' nodules are formed due to proliferation of the pigment epithelium (of the iris, ciliary body and choroid) associated with invasion by the lymphocytes and epitheloid cells.

Clinical Picture
- **Prodromal stage:** Sensitivity to light (photophobia) transient indistinctness of near objects is *the earliest symptoms.*
- *First sign* may be presence of retrolental flare or the presence of a keratic precipitates (KPs) at back of cornea.
- **Fully-developed stage:** has typical signs and symptoms consistent with acute plastic iridocyclitis.
- **Dalen Fuch's Nodules** are characteristic of SO.
- **Exciting (injured) eye:** Keratic precipitates may be present at the back of cornea
- **Sympathizing (sound) eye:** Usually involved after 4-8 weeks of injury in the other eye.
- **Treatment** – Early excision of the injured eye.
  - Topical cycloplegics + IV/oral steroids are also used for treatment.

Ophthalmology

211. Ans. (c) Penetrating injury to Ciliary body

Ref: A.K. Khurana, 6th ed. pg. 163, 437

Please refer to above explanation.

212. Ans. (b) Hammer and chisel

Ref: A.K. Khurana, 6th ed. pg. 163, 437

213. Ans. (b) Trauma

Ref: A.K. Khurana, 6th ed. pg. 91, 335

SUBCONJUNCTIVAL HEMORRHAGE

- A subconjunctival hemorrhage is blood that is located between the conjunctiva and the underlying sclera.
- This results from rupture of small vessels bridging the potential space between the episclera and the conjunctiva. Blood dissecting into this space can produce a spectacular red eye, but vision is not affected and the hemorrhage resolves without treatment.

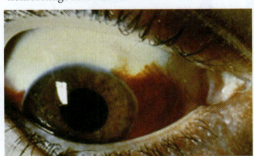

- Subconjunctival hemorrhage is usually spontaneous **but can result from blunt trauma**, eye rubbing, or vigorous coughing. Occasionally it is a clue to an underlying bleeding disorder.
- **Sx:** The most obvious sign of a subconjunctival hemorrhage is a bright red patch on the white (sclera) of your eye.
- Despite its bloody appearance, a subconjunctival hemorrhage should **cause no change in vision**, no discharge from eye and no pain.
- **Note:** *If trauma is not is option, the next best option you can choose is pertusis or chronic cough.*

214. Ans. (b) Optic disc

- Optic disc is not involved in papillary light reflex.
- Pathway of papillary light reflex:

Retina → Optic Nerve → Optic Chiasma → Optic Tract → Prerectal Nucleus → Edinger Westphal Nucleus → Inferior Division of 3rd Nerve → Ciliary Ganglion → Short Ciliary Nerves → Sphincter Pupillae

215. Ans. (d) Exophthalmos

Ref: A.K. Khurana, 6th ed. pg. 422-23, Khurana's, 4th ed. pg. 397-398

- *Blowout fractures mainly involve orbital floor and medial wall.*
- *It usually result from trauma to the oribit by a relatively large, often rounded object, such as tennis ball, cricket ball etc.*
- *With a resultant fracture of the weakest point of the orbital wall.*

Classification

- **Pure blow-out fractures:** Not associated with involvement of the orbital rim.
- **Impure blow-out fractures:** Associated with other fractures about the middle third of the facial skeleton.

Clinical Feature

- Periorbital oedema and blood extravasation in and around the orbit
- Emphysema of the eyelids occurs more frequently with medial wall than floor fractures.
- Paraesthesia and anaesthesia
- Ipsilateral epistaxis
- Proptosis and Ptosis
- Enophthalmos; NOT Exophthalmos
- Diplopia
- **Plain x-rays** (Water's view): Fragmentation and irregularity of the orbital floor; depression of bony fragments and *'hanging drop/tear drop'* opacity of the superior maxillary antrum from orbital contents herniating through the floor.

216. Ans. (b) Neurofibromatosis

Ref: A.K. Khurana, 6th ed. pg. 309-10

- In some patients who have neurofibromatosis type 1, multiple uveal nevi develop in both eyes. These lesions must be differentiated from the small, tan, melanocytic iris lesions (**Lisch nodules**) that arise multifocally from the anterior surface of the iris.
- Lisch nodules appear to be nodular aggregates of dendritic melanocytes and not true nevi.
- They usually become evident by the age of 10–15 years and are *highly characteristic of NF-1.*

217. Ans. (b) Basal carcinoma

Ref: A.K. Khurana, 6th ed. pg. 384

BASAL CELL CANCER OR RODENT ULCER

- It is the most common malignant tumor of the eyelid.
- Most common site of origin of BCC: Lower eyelid followed by medial canthus.

- Noduloulcerative basal cell cancer is the most common presentation
- The treatment is done by surgical excision with primary repair.

218. Ans. (b) Pleomorphic adenoma

Ref: A.K. Khurana, 6th ed. pg. 399-400

- Most common Epethilial tumor of lacrimal gland: Pleomorphic Adenoma (MC benign lacrimal gland tumor)
- Most common malignant eyelid tumor: Basal cell CA > Squamous cell CA
- Most common benign eyelid tumor: Papilloma

219. Ans. (b) Brain

Ref: A.K. Khurana, 6th ed. pg. 303-304

- The child is usually brought to the surgeon on account of a peculiar white reflex from the pupil, sometimes called leucocoria 'amaurotic cat's eye'
- Other modes of presentation include a convergent or divergent squint, cataract, buphthalmos, a hypopyon or proptosis,
- If left untreated retinoblastoma runs through the same stages as melanoma of the choroid:
  - Quiescent stage, lasting from six months to a year
  - Glaucomatous stage
  - Stage of extraocular extension
  - Stage of metastasis
- Metastasis first occurs in the pre-auricular and neighbouring lymph nodes, later in the cranial and other bones.
- **Direct extension by-continuity to the optic nerve [which is affected early) and Brain is more common, while metastases in other organs, usually the liver are relatively rare.**
- Clinically cauliflower-like mass-arising from the retina is seen extending into the vitreous. There is neovascularization on the surface with white areas of calcification. Vitreous or anterior chamber seedings are seen as fluffy whitish-grey deposits. The endophytic type of retinoblastoma presents as an exudative retinal detachment.

220. Ans. (a) Esotropia

Ref: A.K. Khurana, 6th ed. pg. 303-304

NEURO-OPHTHALMOLOGY

221. Ans. (b) Pituitary adenoma

Ref: A.K Khurana's Ophthalmology, 6th ed. pg. 313-14

Type of visual field defect

1. **Unilateral blindness:** U/L optic nerve lesion
2. **Bitemporal hemianopia:** Optic chiasmal lesion *(ex: Pituitary adenoma).*
   - **Binasal hemianopia:** 2 seaparate lesion at chiasma laterally
4. **Homonymous hemianopia:** Lesion at U/L optic tract.
5. **Superior quadrantopia:** Temporal lobe lesion *(pie on the sky).*
6. **Inferior quadrantopia:** Parietal Lobe lesion *(pie on the floor)*
7. **Homonymous hemianopia with macular sparing:** Occipital lobe lesion

Site of lesion

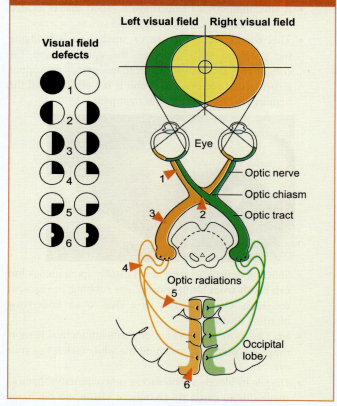

222. Ans. (b) Red green

Ref: A.K. Khurana, 6th ed. pg. 329

- Optic neuritis, the most serious adverse effect reported due to ethambutol toxicity, typically presents as reduced visual acuity, central scotoma, and loss of the ability to see green (or, less commonly, red).
- *Please refer to pharmacology section for detailed discussion on ATT and their side effect.*

223. Ans. (d) Fasanella servat operation

Ref: A.K. Khurana, 6th ed. pg. 381

- **Fasanella-servat operation** or Tarso-conjunctivo-mullerectomy is the surgery of choice for ptosis due to Horner syndrome: as the ptosis in Horner syndrome is mild (2 mm) and is due to Muller's muscle dysfunction (sympathetic supply)
- **Sling surgery** is done in severe ptosis with poor Levator action. Here the ptosis is mild so sling is not advised
- Levator resection upto 15 mm strengthens levator muscle and is done to correct mild degree of ptosis. If fasanella Servat operation is not provided, that it is the best correct option.

224. **Ans. (b) Lateral rectus**

- In raised intracranial tension, the nerves affected are the ones which have long intracranial course leading to false localizing signs. Since the CN VI emerges straight from the brainstem (while others originate obliquely), this nerve is more liable to get affected in increased intracranial pressure.
- CN VI supplies, lateral rectus muscle. Hence lateral rectus muscle is the first one to be affected in increased ICP.

225. **Ans. (d) Homonymous hemianopia with macular sparing**

Ref: Harrison's, 19th ed. pg. 198-199

Please look at the diagram carefully to understand the visual pathway and its corresponding pathology.

- Unilateral optic nerve lesion: Unilateral blindness
- **Binasal hemianopia:** Bitemporal optic chiasma lesion. Two different lesions compressing the chiasma from the lateral parts.
- **Bitemporal hemianopia:** Binasal retinal damaged à **optic chiasmal lesion.** Commonest lesion is *pituitary adenoma.*
- **Homonymous hemianopia:** Lesion at optic tract AND optic radiation
- **Homonymous superior quadrantonopia:** All superior quadrantonopia goes to the temporal lobe *(pie in the sky).*
- **Homonymous inferior quadrantonopia:** All inferior quadrantonopia goes to the parietal lobe *(Pie on the floor).*
- **Homonymous hemianopia w/ macular sparing:** Lesion in occipital cortex lesion.

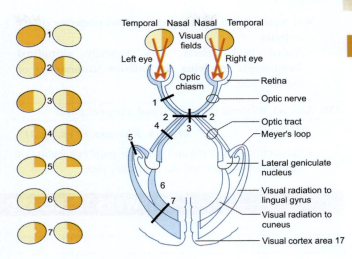

226. **Ans. (d) Homonymous hemianopia**

Ref: Harrison's, 19th ed. pg. 198-199

Please refer to above explanation.

227. **Ans. (c) Left optic tract**

Ref: Harrison's, 19th ed. pg. 198-199

228. **Ans. (d) Bitemporal hemianopia**

Ref: Harrison's, 19th ed. pg. 198-199

"**Bitemporal hemianopia** is usually caused by tumors in the region of the sells turcica, pressure by a suprasellar aneurysm or by chronic arachnoiditis; these press upon the chiasma so that the fibers going to thenasal halves of each retina are destroyed. **Tumors of the pituitary body**[Q] are most common.

229. **Ans. (c) Diabetes**

Ref: Harrison's, 19th ed. pg. 202

- **Isolated third nerve palsy with pupillary sparing** is seen in **diabetic neuropathy** involving cranial nerves
- Other causes which can also cause pupillary sparing oculomotor palsy are **Vascular diseases** and HTN.

230. **Ans. (b) AION (Anterior Ischemic Optic Neuropathy)**

Ref: Harrison's, 19th ed. pg. 202

- Anterior Ischemic Optic Neuropathy refers to a segmental or generalized infarction of anterior part of the optic nerve

FMGE Solutions Screening Examination

- It occurs due to occlusion of the **short posterior ciliary arteries**
- Visual field defects show typically **altitudinal hemianopia involving the inferior (commonly)** or superior half.

231. Ans. (c) Bilateral constricted and irregular pupil

Ref: A.K. Khurana, 6th ed. pg. 317

- Bilaterally constricted and irregular pupil is a feature of Argyll Robertson Pupil aka Prostitue's pupil

Argyll (Neurosyphillis)	Adie's
• Bilateral constricted and irregular pupil • Light reaction: -ve • Accomodation: + ve • Aka prostitute's pupil	• Seen post viral illness → inflammation of ciliary ganglion → sympathathetic stimulation • Dilated pupil, other is N. • NO RESPONSE TO LIGHT • Accomodation slow • Pupil is super sensitive to pilocarpine

ANSWERS TO BOARD REVIEW QUESTIONS

232. Ans. (b) 6.5 ml

Ref: Ocular pathology by Myron Yanoff, Joseph William Sassan p. 529

233. Ans. (d) 200,000 IU per dose

Ref: Khurana, 4th ed. pg. 436

234. Ans. (d) Strabismus

Ref: Yanoff and ducker pg. 1311

235. Ans. (c) CRVO

Ref: Neuro-ophthalmology: the practical guide by Leonard A. Levin p 101, khurana 4th ed p-298

236. Ans. (a) Scotoma

Ref: Optic Nerve Disorders: Diagnosis and Management by Jane W. Chan p. 151

237. Ans. (b) Optic nerve glioma

Ref: Pediatric Ophthalmology: A clinical Guide by Gallin p. 105

238. Ans. (a) Enterovirus 70

Ref: Khurana, 4th ed. pg. 70; Harrison's 18th ed ch-191

239. Ans. (c) Diabetes

Ref: Parson's, 20th pg. 297

240. Ans. (a) The posterior limit of Descemet's membrane of cornea

Ref: Khurana, 4th ed pg. 90

241. Ans. (c) Second

Ref: Ganong, 22nd ed. ch-8

242. Ans. (b) 3/60

Ref: Khurana, 4th ed. pg. 444

243. Ans. (a) Sarcoidosis

244. Ans. (b) Loss of accommodation

245. Ans. (b) Pars plicata

246. Ans. (c) Vitamin C

247. Ans. (a) Optic neutitis

248. Ans. (a) Nuclear

249. Ans. (c) Pupillary block

250. Ans. (a) Increase uveo-scleral outflow

251. Ans. (b) Corneal surface

252. Ans. (a) Simple

253. Ans. (b) Hypertensive retinopathy

254. Ans. (d) Choroiditis

255. Ans. (c) Purkinje shift is all colours seen as grey in bright light

256. Ans. (b) Ceftriaxone

Ophthalmology

1117

257. Ans. (c) Central cataract

258. Ans. (b) Posterior lenticonus

259. Ans. (d) ATT with steroids given

260. Ans. (a) CRVO

261. Ans. (b) Direct ophthalmoscopic screening at 32 weeks post conceptional age

262. Ans. (a) EOG

263. Ans. (a) Pars plana vitrectomy

264. Ans. (d) All of the above

265. Ans. (a) Angle closure glaucoma

266. Ans. (b) Retinal detachment

267. Ans. (b) Osteosarcoma

268. Ans. (d) Hydrogel

269. Ans. (a) Congenital rubella

270. Ans. (c) Vitreous loss

271. Ans. (a) Infective endocarditis

272. Ans. (a) Myopia

273. Ans. (a) 3 years

274. Ans. (a) 4 weeks

275. Ans. (a) Tuberous sclerosis

276. Ans. (d) Jaeger chart

277. Ans. (c) Diabetic retinopathy

278. Ans. (c) Exopthalmos

279. Ans. (d) Eye patching

280. Ans. (a) Between deep stroma and descemet membrane

281. Ans. (a) Homonymous hemianopia

282. Ans. (b) Moraxella axenfeld

283. Ans. (a) Enterovirus 70

284. Ans. (d) White ropy discharge

285. Ans. (a) Limbus

286. Ans. (a) Staphylococcus aureus

287. Ans. (b) Herpes simplex

288. Ans. (b) Keratoconus

289. Ans. (a) Fifth

290. Ans. (a) Retinitis pigmentosa

291. Ans. (a) Papilledema

292. Ans. (a) Foster kennedy

293. Ans. (a) Elevation and intortion

294. Ans. (b) Latent squint in distant vision

295. Ans. (a) Inflammation of gland of zeis

296. Ans. (b) Madarosis

297. Ans. (a) Leprosy

298. Ans. (a) Sjogren syndrome

299. Ans. (b) Vernal conjunctivitis

300. Ans. (b) Lens cortex

301. Ans. (b) Retinoblastoma

302. Ans. (b) Corneal ulcer

303. Ans. (b) CMV retinitis

304. Ans. (b) Rheumatoid arthritis

305. Ans. (a) Anterior ischemic optic neuritis

306. Ans. (a) Retinoblastoma

307. Ans. (a) Indirect ophthalmoscopy

308. Ans. (c) Myopia

Explanations

309. Ans. (a) Granuloma uveitis

310. Ans. (a) Iron deposition

311. Ans. (c) Arcus senilis

312. Ans. (b) 1.5 mm

> Ref: Kanski 7th ed. chapter 10, Glaucoma: Science and Practice By John Morrison, Irvin Pollack p. 91

313. Ans. (a) Bacterial

> Ref: Parson's, 20th ed. pg. 173

Due to reduced incidence of TB, hypersensitivity to S.aureus is the leading cause.

314. Ans. (a) Pigmentary glaucoma

> Ref: Khurana, 4th ed. pg. 237

315. Ans. (a) Diabetes mellitus

> Ref: Khurana, 4th ed. pg. 256

316. Ans. (a) Solar eclipse

> Ref: Khurana, 4th ed. pg. 263

317. Ans. (a) Retinal detachment

> Ref: Oxford Handbook of Ophthalmology, pg. 418

318. Ans. (a) Limbus

> Ref: Khurana, 4th ed. pg. 111

319. Ans. (a) Posterior capsule

> Ref: Khurana, 4th ed. pg. 191

320. Ans. (a) Melanoma of choroid

> Ref: Kanski, 5th ed. pg. 331, 334, 577-86

321. Ans. (c) Pseudomonas

> Ref: Yanoff & Ducker-ophthalmology, 2nd ed. pg. 04, Khurana, 4th ed. pg. 92

322. Ans. (a) Anatomical and visual axis

> Ref: Kanski's, 7/e, chapter 18

323. Ans. (c) B scan

> Ref: Kanski 7/e, chapter 9, Textbook of ophthalmology by H.V. nema, p 525

324. Ans. (a) Fundoscopy

> Ref: Kanski 7/e, chapter 11, Intraocular drug delivery by glenn J. Jaffe p 330

325. Ans. (c) Intermediate uveitis

> Ref: Khurana 4/e, p 216, 161

326. Ans. (c) Neurofibromatosis

> Ref: Khurana 4/e, p 131, Yanoff 2/e, p 518

327. Ans. (c) Premature newborn

> Ref: Khurana 4/e, p 131, Yanoff 2/e, p 518

328. Ans. (d) Episcleritis

> Ref: Kanski 7/e, chapter 8, 11, vaugham and asbury's general ophthalmology 17/e, chapter 16

329. Ans. (a) High myopia

> Ref: Kanski 7/e, chapter 3, Khurana 4/e, p 531, 535

330. Ans. (d) Post transplant astigmatism

> Ref: Kanski 7/e, chapter 7, Khurana 4/e, p 124

331. Ans. (a) Chromosome 3

> Ref: The retina and its disorders edited by joseph besharse, dean bok Elsevier 2011 p 141

332. Ans. (a) Anterior staphyloma

> Ref: Khurana 4/e, p 510

333. Ans. (a) Idiopathic

> Ref: Yanoff 2/e, p 1115, Review of ophthalmology by William B. Trattler, peter K. Kaiser, Neil J. Friendman 2012, p 299, Esentials of ophthalmology by Neil J. Friedman 1st 2007, p 195

334. Ans. (a) Cataract

> Ref: Khurana 4/e, p 428

335. Ans. (b) Edinger-westphal nucleus

> Ref: Khurana 4/e, p 292

336. Ans. (d) Diptheroids

> Ref: Textbook of microbiology by vasanthakumari p 452

337. Ans. (a) Endothelium

> Ref: Khurana 6/e, p 100

Ophthalmology

338. Ans. (a) Myopia

Ref: Khurana 4/e, p 275, Kanski 7/e, Chapter 16, Parson's 21/e, p 326

339. Ans. (b) Iridocyclitis

Ref: Khurana 4/e, p 163, Parson 21/e, p 229

340. Ans. (a) Acute angle-closure glaucoma

Ref: Parson 21/e, p 290, Yanoff Ducker 3/e, p 1165

341. Ans. (c) Interior rectus

Ref: Khurana 4/e, Chapter 391, Kanski 7/e, chapter 3

342. Ans. (d) Nd:YAG

Ref: Khurana, pg. 431

343. Ans. (c) Sympathetic nerves

Ref: Khurana 4/e, p 340, Gray's anatomy 40/e, p 691

344. Ans. (b) Surface ectoderm

Ref: Yanoff and ducker-ophthalmology 2/e, p 22-23, parson 20/e, p 5, Khurana 4/e, p 10

345. Ans. (b) Retina

Ref: Gray's anatomy 39/e, chapter 43

346. Ans. (c) Specular microscope

Ref: Yanoff 3/d, p 83

347. Ans. (b) 2500/mm²

Ref: Khurana 4/e, p 90, Parson 21/e, p 120

348. Ans. (a) <3/60

Ref: http://www.who.int/blindness/en/

- According to WHO definition of blindness is vision <3/60
- India has also adopted the same definition (Inability to count fingers from a distance of 3 meters)
- **Ultimate WHO goal:** Reduce blindness prevalence (in India) to 0.3% of total population by 2020.

ANSWERS TO IMAGE-BASED QUESTIONS

349. Ans. (b) Pterygium

350. Ans. (a) Hypopyon

351. Ans. (a) Retinitis pigmentosa

The image shows a fundus with bony spicules and a pale disc with thinned out blood vessels suggestive of diagnosis of Retinitis Pigmentosa.

352. Ans. (b) Dot blot haemorrhages

The fundus shows dot in the middle and blotted ink appearance of fundus haemorrhage suggestive of diagnosis of diabetic retinopathy.

16

Dermatology

MOST RECENT QUESTIONS 2019

1. A 25-year-old female presents with history of fever and oral ulcers and has developed erythematous lesions on her face. Comment on the diagnosis.

   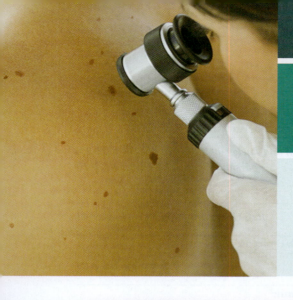

   a. SLE
   b. Dermatomyositis
   c. Melasma
   d. Rosacea

2. The following lesion was noticed in a patient with history of involuntary weight loss. What is the diagnosis?

   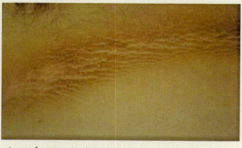

   a. Acanthosis nigricans
   b. Leser-Trélat sign
   c. Actinic keratosis
   d. Intertriginous Candida

3. Which is not correct about the lesion shown?

   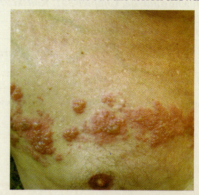

   a. The lesions are infectious to seronegative individuals
   b. Can be associated with meningoencephalitis
   c. Bilaterally symmetrical dermatomal vesicular eruption
   d. Geniculate ganglion is involved in Ramsay Hunt syndrome

4. The shown instrument is:

   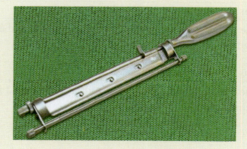

   a. Single cutting razor
   b. Double cutting razor
   c. Humby's knife
   d. Finochietto knife

5. Most appropriate Management to reduce recurrence of keloid:
   a. Intralesional steroids   b. Surgery
   c. Cryotherapy   d. Electrocoagulation

Dermatology

6. An infant presents with the condition as shown below after a pharyngeal infection. The shown condition is:

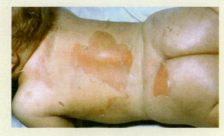

   a. Staphylococcal scalded skin syndrome
   b. Epidermolysis bullosa simplex
   c. Impetigo contagiosa
   d. Pemphigus foliaceus

7. The shown penile lesion is:

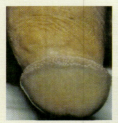

   a. Genital wart
   b. Pearly penile papule
   c. Balanitis
   d. Sebaceous gland prominence

8. The shown lesions are:

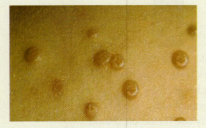

   a. Molluscum contagiosum
   b. Chicken pox
   c. Pemphigus
   d. Common warts

9. Identify condition in the shown image:
   (Recent Pattern Question 2018-19)

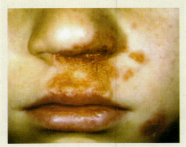

   a. Impetigo
   b. Chickenpox
   c. Pemphigus
   d. Traumatic crust

10. Common neurological tumour associated with NF-2:
    (Recent Pattern Question 2018-19)
    a. Acoustic neuroma
    b. Optic glioma
    c. Café-Au-Lait macules
    d. Meningioma

11. What are these colored divisions on body called:
    (Recent Pattern Question 2018-19)

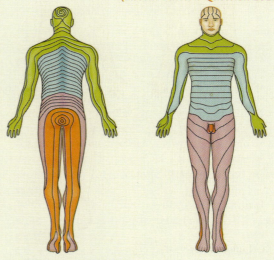

    a. Lymphatic development
    b. Dermatomes
    c. Blaschko Lines
    d. Vascular development

12. Which of the following is NOT seen in congenital syphilis:
    (Recent Pattern Question 2018-19)
    a. Maculopapular skin lesion
    b. Hutchison teeth
    c. Bow legs
    d. Gumma ulcers

13. Which of the following is used for treatment of Vitiligo?
    (Recent Pattern Question 2018-19)
    a. Retinoids
    b. Systemic steroids
    c. Psoralen PUVA
    d. Nd-YAG laser

14. Tzanck smear as shown in the image shows:

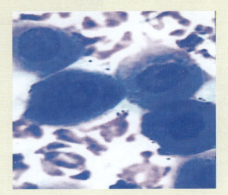

    a. Acanthosis
    b. Acantholytic cells
    c. Smudge cells
    d. Anaplasia

FMGE Solutions Screening Examination

15. Name the horizontal lines shown in the image:
    (Recent Pattern Question 2018-19)

    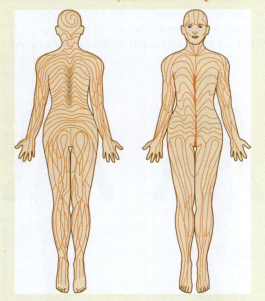

    a. Langer lines
    b. Blaschko lines
    c. Kraissl lines
    d. Borges lines

16. In which condition is Nikolsky's sign positive and bulla spread sign seen? *(Recent Pattern Question 2018)*
    a. Dermatitis herpetiformis
    b. Pemphigus vulgaris
    c. Bullous pemphigoid
    d. Erythema multiforme

17. Identify the given image: *(Recent Pattern Question 2018)*

    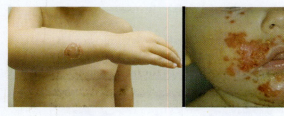

    a. Chicken pox
    b. Eczema
    c. Molluscum contagiosum
    d. Impetigo

18. Fordyce's spots involves: *(Recent Pattern Question 2018)*
    a. Sweat gland
    b. Mucus gland
    c. Sebaceous gland
    d. Moll glands

19. The shown image is the causative agent for:
    (Recent Pattern Question 2018)

    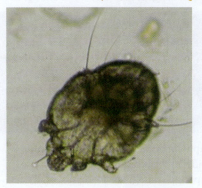

    a. Scabies
    b. Pediculosis
    c. Molluscum contagiosum
    d. Pthirus pubis

20. Identify the type of nevus:
    (Recent Pattern Question 2018)

    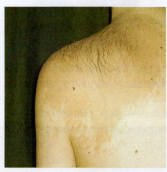

    a. Café au lait macule
    b. Plexiform neurofibroma
    c. Becker nevus
    d. Nevus of Ota

21. Identify the lesion on trunk:
    (Recent Pattern Question 2018)

    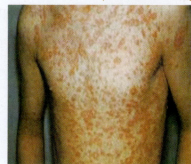

    a. Pityriasis alba
    b. Pityriasis rosea
    c. Pityriasis versicolor
    d. Chicken pox

Dermatology

22. Possible diagnosis based on wood lamp examination?
    (Recent Pattern Question 2017)

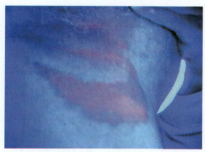

   a. Psoriasis
   b. Erythrasma
   c. Pityriasis versicolor
   d. Tinea versicolor

23. Identify the type of nevus: *(Recent Pattern Question 2017)*

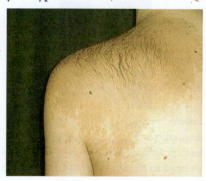

   a. Becker nevus
   b. Nevus of ota
   c. Café au lait macule
   d. Plexiform neurofibroma

24. Identify the lesion present on trunk of patient:
    (Recent Pattern Question 2017)

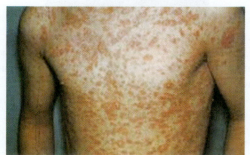

   a. Pityriasis alba
   b. Pityriasis rosea
   c. Pityriasis versicolor
   d. Pityriasis rubra pilaris

25. A middle age patient presented to you with the shown type of baldness. Diagnosis: *(Recent Pattern Question 2017)*

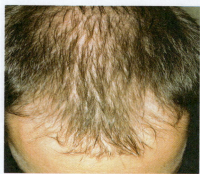

   a. Alopecia areata
   b. Telogen effluvium
   c. Male pattern baldness
   d. Cicatricial hair loss

26. Pemphigus foliaceous is a condition which is seen due to antibody against: *(Recent Pattern Question 2017)*
   a. Desmoglein 1   b. Desmoglein 2
   c. Desmoglein 3   d. Desmoglein 4

27. Pemphigus vulgaris can be seen due to antibodies against desmosomal cadherin cell binding protein:
    (Recent Pattern Question 2017)
   a. Desmoglein 1   b. Desmoglein 3
   c. Both   d. None

28. Row of tombstone is seen in which skin disorder:
   a. Pemphigus vulgaris *(Recent Pattern Question 2017)*
   b. Pemphigus foliaceous
   c. Paraneoplastic pemphigus
   d. Bullous pemphigoid

29. The shown immunofluroscence pattern in skin biopsy is suggestive of: *(Recent Pattern Question 2017)*

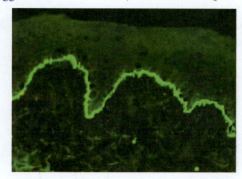

   a. Pemphigus vulgaris
   b. Pemphigus foliaceous
   c. Paraneoplastic pemphigus
   d. Bullous pemphigoid

FMGE Solutions Screening Examination

30. Identify the lesion: *(Recent Pattern Question 2017)*

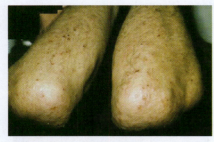

   a. Erythema marginatum
   b. Dermatitis herpetiformis
   c. Psoriasis
   d. Dermatomyositis

31. Hertoghie's sign is seen in:
   (Recent Pattern Question 2017)
   a. Contact dermatitis   b. Atopic dermatitis
   c. Seborrheic dermatitis d. Neurodermatitis

32. A young girl having low intelligence presented as shown below. There is history of epilepsy. Diagnosis:

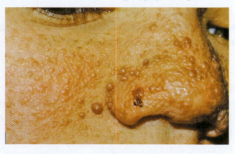

   a. Neurofibromatosis   *(Recent Pattern Question 2017)*
   b. Tuberous sclerosis
   c. Systemic lupus eythematous
   d. Systemic sclerosis

33. A patient presented with blue marks on face as shown in image. Most likely diagnosis:
   (Recent Pattern Question 2017)

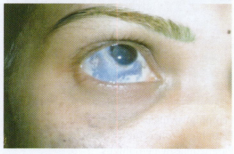

   a. Nevus Ito
   b. Nevus ota
   c. Blue nevus
   d. Tuberous sclerosis

34. A patient presented with lesions in interdigital clefts. The oral drug used is? *(Recent Pattern Question 2017)*

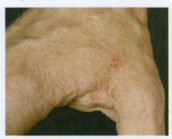

   a. Permethrin   b. Ivermectin
   c. Benzyl benzoate d. Sulphur

35. A baby presents with fever, erythema around face and rash all over body. Treatment to be initiated:
   (Recent Pattern Question 2017)

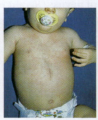

   a. Acyclovir   b. Valcyclovir
   c. Raltegravir   d. Antipyretics

36. A patient presents with lesion on occipitotemporal region of head as shown in image. Possible diagnosis:
   (Recent Pattern Question 2017)

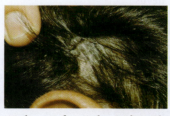

   a. Dermatitis herpeteformis b. Lichen planus
   c. Tinea captitis   d. Traumatic alopecia

37. Patient presented with patchy rash involving trunk and back as shown in image. Diagnosis is?
   (Recent Pattern Question 2017)

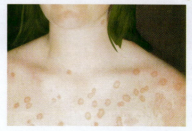

   a. Candida   b. Tinea corporis
   c. Tinea versicolor d. Tinea capitis

Dermatology

38. Possible diagnosis is? *(Recent Pattern Question 2017)*

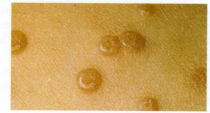

   a. Molluscum contagiosum b. Pityriasis versicolor
   c. Pityriasis rosea   d. Tinea corporis

39. A 60-year-old lady presents with lesion on upper eyelid as shown in image. Diagnosis is?
   (Recent Pattern Question 2017)

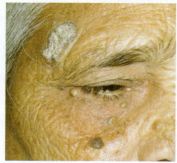

   a. Kerato-acanthoma   b. Basal cell cancer
   c. Bowen' disease   d. Psoriasis

40. A hypothyroid female patient presents with alopecia. Diagnosis is? *(Recent Pattern Question 2017)*
   a. Alopecia areata   b. Androgenic alopecia
   c. Telogen effluvium d. Traumatic alopecia

41. Acrodermatitis enterohepatica occurs due to?
   (Recent Pattern Question 2017)
   a. Copper deficiency b. Zinc deficiency
   c. Iron deficiency   d. Folic acid deficiency

42. Malassezia furfur is a causative organism for:
   (Recent Pattern Question 2017)
   a. Tinea versicolor   b. Tenia coli
   c. Tinea capitis   d. Tinea corporis

43. In the shown lesion scratching leads to bleeding followed by further formation of similar lesion is suggestive of?
   (Recent Pattern Question 2017)

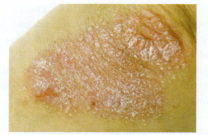

   a. Pityriasis versicolor b. Psoriasis
   c. Lichen vulgaris   d. Psoriasis

44. 25-year-old Truck driver with repeated Herpes infection presents with following skin lesions. Diagnosis is:
   (Recent Pattern Question 2017)

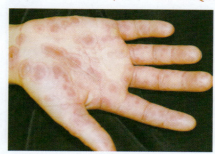

   a. Hand foot mouth disease b. Steven Johnson syndrome
   c. Erythema multiforme   d. Dermatitis herpetiformis

45. True about chickenpox rash are all EXCEPT:
   (Recent Pattern Question 2016)
   a. Superficial   b. Pleomorphic
   c. Centripetal   d. Palms and soles involved

46. A 25-year-old patient present with violaceous lesion on arms. What is the likely diagnosis:
   (Recent Pattern Question 2016)

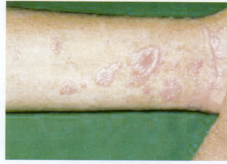

   a. Psoriasis   b. Pityriasis rosea
   c. Lichen planus   d. Dermatophytosis

47. What is the diagnosis of the given image?
   (Recent Pattern Question 2016)

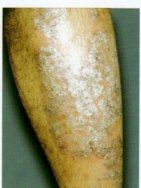

   a. Lichen planus   b. Lichenoid dermatitis
   c. Psoriasis   d. Pityriasis rosea

FMGE Solutions Screening Examination

48. Best treatment of 24-year-old female with the following lesions? *(Recent Pattern Question 2016)*

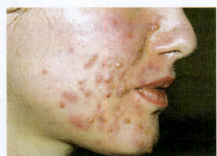

   a. Steroids
   b. Isotretinoin
   c. Tetracycline
   d. Erythromycin

49. Patient present with axillary frecking (as shown in image). Diagnosis: *(Recent Pattern Question 2016)*

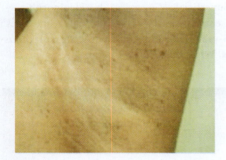

   a. Neurofibromatosis
   b. Tuberous sclerosis
   c. Ichthyosis vulgaris
   d. Von Hippel–Landau

50. What is the likely diagnosis? *(Recent Pattern Question 2016)*

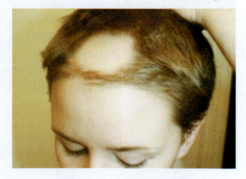

   a. Alopecia areata
   b. Androgenic alopecia
   c. Telogen effluvium
   d. Tinea capitis

51. Sunscreen lotion contains: *(Recent Pattern Question 2016)*
   a. Mercury
   b. Selenium
   c. Sulfide
   d. Zinc oxide

52. Average weight of skin:
   a. 5 kg
   b. 10 kg
   c. 15 kg
   d. 18 kg

53. Deepest layer of epidermis:
   a. Stratum corneum
   b. Stratum spinosum
   c. Stratum granulosum
   d. Stratum germinatum

54. Synthesis of keratin mainly takes place in this layer of epidermis:
   a. Stratum basale
   b. Stratum cornuem
   c. Stratum cranulosum
   d. Stratum spinosum

55. Hyperkeratosis is:
   a. Thinning of stratum corneum
   b. Thickening of stratum corneum
   c. Thinning of stratum basale
   d. Thickening of stratum basale

56. Odland bodies are seen in this layer of epidermis:
   a. Stratum cornuem
   b. Stratum granulosum
   c. Stratum spinosum
   d. Stratum basale

57. Principal cell of epidermis:
   a. Melanocytes
   b. Langerhan cell
   c. Keratinocytes
   d. Merkel cell

58. Langerhan cell present in which layer of epidermis:
   a. Basale
   b. Cornuem
   c. Granulosum
   d. Spinosum

59. Merkel cells are present in which of the following layers on epidermis:
   a. Basale
   b. Cornuem
   c. Granulosum
   d. Spinosum

60. Acantholysis is:
   a. Lysis of basale cell layer
   b. Separation of keratinocytes
   c. Thickening of granular layer
   d. Thickening of corneum layer

61. Acanthosis is:
   a. Separation of keratinocytes
   b. Thickening of granular layer
   c. Thickening of corneum layer
   d. Thickening of prickle cell layer

62. Parakeratosis is:
   a. Absence of nucleus in stratum corneum
   b. Persistence of nucleus in stratum corneum
   c. Thickening of corneum layer
   d. Thickening of prickle cell layer

63. Skin turnover time in case of psoriasis:
   a. 2 days
   b. 4 days
   c. 8 days
   d. 10 days

64. A person starts to sweat on forehead and gets a runny watery nose whenever he eats hot and spicy meals. This kind of sweating is:
   a. Mental sweating
   b. Physical sweating
   c. Thermogenic sweating
   d. Gustatory sweating

65. True about fordyce spot:
   a. Axilla is most common site
   b. Lips are most common site
   c. Blockage of eccrine gland ducts
   d. Blockage of apocrine gland ducts

Dermatology

66. **Most common site of fordyces spot:**
    a. Lips
    b. Below tongue
    c. Axilla
    d. Groin

67. **True about macule:**
    a. Flat lesion >2 cm
    b. Flat lesion <2 cm
    c. Elevated lesion >2 cm
    d. Elevated lesion <2 cm

68. **Size of papule:**
    a. <5 cm
    b. <5 mm
    c. <0.5 mm
    d. <0.05 cm

69. **A papule that is raised, non-purulent is most probably due to:**
    a. Insect bite
    b. Urticaria
    c. Angioedema
    d. Erythema nodosum

70. **Green color at bruise site is due to:**
    a. Hemotidin
    b. Bilirubin
    c. Hemosiderin
    d. Biliverdin

71. **All of the following statements are true about Propniobacterium acnes EXCEPT:**
    a. Normal flora of skin
    b. Causes acne vulgaris
    c. Sulfur granules in the purulent sinuses are characteristic
    d. Can be found in G.I. tract also

72. **Deposition of IgA in dermoepidermal junction. What could be probable diagnosis:**
    a. Nummular eczema
    b. Pemphigus vulgaris
    c. Bullous pemphigoid
    d. Dermatitis herpetiformis

73. **Acantholytic cells are seen in?**
    a. Pemphigus vulgaris
    b. Bullous pemphigoid
    c. Cicatricial pemphigoid
    d. Dermatitis herpetiformis

74. **Pemphigus vulgaris is caused by:**
    a. Bacteria
    b. Virus
    c. Autoimmune
    d. Fungal

75. **Pemphigus bullae are located at:**
    a. Subepidermal
    b. Intraepidermal
    c. Subdermal
    d. All of the above

76. **Subepidermal lesions are seen in?**
    a. Pemphigus vulgaris
    b. Pemphigoid bullae
    c. Burns
    d. Bullous impetigo

77. **Intraepidermal bulla are seen in:**
    a. Bullous pemphigoid
    b. Pemphigus vulgaris
    c. Bullous impetigo
    d. Dermatitis herpetiformis

78. **All are true about pemphigus bullae except:**
    a. Flaccid bullae located intradermal area
    b. Nikolsky sign absent
    c. Usually involves mucosa
    d. Acantholysis present

79. **Intercellular antibodies deposition on immunofluorescence is seen in:**
    a. Psoriasis
    b. Pemphigus
    c. Pemphigoid
    d. Prophyria

80. **Drug of choice for dermatitis herpetiformis:**
    a. Dapsone
    b. Rifampicin
    c. Ketokonazole
    d. Azithromycin

81. **Darrier sign is seen in:**
    a. Atopic dermatitis
    b. Pemphigus vulgaris
    c. Urticaria pigmentosa
    d. Bullous pemphigoid

82. **Most common site of angioedema:**
    a. Hands
    b. Lips
    c. Skin
    d. Eyelid

83. **Angioedema is characterized by swelling of the**
    a. Subcutaneous tissue
    b. Epidermis
    c. Dermis
    d. Blood vessels

84. **All are true about Xeroderma Pigmentosa except:**
    a. Due to deficiency of IgA
    b. Has marked sensitivity to UV light
    c. Due to defective DNA repair
    d. Autosomal recessive

85. **Acrodermatitis enteropathica is due to deficiency of:**
    a. Iron
    b. Copper
    c. Zinc
    d. Magnesium

86. **All are true about Keloid except:**
    a. May be familial
    b. Appears mostly on sternum
    c. Subsides over time
    d. Hyperkeratotic

87. **Which of the following presents with hypopigmented patches:**
    a. Blue nevus
    b. Nevus ito
    c. Nevus becker
    d. Nevus Anemicus

88. **Dermatophytes are**
    a. Tinea versicolor
    b. Trichophyton rubrum
    c. Sporothrix
    d. All of the above

89. **Which of the following structure is affected by dermatophytes:**
    a. Skin
    b. Hair
    c. Nail
    d. All of the above

90. **Trichophyton infects:**
    a. Skin + nail
    b. Skin + hair
    c. Hair + nail
    d. Skin + hair + nail

91. **Which of the following infects skin and hair:**
    a. T. verrucosum
    b. M. Gypseum
    c. Both
    d. None

92. **A case of 12-years-old boy presents to you with boggy swelling and easily pluckable hair. What would be the probable diagnosis:**
    a. Lichen planus
    b. Tinea capitis
    c. Epidermophytosis
    d. Alopecia areata

93. **An adult male presented 4 weeks after intercourse with fever, rubbery consistency ulcer, inguinal lymphadenopathy. Causative organism:**
    a. LGV
    b. Syphillis
    c. Chancroid
    d. HIV

FMGE Solutions Screening Examination

94. Painful ulcer on glans penis is seen in:
    a. Syphilis
    b. Lymphogranuloma venerum
    c. Chancroid
    d. Chancre
95. School of fish appearance is seen in?
    a. Bacterial vaginosis
    b. Hemophilus Ducreyi
    c. Gonococcus
    d. Chlamydia
96. Moth eaten alopecia is caused by:
    a. Secondary syphilis
    b. Primary syphilis
    c. Tertiary syphilis
    d. Early relapsing syphilis
97. All cause genital ulcer except:
    a. Gonorrhoea
    b. Chancroid
    c. HSV
    d. LGV
98. Child with recurrent mouth ulcer which usually begin as a round yellowish elevated spot surrounded by a red halo and heals within 7–10 days:
    a. Gingivitis
    b. Aphthous ulcers
    c. Malignancy
    d. Herpetic ulcer
99. Alopecia areata is due to defect of this stage of hair growth:
    a. Anagen effluvium
    b. Telogen effluvium
    c. Catagen
    d. None
100. Infection caused by human papilloma virus is called as?
    a. Condylama lata
    b. Condyloma acuminata
    c. Verrucous wart
    d. Plantar wart
101. Which of the following is the causative organism of Verruca vulgaris:
    a. CMV
    b. Human immunodeficiency virus
    c. Human papilloma virus
    d. Ebstein barr virus
102. All of the following tests are used for diagnosis of leprosy EXCEPT:
    a. Clinical examination
    b. Lepromin test
    c. Slit skin smear
    d. Skin biopsy
103. Thalidomide is mostly effective in:
    a. Nerve Abscess
    b. Type I Lepra reaction
    c. Type II Lepra reaction
    d. Both type I and II leprae reaction
104. TB presents with all of the following skin conditions, except:
    a. Lupus vulgaris
    b. Scrofuloderma
    c. Erythema nodosum
    d. Lichen scrofulosorum
105. Lichen planus is associated with:
    a. Koilonychia
    b. Tinea versicolor
    c. Psoriasis
    d. Pterygium of nail
106. Bandlike infiltrate of lymphocytes at the dermoepidermal junction, and "saw-tooth" rete ridges are diagnostic histological features of:
    a. Lichen planus
    b. Lupus erythematosus
    c. Psoriasis vulgaris
    d. Seborrhoeic dermatitis
107. Treatment of choice in severe cystic acne:
    a. Isotretinoin
    b. Tretinoin
    c. Benzoyl peroxide
    d. Azelaic acid
108. Oral treatment of acne is:
    a. Ivermectin
    b. Benzyl peroxide
    c. Doxycycline
    d. Adapalene
109. Target or Iris lesion are seen in:
    a. Urticaria
    b. Erythema multiformae
    c. Scabies
    d. Lichen planus
110. Annular herald patch is seen in:
    a. Lichen planus
    b. Psoriasis
    c. Pityriasis alba
    d. Pityriasis rosea
111. Pityriasis alba is a type of:
    a. Vitiligo
    b. Atopic eczema
    c. Photoallergy
    d. Infection
112. A girl presented with the lesions shown below: treatment of choice:

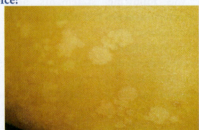

    a. Topical imidazole
    b. Terbinafine
    c. Fluconazole
    d. Selenium sulphide
113. Pityriasis Versicolor is caused by:
    a. Tinea rubrum
    b. Malassezia furfur
    c. Tinea capitis
    d. Varicella
114. Nikolsky sign is seen in:
    a. Herpes simples
    b. Herpes zoster
    c. Pemphigus vulgaris
    d. All of the above
115. Diagnose the following:

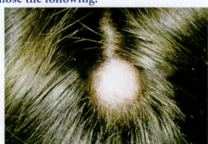

    a. Melanoma
    b. Sebaceous cyst
    c. Basal cell carcinoma
    d. Papulo-squamous disorder
116. Erythrasma is caused by
    a. Corynebacterium minutissimum
    b. Corynebacterium Jeikeium
    c. Corynebacterium parvum
    d. Corynebacterium amycolatum

BOARD REVIEW QUESTIONS

Dermatology

117. Substance common in skin, hair and nail is?
- a. Vimentin
- b. Keratin
- c. Laminin
- d. Nectin

118. Stratum lucidum is present between which two layers?
- a. Corneum and granulosum
- b. Granulosum and spinosum
- c. Spinous and basale
- d. Basal and subbasale

119. Which of the following is not a component of sebum?
- a. Cholesterol
- b. Wax
- c. Glycerides
- d. Propylene

120. Which of the following drug causes pigmentation of skin?
- a. Minocycline
- b. Penicillin
- c. Furosemide
- d. Amefostine

121. Most common cause of TEN?
- a. Drugs
- b. Herpes simplex
- c. Autoimmune
- d. Porphyria

122. Diascopy is done for?
- a. Change in color of lesion on wood's light exposure
- b. Scraping of lesion for KOH mount
- c. Change in color of lesion on pressure with glass slide
- d. Aspiration of lesion for inflammatory exudates

123. Civatte bodies are seen in
- a. Linchen planus
- b. Tinea cruris
- c. Psoariasis
- d. SSSS

124. Cradle cap is
- a. Atopic dermatitis
- b. Seborrheic dermatitis
- c. Vernix caseosa
- d. Urticarial dermatitis

125. Incorrect about scabies
- a. Burrows are pathognomonic
- b. Itch mites buries in stratum corneum
- c. High yield Lesions on palms and face
- d. Ivermectin blocks glutamate driven chloride lesions

126. Tinea corporis gladiatorum involves
- a. Glans penis
- b. Trunk
- c. Scalp
- d. Nails

127. Merkel cells are seen in
- a. Epidermis
- b. Dermis
- c. Hypodermis
- d. All of the above

128. First cutaneous manifestation in leprosy
- a. Hypopigmented macule
- b. Hypoanesthetic macule
- c. Painless bun in hand
- d. Inverse ptosis

129. Sausage digits are seen in
- a. Bronchiectasis
- b. Psoriatic arthritis
- c. Scleroderma
- d. Koenen tumors

130. Mechanic hands are seen in
- a. Guttate psoriasis
- b. Scleroderma
- c. Dermatomyositis
- d. Pustular psoriasis

131. Infection caused by human papilloma virus:
- a. Condylamalata
- b. Condyloma acuminata
- c. Verrucous wart
- d. Plantar wart

132. Thalidomide is mostly effective in:
- a. Nerve Abscess
- b. Type I Lepra reaction
- c. Type II Lepra reaction
- d. Both type I and II leprae reaction

133. Deposition of IgA in dermo-epidermal junction. What could be probable diagnosis:
- a. Nummular eczema
- b. Pemphigus vulgaris
- c. Bullous pemphigoid
- d. Dermatitis herpetiformis

134. Pathergy test is used for
- a. Sarcoidosis
- b. Scleroderma
- c. Behçet disease
- d. Kaposi sarcoma

135. Nikolsky sign is absent in
- a. Pemphigus vulgaris
- b. Bullous pemphigoid
- c. Toxic epidermal necrolysis
- d. Necrolytic migratory erythema

136. Target lesion are seen in
- a. Erythema multiforme
- b. TSS
- c. Acanthosisnigricans
- d. All of the above

137. Pterygium of nail is seen in?
- a. Psoriasis
- b. Pemphigus
- c. Pemphigoid
- d. Lichen planus

138. Oil drop sign of nail is seen in?
- a. Lichen planus
- b. Dermatophytes
- c. Lupus vulgaris
- d. Psoriasis

FMGE Solutions Screening Examination

139. Necrobiosis Lipoidica diabeticorum is seen in?
    a. Sarcoidosis   b. Renal cell carcinoma
    c. Diabetes mellitus   d. Leprosy
140. Darrier's sign is seen in?
    a. Urticaria pigmentosa b. Xanthogranuloma
    c. ALL   d. All of the above
141. Follicular hyperkeratosis is related to deficiency of?
    a. Vitamin A   b. Vitamin C
    c. Zinc   d. Vitamin E
142. Carpet track sign is seen in?
    a. Lupus vulgaris   b. Lupus pernio
    c. DLE   d. SLE
143. Fat is present in relation to which anatomical structure?
    a. Epidermis   b. Dermis
    c. Subcutaneous tissue d. Nail bed
144. Groove sign is seen in?
    a. Chancroid   b. Syphilis
    c. LGV   d. Psoriasis
145. Gottron's papules ae seen in?
    a. SLE   b. MTCD
    c. Dermatomyositis   d. Rheumatoid arthritis
146. Dry ice is?
    a. Methane hydrate   b. Liquid nitrogen
    c. Solid carbon dioxide d. Frozen water
147. Linear deposition of IgG and C3 in lamina lucida is seen in?
    a. Dermatitis herpetiformis
    b. Pemphigus vulgaris
    c. Pemphigus foliaceus
    d. Bullous pemphigoid
148. Tomb stone appearance is seen in?
    a. Bullous pemphigoid   b. Pemphigus vulgaris
    c. Linear IgA disease   d. Dermatitis herpetiformis
149. Wickham's striae is seen in?
    a. Lichen planus   b. Psoriasis
    c. Prurigo   d. DLE
150. Vagabond's disease is caused by?
    a. Scabies   b. Herpes genitalis
    c. Pediculosis corporis d. Ant bite reaction
151. Koebners phenomenon is seen in?
    a. Acne vulgaris   b. Pemphigus vulgaris
    c. Psoriasis   d. Ichthyosis
152. Obliteration of apocrine duct leads to?
    a. Fordyce's disease   b. Fox fordyce's disease
    c. Moll's gland   d. Pearly benign papules
153. Norwegian scabies is seen in?
    a. Children
    b. Pregnant women
    c. Patients on chemotherapy
    d. Infants
154. Groove sign is seen in?
    a. Chancroid   b. Syphilis
    c. LGV   d. Psoriasis
155. Melanocytes are located in which layer?
    a. Stratum malphigii
    b. Stratum basale
    c. Stratum corneum
    d. Stratum granulosum
156. Coarse pitting of nails is seen in?
    a. Psoriatic carthiritis
    b. Dermatitis herpetiformis
    c. Bullous pemphigoid
    d. Pemphigus vulgaris
157. Fungus causing hair skin and nail infection is?
    a. T. rubrum   b. E. floculossum
    c. M. Canis   d. M. Ayouni
158. Pathognomic lesion of scabies is?
    a. Papules   b. Vesicle
    c. Burrow   d. Pits
159. Christmas tree arrangement of skin lesion is seen in?
    a. P. versicolor   b. P. rosea
    c. P. folliculitis   d. Tineacorporis
160. Buschke ollendorf sign is seen in?
    a. Gonorrhoea   b. Congenital syphilis
    c. Secondary syphilis   d. Herpes genitalis
161. Salt and pepper skin is seen in?
    a. Dermatomyositis   b. SLE
    c. Scleroderma   d. Syphilis
162. Apple jelly nodules are seen in?
    a. Lupus vulgaris
    b. Scrofuloderma
    c. Chancre
    d. Atypical mycobacterial infection
163. Munro's micro abscess is seen in?
    a. Psoriasis   b. DLE
    c. Lichen planus   d. Mycosis fungoides
164. All are causes of erythema multiforme EXCEPT:
    a. Chronic renal failure
    b. Infectious mononucleosis
    c. Mycoplasma
    d. Collagen vascular disease
165. Saucer right side up is a characteristic feature of this type of leprosy:
    a. Borderline borderline b. Tuberculoid
    c. Borderline tuberculoid d. Intermediate
166. Swiss cheese lesion is a characteristic feature seen in this type of leprosy:
    a. Borderline borderline b. Tuberculoid
    c. Borderline tuberculoid d. Intermediate

Dermatology

IMAGE-BASED QUESTIONS

167. Identify the instrument

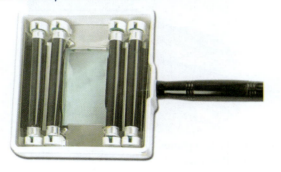

a. Infra-red lamp b. UV rays lamp
c. Wood lamp   d. Slit lamp

168. This finding is characteristic of?

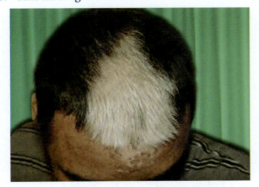

a. Leucoderma   b. Piebaldism
c. Nevus anemicus d. Nevus achromicus

169. This test is used is for diagnosis of ?

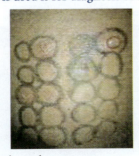

a. Behçet's syndrome
b. Contact dermatitis
c. Pyoderma gangreosum
d. Atopic dermatitis

170. These typical lesions are present in?

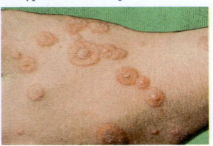

a. Pemphigus
b. Bullous pemphigoid
c. Erythema multiforme
d. Dermatitis herpetiformis

171. This classical presentation is of ?

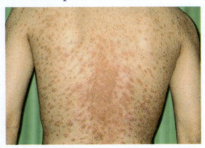

a. Pityriasis rosea
b. P. alba
c. P. rubra
d. P. versicolor

172. What is the treatment of choice for this condition?

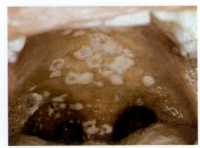

a. Anti-histaminic
b. Steroid
c. Clotrimazole paint
d. Selenium sulphide

173. All are correct about the lesion shown except?

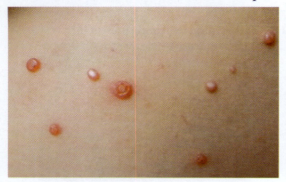

a. Molluscum contagiosum
b. Caused by RNA virus
c. Propagate via auto-inoculation
d. Not seen in soles or palms

176. The image shows?

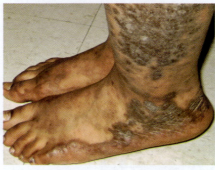

a. Lichen planus
b. Psoriasis
c. Tinea corporis
d. Pityriasis versicolor

174. A patient develops honey colored pustules on the skin. The diagnosis is?

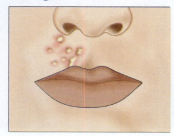

a. Impetigo
b. Staphylococcal scalded skin syndrome
c. Carbuncle
d. Sycosis barbae

177. The image shows which skin lesion?

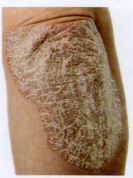

a. Lichen planus   b. Psoriasis
c. Tinea corporis   d. Pityriasis versicolor

175. The image shows?

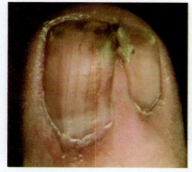

a. Pterygium nail   b. Tinea unguium
c. Botryomycosis   d. Onchomycosis

178. Multiple painful bleeding ulcers with inguinal bubo is seen with

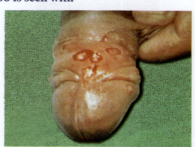

a. Chancre   b. Granuloma inguinale
c. Lymphogranuloma venerum
d. Chancroid

179. All are true about the lesions shown except?

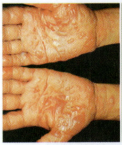
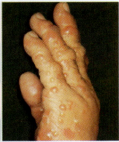

a. Itchy lesions on palms
b. Potent topical steroids resolve most cases
c. Associated with anhidrosis
d. Painful deep seated vesicles

182. The given image shows?

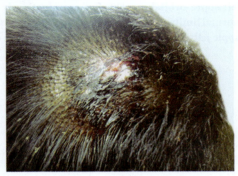

a. Favus
b. Kerion
c. Seborrheic
d. Scutula

180. The image shows presence of?

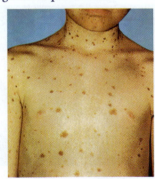

a. Lentiginosis
b. Freckles
c. Shagreen patch
d. Congenital nevus

183. Which of the following is not effective against this condition?

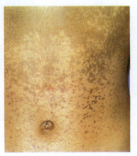

a. Topical ketoconazole
b. Griseofulvin
c. Topical selenium sulphide
d. Topical sulfur preparations

181. Identify the type of leprosy based on shown lesion:

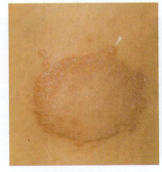

a. Borderline borderline
b. Tuberculoid
c. Borderline tuberculoid
d. Intermediate

184. All are true about the lesion shown *except*?

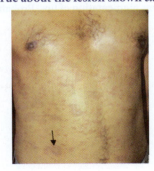

a. HHV-7
b. Herald patch
c. Predominantly occurs on genitals
d. Spontaneous healing

FMGE Solutions Screening Examination

185. A 25-year-old woman presents with skin lesion on left supra-orbital margin. Eye examination is within normal limits. CXR done was normal. Diascopy shows apple jelly nodules. The image shows presence of?

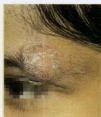

a. Lupus vulgaris b. Lupus Pernio
c. Erythema marginatum
d. Leprosy

186. The image shows presence of?

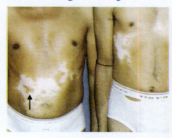

a. Vitiligo
b. Piebaldism
c. Xeroderma pigmentosum
d. Incontinentia pigmenti

187. A 20-year-old man with history of melena and abdominal pain has pigmentation of lips. Probable diagnosis is?

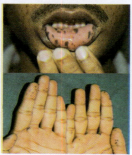

a. Incontinentia pigmenti
b. Cronkhite Canada syndrome
c. Brooke Spiegler syndrome
d. Peutz Jeghers syndrome

188. The image shows presence of?

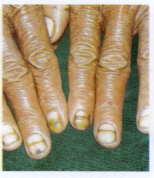

a. Muehrcke's nails b. Lindsay nails
c. Leukonychia d. Beau's lines

189. The image shows presence of?

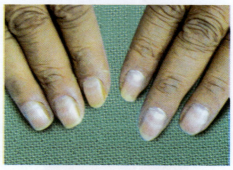

a. Muehrcke's nails b. Lindsay nails
c. Leukonychia d. Beau's lines

190. A 25-year-old young adult female presents with following lesions in axilla, as shown by the arrow:

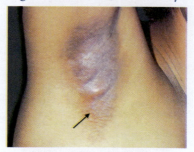

a. Hidradenitis suppurativa
b. Fordyce spot
c. Acne fulminans
d. Acne conglobate

Dermatology

191. The given KOH mount of patient shows?

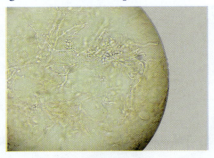

a. Spaghetti and meat ball appearance
b. Budding yeasts and pseudohyphae
c. Clusters of pigmented cells
d. Septate hyphae

194. A 28-year-old lady has asymptomatic dome shaped small lesions on a forehead for last 2 months. She has a 2-year-old daughter with similar lesions. What is the causative agent?

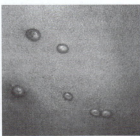

a. Papillomavirus b. Poxvirus
c. Herpes virus   d. Coxsackie virus

192. A 20-year-old patient presents with an extremely itchy lesion on one arm. Diagnosis is?

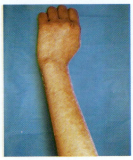

a. Tinea corporis   b. Tinea imbricata
c. Tinea incognito d. Tinea manuum

195. A patient after a trip to Bangkok developed fever and perioral vesicles. What is the diagnosis?

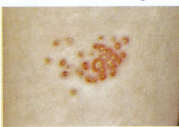

a. Herpes simplex
b. Impetigo
c. Molluscum contagiosum
d. Bullous pemphigoid

193. These lesions are seen in which of the following?

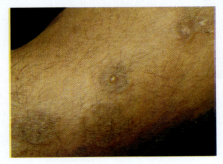

a. Erythema infectiosum
b. Erythema nodosum
c. Erythema induratum
d. Erythema multiforme

196. Identify the lesion:

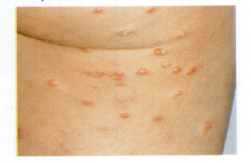

a. Molluscum contagiosum
b. Herpes simplex
c. Pityriasis rosea
d. Gianotti-Crosti syndrome

197. A 13-year-old boy presents with patchy depigmented skin on the right flank and upper thigh in segmental distribution. The depigmentation started 1 year back but has been static for last 4 months. Mother reports use of topical steroids which was ineffective. Diagnosis is?

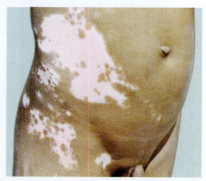

a. Piebaldism
b. Segmental vitiligo
c. Hypomelanosis of Ito
d. Hypopigmented streaks

198. Identify the lesion:

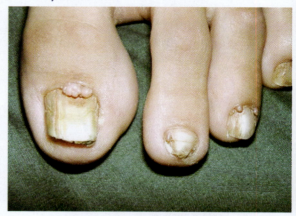

a. Koenen tumor
b. Onychomycosis
c. Onychodystrophy
d. Onychogryphosis

199. All of the following statements regarding this image are true *EXCEPT*:

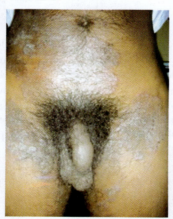

a. Dhobi itch
b. Jock itch
c. More common in tropics
d. Caused by *Candida*

Answers to Image-Based Questions are given at the end of explained questions

Dermatology

ANSWERS WITH EXPLANATIONS

1137

MOST RECENT QUESTIONS 2019

1. Ans. (a) SLE

Ref: Harrison 20th ed. page 2518-2519

- The image shows an erythematous rash sparing the nasolabial folds which coupled with clinical history points to diagnosis of SLE.
- Choice B leads to heliotrope rash involving the upper eye lid and proximal muscle weakness.
- Choice C presents as grey-brown patches, usually on the face on the cheeks, bridge of the nose, forehead, chin, and above the upper lip. It can also appear on sun-exposed parts of body, such as the forearms and neck.
- Choice D presents as redness, and can slowly spread beyond the nose and cheeks to the forehead and chin. There will be flushing, visible blood vessels and acne like breakouts.

2. Ans. (a) Acanthosis nigricans

Ref: Fitzpatrick Colour Atlas and Synopsis of Clinical Dermatology page 88

- The image shows presence of *asymmetric, velvety hyperpigmentation* at the back of the neck of the patient suggestive of diagnosis of acanthosis nigricans. It is seen in patients with impaired glucose tolerance and internal malignancy.
- Choice B is seen in patients with internal malignancy but has multiple pigmented skin lesions.
- Choice C is a crusty, scaly growth caused by damage from exposure to ultraviolet (UV) radiation.
- Choice D has red inflamed lesions and is hence ruled out.

3. Ans. (c) Bilaterally symmetrical dermatomal vesicular eruption

Ref: Harrison 20th ed. page 1355

- The image shows lesions of Herpes Zoster that develop unilaterally in a single dermatome.
- Choice A is correct since seronegative individuals on contact with these patients can develop chicken pox.
- Choice B is correct since neurological complication can develop in the form of meningoencephalitis.
- Choice D is correct since Ramsay Hunt syndrome leads to eruption in external auditory canal and the geniculate ganglion of sensory division of facial nerve is involved.

4. Ans. (c) Humby's knife

- The shown instrument is used in plastic surgery for skin feeling during grafting procedure. The instrument is Humby's knife.

5. Ans. (a) Intralesional steroids

- In patients with recurrent keloids, intralesional steroids are often very effective.
- Uniform protocol of corticosteroid injections and ointment application reduces recurrence rate of keloid drastically.
- Book says: "Intralesional steroids have been the mainstay of treatment of keloids"
- MC used steroid: Triamcinolone acetonide in concentration 10–40 mg/mL, administered intra-lesionally with 25–27 G needle at 4–6 weeks interval.
- Other modalities that can be used (less effective)
  - Silicon gel sheets and silicone occlusive dressing
  - Topical corticosteroid impregnated tape
  - Cryotherapy
  - Radiation therapy

6. Ans. (a) Staphylococcal scalded skin syndrome

- Staphylococcal Scalded Skin Syndrome aka Dermatitis Exfoliativa Neonatorum
- **Cause:** Toxin producing Staph Aureus (exfoliative toxins A and B)
- **Characterized** by erythema and widespread loss of superficial epidermal layers, resembling burn
- **Symptoms:**
  - After staphylococcal infection like otitis, pharyngitis or conjunctivitis → fever with ery-thema resembling scarlet fever
  - It later becomes small unstable blisters → erodes quickly and leads to widespread skin loss (generalized).
  - Blister contains stratum corneum (in TEN, full thickness epidermal damage), subcorneal blisters and acantholysis.
- **Treatment**: Fluid replacement + Antibiotics

7. Ans. (b) Pearly penile papule

Ref: Dermatology Essentials E-Book, P 936

- The shown condition is pearly penile papule (PPP)
- Patients with pearly penile papule usually present with concern that they might have genital warts.
- PPP are benign, 1–2 mm dome shaped spots, asymptomatic angiofibromas that occur in rows, circumferentially around the coronal sulcus of penis.

Explanations

- **Incidence:** 8–30%; MC in 3rd decade
- Mostly seen in circumcised males. It is not related to HPV
- **NOTE:** Warts are not as linear or as clearly defined as PPP.
- **Treatment:**
  - Usually not required; Reassurance
  - For lesion removal: Podophyllin application, cryotherapy, Electrodesiccation and curettage and CO_2 laser.

Extra Mile

- **Balanitis:** It is inflammation of glans of penis or prepuce due to poor personal hygiene by Candida species, streptococci, HPV, HSV, Gardnerella etc.

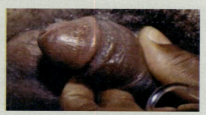

BALANITIS

- Sebaceous gland prominence

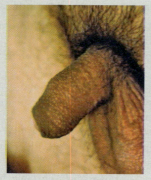

- Psoriasis of glans and shaft of penis

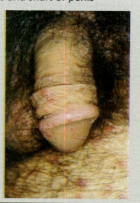

8. Ans. (a) Molluscum contagiosum

- Molluscum contagiosum caused by large DNA virus of pox group.
- Characterized by multiple, umbilicated pearly lesion
- More common in childhood and on face
- It tends to resolve spontaneously
- Lesion occurring on genitalia or lower abdomen in adult are almost always sexually transmitted.
- **HPE:** Molluscum bodies—multinucleated giant cell in the central keratinous core of lesion of giemsa stain.
- **Treatment:** Cryotherapy or KOH or Phenol application

9. Ans. (a) Impetigo

Ref: Pediatric Dermatology E book by Lawrence Schachner p 1338

- Impetigo is a highly contagious bacterial infection of superficial layer of epidermis.
- **MCC:** *Staphylococcus aureus* and *Streptococcus*.
- **It occurs in two forms:**
  1. **Non-bullous impetigo:** Caused by *Staphylococcus aureus*. Most commonly affects child age group and characterized by honey colored crust (*as seen in this patient*).
  2. **Bullous impetigo:** Can be caused by *Staphylococcus aureus* or *Streptococcus*. Common in all age groups.

10. Ans. (a) Acoustic neuroma

Ref: Neurofibromatoses in Clinical Practice, P 47-48

- Neurofibromatosis is a type of autoimmune skin disorder, and is associated with several other systemic conditions/tumors.
- Acoustic neuroma is the most common neural tumor associated with NF-2

TABLE: Differences between NF1 and NF2

NF1	NF2
Common (90% of all NF cases)	Much less common (10% of all NF cases)
Chromosome 17 mutations	Chromosome 22 mutations
Almost always diagnosed by age 10	Usually diagnosed in second to fourth decades
Cutaneous lesions common (>95%) - Cafe au lait spots - Lisch nodules - Cutaneous NFs (often multiple) - Plexiform NFs (pathognomonic)	Cutaneous, eye lesions less prominent - Mild/few cafe au lait spots Juvenile subcapsular opacities

Contd...

Dermatology

NF1	NF2

• CNS lesions less common (15-20%)
  ▪ T2/FLAIR hyperintensities (myelin vacuolization; lesions wax, then wane)
  ▪ Astrocytomas (optic pathway gliomas—usually pilocytic—other gliomas)
  ▪ Sphenoid wing, dural dysplasias
  ▪ Moyamoya
  ▪ Neurofibromas of spinal nerve roots
	• CNS lesions in 100%
	  ▪ Bilateral vestibular schwannomas (almost all)
	  ▪ Nonvestibular schwannomas (50%)
	  ▪ Meningiomas (50%)
	  ▪ Cord ependymomas (often multiple)
	  ▪ Schwannomas of spinal nerve roots

Extra Mile

Diagnostic criteria of NF1

Two or more of the following:
- At least six café-au-lait macules (>5 mm diameter in prepubertal individuals and >15 mm in postpubertal individuals)
- Freckling in axillary or inguinal regions
- Optic glioma
- At least two Lisch nodules (iris hamartomas)
- At least two neurofibromas of any type, or one plexiform neurofibroma
- A distinctive osseous lesion (sphenoid dysplasia or tibial pseudarthrosis)
- A first degree relative with NF1

TABLE: Diagnostic criteria for NF-2

Main criteria
Bilateral vestibular schwannomas or
First-degree relative with neurofibromatosis type 2 plus 1. Unilateral vestibular schwannomas or 2. Any two of the following: Meningioma, glioma, schwannoma, or juvenile posterior lenticular opacities

11. Ans. (b) Dermatome

Ref: PubMed

- The shown division is dermatomal division
- Dermatome is the area of the skin of the human anatomy that is mainly supplied by branches of a single spinal sensory root.

- Blaschko lines or the lines of Blaschko are thought to represent pathways of epidermal cell migration and proliferation during the development of the fetus.
- These lines are invisible but many inherited and acquired diseases of skin manifest themselves according to these patterns creating the visual appearance of these lines.

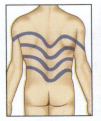 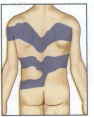
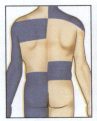 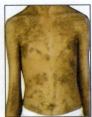

12. Ans. (c) Bow legs

Ref: Avery's Neonatology: Pathophysiology & Management of the New born, P 1040-41

FEATURES OF CONGENITAL SYPHILIS:

- Skin lesion: Maculopapular rash
- Hepatosplenomegaly and lymphadenopathy
- Failure to thrive
- Anaemia, jaundice
- Gummatous ulcer
- Saddle nose, prominent forehead
- Interstitial keratitis
- CN-VIII involvement: SNHL
- Syphilitic rhinitis- purulent nasal discharge
- Dental deformities: Hutchinson's teeth

Extra Mile

Hutchinson triad:
- Interstitial keratitis
- SNHL
- Hutchinson teeth

13. Ans. (c) Psoralen PUVA

Ref: Bhutani Atlas of Dermatology, 6th ed. pg. 209-210

- Vitiligo is an acquired autoimmune condition targeting melanocytes and presents with localized or widespread white depigmented patches.
- Thyroid dysfunction is the most common association.

TREATMENT OF VITILIGO

- Mainstay of therapy: Psoralen with UVA (PUVA)
- No therapy is effective alone
  - Topicals
    - Corticosteroids
    - Immunomodulators

FMGE Solutions Screening Examination

- Light Therapy:
  - UVA or UVB 2
  - UVA + Psoralen = PUVA (Topical and Systemic)
  - UVB = Laser
- Systemic Treatment: NOT USED
- Surgical Rx:
  - Melanocyte Transplant
  - Skin Grafts Transplant
- Bleaching Agents: Depigment all skin

14. Ans. (b) Acantholytic cells

Ref: Fitzpatrick Colour Atlas, 8th ed. pg. 681

- The image shows Acantholytic cells with ground glass nuclei consistent with tzanck cells.
- *Acantholysis is defined as the loss of coherence between epidermal cells due to the breakdown of their intercellular bridges.* In contrast Acanthosis implies thickening of skin due to diffuse epidermal hyperplasia.

Extra Mile

- **Hyperkeratosis:** Hyperplasia of the stratum corneum with abnormal keratin.
- **Papillomatosis:** Surface elevation caused by hyperplasia and enlargement of dermal papillae.
- **Parakeratosis:** Keratinization characterized by retention of the nuclei in the stratum corneum. On squamous mucosal membranes, such as buccal mucosa parakeratosis is normal.
- **Spongiosis:** Intercellular edema of the epidermis

15. Ans. (b) Blaschko lines

Ref: Fitzpatrick Dermatology, 9th ed. pg. 302

- The image shows lines of Blaschko which represent a pattern assumed by many different nevoid and acquired skin diseases on the human skin and mucosae.
- They represent *normal developmental growth pattern of skin*
- These lines do not correspond to any known nervous, vascular or lymphatic structures.
- *Langer's lines* correspond to alignment of *collagen fibers* in the dermis. They are used to determine direction with the human skin along which the skin has the least flexibility.
- *Kraissl lines* differ from Langer's lines in that unlike Langer's lines, which are defined in term of collagen orientation, Kraissl's lines are oriented *perpendicular to the action of the underlying muscles.*
- *Borges lines are relaxed skin tension lines.* The relaxation is achieved by joint mobilization, muscle contraction, or pinching.

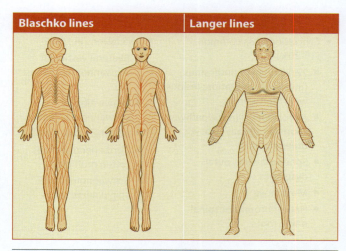

16. Ans. (b) Pemphigus vulgaris

Ref: TB of Dermatology, leprology & Venereology Devinder Mohan Thappa E book Chapter 4

- **Pemphigus vulgaris:** The antibodies are directed against Desmoglein 3 (*which binds the epidermal cells together*), causing loss of cell to cell adhesion.
  - In mucosal *Proteus vulgaris*: Antibody against only DSG3
  - In mucocutaneous *P. vulgaris*: Antibody against DSG 1 and 3
- **Upon examination and HPE following findings are seen:**
  - Bulla spread sign, Nikolsky's sign, acantholytic cells.
  - HPE shows suprabasal blister with row of tomb stone appearance.
  - Direct immunofluorescence shows intraepidermal IgG deposits in fishnet pattern.

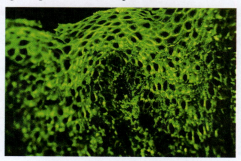

- **Bullous pemphigoid:** Most common autoimmune bullous disease. Presence of large, tense bullae. Common in elderly.
- **Dermatitis herpetiformis:** Gluten sensitive enteropathy. Very commonly (70–100%) have coeliac disease. Its dermal manifestation is severe itching. HPES shows IgA deposited in dermal papilla.
  - **Rx:** Gluten free diet and dapsone (DOC) is used for treatment.

Dermatology

- **Erythema multiforme:** Most commonly caused by HSV virus. Others causes can be malignancy, drug, mycoplasma, idiopathic. Has a characteristic target lesion.

> **Extra Mile**

TABLE: Autoimmune bullous diseases—target antigens

Disease	Target antigens
Pemphigus foliaceus	Desmoglein 1
Herpetiform pemphigus	Desmoglein 1
IgA pemphigus (SPD type)	Desmocollin 1
IgA pemphigus (IEN type)	Desmoglein 1 or 3
Pemphigus vulgaris	Desmoglein 3
Epidermolysis bullosa acquisita	Type VII collagen

17. Ans. (d) Impetigo

Ref: Pediatric Dermatology E book by Lawrence schachner p 1338

- Impetigo is a highly contagious bacterial infection of superficial layer of epidermis. It is caused most commonly by *Staphylococcus aureus* and *Streptococcus*.
- It occurs in 2 forms:
  - **Non-bullous impetigo:** Caused by *Staphylococcus aureus*. Most commonly affects child age group and characterized by honey colored crust (*as seen in this patient*).
  - **Bullous impetigo:** Can be caused by *Staphylococcus aureus* or *Streptococcus*. Common in all age groups.

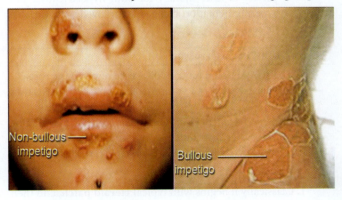

18. Ans. (c) Sebaceous gland

Ref: Illustrated Synopsis of Dermatology & Sexually transmitted diseases E book by Neena Khanna P123

- Fordyce spot is ectopic sebaceous gland.
- **Most common site:** Upper lip and buccal mucosa.
- Usually asymptomatic condition. No treatment required.

> **Extra Mile**

- **Fox Fordyce disease:** Keratin obstruction of apocrine ducts
- **Hidradenitis suppurativa:** Keratin obstruction of apocrine ducts extending into hair follicles. Also known as inverse acne.
  - Most common site axilla.
- **Acne vulgaris:** Obstruction of pilosebaceous gland.
- **Miliaria:** Occlusion of eccrine gland due to *Staphylococcus epidermidis*.

19. Ans. (a) Scabies

Ref: Illustrated Synopsis of Dermatology & Sexually transmitted diseases E book by Neena Khanna P 14-15

- Scabies is a contagious skin infestation caused commonly by female mite sarcoptes scabiei (*the shown image*).
- Incubation period 3-4 weeks.
- **In infant scabies:** Face, palms and soles involved.
- S shaped burrow is pathognomonic of scabies infestation.
- Adult scabies spares face.
- Scabies is one of the water washed disease, involves axillae, elbow, flexures, wrist, finger, webs, umbilicus, lower abdomen and genitalia. These involved areas if joined with an intersecting lines is known as circle of hebra.
- **DOC:** 5% permethrin.
- **Oral DOC for scabies:** Ivermectin.

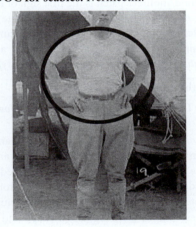

Circle of hebra

> **Extra Mile**

- **Pediculosis (vagabond disease)**
  1. Head louse : *P. capitis*
  2. Body louse : *P. corporis*
  3. Pubic/crab louse : Pthirus pubis DOC is 1% permethrin.
- **Molluscum Contagiosum**
  - Caused by Pox virus. Pearly white papules with umbilication. Common in children on face. Inclusion body known as molluscum body or *Henderson Peterson body*.

FMGE Solutions Screening Examination

20. Ans. (c) Becker nevus

Ref: Illustrated Synopsis of Dermatology & Sexually transmitted diseases E book by Neena Khanna P35

- Becker's nevus, also called pigmented hairy epidermal nevus, is a cutaneous hamartoma that can have increased epidermal (melanocyte), dermal (smooth muscle), and appendageal (hair follicle) components.
- Classically, Becker's nevus is first noticed around puberty on the shoulders and chest in males. The prevalence in postpubertal males is approximated to be 0.5%, or 1 in 200.
- It may involve only surface of body in women.

Note:
- **Nevus of Ota:** Seen usually around eyes.
- Café au lait macule is light brown macule commonly seen on trunk and has smooth edges.

21. Ans. (b) Pityriasis rosea

Ref: Illustrated Synopsis of Dermatology & Sexually transmitted diseases E book by Neena Khanna P39

- Pityriasis rosea is a noncontagious, erythematous skin lesion, caused by human herpesvirus 6 and 7.
- Classically it begins with typical **Herald patch** (single red and scaly), and then becomes generalized patch.
- Sometimes, these patches are also referred to as Cigarette paper scales.
- Herald/mother's patch is the first sign of Pityriasis rosea.
- *Fir-tree or Christmas-tree appearance* due to distribution of lesion along the line of cleavage on trunk.
- Mainly involves trunk. Spares palm and soles (*this feature differentiates it from secondary syphilis*)

22. Ans. (b) Erythrasma

Ref: Dermatology by Jean L. Bolognia, Joseph L. Jorizzo, Ronald P.

- *Erythrasma* is a superficial, localized, mild and often chronic skin infection caused by *corynebacterium minutissimum*.
- The growth of the organism is favoured by moist, occluded intertriginous areas, including groin, axilla, intergluteal fold and inframammary and periumbilical areas.
- These lesions are irregular in shape and size, red, well defined patches covered with fine scales and wrinkling.
- The infection begins as a proliferation of C minutissimum within the stratum corneum.
- **Under wood's lamp examination:** Bright coral red fluorescence.
- This *bright coral red fluorescence under wood's lamp* is as a *result of porphyrin production* by the bacteria. It is considered as the best way to make diagnosis.

Extra Mile

- Tinea versicolor may resemble erythrasma, but does not tend to localize to body folds.

23. Ans. (a) Becker nevus

Ref: Diagnostic Pathology: Nonneoplastic Dermatopathology pg. 477

Becker's nevus, also called *pigmented hairy epidermal nevus*, is a cutaneous hamartoma that can have increased epidermal (melanocyte), dermal (smooth muscle), and appendageal (hair follicle) components. Classically, Becker's nevus is first noticed around puberty on the shoulders and chest in males, but may be congenital, involve any area of the body, and occur in women. The prevalence in postpubertal males is approximated to be 0.5%, or 1 in 200.

Epidemiology
- Age
  - Most often presents in adolescence following puberty
- Sex
  - Much more common in males (M:F = 6:1)

Site
- Often seen on shoulder girdle or trunk

Presentation
- Well-demarcated, irregular, tan to dark brown, slightly raised plaque, often with hypertrichosis
- Usually solitary, wide variety in size though typically >1 cm
- Rarely associated hypoplasia of ipsilateral breast/arm, scoliosis, spina bifida, or with accessory areola/scrotum **(Becker nevus syndrome)**

Treatment
- As lesions generally asymptomatic, no treatment is required
- Laser therapy
  - Variety of laser therapy for both hypertrichosis and hyperpigmentation has been employed with variable success.

24. Ans. (b) Pityriasis rosea

- The shown lesion on trunk is a case of pityriasis rosea.
- **Pityriasis rosea** is a common skin problem that causes a rash.
- *Multiple round to oval erythematous patches* with fine central scales distributed along the skin tension lines of cleavage on the trunk in *Christmas (fir) tree pattern*.

Characteristic features

1. Classically it begins with typical **Herald patch,** and then becomes generalized patch.
2. Herald/mother's patch is the first sign of Pityriasis rosea.
3. *Fir-tree or Christmas-tree appearance* due to distribution of lesion along the line of cleavage on trunk.
4. Cigarette paper scales
5. Mainly involves trunk; *spares palms & soles (this feature differentiate it from secondary syphilis which commonly involves palms & soles).*

Dermatology

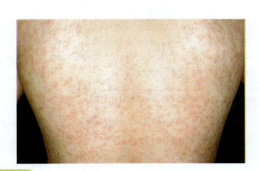

25. Ans. (c) Male pattern baldness

- The shown image is a case of *male pattern baldness*.
- Male pattern hair loss is an androgen dependent process.
- In majority of cases, this balding is patterned. The two major components being *frontotemporal recession* and *loss of hair over the vertex*.

> **Extra Mile**

Alopecia areata: Autoimmune disease characterized by patchy hair loss with no visible signs of inflammation, exclamation mark hair and geometric pitting of the nails

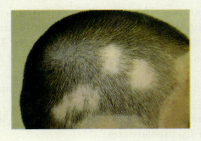

Telogen effluvium: This type of hair loss happens when hair follicles are fluctuated into the telogen or resting phase prematurely.
There are large amount of hair that begin to fall prematurely at the same time secondary to certain stress like chronic illness, pregnancy, depression, etc. Mostly seen in female.

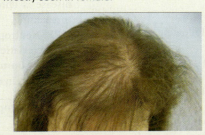

Cicatricial alopecia
Occurs due to inflammatory disorders that cause permanent destruction of pilosebaceous unit and irreversible hair loss

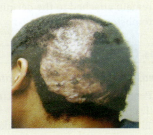

26. Ans. (a) Desmoglein 1

Ref: Inflammatory Dermatopathology: A Pathologist's Survival Guide, pg. 159

- Pemphigus foliaceous is a condition which arises due to antibody against desmoglein 1 (*remember F = First*)
- *Desmogleins* along with *desmocollins* connect two cells of epidermis. It is expressed in different layers of skin and mucosa.
- Desmogleins have several isoforms and if antibody forms against them, it will lead to different disease entitiy.

Desmogleins	DSG 1	DSG 3
Location	Epidermis, *subcorneal layer* It is not expressed in mucosal layer	Epidermis, *stratum basale* It is expressed in mucosal layer as well
Associated disease if antibody formed (IgG antibody)	Pemphigus foliaceous (subcorneal blister)	Pemphigus vulgaris (can involve DSG 1 as well)

27. Ans. (c) Both

Ref: Inflammatory Dermatopathology: A Pathologist's Survival Guide P 159

The antibodies in *pemphigus vulgaris* are directed against *desmoglein* 3, a desmosomal cadherin that mediates cell binding. Desmoglein 3 is expressed in greater concentration in the lower epidermis, the location of the suprabasal acantholytic blister of pemphigus vulgaris.

- More than half of sera from patients with pemphigus vulgaris also have circulating antibodies against desmoglein 1.
- Established lesions of pemphigus vulgaris demonstrate suprabasilar acantholysis with frequent involvement of follicular external root sheaths
- The basal keratinocytes separate from one another but remain attached to the dermis, reminiscent of a "row of tombstones"

28. Ans. (a) Pemphigus vulgaris

Please refer to above explanation

- Pemphigus vulgaris is characterized by following signs:
  1. Bulla spread sign
  2. Perilesional and distant nikolsky sign
  3. Tzanck smear: Acantholytic cell
- Histopathology shows suprabasal blister with row of tomb stone appearance of basal cells.
- Direct immunofluorescence from perilesional skin demonstrated intraepidermal IgG deposites in a *fishnet pattern*.

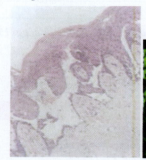
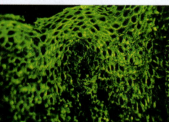

FIGURE: Pemphigus vulgaris, shows suprabasal cleavage with acantholysis. "Row of tomb stones appearance" can be seen in the floor of bulla

29. Ans. (d) Bullous pemphigoid

Ref: Mayo Clinic Internal Medicine Board Review, pg.162

- Bullous pemphigoid is the *most common autoimmune bullous disease*.
- It occurs predominantly in elderly population.
- It presents as *large, tense bullae* with a predilection for flexural areas.
- Immunofluroscence testing is important for its diagnosis.
- Almost all cases have deposition of C3 and IgG in a *linear pattern at the basement membrane zone* (as shown in the image of question).

30. Ans. (b) Dermatitis herpetiformis

Ref: Bhutani Atlas of Dermatology, 6th ed. pg. 179

- Dermatitis herpetiformis is a condition seen in middle aged patients with male predilection.

Clinical Features

Dermatitis herpetiformis is an immunopathologic vesiculobullous disease of skin rarely showing oral manifestations. The condition represents the *cutaneous expression of gluten enteropathy* (gliadin sensitivity). The skin lesions are *pruritic* and are located primarily on the extremities and buttocks. They are *vesicular with a tendency to rupture and desquamate*. Oral bullae may be encountered and many patients present with aphthous like ulcers. The disease is chronic, lasting for many years, yet is not life threatening.

HPE: Neutrophilic microabscess in dermal papillary tip is **characteristic**.

Direct immunofluorescence: Shows granular IgA deposition in dermal papillary area.

31. Ans. (b) Atopic dermatitis

- **Hertoghe's sign** is lateral thinning of the eyebrows. It is seen in condition like atopic dermatitis.

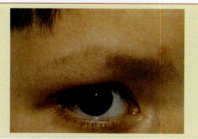

- **Dennie morgan fold:** A deep fold that can be found under the lower lid. Also seen in atopic dermatitis.

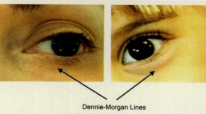

32. Ans. (b) Tuberous sclerosis

Ref: Harrison's, 19th ed. pg. 359

- **Triad of tuberous sclerosis** is remembered with simple mnemonic **EpiLoA**: **Ep**ilepsy, **Lo**w IQ, and **a**denoma sebaceum.

Dermatology

- The patient in image presented with adenoma sebaceum and other triad of tuberous sclerosis.
- The **earliest cutaneous sign** tuberous sclerosis, is macular hypomelanosis, referred to as an *ash leaf spot*.
- Examination of the patient for additional cutaneous signs such as multiple angiofibromas of the face *(adenoma sebaceum)*, ungual and gingival fibromas, fibrous plaques of the forehead, and connective tissue nevi *(shagreen patches)* is recommended.
- Internal manifestations include seizures, mental retardation, central nervous system (CNS) and retinal hamartomas, pulmonary lymphangioleiomyomatosis (women), renal angiomyolipomas, and cardiac rhabdomyomas.

33. Ans. (b) Nevus ota

Ref: Oski's Pediatrics, Principle and Practice, pg. 829

- *Nevus of Ota*, is a hamartoma of dermal melanocytes.
- It is a bluish or gray-brown patch of pigmentation that occurs on the skin of the face, usually in the distribution of the first and second branches of the trigeminal nerve. Perhaps two-thirds of affected infants have an *associated ipsilateral bluish discoloration of the sclera*.
- Histologically, a nevus of Ota is *identical to a mongolian spot* and likely results from errors in migration spot, however, the nevus of Ota does not undergo spontaneous regression. If scleral pigmentation is present, glaucoma may occur.
- Malignant degeneration occurring within a nevus of Ota is rare. Management options for the nevus include the use of a covering cosmetic or treatment with a pigmented lesion laser.

Nevus of Ito: A patch of hyperpigmentation similar to the nevus of Ota but *occurring over the shoulders*, in the supraclavicular areas, and on the sides of the neck, the upper arms, and the scapulae is known as the *nevus of Ito*. These lesions persist throughout life. Treatment options are analogous to those for the nevus of Ota.

34. Ans. (b) Ivermectin

Ref: KDT, 6th ed. pg. 864

Explanation:

- The image shows lesions in inter-digital clefts suggestive of scabies.
- Scabies is caused by an ectoparacite sarcoptes scabiei. It is highly contagious. The mite burrows through the epidermis, laying eggs which form papules that itch intensely.
- Most common site of entry—finger webs.

- Drugs used are:
  - **Permethrin:** Broad spectrum and potent insecticide, currently most efficacious.
    - It is preferred topical drug for scabies.
    - **MOA:** It causes neurological paralysis in insects by delaying depolarization.
    - Single application needed in most cases.
    - Very less toxicity; 100% cure rate.
  - **Lindane:** Another broad spectrum insecticide. Efficacy lower than permethrin.
    - **MOA:** Kills lice and mites by penetrating through their chitinous cover and affecting the nervous system.
  - **Benzyl benzoate:** Oily liquid with a faint aromatic smell.
    - It is applied over face and neck after a bath. A second coat is applied next day which is washed after 24 hours.
  - Crotamiton
  - Sulfur

> **Extra Mile**
>
> - **Ivermectin:** Highly effective in scabies pediculosis and Norwegian scabies
>   - It is the only orally administered drug which is used for scabies (ectoparasitosis). Oral DOC for scabies.
>   - A single dose of 0.2 mg/kg has cured almost 90–100% of population.
>   - *It is contraindicated in children <5 years, pregnant and lactating women.*

35. Ans. (d) Antipyretics

Ref: Primary Care Dermatology, An Issue of Primary Care, pg. 526

- The shown image is a case of roseola infantum also known as 6th day disease.
- Roseola infantum, also known as 3-day fever, is characterized by high-grade fever followed by abrupt defervescence and onset of a rash. It is the most common exanthem before age 2. It is typically seen in children between the ages of 6 months and 4 years, with a peak age of acquisition between 9 and 21 months.
- *It is most commonly caused by human herpes virus (HHV) –6 and less commonly by HHV-7, enterovirus, adenovirus, and parainfluenza virus.*
- The modes of transmission and incubation periods vary depending on the etiologic agent. In most patients with roseola caused by HHV-6 the average incubation period is 9–10 days. Usually by the time the rash appears, viremia has already resolved.

36. Ans. (c) Tinea captitis

Ref: Harrison's, 19th ed. pg. 355

- The image shows a boggy scalp of Tinea capitis

Tinea capitis	Varies from scaling with minimal hair loss to discrete patches with "black dots" (broken infected hairs) to boggy plaque with pustules (kerion)	Invasion of hairs by dermatophytes, most commonly *Trichophyton tonsurans*	Oral griseofulvin or terbinafine plus 2.5% selenium sulfide or ketoconazole shampoo; examine family members
Traumatic alopecia	Broken hair, often of varying lengths irregular outline	Traction with curlers, chemicals (e.g., hair straighteners) Mechanical pulling (trichotillomania)	Discontinuation of offending hair style of chemical treatments; require observation of shaved hairs (for growth) or biopsy, possibly followed by psychotherapy

37. Ans. (b) Tinea corporis

Ref: Oski's Essential Pediatrics, pg. 155

- The annular lesion with central clearing, is most likely indicative of tinea corporis.
- The infection of nonhairy areas of the skin by dermatophytes is limited to the epidermis, only the most superficial layers of the skin are involved. The rings are generally erythematous. As the inflammation spreads, the active infection in the center of the lesions is destroyed, and this area clears, frequently resulting in the picture of an advancing border with central clearing.
- The organism responsible for most cases of tinea corporis is *Trichophytom tonsurans. Microsporum canis, Microsporum audouinii,* and *Trichophyton mentagrophytes* infections are also seen.

38. Ans. (a) Molluscum contagiosum

Ref: Harrison's, 19th ed. pg. 220e-1

- Vesicle with central umbilication is most likely suggestive of molluscum contagiosum.
- Molluscum contagiosum is a cutaneous poxvirus infection characterized by multiple umbilicated flesh-colored or hypo-pigmented papules.
- Molluscum contagiosum is highly prevalent among children and is the most common human disease resulting from poxvirus infection.
- Swimming pools are a common vector for transmission.

39. Ans. (b) Basal cell cancer

Ref: Harrison's, 19th ed. pg. 501

The image shows a lesion on face showing *raised and beaded appearance*. It is suggestive of diagnosis of BCC. The *most common site* is the face with a line drawn between angle of mouth and ear Lobule–*Onghren's line*.

40. Ans. (a) Alopecia areata

Ref: Harrison's, 19th ed. pg. 355

	Clinical	Pathogenesis	Treatment
Telogen effluvium (choice C)	• Diffuse shedding of normal hairs • Follows major stress (high fever, severe infection) or change in hormone levels (postpartum) • Reversible without treatment	Stress causes more of the asynchronous growth cycles of individual hairs to become synchronous; therefore, larger numbers of growing (anagen) hairs simultaneously enter the dying (telogen) phase	Observation, discontinue any drugs that have alopecia as a side effect, must exclude underlying metabolic causes, e.g. hypothyroidism, hyperthyroidism

Contd...

Dermatology

	Clinical	Pathogenesis	Treatment
Androgenetic alopecia (male pattern; female pattern) (choice B)	• Miniaturization of hairs along the midline of the scalp • Recession of the anterior scalp line in men and some women	• Increased sensitivity of affected hairs to the effects of androgens • Increased levels of circulating androgens (ovarian or adrenal source in women)	If no evidence of hyperandro-genemia, then topical minoxidil finastheride[Q] spironolactone (women); hair transplant
Alopecia areata (choice A)	• Well-circumscribed, circular areas of hair loss, 2–5 cm in diameter • In extensive cases, coalescence of lesions and/or involvement of other hair-bearing surfaces of the body • Pitting or sandpapered appearance of the nails	The germinative zones of the hair follicles are surrounded by T lymphocytes **Occasional associated disease: hyperthyroidism, hypothyrodidism, vitiligo. Down syndrome**	Topical anthralin or tazarotene; intralesional glucocorticoids; topical contact sensitizers
Traumatic alopecia (choice D)	Broken hairs, often of varying lengths irregular outline	• Traction with curlers, rubber bands braiding • Exposure to heat or chemical (e.g. hair straighteners) • Mechanical pulling (trichotillomania)	Discontinuation of offending hair style or chemical treatments; diagnosis of trichotillomania may require observation of shaved hairs (for growth) or biopsy, possibly followed by psychotherapy

41. Ans. (b) *Zinc deficiency*

Ref: Harrison's, 19th ed. pg. 96e-9

Acrodermatitis enteropathica (AE)

- *AE is characterized by abnormalities in zinc absorption* due to defect in intestinal zinc transporter *which leads to zinc deficiency.*
- It is a rare autosomal recessive (AR) disorder which classically present during infancy on weaning from breast milk to formula or cereal which have lower zinc bioavailability than breast milk.
- **Classical features of AE include:** *(Mnemonic-"DEAL")*
  - **D**iarrhea, **D**epression
  - **E**czematous erosive dermatitis
  - **A**lopecia (non scarring), **A**pathetic look
  - **L**ethargy, irritability, whining and crying.

42. Ans. (a) *Tinea versicolor*

Ref: Harrison's, 19th ed. pg. 350

- *Malassezia furfur*, a normal inhabitant of the skin is a nondermatophytic, dimorphic fungus is a causative organism for *Tinea versicolor.*
- The expression of infection is promoted by heat and humidity. The typical lesions consist of oval scaly macules, papules, and patches concentrated on the chest, shoulders, and back.

- On dark skin the lesions often appear as hypopigmented areas, while on light skin they are slightly erythematous or hyperpigmented.
- A KOH preparation from scaling lesions will demonstrate a confluence of short hyphae and round spores ("spaghetti and meatballs").

43. Ans. (d) *Psoriasis*

Ref: Harrisons, 19th ed. pg. 347

- The silver scaly lesion as shown in the patient in the given image is more likely a case of psoriasis.

PSORIASIS

- Psoriasis is one of the most common dermatologic diseases, affecting up to 2% of the world's population.
- **Clinical feature:** Characterized by—
  - Erythematous, sharply demarcated papules and rounded plaques covered by silvery micaceous scale. The skin lesions of psoriasis are variably pruritic.
  - *Koebner* or isomorphic phenomenon: Traumatized areas often develop lesions of psoriasis.

44. Ans. (c) **Erythema multiforme**

Ref: Harrison's, 19th ed. pg. 134

- The shown target lesions on palm are diagnostic of erythema multiforme.
- The classic target lesions of *erythema multiforme* appear symmetrically on the elbows, knees, palms, soles, and face.

FMGE Solutions Screening Examination

- In severe cases, these lesions spread diffusely and involve mucosal surface.
- Choice B, Steven JOhnson syndrome is ruled out due to presentation of vesico-bullous lesions

Disease	Etiology	Description	Group affected /Epidemiologic factor	Clinical syndrome
Hand-foot-and-mouth disease (Choice A)	Coxsackievirus A16 most common cause	Tender vesicles, erosions in mouth; 0.25 cm papules on hands and feet with rim of erythema	Summer and fall; primarily children <10 years old; multiple family members	Transient fever
Erythema multiforme (EM) (Choice C)	• Infection • Drugs • Idiopathic	• Target lesions (central erythema surrounded by area of clearing and another rim of erythema) up to 2 cm, symmetric on knees, elbows, palms, soles. • When extensive and involving mucous membranes, it is termed as EM major	Herpes simple virus or *Mycoplasma pneumoniae* infection; drug intake (i.e., sulfa, phenytonia, Penicillin)	50% of patients <20 years old; EM major, which can be confused with Stevens-Johnson syndrome (but EM major lacks prominent skin sloughing)

45. Ans. (d) Palms and soles involved

Ref: Robbins, 9th ed. pg. 358

- IP of chickenpox- **10–21 days**
- Infectious period is **2 days before to 5 days after** the onset of rash
- **Chickenpox** is caused by VZV and reactivation of latent VZV causes shingles (also called *herpes zoster*).
- Like HSV, VZV infects mucous membranes, skin, and neurons and causes a self-limited primary infection in immunocompetent individuals.

Small pox	Chicken pox
• Face involved	• Involves trunk mainly
• Centrifugal; involves palms and soles	• Centripetal; palm and soles not involved
• Umbilicated, deep lesion	• Superficial lesion
• Same stage at one point of time	• Pleomorphic rash
• Extensor aspect involved/axilla, mucous not involved	• Axilla, mucosa involved
• Heals slowly	• Rapid healing
• Scab formation 10–14 days	• Scab formation 4–7 days

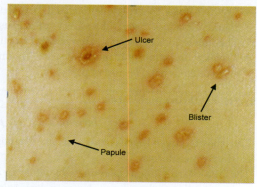

46. Ans. (c) Lichen planus

Ref: Harrisons, 19th ed. pg. 349

LICHEN PLANUS

- Lichen planus (LP) is a *papulosquamous disorder* that may affect the skin, scalp, nails, and mucous membranes.
- The primary cutaneous lesions of LP are pruritic, **polygonal, flat-topped, violaceous papules**.
- **Most common site** can occur anywhere but have a predilection for the **wrists, shins,** lower back, and genitalia.

Characteristic Feature

1. **Wickham's striae:** A network of gray lines on the surface of papules.
2. **Lichen planopilaris:** Involvement of the **scalp may lead to scarring alopecia**, and nail involvement may lead to permanent deformity or loss of finger nails and toe nails.
3. Lichen planus commonly involves mucous membranes, particularly the buccal mucosa (Erosive stomatitis) which may persist for years and linked to an *increased risk of oral squamous cell carcinoma.*
4. **LP may be associated with hepatitis C infection.** The course of LP is variable, but most patients have **spontaneous remissions 6 months to 2 years** after the onset of disease.

Treatment of choice: Topical glucocorticoids.

Dermatology

1149

3. **Guttate psoriasis (eruptive psoriasis):** This is **most common in children** and young adults.
   - Patients present with many small erythematous, scaling papules, **frequently after upper respiratory tract** infection with β-hemolytic streptococci.
4. **Pustular psoriasis:** Usually localized to the **palms and soles**, or may be generalized. Can present with fever and or pustular eruptions.

Treatment

- **Limited psoriasis:** Topical glucocorticoids, Calcipotriene (topical vitamin D analogue), retinoid (tazarotene).
- Widespread psoriasis:
  - **UV light:** Ultraviolet B (UVB), narrow band UVB, and ultraviolet A (UV A) light with either oral or topical **psoralens (PUVA)** is used.
  - **Methotrexate** is an effective agent, especially in patients with psoriatic arthritis.

Note: *Oral glucocorticoids should not be used for the treatment of psoriasis due to the potential for development of life-threatening pustular psoriasis when therapy is discontinued.*

---

48. Ans. (c) Tetracycline

Ref: Harrisons, 19th ed. pg. 352

■ ACNE VULGARIS

- It is a self-limited disorder primarily of teenagers and young adults.
- Increase in sebum production by sebaceous glands after puberty is a the permissive factor for the disease expression.
- **Clinical hallmark of acne vulgaris:** Comedone, which may be closed (*whitehead*) or open (*blackhead*).
- **The earliest lesions seen in adolescence** are generally mildly inflamed or noninflammatory comedones on the forehead.
- **Most common location for acne** is the face, but involvement of the chest and back is common.

Treatment of Acne

- **Minimal to moderate pauci-inflammatory disease** respond adequately to local therapy alone: Topical agents such as retinoic acid, benzoyl peroxide, or salicylic acid.
- *Given the image, it is obvious that the case is not a minimal to moderate case of acne vulgaris. It is more likely moderate to acne vulgaris with inflammatory papules, pustules and comedones.*
- **Harrisons states:** *"Patients with moderate to severe acne with a prominent inflammatory component will benefit from the addition of systemic therapy, such as tetracycline in doses of 250–500 mg BD or doxycycline in doses of 100 mg BD"*

Extra Mile

TABLE: Papulosquamous disorders

	Clinical features	Other notable features	Histologic features
Psoriasis	Sharply demarcated, erythematous plaques with *mica-like scale;* predominantly on elbows, knees, and scalp; atypical forms may localize to intertriginous areas; eruptive forms may be associated with infection	May be aggravated by certain drugs, infection; severe forms seen in association with HIV	Acanthosis, vascular proliferation
Lichen planus	*Purple polygonal papules marked by severe pruritus;* lacy white markings, especially associated with mucous membrane lesions	Certain drugs may induce; thiazides antimalarial drugs	Interface dermatitis

---

47. Ans. (c) Psoriasis

Ref: Harrisons, 19th ed. pg. 347

- The silver scaly lesion on the skin of the patient in the given image is more likely a case of psoriasis.

■ PSORIASIS

- Psoriasis is one of the most common dermatologic diseases, affecting up to 2% of the world's population.
- **Clinical feature:** Characterized by—
  - Erythematous, sharply demarcated papules and rounded plaques covered by silvery micaceous scale. The skin lesions of psoriasis are variably pruritic.
  - *Koebner* or isomorphic phenomenon: Traumatized areas often develop lesions of psoriasis.

Types of Psoriasis

1. **Plaque-type:** It is the **most common variety** of psoriasis.
   - Patients present with stable, slowly enlarging plaques, which remains unchanged for long periods of time.
   - The **most commonly involved areas are** the elbows, knees, gluteal cleft, and scalp. Involvement tends to be **symmetric**.
2. **Inverse psoriasis** affects the intertriginous regions, including the axilla, groin, submammary region, and navel.

Explanations

FMGE Solutions Screening Examination

- **If patients with** severe nodulocystic acne are unresponsive to the therapies discussed above: Treatment with the synthetic retinoid isotretinoin is the choice. Its dose is based on the patient's weight, and it is given once daily for 5 months.
- Isotretinoin gives excellent result, but its teratogenic side effects limits its use in reproductive age group females.

49. Ans. (a) Neurofibromatosis

Ref: Harrisons, 19th ed. pg. 2331

NF-1 is diagnosed when *any two of the following seven signs are present*:

1. Six or more café au-lait macules. *Café au-lait spots are the* **hallmark of** *neurofibromatosis and are present in almost 100% of patients.*
2. Axillary or inguinal freckling consisting of multiple hyperpigmented areas 2–3 mm in diameter.
3. Two or more iris Lisch nodules. Lisch nodules are hamartomas located within the iris and are best identified by a slit-lamp examination.
4. Two or more neurofibromas or one plexiform neurofibroma.
5. Osseous lesion such as sphenoid dysplasia (which may cause pulsating exophthalmos) or cortical thinning of long bones with or without pseudoarthrosis.
6. Optic gliomas are present in ≈15% of patients with NF-1.
7. First Degree relative with NF-1

50. Ans. (a) Alopecia areata

Ref: Harrisons, 19th ed. pg. 354-55

- **Alopecia is of two types:** Scarring and Nonscarring.

Scarring alopecia	Nonscarring alopecia
It is associated **with fibrosis, inflammation,** and loss of hair follicles.	In this type **the hair shafts are absent** or miniaturized, but the **hair follicles are preserved** *(reversible condition)*
Most common causes of scarring alopecia are primary cutaneous disorder such as *lichen planus, folliculitis decalvans, chronic cutaneous (discoid) lupus,* or *linear scleroderma (morphea).*	**The most common causes** of nonscarring alopecia include 1. *Androgenetic alopecia* 2. *Telogen effluvium* 3. *Alopecia areata* 4. *Tinea capitis*, and the early 5. Phase of *traumatic alopecia.* 6. SLE

Extra Mile

- SLE has non-scarring alopecia
- This non-scarring alopecia coincides with flare up of systemic disease and presents as lupus hairs.
  - Discoid lupus erythematosus has scarring alopecia
  - Linear scleroderme [Morphea] has scarring alopecia

51. Ans. (d) Zinc oxide

Ref: Robbins, 9th ed. pg. 391

- Sunscreens are rated for their photoprotective effect by their sun protection factor (SPF).
- The SPF is simply **a ratio of the time required to produce sunburn erythema with and without sunscreen application.**
- The SPF of most sunscreens reflects protection from UV-B but not from UV-A.
- US. Food and Drug Administration (FDA) has recognized category-I ingredients as safe and effective. Those ingredients are listed in the table below:

FDA CATEGORY I MONOGRAPHED SUNSCREEN INGREDIENTS

Ingredients	Maximum concentration, %
p-Aminobenzoic acid (PABA)	15
Avobenzone	3
Cinoxate	3
Dioxybenzone (benzophenone-8)	3
Ecamsule	15
Homosalate	15
Methyl anthranilate	5
Octocrylene	10
Octyl methoxycinnamate	7.5
Octyl salicylate	5
Oxybenzone (benzophenone-3)	6
Padimate O (octyl dimethyl PABA)	8
Phenylbenzimidazole sulfonic acid	4
Sulisobenzone (benzophenone-4)	10
Titanium dioxide	25
Trolamine salicylate	12
Zinc oxide	25

52. Ans. (a) 5 kg

- Average weight of skin is ~4 kg. Skin is considered to be the largest organ of the body.
- It is 12-15% of the total body weight.
- *Given these options, 5 kg is closest and best choice.*

53. Ans. (d) Stratum germinatum

Ref: Fitzpatrick, 7th ed. pg. 384

- Epidermis of the skin has 4 layers:
  1. **Stratum basale/Germinatum:** Deepest most layers having single row **columnar** epithelial cells. It is actively dividing layer.

2. **Stratum spinosum:** Also known as prickle cell layer. Polygonal in shape. *Synthesis of keratin mainly takes place here.*
3. **Stratum granulosum:** Diamond shaped. *Microscopically there is presence of* **keratohyaline granules and Odland bodies** *(membrane coating granules)*
4. **Stratum corneum:** Also known as horny cell layer. Most superficial layer of skin. This layer is a nuclear dead cell layer.

- **Note:** *Stratum lucidum is the 5th layer of skin found on palm and soles. It is located between stratum granulosum and corneum.*

Extra Mile

- **Stratum corneum** develops last. Therefore this layer is absent in premature babies
- **Stratum corneum** is dead layer of epidermis
- **Hyperkeratosis:** Thickening of stratum corneum.

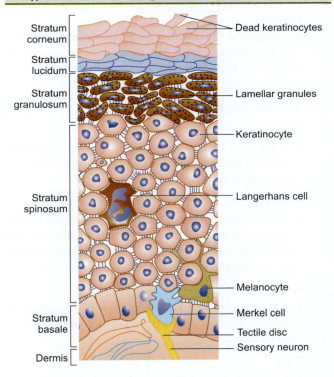

54. Ans. (d) Stratum spinosum

Ref: Fitzpatrick, 7th ed. pg. 384

55. Ans. (b) Thickening of stratum corneum

Ref: Fitzpatrick, 7th ed. pg. 384

56. Ans. (b) Stratum granulosum

Ref: McGraw Hill Speciality Board Review Dermatology 2nd ed. pg. 561

57. Ans. (c) Keratinocytes

Ref: Fitzpatrick, 7th ed. pg. 100

CELLS OF EPIDERMIS

- **Keratinocytes:** These are considered as the principal cells of epidermis. They proliferate in basal layer and differentiation occurs in spinosum and granulosum layer which further matures fully and dies in corneum. (keratinocytes are present in all 4 layers of epidermis)
- **Melanocytes and Merkel cell:** Present in stratum basale.
  - **Melanocytes** synthesize melanin pigment and transfer to keratinocytes
  - **Merkel cells** for touch sensation. Also known as touch cells
- **Langerhan cell** found in stratum spinosum and act as **antigen presenting cells** (macrophages).
  - They contain **tennis racquet shaped granules** also known as **Bierbeck granules.**

58. Ans. (d) Spinosum

Ref: Fitzpatrick, 7th ed. pg. 384

59. Ans. (a) Basale

Ref: Fitzpatrick, 7th ed. pg. 62

60. Ans. (b) Separation of keratinocytes

Ref: Harrison, 19th ed. pg. 370

- Keratinocytes are connected to one another by intracellular desmosomal bridges.
- If there is loss of these desmosomal bridges, it will lead to **separation of keratinocytes** and the condition is known as **acantholysis.**
- If separation continues, there will be intracellular edema, and the condition is known as **Ballooning.**

Extra Mile

- Degeneration of stratum basale is seen in: Lichen planus
- **Acanthosis:** Thickening of stratum spinosum
- **Hypergranulosis:** Thickening of stratum granulosum
- **Hyperkeratosis:** Thickening of stratum corneum
- **Parakeratosis:** Persistence of nucleus in stratum corneum layer

61. Ans. (d) Thickening of prickle cell layer

Ref: Harrison, 19th ed. pg. 370

- **Acanthosis:** Thickening of stratum spinosum aka prickle cell layer.

62. Ans. (b) Persistence of nucleus in stratum corneum

- Stratum corneum is the most superficial layer of the skin and is devoid of nucleus.

FMGE Solutions Screening Examination

- Parakeratosis is retention of nucleus in stratum corneum
- If there is presence of nucleus in this layer it can be a normal case or can be associated with some pathology.
- **Normally** nucleus in cornuem persists in vagina and in mucous membrane of mouth.
- **Pathologies having nucleus in stratum corneum:** seborrheic dermatitis, squamous cell CA, Actinic keratosis, psoriasis, etc.

63. Ans. (b) 4 days

Ref: Neena Khanna: Synopses of Dermatology 4th ed. pg. 52

- Normal skin turnover from basal cell layer to corneum layer takes around **4–5 weeks**.
- **In conditions like psoriasis**, the mitotic activity is increased and the turnover time is highly reduced to 3–7 days with an **average of 4 days**.

64. Ans. (d) Gustatory sweating

Types of Sweating

- **Gustatory sweating:** Sweating on scalp, forehead and nose in response to hot and spicy meals.
- **Mental sweating:** Occurs in response to emotional stimuli like. For example, mental stress, emotional stress. Sweating usually noticed on palms, soles and axilla.
- **Thermogenic sweating:** Sweating in response to pre-optic stimulation of hypothalamus in order to maintain the body temperature.

65. Ans. (b) Lips are most common site

Ref: Harrison, 19th ed. pg. 127

- **Fordyce's spots** are ectopic sebaceous glands.
  - MC site: **Lips > oral mucosa > Vulva and Penis (Tysons gland)**
  - **MC age group:** Puberty
  - M > F
  - **Characterized as** discrete pin headed size, yellowish maculo-papular lesions in mucus membrane of lips and oral cavity.
  - **Mimicks** or are very often confused as **koplik's spot of measles.**

> **Extra Mile**
>
> - **Obstruction of eccrine sweat gland ducts:** Miliaria
> - **Obstruction of apocrine sweat gland ducts:** Fox fordyces spot/disease aka Apocrine Miliaria
> - **MC site of fox fordyces disease:** Axilla
> - **MC age group of fox fordyces spot:** 13–35 years *(Females are MC affected).*

66. Ans. (a) Lips

Ref: Harrison, 19th ed. pg. 240 table 45.2/

67. Ans. (b) Flat lesion <2 cm

Ref: Harrison's, 19th ed. pg. 319

DESCRIPTION OF PRIMARY SKIN LESIONS

Macule
- A flat, colored lesion, <2 cm in diameter, not raised above the surface of the surrounding skin. A "freckle" or ephelid, is a prototypical pigmented macule.

Patch
- A large (>2 cm) flat lesion with a color different from the surrounding skin. This differs from a macule only in size.

Papule
- A small, solid lesion, <0.5 cm in diameter, raised above the surface of the surrounding skin and thus palpable (e.g. a closed comedone, or white-head in acne).

Nodule
- A larger (0.5–5.0 cm), firm lesion raised above the surface of the surrounding skin. This differs from a papule only in size (e.g. a large dermal nevomelanocytic nevus).

Tumor
- A solid, raised growth >5 cm in diameter.

Plaque
- A large (>1 cm), flat-topped, raised lesion; edges may either be distinct (e.g,. psoriasis) or gradually blend with skin (e.g. in eczematous dermatitis).

Vesicle
- A small, fluid lesion, <0.5 cm in diameter, raised above the pane of surrounding skin. Fluid is often visible, and the lesions are translucent (e.g. vesicles in allergic contact dermatitis caused by Toxicodendron [poison ivy]).

Pustule
- A vesicle filled with leukocytes. Note: The presence of pustules does not necessarily signify the existence of an infection.

Bulla
- A fluid-filled raised often translucent lesion >0.5 cm in diameter.

Wheal
- A raised erythematous, edematous papule of plaque, usually representing short-lived vasodilatation and vasopermeability.

Telanglectasia
- A dilated, superficial blood vessel.

Dermatology

68. Ans. (b) <5 mm

Ref: Harrison's 19ᵗʰ ed. pg. 319

Please refer to above explanation

69. Ans. (a) Insect bite

- **Insect bite:** Presents as papule. It can be painful or painless
- **Angioedema:** Edema of subcutaneous and submucosal tissue can be due to allergic reaction.
- **Urticaria** is an auto-inflammatory condition. MC symptom is itching.
- **Erythema Nodosum:** Inflammation of submucosal fatty cells.

70. Ans. (d) Biliverdin

- Bruise is a skin contusion which is also known as hematoma of skin
- Capillaries and sometimes venules are damaged by trauma, allowing blood to seep, hemorrhage, or extravasate into the surrounding interstitial tissues.
- Larger bruises may change color due to the breakdown of hemoglobin from within escaped RBC in the extracellular space.
- The striking colors of a bruise are caused by the Phagocytosis and sequential degradation of hemoglobin to biliverdin to bilirubin to hemosiderin.
- The color changes noted at the site of bruise is secondary to:

- **Hemoglobin** itself producing a red-blue color
- **Biliverdin producing a green color**
- **Bilirubin** producing a yellow color
- **Hemosiderin** producing a golden-brown color

71. Ans. (c) Sulfur granules in the purulent sinuses are characteristic

Ref: Harrison, 19ᵗʰ ed. pg. 1090

- **Propionibacterium acne** is a Gram-positive bacterium, which is a normal flora of the skin.
- It can also cause chronic blepharitis and endophthalmitis.
- It is basically linked to the skin condition acne.
- Aside from skin it lives primarily on fatty acids in sebum secreted by sebaceous glands in the follicles.
- It may also be found throughout the gastrointestinal tract in humans.
- The antibiotics most frequently used to treat acne vulgaris are: Erythromycin, clindamycin, doxycycline and minocycline.
- *Actinomyces israelii is an opportunistic pathogen which causes actinomycosis.*
- Its lesions are often characterized as "wooden." Sulfur granules form in a central purulence surrounded by neutrophils is very characteristic of actinomycosis.

72. Ans. (d) Dermatitis herpetiformis

Ref: Harrison, 19ᵗʰ ed. pg. 373

Diagnosis of Dermatitis Herpetiformis is confirmed by a simple blood test for IgA antibodies, and by a skin biopsy in which the *pattern of IgA deposits in the dermo-epidermal junction*, revealed by direct immunofluorescence.

> **Extra Mile**

TABLE: Differentiating Dermatitis Herpetiformis, Pemphigus and Pemphigoid Vulgaris

Feature	Dermatitis herpetiformis	Pemphigus vulgaris	Pemphigoid
Lesion	Intensely itchy vesicles, papulovesicles	Thin walled, delicate, flaccid bullae / blister that rapidly rupture & erode	Large, tense often blood stained blisters
Area of predeliction	Knees, elbows, scalp, buttock, & around axilla	Upper part of body Buccal mucosa is commonly involved	Lower part of body Mucosa not involved
Associated with	G.I. absorptive defect due to gluten enteropathy	• Acantholysis • Nikolsky sign	–

Lab finding	• Small intestine biopsy: partial villous atrophy
	• Lesion biopsy: Subepidermal blisters
	• IgA & neutrophils in papillary tips
		• Lesion biopsy:
		  ▪ **Acantholysis**
		  ▪ ***Intraepidermal blisters***
		  ▪ Row of tomb stone
		  ▪ IgG, C_3 complement deposition between epidermal cells.
			• Lesion biopsy:
			  ▪ **Subepidermal blisters**
			  ▪ Subepidermal collection of IgG, C_3-complement, eosinophils, polymorphs.

Treatment	• Gluten free diet • *Dapsone (DOC)*	• Systemic steroid • Immunosuppresant	• Systemic steroid • Immunosuppresant

FMGE Solutions Screening Examination

73. Ans. (a) Pemphigus vulgaris

Ref: Harrison, 19th ed. pg. 370

- The rounded keratinocytes with hyperchromatic nuclei and perinuclear halo (due to condensing of cytoplasm in periphery) are called **acantholytic cells.**
- It is seen in case of pemphigus vulgaris
- **Acantholytic cells** can be demonstrated in bed side by **Tzanck test.**

74. Ans. (c) Autoimmune

Ref: Harrison, 19th ed. pg. 370

PEMPHIGUS

- *Pemphigus is an autoimmune blistering disorder*
- It results from the loss of integrity of normal intercellular attachments with the epidermis.
- Commonly affects indicividuals of age between 40-60.
- Equal prevalence among males and females.
- There are five variants of pephigus:
  - *Pemphigus Vulgaris:* Most common type
  - *Pemphigus Foliaceous:* Superficial pemphigus
  - *Pemphigus VegetAns.* Least common type
  - *Pemphigus Erythematous*
  - *Fogo Selvagem:* An endemic form of pemphigus foliaceus.
- *Refer to above table*

75. Ans. (b) Intraepidermal

Ref: Harrison, 19th ed. pg. 371-72

- Pemphigus has intraepidermal bullae and Pemphigoid has subepidermal bullae

TABLE: Difference between Pemphigus and Pemphigoid Bullae

Features	Pemphigus	Pemphigoid
Row of Tomb stone	Present	Absent
Nikolsky Sign	Present	Absent
Bullae location	Intraepidermal – flaccid Bullae	Subepidermal & tense Bullae
Mucosa involvement	Present (common)	Absent or less common
Acantholysis	Present	Absent
Prognosis	Poor	Good

76. Ans. (b) Pemphigoid bullae

Ref: Harrison, 19th ed. pg. 371-72

- Pemphigus has intraepidermal bullae
- Pemphigoid has subepidermal bullae
- *Refer to the previous answer for detailed explanation.*

77. Ans. (b) Pemphigus vulgaris

Please refer to above explanation.

78. Ans. (b) Nikolsky sign absent

Ref: Harrison, 19th ed. pg. 370

Nikolsky sign is present in pemphigus bullae. It is absent in pemphigoid bullae.

79. Ans. (b) Pemphigus

Ref: Neena Khanna, 3rd pg. 61-6

- In Pemphigus, there is production of **IgG auto antibodes** against polypeptide complexes present in the **intercellular substance of epidermis.**
- Lesional sites show a characteristic **Fish net like pattern of intercellular IgG** deposits in the intercellular area.

80. Ans. (a) Dapsone

Ref: Katzung, pg. 1468

- **Dermatitis herpetiformis** is a chronic blistering skin condition, characterized by blisters filled with a watery fluid.
- DH is neither related to nor caused by herpes virus: the name means that it is a skin inflammation having an appearance similar to herpes.
- It characterized by intensely itchy, chronic papulovesicular eruptions, usually distributed symmetrically on extensor surfaces (buttocks, back of neck, scalp, elbows, knees, back, hairline, groin, or face).
- **Diagnosis** is confirmed by a simple blood test for IgA antibodies, and by a skin biopsy in which the pattern of IgA deposits in the dermo-epidermal junction, revealed by direct immunofluorescence.
- **Treatment:** dapsone is considered as drug of choice for DH.
- In case of intolerance to dapsone, other drugs which can be used are: Colchicine, Tetracycline, Sulfapyridine.

81. Ans. (c) Urticaria pigmentosa

Ref: Harrison, 19th ed. pg. 367

- **Urticaria pigmentosa:** Excess of mast cells in many tissues lead to numerous red-brown/pink papules over trunk & limbs. Present as red/pink nodules in infants & young children but disappear later in childhood.
- **Atopic dermatitis**: WHITE DERMATOGRAPHISM: running a blunt object as key on affected skin produces a white line.

Dermatology

- **Pemphigus vulgaris:** Manual pressure on the skin elicits the separation of epidermis called NIKOLSKY SIGN.
- **Bullous pemphigoid:** Utricarial/eczematous prodrome with faint dusky erythema in a figurative pattern.

82. Ans. (b) Lips

Ref: Harrison, 19th ed. pg. 363; Harwood Clinical Practice pg. 855

- Angioedema is the swelling of deep dermis, subcutaneous, or submucosal tissue due to vascular leakage.
- Acute episodes often involve the eyelids, lips, tongue, larynx, GI tract and face; however, angioedema may affect other parts of body, including respiratory and gastrointestinal (GI) mucosa.
- Most common site of angioedema lips.
- Laryngeal swelling can be life-threatening.

> **Extra Mile**
>
> - **Angioneurotic edema (swelling of face & lips) in presence of intense pruritis and evidence of vascular collapse (hypotension)** suggest a diagnosis of **anaphylaxis.**

83. Ans. (a) Subcutaneous tissue

Ref: Harrison, 18th ed. pg. 2711

84. Ans. (a) Due to deficiency of IgA

Ref: Harrison, 19th ed. pg. 386

- Disease entity which is caused due to deficiency to zinc is Acrodermatitis Enteropathica

XERODERMA PIGMENTOSA

- It is an *autosomal recessive skin disorder* with cellular hypersensitivity to ultraviolet radiation & certain chemical agents and cancer chemotherapeutic agents like cisplatin, carmustine etc.
- Covalent linkage between adjacent pyrimidines in DNA is damaged by UV rays & chemicals.
- In normal circumstances, damaged DNA is repaired by nucleotide excision & repair pathway (NER) but in case of Xeroderma Pigmentosa, *NER is defective* leading to clinical signs and symptoms.

Clinical Presentation of XP Includes

1. **Skin involvement**
   - Hallmark of XP is *Photosensitivity* which causes acute sunburn reaction on minimal UV exposure.
   - Skin is like dry parchment and pigmented, which gives the name Xeroderma Pigmentosa.

2. **Ocular involvement**
   - Loss of lashes
   - Conjuctival infection
   - Keratitis
3. **Neurological involvement**
   - Mild case: Hyporeflexia
   - Severe cases: Mental retardation, sensorineural deafness, spasticity & seizures.

85. Ans. (c) Zinc

Ref: O.P. Ghai, 8th ed. pg. 121

ACRODERMATITIS ENTEROPATHICA (AE)

- *AE is characterized by abnormalities in zinc absorption* due to defect in intestinal zinc transporter *which leads to zinc deficiency.*
- It is a rare autosomal recessive (AR) disorder which classically present during infancy on weaning from breast milk to formula or cereal which have lower zinc bioavailability than breast milk.
- **Classical features of AE include:** *(Mnemonic-"DEAL")*
   - **D**iarrhea, **D**epression
   - **E**czematous erosive dermatitis
   - **A**lopecia (non scarring), **A**pathetic look
   - **L**ethargy, irritability, whining & crying.

86. Ans. (c) Subsides over time

Ref: Manipal Manual of Surgery, 4th ed. pg. 9

- Keloids can be remembered as *"scars that don't know when to stop."*
- A keloid, sometimes referred to as a keloid scar, is a tough heaped-up scar that rises quite abruptly above the rest of the skin.
- It can appear few day to few weeks after surgery.
- It usually has a smooth top and a pink or purple color. Keloids are irregularly shaped and tend to enlarge progressively.
- *Unlike scars, keloids do not subside over time.* Instead it spreads and includes normal skin also.
- Keloid scars are made of dense collagen fibres.
- Recurrence is possible after local excision.
- It can be familial.
- *Most common site of keloid: Sternum.*
- It can be treated by intrakeloid injection of Triamcinolone.
- Best cure of keloid is achieved by excision and radiotherapy.

FMGE Solutions Screening Examination

87. Ans. (d) Nevus Anemicus

Ref: Neena Khanna Synopsis of Dermatology, 4th ed. pg. 147

NEVUS ANAEMICUS

- Nevus is circumbscribed malformation of skin.
- Nevus anemicus is a congenital anomaly that presents clinically as a hypopigmented macule or patch.
- It usually presents at birth and is unilateral.
- It does not increase in size
- Pressure with glass slide makes the lesion disappear & indistinct from surrounding skin.

Extra Mile

Nevus anemicus	Functional development defect in vascular filling, characterized by pale round flat lesions.
Becker nevus	Irregular pigmentation of shoulder, upper chest or scapular area.
Ito nevus	Pigmentation of skin innervated by lateral branches of the supraclavicular nerve.
Ota nevus	Occulodermal melanosis
Freckles	Yellowish or brownish macules of hyperpigmentation, seen on the exposed parts of the skin.

88. Ans. (b) Trichophyton rubrum

Ref: Harrison, 17th ed. pg. 1309

DERMATOPHYTOSIS OR RING WORM (TINEA) INFECTION

- Dermatophytes include a group of fungi (ring worm) that under most conditions have the ability to infect & survive only on dead keratin; that is the superficial topmost layer of skin (stratum corneum or keratin layer), hair and nails.
- They cannot survive on mucosal surfaces (e.g. mouth or vagina) where the keratin layer does not form.
- The ring worm fungi belongs to 3 genera:

Trichophyton	Microsporum	Epidermophyton

• Infects skin, hair & nail
• Infecting species include:
  ▪ Trichophyton rubrum
  ▪ Mentagrophyte
  ▪ Violaceum
  ▪ Verrucosum
  ▪ Schoenleinii
	• *Infects skin and hair* but does not involve nails
	• Several infecting species include: Microsporum audounii, M. gypseum and M. canis
		Infect skin & nails but does not involve hair Only infecting species is Epidermophyton floccosum.

Mnemonic
- **TSH-N** *(Trichophyton infects Skin, Hair and Nail)*
- **MSH** *(Microsporum infects Skin and Hair)*
- **ESN** *(Epidermophyton infects Skin and Nail)*

89. Ans. (d) All of the above

Please refer to above explanation

90. Ans. (d) Skin + Hair + Nail

Ref: Roxburg, 17th ed. pg. 39

- Trichophyton Infects skin, hair & nail.
- Infecting species include:
  ▪ Trichophyton rubrum, mentagrophytes, violaceum, verrucosum and Schoenleinii.

91. Ans. (c) Both

- In the given choices, T. verrucosum and M.Gypseum both infect skin and hair.

Please refer to above explanation

92. Ans. (b) Tinea capitis

Ref: Roxburg, 17th ed. pg. 41

- **Tinea capitis** is most commonly caused by Microsporum canis.
- Second MCC of tenia capitis is trichophyton tonsurans.
- It is never caused by epidermophyton as it does not involve hair.
- It presents with localized non-cicatricial alopecia, itching, scaling with or without boggy swelling of scalp & *easily pluckable hair.*
- Tenia capitis is diagnosed by potassium hydroxide (KOH) wet mounts of hair & scale.
- **Treatment:** Griseofulvin is DOC

93. Ans. (a) LGV (b) Syphillis

Ref: Neena Khanna Synopsis of Dermatology, 4th ed. pg. 322

- LGV is a STD, caused by chlamydia presents classically with painless lymphadenopathy.
- Mnemonic to remember LGV:
  ▪ **ABCDEFG:** Asymptomatic, Bubo, Chlamydia, Doxy, Esthiomine, Fries test, Groove sign
- Syphilis: Genital ulcer (Hard Chancre: Single, clean based, indurated, non tender, does not bleed on touch)

Disease	Ulcer	Lymph node
Syphilis	Painless	Painless
Chancroid	Painlful	Painful
LGV	Painless	Painful (Bubo)

Dermatology

94. Ans. (c) Chancroid

Ref: Harrison, 19th ed. pg. 881, 1134

- **Chancroid** is a bacterial STD caused by H.Ducreyi. It is characterized by **painful sores** on the genitalia. Chancroid is known to spread from one individual to another solely through sexual contact.

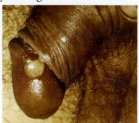

- A **chancre** on the other hand is a painless ulceration/sore most commonly formed during the primary stage of syphilis.

95. Ans. (b) Hemophilus Ducreyi

Ref: Harrison, 19th ed. p-1012

- **School of fish appearance** stained smear from genital lesions in cases of chancroid. Causative agent of chancroid is Hemophilus ducreyi.
- H. Ducreyi a major cause of genital ulceration in developing countries characterized by painful sores on the genitalia. Another early symptom is dark or light-green shears in excrement.
- Chancroid starts as an erythematous papular lesion that breaks down into a painful bleeding ulcer with a necrotic base and ragged edge.
- **H. ducreyi can be cultured on chocolate agar.**

96. Ans. (a) Secondary syphilis

Ref: Harrison, 19th ed. pg. 1132

- **Hallmark features of SECONDARY SYPHILIS:** asymptomatic, bilateral symmetrical pleomorphic maculo-papular rash on palms and soles, non-tender lymphadenopathy.
- **Other findings:** Condyloma Lata, *Moth Eaten Alopecia* arthritis, proteinuria.
- **Features that are never seen:** Vesico-bullous lesions, intense pruritus, Interstitial Keratitis.

97. Ans. (a) Gonorrhoea

Ref: Harrison, 19th ed. pg. 1107-08

- Gonorrhea is STD caused by Neisseriae gonorrhea. It doesn't present with genital ulcer.
- Patient presents with *greenish yellow or whitish discharge from the vagina*, lower abdominal or, pelvic pain, burning when urinating, conjunctivitis, swelling of the vulva (vulvitis), burning in the throat (due to oral sex), swollen glands in the throat (due to oral sex)

- A **genital ulcer** is located on the genital area, usually caused by a sexually transmitted disease such as genital herpes, syphilis, chancroid, or chlamydia trachomatis.
- Genital ulcers are not strictly a sign of an STD. They can occur in patients with Behcet's syndrome, lupus, and some forms of rheumatoid arthritis (all non-communicable diseases).
- Genital tuberculosis, often caused by direct genital contact with infected sputum, can also present as genital ulcer.

TABLE: Causes of Genital Ulcer

Bacterial	Viral	Parasitic	Non-infectious
• Hemophilus Ducreyi • Treponema pallidum • Chlamydia trachomatis • Donovanosis • Balanitis	• Herpes simplex • Varicella zoster • EBV • Cytomegalovirus	• Sarcoptes scabiei • Phthirus pubis • Entamoeba histolytica • Trichomonas vaginalis	• Trauma • Pyoderma gangrenosum • Reiter's syndrome • Wegener granulomatosis • Neoplasms

98. Ans. (b) Aphthous ulcers

Ref: Harrison's, 19th ed. pg. 239

- Apthous ulcers are also called as canker sores/apthous stomatitis and present as round ulcer with yellowish base and surrounded by a red halo.
  - The usual sites are oral mucosa on the insides of lips, cheeks or below the tongue.
  - Most of apthous ulcers are <5mm in size and heal within 1-2 weeks.
  - *Painless* recurrent apthous ulcers are seen in SLE
  - *Painful* recurrent apthous ulcers in oral cavity and genitilia is seen are in Behcet disease

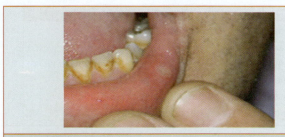

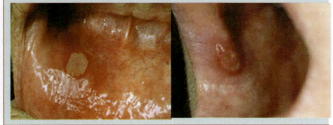

FMGE Solutions Screening Examination

99. Ans. (a) Anagen effluvium

Ref: Fitzpatrick Dermatology, 7th ed. pg. 763

- **Alopecia areata is an autoimmune disorder, in which anagen is prematurely arrested**. It presents as non-inflamed bald patches on scalp.
  - **Pathognomonic feature:** *Exclamation mark hairs*, which taper as they approach scalp.
  - **Treatment:** depends on extent of disease. Localized condition: Intra lesional steroids. In extensive condition application of diphencyprone is effective.
- **Telogen Effluvium:** Hair follicles are usually not involved in this phase, if synchronised into telogen resting mode, they will be shed in about 3 months later. It might be seen in severe stress, high fever, child birth, surgery.
- **Catagen:** It is a resting phase of hair follicle development and lasts for 3–4 weeks. Hair protein synthesis stops and follicle retreats towards the surface. 10–20% Scalp hair are in this phase.

100. Ans. (b) Condyloma acuminata

Ref: Fitzpatrick Dermatology, 8th ed. pg. 862

WARTS

- Caused by Human Papilloma virus (HPV). It is the most common virus induced tumor and shows Koebner's phenomenon.
- Condyloma Acuminata are genital warts caused most commonly by human papilloma virus type 6 and 11.
- **DOC:** 20% podophyllin or glutaraldehyde.
- **Treatment of choice in pregnancy:** Cryotherapy. If not available: Trichloroacetic acid
- *Most common cutaneous wart: Verruca Vulgaris*

Extra Mile

Warts	Seen in
Plane wart	Verruca plana
Filiform wart	Verruca filiformis
Plantar wart	Verruca plantaris or myrmecia wart
Veneral wart	Condylomata accuminata
Massive wart	Buschke lowen stein tumor
Condyloma lata	Treponema Pallidum

101. Ans. (c) Human papilloma virus

Ref: Fitzpatrick Colour Atlas, 7th ed. pg. 639

- Causative organism of Verruca vulgaris is human papilloma virus.

- Most common types of HPV associated with warts

Warts	Seen in
Common warts	HPV types 2 and 4
Myrmecia (Deep palmoplantar warts)	HPV 1
Flat warts	HPV 3, 10, 28
Butcher warts	HPV type 7
Focal epithelial hyperplasia (Heck disease)	HPV type 13, 32

102. Ans. (b) Lepromin test

Ref: Harrison, 19th ed. pg. 1126

- **Lepromin test** has only prognostic significance because it tells about cell mediated immunity & classifies the type of disease.
- It has no diagnostic value.

Diagnosis of Leprosy
- **Clinical examination**
  - Sensory testing
  - Peripheral nerve examination
- **Demonstration of acid fast bacilli**
  - In skin smear prepared by slit & scrape method
  - Nasal swabs by modified ziehl–nelson method
- Nerve biopsy
- Foot pad culture (in mouse)
- **Skin biopsy**
  - Periappendiceal lymphocytosis
  - Virchow (lepra/foam) cells are diagnostic

103. Ans. (c) Type II Lepra

Ref: Harrison, 19th ed. pg. 1127-28

Type I Leprae Reaction: Reversal Reaction	Type II Leprae Reaction: Erythema nodosum Leprosum
Type IV delayed Hypersensitivity reaction	Type III Hypersensitivity (Jarisch-Herxheimer) reaction
Found in TT (tuberculoid type)	Found in LL (Lepromatous Leprosy)
Thalidomide has no role	*Thalidomide is most effective drug*
DOC is corticosteroid	DOC is corticosteroid

- **Remember:** *Thalidomide is absolutely contraindicated in women of child bearing age due to chances of phocomelia (seal limb deformity)*

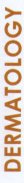

Dermatology

104. Ans. (c) Erythema nodosum

Ref: Harrison, 19th ed. pg. 132

Lupus Vulgaris: Can be endogenous & exogenous. Presents with non itchy annular plaque or long standing duration with atrophy. Apple jelly nodules are present in 10% of cases

Scrofuloderma: Contagious spread of TB may be from underlying lymphnodes, fascia or bone.

Most common site is cervical *lymph nodes*.

Ulcer with bluish edges with undermined edges. After healing puckered scarring marks will develop.

Lichen Scrufulosorum: Seen in children. Multiple grouped white papules all over the body, most commonly trunk. It is a source of TB lymphadenitis.

Erythema nodosum: It is a panniculitis that presents as a painful red nodule on lower limbs. It is due to C1 deposition in vessels of subcutis.

Causes: Idiopathic, Bacterial, fungal , viral infection, drugs (sulphonamides, contraceptives), IBD, Sarcoidosis, Behcet's disease.

105. Ans. (d) Pterygium of nail

Ref: Fitzpatrick Color Atlas, 7th ed. pg. 1008-09

- **Lichen planus** (LP) is a disease of the skin and/or mucous membranes that resembles lichen.
- It is an autoimmune disorder.
- Lichen planus may be categorized as affecting mucosal or cutaneous surfaces.
- **Cutaneous forms** are those affecting the skin, scalp, and Nails
- *Pterygium of nail is characteristically seen in lichen planus.*
- Koilonychia is found in Iron deficiency anemia (not megaloblastic anemia).

🔵 **Extra Mile**

TABLE: Patterns of Nail Involvement in different Conditions

• Iron deficiency anemia	• Koilonychia
• Arsenic poisoning	Mee's Line
• Lichen planus	Pterygium, Onychia, Onychorrhexis, Pitting
• Psoriasis	Pitting of nail (thimble nail) Oil drop nails Onycholysis: Detachment of nail plate

106. Ans. (a) Lichen planus

Ref: Harrison, 19th ed. pg. 349

The Characteristic Features of Lichen Planus are:

- Hyperkeratosis with absence of parakeratosis(which is a mode of keratinization characterized by the retention of nuclei in the stratum corneum)

- Hypergranulosis (which is thickening of the granular layer) with Basal cell degeneration
- *Presence of irregular acanthosis with saw-tooth appearance of the rete-ridges.*
- Presence of upper *dermal band-like lympho-histiocytic infiltrate* that impinges on the epidermis, leading to obliteration of the dermo-epidermal interface
- Presence of *Civatte bodies* (also known as colloid bodies and hyaline bodies), representing degenerated, apoptotic keratinocytes.

107. Ans. (a) Isotretinoin

Ref: Katzung, 1308, 1455; KDT 854

108. Ans. (c) Doxycycline

Ref: Dermatology Secrets, 7th ed. pg. 1295

- Oral treatment of acne is doxycycline.
- Ivermectin is oral DOC for scabies.
- Benzyl peroxide and Adapalene are available in ointment form.

109. Ans. (b) Erythema Multiforme (EM)

Ref: Harrison, 19th ed. pg. 129, 134

- It is an acute self limited, usually mild and often relapsing mucocutaneous syndrome
- MCC is infection with Herpes simplex virus.
- 2nd MCC: Mycoplasma pneumonia.

Clinical Presentation

- Occurs in all ages but mostly in adolescents & young adults, with a slight male preponderance.
- Characteristic **Target/Iris/Bull's eye/Annular lesion.**
- Most occur in symmetric acral distribution on extensor surface of extremities (hand, feet, elbow & knees), face & neck and appear less frequently on thigh, buttocks & trunk.
- Influenced by mechanical factors (Koebner's phenomenon) & actinic factors (predilection of sun exposed sites).

110. Ans. (d) Pityriasis rosea

Ref: Harrison 19th ed. pg. 349

- **Pityriasis rosea:** is a common skin problem that causes a rash.
- Multiple round to oval erythematous patches with fine central scales distributed along the skin tension lines of cleavage on the trunk in Christmas (fir) tree pattern.

Characteristic Features

- Classically it begins with typical Herald patch, and then becomes generalized patch.
- Herald/mother's patch is the first sign of Pityriasis rosea.

- *Fir-tree or Christmas-tree appearance* due to distribution of lesion along the line of cleavage on trunk.
- Cigarette paper scales
- Mainly involves trunk; *spares palms & soles (this feature differentiates it from secondary syphilis which commonly involves palms & soles).*

111. Ans. (b) Atopic eczema

Ref: Sauer's Manual of Skin Diseases, 10th pg. 372

- Pityriasis alba is a variant of **atopic eczema** occurring in ethnic children. It is more noticeable in summer months. The loss of color is temporary and is not related to vitiligo.
- It should preferably be treated with immunomodulators than steroids (the latter cause further hypopigmentation)

Differentials of Hypopigmented Patch		
Pityriasis alba (Simplex)	**Pityriasis Versicolor**	**Indeterminate Leprosy**
• Recurrent • Scaly hypopigmented macule mostly in **cheeks** and other part of face primarily in young children before puberty	• Scaly macule • Hands & lower limbs usually not involved • Rare in children & common in young adult • On upper trunk and shoulders (MC)	• **Epidermal Atrophy** • **Non scaly** • Resident of high leprosy prevalence state:-Bihar,-Tamilnadu, Orissa etc. • Anesthesia+

112. Ans. (a) Topical imidazole

- The shown picture is diagnosed as: Tinea/ring worm
- Topical imidazole derivative is most effective in treatment of this condition.
- Oral griseofulvin and selenium sulphide is also given

113. Ans. (b) Malassezia furfur

Ref: Fitzpatrick Dermatology, 8th ed. pg. 806

TINEA/PITYRIASIS VERSICOLOR

- *Caused by Malassezia furfur.* Most common species in India: Malassezia globosa
- It is usually seen in young adults and clinically presents with multiple small, scaly, hypopigmented macules that develop insidiously over the skin of chest & back.

Diagnosis
- **Examination of scales in 10% KOH:** Shows short hyphae & round spores *(spaghetti & Meat Ball appearance).*
- Wood lamp examination show apple green fluorescence.
- Skin surface biopsy

Treatment
- Whitfield's ointment (3% salicylic acid + 6% Benzoic acid), Selenium disulphide, Sodium thiosulphate.
- Topical Miconazole/Ketoconazole/Itraconazole; Clotrimazole,
- Systemic Keto/Itraconazole
- *Griseofulvin is not effective in case of pityriasis versicolor.*

> **Extra Mile**
> - *Griseofulvin is used systemically for dermatophytosis (tinea infection).*
> - *Griseofulvin is ineffective topically.*
> - *Griseofulvin has no role in treatment of T. versicolor & candida.*

114. Ans. (d) All of the above

Ref: Fitzpatrick, 7th ed. pg. 352

NIKOLSKY SIGN

- It is shearing away or dislodgement or sheet like removal of epidermis on applying lateral (tangential) pressure on normal skin.
- It results in formation of new bullae on stroking normal skin or if applied pressure to pre existing bullae, results in spread of bullae *(bullae spread sign).*
- Nikolsky sign is noted in blistering disorder in which pathology is above the basement membrane zone which is seen in:
  1. Pemphigus all types (except pemphigoid)
  2. Epidermal necrolysis – Stevens Johnson syndrome
  3. Toxic epidermal necrolysis (TEN or Lyell syndrome involving >30% BSA)
  4. Staphylococcal scalded skin syndrome (SSSS)
  5. Epidermolysis bullosa simplex & dystrophic Herpes, Leukemia etc.

115. Ans. (b) Sebaceous cyst

Ref: Fitzpatrick Color Atlas, 7th ed. pg. 173

116. Ans. (a) Corynebacterium minutissimum

Ref: Fitzpatrick Color Atlas, 7th ed. pg. 2146

- **Erythrasma is usually caused by C. Minutissimum**, which produces *coral red fluorescence with wood lamp*, owing to production of porphyrins. Erythrasama produces dry, reddish-brown slightly scaly and asymptomatic eruption that affects body folds.
- **C. Parvum** (propionibacterium acnes) causes excessive sebum production and lead to formation of acnes.
- **C. Amycolatum** has been shown to cause pneumonia, peritonitis, empyema, infectious endocarditis.
- **C. Jeikeium** typically causing opportunistic infection in the bone marrow transplant patients.

Dermatology

ANSWERS TO BOARD REVIEW QUESTIONS

117. Ans. (b) Keratin

Ref: Bolognia Dermatology, ch: 55

118. Ans. (a) Corneum and granulosum

Ref: Rooks, 8th ed. ch:3

119. Ans. (d) Propylene

Ref: Rooks, 8th ed. ch: 42.5

120. Ans. (a) Minocycline

Ref: Harrison's, 18th ed ch: 53

121. Ans. (a) Drugs

Ref: Harrison's, 18th ed ch: 53

122. Ans. (c) Change in color of lesion on pressure with glass slide

Ref: Harrison's, 18th ed. ch: 53

123. Ans. (a) Lichen Planus

Ref: Pathology of head neck, pg. 83

124. Ans. (b) Seborrheic dermatitis

Ref: Clinical Dermatology, 6th ed. pg. 302

125. Ans. (c) High yield Lesions on palms and face

Ref: Harrison, 19th ed. / 2744; Essential adult Dermatology pg. 308-09

126. Ans. (b) Trunk

Ref: Sports Dermatology, pg. 73

127. Ans. (a) Epidermis

Ref: Harrison's, 19th ed. pg. 502

128. Ans. (b) Hypoanesthetic macule

Ref: Harrison's, 19th ed. pg. 1124-25

129. Ans. (b) Psoriatic arthritis

Ref: Harrison's, 19th ed. / 348

130. Ans. (c) Dermatomyositis

Ref: Harrison's, 19th ed. / 374-375

131. Ans. (b) Condyloma acuminata

Ref: Harrison's 19th ed. / 1199, 544

132. Ans. (c) Type II Lepra reaction

Ref: Harrison's 19th ed. / 716-17

133. Ans. (d) Dermatitis herpetiformis

Ref: Harrison's 19th ed. / 373

134. Ans. (c) Behçet disease

Ref: Harrison's 19th ed. / 2194-95

135. Ans. (b) Bullous pemphigoid

Ref: Harrison's 19th ed. / 373

136. Ans. (a) Erythema multiforme

Ref: Harrison's 19th ed. / 129, 134

137. Ans. (d) Lichen planus

Ref: Roxburg 17th ed p 144, Rooks 7th ed p 42.1-42.14

138. Ans. (d) Psoriasis

Ref: Lippincott's Primary Care Dermatology p 47, Baran and Dawber's Disease of the Nails ad their Management by Robert Baran, David A. R. de Berker, Mark Holzberg, Luc Thomas ch-6

139. Ans. (c) Diabetes mellitus

Ref: Rooks 8th ed p 60.13, Diabetic Foot: A Clinical Atlas by Pendsey p 89

140. Ans. (d) All of the above

Ref: Rooks 8th ed p 22.31

141. Ans. (a) Vitamin A

Ref: Roxberg dermatology p 291, Harper 28th ed p 468 Table 44-1

142. Ans. (c) DLE

Ref: Rooks 8th ed. p 51.4

143. Ans. (c) Subcutaneous tissue

Ref: Rooks 8th ed p 3.53, Roxburgh's common skin diseases 17th ed p. 1

Explanations

144. Ans. (c) LGV
Ref: Greenberg's Text-Atlas of Emergency Medicine by Micheal I. Greenberg p 367, Nord Guide to Rare Diseaes p. 8

145. Ans. (c) Dermatomyositis
Ref: Harrison's 17th edch: 388

146. Ans. (c) Solid carbon dioxide
Ref: Rook's 8/e, p 77.39

147. Ans. (d) Bullous pemphigoid
Ref: Rook's dermatology 7/e, p 41.3-41.19

148. Ans. (b) Pemphigus vulgaris
Ref: Rook's dermatology 7/e, p 41.3-41.19

149. Ans. (a) Lichen planus
Ref: Rook's 8/e, p 41.14

150. Ans. (c) Pediculosis corporis
Ref: Rook's 8/e, p 38.22

151. Ans. (c) Psoriasis
Ref: Rook's 8/e, p 5.8

152. Ans. (b) Fox fordyce's disease
Ref: Rook's text book of dermatology 7/e, p 45.23, 8/e, p 71.11

153. Ans. (c) Patients on chemotherapy

154. Ans. (c) LGV
Ref: Rook's 8/e, p 34.33, Greenberg's Text-Atlas of emergency medicine by Michael I. Greenberg p. 367, Nord guide to rare diseases, p 8

155. Ans. (b) Stratum basale
Ref: Bolognia 2/e, ch:64

156. Ans. (a) Psoratic arthiritis
Ref: Rook's 8/e, p 65.13

157. Ans. (a) T. rubrum
Ref: Ananthnarayan 8/e, p 604, jawetz 24/e, ch 45 Table 45-2, Rook's 7/e, p 36.33

158. Ans. (c) Burrow
Ref: Rook's 8/e, pg. 38.36.39

159. Ans. (b) P. rosea
Ref: Rook's 8/e, pg. 38.81

160. Ans. (c) Secondary syphilis
Ref: Textbook of Sexually Transmitted Diseases 2/e, pg. 205

161. Ans. (c) Scleroderma
Ref: Rook's 8/e, pg. 51.96

162. Ans. (a) Lupus vulgaris
Ref: Rook's 8/e, pg. 31.14

163. Ans. (a) Psoriasis
Ref: Rook's 7/e, pg. 35.1

164. Ans. (a) Chronic renal failure
Ref: Bhutani's Colour Atlas, 6th ed. p-125

Triggers for Erythema Multiforme
- Infections like HSV 1 and 2, VZ virus, Infectious mononucleosis, Hepatitis B, Mycoplasma
- Collagen vascular disease
- Malignancy
- Idiopathic
- Drugs

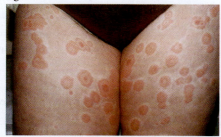

165. Ans. (b) Tuberculoid
- Saucer right side up is a feature of tuberculoid leprosy. It is so called because its borders are well defined and raised and depressed center (**Saucer right side up**)
- **Sensation:** Total anesthesia
- **Hair:** Total loss
- **Surface:** Dry and scaly

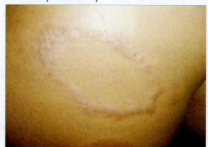

Tuberculoid leprosy: Annular, erythematous anaesthetic patch with well defined and raised borders and SSS Negative

166. **Ans. (a)** Borderline borderline

Borders:
- Both well-defined and ill-defined lesions coexist (**polymorphic**) **in equal number.**
- **Bizarre geographical** lesion
- **Annular** lesions
- **Swiss cheese** or **punched out** lesions are characteristic
- Sensation: Mild-moderate hypesthesia

- Hair: mild loss
- Surface: dry/shiny

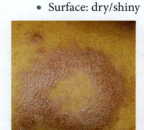
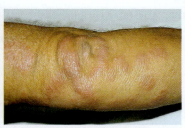

ANSWERS TO IMAGE-BASED QUESTIONS

167. **Ans. (c)** Wood's Lamp
- Woods lamp emits long-wave UV radiation (UVR), also called black light.
- This is generated by a high pressure mercury arc fitted with a compound filter made of barium silicate with 9% nickel oxide, the "Wood's filter."
- This filter is opaque to all light rays except a band between 320 and 400 nm with a peak at 365 nm.
- The output of Wood's lamp is generally low (<1 mw/cm^2). The fluorescence of normal skin is very faint or absent.
- It is useful for diagnosis of tinea capitis, Pityriasis Versicolor, Erythrasma, Acne vulgaris, Vitiligo and Porphyria.

168. **Ans. (b)** Piebaldism

It is an autosomal dominant disorder with melanocyte development defect. The presenting feature which is shown in the image is a white forelock of hair and multiple hypopigmented macules.

169. **Ans. (b)** Contact dermatitis

170. **Ans. (c)** Erythema multiforme

The image shows presence of target lesions diagnostic of Erythema Multiforme.

171. **Ans. (a)** Pityriasis rosea

The Picture shows inverted Christmas tree appearance of lesions suggestive of diagnosis of Pityriasis rosea.

The essential clinical features are the following:
- Discrete circular or oval lesions
- Scaling on Most Lesions
- Peripheral Collarette scaling with central clearance on at least two lesions.

172. **Ans. (c)** Clotrimazole paint

The image shows presence of oral thrush caused by candida Albicans, and is best managed by topical application of Clotrimazole.

173. **Ans. (b)** Caused by RNA virus
- The image shows lesion of molluscum contagiosum which are lesions are flesh-colored, dome-shaped, and pearly in appearance. They are often 1–5 mm in diameter, with a dimpled center. *The lesions are caused by pox virus which is a DNA virus.*
- Molluscum contagiosum is most common in children who become infected through direct skin-to-skin contact or indirect skin contact with fomites, such as bath towels, sponges and are commonly seen in intertriginous areas.

174. **Ans. (a)** Impetigo

The usual organism is streptococcus pyogenes > *Staphylococcus aureus*

175. **Ans. (a)** Pterygium nail
- The image shows a triangular or wing like appearance in the middle of the nail. Pterygium forms if there is scar tissue in the nail matrix.
- Since the nail matrix at that particular site cannot manufacture nail plate, the proximal nail fold skin grows out with the skin of the nail bed, giving rise to the triangular formation.

176. **Ans. (a)** Lichen planus
- The image shows presence of purple polygonal plaques on the legs and dorsum of feet of the patient diagnostic of lichen planus.
- "6 Ps" of lichen planus: planar (flat-topped), purple, polygonal, pruritic, papules, and plaques

177. **Ans. (b)** Psoriasis

178. **Ans. (d)** Chancroid

179. **Ans. (c)** Associated with anhidrosis

Ref: Bhutani's Colour Atlas, 6th ed. pg. 105

- The image shows presence of vesicular sago like grains on palms and sides of fingers diagnostic of pompholyx.

FMGE Solutions Screening Examination

- It is associated with hyperhidrosis and more common in summers.

180. Ans. (a) Lentiginosis

Ref: Bhutani's Atlas of Dermatology, 6th ed. pg. 332-33

- The image shows presence of irregular dark macules all over the trunk, neck of the patient. This is seen with lentiginosis.
- Freckles are seen on sun exposed parts of the body with ill-defined edges and darken on sunlight exposure.
- Shagreen patch has *peau d'orange* appearance and is single lesion usually in patients of tuberous sclerosis.
- Congenital nevi have pigmented macules which become nodular and are bilaterally symmetrical.

181. Ans. (c) Borderline tuberculoid

- The shown image is a case of borderline tuberculoid (BT) based on Ridley Jopling classification. They are usually single or few around 3–10 at times.
- It is characterized by well-defined borders but with areas of poor definition (serrated), known as **satellite lesions** near margins.
- In this type of leprosy following characters are seen:
  - Sensation: Significant hypoesthesia
  - Hair: Significant loss
  - Surface: Significant dry or sometimes scaly
  - Size: From large to small

182. Ans. (b) Kerion

Ref: IAP Atlas, 2nd ed. pg. 378

- The image shows a boggy swelling with plaques that drain serous fluid causing crusting in hair.
- This is diagnostic of kerion. In this condition, hair can be easily pulled out.
- Favus causes yellow colored scutula and scarring alopecia.

183. Ans. (b) Griseofulvin

Ref: Bhutani's Colour Atlas, 6th ed. pg. 17

- The image shows presence of discrete hypopigmented scaly macules on anterior abdominal wall and chest suggestive of diagnosis of pityriasis versicolor.

Management of Pityriasis Versicolor

- Lotions or shampoos containing sulfur, salicylic acid, or selenium sulfide will clear the infection if used daily for 1–2 weeks and then weekly thereafter.
- Treatment with some oral antifungal agents is also effective, but they do not provide lasting results and they are not FDA-approved for this indication.
- Ketoconazole, itraconazole and fluconazole are used.

- Griseofulvin is not effective, and terbinafine is not reliably effective for tinea versicolor.

184. Ans. (c) Predominantly occur on genitals

Ref: Bhutani's Colour Atlas, 6th ed. pg. 155

The image shows multiple erythematous plaques on the trunk with herald patch (marked with arrow) in the right iliac fossa. Pityriasis rosea has a viral etiology and is caused by HHV-7.

185. Ans. (a) Lupus vulgaris

Ref: Bhutani's Colour Atlas, 6th ed. pg. 73

- The image shows presence of erythematous brown macule on left supraorbital margin. Since CXR is normal, sarcoidosis is less likely.
- Diascopy should nail the diagnosis in favour of lupus vulgaris with apple jelly appearance.
- Lupus vulgaris is seen in patients with good immunity.

186. Ans. (b) Piebaldism

Ref: Bhutani's Atlas of Dermatology, 6th ed. pg. 307

- The image shows depigmented areas on ventral aspect of trunk with multiple islands exhibiting hyperpigmentation. The image on the right shows a white forelock of hair. Thus the diagnosis is piebaldism.
- The pattern of inheritance is autosomal dominant with defective gene located to chromosome 4.
- It occurs due to defective migration and differentiation of melanoblasts from neural crest.

187. Ans. (d) Peutz Jeghers syndrome

Ref: Bhutani's Atlas of Dermatology, 6th ed. pg. 306

The image shows presence of lentiginosis around lips and fingers. The history of melena points to concomitant GIT lesion. This is seen in Peutz Jehgers syndrome characterized by hamartomatous polyps mostly located in jejunum.

188. Ans. (d) Beau's lines

Ref: Bhutani's Atlas of Dermatology, 6th ed. pg. 277

- The image shows presence of transverse ridges in each of the nails which has occurred due to temporary cessation of nail plate growth.
- The color of proximal and distal part is same, effectively ruling out choice (b) Lindsay nails where the proximal half is white and distal half is pink/brown or red.
- Choice (a) Muehrcke's nails is ruled out as it has white bands parallel to lunula with intervening pink area.
- Choice (c), Leukonychia is ruled out as it has a uniform pallor of nail bed and the nail appears white.

Dermatology

189. Ans. (a) Muehrcke's nails

Ref: Bhutani's Atlas of Dermatology, 6th ed. pg. 277

The image shows Muehrcke's nails characterized by white bands which run parallel to lunula. This is seen in nutritional deficiency states (Hypoalbuminemia) and goes across the entire nail plate. The intervening normal area is pink interspersed with white bands.

190. Ans. (a) Hidradenitis suppurativa

Ref: Bhutani's Atlas of Dermatology, 6th ed. pg. 266

- **Hidradenitis suppurativa:** Keratin obstruction of apocrine duct extending into hair follicles. Lesions similar to acne but in apocrine area hence called inverse acne.
- Most common site is axilla.
- Rx retinoids, broad spectrum antibiotics
- **For fordyce disease:** Keratin obstruction of apocrine duct lesser than hidradenitis
- Only in flammatory papules in apocrine area
- **Acne conglobata:** Nodules and discharging sinus on buttocks, chest back. Rx oral steroids, oral isotretinoin.
- **Fordyce spot:** Ectopic sebaceous buccal gland.
- Site upper lips > Mucosa.

191. Ans. (b) Budding yeasts and pseudohyphae

Ref: Bhutani Atlas of Dermatology, 6th ed. pg. 29

The image shows KOH mount showing pseudohyphae in branching pattern and budding yeasts seen in *candida* infection.

192. Ans. (b) Tinea imbricata

Ref: Bhutani Atlas of Dermatology, 6th ed. pg. 18-19

- The image shows multiple scaly lesions with a clear intervening skin in between suggestive of diagnosis of Tinea imbricata.
- It is caused by Trichophyton concentricum and is highly pruritic.
- Choice A, Tinea corporis is classic ringworm and presents with large plaque with central clearing.
- Choice C, Tinea incognito is a tinea infection modified by steroid application
- Choice D, Tinea manuum will involve the palms.

193. Ans. (d) Erythema multiforme

Ref: Bhutani Atlas of Dermatology, 6th ed. pg. 77-78

The image shows presence of target lesions suggestive of erythema multiforme which is acute, self-limited, and is considered to be a type IV hypersensitivity reaction associated with certain infections, medications, and other triggers. The papules evolve into pathognomonic target or iris lesions that appear within a 72-hour period and begin on the extremities.

194. Ans. (b) Poxvirus

Ref: Bhutani Atlas of Dermatology, 6th ed. pg. 45-46

- The image shows multiple, rounded, dome-shaped, pink, waxy papules that are umbilicated and contain a caseous plug. The diagnosis is Molluscum contagiosum and is caused by pox virus.
- Molluscum contagiosum is most common in children who become infected through direct skin-to-skin contact or indirect skin contact with fomites.

195. Ans. (a) Herpes simplex

Ref: Bhutani Atlas of Dermatology, 6th ed. pg. 48-49

- Notice the grouped vesicles with lesions showing umbilication which is a presentation of primary herpes gingivostomatitis.
- Primary episode is quite distressing for the patient with fever, constitutional symptoms and small eroded painful lesions on lips oral mucosa and perioral area.
- Impetigo presents with honey colored crusts on the skin and is ruled out.
- Molluscum contagiosum is caused by pox virus infection and produces crops of dome shaped papules with umbilicated center which are asymptomatic.
- In the given question the patient has fever and location of vesicles is perioral and a trip to a place known for sex tourism favors diagnosis of herpes simplex.

196. Ans. (a) Molluscum contagiosum

Ref: Bhutani Atlas of Dermatology, 6th ed. pg. 45-46

197. Ans. (b) Segmental vitiligo

Ref: Bhutani Atlas of Dermatology, 6th ed. pg. 209

- Vitiligo is an acquired autoimmune condition targeting melanocytes and presents with localized or widespread white depigmented patches. Thyroid dysfunction is the most common association.
- Piebaldism is an autosomal dominant condition characterized by white forelock and circumscribed depigmented patches affecting the body. It is caused by a defect in proliferation and migration of melanocytes during embryogenesis. Unlike vitiligo, it is congenital and nonprogressive. In the question the depigmentation started at age the of 12 years and the patient presented at 13 years.

- Nevoid hypomelanosis is characterized by hypopigmented patches or streaks which follow the lines of Blaschko. They are present at birth and may develop in the first 2 years of life.

198. Ans. (a) Koenen tumor

Ref: Bhutani Atlas of Dermatology, 6th ed. p-299

Koenen tumor is seen in tuberous sclerosis and is subungual fibroma.

Tuberous sclerosis is inherited as an autosomal dominant trait with variable penetrance and a prevalence of 1/6,000 people. Molecular genetic studies have identified two foci for the TS complex. The *TSC1* gene is located on chromosome 9q34, and the *TSC2* gene is on chromosome 16p13.

199. Ans. (d) Caused by *Candida*

Ref: Bhutani Atlas of Dermatology, 6th ed. pg. 19

The image shows tinea cruris-ringworm of the groin which is also called as "jock's itch"/"Dhobi itch". It is common in the tropics.

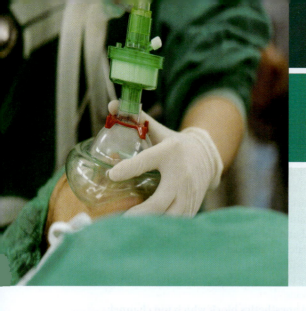

17
Anesthesia

MOST RECENT QUESTIONS 2019

1. In CPR, number of chest compression per minute in an adult:
   a. 30–50 per minute
   b. 50–72 per minute
   c. 100–120 per minute
   d. 120–200 per minute
2. Spinal anaesthesia in an adult is given at this level:
   a. T12–L1
   b. L1–L2
   c. L3–L4
   d. L5–S1
3. Colour of nitrous oxide cylinder is?
   a. Blue
   b. Blue body with white shoulder
   c. White
   d. Black
4. The duration of spinal anaesthesia is based directly on:
   a. Dose
   b. Height
   c. Age
   d. Total body fat
5. On repeated use, which of the following inhalational anaesthetic agent can cause hepatitis:
   a. Isoflurane
   b. Halothane
   c. Sevoflurane
   d. Ether
6. Which of the following is used for day care surgery?
   a. Ketamine
   b. Thiopentone
   c. Propofol
   d. Etomidate

LOCAL ANESTHETICS AND INSTRUMENTS

7. Drug used for Hypotensive episode during spinal anaesthesia: *(Recent Pattern Question 2018-19)*
   a. Nor adrenaline
   b. Phenelzine
   c. Ephedrine
   d. Na+ Nitroprusside
8. Shortest acting local anaesthetics agent:
   (Recent Pattern Question 2018-19)
   a. Bupivacaine
   b. Lidocaine
   c. Tetracaine
   d. Prilocaine
9. True about nasal cannula:
   (Recent Pattern Question 2018-19)
   a. 10 L oxygen flow, variable performance device
   b. Low flow, fixed performance device
   c. Low flow, variable performance device
   d. High flow fixed performance device
10. Which of the following ligament is pierced during lumbar puncture right before entering dura mater?
    (Recent Pattern Question 2018)
    a. Supraspinous ligament
    b. Interspinous ligament
    c. Infraspinous ligament
    d. Ligamentum flavum
11. Which of the following local anesthetics causes methemoglobinemia? *(Recent Pattern Question 2018)*
    a. Lignocaine
    b. Benzocaine
    c. Chloroprocaine
    d. Dibucaine
12. Correct sequence of resuscitation is:
    (Recent Pattern Question 2018)
    a. Early assessment, CPR, defibrillator, advance life saving
    b. CPR, early assessment, defibrillator, advance life saving
    c. CPR, defibrillator, early assessment, advance life saving
    d. Early assessment, defibrillator, CPR, advance life saving
13. Which fibers are mainly affected by Local anesthesia?
    (Recent Pattern Question 2017)
    a. A beta
    b. A delta
    c. B fibers
    d. C fibers
14. Tourniquet applied in Bier's block can provide anesthesia for? *(Recent Pattern Question 2017)*
    a. ½ hour
    b. 1 hour
    c. 2 hours
    d. 3 hours
15. Which is true about Cracking of cylinder valve?
    (Recent Pattern Question 2017)
    a. Should be performed rapidly and for prolonged duration
    b. Momentarily opening it to blow away foreign matter from the outlet
    c. It increases the likelihood of flash fire
    d. It refers to a fracture of stem of the valve
16. What is the use of soda lime in anesthesia machine?
    a. In vaporizers *(Recent Pattern Question 2017)*
    b. In oxygen concentrators
    c. In breathing circuits to absorb CO_2
    d. To treat metabolic abnormality
17. The purpose of cuff in endotracheal tube is?
    (Recent Pattern Question 2017)
    a. To reduce incidence of pressure necrosis
    b. To prevent pneumothorax
    c. To prevent the tube from slipping out
    d. To prevent regurgitation of gastric contents

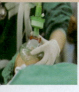

FMGE Solutions Screening Examination

18. Capnography monitors: *(Recent Pattern Question 2017)*
    a. Concentration of inhaled O_2
    b. Concentration of exhaled CO_2
    c. Concentration of electrolyte
    d. Blood pressure blood flow to the peripheral organs
19. What is this instrument used for:

    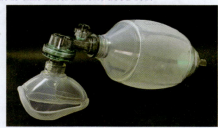

    a. Ventilation
    b. Feeding
    c. TURP
    d. Cholestomy
20. Laryngeal Mask Airway (LMA) is used for?
    a. Maintenance of the airway
    b. Facilitating laryngeal surgery
    c. Prevention of aspiration
    d. Removing oral secretions
21. A patient is on mechanical ventilation in Intensive Care unit (ICU), ventilator show alarms for increase in both peak and plateau pressure during inspiration. This indicates:
    a. Obstruction of tracheal tube
    b. Decrease in distensibility of lungs and chest wall
    c. Acute bronchospasm
    d. Increase compliance of lungs
22. Oxygen cylinder color:
    a. Black body white shoulder
    b. White body black shoulder
    c. Brown body and shoulder
    d. Blue body and shoulder
23. Pin index system for oxygen?
    a. 1,5
    b. 2,5
    c. 4,5
    d. 3,5
24. Pin index system for nitrous oxide?
    a. 1,6
    b. 2,5
    c. 3,5
    d. 1,5
25. Pin index safety mechanism in anesthesia machines are basically used to:
    a. Prevent wrong attachment of cylinder
    b. Prevent incorrect attachment of anesthesia machines
    c. Prevent wrong inhalational drug delivery
    d. Prevent incorrect anesthesia face mask attachment
26. ETT is not useful for:
    a. Pneumothorax
    b. Pulmonary toilet
    c. Obstruction
    d. Decreased level of consciousness
27. American society of anesthesiologist scoring is used to assess?
    a. Oral cavity for intubation
    b. Overall health status of patient
    c. Risk actor
    d. Pain scale
28. Local anesthesia acts by blocking
    a. Calcium channel
    b. Sodium channel
    c. By blocking both sodium and calcium
    d. None
29. Local anesthetics block which ion channel:
    a. K^+
    b. Ca^+
    c. Na^+
    d. Cl^-
30. Anesthetic agent with vasoconstrictor is contraindicated in:
    a. Spinal block
    b. Regional block
    c. Epidural block
    d. Ring block
31. Which of the following doesn't belong to ester group of local Anesthetics:
    a. Chlorprocaine
    b. Tetracaine
    c. Benzocaine
    d. Dibucaine
32. Which of the following is an ester:
    a. Chlorprocaine
    b. Bupivacaine
    c. Dibucaine
    d. Prilocaine
33. Which of the following is an ester:
    a. Prilocaine
    b. Bupivacaine
    c. Lignocaine
    d. Procaine
34. All are esters EXCEPT:
    a. Prilocaine
    b. Cocaine
    c. Tetracaine
    d. Chlorprocaine
35. Which of the following statement is true about ether as an anesthetic agent?
    a. Used with muscle relaxant
    b. Slow induction
    c. High risk of cardiac arrhythmia
    d. Recovery faster
36. Most cardiotoxic local Anesthetic:
    a. Dibucaine
    b. Bupivacaine
    c. Lignocaine
    d. Chlorprocaine

MUSCLE RELAXANTS AND ANALGESICS

37. The shortest acting opioid is:
    (Recent Pattern Question 2018)
    a. Fentanyl
    b. Sulfentanil
    c. Remifentanil
    d. Alfentanyl

38. The drug shown can be given by all of the following routes EXCEPT: *(Recent Pattern Question 2018)*

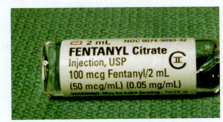

    a. Epidural
    b. Intravenous
    c. Intrathecal
    d. Intradermal

39. Hoffman degradation is seen in metabolism of?
    (Recent Pattern Question 2017)
    a. Atracurium
    b. Pancuronium
    c. Vecuronium
    d. Nitrous oxide

40. A 60-year-old patient undergoing surgery has serum bilirubin = 8.9 mg% and serum creatinine = 1.9 mg%. Which anesthetic drug is preferred?
    (Recent Pattern Question 2017)
    a. Atracurium
    b. Nitrous oxide
    c. Vacuronium
    d. Mivacurium

41. Malignant hyperthermia is due to defect in which receptor? *(Recent Pattern Question 2017)*
    a. Succinylcholine receptor
    b. Ryanodine receptor
    c. Kainate receptor
    d. AMPA receptor

42. Which is the fastest non depolarising muscle relaxant?
    (Recent Pattern Question 2017)
    a. Mivacurium
    b. Rocuronium
    c. Succinylcholine
    d. Atracurium

43. Side effect of alfentanil:
    a. Chest wall rigidity
    b. Hypertension
    c. Convulsion
    d. Hallucination

44. Muscle rigidity by fentanyl is due to which receptor:
    a. Mu (μ)
    b. Kappa (k)
    c. Delta (δ)
    d. Sigma (σ)

45. Which of the following drug causes malignant hyperthermia:
    a. Mivacurium
    b. Pancronium
    c. Succinylcholine
    d. Atracurium

46. Malignant hyperthermia is caused by:
    a. Ryanodine receptor
    b. Nicotinic receptor
    c. Muscarinic receptor
    d. NMDA receptor

47. All are true about Succinylcholine EXCEPT:
    a. Shortest acting muscle relaxant
    b. Neostimine antagonizes its action
    c. Responsible for post-op muscle pain
    d. Depolarizing agent

48. Which of the following is shortest acting non depolarizing Muscle Relaxant?
    a. Vecuronium
    b. Mivacurium
    c. Succinylcholine
    d. Atracrium

49. Which of the following is not an effect of Suxamethonium?
    a. Hyperkalemia
    b. Increased intragastric pressure
    c. Tachycardia
    d. Myalgia

50. Longest acting neuromuscular blocking agent is
    a. Atracuronium
    b. Vecuronium
    c. Doxacuronium
    d. Pancuronium

GENERAL ANESTHETIC, IV/INHALATION AGENTS

51. An anaesthetic agent causing Hepatitis:
    (Recent Pattern Question 2018-19)
    a. Halothane
    b. Etomidate
    c. Prilocaine
    d. Bupivacaine

52. MC gas used for pneumoperitoneum?
    (Recent Pattern Question 2018-19)
    a. Carbon dioxide
    b. Oxygen
    c. Air
    d. Nitrogen

53. Drug used to control secretions in general anesthesia?
    a. Hyoscine
    b. Glycopyrrolate
    c. Pethidine
    d. Lorazepam

54. Anesthetic agent of choice in pediatric patients:
    a. Ketamine
    b. Desflurane
    c. Sevoflurane
    d. Propofol

55. Best Anesthetic drug to be given in day care surgery:
    a. Ketamine
    b. Sevoflurane
    c. Desflurane
    d. Propofol

56. Regarding propofol, which one of the following is false:
    a. It is used as an induction agent
    b. It possess anti-pruritic action
    c. It is painful on injecting intravenously
    d. It has strong tendency to cause vomiting

57. Postanesthetic nausea and vomiting is uncommon with:
    a. Propofol
    b. Halothane
    c. Fentanyl
    d. Sufentanil

58. Which one of the following is the fastest acting inhalational agent?
    a. Halothane
    b. Ether
    c. Isoflurane
    d. Sevoflurane

59. In renal failure, IV anesthetic used is?
    a. Atracurium
    b. Vivacurium
    c. Pancuronium
    d. Cisatracurium

60. All of the following drugs will cause malignant hyperthermia EXCEPT?
    a. Nitrous oxide
    b. Desflurane
    c. Isoflurane
    d. Sevoflurane

FMGE Solutions Screening Examination

61. Drug producing dissociative anesthesia:
    a. Propofol   b. Enflurane
    c. Ketamine   d. Sevoflurane
62. All of the following are pharmacological effects of ketamine, EXCEPT:
    a. It causes profound analgesia
    b. It causes severe fall in blood pressure
    c. It causes amnesia
    d. It increases cerebral blood flow
63. Which of the following anesthetic agent is contraindicated in a patient with raised intracranial pressure:
    a. Etomidate   b. Thiopentone
    c. Propofol   d. Ketamine
64. Ketamine not used in:
    a. Full stomach   b. Increased ICT
    c. Pediatric patient d. Asthma patient
65. Which anesthetic agent is contraindicated in porphyria:
    a. Propofol   b. Ketamine
    c. Thiopentone   d. Etomidate
66. Absolute contraindication to thiopentone:
    a. Cardiotoxicity
    b. Acute intermittent phorphyria
    c. Malignant hyperthermia
    d. Methhemoglobinemia
67. Chloroform is:
    a. Hepatotoxic   b. Cardiotoxic
    c. Both   d. None
68. High spinal anesthesia is characterized by?
    a. Hypertension, tachycardia
    b. Hypertension, bradycardia
    c. Hypotension, tachycardia
    d. Hypotension, bradycardia

PRE-OP ANESTHETIC PREPARATION

69. Pre anesthetic evaluation of airway intubation in an elderly lady is done by:
    a. ASA scoring *(Recent Pattern Question 2018-19)*
    b. Mallampati scoring
    c. Aldrete scoring system
    d. Wilson scoring system

70. Thiopentone is preferred as an induction agent because of? *(Recent Pattern Question 2017)*
    a. Smoothness of induction b. Rapid recovery
    c. Both   d. None
71. Which is not a complication of giving anesthesia to a chronic smoker?
    a. Intra-operative bronchospasm
    b. Increased mucosal clearance
    c. Atelectasis
    d. Post-operative pneumonia

INTRA-OP AND POST-OP PATIENT CARE

72. The proper ET tube position is best confirmed by: *(Recent Pattern Question 2018-19)*
    a. Mapleson circuit b. Capnography
    c. Laryngeal mask airway d. Bag mask ventilation
73. Instructions for routine intubation are all EXCEPT:
    a. Head tilt   b. Chin lift
    c. Cricoid pressure d. Jaw thrust
74. According to ASA what is the initial management for cardiac arrest:
    a. Secure airway   b. Carotid pulse palpation
    c. IV adrenaline   d. Cardiac compression
75. Sellick's maneuver is used for?
    a. To prevent alveolar collapse
    b. To prevent gastric aspiration
    c. To facilitate Respiration
    d. To reduce dead space
76. Factors favoring fat embolism in a patient with major trauma?
    a. Hypovolemic shock b. Respiratory failure
    c. Diabetes   d. Mobility of fracture

MISCELLANEOUS

77. Heimlich maneuver is performed to dislodge foreign body located in *(Recent Pattern Question 2017)*
    a. Oesophagus   b. Bronchus
    c. Trachea   d. Upper stomach

BOARD REVIEW QUESTIONS

78. Hallucinations are seen with?
    a. Propofol   b. Sevoflurane
    c. Ketamine   d. Isoflurane
79. Succinylcholine causes?
    a. Severe hyperkalemia b. Paraplegia
    c. Liver failure   d. Renal failure

80. Mendelson's syndrome is due to?
    a. Hypersensitivity reaction to anesthetic agent
    b. Gastric contents aspiration
    c. Faulty intubation
    d. Asphyxia due to tracheal stenosis

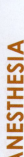

Anesthesia

81. Anesthetic agent not metabolized by body is?
   a. N20
   b. Gallamine
   c. Sevofluorane
   d. Halothane

82. Compression depth in CPR in adults is?
   a. 1 inch
   b. 2 inch
   c. 3 inch
   d. 4 inch

83. What is true about laryngeal mask airway?
   a. Prevents aspiration
   b. Used in oral surgeries
   c. Used in laryngeal surgeries
   d. Maintains airway

84. Lignocaine is used as?
   a. 0.5% jelly, 1 % injection   b. 1% jelly, 2 % injection
   c. 2% jelly, 4% injection   d. 4% jelly, 5% injection

85. PIN index of nitrous oxide is?
   a. 1-5
   b. 2-5
   c. 3-5
   d. 1-6

86. The muscle relaxant that can be given in renal disease is?
   a. Doxacurium
   b. Pancuronium
   c. Vecuronium
   d. Gallium

87. Fastest onset skeletal muscle relaxant is?
   a. Vecuronium
   b. Rocuronium
   c. Mivacurium
   d. Atracurium

88. Hoffman elimination is seen in:
   a. Cisatracurium
   b. Mivacurium
   c. Pipecuronium
   d. Vecuronium

89. All are true about halothane EXCEPT?
   a. Amber coloured bottles   b. Arrythmogenic
   c. Hepatitis
   d. Bronchospasm

90. Mallampati classification in which tonsillar pillars, uvula is not seen?
   a. Class I
   b. Class II
   c. Class III
   d. Class IV

91. Most efficient Mapelson circuit for spontaneous ventilation?
   a. Mapelson A
   b. Mapelson B
   c. Mapelson C
   d. Mapelson D

92. Shortest acting spinal Anesthetic agent?
   a. Lidocaine
   b. Bupivacaine
   c. Tetracaine
   d. Ropivacaine

93. High spinal anesthesia leads to:
   a. Bradycardia and Hypotension
   b. Bradycardia and increased BP
   c. Tachycardia and increased BP
   d. Tachycardia and decreased BP

94. Meyer Overton rule is for?
   a. Inhalational Anesthetics
   b. Local Anesthetics
   c. Depolarising neuromuscular blockade
   d. Non depolarising neuromuscular blockade

95. Celiac block is given for?
   a. Abdominal malignant growth
   b. Chest pain
   c. Sciatica
   d. Perineal pain

96. Side effect of alfentanil:
   a. Chest wall rigidity
   b. Hypertension
   c. Convulsion
   d. Hallucination

97. Muscle rigidity by fentanyl is due to which receptor
   a. Mu (μ)
   b. Kappa (k)
   c. Delta (δ)
   d. Sigma (σ)

98. Anesthesia of choice in pediatric patients:
   a. Ketamine
   b. Desflurane
   c. Sevoflurane
   d. Propofol

99. Which one of the following is the fastest acting inhalational agent?
   a. Halothane
   b. Ether
   c. Isoflurane
   d. Sevoflurane

100. In renal failure, IV anesthetic used
   a. Atracurium
   b. Vivacurium
   c. Pancuronium
   d. Cistracurium

101. Which Anesthetic agent is contraindicated in porphyria
   a. Propofol
   b. Ketamine
   c. Thiopentone
   d. Etomidate

102. Absolute contraindication for thiopentone
   a. Cardiotoxicity
   b. Acute intermittent phorphyria
   c. Malignant hyperthermia
   d. Methemoglobinemia

103. According to ASA what is the initial management for cardiac arrest:
   a. Breathing
   b. Carotid pulse palpation
   c. IV adrenaline
   d. Chest compressions

104. First sensation to be lost in local anesthetic use is?
   a. Touch
   b. Pain
   c. Temperature
   d. Pressure

105. Longest acting local Anesthetic drug is?
   a. Procaine
   b. Prilocaine
   c. Lignocaine
   d. Bupivacaine

106. Hoffmann elimination is seen with?
   a. Gallamine
   b. Thiopentone
   c. Atracurium
   d. Lignocaine

107. Which day is considered as "World anesthesia day"?
   a. 16th September
   b. 16th October
   c. 16th November
   d. 16th December

108. Agent causing malignant hyperthermia is?
   a. Succinylcholine
   b. N_2O
   c. Dantrolene sodium
   d. Gallamine

109. Ketamine is not given in?
   a. Hypertensive patients
   b. Hypovolemic patients
   c. Septic
   d. Asthmatic patients

Questions

1171

FMGE Solutions Screening Examination

IMAGE-BASED QUESTIONS

110. The image shows which cylinder?

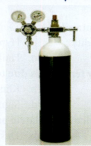

a. Oxygen Cylinder
b. Nitrous oxide cylinder
c. Cyclopropane cylinder
d. Halothane cylinder

111. Name the following instrument used in giving anesthesia

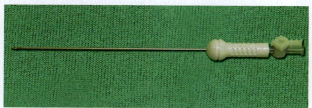

a. Intravenous regional anesthesia access needle
b. Vere's Needle
c. Lumbar puncture needle
d. Hypodermic needle

112. The diagrams of a correctly positioned proseal-type Laryngeal Mask Airway is provided below. Above what site is the arrow marked area of the airway positioned?

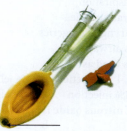

a. Carina
b. Upper end of trachea
c. Vocal cords
d. Above esophagus

113. The following procedure is being performed. Identify the markings.

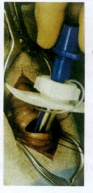 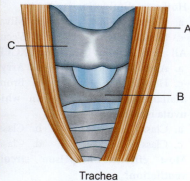

a. A = Sternomastoid muscle, B = Cricoid cartilage, C = T Thyroid cartilage
b. A = Cricoid cartilage, B = Sternomastoid muscle, C = Thyroid cartilage
c. A = Thyroid cartilage, B = Cricoid cartilage, C = Sternomastoid muscle
d. A = Sternomastoid muscle, B = Thyroid cartilage, C = Cricoid cartilage

114. All are correct about the image shown excpet:

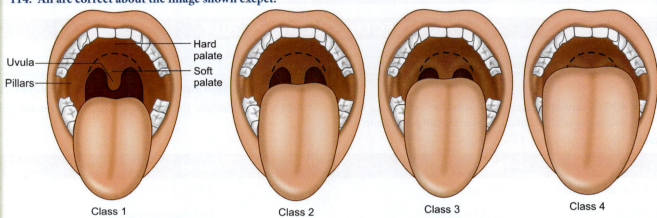

a. Mallampati classification
b. Helps in tidentifying cases with difficult orotracheal intubation
c. Not influenced by tongue mobility and size
d. Has limited utility in patients reduced neck extension

115. What is the size of this shown pink color canula: *(2018)*

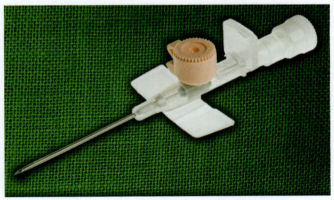

a. 16G b. 18G c. 20G d. 22G

Answers to Image-Based Questions are given at the end of explained questions

FMGE Solutions Screening Examination

ANSWERS WITH EXPLANATIONS

MOST RECENT QUESTIONS 2019

1. **Ans. (c) 100–120 per minute**

   Ref: American Red Cross CPR Guidelines 2018-19

   - CPR is cardiopulmonary resuscitation. According to latest 2018-19 CPR guidelines, the number of chest compression per minute in adult or infant is same i.e. 100 per minute.

   TABLE: American Red Cross- New CPR Guidelines 2019

	Adult	Infant
Depth of compression	At least 2"	1 ½"
Breathing	Look for chest rise Deliver breaths over 1 second	Look for chest rise Deliver breaths over 1 second
Compression to breath ratio	30 : 2	30 : 2
Compression rate	100-120/minute (until help/paramedics arrive)	100/minute
Site of chest compression	One hand should be placed on the breast bone in the center of the chest, second hand should be placed on first while keeping fingers off the chest (Image)	Use 2–3 fingers in the center of the chest on the lower half of the breast bone to compress the chest about 1 ½" (Image)

2. **Ans. (c) L 3–L4**

   Ref: Basic Clinical Anaesthesia by Paul K P 217

   - Spinal anaesthesia is required mainly in lower abdominal surgery such as inguinal herniorrhaphy, appendectomy, abdominal hysterectomy or caesarean delivery.
   - It is preferably given at L3–L4
   - Above L3 there is a risk of traumatic damage to spinal cord

Anesthesia

1175

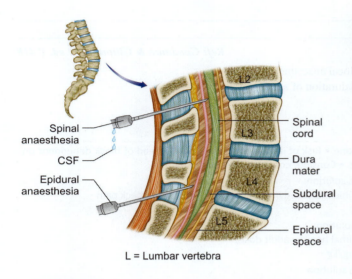

L = Lumbar vertebra

3. Ans. (a) Blue

TABLE: Color coding of different gas cylinders

Gas	Shoulder	Body
Oxygen	White	Black
Nitrous oxide	Blue	Blue
Cyclopropane	Orange	Orange
Carbon dioxide	Grey	Grey
Air	White	Grey
Nitrogen	Black	Black
Entonox	White	Blue

4. Ans. (b) Height

Ref: https://www.ncbi.nlm.nih.gov/pmc/articles/PMC4823409

- Study states: Final level of block can be predicted by patient height and weight.
- The data shows that the time to attain a suitable sensory level for surgery and duration of action correlates incrementally with height and inversely related to weight.

5. Ans. (b) Halothane

Ref: Katzung 14th ed. P 449

- Halothane is known anaesthetic agent to produce hepatotoxicity (Halothane hepatitis).
- **Incidence:** 1 in 20,000 to 35,000. Seen on repeated exposure with halothane and NOT with other inhalational agents like isoflurane, enflurane, desflurane etc.
- **Proposed MOA for hepatotoxicity:** formation of reactive metabolites that either cause direct hepatocellular damage (e.g., free radicals) or initiate immune mediated responses.

> **Extra Mile**
> - Inhalational agents like halothane, enflurane, desflurane, sevoflurane are known to depress cardiac contractility → decrease MAP (mean arterial pressure)
> - They also known to increase myocardial sensitivity to epinephrine

6. Ans. (c) Propofol

Ref: Katzung 14th ed. P 450

- Propofol is a preferred alternative to inhaled anaesthetics. Given by continuous infusion
- It is preferred anaesthetic agent in day care surgery
- **Preferred day care anaesthetic agents:** Propofol, Alfentanil, Isoflurane and congener, Mivacurium *(Mn: PAIM)*
- IV anaesthetic agent of choice in malignant hyperthermia: **Propofol**
- Agent of choice in induction in children: **Sevoflurane**
- Agent of choice in CHF and shock patients: **Ketamine**
- Agent of choice in aneurysm surgery and cardiac disease: **Etomidate**

LOCAL ANESTHETICS AND INSTRUMENTS

7. Ans. (c) Ephedrine

Ref: Goodman & Gillman 13th ed. P 415

- Hypotension is commonly associated with spinal anaesthesia.
- Treatment of hypotension is usually warranted when the BP decrease to about 30% of resting values.
- Aim of therapy: To maintain brain and cardiac perfusion and oxygenation

Treatment of hypotensive episode:
- Prior to spinal anaesthesia a bolus of fluid (500-1000 ml) is administered
- Usual cause of hypotension is decreased venous return, possibly complicated by decreased heart rate, drugs with preferential vasoconstrictive and chronotropic properties are preferred.
- **Drug of choice:** Ephedrine, 5–10 mg intravenously.
- **Other treatment options:** Phenylephrine, Oxygen, fluid infusion, administration of vasoactive drugs.

> **Extra Mile**
> - Noradrenaline, a sympathomimetic agent, itself causes reflex bradycardia.
> - Phenelzine is one of the MAO inhibitor, has no role
> - Na+ Nitroprusside: strong vasodilator. It can precipitate hypotension

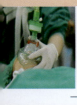

8. Ans. (b) Lidocaine

Ref: Goodman & Gillman 13th ed. P 418

- Among the given choices, lidocaine is the shortest acting local anaesthetic agent.
- Lidocaine can be used as several forms of anaesthesia and duration of action varies:
  - Local anaesthesia: ~ 30 min
  - Nerve block: 60 – 90 min
  - Spinal/Epidural anaesthesia: 60 – 90 min

EPIDURAL ANESTHESIA • Use with epinephrine- containing test done • Risk of intravenous injection • Spread of block dependent on dose and volume injected •Epidural catheter allows repeated dosing • Consider coagulation status of patient

Chloroprocaine	• Short duration • Epinephrine prolongs action	• 2-3% solution • Possible increased incidence of post procedure back pain
Lidocaine	• Intermediate duration • Epinephrine prolongs action	• 2% solution • Maximal healthy adult dose, ~4 mg/kg
Bupivacaine	• Long duration	• 0.5% solution • Maximal healthy adult dose, ~2-3 mg/kg
Ropivacaine	• Long duration	• 0.5-1.0% solution • Maximal healthy adult dose, ~2-3 mg/kg • May have less toxicity than equi- efficacious dose of bupivacaine

SPINAL ANESTHESIA • Dose and baricity of anesthetic strongly influences spread •Addition of opioids can prolong analgesia • Consider coagulation status of patient

Lidocaine	• Short duration (60-90 min)	• ~25-50 mg for perineal and lower extremity surgery • Association of spinal lidocaine with transient neurological symptoms
Tetracaine	• Long duration (210-240 min)	• Duration increased by epinephrine • ~5 mg for perineal surgery • ~10 mg for lower extremity surgery
Bupivacaine	• Long duration (210-240 min)	• ~10 mg for perianal and lower extremity surgery • 15-20 mg for abdominal surgery

Note: The shortest acting local anesthetic is chloroprocaine. Book states: *"The onset and duration of action of spinal chloroprocaine are even shorter than those of lidocaine"*
- Tetracaine is a long-acting amino ester.
- Prilocaine is an intermediate-acting amino amide.
  (Goodman & Gillman 13 edition page 412)
- Bupivacaine is also a long acting local anaesthetic.

9. Ans. (c) Low flow, variable performance device

Ref: Airway Management P 88;
Emergency Care and transportation of Sick and injured, P 208

- Nasal cannula is an oxygen delivery system
- It is used for low-medium concentration of oxygen for the patients with mild to moderate respiratory distress (used when patient cannot tolerate mask)
- Can be used continuously with meals and activity

- **Flow rate:**
  - **Adult:** 4 – 6 L/m (delivers up to 40% FiO_2)
  - **Child:** < 3 L/m
  - **Infant/toddler:** < 2 L/m
  - Flow rate > 4L can cause irritation and dryness
- Depth and rate of breathing affect amount of oxygen reaching the lungs
- **Formula for FiO_2 calculation:**
  - 20% + (4 × oxygen litre flow)

OXYGEN DELIVERY DEVICES

Low flow (variable performance devices)	Reservoir system (variable performance devices)	High flow (fixed performance devices)
• Nasal cannula • Nasal catheter • Transtracheal catheter	• Reservoir cannula • Simple face mask • Partial rebreathing mask • Non rebreathing mask • Tracheostomy mask	• Ventimask • Aerosol mask • T-piece with nebulisers

Extra Mile

OXYGEN DEVICES AND THEIR FLOW RATES

- **Masks:**
  - Simple mask: Flow rate 5 – 10 L/m. Delivers 35-40% FiO_2
  - Partial rebreathing mask: Flow rate 10 – 12 L/m. Delivers 50 – 60% FiO_2
  - Non breathing mask: Flow rate 10 – 15 L/m. Delivers up to 90% FiO_2
- **Enclosure systems:**
  - Hoods: Flow rate 10 – 15 L/m. Delivers 80 – 90% FiO_2
  - Tents: using high flow rate can deliver up to 50% FiO_2

10. **Ans. (d) Ligamentum flavum**

> *Ref: Clinical Neuroanatomy by Richard; S Snell, P 29*

Structures which are pierced while doing lumbar puncture:

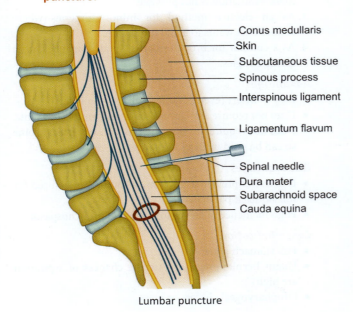

Lumbar puncture

- Skin → Subcutaneous tissue → Supraspinous ligament → Interspinous ligament → Ligamentum flavum → Dura mater → Arachnoid membrane

Needle Used

- **Dura cutting needle/Quincke's needle:** More traumatic
- **Dura separating needle/Whitacre needle:** Atraumatic. Less incidence of postpuncture headache
- **Size:** 25G (Preferred)

11. **Ans. (b) Benzocaine**

> *Ref: Handbook of Local Anesthetics, By Stanley F. Malamed; E-book, P 153*

- Local anesthetics causing methemoglobinemia are: Benzocaine and prilocaine (prilocaine mainly in neonates).
- **Dibucaine:** Longest acting, most potent and most toxic LA.
- **Chloroprocaine:** Shortest acting LA.
- **LA highest incidence of malignant hyperthermia:** Lignocaine
- **Inhalational agent having highest incidence of malignant hyperthermia:** Halothane

12. **Ans. (a) Early assessment, CPR, defibrillator, advance life saving**

> *Ref: ABC of Resuscitation by Jasmeet Soar, Gavin D Perkins; Jerry Nolan, Ch 9*

In an unresponsive patient:

- **Assess** pulse and breathing, on carotid artery for less than 10 seconds, if there is absent pulse, **start CPR**.
  - **Site of chest compression:** At the center of chest, lower half of sternum
  - **Depth of compression:** 2 inches or 5 cm
  - Rate 100/min
  - **Number of chest compression given per cycle of CPR:** 30
  - Maintain patent airway by head tilt, chin lift, jaw thrust
- Defibrillator is used next
- Call for advance life support help.

13. **Ans. (b) A delta**

Susceptibility order of nerve fibers are as follows:

- **Pressure:** Aα > Aβ > Aγ > Aδ > B > C
- **Local anesthetic:** Aγ & Aδ >> Aa & Aβ >> B >> C
- **Hypoxia:** B > A > C
- **Paresthesias** (inappropriate sensations such as burning or prickling) usually seen when A-delta is involved.

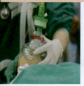

FMGE Solutions Screening Examination

14. Ans. (b) 1 hour

Ref: Morgan Clinical Anesthesia, 4th ed. pg. 341

- Bier's block can provide intense regional anesthesia for 45-60 minutes and short surgical procedures can be done on forearm, hand and leg.
- The procedure is usually done for *carpal tunnel release*.

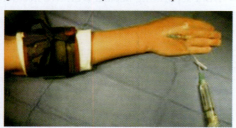

- An intravenous Catheter is inserted on the dorsum of the hand and *double pneumatic tourniquet* is placed on the arm.
- The extremity is elevated and exsanguinated by wrapping an *esmarch elastic bandage* from a distal to proximal direction.

15. Ans. (b) Momentarily opening it to blow away foreign matter from the outlet

Ref: Objective Anesthesia Review: A Comprehensive Textbook for Examinees, pg. 358

Before connecting the cylinder to the anesthesia machine the protective cap should be removed and the valve should be opened slowly and briefly. While opening the valve the port should point away from the user or other personnel. This is known as cracking the valve. *It helps to clear dust and other foreign materials from the valve outlet before it is connected to the machine.* It reduces the possibility of fires and explosions when the valve is opened after connecting it to the machine. It also prevents the dust from being blown into the machine and clogging the filters.

16. Ans. (c) In breathing circuits to absorb CO_2

Ref: Ajay Yadav's Textbook of Anesthesia, pg. 29-30

- Soda lime is mixture of
  1. Calcium hydroxide 94%
  2. Sodium hydroxide 5%
  3. Potassium hydroxide 1%.
- They react with CO_2 to form calcium carbonate.
- Soda lime also contains small amounts of silica to make the granules less likely to disintegrate into powder and a chemical dye which changes color with change in pH.
- As more CO_2 is absorbed the pH decreases and the *color of the dye changes from pink to yellow/white* (Clayton yellow-pH indicator).

17. Ans. (d) To prevent regurgitation of gastric contents

- Cuffs prevent leakage between the endotracheal tube and the trachea-both leakage of gas outwards during IPPV and of gastric contents, blood and mucus into the lungs.

18. Ans. (b) Concentration of exhaled CO_2

- Capnography–Measures end tidal CO_2 in inspired and expired gases.
- End tidal CO_2 is a reliable estimate of $PaCO_2$ in most settings.

19. Ans. (a) Ventilation

Ref: Miller's Anesthesia, 7th ed. pg. 2139

- AMBU Bag stands for *Ambulatory Breathing Unit*.
- It is a self-refilling bag-valve-mask unit with 1-1.5L capacity, used for ventilating and oxygenating intubated patients, allowing both spontaneous and artificial respiration.

20. Ans. (a) Maintenance of the airway

Ref: Miller's Anesthesia, 7th ed. pg. 1683

It is placed blindly in oropharnyx and the cuff is inflated with large volume of air (**30 to 40 ml** for adult size). Inflated cuff seals the lateral and posterior pharyngeal walls and patient can be ventilated through ventilation ports.

Indications
1. As an alternative to intubation where difficult intubation is anticipated
2. Securing airway in emergency where intubation and mask ventilation is not possible.
3. As an elective method for minor surgeries where anaesthetist wants to avoid intubation.
4. As a conduit for bronchoscopes, small size tubes, gum elastic bougies.

Advantages
- Easy to insert (even paramedical staff can insert].
- Does not require any laryngoscope and muscle relaxants.
- Does not require any specific position of cervical spine so can be used in cervical injuries.

Disadvantages
- It does not prevent aspiration so should not be used for full stomach patients.
- High incidence of laryngsospasm and bronchospasm.

Contraindications
- Full stomach patients.
- Hiatus hernia, pregnancy (where chances of aspiration are high)
- Oropharyngeal abscess or mass.

Anesthesia

- Patients who are vulnerable to go in bronchospasm.

21. Ans. (a) Obstruction of tracheal tube

Ref: Handbook of Mechnical Ventilation, 2ⁿᵈ ed.

Setting-off of an alarm for peak inspiratory pressure during ventilation indicates an endotracheal tube kinking/ obstruction

Complications of Intubation

Perioperative

1. Esophageal intubation: This is a hazardous complication. If not detected in time, can cause severe hypoxia and even death.
2. lschemia, edema and necrosis at local site (especially with red rubber tubes).
3. Aspiration (if cuff is not properly inflated).
4. Bronchial intubation and collapse of other lung.
5. **Tracheal tube obstruction by secretions, kinking.**
6. Accidental extubation
7. Trauma to gums, lip, epiglottis, pharynx, larynx and nasal cavity (in nasal intubation).
8. Reflex disturbances like laryngospasm, bronchospasm, breath holding.
9. Cardiac arrhythmias, hypertension or even cardiac arrest.

22. Ans. (a) Black body white shoulder

Ref: Miller's Anesthesia, 7ᵗʰ ed. pg. 675

Gas	Color Code		Pin index position
	Body	**Shoulder**	
Oxygen	*Black*	*White*	2, 5
Nitrous oxide	Blue	Blue	3, 5
CO_2	Gray	Gray	1, 6
Helium	Brown	Brown	2, 5
Air	Grey	White/black quartered	1, 5

23. Ans. (b) 2, 5

Ref: Miller's Anesthesia, 7ᵗʰ ed. pg. 675

- Pin index for oxygen is 2, 5.
- Cylinder of oxygen is black body with white shoulder.
- *Please refer to previous answer for explanation.*

24. Ans. (c) 3, 5

Ref: Miller's Anesthesia, 7ᵗʰ ed. pg. 675

Please refer to above table

25. Ans. (a) Prevent wrong attachment of cylinder

Ref: Miller's Anesthesia, 7ᵗʰ ed. pg. 675

- Each gas cylinder has two holes in its cylinder valve that mate with corresponding pins in the yoke of anesthesia machine.
- Each cylinder has a particular pin code and unless the correct cylinder valve is attached, the pins & holes will not coincide.
- Thus it is practically impossible to fit any cylinder to wrong yoke.
- To discourage incorrect cylinder attachment a pin index safety system has been adopted
- To prevent misconnection, gas cylinder valve blocks have holes drilled in 2 of 6 positions (a single hole in entonox)
- The pin index safety system is also ineffective if yoke pins are damaged or cylinder is filled with wrong gas or using extra sealing washers.

26. Ans. (a) Pneumothorax

Ref: Miller's Anesthesia, 7ᵗʰ ed. pg. 288

ETT is Endotracheal Tube Toilet

- It involves clearance of airway secretions, and is a normal process needed for the preservation of airway patency and the prevention of respiratory tract infection.
- Impaired clearance of airway secretions like in patients with depressed level of consciousness can result in atelectasis and pneumonia, and may contribute to respiratory failure.
- The primary indications for tracheal suctioning is to remove secretions in order to enhance oxygenation or to obtain samples of lower respiratory tract secretions for diagnostic tests. In the end, perform tracheal suctioning after endotracheal intubation to clear the airway of aspirated material or secretions or to enhance oxygenation in a tracheostomy patient with respiratory insufficiency.
- Perform bronchopulmonary toilet when secretions are visible in the endotracheal tube or at the orifice of the tracheostomy tube. Perform tracheal suctioning when the patient has coarse rales, rhonchi, or tubular breath sounds; acute or worsening dyspnea; or arterial oxygen desaturation.

27. Ans. (b) Overall health status of patient

Ref: Fundamentals of Anesthesia, 3ʳᵈ ed. pg. 4

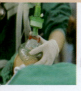

FMGE Solutions Screening Examination

ASA Physical Status Scale

Class	Physical status
1	Healthy patient with no organic or psychological disease process.
2	Mild disease/mild systemic illness but no functional limitation
3	Systemic illness with functional limitation
4	A patient with severe systemic disease which is a constant threat to life (e.g. unstable angina)
5	A moribund patient unlikely to survive with or without surgery.
6	Brain dead patient (for organ transplant)

28. Ans. (b) Sodium channel

Ref: Miller's Anesthesia, 7th ed. pg. 353

- The local anesthesia (LA) acts by blocking sodium channel. With this blockage, there is decrease in entry of Na+ ions during action potential (AP). As the LA concentration is increased, the rate of rise of AP and maximum depolarization decreases, causing slowing of conduction.
- A time comes when local depolarization fails to reach the threshold potential and conduction block ensues.
- Exposure to higher concentration of calcium reduces the inactivation of Na+ channels and lessens the degree of block.

Extra Mile

- Lignocaine is most commonly used local Anesthetic.
- It is **drug of choice** for treatment of **ventricular arrhythmias** but due to digitalis toxicity but it is ineffective *in atrial arrhythmias.*

29. Ans. (c) Na+

Ref: KDT, 6th ed. pg. 353

30. Ans. (d) Ring block

Ref: Morgan, clinical Anesthesiology, 4th ed. pg. 34

- Vasoconstrictor should not be added for ring block of hand, finger, toes, penis, pinna as all these organs are supplied by end arteries and ischemic damage may occur
- Adrenaline is most commonly used vasoconstrictor.
- Felypressin is preferred in cardiovascular disease patient.

31. Ans. (d) Dibucaine

Ref: KDT, 6th ed. pg. 352

- Dibucaine is amide group of local anesthetics.

TABLE: Ester and amides

Ester (one 'I' in name)	Amides (2 'I' in name)
• Cocaine • Benzocaine • Chlorprocaine • Tetracaine	• Lignocaine • Bupivacaine • Prilocaine • Dibucaine • Etidocaine

- All LA causes causes vasodilation and hypotension, except Cocaine. It causes vasoconstriction and significant rise in BP.

32. Ans. (a) Chlorprocaine

Please refer to previous question for explanation.

33. Ans. (d) Procaine

Ref: KDT, 6th ed. pg. 352

Please refer to above explanation

34. Ans. (a) Prilocaine

Ref: KDT, 6th ed. pg. 352

35. Ans. (b) Slow induction

Ref: KDT, 6th ed. pg. 371

- Blood gas coefficient of ether is 12 which means ether has **slow induction & slow recovery**.
- Irritant vapour, which can readily induce laryngeal spasm and make induction even slower and stimulates salivary and bronchial secretions, *So atropine as pre medication is required.*
- Ether is highly inflammable and causes explosion with cautery. It should not be used when diathermy is needed in the airways because of risk of fire or explosion. *Muscle relaxants need not be used as ether itself produces excellent relaxation.*
- Ether liberates catecholamines and tends to maintain blood pressure. *Cardiac arrythmias occur rarely* with ether and there is no sensitization of myocardium to circulating catecholamines.
- Adrenaline is relatively safe with ether. Bronchial smooth muscle is relaxed.

36. Ans. (b) Bupivacaine

Ref: KDT, 6th ed. pg. 357

- Bupivacaine is a local anesthetic agent from Amide group.
- It is most cardiotoxic LA.
- Shortest acting LA: Chlorprocaine
- Longest acting LA: Dibucaine
- Most commonly used LA: Lignocaine
- Local anesthetic which causes methhemoglobinemia: Prilocaine

Anesthesia

MUSCLE RELAXANTS AND ANALGESICS

37. Ans. (c) Remifentanil

Ref: Smith and Aitken's Textbook of Anesthesia; E-book, P 460

- Remifentanil is shortest acting opioid due to its metabolism by plasma esterase. Dose reduction is not necessary in hepatic or renal disease.
- **Most potent opioid:** Sulfentanil.
- Alfentanyl is opioid of choice for day care surgery.
- **Opioid causing neuroleptic analgesia:** Fentanyl + droperidol
- **Opioid causing neuroleptic anesthesia:** Fentanyl + droperidol + N_2O.

38. Ans. (d) Intradermal

Ref: Pain Assessment and Pharmacological Management; E-book, P 369

- Fentanyl can be given by intravenous, intrathecal, epidural and transdermal patch.
- Side effects of fentanyl are muscle rigidity, respiratory depression and bradycardia.

39. Ans. (a) Atracurium

Ref: Essentials of Clinical Anesthesia, pg. 139

- *Hoffman degradation is simply spontaneous breakdown of the molecule at physiologic pH and temperature.* This process occurs despite renal or hepatic failure, and therefore the duration of action of atracurium and cisatracurium is essentially unchanged inpatient with renal or hepatic impairment.
- Therefore, Atracurium and Cisatracurium can be given in renal failure and hepatic failure.

40. Ans. (a) Atracurium

Ref: Broody's Human Pharmacology, pg. 144

- Since in this case, there is both renal and hepatic impairment, the anesthetic agents have to be given very carefully. Agent of choice in such cases is atracurium.
- Prolonged neuromuscular block has been reported in these patients with pancuronium, vecuronium, rocuronium, and tubocurarine. These drugs are all H_2O-soluble compounds that depend on glomerular filtration, tubular excretion, and tubular reabsorption for clearance. The large volume of distribution in an edematous renal patient, a reduced renal clearance, and decreased plasma protein binding can cause prolonged elimination. The drug of choice in patients with renal disease is atracurium because of its unique degradation that is unaffected by renal or hepatic dysfunction.

- Hepatic disease also prolongs the duration of neuromuscular blockade. The liver is especially important in the metabolism of steroid-type relaxants such as vecuronium and rocuronium. In patient with cholestasis or cirrhosis, uptake of drug into the liver is decreased; thus plasma clearance is also decreased, leading to a prolonged effect. Because butyrylcholinesterase is produced in the liver, in patients with hepatic disease a decrease in enzyme production may prolong the effect of succinylcholine. Again, because the liver is not involved in the elimination of atracurium, it is the drug of choice in patient with hepatic failure.

41. Ans. (b) Ryanodine receptor

Ref: Miller's Anesthesia, 2015 ed. pg. 1314

- Malignant hyperthermia is a condition that is usually triggered by exposure to certain drugs used for general anesthesia, specifically the volatile anesthetic agents and the neuromuscular blocking agent succinylcholine.
- **Succinylcholine** is depolarizing/non competitive M.R. with shortest duration of action (3-5 minutes) due to rapid hydrolysis by pseudo cholinesterase.
- It causes dual/biphasic block. It causes hyperkalemia, increased intraocular & intragastric pressure and temperature which leads to *malignant Hyperthermia.*
- Susceptibility to MH is often inherited as an *autosomal dominant disorder*, for which there are at least 6 genetic loci of interest, most prominently the **Ryanodine receptor gene (RYR1).**
- **DOC for malignant hyperthermia:** Dantrolene
- Propofol is the intravenous Anesthetic of choice in the patients with **malignant hyperthermia.**

> **Extra Mile**
>
> - Glutamate-activated ion channels have been classified, based on selective agonists, into three categories: AMPA receptors, Kainate receptors, and NMDA receptors. AMPA and Kainate receptors are relatively nonselective monovalent cation channels involved in fast excitatory synaptic transmission, whereas NMDA channels conduct not only Na+ and K+ but also Ca++ and are involved in long-term modulation of synaptic responses (long-term potentiation).

42. Ans. (b) Rocuronium

- Fastest acting NDMR- **Rocuronium**
- Longest acting NDMR- **Pancuronium**
- Shortest acting NDMR *(Non-depolarizing muscle relaxant)*-MIVACURIUM.
- Shortest acting depolarizing muscle relaxant: Sch
- *Overall shortest acting* muscle relaxant: Sch.

Explanations

1181

FMGE Solutions Screening Examination

43. Ans. (a) Chest wall rigidity

Ref: Miller's Anesthesia, 7th ed. pg. 806

- **Alfentanil** is a short-acting synthetic opioid analgesic drug, used for anesthesia in surgery. It is an analogue of fentanyl, with lower potency.
- **Adverse side effect of alfentanil:** Chest wall rigidity, followed by others like respiratory depression, arrhythmia, Bradycardia, hypertension, blurred vision etc.

Extra Mile

- *Remifentanyl, Alfentanyl & Sufentanil have short duration of action so can be used as outpatient anesthetic agents*
- *Best anesthetic agent for OPD patients: Alfentanyl*

44. Ans. (a) Mu (μ)

Ref: Miller's Anesthesia, 7th ed. pg. 914

Opioid receptors are of four variety – mu (μ), Kappa (k), delta (δ) & sigma (σ)

Receptor	Clinical effect	Agonist
Mu (μ) (μ₁) (μ₂)	Muscle rigidity Physical dependence Supraspinal analgesia Respiratory depression	Fentanyl Morphine β – Endorphin
Kappa (k)	Sedation Spinal analgesia	Morphine Nalbuphine Dynorphin (endogenous opioid) Butorphanol oxycodone
Delta (δ)	Analgesia Behavioral Epileptogenic	Leu – Enkephalin β – Endorphin
Sigma (σ)	Dysphoria Hallucination Respiratory stimulation	Pentazocine Nalorphine Ketamine

45. Ans. (c) Succinylcholine

Ref: Miller's Anesthesia, 7th ed. pg. 866

- Malignant hyperthermia is a condition that is usually triggered by exposure to certain drugs used for general anesthesia, specifically the volatile anesthetic agents and the neuromuscular blocking agent succinylcholine.
- **Succinylcholine** is depolarizing/non competitive M.R. with shortest duration of action (3-5 minutes) due to rapid hydrolysis by pseudo cholinesterase.
- It causes dual/biphasic block. It causes hyperkalemia, increased intraocular & intragastric pressure and temperature which leads to **malignant Hyperthermia**.

- Susceptibility to MH is often inherited as an autosomal dominant disorder, for which there are at least 6 genetic loci of interest, most prominently the **Ryanodine receptor gene (RYR1)**.
- **DOC for malignant hyperthermia:** Dantrolene

46. Ans. (a) Ryanodine receptor

Please refer to above explanation

47. Ans. (b) Neostimine antagonizes its action

Ref: KDT, 6th ed. pg. 344

Reversal of Muscle Relaxation

- Depolarizing (Non Competitive) muscle relaxants are not antagonized.
- Nondepolarizing (competitive) muscle relaxants are antagonized by Acetyl choline or Anticholinesterase: Neostigmine, Pyridostigmine, Edrophonium
- In order to prevent muscarinic effects atropine is given in combination.

48. Ans. (b) Mivacurium

Ref: KDT, 6th ed. pg. 343

- Shortest acting non-depolarizing muscle relaxant: Mivacurium.
- **Duration of action** 15–20 minutes
- Shortest acting depolarizing muscle relaxant: Sch
- Overall shortest acting muscle relaxant: Sch.
- Shortest acting local Anesthetic: chlorprocaine
- Sch duration of action 6–10 minutes

Classification of Muscle Relaxants

Neuro Muscular Blocking agent	
Depolarizing (Non-competitive) muscle relaxant	Non-depolarizing (Competitive) muscle relaxant
1. Suxamethonium 2. Succinyl choline 3. Scoline Decamethonium	1. Gallamine, 2. D-tubocurarine, Atracurium, 3. Mevacurium 4. Vecuronium 5. Pancuronium 6. Rocuronium

49. Ans. (c) Tachycardia

Ref: KDT, 6th ed. pg. 342

Summary of Effect of Sch

CARDIOVASCULAR SYSTEM

- It produces muscarinic effects similar to acetylcholine. It can cause profound *bradycardia*, so atropine should be given prior to use of succinylcholine (especially in children).

Anesthesia

HYPERKALEMIA

- This is due to excessive muscle *fasciculations*. Ventricular arrhythmias can occur due to hyperkalemia. In a normal subject serum potassium increases by 0.5 mEq/L.
- It also causes muscle pain/soreness

CNS

- Sch *increases intracranial tension* due to contraction of neck muscles and blocking venous outflow (jugular veins) from cranium. This rise in ICT can be prevented by precurarization.

EYE

- Ocular muscles which are multiple, undergo tonic contraction after administration of succinylcholine *increasing the intraocular tension (IOT)*.This increase in intraocular tension can not be avoided by precurarization (precurarization is the technique in which one tenth dose of nondepolarizing muscle relaxant is given 3 minutes prior to succinylcholine).

GIT

- *Intragastric pressure is increased* due to contraction of abdominal muscles and this increases intragastric pressure which *can cause aspiration* in vulnerable individuals..Normally intragastric pressure of > 28 cm of H_2O is required to overcome the competency of gastroesophgeal junction but in conditions like pregnancy, hiatus hernia, ascites, pressure >15 cm of H_2O can cause aspiration. So precurarization is necessary in these conditions.
- Increased salivation.
- Increased gastric secretions.
- Increased peristalsis.

Remember

- **Malignant hyperthermia:** SCh is the most commonly implicated drug.
- **Anaphylaxis:** Severe hypersensitivity reaction can occur with succinylcholine.
- **Masseter spasm:** SCh can cause masseter spasm especially in children and patient's susceptible to malignant hyperthermia.

50. Ans. (c) Doxacuronium

Ref: KDT, 6th ed. pg. 343

- Doxacuronium is the longest acting neuromuscular blocking agent. Duration of action of doxacuronium is 120 minutes.

- Atracuronium duration of action- 45 minutes
- Vecuronium duration of action- 25–40 minutes
- Pancuronium duration of action 85–100 minutes

Extra Mile

- Most potent skeletal muscle relaxant: **Doxacuronium**
- Least potent skeletal muscle relaxant: **Succinylcholine**
- Least potent non-depolarizing muscle relaxant: **Rocuronium**
- Most commonly used muscle relaxant for routine surgery: **Vecuronium**

GENERAL ANESTHETICS, IV/INHALATIONAL AGENTS

51. Ans. (a) Halothane

Ref: Goodman & Gillman 13th ed. P 395

- Halothane is one of the light sensitive anaesthetic agent, marketed in amber color bottles
- **Side effect:** Fulminant hepatic necrosis (halothane hepatitis).
- **Incidence:** ~1 in 10,000 patients receiving halothane
- **Fatality:** 50%
- Halothane hepatitis is a syndrome which is characterized by fever, anorexia, nausea, vomiting and can be accompanied by a rash and peripheral eosinophilia.
- Halothane hepatitis may be the result of an immune response to hepatic proteins that become trifluoroacetylated as a consequence of halothane metabolism.

Extra Mile

Important side effects
- **Lidocaine:** Methemoglobinemia, cauda equine syndrome
- **Prilocaine:** Methemoglobinemia
- **Etomidate:** Adrenal suppression
- **Bupivacaine:** Most cardiotoxic LA, ventricular arrhythmia
- **Ketamine:** Dissociative anaesthesia, hypertension and tachycardia
- **Nitrous oxide:** Bone marrow depression, diffusion hypoxia

52. Ans. (a) Carbon dioxide

Ref: Page 582: Morgan Clinical Anaesthesia

Laparoscopic surgery involves insufflation of carbon dioxide into the peritoneal cavity producing a pneumoperitoneum. This causes an increase in intra-abdominal pressure (IAP). Carbon dioxide is insufflated into the peritoneal cavity at a rate of 4–6 litre min^{-1} to a pressure of 10–20 mm Hg. The pneumoperitoneum is maintained by a constant gas flow of 200–400 ml min^{-1}.

Explanations

FMGE Solutions Screening Examination

53. Ans. (b) Glycopyrrolate

Ref: Ajay Yadav's Anesthesia, 4th ed. pg. 48

- **To control secretions, anti-cholinergics are used:** Glycopyrrolate, Atropine and Scopolamine.
- Glycopyrrolate is preferred over atropine and scopolamine because it doesn't cross blood brain barrier. *Therefore it is devoid of central side effects.*

Drugs Used for Premedication:

- **Sedative/Anti-anxiety:**
  - Lorazepam MC used
  - Midazolam in day care surgery
- **Anti-emetics:** Hyoscine *(Most potent)*, Ondensatron, Metoclopramide
- **To decrease pain:** Morphine and Pethidine

54. Ans. (c) Sevoflurane

Ref: KDT, 6th ed. pg. 373-374

SEVOFLURANE

- Induction and emergence of anesthesia is rapid with sevoflurane.
- Absence of pungent smell makes it pleasant and administrable through face mask and is **considered as anesthesia of choice in pediatric patient.**
- Side effect: Respiratory depression and Arrhythmia.

DESFLURANE

- Desflurane is one of the inhalation (volatile liquid) anesthetic agents.
- It is fastest acting but less soluble than isoflurane.
- It has the most pungent odor, which make it unsuitable for induction.
- It irritates air passage, which may induce coughing, laryngeal spasm.

PROPOFOL

- Anesthesia of choice for **day care surgery.**
- Short acting, action diminishes the same day.
- Advantage: has anti emetic property. It is safe in porphyria.
- **Disadvantages:** Causes myocardial depression and hypotension.

KETAMINE

- Has maximum analgesic property.
- Produces **dissociative anesthesia.**
- Induction agent of choice in asthma patient.

55. Ans. (d) Propofol

Ref: KDT, 6th ed. pg. 373-374

PROPOFOL

- Anesthesia of choice for **day care surgery.**
- Short acting, action diminishes the same day.
- **Advantage:** Has anti emetic property. *It is safe in porphyria.*
- **Disadvantages:** Causes myocardial depression and hypotension.

56. Ans. (d) It has strong tendency to cause vomiting

Ref: KDT, 6th ed. pg. 375

Salient Features of Propofol

- It is a **milky white powder** that is **preservative free.** Therefore, it must be used within 6 hours.
- It is an **oil based preparation**, therefore injection is *painful.*
- Onset of action: 15 seconds
- Duration of action: 5-10 min. (due to redistribution)
- Due to rapid action, post anesthetic nausea and vomiting is uncommon with propofol
- It possesses very **strong antiemetic and antipruritic action.**
- It *decreases blood pressure* and impairs baroreceptor reflexes.
- It produces more severe and prolonged *respiratory depression* than thiopentone.
- It has no *muscle relaxant property.*
- It has cerebroprotective activity but does not possess anticonvulsant activity. Rather, **myoclonic jerking and muscle twitching** can be seen with the use of propofol.
- It is the intravenous Anesthetic of choice for **day care surgery.**
- It is also the intravenous Anesthetic of *choice for sedation in ICU.*
- Propofol is the intravenous Anesthetic of choice in the patients with **malignant hyperthermia.**
- Along with opioids (alfentanil or fentanyl) *propofol is the agent of choice for total intravenous anesthesia (TIVA).*
- Propofol infusion syndrome (on long term use as a continuous infusion >48 hours) leads to acute cardiac failure, hepatomegaly, lipemia, rhabdomyolysis.

57. Ans. (a) Propofol

Please refer to above explanation

58. Ans. (d) Sevoflurane

Ref: KDT, 6th ed. pg. 373-74

- Non pungency & rapid increase in alveolar anesthetic concentration, makes sevoflurane an excellent choice for smooth & rapid inhalational induction in pediatrics & adult population.

Anesthesia

- *Induction and recovery are very fast in desflurane.* Due to its short action it is commonly used as *anesthesia for OPD.*
- Blood gas partition coefficient of sevoflurane is lesser than halothane and isoflurane *(halothane-2.3, isoflurane-1.4, sevoflurane-0.69, desflurane 0.42),* which makes it *fastest acting inhalational agent among the choices.*

---

59. Ans. (a) Atracurium

Ref: KDT, 6th ed. pg. 345

- Atracurium and Cisatracurium undergoes spontaneous degradation by Hoffmann elimination. *So its pharmacokinetics are independent of renal and hepatic functions.* Therefore, it can be given in renal failure.
- Muscle relaxant of choice in renal failure: **Atracurium**
- Muscle relaxant of choice in renal and, or hepatic failure: **Cis-atracurium**
- Muscle relaxant in which Hoffman elimination is seen: **Atracurium, Cis-atracurium**

---

60. Ans. (a) Nitrous oxide

Ref: KDT, 6th ed. pg. 370-71

- Malignant hyperthermia (MH) is a life-threatening clinical syndrome of hypermetabolism involving the skeletal muscle.
- It is triggered in susceptible individuals primarily by the volatile inhalational anesthetic agents and the muscle relaxant succinylcholine.
- The most common triggering agents are volatile anesthetic agents such as: Halothane, Sevoflurane, Desflurane, Isoflurane, Enflurane or the depolarizing muscle relaxants suxamethonium and dexamethonium.
- *Anesthetic agents which are considered safe* include local anesthetics:
  - Lidocaine, bupivicaine, mepivacaine, opiates (morphine, fentanyl), ketamine, barbiturates, *nitrous oxide,* propofol, etomidate and benzodiazepines.
- Non-depolarizing muscle relaxants which are safe:
  - Pancuronium, cisatracurium, atracurium, mivacurium, vecuronium and rocuronium also do not cause malignant hyperthermia.

---

61. Ans. (c) Ketamine

Ref: Katzung, 9th ed. pg. 1604; KDT, 6th ed. pg. 376

- Ketamine is the only intravenous anesthetic that possesses analgesic properties and produces cardiovascular stimulation.
- It causes *"dissociative anesthesia"* which is characterized by profound analgesia, immobility, amnesia and feeling of dissociation from one's own body and the surrounding.
- **In addition it also causes:**
  - Hallucination

- Delusion and illusion.
- Profound analgesia
- **Ketamine increases all pressures like:**
  - BP (hypertension)
  - Intracranial tension (ICT)
  - Intraocular pressure (IOP)
- It is **contraindicated** in intracerebral mass/hemorrhage.

Extra Mile

About Ketamine: (Remembered as:)

K	Kids: can be given to kids
E	Emergence reaction: s/e occurring during recovery
T	Thalamo-cortical junction affected: Dissociative Anesthesia
A	Analgesia strongest
M	Meal: can be given with full stomach
I	Increase: BP/IOP/ICT
N	NMDA receptor blocker
E	Excellent bronchodilator: inducing agent of choice in asthma patient.

Extra Mile

- **PROPOFOL** causes myocardial depression and fall in BP.

---

62. Ans. (b) It causes severe fall in blood pressure

Ref: KDT, 6th ed. pg. 376

Ketamine causes increase in blood pressure.

Please refer to above explanation

---

63. Ans. (d) Ketamine

Ref: KDT, 6th ed. pg. 376

- *Please refer to above explanation.*
- Ketamine causes increase in all pressure i.e. intracranial, intraocular, intragastric and intravascular pressure.
- Therefore, it is not used in raised ICT/IOT & hypertension as it may increase the pressure to morbid levels.
- Anesthetic agents of choice in head injury/increased ICP are:
  - Thiopentone *(cerebro protective)*
  - Propofol
  - Etomidate *(protection against circulatory depression)*
  - Isoflurane

---

64. Ans. (b) Increased ICT

Ref: Katzung, 9th ed. 1604; KDT, 6th ed. pg. 376

1185

Explanations

FMGE Solutions Screening Examination

65. Ans. (c) Thiopentone

Ref: KDT, 6th ed. pg. 374

- Thiopentone is an ultrashort acting thiobarbiturate because of rapid redistribution.
- It has poor analgesic property.
- I/v injection is very painful. Therefore it is contraindicated unless opioids or N_2O has been given.
- Contraindicated in porphyria patients

> **Extra Mile**
> - Etomidate is contraindicated in adrenal insufficiency.
> - *Anesthetic drug safe in patients with porphyria: Propofol*

66. Ans. (b) Acute intermittent phorphyria

> **Extra Mile**
> - Thiopentone is C/I in acute intermittent porphyria.
> - Etomidate is C/I in adrenal insufficiency.
> - LA which causes meth-hemoglobinemia: Prilocaine
> - Malignant hyperthermia is caused by: Succinylcholine
> - DOC for malignant hyperthermia: Dantrolene

67. Ans. (c) Both

Ref: Principles of Anesthesia, 4th ed. pg. 73

Chloroform is both hepatotoxic and cardiotoxic.

68. Ans. (d) Hypotension, bradycardia

Ref: KDT, 6th ed. pg. 360

Systemic Effects (Physiological Alterations) of Central Neuraxial Blocks

■ CARDIOVASCULAR SYSTEM

The most prominent effect is hypotension which is because of the following factors:
- Venodilatation which is because of sympathetic block which maintains the venous tone.
- Dilatation of post arteriolar capillaries which is again because of loss of sympathetic tone.
- **Decreased cardiac output which is because of:**
  - **Decreased venous return:** Due to blood pooling in veins of lower limb and lower abdomen.
  - **Bradycardia:** Bradycardia can occur as a result of:
    - Decreased atrial pressure because of decrease venous return (Bainbridge reflex) and
    - Direct inhibition of cardioaccelerator fibers (T1 to T4).
- Paralysis of nerve supply to adrenal glands with consequently decreased catecholamine release.
- Direct absorption of drug into systemic circulation.
- Compression of inferior vena cava and aorta by pregnant uterus, abdominal tumors (supine hypotension syndrome).

■ NERVOUS SYSTEM

- Autonomic fibers (mediated by C fibers) are most sensitive and they are blocked earliest followed by sensory and then motor fibers. So, sequence of block is Autonomic - Sensory - Motor. The recovery occurs in reverse order although number of studies have suggested return of autonomic activity before sensory.

PRE-OP ANESTHETIC PREPARATION

69. Ans. (b) Mallampati scoring

Ref: Airway management, An Issue in Anaesthesiology clinic, P 284

- Mallampati scoring is used to predict the ease of endotracheal intubation

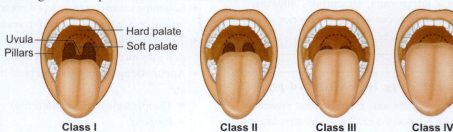

- Class I : Uvula, fauces, soft palate, pillars visible
- Class II : Uvula, soft palate, fauces visible
- Class III : Base of uvula visible, soft palate
- Class IV : Only hard palate visible

ANESTHESIA

Anesthesia

ASA SCORING

- **American Society of Anesthesiologist** classification system developed to categorize patient's physiological status that helps in predicting the operative risk.

ASA Classification	Description	Example	Perioperative mortality risk
1	A normal healthy patient		0.1%
2	Patient with mild systemic disease	Controlled epileptic patient	0.2%
3	Patient with severe systemic disease	Poorly controlled diabetes mellitus	1.8%
4	Patient with severe systemic disease that is constant threat to life	Dyspnoeic patient	7.8%
5	A moribund patient who is not expected to survive without operation	Hypovolemic shock	9.4%
6	Declared brain dead, whose organs are being removed for donation		

Extra Mile

- **Aldrete/Modified aldrete scoring system:** For determination of discharge of patient from anaesthesia care unit
- **Wilson scoring system:** For ease of laryngoscopy *(score < 5= easy laryngoscopy; Score > 7= Severe difficulty in laryngoscopy)*
- **P-POSSUM scoring system:** For predicting the mortality of neurosurgical patients

70. Ans. (c) Both

Thiopentone is preferred as an induction agent because of:
- Ease and rapidity of induction
- Absence of stage of delirium
- Rapid recovery
- Ability to increase depth rapidly

71. Ans. (b) Increased mucosal clearance

Ref: Handbook of Clinical Anesthesiology 3rd ed. by Brian Pollard 120

- From an anesthesiologist's perspective, smoking increases the relative risk of postoperative pulmonary complications by up to six times.
- A common concern is the increased risk of laryngospasm and bronchospasm.
- *Smoking increases airway mucous production and impairs ciliary function resulting in poor sputum clearance. This in combination with smoke-induced impairment of immune function, increases the likelihood of developing postoperative pneumonia.*
- **The pre-operative effect of smoking on respiratory system are:**
  - Hyper-reactive airways especially small airways
  - Reduced muco-ciliary clearance
  - Increased mucus secretion
  - Altered surfactant and permeability
  - V/Q mismatch

INTRA-OP AND POST-OP PATIENT CARE

72. Ans. (b) Capnography

Ref: www.capnography.com

CAPNOGRAPHY

- Best/confirmatory sign of endotracheal intubation
- Measures end tidal CO_2 in inspired and expired gases
- It is the most reliable tool to confirm placement of an advanced airway, both for endotracheal (ET) tubes and supraglottic-airway devices.
- When a device is placed correctly, a waveform and end-tidal CO_2 ($ETCO_2$) reading appear within seconds after the first ventilation is delivered to the patient.
- **Characteristics of normal capnogram:**
  - Rapid increase from B to C
  - Horizontal (rising) plateau from C to D
  - Rapid decrease from D to E

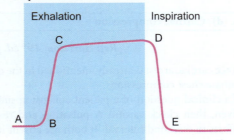

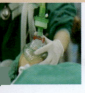

- **Phases of capnograph:**
  - **Phase I:** Inspiratory baseline (beginning of expiration)
  - **Phase II:** Expiratory upstroke (mixing of alveolar gas with dead space)
  - **Phase III:** Alveolar plateau
  - **Phase IV:** Inspiratory down stroke

TYPES OF CAPNOGRAM

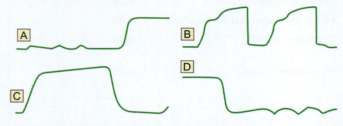

A	Near flat-line of apnea to normal rounded rectangle
B	Irregular top indicating problem with airway placement
C	Near-normal shape indicates successful airway placement
D	Sudden drop indicating displacement of airway or cardiac arrest

> **Extra Mile**
>
> **Some typical capnograph appearances**
> - **Shark fin appearance:** Bronchospasm/COPD
> - **Biphasic/Dual waveform aka curare cleft:** Endobronchial intubation
> - **Tooth like hump at the end of expiratory phase aka cardiogenic oscillation:** Heart beating against lungs
> - **Steeple sign capnogram:** Due to loose connection between sampling tube and monitor
> - **Tail/Pig tail capnogram:** Slit in sampling tube

73. Ans. (c) Cricoids pressure

Ref: Miller's Anesthesia, 7th ed. pg. 2430

- Cricoid pressure is called Sellick's manuever
- It is a method of preventing regurgitation in an anesthesized patient during rapid endotracheal intubation by applying pressure to the cricoid cartilage.
- It is indicated *only for high risk cases* where patient is not fasting example: Upper GI surgery, obstetric anesthesia.
- Studies have not shown any mortality reduction.

74. Ans. (d) Cardiac compression

Ref: Harrison, 19th ed. pg. 1768

- Since cardiac arrest is already, mentioned in the question, initiate chest compressions.
- If a clinical question of a patient collapsing suddenly is given, then check carotid A pulsation and respiratory efforts in 6 second interval. If both are absent it implies cardio-respiratory arrest. Then perform CPR.

75. Ans. (b) To prevent gastric aspiration

Ref: Miller's Anesthesia, 7th ed. pg. 2430

- Sellick's manuever is a method of preventing regurgitation of an anesthesized patient during endotracheal intubation by applying pressure to the cricoid cartilage.
- Or in other words, Sellick's maneuver is application of *backward pressure on cricoid cartilage to prevent gastric aspiration (Mendelson's syndrome).*

76. Ans. (d) Mobility of fracture

Ref: Textbook of Neurosurgery, 3rd ed. pg. 2713

Factors Favoring Fat Embolism

Traumatic	Non-traumatic
• Fracture of long bones eg. Femur • Reaming • Mobility of fracture	• Diabetes • Fatty liver • Pancreatitis • Sickle cell anemia • Decompression sickness • Extensive burns • Inflammation of bone & soft tissue • Oil or fat introduced to body

MISCELLANEOUS

77. Ans. (c) Trachea

Ref: Emergency Procedure and Techniques, pg. 48

HEIMLICH MANEUVER

The primary indication for use of the Heimlich maneuver is *upper airway obstruction due to a bolus of food* or any aspirated foreign material unrelieved by coughing and traditional means that now is causing complete airway obstruction and threatening asphyxiation.

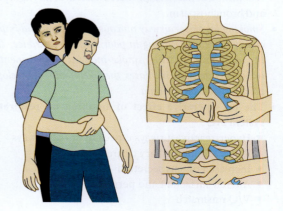

Anesthesia

ANSWERS TO BOARD REVIEW QUESTIONS

78. Ans. (c) Ketamine

Ref: *Anesthesia for Medical Students by Sullivan 1999 ed. pg. 83*

79. Ans. (a) Severe hyperkalemia

Ref: *Miller 4th ed. Ch: 9*

80. Ans. (b) Gastric aspiration

Ref: *Fundamentals of Anesthesia by Tim Smith 3rd edn. pg. 5*

81. Ans. (a) N20

Ref: *Miller's 7th ed. ch: 24*

82. Ans. (b) 2 inch

Ref: *2015 AHA Guidelines*

83. Ans. (d) Maintains airway

Ref: *Ajay Yadav, 2nd ed. p-36*

84. Ans. (c) 2% jelly, 4% injection

Ref: *Morgan's 4th ed. p-270, KDT 6th ed. p-357*

85. Ans. (c) 3-5

Ref: *Morgan 4th ed. p-2*

86. Ans. (c) Vecuronium

Ref: *Fundamentals of anesthesia by Tim Smith p-618*

Vecuronium is primarily eliminated by hepatic mechanisms. Since 30% of dose is excreted unchanged in urine, the elimination half life of drug is increased.

87. Ans. (b) Rocuronium

Ref: *Lee 13th ed. p-188, Miller's 6th ed. p-492-535*

88. Ans. (a) Cisatracurium

89. Ans. (d) Bronchospasm

90. Ans. (c) Class III

91. Ans. (a) Mapleson A

92. Ans. (a) Lidocaine

93. Ans. (a) Bradycardia and hypotension

94. Ans. (a) Inhalational Anesthetics

95. Ans. (a) Abdominal malignant growth

96. Ans. (a) Chest wall rigidity

97. Ans. (a) Mu (μ)

98. Ans. (c) Sevoflurane

99. Ans. (d) Sevoflurane

100. Ans. (a) Atracurium

101. Ans. (c) Thiopentone

102. Ans. (b) Acute intermittent phorphyria

103. Ans. (d) Cardiac compression

104. Ans. (b) Pain

Ref: *Oral and Maxillofacial Surgery, 3rd ed. Elsevier pg. 77*

The classical order of sensation loss during local anesthesia is:
1. Pain
2. Temperature
3. Touch
4. Deep pressure
5. Motor (Recovery is in reverse order)

The order of sensation loss in spinal anesthesia is cold/warm followed by pin-pnick, pain.

105. Ans. (d) Bupivacaine

Ref: *Morgan's Anaesthesiology 4/e, p 269*

106. Ans. (c) Atracurium

Ref: *Lee Synopsis of Anesthesia 12/e, p 215*

107. Ans. (b) 16th October

Ref: *Miller's 7/e, ch-1*

108. Ans. (a) Succinylcholine

Ref: *Goodman and Gillman p 152, 11/e, 352-54*

109. Ans. (a) Hypertensive patients

Ref: *Miller's 7/e, Ch 26*

FMGE Solutions Screening Examination

ANSWERS TO IMAGE-BASED QUESTIONS

1190

110. Ans. (a) Oxygen cylinder

	Body color	Shoulder color
Oxygen	Black	White
Nitrous oxide	Blue	Blue
Carbon dioxide	Grey	Grey
Air	Grey	White/black quarters
Entonox	Blue	Alternate blue and white quarter shoulder
Helium	Brown	Brown

111. Ans. (b) Veres needle

It is used to create pneumoperitoneum before laparoscopic surgery for insufflation of carbon Dioxide.

112. Ans. (d) Above esophagus

113. Ans. (a) Sternomastoid muscle, B = Cricoid cartilage, C = Thyroid cartilage

114. Ans. (c) Not influenced by tongue mobility and size

115. Ans. (c) 20G

- The shown pink canula is 20G in size with flow rate of 55–60 mL/min.
- The canula is ~1mm in diameter and 32 in length.

Theoretical Maximum flow rates		
Colour	Gauge	Flow
Yellow	24G	13 ml/min
Blue	22G	30 ml/min
Pink	20G	55 ml/min
Green	18G	80-100 ml/min
White	17G	135 ml/min
Grey	16G	180 ml/min
Orange or Brown	14G	270 ml/min

ANESTHESIA

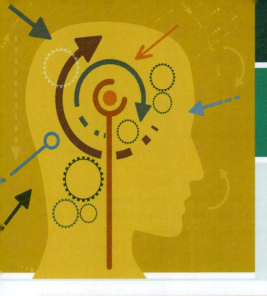

18

Psychiatry

MOST RECENT QUESTION 2019

1. A 24-year-old lady presented with sudden onset chest pain like heart attack, palpitations lasting for about 20 minutes. There has been previous recurrent episode of same. She says there were 3 similar episodes last month:
   a. Acute psychosis
   b. Panic attack
   c. Post-traumatic stress disorder
   d. Mania

SCHIZOPHRENIA AND PSYCHOSIS

2. Management of violent patient in psychiatry is treated with all EXCEPT: *(Recent Pattern Question 2018-19)*
   a. BZD
   b. CBT
   c. ECT
   d. Haloperidol

3. Negative symptoms of schizophrenia are all EXCEPT: *(Recent Pattern Question 2018-19)*
   a. Overactivity
   b. Anhedonia
   c. Alogia
   d. Apathy

4. Capgras syndrome is? *(Recent Pattern Question 2017)*
   a. Familiar person replaced by impostor
   b. Nonfamiliar person appears to be familiar
   c. Wife cheating with another man
   d. Famous person is in love with patient

5. Fregoli syndrome is: *(Recent Pattern Question 2017)*
   a. Familiar person replaced by impostor
   b. Nonfamiliar person appears to be familiar
   c. Wife cheating with another man
   d. Famous person is in love with patient

6. Which of the following atypical antipsychotic agents is associated with the most weight gain?
   (Recent Pattern Question 2017)
   a. Olanzapine
   b. Ziprasidone
   c. Aripiprazole
   d. Quetiapine

7. Which of the following is seen in Catatonia
   (Recent Pattern Question 2016)
   a. Cataplexy
   b. Echolalia
   c. Positivism
   d. Disobedience

8. An old patient was brought to the hospital with the history of auditory hallucinations. He states that, some unknown peoples are conspiring against him. He hears them talking on his every actions continuously. What could be the most likely diagnosis?
   a. Dementia
   b. Delusional disorders
   c. Schizophrenia
   d. Acute psychosis

9. A patient is brought to your clinic with complaint of unrealistic behavior from last 5–6 months. Family members mentioned about loss of his wife few years back. They also mentioned about his talking behavior in absence of everyone and sometimes muttering to himself loudly inside his room. The most likely diagnosis is
   a. Major depression
   b. Schizophrenia
   c. Conversion disorder
   d. Delusion

10. A schizophrenia patient refuses to take drugs, because he complains that he is persistently hearing people talking in spite of taking the medications. Which drug will be most suitable for his condition?
    a. Chlorpromazine
    b. Clozapine
    c. Resperidone
    d. Fluphenazine

11. A 43-year-old male is diagnosed with Schizophrenia but he refused to take treatment. Which of the following antipsychotic drug is the treatment of choice for this patient?
    a. Clozapine
    b. Risperidone
    c. Olanzapine
    d. Fluphenazine

12. Clinical manifestation of Schizophrenia are all of the following EXCEPT:
    a. Delusion
    b. Altered sensorium
    c. Auditory hallucinations
    d. Catatonia

13. Which of the following is not a characteristic symptom/sign of schizophrenia:
    a. Inappropriate affect
    b. Disturbance of thought process
    c. Visual hallucinations
    d. Auditory hallucinations

14. Prognosis in Schizophrenia is less favorable if:
    a. Occurs in women
    b. History of depression
    c. Gradual onset
    d. Acute onset

FMGE Solutions Screening Examination

15. Schizophrenia with worst prognosis:
    a. Paranoid   b. Catatonic
    c. Hebephrenic   d. Simple
16. A patient was caught by police for fighting with classmates because he thought they were planning to kill him. He states that his dead grandfather talks to him every now and then for last one month. He is delusional from past few weeks also. What will be the most likely diagnosis:
    a. Delusional disorder
    b. Post traumatic stress disorder
    c. Mania
    d. Schizophrenia
17. A 13 year young boy is brought by his parents with history of frequent fighting at school, disciplinary problems, stealing money, assaulting his batch mates and being weak in studies. What is the most appropriate diagnosis for this child:
    a. Attention deficit hyperactivity disorder
    b. Conduct disorder
    c. Autism
    d. Nothing abnormal (teenage phenomenon)
18. Which of the following is *not* Bleuler's 4 A's of Schizophrenia:
    a. Association   b. Inappropriate Affect
    c. Automatism   d. Ambivalence
19. All of the following are Schneider's first rank symptoms EXCEPT:
    a. Running commentary   b. Primary delusion
    c. Thought insertion   d. Delusion of guilt
20. Antipsychotic drugs relieve positive symptoms of schizophrenia by targeting which of the following neurotransmitters:
    a. Acetylcholine   b. GABA
    c. Dopamine   d. Serotonin

DEPRESSION, SUICIDE AND ADJUSTMENT DISORDER

21. **Double depression is:** *(Recent Pattern Question 2018-19)*
    a. Major depressive disorder from 2 years
    b. Major depression with OCD
    c. Depression with dysthymia
    d. Depression with anxiety attack
22. Indoor management of anorexia nervosa is done on priority in patients with: *(Recent Pattern Question 2018)*
    a. Forced eating symptoms
    b. Weight loss >75%
    c. Amenorrhea
    d. Depression

23. Copycat suicide is seen at age of:
    (Recent Pattern Question 2018)
    a. Adolescence   b. Child age
    c. Adult age   d. Old age
24. What would be the choice of initial treatment when a 65-year-old man with carotid artery stenosis develops severe depression and hypersomnia:
    (Recent Pattern Question 2017)
    a. Amitriptyline   b. Doxepin
    c. Nortriptyline   d. Phenelzine
25. The most common psychiatric disorder associated with stroke is: *(Recent Pattern Question 2017)*
    a. Psychosis   b. Bipolar disorder
    c. Depression   d. Mania
26. Dysthymia is seen in *(Recent Pattern Question 2016)*
    a. Bipolar Mood disorder
    b. Major depressive disorder
    c. Minor depressive disorder
    d. Persistent depressive disorder
27. Which of the following is true about depression:
    a. Increased Serotonin and Norepinephrine
    b. Increased serotonin decreased Norepinephrine
    c. Decreased serotonin and Norepinephrine
    d. Decreased serotonin increased Norepinephrine
28. Neurotransmitters mainly involved in depression are:
    a. Serotonin and Dopamine
    b. Serotonin and GABA
    c. Dopamine and GABA
    d. Serotonin and Norepinephrine
29. All of the following are the feature of masked depression EXCEPT
    a. Body aches and pains   b. Gastrointestinal symptoms
    c. Functional impairment   d. Depressed mood
30. What is the most common cause of DALY'S in world?
    a. Schizophrenic   b. Mania
    c. Depressive Disorder   d. Alzheimer's
31. In clinical practice, most common psychiatric illness seen is:
    a. Maniac disorder   b. Schizophrenia
    c. Depressive disorder   d. Bipolar disorder
32. A 40 year man is diagnosed with terminally ill cancer. He is not able to digest the fact. He previously indulged with his children like playing with his daughter, dropping her at school, but now he is not pleasurable in such events. He even stopped meeting friends and has difficulty in sleeping also. What could be the possible diagnosis:
    a. Post traumatic stress disorder
    b. Adjustment disorder
    c. Major depression
    d. Sleep disorder

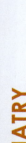

Psychiatry

33. A patient who after getting fired from her job prefers to stay isolated, has anhedonia and also lost weight. She thinks that because of her worthlessness she got fired. What could be the possible diagnosis:
    a. Adjustment disorder
    b. Major depressive disorder
    c. Post traumatic stress disorder
    d. Sleep disorder

34. The son of a construction worker died at his work place. After that he is neither going out, nor eating food properly. His wife consulted a physician and stated that he has been doing this for over 2 months. What is the most likely diagnosis:
    a. Adjustment disorder   b. PTSD
    c. Severe depression   d. Bipolar

35. Suicide is least commonly seen in:
    a. Female   b. Old age
    c. Living alone   d. Depression

36. Most common cause of impotency in male:
    a. Generalized disorder   b. Local disorder
    c. Psychogenic   d. Somatic disorder

PERSONALITY DISORDER/OCD

37. In nondiabetic nonhypertensive patient having some extra beats in pulse. Doctor informed it is benign. But patient is still going for investigations from doctor to doctor. This is a type of: *(Recent Pattern Question 2018)*
    a. Conversion disorder   b. Hypochondriac disorder
    c. Somatoform pain   d. Depression

38. A 6-year-old child with no interest in daily activity and not engaging with other children of his age group is likely to be suffering from:
    (Recent Pattern Question 2018)
    a. Autism   b. ADHD
    c. Depression   d. Bipolar disorder

39. What is the drug of choice for OCD:
    (Recent Pattern Question 2017)
    a. Buspirone   b. Risperidone
    c. Fluoxetine   d. Clomipramine

40. Goal directed repetitive behaviour is seen in
    (Recent Pattern Question 2017)
    a. Depression   b. OCD
    c. Mania   d. Schizophrenia

41. Psychological separation of a mental function from the rest of the personality is called as?
    (Recent Pattern Question 2017)
    a. Isolation   b. Dissociation
    c. Acting out   d. Paranoia

42. Skinnerian conditioning is:
    (Recent Pattern Question 2016)
    a. Pavlov method   b. Classical conditioning
    c. Operant conditioning   d. Stimulus response

43. A 25-year-old man has presented to you with sexual indulgence and increased alcohol consumption, irritability and decreased sleep, from last 10 days. The family members stated that he was career oriented remained wide awake and had prolonged periods of activity without getting fatigued. What would be the most likely diagnosis:
    a. Schizophrenia
    b. Mania
    c. Impulsive control disorder
    d. Alcohol dependence

44. Which one of the following is not a characteristic feature of mania?
    a. Elated mood
    b. Increased energy
    c. Heightened concentration
    d. Impaired judgment

45. True about obsession:
    a. Ego dystonic
    b. Ego syntonic
    c. Feel pleasure and enjoy
    d. Must be followed by compulsion

46. Which of the following is part of the treatment for OCD:
    a. MAO inhibitor
    b. Exposure and response prevention
    c. Diazepam
    d. Neurosurgery

47. Treatment of choice for phobia:
    a. Behavior therapy   b. Psychotherapy
    c. Relaxation therapy   d. Covert sensitization

48. Which of the following best explains behavioral therapy in phobia?
    a. Exposure and response prevention followed by flooding
    b. Systemic desensitization followed by exposure and response prevention
    c. Exposure and response prevention followed by systemic desensitization
    d. Flooding followed by systemic desensitization

49. All of the following is good prognostic factor for bipolar disorder EXCEPT:
    a. Acute onset
    b. Early age of onset
    c. Early responsive treatment
    d. Associated with depression

50. Lithium most commonly used in:
    a. Bipolar disorder   b. Depressive disorder
    c. Personality disorder   d. Headache

1193

Questions

FMGE Solutions Screening Examination

51. Which one of the following is *not* used in therapy of bipolar affective disorders:
    a. Lithium carbonate
    b. Sodium valproate
    c. Phenytoin sodium
    d. Olanzapine

52. A sensitive person, gets affected easily and has difficulty in controlling anger and doesn't meet people. What is the personality defect:
    a. Maniac
    b. Schizoid personality
    c. Borderline
    d. Paranoid personality

53. Anorexia nervosa is an eating disorder characterized by all EXCEPT:
    a. Menorrhagia
    b. Salivary gland enlargement
    c. Acrocyanosis
    d. Bradycardia

54. A 20-year-old man was found in a city far away from his home town, working in a factory. He was unable to tell about his previous life. Which of the following is the likely diagnosis:
    a. Post traumatic stress disorder
    b. Body dysmorphic disorder
    c. Dissociative fugue
    d. Dissociative identity disorder

55. A 21-year-old girl is disturbed that her nose is too big. She is convinced that it is disfiguring though no one else can see that way. What is the likely diagnosis:
    a. Delusional disorder
    b. Obsessive compulsive disorder
    c. Body dysmorphic disorder
    d. Specific phobia

DELIRIUM, DEMENTIA AND ALZHEIMER'S DISEASE

56. Most commonly psychiatric illness seen in medico-surgical patient: *(Recent Pattern Question 2018-19)*
    a. Depression
    b. Schizophrenia
    c. Delirium
    d. Dementia

57. Most common acute organic mental disorder: *(Recent Pattern Question 2018-19)*
    a. Delirium
    b. Dementia
    c. Amnesia
    d. Anxiety disorder

58. Clouding of consciousness is seen in:
    a. Dementia
    b. Delirium
    c. Schizophrenia
    a. Depression

59. Which of the following present with loss of consciousness:
    a. Schizophrenia
    b. Dementia
    c. Mania
    d. Organic brain syndrome

60. All are true about Dementia EXCEPT:
    a. Impaired memory
    b. Loss of consciousness
    c. Normal wake-sleep cycle
    d. Deterioration of personality

61. Dementia pugilistica occurs due to?
    a. Old age
    b. Trauma
    c. Antiepileptic drugs
    d. Hydrocephalus

62. Drug used in alzheimer's disease are all EXCEPT:
    a. Biperidin
    b. Donepezil
    c. Rivastigmine
    d. Memantine

63. Reversible dementia is seen in all EXCEPT:
    a. Wernicke's encephalopathy
    b. Alzheimer's
    c. Hypothyroidism
    d. Head trauma

SUBSTANCE ABUSE

64. Drug of choice for alcohol poisoning: *(Recent Pattern Question 2018)*
    a. Disulfiram
    b. Methycobalamin
    c. Fomepizole
    d. Benzodiazepine

65. Disulfiram is a type of: *(Recent Pattern Question 2018)*
    a. Aversion therapy
    b. Anticraving therapy
    c. Maintenance therapy
    d. Alcohol withdrawal therapy

66. Date rape drug *(Recent Pattern Question 2016)*
    a. Diazepam
    b. Lorazepam
    c. Temazepam
    d. Flunitrazepam

67. Grass/Weed/pot slang is used for *(Recent Pattern Question 2016)*
    a. Cocaine
    b. Cannabis
    c. LSD
    d. Opioid

68. Trip word in LSD is defined as *(Recent Pattern Question 2016)*
    a. Occasional use with long absistence
    b. Frequent use with short absistence
    c. Single use for lifetime
    d. Occasional use with short abstinence

69. Alcohol withdrawal presents with all EXCEPT:
    a. Hallucinations
    b. Tremors
    c. Bradycardia
    d. Sweating

70. After cessation of drinking in a person dependent on alcohol, when does the risk of alcoholic seizures peak
    a. 6-8 hours after cessation of alcohol
    b. 8-12 hours after cessation of alcohol
    c. 12-24 hours after cessation of alcohol
    d. 24-48 hours after cessation of alcohol

Psychiatry

71. The treatment of acute alcohol intoxication is based on which of the following?
    a. Severity of respiratory and CNS depression
    b. Age and sex of the patient
    c. Medical fitness of the patient
    d. Amount of breath odour

72. Which of the following is *not* a form of cannabis?
    a. Bhang
    b. Charas
    c. Cocaine
    d. Ganja

73. Early and rapid addiction is seen with:
    a. Smoking
    b. Chewing betal seeds
    c. Alcohol
    d. Narcotics

74. "Bad-trip" is associated with:
    a. Bhang
    b. Ganja
    c. Cocaine
    d. LSD

75. IQ range of Severe Mental Retardation:
    a. Below 20
    b. 21-34
    c. 21-40
    d. 35-49

BOARD REVIEW QUESTIONS

76. A lady washes her hands 40 times per day for no apparent reason. Cognitive behavior therapy for her treatment should include?
    a. Response prevention
    b. Aversion
    c. Thought stopping
    d. Desensitization

77. All are first rank symptoms of schizophrenia EXCEPT?
    a. Voices commenting
    b. Thought broadcasting
    c. Delusion of persecution
    d. Somatic passivity

78. Which of the following is not a component of 4A's of schizophrenia?
    a. Autism
    b. Affect
    c. Auditory hallucination
    d. Ambivalence

79. Term "Dementia precox" was coined by?
    a. Sigmund freud
    b. Bleuler
    c. Kraepelin
    d. Schneider

80. Kleptomania is?
    a. Fear of heights
    b. Impulse control disorder
    c. Compulsive eating disorder
    d. None of the above

81. Outside environment seems strange in?
    a. Déjà vu phenomenon
    b. Derealisation
    c. Jamais vu phenomenon
    d. Mania

82. Dialectical behaviour therapy is used for?
    a. Personality disorder
    b. Somatoform disorder
    c. Schizophreniform disorder
    d. Schizophrenia

83. Akathasia is?
    a. Increase sense of Restlessness and anxiety
    b. Buco-linguo-masticatory triad
    c. Involuntary distal movement
    d. Increase sensation of worthlessness and anxiety

84. CAGE questionnaire is used for?
    a. Sex addiction
    b. Alzheimer's disease
    c. Alcohol addiction
    d. Opioid addiction

85. Fear of being alone in a crowd or fear of travelling alone in a bus?
    a. Agoraphobia
    b. Generalised anxiety disorder
    c. Dissociative fugue
    d. Obsessive compulsive disorder

86. Most common symptom of psychiatric illness?
    a. Anxiety
    b. Depression
    c. Schizophrenia
    d. Somatoform illness

87. Not a negative symptom in schizophrenia
    a. Anhedonia
    b. Decreased emotional expression
    c. Diminished social engagement
    d. Delusions

88. Not a feature of side effects of lithium?
    a. Neutrophilia
    b. Hypothyroidism
    c. Polyuria
    d. Steven Johnson syndrome

89. Prognosis in Schizophrenia is less favorable if:
    a. Occurs in women
    b. History of depression
    c. Gradual onset
    d. Acute onset

90. Which of the following is *not* Bleuler's 4 A's of Schizophrenia:
    a. Association
    b. Inappropriate affect
    c. Automatism
    d. Ambivalence

91. Son of a construction worker died at his work place. After that he is not going out, not eating food properly. His wife consulted physician and states that he has been doing this over 2 months. What is the most likely diagnosis:
    a. Adjustment disorder
    b. PTSD
    c. Severe depression
    d. Bipolar

92. Suicide least commonly seen in:
    a. Female
    b. Old age
    c. Living alone
    d. Depression

FMGE Solutions Screening Examination

93. True about obsession?
    a. Ego dystonic
    b. Ego syntonic
    c. Feel pleasure and enjoy
    d. Must be followed by compulsion
94. Clouding of consciousness seen in:
    a. Dementia   b. Delirium
    c. Schizophrenia   d. Depression
95. Which of the following presents with loss of conciousness:
    a. Schizophrenia   b. Dementia
    c. Mania   d. Organic brain syndrome
96. In case of Alzheimer's disease Dementia pugilistica occurs due to:
    a. Old age   b. Trauma
    c. Antiepileptic drugs d. Hydrocephalus
97. Alcohol withdrawal presents with all EXCEPT:
    a. Hallucinations   b. Tremors
    c. Bradycardia   d. Sweating
98. "Bad-trip" is associated with:
    a. Bhang   b. Ganja
    c. Cocaine   d. LSD
99. IQ range of moderate mental retardation:
    a. Below 20   b. 21-34
    c. 21-40   d. 35-49
100. Bright light therapy is used for?
    a. Seasonal affective disorder
    b. Schizophrenia
    c. Adjustment disorder
    d. Anxiety
101. Treatment of depression with suicidal tendencies is?
    a. Clozapine   b. Mitrazapine
    c. ECT   d. Olenzapine
102. DALY lost due to mental diseases is?
    a. 10%   b. 14%
    c. 18%   d. 28%
103. Ganser syndrome is related to?
    a. Approximate answer b. Ataxia
    c. Confusion   d. Repeated answers
104. Treatment of a child suffering from ADHD with Tourette's syndrome is?
    a. Atomoxetine   b. Methylphenidate
    c. Amphetamine   d. Guanfacine
105. About narcolepsy all are true EXCEPT?
    a. Associated with cataplexy
    b. Equal in male and female
    c. NREM disorder
    d. Hypnogogic hallucinations
106. True about good sleep hygiene is?
    a. Same time for sleeping and waking up daily
    b. Heavy exercise in evening
    c. Heavy dinner at night
    d. Small naps in day

107. Which of the following is not a perceptual disorder?
    a. Imagery   b. Illusion
    c. Hallucinations   d. Synaesthesia
108. Cause of death in retts syndrome is?
    a. Hypoglycemia   b. Cardiac arrythmia
    c. Seizures   d. Respiratory failure
109. An IQ of 50-60 is which type of mental retardation?
    a. Mild   b. Moderate
    c. Severe   d. Very severe
110. Which defense mechanism is seen in panic disorder?
    a. Personalisation   b. Reaction formation
    c. Catastrophisation d. Derealization
111. If both parents are suffering from schizophrenia then what chance does the offspring have of being schizophrenic?
    a. 4%   b. 14%
    c. 40%   d. 50%
112. Aversion therapy is used for?
    a. Depression   b. Mania
    c. Paraphilia   d. Suicidal tendencies
113. Minimum time period to diagnose depression with daily manifestation is?
    a. 1 weeks   b. 2 weeks
    c. 4 weeks   d. 8 weeks
114. Delusion is a disorder of?
    a. Thought   b. Personality
    c. Memory   d. Cognition
115. Which of the following is a symptom of opioid withdrawal?
    a. Pupillary constriction b. Piloerection
    c. Hypotension   d. Constipation
116. Pseudodementia is seen in?
    a. Depression   b. Schizophrenia
    c. Parkinson's disease d. Dissociative disorder
117. A child with schizophrenia was on medications. Suddenly he developed neck stiffness and spasm. Best treatment of such a case is?
    a. Benztropine   b. Lorazepam
    c. Diphenhydramine   d. Propranolol
118. Delusion that an identical looking individual has been replaced by imposter is?
    a. De clerambault's syndrome
    b. Capgras syndrome
    c. Cotard's syndrome
    d. Ekbom's syndrome
119. Which of the following is classified as mood stabilizing drug?
    a. Valproate   b. Clonazepam
    c. Desvenlafaxine   d. Amitriptyline
120. Squeeze technique is used for: (2018)
    a. Premature ejaculation b. Azoospermia
    c. Depression   d. Anxiety

Psychiatry

ANSWERS WITH EXPLANATIONS

MOST RECENT QUESTION 2019

1. Ans. (b) Panic attack

Ref: Harrison's 19th ed. P 3262

- Panic disorder is defined by the presence of recurrent and unpredictable panic attacks, which are distinct episodes of intense fear and discomfort associated with a variety of physical symptoms like chest pain, fear of impending doom, palpitation, sweating, trembling, paresthesias, GI distress etc,
- **Diagnostic criteria:** 1 month of concern or worry about the attack or behavioural change related to them
- Lifetime prevalence of panic disorder is 2–3%
- Symptoms are always sudden onset, in an unexpected fashion, developing within 10 minutes and usually resolving within an hour.
- Frequency of panic attack varies: ranging from once a week to clusters to attacks separated by months of well being

SCHIZOPHRENIA

2. Ans. (b) CBT

Ref: Kaplan's Textbook of Psychiatry Ch 29.2

- Violence is one of the common psychiatric emergencies. It is characterized by physical aggression of one person on another.
- It is most commonly associated with psychotic disorder and personality disorders.

Management

- Physical restraint *(only if necessary)*.
- Give injection of Haloperidol (5 mg IM/IV) with or without lorazepam (2 mg IV). Repeat every 2 hours if necessary.
- Hospitalization → Referral to psychiatric services for further management
- In acute cases ECT can also be used.
- **Note:** CBT is not done in any of the acute psychiatric illness including depression.

3. Ans. (a) Overactivity

Ref: Kaplan's Textbook of Psychiatry Ch 12.8

NEGATIVE SYMPTOMS OF SCHIZOPHRENIA

- Affect flattening/blunting
- Alogia (poverty of speech/content)
- Avolition/apathy (lack of interest/motivation)
- Anhedonia (a sociality)
- Lack of attention

NOTE

- Over activity is NOT a negative symptom of schizophrenia.
- Example of positive symptoms: Conceptual disorganization, delusions, auditory hallucination or hallucinations
- Negative symptoms are associated with poor prognosis, while positive symptoms are associated with good prognosis.

4. Ans. (a) Familiar person replaced by impostor

Ref: Patient based approach to cognitive neurosciences pg. 155

Capgras syndrome: Chronic paranoid psychosis who is convinced that multiple persons, including members of family, had been replaced by imposters.

5. Ans. (b) Nonfamiliar person appears to be familiar

Ref: Patient based approach to cognitive neurosciences pg. 155

- **Fregoli syndrome** involves the belief that a person who appears to be well known to the patient is really impersonating.
- Christodoulou suggested that capgras syndrome is characterized by a "hypoidentification" of a person known by the patient, who is felt to be an imposter, while Fregoli syndrome was the manifestation of "hyperidentification" in which a known person could be seen in the disguise of others.

6. Ans. (a) Olanzapine

- Most common atypical antipsychotics associated with weight gain is: **Clozapine, Olanzapine**
- Other drugs associated with weight gain are Quetiapine, Risperidone and Asenapine, sertindole.

7. Ans. (b) Echolalia

Ref: Harrison's, 19th ed.

FMGE Solutions Screening Examination

- Catatonia is a syndrome. It is a state of neurogenic motor immobility and behavioral abnormality manifested by stupor.
- It can be a part of medical illness or a psychiatric illness.
- Signs and symptoms:
  - **Echolalia:** Repetition of words or sentences heard by patient. Ex: what is this color? Patient replies: what is this color.
  - **Echopraxia:** Repetition of action
  - **Rigidity**
  - **Negativism:** Opposition or no response to instructions or external stimuli
  - **Automative obedience:** Excessive obeying of command without thinking of its consequence
  - **Catalepsy:** Waxy flexibility
  - **Posturing:** Spontaneous and active maintenance of a posture against gravity
  - **Mitgehen:** Excessive movement with slight pressure
  - **Gegenhalten:** Resistance of movement with proportional force
  - **Staring:** Persistent glaring/staring at one place

DIAGNOSIS

- **According to ICD 10:** Any one symptom if present is diagnostic
- **DSM 5 says:** Any 3 symptoms present is diagnostic

Treatment: IV Lorazepam

Note: *Cataplexy* is symptom of *narcolepsy*, while catalepsy is a feature of catatonia.

---

8. Ans. (c) Schizophrenia

Ref: Harrison, 19th ed. pg. 2720

- Hallucinatory voice commenting (keeping up a running commentary) on one's behavior, thought or action in the third person *(third person hallucination)* is a classical presentation of schizophrenia.
- The patient presented here presents with 3rd party auditory hallucination, which is a very characteristic finding of Schizophrenia.

TABLE: Diagnostic criteria for schizophrenia according to DSM-IV and ICD 10

	DSM-IV	**ICD-10**

≥ 1 criteria for 1 month	• Bizzare delusions
	• Hallucinations consist of:
	  ▪ Hallucinatory voice commenting (keeping up a running commentary) on one's behavior, thought or action in the third person *(third person hallucination)*
	  ▪ Voices discussing or arguing i.e. hallucinations of two or more voices discussing or conversing with each other
		• Thought echo/ insertion/withdrawal/ broadcasting
		• Delusion of control
		• Hallucinatory voices
		• Persistent delusions

	DSM-IV	**ICD-10**
Or ≥ 2 Criteria	• Delusions • Hallucinations • Negative symptoms i.e. affective flattening, alogia or avolition • Grossly disorganized or catatonic behavior • Disorganized speech (eg frequent incoherence or derailment)	• Thought block/ disorder • Persistent hallucinations • Negative symptoms • Catatonia
Time course	• Symptom for 1 month + 6 months social/occupational disturbance	• 1 month (most of the time)
Exclusions	• Brief mood disturbance or schizoaffective disorder • Direct effect of drug abuse/ medication/medical condition	• Schizoaffective disorder or extensive depressive/manic symptoms • Drug intoxication/withdrawal, overt brain disease.

- Negative symptoms respond poor to treatment *(poor prognosis)* while positive symptoms are well responsive to treatment *(better prognosis)*.

Positive Symptoms	**Negative Symptoms**
• Hallucination • Delusion • Illusion • Thought disorder • Aggressive behavior • Irrational conclusion	• Anhedonia: loss of interest in things which were interesting before. • Avolition: lack of desire to achieve goal • Alogia: poverty of speech • Attention deficit and cognition deficit • Social withdrawal/poor socialization skill • Emotional blunting

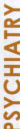

Psychiatry

9. Ans. (b) Schizophrenia

Please refer to above explanation

10. Ans. (b) Clozapine

Ref: Harrison, 19th ed. pg. 2271, 2617

- The patient here is a case of resistant schizophrenia as the auditory hallucination is not responding to treatment. As we know that:
  - *Auditory hallucinations are first symptom to go with treatment and also 1st symptoms to reappear after drug resistance.*
- **Clozapine is:**
  - A reserve drug for resistant schizophrenia
  - Drug with least extra pyramidal side effects (extardive dyskinesia)
  - Major side effect of clozapine is agranulocytosis, sedation, sialorrhea, weight gain

> **Extra Mile**

Antipsychotic	
Longest acting	Fluphenazine (2-4 weeks)
With antidepressant action	Flupenthixol
Least extrapyramidal side effect	Risperidone
Least potent	Chloropromazine (CPZ)
Least Hypotensive & Least Antiemetic	Molindone

11. Ans. (d) Fluphenazine

Ref: Harrison, 19th ed. pg. 2722

Fluphenazine can be given as monthly intramuscular depot preparation. Thus it is preferred in non-compliant patients.

Important Points Regarding Anti-Psychotic Agents

- Fluphenazine (enanthate and decanoate) and haloperidol (decanoate) are long-acting injectable (s.c. or i.m) forms of typical antipsychotics.
- **Risperidone** is the first atypical antipsychotic available in *long-acting injectable form.*
- Most commonly used antipsychotic by *intravenous* route is **haloperidol**
- **Ziprasidone, aripiprazole, asenapine and iloperidone** has *negligible risk to cause metabalic adverse effects* (weight gain, hyperlipidemia and new onset diabetes mellitus)
- **Asenapine, paliperidone and ziprasidone** has greatest potential to *prolong QT interval.*
- Asenapine → available as sublingual

12. Ans. (b) Altered sensorium

Ref: Harrison, 19th ed. pg. 2270-71

- Schizophrenia is a formal thought disorder, characterized by third person hallucination & inappropriate emotion (affect)
- Altered consciousness (sensorium) is a characteristic feature seen in delirium *(not in szchizophrenia)*

Characteristics

- Only 3rd person hallucinations are characteristic of schizophrenia.
- Third person hallucination means: Two or more voices talking to one another, discussing about the patient; and giving a running commentary on his actions or thoughts.
- *Auditory hallucination is most characteristic of Schizophrenia.*

13. Ans. (c) Visual hallucinations

Ref: Harrison, 19th ed. pg. 2270-71

14. Ans. (c) Gradual onset

Ref: Harrison, 19th ed. pg. 2271

Prognostic Factor of Schizophrenia

Good prognostic factor	Bad prognostic factor
• *Female sex*	• Male sex
• Acute onset (late onset)	• Gradual onset (early onset)
• No family history of schizophrenia	• Family history of schizophrenia
• History of depressive order	• Emotional blunting
• Premorbid personality	• Negative symptoms
• Positive symptoms	

15. Ans. (c) Hebephrenic

Ref: Harrison, 19th ed. pg. 2271

- Surprisingly, the name simple doesn't fit with the better prognosis. It has the worst prognosis among the types of schizophrenia.

TABLE: Types of Schizophrenia

Paranoid	Hebephrenic	Simple
• Most common type. • Late onset. • It has more positive and less negative symptom • Has better prognosis	• Early onset • Personality and emotions get affected • Worst prognosis	• No positive symptom at all • Only negative symptoms • **Poor prognosis**
	Catatonic Due to imbalance of NT, there is hyperactivity and hypoactivity. BEST prognosis	**Undifferentiated** • Can't be categorized in one particular category. • Has >1 category.

Explanations

FMGE Solutions Screening Examination

16. Ans. (d) Schizophrenia

Ref: Harrison, 19th ed. pg. 2270-71

- Patient in the given case is delusional and has disorganized behavior with his classmates.
- He even hears his dead grandfather talking to him (auditory hallucination), which is a very characteristic finding of schizophrenia.
- In case of delusional disorder, hallucinations are rare, and in case they are present, they are usually tactile or olfactory

TABLE: Differentiating Delusions of Different Causes

Delusion due to Delusional disorder	Delusion due to Schizophrenia
• Delusions are non bizarre (ie involving situations that occur in life as being followed, deceived, infected, loved etc)	• Bizarre delusions
• Behaviour & personality is normal except in the delusional area	• Behaviour & personality is deteriorated in almost all areas
• Hallucinations are very rare & if occur are of tactile or olfactory variety	• Hallucinations are very common • Auditory variety is most common • *3rd person hallucination* is characteristic

17. Ans (b) Conduct disorder

Ref: Ahuja 5th ed. pg. 173, Kaplan, 9th ed. pg. 1234-6

The child is not normal and suffers from conduct disorder.

TABLE: Differentiation between different disorders mentioned in the question

Autism	Attention Deficit Disorder	Conduct Disorder
There is marked impairment of reciprocal social and interpersonal interaction: ***Absence of social smile*** • ***Absence of fear*** • Lack of attach-ment to parents and absence of separation anxi-ety • ***Lack of friends***	More common in males, the onset occurs before the age of 7 years, characterized, by: • *Poor attention span with distractibility* • *Hyperactivity* • *Impulsivity* • *Moving about here and there*	There is violation of rights and rules like: • **Frequent lying** • **Stealing** or robbery Running away from home & school • **Physical violence** • Cruelty • Poor at studies

18. Ans. (c) Automatism

Ref: Kaplan & Saddock, 10th ed. pg. 468

- Autism, NOT automatism is part of Bleuler's four A's
- Eugene Blueler's Fundamental symptoms of schizophrenia (*4 A's of Blueler*):
  - **Ambivalence**–Inability to decide for or against (confusion)
  - **Autism**–Withdrawal into self
  - **Association disturbance**–Loosening of association, thought disorder
  - **Affect disturbance**–Inappropriate affect

19. Ans. (d) Delusion of guilt

Ref: Harrison, 19th ed. pg. 2271

- **Schneider's first rank symptoms of schizophrenia include**: Hallucination, Delusion (*primary delusion, NOT delusion of guilt*), Passivity (made) phenomenon, and thought alienation phenomenon.
- *Presence of one symptom is diagnostic of schizophrenia.*

Hallucination

- Hearing Audible thought
- Voice heard arguing or discussing or both
- Voice commenting on one's action
- Hallucinations in form of commentary
- 3rd person hallucination
- Somatic hallucination

Thought alienation phenomenon

- Thought withdrawal
- Thought insertion
- Thought broadcasting

Passivity

- Made feeling (affect)
- Made impulse
- Made volition
- Somatic passivity

Delusional perception

- Primary delusion

20. Ans. (c) Dopamine

Ref: Harrison, 19th ed. pg. 215

- Antipsychotics targeting positive symptoms probably act by *blocking the postsynaptic dopamine (D$_2$) receptors in the mesolimbic system*. Other receptors such as 5-HT, muscarinic receptors and GABA are also probably important. Atypical antipsychotics are also called as Serotonin Dopamine Antagonists (SDAs) due of their action on both dopamine and 5-HT.

Psychiatry

- Overactivity of DA receptor causes positive symptoms
- Their blockage of D2 antagonist relieves from positive symptoms
- Underactivity of NMDA receptor is responsible for negative symptoms.

DEPRESSION, SUICIDE AND ADJUSTMENT DISORDER

21. Ans. (c) Depression with dysthymia

Ref: Harrison's 20th ed. P 3269

- Prolong/persistent disorder is known as dysthymia. Therefore dysthymia is also known as persistent depressive disorder.
- It consist of a pattern of chronic (at least 2 years), ongoing depressive symptoms that are usually less severe than we seen in major depression.
- Often times the conditions like depression and dysthymia occur together and is difficult to separate.
- This persistence of depression with dysthymia is known as double depression.

22. Ans. (b) Weight loss >75%

Ref: Treatment manual for anorexia nervosa; 2/ed. P 277-278

- Anorexia nervosa (AN) is a type of eating disorder marked by an inability to maintain a normal healthy body weight, often dropping below 85% of ideal body weight (IBW).
- Bulimia nervosa (BN) is characterized by recurrent episodes of binge eating in combination with some form of inappropriate compensatory behavior.
- Indian patients chiefly present with refusal to eat, persistent vomiting, marked weight loss, amenorrhea and other somatic symptoms, but do not show over activity or disturbances in body image seen characteristically in anorexia nervosa.
- Nutritional rehabilitation along with some form of re-educative psychotherapy remains the mainstay of management of anorexia nervosa.
- In bulimia nervosa, both fluoxetine and cognitive behavior therapy have been found to be effective.

23. Ans. (b) Child age

Ref: Dying, Death and Bereavement; P 323

- A copycat suicide is defined as an emulation of another suicide that the person attempting suicide knows about either from local knowledge or due to accounts or depictions of the original suicide on television and in other media.
- It is commonly seen among teenagers.

24. Ans. (c) Nortriptyline

- Elderly patients are often sensitive to the hypotensive, sedative and anticholinergic effects of antidepressants, and this patient is at special risk for hypotension because of his carotid artery stenosis. Nortryptiline is *least likely* to cause these side effects.

25. Ans. (c) Depression

Ref: Comprehensive Clinical Psychiatry, Theodore, 2nd ed. pg. 221

- Depression is more commonly associated with frontal lobe lesions
- Left frontal lobe lesions are more commonly associated than the right frontal lobe.
- Depression occurs in 30 to 50% of stroke patients within two years of the event.
- Mania is less common and it occurs almost exclusively with right hemisphere lesions. Many of the patients who develop mania have a family history of affective disorders.

26. Ans. (d) Persistent depressive disorder

Ref: Harrison's, 19th ed. pg. 2706

- Persistent depressive disorder, also called dysthymia is a continuous long-term (chronic) form of depression.
- **Dysthymia** is, sometimes called **neurotic depression, dysthymic disorder**, or **chronic depression**, is a mood disorder consisting of the same cognitive and physical problems as in depression, with **less severe but longer-lasting symptoms.**

27. Ans. (c) Decreased serotonin and Norepinephrine

Ref: Harrison 19th ed./2714-2715

- Depression is one of the mood disorders
- It is considered as second most common psychiatric disorder.
- Most commonly seen in middle age females. M:F ratio= 1:2
- *Neurotransmitters involved are serotonin a NE and DA. All 3 are decreased.*

FMGE Solutions Screening Examination

Diagnostic Criteria of Depression

Major Criteria	Minor Criteria
Persistent sadness of mood	Loss of appetite
Loss of pleasure in activities	Sleep disturbance
Easy fatiguability	Decreased libido
	Decreased concentration
	Ideas of guilt, worthlessness, hopelessness
	Suicidal ideas

Depression Category on Basis of Severity

- Mild Depression   : 2 major + 2 minor
- Moderate Depression : 2 major + 3 minor
- Severe Depression   : 2 major + 4 minor

Extra Mile

Disease	Related Neurotransmitter
Alzheimer's disease	Acetyl choline decreased
Depression	Norepinephrine, Serotonin (5-HT) & dopamine are DECREASED
OCD	Serotonin (5 HT) decreased
Schizophrenia	Dopamine, Serotonin increased Glutamate decreased

28. Ans. (d) Serotonin and Norepinephrine

Please refer to the previous answer for explanation.

29. Ans. (d) Depressed mood

Ref: Ahuja, 5th ed. pg. 81,109-110

- Masked depression means hidden depression which practically means that the patient is having a depression which manifests in somatic symptoms like vague body aches, bowel complaints and inability to carry out normal activities. However, the mood is not seems to be depressed.

30. Ans. (c) Depressive Disorder

- DALY's is Disability Adjusted Life years.
- It is a measure of the burden of disease in a population and the effectiveness of the intervention.
- DALYs express years of life lost to premature death and years lives with disability adjusted for the severity of the disability.
- One DALY is "one lost year of healthy life"
- *According to Park 23rd ed. Most common cause of DALY's is depressive disorder.*

31. Ans. (c) Depressive disorder

Ref: Kaplan Synopsis 10th ed. pg. 528-30

- Most common psychiatric disorder and worldwide: **Anxiety disorders > depression**
- Female is most commonly affected as compared to males
- Depression is the most common psychiatric disorder associated with severe medical illness like hypothyroidism, cancer, AIDS, post MI, stroke etc.

32. Ans. (c) Major depression

Ref: Harrison, 19th ed. pg. 2714

- Major depression is the second most common psychiatric disorder world wide & in India with highest life time prevelance (17%), *most commonly involving middle (old) age females.* Independent of culture or country, is *two fold greater prevalent in females than in males.*
- It is the most common psychiatric disorder associated with severe medical illness as myxedema (hypothyroidism, cancer, AIDS, post partum, post MI and post surgery etc.)
- In depression monoamine neurotransmitters (monoaminergic NTs) NE and serotonin (and dopamine also) are reduced.
- For diagnosing Major depression
  - > 1 essential criteria
    - Depressed /low mood
    - Loss of interest or pleasure
  - > 4 of the following for > same 2 weeks
    - Appetite or weight loss
    - Sleep loss
    - Psychomotor activity (not meeting friends)
    - Concentration loss
    - Low energy (feeling of fatigue, weakness)
    - Feeling of worthlessness or guilt
    - Suicidal thoughts
- Patient given in the question fits in the critera:
- **1st criteria:** He has depressed mood and loss of interest or pleasure in dropping his daughter at school
- **In 2nd criteria**: Difficulty in sleeping, Not meeting with friends, decrease in energy.

Extra Mile

MC psychiatric disorder is Anxiety spectrum disorders > depression

Ref: Harrison 19th ed. pg. 2708

33. Ans. (b) Major depressive disorder

Ref: Harrison, 19th ed. pg. 2714-15

Please refer to above explanation.

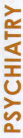

Psychiatry

34. Ans. (a) Adjustment disorder

Ref: Kaplan & Sadock, 10th ed. pg. 790

- Adjustment disorder is a short-term condition that occurs when a person is *unable to cope with, or adjust to, a particular source of stress*, such as a major life change, loss, or event.

Diagnostic Criteria

- Development of emotional or behavior symptoms *in response to identifiable stressor (not of an unusual or catastrophic type)*, **occurring within 3 months of onset of stressor** & does not persist for > 6 months if stressor is terminated.
  - Marked distress that is in excess of what would be expected
  - Significant impairment in social or occupational life
- *In this question, the examiner wanted us to mis-diagnose as severe depression, but the arousal of symptoms, i.e. within 3 months of stressor favours diagnosis of adjustment.*
- The type of stress that can trigger adjustment disorder varies depending on the person, but can include:
  - Ending of a relationship or marriage
  - Losing or changing job
  - **Death of a loved one** (*as seen in this case*)
  - Developing a serious illness (yourself or a loved one)
  - Being a victim of a crime
  - Having an accident
  - Undergoing a major life change (*such as getting married, having a baby, or retiring from a job*)
  - Living through a disaster, such as a fire, flood, or hurricane.
- A person with adjustment disorder develops emotional and/or behavioral symptoms as a reaction to a stressful event. **These symptoms generally begin within three months of the event and rarely last for longer than six months after the event or situation.**
- Adjustment disorder is not the same as post-traumatic stress disorder (PTSD). *PTSD generally occurs as a reaction to a life-threatening event and tends to last longer.* Adjustment disorder, on the other hand, is *short-term*, rarely lasting longer than six months.

35. Ans. (a) Female

Ref: Kaplan & Sadock, 10th ed. pg. 428

- Mood disorders (major depression) and alcohol dependence are two most common causes of suicide.
- Men **COMMIT** suicide four times as often as women. Women **ATTEMPT** suicide four times as often as men. Women usually take psychoactive substance while men use firearms.

- **Suicidal risk is much more in presence of following risk factors:**
  - *Early in illness* (than later), **more commonly in men (than women) of middle or old age (>40 years).**
  - Single, separated, divorced, widowed, or recently bereaved, social isolation, unemployed.
  - *At the onset or end of depressive episode (i.e. depression in involution). Early* treatment particularly with SSRIs may increase suicidal feelings & attempts. As with other psychiatric patients, the months after discharge from a hospital are time of high risk. Subtherapeutic doses may increase risk.
- Presence of *marked haplessness.*
- At the peak of depression, the patient is either too retarded or depressed to commit suicide. *So, early stages of depression, during recovery (involution) from depression and 3 months period from recovery is high risk period for suicide.*

Suicide	
Biological factors	**Most important risk factors**
- Decreased *central serotonin (5 HT)* plays an important role in suicide - Decreased concentrations of serotonin metabolite *5-HIAA in CSF*	- Psychosis - Substance abuse - Personality disorder - Hypochondriac
Most important causes: - *Major depression* - *Substance abuse* - *Schizophrenia*	

36. Ans. (c) Psychogenic

Ref: Kaplan & Sadock 10th ed. pg. 693

- Most common cause of impotency in male is psychogenic.

PERSONALITY DISORDER/OCD

37. Ans. (b) Hypochondriac disorder

Ref: Handbook of outpatient treatment of adults: Non psychotic mental disorder; P 300

- **Hypochondriasis** is a condition in which a person is inordinately worried about having a serious illness. The person is preoccupied with thoughts of a serious life threatening diagnosis or medical illness.
- **Somatoform pain:** Only pain of one location of long standing duration.
- **Conversion disorder:** Anxiety due to conflict.

38. Ans. (a) Autism

Ref: Textbook of autism spectrum disorders, edited by Eric Hollander e.g.al; P 99-102

- **Autism:** Impairment in social communication and interaction, language development delay, restrictive repetitive stereotyped behavior.
- **ADHD:** Child is hyperactive, impulsive, attention deficit.

39. Ans. (c) Fluoxetine

- The drugs of choice for OCD are SSRI or clomipramine (2nd drug of choice)
  - **SSRIs:** *Fluoxetine, Fluvoxamine, Paroxetine, Sertraline, Citalopram, Escitalopram*
- Exposure and Response Prevention is a part of cognitive and behavior therapy for OCD.
- Combination of behavior therapy & drug therapy gives best results for treatment of OCD.

40. Ans. (b) OCD

- O.C.D does not arise from any cognition bias but a goal directed dysfunction that interacts with anxiety and irrational belief. They cannot exert necessary control over their actions to realize this goal.

41. Ans. (b) Dissociation

Ref: Ahuja 5th ed. pg. 213

- Dissociation is a neurotic/immature defence mechanism characterized by involuntary splitting or suppression of a mental function or a group of mental function from rest of the personality in a manner that allows expression of forbidden unconscious impulses without having any sense of responsibility for actions.

42. Ans. (c) Operant conditioning

Ref: PubMed

- B.F. Skinner (1904–1990) is often referred to as the **father of operant conditioning.** This conditioning is based on behavioural change with reinforcement or punishment.

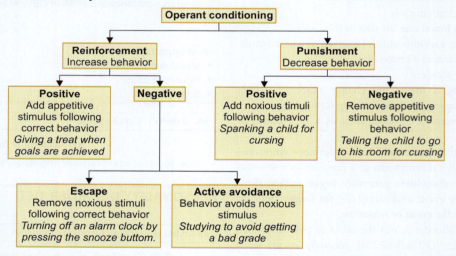

Note: Classical conditioning differs from operant or instrumental conditioning: in classical conditioning, behavioral responses are elicited by antecedent stimuli (e.g: chocolate wrapper stimulate salivation), whereas in operant conditioning behaviors are strengthened or weakened by their consequences (i.e., reward or punishment).

43. Ans. (b) Mania

Ref: Kaplan & Sadock, 10th ed. pg. 2717

DSM- IV Diagnostic Criteria of Mania

- Abnormally & persistently elevated, expansive, or irritable mood lasting for at least 1 week or any duration, if requires hospitalization.
- > 3 are needed
  - Inflated self esteem or grandiosity
  - Decreased need for sleep (≤ 3 hours)
  - More talkative or pressure to keep talking
  - Flight of ideas or subjective experience that thoughts are racing

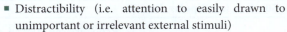

- Distractibility (i.e. attention to easily drawn to unimportant or irrelevant external stimuli)
- Increase in goal-directed activity (social spiritual religious, sexual) or psychomotor agitation
- Excessive involvement in pleasurable activities *(eg. unrestrained buying sprees, foolish business investments, donations or sexual indiscretions)* that have a high potential for painful consequences.

Why Mania: This patients satisfies the criteria and his conditions fits into it.

- The patient is irritable for 10 days (i.e. criteria A-abnormally & persistently elevated mood for atleast 1 week). There are ≥ 3 criteria B features: increased sexual indulgence & alcohol consumption *(excessive involvement in pleasureable activity),* decreased need for sleep and career oriented prolonged work without getting tired.

44. Ans. (c) Heightened concentration

Please refer to above explanation

45. Ans. (a) Ego dystonic

Ref: Kaplan & Sadock 10th ed./279

- The idea in OCD is Egodystonic or ego-alien (foreign to one's own personality), NOT ego syntonic.
- Persons with OCD are stubborn, rigid, overconscious, scrupulous & inflexible about matters of morality & ethics (not indecisive).
- *Shows perfection that interferes with task completion*
- Is excessively devoted to work and productivity to the exclusion of leisure activities & friendships. Is reluctant to delegated task or work to others. Adopts a miserly spending style.

Obsession	Compulsion
• Fear something terrible may happen (fire, death, or illness of loved one, self or others • Concern or need for symmetry, order or exactness • Concern or disgust with bodily wastes or secretion (urine, stool, saliva), dirt, germs, environmental toxins • Scrupulosity (excessive praying or religious concerns out of keeping with patients background) • Forbidden or perverse sexual thoughts, images or impulses • Believes in Luck & unlucky numbers. • Intrusive nonsense sounds, words or music	• Excessive hand washing, checking, cleaning, ordering, arranging, counting etc.

46. Ans. (b) Exposure and response prevention

Ref: Harrison, 19th ed. pg. 2713

Exposure and Response Prevention is a part of cognitive and behavior therapy for OCD.

MANAGEMENT OF OBSESSIVE COMPULSIVE DISORDER

Behaviour Therapy (BT)

- *It is treatment of choice for OCD*
- Exposure & response prevention is the preferred & principal approach. It is most effective in obsessional rituals (i.e. compulsions)
- In this form of therapy, the patient is asked to endure, in a graduated manner, the anxiety that a specific obsessional fear provokes while refraining from compulsions that allay (reduce) that anxiety. The principle behind success of treatment are based on habituation based on response prevention.

Pharmacotherapy

- The drug of choice for OCD are SSRI or clomipramine (2nd drug of choice)
  - SSRI's
    - ♦ FLUXOETINE, FLUVOXAMINE, PAROXETINE, SERTRALINE, CITALOPRAM, ESCITALOPRAM
- Combination of behavior therapy & drug therapy gives best results for treatment of OCD.
- **Clomipramine:** It is the most selective for serotonin reuptake versus norepinephrine re-uptake & exceeds in the respect only by SSRI's.
- **2nd line drugs:** If treatment with SSRIs or clomipramine is unsuccessful, valproate lithium or carbamazepine are used.

Psychotherapy

- To treat OCD, Psychoanalytic prolonged insight oriented or exploratory & interpretative psychotherapy is used in educated & psychologically oriented patients.
  - **ECT:** is used in severe depression with OCD
  - **Psychosurgery:** It is indicated only for most chronic, treatment resistant cases that have resisted (IPD or OPD) treatment (including drug of behavior therapy) for at least a year.

47. Ans. (a) Behavior therapy

Ref: Kaplan & Sadock, 10th ed. pg. 605

BEHAVIOUR THERAPY

It is the treatment of choice in phobia, which may of following types

- *Exposure & Response prevention is 1st line of behavior therapy*
- Flooding (implosion or intensive exposure)

FMGE Solutions Screening Examination

- Systemic desensitization: Progressive exposure to anxiety evoking stimulus .
- Relaxation techniques

Medications

- Anxiolytic drugs
- Tricyclic antidepressant
- SSRI
- MAO inhibitors

COVERT SENSITIZATION

- It is an aversion therapy, used for the treatment of conditions which are pleasant but undersirable. Eg. Alcohol dependence, and sexual deviations like homosexuality & transvestism etc.
- The main aim of aversion therapy is pairing of pleasant stimulus with an unpleasant response so that pleasant stimulus becomes unpleasant by association.

48. Ans. (c) Exposure and response prevention followed by systemic desensitization

Ref: Harrison, 19th ed. pg. 2712-13

BEHAVIOUR THERAPY

- It is the treatment of choice in phobic disorders and several other psychiatric illness. Exposure and response prevention followed by systemic desensitization behavior therapy is the treatment of choice in phobia. It can be of following types:
- Exposure & Response prevention is **1st line of behavior therapy**
- Systemic desensitization: progressive exposure to anxiety evoking stimulus *(2nd line)*
- Flooding (implosion or intensive exposure)
- Relaxation techniques

49. Ans. (b) Early age of onset

Good Prognostic Factors	Poor Prognostic Factors
• Acute or abrupt onset • Typical clinical features • Severe depression • Well-adjusted premorbid personality • Good response to treatment	• Co-morbid medical disorder, personality disorder or alcohol dependence • Double depression (acute depressive episode superimposed on chronic depression or dysthymia) • Catastrophic stress or chronic ongoing stress • Unfavourable early environment and *early age of onset* • Marked hypochondriacal features, or mood incongruent psychotic features • Poor drug compliance

50. Ans. (a) Bipolar disorder

Ref: Harrison, 19th ed. pg. 2717

- **DOC for prophylaxis of bipolar disorder- Lithium**
- DOC for acute mania: Benzodiazepines + atypical antipsychotic
- Lithium can also be used in treatment of neutropenia, Cluster headache and major depression episodes.
- **Therapeutic level of lithium: 0.8 – 1.2 mEq/L**
- **Toxicity seen after >1.5 mEq/L**
- Most common side effect of lithium: Coarse tremor
- **Side effects of lithium (Mn: LITTH)**
  - Leukocytosis
  - Insipidus (DI)
  - Tremor, teratogenic (MC-Ebstein anomaly)
  - Hypothyroidism
- Lithium is contraindicated in 1st trimester of pregnancy. It can cause congenital heart defect- **Ebstein anomaly.**

51. Ans. (c) Phenytoin sodium

Ref: Harrison, 19th ed. pg. 2718, 4665e-2

- Lithium has traditionally been the drug of choice for the treatment of manic episode (acute phase) as well as for prevention of further episodes in bipolar mood disorder. It has also been used in treatment of depression with less success.
- Antipsychotics are an important adjunct in the treatment of mood disorder. The commonly used drugs include risperidone, obnzapine, quetiapine, haloperidol, and aripiprazole.

The other mood stabilizers which are used in the treatment of bipolar mood disorders include;

- Sodium valproate
- Carbamazepine and Oxacarbazepine
- Benzodiazepines Lorazepm (IV and orally) and clonazepam
- Lamotrigine

52. Ans. (c) Borderline

Ref: Harrison, 19th ed. pg. 2720

Personality disorders and their clinical manifestation:

- **Borderline:** Pervasive pattern of unstable and intense interpersonal relationship, difficulty in controlling anger hence avoids meeting people.
- **Paranoid:** Generalized mistrust and suspiciousness
- **Schizoid:** Markedly detached from others. Excessive preoccupation with fantasy and introspection and emotional coldness.

53. Ans. (a) Menorrhagia

Ref: Harrison, 17th ed. pg. 471-7

Psychiatry

Amenorrhea _(and not menorrhagia)_ is seen in 100% patients of anorexia nervosa. It is a mandatory finding diagnostic criterion to be fulfilled for anorexia nervosa.

	Anorexia nervosa	Bulimia nervosa
Feature	Refusal to maintain body weight above a minimal normal	Irresistible craving for food with episodes of over eating in less time (Binge eating)
Method of weight control		Attempts to counter act the effects of over eating by self-induced vomiting: • Purgative abuse, • Periods of starvations • Appetite suppressants
Ritualised excercise	Common	Rare
Amenorrhea	**100%**	50%
Decreased Vitals ↓ BP, ↓ Pulse	**Common**	Uncommon
Hypothermia	**Common**	Rare
Skin changes (Hirsutism)	**Common**	Rare
Medical Complications	Hypokalemia Cardiac arrythmias	Hypokalemia Cardiac arrythmias

54. Ans. (c) Dissociative fugue

DISSOCIATIVE FUGUE

- Dissociative fugue is characterized by _episodes of wandering away (usually away from home)._ During the episode, the person usually _adopts a new identity_ with _complete amnesia for the earlier life._ The onset is usually sudden, often in the presence of severe stress. The termination too is abrupt and is followed by amnesia for the episode, but with recovery of memories of earlier life.

MULTIPLE PERSONALITY (DISSOCIATIVE IDENTITY) DISORDER

- In this dissociative disorder, the person is dominated by two or more personalities, of which only one is being manifest at a time. These personalities are usually different, at times even opposing.

POST-TRAUMATIC STRESS DISORDER

- Arises as a delayed and/protracted response to an exceptionally stressful or catastrophic life event or

situation, which is likely to cause pervasive distress in 'almost any person' (e.g. disasters, war, rape or torture, serious accident). The symptoms of PTSD may develop, after a period of latency, within six months after the stress or maybe delayed beyond this period

- PTSD is characterized be recurrent and intrusive recollections of the stressful event either in flashbacks or in dreams.

55. Ans. (c) Body dysmorphic disorder

- Body dysmorphic disorder is a somatoform disorder, wherein the affected person is concerned with body image
- It manifests as excessive concern about and preoccupation with a perceived defect of their physical features.
- The person is under an impression that they have a defect in either one feature or several features of their body, which causes psychological distress that causes clinically significant distress or impairs occupational or social functioning.
- _This condition co-exists with emotional depression and anxiety, social withdrawal or social isolation._

DELIRIUM, DEMENTIA AND ALZHEIMER'S DISEASE

56. Ans. (c) Delirium

Ref: Kaplan's Textbook of Psychiatry Ch 10.2

- Delirium is the most common psychiatric condition seen in medico-surgical patient.

TABLE: Delirium incidence and prevalence in different scenarios

Population	Prevalence Range (%)	Incidence Range (%)
General medical inpatients	10-30	3-16
Medical and surgical inpatients	5-15	10-55
General surgical inpatients	N/A	9-15 postoperatively
Critical care unit patients	16	16-83
Cardiac surgery inpatients	16-34	7-34
Orthopedic surgery patients	33	18-50
Emergency department	7-10	N/A
Terminally ill cancer patients	23-28	83
Institutionalized elderly	44	33

Explanations

_1207_

FMGE Solutions Screening Examination

57. Ans. (a) Delirium

Ref: Kaplan's Textbook of Psychiatry Ch 12.2

- Delirium is also known as organic brain syndrome/acute brain failure/cerebral insufficiency.
- Delirium is occasionally termed to denote the acute form organic mental syndrome. It is most common organic mental disorder seen in clinical practice.

58. Ans. (b) Delirium

Ref: Harrison, 19th ed. pg. 166

DELIRIUM

- It is characterized by global impairment of consciousness *(clouding of consciousness),* resulting in reduced levels of alertness, attention & perception of environment along with acute onset of fluctuating cognitive impairment.
- It is the commonest organic mental disorder

Clinical Features & Diagnosis

- Global impairment of consciousness & attention is the hallmark/cardinal feature of Delirium. It manifests as:
  - Diminished ability to focus, sustain or shift attention.
  - Reduced levels of alertness, attention, and perception of environment.
  - Drowsiness (mental slowness), distractibility & disorientation.
- Global impairment of cognition is manifested as:
  - Disorientation (in time, place and person)
  - *Disturbance of immediate & recent memory*
  - *Remote memory is intact.*

59. Ans. (d) Organic brain syndrome

ORGANIC BRAIN SYNDROME

- It is also known as organic brain disease which is decreased mental function due to a medical disease, other than a psychiatric illness.
- Cognitive or higher mental functions *(i.e. consciousness, orientation & abstract thinking)* are impaired in organic brain syndrome.

60. Ans. (b) Loss of consciousness

Ref: Harrison, 19th ed. pg. 170, 173

- Impairment of higher mental function is noted in case of dementia, but there is NO impairment of consciousness.
- Impairments in dementia (Mn: *A Thinking Memorable Intelligent Judge Can't be Impulsive)*
  - Abstract thinking
  - Memory *(recent > remote)*
  - Intellectual function
  - Judgment
  - Continence (fecal & urinary)
  - Impulse control (catastrophic reaction)
  - Personality & personal care
- Memory impairment (ex. Forgetfulness) is typically an early & prominent feature in dementia
- No matter how severe the dementia, patients show no impairment in their level of consciousness.
- Hallucinations & Delusion can occur in 20-40% of patients with dementia.

Feature of Cortical & Subcortical Dementia

Features	Cortical Dementia	Subcortical Dementia
Site	Cortex (frontal, parietal, temporal, occipital, hippocampus)	Subcortical grey matter
Memory impairment	• Severe, early • Recall helped very little by cues	• Mild to moderate • Recall helped partially by cues & recognition tasks
Mathetical skills	• Impaired early (Acalculia)	• Preserved
Language	• Early, Dysphasia (Aphasia)	• Normal & Anomia (in severe cases)
Speech	• Articulate until late	• Dysarthria
Personality	• Indifferent	• Apathetic, inert

Etiology of Dementia

1. Decreased level of NE in locus cereuleus
2. Decreased level of Acetylcholine in Nucleus basalis of meynert
3. In moderate to severe dementia: *Increased* level of Glutamate.

61. Ans. (b) Trauma

Ref: Harrison, 19th ed. pg. 173

- Dementia Pugilistica is also known as punch drunk syndrome. It is a form of dementia usually secondary to some trauma to head.

ALZHEIMER'S DISEASE

- Alzheimer's disease, the most common cause of dementia.
- It initially presents with minor forgetfulness & gradually progressive short term memory loss
- The memory is lost for recent events first with a delayed loss of long term memory mainly affecting episodic memory.

- **Feature of Alzheimer dementia are**
  - *Memory impairment without impairment of consciousness*
  - Aphasia: Language disturbace
  - Apraxia: Impaired ability to carry out motor activities despite intact motor function
  - Agnosia: Failure to recognize or identify objects despite intact sensory function
  - Agnosia: Failure to recognize or identify objects despite intact sensory function
  - Anosognosia (*Unware of his problem*), Prosopognosia (*difficulty in identifying known faces*)
  - Disturbance in executive functioning (i.e planning organizing, sequencing, abstracting)
  - Focal neurological signs (ex asymmetrical hyper-reflexia or weakness)

Extra Mile

Neuropathological findings of Alzheimer's disease

Gross	Microscopic
• Diffuse atrophy with flattened cortical sulci & enlarged cerebral ventricles	• Senile (Amyloid) plaques • *Neurofibrillary tangles* • Neuronal – loss (especially in cortex & hippocampus) • Synaptic loss • Granulovascular degeneration of the neurons

Remember

Neurofibrillary tangles are not unique to Alzheimer's disease but also occur in Down's syndrome, Dementia pugilistica (punch-drunk syndrome), Parkinson dementia complex.

62. Ans. (a) Biperidin

Ref: Harrison, 19th ed./2601-02

- Alzheimer's disease is most common cause of dementia.
- Cause → Decreased level of Ach in nucleus basalis of meynert

Drugs Used in the Treatment of Alzheimer's are:

- Acetycholine esterase inhiitors: (It increases Ach level)
  - Donepezil
  - Tacrine (Hepatotoxic; not used)
  - Galantamine
- **Rivastigmine:** Carbamate derivative of physostigmine
- **Memantine:** NMDA glutaminergic antagonist
- Biperidin is an anti cholinergic drug used to treat parkinsonism.

63. Ans. (b) Alzheimer's

Ref: Harrison's 18th ed. 3300-07

- Alzheimer's disease is most common cause of irreversible dementia.

TABLE: Reversible vs Irreversible dementia

Reversible	Irreversible

• Vitamin deficiency
  ■ B1- Wernicke's
  ■ B12- SCID
  ■ Nicotinic acid- Pellagra
	Alzheimer's

Endocrine (**Hypothyroidism,** *adrenal insufficiency, cushing's*)	Vascular dementia (Multi-infarct)
• Head trauma and diffuse brain damage • Haemorrhage-*subdural, epidural, normal pressure hydrocephalus*	Leucoencephalopathy
Primary metastatic brain tumor	Metabolic disorder (*Wilson's disease, Leigh disease, Leucodystrophy*)
• Toxic dementia (**MCC of reversible dementia**)	Degenerative disorder 1. *Parkinsonism* 2. *Pick's disease* 3. *Prion's disease,* 4. *Multiple sclerosis* 5. *Huntington's disease* 6. *Diffuse lewy body dementia*

SUBSTANCE ABUSE

64. Ans. (c) Fomepizole

Ref: Safe and effective medication use in emergency department, By victor cohen; P 120

- The primary antidotal treatment of methanol or ethylene glycol involves blocking alcohol dehydrogenase, this enzyme is inhibited by fomepizole or ethanol.

65. Ans. (a) Aversion therapy

Ref: Principles of addiction medicine; P 843

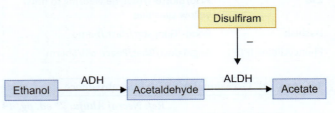

- Disulfiram acts by inhibiting aldehyde dehydrogenase, which causes accumulation of acetaldehyde.

FMGE Solutions Screening Examination

- This accumulation of acetaldehyde leading to distressing symptoms like hot flushes, pulsatile headache, respiratory difficulty, nausea, vomiting, sweating, orthostatic syncope, chest pain, hypotension, confusion and blurred vision.
- This particular reaction produces aversion from intake of alcohol.

  Anticraving medication: Naltrexone, acamprosate, baclofen, fluoxetine, topiramate.

66. Ans. (d) Flunitrazepam

Ref: Harrisons, 19th ed. pg. 469e1; PubMed

- **Flunitrazepam (Rohypnol)** is a tasteless, odorless benzodiazepine derivative primarily used to treat insomnia, but it has significant abuse potential because of its strong hypnotic, anxiolytic, and amnesia-producing effects. It is a club drug commonly referred to as a **"date-rape drug" or "roofies."**
- Earlier, it was used in some countries to treat severe insomnia and in fewer, early in anesthesia.
- **Mechanism of action:** The drug enhances GABAA receptor activity.
- **Toxicity/overdose:** Treated with **flumazenil**, a benzodiazepine receptor antagonist.

Extra Mile

- Commonly abused club drugs include flunitrazepam, GHB (Gamma Hydroxybutyrate), and ketamine
- GHB and ketamine can be identified in blood.
- Flunitrazepam can be identified in urine and hair samples.

67. Ans. (b) Cannabis

Ref: Pub Med

TABLE: Common abused substances and their slang names

Abused substance	Slang names
Cannabis/Marijuana	Aunt mary/Dope/Ganja/Grass/Green/Joint/Pot/weed
Cocaine	Coke/snow/toot/coca
Heroin	Brown sugar/china white/Dope/Junk/Hell dust/Smack
LSD	Acid/Blotters/Blue heaven/micro dots/yellow sunshine
Hashish	Boom/Gangster/Hash/hemp
Phencyclidine (PCP)	Angel dust/Boat/Peace pill/Sherm

68. Ans. (a) Occasional use with long absistence

Ref: Neeraj Ahuja, 7th ed. pg. 49

- The textbook quotes: *"Although tolerance as well as psychological dependence can occur with LSD use, no physical dependence or withdrawal syndrome is reported. A common pattern of LSD use is a trip (occasional use followed by a long term period of abstinence)"*.

69. Ans. (c) Bradycardia

Ref: Harrison, 19th ed. pg. 2727

- The symptoms which arises when an alcoholic reduces or stops alcohol consumption after prolonged periods of excessive alcohol intake.
- *In case of alcohol withdrawal there is hallucinations,, tremors, sweating and tachycardia, NOT bradycardia.*
- **Clinical presentation**
  - Hangover next morning: *Most common withdrawal syndrome*
  - Mild tremors *(Most Common symptom)*
  - Nausea, vomiting
  - Weakness, insomnia, anxiety
  - Delirium tremens: Most severe withdrawal syndrome
  - Alcoholic seizures (Rum fits)
  - Alcoholic hallucinosis

TABLE: Appearance of Alcohol withdrawal symptoms

Time	Symptoms
6-12 hours	Minor withdrawal symptoms: Insomnia, tremulousness, anxiety, GIT upset, headache, diaphoresis, palpitations, anorexia
12-24 hours	Alcoholic hallucinosis; visual, auditory, or tactile hallucination
24-48 hours	*Withdrawal seizures:* Generalized tonic-clonic seizures
48-72 hours	Derlirium tremens; visual hallucinations, disorientation, *tachycardia*, hypertension, low-grade fever, agitation, diaphoresis

70. Ans. (d) 24–48 hours after cessation of alcohol

Ref: Harrison, 19th ed. pg. 2727

71. Ans. (a) Severity of respiratory and CNS depression

Ref: Harrison, 19th ed. pg. 2727

- CNS depression predisposes to chances of aspiration due to suppression of airway defence mechanisms. Hence it is the most important parameter determining hospitalization in acute intoxication of any etiology.

Acute Alcohol intoxication:

- After a brief period excitation, there is a generalized central nervous system depression with alcohol use.
- With increasing intoxication, there is increased reaction time, slowed thinking, distractibility and poor motor control.
- Later, dysarthria, ataxia and incoordination can occur. There is progressive loss of self control with frank disinhibited behavior.

Psychiatry

- The duration of intoxication depends on the amount and the rapidity of ingestion of alcohol. Usually the signs of intoxication are obvious with blood levels of 150–200 mg %. With blood alcohol levels of 300–450 mg % increasing drowsiness followed by coma and respiratory depression develop.

72. Ans. (c) Cocaine

Ref: Harrison, 19th ed. pg. 469e-1

- Cannabis and its products contain (-) D-9 TetraHydro Coannabinol (Δ9-THC).
- It is obtained from Indian hemp plant known as cannabis Sativa.
- Different parts of plants have different product:
  - Dried leaves: *Bhang*
  - Dried female inflorescence: *Ganja*
  - Resinous extract from flowering tops: *Charas /Hashish*
  - *Marijuana/Marihuana: other name for cannabis*
- In case of cannabis abuse there is an episode of acute violent behavior for which the person claims amnesia. This is known as ***Run Amok.***

Extra Mile

Substance	Characteristic clinical feature
• Cocaine	Magnus symptoms (cocaine bugs or Tactile hallucination)
• Cannabis	• Run Amok • Amotivation syndrome • Flashbacks
• Alcohol	• Mc-Evan's sign Morbid jealousy
• LSD	• Bad Trips • Flash backs
• Amphetamine	Paranoid Halucinatory syndrome (like paranoid schizophrenia)
• Phencyclidine (Angel dust)	Dissociative anesthesia

73. Ans. (a) Smoking

Ref: Harrison, 19th ed. pg. 17, 266e-4

- **Alcohol is the most common substance abused in India and worldwide.**
- **Early and rapid addiction has been seen with SMOKING**
- **Most common illicit drug/substance abused: Cannabis > Amphetamine (2nd MC).**
- **Nicotine (tobacco/smoking):** Highly addictive and heavily used drug/substance

74. Ans. (d) LSD

Ref: Harrison, 19th ed. pg. 469e-4

- LSD intoxication causes *bad trips*, which is acute panic reaction in which the individual experience a loss of control over his self.
- Spontaneous recurrence of LSD, or sometimes cannabis use experience even during a withdrawal state is known as *Flash back.*

75. Ans. (b) 21–34

Ref: O.P. Ghai 8th ed./584-85

Categories of mental retardation based on IQ levels

Mental retardation	IQ range
Mild MR	50-69
Moderate MR	35-49
Severe MR	21-34
Profound MR	20 or below

ANSWERS TO BOARD REVIEW QUESTIONS

76. Ans. (a) Response prevention

Ref: Kaplan and Sadocks 10th ed p 953

77. Ans. (c) Delusion of persecution

Ref: Kaplan 10th ed p 468

78. Ans. (c) Auditory hallucination

Ref: Kaplan and Sadocks Synopsis of Psychiatry, 10th ed ch-13

79. Ans. (c) Kraepelin

Ref: Kaplan 10th ed p 467

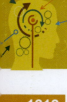

80. Ans. (b) Impulse control disorder
    Ref: Kaplan and Sadocks 10th ed p 25

81. Ans. (b) Derealisation
    Ref: Kaplan and Sadocks 10th ed ch-20, Oxford Handbook of Psychiatry by davidSemple, Roger Smyth, Jonathan Burns p 372

82. Ans. (a) Personality disorder

83. Ans. (a) Increase sense of Restlessness and anxiety

84. Ans. (c) Alcohol addiction

85. Ans. (a) Agoraphobia

86. Ans. (a) Anxiety

87. Ans. (d) Delusions

88. Ans. (d) Steven Johnson syndrome

89. Ans. (c) Gradual onset

90. Ans. (c) Automatism

91. Ans. (a) Adjustment disorder

92. Ans. (a) Female

93. Ans. (a) Ego dystonic
    - Ego-syntonic refer to instincts or ideas that are *acceptable* to self and compatible with one's values and ways of thinking. Example for a thief, stealing would be considered ego-syntonic. Another such example is anorexia nervosa.
    - Ego-dystonic refers to behaviour, ideas which are distressing, *unacceptable* or to one's self concept. Example millionaire thinking of begging for food or obsessive compulsive disorder.

94. Ans. (b) Delirium

95. Ans. (d) Organic brain syndrome

96. Ans. (b) Trauma

97. Ans. (c) Bradycardia

98. Ans. (d) LSD

99. Ans. (d) 35–49

100. Ans. (a) Seasonal affective disorder
    Ref: Principles and Practice of Psychopharmacotherapy by Pavuluri p. 244

101. Ans. (c) ECT
    Ref Kaplan Synopsis 10th ed. p. 557

102. Ans. (b) 14%
    Ref: http://www.who.int

103. Ans. (a) Approximate answer
    Ref: Kaplan and Sadocks Concise Textbook of clinical psychiatry 3rd ed. p. 302

104. Ans. (b) Methylphenidate
    Ref: Nelson 19th ed. p. 111

105. Ans. (c) NREM disorder
    Ref: Kaplan and sadock's 10/e, chapter 24.2

106. Ans. (a) Same time for sleeping and waking up daily
    Ref: With text

107. Ans. (a) Imagery
    Ref: Kaplan and Sadock's 10/e, Kaplan p. 233

108. Ans. (d) Respiratory failure
    Ref: Nelson's 18/e, chapter 599

109. Ans. (a) Mild
    Ref: Current Diagnosis and Treatment in Osychiatry p. 543

110. Ans. (b) Reaction formation
    Ref: Kaplan and Sadock's 10/e, chapter 16.2

111. Ans. (c) 40%
    Ref: Kaplan and Sadock's 10/e, Table 13-3

112. Ans. (c) Paraphilia
    Ref: Kaplan and Sadock's 10th ed. p. 953

113. Ans. (b) 2 weeks
    Ref: American Psychiatric Association, Diagnostic and Statistical Menual of Mental Disorders, 4/e

Psychiatry

114. Ans. (a) Thought

Ref: Kaplan 9th ed. /281

115. Ans. (b) Piloerection

Ref: Kaplan and Sadock's Synopsis of Psychiatry 10/e, chapter 12.10

116. Ans. (a) Depression

Ref: Kaplan and Sadock's Synopsis of Psychiatry: Behavioral Sciences Clinical Psychiatry 10th ed. /339, Table 10.3-11

117. Ans. (a) Benztropine

Ref: Handbook of Psychiatric Drug Therapy by Lawrence 3th ed. p. 869)

118. Ans. (b) Capgras syndrome

Ref: Kaplan and sadock's 10th ed. /508-510

119. Ans. (a) Valproate

Ref: Goodman Gillman 11th ed. /317-318

120. Ans. (a) Premature ejaculation

Squeeze technique is used in premature ejaculation

19
Radiology

MOST RECENT QUESTIONS 2019

1. Comment on the diagnosis of CT chest shown below.

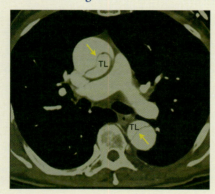

   a. Aortic dissection
   b. Pulmonary embolism
   c. Cardiac myxoma
   d. Aortic aneurysm

2. Which is used for calculation of ejection fraction?
   a. MUGA
   b. SPECT using thallium 201
   c. PET myocardial perfusion imaging
   d. Sestamibi scan with pharmacological stress

3. The shown radiograph is a case of:

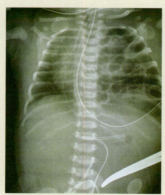

   a. Diaphragmatic hernia
   b. Intestinal obstruction
   c. Pleural effusion
   d. Pneumonia

4. Maximum radiation exposure:
   a. X-ray abdomen
   b. HSG
   c. IV Angiography
   d. Barium enema

5. All of the following areas are scanned in FAST except:
   a. Pericardium
   b. Pleural cavity
   c. Spleen
   d. Liver

6. In the shown lateral view of chest X-ray, what is the structure marked with X or white arrow head?

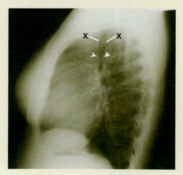

   a. Esophagus
   b. Pulmonary artery
   c. Trachea
   d. Left atrium

7. A patient presented with complaints of low grade fever with dyspnoea. The shown X-ray is suggestive of:

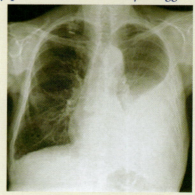

   a. Consolidation
   b. Exudative pleural effusion
   c. Pneumothorax
   d. Hydropneumothorax

BASIC RADIOLOGY PRINCIPLES AND RADIOTHERAPY

8. Which of the following investigations work on the same principle? *(Recent Pattern Question 2018-19)*
   a. CT and MRI
   b. CT and X-ray
   c. USG and HIDA scan
   d. MRI and PET scan
9. Which of the following investigation must be performed before giving contrast to the patient? *(Recent Pattern Question 2018)*
   a. K.F.T
   b. L.F.T
   c. Urine specific gravity
   d. Serum electrolytes
10. What is the gold standard investigation of choice for deep vein thrombosis? *(Recent Pattern Question 2017)*
    a. Double contrast duplex
    b. Venography
    c. CT scan
    d. MRI
11. The shown image modality is: *(Recent Pattern Question 2017)*

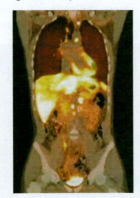

    a. PET- CT scan
    b. PET–MRI
    c. CECT
    d. X-ray
12. What is this image called *(Recent Pattern Question 2016)*

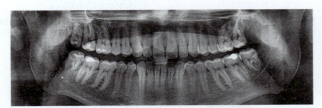

    a. Orthopantogram
    b. Lateral cephalogram
    c. Towns view
    d. Stenver view
13. Loss of proton and electron both when rays travel through the body:
    a. Compton effect
    b. Loss of linear energy
    c. Loss of biological dose
    d. Photoelectric effect
14. Maximum penetrating rays:
    a. Alpha
    b. Beta
    c. Gamma
    d. Delta
15. Unit of radiation exposure:
    a. Rad
    b. Gray
    c. Sievert
    d. Roentgen
16. Iridium 192 half life is?
    a. 2.7 days
    b. 8 days
    c. 74 days
    d. 16 hours
17. Radioiodine 131 half life is?
    a. 8 days
    b. 15.7 days
    c. 74.3 days
    d. 13 hours
18. Half- life of cobalt-60 is?
    a. 53 years
    b. 5.3 years
    c. 0.53 years
    d. 7.8 years
19. Half- life of radium 226 is?
    a. 15.9 years
    b. 159 years
    c. 1620 years
    d. 15900 years
20. Radioisotope used for thyroid treatment of metastasis/ablation
    a. I-123
    b. I-131
    c. I-83
    d. I-90
21. The radioisotope used for ablation of thyroid gland is
    a. Iodine 123
    b. Iodine 125
    c. Iodine 131
    d. Technetium 99 pertechnate
22. Which of the following is not used as a Radioisotope:
    a. Iodine-131
    b. Caesium-137
    c. Iridium-192
    d. Iodine-135
23. Who discovered gamma knife?
    a. Rutherford
    b. Roentgen
    c. Leksell
    d. John R Adler
24. PET scan isotope is:
    a. Phosphorus-32
    b. 18-fluoro-deoxyglucose
    c. Iridium-77
    d. Radium-226
25. Ionizing radiation with maximum penetration is:
    a. Alpha particles
    b. Beta particles
    c. Gamma rays
    d. Microwaves
26. Purely beta emission comes from:
    a. P 32
    b. I 131
    c. Cobalt 60
    d. Ra 226
27. Occupational radiation exposure allowed per year to Indian population?
    a. 2 mSv
    b. 5 mSv
    c. 10 mSv
    d. 20 mSv
28. Which of the following is a functional investigation:
    a. CT scan
    b. MRI
    c. USG
    d. PET scan
29. Gadolinium is a contrast agent used for:
    a. CT - angiography
    b. Bronchography
    c. MRI - Imaging
    d. Contrast Sonography
30. Absolute contraindication for MRI:
    a. Pacemaker
    b. Claustrophobia
    c. Penile prosthesis
    d. Joint replacement

FMGE Solutions Screening Examination

31. Correct regarding B-scan on ultrasound is
    a. 2D image   b. 3D image
    c. Visualizing blood flow d. All of above
32. Which phase of the cell cycle is most sensitive to radiotherapy:
    a. G2M phase   b. S phase
    c. M phase   d. G_2 phase
33. Most common complication of radiotherapy of head and neck cancer?
    a. Dryness of mouth   b. Jawbone necrosis
    c. Odynophagia   d. Bleeding
34. The most radio sensitive tumor amongst the following is:
    a. Small cell lung cancer   b. Seminoma
    c. Soft tissue sarcoma   d. Osteosarcoma
35. Maximum radiation exposure occurs in:
    a. Bone scan   b. MRI
    c. CT scan   d. X-ray
36. Which of the following is a non-iodinated contrast?
    a. Gadolinium   b. Visipaque
    c. Iopamidol   d. Ditriazoate
37. All of the following about MRI are correct EXCEPT:
    a. MRI is useful for localizing small lesions in the brain
    b. MRI is useful for evaluating bone marrow
    c. MRI is better for calcified lesions
    d. MRI is contraindicated in patients with pacemakers

UROLOGY AND BONE IMAGING

38. Which of the following is a gold standard investigation for diagnosis of renal stone? *(Recent Pattern Question 2018)*
    a. USG
    b. Helical CT with Non-contrast
    c. Helical CT with Contrast
    d. MRI
39. Identify the bone marked with arrow:
    (Recent Pattern Question 2017)

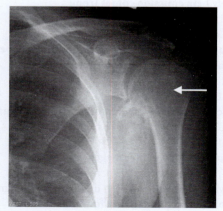

    a. Radius   b. Ulna
    c. Humerus   d. Clavicle

40. On IVP this image was obtained. What is the diagnosis?
    (Recent Pattern Question 2017)

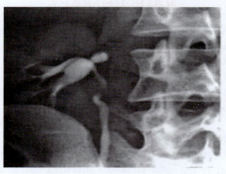

    a. Horse shoe kidney
    b. Duplex collecting system
    c. Cross fused ectopic kidney
    d. Polycystic kidney
41. MRI spine shows following finding. What is the diagnosis? *(Recent Pattern Question 2017)*

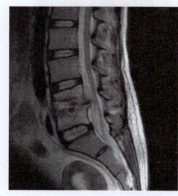

    a. Osteoporosis   b. Metastasis
    c. TB spine   d. Osteopetrosis
42. X-ray pelvis image is shown. What is the structure marked with arrow? *(Recent Pattern Question 2017)*

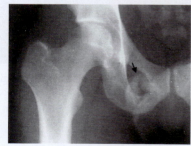

    a. Acetabulum   b. Obturator foramen
    c. Ischial foramen d. Symphysis pubis
43. Ring sign is seen on urography. What is the diagnosis of the patient is? *(Recent Pattern Question 2017)*
    a. Hydronephrosis   b. Polycystic kidney
    c. Papillary necrosis d. Renal cell carcinoma

44. Which of the following condition is most predisposed for contrast nephropathy:
    a. Diabetes
    b. Hypertension
    c. Malignant hypertension
    d. Hypertensive glomerulosclerosis
45. Which of the following cancer is LEAST LIKELY to occur secondary to radiation exposure:
    a. Hepatocellular CA
    b. Renal cell CA
    c. Stomach CA
    d. Colon CA
46. Ring sign is seen on Urography film in a diabetic is due to?
    a. Hydronephrosis
    b. Polycystic kidney
    c. Papillary necrosis
    d. Emphysematous pyelonephritis
47. Spider leg sign on IVP suggests:
    a. Renal stone
    b. Polycystic kidney
    c. Hypernephroma
    d. Hydronephrosis
48. Spider-leg deformity of pelvicalyceal system on intravenous urography (IVU) is a constant feature of:
    a. Tuberculosis
    b. Renal cell carcinoma
    c. Polycystic disease
    d. Wilm's tumor
49. Adder head on I.V.P. is seen in:
    a. Ureterocoele
    b. Cystocele
    c. Enterocele
    d. Omentocele
50. Which of the following investigation is preferred for diagnosis of vesicoureteric reflux:
    a. Intravenous urography
    b. Micturating cystourethrogram
    c. Retrograde pyelography
    d. Ultrasonography
51. Crew cut appearance on X ray skull is seen in:
    a. Thalassemia
    b. Megaloblastic anemia
    c. Autoimmune hemolytic anemia
    d. Dimorphic anemia
52. Bone within a Bone appearance is seen in:
    a. Osteo-necrosis
    b. Osteoporosis
    c. Osteopetrosis
    d. Osteomyelitis
53. 'Hair on end' appearance in skull X-ray is characteristic of:
    a. G6PD deficiency
    b. Sickle cell anemia
    c. Rickets
    d. Scurvy
54. Martel sign is seen in
    a. Gout
    b. Ankylosing spondylitis
    c. Osteoarthritis
    d. Rheumatoid arthritis
55. Nuchal thickness is evaluated in:
    a. Ante natal USG first trimester
    b. Prenatal USG screening
    c. Antenatal USG second trimester
    d. Antenatal USG third trimester

ABDOMEN IMAGING

56. Investigation of choice for acute cholecystitis is:
    (Recent Pattern Question 2018-19)
    a. H.I.D.A scan
    b. USG
    c. CT scan
    d. Biopsy
57. Investigation of choice for GERD:
    (Recent Pattern Question 2018-19)
    a. USG
    b. HIDA
    c. Manometry
    d. 24-hour pH monitoring
58. Comment on the diagnosis of the image shown below
    (Recent Pattern Question 2018)

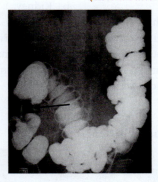

    a. Apple core appearance
    b. Claw sign
    c. Coffee bean appearance
    d. String sign of kantor
59. Name the structure marked with arrow:
    (Recent Pattern Question 2017)

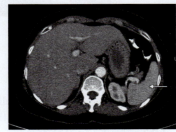

    a. Right kidney
    b. Left kidney
    c. Spleen
    d. Stomach
60. A 7-year-old child presented with abdominal pain, fever and jaundice. CT abdomen is given below. What is the most likely diagnosis? *(Recent Pattern Question 2017)*

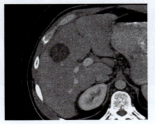

    a. Amebiasis
    b. Hemangioma
    c. Hepatoma
    d. Hydatid cyst

FMGE Solutions Screening Examination

61. Identify the organ shown with an arrow
    (Recent Pattern Question 2016)

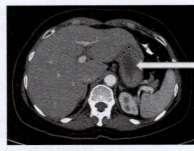

   a. Spleen b. Kidney
   c. Stomach d. Liver

62. Most useful investigation of choice for liver abscess is
    a. Exploratory laparotomy b. Ultrasound
    c. Liver enzymes d. Parasite in the stool

63. Normal thickness of gallbladder wall:
    a. 1 mm b. 1 cm
    c. 3 mm d. 5 cm

64. Thumb print on barium is seen in:

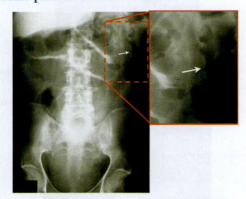

   a. Volvulus b. Ischemic colitis
   c. Crohn's disease d. Intussusception

65. Diagnosis of the given X-ray of abdomen:

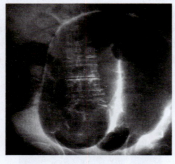

   a. Small intestine obstruction
   b. Pneumointestinalis
   c. Sigmoid volvulus
   d. Intussusception

66. Double bubble sign is seen in:
    a. Duodenal atresia
    b. Jejunal atresia
    c. Ileal atresia
    d. Hypertrophic pyloric stenosis

67. Double barrel sign is seen in?
    a. Primary Sclerosing cholangitis
    b. Primary Biliary cirrhosis
    c. Obstructive jaundice
    d. Duodenal atresia

68. Cobble stoning of intestine with string sign of kantor is seen in :
    a. Crohn's disease b. Ulcerative colitis
    c. Ischemic colitis d. Amoebic colitis

69. Pipe stem colon on barium enema is seen with:
    a. Crohn's disease b. Ulcerative colitis
    c. Ischemic colitis d. Irritable bowel syndrome

70. Target sign is seen in:
    a. Ischemic colitis b. Meckel's Diverticulum
    c. Intussusception d. Volvulus

71. Cork screw appearance on barium swallow is seen in:
    a. Achalasia cardia
    b. Diffuse esophageal spasm
    c. Zenker's diverticulum
    d. Scleroderma

72. IOC for neonatal hypertrophic pyloric stenosis:
    a. X-ray b. CT scan
    c. MRI d. Ultrasound

73. Saw tooth appearance is seen in:
    a. Diverticulosis b. Cholecystitis
    c. Appendicitis d. Hiatus hernia

74. Apple core appearance on barium enema is seen in?
    a. Carcinoma colon b. TB caecum
    c. Crohns disease d. Ulcerative colitis

75. IOC acute pancreatitis:
    a. Contrast CT b. USG
    c. Serum lipase d. Serum amylase

76. Sentinel loop on X-ray:
    a. Meckel's diverticulum
    b. Acute cholecystitis
    c. Acute mesenteric adenitis
    d. Acute pancreatitis

77. A patient presents with right hypochondrium pain. Which of the following investigations should be done:
    a. CT b. MRI
    c. USG d. Cholecystogram

78. RTA brought in casualty. On examination liver rupture is suspected. Which of the following investigation is to be done first?
    a. CT b. MRI
    c. USG d. Peritoneal lavage

79. **Identify the image:**

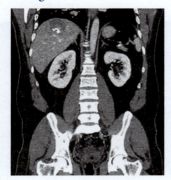

    a. Digital X-Ray   b. CT
    c. PET scan   d. USG

THORAX IMAGING

80. **Identify the pathology in the given X-ray:**
(Recent Pattern Question 2018-19)

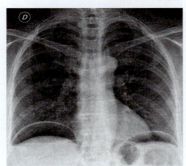

    a. Pneumothorax   b. Pneumoperitoneum
    c. Hydrothorax   d. Normal X-ray

81. **The following image shows:**
(Recent Pattern Question 2018-19)

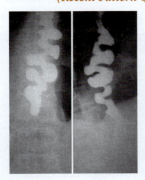

    a. Achalasia cardia
    b. Diffuse oesophageal spasm
    c. Carcinoma Oesophagus
    d. Schatzki's Ring

82. **The Lateral view X-ray lung shows:**
(Recent Pattern Question 2018)

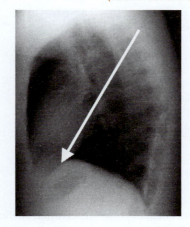

    a. Major fissure   b. Minor fissure
    c. Azygos fissure   d. Transverse fissure

83. **Comment on the diagnosis:**
(Recent Pattern Question 2017)

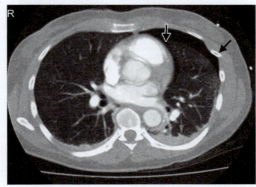

    a. Hydrothorax   b. Pneumothorax
    c. Pleural effusion   d. Hydropneumothorax

84. **CT chest is as shown below. What is the diagnosis?**
(Recent Pattern Question 2017)

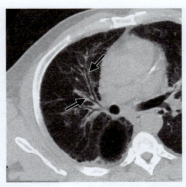

    a. Bronchiectasis   b. Pneumonia
    c. Pulmonary TB   d. COPD

FMGE Solutions Screening Examination

85. The shown investigation is:
(Recent Pattern Question 2017)

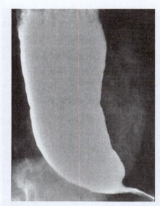

a. Barium enema
b. Barium swallow
c. Plain X-ray
d. Fluoroscopy

86. Identify the pathology in the given chest X-ray:
(Recent Pattern Question 2017)

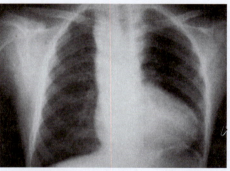

a. Tetralogy of Fallot
b. Transposition of great arteries
c. Pericardial effusion
d. Total anomalous pulmonary veinous return

87. In the CECT shown below what is the structure marked with arrow?
(Recent Pattern Question 2017)

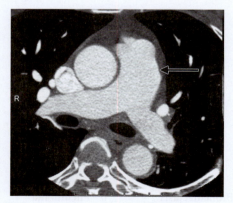

a. Aorta
b. Trachea
c. Descending aorta
d. Main pulmonary artery

88. The arrow at CXR points to?
(Recent Pattern Question 2017)

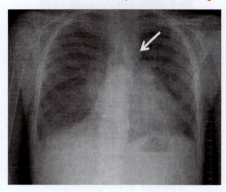

a. Left atrium
b. Left atrial appendage
c. Lingular lobe lung
d. Aortic knuckle

89. The following image shows
(Recent Pattern Question 2016)

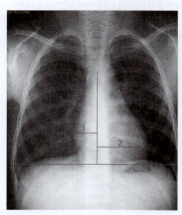

a. Pulmonary edema
b. CT ratio being measured
c. Atelectasis
d. Bronchiectasis

90. In a patient with bronchopneumonia lung, finding on CXR
(Recent Pattern Question 2016)

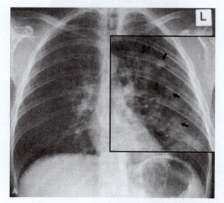

a. Patchy consolidation
b. Diffuse consolidation
c. Mediastinal shift
d. Massive pleural effusion

91. All of the following are true in chest X-ray PA view EXCEPT:
    a. Right ventricle forms the right heart border
    b. Left ventricle forms the left heart border
    c. Cardiothoracic ratio in adults is normally 50% or less than that
    d. Right atrium forms the right heart border
92. Trans-esophageal echocardiography is better than trans-thoracic Echocardiography because of better evaluation of?
    a. Diastolic dysfunction
    b. Left ventricular hypertrophy
    c. Systolic function
    d. Left atrial appendage clots
93. Most common congenital cardiac anomaly diagnosed in adulthood:
    a. ASD   b. VSD
    c. PDA   d. TAPVR
94. Box shaped heart is seen in which of the following condition:
    a. Coaractation of aorta   b. Pericardial effusion
    c. Tetralogy of fallot   d. Ebstein anomaly
95. Curschmann spirals and flattening of diaphragm is seen in:
    a. Asthma   b. COPD
    c. Silicosis   d. Pulmonary embolism
96. Flexible Bronchoscope contains holes for all of these functions EXCEPT?
    a. Ventilation
    b. Drainage of secretion
    c. For biopsy
    d. To remove foreign body
97. Hampton hump is seen in:
    a. Pulmonary TB
    b. Bronchogenic carcinoma
    c. Pulmonary embolism
    d. Pulmonary hemorrhage
98. Westermark's sign is seen in:
    a. Pulmonary embolism
    b. Pulmonary sequestration
    c. Pulmonary alveolar proteinosis
    d. A.B.P.A (Allergic Broncho-pulmonary Aspergillosis)
99. Continuous diaphragm sign is seen on X-ray. Diagnosis is?
    a. Pneumopericardium
    b. Pneumomediastinum
    c. Pneumothorax
    d. Pericardial abscess
100. Air Bronchogram is seen in:
    a. Pneumonia
    b. Pleural effusion
    c. Pneumothorax
    d. Pneumo-peritoneum

101. IDENTIFY: (X-ray chest showing big mass on left upper lobe, touching sternum)

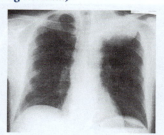

    a. Lung carcinoma   b. Hydatid cyst
    c. Lung Abscess   d. Aspergilloma
102. Golden S sign is seen in:

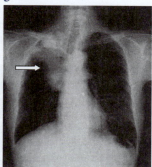

    a. Bronchogenic carcinoma with collapse of lung
    b. Traction Bronchiectasis with apical scarring
    c. Emphysema with increased lucency and flattened diagphragm
    d. Pulmonary edema
103. Pop-corn calcification is seen with?
    a. Pulmonary tuberculosis   b. Pulmonary hamartoma
    c. Klebsiella infection   d. Foreign body

NEUROLOGY IMAGING

104. Identify the pathology in the shown CT:
     (Recent Pattern Question 2018-19)

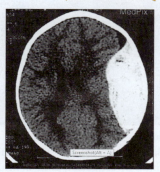

    a. Intraventricular bleed
    b. Massive Epidural hemorrhage
    c. Subdural hemorrhage
    d. Subarachnoid haemorrhage

FMGE Solutions Screening Examination

105. Identify the image given below
    (Recent Pattern Question 2018)

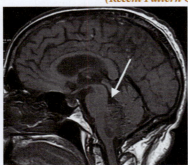

   a. Lateral ventricle   b. Corpus callosum
   c. 3rd ventricle   d. 4th ventricle

106. Angiography of brain blood vessels of brain as is shown in image. Identify the artery marked with arrow?
    (Recent Pattern Question 2017)

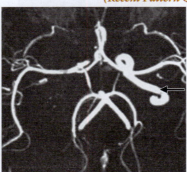

   a. Anterior communicating artery
   b. Posterior cerebral artery
   c. Middle cerebral artery
   d. Internal carotid artery

107. In the given imaging, what is the structure marked with arrow?   *(Recent Pattern Question 2017)*

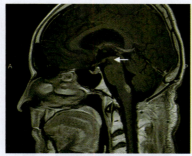

   a. Midbrain   b. Pons
   c. Medulla   d. Cerebellum

108. Most common investigation done in brain tumor
    (Recent Pattern Question 2016)
   a. CT   b. MRI
   c. Digital X-ray d. USG

109. IOC for sub-arachnoid hemorrhage
   a. CT scan   b. MRI
   c. Lumbar puncture d. MRA

110. Extradural hemorrhage is seen as:

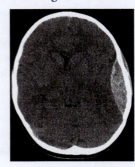

   a. Hypodense bi concave   b. Hypodense bi convex
   c. Hyperdense bi concave d. Hyperdense bi convex

111. Intracranial calcification is best diagnosed by:
   a. Plain X-ray skull   b. CT scan
   c. FDG-PFT scan   d. MRI

112. The investigation of choice for meningeal carcinomatosis in CNS is:
   a. Enhanced MRI   b. SPECT
   c. PET   d. NCCT

MAMMOGRAPHY

113. The most appropriate technique for mammography is:
   a. Spot Compression view b. Medial lateral oblique view
   c. Lateral view   d. Bird's eye view

114. Which one of the following statements regarding mammography is FALSE:
   a. It can detect 95 % of early breast cancers
   b. Normal mammogram rules out breast cancer
   c. The sensitivity of this investigation increases with age as the breast becomes less dense.
   d. Mammography is a safe investigation even after radiation exposure.

OBSTETRICAL IMAGING

115. Father of obstetrical ultrasound:
   a. Ion Donald
   b. John Wild
   c. Doppler John
   d. Hounsfield

116. By ultrasonography, the earliest sign of conception is:
   a. Small white gestational ring
   b. Presence of foetal pole
   c. Presence of yolk sac
   d. Presence of cardiac pulsations

BOARD REVIEW QUESTIONS

Radiology

1223

117. **Half-life of tritium is?**
   a. 6 hours
   b. 3 days
   c. 10 months
   d. 12 years

118. **Colon cut off sign is seen in?**
   a. Carcinoma colon
   b. Pancreatitis
   c. Sigmoid valvulus
   d. Diverticulosis

119. **Chain of lakes appearance is seen in?**
   a. Chronic pancreatitis
   b. Acute pancreatitis
   c. Gall stone ileus
   d. Sub-acute intestinal obstruction

120. **Double atria shadow is a feature of enlargement of?**
   a. Left atria enlargement
   b. Right atrial enlargement
   c. Right ventricular enlargement
   d. Left ventricular enlargement

121. **Palla sign is?**
   a. Enlarged right descending pulmonary artery
   b. Enlarged left descending pulmonary artery
   c. Bilateral wedge shaped lung infarction
   d. Elevated hemi-diaphragm

122. **Bulging fissure sign is seen in**
   a. Friedlander's pneumonia
   b. Pneumonia alba
   c. Psittacosis
   d. Broncho-alveolar carcinoma

123. **Earliest radiological feature of raised ICT in children?**
   a. Sutural diastasis
   b. Posterior clinoid erosion
   c. Silver beaten appearance
   d. Sella erosion

124. **MRI finding of face of panda appearance is seen in**
   a. Wilson disease
   b. Menke disease
   c. Huntington chorea
   d. Parkinsonism

125. **Snow storm appearance on antenatal USG is seen in**
   a. Hydatiform mole
   b. Miliary TB
   c. Arnold chiari malformation
   d. Beckwith Wiedemann syndrome

126. **Investigation of choice for diagnosis of dysphagia lusoria**
   a. CT angiography
   b. Barium swallow
   c. Esophageal manometry
   d. Barium meal follow through

127. **String of beads sign is seen in**
   a. Crohn's disease
   b. Fibromuscular dysplasia
   c. Chronic pancreatitis
   d. Intestinal ileus

128. **Bat wing appearance on CT scan is seen in**
   a. Joubert syndrome
   b. Pulmonary edema
   c. Pulmonary artery syndrome
   d. SVC syndrome

129. **All are true about MRI EXCEPT?**
   a. Complex interaction of protons with magnetic fields
   b. Preferred contrast agent is gadolinium
   c. Cerebral edema is better seen on T2W
   d. FLAIR sequence shows low brain intensity

130. **PET scan uses**
   a. 18-Fluorodeoxy-glucose
   b. 18-Fluorinated Glucose
   c. Iodinated contrast
   d. Gadolinium contrast

131. **M.U.G.A scan is used for diagnosis of?**
   a. Ejection fraction
   b. GFR
   c. Cerebral oxygen uptake
   d. Pulmonary function test

132. **Investigation of choice for Zollinger Ellison syndrome?**
   a. Endoscopic ultrasound
   b. Secretin study
   c. Basal acid output
   d. Upper GI endoscopy

133. **Double barrel sign is seen due to?**
   a. Dilated CBD
   b. Dilated Portal vein
   c. Dilated Common Hepatic duct
   d. Dilated left hepatic duct

134. **In the X-ray image,**
   a. Fat is darker than water
   b. Calcium is darker than air
   c. Bone is darkest
   d. Heart is darker than vertebra

135. **The degree of blackness of a film is called**
   a. Spatial resolution
   b. Contrast
   c. Density
   d. Sharpness

136. **Continuous diaphragm sign is seen in**
   a. Pneumothorax
   b. Pneumo-mediastinum
   c. Pneumo-peritoneum
   d. Subcutaneous emphysema

137. **Stratosphere sign is seen in:**
   a. Pneumothorax
   b. Pleural effusion
   c. Pneumonia
   d. Consolidation

138. **Reigler sign is seen in**
   a. Pneumoperitoneum
   b. Pneumothorax
   c. Renal abscess
   d. Retroperitoneal haemorrhage

139. **Water lily sign in lung is seen with?**
   a. Echinococcus
   b. Paragonimus
   c. Ankylostoma
   d. Angiostrongyloides

140. **Egg on side appearance of heart is seen in the radiograph of?**
   a. TAPVC
   b. TGA
   c. ASD
   d. VSD

141. **Radionuclide scan done for Parathrroid adenoma is?**
   a. Sesta MIBI scan
   b. Iodine-123 scan
   c. 99mTc-sulphur colloid
   d. Gallium scan

142. **Milliary shadow in chest X ray is seen in all EXCEPT:**
   a. Milliary tuberculosis
   b. Tropical eosinophillia
   c. Asbestosis
   d. Metastasis

Questions

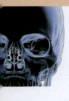

FMGE Solutions Screening Examination

143. Radioisotope used in PET scan is?
    a. Tachnetium 99m
    b. Iodine 123
    c. Iodine 131
    d. Fluoride-18
144. How much area is covered by spiral CT in 30 seconds?
    a. Entire organ
    b. Entire abdomen
    c. Entire trunk
    d. Whole body
145. Best investigation for diagnosing abdominal aortic aneurysm is?
    a. USG
    b. CT angiography
    c. Classical radiography
    d. Non contrast CT scan
146. Which of the following is the investigation of choice for dissecting aortic aneurysm?
    a. CECT
    b. PET
    c. MRI
    d. TEE
147. Dawson finger in brain seen in which condition?
    a. Cortical vein thrombosis
    b. Multiple sclerosis
    c. Lacunar infarcts
    d. Alzhemir's disease
148. Kerley B lines are seen in which part of chest X-ray?
    a. Upper portion
    b. Mid portion
    c. Peripheral lower
    d. Upper peripheral zone
149. Figure of 8 sign on X-ray is seen in?
    a. TAPVC
    b. TGA
    c. TOF
    d. Ebstein's anomaly
150. Investigation of choice for subdural hemorrhage is?
    a. Angiography
    b. NCCT
    c. CECT
    d. MRI

Radiology

IMAGE-BASED QUESTIONS

151. Comment on the diagnosis.
(Most Recent Question 2019)

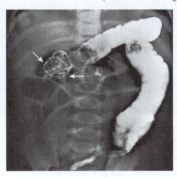

a. Intussusception   b. Malrotation
c. Duodenal atresia d. Ileal atresia

154. The following CT shows:

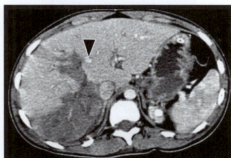

a. Liver laceration   b. Kidney cyst
c. Pancreas contusion d. Perforation peritonitis

152. Identify the lesion shown in the CT head of an unconscious unresponsive patient with GCS of 5.

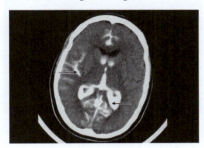

a. SAH and IVH
b. Brain tumor
c. Hydrocephalus
d. Extradural and subdural hemorrhage

155. CT head shows?

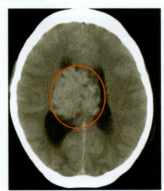

a. Brain tumor   b. Brain infarction
c. S.A.H   d. I.V.H

153. Identify the lesion shown in the CT head of an unconscious unresponsive patient with GCS of 5.

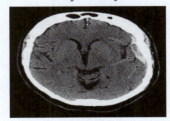

a. Extradural hemorrhage
b. Subdural hemorrhage
c. Subarachnoid hemorrhage
d. Intraventricular hemorrhage

156. The following IVP shows presence of?

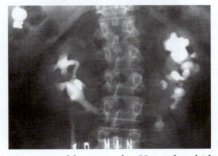

a. Drooping lily sign b. Horseshoe kidney
c. Duplication of kidney
d. Normal scan

157. The cholangiogram shows?

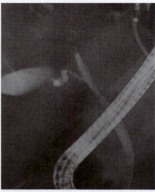

   a. Klatskin tumor   b. Gall stones
   c. Choledocholithiasis   d. Porcelain gallbladder

158. A 3-year-old non-vaccinated child presented with fever and fast breathing. His mother told that he has recently developed measles rash. CXR shown below is indicative of which infection?

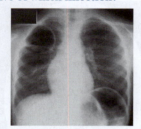

   a. Staphylococcus aureus
   b. Staphylococcus albus
   c. Streptococcal pneumoniae
   d. Streptococcal viridans

159. A neonate with Down syndrome is having bilious vomiting

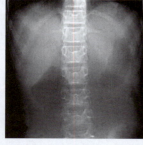

   a. Duodenal atresia
   b. Congenital hypertrophic pyloric stenosis
   c. Ileal atresia
   d. Anorectal malformation

160. A 40-year-old intravenous drug abuser presents with Vomiting, Jaundice and Right Hypochondrium pain. USG abdomen shows presence of?

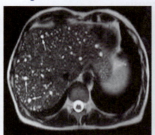 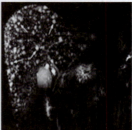

   a. Amoebic liver abscess
   b. Acute viral hepatitis
   c. Acute cholecystitis
   d. Hepatocellular carcinoma

161. Neonate with respiratory distress 6 hours after birth. CXR was performed. Diagnosis is?

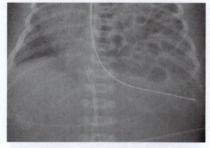

   a. Meconium aspiration syndrome
   b. Congenital Pneumonia
   c. Bochdalek Hernia
   d. Transient Tachypnea of Newborn

162. A 3 days old neonate with abdominal distention and non-passage of stool. The X-ray done shown below is called?

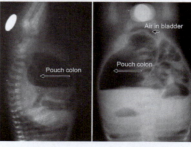

   a. Invertogram   b. Infantogram
   c. Babygram
   d. Double contrast barium study

Radiology

163. Neonate with anoxic spells and single S2. CXR shows all EXCEPT?

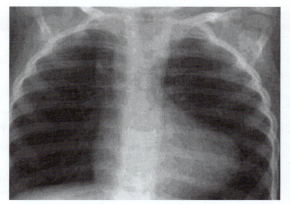

a. Boot shaped heart
b. Pulmonary plethora
c. Right sided aortic arch
d. Right ventricular hypertrophy

165. The marked structure in chest X-ray is: *(2018)*

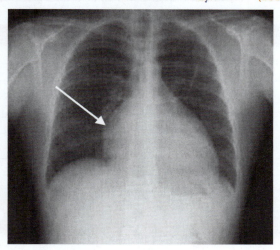

a. Inferior vena cava b. Right atrium
c. Right ventricle   d. Superior vena cava

164. In the shown image, what is the marked line with B is which fissure: *(2018)*

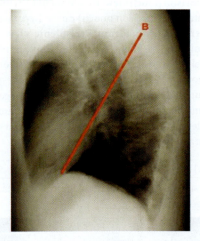

a. Minor fissure   b. Major fissure
c. Transverse fissure d. Azygous fissure

166. In the shown X-ray what is the name of structure marked: *(2018)*

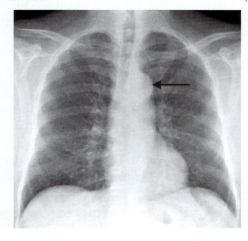

a. Aortic knob   b. Left atrium
c. SVC   d. Pulmonary trunk

Answers to Image-Based Questions are given at the end of explained questions

FMGE Solutions Screening Examination

ANSWERS WITH EXPLANATIONS

MOST RECENT QUESTIONS 2019

1. Ans. (a) Aortic dissection

Ref: Harrison 20th ed. pg. 1921

The given image is of a CT chest showing intimal flap of aortic dissection and involves both ascending and descending aorta.

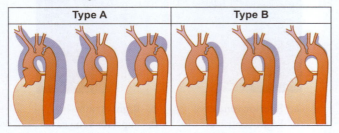

2. Ans. (a) MUGA

Ref: Harrison 20th ed. pg. 675

MUGA or Multiple Uptake Gated Acquisition Angiography and is used to asses LV function and Volume. Choices B, C and D are used for angiographically significant Coronary artery disease.

3. Ans. (a) Diaphragmatic hernia

- The shown image is suggestive of diaphragmatic hernia.
- Intestinal loop in thoracic cavity and absence of bowel loops in abdomen is highly suggestive of diaphragmatic hernia.

4. Ans. (d) Barium enema

Ref: Radiation dose in X-ray and CT exams; https://www.radiologyinfo.org/en/pdf/safety-xray

TABLE: Radiation exposure in different investigations

Procedure	Mean effective dose (mSv)
Chest X-ray (PA View)	0.02
Chest X-ray (PA + Lateral view)	0.1
Mammogram	0.4
Abdomen X-ray	0.7
HSG	0.9 – 1.3
CT Brain	2.2
IVP	3
ERCP	4
Coronary angiography	7 (2–16)
Barium enema	8 (2–18)

Contd...

Procedure	Mean effective dose (mSv)
CT Colonography	6
CT Abdomen and Pelvis	10
Thallium scan	16.9

5. Ans. (b) Pleural cavity

Ref: Principle and Practice of Trauma Care by SK Kochar, P 51

- FAST scan is Focused Assessment with Sonography for Trauma
- It is a rapid, decision making scan done on the patients immediately at the time of trauma. It has sensitivity of ~90% and specificity of ~95%.
- Aim of this scan is to identify intraperitoneal free fluid (to rule out hemoperitoneum), which helps in precise decision making on immediate transfer of patient to operation theatre.
- Four regions that are mainly assessed by FAST scan are:
  1. **Pericardial/Subxiphoid view:** To rule our pericardial effusion
  2. **Right upper quadrant view/Perihepatic view/ Morison pouch view:** to rule out fluid in the hepatorenal interface (morison pouch) due to hepatorenal trauma
  3. **Left upper quadrant/Perisplenic view:** To rule out fluid in perisplenic space due to spleen trauma
  4. **Pelvic/Suprapubic view:** This space (pouch of Douglas) is most dependent peritoneal space. It rules out bladder or other pelvic organ damage.
- Extension of FAST is eFAST, which includes scanning of pleural space also, to rule out any injury to lungs or pleural effusion.

6. Ans. (c) Trachea

- The structure in CXR lateral view is trachea. Refer to the image below

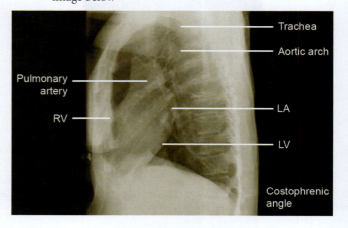

Radiology

7. Ans. (b) Exudative pleural effusion

- The given X-ray shows massive pleural effusion. Since there is history of low grade fever and dyspnea, this can be secondary to some underlying pathology, producing exudative effusion.

BASIC RADIOLOGY PRINCIPLES AND RADIOTHERAPY

8. Ans. (b) CT and X-ray

- Out of given choices, CT and X-ray work on the same principle.
  - X-rays passed through the body are either absorbed or attenuated (weakened) at different levels
  - The image contains shadow of the dense tissues of body
  - If 3D image required, as in CT, a detector is placed opposite to radiation source → take pictures from different angles → reconstruction of image by computer.

Extra Mile

- **Working principle of other radiological procedures:**
  - **Ultrasound:** Uses sound waves (Piezoelectric effect)
  - **MRI:** Uses magnetic fields/radio-frequency waves
  - **Nuclear medicine:** Uses gamma rays
  - **PET scan:** Uses short-lived positron emitting isotopes (each positron gives two gamma rays)

9. Ans. (a) K.F.T

Ref: Harrison: 19th ed, P 1803

The contrast can lead to development of renal shutdown due to contrast nephropathy. Serum creatinine should be checked before any contrast study is performed. Adequate hydration of the patient can prevent such a mishap. Drug of choice for management of contrast nephropathy is N-acetyl Cysteine.

10. Ans. (b) Venography

- Duplex ultrasound is the **initial investigation of choice** in nearly all patients with suspected DVT.
- Its reliability is dependent upon the skill of the user.
- Major axial veins of the lower limb are well displayed.
- It has a sensitivity of 98.7% and specificity of 100% for above-knee DVT and a sensitivity of 85.2% and specificity of 98.2% for below-knee DVT.
- **Gold standard/Best test** for venous occlusion is **invasive venography.**

11. Ans. (a) PET-CT scan

- The shown image is of PET-CT.

- Shown below are three images. First image is of CT scan, second image PET scan. When these two images are superimposed, the image is said to be PET-CT.

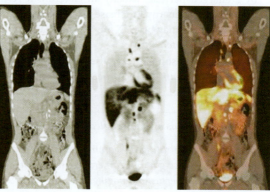

12. Ans. (a) Orthopantogram

- **An orthopantogram is a panoramic or wide view X-ray of the lower face,** which displays all the teeth of the upper and lower jaw on a single film. It demonstrates the number, position and growth of all the teeth including those that have not yet surfaced or erupted.
- **A lateral cephalogram is a lateral or side view X-ray of the face,** which demonstrates the bones and facial contours in profile on a single film (*image*).

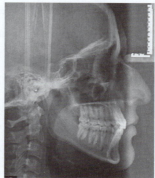

Figure: Lateral cephalogram

- **Towns view and stenver view** is used to visualize the petrous part of the pyramids, the dorsum sellae and the posterior clinoid processes, which are visible in the shadow of the foramen magnum.

13. Ans. (a) Compton effect

Ref: Comprehensive Biophysics, 2014 ed. pg. 1

When X-rays travel through the body it can cause 2 effects:

- Photoelectric effect and Compton effect.
- The *photoelectric effect* is the observation that many metals emit electrons when light shines upon them.

FMGE Solutions Screening Examination

Compton Effect

- *Compton scattering* is the inelastic *scattering* of a photon by a charged particle, usually an electron. It results in a decrease in energy (increase in wavelength) of the photon (which may be an X-ray or gamma ray photon), called the *Compton effect*.
- This is the reason, it is advised to wear lead apron *(thickness- 0.5 mm)* in the procedure room.

14. Ans. (c) Gamma

Ref: Essentials of Radiological Science, 2nd ed. pg. 10

- Maximum penetrating is gamma rays, therefore least dangerous. Hence gamma camera is used therapeutically for myocardial perfusion imaging.
- Least penetrating is alpha rays, therefore most dangerous

15. Ans. (d) Roentgen

Ref: Essentials of Radiological Science, 2nd ed. pg. 3

- Unit of radiation exposure- **Roentgen** (SI = Coloumb/kg)
- Unit of absorbed radiation **RAD** (SI = GRAY)
- Unit of biologic effect of radiaiton **Rem** (SI = Sievert)

16. Ans. (c) 74 days

Ref: Basic Radiological Physics, 2nd ed. pg. 180

- Iridium-192, emits gamma rays. It has energy of 0.4 MeV.
- T1/2 of iridium 192: 74 days

Important Half Life of Radionuclides

- **Gold-198:** 2.7 days
- **Iodine-123:** 13.3 hours
- **Iodine-131:** 8 days
- **Phosphorus-32:** 14.3 days
- **Yttrium 90:** 64 hours
- **Cobalt-60:** 5.26 years
- **Caesium-137:** 30 years
- **Radium-226:** 1620 years

17. Ans. (a) 8 days

Ref: Basics Radiological Physics, 2nd ed. pg. 180

Please refer to above explanation

18. Ans. (b) 5.3 years

Ref: Basics Radiological Physics, 2nd ed. pg. 180

Please refer to above explanation

19. Ans. (c) 1620 years

Ref: Basics Radiological Physics, 2nd ed. pg. 180

Please refer to above explanation

20. Ans. (b) I -131

Ref: Sutton, 7th ed. pg. 1504

- **Iodine-131** has a radioactive decay half-life of about eight days.
- Iodine-131 exhibits a beta mode of decay, and leads to death in cells that it penetrates up to several millimeters and hence is useful for thyroid ablation.
- **I-123** has a half-life of 13.22 hours and is a radioactive isotope of iodine used in nuclear medicine imaging, including single photon emission computed tomography.

21. Ans. (c) Iodine 131

Ref: Sutton, 7th ed. pg. 1504

22. Ans. (d) Iodine-135

Ref: Essentials of Radiological Science, 2nd ed. pg. 15

- **Iodine-131** is used to treat the thyroid for cancers and other abnormal conditions such as hyperthyroidism
- **Iridium-192** can be implanted into cancers of the tongue.
- **Iodine-135** is an isotope of iodine which is an important isotope from the viewpoint of nuclear reactor physics. It is produced in relatively large amounts as a fission product, and decays to xenon-135, *which is a nuclear poison.*
- **Caesium-137** is another example of an implantable radioactive isotope used in the treatment of uterine or vaginal cancers.
- **Radium-223:** This is a new radioisotope used in treatment for secondary cancer in the bones.
- **Strontium-89 and samarium-153:** Used for treatment of secondary bone CA.

23. Ans. (c) Leksell

- The *Gamma Knife* is an advanced radiation treatment for adults and children with small to medium brain tumors. This surgery sometimes referred to as **stereotactic radio surgery** (SRS), is a non-invasive method for treating brain disorders. It is the delivery of a single, high dose of irradiation to a small and critically located intra-cranial volume through the intact skull.
- **Prof Rutherford**- Father of nuclear physics
- John R. Adler- Cyberknife therapy
- Wilhelm Röentgen- discovered X-rays.

Radiology

24. Ans. (b) 18-Fluoro-deoxyglucose

Ref: Harrison, 19th ed. pg. 102e-12

- Radionuclides used in PET scanning are typically isotopes with short half-lives such as carbon-11 (~20 min), nitrogen-13 (~10 min), oxygen-15 (~2 min), fluorine-18 (~110 min), or rubidium-82(~1.27 min).
- These radionuclides are incorporated either into compounds normally used by the body such as glucose (or glucose analogues), water, or ammonia, or into molecules that bind to receptors or other sites of drug action. Such labelled compounds are known as radiotracer.
- *At present, however, by far the most commonly used radiotracer in clinical PET scanning is fluorodeoxy-glucose (also called FDG or fludeoxy-glucose), an analogue of glucose that is labeled with fluorine-18.*
- This radiotracer is used in essentially all scans for oncology and most scans in neurology, and thus makes up the large majority of all of the radiotracer (>95%) used in PET and PET/CT scanning.

25. Ans. (c) Gamma rays

Ref: Essentials of Radiological Science, 2nd ed. pg. 10

- **Alpha** particles are emitted from the nuclei of radioactive atoms and have high speeds and high energy and are the least penetrating. Their maximum range in air is about 10 cm and can be stopped by the outer layer of skin. If they enter the body, alpha emitters are hazardous to human health. As they disintegrate, they can damage tissue. The normal route of entry by alpha particles are inhalation, digestion and through wounds.
- **Beta** particles are also emitted from the nuclei of radioactive atoms, but they are much smaller in mass than alpha particles and have considerably more penetrating power. Beta emitters are capable of penetrating wood to 4 cm and the human body to 1 cm. Like alpha emitters, they are internal radiation hazards and have the same routes of body entry. They can be stopped by ordinary wall or a 1.3-cm thick sheet of aluminum.
- *Gamma radiation originates in the nucleus of an atom. It can penetrate deeply into tissue, and may produce burns similar to deep sunburn, alter genes to cause mutations, and reduce the white blood cell count and encourage infections.*
- **X-rays** cause cancer by inducing mutations. X-rays are a form of electromagnetic radiation that is produced when high-speed electrons strike the target material inside the X-ray tube. The quality of the X-ray, which is the power to penetrate through matter, depends upon the wavelength and the material being irradiated. Hard X-rays with short wavelengths will penetrate thick steel plate. Soft X-rays with long wavelengths are less penetrating.

- **Neutrons** are particles released upon the disintegration of radioactive isotopes. Neutron particles are highly penetrating and require heavy shielding. They are capable of penetrating the human body to several centimeters. Within the body the neutrons release excess energy which can cause tissue damage. Secondary releases of energy may also occur from alpha, beta, and gamma emitters released from the neutrons.

26. Ans. (a) P 32

- **Radioactive phosphorus:** Pure beta emission
  - Used in Bone tumor and polycythemia
- **Cobalt 60**- emits gamma rays
- **Radium-226**- Emits α, β, γ

27. Ans. (d) 20 mSv

Natural Radiation exposure	2.5 mSv
Yearly dose limit for public	1.0 mSv
Yearly dose limit for occupational workers	**20 mSv**
Dose level at which chromosomal aberrations can be measured	100 mSv
Dose at which nausea, vomiting may start	Approx 1000 mSv (1 Sv)
Dose level for 50% death of exposed population in 60 days	Approx 4,000 mSv (4Sv)

- The U.S. Nuclear Regulatory Commission (NRC) guidelines mandate-
  - To limit human-made radiation exposure for individual members of the public to 100 mrem (1 mSv) per year
  - To limit occupational radiation exposure to adults working with radioactive material to 5,000 mrem (50 mSv) per year
- The radiation exposure of occupationally exposed individuals is carefully monitored with the use of pocket-pen-sized instruments called dosimeters.

28. Ans. (d) PET scan

- Positron emission tomography (PET) is a nuclear medical imaging modality that produces a three-dimensional image of functional processes in the body.
- The most common indication for a PET scan is to detect *cancer metastasis.*
- The technique operates on the principle of detecting gamma rays emitted indirectly by a positron-emitting radionuclide (tracer).
- Three dimensional imaging is done with the aid of a CT X-ray scan performed on the patient during the same session.

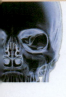

FMGE Solutions Screening Examination

- The biologically active molecule chosen for PET is FDG (*18-Fluoro deoxy glucose*), an analogue of glucose, the concentrations of tracer imaged will indicate tissue metabolic activity by virtue of the regional glucose uptake.
- **Also remember:** Functional magnetic resonance imaging or functional MRI (fMRI) is an imaging procedure that measures brain activity by detecting associated changes in blood flow. This technique relies on the fact that cerebral blood flow and neuronal activation are coupled. It is used for diagnosis of alzeihmer's disease

29. Ans. (c) MRI-Imaging

Ref: Harrison, 19th ed. pg. 440

- **The most commonly used compounds for contrast enhancement are gadolinium-based** and they improve the visibility of internal body structures in magnetic resonance imaging.
- MRI contrast agents alter the relaxation times of atoms within body tissues where they are present after oral or intravenous administration.
- This relaxation emits energy which is detected by the scanner and is mathematically converted into an image.
- *Gadolinium containing MRI* contrast agents are used for enhancement of vessels in MR angiography or for brain tumor diagnosis which is associated with the degradation of the blood-brain barrier.

30. Ans. (a) Pacemaker

Ref: Harrison, 19th ed. pg. 440e-t

Contraindications of MRI

Absolute contraindication	Relative contraindication
• Pacemaker • Metallic foreign body in the eye • Deep brain stimulator • Swan-Ganz catheter • Bullets or gunshot pellets • Cerebral aneurysm clips • Cochlear implant • Magnetic dental implants	• AAA stent • Stapes implant • Implanted drug infusion device • Neuro or bone growth stimulator • Surgical clips, wire sutures, screws or mesh • Ocular prosthesis • Penile prosthesis • Joint replacement or prosthesis • Other implants, in particular mechanical devices

31. Ans. (a) 2D image

Modes of Ultrasound used in Medical Imaging

Mode	Principle	Application in practice
A-mode: (amplitude mode)	Simplest type of ultrasound. Single transducer scans a line through the body with the echoes plotted on screen as a function of depth	Therapeutic ultrasound aimed at a specific tumor or calculus to allow for pinpoint accurate focus of the destructive wave energy
B-mode (brightness mode)	Horizontal array of transducers scan a plane through the body that can be viewed as a two-dimensional image on screen.	Commonly known as 2D mode now
C-mode	C-mode image is formed in a plane normal to a B-mode image	Selects data from a specific depth from an A-mode line is used; then the transducer is moved in the 2D plane to sample the entire region at this fixed depth.
M-mode (motion mode) ultrasound	Pulses are emitted in quick succession and either an A-mode or B-mode image is taken.	Used to determine the velocity of specific organ structures like in valvular heart disease.
Doppler mode	Makes use of the Doppler effect in measuring and visualizing blood flow	Used in evaluation of buergers disease and valvular heart disease.

Also remember
Types of Doppler

- **Color Doppler**: Velocity information is presented as a color-coded overlay B-mode image
- **Pulsed wave (PW) Doppler**: Doppler information is sampled from only a small sample volume (defined in 2D image), and presented on a timeline.
- **Duplex**: a common name for the simultaneous presentation of 2D and (usually) PW Doppler information.

32. Ans. (a) G2M phase

- Dividing cells are most sensitive to radiotherapy. The phase that is most sensitive to radiation is G2M.

Remember the Sensitivity in this Order

G2M > G2 > M > G1 > early S > Late S

33. Ans. (a) Dryness of mouth

DRYNESS OF MOUTH is the most common complication noted in patients undergoing radiotherapy of head and neck CA.

Radiology

> **Extra Mile**
> - Most radiosensitive tissue: **Bone Marrow**
> - Least radiosensitive: **Nervous tissue**
> - Most radiosensitive cell: **Lymphocyte**
> - Least radiosensitive cell: **Platelets**
> - Most sensitive phase of cell cycle: **G2-M phase**
> - Least radiosensitive: **Late S2**
> - Most readiosensitive cancer of head and neck: **Nasopharyngeal carcinoma**

34. Ans. (b) Seminoma

Ref: Devita, 7th ed. p-1907

- **Most radiosensitive tumor:** HL > Ewing's
- **Most radiosensitive tumor of head and Neck:** Nasopharyngeal CA > Glottic CA

Radiosensitivity of tumors			
Highly sensitive	**Moderate sensitive**	**Relatively Resistant**	**Highly Resistant**
• Ewing's sarcoma • Lymphoma • Wilms tumor • Multiple Myeloma • Seminoma	• Nasopharyngeal CA • Dysgerminoma • Medulloblastoma • Small Cell Cancer lung • Breast Cancer • Ovarian Cancer • Basal cell cancer • Nasopharyngeal Cancer • Dysgerminoma • Small Cell Cancer lung • Breast Cancer • Ovarian Cancer • Basal cell cancer	• Renal cell CA • Rectal/ colon cancer • Bladder Carcinoma • Soft tissue sarcoma Squamous cell carcinoma of lung • Cervix cancer	• Hepatoma • Melanoma • Pancreatic cancer • Osteosarcoma

35. Ans. (a) Bone scan

Ref: Review of Radiology by Sumer Sethi, 5th ed. pg. 23.

- Radiation exposure for **CT Head** is equivalent to **115 CXR.**
- **CT whole Body is around** 400 CXRs.
- Radiation exposure of **Bone Scan** is equivalent to **200 CXR**.

36. Ans. (a) Gadolinium

- Gadolinium is a lanthanide.
- Gd-DTPA is classed as an acyclic, ionic gadolinium contrast medium.
- Its paramagnetic property reduces the T1 relaxation time.
- *Gadolinium* based agents *may cause* a toxic reaction known as *nephrogenic systemic fibrosis (NSF)* in patients with severe kidney problems.
- Rest all are iodinated contrast agents.

37. Ans. (c) MRI is better for calcified lesions

MRI Versus CT

- CT is superior to MRI for calcification **and acute intracranial haemorrhage.**
- Cortical bone is better evaluated by CT.
- **MRI is better for brain,** spine pathologies other than head injury, stroke, calcification, brain haemorrhage.
- MRI is better for bone marrow.
- **MRI is contraindicated in pacemakers,** cochlear implants, and metallic foreign bodies in sensitive locations.

UROLOGY AND BONE IMAGING

38. Ans. (b) Helical CT with Non-contrast

Ref: SRB Manual of Surgery, 5th ed. P 1190, 1107

- The best investigation for kidney stone and ureteric stone is non-contrast helical CT abdomen.
- The limitation of USG is that it is less sensitive and can scan only the kidney and proximal ureter.
- Helical CT can detect stones as small as 1 mm which can be missed by other modalities.

> **Extra Mile**
> IOC for Ureteric Stones is helical Non-contrast CT abdomen
> IOC for Polycystic kidneys is non-contrast CT/ MRI. Contrast may be used depending on level of renal function.
> Always check serum creatinine before giving contrast

FMGE Solutions Screening Examination

39. Ans. (c) Humerus
- The structure shown in the image is humerus
- A very common tumor of humerus upper end is unicameral bone cyst/simple bone cyst, which is characterized radiologically by *trap door sign or falling leaf sign*

40. Ans. (b) Duplex collecting system
- The shown IVP finding in image is known as drooping lily sign, which is a characteristic finding of duplex ureter.

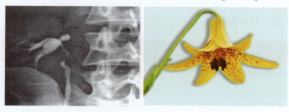

- The **drooping lily sign** is a radiological sign in patients with a duplicated collecting system. It refers to the inferolateral displacement of the opacified lower pole. The size of calyces in kidney is also smaller.

41. Ans. (c) TB spine
- Notice the vertebral body collapse, which is diagnostic of pott spine.
- IOC for Pott's spine: MRI
- The **earliest sign** of infection are local **osteoporosis of two adjacent vertebra and narrowing of intervertebral disc space**, with fizziness of end plates.
- Progressive disease is associated with signs of bone destruction and collapse of adjacent vertebral bodies into each other.

42. Ans. (b) Obturator foramen
(Revise the pelvic anatomy as shown on X-ray from this image given below)

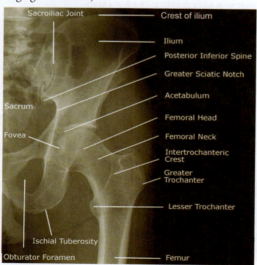

43. Ans. (c) Papillary necrosis
- *Ring sign appearance by CT urography* or IVP shows radio-contrast outlines of sloughed renal papillae in *papillary necrosis*, which often have a triangular shape. Also remember:
- **Cortical ring sign:** A circular shadow cast by a rotated scaphoid in scapho-lunate subluxation which is due to scaphoid's abnormal orientation.

44. Ans. (a) Diabetes

Ref: Harrison, 19th ed. pg. 270e-9
- Contrast nephropathy is defined as a condition arising after an investigation using contrast agent.
- *A rise in serum creatinine level above 25%* from baseline within 48-72 hours of procedure *indicates contrast nephropathy*.
- Out of the given condition diabetes is most predisposed for contrast induced nephropathy.

45. Ans. (b) Renal cell CA

Ref: Harrison, 19th ed. pg. 263e-7

Cancers associated with high dose exposure include leukemia, breast, bladder, colon, liver, lung, esophagus, ovarian, multiple myeloma, and stomach cancers.

46. Ans. (c) Papillary necrosis

Ref: Harrison, 19th ed. pg. 1860

Refer to above explanation

47. Ans. (b) Polycystic kidney

Ref: Radiological and Imaging Secrets, 2nd ed. pg. 79
- Polycystic kidney autosomal dominant and recessive forms multiple cysts that deform the pelvi-calyceal system resulting in spider leg sign.
- MC extra-renal malformation in polycystic kidney disease = Hepatic cysts
- MC Cardiac malformation in polycystic kidney disease = Mitral valve prolapse
- MC GIT malformation in polycystic kidney disease = colonic diverticulosis

> **Extra Mile**
>
> **Remember these Important Radiological Signs in Urology**
> - Spider leg appearance—polycystic kidney
> - Cobra head appearance—ureterocele
> - Flower vase appearance of ureters—horse shoe kidney
> - Sandy patches—schistosomiasis of bladder
> - Soap bubble appearance—hydronephrosis

48. Ans. (c) Polycystic disease

49. Ans. (a) Ureterocoele

Ref: SRB Manual of Surgery, 4th ed. pg. 1279

The *adder head/cobra head sign* refers to dilatation of the distal ureter, surrounded by a thin lucent line, which is seen in patients with an adult-type *ureterocoele*. The presence of this cobra head appearance is an indicator of ureterocele.

A ureterocele is a submucosal cystic dilation of the terminal segment of the ureter.

50. Ans. (b) Micturating cystourethrogram

Ref: SRB Manual of Surgery, 4th ed. pg. 1118

Steps in MCU

- Catheterization to fill the bladder with a radio-contrast agent, typically cystografin.
- Under fluoroscopy, we can see the contrast entering the bladder.
- If the contrast moves into the ureters and back into the kidneys, the radiologist makes the diagnosis of vesicoureteral reflux.

Indication of MCU

1. All males with recurrent UTIs, or abnormality on ultrasound if first UTI urinary tract infection
2. First episode UTI in females <3 years of age
3. Febrile UTIs in females <5 years of age
4. Older females with pyelonephritis or recurrent UTIs
5. Suspected obstruction (e.g. Bilateral hydronephrosis)
6. Suspected bladder trauma or rupture
7. Stress incontinence (urine)

51. Ans. (a) Thalassemia

Ref: Harrison, 19th ed. pg. 637

- Crew cut appearance in thalassemia occurs due to expansion of the marrow on account of extra-medullary hematopoiesis.
- The widened diploic spaces on X-ray skull lateral view appears as Crew cut or hair on end appearance.

52. Ans. (c) Osteopetrosis

Ref: Harrison, 19th ed. pg. 426e-4

- **Bone within a bone** describes the bones that appear to have another bone within them.
  Causes: P.O.S.T-C.G.D
  - **P**aget's disease of bone
  - **O**steopetrosis
  - **S**ickle cell disease
  - **T**halassemia
  - **C**affey's disease
  - **G**aucher's disease
  - **G**rowth recovery lines (after infancy)
  - **H**ypervitaminosis **D**

53. Ans. (b) Sickle cell anemia

- Hair on end appearance of the skull is a characteristic feature of chronic haemolysis usually seen in patients with thalassemia and sickle cell anaemia. It results from accentuated vertical trabeculae between the inner and outer tables of the skull because of excessive bone marrow hyperplasia.

Conditions where 'Hair on End Appearance' is seen:
Mnemonic: HI NEST

- Hereditary spherocytosis
- Neuroblastoma
- Enzyme deficiency (e.g. G-6-P deficiency causing haemolytic anaemia)
- Sickle cell disease
- Thalassemia major

54. Ans. (a) Gout

Ref: Harrison Rheumatology, 2006 ed. pg. 261

- **Martel sign or rat bite sign**- Sharply marginated, bony erosions from a long-standing soft-tissue tophus, seen in X-Ray in a patients with gout.

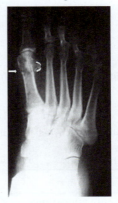

55. Ans. (c) Ante-natal USG second trimester

- The **nuchal thickness** is a parameter that is measured in a second trimester scan (18–22 weeks) *and it is not to be mixed with nuchal translucency (which is measured in the first trimester at 11-14 weeks).*
- The **nuchal thickness** is measured in a second trimester scan.
- Nuchal translucency scan is performed between 11 and 14 weeks of gestation, because the accuracy is best in this period.

FMGE Solutions Screening Examination

- The scan is obtained with the fetus in sagittal section and a neutral position of the fetal head
- The head of the fetus should neither be hyper-flexed nor extended, either of which can influence the nuchal translucency thickness.
- Both are used for diagnosis of Trisomy 21 prenatally.

ABDOMEN IMAGING

56. Ans. (b) USG

- **USG is IOC for:**
  - Acute cholecystitis
  - Cholelithiasis, Renal stone
  - Intrauterine pathology
  - Intrauterine assessment of foetus
  - To see minimal pleural fluid/ascitic fluid
  - Hydrocephalus in infants
  - Congenital hypertrophic pyloric stenosis (CHOPS)
- Most sensitive and specific test for cholecystitis: HIDA scan

57. (d) 24-hour pH monitoring

- **IOC for GERD:** 24-hour pH monitoring
- It is the **most accurate/most sensitive/Gold standard** test for measuring pattern, frequency and duration of reflux episodes.
- It quantifies the actual time the esophageal mucosa is exposed to gastric juice

> **Extra Mile**
>
> - **Manometry:** IOC for motility disorders of esophagus (Ex: Achalasia cardia, diffuse esophageal spasm, corkscrew esophagus).
> - **Uses of HIDA scan:**
>   - Biliary atresia
>   - Neonatal hepatitis (parenchymal liver disease)
>   - Abnormal biliary leakage
>   - Acute/Chronic cholecystitis

58. Ans. (a) Apple core appearance

Ref: SRB Manual of Surgery: 5th ed, P 905

- The image shows an appearance of an annular *constricting* carcinoma of the bowel, usually the colon form the circumferential involvement of lumen.
- The string sign of Kantor is seen in Crohn's disease at the junction of ileum entering into the caecum. In this image small intestine is not visualized.
- Claw sign is seen on barium enema in intussusception.
- Coffee bean sign is seen on X-ray abdomen in case of sigmoid volvulus.

59. Ans. (c) Spleen

Check out the structures on CT scan and their names in given image.

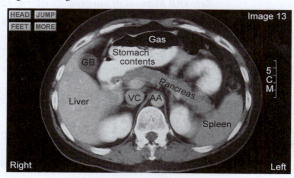

60. Ans. (d) Hydatid cyst

- **Hepatic hydatid disease** is a parasitic zoonosis caused by the *Echinococcus* tape worm. In the liver, two agents are recognised as causing disease in the human:
  - *Echinococcus granulosus*
  - *Echinococcus multilocularis*
- In the human manifestation the disease caused by echinococcus is most commonly localized to liver (in 75% of cases), followed by lungs (in 5–15% of cases) and other organs in the body such as the spleen, brain, heart, and kidneys (in 10–20% of cases).
- If the patient has cysts in the liver, symptoms abdominal discomfort, hepatomegaly with an abdominal mass, jaundice, fever and/or anaphylactic reaction.

Radiographic features:

- **Plain radiograph:** Shows a curvilinear or ring calcific shadow overlying the liver due to calcification of the pericyst.
- **Ultrasound:** Multiseptate cyst with "daughter" cysts and echogenic material between cysts.
- **CT scan:** Septation and daughter cysts may be visualised. The **water-lily sign** indicates a cyst with floating, undulating membrane, caused by a detached endocyst. It may also show hyperdense internal septa representing a **spoke wheel pattern** within a cyst.

> **Extra Mile**
>
> - Definitive host of echinococus granulosus: Dog
> - Intermediate host of echinococus granulosus: Sheep
> - **Accidental host for echinococus granulosus is Man.**
> - MCC of amoebic liver abscess is **Entamoeba histolytica.** This condition is mostly associated with alcoholic liver diseases (in ~ 80% of cases). M:F = 10:1
> - MCC of pyogenic liver abscess in E. coli. associated with alcoholic liver disease in 20–30% cases. M:F = 1.5:1

Radiology

61. Ans. (c) Stomach

For explanation, read the CT image

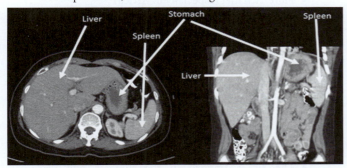

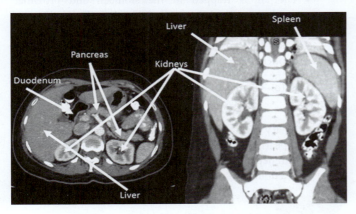

- Multiple questions have been framed on this image in last many exams.

62. Ans. (b) Ultrasound

Ref: Bailey & Love, 25th ed. pg. 69

- On ultrasound, an abscess cavity in the liver is seen as a hypoechoic or anechoic lesion with ill-defined borders; internal echoes suggest necrotic material or debris. **The investigation is very accurate and is used for aspiration, both diagnostic and therapeutic.**
- Where there is doubt about the diagnosis, a computerized tomography (CT) scan may be helpful.

> **Extra Mile**
>
> **Diagnostic pointers for infection with Entamoeba histolytica**
>
> - Bloody mucoid diarrhoea in a patient from an endemic area or following a recent visit to such a place
> - Upper abdominal pain, fever, cough, malaise
> - In chronic cases, a mass in the right iliac fossa = *amoeboma*
> - Sigmoidoscopy shows typical ulcers—biopsy and scrapings may be diagnostic
> - Serological tests are highly sensitive and specific outside endemic areas
> - **Ultrasound and CT scans are the imaging methods of choice.**

63. Ans. (c) 3 mm

Ref: Clinical Sonography, 4th ed. pg. 88

- GB wall thickness Measured in the side in contact with the liver with the help of ultrasonography.
- Normally it is up to 3 mm.
- From 3–5 mm: suspicion of wall thickness
- More than 5 mm >>> It is a thick wall gall bladder which is seen in:

1. Cholecystitis (acute-chronic)
2. Ascites
3. Hepatitis (viral)
4. Schistosomiasis

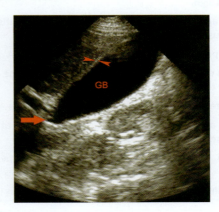

> **Extra Mile**
>
> **Size of GB**
> - Long axis 6-12 cm, short axis 3-5 cm
> - Contracted < 5 cm
> - Distended > 12 cm

64. Ans. (b) Ischaemic colitis

Ref: Harrison, 19th ed. pg. 267, 1857

- **Ischaemic colitis** occurs due to inflammation of the colon secondary to vascular insufficiency and ischaemia. Abdominal radiographic findings are include-
  - **'Thumb-printing' sign is due to mucosal edema and hemorrhage**
  - Ileal Distention
  - Localized intramural gas

TABLE: Radiological findings and their respective pathology

Barium enema findings	Associated pathology
Apple core deformity Irregular filling defect	Colon CA
Bird beak sign, Ace of spades	Volvulus

Contd...

FMGE Solutions Screening Examination

Barium enema findings	Associated pathology
Bird beak appearance	Achalasia cardia
Claw sign Coiled spring sign	Intussusception
Coffee bean sign	Sigmoid volvulus
Corkscrew appearance Nut cracker esophagus Curling esophagus	Diffuse esophageal spasm
Dilated proximal zone with narrow distal zone of coning	Hirschsprung disease
Inverted 3 sign of Frosberg Widening of C loop of duodenum/ Antral pad sign.	Pancreas head CA
Lead pipe appearance Loss of haustrations	Ulcerative colitis
Rat tail appearance	Esophageal CA
String sign of kantor Raspberry thorn ulcers	Crohn's disease
Smooth irregular filling defects	Colonic polyps
Saw tooth appearance Champagne glass sign	Diverticulosis of colon
String sign	Congenital hypertrophic pyloric stenosis
Thumb print sign	Ischemic colitis

65. Ans. (c) Sigmoid volvulus

Ref: SRB Manual of Surgery, 4th ed. pg. 1329

- The given image shows coffee bean sign, which is seen in sigmoid volvulus.

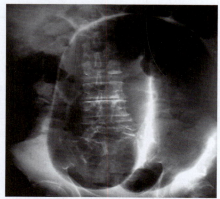

- It is a cause of large bowel obstruction and occurs when the sigmoid colon twists on the sigmoid mesocolon.

Clinical Presentation
- Constipation
- Abdominal bloating
- Nausea and/or vomiting

Causes
- Chronic constipation and/or laxative abuse
- Fibre-rich diet (especially in Africa)
- Chagas disease (especially in South America)

Treatment
- Rectal tube insertion is successful in treating 90% of cases.
- The most serious complication is bowel ischaemia.

66. Ans. (a) Duodenal atresia

Ref: SRB manual of Surgery, 4th ed. pg. 1280

- The diagnosis of duodenal atresia on X ray abdomen shows two large air filled spaces, called "**double bubble**" sign.
- The air is trapped in the stomach and proximal duodenum, which are separated by the pyloric sphincter, creating the appearance of two bubbles visible on X-ray.
- Since the closure of the duodenum is complete in duodenal atresia, no air is seen in the distal duodenum.

67. Ans. (c) Obstructive jaundice

Ref: Abdominal Ultrasound, 3rd ed. pg. 82

- Biliary dilatation is also easily seen on ultrasound, appearing as an extra tube running alongside the intrahepatic portal veins and hence gives an appearance of a double barrel gun aka *double-barrel sign*.

> **Extra Mile**
>
> **Some important radiological signs**
> - **Double bubble sign** is seen in (LAD): Ladd band/malrotation, Annular pancreas, Duodenal atresia
> - **Single bubble appearance**: pyloric stenosis
> - **Thumb print sign**: ischemic colitis
> - **Multiple air fluid level**: Ileal/Jejunal obstruction

68. Ans. (a) Crohn's disease

- **Cobble stone mucosa** is appearance of the intestinal mucosa in Crohn's disease **to the endoscopist,. Cobblestoning refers to the uniform nodules–due to the sub-mucosal fibrosis.**
- **String sign of Kantor is due to involvement of** the terminal ileum in Crohn's disease.
- It is caused by severe spasm due to irritability of the loop producing the appearance of a frayed cotton string.
- Subsequently the wall of the ileum may become fibrotic and the lumen fixed in diameter.

69. Ans. (b) Ulcerative colitis

Barium Enema Findings in Ulcerative Colitis

- *Earliest finding on air-contrast Barium enema is loss of and fine mucosal granularity.*

Radiology

- *Pseudo-polyps which are scattered islands of edematous mucosa in vast expanse of ulcerated mucosa*
- Double-tracking- long, longitudinal ulcers in submucosa
- Bowel margins appear spicule like from tiny, multiple ulcerations
- Collar button ulcers-from undermining
- Shortening of the colon-may be from spasm of longitudinal muscles or from irreversible fibrosis (lead-pipe colon/ pipe stem colon)
- Loss of haustrations on left side of colon.

70. Ans. (c) Intussusception

Ref: SRB Manual of Surgery, 4th ed. pg. 996

- Target sing is seen in intussusception.
- Other signs which is seen in case of Intussusception are: Coiled spring appearance, claw sign.
- The appearance is generated by concentric alternating echogenic and hypo-echogenic bands. The echogenic bands are formed by mucosa and muscularis whereas the submucosa is responsible for the hypo-echoic bands.

Also Remember

- The **pseudo kidney** of intussusception refers to the longitudinal ultrasound appearance of the intussuscepted segment of bowel.
- **Coffee bean sign:** Sigmoid volvulus
- **Whirlpool sign on USG:** Midgut volvulus
- **Thumb print sign:** Ischemic colitis
- **Saw tooth appearance on barium enema:** Diverticula of colon
- **Seagull/Mercedez Benz/Crow Feet Sign:** Radiolucent gall stone with gas
- **Bird's beak appearance on barium swallow:** Achalasia cardia
- **Bird's beak appearance on barium enema:** Volvulus
- **Corkscrew appearance on barium swallow:** Diffuse esophageal spasm.
- **Beak sign; Double track or Tram track sign; Shoulder sign; String sign:** Hypertrophic pyloric stenosis.

71. Ans. (b) Diffuse esophageal spasm

Ref: SRB Manual of Surgery, 4th ed. pg. 1323

- **Cork screw appearance** on barium swallow is seen with diffuse esophageal spasm.
- **Bird beak appearance** is seen with achalasia cardia.
- **Rat tail appearance** as per bailey and love is seen with carcinoma esophagus.

72. Ans. (d) Ultrasound

Ref: SRB Manual of Surgery, 4th ed. pg. 877

- Ultrasound abdomen is the investigation of choice for diagnosing hypertrophic pyloric stenosis.

- It is reliable, highly sensitive, highly specific, and easily performed.
- The mandatory measurements include pyloric muscle thickness and pyloric channel length.
- *Muscle wall thickness 3 mm or greater and pyloric channel length 14 mm or greater are considered abnormal in infants younger than 30 days.*

73. Ans. (a) Diverticulosis

Ref: SRB Manual of Surgery, 4th ed. pg. 952

- *Most common site of diverticulosis is the sigmoid colon in as many as 95% of patients with cecum being involved in 5% of patients.*
- *Reasons for sigmoid colon being the main site of diverticulosis and leading to saw tooth appearance-*
  - Sigmoid colon is the narrowest portion of the colon, and generates the highest intra-segmental pressures
  - Combination of numerous haustra and dehydrated stool in the sigmoid colon leads to segmentation, in which the sigmoid colon functions as multiple small compartments.

Also Remember

TABLE: Pathologies and their radiological findings

Diverticulosis	Saw tooth appearance on barium enema
Intussusception	Claw sign on barium sign
Volvulus	Coffee bean sign /bird of prey sign
Ischemic colitis	Thumb printing sign

74. Ans. (a) Carcinoma Colon

Ref: Bailey, 26th ed. pg. 70

- On double contrast barium enema of the rectum and distal sigmoid colon demonstrates a typical annular constricting carcinoma of the colon with overhanging edges on both the proximal and distal margins forming a so called "apple-core" lesion.

75. Ans. (a) Contrast CT

Ref: Bailey, 26th ed. pg. 192, 1121

- CECT can be used to assess the severity of acute pancreatitis and to estimate the prognosis. Balthazar et al developed a grading system in which patients with acute pancreatitis are classified into one of the following 5 grades:
  - **Grade A** - Normal-appearing pancreas
  - **Grade B** - Focal or diffuse enlargement of the pancreas
  - **Grade C** - Pancreatic gland abnormalities associated with peri-pancreatic fat infiltration
  - **Grade D** - A single fluid collection
  - **Grade E** - Two or more fluid collections

FMGE Solutions Screening Examination

76. Ans. (d) Acute pancreatitis

Ref: Bailey, 26th ed. pg. 1128-29

- The most commonly recognized radiologic signs associated with acute pancreatitis include the following:
  - Air in the duodenal C-loop
  - *The sentinel loop sign,* which represents a focal dilated proximal jejunal loop in the left upper quadrant.
  - *The colon cut-off sign*, which represents distention of the colon to the transverse colon with a paucity of gas distal to the splenic flexure.

77. Ans. (c) USG

Ref: Bailey, 26th ed. pg. 1100

78. Ans. (c) USG

Ref: Bailey, 26th ed. pg. 109

- In any case of bunt abdominal trauma, first investigation to be performed is ultrasonography.
- In emergency situation, USG technique used is FAST (Focussed Assessment with Sonography for Trauma).
- In FAST, the radiologist, immediately performs the USG abdomen keeping in mind to assess the four major areas to see any collection of fluid due to abdominal organ rupture.
- **Four areas assessed in FAST:** Perihepatic area, Perisplenic area, Pericardial area, Pelvis
- **Updated modality of FAST is eFAST (Extended FAST):** Pleural areas are also assessed along with superior mediastinal area.

79. Ans. (b) CT

THORAX IMAGING

80. Ans. (b) Pneumoperitoneum

- **IOC for pneumoperitoneum:** Chest X-ray PA view in erect position (including diaphragm)

RADIOLOGICAL SIGNS OF PNEUMOPERITONEUM

- **Gas under diaphragm sign:** Accumulation of gas under right side hemidiaphragm
- **Mustache sign**/Cupola sign/Saddle bag sign
- **Rigler sign:** Air outlining both internal and external intestinal wall
- **Urachus sign:** Air outlining middle umbilical ligament
- **Inverted V sign:** Air outlining both umbilical ligaments
- **Falciform ligament sign:** Air surrounding falciform ligament (becomes prominent).

81. Ans. (b) Diffuse oesophageal spasm

- The finding shown in image is corkscrew esophagus, which is seen in patients with diffuse esophageal spasm (due to uncoordinated activity of esophageal smooth muscles).
  - This is possible due to fragmental degeneration of vagal nerve fibres
  - Simultaneous and repetitive contraction in esophagus body with normal lower esophageal sphincter.
- **Clinical feature:**
  - Chest pain, Non-progressive dysphagia with solids and liquids and non exertional chest pain, which responds to nitro-glycerine.
- **IOC for DES:** Manometry
- **Upon barium swallow:** Corkscrew appearance
- Similar to DES, there is **nutcracker esophagus** where there is high-amplitude peristalsis (>80 mm Hg) for increased duration.

> **Extra Mile**
>
> Other radiological findings of esophageal pathology
> - **Barium swallow:** Bird beak/Pencil tip: Achalasia cardia
> - **Barium swallow-rat tail appearance (with filling defect):** Achalasia cardia
> - **Barium swallow:** Worm eaten appearance: Esophageal varices

82. Ans. (a) Major fissure

Ref: Fundamentals of Radiology by Squire, P 136

The image shows left lung with *major* fissure separating the left upper lobe from the lower lobe.

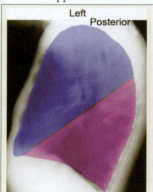 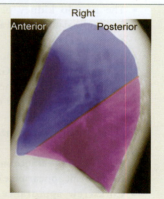

Notice the major fissure in left lung segregating the upper and lower lobes. Compare with the image given below.

Notice the major fissure and minor fissures in right lung. Compare with the image given below.

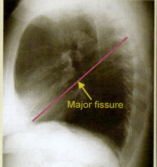 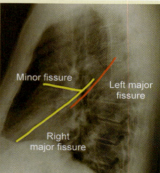

Azygos fissure is seen as a curvilinear density in upper right lung, convex towards the chest wall. Azygos lobe is found as an anatomic variant in 1% of population.

Radiology

> **Extra Mile**
> - Shift in the position of fissures is seen in segmental atelectasis
> - **Comet tail sign:** Rounded atelectasis
> - **S sign of golden:** Upper lobe atelectasis

83. Ans. (b) Pneumothorax

- The shown CT scan clearly shows air in the pleural cavity (arrow) around left lung. This condition is pneumothorax.
- In case of pleural effusion, the water will appear relatively white and at lower aspect on CT (*due to gravity*).

84. Ans. (a) Bronchiectasis

- The shown image of CT, is suggestive of bronchiectasis, characterized by tram *track sign of airways*.
- Bronchiectasis is an abnormal dilatation of airway.
- **Radiological findings:**
  - Tram track sign
  - Cluster of grape appearance
  - Signet ring sign

85. Ans. (b) Barium swallow

- The given imaging here is barium swallow, showing achalasia cardia.
- Barium swallow is done for esophageal pathology.
- Barium meal is for stomach and first part of duodenum.
- Barium meal follow through is for small intestine.
- Barium enema is for colon.

86. Ans. (a) Tetralogy of Fallot

- The given image shows boot shaped heart, which is a characteristic finding seen in Tetralogy of Fallot.

Also Remember
Radiological findings of congenital heart disease:

- Figure of '8' appearance or Snowman appearance: **TAPVR (type I)**
- "Egg on its side" or "Apple on a stem" appearance: TGA (transposition of great arteries)
- **"Boot-shaped Heart"** /Classic coeur en sabot: TOF
- Box/Balloon shaped heart: Ebstein Anomaly
- '3 sign' and inferior rib notching on CXR: Coarctation of Aorta

87. Ans. (d) Main pulmonary artery

(Revise the chest CT anatomy from the image given below)

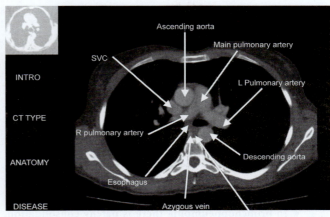

88. Ans. (d) Aortic knuckle

- Right border of heart is formed by—
  - Superior vena cava
  - The right atrium
  - Small part of inferior vena cava
- Left heart border is formed by—
  - Aortic nuckle
  - The pulmonary bay
  - The auricle of left atrium
  - The left ventricle.

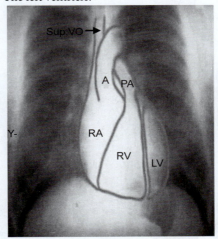

89. Ans. (b) CT ratio being measured

Cardiothoracic ratio

- It is a estimation of cardiac size
- Vertical line is drawn through the midsternal line
- Maximal distances of the right and left heart borders from the midsternal line are added
- Greatest transverse diameter of thorax is obtained
- Normal value = ≤50%

FMGE Solutions Screening Examination

1242

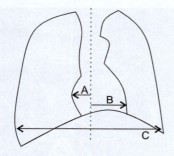

FIGURE: Cardiothoracic ratio

90. Ans. (a) Patchy consolidation

- In **bronchopneumonia** there is patchy consolidation, no mediastinal shift.
- In **lobar pneumonia there is diffuse consolidation.**
- In collapse, there is mediastinal shift on the same side.
- In pleural effusion, there is contralateral mediastinal shift.

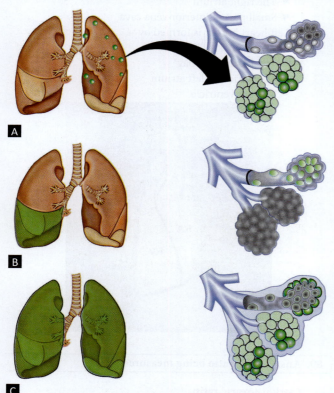

FIGURE: (A) Bronchopneumonia; (B) Lobar pneumonia; (C) Interstitial pneumonia

91. Ans. (a) Right ventricle forms the right heart border

Ref: Essential Radiology, 2nd ed. pg. 22

- **Right ventricle is not a border forming structure in PA view.** However, it forms anterior border in lateral view of Chest X-ray.

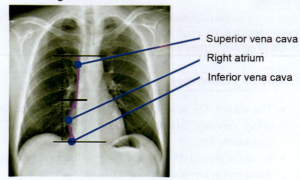

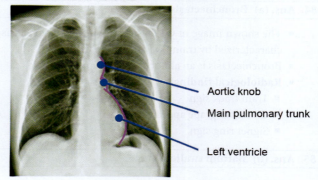

FIGURE: Heart border forming structures

92. Ans. (d) Left atrial appendage clots

Ref: Harrison, 19th ed. pg. 270e-2

T.E.E. is preferred over the routine Trans-thoracic echocardiography for the following situations:

1. Internal heart structures and path of blood flow in congenital heart disease is better evaluated.
2. To evaluate the effects of surgical intervention to the heart, such as repair of congenital heart defects.
3. When T.T.E is indicated, but circumstances (i.e., pulmonary disease like emphysema) that may interfere with the ability to obtain adequate images.
4. Mitral valve disease
5. Blood clots or masses inside the heart
6. Aortic Dissection
7. Implanted prosthetic heart valves
8. To evaluate for blood clots in the heart prior to cardioversion or ablation procedures.

93. Ans. (a) ASD

Ref: Harrison, 19th ed. pg. 1520

Radiology

ATRIAL SEPTAL DEFECT (ASD)

- In atrial septal defect there is congenital defect in the interatrial septum.
- *It is Most common CHD diagnosed in adulthood*

TYPES Based on Defects with Different Locations Functionally the same

- *Primum*- lower part of the septum
- *Secundum*- located near the foramen ovale or fossa ovalis
- *Sinus venosus*- caval location
- *Coronary sinus- least common* → near SVC entry

Also Remember

- Most common CHD **diagnosed in infancy- VSD**
- 2nd OVERALL MOST COMMON CONGENITAL CARDIAC ANOMALY- **VSD**
- In VSD all chambers are enlarged EXCEPT: **Right Atrium**
- MC cyanotic congenital heart disease: **Tetralogy of Fallot (TOF)**
- **2nd most common cyanotic CHD after TOF- TGA**
- **Most common cause of cyanosis in neonate: Transposition of Great arteries**
- Most common cause of congenital heart disease beyond the neonatal period: **Tetralogy of Fallot**

Radiological Features:

- All chambers are enlarged in ASD EXCEPT Left ventricle.
- **Increased vascularity:** Pulmonary artery over loading.
- Enlarged main (dilated MPA) and central pulmonary arteries

---

94. Ans. (d) Ebstein anomaly

Ref: Pediatric Radiology, 1st ed. 57

- **Ebstein anomaly** is a congenital heart defect in which the septal and posterior leaflets of the tricuspid valve are displaced towards the apex of the right ventricle of the heart.
- **It causes atrialization of right ventricle.**

Radiographic Features In Different Congenital Heart Diseases:

- Figure of '8' appearance or Snowman appearance: **TAPVR (type I)**
- Egg on its side" or "Apple on a stem" appearance: TGA
- **Boot-shaped Heart"** /Classic coer en sabot: TOF
- **Box/Balloon shaped heart:** Ebstein Anomaly
- **'3 sign' on CXR:** Coaractation of Aorta

---

95. Ans. (a) Asthma

Ref: Harrison, 19th ed. pg. 1675

- Flattening of diaphragm is seen with obstructive airway diseases due to the process of air trapping.

- The point that clinches the diagnosis in favor of asthma is the curschmann spirals which represent the cast of the airways formed by mucus plugs in small airways in these patients.

---

96. Ans. (d) To remove foreign body

Ref: Harrison, 19th ed. pg. 1667
Foreign body is removed by rigid bronchoscopy.

Indications for Rigid Bronchoscopy

- Bleeding or hemorrhage
- Foreign body extraction
- Deeper biopsy specimen when fiber-optic specimen is inadequate
- Dilation of tracheal or bronchial strictures, relief of airway obstruction, insertion of stents, and pediatric bronchoscopy.
- It is also used for tracheobronchial laser therapy or other mechanical tumor ablation.

---

97. Ans. (c) Pulmonary embolism

Ref: Harrison, 19th ed. pg. 1633
HAMPTON HUMP is a radiologic sign which consists of a shallow wedge-shaped opacity in the periphery of the lung with its base against the pleural surface.

---

98. Ans. (a) Pulmonary embolism

Ref: Harrison, 19th ed. pg. 1633
Westermark sign is due to focus of oligemia in pulmonary embolism (PE). The sign develops due to following reasons:
- Dilation of the pulmonary arteries proximal to the embolus
- Collapse of the distal vasculature creating the appearance of a sharp cut off on chest X ray
The chest X-ray is normal in the majority of PE cases, the Westermark sign is seen in 2% of patients

---

99. Ans. (b) Pneumomediastinum

Ref: Harrison, 19th ed. pg. 1720

- Normally the central portion of the diaphragm is not discretely visualised on chest X-ray as it merges with the cardiac borders.
- However if the diaphragm can be seen continuously across the midline then this is diagnostic of free gas within the mediastinum, pericardium or peritoneal cavity.
- **Continuous diaphragm sign** is seen in pneumo-mediastinum.

---

100. Ans. (a) Pneumonia

Ref: Harrison, 19th ed. pg. 806

- **Air bronchogram** refers to the phenomenon of air-filled bronchi (*dark*) being made visible by the opacification of surrounding alveoli (*grey - white*).

FMGE Solutions Screening Examination

- It is almost always caused by a pathologic airspace (alveolar) process, in which something other than air fills the alveoli.
- Air bronchograms will not be visible if the bronchi themselves are opacified (e.g. by fluid).
- Air bronchograms can be seen with several processes, including the following:
    - *Pulmonary consolidation* (pneumonia)
    - Pulmonary oedema
    - Non-obstructive atelectasis
    - Severe interstitial lung disease

101. Ans. (a) Lung carcinoma

Ref: Harrison, 19th ed. pg. 511

Findings in Chest X-ray Suggestive of Lung Cancer-
- Central lesions appear as a bulky hilum, representing the tumor and local nodal involvement.
- In contrast a more peripheral location may appear as a rounded or spiculated mass.
- Cavitation may be seen as an air-fluid level.
- Destruction of the adjacent rib or evidence of soft tissue growing into the soft tissues superficial to the ribs as seen in the above case where lung CA is in the right upper lobe.

HYDATID CYSTS

It result from infection by the *Echinococcus* worm, and can result in cyst formation anywhere in the body.
- **Most common organ involved**: Liver > Lung

There are several clinical signs in hydatid disease:
- **Cumbo sign**: Air is seen between the pericyst and the laminated membrane of the cyst.
- **Serpent sign**: Internal rupture of the cyst with collapse of membranes of parasite into the cyst.
- **Spin sign/whirl sign**: Detached membranes with small pleural reaction seen in hydatid cyst of lung.
- **Empty cyst sign**: May be seen after complete evacuation of parasitic membranes.

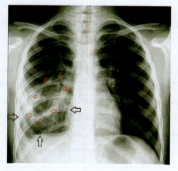

LUNG ABSCESS
- A **lung abscess** is a circumscribed collection of pus within the lung.

- Most commonly seen in superior segment of lower lobes or posterior segments of lower lobes.
- **X-ray:** The classical appearance of a pulmonary abscess is a cavity containing an air-fluid level.
- **IOC for abcess:** Contrast CT.

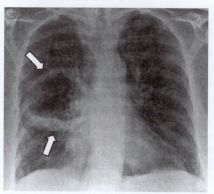

ASPERGILLOMA
- **Aspergillomas** are mass-like fungus balls that are typically composed of *Aspergillus fumigatus* and is a non-invasive form of pulmonary aspergillosis
- **CXR:** Aspergillomas typically appear as rounded or ovoid soft tissue attenuating masses located in a surrounding cavity and outlined by a crescent of air.
- **CT**: Appearances are those of a well formed cavity with a central soft tissue attenuating rounded mass surrounded by an *air crescent sign or a Monad sign*.

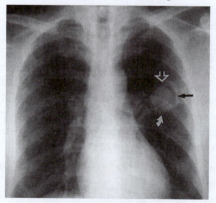

102. Ans. (a) Bronchogenic carcinoma with collapse of lung

- The Golden S sign (reverse S sign of Golden.) is seen in PA chest radiographs with right upper lobe collapse.
- It is caused by a central mass obstructing the upper lobe bronchus and should raise suspicion of a primary bronchogenic carcinoma.
- The right upper lobe appears dense and shifts medially and upwards with a central mass expanding the hilum. The combination of two changes together form a reverse S shape.

Radiology

NEUROLOGY IMAGING

104. Ans. (b) Massive Epidural hemorrhage

TABLE: Difference between different kinds of intracranial bleed

	Epidural hemorrhage	Subdural hemorrhage	Subarachnoid hemorrhage
Site	Above dura (between brain and skull)	Below dura (between dura and arachnoid mater)	Below arachnoid (between arachnoid and Pia mater)
Source of bleed	Middle meningeal artery	Cortical bridging vein tear	Circle of Willis
CT appearance	Biconvex white/Lenticular	Concavo-convex/Moon crescent	Star shaped opacity
Image			

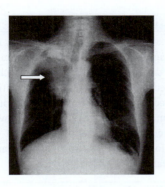

103. Ans. (b) Pulmonary hamartoma

Ref Robbins, 8th ed. pg. 1433

- Lung hamartoma is a lesion seen as rounded focus of radio-opacity called as coin lesion or as popcorn lesion on X-ray.
- It is a benign neoplasm rather than a lung malformation and the finding of chromosomal aberration **6p21 or 12q14**, indicates a **clonal origin**.
- **Note:** Popcorn calcification on mammography: FIBROADENOMA

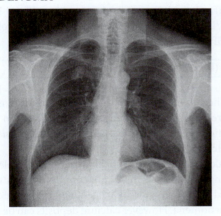

FIGURE: Popcorn calcification in lung-pulmonary hamartoma

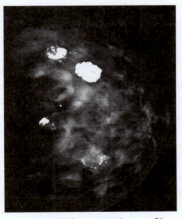

FIGURE: Popcorn calcification in breast-fibroadenoma

105. Ans. (d) 4th ventricle

Ref: Fundamentals of Radiology by Squire, P 532

- The image shows the arrow pointed at fourth ventricle just posterior to brainstem and anterior to cerebellum.
- CSF flows via cerebral aqueduct (between third and fourth ventricles) into the fourth ventricle.
- It then leaves the ventricular system via two foramina of *luschka* at sides of inferior aspect of cerebellum and foramen of *magendie* at the back of inferior cerebellum.
- CSF then flows above the cerebral hemispheres within the subarachnoid space and is *absorbed by arachnoid granulations* at superior sagittal sinus.

106. Ans. (d) Internal carotid artery

- The shown image is angiographic image of Circle of Willis.
- The artery marked with arrow is internal carotid artery.
  (Keywords in image: PCA, posterior cerebral artery; PCoA, posterior communicating artery; ACA, anterior cerebral artery; ACoA, anterior communicating artery; MCA, middle cerebral artery; ICA, internal carotid artery).

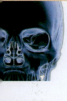

FMGE Solutions Screening Examination

1246

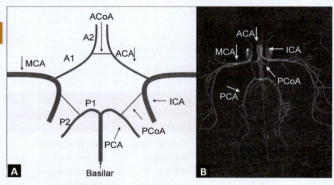

107. Ans. (a) Midbrain

(Revise the brainstem anatomy from the image shown below.)

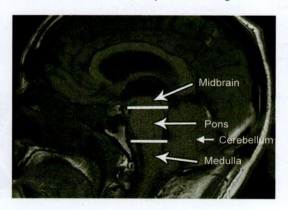

108. Ans. (b) MRI

IOC for certain conditions:

Conditions	Investigation of choice
Interstitial lung disease, bronchiectasis, fibrosis	HRCT
Gall stone, pleural effusion	USG
Spinal cord Neural tissue Chronic subarachnoid haemorrhage Stress fracture Femur neck fracture Bone marrow study	MRI
Cortical bone Calcification Acute head Injury Skull fracture Pelvic fracture	CT scan
Characterization of renal stone calculi	Dual source CT
Chronic pancreatitis	MRCP

109. Ans. (a) CT scan

Ref: Harrison, 19th ed. pg. 1786

- The diagnosis of subarachnoid hemorrhage (SAH) usually depends on a high index of clinical suspicion combined with radiologic confirmation via urgent computed tomography (CT) scan without contrast.
- Traditionally, a negative CT scan is followed with lumbar puncture (LP). However, non-contrast CT followed by CT angiography (CTA) of the brain can rule out SAH with greater than 99% sensitivity.

110. Ans. (d) Hyperdense bi convex

Ref: Harrison, 19th ed. pg. 457e-2

- In extradural hematoma or epidural hematoma, the tightly attached dura is stripped from the inner table of the skull, producing a characteristic **lenticular shaped hemorrhage** on noncontrast CT scan.
- **Epidural hematomas are usually caused by tearing of the middle meningeal artery** following fracture of the temporal bone.
- And the acute hematomas are hyperdense on NCCT and are hypodense only when they are chronic and becomes difficult to differentiate the chronic epidural hematoma (B/L and U/L) from hygromas which are collection of CSF from the rent of sub arachnoid space.

111. Ans. (b) CT scan

Ref: Harrison, 19th ed. pg. 426e-7

- When the Hounsfield units (Hu) exceed an established threshold (100 Hu), the source is believed to be calcification. **CT imaging is the gold standard in detecting calcification.**
- Calcifications of the pineal gland, choroid plexus, basal ganglia anal dura mater are commonly seen with aging and are usually not associated with pathological clinical phenomena. However calcium deposits can be associated with several intracranial pathologies including tumors, cerebrovascular diseases, congenital conditions, trauma and endocrine/metabolic disorders.

112. Ans. (a) Enhanced MRI

Ref: Multiple Journals

- Leptomeningeal carcinomatosis (LC) refers to *diffuse seeding of the leptomeninges by tumor metastases*.
- LC occurs in an estimated 20% of patients diagnosed with cancer and is most commonly found in breast carcinoma, lung carcinoma, and melanoma in adults and hematogenous malignancies and primitive neuroectodermal tumor (PNET) in children.
- *Contrast-enhanced MRI of the brain and spine is the imaging modality of choice* because of its safety, excellent contrast resolution, and multiplanar abilities.

Radiology

MAMMOGRAPHY

113. Ans. (b) Medial lateral oblique view

Ref: Harrison, 19th ed. pg. 525

***There are numerous** mammography views that can broadly be split into two groups*

- **Standard views**- Medio-Lateral, Medio-lateral oblique, Craniocaudal
- **Supplementary views** - Additional information or problem solving
  - The **mediolateral oblique (MLO) view** is one of standard mammographic views. It is the most important projection as it allows to depict most breast tissue.
  - **The Mediolateral view** loses significant tissue volume in the upper outer quadrant of the breast where statistically the most breast cancers are found. By doing an MLO view you get extra tissue without extra exposure.

114. Ans. (b) Normal mammogram rules out breast cancer

Ref: Bailey & Love, 25th ed. pg. 828

- Soft tissue radiographs are taken by placing the breast in direct contact with ultrasensitive film and exposing it to low-voltage, high amperage X-rays.
- *The dose of radiation is approximately 0.1 cGy and, therefore, mammography is a very safe investigation.*
- *The sensitivity of this investigation increases with age as the breast becomes less dense.*
- In total, 5% of breast cancers are missed by population-based mammographic screening programmes; even in retrospect, such carcinomas are not apparent. Thus, a **normal mammogram DOES NOT exclude the presence of carcinoma.**
- Digital mammography allows manipulation of the images and computer aided diagnosis.
- **Tomo-mammography** is also being assessed as a **more sensitive** diagnostic modality

OBSTETRICAL IMAGING

115. Ans. (a) Ion Donald

- Father of USG: **JOHN WILD**
- Father of Obstetrical USG: **ION DONALD**
- Father of Doppler: **Doppler John**
- Father of CT Scan: Godfrey Hounsefield
- Father of X-Ray: Roentgen
- Father of MRI: **Laterbuer and Mansfield**

116. Ans. (a) Small white gestational ring

Ref: Rosen's Emergency Medicine, 7th ed. pg. 175

- Although the blastocyst begins to implant in the endometrium at 3 weeks menstrual age (1 week after conception), **the first definitive ultrasound sign of pregnancy is the "gestational sac."** This is a sonographic not an anatomic term.
- Before the appearance of the gestational sac, the endometrium is markedly echogenic and the arcuate vessels are somewhat prominent. This, however, is non-diagnostic and can often be seen in the normal late secretory phase. In ultrasound images, the gestational sac appears as a thick echogenic ring surrounding a sonolucent center.
- Sonographically, the chorionic sac (gestational sac) is embedded in the depth of the thick endometrium (decidua) and appears on one side of the cavity line, not in the middle of it. This sonolucent center is actually the fluid-filled chorionic sac.
- **The sac grows @1 mm/day in mean diameter during early pregnancy.** With further growth, first the yolk sac and later the embryo become visible sonographically inside the chorionic cavity. The yolk sac has a very bright echogenic rim around a sonolucent center. When it first appears at <5 weeks, it may only be **1 to 3 mm** in diameter
- Discriminatory size of the gestational sac for trans-vaginal visualization of the yolk sac is reported from 5 to

ANSWERS TO BOARD REVIEW QUESTIONS

117. Ans. (d) 12 years

Ref: Wofgang, 5th ed. pg. 1065

118. Ans. (b) Pancreatitis

Ref: Wofganag, 5th e p-846/748, Blueprints Radiology, 2e- p-55

119. Ans. (a) Chronic pancreatitis

Ref: Sutton's Radiology, 7th ed. volume 1 pg. 798, Sabiston Textbook of Surgery, 18th ed. ch

120. Ans. (a) Left atria enlargement

121. Ans. (a) Enlarged right descending pulmonary artery

122. Ans. (a) Friedlander's pneumonia

123. Ans. (a) Sutural diastasis

124. Ans. (a) Wilson disease

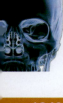

FMGE Solutions Screening Examination

125. Ans. (a) Hydatiform mole
126. Ans. (a) CT angiography
127. Ans. (b) Fibromuscular dysplasia
128. Ans. (a) Joubert syndrome
129. Ans. (d) FLAIR sequence shows low brain intesnsity
130. Ans. (a) 18- Fluorodeoxy-glucose
131. Ans. (a) Ejection fraction
132. Ans. (a) Endoscopic ultrasound
133. Ans. (a) Dilated CBD
134. Ans. (a) Fat is darker than water
135. Ans. (c) Density
136. Ans. (b) Pneumomediastinum
137. Ans. (a) Pneumothorax
138. Ans. (a) Pneumoperitoneum
139. Ans. (a) Echinococcus
140. Ans. (b) TGA

Ref: Pediatrics Radiology: The Requisites by Johan G. Blickman, Bruce R. Parker, M.D., Patrick D. Barnes pg. 52

141. Ans. (a) Sesta MIBI scan

Ref: Grainger and Allison, 4th ed. pg. 1380

142. Ans. (c) Asbestosis

Ref: PJ Mehta, 14th ed. pg. 309

143. Ans. (d) Fluoride-18

Ref: Sutton's Radiology, 7th ed. pg. 1826

144. Ans. (d) Whole body

Ref: Molecular anatomic imaging: PET-CT and Spect-Ct integrated Modality imaging by Gustav konrad von schulthessch 6

145. Ans. (b) CT angiography

Ref: Interventional Cardiology by Sinha, pg. 134, Harrison's 17/e, chapter 242

146. Ans. (d) TEE

Ref: Sutton 7/e, vol-1, p-278, 309, Oxford handbook of cardiology by punitramrakha p-768

147. Ans. (b) Multiple sclerosis

Ref: Sutton 7/e, volume 2, p-1799

148. Ans. (c) Peripheral lower

Ref: Sutton 7th ed. /289

149. Ans. (a) TAPVC

Ref. Sutton 7/e different pages, pediatric radiology: The requisites by Johan G. Blickman, Bruce R. Parker, M.D., Patrick D. Barnes p-52

150. Ans. (b) NCCT

Ref: Appendix-81 for "Traumatic Intracranial Hemotomas

ANSWERS TO IMAGE-BASED QUESTIONS

151. Ans. (a) Intussusception

Ref: Nelson 20th ed. pg. 1813

The image shows presence of "coiled spring" sign which is seen when an intussusception has occurred. These ring shadows represent contrast reflux within the lumen between the walls of the intussusceptum and intussuscipiens.

152. Ans. (a) SAH and IVH

The NCCT shows presence of hyperdensity in the area of slyian fissure (right side black arrow) indicating Subarachnoid hemorrhage. The presence of hyperdensity in ventricles indicated concomitant intraventricular hemorrhage (left side white arrow).

153. Ans. (b) **Subdural hemorrhage**

The concavo convex bleed is marked by three arrows indicating, subdural hemorrhage.

154. Ans. (a) Liver laceration

The image shows a hematoma seen in the posterior part of liver (black area).

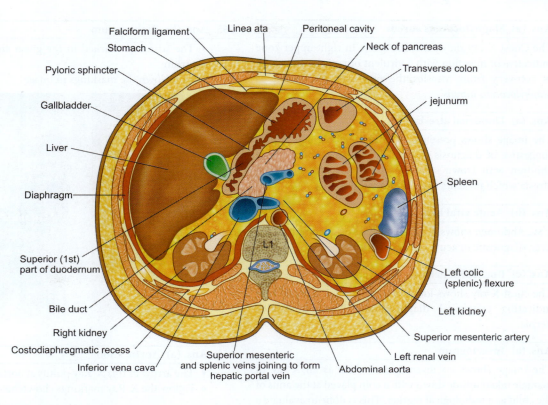

155. Ans. (a) Brain tumor

The image shows a brain tumor obliterating the ventricular system.

156. Ans. (b) Horseshoe kidney

157. Ans. (a) Klastskin tumor

The image shows the endoscope in the middle and the biliary tree. You can notice the contrast in gall bladder (9 o'clock) and cystic duct where it is meeting the common hepatic duct. However the left and right hepatic ducts are not visible indicating a tumor causing obstruction to flow of contrast.

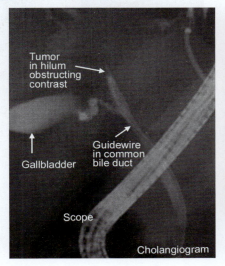
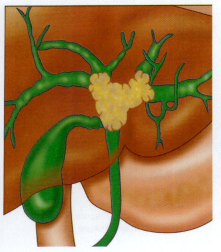

FMGE Solutions Screening Examination

158. Ans. (a) Staphylococcus aureus

The Chest X-ray shows a cystic cavity in right upper zone indicative of infection with a virulent organism. In setting of recovery from measles the organism responsible is *Staphylococcus aureus*.

159. Ans. (a) Duodenal atresia

The image shows presence of double bubble appearance suggestive of diagnosis of duodenal atresia. About 8% of children with Down syndrome are born with duodenal atresia which presents with bilious vomiting.

160. Ans. (b) Acute viral hepatitis

USG Abdomen shows presence of starry sky pattern of the liver, diagnostic of acute viral hepatitis

161. Ans. (c) Bochdalek hernia

The chest X-ray shows loops of bowel on left side of chest indicating congenital diaphragmatic hernia/Bochdalek hernia.

162. Ans. (a) Invertogram

The image shows an invertogram which is an X-ray of neonate taken upside down with a coin placed at the anus of the child as a radiological marker. This is done to evaluate a child with anorectal malformations.

163. Ans. (b) Pulmonary plethora

The CXR shows an enlarged heart with boot shaped configuration and reduced vascularity of lungs. The clinical diagnosis is Tetralogy of Fallot, and due to subpulmonic stenosis it presents with pulmonic oligemia.

164. Ans. (b) Major fissure

- The shown image shows major fissure or oblique fissure.

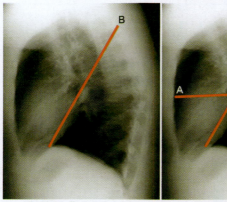
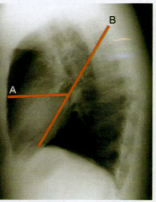

B: Major fissure L Lung

A: Minor Fissure R Ling
B: Major fissure L Lung

165. Ans. (b) Right atrium

- The structure marked in the given chest XRay is right atrium
- Note down the markings in image

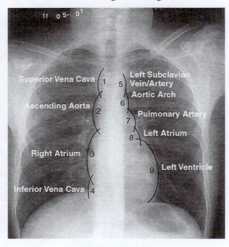

166. Ans. (a) Aortic knob

- The arrow in this X-Ray points at aortic knob
- Follow the X-Ray markings shown below

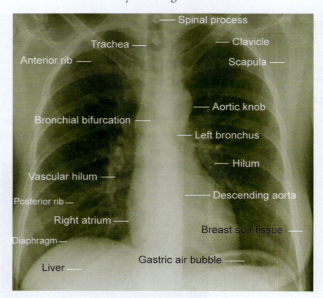

Key Points

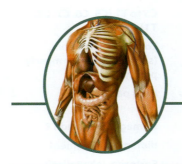

Anatomy

- Upper lateral cutaneous nerve is a branch of: **Axillary nerve**
- An injury to anatomical snuff box causes fracture of this bone: **Scaphoid**
- Muscle of arm causing flexion, adduction and medial rotation: **Pectoralis Major**
- Testicular artery is a branch of: **Abdominal aorta**
- Inferior scapular angle lies at which level: **T8**
- Muscle causing adduction at hip joint: **Gluteus medius**
- Deep inguinal ring is formed in: **Transversalis fascia**
- Nerve damage that can cause hypothenar muscle wasting and loss of sensation of medial one and half digits: **Ulnar nerve**
- Failure of closure of rostral neuropore at 25th day leads to: **Anencephaly**
- Parotid gland is supplied by this nerve: **Glossopharyngeal nerve**
- Killian's Dehiscence is formed due to: **Inferior constrictor muscle**
- Muscle biceps brachii inserts into: **Radial tuberosity**
- Nerve supplying area between great toe and 2nd toe: **Deep Peroneal nerve**
- Dermatome supplying area of nipples: **T4**
- Dermatome Supplying area of umbilicus: **T10**
- Retraction of scapula is done by: **Middle fibers of trapezius muscle**
- Nerve supplying cornea: **Trigeminal nerve**
- Longest extraocular muscle: **Superior Oblique (7.7 cm)**
- Shortest extraocular muscle: **Medial rectus (5.5 cm)**

TABLE: Important bone and their nutrient arteries

Bone	Nutrient artery
Femur	Branch of Femoral artery → **Profunda femoris artery**
Tibia	Posterior tibial artery
Fibula	Branch of posterior tibial artery → **Peroneal artery**
Clavicle	Subscapular artery
Radius and Ulna	Anterior interosseous artery
Humerus	Profunda brachii artery

TABLE: Branches of subcalvian artery

1st part	VIT-CD • Vertebral artery • Internal mammary artery • Thyrocervical trunk
2nd part	Costocervical trunk
3rd part	Dorsal scapular artery

TABLE: Weight of some important organs

Organ	Weight
• Pituitary	0.5–0.6 gram (500–600 mg)
• Brain	Males: 1.4 kg Females: 1.27 kg
• Thyroid gland	20–40 gram
• Kidney	130–160 gram
• Adrenal gland	5–6 gram
• Prostate gland	15–20 gram

TABLE: Length of important anatomical structure

Organ	Length
• Fallopian tube	10–12 cm
• Bile duct • Appendix • Gallbladder	8 cm Mn: BAG

Contd...

FMGE Solutions Screening Examination

Organ	Length
• Spinal cord • Thoracic duct • Transverse colon • Umbilical cord • Femur • Deferens (Vas Deferens)	45 cm **Mn: STTUFeD**
• Sigmoid colon • Esophagus • Duodenum • Descending colon • Ureter • Urethra (male)	25 cm **Mn: SEDDUU**
• Inguinal canal • Optic nerve • Urethra (Female)	4 cm **Mn: I lOve U**

TABLE: Glands of face and their duct

Gland	Duct	Nerve	Development	Acini histology
Parotid gland	Stensen duct (opens opposite to upper 2nd molar)	CN V (auriculotemporal branch)	Ectodermal	Serous acini
Submandibular gland	Wharton's duct (open on sides of frenulum at the floor of mouth)	CN VII (chorda tympani branch)	Endodermal	Mixed (serous > Mucinous)
Sublingual gland	Bartholin's and Rivinus duct (open at floor of mouth)	CN VII (chorda tympani branch)	Endodermal	Mixed (Mucinous > serous)

OFTEN ASKED ONES

• Most frequently fractured bone of body	Clavicle
• First bone to ossify	Clavicle
• Only long bone which has no medullary cavity	Clavicle
• All long bone ossify in cartilage EXCEPT clavicle. *It ossifies in membrane*	Clavicle
• Most frequently dislocated carpal bone	Lunate
• Most frequently fractured carpal bone	Scaphoid

• Nerve supply of deltoid	Axillary nerve
• MC fractured carpal bone	Scaphoid (boat shaped)- 2nd MC site of avascular necrosis
• Ape thumb deformity	Median nerve (opponens pollicis muscle paralyzed)
• Musician's nerve	Ulnar nerve (root value C8, T1)
• Labourer's nerve/ eye of the hand	Median nerve
• Root value of radial nerve	C5 to T1 (C5, C6, C7, C8, T1)
• Winging of scapula	Long thoracic nerve (serratus anterior muscle paralyzed)
• Police man tip hand/porter's tip hand	Erb's paralysis
• Klumpke's paralysis	Damage to C8 and T1
• Strongest ligament of body	Iliofemoral ligament
• Longest muscle of body	Sartorius (aka tailor's muscle)
• Nerve supply of gluteus maximus	INFERIOR gluteal N. (L5, S1, S2) Mn: 512
• Nerve supply of gluteus medius and minimus	SUPERIOR gluteal N. (L4, L5, S1) Mn: 451
• Vessel used in coronary artery bypass graft (CABG)	Internal Mammary Artery
• Muscle which is known as peripheral heart	Soleus
• Locking of the knee by	Quadriceps femoris muscle (occurs at last stage of extension)
• Unlocking of the knee by	Popliteus muscle (occurs at first stage of flexion)
• Sternal angle and bifurcation of trachea at	T4 level
• Arch of aorta begins and terminates at	T4 level
• Police man of abdominal cavity	Greater omentum
• Muscle of horror	Platysma
• Nerve supply of upper eyelid and TIP of nose	V1 (ophthalmic branch of trigeminal)
• Most commonly nerve paralyzed	Facial N (longest intraosseous course)
• Emergency tracheostomy at	Tracheal ring 2–3

Contd...

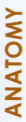

Contd...

Anatomy

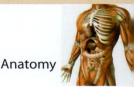

Key Points

Ova released in form of	**Secondary oocyte**
Blastocyst formation	**5th day after fertilization**
Implantation occurs	**6th day after fertilization, completes on 10th day.**
Liver has 8 segments.	**Caudate lobe-segment 1; Quadrate lobe-segment 4**
Narrowest part of esophagus	**Cricopharynx at the root of neck**
Test which is done to check gluteus medius and minimus	**Trendelenburg test**
Trigone of bladder develops	**From mesonephric duct (mesodermal in origin)**
Pouch of Douglas	**Between rectum and uterus**
Parotid gland duct	**Stensen's duct**
Submandibular gland duct	**Wharton's duct**
Muscle which opens Eustachian tube while yawning	**Tensor veli palatini and levator veli palatini**
Ovarian artery/testicular artery is a branch of	**Abdominal aorta**
Most common fracture of humerus	**Supracondylar fracture**
Muscle not attached to apex of orbit	**Inferior oblique**
Which bone does not contribute to Medial wall of orbit	**Zygoma**
Which layer of scalp is vascular	**Subcutaneous tissue**
Magendie foramen drains CSF from:	**4th ventricle**
Closure of neural tube begins at	**Cervical end (if choice given is "multiple sites" then it is the best answer)**
Junction of anterior and posterior horn of lateral ventricle is called:	**Trigone and lateral ventricle**
Infection of CNS spreads in inner ear through	**Cochlear Aqueduct**
Posterior communicating artery is a branch of	**Middle Cerebral Artery**
The chorda tympani nerve arises from	**Facial nerve**
Broca's area is located in	**Inferior frontal gyrus**
Lower angle of scapula lies at	**Level of T 7**
Nerve injured with fracture of surgical neck of humerus	**Axillary**

Nerve injured with fracture of shaft of humerus	**Radial**
Nerve injured with fracture of medial humeral epicondyle	**Ulnar**
Muscle that initiates abduction of arm	**Supraspinatus**
Most commonly torn tendon of rotator cuff	**Supraspinatus**
"Claw" hand is due to paralysis of which muscle group	**Lumbricals**
Innervation to nail bed of ring finger	**Ulnar and median**
Innervation to nail bed of middle finger	**Median nerve**
Dermatome of thumb	**C6**
Spinal levels of axillary nerve	**C5 and C6**

- Sprengel's deformity is associated with this bone: **Scapula (failure of normal scapular descent during development)**
- Largest branch of brachial plexus: **Radial nerve**
- Largest branch of lumbar plexus: **Femoral nerve**
- Erb's point anatomical location at junction of: **C5, C6**
- Klumpke's paralysis involves: **C8, T1**
- This nerve injury can cause wasting of intrinsic muscles of hand: **Ulnar nerve**
- Guyon's canal is in relation to this nerve: **Ulnar nerve**
- Paralysis of this muscle can cause "Dropped shoulder": **Trapezius**
- Power grip of hand is mainly due to: **Long Flexors**
- Cephalic veins drain into: **Axillary vein**
- Upper outer quadrant of breast is drained by this lymphatic: **Anterior axillary**
- Main blood supply of the femoral head: **Medial circumflex femoral artery**
- Nutrient artery of the femur: **Profunda femoris artery**
- Nutrient artery of tibia: **Posterior tibial artery**
- Nutrient artery to fibula: **Peroneal artery**
- Ligament which supports talus: **Spring ligament**
- Strongest flexors of the hip: **Psoas major and iliacus muscle (iliopsoas muscle)**
- Chief nerve of medial compartment of thigh: **Obturator nerve**
- Nerve root value of sciatic nerve: **L4, 5, S1, 2, 3**
- Nerve root of posterior cutaneous nerve of thigh: **S1, 2, 3**
- Nerve root value of pudendal nerve: **S2, 3, 4**
- Nerve root value of medial cutaneous nerve of thigh: **L2, L3**

Contd...

Contd...

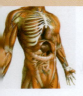

FMGE Solutions Screening Examination

- Hunterian perforators also known as adductor canal perforators are seen in: **Mid-thigh**
- Triceps surae nerve is: **Gastroc-soleus**
- Pressure change in calf compartment during heel touch phase of walking: **Remains same (no change in pressure)**
- Motor nerve supply of diaphragm: **Phrenic nerve**
- **Sensory nerve supply of diaphragm:**
  - Central part: Phrenic nerve
  - Peripheral part: Lower 6 intercostal nerves
- Most common site of morgagni hernia: **Posterolateral part of diaphragm** (*Right anterior being the most common site*)
- Intercostobrachial nerve is a branch of: **2nd intercostal nerve**
- Azygos lobe is a part of this organ: **Lung**
- **Trautmann's triangle** (transmits infection from temporal bone to cerebellum):
  - Bony labyrinth (anteriorly)
  - Sigmoid sinus (posteriorly)
  - Superior petrosal sinus (above)
- **Triangle of safety** (an important landmark of chest tube insertion)
  - Anterior border of latissimus dorsi
  - Lateral border of pectoralis major
  - Imaginary horizontal level of the nipple
- Triangle of Doom
  - Medially: Vas Deferens
  - Laterally: Gonadal vessels
  - Posteriorly: Peritoneal edge
- **Triangle of Doom contains:** External iliac vessels, Deep circumflex iliac vein, femoral nerve and genital branch of genitofemoral nerve
- **Triangle of pain** (contain femoral branch of genitofemoral nerve, lateral cutaneous nerve of thigh)
  - Medially: Gonadal vessels
  - Laterally: Iliopubic tract
- **Passaro (Gastrinoma) triangle:** Seen at upper abdomen
  - Apex: Junction of cystic duct and CBD
  - Inferior part: Junction of D2 and D3
  - Left lateral point: Pancreatic neck & Body junction
- **Koch's triangle** is formed by:
  - Superiorly: Tendon of todaro
  - Inferiorly: Tricuspid valve septal leaflet
  - Basally: Coronary sinus orifice
- Koch's triangle is a part of: **AV node**
- Blood supply of the Koch's triangle: **Right coronary artery**
- Blood supply of SA node: **Right coronary artery**
- Valve guarding coronary sinus: **Thebesian valve**
- Thoracic duct is also known as: **Van horne canal, Pecquet duct**
- Transtubercular plane lies at which level: **L5**

- Length of inguinal canal: **4 cm**
- Cisterna chyli is situated in: **Abdomen**
- Labia majora is developed from: **Genital swelling**
- Helicine artery is a branch of: **Deep artery of penis**
- Nerve supply of perineum is: **Pudendal nerve**
- Anatomical support of prostrate is: **Pubococcygeus**
- Blood supply of liver: **80% portal vein, 20% hepatic artery**
- Stave cells are seen in: **Spleen**
- Most common congenital anomaly of pancreas: **Pancreas divisum**
- Ligament which contains splenic artery: **Splenorenal ligament**
- Angle of mandible is supplied by: **Greater auricular nerve**
- Tip of nose is supplied by: **Ophthalmic nerve (external nasal branch)**
- Metopic suture: **Separates two half of the frontal bone**
- Metopic suture closes at: **6 years**
- Muscle of grinning: **Risorius muscle**
- Common carotid artery bifurcates at: **C4 level (at upper border of thyroid cartilage)**
- Middle meningeal artery is a branch of: **Maxillary artery (1st part of maxillary artery)**
- Anterior choroidal artery is a branch of: **Internal carotid artery**
- Chassaignac tubercle is: **Carotid tubercle on C6 vertebra**
- Ligament of berry function: **Connects thyroid lobe to cricoid lobe**
- Herring bodies are seen in: **Posterior pituitary (ADH and oxytocin both stored here)**
- Otic ganglion supplies this gland: **Parotid gland**
- Gerlach tonsil is also named as: **Tubal tonsil**
- Passavant's ridge is formed by: **Palatopharyngeus and superior constrictor muscle**
- Gillette space corresponds to: **Retropharyngeal space**
- Smallest cranial nerve: **Trochlear nerve**
- Broca's area located at: **Posterior end of superior temporal gyrus (Area 44, 45)**
- Wernicke's area is located at: **Superior temporal gyrus (Area 22)**
- Organs devoid of lymphatics: **Brain, choroid, internal ear, glottis**

- Most prominent spinous process in the spine? **Vertebra prominens (C7)**
- Muscles comprise the erector spinae? **Iliocostalis, Longissimus, Spinalis**

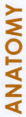

ANATOMY

1254

Contd...

Contd...

Anatomy

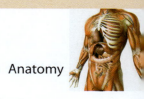

- Pairs of spinal nerves exit from the spinal cord? **31 pairs**
- Region where the manubrium and the body of the sternum articulate? **Sternal angle of Louis**.
- Muscles are innervated by the axillary nerve? **Deltoid and teres minor**
- Foot drop is caused by damage to which nerve? **Common peroneal nerve**
- Artery of the anterior compartment of the leg? **Anterior tibial artery**
- Nerve supplying the lateral compartment of the leg? **Superficial peroneal nerve**
- What is the prominent "bump" on the lateral aspect of the knee? **Head of the fibula**
- What is the part of the lung that extends above the level of the first rib? **The cupula**
- Right lung has how many lobes? **Three**
- Left lung has how many lobes. **Two**
- What is the only valve in the heart that has two cusps? **Mitral (bicuspid) valve**
- Which vein travels with the right coronary artery? **Small cardiac vein**
- What attaches the cusps of the valves to the papillary muscles in the heart? **Chordae tendineae**
- First branch off the abdominal artery? **Inferior phrenic artery**
- At what vertebral level is the hyoid bone found? **C3**
- Ophthalmic artery is a branch of? **Internal carotid artery**
- Where does the inferior mesenteric vein drain? **The splenic vein**
- The folds of the mucosa of the stomach are known as? **Rugae**
- Mucosal folds of small intestine starting 2nd part of duodenum: **Valvulae conniventes also known as Kerckring folds**
- Artery of the embryonic foregut? **Celiac artery**
- **Portal triad** comprised of? **1. Common bile duct 2. Hepatic artery 3. Portal vein**
- Structure which separate the anatomic right and left lobes of the liver? **Ligamentum teres and ligamentum venosum**
- Rectouterine pouch is also known as? **Pouch of Douglas**
- Broad ligament of the uterus is comprised of? **1. Mesosalpinx 2. Mesovarium 3. Mesometrium**
- What two muscles are tested to see if CN XI is intact? **Trapezius and sternocleidomastoid**
- Only organ in the body supplied by preganglionic sympathetic fibers? **Adrenal medulla**

Contd...

- Location of seminal vesicle? **On the posterior aspect of the urinary bladder**
- Opening of parotid (Stenson's) duct in the oral cavity? **Opposite the second upper molar tooth**
- Function of the arachnoid granulations in brain? **Resorb CSF into the blood**
- Only muscle of the tongue not innervated by the hypoglossal nerve? **Palatoglossus**
- Fundus of stomach is supplied mainly by: **Splenic artery**
- Content of anatomical snuff box: **Radial artery**
- Ovarian artery is a branch of: **Abdominal aorta**
- **Ventral Branches of Abdominal Aorta:**
  - Celiac trunk
  - Superior mesenteric artery
  - Inferior mesenteric artery
- Direct branch of Inferior mesenteric artery: **Superior rectal artery**
- Left adrenal gland is **crescentic/semilunar**
- Right adrenal gland is **pyramidal** in shape
- The average weight of adrenal gland: **4–6 g**
- **Structures and level of piercing in diaphragm:** *(Mn: I ate, 10 Eggs, At 12)*
  - IVC: T8
  - Esophagus: T10
  - Aorta: T12
- Base of the heart is formed by: **Left atrium**
- Nerve supplying serratus anterior muscle: **Long thoracic nerve**
- Inferior vena cava formed at: **L5 level**
- Muller muscle supplied by which nerve: **Sympathetic nerve**
- Arnold nerve is a branch of: **Vagus Nerve**
- Left gonadal vein drain into: **IVC**
- Muscle of upper limb which cover both elbow and shoulder joint: **Long head of triceps brachii**
- **Supination and pronation** of upper limb is due to: **Radioulnar joint**
- Efferent cremasteric reflex is carried by: **Genitofemoral nerve**
- Collecting duct is derived from: **Ureteric bud**
- Most common fracture of humerus- **Supracondylar fracture**
- **Police man** of abdominal cavity- **Greater omentum**
- Nerve supply of upper eyelid and TIP of nose- **V1 (ophthalmic branch of trigeminal).**
- Disc are NOT found between: **C1 and C2; Sacrum-Coccyx**
- Critical vascular zone of spinal cord: **T4–T9**
- Extension of artery of Adamkiewicz is between: **T9–T11**
- Filum terminale is derived from: **Pia mater**

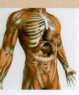

FMGE Solutions Screening Examination

TABLE: Cranial nerves in a nutshell

• Largest cranial nerve	Trigeminal Nerve (CN V)
• Smallest cranial nerve	Trochlear nerve (CN IV)
• Longest intracranial course	Trochlear nerve (CN IV)
• The only cranial nerve to emerge from the dorsal surface of the Brain stem	Trochlear N
• Cranial N. with longest intraosseous course	Facial nerve (CN VII)
• Most common cranial nerve involved in Raised ICT	Abducens N (CN VI)

TABLE: Important vertebral levels (also mentioned inside in explanations section)

• Bifurcation of common carotid artery	C3
• Thyroid Cartilage	C5
• Cricoid Cartilage	C6
• Arch of Aorta	T4
• Tracheal bifurcation (standing)	T6
• Xiphoid process	T9
• Transpyloric plane	L1
• Origin of renal artery	L2
• Subcostal plane	L3
• Bifurcation of abdominal aorta	L4
• Transtubercular plane	L5
• Formation of IVC	L5

TABLE: Ribs at a glance

Rib nomenclature	Rib number
• False ribs	8–12
• True ribs also known as vertebrosternal ribs	1–7th ribs
• Floating ribs	11th and 12th
• Typical ribs	3rd to 9th (individual identification is not possible)
• Atypical ribs	1st, 2nd, 10th, 11th, 12th (can be identified individually)
• Longest rib	7th rib
Strongest rib Shortest rib Widest rib	1st rib
Most oblique rib	9th rib

TABLE: Deep tendon reflexes and their spinal cord level

Reflex/Jerk	Spinal level	Nerve Involved
Biceps Jerk	C5-6	Musculocutaneous
Brachioradialis	C5-6	Radial
Supinator	C5-6	Radial
Triceps	C7-8	Radial
Knee/patella jerk	L3-4	Femoral
Ankle jerk	S1-2	Tibial

TABLE: Normal prostrate anatomy: Has 5 lobes

Lobe	Importance
Anterior	–
Posterior	MC site of prostrate CA
Median	MC site for BPH
Lateral- 2	Site for prostatic adenoma in elderly

STRUCTURE WITH NO LYMPHATICS (BASEC)

- Brain & spinal cord
- Articular cartilage
- Splenic pulp, bone marrow
- Epidermis, Hairs, Nails
- Cornea

FASCIA

- Membranous layer of superficials fascia of perineum: **COLLES FASCIA**
- Deep fascia of thighs: **FASCIA LATA**
- Deep fascia of penis: **BUCK'S FASCIA**
- separates post surface of prostate from rectum: **FASCIA OF DENOVILLIER**
- Condensation of pelvic fascia behind rectum: **FASCIA OF WALDAYER**
- Below umbilicus superf. Fatty layer.: **FASCIA OF CAMPER**
- Below umbilicus deep membraneous layer: **FASCIA OF SCARPA**

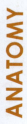

Anatomy

"Since there are multiple questions on aortic and iliac branches, here's the summarized table for the ease of creating an image".

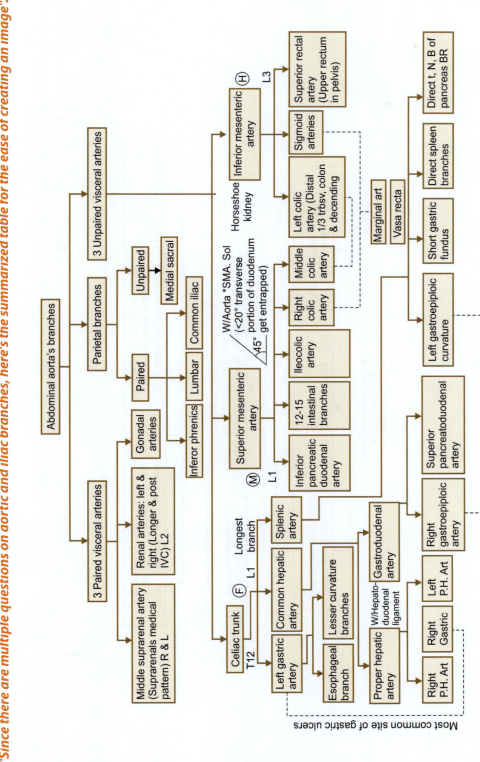

Key Points

FMGE Solutions Screening Examination

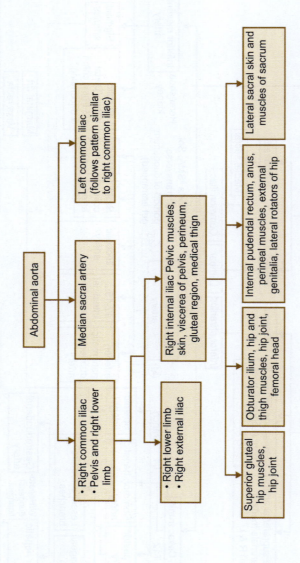

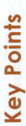

Physiology

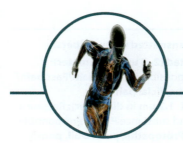

SENSORY SPINAL TRACTS

Tract	Sensation carried
• Ventral/anterior STT	• Crude touch/itching, tickle pressure, sexual sensation, Detection of pressure (Barognosis)
• Lateral STT	• Pin prick/pain, temp
• Fasciculus gracilis (medial) sacral, lumbar region	• Fine touch, vibration, fine pressure, conscious proprioception, stereognosis, 2-point discrimina
• Fasciculus cuneatus (lateral) (thoracic, cervical region)	• Vibration joint/position sense
• CST	• Smoothness and coordination of movt (Skilled movements)

IMPORTANT RECENT ONES

Histamine is produced by	Mast cell
Prolactin is inhibited by	Dopamine
Highest percent of blood is present in this vessel	Veins
Maximum surface area for this vessel	Capillaries
Maximum resistance for this vessel	Arterioles

TABLE: Breathing Patterns

	Condition	Description	Causes
∿∿∿	Eupnea	Normal breathing rate and pattern	Fever, anxiety, exercise, shock
	Tachypnea	Increased respiratory rate	Sleep, drugs, metabolic disorder, head injury, stroke
	Bradypnea	Decreased respiratory rate	
___	Apnea	Absence of breathing	Deceased patient, head injury, stroke
∿∿∿	Hyperpnea	Normal rate, but deep respirations	Emotional stress, diabetic ketoacidosis
∿ⱴⱴ	Cheyne-Stokes	Gradual increases and decreases in respirations with periods of apnea	Increasing intracranial pressure, brain stem injury
∧∧∧	Biot's	Rapid, deep respirations (gasps) with short pauses between sets	Spinal meningitis, many CNS causes, head injury
∧∧∧∧∧	Kussmaul's	Tachypnea and hyperpnea	Renal failure, metabolic acidosis, diabetic ketoacidosis
⋁⋁⋁⋁	Apneustic	Prolonged inspiratory phase with shortened expiratory phase	Lesion in brain stem

CUTANEOUS MECHANORECEPTORS

Four types of mechanoreceptors for sensing touch and pressure

- **Meissner's corpuscles:** Texture and slow vibrations (5-40 Hz)
- **Merkel's cell (slow adapting):** Sustained pressure and touch
- **Ruffini corpuscles (slow adapting):** Sustained pressure
- **Pacinian corpuscles (rapidly adapting):** Deep pressure and fast vibrations (60–300 Hz)

1259

Key Points

Mechanoreceptors/Exteroceptors

Type of receptor	Location	Sensory modality	Nerve fibres
Non-encapsulated receptors			
Free nerve ending	Epidermis, cornea, gut, dermis, ligaments, joint capsules, bone, dental pulp	Pain, crude touch, pressure, heat/cold	AδC
Merkel disc	Hairless skin	Touch	Aβ
Hair follicle receptors	Hairy skin	Light movement on skin (Touch)	Aβ
Meissner's corpuscles	Dermal papillae in finger tips (skin of palm/sole), Basis of **BRAILLE**, Topognosis, Texture	Fine well localized touch, tactile, Vibration <80Hz	Aβ
Pacinian corpuscles	Dermis ligaments, joint capsules, peritoneum, ext. genitalia	Fast Vibration, Deep pressure	Aβ
Ruffini ending	Dermis of hairy skin	Stretch (sustained pressure)	Aβ
NM spindles	Skeletal muscle	Stretch–muscle length	Aα Aβ
Neurotendinous spindles	Tendons	Compression-muscle tension	Aα

NOCICEPTORS

- **Mechanical nociceptors:** Respond to strong pressure from a sharp object
- **Thermal nociceptors:** Activated by skin temperature above 42*C or severe cold
- **Chemical nociceptors:** Responds to various chemical such as bradykinin, Histamine, high acidity
- **Polymodal nociceptors:** Responds to combination of these stimuli

PAIN FIBERS

Impulses from nociceptors transmitted via two fibers:
- A delta fibers-thin myelinated (2–5 um in diameter): Release glutamate and is responsible for **First pain/Fast pain/Epicritic pain**. Localized, superficial pain.
- C fibers- Unmyelinated (0.4–1.2 um in diameter): Release a combination of glutamate and substance P and is responsible for **second pain/slow pain/Protopathic pain**. Dull, poorly localized, Visceral pain.

SOMATOSENSORY PATHWAYS AND THEIR PRIMARY FUNCTION

- **Dorsal column pathway:** Fine touch, vibration and proprioception, two point discrimination
- **Ventrolateral spinothalamic tract:** Pain and temperature, Crude touch, Detection of pressure (**Barognosis**)
- **Spinocerebellar tract:** Skilled movement
- **Corticospinal tract:** Tone and pressure (anterior CST), fine skill movement, precision (lateral CST)

TABLE: Cell cycle

• **Order of cell cycle:** G1 → S → G2 → M → G1 → G0
• DNA and centromere doubling seen in this phase of cell cycle: **S phase**
• Cell division/doubling of cell seen in this phase of cell cycle: **M phase**
• **Cell hypertrophy is due to:** Arrest of cell cycle before G2 phase (S–G2 phase)
• **Cell hyperplasia is due to:** Arrest of cell cycle before going into quiescent phase (G0) → Increase in number of cells
• Most sensitive phase of cell cycle for radiation injury: **G2-M phase**

TABLE: Cell and cell membrane

Thickness: **7–10 nm**
Main constituent is the **protein.** Protein: **50–60%** Lipid: **30–40%**
Protein: **Lipid ratio is 2:1**
Lipids are regular but asymmetrically arranged.
Membrane lipids are **amphiphatic**.
They are arranged as a **bilayer**.
Signal transduction and enzyme activation are the functions of **Phospholipid part.**
The Fluidity of the cell membrane is increased by **Poly unsaturated fatty acids.**

Contd...

Physiology

- RBC membrane is especially having **spectrin** (maintains integrity) and **glycophorin**.
- **Lipid bilayer** acts as a **gel**.
- **Resting membrane potential is due to: K⁺**
- Resting membrane potential is close to **isoelectric potential of:** Cl⁻ (i.e. - 70 mV)
- **IPSP** is due to **Cl⁻ influx or K efflux or both**
- **EPSP** is due to **Na influx**
- **For action potential**; threshold stimulus is required
- **Nerve conduction** follows All or None phenomenon.
- Action Potential
- Axon hillock and initial axon segment has the lowest threshold potential in a **nerve fiber**.
- **Nerve impulse** travels in the direction only at synapse.
- RMP is due to - **Potassium**
- IPSP is due to **Chloride/K⁺**
- Amplitude is due to **Na**
- Equilibrium potential of an ion is calculated by: **Nernst equation**
- **Nernst potential across cell membrane**
  For K⁺ ion: – 90 mV
  For Na⁺ ion: + 60 mB
  For Cl⁻ ion: – 70 mV

TABLE: Cell organelles

Nissl bodies: Group of ribosomes in neurons which are utilized for protein synthesis
Synthesis of lipids occurs in **Agranular Endoplasmic Reticulum.**
Synthesis of proteins occurs in **Rough ER.**
Intracellular sorting and packing is done in **Golgi complex.**
Cell shape and motility are a function of **Microtubules.**
Catabolism of H_2O_2 is a function of **Peroxisomes.**
Site of ATP synthesis is **Mitochondria.**

GOLDEN POINTS (INCLUDES RECENT PATTERN QUESTIONS)

- Pacinian corpuscles consist of unmyelinated endings with a sensory nerve fiber of 2 um in diameter
- Surfactant is produced by: **Type II cells (Granular pneumocytes)**
- Alveoli are mainly lined by: **Type I cells (95% surface area)**
- Type II alveolar cells make up only 5% of surface area, they represent approximately 60% of epithelial cells in alveoli
- Brunner gland secretes: **Alkaline mucus**

Contd...

- Pyloric gland secretes: **Thin viscid Mucus (protects stomach wall from digestion by gastric enzymes)**
- Part of intestine secreting enteropeptidase: **Duodenum (activates trypsinogen)**
- Most abundant form of vitamin D in plasma: **25-Hydroxyvitamin D [25(OH)D]**
- Vitamin D form found in skin: **7-Dehydrocholesterol**
- Upon exposure to UV light 7-dehydrocholesterol is converted to Vitamin D3 (Cholecalciferol)
- Most common form of supplemental vitamin A used: **Al-trans retinyl acetate**
- Largest protein in body: **Titin**
- Volume remained in lung after normal expiration: **Functional residual capacity**
- Volatile acids in plasma is buffered by: **Hemoglobin**
- Vibration sense is carried by: **Pacinian corpuscles**
- Bohr's effect: **OHDC is inversely proportional to both acidity and to concentration of CO_2**
- Haldane effect: **Oxygenation of blood in the lungs displaces carbon dioxide from hemoglobin which increases the removal of carbon dioxide**
- Heart rate if Purkinje fibers became the pacemaker of the heart: **15–40 bpm**
- If SA node discharges at 0.00s, when will it normally arrive at the AV bundle (bundle of His): **0.12 second (0.03 from atria + 0.09 from AV node)**
- Structure with the slowest rate of conduction of the cardiac action potential: **AV bundle**
- Frank starling law of the heart: **Increase in venous return causes increased cardiac output**
- Mean systemic filling pressure: **7 mm Hg**
- Nephrons reaches to adult value at: **36 weeks gestation**
- Below this age BP of 120/80 is considered as hypertension: **<12 years**
- In newborn, renal tubular concentrating capacity reaches adult value at: **1 year**
- Normal GFR as adult value is reached at: **2 years**
- Best method of estimating creatinine assay: **Enzyme assay**
- **Total body water** is 60–70% of total body weight
- 2/3rd of fluid is Intra Cellular Fluid; 1/3rd is Extra Cellular Fluid.
- Evans blue dye is used to measure: **Plasma volume**
- Normal pH of blood: **7.35–7.45**
- Normal plasma protein ratio: **1.7:1**
- Life span of normal RBC: **120 days**
- Platelets are stored at: **Room temperature**
- Mentzer index: **Used to differentiate iron deficiency anemia from beta thalassemia**

FMGE Solutions Screening Examination

TABLE: Measurement of body fluid

Total body water Mn: DATA	D_2O (Deuterium oxide/heavy water)- MC used Aminopyrene, Tritium oxide, Antipyrine,
ECF volume Mn: No SIM	Sucrose Insulin (most accurate) Mannitol Na^+ Thiosulfate
ICF volume	**Indirect method:** ICF = TBW – ECF *(best done by D_2O – Inulin)*
Interstitial fluid	**Indirect method:** ISF = ECF – Plasma volume
Plasma volume Mn: AB-P	Albumin (Radiolabeled I^{125}), Evans Blue
Total blood volume	Plasma volume x 100/100-Hct

TABLE: $Na^+ K^+$ ATPase pump

- Na K ATPase pump is an active, electrogenic pump moves 3 Na^+ ions outside and in place 2 K^+ ions inside utilizing ATP. It helps in intrusion of K^+.
- It accounts for 20% of energy utilized by cells.
- Thus its coupling ratio is 3:2
- Extracellular binding site is Ouabain binding site
- Its activity is inhibited by ouabain and related cardiac glycosides (digitalis)
- It is a P type ATPase (super family of cation transporters)
- Also called E1/E2 type ATPase responsible for carrying ions across cell membranes.
- **Type:** Heterodimer heterogeneous (α & β subunit)

It is an example of active transport

- Generation of Action Potential by
- Nerve cells not neuroglia
- Muscles
- Contractile tissue
- Glands

TABLE: Important RMP

RBC	– 12 mV
Rods & cones	– 40 mV
SA node	– 55 mV
Smooth muscle	– 50 to –60 mV
Cardiac muscle (Single Fiber)	– 85 to – 95 mV
Skeletal muscle	– 90 mV
Nerve fibre	– 90 mV
Inner hair cells	– 150 mV

NEUROTRANSMITTERS

Purines
- Adenosine
- ATP

Lipids and Gases
- Nitric oxide (NO)
- Carbon monoxide
- Cannabinoids

Biogenic Amines
- Catecholamines: Dopamine, norepinephrine and epinephrine
- Indolamines
- Serotonin and Histamine

Amino Acids
- GABA
- Glycine
- Aspartate
- Glutamate

Neuropeptides
- Substance P
- Endorphins and Enkephalins
- Somatostatin, gastrin, cholecystokinin, oxytocin, vasopressin, luteinizing hormone releasing hormone (LHRH)

TABLE: Blood brain barrier (BBB)

- Membranes are generally **asymmetrical**
- Plasma membranes is composed mainly of **proteins**
- Protein content: **55%**
- Phospholipid: **25% × 42%**, 3% carbohydrate
- Function of phospholipid is **transduction of signals and enzyme activation.**
- Lipids and Proteins in cell membrane interact by **Hydrogen bonds.**
- Fluidity of membranes depends in **lipid content.**
- **Saturated fatty acids** increase transition temperature and decrease fluidity
- **Unsaturated Fatty acids** decrease transition temperature and increase fluidity
- Cerebral blood vessels are unique in that the junctions between vascular endothelial cells are nearly fused. The paucity of pores is responsible for what is termed the **Blood Brain Barrier**
- The lipid barrier allows the passage of lipid soluble substances but restrict movements of those that are ionized or have large molecular weight.
- CO_2, O_2 and lipid soluble substances (such as most anesthetics) freely enter the brain, whereas most ions, proteins and large substances such as mannitol penetrate poorly.

Contd...

Physiology

- Water moves freely across the BBB.
- **Mannitol** an osmotically active substance that does not normally cross the BBB, cause a sustained decrease in brain water content and is often used to decrease brain volume.
- BBB may be disrupted by severe Hypertension, tumors, trauma, stroke, infection, marked hypercapnia, hypoxia and sustained seizure activity.

TABLE: Important tests

Decline in serum Ca²⁺ levels show signs of increasing neuromuscular hyperexcitability followed by hypocalcemic tetany.
  Lab values: Decreased serum Ca²⁺
            Increased serum phosphate
            Decreased urinary Phosphate excretion

Clinical tests for endocrine abnormalities: Radioimmunoassays for T4, T3, TSH, cortisol, Ca²⁺, etc.

Glucose Tolerance test: Check a fasting blood sugar level, then have patient drink a 75 g glucose solution. Re-draw blood at 30 min, 1 hr., and 2 hrs. If blood glucose level is >200 mg/dL at 2 hours, then highly suggestive of diabetes.

Dexamethasone suppression test: Dexamethasone, a synthetic steroid, is given to the patient at 11 p.m. The following day blood samples are collected at 4 p.m. and 11 p.m. The normal response is a decrease in circulating adrenal steroid hormones. Those with Cushing's will have continued elevated levels.

Radioiodine injection: Hyperthyroidism will show an increase uptake.

TABLE: Cells of stomach and their function

- G cells secretes - **Gastrin**
- I cells secretes - **CCK**
- S cells secretes - **Secretin**
- D cells secretes - **Somatostatin**
- Parietal cells secretes - **Intrinsic factor**
- Chief cells secretes - **Pepsin**

IMPORTANT PHYSIOLOGICAL FACTS

In nephron most of the reabsorption occurs at which portion: **PCT (~75%)**

Length of proximal convoluted tubule: **15 mm**

Length of distal convoluted tubule: **5 mm**

Length of collecting duct: **20 mm**

Location of macula densa: **DCT**

ADH produced by- **Supraoptic nucleus of hypothalamus**

Contd...

Oxytocin produced by: Paraventricular nucleus of hypothalamus

Teeth grinding is seen in which stage of sleep: **NREM II**

Night terror is seen in which stage of NREM: **Stage III & IV**

Sleep walking is seen in which stage of NREM: **Stage III & IV**

Other name of alpha wave: **Berger wave (discovered by Hans Berger)**

Best test for sleep disorder: **Polysomnography**

Bohr's effect: Fall in pH due to increase **pCO₂**, decreases oxygen affinity of Hb
Haldane effect: Binding of O₂ to Hb reduces affinity of Hb to **CO₂**.

Most important stimulus for central chemoreceptor: ↑ **PaCO₂ (Inc CO₂, Dec O2)**

Most important stimulus for peripheral chemoreceptor: ↓ **PO₂**, ↑ **CO₂**

The partial pressure of O₂ (PaO₂) at sea level: **160 mm Hg.**
The partial pressure of CO₂ (pCO₂) at sea level: **0.23 mm Hg.**
Mean pulmonary arterial pressure: **16 mm Hg**

Mean pulmonary capillary pressure averages about: **7 mm Hg**.
Mean pressure in the aorta: **100 mm Hg.**
GLUT receptor located on sperm: **GLUT 5**

Alpha cells of pancreas secretes: **Glucagon**
Beta cells of pancreas secretes: **Insulin and amylin**
Delta cells of pancreas secretes: **Somatostatin**

Starch is hydrolyzed in mouth by: **Ptylin**

TABLE: Sleep waves

Wave *(Mn: D-TAB)*	Condition	Frequency
• Delta wave	Deep sleep	0.5 – 3 Hz
• Theta wave	Light sleep	4 – 7 Hz
• Alpha wave	Relaxed, awake	8 – 13 Hz
• Beta wave	Excited, active	14 – 30 Hz

TABLE: Sleep stages

Stage	EEG waves	Eye movement
Awake/alert	Beta (eye open) Alpha (eye closed)	Irregular
I-NREM	Alpha + Theta waves	Burst of rolling
II-NREM	Theta waves Sleep spindles K- complex	Alpha like burst
III-NREM	Theta, Delta synchronization	Fixed
IV-NREM	Delta (slowest wave)	Fixed
REM (paradoxical sleep)	Mixed frequency, Low voltage (theta, alpha > Beta)	Darting movements Active dreaming (+) Nightmares

Key Points

FMGE Solutions Screening Examination

TABLE: Important reflexes

Reflex	Stimulus	Response
Cushing reflex	Inc ICT (> 33 mm Hg)	Inc BP, Bradypnea, Bradycardia
Bainbridge reflex	Atrial distention due to rapid infusion of blood/Saline	Reflex tachycardia
Bezold-Jarisch coronary chemoreflex	5HT injection, Nicotine in coronary artery	Apnea, ↓BP, ↓HR
Hering-Breuer inflation reflex	Steady lung inflation	↑ Expiration
Hering-Breuer inflation reflex	Marked deflation of lung	↓ Expiration

TABLE: Muscle fiber types

Type I	Type II
Oxidative, slow fibers	Glycolytic, fast fibers
Easily excited	Difficult to excite
Less fatigability	More fatigability
Slow glycogen depletion	Fast glycogen depletion
Used in marathon runner	Used in sprinter (100 meter) runner
Major fuel: **ATP**	Major fuel: **Phosphate**

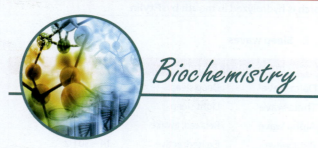

AMINO ACID CLASSIFICATION

• Simple	Glycine, Alanine
• Branched chain	Leucine, Isoleucine, Valine
• Sulphur containing	Cysteine, Methionine
• Hydroxyl containing	Serine, Threonine
• Amide	Glutamine, Asparagine
• Acidic AA	Aspartic acid, Glutamic acid
• Basic AA	Histidine, Arginine, Lysine
• -OH containing	Serine, Threonine, Tyrosine
• Serine analog drugs	Cycloserine, Azaserine

Wernicke encephalopathy is due to deficiency of	• Thiamine
Strenuous exercise is not done in this glycogen storage disease	• Mc Ardle disease
Vitamin which is most potent anti-oxidant	• Vitamin E
Vitamin which helps in iron absorption	• Vitamin C
AA that accelerate ageing	• Homocysteine
AA that decreases ageing	• Cysteine, Taurine
Bend in DNA structure	• Glycine
AA which absorbs UV light	• Tryptophan (Max), Tyrosine, Phenylalanine
MC type of albinism	• OCA 2 (Oculocutaneous Albinism type II)

- Keshan disease is due to deficiency of: **Selenium**
- Kashin-Beck disease: **Due to excess of selenium**
- Menkes disease: **Due to deficiency of copper**
- Acrodermatitis enteropathica: **Due to deficiency of zinc (AR condition)**
- Vitamin having only animal source: **Vitamin B12**
- Vitamin having antioxidant property: **Vitamin E**
- Physiological uncoupler: **Thyroid hormones, unconjugated bilirubin, long chain fatty acid**
- Sickle cell anemia is caused by point mutation in β globin chain
- At 6th position the hydrophilic **glutamic acid gets replaced with valine** (Hydrophobic)
- Hyperammonemia type 1 is due to deficiency of this enzyme: **Carbamoyl Phosphate Synthase I**
- Tomcat urine smell is seen in: **Multiple carboxylase deficiency**
- Boiled cabbage urine smell is seen in: **Hypermethioninemia**
- Smallest and simplest amino acid: **Glycine**
- Storage form of folate: **N-methyl folate**
- Energy for the urea cycle come from: **Fat metabolism**
- Precursor of all sphingolipids: **Ceramide**
- Type of bilirubin is found in neonatal jaundice: **Indirect or unconjugated**
- This amino acid is a phenol: **Tyrosine**
- This vitamin is an important component of rhodopsin: **Vitamin A**
- Part of the 30s ribosome binds to the Shine-Dalgarno sequence: **16s subunit**
- This test is used to determine whether a gene is expressed: **Northern blotting**

Contd...

Biochemistry

- This complex of the ETC contains Cu⁺: **Complex 4**
- Inhibitors of complex IV of the ETC: **1. Cyanide, 2. CO, 3. Azide**
- Gluconeogenesis is inhibited by: **Insulin**
- **Gluconeogenesis** occurs in both cytoplasm and mitochondria
- Mercaptopurine is – **Nucleotide analogue**
- Source of ATP in RBC cell: **EMP pathway**

- Net ATP produced in anaerobic glycolysis: **2 ATP**
- Net ATP produced in aerobic glycolysis: **7 ATP**
- Cancer cells derive nutrition from **glycolysis**.
- Allosteric inhibition is seen in: **G-6-P, F-6-P**
- Erythrocytes lack **mitochondria** (all the cell organelles)
- Fluoroacetate inhibits aconitase enzyme: **Non-competitive reaction**
- Arsenite inhibits alpha-**Ketoglutarate dehydrogenase** enzyme–**Noncompetitive reaction**.
- Malonate inhibits succinate dehydrogenase enzyme– **Competitive reaction**
- Internal respiration is **exergonic** and **catabolic** and it uses **cytochromes b, c1, c, a, a3**
- Von Gierke's disease is due to **G-6-P Deficiency**
- Pompe's disease lysosomal a1-4, a1-6 glucosidase acid maltase deficiency.
- **Mc Ardle's disease** is muscle phosphorylase deficiency.
- **Acetyl CoA** is not a substrate for gluconeogenesis and cannot be converted back to glucose directly.
- **Gaucher disease** is due to Beta Glucocerebrosidase deficiency.
- Foam cells and sphingomyelinase deficiency is seen in **Niemann-Pick disease**
- Type 1 familial hypolipoprotinemia is due to deficiency of **lipoprotein lipase deficiency**.
- Palmitoleic acid is derivative of which family: **ω7 family**
- Lipoprotein which transport cholesterol from liver to plasma: **VLDL**
- Most important apoprotein in HDL: **Apo A-I**
- Most important apoprotein in chylomicrons: **Apo B-48**
- De novo synthesis of fatty acids occurs in the **cytosol**
- Malic enzyme forms malic acid from pyruvic acid in the presence of CO_2 **& NADPH.**
- Long chain fatty acid penetrate the inner mitochondrial membrane only in combination with **carnitine**.
- Beta-oxidation of odd chain fatty acid produces **acetyl CoA propionyl CoA**.

- Refsum's disease occurs due to deficiency of **phytanic alpha oxidase**.
- Alkaptonuria deficiency is: **Homogentisate oxidase**
- **Liver** is the only organ which produces ketone bodies (but never utilizes it)
- **Gout** is metabolic disorder of purine metabolism.
- Mutation in sickle cell disease: **Base pair substitution**
- **LDL** has maximum cholesterol content
- Conversion of norepinephrine to epinephrine: **Demethylation**
- Enzyme required for demethylation: **Phenylethanolamine-N-methyltransferase**
- Enzyme is used to convert phenylalanine to tyrosine: **Phenylalanine hydroxylase**
- Beta oxidation of odd chain fatty acid produces: **Acetyl CoA and Propionyl CoA**
- Complete HGPRT deficiency cause **Lesch-Nyhan syndrome**
- Partial HGPRT deficiency causes **Kelley-Seegmiller syndrome**
- Normal growth require **proto-oncogenes** not oncogenes
- DNA ligase and primase are used in **DNA replication**
- The **sigma sub unit** enables RNA polymerase to recognize promoter regions on DNA.
- **Template** is required for protein and nucleic acid synthesis
- Alzheimer's, cystic fibrosis and prion diseases occur due to **protein misfolding**
- **Microsatellites** are tandem repeats of one to six nucleotide scattered throughout the genome.
- After digestion by restriction endonucleases the DNA ends can be ligated by **DNA-ligase**.
- **DNA microarrays** is used for detection in DNA sequences and Gene expression.
- Proline and glycine have the least tendency to form **Alpha-helix**.
- Structural proteins are usually fibrous proteins, transport and functional protein are usually **globular**
- Simple globular proteins are **albumin and globulin**.
- Adenyl cyclase, guanylate cyclase and glycogen synthase enzymes are activated by **calcium and calmodulin**.
- **Phenylketonuria** is caused by deficiency of phenylalanine hydroxylase & dihydrobiopterin reductase.
- **Alkaptonuria** is due to defective homogentisate 1, 2-dioxygenase.
- Maple syrup urine disease is deficiency of branched chain **alpha keto acid dehydrogenase**.
- **Succinyl CoA** is formed by valine, isoleusine, methionine.

Contd...

Contd...

Key Points

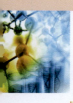

FMGE Solutions Screening Examination

- **Niacin** in biologically active form of NAD+ & NADP+.
- **Vit A** intoxication leads to demineralization of bone, hypercalcemia, hyperostosis.
- **ATP** is used in a set of reactions that converts chemical energy into light energy.
- **Cobalt** containing vit B12 is found only in food of animal origin and is absorbed from distal ileum.
- **Vitamin B12** & **folic acid** supplements treat pernicious anemia by increasing DNA synthesis in bone marrow
- Niacin sparing amino acid: **Tryptophan**
- Which bases are purine? **Adenine and Guanine**
- Which bases are pyrimidines? **Cytosine, Uracil, Thymine**
- What enzyme is deficient in Severe Combined Immunodeficiency Disease (SCID)?
- Adenosine Deaminase
- The start codon AUG codes for which amino acid? **Methionine**
- Which RNA is the most abundant?: **rRNA – (Mn: r = rampant)**
- Which RNA is the longest? **mRNA – (Mn: M = massive)**
- Which RNA is the smallest? **tRNA – (Mn: t = tiny)**
- Which organelle is the site for labeling specific proteins for the lysosome? **Golgi apparatus**
- What type of collagen makes the basement membrane? **Type IV**
- Collagen is loaded with tons of which amino acids? **Proline and Lysine**
- What enzyme is deficient in Fructose Intolerance? **Aldolase B**
- What enzyme is deficient in Essential Fructosuria? **Fructokinase**
- Tyrosinemia types and Enzyme defect
  - I: **Fumarylacetoacetate hydroxylase** (hepatorenal)
  - II: **tyrosine transaminase** (oculocutaneous)
  - III: **PHPP hydroxylase** (neonatal)

Nitisinone acts by inhibiting this enzyme Tyrosine → PHPP → Homogentisic acid	**Parahydroxyphenyl Pyruvate Hydroxylase** To treat hereditary tyrosinemia type I, Alkaptonuria
Folate trap is due to deficiency of	B12
Folate trap increases the risk of this disease	Acute coronary syndrome
Calcium acts as cofactor for which enzymes	Lipase, Lecithinase
Copper acts as cofactor for this enzyme	Cyt C oxidase, Lysil oxidase, AA oxidase, SOD, Tyrosinase
Iron acts as cofactor for this enzyme	Succinate DeH
Zinc acts as cofactor for these enzymes	ALD, ALP, ALA dehydratase, carbonic anhydrase, LDH

TABLE: Special group attached with amino acids

Amino Acid	Special group
Arginine	Guanidinium
Phenylalanine	Benzene
Tyrosine	Phenol
Histidine	Imidazole
Proline	Pyrrolidine
Methionine	Thioether linkage
Tryptophan	Indole
Cysteine	Thioalcohol (-SH)

TABLE: Pathways and their rate limiting enzymes

Pathway	Rate limiting enzyme
• Glycolysis	Phosphofructokinase
• Glycogenesis	Glycogen synthase
• Glycogenolysis	Phosphorylase
• Cholesterol synthesis	HMG - COA Reductase
• Ketone body formation	HMG - COA synthase
• Bile acid synthesis	7-a-hydroxylase
• Fatty acid synthesis	Acetyl COA carboxylase
• Uric acid synthesis	Xanthine oxidase
• Urea cycle	CPS I
• Pyrimidine synthesis	CPS II

TABLE: Cycles and their location

Mitochondria Mn: KEBOK	Cytoplasm	Both mitochondria and cytoplasm
Krebs cycle	Glycolysis	Gluconeogenesis
ETC	Glycogenesis	Urea synthesis
Bet oxidation of FA	Glycogenolysis	Heme synthesis
Oxidative phosphorylation	HMP Shunt	
Ketogenesis	FA synthesis	
	Cholesterol synthesis	
	Bile acid/Salt synthesis	

TABLE: GLUT receptors, their location and function

Receptor	Location on tissue	Function
GLUT 1	Brain, kidney, colon, placenta, RBC	Glucose uptake
GLUT 2	Liver, pancreatic beta cell, small intestine, Kidney	Rapid uptake or release of glucose

Contd...

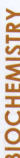

Biochemistry

Receptor	Location on tissue	Function
GLUT 3	Brain, kidney and placenta	Glucose uptake
GLUT 4	Heart, skeletal muscles, adipose tissue	Insulin-stimulated glucose uptake
GLUT 5	Small intestine	Absorption of glucose

TABLE: Lysosomal storage disease and deficient enzymes

- Hurler's syndrome: **Alpha-L-iduronidase deficiency**
- Hunter's syndrome: **Iduronate-2-sulfatase deficiency**
- Gaucher's: **Glucocerebrosidase deficiency**
- Farber's disease: **Ceramidase deficiency**
- Fabry disease: **Alpha Galactosidase-A**
- Tay-sachs: **Hexosaminidase A deficiency**
- Sandhoff disease: **β-Hexosaminidase A and B**
- Metachromatic leukodystrophy: **Arylsulfatase A enzyme deficiency**
- Krabbe disease: **Galactocerebrosidase**

MAJOR APOLIPOPROTEINS

- **Chylomicron:** A, B48, CII, E *(least protein, max size, max density)*
- **VLDL:** Apo B100, CII, E
- **LDL:** Apo B100
- **HDL:** Apo A1

TABLE: Source of energy during starvation

STAGE	I	II	III
Duration	1st 2–3 days	Up to 2 weeks (longest)	<1 week
Energy source	Carbohydrate	Fats	Proteins
Metabolism	Initially Glycogenolysis then gluconeogenesis	Lipolysis and ketone body formation	Breakdown of protein

TABLE: Amino acid at a glance: total AA = 20 in number

Essential AA (8): *Can't be synthesized.* *(Mn: TV TILL 8 PM)*	Semi-essential AA: *Can be synthesized under normal condition as per demand.*	Non-Essential AA: *synthesized in body readily*
Threonine, Valine, Tryptophan, Isoleucine, Lysine, Leucine, Phenylalanine, Methionine	Histidine Arginine	The remaining 10 AA are Non-essential.

TABLE: Vitamin B, their other names and disease entities due to deficiency

Vitamin	Other name	Deficiency causes
Vit B1	Thiamine	***Beriberi,*** *Wernicke's encephalopathy*
Vit B2	Riboflavin	Angular stomatitis, cheilosis, dermatitis, Glossitis
Vit B3	Niacin	Pellagra (4D's- Dementia, Diarrhea, Dermatitis, Death)
Vit B5	Pantothenic acid	Burning foot syndrome, Leiner disease
Vit B6	Pyridoxine	Peripheral neuropathy, Sideroblastic anemia, Pellagra, Homocystinuria, Hartnup disease
Vit B7	Biotin	Multiple carboxylase deficiency
Vit B9	Folic acid	Megaloblastic anemia, Neural tube defect
Vit B12	Cyano-cobalamin	Megaloblastic anemia, subacute combined degeneration (SACD)

TABLE: Forms of Vitamin K

Feature	Vitamin K1	Vitamin K2	Vitamin K3
Aka	Phylloquinone	Menaquinone	Menadione
Source	Several green vegetables and prepared synthetically	Synthesized by GI bacteria, supplies 50% human requirement	Synthetic, Analog of 1, 4-naphthoqui-none
Solubility	Fat soluble	Fat soluble	Diphosphate salt is Water soluble

TABLE: Urea cycle and their associated enzyme defect

Disease condition	Enzyme defect
• Hyperammonemia I	CPS I defect
• Hyperammonemia II	OTC defect
• Citrullinemia I	Argininosuccinate synthase
• Argininosuccinic aciduria	Argininosuccinate lyase
• Hyperargininemia	Arginase
• HHH Syndrome	Ornithine transporter defect

TABLE: Inborn error of metabolism and urine odor

IEM	Urine odor
• Swimming pool	Hawkinsinuria
• PKU	Mousy/musty

Contd...

FMGE Solutions Screening Examination

IEM	Urine odor
• Glutaric acidemia	Sweaty feet, acrid
• Isovaleric acidemia	Sweaty feet, acrid
• MSUD	Maple syrup
• Hypermethioninemia	Boiled cabbage
• Trimethylaminuria	Rotting fish
• Tyrosinemia	Boiled cabbage, rancid butter

TABLE: Maple syrup urine disease types and their associated enzyme defect

Gene	Component	MSUD types
E1a	Branched chain alpha keto acid decarboxylase	Type Ia MSUD
E1b	Branched chain alpha keto acid decarboxylase	Type Ib MSUD
E2	Dihydrolipoyl transacylase	Type II MSUD
E3	Dihydrolipoamide dehydrogenase	Type III MSUD

TABLE: Inhibitors of electron transport chain

Complex	Inhibitors
• Complex I	Rotenone, Piericidin A, Amobarbital
• Complex II	Malonate, TTFA
• Complex III	BAL, Antimycin A, Naphthoquinone
• Complex IV	Na azide, HCN, CO
• Complex V	Atractyloside, Oligomycin

IMPORTANT TESTS AND THEIR APPLICATION

- **Murexide test:** Uric acid
- **Rothera test:** Ketone body
- **Biuret test:** Detect maximum 2 peptide bond
- **Hopkins cole test:** Tryptophan
- **Millions test:** Tyrosine
- **Gerhardt test:** Acetoacetic acid
- **Hay test:** Bile salt
- **Fouchet's test:** Bile pigment
- **Ehrlich test:** Urobilinogen
- **Molisch test:** for CHO
- **Guthrie FeCl$_3$ test:** PKU
- **Ames test:** Carcinogenicity due to salmonella typhimurium

TABLE: Must know points about porphyria

- MC type of porphyria: **Porphyria cutanea tarda**
- MC acute porphyria: **Acute intermittent porphyria**
- MC porphyria in child: **Erythropoietic protoporphyria**
- Erythropoietic porphyria: **Usual clinical presentation photosensitivity**
- Hepatic porphyria with cutaneous manifestation: **PCT**

FLOWCHART: Porphyria and their enzyme defect

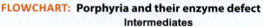

Intermediates	Enzymes	Diseases
Glycine + Succinyl CoA ↓ δ-Aminolevulinic acid	δ-Aminolevulinic acid synthase	Sideroblastic anemia (X-linked)
↓ Porphobilinogen	δ-Aminolevulinic acid dehydratase	ALAD-Deficient Porphyria
↓ Hydroxymethylbilane	Porphobilinogen deaminase	Acute intermittent porphyria
(Nonenzymatic) → Uroporphyrinogen I → Coproporphyrinogen I / Uroporphyrinogen III	Uroporphyrinogen III cosynthase	Congenital erythropoietic porphyria
↓ Coproporphyrinogen III	Uroporphyrinogen decarboxylase	Porphyria cutanea tarda
↓ Protoporphyrinogen IX	Coproporphyrinogen Oxidase	Hereditary coproporphyria
↓ Protoporphyrin IX Fe^{2+}	Protoporphyrinogen oxidase	Variegate porphyria
↓ Heme	Ferrochelatase	Erythropoietic protoporphyria

Photo courtesy of UTMB Preventative Medicine & Community Health, Porphyria Laboratory, University of Texas Medical Branch, Galveston Texas

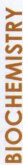

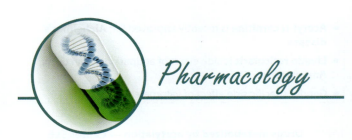

Pharmacology

PHARMACOLOGY—AT A GLANCE

- Phase of clinical trial which recruits healthy human volunteers: **Phase 0**
- Clinical trial to assess safety and non-toxicity: **Phase I**
- Number of patients in Phase II clinical trial: **20–200**
- Ethical clearance is not required for which phase of clinical trial: **Phase 4**
- Drugs are tested on healthy human volunteers in which phase of clinical trial: **Phase 1 and Phase 0**
- Phase which is dealing with microdosing: **Phase 0**
- Phase V clinical trial is: **Pharmacoepidemiology**
- **Maximum** parasympathetic outflow by which cranial nerve: **CN-X**
- 100% Bioavailability is seen with this route: **I.V. route**
- **Area under curve** denotes: **Bioavailability**
- **Bioavailability** is the fraction of administered drug that reaches the systemic circulation in the unchanged form.
- **Absorption and first pass mechanism** are two important Determinants of bioavailability.
- Shortest acting steroid: **Hydrocortisone**
- Formoterol and Indacaterol: **Long acting Beta 2 agonist (Bronchodilator)**
- Antiepileptic with highest teratogenic potential: **Sodium Valproate**
- Drug of choice for cardiogenic shock: **Dobutamine**
- DOC for neurogenic diabetes insipidus: **Desmopressin**
- Shortest acting mydriatic agent: **Tropicamide (t1/2: 6 hrs)**
- Cycloplegic agent of choice in child: **Atropine 1% ointment**
- Fastest acting insulin: Insulin **Aspart**
- Peakless insulin: **Glargine**
- Physiological antagonism of Histamine: **Adrenaline**
- Preferred agent for treatment of ventricular arrhythmia: **Lignocaine**
- DOC for diabetic diarrhea: **Clonidine**
- DOC for brucellosis: **Doxycycline**
- DOC for Schistosomiasis: **Praziquantel**

Contd...

- DOC for nasal carriers of MRSA: **Mupirocin**
- DOC for motion sickness: **Hyoscine**
- Side effect of aminoglycoside: **Nephrotoxicity and Ototoxicity**
- DOC for malignant hyperthermia: **Dantrolene**
- Cardiotoxic anesthetic agent: **Etomidate**
- Cevimeline is used for: **Xerostomia in Sjögren's syndrome**
- Urine should be alkalinized for acid drug poisoning and acidified for **alkaline poisoning**.
- Drugs having **steep DRC** have narrow therapeutic index
- **Pharmacovigilance** is the science and activities relating to the detection, assessment, understanding and prevention of adverse effect of any other possible drug related problems.
- **Ach** is the principle neurotransmitter at neuromuscular junctions as well as pre-ganglionic fibers.
- Rate limiting step in the **biosynthesis of ach: Uptake of choline**
- Most common class of drug for causing first dose effect: **selective alpha-1 blocker (e.g.: Prazosin)**
- Irreversible alpha-1 adrenoceptor antagonist: **Phenoxybenzamine (DOC for pheochromocytoma)**
- Retrograde ejaculation is a known side effect of: **Alpha 1 blockers (Prazosin, Phentolamine)**
- Vasomotor reversal of dale is seen due to: **Alpha blocker followed by Epinephrine**
- Beta blocker which releases Nitric oxide: **Celiprolol, Nebivolol, Nipradilol** *(CNN)*
- DOC for beta blocker poisoning: **Glucagon**
- DOC for organophosphate poisoning: **Atropine**
- DOC for atropine poisoning: **Physostigmine**
- Pin-point pupil is seen in poisoning with: *(Mn: POMP)*
- Pontine hemorrhage, Organophosphate, Morphine and Phenol poisoning
- **Streptomycin** is contraindicated throughout pregnancy
- Side effect of Streptomycin: Nephrotoxic, Ototoxic, Neuromuscular Junction Blocker
- Low molecular weight heparin affects which factor: **Factor Xa >> IIa**
- All ACE inhibitors are prodrug EXCEPT **Captopril and Lisinopril**
- **Febuxostat:** Anti-gout and Xanthine Oxidase inhibitor
- **Drugs causing disulfiram like reaction:**
- Griseofulvin, Metronidazole, Chlorpropamide, Cefoperazone, Cefotetan, Trimethoprim
- **Atropine** is the antidote for–Organophosphate and carbamate poisoning.

Contd...

Key Points

1269

FMGE Solutions Screening Examination

- **Oximes** are used for Organophosphate poisoning
- Cystoid macular edema in aphakic is caused by **Dipivefrine**.
- New drug approved for over active bladder stimulating β3 receptors – **Mirabegron**.
- DOC for narcolepsy – **Modafinil**
- Antidepressant used for smoking cessation: **Bupropion**
- Treatment of alopecia in males – **Minoxidil**
- Vasopressor of choice in pregnancy – **Ephedrine**
- Most cardio selective Beta blocker – **Nebivolol**
- Longest acting Beta blocker – **Nadolol**
- Maximum membrane stabilizing activity Beta blocker – **Propanolol**
- Earliest appearing adverse effect of digitalis – **Nausea and vomiting**
- Only oral inotropic drug- **Digoxin**
- Most widely used Beta blocker for Congestive heart failure – **Carvedilol**
- **Beta Blockers With Partial Agonistic Activity** (*Remembered as COntain Partial Agonistic Activity*): Celiprolol, Oxprenolol, Pindolol, Alprenolol, Acebutolol
- MOA of hyoscine – **M3 blocker**
- **Mannitol** – Indicated in cerebral edema and is contraindicated in cerebral hemorrhage
- Oral mannitol side effect – **Osmotic diarrhea**
- Zileuton – **LOX inhibitor**
- Selective COX-2 inhibitor: **Etoricoxib**
- **Sodium Cromoglycate** – Mast cell stabilizer
- Most common adverse effect of beta 2 agonist (eg: Salbutamol) – **Tremors**
- **Abciximab** – GpIIb/IIIa blocker
- DOC for GIST & CML– **Imatinib**
- DOC Benign Prostatic hypertrophy: **Tamsulosin**
- MOA finasteride – **5 alpha reductase inhibitor**
- Long acting somatostatin analogue – **Octreotide**
- Funny current blocker drug: **Ivabradine**
- Phosphodiesterase 3 inhibitor used in heart failure: **Amrinone, Milrinone**
- Recently approved PDE3 inhibitor which is also a myocardial Calcium sensitizer: **Levosimendan**
- Cerebroselective calcium channel blocker: **Nimodipine**
- Ranolazine is recently approved for: **Angina**
- Mechanism of action of **Fasudil**: Rho kinase inhibitor
- **Edaravone** is recently approved drug for: **Amyotrophic lateral sclerosis**

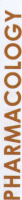

- **Acetyl-N carnitine** is recently approved for: **Alzheimer's disease**
- **Livedo reticularis is** side effect of antiparkinsonian drug: **Amantadine**
- Gender specific side effect of valproate: **PCOS**

TABLE: Drugs metabolized by acetylation → Causes SLE

These drugs are remembered as CHIPS-ABC drugs:
• Clonazepam
• Hydralazine
• Isoniazid
• Procainamide
• Sulfonamides
• Acebutolol, Amrinone, ASA
• Benzocaine
• Caffeine

TABLE: Drugs which are enzyme inducers and enzyme inhibitors

Enzyme inducers	Enzyme inhibitors
• Griseofulvin • Phenytoin • Rifampicin • Smoking • Carbamazepine • Phenobarbitone • Barbiturate • DDT	• Phenylbutazone • Erythromycin • Allopurinol, Amiodarone • Ciprofloxacin • Omeprazole • Cimetidine • Ketoconazole • Valproate
Remembered as: *GPRS Cell Phone Battery Dead*	Mn: PEACOCK Vala

TABLE: Anti-muscarinic drugs used in ophthalmology

Drug	Duration of effect (days)
Atropine	7–10
Scopolamine	3–7
Homatropine	1–3
Cyclopentolate	1
Tropicamide	0.25 days (6 hrs)

TABLE: Side effect of antiepileptic drugs

Drug	Side effect
• Na + Valproate	Hepatotoxicity, Reversible Alopecia, Weight Gain, Tremor, PCOS, Most teratogenic (neural tube defect)
• Phenytoin	Gum hypertrophy, Fetal hydantoin syndrome, megaloblastic anemia

Contd...

Pharmacology

Drug	Side effect
• Carbamazepine	Bone marrow suppression, agranulocytosis, SJS
• Topiramate	Renal stone, Weight loss
• Zonisamide	Renal stone, Weight loss
• Vigabatrin	Visual field defect, Weight gain

TABLE: Drugs of choice *for some commonly asked malignancies: (Harrison 19th ed.)*

Malignancy	First line drugs
Chronic Lymphatic leukaemia	Fludarabine
Chronic Myeloid leukaemia	Imatinib
Hairy cell leukemia	Cladribine
Multiple myeloma	Bortezomib
Choriocarcinoma	Methotrexate
Prostate carcinoma	Bicalutamide/Flutamide

TABLE: Some common side effects of anti-CA drugs

- **Busulfan** & **Bleomycin** – Pulmonary Fibrosis
- **Doxorubicin & Daunorubicin:** Cardiotoxicity
- **Cisplatin** – Ototoxic, Nephrotoxic, Vomiting
- **Vincristine** & **Vinblastine** – Peripheral Neuropathy
- **Ifosfamide, Cyclophosphamide:** Hemorrhagic cystitis
- **6 Mercaptopurine:** Hepatotoxicity

SOME IMPORTANT DRUG OF CHOICE

DOC for acute severe asthma	Salbutamol
DOC for nephrogenic diabetes insipidus	Thiazides
DOC for central diabetes insipidus	Desmopressin
DOC for morning sickness	Doxylamine
DOC for cisplatin induced vomiting	Ondansetron
DOC for delayed vomiting due to cisplatin	Aprepitant
DOC for motion sickness	Hyoscine
DOC for levodopa induced vomiting	Domperidone
DOC for hypertensive emergencies	Nicardipine
DOC for hypertensive emergency in pregnancy	Labetalol
DOC for anaphylactic shock	Adrenaline
DOC for cardiogenic shock with oliguric renal failure	Dopamine
DOC for carcinoma pancreas	Gemcitabine

Contd...

DOC for hairy cell leukemia	Cladribine
DOC for CLL	Fludarabine
DOC choriocarcinoma	Methotrexate
Drug of choice for cyclophosphamide induced hemorrhagic cystitis	Mesna
DOC for glioma	Nitrosourea
DOC colorectal cancer	5 FU
Disulfiram like reaction anti-cancer drug	Procarbazine
Hodgkin's new Regimen (ABVD)	Adriamycin Bleomycin Vinblastine Dacarbazine
Non-Hodgkin's Lymphoma Regimen (R-CHOP)	+/- Rituximab Cyclophosphamide Hydroxydaunorubicin (doxorubicin) Oncovin (Vincristine) Prednisolone
DOC for liver fluke	Triclabendazole
DOC for Dog tape worm/ Echi. Granulosus	Albendazole
DOC for Filarial worm	Diethylcarbamazine (DEC)
DOC for strongyloides and onchocerca	Ivermectin
Oral DOC for scabies	Ivermectin
DOC for scabies	5% Permethrin
DOC for Platyhelminthes	Praziquantel or Niclosamide
Oral DOC for kala-azar	Miltefosine
DOC for Chagas disease	Benznidazole
DOC for dermatophytosis	Systemic Griseofulvin + Topical azole
DOC for candida	Fluconazole
DOC for Aspergillosis	Voriconazole
DOC for P. vivax	Chloroquine
DOC for P. falciparum	ACT
DOC for cerebral malaria	Artesunate
DOC for cerebral malaria during pregnancy	Quinine
DOC in Alzheimer's disease	Donepezil
Drug used in for Alzheimer's disorder	Galantamine/ Rivastigmine/ Donepezil/Memantine

Contd...

Key Points

1271

FMGE Solutions Screening Examination

DOC for OCD	**Fluoxetine**
Newly diagnosed Parkinson disease patient should be started first on:	**Rasagiline** (due to its neuroprotective action- Studies)
DOC for parkinsonism in young	**Ropinirole and Pramipexole**
DOC for drug induced parkinsonism	**Benzhexol**
DOC for paroxysmal supra ventricular tachycardia	**Adenosine**
DOC for Supraventricular Tachycardia	**Verapamil**
DOC for Atrial Fibrillation	**Esmolol**
DOC for digitalis induced ventricular arrhythmia	**Lignocaine**
DOC for torsades de pointes	**Mg⁺**
DOC for morphine poisoning	**Naloxone**
DOC for alcohol withdrawal syndrome	**Benzodiazepines (Chlordiazepoxide)**
DOC for mania	**Lithium**

TABLE: Drug of choice for different seizures

Absence seizures (petit mal)	Na+ valproate
GTCS (Grand mal)	Lamotrigine > Na⁺ Valproate
Focal seizure	Carbamazepine
Myoclonic seizures	Na⁺ Valproate > Lamotrigine
Infantile/salaam seizure	ACTH
Infantile spasm with tuberous sclerosis	Vigabatrin
Febrile seizures	Diazepam (per rectal)
Status epilepticus	Lorazepam (IV)
Eclamptic seizure	Magnesium sulfate
Seizure during pregnancy	Lamotrigine
Neonatal seizure	Phenobarbitone

TABLE: Diuretics their MOA and site of action

Diuretic class	Drugs	MOA	Site of action
Osmotic diuretic	Mannitol	Inhibit water and solute reabsorption	All part of tubule, but mainly proximal tubule
Loop diuretics	Furosemide Torsemide	Inhibit Na⁺-K⁺-2 Cl co-transport	Thick ascending loop of Henle

Contd...

Diuretic class	Drugs	MOA	Site of action
Thiazide diuretic	Hydrochloro-thiazide Benzthiazide Chlorthalidone Indapamide	Inhibit Na⁺- Cl⁻ co-transport	Distal tubule
K⁺ sparing diuretic	Spironolactone Triamterene Amiloride	Decrease Na⁺ reabsorption Decrease K⁺ secretion	Collecting tubule
Carbonic anhydrase inhibitor	Acetazolamide	Inhibit H⁺ secretion and HCO₃ reabsorption, which reduces Na⁺ reabsorption	Proximal tubule

TABLE: Typical antipsychotics and its action on its D receptor

Typical antipsychotics	
Strong D2 blocker	Haloperidol-has maximum risk of EPS Droperidol
Weak D2 blocker	Chlorpromazine Thioridazine – has minimum risk of EPS
Intermediate D2 blocker	Fluphenazine Prochlorperazine

TABLE: Antimicrobials with their mechanism of action

Drugs which inhibit cell wall formation	Drugs which inhibit protein synthesis
Cycloserine Vancomycin Fosfomycin Bacitracin Beta lactam	Tetracycline Chloramphenicol Macrolides (Erythro, Clarithro, Azithro) Clindamycin Streptogramins (Quinupristin + dalfopristin)
Remembered as: <u>C</u>ell <u>V</u>all o<u>F</u> <u>B</u>acteria	<u>T</u>he <u>C</u>hild <u>M</u>ay <u>C</u>limb <u>S</u>tairs

TABLE: Antimicrobials and their side effects

Antimicrobial drugs	Side effects
Chloramphenicol	• Bone marrow suppression • Grey baby syndrome
Tetracycline	• Teeth discoloration and bone growth suppression • Phototoxicity • Fanconi syndrome (in case of expired tetracycline) • Vestibular dysfunction

Contd...

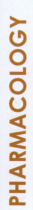

Pharmacology

Antimicrobial drugs	Side effects
Vancomycin	• Red man syndrome • Nephrotoxic and ototoxic
Clindamycin	• Pseudomembranous colitis
Erythromycin estolate	• Cholestasis
Aminoglycosides	• Nephrotoxicity and Ototoxicity

TABLE: Choice of drugs for common problems during pregnancy/safe and unsafe drugs during pregnancy

Drug class (condition)	Unsafe drugs	Safer alternative
Antibacterials	Fluoroquinolones Tetracycline Doxycycline Chloramphenicol Streptomycin Kanamycin Tobramycin	Penicillin G; Ampicillin Amoxicillin-Clavulanate Cloxacillin, Piperacillin Cephalosporins Erythromycin
Antitubercular	Pyrazinamide, Ethambutol Streptomycin	Isoniazid Rifampicin
Anti hypertensives	ACE inhibitors Angiotensin (R) blocker Diuretics Propranolol and nitroprusside	Methyldopa Hydralazine Atenolol, Metoprolol, Pindolol Nifedipine
Antithyroid drugs	Carbimazole Radioactive iodine Iodide	Propylthiouracil (PTU)

TABLE: Recommended doses of antitubercular drug

Drug	Daily dose		3 x per week dose	
	mg/kg	For >50 kg	mg/kg	For >50 kg
Isoniazid (H)	5 (4-6)	300 mg	10 (8-12)	600 mg
Rifampin €	10 (8-12)	600 mg	10 (8-12)	600 mg
Pyrazinamide (Z)	25 (20-30)	1500 mg	35 (30-40)	2000 mg
Ethambutol (E)	15 (15-20)	1000 mg	30 (25-35)	1600 mg

TABLE: Important side effects of antitubercular drugs

Peripheral neuropathy (*due to vit B6 deficiency*): **Isoniazid**	
Orange color urine- **Rifampicin**	

Contd...

Flu-like symptoms- **Rifampicin**	
Hyperuricemia/gout- **Pyrazinamide**	
Optic neuritis/Red green color blindness- **Ethambutol**	
Nephrotoxic, Ototoxic, Neuromuscular Junction Blocker- **Streptomycin**	
Most hepatotoxic ATT: **Pyrazinamide**	
Hypothyroidism: **Ethionamide and PAS**	
Psychotic symptoms: **Cycloserine**	

TABLE: Antiplatelet drugs and their target of inhibition

Antiplatelet drugs	Target of inhibition
Aspirin	Inhibit TXA_2 (Thromboxane A_2) release
Terutroban	TXA_2 receptor blocker
Clopidogrel and Ticlopidine	Inhibit ADP receptor P2Y12 irreversibly
Cangrelor, Ticagrelor	Reversible inhibitor of P_2Y_{12}
Abciximab Tirofiban Eptifibatide	Inhibit GP IIb/IIIa
Atopaxar, Vorapaxar	Thrombin Inhibitor
Heparin	AT3 mediated IIa and Xa inhibition
Low molecular weight heparin (Enoxaparin, Dalteparin, Tinzaparin)	AT3 mediated Xa >> IIa inhibition
Fondaparinux	AT3 mediated Xa inhibition
Hirudin, Lepirudin	Direct thrombin inhibitor

TABLE: Oral hypoglycemic agents

Drugs		Remark
Oral glucose-lowering agents		
Biguanides (Metformin)	• Therapy of type 2 diabetes • Usually initial agent in type 2 diabetes	• Reduce hepatic glucose production • Weight neutral • Do not cause hypoglycemia • Adverse events include diarrhea, nausea, lactic acidosis (black-box warning) • Use cautiously in renal insufficiency, • Avoid use in patents with hepatic dysfunction

Contd...

Key Points

1273

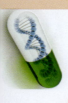
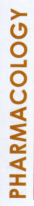

FMGE Solutions Screening Examination

Drugs		Remark
α-Glucosidase inhibitors Acarbose, miglitol, voglibose	• Therapy of type 2 diabetes	• Reduce carbohydrate breakdown in GI tract • **Adverse effects:** GI flatulence, elevated liver function tests • Can be combined with other agents • Relatively modest glucose lowering
Dipeptidyl peptidase 4 inhibitors Sitagliptin, Saxagliptin, Linagliptin, Alogliptin, Vildagliptin	• Therapy of type 2 diabetes	• Prolong action of GLP-1; Promotes insulin secretion • Can be combined with other agents • Relatively modest glucose lowering
Insulin secretagogues: Sulfonylureas **Second generation:** Glyburide, Glibenclamide, Glipizide, and other	• Therapy of type 2 diabetes	• Stimulate insulin secretion • Major adverse events is hypoglycemia • Adjustments needed in renal/liver disease • 2nd gen are more potent, may have better safety profile than first-generation agents. • Can be combined with other agents • Modest weight gain
Insulin secretagogues-nonsulfonylureas Repaglinide, nateglinide	• Therapy of type 2 diabetes	• Increase insulin secretion, quicker onset and shorter duration than sulfonylureas • Major adverse event: Hypoglycemia
SLGT2 inhibitors Canagliflozin, Dapagliflozin, Empagliflozin	• Therapy of type 2 diabetes	• Prevent glucose reabsorption and promote renal glucose excretion • Mild weight loss and BP reduction • Do not cause hypoglycemia • May increase rate of lower urinary tract and genital mycotic infections, hypotension, and DKA

Contd...

Drugs		Remark
Thiazolidinediones Rosiglitazone, Pioglitazone	• Therapy of type 2 diabetes	• Increase insulin sensitivity • Adverse effects: Peripheral edema, CHF, weight gain, fractures, macular edema • Use with caution in CHF, liver disease
GLP-1 agonists Albiglutide, dulaglutide, exenatide, liraglutide	• Therapy of type 2 diabetes	• Increase Insulin secretion, Decrease gastric emptying, Decrease glucagon • Injected subcutaneously • Often associated with weight loss • Adverse events include nausea • Do not use with agents that decrease GI motility • Risk of hypoglycemia with insulin
Amylin analogue Pramlintide	• Adjunctive therapy with insulin in type 1 and type 2 diabetes	• Slows gastric emptying, decreases glucagon • Injected subcutaneously • Decrease postprandial glycemia • Often associated with weight loss • Risk of hypoglycemia with insulin

TABLE: Hypolipidemic drugs

Drug	Mechanism of action
Statins (simvastatin, rosuvastatin)	HMG-CoA reductase inhibitor
Fibrates (clofibrate, fenofibrate, gemfibrozil)	PPAR-alpha agonist
Cholestyramine, colestipol, colesevelam	Bile acid sequestrant
Ezetimibe	Inhibit cholesterol absorption

Contd...

Pharmacology

Drug	Mechanism of action
Alirocumab, evolocumab	PCK-K9 inhibitor
Lomitapide	Microsomal TG transfer protein inhibitor
Torcetrapib, anacetrapib	Cholesteryl Ester Transfer Protein inhibitor
Mipomersen	Apolipoprotein B 100 synthesis inhibitor
Volanesorsen	Apolipoprotein C-III synthesis inhibitor

TARGETED ANTI-CA THERAPY

Class	Drugs	Use
Proteosome inhibitor	BORTEZOMIB, CARFILZOMIB, IXAZOMIB — it inhibits NF-KB which does the cell division	MM
PARP inhibitor	OLAPARIB, RUCAPARIB, NIRAPARIB	BRCA # Ovarian CA
CDK inhibitor	Inhibits CDK 4 and 6 both	Breast CA
Tyrosine kinase inhibitor	Imatinib	DOC for CML & GIST
	Lapatinib	Breast CA
	Sorafenib	Hepatocellular CA
	Sunitinib	Renal cell CA
	Vandetanib	Medullary CA thyroid

IMPORTANT MAB AND THEIR USE

• Palivizumab	RSV
• Eculizumab	PNH
• Omalizumab, Mepolizumab, Reslizumab	Bronchial asthma
• Daratumumab	MM
• Cetuximab	Recurrent head & neck CA
• Rituximab	CLL and NHL

DRUG USED IN MEDICALECTOMIES

• Labyrinthectomy	Gentamicin
• Adernalectomy	Mitotane, Metyrapone, Aminoglutetheimide, Ketocon
• Prostatectomy (Androgen Ablation)	Bicalutamide (LHRH agonist)
• Castration (orchidectomy/oophorectomy)	GnRH analogue (Goserelin, Buserelin, Leuprolide)
• Pancreatectomy	Streptozotocin, Alloxan

AGENTS USED IN GOUT AND RHEUMATOID ARTHRITIS

• DOC for acute gouty arthritis	• **NSAIDS (except Aspirin)**
• DOC for chronic gout	• **DOC: Allopurinol (Xanthine oxidase inhibitor)** • **Febuxostat (if allergy w/ Allopurinol)**
• Uricosuric agent used in gouty arthritis	• **Probenecid, Sulfinpyrazone, Lesinurad, Benzbromarone**
• DOC for Rheumatoid arthritis	• **Mtx**
• Calcineurin inhibitor causing gum hypertrophy and Hirsutism	• **Cyclosporine**
• Fastest acting anti rheumatoid agent	• **Leflunomide**
• **TNFα inhibitor**	• Adalimumab, certolizumab, Etanercept, Infliximab, Golimumab
• IL-1 R#	• ANAKINRA
• IL-2#	• DACLIZUMAB • BASILIXIMAB
• IL-6 R#	• TOCILIZUMAB
• **Costimulation inhibitor**	• Abatacept • Belatacept (b/w CD 80 & 28)
• **Calcineurin inhibitor:**	• **Cyclosporine, Tacrolimus**
• **Mtor inhibitor**	• **SIROLIMUS, EVEROLIMUS**

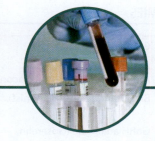

Pathology

• Number of DNA base pairs in human genome	3.2 billion DNA Base pairs
• Total Number of genome that is encoding protein in human	20,000
• Mobile genetic element/Jumping genes	Transposons (1/3rd of human genome)
• Person to person variation (susceptibility to diseases, drug action) in genome	1.5% (represents 15 million base pairs)
• MC forms of DNA variation	SNP and CNV (single nucleotide polymorphism and Copy number variation)
• Function of PDGF	Chemotactic for neutrophils, macrophages Stimulate proliferation of fibroblast Stimulate ECM protein synthesis
• MC adhesion molecule for Diapedesis	PECAM/CD 31
• VEGF that stimulate embryonic vessel development	VEGF-B
• VEGF that causes Lymphangiogenesis	VEGF-C and D
• Maximum volume of cell contributed by	Cytosol (54%)
• Number of mitochondria/cell	1700
• Most abundant glycoprotein in basement membrane	Laminin

IMPORTANT POINTS ON NECROSIS

• MC type of necrosis/cell death due to sudden occlusion of blood supply	Coagulative necrosis
• Primary mechanism of coagulative necrosis	Denaturation of I/C proteins
• Primary mechanism of liquifactive necrosis	Enzymatic digestion of cell
• Solid organ where ischemic necrosis is liquifactive	Brain
• Variants of coagulative necrosis	Caseous necrosis, gangrene
• Caseous necrosis is caused by	TB (most common), syphilis, fungal (Histoplasmosis, Coccidioidomycosis)
• Malignant hypertension causes this type of necrosis	Fibrinoid necrosis

NECROPTOSIS VS PYROPTOSIS

• **Necroptosis** (programmed necrosis)	• Resembles necrosis morphologically and apoptosis mechanistically • Caspase independent programmed cell death → Triggered from signaling by RIP1 and RIP3 complex → reduces mt.ATP gen, production of ROS, inc permeability of lysosomal membrane → cellular swelling and membrane damage **Necroptosis is seen in: (RAPS)** • Reperfusion injury • Acute pancreatitis • Parkinson's disease • Steatohepatitis • Backup defence against CMV (they encode caspase inhibitors)
• **Pyroptosis**	• Occurs in cells infected with microbes • Involves activation of caspase-1 → Activate IL-1 • IL 1 and IL11 → causes cell death of infected death • Characterized by swelling of cells, loss of plasma membrane integrity, and release of inflammatory mediators

Most common mediastinal tumor: Thymoma (anterior mediastinum)
Most common middle mediastinal tumor: Lymphoma
Most common middle mediastinal mass: Pericardial cyst
Cancer associated with Epstein-Barr virus:
- Nasopharyngeal Carcinoma
- Burkitt's lymphoma
- Hodgkin's disease

Caseous necrosis is seen in organ in which organ: Lung (Tuberculosis)
Viral infection causing genial CA: HPV

Contd...

Pathology

Trilateral retinoblastoma involves: Bilateral eye retinoblastoma plus pinealoblastoma

Most common source of brain metastasis: Lung

Thyroid CA associated with pheocromocytoma and hyperparathyroidism: Medullary cancer thyroid (MEN IIa)

India ink is used for diagnosing: Cryptococcus neoformans

Patau syndrome is: Trisomy 13

Edward syndrome: Trisomy 18

Down syndrome: Trisomy 21

Pitting is: Removal of nuclei from old RBC's by the spleen without destroying the cell, and the cell send back plasma circulation.

Culling is defined as: Removal of abnormal RBC form the blood by spleen

Removal of worm out and abnormal RBC's and platelets from the bloodstream by phagocyte cells in the spleen is: Phagocytosis

Highly aggressive lung cancer with rapid doubling capability and metastasis: Small cell lung CA

Type of necrosis seen in Brain pathology: Liquefactive necrosis

MC urinary bladder CA: Transitional cell CA

GITTRE CELLS are modified CNS macrophages

Acrocentric chromosomes are: 13, 14, 15, 21, 22, Y

Pregnancy tumor of gums: Granuloma pyogenicum

Grawitz tumor is also known as Hypernephroma/RCC

HPE finding of type IV lupus nephritis: Wire loop lesions

Noonan syndrome has phenotype similar to: Turner syndrome

Largest gene: Dystrophin gene

Partial trisomy of chromosome 22: Cat eye syndrome

Garland triad aka 1-2-3 sign is suggestive of: Thoracic sarcoidosis

Coast of California sign is seen in: Neurofibromatosis

Accordion sign seen in: Pseudomembranous colitis

Rosenthal fibers in affected brain is characteristic of-Alexander's disease

Bear paw sign is seen in: Xanthogranulomatous pyelonephritis

Subendothelial Deposits are seen in SLE patients

- Necroptosis resembles necrosis morphologically and apoptosis mechanistically as a form of programmed cell death.
- Necroptosis is triggered by ligation of TNFR1, and viral proteins of RNA and DNA viruses.
- Pyroptosis occurs in cells infected by microbes. It involves activation of caspase-1 which cleaves the precursor form of IL-1 to generate biologically active IL-1. Caspase-1 along with closely related caspase-11 also cause death of the infected cell.

Contd...

- Autophagy is an adaptive response to enhanced nutrient deprivation and involves sequestration of cellular organelles into cytoplasmic autophagic vacuoles (autophagosomes) that fuse with lysosomes and digest the enclosed material.
- Location of selectins
  - **L- selectin:** Leucocytes, monocytes, T cell, B cell
  - **E selectin:** Endothelium activated by cytokines
  - **P selectin:** endothelium activated by cytokines (TNF, IL1), Histamine, platelets

Chédiak-Higashi syndrome: Decreased leukocyte functions because of mutations affecting protein involved in lysosomal membrane traffic

Chronic granulomatous disease: Due to decreased oxidative burst

TABLE: Classification of Ehlers-Danlos syndromes

EDS Type	Clinical findings	Inheritance
Classic (VII)	Skin and joint hypermobility, atrophic scars, easy bruising	Autosomal dominant
Hypermobility (III)	Joint hypermobility, pain, dislocations	Autosomal dominant
Vascular (IV)	Thin skin, arterial or uterine rupture, bruising, small joint hyperextensibility	Autosomal dominant
Kyphoscoliosis (VI)	Hypotonia, joint laxity, congenital scoliosis, ocular fragility	Autosomal dominant
Arthrochalasis (VIIa, b)	Severe joint hypermobility, skin changes (mild), scoliosis, bruising	Autosomal dominant
Dermatosparaxis (VIIc)	Severe skin fragility, cutis laxa, bruising	Autosomal dominant

TABLE: Examples of trinucleotide repeat mutations

Disease	Repeated nucleotide	Number of repeats
Fragile X syndrome	CGG	55-200 (pre); >230 (full)
Friedreich ataxia	GAA	34-80 (pre); >100 (full)
Myotonic dystrophy	CTG	34-80 (pre); >100 (full)
Spinobulbar muscular atrophy (Kennedy disease)	CAG	38-62
Huntington disease	CAG	36-121

Key Points

FMGE Solutions Screening Examination

TABLE: Mechanisms of hypersensitivity reactions

Type	Immune mechanisms	Prototypical disorders
Immediate (type I) hypersensitivity	Production of IgE antibody → immediate release or vasoactive amines and other mediators from mast cells; later recruitment of inflammatory cells	Anaphylaxis; allergies; bronchial asthma (atopic forms)
Antibody-mediated (type II) hypersensitivity	Production of IgG → binds to antigen on target cell or tissue → phagocytosis or lysis or target cell by activated complement or Fc receptors; recruitment or leukocytes	Autoimmune hemolytic anemia; goodpasture syndrome
Immune complex—mediated (type III) hypersensitivity	Deposition of antigen-antibody complexes → complement activation → recruitment of leukocytes by complement products and Fc receptors → release of enzymes and other toxic molecules	Systemic lupus erythematosus; some forms of glomerulonephritis; serum sickness; Arthus reaction
Cell-mediated (type IV) hypersensitivity	Activated T lymphocytes → (1) release of cytokines, inflammation and macrophage activation; (2) T cell-mediated cytotoxicity	Contact dermatitis; multiple sclerosis; type 1 diabetes; tuberculosis

NEPHROPATHY AND HPE FINDINGS

HPE finding	Associated abnormality
Subepithelial Humps	Acute Poststreptococcal Glomerulonephritis
Linear Subendothelial deposits	Goodpasture syndrome (Type II)
Mesangial deposits	IgA Nephropathy
Spike and dome shaped deposits	Membranous nephropathy
Subendothelial humps	Membranoproliferative glomerulonephritis
Holly leaf mesangial deposits	FSGS

MEN SYNDROMES

Type (Chromosomal location)	Tumors	Remark
MEN 1 (11q13)	• Parathyroid adenoma (90%) • Entropancreatic tumors (30-70%) • Pituitary adenoma (15-50%)	• Overall MC type of MEN1 is Parathyroid adenoma • MC enteropancreatic tumor is: Gastrinoma (>50%) • VIPoma is least common type of enteropancreatic tumor (<1%) • MCC of pituitary adenoma is Prolactinoma
MEN 2A	• Medullary CA thyroid (90%) • Pheochromocytoma (10-50%) • Parathyroid adenoma (>25%)	
MEN 2B Aka MEN 3	• Medullary CA thyroid (>90%) • Pheochromocytoma (>50%) • Associated abnormalities (40-50%) • Mucosal neuroma • Marfanoid habitus • Megacolon • Medullated corneal nerve fibers	
MEN 4	• Parathyroid adenoma • Pituitary adenoma • Reproductive organ tumors *(testicular cancers, neuroendocrine cervical CA).*	

- Most common cause of cell injury is – **Hypoxia**
- Most common cause of hypoxia – **Ischemia**
- Most common and sensitive cells in the body damaged due to hypoxia – **Neurons**
- Cytochrome C plays an important role in: **Apoptosis**
- Not a cellular adaptation: **Necrosis**.
- Barrett's esophagus is an example of: **Metaplasia**.
- Myelin figures are derived from: **Damaged cell membrane**.
- H_2O_2 is produced as well as destroyed in: **Peroxisome**.
- **CNS** – liquefactive necrosis (only solid organ where liquefactive necrosis seen)
- **TB**- caseous necrosis
- Most characteristic **feature of apoptosis** – Absence of inflammation and intact cell membrane
- Important indicator of free radical injury – **Lipofuscin** (alveolar wall)
- Myositis ossificans – Connective tissue metaplasia

Contd...

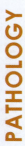

Pathology

- Most common site for metastatic calcification – **Lungs**
- **Haber-Weiss reaction is:** Generation of free radical from H_2O_2.
- **Fenton Reaction** – $H_2O_2 + Fe^{2+} \rightarrow Fe^{2+} + OH + OH$
- The most common fixative for light microscope is – **10% neutral buffered formalin**
- The most common fixative for electron microscope is – **Glutaraldehyde**
- Hall mark of acute inflammation – **Increased vascular permeability**
- Formation of endothelial gaps – **Mechanism of increased vascular permeability**
- Rolling of neutrophils done by – **Selectins**
- Leukocytes with giant granules in peripheral blood smear seen in – **Chédiak–Higashi syndrome**
- Eosinophils have major basic protein which is toxic to **parasites**
- Most important chemical mediators of acute inflammation – **Histamine**
- Most potent **microbicidal system** – oxygen dependent MPO system, NADPH oxidase / Respiratory burst
- Most important fibrogenic agent → **TGF – beta**
- **SRS** – A components – LTB4 & LTC4
- Most common complement deficiency associated with **Streptococcal septicemia** and **lupus** like syndrome in children – Deficiency of C2
- Chemotactic for neutrophils – **IL 8**
- Most common type of inflammation - **Catarrhal inflammation**
- **Vitamin K** dependent clotting factors – 2, 7, 9, 10, protein C & S
- **Functions of bradykinin**
  - Contraction of smooth muscles (bronchospasm, vasospasm of muscular arteries)
  - Pain
  - Dilation of the venules
- Monocytes and macrophages are the primary leukocytes in **chronic inflammation**
- Epithelioid cells are macrophages activated by **INF – Gamma**
- Granulation tissue is the hallmark of – **Fibrogenic repair**
- Severe generalized edema is called – **Anasarca**
- Hemosiderin laden macrophages (heart failure cells) found in **Lung**
- **Bernard–Soulier syndrome** – A defect in the glycoprotein factor results in defective platelet adhesion

Contd...

- **Virchow triad** – Endothelial cell injury + alteration of blood flow+ hypercoagulability
- **Thrombin** is procoagulant but thrombin-thrombomodulin complex is anticoagulant
- Most common inherited cause of hypercoagulability – **Leiden mutation** (factor 5 mutation)
- **Lines of Zahn** are produced by the alternating pale layers of platelets mixed with some fibrin and dark layers containing more red cells
- Most common site for **DVT – Deep veins below the knee**
- **Chargaff's rule** – amount of purine is equal to pyrimidine (A + G = C + T)
- Most common death in Marfan syndrome – **Aortic Dissection**
- Autosomal recessive diseases are most common type of mendelian mode of inheritance
- **In AR inheritance**, both parents must have mutant gene
- Essential amino acid in PKU – **Tyrosine**
- **Uniparental Disomy** – Should be suspected in an individual manifesting a recessive disorder, where only one parent is a carrier
- **PGF2a is a vasoconstrictor** where PGD2, PGE2 are vasodilators
- The chief cell responsible for scar contraction is **myofibroblast**
- **Heart failure cells are:** Hemosiderin laden macrophages.
- Heart failure cells seen in: **Lungs**
- Platelet aggregation requires: **Glycoprotein IIb-IIIa**
- Fibrin is degraded by: **Plasmin**
- **Virchow's triad of thrombosis include:** Vascular (endothelial) injury; abnormal blood flow (stasis or turbulence); hypercoagulability.
- Virchow's fifth sign of inflammation is: **Loss of function**
- **Leiden factor is:** Mutated factor V.
- Most common source of embolism: **DVT (deep vein thrombosis).**
- **Red aka hemorrhagic infarcts are seen in:** Ovary, lung, small intestine.
- **Pale aka white infarcts are seen in:** Heart, spleen, liver, kidney, brain.
- In inflammation Rubor is due to: **Arteriolar dilatation**.
- **Hallmark of acute inflammation:** Increased vascular permeability.
- Which Cells primarily involved in acute inflammation: **Neutrophils**.

Contd...

Key Points

FMGE Solutions Screening Examination

- Major microcirculation involved in acute inflammation: **Venules**.
- Cell-matrix adhesion is mediated by: **Integrins**.
- Major cells which are involved in chronic inflammation: **Macrophages**.
- **Life span of neutrophils:** 4–8 hours (in blood) and 2–5 days (in tissues).
- Phagocytic cells in brain (CNS): **Microglia**.
- Oxygen dependent killing in phagocytes is through: **NADPH oxidase**.
- **Chédiak–Higashi syndrome** is a defect of: **Phagocytosis**.
- Most abundant glycoprotein in basement membrane: **Laminin**.
- **Warthin finkeldey** giant cells are seen in measles
- **Reed–sternberg cells** seen in **hodgkin's lymphoma**
- Most common site for keloid – **Sternum**
- Triplet repeat of CCG nucleotides seen in-**Fragile X syndrome**
- There is presence of CAG repeats associated with – **Huntington's chorea**
- **Gonadal/Germline mosaicism** seen in – osteogenesis imperfecta and tuberous sclerosis
- Diagnosis of choice for **Fragile X Syndrome** – PCR
- White spots on the iris known as brushfield spots seen in **Down syndrome**
- Mitotic non-disjunction is responsible for development of **mosaicism**
- Patients of Down syndrome having predisposition for **Hirschsprung's disease**, **duodenal atresia** and **Alzheimer's disease**.
- **Robertsonian translocation** seen in about 4% cases of Down syndrome
- **AML M7** variety is associated with Down syndrome
- Maternal meiotic non-dysjunction is most common cause of **down syndrome**
- **Triple test and Quadruple screen** test is used for screening of Downs syndrome at 15–20 weeks of pregnancy
- Maternal serum of alpha fetoprotein + estriol + hCG are the components of triple test this are low in **Edward syndrome**
- **AFP** is increased in neural tube defects but reduced in Edward and down syndromes
- **Patau syndrome** is trisomy 13, features are polydactyly cleft lip and holoprosencephaly.
- **Edward syndrome** is trisomy 18, features are micrognathia overlapping flexed fingers.

- **Cat eye syndrome** is a partial trisomy of chromosome 22 and is coined due to the particular appearance of the ventricular colobomas in the eyes.
- **Klinefelter syndrome** is male chromosomal disorder of chromosome 47, XXY, there is decrease in testosterone and inhibin but increase in LH and FSH.
- **Noonan syndrome** is autosomal congenital disorder mostly mutation in genes on chromosome 12.
- Trisomy 7 mostly occur due to mitotic non – Disjunction.
- Trisomy 18 is more commonly seen in **2nd meiotic division**.
- **Lyon's hypothesis** says inactivation of either maternal or paternal x chromosome among all the cells of blastocyst by about 16th day of embryonic life
- **Barr bodies** are absent in normal males and turner syndrome but female has 1 Barr body.
- Benign tumor developing from all three germ layers – **Teratoma**
- Lesion with normal differentiation at abnormal site – **Choristoma**
- Hallmark of malignant transformation – **Anaplasia**
- **Hamartoma** – Abnormal differentiation in normal site
- **Malignant tumors** have upregulation of telomerase activity
- HNPCC is AD but is due to defective **DNA repair**
- Cell cycle sequence **G1-S-G2-M-G0**
- The initiation of DNA replication involve the formation of an active complex between **Cyclin E** and **CDK2**
- The main mediator that propels the cell beyond prophase is – **Cyclin B CDK1 complex**
- Proto-oncogenes were discovered by **Harold Varmus** and **Michael Bishop**
- The point mutation of **Ras family gene** is the single most common abnormality of oncogenes in human tumors
- **MYC** is associated with conflict model in carcinogenesis
- **K-RAS**- Colon, lung & pancreatic tumors
- **N-RAS** – Melanoma, AML
- **H-RAS** – Bladder and kidney tumors
- **C-MYC** – Burkitt's lymphoma
- **L-MYC** – Small cell lung cancer
- **N-MYC** – Neuroblastoma
- **RB gene** was the first tumor suppressor gene to be discovered
- **RB gene** is present on chromosome 13q14
- Retinoblastoma is associated with **Knudsen two hit hypothesis**

Contd...

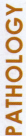

Contd...

Pathology

- **P53 gene** is the most commonly mutated gene in human cancer
- The nonmutated P53 gene is also called as – **Wild type**
- **Toll – like** receptor causes the activation of NF – Kappa beta and AP-1
- **CD45** is also called a leukocyte common antigen (LCA)
- Antigen presenting cells include – B-cells macrophages and dendritic cells
- HEV are lined by simple cuboidal cells as opposite to regular venules lined by **endothelial cells**.
- Pan B cell – **CD 19**
- **Isotype switching** – Change in the class of the antibody produced by the plasma cell
- **IgM** and **IgG** are responsible for activation of classical pathway
- **IgA, IgE** and **IgD** are responsible for activation of alternate pathway
- **NK cells** are unique as they are capable of direct cell lysis
- **MHC is** located on short arm of chromosome 6
- **MHC 1** molecule is present on all the nucleated cells and platelets
- **MHC 2** molecule is present on all the APC'S (Antigen Presenting Cells)

Crumpled tissue paper app	Gaucher's disease (massive splenomegaly)
Hunner ulcer	Interstitial cystitis
Cushing ulcer	Stomach ulcer due to raised ICP
Curling ulcer	Ulcer in D1 portion d/t burns
Cameron ulcer	Hiatus hernia

IMPORTANT ONE LINERS

- Foam Cells are: **Lipid Laden Macrophages**
- Artery not involved in atherosclerosis: **Pulmonary trunk**.
- Most common cause of aortic aneurysm: **Atherosclerosis**.
- Infection causing atherosclerosis: **Chlamydia pneumoniae, herpes virus (CMV)**.
- Tree bark calcification is seen in: **Syphilitic aneurysm**.
- Pulseless disease is: **Takayasu arteritis**.
- Most common benign vascular tumor: **Hemangioma**.
- Kaposi's sarcoma is associated with: **HHV-8**.

Contd...

- Characteristic of rheumatic carditis: **Pancarditis**.
- Most commonly involved valve in Rheumatic fever: **Mitral valve**.
- McCallum plaque is seen in: **Rheumatic carditis** (on left atrium).
- Most common cause of constrictive pericarditis: **TB**.
- Gitter cells are: **Microglia**
- Maximum decrease in CSF chloride: **TB meningitis**.
- Characteristic pathological feature of parkinsonism: **Lewy bodies**.
- Most common cause of intracerebral (intraparenchymal) hemorrhage: **Hypertension**.
- Important features of **Dandy-Walker syndrome**: Agenesis of cerebellar vermis and corpus callosum, cystic enlargement of 4th ventricle, hydrocephalus.
- Most common cerebellar tumor in children: **Astrocytoma**
- Most common cerebellar tumor in children: **Astrocytoma**
- Wermer's syndrome is: **MEN-I**.
- Sipple's syndrome is: **MEN-IIA**.
- Orphan Annie eye nuclei is characteristic of this thyroid CA: **Papillary thyroid carcinoma**.
- Most common thyroid carcinoma: **Papillary carcinoma**.
- Weight range of adrenal in Cushing s disease: **25-40 gm**.
- **Nesidioblastoma** is due to: Hyperplasia of pancreatic beta cells.
- Tadpole cells are seen in: **Rhabdomyosarcoma**.
- Brown tumor of bone is seen in: **Hyperparathyroidism**.
- Most common mutation in Ewing's sarcoma: **Translocation t 11:22**.
- Tophus is pathognomonic for: **Gout**.
- Bilateral breast cancer: **Lobular carcinoma**.
- Most common breast cancer: **Invasive ductal carcinoma**.
- Most common gene involved in breast cancer (overall): **P53**.
- Most common gene involved in familial breast cancer: **BRCA-1**.
- Call-Exner bodies are seen in: **Granulosa-theca cell tumor**.
- Most common testicular tumor and testicular germ cell tumor: **Seminoma.**
- Definitive marker for hepatoblastoma: **AFP**.
- Canals of herring are present in: **Liver**.
- 'Comet tail artefact' with thickening of gallbladder wall: **Adenomyomatosis**.
- 'Onion skin' fibrosis of bile duct is seen in: **Primary sclerosing cholangitis**.

Contd...

Key Points

FMGE Solutions Screening Examination

- **Nutmeg liver is seen in**: Right sided heart failure (chronic passive congestion).
- **Rate limiting step in bilirubin metabolism**: Excretion of conjugated bilirubin into canaliculi.
- **Most common site of intestinal amebiasis**: Cecum and ascending colon.
- Pipe-stem appearance is seen in: **Ulcerative colitis**.
- Most specific marker of GIST: **C-Kit (CD 117)**.
- Most common site of GIST: **Stomach**.
- Most common site of gastric carcinoma: **Pylorus and antrum**.
- **Most common complication of peptic ulcer**: GI bleeding (e.g. Haematemesis).
- **Most common site of peptic ulcer**: 1st part of duodenum.
- **Most common symptoms of bladder cancer**: Painless hematuria.
- Michaelis-Gutmann bodies are seen in: **Malakoplakia**.
- Kimmelstiel-Wilson lesion is characteristic of: **Diabetic nephropathy**.
- **Hallmark of IgA nephropathy**: Hematuria after 1-2 days of an upper respiratory tract infection.
- Most common cause of nephrotic syndrome in adults: **Membranous GN**.
- Crescent formation is characteristic of: **RPGN**.
- Most common cause of nephritic syndrome: **RPGN**.
- Tamm–Horsfall protein is produced by: **Loop of Henle**.
- Carcinoid tumors arise from: **Enterochromaffin cells**.
- Marker of squamous cell carcinoma of lung: **Cytokeratin**.
- Most common lung carcinoma: **Adenocarcinoma**.
- Potato nodes are seen in: **Sarcoidosis**.
- Bilateral hilar lymphadenopathy with non-caseating granuloma: **Sarcoidosis**.
- Most common form of emphysema seen clinically: **Centriacinar emphysema** (centrilobular emphysema).

HEPATITIS

Mnemonic for failure: causes of acute liver
A: Acetaminophen, hepatitis A, autoimmune hepatitis
B: Hepatitis B
C: Hepatitis C, cryptogenic
D: Drugs/toxins, hepatitis D
E: Hepatitis E, esoteric causes (Wilson disease, Budd-Chiari)
F: Fatty change of the microvesicular type (fatty liver of pregnancy, valproate, tetracycline, Reye syndrome)

Contd...

TABLE: The hepatitis viruses

Virus	Hepatitis A	Hepatitis B	Hepatitis C	Hepatitis D	Hepatitis E
Type of virus	ssRNA	Partially dsDNA	ssRNA	Circular defective ssRNS	ssRNA
Viral family	Hepatovirus; related to picornavirus	Hepadnavirus	Flaviviridae	Subviral particle in Delta Viridae family	Hepevirus
Route of transmission	Fecal-oral (contaminated food or water)	Parenteral, sexual contact, perinatal	Parenteral; intranasal cocaine use is a risk factor	Parenteral	Fecal-oral
Mean Incubation period	2 to 6 weeks	2 to 26 weeks (mean 8 weeks)	4 to 26 weeks (mean 9 weeks)	Same as HBV	4 to 5 weeks
Frequency of chronic liver disease	Never	5%–10%	>80%	10% (co-infection); 90%–100% for superinfection	In Immunocompromised hosts only
Diagnosis	Detection of serum IgM antibody	Detection of HBsAg or antibody to HBcAg; PCR for HBV DNA	3rd-generation ELISA for antibody detection; PCR for HCV RNA	Detection of IgM and IgG antibodies; HDV RNA serum; HDAg In liver	Detection of serum IgM and 10 antibodies; PCR for HEV RNA

Pathology

TABLE: Hereditary hyperbilirubinemia

Disorder	Inheritance	Defects in bilirubin metabolism	Liver pathology	Clinical course
Unconjugated hyperbilirubinemia				
Crigler-Najjar syndrome type I	Autosomal recessive	Absent UGT1A1 activity	None	Fetal in neonatal period
Crigler-Najjar syndrome type II	Autosomal dominant with variable penetrance	Decreased UGT1A1 activity	None	Generally mild, occasional kernicterus
Gilbert syndrome	Autosomal recessive	Decreased UGT1A1 activity	None	Innocuous
Conjugated hyperbilirubinemia				
Dubin-Johnson syndrome	Autosomal recessive	Impaired biliary excretion of bilirubin glucuronides due to mutation in canalicular multidrug resistance protein 2 (MRP2)	Pigmented cytoplasmic globules	Innocuous
Rotor syndrome	Autosomal recessive	Decreased hepatic uptake and storage? Decreased biliary excretion?	None	Innocuous

UGT1A1, Uridine diphosphate-glucuronyl transferase family, peptide A1

HODGKIN'S LYMPHOMA

	Classical				Non-Cl:
	Nodular sclerosis	Mixed cellularity	Lymphocyte rich	Lymphocyte depleted	Lymphocyte predominant
Incidence	MC type	MC type in India		a/w HIV	
RS cell	Variant = lacunar cell	Max no. of RS cell	**Least no. of RS cell**	3 types of RS cell	Popcorn cell
CD marker	15 + and 30+	15 + and 30+	15 + and 30+ CD 20-ve	15 + and 30+	CD 20+ 15 and 30 -ve
Prognosis	Excellent	Very good	Good to Excellent	Poor	Excellent

Types of Graft Rejection

	Acute	Hyperacute	Chronic
Duration	5 days to 3 months	Immediately within minutes or hours	Occurs after months or years
Mechanism	Involves humoral (antibodies) and Cellular (T cell) rejection	Due to preformed antibodies (humoral)	Involves T cell (cellular rejection)
Hypersensitivity	IV	II	IV and III

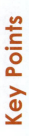

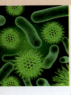

FMGE Solutions Screening Examination

• Antoni A and B	Schwannoma, Sarcoidosis, Sporotrichosis (Gardner's disease)
• Asteroid body	Sporotrichosis
• Azzopardi effect	Oat cell lung CA
• Banana bodies	Farber disease (Dec Ceramidase)
• Birbeck granules	Histiocytosis X
• Cigar bodies	Sporotrichosis
• Caterpillar cell/ Anitschnow cell	Aschoff Nodule (RF)
• Caterpillar body	Porphyria
• Civatte bodies	Lichen planus
• Councilman body	Acute viral hepatitis, YF
• Donovan body	Granuloma inguinale
• Dutcher body	Multiple myeloma
• Guarneri body	Small pox
• Gamma gandy body	Portal HTN, sickle cell disease
• Globi bodies	Leprosy
• Globoid cell	Krabbe disease
• Hirano bodies	Alzheimer's
• Hurthle cell	Hashimoto's thyroiditis
• Kamino bodies	Nevus
• Marquee bodies	Kala-azar-Leishmania donovani
• Odland bodies	Normal skin body
• Orphan annie nuclei	Papillary CA thyroid
• Psamomma bodies	Papillary CA thyroid, Serous cystadenoma, Meningioma (PSM)
• Russell bodies	MM
• Schaumann bodies	Sarcoidosis
• Zellballen bodies	Chemodectoma/Paraganglioma

Staining Method	
Z–N stain	Acid fast stain for mycobacteria, Nocardia
Kinyoun stain	Cold acid fast stain cryptosporidium parvum, Mycobact, Nocardia
Albert stain	Metachromatic stain for C. diphtheriae

Colony Appearance	
• Thumb print app	Bordetella pertussis
• School of red fish	H. ducreyi (Chancroid)
• Fried egg colony	Mycoplasma hominis
• Poached egg colony	C. diphtheriae (Mitis) In tellurite agar
• Frog head colony	C. diphtheriae (intermedius)
• Nagler reaction	Cl. perfringens
• Medusa head	Bacillus anthracis
• Draughtsman colony	Strep. pneumoniae

TABLE: Agglutination tests and their uses

Agglutination test	Used mainly for
Direct agglutination test	Determination of blood group Bacterial agglutination test for serotyping and serogrouping. **E.g.: Vibrio Cholera, Salmonella Sp.**
Slide agglutination test	Used for serotyping of salmonella **VDRL for syphilis**
Tube agglutination test	Aka standard agglutination test. Used for serological diagnosis of typhoid, brucellosis and typhus fever. **E.g.: Widal Test, *Weil–Felix reaction*, and Kahn test**
Passive agglutination test	Rheumatoid factor **ANA for SLE** Antibody to Trichinella spiralis and antibody to group A strep.

- Sporulation of bacteria seen in which phase: **Stationary phase**
- Doubling of bacteria seen in this phase: **Exponential phase**
- Bacterial cell wall is made up of: **Peptidoglycan**
- Fungal cell wall is made up of: **Chitin**
- Eukaryotic ribosomes are **80s ribosomes** (60s + 40s subunits)
- Prokaryotic ribosomes are **70s ribosomes** (50s + 30s subunits)
- **Staph. aureus** is the most common organism causing hospital acquired wound infections/surgical wounds

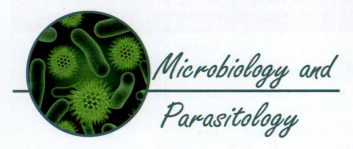

Microbiology and Parasitology

Culture Media	
VR media	V. cholerae alkaline peptone water
Stuart transport medium	Resp. specimen
Enrichment media	Selenite F broth, Salmonella, Shigella
Enriched media	Blood agar chocolate agar
Selective media	Wilson Blair medium Salmonella
Potassium tellurite blood agar	C. diphtheriae

Contd...

Microbiology and Parasitology

- **Hot air oven utilizes** 180°C for 1 hour, used for lab glass wares/glass syringes
- **Autoclaving**-attain temperature of 122°C under 15lb/sq inch pressure
- **Formaldehyde** gas is used for fumigation of OT/labs/rooms/woollen blankets
- **Bacillus stearothermophilus** is a thermophile organism whose spores are extremely heat resistant.
- **Bacillus subtilis** is the biological indicator for testing dry heat sterilizers, ethylene oxide sterilizers
- **Bacillus subtilis** is used in Guthrie test
- **Clostridium botulinum** spores are the most heat resistant organism and require 120°C 4 min or 100°C 330 min
- Proteus strains are used as antigens for **Weil–Felix reactions**
- **Classical pathway** is activated by IgM, IgG and immune complexes
- **Alternate pathway** is activated by bacterial endotoxin, zymogen, IgA and IgG4, cobra venom
- Most important **opsonizing complement-C3b**
- Most important chemotactic: **C5a**
- Proinflammatory cytokines that are present with dominance of **CMI-IL2, INF gamma, TNF alpha, IL1**
- Anti-inflammatory cytokines that are present with dominance of humoral immunity: **IL4, 5, 6, 10**
- Bruton agammaglobulinemia is X linked disease characterized by defective opsonization due to deficiency of **opsonizing antibodies**
- **Ataxia telangiectasia** is AR disorder characterized by triad of *cerebellar ataxia + oculocutaneous telangiectasia and immunodeficiency.
- **Chédiak–Higashi syndrome:** AR disorder associated with mutation in LYST gene
- **SCID**- due to lack of combined T cell, B cell, NK cells
- Most common primary tumor of anterior mediastinum is **Thymoma**
- **Nagler's reaction** is seen in clostridium perfringens, it is due to alpha toxin
- Most common species of pseudomonas causing intravenous catheter related infection: **Pseudomonas maltophilia**
- Most common organism implicated in osteomyelitis: **Staph. aureus**
- Most common cause of Hand foot mouth disease- **coxsackievirus A16**
- Most common viruses implicated in encephalitis- **Echoviruses**
- **Leptospirosis**-triad of fever, jaundice, renal failure,
- Gas gangrene most commonly caused by clostridium **perfringens (clostridium welchii)**

- Pikes media is transport media for **streptococcus pyogenes**
- Culture media for corynebacterium diphtheriae is - **Loeffler's serum slope**
- Culture media for neisseria gonorrhoeae is - **Thayer Martin medium**
- Fir tree appearance of colonies on culture shown by - **Bacillus anthrax**
- Daisy head appearance of colonies on culture shown by **C. diphtheria**
- Fried egg colonies- **Mycoplasma**
- Darting motility shown by - **vibrio cholera**
- Swarming motility - **cl. tetani, proteus**
- Tumbling motility - **Listeria monocytogenes.**
- HACEK group of organisms
    - **H**-haemophilus species
    - **A**-actinobacillus actinomycetemcomitans
    - **C**-cardiobacterium hominis
    - **E**-eikenella corrodens
    - **K**-kingella kingae
- Weil Felix reaction is used for diagnosis of rickettsial disease
- **Toxins inhibiting protein synthesis:** Diphtheria, pseudomonas, shiga toxin
- MCC of traveler's diarrhea - **ETEC**
- Sereny test is an invasive test for Shigella
- Causative organism for trench fever - **Bartonella Quintana**
- **Mycoplasma** are also known as PPLO/eaton agent
- All DNA viruses are usually double stranded except **parvovirus (single stranded)**
- All RNA viruses are single stranded except **reovirus**
- Largest virus-pox virus, smallest virus-**parvovirus**
- HP body seen in: **Molluscum contagiosum**
- Negri bodies: **Rabies**
- Small pox- **Guarnieri bodies**
- **Primary infection with VZV** in non immune individuals causes-Chicken pox. Reinfection with VZV in immunocompromised individuals causes-herpes zoster (shingles)
- Swimming pool conjunctivitis - **Adenovirus** type 3, 7, 14
- Enterovirus 70- causes acute **Hemorrhagic conjunctivitis.**
- MCC of diarrhea in infants - **Rotavirus**
- Genital warts - **HPV 6, 11**
- **Antigenic drift in influenza** is due to point mutation under selection pressure of community
- **Antigenic shift in influenza** is due to genetic reassortment of human with avian/animal viruses → antigenic variations
- Yeast like organism-**Candida**
- Septate hyphae is seen in **Aspergillus**

Contd...

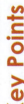

Key Points

FMGE Solutions Screening Examination

- Most common fungal infection seen in immunocompetent host - **Aspergillus**
- Most common opportunistic fungal infection in HIV/AIDS patient - **Candida**
- Prominent polysaccharide capsule is seen in **Cryptococcus**
- Most common fungus producing meningitis in immunocompromised host is **Cryptococcus**
- Only rickettsia which can be cultured is - **R. Quintana**
- Enterotoxins are not produced by - **Streptococcus**
- Casoni test is done in case of - **Hydatid cyst**
- Most common Protozoan parasite is **toxoplasma gondii**
- Mega esophagus is seen in **Chagas' disease**
- Smallest tapeworm - **echinococcus granulosus**
- Dwarf tapeworm is **H. nana**
- Longest tapeworm - **T. saginata**
- Cutaneous larva migrans- are caused by Ancylostoma **Braziliense**
- Bile stained eggs in stool is seen in ascaris, trichuris
- **Dumbbell** shaped eggs seen in case of: **Trichuris trichiura**
- Not commonly seen in ascariasis - **Anemia**
- Cystic stage is not seen in - **Trichomonas vaginalis.**
- Cellulitis is caused by: **Streptococcus**
- Pyoderma most commonly caused by staph aureus
- Cetrimide agar isolate which of the following bacteria: **Pseudomonas**
- Thayer martin agar is for: **N. meningitis**
- Traveller's diarrhea is caused by: **ETEC**
- HUS is caused by which strain of E. coli: **EHEC (0157: H7)**
- Incubation period of Diphtheria: **2–5 days**
- IP of chicken pox- **10-21 days**
- Infectious period of chicken pox is 2 days before to 5 days after the onset of rash
- Which protein attached to surface of bacteria and phagocytized: **Antibody**
- Food poisoning 2 hours after intake of food: **Staph. aureus**

TABLE: Some important motilities to note

Tumbling motility	Listeria
Swarming motility	Proteus
Gliding motility	P. aeruginosa, mycoplasma
Darting motility	Campylobacter, Vibrio Cholera
Falling leaf motility	Giardia
Shooting star motility	Vibrio
Cork screw motility	T. pallidum
Lashing motility	Borrelia

TABLE: Various shapes of bacteria

Shape	Associated bacteria
Club shape	Cornyebacteria
Lanceolate	Pneumococci
Half-moon/lens	Meningococci
Kidney shape	Gonnococci
Comma	Vibrio and campylobacter
Drumstick appearance	Clostridium tetani
Chinese letter pattern	Corynebacterium diphtheria
D-shaped	Neisseria meningitides
Kidney shaped appearance	N. Gonorrhoeae
Flame shaped appearance	Strep. pneumoniae

TABLE: Types of food poisoning caused by bacillus cereus

Diarrhea type-main symptom	Emetic type-main symptom
Associated with wide range of food intake including meat, puddings etc. **I.P. 8–16 hours** Occurs due to heat labile enterotoxin	Associated with intake of Chinese fried rice **I.P.** 1–5 hours Due to pre-formed, heat stable toxin

TABLE: Clostridium microbes that causes food poisoning

Clostridium perfringens type A: Gastroenteritis
Clostridium perfringens type C: Necrotising enteritis
Clostridium botulinum: Botulism
Clostridium difficile: Acute colitis

TABLE: Viral inclusion bodies and their sites

Intracytoplasmic	Intranuclear	Intracytoplasmic + Intranuclear
Negri bodies in Rabies **Guarnieri bodies** in Small pox **Henderson-Peterson bodies** in Molluscum contagiosum	**Cowdry type A in Herpes simplex virus** and Varicella zoster virus and Torres bodies in Yellow fever **Cowdry type B** in Polio and adenovirus	**Warthin finkeldey bodies** in *Measles*

MICROBIOLOGY AND PARASITOLOGY

Forensic Medicine

TABLE: Rickettsial diseases, their causative agents and vector

Disease	Cause	Vector
Epidemic typhus	R. prowazekii	Louse
Endemic typhus	R. typhi	Rat flea
Scrub Typhus	R. tsutsugamushi	Trombiculid mite
Indian tick typhus	R. conorii	Tick
RMSF	R. rickettsia	Tick
Trench fever	Bartonella quintana	None
Q fever	Coxiella	None but rarely soft tick

TABLE: Some or important points about Immunoglobulin (Ig)

Ig having maximum molecular weight: **IgM**	
First antibody produced by newborn: **IgM**	
All immunoglobulin are heat stable except: **IgE**	
Ig present in **breast milk**: **IgA**	
Ig present **in oral cavity**: **IgA**	
Ig with **maximum half-life**: **IgG**	
Ig with **minimum half-life**: **IgE**	
Ig having **maximum serum concentration**: **IgG**	
Ig having **least serum concentration**: **IgE**	

TEST FOR HIV
- Ser. Elisa – (Screening)
- Western blot – (Confirmatory)
- PCR RNA – IOC
- PCR DNA – IOC for window period
- Viral culture – Efficiency of antiviral

PARASITIC EGGS

Bile stained	Non-bile stained
• Ascaris • Trichuris	• Necator americanus • Enterobius vermicularis • H. nana • Ancylostoma duodenale

FLOATING VS NON FLOATING EGGS IN SATURATED SALT SOLUTION

Floats (FATEH)	Sink/Doesn't Float (STUF)
• Fertilized eggs of Ascaris • Ancylostoma duodenale • Trichuris trichiura • Enterobius vermicularis • H. nana	• Strongyloides stercoralis • Taenia solium/saginata • Unfertilized eggs of ascaris • Fasciola hepatica

TABLE: Important to know

• Sclerotic bodies are seen in	Chromoblastomycosis
• Organism present as cluster of round yeast cell with short, stout hyphae which is branched or curved	Tinea nigra
• Culture colonies are creamy white, smooth and with yeast odour	Candida albicans
• Culture shows round colonies with "cut-glass" appearance in transmitted light/inverted Fir tree app:	Bacillus anthrax
• Largest protozoa	Syringammina Fragilissima (20 cm)
• Largest liver fluke	Fascioloides magna
• Largest nematode	Ascaris

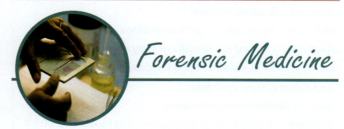

Forensic Medicine

Blood stain specific test: **Hemin test**
Plaintiff is: A person who files case in civil court
Grounds for MTP (Act 1971): • **Therapeutic:** Risk to pregnant women • **Eugenic:** Risk for child to be born • **Humanitarian:** Pregnancy caused by rape • **Socioeconomic:** Pregnancy due to contraceptive failure
Most common type of finger print: **Loops**
Postponement of hanging of pregnant lady is defined by which CrPC: **416**
IPC for marital rape: **IPC 376 A**
Declaration of Geneva is related with: **Hippocratic oath**
Declaration of Helsinki: Ethical principles for medical research involving human subjects
Declaration of Tokyo: International guidelines for physicians concerning torture and other cruel, inhuman or degrading treatment or punishment in relation to detention and imprisonment
Declaration of Lisbon: **Deals with the rights of the patient**
Declaration of Malta: **Hunger strikers**
Blanket consent is taken: **While admission to do any surgery**
Best bone specimen for sex differentiation: **Pelvis**

Contd...

FMGE Solutions Screening Examination

Davidson body is sued to determine:	**Sex**
Pearson formula is used for:	**Stature**
Rugoscopy is study of:	**Palate prints**
Locard system is:	**Poroscopy**
Galton's system is used for:	**Dactylography**
Instantaneous rigors is seen in:	**Cadaveric spasm**
Time of floating of dead body in drowning in summer:	**24 hours**
For toxicology sampling, best site for blood collection:	**Femoral vein**
Hara-kiri is suicide by stabbing in:	**Abdomen**
In blast injury which organ injured first:	**Tympanic membrane > Lung**
Kennedy phenomenon is seen in:	**Gunshot injury**
Pond's fracture is commonly seen in which age group:	**Children**
Telefono is:	**Beating on ears**
Outer covering of diatom is made of:	**Silica**
Raygat's test is used for:	**Specific gravity of lung**
Latte's crust of blood stain is used to detect:	**Blood group**
Angel dust is:	**Phencyclidine**
Borax is:	**Gastrointestinal irritant**
Widmark's formula helps in measurement of blood level of:	**Alcohol**
McEwan's sign is seen in:	**Alcoholic intoxication**
White vitriol is:	**Zinc sulfate**
Blue vitriol is:	**Copper sulfate**
Lee-Jones test is used for:	**Cyanide**
Trousseau sign is positive in which poisoning:	**Oxalic acid**
Odor of cyanide is:	**Bitter almond**

Sexual asphyxia is associated with –	**Masochism & Transvestism**
Arborescent or Filigree burns (Lichtenberg's flowers pattern) are seen in –	**lightening**
Crocodile/Flash burns/joule burns/arc eye burn are seen in-	**Electrocution**
Poisoning which does not affect diffusion at tissue level –	**Curare** (It affects conduction at N-M level)
Chicken fat clot is never a characteristic feature of	**antemortem wounds**
Defense attitude/boxer's attitude/pugilistic attitude is seen in	**burns**
Gettler's test is used in death due to drowning	
Podogram – study of footprints	
Finger printing bureau of the world was established at writer's building at Calcutta in year 1897	

Rounded (horse shoe shaped) nasal openings, orbits, palate:	**Mongols**
Triangular (narrow & elongated) nasal openings, orbits, palate:	**Europeans**
Quadrangular (square or rectangular) nasal openings, orbits, palate:	**Negros**
Bertillon system (anthropometry) is applicable after age of	**21 years**
Quetelet's rule of biological variation: No two hands have similar finger prints	
Criminals may attempt to **mutilate finger prints** by applying CO_2 now, corrosive agents, burns, eroding against hard surface	
Infrared photography: Makes old tattoos readily visible	
First temporary teeth to appear is lower central incisor, first permanent (secondary) teeth to appear is 1st molar.	
Angle of mandible is obtuse in infancy and old age.	
Heart shaped pelvic inlet is seen in males & is widest in its posterior part, in females it is oval, widest most anteriorly than in males.	
Whiplash injury results from acute hyperextension of cervical spine in region C4-C6 vertebrae	
Ring fracture is any fracture round the foramen magnum	
Brush burn/Friction burn/gravel rash are type of graze	
Gun powder a term usually used for black power consists of pot nitrate: 75%, charcoal: 15 %, sulphur: 10%	
MC organ to be damaged in under water blast is **Gastrointestinal tract.**	
Zenker's degeneration: Electrical injury produced in muscle	
Cause of death in judicial hanging is **fracture of C2-3 or C3-4 vertebrae**	
Frequency of hyoid fracture: Throttling > strangulation > Hanging.	
Most reliable micro-chemical test for detecting blood in both recent & old stains: **Spectroscopic test**	
Res Ipsa Loquitur: Thing or facts speak for itself	
Corpus delicti: Body of offense.	
Novus actus interveniens: A person is not only responsible for his action but also for logical consequences of actions.	
Atavism: The child does not resemble its parents but its grandparents.	
Autopsy of the spinal cord is most commonly done through posterior approach	
Subpoena/Summon: A document compelling attendance.	
Albuminuria is seen with krait bite; **Hematuria** is seen in viper bite; **Myoglobinuria** is seen in sea snakes	
Fatal period in drowning: **Death in fresh water:** 4-5 minutes **Death in salt water:** 8-10 minutes	

Contd...

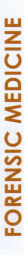

Forensic Medicine

Barberio's test is used for identification of: **Semen**

Test to distinguish human vs. animal blood - **Precipitin Test.**

Snake bite:
Cobra & krait: Neurotoxic
Sea snake: Myotoxic
Viper: Vasculotoxic, Hemotoxic

TABLE: Some important IPC's on Hurt (*very potential topic*)

Sec 319	Hurt
Sec 320	Grievous hurt
Sec 321	Voluntarily causing hurt
Sec 322	Voluntarily causing grievous hurt
Sec 325	Punishment for voluntarily causing grievous hurt
Sec 326	Punishment for voluntarily causing grievous hurt by a dangerous weapon

Dowry death investigation is done by: **Magistrate**

IPC for perjury: **IPC 191**

Punishment for perjury: **IPC 193**

Sexual gratification by contact. Ex: rubbing genitalia on another person: **Frotteurism**

Blood alcohol level while driving: **30 mg%**

Phytobezoar is: **Intake of indigestible plant materials**

A female forges to have a child, whereas she doesn't have. It is **Suppositious child**

A child who is born to an unmarried women: **Illegitimate child**

TABLE: Types of hair on basis of medulla

Ladder or lattice type: **Animals**
Discontinuous type: **Animals**
Interrupted type: **White race, Caucasians**
Fragmented type: **Fetus, newborn**

TABLE: Different metallic poisoning and their effect on hair and skin

Poisoning	Color of hair and skin
Arsenic (As)	• Yellow color of skin, hair & mucous membrane • Milk rose (Brownish pigmentation)/Rain drop pigmentation • Black foot disease
Copper (Cu)	• Jaundiced skin • Green - Blue skin, hair & perspiration • Green – Purple line on gums
Mercury (Hg)	• Blue-black line on gums with jaw necrosis and loosening of tooth • Brown deposits on anterior lens capsule (mercurialentis) • Acrodynia (pink disease)
Lead (Pb)	• Blue stippled burtonian line on gums, especially on upper jaw.

TABLE: Poisoning and organ preserved

Poisoning	Organ preserved
Strychnine poisoning	Spinal cord (entire length)
Pesticides and Insecticides poisoning	Fat
CO, Cyanide, Organophosphates, Opiates, Barbiturates, Alkaloids and Strychnine poisoning (*Mn: COOBAS*)	Brain
Arsenic, Radium and Thallium poisoning (*Mn: ART*)	Bone

TABLE: Poisoning and their Antidote

Poisoning	Antidote/treatment
Oxalic acid (ink remover)	Calcium gluconate
Phosphorus	Copper sulfate
Organophosphorus	Atropine
Datura	Physostigmine
Arsenic	BAL, DMSA
Mercury	BAL, DMSA
Lead (Plumbism)	EDTA, DMSA
Alcohol	Ethyl alcohol
Opium (Afeem)	Naloxone
Heroine/Brown sugar/ Junk/ Smack	Amyl nitrite
Bhang/Ganja/Charas	Diazepam
Strychnine	Diazepam
Copper	Potassium ferro ferricyanide
Cyanide	Hydroxocobalamin

TABLE: Gun powders types and its constituent

Black gun powder	Smokeless powder
Consists of: Potassium nitrate 75% Sulfur 10% Charcoal 15%	**Consists of:** • *Nitrocellulose* (single base; gun cotton) • Nitroglycerine + Nitrocellulose • Nitroglycerine + Nitrocellulose + Nitroguanidine (triple base)

Key Points

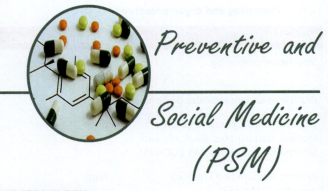

Preventive and Social Medicine (PSM)

UPDATES IN PSM

• Ayushman Bharat Programme (ABP)	Health protection scheme (covers insurance of 5L)
• 2 major initiatives under ABP	Health and Wellness centre, National Health Protection Scheme
• Aim of health and wellness Centre	"bring health care closer to home" (1.5 L in number)
• Nobel prize in physiology to Jeffrey C Hall et al	Discovery of molecular mechanism controlling circadian rhythm
• Theme for world health day 7 Apr 2019	Universal health coverage- everyone everywhere
• Definition of blindness	Person unable to count fingers from 3 meter distance
• NPCB now new term	NPCB and Visual impairment
• Goal to reduce blindness by 2020	0.3% (now 1%)
• HDI	0.55
• GFR	2.3
• Sex ratio in India	940/1000
• Age 0 – 6 year sex ratio	914/1000
• Highest sex ratio	Kerala
• Birth and death rate	21.6 and 7 respectively
• What is PENCIL portal	Electronic platform for effective enforcement for no child labor under ministry of labour and Employment
• 2 new contraceptives launched by health ministry	Antara (Inj) and Chhaya (pill) MPA: Methylprogesterone Acetate
• JEET program	Joint Effort for Elimination of TB
• SAPNA model	A local school going girl, a role model for leprosy elimination (MEENA- UNICEF)

Contd...

• World malaria day	25 April 2019
• Mosquirix vaccine (RTS,S)	First approved malaria vaccine (available in Malawi for 5 mo to 2 years child)
• Pre-exposure prophylaxis if rabies	I/D: 2 site on 0 and 7 day IM: 1 site on 0 and 7 day
• Rabies Ig is given in this category of bite	Category III
• Td vaccine advantage	Freeze and heat resistant, open vial policy is applicable. Shelf life- 24 – 36 month
• Characteristics of mentally healthy person	• Feels comfortable, secure and adequate about himself • Feels right towards other • Able to meet demands of life
• NITI Aayog (replaced planning commission on 1st Jan 2015)	**National Institution for Transforming India** • Provides a critical directional and strategic input into the development process. "Think tank" • Monitor and evaluate the implementation of programmes • Focus on technology upgradation and capacity building
• 3 years action agenda of NITI Aayog (2018-18 to 2019-20)	• The Aayog was told to prepare: • 15 year vision, 7 year strategy and Three Year Action agenda documents • Proposed agenda is attached at the end of this sec:
• Proposed ICD 11 to be presented in 2019 contains how many chapters	26
• EYE strategy for	Elimination Yellow Fever Epidemic (by WHO, UNICEF)

IMPORTANT ONE LINERS

Father of Medicine/First true Epidemiologist – **Hippocrates**
'Epidemiological Triad' comprises of – Agent, Host and Environment
Extermination of organism is – **Eradication**
Action taken prior to onset of disease is - **Primary Prevention**
Early diagnosis and treatment – **Secondary Prevention**
Ivory Towers of disease – **Large hospitals**
Prevalence is a ratio not rate

Contd...

Preventive and Social Medicine (PSM)

Total no of deaths /total no of cases – **Case fatality**

Observe deaths/expected deaths is – **Standardized mortality ratio (SMR)**

Cohort study is forward looking /prospective study

Relative risk is incidence among exposed /incidence among non-exposed

Framingham heart study is a cohort study

First case to come to notice of investigator is **index case**

Gap between primary case and secondary case is **serial interval**

First vaccine to be discovered is **smallpox vaccine** (Edward Jenner)

Risk of cold chain failure is greatest at- **subcenter/village level**

Bleaching powder – 33% available chlorine

Most effective sterilizing agent is – **Autoclaving**

Sensitivity identifies – true positives, specificity identifies - True Negative.

Usefulness of a screening test is given by – **Sensitivity**

Koplik's spots are diagnostic of – **Measles** (upper 2nd molar)

DOTS is – Directly Observed Treatment, Short Course Chemotherapy

HBeAg is marker of – Infectivity/Viral replication

SARS is caused be – Coronary virus

DANISH 1331 strain for – BCG vaccine

Chandlers Index for hookworms is – Average number of Eggs/g of stool

Only communicable disease of man that is always fatal – **Rabies**

Slim disease is – **AIDS**

MC cause of heart disease in 5-30 years old is – **Rheumatic fever**

WHO blindness is - **<3/60**

Prevalence of blindness in India – **1%**

MC complaint of IUD insertion is – **bleeding**

MTP Act, 1971 was passed in – **April 1972**

3 most important MCH problems – **Malnutrition, Infection** and **Unregulated fertility**

Tocopherols are – **Vitamin E**

Richest source of vitamin-C – **Amla** (Indian Gooseberry)

Adult Pregnant females are anemic if – **Hb < 11 g%**

IQ calculation by = Mental Age/Chronological Age × 100

Disinfecting action of chlorine is due to – **Hypochlorous acid**

Residual level of chlorine in water – **0.5 mg × Contact period 1 hr**

Paris green is a – **Stomach Poison**

Sickness benefit under ESI Act, 1948 – **91 days**

World Health day – **7th April**

17 D strain – **Yellow fever vaccine**

DOC for lymphogranuloma venereum – **Doxycycline**

Hepatitis A & E transmission – **Faecal-oral route**

DOC cholera in pregnancy – **Furazolidone**

Tourniquet test (dengue) is +ve - >20 petechial spots/sq. inch in cubital fossa

8th Day Disease – **Tetanus neonatorum**

The Factory Act and ESI Act were passed in – **1948**

No plant source for vitamins – **B$_{12}$ and D**

Milk is poor in – **Vit C and iron**

Multi-purpose Workers introduced by - **Kartar Singh Committee**

DOTS Plus refers to – **MDR TB treatment (Cat. IV)**

Midday meal program provides – **1/3 calories and ½ proteins**

MC side effect of Depot contraceptives – **Irregular menstrual bleeding**

Q-fever is caused by **Coxiella burnetii**

Carcinoma protected by OCP's – **Ovarian carcinoma**

Mortality is included in – **NRR** (Net reproduction rate)

Health worker in Malaria control must visit all houses every – **Fortnight**

Hepatitis B vaccine is type of – **killed vaccine**

Vaccine strain for swine flu vaccine in India – **A7/California**/2009

Normal IQ is – 90 to 109

Amplifier host of Japanese encephalitis – **Pigs**

In ORS, Na$^+$ absorption is due to – **Glucose**

Plasmodium discovered by – **Laveran**

MDR TB is – Resistance to INH and Rifampicin

Denominator of GFR – Women in reproductive age group (15-49 years)

Most abundant Ig in breast milk – **IgA**

Most important step after disaster – **Chlorination of water**

Category 9 biomedical waste is – **Incineration ash**

Rural health Scheme was recommended by – **Srivastava Committee**

In DOTS diagnosis is based on – **Sputum smears**

Maximum tolerable sound level to human ears – **85 dB**

Wasted sharps biochemical waste category – **Four**

OPV vaccine doses in immunization program – 5

Contd...

Contd...

Key Points

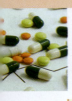

FMGE Solutions Screening Examination

PREVENTIVE AND SOCIAL MEDICINE (PSM)

- Least priority color in triage – **Black**
- Marc Koska discovered – **K1 auto-disable syringes**
- Sufficiency of pasteurization is tested by – **Phosphatase test**
- MC organism of food poisoning – **Staphylococcus**
- 1994 epidemic in India was – **Plague**
- Father of Modern Toxicology – **Mathieu Orfila**
- Main aim of vision 2020 – **Eliminate avoidable blindness**
- Doors + windows area in school area - **>25% floor area**
- Web of causation proposed by – **McMahon and Pugh**
- Prophylactic treatment of rheumatic heart disease – **Benzathine penicillin**
- Ambulatory patients in triage – **Cat III (Green)**
- MDG Goal 4 is to reduce child mortality by – **Two-thirds by 2015**
- Blood screening before transfusion – **HIV/HBV/HCV/Malaria/Syphilis**
- Failure rate of condoms – **2-14 per HWY**
- India is in Demographic cycle – **Stage 3** (Declining Birth rate and Declining Death rate)
- Avian influenza DOC – **Oseltamivir 150 mg BD × 5 days**
- Normal distribution curve is – **Bell shaped symmetric**
- MPW is located at – **Subcenter level**
- International Conference at Alma-Ata (1978) gave concept of – **primary health care**
- MC disorder to be screened in neonates – **Neonatal hypothyroidism**
- Richest source of vit-A/D is – **Halibut liver oil**
- Under RNTCP, Case finding is – **Passive**
- Annual growth rate for India – **1.93%**
- Yaws is caused by- **Treponema pertenue**
- For every 1 clinical case of Poliomyelitis, there are – **1000 sub-clinical cases**
- Small Pox was declared Eradicated on- **8th May, 1980**
- Only Non-steroidal OCP – **Centchroman (Saheli)**
- MCC of blindness – **Cataract**
- Elimination level for leprosy – **<1/10, 000**
- Polio stool samples are transported in – **Reverse cold chain (+2°C to +8°C)**
- Reverse smoking causes: **Carcinoma of hard palate**
- ORS solution should be used within – **24 hours**
- Year of great divide: **1921**
- MCC of MMR in India: **Postpartum hemorrhage**
- MC direct cause of MMR: **PPH**
- MC indirect cause of MMR: **Anemia**
- Gap between primary case and secondary case: **Serial interval**
- Total amount of iron given during the pregnancy: **1000 mg**
- Best contraceptive for a lactating female: **Progesterone only pill**
- Ebola virus is spread by: **Through contact of body fluids**
- Vitamin D richest source is: **Fish liver oil**
- Chronic malnutrition is assessed by: **Height/age**
- Refrigerated breast milk can be kept for: **24 hours**
- In cholera epidemic which step should be first taken: **Safe water supply and sanitation**
- Toxin in Epidemic dropsy is: **Sanguinarine**
- Beds in CHC: **40**
- Iodized salt is given in an area endemic of Goiter. Type of prevention: **Specific protection**
- Graph showing Sharp rise and sharp fall in number of cases: **Point source epidemics**
- Changes in occurrence of a disease over a long period of time: **Secular trend**
- Lead time: **Delay between initiation and completion of a process**

TABLE: Levels of prevention

Level of prevention	Timing	Mode of prevention
Primordial	Before emergence of risk factor	–
Primary	Risk factor present but NO disease yet	Health promotion Specific protection
Secondary	When probably Disease has started	Early diagnosis Treatment
Tertiary	Disease in progression	Disability limitation Rehabilitation

TABLE: Vaccines and their associated strain

Vaccine	Strain
Anti HIV	Ankara strain (under trial)
Anti-malarial	Lytic cocktail (SPF 66)
BCG	DANISH 1331
Japanese Encephalitis	Nakayama Strain (killed) SA 14-14-2 (live)- Currently used
Killed H1N1	California strain
Measles	Edmonston strain
Mumps	Jeryl Lynn Strain
Rabies	Fixed viral strain
Rubella	RA 27/3 strain
Varicella	Oka strain
Yellow fever	17 D strain

Contd...

Preventive and Social Medicine (PSM)

TABLE: Some common infectious diseases and their incubation period

Disease	Causative organism	Incubation period
Mumps	RNA Myxovirus	14 to 21 days
Influenza	Orthomyxovirus	18 to 72 hours
Measles (Rubella)	RNA Paramyxovirus	10 to 14 days
Chickenpox	Human Herpes Virus 3	14 to 16 days

TABLE: Common mosquitos and their associated diseases

Anopheles (Sophisticated mosquito)	Culex (nuisance mosquito)	Aedes (tiger mosquito)	Mansonoides
Malaria	• Japanese encephalitis • West Nile fever • *Bancroftian filariasis* • Viral hemorrhagic	• Yellow fever • Rift valley fever • Chikungunya fever • Dengue • Dengue haemorrhagic fever	• Brugian filariasis

TABLE: Some national health programs and their respective years

National Mental Health Programme: **1987**
National Family Planning Programme: **1951**
National Tuberculosis Programme (NTP): **1962**
Revised National TB Control Programme (RNTCP): **1992**
National AIDS Control Programme (NACP): **1987**
National Malaria Control Programme (NMCP): **1953**
National Leprosy Control Program: **1955**
Integrated Child Development Services scheme (ICDS): **1975**
National Programme for Control of Blindness (NPCB): **1976**

TABLE: IQ scoring of mental retardation

Mental status	IQ range
Normal IQ	70 and below
Mild mental retardation	50–69
Moderate MR	35–49
Severe MR	21–34
Profound MR	20 and below

TABLE: Food adulteration diseases and their toxins

Disease	Toxin	Adulterant
Lathyrism	BOAA	Khesari Dal
Epidemic dropsy	*Sanguinarine*	*Argemone oil*
Endemic ascites	Pyrrolizidine alkaloids	Crotalaria seeds
Ergotism	Ergot/clavine alkaloids	Claviceps fusiformis
Aflatoxicosis	Aflatoxins	Aspergillus flavus

TABLE: Interpretation of Chandler's index

Average number of eggs/g of stool	Interpretation
<200	No significance
200–250	Potential danger
250–300	Minor public health problem
>300	Major public health problem

MODIFIED KUPPUSWAMI SCALE

It includes 3 components:
- Education status of head
- Occupation status of head
- Income per capita.

Total score of 3 components	Socioeconomic class
26–29	Upper
16–25	Upper-middle
11–15	Lower-middle
05–10	Upper-lower
03–04	Lower

TABLE: Triage color code and their significance

Category	Color	Remarks/steps
Category 1	Red	**Highest priority** - Patient immediate resuscitations or lifesaving surgery (0 to 6 hours)
Category 2	Yellow/blue	High possible resuscitation or life-saving surgery (within 6 to 24 hours)
Category 3	Green	Ambulatory/low minor injuries; non-life threating
Category 4	Black	Dead, Moribund; least priority

FMGE Solutions Screening Examination

TABLE: Biomedical waste management

Color Category	Type of biomedical waste	Treatment options
Yellow	• Human & animal anatomical waste • Soiled waste (with blood, body fluid) • Expired/Discarded/cytotoxic medicine • Chemical waste • Chemical liquid waste • Discarded linen, mattress, beddings contaminated with blood or body fluids	Incineration/Deep burial Non-chlorinated chemical disinfection
Red	• Recyclable contaminated waste ▪ Disposable items such as tubes, bottles, IV sets, urine bags, syringes without needle, gloves	Autoclaving or microwaving/hydroclaving followed by shredding
White/Translucent (puncture/leak proof container)	• Waste sharps including metals: Needles, blades or any contaminated sharp object	Autoclaving or dry heat sterilization followed by shredding and mutilation
Blue	• Glassware: included medicine vials except those contaminated with cytotoxic waste • Metallic body implants	Disinfection (by soaking waste with detergent and sodium hypochlorite)/Autoclaving/Microwaving/Hydroclaving

INSTRUMENT OF IMPORTANCE PUBLIC HEALTH

Instruments	Use
• Ice Lined Refrigerator	Cold chain temperature maintenance
• Dial Thermometer	Cold chain temperature monitoring
• Horrocks apparatus	Chlorine demand estimation in water
• Chloroscope	Measuring level of residual chlorine in drinking water

Contd...

Instruments	Use
• Winchester Quart/Quart Bottle	Assess physical & chemical quality of drinking water
• Kata Thermometer	Assess cooling power and velocity of air
• Psychrometer	Humidity
• Anemometer	Assess air & wind velocity
• Hygrometer/Sling Psychrometer	Assess air humidity
• Salter's Scale	Field instrument to assess lbw
• Stadiometer	Height of adult
• Shakir's Tape	Mid arm circumference

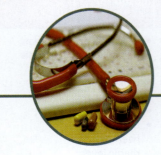

SPECIFIC GRAVITY

• Specific gravity of ascitic fluid/Edema	<1.012 (transudate); >1.020 (exudate)
• Effusion fluid	<1.016 (transudate); >1.016 (exudate)
• Urine	1.015–1.025
• Hydatid fluid	1.005–1.009

TABLE: Classification of weight status and disease risk

Classification	Body mass Index (kg/m²)	Obesity class	Disease Risk
Under weight	<18.5	–	–
Healthy weight	18.5–24.9	–	–
Over weight	25.0–29.9	–	Increased
Obesity	30.0–39.9	I	High
Obesity	35.0–39.9	II	Very high
Extreme obesity	≥40	III	Extremely high

Medicine

TABLE Ethnic-specific cut point values for waist circumference

Ethnic group	Waist circumference
Europeans	
Men	>94 cm (>37 in)
Women	>80 cm (>31.5 in)
South Asians and Chinese	
Men	>90 cm (>35 in)
Women	>80 cm (>31.5 in)
Japanese	
Men	>85 cm (>33.5 in)
Women	>90 cm (>35 in)
Ethnic south and central Americans	Use south asian recommendations until more specific data are available
Sub-Saharan Africans	Use European data until more specific data are available
Eastern Mediterranean and Middle Eastern (Arab) Populations	Use European data until more specific data are available

TREMORS

• Physiological tremors	Anxiety, Fright (8–12 Hz)
• Resting tremor, Pin rolling	PD (4–6 Hz)
• Intentional tremor	Cerebellar lesion <4 Hz
• Essential/Fine tremor	Hyperthyroidism Rosenbach sign: Fine tremor of closed eyelids
• Flapping tremor/Asterixis	Hepatic and metabolic tremor
• Perioral tremor	Rabbit synd. General paresis of insane

Most common type of headache: **Tension headache**

Most common type of headache in males: **Cluster headache**

Most common type of seizure in neonate: **Subtle seizure**

Most common type of seizure in adults: **GTCS**

Most common cause of meningitis in neonate: **Klebsiella > Staph. Aureus**

Most common primary malignant brain tumor: **Glioma**

Most common benign brain tumor: **Meningioma**

IOC for Addison's disease: **ACTH stimulation test**

IOC Conn's syndrome: **Plasma renin/Aldosterone ratio**

Congenital adrenal hyperplasia: **21a- Hydroxylase**

Contd...

Best test for short term control of diabetes: **Serum Fructosamine**

Curschmann's spirals are seen in **Bronchial asthma**

Pink frothy sputum is seen in **Pulmonary edema**

Most common cause of acute bacterial endocarditis: *Staph aureus*

Most common cause of sub-acute bacterial endocarditis: *Step viridans*

Most common cause of prosthetic valve endocarditis: **CONS**

Libman sacks endocarditis is seen with: **SLE**

Strongest layer of GIT: **Sub mucosal layer**

Pacemaker of GIT: **Cells of Cajal**

Most common cause of hemoptysis: **Pulmonary TB**

Most common cause of hematemesis: **PUD**

IOC of GERD: **24-hour pH monitoring**

Marker of eradication of H. Pylori: **Urea breath test**

DOC of IBD: **Sulfasalazine**

Hepatitis B antigen first to appear in blood: **HBsAg**

Hepatitis B antigen which never appears in blood: **HBcAg**

Pseudochylous ascites is seen in: **Malignant ascites**

Pseudo-lymphoma is seen in: **Sjögren's syndrome**

Most common type of nephrotic syndrome in adults: **Focal segmental glomerulosclerosis**

Most common type of nephrotic syndrome in children: **Minimal change disease**

Most sensitive marker of SLE: **ANA (Antinuclear antibody)**

Investigation of choice for SLE: **ds- DNA**

Antibody causing psychosis in SLE: **Anti-Ribosomal-P antibody**

IOC for antiphospholipid antibody syndrome: **Anti-B2 Glycoprotein antibody**

Earliest clinical feature of scleroderma: **Raynaud's phenomenon**

Interstitial pneumonia is most frequently due to influenza virus

Bulging fissure on CXR is seen in: **Klebsiella pneumonia**

Most common site of Bronchiectasis: **Left Lower lobe**

Most common clinical presentation of lung CA: **Cough**

Glucose fever is relates with: **Aldosterone**

Partial pressure of oxygen in alveoli: **103 mm Hg**

CSF glucose compared to blood glucose: 60–70% of concentration of blood

Resistant hypertension: **Resistance to 3 or more anti-hypertensive drugs including thiazides**

Contd...

Key Points

FMGE Solutions Screening Examination

- Antibody incriminated causing Henoch-Schonlein purpura: **IgA**
- Iron is absorbed from: **Duodenum with fast clearance**
- **Thalassemia:** Autosomal Recessive
- **Diarrhea** can present with hypokalemia and Metabolic acidosis
- Seborrheic dermatitis, cellulitis, alopecia and apathy is seen in: **Biotin deficiency**
- RBC cast is present in: **Acute Glomerulonephritis**
- In Wilson disease, chelation is done by: **ZINC**
- In hemochromatosis, all organs are affected except: **CNS**
- CNS bleed in boxers: **Subdural hemorrhage**
- LE cells are seen in: **SLE**
- Emphysema seen due to chronic smoking: **Centriacinar emphysema**
- Wegener's granulomatosis is diagnosed by: **c-ANCA**
- DOC for enteric fever: **Ceftriaxone**
- DOC for listeria meningitis: **Ampicillin**
- DOC for Herpes simplex encephalitis: **Acyclovir**
- Mottling of lung is seen in: **Silicosis**
- Antibody in Goodpasture syndrome: **Anti-GBM**
- Most common Callum patch in rheumatic heart disease is seen in: **Left Atrium**
- Canon A wave is seen in: **Complete Heart Block**
- Most common cause of mitral stenosis: **Rheumatic fever**
- In case of severe MS how much left atrial pressure required to maintain a normal cardiac output: **~25 mm Hg**
- **Malar flush** with **pinched and blue facies** are clinical findings in case of: **Severe Mitral stenosis**
- **Carvallo's sign is seen in: Functional tricuspid regurgitation (TR)** secondary to severe pulmonary hypertension
- **Carvallo's sign:** Functional TR may be audible along the left sternal border. **This murmur is usually louder during inspiration and diminishes during forced expiration**

TABLE: Congenital heart diseases and their CXR finding

Total anomalous pulmonary venous connection	Figure of 8 or snowman heart
Transposition of great arteries	Egg on side appearance
TOF	Boot shaped heart
Ebstein anomaly	Box shaped heart
Coarctation of aorta	'3' sign

TABLE In HIV positive individuals/AIDS

Most common malignancy	Kaposi sarcoma (70%)
Most common cause of seizures	HIV encephalopathy > Toxoplasmosis
Most common fungal infection	Cryptococcus neoformans
Most common lymphoma (NHL)	B- cell immunoblastic lymphoma (CMS lymphoma)
Most common cause of blindness	CMV retinitis
Most common eye lesions	Cotton wool spots, HIV keratitis
Most common opportunistic infection	Pneumocystis carinii (Tuberculosis in India)
Most common CXR finding in TB with HIV	Miliary shadows
Most common electrolyte abnormality	Hyponatremia, SIADH

TABLE: ECG basics

ECG finding	Significance
P wave	Atrial depolarization
QRS	Ventricular depolarization
T wave	Ventricular repolarization
U wave	Delayed repolarization of papillary muscles
PR interval	Spread of impulse from SAN to AVN
ST segment	Isoelectric segment

TABLE: S1 heart sounds and its variables

Loud S1	Soft S1	Variable S1	Reversed split S1
Normal in children	Sinus bradycardia	AV dissociation	Mitral stenosis
Anemia	Prolonged PR interval	Atrial fibrillation	Left atrial myxoma
Pregnancy	Severe MR	Complete heart block	Left bundle branch block
Sinus tachycardia	Chronic severe MR	Multiple ectopics	
Thyrotoxicosis,	Acute MI	Ventricular tachycardia	
Beriberi	Myocarditis	Atrial flutter with varying block	
AV fistula	Ventricular aneurysm		
Mitral and tricuspid stenosis	Cardiomyopathy		
Short PR interval	Calcified MS		

Medicine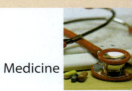

TABLE: Heart sounds and murmurs

Mid-systolic murmur	Pansystolic murmur	Late systolic murmur	Early diastolic murmur	Mid-diastolic murmur	Continuous murmurs
AS PS HOCM TOF ASD	MR VSD TR	MVP OCM	AR PR Graham Steell murmur (pulmonary incompetence due to pulmonary HT and MS)	MS Austin flint (aortic regurgitation) TS Carey-Coombs murmur (Rheumatic fever)	PDA Coronary AV fistula ASD Mammary souffle Anomalous left coronary artery Ruptured aneurysm of sinus of Valsalva Proximal coronary artery stenosis Aortopulmonary window

TABLE: Mediastinal masses: Most common lesions are

Anterior mediastinum	Middle mediastinum	Posterior mediastinum
Thymoma (Most common) Lymphomas Teratomatous neoplasms Thyroid masses	Pericardial cyst (Most common mediastinal mass) Lymphoma (MC mediastinal tumor) Vascular masses Granulomatous disease Bronchogenic cysts	Neurogenic tumors Meningoceles Meningomyeloceles Gastroenteric cysts Esophageal diverticula

TABLE: Anemia and their causes

Microcytic Hypochromic anemia	Normocytic Normochromic	Macrocytic anemia
Sideroblastic anemia Iron deficiency Thalassemia Anemia of chronic disease Lead poisoning	CRF A.I.H.A HL/NHL C.L.L Aplastic anemia	CLD Hypothyroidism Aplastic anemia Decrease B_{12} and Folic acid level

TABLE: Extravascular and intravascular hemolysis

Extravascular hemolysis	Intravascular hemolysis
Hereditary Spherocytosis Thalassemia Sickle cell anemia	Cold agglutinin syndrome G6PD (XLR)
Haptoglobin level normal	Haptoglobin level decreases or absent

TABLE: Common hematological malignancies

Disease	Finding	IOC	TOC
Polycythemia vera	Hb >19 gm%	Urinary erythropoietin level	Venesection (phlebotomy)
CML	Ph (9:22)	Flow cytometry	Imatinib
Essential thrombocytosis	Platelets conc: ↑↑	Platelets conc:	Hydroxyurea
Myelofibrosis	Tear drop RBC	BM Biopsy	BM Tx

TABLE: Intracranial bleed and their CT findings

Subdural hematoma	Concavo-convex bleed hyper-density
Extradural hemorrhage	Biconvex /flame shaped hyper-density
Subarachnoid hemorrhage	Intraventricular bleed/blood in sylvian fissure
Intraparenchymal bleed	Mostly a lesion or hyperdensity in basal ganglia secondary to hypertension.

Key Points

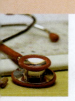

FMGE Solutions Screening Examination

TABLE: CSF findings in common infections

CSF	Normal	Acute bacterial meningitis	Tubercular meningitis	Viral meningitis	Guillain–Barre syndrome	Fungal meningitis
Pressure	50–180 mm H_2O	Increased	Increased	Increased	Normal	Elevated
Color	Clear	Turbid	Straw	Clear	Normal	
Cells	0–4 lymphocytes/cu.mm	>1000	>100	>25	Normal	25–500
Sugar	2/3rd of blood sugar	Decreased	Decreased	Normal	Normal	Low
Protein	15–45 mg %	Increased	Increased	Increased	Increased (albumin-cytological disassociation)	Normal/elevated

TABLE: Differences between lower and upper motor neuron lesion

	LMN	UMN	Extra pyramidal damage
TONE	Decreased tone/flaccidity	Increased spasticity	Decreased rigidity
DTR	Areflexia	Brisk reflex	Normal
Special features	Fasciculations + wasting	Babinski's sign + No wasting	Chorea, athetosis, hemiballismus
Superficial reflex	Present	Absent	–
Example	Motor neuron disease	Cerebral malaria	Punch drunk syndrome

TABLE: Modified Jones Criteria

Major criteria	Minor criteria	Essential criteria
Carditis	Fever	ASO titer > 333 IU for children 5–15 years
Arthritis	Arthralgia	Throat swab positive for group A beta hemolytic streptococcus
Sydenham chorea	Laboratory parameters Increased PR interval CRP positive Leukocytosis Increased ESR	
Erythema marginatum		
Subcutaneous nodules		

TABLE: Hormonal levels in some common adrenal pathologies

Aldosterone	↑Conn's ↓Addison's
Cortisol	↑Cushing syndrome
Sex steriods	↑Congenital adrenal hyperplasia ↓Hypogonadism

TABLE: Common infections and their causative organism

Infection	Causative organism
Lobar pneumonia/Community acquired Pneumonia	Pneumococcus

Contd...

Infection	Causative organism
Nosocomial pneumonia	*Staph. aureus*
HIV associated pneumonia	*P. Jiroveci*
Meningitis adults (sporadic)	Pneumococcus
Meningitis adults (epidemic)	*Neisseria meningitidis*

TABLE: Anion gaps

Normal anion gap (Mn: FUSED CAR)	Increased anion gap (Mn: MUDPILES)	Decreased anion gap (Mn: BPH-M)
F- Fistula pancreatic U-Ureterosigmoidostomy S- Small bowel fistula E- Extra chloride D- Diarrhea C- Carbonic anhydrase Inhibitor (acetazolamide) A- Adrenal insufficiency R- Renal tubular acidosis	M - Methanol U - Uremia D - DKA/AKA/SKA (diabetic/alcoholic/starvation) P - Paraldehyde / phenformin I - Iron / INH L - Lactic acidosis E - Ethylene glycol S - Salicylates	Bromide intoxication Plasma cell dyscrasia Hypoalbuminemia Monoclonal protein

TABLE: Important casts

Hyaline cast: Present normally in urine
RBC cast: Seen in acute glomerulonephritis
WBC cast: Seen in interstitial nephritis, pyelo nephritis
Brood granular casts: Seen in chronic renal failure

Medicine

TABLE: Tumor markers

Tumor markers	Cancer	Non-neoplastic conditions
Hormones		
Human chorionic gonadotropin	Gestational trophoblastic disease, gonadal gem cell tumor	Pregnancy
Calcitonin	Medullary cancer of the thyroid	
Catecholamines	Pheochromocytoma	
Oncofetal antigens		
α Fetoprotein	Hepatocellular carcinoma, gonadal germ cell tumor	Cirrhosis hepatitis
Carcinoembryonic antigen	Adenocarcinomas of the colon, pancreas, lung, breast, ovary	Pancreatitis, hepatitis, inflammatory bowel disease, smoking
Enzymes		
Prostatic acid phosphatase	Prostate cancer	Prostatitis, prostatic hypertrophy
Neuron-specific enolase	Small-cell cancer of the lung, neuroblastoma	
Lactate dehydrogenase	Lymphoma, Ewing's sarcoma	Hepatitis, hemolytic anemia, many others
Tumor-associated proteins		
Prostate-specific antigen	Prostate cancer	Prostatitis, prostatic hypertrophy
Monoclonal immunoglobulin	Myeloma	Infection, MGUS
CA-125	Ovarian cancer, some lymphomas	Menstruation, peritonitis, pregnancy
CA 19–9	Colon, pancreatic, breast cancer	Pancreatitis, ulcerative colitis
CD30	Hodgkin's disease anaplastic large-cell lymphoma	–
CD 25	Hairy cell leukemia, adult T cell leukemia/ lymphoma	–

TABLE: Suspected carcinogens

Tumor markers	Cancer
Carcinogens	Associated cancer of neoplasm
Alkylating agents	Acute myeloide leukemia, bladder cancer
Androgens	Prostate cancer
Aromatic amines (dyes)	Bladder cancer
Arsenic	Cancer of the lung, skin
Benzene	Acute myelocytic leukemia
Chromium	Lung cancer
Diethylstilbestrol (prenatal)	Vaginal cancer (clear cell)
Epstein-Barr virus	Burkitt's lymphoma, nasal T cell lymphoma
Estrogens	Cancer of the endometrium, liver, breast
Ethyl alcohol	Cancer of the breast, liver esophagus, head and neck
Helicobacter pylori	Gastric cancer, gastric MALT lymphoma
Hepatitis B or C virus	Liver cancer
Human immunodeficiency virus	Non-hodgkin's lymphoma, kaposi's sarcoma, squamous cell carcinomas (especially of the urogenital tract)
Human papilloma virus	Cancers of the cervix, anus, oropharynx
Human T cell lymphotropic virus type 1 (HTLY-1)	Adult T cell leukemia/lymphoma
Immunosuppressive agents (azathioprine cyclosporine, glucocorticoids)	Non-hodgkin's lymphoma
Ionizing radiation (therapeutic or diagnostic)	Breast, bladder, thyroid, soft tissue, bone, hematopoietic and many more
Nitrogen mustard gas	Cancer of the lung, head and neck, nasal sinuses
Nickel dust	Cancer of the lung, nasal sinuses
Phenacetin	Cancer of the renal pelvis and bladder
Polycyclic hydrocarbons	Cancer of the lung, skin (especially squamous cell carcinoma of scrotal skin)
Radon gas	Lung cancer
Schistosomiasis	Bladder cancer (squamous cell)
Sunlight (ultraviolet)	Skin cancer (squamous cell and melanoma)
Tobacco (including smokeless)	Cancer of the upper aerodigestive tract, bladder
Vinyl chloride	Liver cancer (angiosarcoma)
Agents that are thought to act as cancer initiators and/ or promoters	

Key Points

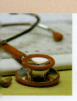

FMGE Solutions Screening Examination

TABLE: A comparison of syndromes of obesity—hypogonadism and mental retardation

Feature	Syndrome				
	Prader-Willi	Laurence-Moon-Biedl	Ahlstrom's	Cohen's	Carpenter's
Inheritance	Sporadic; two-thirds have defect	Autosomal recessive	Autosomal recessive	Probably autosomal recessive	Autosomal recessive
Stature	Short	Normal; infrequently short	Normal; infrequently	Short or tall	Normal
Obesity	Generalized Moderate of severe onset 1–3 years	Generalized Early onset, 1–2 years	Truncal Early onset, 2–5 years	Truncal Mid-childhood, age 5	Truncal, gluteal
Craniofacies	Narrow bifrontal diameter almond-shaped eyes strabismus v-shaped mouth high-arched palate	Not distinctive	Not distinctive	High nasal bridge Arched palate Open mouth Short philtrum	Acrocephaly Flat nasal bridge High-arched palate
Limbs	Small hands and feet hypotonia	Polydactyly	No abnormalities	Hypotonia Narrow hands and feet	Polydactyly Syndactyly Genu valgum
Reproductive status	1° Hypogonadism	1° Hypogonadism	Hypogonadism in males but not in females	Normal gonadal function or hypogonadotropic hypogonadism	2° Hypogonadism
Other features	Enamel hypoplasia Hyperphagia Temper tantrums Nasal speech			Dysplastic ears Delayed puberty	
Mental retardation	Mild to moderate		Normal intelligence	Mild	Slight

IMPORTANT TO KNOW

• Light's criteria is used to determine	Exudative vs transudative pleural fluid
• MCC of pleura effusion	CHF
• MCC of exudative pleural Effusion	TB
• Comprehension and Fluency and in Broca's and Wernicke's aphasia	BCWF **Broca:** Comprehension preserved **Wernicke:** Fluency preserved
• Triad of Miller Fisher syndrome	Acute ext Ophthalmoplegia Areflexia Ataxia
• Useless hand syndrome of oppenheimer	MS (MRI: Dawson finger sign)

• Charcot's triad of MS	Intentional tremor, Nystagmus, Dysarthria (IND)
• Charcot triad of Ascending cholangitis	RUQ pain, fever, jaundice
• Ashleaf spot, Shagreen patch seen in	Tuberous sclerosis/Koenen tumor
• Vogt triad of tuberous sclerosis	Seizure, MR, facial angiofibroma
• DAS 28 score is used for	To assess severity of RA
• Anti Histone A/B is specific for	Drug induced lupus
• McGinn white sign is seen in	Pulm Embolism (S1Q3T3)
• Sputum containing charcot-leyden crystal, curschmann spirals, Creola bodies	Bronchial Asthma
• Current jelly sputum	Klebsiella pneumoniae

Contd...   *Contd...*

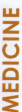

Medicine

• Giant cell/Hecht's pneumonia is seen in	Measles
• Austin flint murmur is heard in	Severe AR
• Osborn wave/ J wave is seen in	Hypothermia
• ST segment in ECG	End to S to beginning of T
• ECG finding of digitalis toxicity	T wave inversion, Inverse check mark sign
• Wenckebach phenomenon is seen in	2nd degree heart block (Mobitz 1) Seen in digitalis toxicity, B# toxicity
• Murmur which is increased in valsalva maneuver	HOCM, MVP
• Aschoff bodies are pathognomonic of this condition	RF
• D Xylose test is used for	Malabsorption (pancreatic vs intestinal cause)
• Fulminant hepatitis rate is maximum in	Hep D superinfection
• Diuretic which can cause barter syndrome	Furosemide
• Nephrocalcinosis is a feature of this type of RTA	Type I
• Hyperkalemia is feature of this type of RTA	Type IV
• MM, Fanconi synd, Wilson's disease can cause this RTA	Type II (MC type of RTA)
• RIFLE criteria is used for	ARF
• Reid index is used in	Chronic bronchitis (>0.4)
• MC cause of BUDDCHIARI syndrome –	polycythemia vera
• MC symptom of portal hypertension –	GI bleeding
• Most specific tumor marker of HCC –	alpha fetoprotein
• MC renal lesion associated with HCV-MPGN -1	MPGN
• MC GN associated with HIV	FSGS
• MC cause of nephrotic syndrome in adult	MGN
• MC type of MI	Ant wall MI
• MC type of HIV in India	HIV 1 subtype C

Contd...

• MC organ affected in amyloidosis	Kidney
• MC cause of death in amyloidosis	Heart
• First enzyme rise in MI	Myoglobin
• First enzyme to diagnosed in MI	CKMB
• Most important enzyme diagnosed MI	Trop I
• MC type of stroke	EMBOLIC
• MC site of hemorrhagic stroke	Putamen
• MC type of fistula in CD	Colocolic
• MC type of incontinence in LMN bladder	over flow incontinence
• MC type of incontinence in UMN balder	urge incontinence
• Ankle Jerk in UMNL	Brisk (and absent in LMNL)
• MC cause of cardiac tamponade	Neoplastic disease, idiopathic pericarditis, uremia
• MC nerve affected intracranial aneurism	III
• MC nerve inv in increased ICP	VI
• MC complication of hemodialysis	HTN
• Least common RCC	chromophobe renal carcinoma
• MCC of chr. renal failure	DM nephropathy
• MCC of HTN	Essential HTN
• MCC Of hematuria	Ig A nephropathy

CHANNELOPATHIES

Disease	Ion channel involved
• Hypokalemic periodic paralysis	Slow Ca+ channel
• Hyperkalemic periodic paralysis	Na+
• Cystic fibrosis, Myotonia congenital	Cl-
• Episodic ataxia-1	K channel
• Episodic ataxia-2, Malignant hyperthermia	Ca+ channel

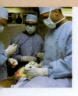

FMGE Solutions Screening Examination

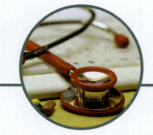

Surgery

Most common site for polymazia is **axilla**	
Amazia refers to absence of stromal and glandular part of breast but presence of nipple and areola	
Tietze disease: Costochondritis, MC involves 2nd costal cartilage	
Mondor's disease – Superficial thrombophlebitis of veins over chest wall and upper abdominal wall	
Fibrocystic disease of breast is usually B/L and common in younger women	

Mastitis
- MC organism: **Staph aureus**
- **Rx** – modified Hiltons method
- **IOC** – USG

Breast cyst
- Well defined **lump**
- **IOC** – USG GUIDED FNAC
- **Rx** – USG guided aspiration

Fibroadenoma
- MC benign **tumor of breast**
- Highly mobile – **Breast mouse**
- MC breast tumor in females less than **30 yrs of age**
- Firm in consistency
- Upon mammography: Popcorn calcification
- **IOC**- FNAC
- **Rx** – Excision

Nipple discharge
- **Bloody** – Duct papilloma (MCC)
- **Greenish** / grumous – Duct ectasia (MCC)
- **Milky** – Galactorrhea (MCC pathologically)
- **Serous** – Fibro cystic disease of breast (MCC)

Duct ectasia
- IOC - Mammography
- Rx – Hadfield's operation

Duct papilloma
- IOC - Mammography
- Rx - Microdochectomy

Cystosarcoma phyllodes
- Huge lump
- Irregular and variable consistency
- IOC –FNAC
- Rx- benign – Wide local excision
- Malignant – Simple mastectomy

Breast cancer
- **Genetic** – BRCA 1, BRCA 2, P53 (Li-Fraumeni syndrome)
- **IOC** – Mammography
- Ductal carcinoma in situ
- MC non-invasive breast cancer
- MC comedo cell pattern
- IOC - Incisional biopsy
- Rx - Simple mastectomy

TABLES: Types of mastectomy

Simple or total mastectomy	Removal of breast tissue, nipple-areola complex, and skin
Extended simple mastectomy	Simple mastectomy + removal of level I axillary LNs.
Modified radical mastectomy	Removes all breast tissue and skin, nipple areola complex, pectoralis major and minor muscles and the level, I, II and III axillary LNs,
Extended radical mastectomy	Radical mastectomy + Removal or internal mammary, LNs
Super radical mastectomy	Radical mastectomy + Removal of internal mammary, mediastinal and supraclavicular LNs

3 IMPORTANT TYPES OF MRM

Patey's	Pectoralis minor removed to dissect level III LN
Auchincloss's	Preservation of both pectoralis major and minor. Level I and II LN dissection
Scanlon's	Pectoralis minor divided to remove level III LN

NOTE: Structure NOT removed in radical mastectomy: Supraclavicular LN

Bile and gallbladder facts
- Maximum capacity gall bladder - **50 mL**
- Concentration of bile: **5-10 times**
- Production of bile: **40 mL/hr**
- Terminal ileum absorbs – **B_{12} & bile salts**

Surgery

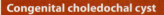

Congenital choledochal cyst
Cyst like dilatation of biliary tree due to weakness of wall
Type 1 is most common
Type 4 is Caroli's disease
IOC – MRCP
Rx: Excision

Cholelithiasis
Pigmented stones: Hemolytic anemia MC cause
Predisposing factor 5f's – fatty, forty, female, fertile and flatulence
IOC-USG abdomen
Rx-laparoscopic cholecystectomy

Acute cholecystitis
IOC – HIDA scan
Rx - Conservative

Chronic cholecystitis
IOC-USG
Rx-Laparoscopy cholecystectomy

Mucocele of gallbladder
Stone in Hartmann's pouch cannot cause mucocele
C/f–lump in Right Upper Quadrant
IOC–USG
Rx-Laparoscopic cholecystectomy

Empyema/pyocele
Clinical feature-Tender lump + fever
IOC–USG
Rx-Cholecystectomy +/- antibiotics

Pneumobilia
Air from D1 passes in gall bladder through fistula, presence of air in biliary tree
Management: Ileostomy with extraction of stone

Acalculous cholecystitis
Cause-Typhoid infection, trauma, septicemia, DM
IOC–HIDA scan
Rx-Usg guided drainage + Antibiotics

Saint's triad
Gallstones
Hiatus hernia
Diverticulosis

Rigler's triad
Small bowel obstruction
Gas within Gall Bladder and or bile ducts
Ectopic gallstone

TABLE: Gallstones
10% gallstones – Radio opaque
90% gallstones – Radio lucent
Gallstones – Mercedes Benz sign, sea gull sign
Limey bile – Sequestration of calcium salts in bile after gradual obstruction of CBD

TABLE: Important tumor staging and classification

Chang staging	Medulloblastoma
Masaoka staging	Thymoma
Shimada index	Neuroblastoma
Rees	Ellsworth classification, Esson prognostic index Retinoblastoma
Bloom–Richardson classification	CA breast
Noguchi's classification	Adenocarcinoma lung
Sullivan modification of MacFarlane system	Adrenocortical CA
Gleason score	CA prostrate
Nevin staging	CA GB
Duke staging	Colorectal ca
Robson staging	RCC
Jackson score	CA penis

Most common Nodes involved:
CA penis: Inguinal nodes
CA testis: Para-aortic LN
On right: Inter aorto-caval LN
On left: Para-aortic LN
CA bladder: Obturator LN
CA prostrate: Obturator LN

Must know facts
Nigro regimen is used for: **Anal Canal CA**
TOC for Duodenal Atresia, Annular pancreas: **Duodenoduodenostomy**
TOC for superior mesenteric artery syndrome: **Duodenojejunostomy**
Length of these instruments:
- Proctoscope 10–12 cm
- Rigid Sigmoidoscope: 25 cm
- Flexible sigmoidoscope: 60 cm
- Colonoscope: 160 cm

Contd...

Key Points

FMGE Solutions Screening Examination

Must know facts

Intracranial bleed:
EDH: Due to tear of middle meningeal artery, appear biconvex on CT, **lucid interval** is present.
SDH: Due to rupture of bridging veins, appear crescentic or concavo - Convex on CT.
Duret hemorrhage is small area of bleeding in ventral and para median part of upper brain stem. Diagnosis: CT or MRI

Bilateral grade 4 or 5 VUR is better treated surgically with ureteric reimplantation.

Berry aneurysm is the most common intra cranial aneurysm

Young women on OCP's are predisposed to **stroke due to venous thrombosis** of sagittal sinus or small cortical veins

Major causes of delayed neurological deficit after CVA: re-rupture, hydrocephalus, vasospasm, hyponatremia.

Commonly used preparation of mannitol: **20% solution, 0.25 g/kg is given IV bolus**

Primary brain injury occurs at the time of injury, secondary brain occurs at some time after impact

MC tumors of brain: **Metastatic/Secondaries**

MC posterior fossa tumor in children: **Astrocytoma**

MC site of Medulloblastoma: **Vermis**

MC spinal tumor: **Metastatic**

MC primary spinal tumor: **Nerve sheath tumor**

MC intra medullary tumor: **Astrocytoma**

MC site of primary spinal tumor: **Intradural extramedullary**

The term " dumbbell" lesion is used to describe **neurofibroma**

Acoustic neuroma can arise from any nerve except optic and olfactory nerve.

Common uses of **stereotactic radiosurgery:** Metastatic tumors, benign lesions of cranial nerve, A-V malformations, trigeminal neuralgia.

Struma ovarii: Benign ovarian tumor containing thyroid tissue, some patients develop thyrotoxicosis.

Lingual thyroid: rounded swelling developed at the back of the tongue at the foramen cecum.

Refetoff syndrome: End organ resistance to T4

Father of thyroid surgery: Theodor Kocher.

The **external laryngeal** nerve runs close to superior thyroid artery and **recurrent laryngeal nerve runs** close to inferior thyroid artery.

Wolff-chaikoff effect: Iodine induced hypothyroidism

Jod-Basedow effect: Iodine induced hyper thyroidism

MC site of thyroglossal cyst: **Sub hyoid**.

Acute suppurative thyroiditis is rare seen in children & caused by streptococcus & anaerobes.

Must know facts

Hashimoto's thyroiditis or Struma Lymphomatosa is MC inflammatory disorder of thyroid and leading cause of hypothyroidism. Auto antibodies are produced against Tg, TPO, TSH-R.

Grave's disease (Diffuse toxic goiter): MC cause of hyperthyroidism caused by stimulatory autoantibodies to TSH–R.

Toxic adenoma (Plummer's disease): single hyper functioning nodule typically occurs in young patients.

Thyroid storm (Thyrotoxic crisis): It is an emergency due to decompensated hyperthyroidism.

Thyroglossal fistula is never congenital

MC postoperative complication after thyroidectomy: **Hemorrhage**.

MC benign tumor of thyroid gland: **Follicular adenoma**.

Papillary carcinoma: MC carcinoma of thyroid associated with history of radiation exposure. It has best prognosis.

Predisposing factor for long standing goiter: **Follicular carcinoma of thyroid**.

Anaplastic CA of thyroid: MC carcinoma with worst prognosis, neck gets frozen with hard fixed mass.

Medullary carcinoma of thyroid is associated with RET oncogene; tumor marker: Calcitonin.

Sub- Acute thyroiditis/granulomatous thyroiditis/de quervain's thyroiditis is associated with viral infection & can occur as a consequence of viral infection. Only painful condition of thyroid

Pemberton's sign is MC associated with Retrosternal goiter.

MC type of kidney stone (85%) is **calcium oxalate**.

Xanthine & uric acid stone are radio lucent.

Struvite stones composed of Ca^+, NH_3, $Mg\,(PO)_4$ and best treated by **PCNL + ESWL**.

Randall's plaques are soft tissue calcification found in the deep renal medulla.

Infectious stones are more common in females.

Stone in upper ureter: Pain referred to testis.

Stone in mid ureter: Pain referred along iliohypogastric nerve to iliac fossa, mimicking appendicitis.

Stone in lower ureter: Pain referred along ilioinguinal nerve to thigh, scrotum and perineum.

Acidic urine is seen in **calcium oxalate, cystine, uric acid**.

Alkaline urine is seen in **calcium phosphate, struvite**.

NCCT is most sensitive investigation for renal calculi.

If Stone <2 cm treatment is **ESWL**.

Stone >2 cm treatment is **PCNL**.

Contd...   *Contd...*

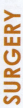

Surgery

Must know facts

MC cause of ureteric obstruction is **Stone**.

MC cause of ureteric colic in hematuria is **Clot**.

Pyelonephritis MC caused by E coli
Clinical feature: Fever, flank pain, vomiting and 80 – 90% of patients have diabetes.

Pyonephrosis MC cause is renal stone
Clinical feature: Anemia, fever, swelling in loin.

M. Tuberculosis reaches the genitourinary organs by hematogenous route from lungs.

Intermittent hydronephrosis (dietl's crisis) associated with swelling in the loin.

MC type of RCC mainly sporadic is **clear cell carcinoma**.

RCC/VHL syndrome: MC sites of distant metastasis are lungs> bone> liver > brain.

MC primary renal tumor of childhood is **wilm's tumor.**

Transitional cell carcinoma accounts for 90% of upper urinary tract cancers.

ADPKD associated with cyst in all sites except brain.

Most common gas produced in intestinal obstruction: N_2

Most common gas produced in Clostridial infection: H_2S

MC gas used to create pneumoperitoneum in laparoscopy: CO_2

MC cause of upper G.I bleeding: **Peptic ulcer**

MC cause of lower G.I bleeding: **Non-specific ulcers**

MCC of jejunostomy feeding: **Diarrhea**

MC site of aortic rupture: **Ligamentum arteriosum**

MCC of leg ulcer: **Venous ulcer**

MC site of fasciotomy: **Calf**

Best treatment for subaponeurotic hematoma: **I & D**

Hardy was first surgeon to do proximal ureteric implantation

Grayhack shunt is shunt for priapism made between corpora cavernosa & corpora spongiosa

TABLE: Strawberry Q' forms

- Strawberry gingivitis: **Wegeners granulomatosis**
- Strawberry cervix: **Trichomonas vaginalis**
- Strawberry gallbladder: **Cholesterolosis**
- Strawberry nasal mucosa: **Sarcoidosis**
- Strawberry nasal mass: **Rhinosporidiosis**
- Strawberry tongue: **Kawasaki disease**

Some most common neoplasm

MC childhood tumor - **Leukemia**
MC childhood leukemia - **ALL**
MC solid tumor of childhood - **Brain tumor**
MC tumor of infancy - **Neuroblastoma**
MC abdominal tumor of child - **Neuroblastoma**

THE SURGICAL MOST COMMON LIST

1305

What is/are the most common...

- MC Cause of acute prostatitis is **E. coli.**
- MC Reason to get treatment for BPH is **symptomatic relief**.
- MC Location for prostate CA is in the **peripheral zone of the prostate gland.**
- MC Renal anomaly is **horseshoe kidney**
- MC Renal inflammatory disorder is **pyelonephritis**
- MC Renal tumor is **renal cell carcinoma**
- MC Source of renal neoplasm is **metastasis**.
- MC Surgery performed on males is **circumcision**
- MC Cause of erectile dysfunction is **vasogenic**
- MC Motility disorder of the esophagus is **achalasia cardia**
- MC Site of peptic ulcer disease is **the first part of the duodenum**
- MC Cause of surgical abdomen is **acute appendicitis.**
- MC Causes of appendix obstruction in the young is **mesenteric lymphadenitis or lymphoid hyperplasia**
- MC Causes of appendix obstruction in older patients is **fecolith and foreign body**.
- MC Tumor of the appendix is **carcinoid**.
- MC Benign tumor of the small bowel is **leiomyoma**.
- MC Primary tumor of the small bowel **adenocarcinoma**.
- MC Malignant tumors of the small bowel are **adenocarcinoma, carcinoid, and lymphoma**.
- MC Small bowel malignancy of children is **lymphoma**.
- MC Surgical condition of the small bowel is **obstruction secondary to adhesions**
- MC Anaerobe in the colon is *Bacteroides* fragilis
- MC Site for metastases from the colon is **the liver**.
- MC Location of colonic obstruction is the **sigmoid colon**.
- MC Cause of colonic obstruction is **adenocarcinoma**.
- MC Site of volvulus is the **sigmoid colon**.
- MC Site of bile duct carcinoma is the **bifurcation of the common hepatic ducts**.
- MC Causes of acute pancreatitis are alcohol consumption and biliary calculi.
- **MC Causes of death in a patient** with pancreatitis are respiratory distress, cardiovascular collapse, coagulopathy and hemorrhage.
- **MC Local complications of acute pancreatitis are paralytic** ileus, sterile peripancreatic fluid collection, and pancreatic abscess.
- MC Best **diagnostic imaging technique** for prostate CA is TRUS

Contd...

Key Points

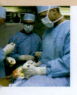

FMGE Solutions Screening Examination

- MC site of carcinoma in oral cavity – **Bucco alveolar complex**
- MC oral cancer – **squamous cell carcinoma**
- Carcinoma tongue MC site – **lateral middle 1/3**
- Carcinoma oral cavity best prognosis – **carcinoma lip**
- MC site of peptic ulcer diseases – **first part of duodenum**
- Second most common site of PUD – **anteropyloric junction**
- Third most site of PUD – **laser curvature of antrum and pylorus**
- MC site of carcinoma stomach – **esophago gastric junction and cardia**
- Maximum conc. of H. pylori – **antrum**
- MC complication of PUD – **Bleeding**
- MC cause of death in PUD – **Perforation**
- Second MC site of gastric carcinoma – **anteropyloric junction**
- MC gastric carcinoma – **adeno carcinoma (histological type)**
- MC benign tumor in small intestine – **adenoma (Ileum)**
- MC malignant tumor in small intestine – **adeno carcinoma (deodeno jejunal junction)**
- MC site of carcinoid tumor in body – **bronchus**
- MC site of carcinoid in intestine – **ileum**
- MC hormone release in carcinoid – **5 HT**
- MC symptom of carcinoid – **flushing and diarrhea**
- MC type of intestinal polyp – **Hyperplastic polyp**
- MC site colorectal carcinoma – **rectum and sigmoid**
- MC effected by metastasis form of colorectal carcinoma – **Liver**
- MC presenting symptom of congenital pyloric stenosis – **vomiting (metabolic alkalosis)**
- MC used surgery in India for duodenal ulcer – **trunkalvegotomoy + drainage**
- MC cause of pernicious anemia – **vitamin B12**
- MC affected part of stomach in pernicious anemia – **fundus and body**
- MC site of leimyomas in GIT – **Stomach**
- MC type of benign tumor of stomach – **leimyomas**
- MC hallmark of Whipplies disease – **SI mucosa macrophages**
- MC test in small intestine malabsorption – **D- xylose absorption test**
- MC CNS manifestation in Whipplies disease - **Dementia**
- MC cause of persistent symptoms of celiac disease – **control intake of gluten**

- MC cause of massive bleeding through PR (55 yrs) - **diverticulosis**
- MC cause painless maroon colored stool - **diverticulosis**
- MC long term affect of radiation on GIT – **telangiectasis**
- MC site of polyp in GIT - **small intestine**
- MC site for Hamartomatous polyp – **small intestine**
- MC site for polyp in Peutz-Jeghers syndrome – **small intestine**
- MC site for polyp in juvenile polyposis – **large intestine**
- MC cause of acute of loss vision – **acute pancreatitis (Purtscher's retinopathy)**
- MC cause of complication of pancreatic pseudocyst – **body and tail of pancreas**
- MC presentation of ZES-PUD+ diarrhea
- MC site of PUD in ZES - **Duodeno bulb (second part of duodenal)**
- MC tumor associated with neurofibroma-1—**optic glioma**
- MC tumor associated with NF-2 – **acoustic neuroma**
- PAUD E ORANGE is seen in – **carcinoma of breast**
- PAUD E ORANGE is due to – **lymphatic obstruction**
- MCC of UTI- **E. coli**
- MCC of renal stone – **Ca+ Oxalate**
- MCC Ca+ oxalate stone – **idiopathic hypercalcemia**
- MCC stag horn calculus- **roteus infection**
- ADPKD cysts not seen in – **lung and brain**
- Best treatment for formed abscess: **I/D**
- Best treatment for TB/cold abscess: **ATT**
- MCC of mycotic aneurysm: **Staph aureus**
- Selmonosky triad is seen in: **Thoracic outlet synd (supraclavicular tenderness, hand paleness on elevation, weakness of 4th and 5th finger)**
- Thrombophlebitis of superficial veins of breast: **Mondor's disease**
- Absence of nipple from breast is condition known as: **Athelia**
- MC type of diaphragmatic hernia: **Posterolateral hernia of Bochdalek**
- Hourglass stomach is seen in: **Pyloric stenosis**
- Cullen sign is seen in: **Hemoperitoneum (periumbilical)**
- Gray turner sign: **Dark bluish/greenish discoloration of flank**
- Karydaki/Bascom's procedure is done in: **Pilonodal sinus**
- Scoring/criteria used in acute pancreatitis: **APACHE score (bed side), Balthazar score (CT severity index), Ranson's criteria**
- Kehr sign is seen in: **Splenic rupture**

Contd...

Contd...

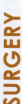

Surgery

- Intra-op fluid of choice for irrigation in BPH: **1.5% isotonic Glycine**
- Post op fluid of choice for irrigation: **0.9% NS**
- For cutting umbilical cord of a newborn baby blade used is: **No. 10**
- Use of fogarty catheter: removal of fresh clot embolus in artery
- Needle used for bone marrow biopsy: **Jamshidi Needle**
- Cleft lip corrected at this age and weight: **10 weeks age/10 pounds weight (Millard criteria)**
- Ogilvie syndrome is: **Acute pseudo colonic obstruction**

TABLE: Salivary gland tumors

Pleomorphic adenoma
- Overall most common tumor of salivary gland
- MC benign salivary gland tumor
- MC tumor of major salivary glands
- MC site is parotid tail (superficial lobe)

Warthin's tumor
- 2nd MC benign tumor of parotid gland
- MC malignant tumor of parotid gland: **Mucoepidermoid CA**
- 2nd MC malignant tumor of parotid gland: **Adenoid cystic CA**
- Most common organism associated with sialadenitis: *Staph. aureus and Strep. viridans*
- Most common salivary gland associated with sialolithiasis: **submandibular gland *(80 %)* > *Parotid gland (20%)***

What is/are the most common...

MC Complication of spinal anesthesia is posture-related headache one day after anesthesia, probably secondary to CSF leakage.

MC Indication for nasogastric tube placement is: **gastric decompression**.

MC Reason for recurrent post-operative ulcer disease is **inadequate vagotomy**.

MISCELLANEOUS

The most common...

MC Suture is over and over.

MC Cause of **hypercalcemia** in a surgical patient is primary and secondary hyperparathyroidism and metastatic bone disease.

MC Cause of **hypermagnesemia** secondary to renal failure.

MC NSAID that decreases platelet function is **aspirin**.

MC Cause of hypovolemic shock is **hemorrhage**.

MC Toe problem is **ingrown toe nails**.

MC Cause of death in children and adults less than 35 years of age is **trauma**.

Contd...

MC Injury to the thoracic cage is **rib fracture**.

MC Hernia in both sexes and all age groups is **bilateral inguinal hernia.**

MC Causes of true aneurysm are acquired **atherosclerosis, congenital fibromuscular dysplasia (Marfans)**

MC Cause of spontaneous, bloody unilateral nipple discharge is **intraductal papilloma.**

MC Cause of hypercalcemia is **hyperparathyroidism**

MC Cause of pre-sinusoidal portal hypertension is **schistosomiasis.**

MC Appliance for compression of bleeding esophageal varices is the **Sengstaken-Blakemore tube.**

MC Cause of secondary hypersplenism is **portal hypertension**.

MC Type of primary liver cancer is **hepatoma**.

MC Benign liver tumor is **hemangioma**

MC Indication for splenectomy is **splenic injury**.

MC Cause of spontaneous splenic rupture is **malaria > mononucleosis.**

MC Hemolytic anemia to respond to splenectomy is **congenital hereditary spherocytosis**.

Indication for aortic/bifemoral bypass graft is **bilateral iliac obstruction**

Cause of renovascular hypertension in children is **fibromuscular dysplasia**.

Site of embolic occlusion is **the femoral artery**.

Benign type of melanoma is **superficial lentigo malignant melanoma**

The variant of Hodgkin's Disease with the best prognosis is **lymphocyte predominant**

The variant of Hodgkin's Disease with the worst prognosis is **lymphocyte depleted**

SOME NAMED SURGERIES

• Patey's operation	Parotidectomy, mastectomy
• Commando operation	CA tongue (Post 1/3rd)
• Nissen's fundoplication, Toupet's partial fundoplication, Belsey mark, Hills	GERD
• Ramsted's operation	Congenital Hypertrophic Obstructive Pyloric Stenosis
• Allison's repair	Hiatus hernia
• Hartmann's operation	Hydrocele (small, medium sized)
• Lords operation	Hydrocele (large sized)

1307

Key Points

FMGE Solutions Screening Examination

IMPORTANT SIGNS

Chvostek's sign	Contraction of facial m/s (masseter spasm) elicited by tapping the facial n. anterior to ear.
Homan's sign	Calf tenderness may be exaggerated by passive dorsiflexion of ankle
Hamman's sign	Mediastinal crunch seen in esophagus rupture.
Trousseau's Phenomenon/sign *(Carpopedal spasm elicited by occlusion of brachial artery with a BP cuff for 3 minutes)*	Seen in hypocalcemia (hypoparathyroidism, alkalotic or latent tetany, hypomagnesemia, hypo and hyperkalemia).
Troisier's sign	Enlargement of Virchow's nodes (left supraclavicular LN) in occult gastric carcinoma etc.
Trousseau's sign	Seen in migratory superficial thrombophlebitis (as in pancreatic CA).
Tinel's sign	Tingling sensation on percussion. It indicates partial lesion or beginning of regeneration of nerve

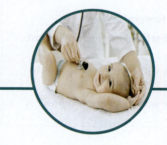

Pediatrics

Infant usually doubles his birth length by **4 ½ yrs of age.**

Most full term infants regain their birth weight by the age of **10 days.**

Central incisors is first to develop and second molar is last to develop in primary dentition.

The circumference of head and chest are almost same by the age of **9 months** to 1 year.

Insulin and insulin like growth factor **stimulate fetal growth**.

First sign of sexual maturation is enlargement of breast in females and testes in boys.

Malnutrition measurement
Acute malnutrition – Weight for height
Chronic malnutrition – Height for age

Contd…

Most vulnerable period of organogenesis is b/w 18-55 days of gestation.

Most common epileptic drug causing Neural tube defects- Valproate

Hyperbilirubinemia in girl babies – Oxytocin induced to mother

Premature closure of ductus in preterm baby – indomethacin

Most common complication during vaginal delivery in diabetic mother – **Shoulder dystocia**

Highest risk of transmission of Hepatitis – At the time of delivery.

Triad of Congenital Rubella – Deafness + cataract + heart defect (PDA)

Triad of congenital Syphilis – Deafness + interstitial keratitis + Hutchinson's teeth

Triad of Toxoplasmosis – Chorioretinitis + intracranial calcification + hydrocephalus

Most common congenital infection is **CMV**

Most common organism causing fetal malformation – **Rubella**

Recurrent abortions and IUGR are usually–not seen in – **Syphilis**

Sabin field man dye test is used to detect immunoglobulin G in toxoplasmosis

Most of the new born pass urine by **12 hours of age** and almost all of them do so by **48 hrs**

Fetal adrenal cortex is largest organ of fetus.

Most common manifestation of acute hypoxemia in a new born- **bradycardia, cardiac systole**.

Early conjugated NNHB with direct bilirubin more than 0.5 mg/dl is noted as neonatal syphilis.

Vitamin E has role in prevention of **PBD** and **ROP**.

Protein required in a new born – **100 kcal/kg**

Breast milk does not provide immunity against **pertussis**.

Minimum time of breast feeding per episode – **15-20 min**.

Vitamin absent in breast milk – Vitamin C > Vitamin D

Mature Breast milk by **day 7**.

Lacta albumin in breast milk - Soft/Golden yellow color stool.

Sucking + swallowing – **34 weeks**.

Earliest fetal breathing movements – **11-16 weeks**

Flag sign – **Kwashiorkor**

Chipmunk faces in case of – **Thalassemia**

Monkey faces in case of– **Marasmus**

Most common cause of congenital hydrocephalus – **Aqueductal stenosis**

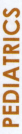

Pediatrics

TABLE: Development of fetus according to age

Social smile develops by **2 months**
Head control develops by **3 months**
4 months – Hand regard
5 months – Ulnar grasp
Child can sit with support by **5 months**
5 months – Lumbar control, Tripod position
7 months – Palmar grasp
7 months – Stranger anxiety
9 months – Wave bye bye
Pincer grasp develops by **9 months** (9-11 months)
Mature pincer grasp at **12 months**
24 months – Can speak in a sentence
2 years - Dry by day
3 years – Dry by night
Can draw- at: • **Circle:** 3 years   • **Square:** 4 years   • **Triangle:** 5 year
36 months – Climb upstairs with alternate feet
Child knows his full name, gender, eats without spilling, dress without supervision- **5 years**
Tells age and sex, uses pronouns, handedness by **3 years**
Child stands without support by **1 year**
Child can build tower of 3 cubes at **15 months**
Child can go up and downstairs with one step at a time by **2 years**.
Parachute reflex develops during **9th** month of life.
A child can skip by the age of **5 years**

TABLE: Fetal birth weight according to maturity

ELBW: < 1 kg
VLBW: < 1.5 kg
LBW: < 10th percentile (<2-5 kg)
Preterm: < 37 weeks
Post-term: >42 weeks

Early sign of puberty in male is enlargement of testes. In females it is determined by: **Thelarche**
Anemia for an infant at Hemoglobin less than **12 gm%**
In neonatal sepsis, acute phase reactant: **CRP**
Acyanotic congenital heart disease: **ASD, VSD, PDA**
Cyanotic congenital heart disease: **TGA, TOF, TAPVR**

TABLE: Apgar score and its interpretation

	Score 0	Score 1	Score 2
Appearance	Blue or pale all over	Blue at extremities	Pink all over
Pulse rate	Absent	<100	>100
(Grimace) Reflex irritability	No response	Grimace	Cry or pull away when stimulated
Activity	None	Some flexion	Flexed arms and legs that resist extension
Respiratory effort	Absent	Weak, irregular, gasping	Strong, lusty cry
Total score: 10	No distress: 7–10	Mild distress: 4–6	Severe distress: 0–3

TABLE: Triple test parameter and its value in different congenital defects

Triple test parameters	Alpha feto protein	Unconjugated estriol	Beta hCG
Down syndrome	Low	Low	High
Edward syndrome	Low	Low	Low
Neural tube defects Omphalocele, multiple gestation	High	Not applicable	Not applicable

- MC enzyme deficiency in CAH -21 HYDROXYLASE
- MC teratogenic effect of steroid-Cleft lip & palate
- MC childhood solid tumor other than brain tumor-Neuroblastoma & germ cell tumor
- MC tumor of newborn-sacrococygeal teratoma
- MC malignency in newborn----neuroblastoma
- MC intrarenal tumor in newborn-mesoblastic nephroma
- MC abdominal mass in neonate-Multicystic kidney
- MC cell seen in broncholitis- Clara cell
- MCC of bronchiolitis –RSV
- Upper segment and lower segment ratio becomes equal at this age: 7 Years
- Most common cause of short stature in childhood in India: Constitutional
- Physiological weight loss in a preterm baby is upto: 15%
- Best indication for successful resuscitation in an Indian child: Inc Heart rate
- Earliest clinical feature of neonatal sepsis: Poor feeding
- Mode of heating in a radiant warmer: Radiation

Key Points

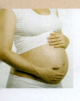
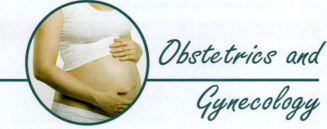

Obstetrics and Gynecology

TABLE: Supports of the genital organs

Level I	Uterosacral ligaments and cardinal ligaments support the uterus and vaginal vault
Level II	Pelvic facias and paracolpos which connects the vagina to the white line on the lateral pelvic wall through arcus tendinous
Level III	Levator ani muscles support the lower one third of vagina

EMBRYOLOGY OF UTERUS

- Mullerian duct present in both sexes and appear at 6 weks
- Mullerian duct disappear in male fetus at 8-9 weeks.
- Remnant of mullerian duct in male are- utriculus masculinus ,appendix of testis.
- Male internal genitalia develop from mesonephric duct/ wolfian duct.
- Remnant of wolfian duct in female – epoophoron(cranial part),paraoophoron (caudal end),gartner duct
- All the remanant of wolfian duct are present in borad ligament.
- 15-20 epoophoron join to form gartner duct
- Mullerian duct give rise to- fallopian tube,uterus,cervix,vagina (upper 2/3) (mesodermal origin)
- Lower 1/3 of vagina is derived from rogenital sinus (endodermal origin)

ANATOMICAL FACTS

- Water under bridge- point where uterine artery(bridge) crosses over the ureter
- Water under the bridge is the most common site for ureter injury.
- This point is 2 cm lateral to cervix and 1.5 cm lateral to internal os.
- During mestruation blood is lost from spiral artery, hence menstrual blood is arterial blood not venous
- Shape of uterus: Pyriform
- **Cavity: Triangular shape cavity on coronal section (Slit shape cavity on sagittal section)**
- Volume:
- 10cc- non pregnant
- 5000cc –term pregnancy (volume of uterus=volume of adult blood approximately
- Weight:
- Nullipara- 50-70 gram
- Multipara- 80 gram
- Term pregnancy- 1 kg
- Immediately after delivery-1 kg

IMPORTANT ONE LINERS

Tubal blockage is most commonly seen with this infection: **Chlamydia**
Fulminant hepatitis in pregnancy most commonly caused by: **HEV**
Constipation in pregnancy is due to this hormone: **Progesterone**
According to American fertility society classification system, unicornuate uterus is classified under this class: **Class II**
Type of molar pregnancy in which fetal tissue is formed: **Partial H Mole**
T shaped uterus seen due to this drug exposure: **Diethylstilbestrol (DES)**
Stage of Cervix cancer reaching involving bladder and rectum: **Stage IVa**
Fruit juice which can prevent UTI: **Cranberry juice (due to its anti-adhesion property)**
Tip of iceberg sign on USG: **Dermoid cyst of ovary**
Karman cannula is used for: **Endometrial aspiration**
In this stage of ovarian carcinoma both ovaries are involved and but the capsule is intact: **IB**
Ovarian Capsule is first involved in this stage of ovarian CA: **Ic**
• MC clinical presentation of genital T. B-**Infertility**
• MC change in fibroid-**Hyaline degeneration**
• MC complication of TAH-**Bleeding**
• MC regime is used inchoriocarcinoma-**MAC regime**
• MC site of metastasis of choriocarcinoma-**Lung**
• MCC of infertility-**Tubalfactor**
• MC C Of tubal disease-**PID**
• MC presentation of treated genital T.B-**Ectopic pregnancy**
• MC complication of ECV is-**fetal distress**
• MC fetal complication of forceps application-**asphyxia**
• MC complication of MTP produce is bleeding-**due to Incomplete evacuation**
• MC type of episiotomy-**mediolateral**
• MC complication of forceps application-**extension of episiotomy**

Contd...

Obstetrics and Gynecology

- MC site for ectopic pregnancy–**Ampulla**
- MC cause of congenital anomaly in baby of diabetic mother–**sacralegenesis**
- MC congenital anamoly in baby of diabetic mother–**neuraltube defect**
- MC problem seen in baby born to diabetic mother–**hypoglycemia**
- MC problem associated in delivery of macrosomia baby–**shoulder dystocia**
- MC cause of PPH–**Uterine atony**
- MC type of PPH–**Primary PPH**
- MC maternal complication of twin vaginal delivery–**atonic PPH**
- MC cause of secondary PPH is–**retained placental bits**
- MC reason for caesarian hysterectomy–**atonic PPH**
- MC indication of forcep is–**prolong second stage of labour**
- MC cancer cervix is squamous cell carcinoma-**95%**
- Most impotant support of uterus-**cardinal ligament**
- Ovlation occure at 14th day before menstration.
- Endomterium before ovulation is k/a proliferative endometrium.
- proliferative endometrium is due to effect of estrogen.
- Endomterium after ovulation is k/a secretory endometrium.
- Secretory endometrium is due to effect of progesterone.
- Major source of progesterone in non pregnant female is carpus luteum,hence secretory phase is also k/a luteal phase

TABLE: Indications of conization

Diagnostic	<li>Entire squamocolumnar junction not visible, large lesion</li><li>Endocervical CIN</li><li>Microinvasion suspected</li><li>Discrepancy between cytology and colposcopy</li>
Therapeutic	In INC II, III
Methods	<li>Cone biopsy</li><li>LLETZ, LEEP (loop electrosurgical excision procedure), NETZ</li>

TABLE: Bethesda system of cytology reporting

Satisfactory cytology—endocervical cells seen
Unsatisfactory

- **Squamous cell abnormalities**
  Atypical squamous cells (ASC)
  - Ascus—atypical cells of undetermined significance
  - ASC-H—cannot rule out high-grade lesion

Contd...

- Low-grade squamous intra epithelial lesion (LSIL)—includes CIN I
- High-grade squamous intraepithelial lesion (HSIL)—includes CIN II, III
- Squamous cell carcinoma
- **Glandular abnormalities**
  Atypical glandular cells
  Adenocarcinoma in situ
  Adenocarcinoma
- **Other malignant neoplasma**

Main support of uterus is **cardinal ligament (aka transverse cervical ligament).**

Broad ligament, infundibulopelvic ligament, ovarian ligaments–**Does not support uterus.**

Most imp muscle of pelvic floor - **Levator ani.**

Uterus, fallopian tube, cervix and upper 2/3 vagina arise from-**mullerian duct/paramesonephric duct (mesodermal origin)**

Lower 1/3 vagina - **Urogenital sinus** (endodermal origin)

Weight of pregnant term uterus - **1 kg**

Wt of uterus immediately after delivery - **1 kg**

Volume of nulliparous uterus = 10 mL, term uterus = 5 liters

Round ligament and ovarian ligaments arise from **gubernaculum**.

Uterus shows both **hypertrophy** and **hyperplasia** during pregnancy.

Endometrium of pregnancy is called **decidua**.

Thickness of endometrium
After menses = .5 mm
Mid cycle = 2–3 mm
Luteal phase = 5-6 mm
At time of implantation = 10–12 mm

Thickness of endometrium is taken at body near fundus by **USG**.

Water under bridge-ureter crossed by **uterine artery**.

Ratio of cervix to corpus:
1:1 - At birth, menopause
1:2 - Post-menarche
1:3 - Reproductive life
2:1 - Pre-menarche

Shape of cervix-round (nullipara), transverse slit like-after deliver/multipara

pH of vagina in adult women - 4–5.5

Vaginal secretions are—cervical secretion, bartholin duct secretion (during coitus)

Epithelial lining-FT (ciliated columnar), uterus (columnar), endocx (high columnar), ectocx (squamous), vagina (st. squamous)

Contd...

FMGE Solutions Screening Examination

MC CA
- Fallopian tube - Adenocarcinoma
- Uterus - Adenocarcinoma
- Cervix - Squamous cell CA
- Vagina - Squamous cell CA
- Vulva - Squamous cell CA

Sentinel LN used for vulva CA (which is superficial inguinal LN).

Bartholin's cyst - MC cyst of vulva, MC due to obstruction and gonococcus infection, causes fluctuant non tender swelling, at Anterior 2/3rd and posterior 1/3rd of junction between labia minova and Hymen.
Rx-Marsupialization

Length of fallopian tube: **10-12 cm.**

Genital tubercle forms - **Clitoris** (in female), **penis** (in male)

Genital swelling – **Labia majora (f)**, **scrotum (m)**

1st polar body - **Released at ovulation**.

2nd polar body-**released after fertilization**.

Ovarian cycle initiated by - **FSH**

Ovulation is due to - **LH** surge, which is due to high level of *estrogen*.

To cause ovulation in ART inj **hCG** is given.

In ART after HCG inj-ovulation occus after **36 hrs**.

Ovulation occurs at **14th day** (irrespective of cycle length)

Carpus luteum (CL) secrets-progesterone (**Mainly**), estrogen, relaxin, inhibin A

Life span of CL - **14 day**

Max function/peak activity of CL- *8th day after* ovulation/22nd day of Cycle.

Steroidogenesis of CL maintained by **LH**

Luteolysis of CL prevented by - **hCG**

Telescoping of glands, pseudostratification - **Proliferative/ estrogenic phase**

Ist Histopathological evidence of ovulation-Sub **nucleolar vacuolation**.

Cork screw glands, stromal edema- **late secretory/ progesterone phase.**

MC cause of 1° amenorrhea-**gonadal dysgenesis** (Turner syndrome)

MC cause of 2° amenorrhea-**ovulatory dysfunction** (PCOD)

Amenorrhea, absent uterus, normal sec sexual characters - **Mullerian agenesis**

Triad of MRKH s* - Mullerian agenesis, renal anomalies, skeletal anomalies.

Amenorrhoea, absent uterus, absent/dec pubic hair-androgen insensitivity s*/testicular feminization s* (XY (s* = syndrome)

BEST test to differentiate MRKH s* vs AIS - **Karyotyping**.

AIS (androgen insensitivity s*)- risk of gonadoblastoma in undescended testis.

MCC cause of Asherman's*- Vigorous curettage done for PPH.

TOC for **Asherman's*** - Hysteroscopic adhesiolysis + IUCD + high dose estrogen.

Imperforated hymen - C/o Amenorrhea, bluish bulging membrane in vagina.

Imperforated hymen-hematocolpos, hematometra, cyclic ab pain. T/t by cruciate incision.

Premature ovarian failure-FSH>40 IU on 2 separate occasion (1 month apart), at age <40 years.

MC used test of ovarian reserve- **sr** FSH (done at day 3)

Streak gonad, high FSH, hypogonadotropic hypogonadism-**Turner syndrome**

Inability to conceive even after 1 yr of unprotected intercourse - **Infertility**.

MC female factor for infertility - **PCOD**

MC male factor for infertility - **Psychogenic**.

Test of ovulation - Sr progesterone level (BEST, done at day 21), TVS (MC USED), endometrial biopsy, cervical mucus, vaginal cytology, basal body temp.

Peri-ovulatory follicle/follicle rupture at - **18-20 mm**

Peri ovulatory uterus show- **Trilaminar sign**.

1st stage of labor - Onset of true labor pain to full cx dilation (i.e. 10 cm)

4th stage of labor - 1 hour observation (post delivery)

True labor pain-progressive dilation, effacement, show, contraction increase in duration frequency and intensity.

1st stage – Nullipara (12 hr), multipara (8 hrs)

Prolonged 1st stage- nulli (20 hrs), multi (14 hrs)

Rate of cervical dilation in active stage
- 1.2 cm/hr - Nulliparous
- 1.5 cm/hr - Multiparous

Rate of descent:
- 1 cm/hr - Nulliparous
- 2 cm/hr – Multiparous

MCC of unstable lie - **Placenta previa.**

MC type of pelvis in female - **Gynecoid (50%)**.

Least common type of pelvis – **Platypelloid (<5%)**.

Pelvis is classified on the basis of **inlet of pelvis**.

Tri-radiate pelvis (VIT D def), rachitic pelvis (rickets)

Vaginal delivery is never possible in naegle's and robert's pelvis.

Slow progress of labor is called **dystocia**.

Contd...

Obstetrics and Gynecology

1313

Contracted inlet- when AP diameter < 10 cm.

Contracted midcavity- when interischial diameter < 8 cm.

Contracted outlet- when intertuberous diameter < 8 cm.

Best predictor for CPD- trial of labor.

Best method to do pelvic assessment – MRI > pelvimetry (manual)

Pacemaker of uterine contraction-at cornu (right > left)

Adequate uterine contraction- 200-220 Monte Video Unit.

MVU- no of contraction in *10 min* × pressure generated in 1 contraction in mm Hg.

Arrest of labor-no change in cervical dilation even after 2 hours of adequate uterine contractions.t/t is LSCS.

MCC cause of vesico vaginal fistula in developing countries-**Obstructed labor.**

Rx for obstructed labor-**LSCS**.

Obstructed labor with IUD- **LSCS** (no role of destructive procedure at all).

MC position of fetal head when it enters pelvis - **LOA (left occipito anterior)**

Direct op position seen in **Anthropoid pelvis**.

MCC of face/brow presentation - **Anencephaly**.

Face/ brow presentation/transverse lie- mcc associated with which type of pelvis-**platypelloid**.

Rx of face presentation - VD (if mentum anterior), LSCS (if mentum post).

Longest diameter of fetal head- mentovertical (14cm) - Brow presentation.

Rx of brow-CS, no role of VD (vaginal delivery).

Grid iron feel - Transverse lie.

Rib cage as presenting part/shoulder presentation-**transverse lie**.

Rx of transverse lie - **LSCS**

MCC of breech- **prematurity/preterm.**

MC type - **Frank breech.**

Worst prognosis/max cord prolapse among breech -**Footling breech.**

Highest risk of cord prolapse among all malpresentation-**trans. Lie**

Stargazer baby-footling breech with hyperextended neck.

Oogonia and spermatogonia are derived from yolk sac.

Folds of Hoboken-umbilical artery.

Day 21-fetal circulation is 1st intact/functional/separated from mother circulation.

MC presentation **cephalic**, MC presenting **part vertex**.

Contd...

Living ligature-middle layer of myometrium.

MCC of 1* PPH - Uterine atony

MCC of 2* PPH - Retained placental tissue

Syntometrine- oxytocin + methergine

Early cord clamping - HIV/Rh -/baby has heart ds/preterm/ premature

MCC of uterine rupture - Previous CS

MCC of APH- Abruptio placenta (1/200 preg), Placenta previa (1/300)

Most imp risk factor for both (AP, PP) - Previous history of the same.

Placenta Previa: Painless, causeless, bright-red, nontender uterus, normal FHS

Abruptio Placenta-painful, h/o trauma, dark altered blood, tender tense uterus, dec FHS

IOC for placenta previa (PP) & abruptio placenta (AP) - **USG**.

Paget's classification used for: **Abruptio placenta**

Macafee's regimen is used for: **Placenta Previa** - (for conservative management).

DOC for lung maturity - Betamethasone 12 mg, IM, 2 doses, 24 hours apart.

Indication for CS in Placenta Previa - Mother unstable, fetal distress, type 3 & 4

Management of Abruptio Placentae - Always termination of pregnancy.

Indication of CS in Abruptio Placentae - Mother unstable, fetal distress.

IOC for adherent placenta - MRI, Rx- **Hysterectomy**.

DOC for chronic hypertension (in preg)- **Methyl dopa**.

DOC for pre-eclampsia - **Labetalol 100 mg bd**

DOC for eclampsia - **MgSO$_4$**

DOC for DM in preg- Insulin. (only FDA approved oral hypoglycemic - Glyburide)

MTP ACT - **Year 1971**.

MTP- opinion of 2 doctors needed if **POG > 12 weeks**.

Minimum age for MTP consent - **18 years**.

Time of cerclage operation - **12-14 weeks**

Decidul cast- pathognomic of ectopic pregnancy.

Recurrent abortion with isolated rise of APTT - **Lupus anticoagulant**.

MCC of thrombocytopenia in preg - **Benign gestational > idiopathic**.

MCC drug used for 2nd Tm abortion - **Prostaglandins**

Rubin criteria is used for-**cervical ectopic**.

Contd...

Key Points

FMGE Solutions Screening Examination

- Spiegelberg criteria-ovarian ectopic, studdiford - **Abdominal ectopic**.
- Follow up of a case of ectopic/molar preg - **Serial hCG level**.
- Most consistent finding in ectopic pregnancy - **Pain**
- Most consistent sign of ectopic pregnancy - **Tenderness**
- MC non tubal site for ectopic - **Ovary**.
- Overall, MC ovarian tumor: **Epithelial cell tumor**
- Most common germ cell ovarian tumor: **Teratoma**
- Most common Malignant germ cell ovarian tumor: **Dysgerminoma**
- Menstrual blood stored in vagina: **Hematocolpos**
- In a diabetic mother, most common fetal complication will be: Congenital heart disease
- In Brow presentation, head of the fetus: **Partial Extension**
- Recurrence of hydatidiform mole accessed by: **β-hCG level**
- Mechanism of action of combined OCP: **Prevent release of ovum from ovary**
- Placental circulation is established by: **21 days**
- Primary treatment for hirsutism in PCOD: **Combined OCP**
- Oxygenated blood from placenta goes to fetal heart via: **Ductus venosus**
- Pace maker of uterine contraction is located at: **Tubal ostia**
- Treatment of choice of Acute hydramnios with fetal distress in pregnancy: **Amniocentesis**
- Cardiac activity in fetus can be assessed via transabdominal scan by: **6 weeks**
- Umbilical cord attached to the margin of placenta: **Battledore Placenta**

TABLE: Diameter of fetal skull

Diameters	Measurement (in cm)	Presentation
Suboccipito-bregmatic	9.5 cm	Vertex
Suboccipito-frontal	10 cm	Vertex
Occipito-frontal	11.5 cm	Vertex
Mento-vertical: Extend from mid-point of chin to the highest point on the saggital suture	14 cm	Brow
Submento-vertical	11.5 cm	Face
Submento-bregmatic	9.5 cm	Face

TABLE: Important vessels and their remnants

Ductus venosus	Ligamentum venosum
Ductus arteriosus	Ligamentum arteriosum
Umbilical arteries	Medial umbilical artery
Left umbilical vein	Ligamentum teres of liver

TABLE: Gestational age and fundal height landmark

Gestational age	Fundal height landmark
12 weeks	Pubic symphysis
24 weeks	Umbilicus
36 weeks	Xiphoid Process of sternum
37–40 weeks	Regression of fundal height between 36 and 32 cm

TABLE: Uterine pressure in a nutshell

Period	Contraction pressure
During the first 30 weeks	20 mm Hg
First stage of labor	40–50 mm Hg
2nd stage of labor	100–120 mm Hg
3rd stage of labor	100–120 mm Hg
Contraction felt clinically	> 10 mm Hg
Contraction associated with pain	15 mm Hg
Pressure required for distending lower uterine segment	15 mm Hg

TABLE: Stages of labor and their respective duration

Stages of Labor	Duration Primipara	Duration Multipara
Stage I: From uterine contraction to full cervical dilatation (10 cm)	12 hours	6 hours
Stage II: Full dilatation to delivery of baby	2 hours	30 minutes
Stage III: Delivery of baby to placental delivery	15 minutes	15 minutes
Stage IV: 1 hour post partum to rule out PPH and vulvar hematoma.	1 hour	1 hour

TABLE: Examination signs during pregnancy

Signs	At AOG
Palmer's sign: Regular and rhythmic uterine contraction	4-8 weeks
Vaginal sign: Softened vaginal wall with copious mucoid discharge	6th week
Goodell's sign: Cervix feels soft and congested	6th week
Hegar's sign: Uterus is enlarged and soft; cervix empty.	6-10 weeks
Osiander sign: Increased pulsation at lateral fornices	8th week
Chadwick's sign or Jacquemier's sign: Dusky hue of the vestibule and anterior vaginal wall (due to local vascular congestion)	8th week
Piskacek's sign: Asymmetrical enlargement of the uterus if there is lateral implantation	8th week

TABLE: Types of abortion and its examination and USG findings

Abortion	Size of uterus	Cervix OS	USG finding
Threatened	Equal to AOG	Closed	Fetus alive
Missed	Smaller than AOG	Closed	Dead fetus
Incomplete	Smaller than AOG	Open	Retained products of conception
Complete	Smaller than AOG	Closed	Uterine cavity empty

TABLE: Division of zygote and types of twinning

Division of zygote on/ after	Types of twining
72 hours/3 days	Dichorionic, Diamniotic
Between 4 and 8 days	Diamniotic, Monochorionic (DAMC)
Between 8 and 12 days	Monoamniotic, Monochorionic (MAMC)
>12 days	Siamese, Conjoined Twins

TABLE: Types of prior uterine incisions and risk of uterine rupture

Prior incision	Rupture rate (percentage)
1. Classical	4–9%
2. T-shaped	4–9%
3. Low-vertical	1–7%
4. Low-transverse	0.2-1.5%

TABLE: Ovarian tumor at a glance

Overall, MC ovarian tumor:	**Epithelial cell tumor**
Overall, MC benign tumor of the ovary:	**Dermoid cyst**
MC benign epithelial tumor of the ovary:	**Serous cystadenoma**
MC malignant ovarian tumor:	**Serous cystadenocarcinoma**
MC germ cell tumor:	Mature Teratoma (Dermoid Cyst)
Most common ovarian tumor associated with pregnancy:	**Dermoid Cyst**
Most common ovarian tumor which undergo torsion:	**Dermoid cyst**
MC malignant germ cell tumor:	**Dysgerminoma**
Ovarian tumor mostly in young age:	**Dysgerminoma**
Ovarian tumor metastasized to contralateral ovary:	**Granulosa cell tumor**

TABLE: Ovarian tumors and their HPE findings

Ovarian tumor	HPE characteristics
Serous cystadenoma	Psamomma bodies
Clear cell tumor	Hobnail cell
Yolk sac tumor	Schiller duval bodies
Granulosa cell tumor	Call exner bodies
Krukenberg tumor	Signet ring cell

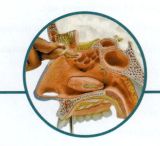

- Auricle is derived from which Branchial arch: **I & II**
- Stapes is derived from which Branchial arch: **II**
- Hyoid bone is derived from: **Branchial arch II & III**
- Auricle is made of how many cartilages: **1 (yellow elastic cartilage)**
- Area of auricle devoid of cartilage: **Lobule and Incisura terminalis**
- Eustachian tube length – 36 mm **(lateral 1/3 is bony and medial 2/3 is cartilage)**
- External auditory canal length – **24 mm (outer 1/3 is cartilage and inner 2/3rd is bony)**
- Layer of tympanic membrane: **3 layers**

Contd...

FMGE Solutions Screening Examination

- Functional area of tympanic membrane: **45–55 mm²**
- Lever ratio between handle of malleus and long process of incus is – **1.3 : 1**
- Ear ossicle which has no muscle attachment: **Incus**
- Origin of tensor tympani muscle on which wall: **Anterior wall (from canal of tensor tympani)**
- Origin of stapedius muscle on which wall: **Posterior wall (Tip of pyramid)**
- While cochlear implant, electrode is placed at: **Scala tympani**
- While cochlear implant, electrode is passed via: **Round window**
- Tuning fork most commonly used for this frequency: **512 Hz**
- Otoacoustic emissions arise from: **Outer cells**
- Best test for screening of hearing in newborn: **Otoacoustic emission**
- Roll over phenomena seen in **Retrocochlear Lesion**
- Bills bar location: **Inner ear**
- Bills bar separates which structure in inner ear: **Facial nerve and Superior vestibular nerve**
- Macewen's triangle or suprameatal triangle is landmark of **mastoid antrum**.
- Organ of Corti contains endolymph, hair cells, and supporting **cells of Hansen's**
- Otolith membrane of macula is made up of **Ca (CO)$_3$** crystals.
- Hamartoma of auricle may result **in cauliflower ear.**
- Most common organism causing cauliflower ear: **Stap aureus**
- Perichondritis of the auricle m/c pathogen is **pseudomonas**
- Normal hearing capacity is from 20 Hz to 20, 000 Hz.
- Moderately severe hearing loss: **56–70 dB**
- Noise induced hearing loss seen maximum at: **5–6 khz**
- **Hennebert sign** is seen in: Meniere's disease
- In case of BPPV, which semicircular canal affected: **Posterior semi-circular canal**
- Acute otitis media most commonly caused by: **Streptococcus pneumonia**
- Bullous myringitis is most commonly caused by: **Adenovirus**
- Wax softened by NaHCO$_3$ solution and syringing by sterile water at body temperature.
- Furunculosis of external ear caused by **staphylococcus.**
- Malignant otitis externa caused by **pseudomonas** seen in diabetics and immune compromised.
- **Central perforation of TM:** Safe CSOM
- **Peripheral perforation of TM** – Unsafe CSOM

- In keratosis obturans external ear canal is filled up by: **Cholesteatoma mass**.
- **Cholesteatoma** is: Old Keratinized mass of squamous cell in middle ear
- **MC site congenital cholesteatoma** - Petrous part of temporal bone
- **MC site of acquired cholesteatoma** – Prussack's space or attic area
- Most **common complication** of CSOM is **brain abscess**
- Most **common intracranial manifestation** of late chronic otitis media: **Brain abscess**
- Most common **extracranial** complication of CSOM: **Mastoiditis**
- Most common organism causing mastoiditis: group A beta hemolytic streptococcus
- Pulsatile tinnitus is seen in **Glomus Tumor**
- Pulsatile otorrhea (aka Lighthouse sign) seen in– ASOM
- **Grommet:** Small tube to drain middle ear
- Most common quadrant preferred for insertion of grommet: **Antero-inferior quadrant**
- Fluctuating hearing loss is seen in – **Ménière's Disease**
- Most common cause of sensorineural hearing loss – **Presby-cusis**
- **Paracusis willisii:** Patient hears better in noisy environment. Seen in case of otosclerosis
- Cohort notch at 2000 Hz seen in **Otosclerosis**
- Loudness of sound is measured by its **Intensity**
- Glomus tumor is a tumor of **paraganglionic cells**
- **Phelp's sign**-Glomus tumor (glomus jugulare)
- Cranial nerve involved in Gradenigo's syndrome: **5th & 6th cranial nerve**
- 3 D's of Gradenigo's syndrome: **Diplopia, Deep pain, Discharge**
- Lyre sign is seen in **Carotid Body** tumor
- Most common tumor of CP angle: **Vestibular schwannoma aka Acoustic neuroma**
- Osteomeatal complex is an important landmark during **FESS**
- Chronic dacryocystitis and mucocele of lacrimal sac are treated by **Dacryocystorhinostomy**
- **Osteomeatal complex includes** – middle meatus, uncinate process and ethmoidal bulla
- Most common site of epistaxis – **Little's area**
- Nasal septum perforation can be a side effect of antiangiogenesis drugs like – **Bevacizumab**
- This illicit drug abuse can cause septal perforation: **Cocaine**

Contd...

ENT

- MC type of DNS present with epistaxis: **Spur**
- Mikulicz cell upon HPE in case of– **Rhinoscleroma**
- Most common organism causing rhinoscleroma: **Klebsiella Rhinoscleromatis**
- Most common organism causing Rhinosporidiosis: **Rhinosporidiosis seeberi**
- Most common sinusitis in children – **Ethmoidal**
- Most common sinusitis in adults – **Maxillary**
- Polyp in adults most commonly arises from which sinus: **Ethmoid sinus**
- Polyp in child most commonly arises from which sinus: **Maxillary sinus**
- Best treatment for polyp: FESS
- **Vidian Neurectomy** is done for: Vasomotor Rhinitis
- Recurrent facial nerve paralysis seen in **Melkerson Rosenthal Syndrome**
- Frog sign, antral sign– **Juvenile angiofibroma**
- Characteristic feature of Juvenile angiofibroma: **Recurrent severe epistaxis in adolescent male.**
- Caldwell-Luc's operation is done for: **Maxillary sinusitis**
- Young's operation is surgical procedure for: **Atrophic rhinitis**
- Most common bone fractured on face: **Nasal septal fracture**
- MC site of fracture on mandible: **Condylar neck**
- **Reinke's space** – seen in glottis area. Often affected by edema causes polypoid degeneration of vocal cords.
- Narrowest portion of larynx in adult: **Glottis**
- Narrowest portion of larynx in child: **Subglottis**
- Intrinsic muscles of larynx is mainly supplied by: **Recurrent laryngeal nerve**
- Only intrinsic laryngeal muscle NOT supplied by RLN: **Cricothyroid muscle**
- Nerve supplying cricothyroid muscle: **Superior laryngeal nerve (external branch)**
- Abductor of vocal cord: **Posterior cricoarytenoid**
- Most common site of vocal cord nodule: **Anterior 1/3rd and Posterior 2/3rd**
- MCC of vocal cord nodule/Singer's nodule: **Vocal abuse**
- Thumb sign on X-ray neck- **acute epiglottitis**
- Steeple sign in X-ray neck: **Croup**
- Most common organism causing acute epiglottitis: **H. influenza B**
- Most common organism causing croup: **Parainfluenza Type I & II**
- Key hole glottis is seen in: **Phonasthenia**

Contd...

- Omega shaped glottis: **Laryngomalacia**
- Turban epiglottis is seen in this case: **TB larynx**
- Mouse nibbled appearance of vocal cord: **TB larynx**
- Most common risk factor for CA larynx: **Smoking**
- Laryngeal papillomatosis most commonly caused by: **HPV 6 & 11**
- **Montgomery tube** – silicon tracheal tube used for surgical management of tracheal stenosis
- **Mobius syndrome:** Bilateral facial nerve paralysis associated with abducens nerve palsy (patients unable to smile and unable to move their eyes from side to side)
- **Choanal atresia:** Persistence of bucconasal membrane; UL > BL
- In choanal atresia membrane is most commonly comprised of: **Bone**
- **McGovern's procedure:** In case of Choanal atresia (placing a wide bore nipple in baby's mouth)
- **Ludwig angina:** Airway obstruction due to laryngeal edema

The most common…

MC benign lesion of the ear is **actinic keratosis**

MC tumor is benign **acoustic neuroma.**

MC cause of vertigo is **vestibular neuritis.**

MC location of **epistaxis in children** is anterior, often traumatic.

MC location of **epistaxis in adults** is posterior, secondary to system causes such as hypertension and atherosclerosis.

MC tumor of the paranasal sinuses is **osteoma**

MC infectious disease in humans is **acute viral rhinitis**

MC noninfectious cause of rhinitis is **allergic** (about 20% of population).

MC medical cause of rhinitis is **decongestant abuse**

MC orbital infection is acute **ethmoidal sinusitis**

MC fungal infection of the oral cavity is **moniliasis**.

MC benign neoplasm of the oral cavity and pharynx is **squamous papilloma**.

MC malignant neoplasm of the oral cavity and pharynx is **squamous cell carcinoma**.

MC benign neoplasm of the parotid gland in children is **hemangioma**

MC malignant neoplasm of the parotid gland is **mucoepidermoid carcinoma**

MC malignant neoplasm of salivary glands (except parotid) is **adenoid cystic carcinoma**.

MC cause of stridor in infant is **laryngomalacia**

Contd...

Key Points

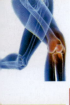

FMGE Solutions Screening Examination

The most common…
MC inflammatory condition of the larynx in adults is **acute laryngitis**.
MC benign tumor of the larynx in children is **squamous papilloma**
MC malignant tumor of the larynx is **squamous cell carcinoma**
MC etiologies of neck masses in children are **congenital and inflammatory**.
MC etiology of neck masses in adults is **neoplasm**.
MC **benign neck tumors** are lipoma and neurogenic tumors (schwannoma, neurofibroma).
MC malignant lateral neck masses in children are **lymphoma and rhabdomyosarcoma**.
MC the **cricoarytenoid muscles** are the only ones that **Abduct the vocal cords**.

Sinus	Condition at Birth	Adult size	First radiological evidence
Maxillary	+ (6–8 mL)	15 years	4–5 months
Ethmoid	+	12 years	1 year
Frontal	–	20 years	6 years
Sphenoid	–	15 years	4 years

TABLE: Larynx anatomy

	Adult larynx	Pediatric larynx
Location	C3 – C6	High in neck At rest: C3 or C4 While swallowing: C1 or C2
Cartilage	Soft	Softer
Thyroid cartilage	Elevated at thyroid angle	Flat
Shape	Cylindrical	Conical
Length of vocal cord	Female: 15–19 mm Male: 17–23 mm	Female: 6 mm Male: 8 mm

TABLE: Male vs female larynx

Male	Female
Length = 44 mm	36 mm
AP = 43 mm	41 mm
Transverse: 36 mm	26 mm

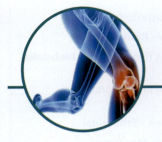

Orthopedics

Term orthopedics was coined by **Nicolas Andry**.
Bone within bone appearance is seen in **osteoporosis**
Short 4th and 5th metacarpal is seen in **pseudo hypoparathyroidism**.
Frankel's line and Wimberger's ring seen in **scurvy**.
Rocker bottom foot is seen in congenital vertical talus and incorrection of CTEV.
Kienbock's disease is avascular necrosis of **lunate**.
Codfish vertebrae is seen in osteoporosis
Triple arthrodesis includes talonavicular, talocalcaneal, calcaneocuboid fusion.
Intra-articular calcification is seen in Charcot's joints.
Quadriceps femoris is main extensor of knee joint.
Knuckle-blender splint: Claw hand
Cock up splint is used for radial nerve palsy.
Locking of knee is seen in bucket handle tear of meniscus.
Mallet finger is avulsion of base of distal phalanx.
Maximum weight for skeletal traction is 20 kg
Chauffeur's fracture involves radial styloid.
K-wire is used for cerclage and fore arm bone fixation.
Barton's fracture involve fracture distal end radius with wrist sublaxation.
Scaphoid is treated by glass holding cast.
MCC of bony ankylosis is pyogenic arthritis.
Onion peeling is seen in Ewing's sarcoma.
MC bone to fracture on face is **nasal bone**
MC site of fracture of mandible is **neck of condyle**.
Earliest X-ray finding of Osteomyelitis: **Periosteal reaction**
Drug of choice for acute gouty arthritis: **Indomethacin**
Deformities in RA
Swan-neck deformity: Hyperextension of the PIP joint with flexion of the DIP joint.
Boutonnière deformity: Flexion of the PIP joint with hyperextension of the DIP joint.
Z-line deformity

Deformities in OA:
- Bouchard's node: Node at PIP
- Heberden node: Node at DIP

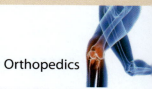

Orthopedics

COMMON FRACTURES AND INJURIES

Fracture	Description
Bankart's fracture	Fracture of anterior glenoid associated with anterior shoulder dislocation
Bennett's fracture	Intra-articular fracture of base of Thumb metacarpal
Boxer's fracture	Fracture of neck of little metacarpal
Bumper fracture	Compression fracture of lateral tibial plateau
Burst fracture	It is a comminuted fracture of the vertebral body where fragments "burst out" in different directions
Chauffeur's #	Intra-articular fracture of radial styloid
Colles' fracture	Distal radius fracture with dorsal angulation, im- impaction and radial drift
Chance fracture aka seat-belt fracture	The fracture line running horizontally through the body of the vertebra and through, the posterior elements
Dashboard fracture	A fracture of posterior lip of the acetabulum, often associated with posterior dislocation of the hip
Duverney fracture	Isolated fracture of the iliac wing
Galeazzi fracture	Radius shaft fracture with dislocation of distal radio-ulnar joint
Gosselin fracture	V-shaped distal tibia fracture extending into the tibial plafond
Hangman's #	Fracture of both pedicles of C2
Hill–Sachs fracture	Impacted posterior humeral head fracture occurring during anterior shoulder dislocation
Jefferson fracture	Fracture of first cervical vertebra
Jones fracture	Fracture of base of 5th metatarsal extending into intermetatarsal joint
Lisfranc fracture	Fracture dislocation of midfoot
March fracture	Stress fracture of 2nd and 3rd metatarsal shaft
Monteggia fracture	Proximal ulna fracture with dislocation of radial head
Moore's fracture	Distal radius fracture with ulnar dislocation and entrapment of styloid process under annular ligament
Pipkin fracture-dislocation	Posterior dislocation of hip with avulsion fracture of Fragment of femoral head by the ligamentum teres

Contd...

Fracture	Description
Pott's fracture	Bimalleolar fracture of the ankle
Cotton's fracture	Trimalleolar ankle fracture
Rolando fracture	Extra-articular comminuted fracture of base of first metacarpal
Runner's fracture	Stress fracture of distal fibula 3–8 cm above the lateral malleolus
Salter–Harris #	Fractures involving a growth plate
Shepherd's fracture	Fracture of the lateral tubercle of the posterior process of the talus
Smith's fracture	Distal radius fracture with volar displacement
Straddle fracture	Bilateral superior and inferior pubic-rani fracture
Whiplash injury	Cervical spine injury where sudden flexion followed by hyperextension takes place

TABLE: Static stabilizer vs dynamic stabilizer of shoulder joint

Static stabilizer	Dynamic stabilizer
Glenoid labrum Glenohumeral ligament Negative pressure in glenoid cavity	Supraspinatus Infraspinatus Teres minor Subscapularis

TABLE: Shoulders pathology and nerve involved

Ant. Shoulder dislocation	Axillary nerve
Surgical neck humerus #	Axillary nerve
Humerus shaft #	Radial nerve
Supracondylar #	Anterior interosseous nerve > median nerve
Cubitus valgus	Tardy ulnar nerve palsy
Medial condyle humerus #	Ulnar nerve

TABLE: Different splint and their uses

Splint	Used in
Knuckle bender splint	Ulnar nerve
Aeroplane splint	Brachial plexus injury
Dennis brown splint	CTEV
Bohler Braun splint	Fracture femur (anywhere from neck to supracondylar region)
Turn buckle splint	VIC (Volkmann ischemic contracture)

Key Points

1319

FMGE Solutions Screening Examination

SOME IMPORTANT SIGNS AND TESTS

Adson's test: For thoracic outlet syndrome
Allen's test: For testing patency of radial and ulnar arteries
Alli's test: For CDH
Anvil test: For testing tenderness of the spine
Ape thumb: For median nerve injury
Apley's grinding test: For meniscus injury
Apprehension test: For recurrent dislocation for the shoulder
Barlow's test: For CDH
Galeazzi sign: For CDH
Galeazzi fracture: Radius shaft fracture with dislocation of distal radioulnar joint
Blue sclera: Osteogenesis imperfect
Bryant's test: For anterior dislocation of the shoulder
Callaways' test: For anterior dislocation of the shoulder
Chvostek's sign: For tetany
Claw hand: For ulnar nerve injury
Coin test: For dorso-lumbar tuberculosis of spine
Cozen's test: For tennis elbow
Drawer test: For ACL and PCL injuries
Anterior: For ACL injury
Posterior: For PCL injury
Finkelstein's test: For de Quervain's tenovaginitis
Foot drop: For common peroneal nerve injury
Froment's sign: For ulnar nerve injury
Gaenslen's test: For SI joint involvement
Gower's sign: For muscular dystrophy
Hamilton–ruler test: For anterior dislocation of the shoulder
Kanavel's sign: For infection in ulnar bursa
Lasegue's test: For disc prolapse
Lachman test: For ACL injury
Ludloff's sign: For avulsion of lesser trochanter
McMurray's test: For meniscus injury
Naffziger's test: Disc prolapse
Ober's test: For tight iliotibial band (e.g. in polio)
O'Donoghue triad: Triad of MCL, ACL & medial meniscus injuries occurring together
Ortolani's test: For CDH
Pivot-shift test: For ACL injury
Policeman tip: For Erb's palsy
Sulcus sign: For inferior dislocation of the shoulder
Thomas's test: For hip flexion deformity
Trendelenburg's test: For unstable hip due to any injury?

IMPORTANT CLASSIFICATION

Neer's: For upper end of humerus fractures
Gustilo: For open fractures
Salter and Harris: For epiphyseal injuries
Lauge Hansen's: For ankle injuries
Pauwel's: For fractures neck of the femur
Garden's: For fractures neck of the femur
Winquist: Femur fracture
Milch: lateral condylar fracture
Campbell: Clavicle fracture
Tile's/Young → Pelvic bone fracture
Thompson and Epstein: Post Hip dislocation
Rockwood: Acromioclavicular Joint injury

RADIOLOGICAL SIGNS

Special views
Judet views: For acetabular fracture
Oblique view of the wrist: For fracture scaphoid
Mortise view: For ankle injuries
Sunset view: For patella - Femoral dysplasia
Von Rosen view: For CDH
Shenton's line: Hip X-ray

Angle
Carrying angle: Elbow
Pauwel's angle: Fracture neck of the femur
Bohler's angle: Fracture of the calcaneum
Kite's angle: Angle in CTEV
Neck-shaft angle: Of the femoral neck

Classic features
Wormian bones: Osteogenesis imperfecta
Sun-ray appearance: Osteosarcoma
Soap-bubble appearance: Osteoclastoma
Onion-peel appearance: Ewing's Sarcoma
Shepherd-Crook deformity: Fibrous dysplasia
Risser's sign: Epiphysis of iliac bone
Aneurysmal sign: TB spine (anterior type)
Tonguing of vertebra: Morquio-Brails disease
Trethowan's sign: Slipped capital femoral epiphysis
Sagging rope sign: Perthe's disease
Patchy calcification: Chondrosarcoma
Fabella: Sesamoid bone in the lateral head of gastrocnemius
Spondylosis: Degenerative spine disease

Orthopedics

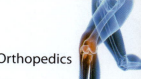

GAITS

Antalgic gait: Occurs in painful condition of lower limb
Trendelenburg gait: Occurs in an unstable hip due to CDH, gluteus medius weakness, etc.
Stiff hip gait: Occurs in ankylosis of the hip
Duck waddling gait: Occurs in bilateral CDH
Scissoring gait: Occurs in CP
High stepping gait: Occurs in foot drop
Circumduction gait: Occurs in hemiplegia
Charlie-Chaplin gait: Occurs in tibial torsion
Sailor's gait: Occurs in bilateral CDH

ORTHOPEDICS—THE MOST COMMON LIST

Location of hip fracture is at the femoral neck and intertrochanter.
Sprained ligament is the anterior talofibular ligament.
Foci of acute hematogenous osteomyelitis are the metaphases of long bones secondary to turbulent flow.
Variety of osteoporosis is the involutional type, often seen in post-menopausal women.
Musculoskeletal morbidity in the elderly is osteoarthritis.
The most movable joint is the glenohumeral joint.
The strongest bone segment is the femoral shaft.

BONE INFECTION—MOST COMMON

Most common organism causing acute osteomyelitis: **Staph. aureus**
MCC of osteomyelitis in **sickle cell anemia patient: Salmonella**
MCC of osteomyelitis in **IV drug abuser: Pseudomonas**
MC organism causing osteomyelitis in **open foot injury: Pseudomonas**
MC organism causing osteomyelitis in **HIV patient: Staph. Aureus**
MC organism causing osteomyelitis in case of **animal bite: Pasteurella Multocida**
MC organism causing osteomyelitis in case of **human bite: Eikenella Corrodens**

TABLE: Radiological appearance of some common bone tumors

Sun burst appearance: Osteosarcoma
Nidu/Seed in cortex: Osteoid osteoma
Onion skin appearance: Ewing's sarcoma
Exostosis (cartilage cap): Osteochondroma
Soap bubble appearance: Giant cell tumor/Osteoclastoma

Tumor	Site
Solitary bone cyst	Upper end of humerus
Aneurysmal bone cyst	Lower limb metaphysis
Osteochondroma	Distal femur
Osteoid osteoma	Femur
Osteoblastoma	Vertebrae
Osteoma	Skull, facial bones
Enchondroma	Short bones of hand
Chordoma	Sacrum
Adamantinoma	Tibial
Ameloblastoma	Mandible
Osteoclastoma	Lower end femur
Fibrous dysplasia	Polyostotic – craniofacial Monostotic – upper femur
Multiple myeloma	Lumbar vertebrae
Osteosarcoma	Lower end femur
Ewings's sarcoma	Femur
Chondrosarcoma	Pelvis
Secondary tumors	Dorsal vertebrae

Some important facts

- **MC type of ant. shoulder D/L:** Subcoracoid (head lies below coracoid process)
- **Blounts disease:** Dysplasia of proximal posteromedial tibial epiphysis
- **Steinberg and Walker Murdoch sign:** Marfans syndrome
- **MC translocation in Ewing's:** t(11:22)
- **David letterman sign/Terry Thomas sign:** Scapholunate dislocation
- **Game keeper's thumb:** Torn ulnar collateral ligament after injury to thumb MCP joint
- **Booadie's Abscess:** Subacute OM
- **Kanavel Sign:** Tenosynovitis
- **Heberden node and Bouchard Node:** OA
- **Swan neck and Boutonniere deformity:** RA
- **Bag of bone sign:** Charcot's Joint (in DM)
- **IOC for CDH:** MRI
- **Screening for CDH:** USG
- **Trethowan's sign:** SCFE
- **Wimberger corner sign:** Cong. Syphillis
- **Froment sign:** Ulnar nerve palsy
- **Phalen test +ve:** Carpal tunnel syndrome
- **Meralgia paresthetica:** Lat cutaneous nerve of thigh
- **Cheiralgia paresthetica:** Superficial radial nerve

Key Points — 1321

FMGE Solutions Screening Examination

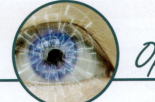
Ophthalmology

EYEBALL AT BIRTH

- **AP diameter:** 16.5 mm (adult size 24 mm by 7–8 years)
- **Corneal diameter:** 10 mm (adult size 11.7 mm 2 years)
- NB hypermetropic by 2–3 D
- Fixation starts at 1 month. Completed by 6 mo
- Macula fully developed by—4–6 mo
- Fusional reflex and accommodation well developed by 4–6 mo
- 3D depth perception/stereopsis—6 years

LENS

- Grow throughout the year
- **Diameter:** 9–10 mm
- **Thickness:** 3.5–5 mm
- **Weight:** 135 mg to 255 mg
- **Total dioptric power:** 18 D (16D – 20D)
- **Refractive index:** 1.39
- **Accommodative power:** 14–16 D at birth; 7–8 D at 25 years and 1–2 D at 50 year

Length of eyeball: **24 mm**	
Volume of orbit: **30 ml**	
Weight of eyeball: **7 gram**	
Volume of eyeball: **6 ml**	
Anterior chamber: **Between iris and cornea (posterior wall)** Posterior chamber: **Between lens and iris**	
Deep anterior chamber in: **Young, Male and Myopes** Shallow anterior chamber in: **Elderly, female and hypermetropes**	
DDO (distant direct ophthalmoscope): **Performed at a distance 22 cm (20–28 cm)**	
Direct ophthalmoscope: Done closest to patient Image is Direct, Erect and Virtual; magnified by 15 times	
Indirect ophthalmoscope: Performed at a distance of 1 m Image is real (true), inverted; magnified by 5 times	
Slit lamp is the best investigation method for diagnosis of vitreous opacities	
Functional assessment of optic nerve is done by **Perimetry**	
Acuity for distant vision is tested by - **Snellen chart**	

Contd...

Acuity for near vision is tested by - **Jaeger type cards**	
Ishihara chart is used for: **Color blindness**	
Retinoscopy Done at a distance 1m. If reflex moves in: **Same direction** - Emmetropia, hypermetropia, myopia<1D **Opposite direction** – Myopia >1D **No movement** - Myopia -1D	
Field of vision is tested by - Perimetry, Bjerrum's screen, confrontation method	
Finchams test: Differentiates colored halos of acute congestive glaucoma from that of acute conjunctivitis	
Gonioscope: The angle of anterior chamber can be examined with the help of a Gonioscope and slit lamp.	
Tonometry: Used for accurate determination of IOT (intraocular tension)	
Arden index: It the ratio between light peak to dark trough. Normally it is 1.85	
Ring scotoma: Seen in retinitis pigmentosa, glaucoma (double arcuate scotoma)	
Roth spots- white centered retinal hemorrhages Seen in **Leukemia, SABE, DM**	
Lens develop from **surface ectoderm**	
Lower and lateral walls of orbit are derived from **visceral mesoderm**	
Total refractive power of eye is **58-60D (Avg-58.6)**	
Total refractive power of cornea **43.78D +/- 1.86D**	
Normal cup-disc ratio-**1:3**	
Maximum refractive index is **at center of lens (1.40)**	
Newborn eye is short axial length is 17.5 mm generally hypermetropic +2.5D and fovea is immature.	
Critical period for the development of fixation of eye reflexes is 2-4 months	
Glycolysis is the main route of metabolism of glucose in the lens.	
IOT ranges from **10-20 mmHg**	
Optic disc - Depressed area of optic disc contains no rods/cones is therefore insensitive to light and called physiological blind spot.	
CME (cystoid macular edema)- shows flower petal appearance of fundus.	
Ink-blot pattern and smoke-stake patterns is seen in: **CSR** (central serous retinopathy).	
CRAO - Cattle truck appearance of retinal veins, cherry red spots.	
Aphakia produces high degree of hypermetropia	
Frequent changes of presbyopic glasses is an early symptom of-**primary open angle glaucoma.**	

Contd...

Ophthalmology

First sign of cavernous involvement /raised ICT IS 6th CN palsy.

Structures passing through optic foramen are - Optic nerve and ophthalmic artery

Bielschowsky sign is for superior oblique palsy.

Sea saw nystagmus of Maddox - Found in para chiasmal lesion.

Argyll-Robertson pupil Light reflex absent, accommodation reflex present Seen in Neurosyphilis, DM, syringomyelia, disseminated sclerosis.

Horner's syndrome: Triad of MIOSIS, IPSILATERAL PTOSIS, ANHYDROSIS.

Marcus gunn pupil is diagnostic of-acute retrobulbar neuritis (optic neuritis)

Parvocellular pathway - Located on layers 3, 4, 5, 6 of retina

Most common cause of viral conjunctivitis-**Adeno virus**

Most common cause of bilateral conjunctivitis in neonates within 3-5days - **Neisseria gonorrhoea.**

Most common cause of severe keratoconjunctivitis in contact lens user - **Acanthamoeba**

Most characteristic lesion of HSV recurrent infection is **the-dendritic ulcer (dendritic keratitis)**

Trachoma-leading preventable cause of blindness

SAFE strategy used for trachoma - Surgery, Antibiotics, Facial hygiene, Environmental change

Corneal transparency is maintained by - **Descemet membrane**

Donor cornea from **cadaveric eye** can be used 6 hours of death. It is stored in **Mc Kaufmanns media** for 4 days.

Corneal ulcers - Ulcer Serpens is due to pseudomonas.

LASIK is absolutely contraindicated in keratoconus

Most common fungus infecting lids - **Candida albicans.**

Posterior staphyloma is due to ectasia at posterior pole, seen in myopia

Anterior staphyloma is due to ectasia of cornea at anterior pole, seen in corneal ulcer perforation.

Sympathetic ophthalmia: retrolental flare is the first sign, Dalen Fuchs nodules

Lens capsule is thinnest at posterior pole.

Ascorbic acid in lens is derived from myo inositol phosphate.

Snow flake/snow storm cataract - Seen in diabetes

Oil drop cataract - Seen in galactosemia

Sunflower cataract - Seen in Wilson's disease

Bread crumb appearance - Seen in complicated cataract

Most common complication of morgagnian cataract-**Phacolytic glaucoma.**

Supero temporal dislocation of lens - Seen in Marfans syndrome

Infero nasal dislocation of lens-seen in **homocystinuria**.

Antero inferior dislocation of lens-**Weill marchesani syndrome**.

Hard contact lenses and IOL lens are made up of **PMMA**

Soft contact lenses are made up of **HEMA (Hydroxyethyl Methacrylate), Silicon Hydrogel**

Earliest filed defects in glaucoma - Central/para central scotoma in bjerrums area.

Most effective surgery for congenital or infantile glaucoma is **goniotomy or trabeculotomy**.

Aphakia - Absence of crystalline lens.power of Aphakic eye is 44 D

Most radioresistant structure in retina-**ganglion cell layer.**

Cotton wool spots (cytoid bodies) are due to focal ischemia in the nerve fiber layer, found in HIV retinopathy.

Flame shaped hemorrhages found in - **Hypertensive and arteriosclerosis retinopathy.**

Field defect in toxic amblyopia - **Centroceacal scotoma.**

TOC for paralytic squint-**surgery**

TOC for amblyopia with unilateral strabismus - **Conventional occlusion (of normal eye)**

TOC for accommodative squint-**correction of refractive errors**.

TOC for concomitant squint-**orthoptic exercises**

Most common intraocular foreign bodies - **Chips of iron and steel**.

Most common cause of intermittent proptosis-**orbital varix (varicose vein in the eye)**

In children:
Most common intraocular tumor - Retinoblastoma
Most common intra orbital tumor - Rhabdomyosarcoma

In adults
MC intraocular tumor - **Malignant melanoma of choroid**
MC intra orbital tumor – **Cavernous Hemangioma**
MC tumor which metastasize to eye - **Neuroblastoma**
MC tumor of eyelids **basal cell carcinoma**
MC tumor of lacrimal gland - **Benign mixed tumor**

Mutations in retinoblastoma are seen at 13q14

MC presentation in retinoblastoma - leukocoria > strabismus.

Vitreous is composed of type II collagen+hyluronic acid.

Trichiasis: Is mis directed eye lashes.
Madarosis: Loss of eye lashes/eyebrows
Tylosis: Thickening of lid margin
Blepharitis: **Inflammation of eyelid**

Fastest acting mydriatic and cycloplegic -**Tropicamide**
Shortest acting mydriatic and cycloplegic -**Tropicamide**
Shortest acting mydriatic without cycloplegia-**phenylephrine.**

Contd...   *Contd...*

Key Points

FMGE Solutions Screening Examination

OPHTHALMOLOGY

- MC congenital color blindness - **Green (deuteranopia)**
- MC cause of blindness in AIDS patients - **CMV retinitis**.
- MC cause of blindness worldwide - **Cataract**
- MC cause of blindness in India - **Cataract**
- MC cause of ocular morbidity - **Refractive errors**
- MC cause of ocular morbidity in youngs - **Refractive errors**
- MC cause of preventable blindness in children - **Vit A deficiency**
- Tear production starts at 6 months
- **Sjogren's syndrome** is due to aqueous deficiency
- MC ocular manifestation of measles - **Vit A deficiency**
- Corneal nerve is visible in - **leprosy, keratoconus**.
- Bluish discoloration of sclera - **osteitis deformans**.
- MC cause of sudden unilateral loss of vision - **Optic neuritis**
- MC treatment modality for acute angle closure glaucoma - **Laser iridotomy**
- Not seen in herpes zoster opthalmicus - **sclero-keratitis**
- Cricket ball injury to eye does not lead to - **Hypopyon**.
- WHO vision 2020 do not include - **epidemic conjunctivitis**.
- Worth 4 dot test is done for: **Binocular vision**
- Jack in a box is seen in: **Aphakia**
- **Tranta's spots**, Ropy discharge is seen in: **Vernal conjunctivitis**
- Interstitial keratitis is seen in: **Syphilis**
- Side effect of oral steroid: **Cataract**
- Side effect of topical steroid: **Glaucoma**
- D/Dx of color haloes:
  - ACG
  - Cataract
  - Mucopurulent conjunctivitis (Not in angular)
  - Vertically fixed mid-dilated pupil seen in: ACG

RECENT ONE'S

- MCC of blindness in India: **Cataract**
- Retrolental Flare is seen in: **Sympathetic Ophthalmitis**
- Ipsilateral CN 3 palsy can lead to: **Weber syndrome**
- Most radiosensitive layer of retina: **Rods and cones**
- Most radioresistant layer of retina: **Ganglion cell layer**
- Ascorbic acid in lens is transported by: **Myoinositol**
- Orbital floor is formed by: **Maxillary bone and palatine bone**
- MC complication after lens extraction in PHPV: **Vitrous Hemorrhage**
- Cornea can be harvested: **Till 6 hours after death**
- Alcaftadine trail used this concentration of drug: **0.25%**
- Definition of blindness according to WHO: **<3/60**

- Vossius ring in eye is due to: **Blunt trauma**
- Alkali injury in eye causes: **Symblepharon**
- **Ankyloblepharon:** Upper and lower lid margin fusion
- Titmus fly test is for: **Stereopsis**
- Jack in the box phenomenon: **Aphakia**
- Anterior lenticonus: **Alport syndrome**
- Posterior lenticonus: **Lowe syndrome**
- Dalen fuch's nodule is seen in: **Sympathetic ophthalmitis**
- Buphthalmos is seen in: **Congenital glaucoma (AR condition)**
- Krukenberg spindle is seen in: **Pigmentary glaucoma (iris pigment on cornea)**
- IOC for indirect ophthalmoscopy: **Indirect ophtha**
- Flame shaped hemorrhages are hallmark of: **Hypertensive retinopathy**
- Flower petal appearance upon fluorescein angiography: **Cystoid macular edema**

OPHTHALMOLOGY—MOST COMMON LIST

WHAT IS/ARE THE MOST COMMON

- MC Refractive surgery is radial keratotomy
- MC Type of glaucoma is chronic open-Angle glaucoma.
- MC Glaucoma-related surgical procedure is trabeculectomy.
- MC Cause of blindness: **Cataract**
- MC etiology of visual loss in patients with diabetes mellitus is macular edema.
- MC Cause of proptosis in children is: **Orbital Cellulitis**
- MC Cause of proptosis in adults is **Grave's Disease**.
- MC Cause of red eye is **Conjunctivitis**.
- MC Cause of ocular venous occlusion is **glaucoma**.
- MC Indication for corneal treatment: **Pseudophakic bullous keratopathy**

TABLE: CN, their respective nucleus location and their function

Cranial nerve	Nucleus location	Function
Oculomotor III	Upper midbrain	Eyeball movements: Extrinsic ocular muscles
Trochlear IV	Lower midbrain	Eyeball movements: Extrinsic ocular muscles
Abducens VI	Pons	Eyeball movements: Extrinsic ocular muscles
Hypoglossal XII	Medulla	Tongue muscles and movements

Contd...

Ophthalmology

TABLE: Few Instruments which are used for ocular examination

Measurement parameter	Instruments used
Corneal thickness	Pachymeter
Corneal curvature	Keratometer
Angle of anterior chamber	Gonioscope
Corneal surface	Placido disc
Corneal endothelium	Specular microscope
Direct ophthalmoscope Remembered as: "DEV"	Routine fundus examination. *"Image formed is Erect and Virtual and magnified, 15 times"*
Indirect ophthalmoscope	For assessment of retinal detachment and other peripheral retinal lesions. *The image is real, inverted and magnified 5 times.*
Perimetry	Optic nerve function

Aqueous humor physiology

- **Protein:** conc less than plasma
- **Glucose:** less than plasma (used by cornea and lens as they are avascular)
- **Acid:** Lactic, Pyruvic, Ascorbic. Conc higher than plasma
- **pH:** 7.2 (lower than plasma)
- **Formed by:** Diffusion (10%), Ultrafiltration: 20% and Active transport: 70%

Must Know Facts

Types of nystagmus	Staphyloma: *an ectatic condition of the eyeball w/ herniation of uveal tissue.*	Proptosis
- **Downbeat:** arnold chiari malformation - **Ocular bobbing-** downbeat ff by slow upbeat: Pontine lesion - **See saw:** Optic chiasma lesion	- **Anterior:** corneal ulcer - **Posterior:** Pathological myopia - **Intercalary:** trauma at limbus - **Ciliary:** Scleritis	- **Sequence of ms involved:** IR > MR > SR> LR - **MCC of B/L proptosis:** thyroid ophthalmopathy - **MCC of U/L proptosis:** thyroid Ophth… - **MCC of B/L proptosis in child:** orbital cellulitis - **MCC of U/L proptosis in child:** ALL

TABLE: WHO classification of xerophthalmia

Class	Signs
X1A	Conjunctival xerosis
X1B	Conjunctival xerosis with bitot's spot
X2	Corneal xerosis
X3A	Corneal xerosis with ulceration
X3B	Keratomalacia

TABLE: Swimming pool related infections

Disease	Causative agent
Swimming pool conjunctivitis	*Adenovirus*
Swimming pool granuloma	*Mycobacterium marinum*
Swimmer's itch	*Schistosoma mansoni S. japonicum*

TABLE: Eye discharge and possible etiological agent

Discharge	Etiological agent
Purulent/mucopurulent	Bacterial conjunctivitis
Watery	Viral conjunctivitis
Ropy	Allergic conjunctivitis
Mucopurulent	Chlamydial conjunctivitis

Causes of Painless and Painful Loss of Vision

Sudden painless loss of vision	Sudden painful loss of vision
Vascular occlusion (CRAO, CRVO) *Retinal detachment* *Vitreous hemorrhage* Ischemic optic neuropathy	Acute iridocyclitis Chemical injuries Mechanical injuries Acute congestive glaucoma Optic neuritis
Gradual painless loss of vision	Gradual painful loss of vision
Progressive pterygium involving the pupil Corneal degeneration Corneal dystrophy Developmental cataracts Senile cataracts Optic atrophy Chorioretinal degeneration Age- related macular degeneration *Diabetic retinopathy* Refractive errors Papilloedema & Papillitis	Chronic iridocyclitis Corneal ulceration Chronic simple glaucoma

1325

Key Points

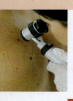

FMGE Solutions Screening Examination

Cherry red spot of retina is seen in—
- CRAO
- Trauma (Blunt trauma, Berlin's edema)
- Neimann pick disease
- Gaucher's disease
- Tay – Sach's disease
- Sand hoff's disease

Mnemonic: Cherry Tree Never Grow Tall in Sand.

TABLE: Comparison of anterior, intermediate and posterior uveitis

	Anterior	Intermediate	Posterior
Aka	Iridocyclitis	Pars Planitis	Chorioretinitis
Cause	Idiopathic	Idiopathic	Toxoplasmosis
Clinical feature	Sudden painless loss of vision	Floaters	Sudden painless loss of vision
Cells	WBC's Keratic precipitate	Snowballs/ snowbanks	Headlight in fog appearance
Treatment	Topical steroids DOC: Cycloplegics	Inj: Triamcinolone	Antimicrobials Systemic steroids

TABLE: Types of cataract and their causes

Type of cataract	Cause
Snow flake/snow storm cataract	Diabetes mellitus/ Down's syndrome
Sunflower/Petals of flower cataract	Wilson's disease Chalcosis (mild reaction to copper) Penetrating trauma (with retention to copper)
Blue dot cortical cataract	Atopic dermatitis Myotonic dystrophy
Vossius ring/Rosette shaped cataract	Blunt trauma
Christmas tree cataract	Myotonic dystrophy
Oil drop cataract Dust like lenticular opacity	Galactosemia
Breadcrumb appearance Polychromatic lusture Rainbow cataract	Complicated cataract/ Secondary cataract
Morgagnian cataract	Hypermature senile cataract

TABLE: Points to know about treatment of glaucoma

First line DOC for ACG: **Mannitol**
TOC for ACG: **Laser iridotomy**
DOC for OAG: PG analogue **(Latanoprost)**
Most powerful anti glaucoma drug: **Latanoprost**
DOC for OAG in India - **Timolol**
Safest anti-glaucoma for children - **Dorzolamide**

TABLE: Lesion in the optic pathway and the type of blindness

Unilateral optic nerve lesion: Unilateral blindness

Binasal hemianopia: Bitemporal optic chiasma lesion. Two different lesions compressing the chiasma from the lateral parts.

Bitemporal hemianopia: Binasal retinal damaged → optic chiasmal lesion. Most common lesion is *pituitary adenoma*.

Homonymous hemianopia: Lesion at optic tract AND optic radiation

Homonymous superior quadrantanopia: All superior quadrantanopia goes to the temporal lobe *(pie in the sky)*.

Homonymous inferior quadrantanopia: All inferior quadrantanopia goes to the parietal lobe *(Pie on the floor)*.

Homonymous hemianopia w/ macular sparing: Lesion in occipital cortex lesion.

Important Nodules

• Dalen fuch nodule	Sympathetic ophthalmitis
• Koeppes nodule	Granulomatous anterior uveitis
• Liesh nodule	NF – 1 and Von Ricklinghausen syndrome
• Foster fuch nodule	Myopia *Foster fuch spot: High myopia*
• Koeppes nodules	Granulomatous uveitis
• Iris nodules	Hansen's disease, NF, fuch heterochromatic iridocyclitis

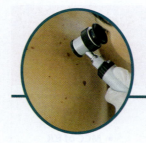

Dermatology

DERMATOLOGY— AT A GLANCE

Average weight of skin: ~ 4 kg
Normal skin turnover **4–5 weeks**
Skin turnover period in case of psoriasis: **4 days**
Epidermis is compared of **4 layers**-Stratum Basale/germinatum, Stratum spinosum, Stratum granulosum, Stratum corneum.
Dermis is composed of collagen, elastic fibers, sweat/sebaceous glands.

Contd...

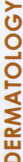

Dermatology

Tzanck smear – Useful in diagnosis of herpes lesion (HSV/VZV multinucleate giant cells)

Tzanck test – Used to differentiate viral lesions of skin from pemphigus.

Body Odor is due to: **Apocrine Gland**

MUST KNOW TERMS

• Cell cycle of keratinocytes	311 hours (28 days)
• Growth rate of scalp hair	0.37 mm/day (90% hair in Anagen phase all time)
• Nail growth rate	**Finger nail:** 1 cm/3 month (0.1 mm/d) **Toe nail:** 1 cm/9 month
• Keratin involved in Epidemolysis bullous simplex	K5 and K14
• Dermis thinnest at	Eyelid and Penis (0.3 mm)
• Type VII collagen defect at basement membrane zone	Epidermolysis bullosa Aquisita
• LIGA disease (Linear IgA bullous disease) due to	BP Ag2
• Bullous pemphigoid is due to this BMZ defect	BP Ag1 and 2
• Herpes gestationis is due this BMZ defect	BP Ag2
• Defect in Hereditary angioedema	C1 esterase inhibitor absent
• Patch test type of HPS reaction	Type IV
• MCC of tinea Unguium	T. Rubrum
• MCC of tinea Mannum	T. Rubrum
• Buddha ears are feature of	Leprosy
• Nevus of ota is seen at this site	Face and Sclera
• Nevus of Ito	Scapular region/ Back
• Becker's lesion	Macular lesion + hair
• Sausage digits are seen in	Psoriatic arthritis
• Dermatitis herpetiformis	Celiac sprue (*anti epidermal transglutaminase A/B*)
• Heliotrope rash/Gottron papule/ Mechanic hand is seen in	Dermatomyositis (anti Jo-1 A/b)
• Elephantiasis face is a feature of	Plexiform NF

Contd...

• Piebaldism+ increased interpupillary distance+ sensory neural deafness	Waardenburg syndrome
• Occlusion due to staph epidermidis in eccrine gland	Miliaria
• Fordyce spot	Ectopic sebaceous gland
• Epidermolysis bullosa simplex	Trauma induced blisters
• Epidermolysis bullosa dystrophica	Absent collagen since birth
• Dilapidated brick wall appearance scene in	Hailey Hailey disease
• Row of tombstone appearance and fishnet pattern seen in	Pemphigus vulgaris
• Desmoglein involved in pemphigus foliaceous	DSG 1
• Desmoglein involved pemphigus vulgaris	DSG 3

COLOR ON WOOD LAMP'S LIGHT

- **Pseudomonas, psoriasis** – Pale blue color
- *Corynebacterium minutissimum* (erythrasma) – Coral red color
- **Erythrasma**- Coral red
- **Tuberous sclerosis** – Ash leaf spots (blue white)
- **Vitiligo** – Chalky white
- **Porphyria cutanea** tarda – Pinkish red (urine)
- **Tinea versicolor** – Golden fluorescence
- **Pityriasis versicolor**: Yellow
- **Squamous cell carcinoma** – Red fluorescence
- **Burrow of scabies**: Green

Fungi which give fluorescence in wood's light are–
M. Canis, M. audouinii, T. schoenleinii.

KOH preparation – Used for diagnosis of Tinea infections

Köbner's isomorphic phenomena seen in:
- Psoriasis
- Lichen planus, lichen nitidus, lichen sclerosus
- Vitiligo
- Kaposi sarcoma
- Pityriasis rubra pilaris
- Necrobiosis lipoidica

Pseudo-isomorphic phenomenon is seen in – **Pityriasis Rubra Pilaris (PRP), molluscum contagiosum, warts**

Nikolsky's sign is seen in–
- Pemphigus
- Staphylococcal scalded skin syndrome (SSSS)
- Toxic shock syndrome
- Porphyria

Contd...

Key Points

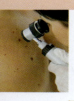

FMGE Solutions Screening Examination

Pseudo-Nikolsky's sign seen in:
- Toxic epidermal necrolysis
- Steven Johnson syndrome
- Erythema multiforme

Dermatomal involvement is seen in–**Herpes zoster**.

Painful lesions are seen in–**Herpes infection**.

Painless lesions are seen in–**Dermatitis herpetiformis (itchy lesions), pemphigoid, pemphigus, erythema multiforme**.

Sub-epidermal lesions are seen in–**Dermatitis herpetiformis, pemphigoid, erythema multiforme.**

Intraepidermal lesions are seen in–**Herpes, pemphigus.**

Lesions involving oral mucosa are seen in–**Secondary and congenital syphilis, pemphigus, Peutz Jegher syndrome, lichen planus.**

MC type of warts–**Verruca vulgaris/common warts.**

MC site of common warts–**Dorsum of hand/finger**

Condyloma acuminate (venereal warts) is associated with HPV 16 and 11.

TOC for anogenital warts in pregnancy is **cryotherapy/laser.**

Molluscum contagiosum is due to infection with pox virus.

Extra-genital molluscal lesions are marker of AIDS in adults.

Darier white disease is Autosomal dominant characterized by warty papules and plaques in seborrheic sites.

Dowling Degos disease is autosomal dominant genodermatosis.

MC bacterial skin infection in children is **Impetigo** in which Honey colored crusts are seen.

MC site of Impetigo is **face**.

MC cause of Impetigo is *Staphylococcus aureus*.

Bullous **pemphigoid** is also known as Senile pemphigoid.

Treatment of bullous pemphigoid is **prednisolone in low doses.**

MC type of pemphigus is **P. vulgaris while the rarest** is **P. vegetans**

P. vulgaris has worst prognosis.

P. vulgaris is diagnosed by **Tzanck** TEST, Fish-net pattern of IgG in epidermis in direct immunofluorescence.

Dermatitis Herpetiformis is recurrent papulovesicular disease with pruritus. Associated with HLA-B8 or DRW3

Max-Joseph spaces, are artificial sub epidermal clefts, often seen in lichen ruber variants of Lichen planus.

Psoriatic arthropathy treated with **Methotrexate (DOC)**

Pityriasis rosea–First feature is Herald patch usually over trunk or upper arm, thigh.

Christmas tree/fir tree pattern seen in **pityriasis rosea.**

Pityriasis versicolor/tinea versicolor caused be **Malassezia furfur.**

"Spaghetti & Meatball" appearance or "Banana & grape" appearance on KOH microscopy: **Pityriasis versicolor**

In **pityriasis rubra** pilaris isolated patches of normal skin are also seen.

Hyperpigmentation is seen in diseases like:
- Addison's disease
- Nelson syndrome
- Hyperthyroidism
- Cushing syndrome
- Ectopic ACTH syndrome
- Freckles

Hypopigmentation is seen in diseases like:
- Vitiligo, piebaldism
- Nevus anemicus
- Nevus depigmentosus
- Pityriasis
- Scleroderma
- Sarcoidosis

Nevus ota, ito, mongolian spots, café au lait spots are causes of local **hypopigmentation.**

Pruritis is hallmark of Atopic dermatitis in which dennie's line and Monk's crawl are seen.

MC presentation of Contact dermatitis is hand **eczema**.

MC cause of air-borne contact dermatitis in India is Allergic Contact Dermatitis due to plant **Parthenium**.

Nummular eczema (discoid dermatitis) is circular/oval coin like pruritic lesions over trunk/extensor surface of limbs in middle age males (M>F).

Asteatotic/xerotic eczema (Winter itch) is inflammatory dermatitis with fine cracks. Seen in summer and involves lower legs in elderly.

Cradle Cap is seen in **Seborrheic Dermatitis.**

Pseudomonas aeruginosa is the MC organism which causes Ecthyma gangrenosum.

Pyoderma Gangrenosum is diagnosed clinically (Morphology of lesions).

MC cause of **Erythema Multiforme** is HSV while MC drug causing it is sulfonamides.

Erythema nodosum is due to infections like streptococcal infection, TB, Leprosy (LL).

Darier sign is seen **Urticaria Pigmentosa**.

Steven Johnson Syndrome is characterized by blisters and epidermal detachment.

In tinea capitis infection of scalp is caused by **trichophyton tonsurans**.

Infection of foot (athlete foot) is caused by **T. rubrum**.

Pistia line is seen in Scarlet fever.

Beau's line is seen in psoriatic arthropathy.

Swimmer's itch – **Bilharziasis/ Schistosomiasis.**

Contd...

Contd...

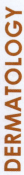

Dermatology

Dhobi's/Jock itch – **Tinea cruris.**

Ground itch – **nematode larvae**

Barber's itch **Syncosis barbae**

Itch mite – **Acarus scabiei** (which transmits Scabies)

Scabies is caused by mite '**Sarcoptes scabiei**".

Pediculosis is caused by **Pediculosis corporis.**

TB-skin caused by **Mycobacterium tuberculosis bovis** and under some conditions by BCG.

Fox-fordyce disease involves axilla and pubis.

Fordyce spots are ectopic sebaceous glands in neonates.

Retinoic acid is DOC in Acne vulgaris, comedonal acne, nodulocystic acne, pustular acne.

Exclamation marks are seen in **Alopecia Areata.**

Half and half nail sign is seen in **Uremia.**

Koilonychia is seen in Iron Deficiency Anemia.

Pterygium, anonychia, pitting is seen in **lichen planus.**

Onycholysis, ridging, pitting, thimble nails are seen in **psoriasis.**

Café-au-lait spots are seen in:
- Neurofibromatosis
- Albright's syndrome & Fibrous dysplasia.
- Watson's syndrome
- Leopard syndrome
- Fanconi's anemia

Leonine facies are seen in:
- LL-Leprosy
- Paget's disease of bone
- Fibrous dysplasia
- Hyperphosphatemia.

Pinch purpura is seen in Primary systemic amyloidosis, EDS, Scurvy.

MC route of transmission of Syphilis is sexual and sometimes transmitted by **BT, transplacental.**

DOC for syphilitic chancre (hard sore) is **BPG 2.4 million U single i.m. dose**

DOC for chancroid (soft sore) is **Single dose of Azithromycin** (or i/m ceftriaxone).

DOC for Lymphogranuloma venereum/inguinale is **Doxycycline or erythromycin for 2 weeks.**

DOC for Donovanosis is **Azithromycin**

Satellite lesions are seen in BT.

Inverted saucer shaped ulcers are seen in **Borderline leprosy.**

Virchow cell is diagnostic of lepromatous leprosy.

Most commonly involved nerve in leprosy: **Ulnar nerve**

Radial nerve is involved last in leprosy but if it is involved complications are more serious.

TABLE: Pathologies arising due to obstruction of sweat gland appendage

Obstruction of eccrine sweat gland ducts: Miliaria
Obstruction of apocrine sweat gland ducts: Fox fordyce spot/disease also known as Apocrine Miliaria
MC site of fox fordyce spot: Axilla
MC age group of fox fordyce spot: 13–35 years (*Females are MC affected*).
Fordice spot are ectopic sebaceous glands.

Classical features of Acrodermatitis Enteropathica include: (*Mnemonic-"DEAL"*)
- **D**iarrhea, Depression
- **E**czematous erosive dermatitis
- **A**lopecia (non scarring), **A**pathetic look
- **L**ethargy, irritability, whining & crying.

TABLE: Difference between pemphigus and pemphigoid bullae

Features	Pemphigus	Pemphigoid
Row of Tomb stone	Present	Absent
Nikolsky Sign	Present	Absent
Bullae location	Intraepidermal – flaccid Bullae	Subepidermal & tense Bullae
Mucosa involvement	Present (common)	Absent or less common
Acantholysis	Present	Absent
Prognosis	Poor	Good

TABLE: The ringworm genera

Trichophyton	Microsporum	Epidermophyton
Infects skin, hair & nail Infecting species include: Trichophyton rubrum mentagrophytes Violaceum Verrucosum schoenleinii	*Infects skin and hair* but does not involve nails Several infecting species include: Microsporum audouinii, M. gypseum and M. canis	*Infect skin & nails* but does not involve hair Only infecting species is Epidermophyton floccosum.
Mnemonic: **TSH-N** (*Trichophyton infects Skin, Hair and Nail*) **MSH** (*Microsporum infects Skin and Hair*) **ESN** (*Epidermophyton infects Skin and Nail*)		

Key Points

1329

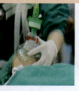

FMGE Solutions Screening Examination

TABLE: Causes of genital ulcer

Bacterial	Viral	Parasitic	Non-infectious
Haemophilus ducreyi Treponema pallidum Chlamydia trachomatis Donovanosis balanitis	Herpes simplex Varicella zoster EBV Cytomegalo-virus	Sarcoptes scabiei Phthirus pubis Entamoeba histolytica Trichomonas vaginalis	Trauma Pyoderma gangreno-sum Reiter's syndrome Wegner's Neoplasms

TABLE: Warts and its associated disease

Warts	Seen in
Plane wart	Verruca plana
Filiform wart	Verruca filiformis
Plantar wart	Verruca plantaris or myrmecia wart
Venereal wart	Condylomata accuminata
Massive wart	Buschke–Löwenstein tumor
Condyloma lata	Treponema Pallidum

TABLE: Differences between syphilis, chancroid and LGV

Disease	Ulcer	Lymph node
Syphilis	Painless	Painless
Chancroid	Painful	Painful
LGV	Painless	Painful (Bubo)

TABLE: Differences between type 1 and type 2 lepra reaction

Type I Leprae Reaction: Reversal reaction	Type II Leprae R: Erythema nodosum leprosum
Type IV delayed HPS reaction	Type III HPS (Jarisch-Herxheimer) reaction
Found in TT (tuberculoid type)	Found in LL (Lepromatous Leprosy)
Thalidomide has no role	Thalidomide is most effective drug.
DOC is corticosteroid	DOC is corticosteroid

IMPORTANT SIGNS

• Carpet Tack Sign	DLE
• Chandelier's sign:	PID in women.
• Antenna sign:	Seen in Keratosis Pilaris
• Buttonholing sign:	NF 1
• Dimpling sign	Dermatofibrosarcoma protuberans
• Asboe Hansen sign	Pemphigus
• Nikolsky sign	Pemphigus, SSSS, TEN
• Auspitz sign/Grattage test	Psoriasis

MUST KNOW TERMS

• Persistence of nuclei in stratum spinosum	Parakeratosis
• Increase in keratinocyte population of spinous layer with thickening of the epidermis	Acanthosis
• Increase in keratinocytes with formation of projections from the surface of the skin	Papillomatosis (Ex: Wart)

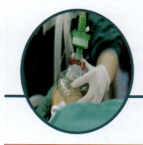

Anesthesia

- Guedels stages of ether anesthesia
  - Stage 1 analgesia
  - Stage 2 delirium
  - Stage 3 surgical anesthesia
  - Stage 4 medullary paralysis.
- Nitric oxide produces second gas effect and fink phenomenon.
- Direct measurement of BP done in **Radial artery.**
- Neuromuscular monitoring performed at **ulnar nerve.**
- Sufentanil is most potent opioid.
- Remifentanil is shortest acting opiod.
- **Alfentanil** is opiod of choice for day care surgery
- Muscle relaxant of choice in shock: **Pancuronium**
- Most cardiostable anesthetic agent: **Etomidate**
- Most cardiostable inhalational agent **Isoflurane**
- Most cerebroprotective inhalational agent **Sevoflurane**
- Whitacre and Sprotte procedure is used for: **Spinal anesthesia**
- **Successful sign of spinal anesthesia:** Flaccid and engorged penis (Reason: Nervi ergentis paralysis)
- **Sequence of block by local anesthesia:** Temperature (cold > Hot) – pain – touch – deep pressure – proprioception
- Nerve fiber Sensitivity to pressure: **A > B > C**
- Nerve fiber sensitivity to hypoxia: **B > A > C**
- Nerve fiber sensitivity to LA: **A gamma, A Delta > Aα & Aβ**
- Anesthetic agents contraindicated in porphyria: **Pentazocine, Etomidate, Thiopentone (PET)**
  - DOC in such condition: **Propofol**

Contd...

Anesthesia

- Protein intake in ICU : **1–1.5 g/kg/day**
- Most common ophthalmic complication during anesthesia: **Corneal abrasion.**
- History of postdural puncture headache is not a contraindication of epidural block
- **Flat Capnogram seen in:**
  - Accidental extubation
  - Dissociation of anesthetic tube
  - Mechanical ventilation failing
- O_2 content of anesthetic mixture: **33%**
- Preanesthetic drug which causes longest amnesia: **Lorazepam**
- Anesthetic with least decrease in systemic vascular resistance: **Halothane**
- MC anaesthetic agent causes Malignant hyperthermia: **Sch**
- LA having highest incidence of malignant hyperthermia: **Lignocaine**
- Inhalational test having highest incidence of malignant hyperthermia: **Halothane**
- Malignant hyperthermia is caused by: **Ryanodine receptor**
- Dextrose fluid is never used for resuscitation
- Opioid given as transdermal: **Fentanyl**

PIN INDEX AND COLOR CODING OF COMMONLY USED GASES

Gas	Color code		Pin index position
	Body	**Shoulder**	
Air	Grey	White/black quartered	1, 5
Oxygen	Black	White	2, 5
Nitrous oxide	Blue	Blue	3, 5
CO_2	Gray	Gray	1, 6
Helium	Brown	Brown	2, 5

AMBU Bag stands for Artificial Maneuver Breathing Unit.

Cyclopropane cylinder is **orange**

ENTONOX cylinder color: **Blue body w/ blue and white shoulder**

Spinal cord extents **from medulla oblongata to lower border** of L1 in adults and lower border of L3 in infants and neonates.

Structures pierced by spinal needle:
Skin → Subcutaneous tissue → supraspinatus ligament → interspinous ligament → Ligamentum flavum → Dura mater → Arachnoid space

Spinal block/sub arachnoid block is given in L3–L4 interspace in adults and L4–L5 in children.

Contd...

Postdural puncture headache presents 12–24 hours of spinal block.

Epidural block is given between dura mater and ligamentum flavum.

Commonly used needle for epidural block is **Tuohys Needle.**

DOC for laryngeal mask insertion is **propofol**

Mallampati grading is used for assessment of size of tongue for laryngoscopy, also for assessment of difficult airway during orotracheal/nasotracheal intubation

Capnography is monitoring of $EtCO_2$ (end tidal CO_2) and it's waveform, normally it is 35–45 mmHg

Normal CVP is **4–7 cmH_2O** (3–12mm Hg is the range)

Seldinger technique is used for catheterization of vein (guide wire technique for central access)

Inotrope of choice for intra operative management of right heart failure due to pulmonary hypertension: **Dobutamine and Milrinone**

Potency of inhalational agent is determined by **MAC (minimum alveolar concentration)**

Methoxyflurane is most potent while **N_2O** is minimum in potency

ENTONOX- 50:50 mixture of **N_2O** and **O_2,** cylinder is blue colored with white shoulder

Induction agent of choice in children **Sevoflurane**

Fastest acting induction agent-**Desflurane**

Bupivacaine is most Cardiotoxic LA

Longest acting LA: **Dibucaine**

Most commonly used LA: **Lignocaine**

Local anesthetic which causes methemoglobinemia: **Benzocaine, Prilocaine, Lignocaine (BPL)**

Most common LA which causes Methemoglobinemia: **Prilocaine**

Thiopentone sodium causes reverse coronary steal phenomenon.

Ketamine produces Dissociative anesthesia

Diazepam causes retrograde amnesia

Anesthesia of choice in day care surgery-**Propofol**

Shortest acting depolarizing muscle relaxant: **Succinylcholine**

Shortest acting NDMR *(Non-depolarizing muscle relaxant)*- **Gantacurium (5-10 min) > Mivacurium (10-15 min)**

Fastest acting NDMR - **Rocuronium**

Longest acting NDMR – **Doxacurium (120 min)**

MC used SMR (skeletal muscle relaxant) in routine surgery -**Vecuronium**

MC used method of brachial plexus block is **supraclavicular block.**

Contd...

Key Points

1331

FMGE Solutions Screening Examination

Mendelson syndrome: regurgitation of gastric contents causes aspiration pneumonitis

Selliks maneuver: to prevent regurgitation, pressure is applied on cricoid cartilage which compresses esophagus against vertebral column.

Drug not useful for induction in infants - **Morphine**

Muscle relaxant of choice in renal failure: **Atracurium**

Muscle relaxant of choice in renal and, or hepatic failure: **Cis-atracurium**

Hoffman elimination is seen in which muscle relaxant: **Atracurium, Cis-atracurium**

Boyle's Machine operates on: **Continuous flow principle**

Venturi mask:
- High flow oxygen delivery device
- Maximum oxygen delivered is 60%

Maximum oxygen delivered by nasal cannula: **44%**

Mapleson circuits type A is Also known as **Magills circuit**
Mapleson circuit type E is known as Ayres T piece best suited for **neonates**.

TABLE: Ester and amides

Ester (one 'I' in name)	Amides (2 'I' in name)
Cocaine Benzocaine Chloroprocaine Tetracaine	Lignocaine Bupivacaine Prilocaine Dibucaine Etidocaine
Remember: Amide group of LA contain "2 i" in their name	

CLASSIFICATION OF MUSCLE RELAXANTS

Neuromuscular blocking agent	
Depolarizing (Non-competitive) MR	Non-depolarizing (Competitive) MR
Suxamethonium/succinyl choline/Scoline Decamethonium	All others, For eg: Gallamine, D-tubocurarine, Atracurium, Mivacurium Ve/ Pan/ro-curonium

ANESTHETIC DOC

Condition	DOC
• Day care	Propofol (i/v), Desflurane (inhalation)
• Epilepsy	Thiopentone
• Neurosurgery	Isoflurane, Thipentone

Contd...

Condition	DOC
• Renal failure/hepatic failure	Isoflurane Cis-atracurium (M/R)
• ECT (Electro convulsive therapy)	Methohexital
• Bronchial asthma, COPD	Ketamine (i/v), Halothane (inhalational)
• Aneurysm surgery, IHD	Etomidate
• Cardiac surgery (preserved LV function)	Isoflurane
• Cardiac surgery (poor LV function)	Opioid
• CHD: Lt to right shunt	Isoflurane/sevoflurane
• Cyanotic HD: Rt to left shunt	Ketamine
• CHF, Shock	Ketamine
• Inhalational agent for induction in children	Sevoflurane
• IVRA (I.V Regional Anesthesia)	Prilocaine > Lignocaine
• TIVA (Total I.V. Anesthesia)	Propofol+Remifentanil

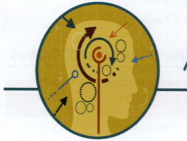

Psychiatry

PSYCHIATRY—AT A GLANCE

Van Gogh syndrome: Dramatic self-mutilation occurring in schizophrenia

Squeeze technique is used for: **Premature ejaculation**

Schizophrenia is a thought disorder

Prevalence of schizophrenia: **1%**

Insight is absent in schizophrenia, mood disorder, delusional disorder

Dementia is not seen in schizophrenia

Not seen in schizophrenia: **Intellectual impairment**

Delusion of Fragmentary–delirium, hebephrenic schizophrenia.

Milieu therapy /family therapy / Therapeutic community – **in schizophrenia**

Contd...

Psychiatry

Drug of choice of schizophrenia: **Olanzapine**

Clozapine is particularly effective in **resistance schizophrenia**

Depersonalization & derealization usually occur together & are seen in – depression, anxiety, schizophrenia, epilepsy.

Pseudo-community, split personality seen in schizophrenia

Morbid jealousy – Mood disorder, alcoholism, drug abuse, epilepsy, schizophrenia

Ambulatory schizophrenia and pseudoneurotic schizophrenia are now included in border line personality disorder.

TABLE: Neurotransmitter levels

Disease	Related neurotransmitter
Schizophrenia	Increased serotonin and Dopamine Decreased Glutamate
Depression	Decreased serotonin, NA, Dopamine
OCD	Decreased serotonin
Alzheimer's disease	Decreased Ach

TABLE: Prognostic factor of schizophrenia

Good prognostic factor	Bad prognostic factor
Female sex Acute onset (late onset) No family history of schizophrenia History of depressive order Premorbid personality	Male sex Gradual onset (early onset) Family history of schizophrenia Emotional blunting

DEPRESSION

- Depression is the **most common psychiatric disorder** in hospitalized patients.
- MC psychiatric illness: **Anxiety**
- **Nihilistic delusion and delusion of guilt** and poverty – Seen in depression.
- Depression is the MC psychiatric disorder in: **Hypothyroidism, AIDS, patients on ocp's, postpartum psychosis**
- OCD leads to **secondary depression**
- DOC for manic depressive disorder: **Lithium**
- Long term use of lithium can cause: **Hypothyroidism**
- **Pseudo depression & nihilistic delusion** are seen in depression.

Insomnia is seen in this withdrawal: **Alcohol withdrawal**

Hypersomnia is seen in **cocaine withdrawal**

Kubler Ross classified 5 stages of death: Denial → Anger → Bargain → Despair → Acceptance.

Contd...

Super ego: Based on moral principle. Ego ideal. E.g.: Mother Teresa, Mahatma Gandhi (idealistic thing)

Ego: Based on reality

Instinct: Inborn, based on principle of pleasure, maternal/paternal instincts

Fibromyalgia is not a somatoform disorder.

CBT does not include: **Interpretation**

Not a defense mechanism – **Transference, derailment**

Generalized anxiety disorder is not an indication for lithium

Angel dust is **Phencyclidine it** produce catatonic syndrome

REM Sleep is characterized by PGO spikes.

NREM stage 2 is characterized by sleep spindles and k-complex.

Muscle hypotonia is most characteristic REM sleep which differentiate it from wakefulness.

Classical tetrad of **Narcolepsy**: Sleep attacks, cataplexy, hypnogogic hallucinations, sleep paralysis.

Illusion: False perception of external object which has real existence.

Impulse: Irresistible desire

Obsessions: recurrent, irrational, intrusive, ego-dystonic and ego-alien ideas.

Overall most common type of hallucination: **Auditory hallucination**

Visual hallucination are mc seen in organic disease

Tactile hallucination are seen in chronic amphetamine poisoning.

Synaesthesia: Stimulus in one modality & hallucination in other modality

Delusion is not a feature **of conversion disorder.**

Delusion of Grandiosity – **MANIA**

Othello syndrome – Jealousy (infidelity)

Induced delusional disorder – Sharing of delusions b/w usually two or occasionally more persons.

Concrete thinking stage **2-7 years**

MC mental disorder in children – **Neurosis**

MC form of pica is **Geophagia.**

Fear of death most commonly at age of **5 years**

Age of onset in **Autism** < 2 ½ years, there is a marked impairment of language

Rett's syndrome
Occurs exclusively in girls
A neuropsychiatric illness, with normal head circumference at birth
Characterized by: Midline hand winging/hand washing stereotypies

Contd...

Key Points

FMGE Solutions Screening Examination

- **In Asperger's syndrome** language is normal AND no delay **in cognitive development** (remember Shahrukh Khan in movie- My Name is Khan)
- Treatment of choice for Hypochondriasis, somatoform disorder Anxiety neurosis, Hysteria – **Supportive Psychotherapy**
- Treatment of choice for phobia – **Behavior therapy**
- Treatment of choice Gilles de la Tourette's syndrome – **Clonidine/Haloperidol**
- EPS are NOT seen with **clozapine**
- **Akathisia** is most common with haloperidol. It is treated by propranolol
- Antidepressant which can be used in t/t of nocturnal enuresis, ADHD, chronic pain: **Imipramine**
- Patients of anorexia nervosa are vulnerable to sudden death due to ventricular **arrhythmias**
- **Delirium** is most common organic disorder
- **Drugs inducing delirium**: Alcohol, heroin, morphine, cannabis, cocaine, LSD.
- **Psychosis** may occur in pregnancy, postpartum, epilepsy
- Main symptom of Korsakoff psychosis: **Confabulation**
- In late phase profound anterograde amnesia & milder retrograde amnesia is found in **delirium & dementia**
- **In acute delirium** sun downing phenomenon is present.
- **In Korsakoff's psychosis** immediate & remote memory is usually retained
- **Amotivation** is lethargy, apathy, loss of interest, anergia, reduced drive, lac of ambition seen in chronic cannabis abuse.
- **Anxiety** is most common psychiatric symptom & generalized anxiety disorder in general population.
- Splitting is a defense mechanism against **BPD**.
- **Sensate focus** technique is used for t/t of impotency
- **Master's and Johnson's technique** is most popular t/t method for psycho sexual dysfunction in which both partners are treated together.
- **Excessive sexual drive** is called satyrism in men and nymphomania in female.
- **Visual hallucination** is characteristic of alcohol withdrawal.
- Most important dependency producing derivatives are **morphine & heroin**.
- ECT most effective in the treatment of major depression with **psychosis, delusion, or suicidal tendency.**
- **ECT is never indicated** in cyclothymia, Dysthymia, Chronic Schizophrenia (with negative symptoms)
- MC complication of direct (modified) ECT: **Fracture T4-T8 spine.**
- **MC complication of modified ECT**: Anterograde & Retro Grade amnesia more of retrograde type.

- Alcohol is the most common substance abused in India and worldwide.
- Most common illicit drug/substance abused: **Cannabis > Amphetamine (2nd MC).**
- DOC for prophylaxis of bipolar disorder - **Lithium**
- DOC for acute mania: **Lithium**
- Therapeutic level of lithium: 0.8 – 1.2 mEq/L
- Toxicity seen after >1.5 mEq/L
- Most common side effect of lithium: **Tremor**
- Most common cause of impotency in male: **Psychogenic**

Antipsychotics

- Recently approved sublingual antipsychotic: **Asenapine**
- Most common side effect of typical antipsychotic: **Extrapyramidal symptoms (EPS)**
- Most common EPS: **Akathisia**
- MC side effect of atypical antipsychotics: **Metabolic/Lipodystrophy syndrome (Weight gain, Inc glucose, altered lipid profile)**
- Atypicals with least weight gain: **Aripiprazole, Ziprasidone**
- Atypicals with max weight gain: **Clozapine**
- Atypicals with least risk of EPS: **Clozapine**
- Typical with least EPS: **Chlorpromazine and Thioridazine**
- Typicals with max risk of EPS: **Haloperidol**
- Atypicals associated with cardiac arrhythmia: **Sertindole, Zotepine**
- Most potent atypical antipsychotic: **Risperidone**
- Atypicals with maximum risk of hyperprolactinemia: **Risperidone**
- Atypical antipsychotic causing corneal opacity: **Chlorpromazine and Thioridazine**
- Known side effects of clozapine: **Agranulocytosis, Sialorrhea, Sedation, weight gain**

TABLE: Eating disorder

	Anorexia nervosa	Bulimia nervosa
Feature	Refusal to maintain body weight above a minimal normal	Irresistible craving for food with episodes of over eating in less time (Binge eating)
Method of weight control		Attempts to counter act the effects of over eating by self-induced vomiting: Purgative abuse, Periods of starvations Appetite suppressants

Contd...

Contd...

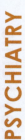

Psychiatry

	Anorexia nervosa	Bulimia nervosa
Ritualized exercise	Common	Rare
Amenorrhea	100%	50%
Decreased Vital aBP, ˉPulse	Common	Uncommon
Hypothermia	Common	Rare
Skin changes (hirsutism)	Common	Rare
Medical Complications	Hypokalemia Cardiac arrhythmias	Hypokalemia Cardiac arrhythmias

FEATURE OF CORTICAL & SUBCORTICAL DEMENTIA

Features	Cortical dementia	Subcortical dementia
Site	Cortex (frontal, parietal, temporal, occipital, hippocampus)	Subcortical grey matter
Memory impairment	Severe, early Recall helped very little by cues	Mild to moderate Recall helped partially by cues & recognition tasks
Mathematical skills	Impaired early (Acalculia)	Preserved
Language	Early, Dysphasia (Aphasia)	Normal & Anomia (in severe cases)
Speech	Articulate until late	Dysarthria
Personality	Indifferent	Apathetic, inert

TABLE: Appearance of alcohol withdrawal symptoms

Time	Symptoms
6–12 hours	Minor withdrawal symptoms: Insomnia, tremulousness, anxiety, GIT upset, headache, diaphoresis, palpitations, anorexia
12–24 hours	Alcoholic hallucinosis; visual, auditory, or tactile hallucination
24–48 hours	*Withdrawal seizures:* generalized tonic-clonic seizures
48–72 hours	Delirium tremens; visual hallucinations, disorientation, *tachycardia*, hypertension, low-grade fever, agitation, diaphoresis

TABLE: Substance abuse and its characteristic clinical feature

Substance	Characteristic clinical feature
Cocaine	Magnus symptoms (cocaine bugs or Tactile hallucination)
Cannabis	Run Amok Amotivational syndrome Flash backs
Alcohol	Mc-Evan's sign Morbid jealousy
LSD	Bad Trips Flash backs
Amphetamine	Paranoid Hallucinatory syndrome (like paranoid schizophrenia)
Phencyclidine (Angel dust)	Dissociative anesthesia

Therapeutic Modes for Diseases

• Milieu therapy Therapeutic community/family therapy	In Schizophrenia
• Bio feedback, Jacobson's relaxation technique, Autohypnosis	In type A behavior/personality (Psychosomatic disorder)
• Semens Seqeeze tech (Masters & Johnson's)	In premature ejaculation
• Abreaction therapy (Amytal interview)	In hysteria & d/g of catatonic syndrome. (Interview with mute, stupor)
• Systemic desensitization	• TOC in Phobias, OCD
• Aversion therapy	• Alcohol dependence, transvestism, homosexuality, hysteria
• Flooding:	• Phobias

Types of Personality

	Clinical features	Increased risk of
Type A	Ambitious, achievement oriented people, often high-achieving career oriented "workaholics", impatient	Coronary heart diseases
Type B	Easy going relaxed individuals	-
Type C	No assertive at all and they always suppress their own desires	Depression, cancer
Type D	Distressed	CHD patient has ↑ Mortality & recurrence from MI

1335

Key Points

Radiology

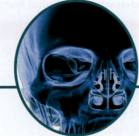

- Father of radiology/X-ray: **W.C. Roentgen** (Discovered on 8 November, 1895)
- Father of USG: **John Wild**
- Father of Obstetrical USG: **Ion Donald**
- Father of Doppler: **Doppler John**
- Father of CT Scan: **Godfrey Hounsfield**
- Father of MRI: **Laterbuer and Mansfield**

Components of X-ray machine:
- Cathode-tungsten
- Anode-tungsten
- Anode in mammography: Molybdenum
- Filter- Al, or Al + Cu or Mo
- Collimator- Pb (Lead)

Radiation Units
- Unit of radiation exposure - **Roentgen** (SI = Coulomb/kg)
- Unit of absorbed radiation - **RAD** (SI = GRAY)
- Unit of biologic effectiveness - **Rem** (SI = Sievert)

Normal distance from which a chest **X-ray** is performed: 180 cm (6 ft")

Thickness of lead jacket – **0.5 mm**

Best X-rays are performed in: 60 – 90 kVp

Minimal amount of pleural fluid required to detect pleural effusion on CXR– **100 – 200 mL**

Best X-ray view to detect minimal effusion is – **Lateral decubitus view of the same side.**

Best investigation to detect minimal fluid – **USG**

FAST Scan is: Focussed Assessment with Sonography for Trauma. Assess four main area to detect fluid in pericardium, RUQ (Morrison pouch), LUQ (Perisplenic), Pelvic area.

Best view to see normal chest- Right lung-LAO; Left lung- RAO

Major part of the radiological hilar shadow – **Pulmonary artery**

In anterior segment of upper lobe is uncommon in **secondary TB.**

Water lily sign or Camalote sign is seen in – **Hydatid lung**

Hounsfield unit of:
- Bone: +1000
- Blood: +40 to +50
- Water: 0
- Fat: - 50 to – 100
- Air: - 1000

Contd...

IOC for bronchiectasis – **HRCT**

Signet-ring sign is seen in **Bronchiectasis**

MC thoracic manifestation of rheumatoid arthritis – **Pleural effusion**

Egg shell calcification is seen in Silicosis, Sarcoidosis

Bat wing appearance on CXR is seen in **Pulmonary edema**.

X-ray signs of Pulmonary embolism- Fleischner's sign, Knuckle sign, Palla's sign.

V/Q mismatch is a sign of pulmonary infarct.

Gold standard investigation of Pulmonary embolism – **Pulmonary angiography**

Golden S sign is seen in **Bronchogenic carcinoma**.

Cannon ball appearance is seen in – **Lung metastasis**

Pop Corn calcification is seen in **Pulmonary Hamartoma**

Bronchial atresia more common in **Left upper lobe**.

Poland syndrome on CXR: **Unilateral hyperlucent lung**

IOC for aortic dissection: **MRI**

Rim sign is seen in: Massive hydronephrosis

Money bag or leather bottle or flask shaped heart is seen in **Pericardial effusion**.

Most sensitive investigation of Pericardial effusion – **Echocardiography-15 ml** can be detected

Pruned tree appearance – Pulmonary arterial hypertension

IOC for Aortic dissection – **MRI**

Champagne glass appearance – **Achondroplasia**

IOC for cardiac tamponade, Pericardial effusion – **2D Echo**

Molten candle wax appearance seen in - **Melorheostosis**

Telephone handle long bones seen in – **Thanatophoric Dwarfism**

Metacarpal sign – Pseudohypoparathyroidism, Turner's syndrome

Pepper-pot skull seen in – **Hyperparathyroidism**

Looser's zones or pseudofractures is the hallmark feature of – **Osteomalacia.**

Rugger jersey spine seen in Renal osteodystrophy, **Osteopetrosis**

Hair on end or crew cut or hair brush appearance seen in – **Thalassemia**

Earliest change in thalassemia – Widening of short bones of hand.

Flask shaped femora seen in- **Thalassemia**

Cotton wool skull seen in – **Paget's disease**

Tram track appearance on skull X-ray: **Sturge weber syndrome**

Most common intracranial calcification: **Pineal Calcification**

Basal ganglia calcification is seen in this condition: Wilson's disease

Erlenmeyer Flask deformity seen in – Metaphyseal dysplasia, Osteopetrosis, Thalassemia

Earliest seen in **Osteomyelitis**- Soft tissue swelling and loss of soft tissue planes.

Hot cross Bun Skull seen in – **Congenital syphilis**

Celery stalk appearance – **Congenital Rubella**

Bone most commonly involved in osteoarthritis – **Patella**

Earliest appearance see in rheumatoid arthritis is – **Periarticular soft tissue swelling**

Cup and pencil appearance seen in **Psoriasis**

Bamboo spine, Romanus sign, Dagger sign, Squaring of vertebrae seen in – **Ankylosing spondylitis**

Codmans triangle, Sunray appearance seen in **Osteosarcoma** Onion peel appearance seen in – **Ewing's sarcoma**

Trap door sign, Fallen fragment sign seen in- **Simple Bone Cyst**

Soap bubble appearance seen in – Giant cell tumor or **Osteoclastoma**

Shepherd Crook deformity femur, Ground glass appearance on X-ray is feature of – **Fibrous Dysplasia**.

Corduroy Cloth appearance on X-ray, Polka dot appearance on CT – **Hemangioma**

Rain drop appearance, punched out lesions on skull is seen in – **Multiple Myeloma**

Inverted napoleon hat sign on AP view, Scotty dog appearance seen in **Spondylolisthesis**

Barium is better for evaluation of motility disorders and for cricopharyngeal dysphagia than endoscopic evaluation.

Pencil tip or bird beak tapering seen in **Achalasia Cardia**

Corkscrew Esophagus seen in – **Diffuse esophageal spasm**

Initial investigation for Hypertrophic Pyloric Stenosis – **USG**

String sign, apple core appearance, Beak sign on barium is seen in – **Hypertrophic Pyloric Stenosis**.

Carman's meniscus sign seen in Malignant ulcer

Double bubble appearance seen in Duodenal atresia, Annular pancreas

Triple bubble sign seen in – **Jejunal atresia**

If coin accidently ingested in esophagus, it will be oriented in coronal plane whereas coins Trachea is oriented saggittally.

Half-life of 18-FDG: **110 minutes**

Best test for avascular necrosis of bone: **MRI**

MC type of ASD in down's syndrome: **Ostium primum**

Overall, MC type of ASD: **Ostium primum**

Widening of C loop of duodenum on barium study: **CA pancreas head**

Contd...

Double duct sign is seen in: **Periampullary carcinoma**

IOC for acute pancreatitis: **CECT**

In chest X-ray Lordotic view is used for:
- **Lung apex pathology**
- Best view for middle lobe examination
- Interlobar fissural examination

IOC for posterior urethral valve: **VCUG (Voiding Cystourethrogram)**

- **Comet tail app on HRCT:** Round Atelectasis
- Hallmark of ureteric TB: **corkscrew ureter**
- Moth eaten calyces on IVP: **Renal TB**
- Ulcer crater sign and Hampton's line: Benign gastric ulcer
- Double atrial shadow is seen in: **LA enlargement**
- Signs of pneumoperitoneum: saddle bag/Mustache/Cupola/ Falciform lig sign/ Rigler sign/urachus sign
- IVP-Spider leg app/swiss cheese appearance: **PCKD**
- IOC for pulm embolism: **CT angio**
- Chamber enlarged in Ebstein anomaly
- MC ASD: **Septum secundum**
- Bulging fissure sign: **Klebsiella Pn**
- CXR finding of Pulm embolism: **Westermark sign, Palla sign, Hampton hump, Fleischner sign**
- Dye used in Bronchography: **Dianosil**
- Scan done for parathyroid adenoma: **Sestamibi scan**
- Radioactive agent used in treatment for ascites: **Gold**
- First sign of radiation exposure: **Erythema**

TABLE: Congenital cardiac conditions and its radiological findings

Lutembacher Syndrome- Congenital ASD with Acquired MS.

Figure of 3 appearance seen in – **Coarctation of Aorta**

Boot shaped heart or Cor-en-sabot seen in – **Tetralogy of Fallot**

Box shaped heart on CXR – **Ebstein anomaly**

Figure of 8 appearance or Snowman appearance seen in – **TAPVC**

Egg on side appearance seen in **TGA**

Most common type of VSD – **Perimembranous**

Most common type of ASD – **Ostium secundum**

Hilar dance on fluoroscopy – **ASD**

Key Points

FMGE Solutions Screening Examination

TABLE: Some important half-life of radionuclides

Gold-198: 2.7 days	
Iodine-123: 13.3 hours	
Iodine-131: 8 days	
Phosphorus-32: 14.3 days	
Yttrium 90: 64 hours	
Cobalt-60: 5.26 years	
Caesium-137: 30 years	
Radium-226: 1620 years	

REMEMBER THESE IMPORTANT RADIOLOGICAL SIGNS IN UROLOGY

- Spider leg appearance → **Polycystic kidney**
- Cobra head appearance → **Ureterocele**
- Flower vase appearance of ureters → **Horseshoe kidney**
- Sandy patches → **Schistosomiasis of bladder**
- Soap bubble appearance → **Hydronephrosis**
- Golf hole ureter → **TB bladder**
- String of purse appearance: **Ureteric TB**

TABLE: Conditions where 'Hair on End Appearance' is seen: Mnemonic: HI NEST

- Hereditary spherocytosis
- Iron deficiency anemia
- Neuroblastoma
- Enzyme deficiency (e.g. G-6-P deficiency causing hemolytic anemia)
- Sickle cell disease
- Thalassemia major

TABLE: Radiological findings and their respective pathology

Barium enema findings	Associated pathology
Apple core deformity / Irregular filling defect	Colon CA
Lead pipe appearance / Loss of haustrations	Ulcerative colitis
String sign of kantor / Raspberry thorn ulcers	Crohn's disease
Smooth irregular filling defects	Colonic polyps
Dilated proximal zone with narrow distal zone of coning	Hirschsprung disease
Saw tooth appearance / Champagne glass sign	Diverticulosis of colon

Contd...

Barium enema findings	Associated pathology
Thumb print sign	Ischemic colitis
Claw sign / Coiled spring sign	Intussusception
Bird beak sign, Ace of spades	Volvulus
Bird beak appearance	Achalasia cardia
Rat tail appearance	Esophageal CA
Corkscrew appearance / Nut cracker esophagus / Curling esophagus	Diffuse esophageal spasm
String sign	Congenital hypertrophic pyloric stenosis
Inverted 3 sign of Forsberg / Widening of C loop of duodenum / Antral pad sign.	Pancreas head CA
Coffee bean sign	Sigmoid volvulus

MRI Head Appearances

• Eye of the tiger	Hallervorden spatz disease
• Face of giant panda	Wilson's disease
• Racing car app	Corpus callosum agenesis
• Humming bird sign, Mickey mouse app	PSP (Progressive Supranuclear Palsy)
• Hot cross bun sign	MSA (Multiple System Atrophy)
• Molar tooth app	Joubert syndrome
• Figure of 8 app	Lissencephaly

TABLE: Radiation exposure in different investigations

Procedure	Mean effective dose (mSv)
• Chest X-ray (PA View)	0.02
• Chest X-ray (PA + Lateral view)	0.1
• Mammogram	0.4
• Abdomen X-ray	0.7
• HSG	0.9–1.3
• CT Brain	2.2
• IVP	3
• ERCP	4
• Coronary angiography	7 (2–16)
• Barium enema	8 (2–18)
• CT Colonography	6
• CT Abdomen and Pelvis	10
• Thallium scan	16.9

OMR Sheet 1 for Model Test Paper-I

1 – 50	51 – 100	101 – 150	151 – 200	201 – 250	251 – 300
1 (A) (B) (C) (D)	51 (A) (B) (C) (D)	101 (A) (B) (C) (D)	151 (A) (B) (C) (D)	201 (A) (B) (C) (D)	251 (A) (B) (C) (D)
2 (A) (B) (C) (D)	52 (A) (B) (C) (D)	102 (A) (B) (C) (D)	152 (A) (B) (C) (D)	202 (A) (B) (C) (D)	252 (A) (B) (C) (D)
3 (A) (B) (C) (D)	53 (A) (B) (C) (D)	103 (A) (B) (C) (D)	153 (A) (B) (C) (D)	203 (A) (B) (C) (D)	253 (A) (B) (C) (D)
4 (A) (B) (C) (D)	54 (A) (B) (C) (D)	104 (A) (B) (C) (D)	154 (A) (B) (C) (D)	204 (A) (B) (C) (D)	254 (A) (B) (C) (D)
5 (A) (B) (C) (D)	55 (A) (B) (C) (D)	105 (A) (B) (C) (D)	155 (A) (B) (C) (D)	205 (A) (B) (C) (D)	255 (A) (B) (C) (D)
6 (A) (B) (C) (D)	56 (A) (B) (C) (D)	106 (A) (B) (C) (D)	156 (A) (B) (C) (D)	206 (A) (B) (C) (D)	256 (A) (B) (C) (D)
7 (A) (B) (C) (D)	57 (A) (B) (C) (D)	107 (A) (B) (C) (D)	157 (A) (B) (C) (D)	207 (A) (B) (C) (D)	257 (A) (B) (C) (D)
8 (A) (B) (C) (D)	58 (A) (B) (C) (D)	108 (A) (B) (C) (D)	158 (A) (B) (C) (D)	208 (A) (B) (C) (D)	258 (A) (B) (C) (D)
9 (A) (B) (C) (D)	59 (A) (B) (C) (D)	109 (A) (B) (C) (D)	159 (A) (B) (C) (D)	209 (A) (B) (C) (D)	259 (A) (B) (C) (D)
10 (A) (B) (C) (D)	60 (A) (B) (C) (D)	100 (A) (B) (C) (D)	160 (A) (B) (C) (D)	210 (A) (B) (C) (D)	260 (A) (B) (C) (D)
11 (A) (B) (C) (D)	61 (A) (B) (C) (D)	111 (A) (B) (C) (D)	161 (A) (B) (C) (D)	211 (A) (B) (C) (D)	261 (A) (B) (C) (D)
12 (A) (B) (C) (D)	62 (A) (B) (C) (D)	112 (A) (B) (C) (D)	162 (A) (B) (C) (D)	212 (A) (B) (C) (D)	262 (A) (B) (C) (D)
13 (A) (B) (C) (D)	63 (A) (B) (C) (D)	113 (A) (B) (C) (D)	163 (A) (B) (C) (D)	213 (A) (B) (C) (D)	263 (A) (B) (C) (D)
14 (A) (B) (C) (D)	64 (A) (B) (C) (D)	114 (A) (B) (C) (D)	164 (A) (B) (C) (D)	214 (A) (B) (C) (D)	264 (A) (B) (C) (D)
15 (A) (B) (C) (D)	65 (A) (B) (C) (D)	115 (A) (B) (C) (D)	165 (A) (B) (C) (D)	215 (A) (B) (C) (D)	265 (A) (B) (C) (D)
16 (A) (B) (C) (D)	66 (A) (B) (C) (D)	116 (A) (B) (C) (D)	166 (A) (B) (C) (D)	216 (A) (B) (C) (D)	266 (A) (B) (C) (D)
17 (A) (B) (C) (D)	67 (A) (B) (C) (D)	117 (A) (B) (C) (D)	167 (A) (B) (C) (D)	217 (A) (B) (C) (D)	267 (A) (B) (C) (D)
18 (A) (B) (C) (D)	68 (A) (B) (C) (D)	118 (A) (B) (C) (D)	168 (A) (B) (C) (D)	218 (A) (B) (C) (D)	268 (A) (B) (C) (D)
19 (A) (B) (C) (D)	69 (A) (B) (C) (D)	119 (A) (B) (C) (D)	169 (A) (B) (C) (D)	219 (A) (B) (C) (D)	269 (A) (B) (C) (D)
20 (A) (B) (C) (D)	70 (A) (B) (C) (D)	120 (A) (B) (C) (D)	170 (A) (B) (C) (D)	220 (A) (B) (C) (D)	270 (A) (B) (C) (D)
21 (A) (B) (C) (D)	71 (A) (B) (C) (D)	121 (A) (B) (C) (D)	171 (A) (B) (C) (D)	221 (A) (B) (C) (D)	271 (A) (B) (C) (D)
22 (A) (B) (C) (D)	72 (A) (B) (C) (D)	122 (A) (B) (C) (D)	172 (A) (B) (C) (D)	222 (A) (B) (C) (D)	272 (A) (B) (C) (D)
23 (A) (B) (C) (D)	73 (A) (B) (C) (D)	123 (A) (B) (C) (D)	173 (A) (B) (C) (D)	223 (A) (B) (C) (D)	273 (A) (B) (C) (D)
24 (A) (B) (C) (D)	74 (A) (B) (C) (D)	124 (A) (B) (C) (D)	174 (A) (B) (C) (D)	224 (A) (B) (C) (D)	274 (A) (B) (C) (D)
25 (A) (B) (C) (D)	75 (A) (B) (C) (D)	125 (A) (B) (C) (D)	175 (A) (B) (C) (D)	225 (A) (B) (C) (D)	275 (A) (B) (C) (D)
26 (A) (B) (C) (D)	76 (A) (B) (C) (D)	126 (A) (B) (C) (D)	176 (A) (B) (C) (D)	226 (A) (B) (C) (D)	276 (A) (B) (C) (D)
27 (A) (B) (C) (D)	77 (A) (B) (C) (D)	127 (A) (B) (C) (D)	177 (A) (B) (C) (D)	227 (A) (B) (C) (D)	277 (A) (B) (C) (D)
28 (A) (B) (C) (D)	78 (A) (B) (C) (D)	128 (A) (B) (C) (D)	178 (A) (B) (C) (D)	228 (A) (B) (C) (D)	278 (A) (B) (C) (D)
29 (A) (B) (C) (D)	79 (A) (B) (C) (D)	129 (A) (B) (C) (D)	179 (A) (B) (C) (D)	229 (A) (B) (C) (D)	279 (A) (B) (C) (D)
30 (A) (B) (C) (D)	80 (A) (B) (C) (D)	130 (A) (B) (C) (D)	180 (A) (B) (C) (D)	230 (A) (B) (C) (D)	280 (A) (B) (C) (D)
31 (A) (B) (C) (D)	81 (A) (B) (C) (D)	131 (A) (B) (C) (D)	181 (A) (B) (C) (D)	231 (A) (B) (C) (D)	281 (A) (B) (C) (D)
32 (A) (B) (C) (D)	82 (A) (B) (C) (D)	132 (A) (B) (C) (D)	182 (A) (B) (C) (D)	232 (A) (B) (C) (D)	282 (A) (B) (C) (D)
33 (A) (B) (C) (D)	83 (A) (B) (C) (D)	133 (A) (B) (C) (D)	183 (A) (B) (C) (D)	233 (A) (B) (C) (D)	283 (A) (B) (C) (D)
34 (A) (B) (C) (D)	84 (A) (B) (C) (D)	134 (A) (B) (C) (D)	184 (A) (B) (C) (D)	234 (A) (B) (C) (D)	284 (A) (B) (C) (D)
35 (A) (B) (C) (D)	85 (A) (B) (C) (D)	135 (A) (B) (C) (D)	185 (A) (B) (C) (D)	235 (A) (B) (C) (D)	285 (A) (B) (C) (D)
36 (A) (B) (C) (D)	86 (A) (B) (C) (D)	136 (A) (B) (C) (D)	186 (A) (B) (C) (D)	236 (A) (B) (C) (D)	286 (A) (B) (C) (D)
37 (A) (B) (C) (D)	87 (A) (B) (C) (D)	137 (A) (B) (C) (D)	187 (A) (B) (C) (D)	237 (A) (B) (C) (D)	287 (A) (B) (C) (D)
38 (A) (B) (C) (D)	88 (A) (B) (C) (D)	138 (A) (B) (C) (D)	188 (A) (B) (C) (D)	238 (A) (B) (C) (D)	288 (A) (B) (C) (D)
39 (A) (B) (C) (D)	89 (A) (B) (C) (D)	139 (A) (B) (C) (D)	189 (A) (B) (C) (D)	239 (A) (B) (C) (D)	289 (A) (B) (C) (D)
40 (A) (B) (C) (D)	90 (A) (B) (C) (D)	140 (A) (B) (C) (D)	190 (A) (B) (C) (D)	240 (A) (B) (C) (D)	290 (A) (B) (C) (D)
41 (A) (B) (C) (D)	91 (A) (B) (C) (D)	141 (A) (B) (C) (D)	191 (A) (B) (C) (D)	241 (A) (B) (C) (D)	291 (A) (B) (C) (D)
42 (A) (B) (C) (D)	92 (A) (B) (C) (D)	142 (A) (B) (C) (D)	192 (A) (B) (C) (D)	242 (A) (B) (C) (D)	292 (A) (B) (C) (D)
43 (A) (B) (C) (D)	93 (A) (B) (C) (D)	143 (A) (B) (C) (D)	193 (A) (B) (C) (D)	243 (A) (B) (C) (D)	293 (A) (B) (C) (D)
44 (A) (B) (C) (D)	94 (A) (B) (C) (D)	144 (A) (B) (C) (D)	194 (A) (B) (C) (D)	244 (A) (B) (C) (D)	294 (A) (B) (C) (D)
45 (A) (B) (C) (D)	95 (A) (B) (C) (D)	145 (A) (B) (C) (D)	195 (A) (B) (C) (D)	245 (A) (B) (C) (D)	295 (A) (B) (C) (D)
46 (A) (B) (C) (D)	96 (A) (B) (C) (D)	146 (A) (B) (C) (D)	196 (A) (B) (C) (D)	246 (A) (B) (C) (D)	296 (A) (B) (C) (D)
47 (A) (B) (C) (D)	97 (A) (B) (C) (D)	147 (A) (B) (C) (D)	197 (A) (B) (C) (D)	247 (A) (B) (C) (D)	297 (A) (B) (C) (D)
48 (A) (B) (C) (D)	98 (A) (B) (C) (D)	148 (A) (B) (C) (D)	198 (A) (B) (C) (D)	248 (A) (B) (C) (D)	298 (A) (B) (C) (D)
49 (A) (B) (C) (D)	99 (A) (B) (C) (D)	149 (A) (B) (C) (D)	199 (A) (B) (C) (D)	249 (A) (B) (C) (D)	299 (A) (B) (C) (D)
50 (A) (B) (C) (D)	100 (A) (B) (C) (D)	150 (A) (B) (C) (D)	200 (A) (B) (C) (D)	250 (A) (B) (C) (D)	300 (A) (B) (C) (D)

ASSESSMENT OF MOCK TEST ON THE BASIS OF SCORES- BY THE AUTHORS

Score	Interpretation	Authors Comments
270 Plus	OUTSTANDING	• Highly appreciable score. Keep doing MCQs
240 – 269	EXCELLENT PERFORMANCE	• Great score. Pay attention on some silly mistakes
210 – 239	VERY GOOD PERFORMANCE	• Keep doing MCQs and continue with revising the notes • Advised not to flow in overconfidence
180 – 209	GOOD PERFORMANCE	• Learn the time management while doing MCQs • Keep moving on same track and avoid overconfidence • Work on anxiety issues if there are any
150 – 179	SATISFACTORY	• You are going well. Continue on the same track • Lacking confidence on studied topics due to lack of revision • Practice more MCQs
130 – 149	UNSATISFACTORY	• You are studying but lacking concept and lack of revision. • Improve on silly mistakes by working on basic subjects • Definite improvement expected
Below 130	POOR SCORE	• Need to work on basic subjects • Conceptual based study is recommended • Do FMGE Solutions to cover 3–4 times with explanations

INSTRUCTIONS FOR FILLING THE SHEET

1. This sheet should not be folded or crushed.
2. Use only blue/black ball pen to fill the circles.
3. Use of pencil is strictly prohibited.
4. Circles should be darkened properly and completely.
5. Cutting & erasing on this sheet is not allowed.
6. Do not use any stray marks on the sheet.
7. Do not use marker, white fluid or any other device to hide the shading already done.

OMR Sheet 2 for Model Test Paper-I

1 – 50	51 – 100	101 – 150	151 – 200	201 – 250	251 – 300
1 Ⓐ Ⓑ Ⓒ Ⓓ	51 Ⓐ Ⓑ Ⓒ Ⓓ	101 Ⓐ Ⓑ Ⓒ Ⓓ	151 Ⓐ Ⓑ Ⓒ Ⓓ	201 Ⓐ Ⓑ Ⓒ Ⓓ	251 Ⓐ Ⓑ Ⓒ Ⓓ
2 Ⓐ Ⓑ Ⓒ Ⓓ	52 Ⓐ Ⓑ Ⓒ Ⓓ	102 Ⓐ Ⓑ Ⓒ Ⓓ	152 Ⓐ Ⓑ Ⓒ Ⓓ	202 Ⓐ Ⓑ Ⓒ Ⓓ	252 Ⓐ Ⓑ Ⓒ Ⓓ
3 Ⓐ Ⓑ Ⓒ Ⓓ	53 Ⓐ Ⓑ Ⓒ Ⓓ	103 Ⓐ Ⓑ Ⓒ Ⓓ	153 Ⓐ Ⓑ Ⓒ Ⓓ	203 Ⓐ Ⓑ Ⓒ Ⓓ	253 Ⓐ Ⓑ Ⓒ Ⓓ
4 Ⓐ Ⓑ Ⓒ Ⓓ	54 Ⓐ Ⓑ Ⓒ Ⓓ	104 Ⓐ Ⓑ Ⓒ Ⓓ	154 Ⓐ Ⓑ Ⓒ Ⓓ	204 Ⓐ Ⓑ Ⓒ Ⓓ	254 Ⓐ Ⓑ Ⓒ Ⓓ
5 Ⓐ Ⓑ Ⓒ Ⓓ	55 Ⓐ Ⓑ Ⓒ Ⓓ	105 Ⓐ Ⓑ Ⓒ Ⓓ	155 Ⓐ Ⓑ Ⓒ Ⓓ	205 Ⓐ Ⓑ Ⓒ Ⓓ	255 Ⓐ Ⓑ Ⓒ Ⓓ
6 Ⓐ Ⓑ Ⓒ Ⓓ	56 Ⓐ Ⓑ Ⓒ Ⓓ	106 Ⓐ Ⓑ Ⓒ Ⓓ	156 Ⓐ Ⓑ Ⓒ Ⓓ	206 Ⓐ Ⓑ Ⓒ Ⓓ	256 Ⓐ Ⓑ Ⓒ Ⓓ
7 Ⓐ Ⓑ Ⓒ Ⓓ	57 Ⓐ Ⓑ Ⓒ Ⓓ	107 Ⓐ Ⓑ Ⓒ Ⓓ	157 Ⓐ Ⓑ Ⓒ Ⓓ	207 Ⓐ Ⓑ Ⓒ Ⓓ	257 Ⓐ Ⓑ Ⓒ Ⓓ
8 Ⓐ Ⓑ Ⓒ Ⓓ	58 Ⓐ Ⓑ Ⓒ Ⓓ	108 Ⓐ Ⓑ Ⓒ Ⓓ	158 Ⓐ Ⓑ Ⓒ Ⓓ	208 Ⓐ Ⓑ Ⓒ Ⓓ	258 Ⓐ Ⓑ Ⓒ Ⓓ
9 Ⓐ Ⓑ Ⓒ Ⓓ	59 Ⓐ Ⓑ Ⓒ Ⓓ	109 Ⓐ Ⓑ Ⓒ Ⓓ	159 Ⓐ Ⓑ Ⓒ Ⓓ	209 Ⓐ Ⓑ Ⓒ Ⓓ	259 Ⓐ Ⓑ Ⓒ Ⓓ
10 Ⓐ Ⓑ Ⓒ Ⓓ	60 Ⓐ Ⓑ Ⓒ Ⓓ	100 Ⓐ Ⓑ Ⓒ Ⓓ	160 Ⓐ Ⓑ Ⓒ Ⓓ	210 Ⓐ Ⓑ Ⓒ Ⓓ	260 Ⓐ Ⓑ Ⓒ Ⓓ
11 Ⓐ Ⓑ Ⓒ Ⓓ	61 Ⓐ Ⓑ Ⓒ Ⓓ	111 Ⓐ Ⓑ Ⓒ Ⓓ	161 Ⓐ Ⓑ Ⓒ Ⓓ	211 Ⓐ Ⓑ Ⓒ Ⓓ	261 Ⓐ Ⓑ Ⓒ Ⓓ
12 Ⓐ Ⓑ Ⓒ Ⓓ	62 Ⓐ Ⓑ Ⓒ Ⓓ	112 Ⓐ Ⓑ Ⓒ Ⓓ	162 Ⓐ Ⓑ Ⓒ Ⓓ	212 Ⓐ Ⓑ Ⓒ Ⓓ	262 Ⓐ Ⓑ Ⓒ Ⓓ
13 Ⓐ Ⓑ Ⓒ Ⓓ	63 Ⓐ Ⓑ Ⓒ Ⓓ	113 Ⓐ Ⓑ Ⓒ Ⓓ	163 Ⓐ Ⓑ Ⓒ Ⓓ	213 Ⓐ Ⓑ Ⓒ Ⓓ	263 Ⓐ Ⓑ Ⓒ Ⓓ
14 Ⓐ Ⓑ Ⓒ Ⓓ	64 Ⓐ Ⓑ Ⓒ Ⓓ	114 Ⓐ Ⓑ Ⓒ Ⓓ	164 Ⓐ Ⓑ Ⓒ Ⓓ	214 Ⓐ Ⓑ Ⓒ Ⓓ	264 Ⓐ Ⓑ Ⓒ Ⓓ
15 Ⓐ Ⓑ Ⓒ Ⓓ	65 Ⓐ Ⓑ Ⓒ Ⓓ	115 Ⓐ Ⓑ Ⓒ Ⓓ	165 Ⓐ Ⓑ Ⓒ Ⓓ	215 Ⓐ Ⓑ Ⓒ Ⓓ	265 Ⓐ Ⓑ Ⓒ Ⓓ
16 Ⓐ Ⓑ Ⓒ Ⓓ	66 Ⓐ Ⓑ Ⓒ Ⓓ	116 Ⓐ Ⓑ Ⓒ Ⓓ	166 Ⓐ Ⓑ Ⓒ Ⓓ	216 Ⓐ Ⓑ Ⓒ Ⓓ	266 Ⓐ Ⓑ Ⓒ Ⓓ
17 Ⓐ Ⓑ Ⓒ Ⓓ	67 Ⓐ Ⓑ Ⓒ Ⓓ	117 Ⓐ Ⓑ Ⓒ Ⓓ	167 Ⓐ Ⓑ Ⓒ Ⓓ	217 Ⓐ Ⓑ Ⓒ Ⓓ	267 Ⓐ Ⓑ Ⓒ Ⓓ
18 Ⓐ Ⓑ Ⓒ Ⓓ	68 Ⓐ Ⓑ Ⓒ Ⓓ	118 Ⓐ Ⓑ Ⓒ Ⓓ	168 Ⓐ Ⓑ Ⓒ Ⓓ	218 Ⓐ Ⓑ Ⓒ Ⓓ	268 Ⓐ Ⓑ Ⓒ Ⓓ
19 Ⓐ Ⓑ Ⓒ Ⓓ	69 Ⓐ Ⓑ Ⓒ Ⓓ	119 Ⓐ Ⓑ Ⓒ Ⓓ	169 Ⓐ Ⓑ Ⓒ Ⓓ	219 Ⓐ Ⓑ Ⓒ Ⓓ	269 Ⓐ Ⓑ Ⓒ Ⓓ
20 Ⓐ Ⓑ Ⓒ Ⓓ	70 Ⓐ Ⓑ Ⓒ Ⓓ	120 Ⓐ Ⓑ Ⓒ Ⓓ	170 Ⓐ Ⓑ Ⓒ Ⓓ	220 Ⓐ Ⓑ Ⓒ Ⓓ	270 Ⓐ Ⓑ Ⓒ Ⓓ
21 Ⓐ Ⓑ Ⓒ Ⓓ	71 Ⓐ Ⓑ Ⓒ Ⓓ	121 Ⓐ Ⓑ Ⓒ Ⓓ	171 Ⓐ Ⓑ Ⓒ Ⓓ	221 Ⓐ Ⓑ Ⓒ Ⓓ	271 Ⓐ Ⓑ Ⓒ Ⓓ
22 Ⓐ Ⓑ Ⓒ Ⓓ	72 Ⓐ Ⓑ Ⓒ Ⓓ	122 Ⓐ Ⓑ Ⓒ Ⓓ	172 Ⓐ Ⓑ Ⓒ Ⓓ	222 Ⓐ Ⓑ Ⓒ Ⓓ	272 Ⓐ Ⓑ Ⓒ Ⓓ
23 Ⓐ Ⓑ Ⓒ Ⓓ	73 Ⓐ Ⓑ Ⓒ Ⓓ	123 Ⓐ Ⓑ Ⓒ Ⓓ	173 Ⓐ Ⓑ Ⓒ Ⓓ	223 Ⓐ Ⓑ Ⓒ Ⓓ	273 Ⓐ Ⓑ Ⓒ Ⓓ
24 Ⓐ Ⓑ Ⓒ Ⓓ	74 Ⓐ Ⓑ Ⓒ Ⓓ	124 Ⓐ Ⓑ Ⓒ Ⓓ	174 Ⓐ Ⓑ Ⓒ Ⓓ	224 Ⓐ Ⓑ Ⓒ Ⓓ	274 Ⓐ Ⓑ Ⓒ Ⓓ
25 Ⓐ Ⓑ Ⓒ Ⓓ	75 Ⓐ Ⓑ Ⓒ Ⓓ	125 Ⓐ Ⓑ Ⓒ Ⓓ	175 Ⓐ Ⓑ Ⓒ Ⓓ	225 Ⓐ Ⓑ Ⓒ Ⓓ	275 Ⓐ Ⓑ Ⓒ Ⓓ
26 Ⓐ Ⓑ Ⓒ Ⓓ	76 Ⓐ Ⓑ Ⓒ Ⓓ	126 Ⓐ Ⓑ Ⓒ Ⓓ	176 Ⓐ Ⓑ Ⓒ Ⓓ	226 Ⓐ Ⓑ Ⓒ Ⓓ	276 Ⓐ Ⓑ Ⓒ Ⓓ
27 Ⓐ Ⓑ Ⓒ Ⓓ	77 Ⓐ Ⓑ Ⓒ Ⓓ	127 Ⓐ Ⓑ Ⓒ Ⓓ	177 Ⓐ Ⓑ Ⓒ Ⓓ	227 Ⓐ Ⓑ Ⓒ Ⓓ	277 Ⓐ Ⓑ Ⓒ Ⓓ
28 Ⓐ Ⓑ Ⓒ Ⓓ	78 Ⓐ Ⓑ Ⓒ Ⓓ	128 Ⓐ Ⓑ Ⓒ Ⓓ	178 Ⓐ Ⓑ Ⓒ Ⓓ	228 Ⓐ Ⓑ Ⓒ Ⓓ	278 Ⓐ Ⓑ Ⓒ Ⓓ
29 Ⓐ Ⓑ Ⓒ Ⓓ	79 Ⓐ Ⓑ Ⓒ Ⓓ	129 Ⓐ Ⓑ Ⓒ Ⓓ	179 Ⓐ Ⓑ Ⓒ Ⓓ	229 Ⓐ Ⓑ Ⓒ Ⓓ	279 Ⓐ Ⓑ Ⓒ Ⓓ
30 Ⓐ Ⓑ Ⓒ Ⓓ	80 Ⓐ Ⓑ Ⓒ Ⓓ	130 Ⓐ Ⓑ Ⓒ Ⓓ	180 Ⓐ Ⓑ Ⓒ Ⓓ	230 Ⓐ Ⓑ Ⓒ Ⓓ	280 Ⓐ Ⓑ Ⓒ Ⓓ
31 Ⓐ Ⓑ Ⓒ Ⓓ	81 Ⓐ Ⓑ Ⓒ Ⓓ	131 Ⓐ Ⓑ Ⓒ Ⓓ	181 Ⓐ Ⓑ Ⓒ Ⓓ	231 Ⓐ Ⓑ Ⓒ Ⓓ	281 Ⓐ Ⓑ Ⓒ Ⓓ
32 Ⓐ Ⓑ Ⓒ Ⓓ	82 Ⓐ Ⓑ Ⓒ Ⓓ	132 Ⓐ Ⓑ Ⓒ Ⓓ	182 Ⓐ Ⓑ Ⓒ Ⓓ	232 Ⓐ Ⓑ Ⓒ Ⓓ	282 Ⓐ Ⓑ Ⓒ Ⓓ
33 Ⓐ Ⓑ Ⓒ Ⓓ	83 Ⓐ Ⓑ Ⓒ Ⓓ	133 Ⓐ Ⓑ Ⓒ Ⓓ	183 Ⓐ Ⓑ Ⓒ Ⓓ	233 Ⓐ Ⓑ Ⓒ Ⓓ	283 Ⓐ Ⓑ Ⓒ Ⓓ
34 Ⓐ Ⓑ Ⓒ Ⓓ	84 Ⓐ Ⓑ Ⓒ Ⓓ	134 Ⓐ Ⓑ Ⓒ Ⓓ	184 Ⓐ Ⓑ Ⓒ Ⓓ	234 Ⓐ Ⓑ Ⓒ Ⓓ	284 Ⓐ Ⓑ Ⓒ Ⓓ
35 Ⓐ Ⓑ Ⓒ Ⓓ	85 Ⓐ Ⓑ Ⓒ Ⓓ	135 Ⓐ Ⓑ Ⓒ Ⓓ	185 Ⓐ Ⓑ Ⓒ Ⓓ	235 Ⓐ Ⓑ Ⓒ Ⓓ	285 Ⓐ Ⓑ Ⓒ Ⓓ
36 Ⓐ Ⓑ Ⓒ Ⓓ	86 Ⓐ Ⓑ Ⓒ Ⓓ	136 Ⓐ Ⓑ Ⓒ Ⓓ	186 Ⓐ Ⓑ Ⓒ Ⓓ	236 Ⓐ Ⓑ Ⓒ Ⓓ	286 Ⓐ Ⓑ Ⓒ Ⓓ
37 Ⓐ Ⓑ Ⓒ Ⓓ	87 Ⓐ Ⓑ Ⓒ Ⓓ	137 Ⓐ Ⓑ Ⓒ Ⓓ	187 Ⓐ Ⓑ Ⓒ Ⓓ	237 Ⓐ Ⓑ Ⓒ Ⓓ	287 Ⓐ Ⓑ Ⓒ Ⓓ
38 Ⓐ Ⓑ Ⓒ Ⓓ	88 Ⓐ Ⓑ Ⓒ Ⓓ	138 Ⓐ Ⓑ Ⓒ Ⓓ	188 Ⓐ Ⓑ Ⓒ Ⓓ	238 Ⓐ Ⓑ Ⓒ Ⓓ	288 Ⓐ Ⓑ Ⓒ Ⓓ
39 Ⓐ Ⓑ Ⓒ Ⓓ	89 Ⓐ Ⓑ Ⓒ Ⓓ	139 Ⓐ Ⓑ Ⓒ Ⓓ	189 Ⓐ Ⓑ Ⓒ Ⓓ	239 Ⓐ Ⓑ Ⓒ Ⓓ	289 Ⓐ Ⓑ Ⓒ Ⓓ
40 Ⓐ Ⓑ Ⓒ Ⓓ	90 Ⓐ Ⓑ Ⓒ Ⓓ	140 Ⓐ Ⓑ Ⓒ Ⓓ	190 Ⓐ Ⓑ Ⓒ Ⓓ	240 Ⓐ Ⓑ Ⓒ Ⓓ	290 Ⓐ Ⓑ Ⓒ Ⓓ
41 Ⓐ Ⓑ Ⓒ Ⓓ	91 Ⓐ Ⓑ Ⓒ Ⓓ	141 Ⓐ Ⓑ Ⓒ Ⓓ	191 Ⓐ Ⓑ Ⓒ Ⓓ	241 Ⓐ Ⓑ Ⓒ Ⓓ	291 Ⓐ Ⓑ Ⓒ Ⓓ
42 Ⓐ Ⓑ Ⓒ Ⓓ	92 Ⓐ Ⓑ Ⓒ Ⓓ	142 Ⓐ Ⓑ Ⓒ Ⓓ	192 Ⓐ Ⓑ Ⓒ Ⓓ	242 Ⓐ Ⓑ Ⓒ Ⓓ	292 Ⓐ Ⓑ Ⓒ Ⓓ
43 Ⓐ Ⓑ Ⓒ Ⓓ	93 Ⓐ Ⓑ Ⓒ Ⓓ	143 Ⓐ Ⓑ Ⓒ Ⓓ	193 Ⓐ Ⓑ Ⓒ Ⓓ	243 Ⓐ Ⓑ Ⓒ Ⓓ	293 Ⓐ Ⓑ Ⓒ Ⓓ
44 Ⓐ Ⓑ Ⓒ Ⓓ	94 Ⓐ Ⓑ Ⓒ Ⓓ	144 Ⓐ Ⓑ Ⓒ Ⓓ	194 Ⓐ Ⓑ Ⓒ Ⓓ	244 Ⓐ Ⓑ Ⓒ Ⓓ	294 Ⓐ Ⓑ Ⓒ Ⓓ
45 Ⓐ Ⓑ Ⓒ Ⓓ	95 Ⓐ Ⓑ Ⓒ Ⓓ	145 Ⓐ Ⓑ Ⓒ Ⓓ	195 Ⓐ Ⓑ Ⓒ Ⓓ	245 Ⓐ Ⓑ Ⓒ Ⓓ	295 Ⓐ Ⓑ Ⓒ Ⓓ
46 Ⓐ Ⓑ Ⓒ Ⓓ	96 Ⓐ Ⓑ Ⓒ Ⓓ	146 Ⓐ Ⓑ Ⓒ Ⓓ	196 Ⓐ Ⓑ Ⓒ Ⓓ	246 Ⓐ Ⓑ Ⓒ Ⓓ	296 Ⓐ Ⓑ Ⓒ Ⓓ
47 Ⓐ Ⓑ Ⓒ Ⓓ	97 Ⓐ Ⓑ Ⓒ Ⓓ	147 Ⓐ Ⓑ Ⓒ Ⓓ	197 Ⓐ Ⓑ Ⓒ Ⓓ	247 Ⓐ Ⓑ Ⓒ Ⓓ	297 Ⓐ Ⓑ Ⓒ Ⓓ
48 Ⓐ Ⓑ Ⓒ Ⓓ	98 Ⓐ Ⓑ Ⓒ Ⓓ	148 Ⓐ Ⓑ Ⓒ Ⓓ	198 Ⓐ Ⓑ Ⓒ Ⓓ	248 Ⓐ Ⓑ Ⓒ Ⓓ	298 Ⓐ Ⓑ Ⓒ Ⓓ
49 Ⓐ Ⓑ Ⓒ Ⓓ	99 Ⓐ Ⓑ Ⓒ Ⓓ	149 Ⓐ Ⓑ Ⓒ Ⓓ	199 Ⓐ Ⓑ Ⓒ Ⓓ	249 Ⓐ Ⓑ Ⓒ Ⓓ	299 Ⓐ Ⓑ Ⓒ Ⓓ
50 Ⓐ Ⓑ Ⓒ Ⓓ	100 Ⓐ Ⓑ Ⓒ Ⓓ	150 Ⓐ Ⓑ Ⓒ Ⓓ	200 Ⓐ Ⓑ Ⓒ Ⓓ	250 Ⓐ Ⓑ Ⓒ Ⓓ	300 Ⓐ Ⓑ Ⓒ Ⓓ

ASSESSMENT OF MOCK TEST ON THE BASIS OF SCORES- BY THE AUTHORS

Score	Interpretation	Authors Comments
270 Plus	OUTSTANDING	• Highly appreciable score. Keep doing MCQs
240 – 269	EXCELLENT PERFORMANCE	• Great score. Pay attention on some silly mistakes
210 – 239	VERY GOOD PERFORMANCE	• Keep doing MCQs and continue with revising the notes • Advised not to flow in overconfidence
180 – 209	GOOD PERFORMANCE	• Learn the time management while doing MCQs • Keep moving on same track and avoid overconfidence • Work on anxiety issues if there are any
150 – 179	SATISFACTORY	• You are going well. Continue on the same track • Lacking confidence on studied topics due to lack of revision • Practice more MCQs
130 – 149	UNSATISFACTORY	• You are studying but lacking concept and lack of revision. • Improve on silly mistakes by working on basic subjects • Definite improvement expected
Below 130	POOR SCORE	• Need to work on basic subjects • Conceptual based study is recommended • Do FMGE Solutions to cover 3–4 times with explanations

INSTRUCTIONS FOR FILLING THE SHEET

1. This sheet should not be folded or crushed.
2. Use only blue/black ball pen to fill the circles.
3. Use of pencil is strictly prohibited.
4. Circles should be darkened properly and completely.
5. Cutting & erasing on this sheet is not allowed.
6. Do not use any stray marks on the sheet.
7. Do not use marker, white fluid or any other device to hide the shading already done.

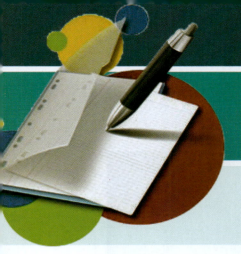

Model Test Paper-I

1. **Medusa head appearance of the colonies is seen in**
   a. Bacillus anthracis
   b. Proteus mirabilis
   c. Clostridium tetani
   d. Pseudomonas aeruginosa

2. **Which of the following is not a component of the crush syndrome?**
   a. Myo-hemoglobinuria
   b. Massive crushing of muscles
   c. Acute tubular necrosis
   d. Bleeding diathesis

3. **Transfer of drug resistance in Staphylococcus is by:**
   a. Transduction
   b. Transformation
   c. Conjugation
   d. Transfection

4. **Which growth factor is involved in fibrosis at lung, liver and kidney after chronic inflammation:**
   a. IL 1
   b. FGF 2
   c. TGF beta
   d. TN

5. **All of the following are enriched media except-**
   a. Blood agar
   b. Chocolate agar
   c. LSS
   d. Tetrathionate broth

6. **All of the following statements about surgical management of gastric lymphomas are true except:**
   a. Stage I gastric lymphomas (small lesions confined to the stomach wall) can be cured completely with surgical therapy alone
   b. Extensive gastric lymphomas that initially are treated with radiation and/or chemotherapy occasionally perforate during treatment and require secondary resection
   c. Patients explored with a presumptive diagnosis of gastric lymphoma should undergo an attempt at curative resection when this is safe and feasible
   d. Without a preoperative diagnosis resection for gastric mass should not be attempted unless lymphoma can be excluded

7. **All of the following statements are true regarding human T cell leukemia virus 1 except:**
   a. It causes adult T cell lymphoma/leukaemia
   b. It has tropism for CD8 + T cell
   c. It has long latent period of about 40 to 60 years
   d. Leukaemia develop in only 3 to 5% of infected individual

8. **At relatively low concentrations, phospholipids form:**
   a. Chylomicrons
   b. Micelles
   c. Monolayer
   d. Bilayer

9. **Choose the correct statement about dronedarone:**
   a. It is more effective than amiodarone
   b. It increases risk of death in patients with permanent atrial fibrillation
   c. QT prolongation is not a risk factor
   d. No need to monitor LFT

10. **Which is the most non-invasive modality to find the chemical environment of the brain?**
    a. PET-CT
    b. MR spectroscopy
    c. CT Angiography
    d. MR PERFUSION

11. **Intraepithelial microabscess seen in psoriasis is called as:**
    a. Pautrier abscess
    b. Munro abscess
    c. Phoenix abscess
    d. None of the above

12. **Lipogranulomatous inflammation is seen in?**
    a. Fungal infection
    b. Tuberculosis
    c. Chalazion
    d. Viral infection

13. **Type 2 Diabetes need screening within what time interval from diagnosis**
    a. Immediately
    b. Within 6 months
    c. Within 5 years
    d. Within one week

14. **All are true about osteoclasts, except:**
    a. Derived from monocyte
    b. Stimulated by PTH
    c. Phagocytosis of foreign bodies
    d. Resorption of bone

15. **Which of the following intrinsic muscles of the thumb attached to 1st metacarpal bone?**
    a. Abductor pollicis brevis
    b. Flexor pollicis brevis
    c. Opponens pollicis
    d. Adductor pollicis

16. **Free edge of Falciform ligament encloses:**
    a. Ligamentum venosum
    b. Portal vein and common bile duct
    c. Ligamentum teres
    d. Right and left gastroepiploic vessel

17. **During moderately intense isotonic exercise all of the following increase except:**
    a. Mean arterial pressure
    b. Heart rate
    c. Respiratory rate
    d. Total Peripheral resistance

FMGE Solutions Screening Examination

18. Lensometer is used to
    a. Measure refractive index of lens
    b. Measure lens thickness
    c. Measure power of spectacles
    d. Measure corneal thickness
19. Rupture of supraspinatus manifest as
    a. Painful movements
    b. Difficulty in initiation of abduction
    c. Difficult abduction after 90°
    d. Flat shoulder
20. Which of the following is the pathognomic sign of active anterior uveitis
    a. Cells in anterior chamber
    b. Hyphema
    c. Keratic precipitates
    d. Snow ball opacities
21. Correct about right and left main bronchi is
    a. Right bronchus is more vertical and broader than the left
    b. Right bronchus is more vertical and has a narrow calibre than the left
    c. Left bronchus is more vertical and broad than right
    d. Left bronchus is more vertical and narrower than right
22. All are sites of insulin administration except?
    a. Dorsum of hands   b. Arms
    c. Lateral aspect of thigh   d. Around umbilicus
23. All are true about diabetic ketoacidosis except?
    a. Raging thirst
    b. It is an early presentation in type 1 DM
    c. Sodium Nitroprusside test is done to detect ketones
    d. Serum bicarbonate > 15 mmol/L
24. All of the following will be seen in the patient shown below except?

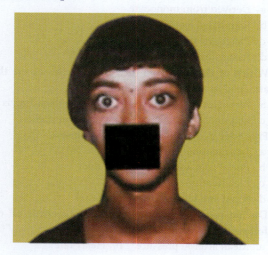

    a. Myxedema   b. Dalrymple sign
    c. Moist warm hands   d. Constipation

25. What is shown in the X-ray skull?

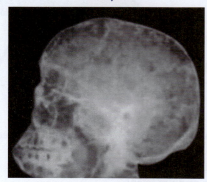

    a. Pepper pot skull
    b. Artifacts
    c. Silver –beaten appearance
    d. Mug shot with pellets
26. The calorie-nitrogen ratio for an infant should be maintained at:
    a. 75:1   b. 100:1
    c. 50:1   d. 150:1
27. Which is not true of cardiopulmonary resuscitation (CPR)?
    a. Closed chest massage is as effective as open chest massage
    b. The success rate for out-of-hospital resuscitation may be as high as 30% to 60%.
    c. The most common cause of sudden death is ischemic heart disease.
    d. Standard chest massage generally provides less than 15% of normal coronary and cerebral blood flow.
28. Smooth muscle is not pain sensitive to:
    a. Cutting   b. Distension
    c. Stretching   d. Torsion
29. All are criteria for identifying 'At Risk' infants except:
    a. Birth weight less than 2.8 kg
    b. Birth order 5 or more
    c. PEM, diarrhoea
    d. Working mother
30. Leiden factor is -
    a. Factor VI   b. Factor VIII
    c. Factor IV   d. Factor V
31. Which of the following statements regarding thyroid physiology are true?
    a. Normally about 20% of T3 is secreted directly from the thyroid gland
    b. The thyroid gland is the only endogenous source of T4
    c. Excess thyroid hormone results in an increase in the number of ATP-dependent sodium pumps on the cell membrane
    d. All of the above

32. Which of the following statement are true regarding asthma?
    a. Occlusion of bronchi and bronchioles by mucus
    b. Curschmann spirals
    c. Charcot laden crystal
    d. All of the above
33. Pulmonary hypertension is defined as a mean pulmonary artery pressure at rest:
    a. 15 mm Hg   b. 25 mm Hg
    c. 35 mm Hg   d. 50 mm Hg
34. Surfactant production in lungs starts at:
    a. 18 weeks   b. 24 weeks
    c. 28 weeks   d. 32 weeks
35. Brunner's glands secrete
    a. Enterogastrones B. C. D.
    b. Bicarbonate-rich secretion
    c. Enzyme-rich secretion
    d. K+-rich secretion
36. A 72-year old man with normal renal functions presents with new onset focal seizures. Which of the following is the best drug to manage the patient?
    a. Sodium valproate   b. Oxcarbazepine
    c. Levetiracetam   d. Pregabalin
37. How much ml of CSF can be safely removed in a routine lumbar puncture?
    a. 10-20 ml   b. 20-30 ml
    c. 30-40 ml   d. 40-50 ml
38. For monitoring warfarin therapy we use:
    a. PT   b. CT
    c. aPTT   d. PT-INR
39. A 64-year-old man complains of pain in the lower chest. A CT scan confirms the presence of a tumor of the lung at T10 level to the left of the midline and invading the surrounding left lung base. Because of the structure most likely involved and penetrating the diaphragm at this level, what could be associated?
    a. Hoarseness
    b. Latissimus dorsi palsy
    c. Budd-Chiari syndrome (hepatic venous outlet obstruction)
    d. Dysphagia
40. Most favoured site for ectopic pregnancy is:
    a. Ovary   b. Abdominal cavity
    c. Fallopian tube   d. Cornual ligament
41. The gold standard for identifying liver lesions by imaging is
    a. Intraoperative ultrasound
    b. Computed tomography (CT) with triple-phase contrast
    c. Magnetic resonance imaging (MRI) with gadoxetate-based contrast
    d. Positron emission tomography (PET) scan
42. All of the following test mentioned below are related to synthetic function of hepatocyte except:
    a. Serum albumin
    b. Prothrombin time
    c. Serum ammonia
    d. Serum γ-glutamyl transpeptidase (GGT)
43. Which of the following is not required in case the second puff is to be taken from an inhaler?
    a. Wash your mouth between 2 puffs
    b. Shake again
    c. Wait for one minute before taking second puff
    d. Keep the mouthpiece dry
44. All of the following diseases are associated with peripheral blood eosinophilia except?
    a. Allergic Bronchopulmonary Aspergillosis (ABPA)
    b. Loeffler syndrome
    c. Pulmonary Eosinophilic Granuloma
    d. Churg Strauss syndrome
45. Increased Reid index is classically associated with?
    a. Chronic Bronchitis   b. Emphysema
    c. Bronchiectasis   d. Interstitial lung disease
46. ESR is a very critical investigation in the diagnosis of TB. Which of the following is true about ESR in TB?
    a. No change in ESR
    b. Confirms recovery from TB
    c. ESR is raised because of increased RBC aggregate
    d. ESR is raised due to decreased RBC size
47. Which of the following is most important molecule for antioxidant pathway in lens?
    a. Glutathione   b. Superoxide dismutase
    c. Catalase   d. Vitamin C
48. What is the complication of the diuretic phase of acute renal failure?
    a. Convulsion
    b. Hyperkalemia
    c. Increased sodium excretion in urine
    d. Metabolic acidosis
49. Within the age group 10 to 35 years, the incidence of carcinoma of the testis in males with intra-abdominal testes is:
    a. Equal to that in the general population.
    b. Five times greater than that in the general population.
    c. Ten times greater than that in the general population.
    d. Twenty times greater than that in the general population.
50. All of the following developmental events are dependent on the production of maternal or fetal glucocorticoids EXCEPT
    a. Induction of thymic involution
    b. Production of surfactant by type II alveolar cells
    c. Functional thyroid
    d. Functional hypothalamo-pituitary axis

FMGE Solutions Screening Examination

51. Osteoclast has specific receptor for:
    a. Parathyroid hormone
    b. Calcitonin
    c. Thyroxin
    d. Vit D3
52. The following type of glomerulonephritis should not be treated with prednisolone?
    a. Minimal change disease
    b. Lipoid nephrosis
    c. Congenital Nephrotic Syndrome
    d. Post-streptococcal GN
53. Regarding HSV 2 infection, which of the following is correct:
    a. Primary infection is symptomatic in developed countries
    b. Recurrent attacks are rare
    c. Encephalitis is commonly caused by it
    d. Newborn acquires the infection via the birth canal
54. Ideal time to start iron therapy in a child with fever, malnutrition and haemoglobin of 7 gm% is?
    a. Immediately
    b. At least 1 month later
    c. When fever goes down
    d. At any time
55. Earliest sign in visual field suggestive of glaucoma:
    a. Isopter contraction
    b. Baring of blind spot
    c. Seidels scotoma
    d. Arcuate scotoma
56. Known gene loci is can be diagnosed by:
    a. FISH
    b. Comparative gene hybridization
    c. PCR
    d. Chromosomal painting
57. Most common site for medulloblastoma is
    a. Medulla
    b. Cerebellum
    c. Cerebral cortex
    d. Pineal gland
58. Which of the following is not functional components of basal ganglia
    a. Substantia nigra
    b. Subthalamus
    c. Red nucleus
    d. Caudate nucleus
59. Cranial nerve most commonly involved in Posterior communicating artery aneurysm is
    a. Oculomotor
    b. Optic
    c. Facial
    d. Trigeminal
60. A 2-year-old boy who attends day care has a fever for 3 days. The fever finally subsides, but then a maculopapular pink rash develops over his trunk and spreads to his arms and face. His mother has not noticed the child scratching at the rash, but says that he does seem more irritable. What is the likely causative agent?
    a. Candida albicans
    b. Chlamydia trachomatis
    c. Escherichia coli
    d. HHV-6
61. Chronic infection by HBV:
    a. Occurs in over 90% of acute infections.
    b. Results in continuous production of infectious virus
    c. Occurs with reduced frequency when HBV is acquired as a perinatal infection
    d. Never resolves spontaneously
62. A 40-year-old woman was involved in a car crash. She was unconscious for 5 minutes. X-ray revealed a depressed fracture in the frontal region. Which of the following statements is true of skull fracture?
    a. It always requires surgical exploration.
    b. It is compound if multiple.
    c. It requires burr holes if compound.
    d. In the anterior cranial fossa, it may produce rhinorrhea.
63. False about Red Cross sign?
    a. Can be used by army medical services
    b. Can be used by members of International red cross Organizations
    c. Can be used by any Medical doctor
    d. Punishable to use without permission
64. All of these drugs are used in treatment of acute gout except:
    a. Allopurinol
    b. Steroids
    c. Colchicine
    d. Naproxen
65. An 85 years old woman presented with bilateral osteoarthritis of the knees. She had no history of previous gastrointestinal disease. Which of the following is the most appropriate initial treatment for her?
    a. Paracetamol
    b. Naproxen
    c. Celecoxib
    d. Dihydrocodeine
66. The most common primary immunodeficiency is:
    a. Common variable immunodeficiency
    b. Isolated IgA immunodeficiency
    c. Wiskott-Aldrich syndrome
    d. AIDS
67. Onion skin spleen is seen in:
    a. ITP
    b. Thalassemia
    c. SLE
    d. Scleroderma
68. Identify

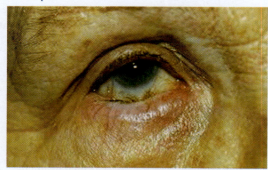

    a. Ectropion
    b. Entropion
    c. Tylosis
    d. Corneal ulcer
69. Iodine salt supplementation is:
    a. Primordial prevention
    b. Tertiary prevention
    c. Primary prevention
    d. Secondary prevention

70. The National Environmental Engineering Research Institute, Nagpur formulated a new type of chlorine tablet which is ____ times better than ordinary halogen tablets:
    a. 2   b. 5
    c. 10   d. 15

71. Economic productive age group for calculating societal dependency ratio is
    a. 15-44 years   b. 15-64 years
    c. > 65 years   d. < 15 years

72. Adenoidectomy is contraindicated in:
    a. Obstructive Sleep Apnoea
    b. Cleft lip
    c. High Arched Palate
    d. Cleft Palate

73. 18 years old man presented with dysphagia, fever and trismus. On examination one side tonsil is enlarged, congested pushing soft palate to other side. All of the following statements about this condition are true except
    a. Abscess is located between Superior Constrictor and Tonsillar Capsule
    b. Trismus seen is due to spasm of Lateral Pterygoid muscles
    c. Single episode of Quinsy is an absolute Indication for Tonsillectomy in children
    d. Interval Tonsillectomy is done after 6 weeks

74. Bone within bone appearance is seen in:
    a. CML
    b. Osteoporosis
    c. Osteopetrosis
    d. Bone infarct

75. "Swiss cheese" nephrogram is a feature of:
    a. Acute ureteral obstruction
    b. Severe hydronephrosis
    c. Polycystic Kidney Disease
    d. Medullary cystic disease of kidney

76. Transfusing blood after prolonged storage could lead to:
    a. Citrate intoxication   b. Potassium toxicity
    c. Circulatory overload   d. Haemorrhagic diathesis

77. The most appropriate drug used for chelation therapy in beta thalassemia major is:
    a. Oral desferrioxamine   b. Oral deferiprone
    c. Intramuscular EDTA   d. Oral Succimer

78. What is the most effective treatment for chronic myeloid leukaemia?
    a. Allogeneic bone marrow transplantation
    b. Heterogeneous bone marrow transplantation
    c. Chemotherapy
    d. Hydroxyurea & interferon

79. Platelets transfusion must be completed in:
    a. 1 hour   b. 2 hours
    c. 3 hours   d. 4 hours

80. The coagulation profile in a 13 year old girl with menorrhagia having von Willebrand's disease is:
    a. Isolated prolonged PTT with a normal PT
    b. Isolated prolonged PT with a normal PTT
    c. Prolongation of both PT and PTT
    d. Prolongation of thrombin time

81. Which of the following is best to prevent rejection after bone marrow transplantation in aplastic anemia?
    a. Anti-thymocyte globulin + cyclosporine
    b. Prednisolone
    c. Cyclosporine
    d. Tacrolimus plus prednisolone

82. Treatment of choice of acute dacryocystitis:-
    a. Massage over lacrimal sac
    b. Syringing and probing
    c. Systemic antibiotics and analgesics
    d. Dacryocystorhinostomy

83. Of the following options, which is not a risk factor for subdural haematoma?
    a. Pregnancy   b. Alcoholism
    c. Dementia   d. Old age

84. Not true regarding inferior walls of orbit
    a. Formed by Maxilla & zygomatic bones
    b. Infraorbital foramen is about 1 cm from orbital rim.
    c. It transmits trigeminal nerves and vessels
    d. Triangular in shape

85. Generally accepted indications for mechanical ventilatory support include
    a. PaO2 of less than 70 kPa and PaCO2 of greater than 50 kPa while breathing room air
    b. Alveolar arterial oxygen tension difference of 150 kPa while breathing 100% O2
    c. Vital capacity of 40–60 mL/kg
    d. Respiratory rate greater than 35 breaths/min

86. The primary mechanism of action of cyclosporine A is inhibition of
    a. Macrophage function
    b. Antibody production
    c. Interleukin 1 production
    d. Interleukin 2 production

87. Grade I lymphedema means?
    a. Pitting edema up to the ankle
    b. Pitting edema up to the knee
    c. Non-pitting edema
    d. Edema disappearing after overnight rest

88. Constipation in children is most commonly due to?
    a. Psychological problems   b. Bad bowel habits
    c. Chagas disease   d. Hirschsprung disease

89. Which of the following is a feature of propaganda?
    a. Knowledge & skills actively acquired
    b. Information centered   c. Appeals to reason
    d. Discipline primitive desires

90. Which of the following indicator denotes the proportion of diseased persons killed by a particular disease?
    a. Case Fatality rate
    b. Proportional mortality rate
    c. Cause-specific death rate
    d. Crude death rate

91. Action of Inferior oblique on adduction is
    a. Elevator   b. Depressor
    c. Extorter   d. Intorter

92. Which of the following is not a feature of chronic progressive external ophthalmoplegia
    a. Starts with bilateral ptosis
    b. May be associated with heart block.
    c. Finally ocular motility palsy
    d. Significant diplopia

93. Amount of squint is different in different directions. This type of squint is called
    a. Comitant squint   b. Incomitant squint
    c. Intermittent squint d. Alternate squint

94. The specimen that is least likely to provide recovery of Trichomonas vaginalis is?
    a. Urine   b. Urethral discharge
    c. Prostatic discharge d. Feces

95. Which of the following is characteristic of the events occurring at an excitatory synapse?
    a. There is a massive efflux of calcium from the presynaptic terminal
    b. Synaptic vesicles bind to the postsynaptic membrane
    c. Voltage-gated potassium channels are closed
    d. Ligand-gated channels are opened to allow sodium entry into the postsynaptic neuron

96. Exposure to ultraviolet light directly facilitates which of the following?
    a. Conversion of cholesterol to 25-hydroxycholecalciferol
    b. Conversion of 25-hydroxycholecalciferol to 1,25-dihydroxycholecalciferol
    c. Transport of calcium into the extracellular fluid
    d. Formation of calcium-binding protein

97. What accompanies sloughing of the endometrium during the endometrial cycle in a normal woman?
    a. An increase in progesterone
    b. The LH "surge"
    c. A decrease in both progesterone and estrogen
    d. An increase in estradiol

98. A female athlete who took testosterone-like steroids for several months stopped having normal menstrual cycles. What is the best explanation for this observation?
    a. Testosterone stimulates inhibin production from the corpus luteum
    b. Testosterone binds to receptors in the endometrium, resulting in the failure of the endometrium to develop during the normal cycle
    c. Testosterone binds to receptors in the anterior pituitary that stimulate the secretion of FSH and LH
    d. Testosterone inhibits the hypothalamic secretion of GnRH and the pituitary secretion of LH and FSH

99. Lesion at which level can cause complete blindness on the side of lesion and loss of reflex in the contralateral side:
    a. Optic nerve
    b. Chiasma
    c. Lateral geniculate body
    d. Occipital lobe

100. True statement regarding postmortem hypostasis is/are -
    a. Also known as rigor mortis
    b. Starts after 8 hours of death
    c. Present all over the body
    d. Starts as blotchy discoloration

101. Which of the following is known as MCH sub-centre
    a. Type A   b. Type B
    c. Type C   d. Type D

102. All of the following are difficult to visualize or examine on Indirect Laryngoscopy except:
    a. Ventricle
    b. Anterior commissure
    c. Pharyngeal Surface of Epiglottis
    d. Subglottis

103. 1 PHC in Hilly areas is established for _____ population?
    a. 3000   b. 30000
    c. 5000   d. 20000

104. IQ is calculated by
    a. Mental age/Chronological age × 100
    b. Mental age-chronological age × 100
    c. Chronological age/ Mental age × 100
    d. Chronological age-Mental age × 100

105. Zenker's diverticulum presents with:
    a. Dysphonia   b. Reflux esophagitis
    c. Dysphagia   d. It is found in stomach

106. Which is true regarding Barrett's esophagus?
    a. Squamous metaplasia of lower esophagus
    b. Seen mainly in females
    c. Premalignant
    d. Respond to conservative management

107. A neonate has been diagnosed with necrotizing enterocolitis with X ray abdomen showing gas in the portal vein. The correct staging of the patients is?
    a. Stage 1   b. Stage 2A
    c. Stage 2B   d. Stage 3

108. The subunits of the heterotrimeric G proteins are called the __, __, and __ subunits.
    a. a, b and c
    b. α, β and θ
    c. α, γ and δ
    d. α, β and γ

109. A 5 year old with history of barefoot walking and open air defecation presents with anemia and swelling around eyes. Which of the following infestation is most likely to be present.
    a. Roundworm
    b. Hookworm
    c. Pinworm
    d. Whipworm
110. Which of the following excludes a diagnosis of irritable bowel syndrome:
    a. Relieved by defecation
    b. Straining during stool passage
    c. Passage of blood per rectum
    d. Changes of stool form
111. In a high risk patient, in active phase of 1st stage of labour, fetal heart rate should be monitored every:
    a. 15 minutes
    b. 30 minutes
    c. 5 minutes
    d. 60 minutes
112. Which of the following is NOT true for Blindness?
    a. Prevalence in India is 6%
    b. WHO cutoff is <3/60
    c. NPCB India cutoff is <3/60
    d. MCC is Cataract in India Prevalence in India
113. Which of the following is not component of three zeros for AIDS control
    a. Zero new infections
    b. Zero number of HIV patients without treatment
    c. Zero AIDS-related deaths
    d. Zero discrimination
114. Which of the following country is the highest TB burden country worldwide
    a. China
    b. India
    c. Pakistan
    d. South Africa
115. All of the following are true about genomic library, EXCEPT
    a. Collection of cloned DNA fragments
    b. Screening is done by oligonucleotide probes
    c. Only exons are present
    d. Vectors are used to carry and replicate the fragments
116. NOT True about Typhoid is
    a. Blood culture is useful in Diagnosis Week 1 onwards
    b. Leads to Rice-watery diarrhoea
    c. Cephalosporins are useful in treatment
    d. Rose spots appear in 2nd week of disease
117. Most common cause of congestive splenomegaly is?
    a. Chronic congestive cardiac failure
    b. Cirrhosis
    c. Hepatic vein occlusion
    d. Stenosis of splenic vein
118. Not transmitted by blood transfusion?
    a. Hepatitis A
    b. Hepatitis B
    c. Hepatitis C
    d. Hepatitis E
119. In hemochromatosis, all are affected EXCEPT:
    a. CNS
    b. Bronze Pancreas
    c. Hyperpigmentation
    d. Restrictive cardiomyopathy
120. Medical treatment in gallbladder stone is amenable for?
    a. Size of stone less than 10 mm
    b. Radiopaque
    c. Calcium bilirubinate oxalate
    d. GB non-functioning
121. Mainly cholecystokinin is secreted by:
    a. Duodenum
    b. Pancreas
    c. Gallbladder
    d. Ileum
122. All of the following are true about simple febrile seizures except?
    a. Antiepileptic treatment is required for at least 1 year
    b. Usually lasts for <15 minutes
    c. Generalized
    d. Antipyretics do not decrease the risk of febrile seizure recurrence
123. Tourniquet test is used for monitoring patients with?
    a. Infectious mononucleosis
    b. Zika Virus infection
    c. Dengue fever
    d. Chikungunya
124. The following statements are correct for Helicobacter pylori except:
    a. It shows positive urease test
    b. It is spiral gram negative flagellate
    c. It can invade tissue to a great depth
    d. It is linked with duodenal ulcer
125. You are in the eye OPD and wish to use a topical beta blocker in a patient. The chosen drug by you should have all the following properties EXCEPT:
    a. Strong local anaesthetic activity
    b. High lipophilicity
    c. High ocular capture
    d. Low systemic activity
126. Ketoconazole should not be given to a patient being treated with astemizole because:
    a. Ketoconazole induces the metabolism of astemizole
    b. Dangerous ventricular arrhythmias can occur
    c. Astemizole inhibits the metabolism of ketoconazole
    d. Astemizole antagonizes the antifungal action of ketoconazole
127. Name the following instrument:

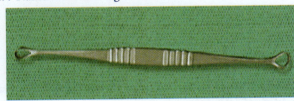

    a. Flushing curette
    b. Uterine curette
    c. Karman's cannula
    d. Cervical dilator

FMGE Solutions Screening Examination

128. Differential expression of the same gene depending on parent of origin is referred to as
    a. Genomic imprinting
    b. Mosaicism
    c. Anticipation
    d. Non-penetrance
129. In firearm injury, Entry wound blackening is due to:
    a. Flame   b. Hot gases
    c. Smoke   d. Unburnt powder
130. ATP is generated in ETC by:
    a. ADP kinase   b. Na⁺ Cl⁻ ATPase
    c. F_0-F_1 ATPase   d. NA⁺ K⁺ ATPase
131. Mechanism of action of uncouplers:
    a. Inhibition of ATP synthesis only not ETC
    b. Inhibition of both ATP synthesis and ETC
    c. Inhibition of only ETC not ATP synthesis
    d. None of the above
132. Glyconeogenesis is
    a. Synthesis of glucose from non-carbohydrate sources
    b. Synthesis of glycogen from glucose
    c. Synthesis of glucose from glycerol
    d. Synthesis of glycogen from non-carbohydrate sources
133. Collagen is composed of all EXCEPT:
    a. Proline   b. Glycine
    c. Hydroxylysine   d. Desmosine
134. Vitamin which is more in Cow's milk than breast milk is:
    a. Vitamin A   b. Vitamin C
    c. Vitamin D   d. None of the above
135. Dietary fibre reduces atherosclerosis by:
    a. Binding to cholesterol   b. ↓VLDL
    c. Forming antioxidants   d. Increasing fluid retention
136. Which one of the following tissues can metabolize glucose, fatty acids, and ketone bodies for ATP production:
    a. Liver   b. Muscle
    c. Brain   d. Red blood cells
137. Human genome contains approximately DNA base pairs
    a. 3.2 billion   b. 2.3 billion
    c. 3.2 million   d. 2.3 million
138. Injectable tetanus toxoid (TT) is an example of:
    a. Active immunity b. Passive Immunity
    c. Native Immunity d. Reaction Immunity
139. Due to recent advances in Health care system, quarantine has been replaced nowadays by:
    a. Active surveillance   b. Passive surveillance
    c. Sentinel surveillance d. Isolation
140. Infant mortality rate, IMR is expressed per:-
    a. 1000 pregnancies   b. 1000 total births
    c. 1000 live births   d. 1000 married women
141. Caloric requirement of adult male worker with moderate levels of activity is:
    a. 2320 Kcal/day   b. 2230 Kcal/day
    c. 2730 Kcal/day   d. 3490 kcal/day
142. Socially attained behavior is:
    a. Culture   b. Acculturation
    c. Socialization   d. Society
143. All are side effects of Oral Contraceptive Pills (OCPs) except:
    a. Breast cancer
    b. Ovarian Cancer
    c. Liver disease
    d. Thromboembolism
144. Chinese letter arrangement of bacilli under microscopy is shown by:
    a. Mycobacterium tuberculosis
    b. Mycobacterium leprae
    c. Clostridium tetani
    d. Corynebacterium diphtheria
145. When correlation between two variables is very strong, the correlation coefficients will be:
    a. >1   b. +1
    c. +0.3   d. -1
146. Most common type of emphysema clinically is:
    a. Panacinar   b. Centriacinar
    c. Paraseptal   d. Segmental
147. Sexual gratification by inflicting pain on partner?
    a. Sodomy   b. Sadism
    c. Necrophilia   d. Bestiality
148. Back examination of polytrauma patient is done by which method:
    a. Logroll
    b. Barrel roll
    c. Chin lift
    d. None
149. Which of the following is not an indication for liver transplantation?
    a. Fatty liver
    b. HIV
    c. Wilson's disease
    d. Primary hyperoxaluria
150. Which gas is used in laparoscopy?
    a. CO_2
    b. N_2O
    c. O_2
    d. N_2
151. Catgut is preserved in:
    a. Glutaraldehyde
    b. Isopropyl alcohol
    c. Iodine
    d. Cetrimide
152. What is the X-ray view used for Superior orbital fissure?
    a. Water's view
    b. Caldwell's view
    c. Lateral skull view
    d. Stenver's Towne's view

MODEL TEST PAPER-I

153. Type of CT Scan used to characterise the chemical composition of kidney stones?
    a. Spiral CT
    b. Multidetector CT
    c. Dual source CT
    d. HRCT
154. Frequency of ultrasound waves in USG
    a. 2000 Hz
    b. 5000 Hz
    c. <2 MHz
    d. >2 MHz
155. Which of the following is NOT found in lipid profile after an overnight fast:

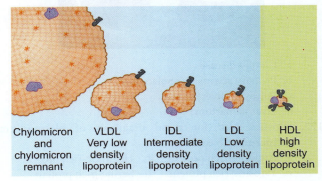

    a. Chylomicrons
    b. VLDL
    c. LDL
    d. HDL
156. All true about postdural puncture headache (PDPH) except-
    a. This is due to loss of CSF and decreased CSF pressure
    b. The incidence of PDPH decreased with increasing age
    c. The headache is less in erect posture increases with supine position
    d. Headache may be accompanied with cranial nerve symptoms
157. This maneuver is described as:

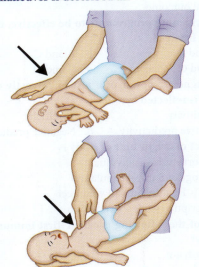

    a. Heimlich maneuver
    b. Chest compression
    c. Charles maneuver
    d. Boyles maneuver

158. A 50 year old female has under gone mastectomy for CA breast. After mastectomy patient is not able to extend adduct and internally rotate the arm. Now supply to which of the following muscle is damaged?
    a. Pectoralis major
    b. Teres minor
    c. Latissimus dorsi
    d. Long head of triceps
159. True about breast cancer in pregnancy:
    a. Occurs in 1 of every 3000 pregnant women
    b. MC non-gynecologic malignancy associated with pregnancy
    c. Ductal carcinoma is MC type, accounting for 75-90% of breast cancer in pregnancy
    d. All of the above
160. All are features of Fournier's gangrene except:
    a. Testicles are involved
    b. Obliterative arteritis seen
    c. Hemolytic streptococci, isolated
    d. Necrotizing fasciitis
161. Candida albicans causes all of the following except
    a. Endocarditis
    b. Meningitis
    c. Mycetoma
    d. Oral thrush
162. Ancylostoma enters the human body by–
    a. Ingestion
    b. Inhalation
    c. Penetration of skin
    d. Inoculation
163. Heat labile immunoglobulin-
    a. IgA
    b. IgG
    c. IgE
    d. IgM
164. Which part of bacteria is most antigenic–
    a. Protein coat
    b. Lipopolysaccharide
    c. Nucleic acid
    d. Lipids
165. Which of the following is agglutination test
    a. Widal test
    b. VDRL
    c. Ascoli's test
    d. Kahn test
166. A three year old child born to a primigravida mother presented with hoarseness. On examination following picture is seen. Which of the following statements is not true about the given condition?

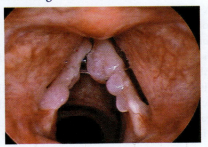

    a. Caused by Human Papilloma Virus 16 and 18
    b. Surgical Excision by Microdebrider is the treatment of Choice
    c. Interferon- α is used as adjuvant therapy to decrease recurrence
    d. Radiotherapy is contraindicated as it may cause malignant transformation

FMGE Solutions Screening Examination

167. A 5-day-old female infant was born with a laryngeal defect. The greater cornuae and the inferior part of the hyoid bone were absent at birth. Failure of development of which of the following embryonic structures has most likely led to these defects?
    a. First Pharyngeal Arch
    b. Second pharyngeal arch
    c. Third pharyngeal arch
    d. Fourth pharyngeal arch

168. The activity of which of the following enzymes is increased in Diabetes Mellitus:
    a. CPT-1
    b. Phosphoenol Pyruvate carboxykinase (PEPCK)
    c. Glucose-6-Phosphatase
    d. All

169. Glucose is a
    a. Ketohexose   b. Ketopentose
    c. Aldopentose   d. Aldohexose

170. A patient with a history of road traffic accident, two months back, presents with complaints of dreams about the accident. He has visualizations of the same scene whenever he visits the place and is afraid to go back to the accident site. Identify the type of disorder that he might be suffering from?
    a. Adjustment disorder   b. PTSD
    c. Anxiety disorder   d. Major depression

171. Drugs not used in Attention deficit hyperactivity disorder is/are:
    a. Clonidine   b. Atomoxetine
    c. Methylphenidate   d. Barbiturate

172. Expression and consequent release of previously repressed emotion is called as:
    a. Regression   b. Dissociation
    c. Abreaction   d. All of the above

173. Cardiac event at the end of isovolumic relaxation phase is:
    a. AV valves open
    b. AV valves close
    c. Corresponds to C wave in JVP
    d. Corresponds to T wave in ECG

174. Choose the correct statement regarding sinus arrhythmia–
    a. It is more pronounced in adults than in children
    b. Increase in heart rate during expiration and decrease in heart rate with inspiration
    c. It is indicative of some dysfunction in the conducting system
    d. It occurs due to alterations in the parasympathetic discharge

175. Best index of platelet function is:
    a. Bleeding time   b. Clotting time
    c. Clot retraction time   d. Prothrombin time

176. CECT Image given suggests:

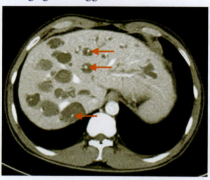

    a. Caroli's disease
    b. Primary sclerosing cholangitis
    c. Polycystic liver disease
    d. Liver hamartoma

177. 'Dipstick test' for rapid diagnosis of plasmodium falciparum is based on:
    a. Arginine-rich protein   b. Histidine-rich protein
    c. Tyrosine-rich protein   d. Serine–rich protein

178. All are true about glycosaminoglycans EXCEPT:
    a. Protein associated with glycosaminoglycans are called core proteins
    b. May be associated with connective tissues
    c. Highly positively charged
    d. Negatively charged
    e. Component of ECM

179. There are several points in the course of a disease process:
    A. Disease onset
    B. Point of first possible detection
    C. Final critical point
    D. Final outcome
    For a screening programme to be effective, it should be applied between:
    a. A and B   b. A and C
    c. B and C   d. C and D

180. The diagnostic power of a test to correctly exclude the disease is reflected by:
    a. Sensitivity   b. Specificity
    c. Positive predictivity d. Negative predictivity

181. Incorrect match or unit of study is
    a. Cohort study - Individual
    b. Ecological Study - Population
    c. RCT - Healthy human volunteer
    d. Descriptive study - Population

182. Which of the following is called 'first immunization' of the baby?
    a. Colostrum
    b. Handing over the baby to mother
    c. OPV
    d. DPT + BCG

183. Area under time and plasma concentration curve signifies:-
    a. Potency
    b. Extent of absorption of drug
    c. Efficacy
    d. Plasma clearance of a drug
184. Which of the following is a recommended step in management of salicylate poisoning?
    a. Chelating agents
    b. Atropine
    c. Alkaline diuresis
    d. Observation
185. Inotropic drugs act by stimulating which of the following receptors:
    a. Alpha 1   b. Alpha 2
    c. Beta 1   d. Beta 2
186. Which of the following is a selective estrogen receptor modulator (SERM)?
    a. Danazol   b. Mifepristone
    c. Raloxifene   d. Dantrolene
187. Drug which reduces both microvascular and macrovascular complications of diabetes mellitus is:-
    a. Tolbutamide b. Repaglinide
    c. Pioglitazone d. Metformin
188. Which of the following is an absolute contraindication for the use of lithium?
    a. Renal failure   b. Glaucoma
    c. Epilepsy   d. Angina
189. Drugs indicated in drug induced vomiting are all except:-
    a. Metoclopramide b. Hyoscine
    c. Ondansetron   d. Chlorpromazine
190. Which of the following statement is true regarding warfarin group of oral anticoagulants?
    a. These interference with the synthesis of vitamin K dependent clotting factors
    b. These can produce anticoagulant effect both in vivo and in vitro
    c. These can produce bleeding like hematuria and cerebral hemorrhage
    d. Their action starts immediately, so are useful for initiation of therapy in deep vein thrombosis.
191. Mechanism of action of methotrexate in chemotherapy is:-
    a. Folic acid antagonism
    b. Pyrimidine antagonism
    c. Purine antagonism
    d. All of these
192. Which of the following is an advantage of adding adrenaline to lignocaine for local anesthetic injection?
    a. Decreases the systemic toxicity
    b. Higher doses can be given
    c. Duration of action can be prolonged
    d. All of the above

193. Most common cause of AVN of the hip is:
    a. Idiopathic   b. Alcoholism
    c. Caissons disease   d. Fracture neck of femur
194. Embalming solution constituents are all EXCEPT:
    a. Ethanol   b. Phenol
    c. Glycerine d. Formalin
195. In the following nutrient arteries to bones, choose the WRONG pair:
    a. Humerus: Profunda brachii
    b. Radius: Anterior interosseous
    c. Fibula: Peroneal
    d. Tibia: Anterior tibial
196. Internal anal sphincter is a part of
    a. Internal longitudinal fibers of rectum
    b. Internal circular muscle fibers of rectum
    c. Puborectalis muscle
    d. Deep perineal muscles
197. Internal pudendal artery is a branch of
    a. Anterior division of internal iliac
    b. Posterior division of internal iliac
    c. Anterior division of external iliac
    d. Posterior division of external iliac
198. Recommended transport medium for stool specimen suspected to contain enteric pathogen is
    a. Amie's medium
    b. Buffered glycerol saline medium
    c. MacConkey medium
    d. Stuart's medium
199. All the following are the examples of enveloped viruses except:
    a. Polio virus
    b. Rubivirus
    c. Molluscum contagiosum virus
    d. Herpes virus.
200. Which of the following is usually the first procedure done for shoulder Dystocia management?
    a. Sharp flexion of hip joints towards abdomen
    b. Suprapubic pressure
    c. 90 degree rotation of posterior shoulder
    d. Emergency C– section
201. Which intravenous anesthetic agent has effect on opioid receptors:
    a. Ketamine   b. Propofol
    c. Thiopentone d. Etomidate
202. Which of the following contraceptive will be effective when used alone on the 15th day of menstrual cycle:-
    a. Copper IUCD
    b. Progesterone only pill or Combined oral contraceptives
    c. Mifepristone
    d. All of these can work if used within 3 days of Unprotected Intercourse
    e. All can be used

203. What is malignant hyperthermia (MH)
    a. Genetic hypermetabolic muscle disease
    b. Genetic hypometabolic muscle disease
    c. Acquired hypermetabolic muscle disease
    d. Acquired hypometabolic muscle disease
204. All of the following can be used for induction of general anesthesia except:
    a. Propofol   b. Thiopentone
    c. Sevoflurane   d. Succinylcholine
205. Calcium is absorbed from:
    a. Duodenum   b. Jejunum
    c. Ileum   d. Colon
206. Which of the following is the diluting segment of the nephron?
    a. PCT
    b. Descending limb of loop of Henle
    c. Thick ascending limb of loop of Henle
    d. Collecting duct
207. Massive blood transfusion is defined as:
    a. Whole blood volume in 24 hours
    b. Half blood volume in 24 hours
    c. 40% blood volume in 24 hours
    d. 60% blood volume in 24 hours
208. Which colour of triage is given the highest priority?
    a. Red   b. Green
    c. Yellow   d. Black
209. D-Dimer is the most sensitive diagnostic test for:
    a. Pulmonary embolism
    b. Acute pulmonary edema
    c. Cardiac tamponade
    d. Acute myocardial infarction
210. Allopurinol is used in organ preservation as:
    a. Antioxidant
    b. Preservative
    c. Free radical scavenger
    d. Precursor for energy metabolism
211. Post-transplant lymphoma is most commonly associated with:
    a. EBV   b. CMV
    c. Herpes simplex   d. HHV-6
212. The most effective bariatric surgery with treatment in the form of weight loss for morbid obesity is:
    a. Roux-en-Y surgery
    b. Biliopancreatic diversion
    c. Vertical banded gastroplasty
    d. Any of the above
213. Most common type of malignant melanoma is:
    a. Superficial spreading
    b. Lentigo maligna melanoma
    c. Nodular
    d. Acral lentiginous
214. Spontaneous regression is seen in:
    a. Port Wine Hemangioma
    b. Strawberry Hemangioma
    c. Cavernous Hemangioma
    d. Arterial angioma
215. Pott's puffy tumor refers to:
    a. Osteomyelitis of the frontal bone
    b. Tuberculosis of the spine
    c. Actinomycosis of maxilla
    d. Osteonecrotic tumor of jaw
216. A clean incised wound heals by:
    a. Primary intention   b. Secondary intention
    c. Excessive scarring   d. None of the above
217. Which of the following is true for shock?
    a. Hypotension   b. Hypoperfusion to tissues
    c. Hypoxia   d. All of the above
218. Non – noxious stimuli perceived as pain is termed as:
    a. Allodynia   b. Hyperalgesia
    c. Hyperesthesia   d. Hyperpathia
219. In children, most common posterior fossa tumor is:
    a. Meningiomas   b. Astrocytoma
    c. Medulloblastoma   d. Glioblastoma multiforme
220. In the perspective of the busy life schedule in the modern society, the accepted minimum period of sexual cohabitation resulting in no offspring for a couple to be declared infertile is:
    a. One year
    b. One and a half-year
    c. Two years
    d. Three year
221. Which of the following is not one of the phases of Implantation of Embryo?
    a. Epithelialization
    b. Apposition
    c. Adhesion
    d. Invasion
222. A pregnant woman with fibroid uterus develops acute pain in abdomen with low grade fever and mild leucocytosis at 28 weeks. The most likely diagnosis is:
    a. Preterm labour
    b. Torsion of fibroid
    c. Red degeneration of fibroid
    d. Infection in Fibroid
223. IUGR is defined when:
    a. Birth weight is below the tenth percentile of the average of gestational age
    b. Birth weight is below 20 percentile of the average of gestational age
    c. Birth weight is below the 30 percentile of the average of gestational age
    d. Weight of baby is less than 1000 gm

224. Which of the following factors is not an important risk factor for tubal ectopic?
    a. A history of tubal surgery
    b. Intrauterine device (IUD) use
    c. In utero diethylstilbestrol (DES) exposure
    d. History of pelvic inflammatory disease
225. Gold standard for diagnosis of endometriosis is:
    a. Laparoscopic visualisation
    b. Histopathological examination
    c. Ultrasound examination
    d. MRI pelvis
226. Which of the following cannot be reason for abnormal bleeding in reproductive age?
    a. Thyroid dysfunction   b. Fibroids
    c. Atrophy   d. Anovulation
227. Apoptosis can occur by change in hormone levels in the ovarian cycle. When there is no fertilization of the ovum, the endometrial cells die because:
    a. The involution of corpus luteum causes estradiol and progesterone levels to fall dramatically
    b. LH levels rise after ovulation
    c. Estradiol levels are not involved in the LH surge phenomenon
    d. Estradiol inhibits the induction of the progesterone receptor in the endometrium
228. A 45 yrs old women present with hot flush after stopping of menstruation. 'Hot Flush' can be relieved by administration of following agents:
    a. Ethinyl estradiol   b. Testosterone
    c. Fluoxymesterone   d. Danazol
229. Myocardial Viability is best evaluated by?
    a. Thallium 201   b. 18 FDG PET
    c. Tc-99m Sestamibi   d. Tc-99m Pyrophosphate
230. Flaring of anterior ends of ribs are seen in?
    a. Neurofibromatosis   b. Hyperparathyroidism
    c. Rickets   d. Coarctation of Aorta
231. A case of carcinoma cervix is found in altered sensorium and is having hiccups, likely cause is:
    a. Septicemia   b. Uremia
    c. Raised ICT   d. None of the above
232. Definitive diagnosis of Hirschsprung's disease is done by?
    a. Rectal Manometry   b. Barium enema
    c. Rectal Biopsy   d. Enteroclysis
233. All are seen with scar dehiscence, except:
    a. Maternal bradycardia b. Fetal bradycardia
    c. Vaginal bleeding   d. Haematuria
234. Hypothalamic amenorrhoea is seen in:
    a. Asherman syndrome
    b. Stein leventhal syndrome
    c. Kallmann syndrome
    d. Down syndrome
235. A girl presents, with cystic swelling at the junction of lower 1/3rd and upper 2/3rd of anterior wall of vagina at 10 O' Clock position. The Diagnosis is:
    a. Bartholin's cyst   b. Gartner's cyst
    c. Adenocarcinoma   d. Vaginal Inclusion Cyst
236. A pregnant lady is diagnosed to be HBsAg positive. Which of the following is the best way to prevent infection to the child.
    a. Hepatitis B vaccine to the child
    b. Full course of Hepatitis B vaccine and immunoglobulin to the child
    c. Hepatitis B immunoglobulin to the mother
    d. Hepatitis B immunization to mother
237. If iodine supplementation in the diet was completely stopped today, thyroid hormone levels in blood will fall to zero after:
    a. 7 days   b. 30 days
    c. 90 days   d. 360 days
238. The thick plate of bone marked with an arrow in the picture below is seen in persistent:

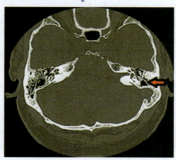

   a. Petrosquamous suture   b. Temporosquamous suture
   c. Petromastoid suture   d. Frontozygomatic suture
239. Which of the following is not true about spread of maxillary sinus carcinoma?
    a. Medial spread occurs to nasal cavity
    b. Anterior spread occurs to facial skin
    c. Posterior spread occurs to orbit
    d. Inferior spread occurs to Alveolus
240. Identify this skin lesion seen in a neonate, noticed first on day 2 of life:

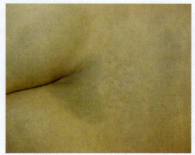

   a. Milia   b. Mongolian spot
   c. Diaper Dermatitis   d. Erythema toxicum

241. What should be used for the treatment of this child with intellectual disability?

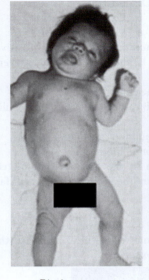
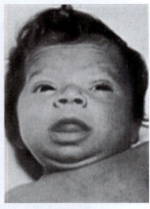

   a. Biotin
   b. Hydroxocobalamin
   c. Pyridoxine
   d. Thyroxine

242. Bone marrow examination of a 2 year old child with massive splenomegaly and pancytopenia showed cells with wrinkled paper appearance of cytoplasm. What could be the possible diagnosis?
   a. Niemann Pick disease
   b. Gaucher disease
   c. Acute Leukemia
   d. Hereditary spherocytosis

243. In primary tuberculosis, all of the following may be seen except:
   a. Cavitation
   b. Caseation
   c. Calcification
   d. Langhans giant cell

244. Most common form of drowning in India:
   a. Suicidal
   b. Homicidal
   c. Accidental
   d. Infanticide

245. Traumatic asphyxia is a type of
   a. Hanging
   b. Ligature Strangulation
   c. Suffocation
   d. Manual strangulation

246. Declaration of venice is related with
   a. Medical ethics
   b. Human experimentation
   c. Terminal illness
   d. Rights of patients

247. Increasing doses of alcohol depresses brain in the following order:
   a. Cerebellum, Frontal lobe, occipital lobe
   b. Frontal lobe, Cerebellum, occipital lobe
   c. Occipital lobe, cerebellum, Frontal lobe
   d. Cerebellum, Occipital lobe, Frontal lobe
   e. Frontal lobe, occipital lobe, cerebellum

248. Masque Ecchymotique is seen in:
   a. Ligature strangulation
   b. Manual strangulation
   c. Traumatic asphyxia
   d. Burking
   e. Chocking

249. A patient presented to ENT OPD with complaints of headache and nasal stuffiness On CT scan Heterogeneous opacification involving multiple sinuses along with Bone erosion (as shown below) was noticed. What would be the most likely diagnosis?

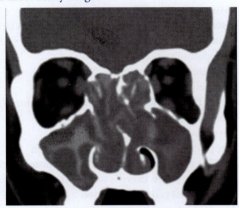

   a. Acute bacterial rhinosinusitis
   b. Chronic Bacterial rhinosinusitis
   c. Allergic Fungal rhinosinusitis
   d. Invasive Fungal Rhinosinusitis

250. In CSF rhinorrhea CSF from middle cranial fossa reaches the nose via:
   a. Sphenoid sinus
   b. Frontal sinus
   c. Cribriform plate
   d. Fovea ethmoidalis

251. The encircled area, in blue, in the given picture is

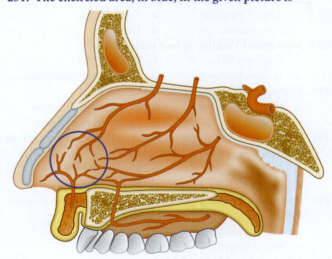

   a. Woodruffs Area
   b. Browne's Area
   c. Little's Area
   d. Kiesselbach's Area

252. In a Normal distribution, statement which is correct is
   a. Mean +/- 2 SD covers 95% values
   b. Mean +/- 3 SD covers 68% values
   c. Mean +/- 1 SD covers 99% values
   d. Mean > Median > Mode

253. Which of the following are referred to as "Ivory Towers of Disease":
    a. Small health centres
    b. Large hospitals
    c. Private practitioners
    d. Health insurance companies
254. In which stage of the demographic cycle is India currently?
    a. High stationary   b. Late expanding
    c. Early stationary   d. Low stationary
255. A family where all of its members are playing a part in its management is known as:
    a. Elementary family   b. New family
    c. 3-Generation family d. Communal family
256. A 30 yrs old female present with hearing loss and following audiogram is obtained. What is her most likely diagnosis?

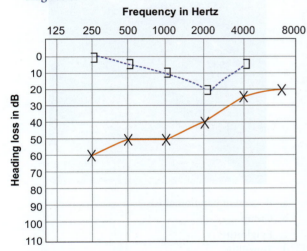

   a. Ototoxicity
   b. Noise Induced Hearing Loss
   c. Otosclerosis
   d. Meniere's Disease
257. Recurrent facial nerve palsy is seen in all except
    a. Melkersson syndrome
    b. Diabetes
    c. Sarcoidosis
    d. Herpes zoster oticus
258. True about Vestibular Schwannoma is
    a. Converging ABLB Laddergram
    b. Recruitment phenomenon is present
    c. High SISI score
    d. Rollover phenomenon is seen
259. Spongiosis involves:
    a. Stratum granulosum
    b. Stratum corneum
    c. Stratum spinosum
    d. Stratum basal

260. A 60 year old man is brought to a psychiatrist with a 10 year history, that he suspects his neighbors and he feels that whenever he passes by they sneeze and plan against him behind his back. He feels that his wife has been replaced by a double and calls police for help. He is quite well-groomed, alert, occasionally consumes alcohol, likely diagnosis is:
    a. Paranoid personality disorder
    b. Paranoid schizophrenia
    c. Alcohol withdrawal
    d. Conversion disorder
261. Nitric oxide acts by increasing:
    a. BRCA 1   b. BRCA 2
    c. Interleukin   d. cGMP
262. VMA is excreted in urine in:
    a. Alkaptonuria   b. Phenylketonuria
    c. Diabetic ketoacidosis d. Pheochromocytoma
263. Which of the following mood stabilizers has anti suicide property?
    a. Lithium   b. Carbamazepine
    c. Valproate   d. Lamotrigine
264. The primary pathology in Athletic Pubalgia is:
    a. Abdominal muscle strain
    b. Rectus femoris strain
    c. Gluteus medius strain
    d. Hamstring strain
265. A patient with tuberculosis of spine first neurological sign is:
    a. Motor loss
    b. Sensory loss
    c. Increased deep tendon reflexes
    d. Bladder involvement
266. A child presents with indurated boggy swelling with crusts and hair loss over scalp as shown in the image. Most likely cause is:

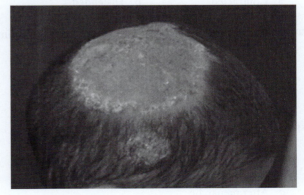

   a. Trichophyton
   b. Epidermophyton
   c. Microsporum
   d. Staph. aureus

267. Identify the implant:

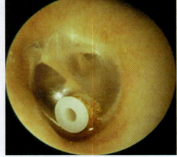

   a. Partial Ossicular Replacement Prosthesis
   b. Total Ossicular Replacement Prosthesis
   c. Piston
   d. Grommet

268. Identify the space marked below by red arrow?

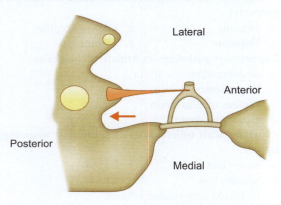

   a. Facial recess   b. Epitympanic recess
   c. Sinus tympani   d. Prussak's space

269. Gallbladder in starvation death is:
   a. Contracted   b. Distended
   c. Mummified   d. Not affected

270. Which of the following cannot be done by a 15 month child?
   a. Walking with support
   b. Transfers objects from 1 hand to another
   c. Builds tower of 2 cubes
   d. Speaks three-word sentences

271. Growth spurt occurs:
   a. Just before appearance of axillary hair
   b. Just before menarche
   c. After 16 years
   d. After menarche

272. The use of highly active antiretroviral therapy is associated with the development of:
   a. Keratitis   b. Uveitis
   c. Retinitis   d. Optic neuritis

273. After a leisure trip, a patient comes with gritty pain in eye and joint pain. What is the most probable diagnosis?
   a. Reiter's syndrome   b. Behcet's syndrome
   c. Sarcoidosis   d. SLE

274. Active immunity is not acquired by:
   a. Infection
   b. Vaccination
   c. Immunoglobulin transfer
   d. Subclinical infection

275. Most common cancer in children less than 10 years:
   a. Leukemia   b. Neuroblastoma
   c. Brain tumor   d. Wilms tumor

276. A 4-year-old child presents to the emergency department with high grade fever, respiratory difficulty and noisy breathing. On examination. X ray of his neck is shown below. The most probable diagnosis is?

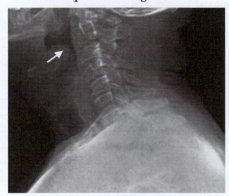

   a. Recurrent papillomatosis
   b. Croup
   c. Epiglottitis
   d. Tonsillitis

277. Drug of choice for a child with first episode nephrotic syndrome is?
   a. Cyclophosphamide   b. Prednisolone
   c. Mycophenolate   d. Cyclosporine

278. Most common cause of urinary tract infection in children is:
   a. Klebsiella pneumoniae   b. Proteus mirabilis
   c. Escherichia coli   d. Pseudomonas aerogenes

279. Drug of choice for neonatal seizures is?
   a. Phenobarbitone
   b. Valproate
   c. ACTH
   d. Lamotrigine

280. Which of the following is not a sign of active rickets?
   a. Frontal bossing
   b. Wrist widening
   c. Hutchinson teeth
   d. Prominence of costochondral junction

281. 18 year old female with hypopigmented patches near both ankles. What is not used for treatment?

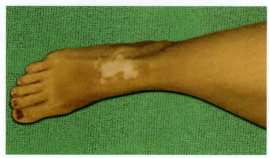

   a. Topical clobetasol
   b. Topical tretinoin
   c. Topical tacrolimus
   d. Topical methoxsalen

282. The ventral surface of the adult heart as seen on gross examination or radiography is comprised primarily of the
   a. Left atrium
   b. Left ventricle
   c. Inferior vena cava
   d. Right ventricle

283. Which of the three primary germ layers forms the histologically definitive endocardium of the adult heart?
   a. Ectoderm
   b. Endoderm
   c. Mesoderm
   d. Epiblast

284. A 39-year-old woman with headaches presents to her primary care physician with a possible herniated disk. Her magnetic resonance imaging (MRI) scan reveals that the posterolateral protrusion of the intervertebral disk between L4 and L5 vertebrae would most likely affect nerve roots of which of the following spinal nerves?
   a. Third lumbar nerve
   b. Fourth lumbar nerve
   c. Fifth lumbar nerve
   d. First sacral nerve

285. Identify the structure depicted below which is the most important source of noradrenergic innervations to cerebral cortex:

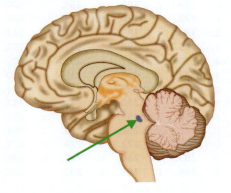

   a. Basal nucleus of Meynert
   b. Locus coeruleus
   c. Raphe nucleus
   d. Amygdala

286. Medial meniscus is more prone to injury because:
   a. It is semi lunar
   b. Attached firmly to tibial collateral ligament
   c. It is avascular
   d. Connected to lateral meniscus by lateral ligament

287. Riders bone is developed in the tendon of:
   a. Gastrocnemius
   b. Adductor longus
   c. Quadriceps femoris
   d. Flexor polices brevis

288. Floor of femoral triangle is formed by all except
   a. Pectineus
   b. Iliacus
   c. Adductor brevis
   d. Adductor longus

289. All of the following are components of a BPP except
   a. Contraction stress test
   b. Amniotic fluid volume
   c. Nonstress test
   d. Fetal tone

290. Which of the following clinical conditions is not an indication for induction of labor?
   a. Intrauterine fetal demise
   b. Severe preeclampsia at 36 weeks
   c. Complete placenta previa
   d. Post term pregnancy

291. You are delivering a 26-year-old G3P2A0L2 at 40 weeks. She has a history of two previous uncomplicated vaginal deliveries and has had no complications this pregnancy. After 15 min of pushing, the baby's head delivers spontaneously, but then retracts back against the perineum. As you apply gently downward traction to the head, the baby's anterior shoulder fails to deliver. McRoberts maneuver is done. The baby finally delivers and the pediatricians attending the delivery note that the right arm is hanging limply to the baby's side with the forearm extended and internally rotated. What is the baby's most likely diagnosis?
   a. Erb palsy
   b. Klumpke's paralysis
   c. Humeral fracture
   d. Clavicular fracture

292. All EXCEPT which of the following are associated with episiotomy dehiscence?
   a. Smoking
   b. Human papilloma virus (HPV) infection
   c. Coagulopathy
   d. Asthma

293. A pregnant patient has a history of multiple substance abuse. She has a little boy that is 2 years old who is slow in school and has difficulty concentrating. Which of the following substances has been associated with behavioral and developmental abnormalities in children?
   a. Tobacco
   b. Cocaine
   c. Caffeine
   d. Marijuana

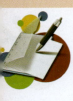

FMGE Solutions Screening Examination

294. You see a 42-year-old patient in your office who is now 5 weeks pregnant with her fifth baby. She is very concerned regarding the risk of Down syndrome because of her advanced maternal age. After extensive genetic counseling, she has decided to undergo a second-trimester amniocentesis to determine the karyotype of her fetus. Prior to performing the procedure, you inform the patient that all of the following are possible complications of the amniocentesis except
    a. Amniotic fluid leakage
    b. Chorioamnionitis
    c. A fetal loss rate of less than 0.5%
    d. Limb reduction defects

295. Contraindications to combination oral contraceptive pill use include which of the following?
    a. Prior acute hepatitis
    b. Prior cervical dysplasia
    c. Prior thromboembolism
    d. Prior simple endometrial hyperplasia

296. Fetal kidneys start producing urine by:
    a. 3 months
    b. 4 months
    c. 5 months
    d. 6 months

297. Ideal time for screening of blood sugar for diabetes in a pregnant female is:
    a. 16-20 weeks
    b. 20-24 weeks
    c. 24-28 weeks
    d. 12-16 weeks

298. Amenorrhea in an 18 year old with a milky discharge from the nipples is a most recognized feature of:
    a. Addison's disease
    b. Hyperprolactinemia
    c. Occult carcinoma
    d. Hypothyroidism

299. Golden colour amniotic fluid is seen in:
    a. Rh incompatibility
    b. Foetal death
    c. IUGR
    d. Foetal distress

300. Primigravida with full term, complains of faintness on lying down and she feels well when turns to side or sitting position. This is due to:
    a. Increased abdominal pressure
    b. IVC compression
    c. Increased intracranial pressure
    d. After heavy lunch

Ans.

1.	a.	2.	d.	3.	a.	4.	c.	5.	d.	6.	d.	7.	b.	8.	c.	9.	b.	10.	b.	11.	b
12.	c.	13.	a.	14.	b.	15.	c.	16.	c.	17.	d.	18.	c.	19.	b.	20.	a.	21.	a.	22.	a.
23.	d.	24.	d.	25.	a.	26.	d.	27.	a.	28.	a.	29.	a.	30.	d.	31.	d.	32.	d.	33.	b.
34.	a.	35.	b.	36.	c.	37.	b.	38.	d.	39.	d.	40.	c.	41.	a.	42.	d.	43.	a.	44.	c.
45.	a.	46.	c.	47.	a.	48.	c.	49.	d.	50.	a.	51.	b.	52.	d.	53.	d.	54.	c.	55.	a.
56.	a.	57.	b.	58.	d.	59.	a.	60.	d.	61.	b.	62.	d.	63.	c.	64.	a.	65.	a.	66.	a.
67.	c.	68.	b.	69.	c.	70.	d.	71.	b.	72.	d.	73.	b.	74.	c.	75.	c.	76.	b.	77.	b.
78.	a.	79.	d.	80.	a.	81.	a.	82.	c.	83.	a.	84.	c.	85.	d.	86.	d.	87.	d.	88.	b.
89.	b.	90.	a.	91.	a.	92.	d.	93.	b.	94.	d.	95.	d.	96.	a.	97.	c.	98.	d.	99.	a.
100.	d.	101.	b.	102.	c.	103.	d.	104.	a.	105.	c.	106.	c.	107.	c.	108.	d.	109.	b.	110.	c.
111.	a.	112.	a.	113.	b.	114.	b.	115.	c.	116.	b.	117.	b.	118.	d.	119.	a.	120.	a.	121.	a.
122.	c.	123.	c.	124.	c.	125.	a.	126.	b.	127.	b.	128.	a.	129.	c.	130.	c.	131.	a.	132.	d.
133.	d.	134.	c.	135.	a.	136.	b.	137.	a.	138.	a.	139.	c.	140.	c.	141.	c.	142.	a.	143.	b.
144.	d.	145.	b.	146.	b.	147.	b.	148.	a.	149.	b.	150.	a.	151.	b.	152.	b.	153.	c.	154.	d.
155.	a.	156.	c.	157.	a.	158.	c.	159.	d.	160.	a.	161.	c.	162.	c.	163.	c.	164.	a.	165.	a.
166.	a.	167.	c.	168.	d.	169.	d.	170.	b.	171.	d.	172.	c.	173.	a.	174.	d.	175.	c.	176.	a.
177.	b.	178.	c.	179.	c.	180.	d.	181.	c.	182.	a.	183.	b.	184.	c.	185.	c.	186.	c.	187.	d.
188.	a.	189.	b.	190.	c.	191.	a.	192.	d.	193.	a.	194.	a.	195.	d.	196.	b.	197.	a.	198.	b.
199.	a.	200.	b.	201.	a.	202.	d.	203.	a.	204.	d.	205.	a.	206.	c.	207.	a.	208.	a.	209.	a.
210.	c.	211.	a.	212.	b.	213.	a.	214.	b.	215.	a.	216.	a.	217.	d.	218.	a.	219.	b.	220.	a.
221.	a.	222.	c.	223.	a.	224.	b.	225.	a.	226.	c.	227.	a.	228.	a.	229.	b.	230.	c.	231.	b.
232.	c.	233.	a.	234.	c.	235.	b.	236.	b.	237.	c.	238.	a.	239.	c.	240.	b.	241.	d.	242.	b.
243.	a.	244.	c.	245.	c.	246.	c.	247.	d.	248.	c.	249.	c.	250.	a.	251.	c.	252.	a.	253.	b.
254.	b.	255.	d.	256.	c.	257.	d.	258.	d.	259.	c.	260.	b.	261.	c.	262.	d.	263.	a.	264.	a.
265.	c.	266.	a.	267.	d.	268.	c.	269.	b.	270.	d.	271.	b.	272.	b.	273.	a.	274.	c.	275.	a.
276.	c.	277.	c.	278.	c.	279.	a.	280.	c.	281.	b.	282.	d.	283.	c.	284.	c.	285.	b.	286.	b.
287.	b.	288.	c.	289.	a.	290.	c.	291.	a.	292.	d.	293.	a.	294.	d.	295.	c.	296.	a.	297.	c.
298.	b.	299.	a.	300.	b.																

OMR Sheet 1 for Model Test Paper-II

1 – 50	51 – 100	101 – 150	151 – 200	201 – 250	251 – 300
1 (A) (B) (C) (D)	51 (A) (B) (C) (D)	101 (A) (B) (C) (D)	151 (A) (B) (C) (D)	201 (A) (B) (C) (D)	251 (A) (B) (C) (D)
2 (A) (B) (C) (D)	52 (A) (B) (C) (D)	102 (A) (B) (C) (D)	152 (A) (B) (C) (D)	202 (A) (B) (C) (D)	252 (A) (B) (C) (D)
3 (A) (B) (C) (D)	53 (A) (B) (C) (D)	103 (A) (B) (C) (D)	153 (A) (B) (C) (D)	203 (A) (B) (C) (D)	253 (A) (B) (C) (D)
4 (A) (B) (C) (D)	54 (A) (B) (C) (D)	104 (A) (B) (C) (D)	154 (A) (B) (C) (D)	204 (A) (B) (C) (D)	254 (A) (B) (C) (D)
5 (A) (B) (C) (D)	55 (A) (B) (C) (D)	105 (A) (B) (C) (D)	155 (A) (B) (C) (D)	205 (A) (B) (C) (D)	255 (A) (B) (C) (D)
6 (A) (B) (C) (D)	56 (A) (B) (C) (D)	106 (A) (B) (C) (D)	156 (A) (B) (C) (D)	206 (A) (B) (C) (D)	256 (A) (B) (C) (D)
7 (A) (B) (C) (D)	57 (A) (B) (C) (D)	107 (A) (B) (C) (D)	157 (A) (B) (C) (D)	207 (A) (B) (C) (D)	257 (A) (B) (C) (D)
8 (A) (B) (C) (D)	58 (A) (B) (C) (D)	108 (A) (B) (C) (D)	158 (A) (B) (C) (D)	208 (A) (B) (C) (D)	258 (A) (B) (C) (D)
9 (A) (B) (C) (D)	59 (A) (B) (C) (D)	109 (A) (B) (C) (D)	159 (A) (B) (C) (D)	209 (A) (B) (C) (D)	259 (A) (B) (C) (D)
10 (A) (B) (C) (D)	60 (A) (B) (C) (D)	100 (A) (B) (C) (D)	160 (A) (B) (C) (D)	210 (A) (B) (C) (D)	260 (A) (B) (C) (D)
11 (A) (B) (C) (D)	61 (A) (B) (C) (D)	111 (A) (B) (C) (D)	161 (A) (B) (C) (D)	211 (A) (B) (C) (D)	261 (A) (B) (C) (D)
12 (A) (B) (C) (D)	62 (A) (B) (C) (D)	112 (A) (B) (C) (D)	162 (A) (B) (C) (D)	212 (A) (B) (C) (D)	262 (A) (B) (C) (D)
13 (A) (B) (C) (D)	63 (A) (B) (C) (D)	113 (A) (B) (C) (D)	163 (A) (B) (C) (D)	213 (A) (B) (C) (D)	263 (A) (B) (C) (D)
14 (A) (B) (C) (D)	64 (A) (B) (C) (D)	114 (A) (B) (C) (D)	164 (A) (B) (C) (D)	214 (A) (B) (C) (D)	264 (A) (B) (C) (D)
15 (A) (B) (C) (D)	65 (A) (B) (C) (D)	115 (A) (B) (C) (D)	165 (A) (B) (C) (D)	215 (A) (B) (C) (D)	265 (A) (B) (C) (D)
16 (A) (B) (C) (D)	66 (A) (B) (C) (D)	116 (A) (B) (C) (D)	166 (A) (B) (C) (D)	216 (A) (B) (C) (D)	266 (A) (B) (C) (D)
17 (A) (B) (C) (D)	67 (A) (B) (C) (D)	117 (A) (B) (C) (D)	167 (A) (B) (C) (D)	217 (A) (B) (C) (D)	267 (A) (B) (C) (D)
18 (A) (B) (C) (D)	68 (A) (B) (C) (D)	118 (A) (B) (C) (D)	168 (A) (B) (C) (D)	218 (A) (B) (C) (D)	268 (A) (B) (C) (D)
19 (A) (B) (C) (D)	69 (A) (B) (C) (D)	119 (A) (B) (C) (D)	169 (A) (B) (C) (D)	219 (A) (B) (C) (D)	269 (A) (B) (C) (D)
20 (A) (B) (C) (D)	70 (A) (B) (C) (D)	120 (A) (B) (C) (D)	170 (A) (B) (C) (D)	220 (A) (B) (C) (D)	270 (A) (B) (C) (D)
21 (A) (B) (C) (D)	71 (A) (B) (C) (D)	121 (A) (B) (C) (D)	171 (A) (B) (C) (D)	221 (A) (B) (C) (D)	271 (A) (B) (C) (D)
22 (A) (B) (C) (D)	72 (A) (B) (C) (D)	122 (A) (B) (C) (D)	172 (A) (B) (C) (D)	222 (A) (B) (C) (D)	272 (A) (B) (C) (D)
23 (A) (B) (C) (D)	73 (A) (B) (C) (D)	123 (A) (B) (C) (D)	173 (A) (B) (C) (D)	223 (A) (B) (C) (D)	273 (A) (B) (C) (D)
24 (A) (B) (C) (D)	74 (A) (B) (C) (D)	124 (A) (B) (C) (D)	174 (A) (B) (C) (D)	224 (A) (B) (C) (D)	274 (A) (B) (C) (D)
25 (A) (B) (C) (D)	75 (A) (B) (C) (D)	125 (A) (B) (C) (D)	175 (A) (B) (C) (D)	225 (A) (B) (C) (D)	275 (A) (B) (C) (D)
26 (A) (B) (C) (D)	76 (A) (B) (C) (D)	126 (A) (B) (C) (D)	176 (A) (B) (C) (D)	226 (A) (B) (C) (D)	276 (A) (B) (C) (D)
27 (A) (B) (C) (D)	77 (A) (B) (C) (D)	127 (A) (B) (C) (D)	177 (A) (B) (C) (D)	227 (A) (B) (C) (D)	277 (A) (B) (C) (D)
28 (A) (B) (C) (D)	78 (A) (B) (C) (D)	128 (A) (B) (C) (D)	178 (A) (B) (C) (D)	228 (A) (B) (C) (D)	278 (A) (B) (C) (D)
29 (A) (B) (C) (D)	79 (A) (B) (C) (D)	129 (A) (B) (C) (D)	179 (A) (B) (C) (D)	229 (A) (B) (C) (D)	279 (A) (B) (C) (D)
30 (A) (B) (C) (D)	80 (A) (B) (C) (D)	130 (A) (B) (C) (D)	180 (A) (B) (C) (D)	230 (A) (B) (C) (D)	280 (A) (B) (C) (D)
31 (A) (B) (C) (D)	81 (A) (B) (C) (D)	131 (A) (B) (C) (D)	181 (A) (B) (C) (D)	231 (A) (B) (C) (D)	281 (A) (B) (C) (D)
32 (A) (B) (C) (D)	82 (A) (B) (C) (D)	132 (A) (B) (C) (D)	182 (A) (B) (C) (D)	232 (A) (B) (C) (D)	282 (A) (B) (C) (D)
33 (A) (B) (C) (D)	83 (A) (B) (C) (D)	133 (A) (B) (C) (D)	183 (A) (B) (C) (D)	233 (A) (B) (C) (D)	283 (A) (B) (C) (D)
34 (A) (B) (C) (D)	84 (A) (B) (C) (D)	134 (A) (B) (C) (D)	184 (A) (B) (C) (D)	234 (A) (B) (C) (D)	284 (A) (B) (C) (D)
35 (A) (B) (C) (D)	85 (A) (B) (C) (D)	135 (A) (B) (C) (D)	185 (A) (B) (C) (D)	235 (A) (B) (C) (D)	285 (A) (B) (C) (D)
36 (A) (B) (C) (D)	86 (A) (B) (C) (D)	136 (A) (B) (C) (D)	186 (A) (B) (C) (D)	236 (A) (B) (C) (D)	286 (A) (B) (C) (D)
37 (A) (B) (C) (D)	87 (A) (B) (C) (D)	137 (A) (B) (C) (D)	187 (A) (B) (C) (D)	237 (A) (B) (C) (D)	287 (A) (B) (C) (D)
38 (A) (B) (C) (D)	88 (A) (B) (C) (D)	138 (A) (B) (C) (D)	188 (A) (B) (C) (D)	238 (A) (B) (C) (D)	288 (A) (B) (C) (D)
39 (A) (B) (C) (D)	89 (A) (B) (C) (D)	139 (A) (B) (C) (D)	189 (A) (B) (C) (D)	239 (A) (B) (C) (D)	289 (A) (B) (C) (D)
40 (A) (B) (C) (D)	90 (A) (B) (C) (D)	140 (A) (B) (C) (D)	190 (A) (B) (C) (D)	240 (A) (B) (C) (D)	290 (A) (B) (C) (D)
41 (A) (B) (C) (D)	91 (A) (B) (C) (D)	141 (A) (B) (C) (D)	191 (A) (B) (C) (D)	241 (A) (B) (C) (D)	291 (A) (B) (C) (D)
42 (A) (B) (C) (D)	92 (A) (B) (C) (D)	142 (A) (B) (C) (D)	192 (A) (B) (C) (D)	242 (A) (B) (C) (D)	292 (A) (B) (C) (D)
43 (A) (B) (C) (D)	93 (A) (B) (C) (D)	143 (A) (B) (C) (D)	193 (A) (B) (C) (D)	243 (A) (B) (C) (D)	293 (A) (B) (C) (D)
44 (A) (B) (C) (D)	94 (A) (B) (C) (D)	144 (A) (B) (C) (D)	194 (A) (B) (C) (D)	244 (A) (B) (C) (D)	294 (A) (B) (C) (D)
45 (A) (B) (C) (D)	95 (A) (B) (C) (D)	145 (A) (B) (C) (D)	195 (A) (B) (C) (D)	245 (A) (B) (C) (D)	295 (A) (B) (C) (D)
46 (A) (B) (C) (D)	96 (A) (B) (C) (D)	146 (A) (B) (C) (D)	196 (A) (B) (C) (D)	246 (A) (B) (C) (D)	296 (A) (B) (C) (D)
47 (A) (B) (C) (D)	97 (A) (B) (C) (D)	147 (A) (B) (C) (D)	197 (A) (B) (C) (D)	247 (A) (B) (C) (D)	297 (A) (B) (C) (D)
48 (A) (B) (C) (D)	98 (A) (B) (C) (D)	148 (A) (B) (C) (D)	198 (A) (B) (C) (D)	248 (A) (B) (C) (D)	298 (A) (B) (C) (D)
49 (A) (B) (C) (D)	99 (A) (B) (C) (D)	149 (A) (B) (C) (D)	199 (A) (B) (C) (D)	249 (A) (B) (C) (D)	299 (A) (B) (C) (D)
50 (A) (B) (C) (D)	100 (A) (B) (C) (D)	150 (A) (B) (C) (D)	200 (A) (B) (C) (D)	250 (A) (B) (C) (D)	300 (A) (B) (C) (D)

ASSESSMENT OF MOCK TEST ON THE BASIS OF SCORES- BY THE AUTHORS

Score	Interpretation	Authors Comments
270 Plus	OUTSTANDING	• Highly appreciable score. Keep doing MCQs
240 – 269	EXCELLENT PERFORMANCE	• Great score. Pay attention on some silly mistakes
210 – 239	VERY GOOD PERFORMANCE	• Keep doing MCQs and continue with revising the notes • Advised not to flow in overconfidence
180 – 209	GOOD PERFORMANCE	• Learn the time management while doing MCQs • Keep moving on same track and avoid overconfidence • Work on anxiety issues if there are any
150 – 179	SATISFACTORY	• You are going well. Continue on the same track • Lacking confidence on studied topics due to lack of revision • Practice more MCQs
130 – 149	UNSATISFACTORY	• You are studying but lacking concept and lack of revision. • Improve on silly mistakes by working on basic subjects • Definite improvement expected
Below 130	POOR SCORE	• Need to work on basic subjects • Conceptual based study is recommended • Do FMGE Solutions to cover 3–4 times with explanations

INSTRUCTIONS FOR FILLING THE SHEET

1. This sheet should not be folded or crushed.
2. Use only blue/black ball pen to fill the circles.
3. Use of pencil is strictly prohibited.
4. Circles should be darkened properly and completely.
5. Cutting & erasing on this sheet is not allowed.
6. Do not use any stray marks on the sheet.
7. Do not use marker, white fluid or any other device to hide the shading already done.

OMR Sheet 2 for Model Test Paper-II

1 – 50	51 – 100	101 – 150	151 – 200	201 – 250	251 – 300
1 Ⓐ Ⓑ Ⓒ Ⓓ	51 Ⓐ Ⓑ Ⓒ Ⓓ	101 Ⓐ Ⓑ Ⓒ Ⓓ	151 Ⓐ Ⓑ Ⓒ Ⓓ	201 Ⓐ Ⓑ Ⓒ Ⓓ	251 Ⓐ Ⓑ Ⓒ Ⓓ
2 Ⓐ Ⓑ Ⓒ Ⓓ	52 Ⓐ Ⓑ Ⓒ Ⓓ	102 Ⓐ Ⓑ Ⓒ Ⓓ	152 Ⓐ Ⓑ Ⓒ Ⓓ	202 Ⓐ Ⓑ Ⓒ Ⓓ	252 Ⓐ Ⓑ Ⓒ Ⓓ
3 Ⓐ Ⓑ Ⓒ Ⓓ	53 Ⓐ Ⓑ Ⓒ Ⓓ	103 Ⓐ Ⓑ Ⓒ Ⓓ	153 Ⓐ Ⓑ Ⓒ Ⓓ	203 Ⓐ Ⓑ Ⓒ Ⓓ	253 Ⓐ Ⓑ Ⓒ Ⓓ
4 Ⓐ Ⓑ Ⓒ Ⓓ	54 Ⓐ Ⓑ Ⓒ Ⓓ	104 Ⓐ Ⓑ Ⓒ Ⓓ	154 Ⓐ Ⓑ Ⓒ Ⓓ	204 Ⓐ Ⓑ Ⓒ Ⓓ	254 Ⓐ Ⓑ Ⓒ Ⓓ
5 Ⓐ Ⓑ Ⓒ Ⓓ	55 Ⓐ Ⓑ Ⓒ Ⓓ	105 Ⓐ Ⓑ Ⓒ Ⓓ	155 Ⓐ Ⓑ Ⓒ Ⓓ	205 Ⓐ Ⓑ Ⓒ Ⓓ	255 Ⓐ Ⓑ Ⓒ Ⓓ
6 Ⓐ Ⓑ Ⓒ Ⓓ	56 Ⓐ Ⓑ Ⓒ Ⓓ	106 Ⓐ Ⓑ Ⓒ Ⓓ	156 Ⓐ Ⓑ Ⓒ Ⓓ	206 Ⓐ Ⓑ Ⓒ Ⓓ	256 Ⓐ Ⓑ Ⓒ Ⓓ
7 Ⓐ Ⓑ Ⓒ Ⓓ	57 Ⓐ Ⓑ Ⓒ Ⓓ	107 Ⓐ Ⓑ Ⓒ Ⓓ	157 Ⓐ Ⓑ Ⓒ Ⓓ	207 Ⓐ Ⓑ Ⓒ Ⓓ	257 Ⓐ Ⓑ Ⓒ Ⓓ
8 Ⓐ Ⓑ Ⓒ Ⓓ	58 Ⓐ Ⓑ Ⓒ Ⓓ	108 Ⓐ Ⓑ Ⓒ Ⓓ	158 Ⓐ Ⓑ Ⓒ Ⓓ	208 Ⓐ Ⓑ Ⓒ Ⓓ	258 Ⓐ Ⓑ Ⓒ Ⓓ
9 Ⓐ Ⓑ Ⓒ Ⓓ	59 Ⓐ Ⓑ Ⓒ Ⓓ	109 Ⓐ Ⓑ Ⓒ Ⓓ	159 Ⓐ Ⓑ Ⓒ Ⓓ	209 Ⓐ Ⓑ Ⓒ Ⓓ	259 Ⓐ Ⓑ Ⓒ Ⓓ
10 Ⓐ Ⓑ Ⓒ Ⓓ	60 Ⓐ Ⓑ Ⓒ Ⓓ	100 Ⓐ Ⓑ Ⓒ Ⓓ	160 Ⓐ Ⓑ Ⓒ Ⓓ	210 Ⓐ Ⓑ Ⓒ Ⓓ	260 Ⓐ Ⓑ Ⓒ Ⓓ
11 Ⓐ Ⓑ Ⓒ Ⓓ	61 Ⓐ Ⓑ Ⓒ Ⓓ	111 Ⓐ Ⓑ Ⓒ Ⓓ	161 Ⓐ Ⓑ Ⓒ Ⓓ	211 Ⓐ Ⓑ Ⓒ Ⓓ	261 Ⓐ Ⓑ Ⓒ Ⓓ
12 Ⓐ Ⓑ Ⓒ Ⓓ	62 Ⓐ Ⓑ Ⓒ Ⓓ	112 Ⓐ Ⓑ Ⓒ Ⓓ	162 Ⓐ Ⓑ Ⓒ Ⓓ	212 Ⓐ Ⓑ Ⓒ Ⓓ	262 Ⓐ Ⓑ Ⓒ Ⓓ
13 Ⓐ Ⓑ Ⓒ Ⓓ	63 Ⓐ Ⓑ Ⓒ Ⓓ	113 Ⓐ Ⓑ Ⓒ Ⓓ	163 Ⓐ Ⓑ Ⓒ Ⓓ	213 Ⓐ Ⓑ Ⓒ Ⓓ	263 Ⓐ Ⓑ Ⓒ Ⓓ
14 Ⓐ Ⓑ Ⓒ Ⓓ	64 Ⓐ Ⓑ Ⓒ Ⓓ	114 Ⓐ Ⓑ Ⓒ Ⓓ	164 Ⓐ Ⓑ Ⓒ Ⓓ	214 Ⓐ Ⓑ Ⓒ Ⓓ	264 Ⓐ Ⓑ Ⓒ Ⓓ
15 Ⓐ Ⓑ Ⓒ Ⓓ	65 Ⓐ Ⓑ Ⓒ Ⓓ	115 Ⓐ Ⓑ Ⓒ Ⓓ	165 Ⓐ Ⓑ Ⓒ Ⓓ	215 Ⓐ Ⓑ Ⓒ Ⓓ	265 Ⓐ Ⓑ Ⓒ Ⓓ
16 Ⓐ Ⓑ Ⓒ Ⓓ	66 Ⓐ Ⓑ Ⓒ Ⓓ	116 Ⓐ Ⓑ Ⓒ Ⓓ	166 Ⓐ Ⓑ Ⓒ Ⓓ	216 Ⓐ Ⓑ Ⓒ Ⓓ	266 Ⓐ Ⓑ Ⓒ Ⓓ
17 Ⓐ Ⓑ Ⓒ Ⓓ	67 Ⓐ Ⓑ Ⓒ Ⓓ	117 Ⓐ Ⓑ Ⓒ Ⓓ	167 Ⓐ Ⓑ Ⓒ Ⓓ	217 Ⓐ Ⓑ Ⓒ Ⓓ	267 Ⓐ Ⓑ Ⓒ Ⓓ
18 Ⓐ Ⓑ Ⓒ Ⓓ	68 Ⓐ Ⓑ Ⓒ Ⓓ	118 Ⓐ Ⓑ Ⓒ Ⓓ	168 Ⓐ Ⓑ Ⓒ Ⓓ	218 Ⓐ Ⓑ Ⓒ Ⓓ	268 Ⓐ Ⓑ Ⓒ Ⓓ
19 Ⓐ Ⓑ Ⓒ Ⓓ	69 Ⓐ Ⓑ Ⓒ Ⓓ	119 Ⓐ Ⓑ Ⓒ Ⓓ	169 Ⓐ Ⓑ Ⓒ Ⓓ	219 Ⓐ Ⓑ Ⓒ Ⓓ	269 Ⓐ Ⓑ Ⓒ Ⓓ
20 Ⓐ Ⓑ Ⓒ Ⓓ	70 Ⓐ Ⓑ Ⓒ Ⓓ	120 Ⓐ Ⓑ Ⓒ Ⓓ	170 Ⓐ Ⓑ Ⓒ Ⓓ	220 Ⓐ Ⓑ Ⓒ Ⓓ	270 Ⓐ Ⓑ Ⓒ Ⓓ
21 Ⓐ Ⓑ Ⓒ Ⓓ	71 Ⓐ Ⓑ Ⓒ Ⓓ	121 Ⓐ Ⓑ Ⓒ Ⓓ	171 Ⓐ Ⓑ Ⓒ Ⓓ	221 Ⓐ Ⓑ Ⓒ Ⓓ	271 Ⓐ Ⓑ Ⓒ Ⓓ
22 Ⓐ Ⓑ Ⓒ Ⓓ	72 Ⓐ Ⓑ Ⓒ Ⓓ	122 Ⓐ Ⓑ Ⓒ Ⓓ	172 Ⓐ Ⓑ Ⓒ Ⓓ	222 Ⓐ Ⓑ Ⓒ Ⓓ	272 Ⓐ Ⓑ Ⓒ Ⓓ
23 Ⓐ Ⓑ Ⓒ Ⓓ	73 Ⓐ Ⓑ Ⓒ Ⓓ	123 Ⓐ Ⓑ Ⓒ Ⓓ	173 Ⓐ Ⓑ Ⓒ Ⓓ	223 Ⓐ Ⓑ Ⓒ Ⓓ	273 Ⓐ Ⓑ Ⓒ Ⓓ
24 Ⓐ Ⓑ Ⓒ Ⓓ	74 Ⓐ Ⓑ Ⓒ Ⓓ	124 Ⓐ Ⓑ Ⓒ Ⓓ	174 Ⓐ Ⓑ Ⓒ Ⓓ	224 Ⓐ Ⓑ Ⓒ Ⓓ	274 Ⓐ Ⓑ Ⓒ Ⓓ
25 Ⓐ Ⓑ Ⓒ Ⓓ	75 Ⓐ Ⓑ Ⓒ Ⓓ	125 Ⓐ Ⓑ Ⓒ Ⓓ	175 Ⓐ Ⓑ Ⓒ Ⓓ	225 Ⓐ Ⓑ Ⓒ Ⓓ	275 Ⓐ Ⓑ Ⓒ Ⓓ
26 Ⓐ Ⓑ Ⓒ Ⓓ	76 Ⓐ Ⓑ Ⓒ Ⓓ	126 Ⓐ Ⓑ Ⓒ Ⓓ	176 Ⓐ Ⓑ Ⓒ Ⓓ	226 Ⓐ Ⓑ Ⓒ Ⓓ	276 Ⓐ Ⓑ Ⓒ Ⓓ
27 Ⓐ Ⓑ Ⓒ Ⓓ	77 Ⓐ Ⓑ Ⓒ Ⓓ	127 Ⓐ Ⓑ Ⓒ Ⓓ	177 Ⓐ Ⓑ Ⓒ Ⓓ	227 Ⓐ Ⓑ Ⓒ Ⓓ	277 Ⓐ Ⓑ Ⓒ Ⓓ
28 Ⓐ Ⓑ Ⓒ Ⓓ	78 Ⓐ Ⓑ Ⓒ Ⓓ	128 Ⓐ Ⓑ Ⓒ Ⓓ	178 Ⓐ Ⓑ Ⓒ Ⓓ	228 Ⓐ Ⓑ Ⓒ Ⓓ	278 Ⓐ Ⓑ Ⓒ Ⓓ
29 Ⓐ Ⓑ Ⓒ Ⓓ	79 Ⓐ Ⓑ Ⓒ Ⓓ	129 Ⓐ Ⓑ Ⓒ Ⓓ	179 Ⓐ Ⓑ Ⓒ Ⓓ	229 Ⓐ Ⓑ Ⓒ Ⓓ	279 Ⓐ Ⓑ Ⓒ Ⓓ
30 Ⓐ Ⓑ Ⓒ Ⓓ	80 Ⓐ Ⓑ Ⓒ Ⓓ	130 Ⓐ Ⓑ Ⓒ Ⓓ	180 Ⓐ Ⓑ Ⓒ Ⓓ	230 Ⓐ Ⓑ Ⓒ Ⓓ	280 Ⓐ Ⓑ Ⓒ Ⓓ
31 Ⓐ Ⓑ Ⓒ Ⓓ	81 Ⓐ Ⓑ Ⓒ Ⓓ	131 Ⓐ Ⓑ Ⓒ Ⓓ	181 Ⓐ Ⓑ Ⓒ Ⓓ	231 Ⓐ Ⓑ Ⓒ Ⓓ	281 Ⓐ Ⓑ Ⓒ
32 Ⓐ Ⓑ Ⓒ Ⓓ	82 Ⓐ Ⓑ Ⓒ Ⓓ	132 Ⓐ Ⓑ Ⓒ Ⓓ	182 Ⓐ Ⓑ Ⓒ Ⓓ	232 Ⓐ Ⓑ Ⓒ Ⓓ	282 Ⓐ Ⓑ Ⓒ Ⓓ
33 Ⓐ Ⓑ Ⓒ Ⓓ	83 Ⓐ Ⓑ Ⓒ Ⓓ	133 Ⓐ Ⓑ Ⓒ Ⓓ	183 Ⓐ Ⓑ Ⓒ Ⓓ	233 Ⓐ Ⓑ Ⓒ Ⓓ	283 Ⓐ Ⓑ Ⓒ Ⓓ
34 Ⓐ Ⓑ Ⓒ Ⓓ	84 Ⓐ Ⓑ Ⓒ Ⓓ	134 Ⓐ Ⓑ Ⓒ Ⓓ	184 Ⓐ Ⓑ Ⓒ Ⓓ	234 Ⓐ Ⓑ Ⓒ Ⓓ	284 Ⓐ Ⓑ Ⓒ Ⓓ
35 Ⓐ Ⓑ Ⓒ Ⓓ	85 Ⓐ Ⓑ Ⓒ Ⓓ	135 Ⓐ Ⓑ Ⓒ Ⓓ	185 Ⓐ Ⓑ Ⓒ Ⓓ	235 Ⓐ Ⓑ Ⓒ Ⓓ	285 Ⓐ Ⓑ Ⓒ Ⓓ
36 Ⓐ Ⓑ Ⓒ Ⓓ	86 Ⓐ Ⓑ Ⓒ Ⓓ	136 Ⓐ Ⓑ Ⓒ Ⓓ	186 Ⓐ Ⓑ Ⓒ Ⓓ	236 Ⓐ Ⓑ Ⓒ Ⓓ	286 Ⓐ Ⓑ Ⓒ Ⓓ
37 Ⓐ Ⓑ Ⓒ Ⓓ	87 Ⓐ Ⓑ Ⓒ Ⓓ	137 Ⓐ Ⓑ Ⓒ Ⓓ	187 Ⓐ Ⓑ Ⓒ Ⓓ	237 Ⓐ Ⓑ Ⓒ Ⓓ	287 Ⓐ Ⓑ Ⓒ Ⓓ
38 Ⓐ Ⓑ Ⓒ Ⓓ	88 Ⓐ Ⓑ Ⓒ Ⓓ	138 Ⓐ Ⓑ Ⓒ Ⓓ	188 Ⓐ Ⓑ Ⓒ Ⓓ	238 Ⓐ Ⓑ Ⓒ Ⓓ	288 Ⓐ Ⓑ Ⓒ Ⓓ
39 Ⓐ Ⓑ Ⓒ Ⓓ	89 Ⓐ Ⓑ Ⓒ Ⓓ	139 Ⓐ Ⓑ Ⓒ Ⓓ	189 Ⓐ Ⓑ Ⓒ Ⓓ	239 Ⓐ Ⓑ Ⓒ Ⓓ	289 Ⓐ Ⓑ Ⓒ Ⓓ
40 Ⓐ Ⓑ Ⓒ Ⓓ	90 Ⓐ Ⓑ Ⓒ Ⓓ	140 Ⓐ Ⓑ Ⓒ Ⓓ	190 Ⓐ Ⓑ Ⓒ Ⓓ	240 Ⓐ Ⓑ Ⓒ Ⓓ	290 Ⓐ Ⓑ Ⓒ Ⓓ
41 Ⓐ Ⓑ Ⓒ Ⓓ	91 Ⓐ Ⓑ Ⓒ Ⓓ	141 Ⓐ Ⓑ Ⓒ Ⓓ	191 Ⓐ Ⓑ Ⓒ Ⓓ	241 Ⓐ Ⓑ Ⓒ Ⓓ	291 Ⓐ Ⓑ Ⓒ Ⓓ
42 Ⓐ Ⓑ Ⓒ Ⓓ	92 Ⓐ Ⓑ Ⓒ Ⓓ	142 Ⓐ Ⓑ Ⓒ Ⓓ	192 Ⓐ Ⓑ Ⓒ Ⓓ	242 Ⓐ Ⓑ Ⓒ Ⓓ	292 Ⓐ Ⓑ Ⓒ Ⓓ
43 Ⓐ Ⓑ Ⓒ Ⓓ	93 Ⓐ Ⓑ Ⓒ Ⓓ	143 Ⓐ Ⓑ Ⓒ Ⓓ	193 Ⓐ Ⓑ Ⓒ Ⓓ	243 Ⓐ Ⓑ Ⓒ Ⓓ	293 Ⓐ Ⓑ Ⓒ Ⓓ
44 Ⓐ Ⓑ Ⓒ Ⓓ	94 Ⓐ Ⓑ Ⓒ Ⓓ	144 Ⓐ Ⓑ Ⓒ Ⓓ	194 Ⓐ Ⓑ Ⓒ Ⓓ	244 Ⓐ Ⓑ Ⓒ Ⓓ	294 Ⓐ Ⓑ Ⓒ Ⓓ
45 Ⓐ Ⓑ Ⓒ Ⓓ	95 Ⓐ Ⓑ Ⓒ Ⓓ	145 Ⓐ Ⓑ Ⓒ Ⓓ	195 Ⓐ Ⓑ Ⓒ Ⓓ	245 Ⓐ Ⓑ Ⓒ Ⓓ	295 Ⓐ Ⓑ Ⓒ Ⓓ
46 Ⓐ Ⓑ Ⓒ Ⓓ	96 Ⓐ Ⓑ Ⓒ Ⓓ	146 Ⓐ Ⓑ Ⓒ Ⓓ	196 Ⓐ Ⓑ Ⓒ Ⓓ	246 Ⓐ Ⓑ Ⓒ Ⓓ	296 Ⓐ Ⓑ Ⓒ Ⓓ
47 Ⓐ Ⓑ Ⓒ Ⓓ	97 Ⓐ Ⓑ Ⓒ Ⓓ	147 Ⓐ Ⓑ Ⓒ Ⓓ	197 Ⓐ Ⓑ Ⓒ Ⓓ	247 Ⓐ Ⓑ Ⓒ Ⓓ	297 Ⓐ Ⓑ Ⓒ Ⓓ
48 Ⓐ Ⓑ Ⓒ Ⓓ	98 Ⓐ Ⓑ Ⓒ Ⓓ	148 Ⓐ Ⓑ Ⓒ Ⓓ	198 Ⓐ Ⓑ Ⓒ Ⓓ	248 Ⓐ Ⓑ Ⓒ Ⓓ	298 Ⓐ Ⓑ Ⓒ Ⓓ
49 Ⓐ Ⓑ Ⓒ Ⓓ	99 Ⓐ Ⓑ Ⓒ Ⓓ	149 Ⓐ Ⓑ Ⓒ Ⓓ	199 Ⓐ Ⓑ Ⓒ Ⓓ	249 Ⓐ Ⓑ Ⓒ Ⓓ	299 Ⓐ Ⓑ Ⓒ Ⓓ
50 Ⓐ Ⓑ Ⓒ Ⓓ	100 Ⓐ Ⓑ Ⓒ Ⓓ	150 Ⓐ Ⓑ Ⓒ Ⓓ	200 Ⓐ Ⓑ Ⓒ Ⓓ	250 Ⓐ Ⓑ Ⓒ Ⓓ	300 Ⓐ Ⓑ Ⓒ Ⓓ

ASSESSMENT OF MOCK TEST ON THE BASIS OF SCORES- BY THE AUTHORS

Score	Interpretation	Authors Comments
270 Plus	OUTSTANDING	• Highly appreciable score. Keep doing MCQs
240 – 269	EXCELLENT PERFORMANCE	• Great score. Pay attention on some silly mistakes
210 – 239	VERY GOOD PERFORMANCE	• Keep doing MCQs and continue with revising the notes • Advised not to flow in overconfidence
180 – 209	GOOD PERFORMANCE	• Learn the time management while doing MCQs • Keep moving on same track and avoid overconfidence • Work on anxiety issues if there are any
150 – 179	SATISFACTORY	• You are going well. Continue on the same track • Lacking confidence on studied topics due to lack of revision • Practice more MCQs
130 – 149	UNSATISFACTORY	• You are studying but lacking concept and lack of revision. • Improve on silly mistakes by working on basic subjects • Definite improvement expected
Below 130	POOR SCORE	• Need to work on basic subjects • Conceptual based study is recommended • Do FMGE Solutions to cover 3–4 times with explanations

INSTRUCTIONS FOR FILLING THE SHEET

1. This sheet should not be folded or crushed.
2. Use only blue/black ball pen to fill the circles.
3. Use of pencil is strictly prohibited.
4. Circles should be darkened properly and completely.
5. Cutting & erasing on this sheet is not allowed.
6. Do not use any stray marks on the sheet.
7. Do not use marker, white fluid or any other device to hide the shading already done.

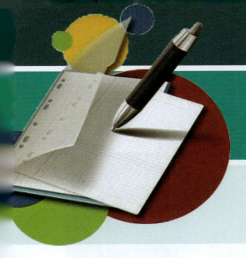

Model Test Paper-II

1. A feature of high-pressure low volume cuffs is?
   a. Higher incidence of postoperative sore throat
   b. Mucosal ischemia
   c. Higher risk of aspiration
   d. Risk of spontaneous extubation

2. Identify the instrument:

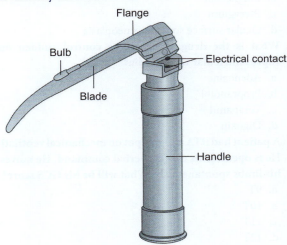

   a. Rigid bronchoscope   b. Laryngoscope
   c. Otoscope   d. Urethroscope

3. Options for "invasive airway" include.
   a. Supraglottic airway devices
   b. Endotracheal intubation
   c. Cricothyrotomy
   d. Combitube

4. The percentage of drug remaining in the plasma after 3 half life is
   a. 6.25%   b. 12%
   c. 6%   d. 12.5%

5. In preoperative interview patient tells you about history of DM II since last 10 years. Which particular investigation will you ask to check for recent control of the disease?
   a. Urine ketones   b. Post prandial sugar
   c. Fasting sugar   d. HBA1c

6. Daily production of CSF is?
   a. 250 ml/day   b. 500 ml/day
   c. 750 ml/day   d. 1000 ml/day

7. The most effective way of preventing tetanus:
   a. Surgical debridement and toilet
   b. Hyperbaric oxygen
   c. Antibiotics
   d. Tetanus toxoid

8. All are true regarding pseudomembranous colitis except:
   a. It is caused by Clostridium difficile
   b. The organism is a normal commensal of gut
   c. It is due to production of phospholipase A
   d. It is treated by vancomycin

9. The Corynebacterium species causing prosthetic valve endocarditis is
   a. C. Jeikeium   b. C. Ulcerans
   c. C. Hoffmannii   d. C. XEROSIS

10. The best method for destroying anthrax spores is:
    a. Dry heat at 140°C for 1 hour
    b. Boiling for 10 minutes
    c. 5% phenol for 6 hours
    d. Formaldehyde 2% for 20 minutes

11. The mu(μ) rhythm on EEG arises from?
    a. Primary visual area
    b. Primary auditory area
    c. Primary sensorimotor area
    d. Primary olfactory area

12. Pruning is:
    a. Programmed elimination during development
    b. Programmed elimination during senility
    c. Programmed elimination during cancer
    d. Programmed elimination during irradiation

13. Copropraxia is seen in:
    a. Dissociative disorder   b. Frontotemporal Dementia
    c. Tourette's disorder   d. Narcolepsy

14. All of the following are features of pathological grief, except:
    a. Onset of grief after 2 weeks
    b. Grief beyond 6 months
    c. Absence of grief symptoms
    d. Fleeting experience of the dead in the initial few days after their death

15. Which of the following symptoms is not part of a panic attack?
    a. Tinnitus   b. Impending doom
    c. Breathing discomfort d. Trembling

FMGE Solutions Screening Examination

16. Which ultrasound imaging mode accurately displays reflector depth?
    a. B-mode
    b. M-mode
    c. C-mode
    d. A-mode
17. Identify the gene that encodes for serine/ threonine kinase & with a loss of function mutation causes Peutz Jeghers syndrome:
    a. SMAD 4
    b. STK 11
    c. WT 1
    d. E cadherin
18. All of the following are paraneoplastic syndrome that can be associated with lung carcinoma except:
    a. Cushing's syndrome
    b. Hypercalcaemia
    c. Hypertrophic osteoarthropathy
    d. Hypoglycemia
19. High level of beta hCG is seen in all except:
    a. Neural tube defect
    b. Germ cell tumor
    c. Gestational trophoblastic disease
    d. Multiple pregnancy
20. Calculate bioavailability of the drug shown in image if AUC(Injected)= 450 and AUC(oral)= 150

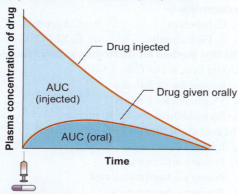

    a. 25.55
    b. 33.33
    c. 35.66
    d. 36.66
21. Toughest layer of cornea that protects against infection to seep through the aqueous humor is
    a. Endothelium
    b. Stroma
    c. Descemet's membrane
    d. Bowman's membrane
22. Identify the sign

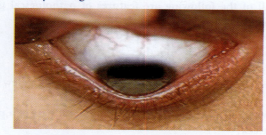

    a. Rizutti Sign
    b. Munson Sign
    c. Bow tie pattern
    d. Bull's eye sign

23. Identify

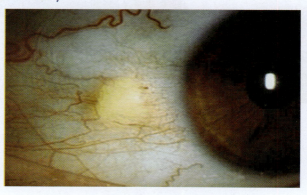

    a. Bitot's spots
    b. Pinguecula
    c. Pterygium
    d. Ocular surface squamous neoplasia
24. What is the drug of choice to control sudden onset supraventricular tachycardia?
    a. Adenosine
    b. Propranolol
    c. Verapamil
    d. Digoxin
25. A patient had RTA and was put on mechanical ventilation. He is opening his eyes on verbal command. He moves all his limbs spontaneously. What will be his GCS score?
    a. 9T
    b. 10T
    c. 11T
    d. 12T
26. Which is the most common mechanism of arrhythmia?
    a. Re-entry
    b. Early after depolarization
    c. Late after depolarization
    d. Automaticity
27. Visual field defect seen in Optic chiasma damage is
    a. Bitemporal hemianopia
    b. Pie in the floor (inferior Quadrantanopia)
    c. Pie in the sky (superior Quadrantanopia)
    d. Binasal Hemianopia
28. Nerve which is NOT directly related to humerus:
    a. Ulnar nerve
    b. Median nerve
    c. Radial
    d. Axillary nerve
29. Thoracic outlet syndrome is best diagnosed by:
    a. MRI
    b. CT
    c. Digital subtraction angiography
    d. Clinical examination

30. Which statement is true about the heart sounds:
    a. S1 is of higher frequency and longer duration as compared to S2.
    b. S2 is of higher frequency and longer duration as compared to S1.
    c. S1 has higher frequency but shorter duration compared to S2.
    d. S2 has higher frequency but shorter duration compared to S1.
31. Most medially located renal structure is:
    a. Renal pyramids   b. Minor calyx
    c. Renal papillae   d. Renal pelvis
32. Finger by which all the muscles in the hand can be tested
    a. Index   b. Ring
    c. Thumb   d. Middle
33. Select the wrong pair of Yolk muscles
    a. RSR LIO   b. RSO LIR
    c. RMR LMR   d. RIR LSO
34. Single skin lesion is seen in which type of leprosy?
    a. TT   b. BL
    c. BT   d. LL
35. All the following are inspiratory muscles except
    a. External intercostal b. Internal intercostal
    c. Diaphragm   d. Elastic recoiling of lungs
36. Which of these is true about trachea?
    a. 20 cm long
    b. Trachea bifurcates at level of T6, in deep inspiration
    c. Lined by stratified columnar epithelium
    d. Tracheal cartilage is circular
37. On breast MRI, which of the following features of a breast mass is more suggestive of a malignant lesion than a benign lesion?
    a. Low-signal internal septations
    b. Lobulated mass which shows no enhancement
    c. Rim-like enhancement of the mass
    d. A focal area of hypointense T2 signal adjacent to the mass
38. Which of the following is the first to improve after surgery for GH producing adenoma?
    a. Impaired glucose tolerance
    b. Hypertension
    c. Cardiomegaly
    d. Soft tissue swelling
39. Which is the first drug to be started in Sheehan's syndrome?
    a. Gonadotropins   b. Estrogen
    c. Thyroxine   d. Corticosteroids
40. Prolactinoma presents with?
    a. Inferior quadrantanopia
    b. Superior quadrantanopia
    c. Priapism
    d. Failure of lactation
41. All are true about Diabetes insipidus except.
    a. Low urine osmolality
    b. Dilutional Hyponatremia
    c. Water deprivation test is used for diagnosis
    d. Polyuria
42. Inactivation of cortisol into cortisone occurs mainly in which organ?
    a. Lungs
    b. Liver
    c. Adrenals
    d. Kidney
43. Conn's syndrome is characterized by all except?
    a. Polyuria   b. Polydipsia
    c. Weakness   d. Anasarca
44. Which is not a feature of MEN 3?
    a. Medullated corneal nerve fibers
    b. Megacolon
    c. Mucosal neuroma
    d. Meningioma
45. In the clinical sign shown below, which is the best test for diagnosis?

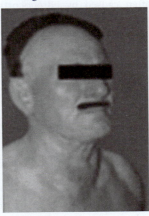 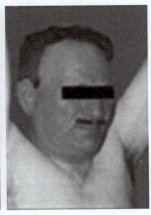

   a. Thyroid Function test b. Thyroid Scan
   c. USG Neck   d. CT neck
46. Reversible Dementia is a feature of?
    a. Hyperparathyroidism   b. Hypothyroidism
    c. Hyperthyroidism   d. Cushing's disease
47. TSH cannot be used for monitoring response to treatment in?
    a. Primary hypothyroidism
    b. Secondary hypothyroidism
    c. Thyroprivic hypothyroidism
    d. Iodine deficiency
48. Blade of grass lesion of found in?
    a. Osteoporosis
    b. Thalassemia
    c. Paget's disease
    d. Carcinoma prostate

FMGE Solutions Screening Examination

49. Which type of diabetes has impaired glucose induced secretion of insulin with preserved β cell mass?
   a. MODY
   b. Wolfram syndrome
   c. Type 1 diabetes
   d. Latent autoimmune diabetes in adults

50. Which of the following changes in the breast is NOT associated with pregnancy?
   a. Accumulation of lymphocytes, plasma cells, and eosinophils within the breast.
   b. Enlargement of breast alveoli.
   c. Release of colostrum.
   d. Accumulation of secretory products in minor duct lumina.

51. Hypercortisolism:
   a. Is most often ACTH-dependent, owing to an ACTH-producing pituitary adenoma.
   b. May be caused by small cell carcinoma of the lung, carcinoid tumors, tumors of the endocrine pancreas, pheochromocytoma, or medullary thyroid carcinoma (MTC).
   c. In children is most often caused by adrenocortical neoplasia.
   d. All of the above

52. Estrogen receptor activity is clinically useful in predicting
   a. The presence of ovarian cancer
   b. The presence of metastatic disease
   c. Response to chemotherapy
   d. Response to hormonal manipulation

53. All of the following statements are true regarding histological features of ARDS except:
   a. In the acute stage, the lungs are heavy, firm, red, and boggy
   b. Alveolar wall are lined by hyaline membrane
   c. In the organizing stage, type I pneumocytes proliferate
   d. In most cases the granulation tissue resolves, leaving minimal functional impairment

54. All of the following statements are true regarding asbestosis except:
   a. Amphiboles are more pathogenic
   b. It begins in a upper zone
   c. Can cause mesothelioma
   d. Pulmonary hypertension in be seen

55. Most common cause of community acquired pneumonia is:
   a. S. Pneumoniae
   b. S. Aureus
   c. M. Pneumoniae
   d. Klebsiella

56. CO_2 is carried in blood mainly by/in:
   a. Dissolved form
   b. Carboxy-Hb
   c. Bicarbonate form
   d. Carbamino-compounds

57. Epilepsy is defined as:
   a. One or more unprovoked seizures
   b. Two or more unprovoked seizures
   c. Three or more unprovoked seizures
   d. Four or more unprovoked seizures

58. Adenocarcinoma is the predominant malignant lesion in which of the following?
   a. Hard palate
   b. Lip
   c. Anterior two-thirds of the tongue
   d. Larynx

59. The most important hepatic function to consider after hepatic resection is:
   a. Hepatic synthetic function.
   b. Detoxification
   c. The liver's role in lipid metabolism.
   d. The liver's role in vitamin metabolism.

60. A patient is found to develop evidence of hepatitis approximately eight weeks after receiving blood transfusions during a surgical procedure. Which of the following statement(s) is/are true?
   a. The virus responsible is most likely hepatitis C
   b. A chronic carrier state will never develop in most patients
   c. There is no role for interferon in the treatment of chronic hepatitis C viral infection
   d. Chronic infection with hepatitis C is not associated with an increased risk of developing hepatocellular carcinoma

61. Which of the following statement(s) is/are true concerning the pathophysiology of variceal hemorrhage?
   a. All patients with portal hypertension will develop esophageal varices
   b. All patients with esophageal varices eventually bleed
   c. Variceal size can predict the incidence of variceal hemorrhage
   d. None of the above

62. Most common skin infection in children is:-
   a. Scabies
   b. Warts
   c. Impetigo contagiosum
   d. Molluscum contagiosum

63. Hypopigmented patches may be seen in:
   a. Becker's nevus
   b. Nevus anemicus
   c. Nevus of Ota
   d. Nevus of Ito

64. All of these are disorders associated with vitiligo except?
   a. Androgenic Alopecia
   b. Hypothyroidism
   c. Addison's disease
   d. Diabetes mellitus

65. Radial keratotomy is done for:
   a. Myopia
   b. Hypermetropia
   c. Corneal scar
   d. All the above

66. Snowflake cataract is seen in:
   a. Myotonic dystrophy
   b. Atopic dermatitis
   c. Diabetes mellitus
   d. Neurofibromatosis

67. Which of these is not true regarding rubella cataract:
    a. Pearly white cataract
    b. May harbor virus inside the lens
    c. Can be associated with cardiovascular anomalies
    d. Reversible
68. Correct sequence of sperm movement is:
    a. Rete testis–straight tubules–efferent tubules
    b. Straight tubules–Rete testis–efferent tubules
    c. Straight tubules–efferent tubules–epididymis
    d. Straight tubules–Rete testis–epididymis
69. A 62-year-old farmer had received chemotherapy for cancer of the head and neck. He has developed classical multidrug resistance (MDR) to which of the following?
    a. Alkylating agents   b. Antimetabolites
    c. Bleomycin   d. Vinca alkaloid
70. The renal arteries arise at which intervertebral level?
    a. T11/T12   b. T12/L1
    c. L1/L2   d. L2/L3
71. The antibody with the highest affinity is
    a. IgG   b. IgA
    c. IgM   d. IgD
72. Paul Bunnel is a type of:
    a. Agglutination reaction   b. CFT
    c. Precipitation   d. Flocculation
73. Membrane attack complex is made up of
    a. C3Bb   b. C3b4b
    c. C3b Bb 3b   d. C5b,6,7,8,9
74. C1 esterase deficiency leads to
    a. Systemic Lupus erythematosus
    b. Angioneurotic edema
    c. Pyogenic infections
    d. Disseminated Neisserial infection
75. Endogenous pyrogens are
    a. IL-1 & TNF-α   b. IL-2 & TNF-α
    c. IL-1 & TNF-β   d. IL-1 & IFN-γ
76. Which of the following has the least failure rate?
    a. CuT   b. LNG IUCD
    c. DMPA   d. OC pills
77. Paralysis of 3rd, 4th, 6th nerves with involvement of ophthalmic division of 5th nerve, localizes the lesion to:
    a. Cavernous sinus   b. Apex of the orbit
    c. Brainstem   d. Base of the skull
78. Which of the following is related to floor of tympanic cavity?
    a. Tensor tympani muscle   b. Eustachian tube.
    c. Internal carotid artery   d. Internal jugular vein
79. All are true about Zenker's diverticulum except
    a. Results due to neuromuscular incoordination
    b. Lies in the anterior wall of pharynx
    c. They are normal in pig
    d. Food may get accumulated

80. Derivatives of urogenital sinus include all except
    a. Bladder   b. Membranous urethra
    c. Prostatic urethra   d. Ejaculatory duct
81. Which is derived from Wolffian duct?
    a. Appendix of testis
    b. Uterus
    c. Appendix of epididymis
    d. Hydatid of morgagni (appendix of testis)
82. Which of the following is not a radiographic feature of pericardial effusion?
    a. 'Flask shaped' cardiac silhouette
    b. Pulmonary oligemia
    c. Pulmonary plethora
    d. Spurious cardiomegaly
83. Visual defect is contralateral homonymous hemianopia with macular sparing. What is the cause for it?
    a. Block in optic tract
    b. Block in optic nerve
    c. Block in optic chiasma
    d. Block in posterior cerebral artery supplying visual cortex
84. Which of the following is not a cerebellar lesion?
    a. Ataxia
    b. Hypertonia
    c. Intentional tremors
    d. Nystagmus
85. Which of the following can cause both superior and inferior rib notching?
    a. Blalock Taussig shunt
    b. Neurofibromatosis-1
    c. Pulmonary atresia with large VSD
    d. Interrupted Aorta
86. The most sensitive and practical technique for detection of myocardial ischemia in the perioperative period is:
    a. Magnetic Resonance Spectrography
    b. Radio-labeled lactate determination
    c. Direct measurement of end-diastolic pressure
    d. Regional wall motion abnormality detected with the trans-esophageal echocardiography (TEE)
87. Which of the following is associated with atresia of the foramen of magendie and foramina of luschka?
    a. Cranium bifidum with meningoencephalocele
    b. Cranium bifidum with meningohydroencephalocele
    c. Arnold – Chiari syndrome
    d. Dandy – Walker syndrome
88. Which is true about the skin disease seen in the picture below?
    a. Most common contagious skin disease in children
    b. Caused by arthropods
    c. Caused by Corynebacterium minutissimum
    d. Idiosyncratic drug reaction

FMGE Solutions Screening Examination

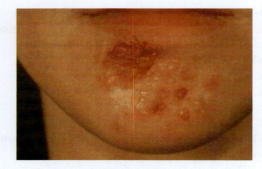

89. Which of these is a Rave drug?
    a. Cannabis   b. Hashish
    c. Ecstasy   d. Heroin
90. Enzyme catalysing the rate-limiting step of glycolysis is:
    a. Hexokinase   b. Phosphofructokinase-1
    c. Phosphoglyceratekinase d. Pyruvate Kinase
91. Which artery does not contribute to Little's area:
    a. Septal branch of facial artery
    b. Anterior ethmoidal artery
    c. Sphenopalatine artery
    d. Posterior ethmoidal artery
92. Fulminant hepatitis is most often seen with-
    a. HCV
    b. HBV
    c. HDV
    d. HEV
93. Following a sudden impact in an accident, a 34-year-old race car driver becomes unconscious and is admitted to the hospital. A CT scan is performed, and a right space-occupying lesion is noted. What is the most likely diagnosis?

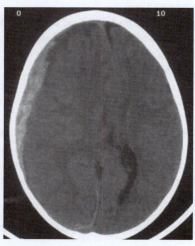

    a. Corpus callosum injury
    b. Pituitary apoplexia
    c. Acute subdural hematoma
    d. Acute epidural hematoma

94. Which of the following is correct regarding "with the rule astigmatism"?
    a. Horizontal Diameter is more
    b. Vertical Diameter is more
    c. Oblique Diameter is more
    d. None of the above
95. Not true regarding atropine
    a. Used as an eye ointment
    b. Used in refraction in children less than 5 yr of age
    c. Fast action
    d. Experimentally used in treatment of myopia
96. Which blood product is best for multiple clotting factor deficiency and active bleeding?
    a. FFP
    b. Whole blood
    c. Packed RBC
    d. Cryoprecipitate
97. Postural tremors are seen in all except?
    a. Alcohol withdrawal
    b. Essential tremors
    c. Generalized paresis
    d. Physiological tremors
98. A patient with ITP on steroids underwent splenectomy. Patient got fever on 3rd post-operative day. Next investigation is likely to reveal?
    a. Left lower lobe consolidation
    b. Port site infection
    c. Focal Intra-abdominal collection
    d. UTI
99. Which statement is most appropriate for DIC?
    a. Increased fibrinogen
    b. Increased D dimer
    c. Resolves if causative factor removed
    d. Absence of bleeding abnormalities rules out DIC
100. Thrombocythemia is characterized by?
    a. Platelets elevation
    b. Low Platelets
    c. Neutrophilia
    d. Monocytosis
101. Which of these is a clotting factor?
    a. Kallikrein
    b. Platelet phospholipid
    c. Calcium
    d. All of these
102. Microcytic Hypochromic anemia is seen in:
    a. Iron deficiency   b. Thalassemia
    c. Hypoproteinemia   d. All of the above
103. Positive predictive value is a function of sensitivity, specificity and
    a. Incidence   b. Prevalence
    c. Negative predictive value d. Accuracy

104. Advantages of dialysis over renal transplantation include
    a. Less expense if the treatment continues for less than 2 years
    b. Increased number of pregnancies in female dialysis patients
    c. Return of normal menses in female dialysis patients
    d. Less anemia in dialysis patients
105. Which committee is known as "The Committee on Multipurpose Workers under Health and Family Planning"
    a. Kartar Singh Committee
    b. Mudaliar committee
    c. Chadah committee
    d. Jungalwalla committee
106. Site most infected in genital warts?
    a. Vulva
    b. Cervix
    c. Vagina
    d. Anus
107. Incubation period of chicken pox is:
    a. 14–18 hours
    b. 3 days
    c. 1 week
    d. 2–3 weeks
108. Protein quantity is assessed by?
    a. Amino acid score   b. NPU
    c. PE ratio   d. None
109. Which of the following portion of optic nerve is longest?
    a. Intraorbital   b. Intraocular
    c. Intracranial   d. Intracanalicular
110. Which of the following is not a primary sign of Vitamin A deficiency?
    a. Corneal xerosis   b. Bitots Spots
    c. Corneal Scar   d. Keratomalacia
111. Economic blindness is defined as
    a. Vision <6/60 to 3/60   b. Vision <3/60 to 1/60
    c. Vision <1/60 to Finger counting
    d. No PL
112. Bow tie optic atrophy is seen in: -

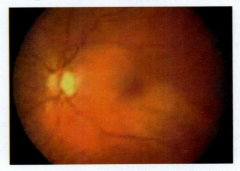

    a. Glaucoma   b. Ischemic optic neuropathy
    c. Chiasma lesion   d. Optic tract lesion

113. 35 year Alcoholic has presented with 2 episodes of hematemesis. On examination his pulse rate is 100/min with BP of 90/60 mm Hg. Per abdomen examination shows spleen palpable 3 cm below costal margin. Which is true about this patient?
    a. Elevated CRP and Low C3
    b. Most common site of bleeding is First part of duodenum
    c. Urgent Elective intubation of patient
    d. The increased pressure of portal vein pressure should be lowered with octreotide
114. All of the following are true regarding G.E.R.D. except?
    a. Occurs during transient relaxation of LES.
    b. Can present with nocturnal cough
    c. Bicarbonate secreted by esophageal mucosa neutralizes the acid
    d. Normal esophageal mucosa on endoscopy excludes G.E.R.D.
115. Gastro-esophageal tear is best detected with:
    a. CT with oral contrast   b. Angiography
    c. UGI endoscopy   d. Barium swallow
116. The following conditions can cause protein-losing enteropathy except?
    a. Ulcerative colitis   b. Irritable bowel syndrome
    c. Celiac disease   d. Lymphoma
117. Malabsorption syndrome features include all, except:
    a. Anemia   b. Constipation
    c. Tetany   d. Steatorrhea
118. Aspirin is given for?
    a. Peptic ulcer disease   b. Transient ischemic attack
    c. Hemorrhagic stroke   d. Protein losing enteropathy
119. Which of the following is regulated by Calcium-Calmodulin complex?
    a. Smooth muscle contraction
    b. Cell division
    c. Endocytosis
    d. All of the above
120. Most common cause of acute pancreatitis is:
    a. Trauma   b. Hyperlipidemia
    c. Alcoholism   d. Viral infection
121. A 20-year-old female presents with excess facial hair and oligomenorrhea, increased levels of free testosterone, and normal ovaries on USG. Most likely diagnosis is:
    a. PCOD
    b. Adrenal hyperplasia
    c. Idiopathic hirsutism
    d. Testosterone-secreting tumor
122. Decreased dietary intake of potassium is incriminated in leading to all except?
    a. Hypertension
    b. Stroke
    c. CHF
    d. Diabetes mellitus

FMGE Solutions Screening Examination

123. Acute hyponatremia becomes symptomatic at:
   a. <135 mEq
   b. <125 mEq
   c. <120 mEq
   d. <110 meq

124. Chronic vomiting leads to?
   a. Metabolic acidosis
   b. Metabolic alkalosis
   c. Respiratory acidosis
   d. Respiratory alkalosis

125. Blast crisis leads to.
   a. Hyperphosphatemia
   b. Hypophosphatemia
   c. Hyperkalemia
   d. Hypokalemia

126. What is the sequence of HIV following entry into a host cell?
   a. RNA – DNA – RNA
   b. RNA – DNA
   c. DNA – RNA
   d. DNA – RNA – DNA

127. Dose of folic acid in prophylaxis of neural tube defects (in micrograms) in a primigravida, without any specific risk factors is?
   a. 40
   b. 400
   c. 4000
   d. None of above

128. Approximate time interval between HIV infection and manifestations of AIDS is?
   a. 7.5 years
   b. 10 years
   c. 12 years
   d. 15 years

129. All of the following patients should be tested for respiratory tuberculosis except?
   a. HIV positive patients with persistent cough
   b. Diabetic patients with persistent cough
   c. Known case of extra-pulmonary TB with persistent cough
   d. Contact with sputum positive patient of TB with persistent cough

130. Burking includes:
   a. Choking
   b. Ligature
   c. Overlying
   d. Traumatic asphyxia

131. Drug of choice for the treatment of peptic ulcer caused due to chronic use of NSAIDs is:
   a. Pirenzepine
   b. Loxatidine
   c. Misoprostol
   d. Esomeprazole

132. Roopmati, a 56-year-old female with lymph-node-positive breast cancer was treated with systemic chemotherapy. Four weeks later, she developed frequent urination, suprapubic pain, dysuria, and hematuria. Which of the following could have prevented this patient's condition?
   a. Folinic acid
   b. Mesna
   c. Dexrazoxane
   d. Amifostine

133. You decide not to prescribe sildenafil in a patient because the patient told you that he is taking an antianginal drug. Which of the following can it be?
   a. Calcium channel blockers
   b. β adrenergic blockers
   c. Organic nitrates
   d. Angiotensin converting enzyme inhibitors

134. Which of the following is NOT associated with thiazide diuretics?
   a. Hypercalciuria
   b. Hyponatremia
   c. Hypokalemia
   d. Hyperuricemia

135. Which of the following statements about imipenem is most accurate?
   a. The drug has a narrow spectrum of antibacterial action
   b. It is used in fixed dose combination with sulbactum
   c. In renal dysfunction, dosage reductions are necessary to avoid seizures
   d. Imipenem is active against methicillin-resistant staphylococci

136. An old woman, Nanda suffered a stroke for which she was given alteplase. She improved considerably. To prevent the recurrence of stroke, this patient is most likely to be treated indefinitely with:
   a. Aspirin
   b. Warfarin
   c. Urokinase
   d. Enoxaparin

137. Mr. Surya Kant was prescribed a first generation H1 antihistamine drug. He should be advised to avoid:
   a. Driving motor vehicles
   b. Consuming processed cheese
   c. Strenuous physical exertion
   d. All of the above

138. Which of the following drugs is most likely to cause hypoglycemia when used as a monotherapy in the treatment of type 2 diabetes?
   a. Acarbose
   b. Glipizide
   c. Metformin
   d. Rosiglitazone

139. All of the following are tumor suppressor genes, EXCEPT
   a. RB
   b. P53
   c. VHL
   d. HER-2

140. Most common upper eyelid tumor is
   a. Squamous cell carcinoma
   b. Sebaceous cell carcinoma
   c. Basal cell carcinoma
   d. Malignant melanoma

141. Reversible loss of polarity with abnormality in size and shape of cells is known as:
   a. Metaplasia
   b. Dysplasia
   c. Hyperplasia
   d. Anaplasia

142. Dystrophic calcification is seen in:
   a. Atheroma
   b. Paget's disease
   c. Renal osteodystrophy
   d. Milk-alkali syndrome

143. Which one of the following is true of antemortem abrasions?
   a. Bright red colour
   b. Exudation of serum is more
   c. Vital reactions are seen
   d. All of the above

144. What is paradox gun:
    a. A shot gun with smooth barrel
    b. A shot gun whose muzzle end is rifled
    c. A shot gun whose muzzle wider
    d. A rifle that fires a single ball
145. In a firearm injury if there is burning, blackening, tattooing around the wound and it is circular in shape, then it is a:
    a. Close shot   b. Close contact shot
    c. Contact shot   d. Distant shot
146. Which of the following is not true about innate immunity?
    a. It is present prior to antigenic exposure
    b. It is relatively non-specific
    c. Memory is seen
    d. It is the first line of defense
147. HLA is located on:
    a. Long arm of chromosome 6
    b. Long arm of chromosome 3
    c. Short arm of chromosome 6
    d. Short arm of chromosome 3
148. Major source of Acetyl CoA:
    a. Triglycerides   b. Fatty acids
    c. Pyruvate   d. Alanine
149. Most important source of ATP:
    a. Oxidative phosphorylation
    b. Substrate level phosphorylation
    c. Aerobic glycolysis
    d. TCA
150. Cyanide is toxic because it:
    a. Inhibits cytochrome oxidase
    b. Forms cyan metHb
    c. Inhibits Na-K ATPase
    d. Inhibits ATP carrier in mitochondria
151. Barbiturates act on ETC complex:
    a. I   b. II
    c. III   d. IV
152. A 30-year-old presents with intractable vomiting and inability to eat or drink for the past 3 days. His blood glucose level is still normal. Which of the following is most important for the maintenance of Blood glucose in this patient?
    a. Liver   b. Heart
    c. Skeletal muscle d. Lysosome
153. Oil drop cataract is produced because of the activity of which enzyme?
    a. Aldose reductase   b. Galactose reductase
    c. Fructose dehydrogenase d. Sorbitol reductase
154. Which lipoprotein has maximum phospholipids?
    a. HDL   b. LDL
    c. VLDL   d. Chylomicrons

155. Vaccine indicated in HIV positive baby of a HIV positive mother is:
    a. Typhoral vaccine   b. Yellow fever vaccine
    c. BCG vaccine   d. Live varicella vaccine
156. Mortality is taken into account while computing:
    a. Total fertility rate   b. Gross reproduction rate
    c. Net reproduction rate   d. General fertility rate
157. Minimum number of post-natal visits to be done by a Healthworker in rural areas is/are:
    a. 1   b. 2
    c. 3   d. 4
158. Breastfeeding must be initiated within:
    a. Half an hour   b. One hour
    c. Two hours   d. Four hours
159. What is the content of pediatric iron folic acid tablet supplied under the reproductive and child health programme?
    a. Iron 60 mg, Folic Acid 500 mcg
    b. Iron 100 mg, Folic Acid 500 mcg
    c. Iron 500 mg, Folic Acid 100 mcg
    d. Iron 20 mg, Folic Acid 100 mcg
160. A group is addressed and a series of lectures is given on a specific health topic; this is a:
    a. Focused group discussion (FGD)
    b. Panel discussion
    c. Symposium
    d. Workshop
161. Primary health centre (PHC) is supposed to provide all except:
    a. Treatment of common ailments
    b. Surgeries for acute emergency conditions
    c. Vaccination
    d. Health education
162. Urine bag is disposed in _____ Biomedical waste management bag:
    a. White   b. Yellow
    c. Red   d. Black
163. Reid's index is increased in which of the following?
    a. Bronchiectasis   b. Bronchial asthma
    c. Chronic bronchitis d. Emphysema
164. Caplan's syndrome is seen in:
    a. COPD   b. Pneumoconiosis
    c. Pulmonary edema d. Bronchial asthma
165. Xanthogranulomatous pyelonephritis is often associated with infection by:
    a. Proteus   b. E. coli
    c. H. Influenza d. Klebsiella
166. Staghorn calculus is made of:
    a. Oxalate
    b. Phosphate
    c. Uric acid
    d. Cystine

FMGE Solutions Screening Examination

167. **Rule of nine to estimate surface area of a burnt patient was introduced by:**
    a. Mortix Kaposi
    b. Wallace
    c. Joseph Lister
    d. Thomas Barclay

168. **During fluid resuscitation in a burns patient using Parkland's formula, volume of fluid given in first 8 hours:**
    a. 25%
    b. 50%
    c. 75%
    d. 100%

169. **All of the following are markers of melanoma except:**
    a. S-100
    b. Cytokeratin-20
    c. HMB-45
    d. Vimentin

170. **Prognostic factor in head injury:**
    a. Age of patient
    b. Glasgow coma scale
    c. Mode of injury
    d. Presence of facial trauma

171. **Most common cause of subarachnoid hemorrhage is:**
    a. Hypertension
    b. AV malformation
    c. Berry aneurysm
    d. Tumors

172. **Most common brain tumor:**
    a. Meningioma
    b. Glioma
    c. Metastasis
    d. Astrocytoma

173. **Kaposi sarcoma is caused by:**
    a. HHV 17
    b. HHV 8
    c. HPV 16
    d. Human simian virus 40

174. **Blood borne spread is a feature of:**
    a. Carcinoma
    b. Sarcoma
    c. Dysplasia
    d. Metaplasia

175. **Which is true about lipoma?**
    a. It is hypoechoic
    b. It is hypointense
    c. It is hypodense
    d. It has Hounsfield units of 200

176. **Which contrast agent is given in perforation peritonitis?**
    a. Iohexol
    b. Iodixanol
    c. Diatrizoate
    d. Metrizoate

177. **Microbubbles are used as contrast in**
    a. X-ray
    b. CT
    c. USG
    d. MRI

178. **A 60-year-old male has bone pain, vertebral collapse, fracture pelvis, the probable diagnosis is:**
    a. Multiple myeloma
    b. Secondaries
    c. TB
    d. Hemangioma of bone

179. **Drug of choice for treatment of acute organophosphate poisoning is:**
    a. Atropine
    b. Pralidoxime
    c. Neostigmine
    d. d-Tubocurarine

180. **All of the following statements are correct about varicocele except:**
    a. Common on the right side
    b. Can present as a later sign of renal cell carcinoma
    c. Has bag of worm like feeling
    d. Can lead to infertility

181. **Fournier's gangrene occurs in the:**
    a. Toes
    b. Scrotum
    c. Fingers
    d. Muscles

182. **Most common testicular tumor in prepubertal adults is:**
    a. Yolk sac tumor
    b. Embryonal cell Ca
    c. Seminoma
    d. Teratoma

183. **A patient, resident of Himachal Pradesh presented with a series of ulcers in a row, on his right leg. The biopsy from the affected area was taken and cultured on Sabouraud's Dextrose agar. What would be the most likely causative organism?**
    a. Sporothrix schenckii
    b. Cladosporium spp.
    c. Pseudallescheria boydii
    d. Nocardia brasiliensis

184. **Pityriasis versicolor is caused by–**
    a. E. floccosum
    b. M. gypseum
    c. M. furfur
    d. T. tonsurans

185. **Man is secondary host for–**
    a. Malaria
    b. Tuberculosis
    c. Filariasis
    d. Relapsing fever

186. **The most important reservoir of Leishmaniasis in India is–**
    a. Dogs
    b. Rodents
    c. Man
    d. Case of post Kala azar dermal Leishmaniasis

187. **IgE is secreted by**
    a. Mast cell
    b. Basophils
    c. Eosinophils
    d. Plasma cells

188. **The arrow is pointing towards which of the following structures?**

    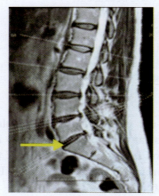

    a. L2-L3 intervertebral disc space
    b. L3-L4 intervertebral disc space
    c. L4-L5 intervertebral disc space
    d. L5-S1 intervertebral disc space

189. **Muscle which acts as tensor of vocal cord is supplied by**
    a. RLN
    b. Internal laryngeal nerve
    c. External laryngeal nerve
    d. Glossopharyngeal nerve

190. A 9-year-old child presented to ENT OPD with Hoarse voice, Croupy cough, Inspiratory stridor & Increasing dyspnea. On palpation of neck, patient also had Bull neck lymphadenopathy. Child also had membrane formed over tonsil, which bleeds on removal. Identify the condition.
    a. Laryngeal TB
    b. Laryngeal diphtheria
    c. Syphilis larynx
    d. Leprosy larynx

191. Most common site of laryngeal involvement in Wegener's granulomatosis is:
    a. Supraglottis
    b. Glottis
    c. Subglottis
    d. Epiglottis

192. All of the following cause grayish white membrane formation on tonsils except
    a. Infectious mononucleosis
    b. Streptococcal tonsillitis
    c. Diphtheria
    d. Ludwig's Angina

193. Cock-up splint is used in management of:
    a. Ulnar nerve palsy
    b. Brachial plexus palsy
    c. Radial nerve palsy
    d. Combined ulnar and median nerve palsy

194. Winging of scapula is due to palsy of:
    a. Long thoracic nerve
    b. Nerve to latissimus dorsi
    c. Spinal accessory nerve
    d. Nerve to rhomboid

195. Nail bed of index finger is supplied by:
    a. Median nerve
    b. Ulnar
    c. Palmar Branch of median nerve
    d. Palmar branch of ulnar nerve

196. Which of the following mucopolysaccharide is responsible for retinal cell- cell attachment?
    a. Keratin sulfate
    b. Dermatan sulfate
    c. Chondroitin sulfate
    d. Heparan sulfate

197. Enantiomers are isomers that differ in structure at which carbon?
    a. Last Carbon
    b. First Carbon
    c. Penultimate Carbon
    d. Carbonyl Carbon

198. Nasolacrimal duct opens into which meatus?
    a. Inferior Meatus
    b. Middle Meatus
    c. Superior Meatus
    d. Supreme Meatus

199. Which of the following promotes rouleaux formation?
    a. Zeta potential on RBC membrane
    b. Fibrinogen
    c. Albumin
    d. Biconcave shape of RBC

200. In blood coagulation, the rate-limiting step is:
    a. Fibrinogen to fibrin conversion by action of thrombin
    b. Conversion of prothrombin to thrombin
    c. Activation of factor X
    d. Action of factor VIII

201. Heme is synthesized in which part of the erythroblastic cells?
    a. Golgi complex
    b. Ribosomes
    c. Endoplasmic reticulum
    d. Mitochondrial matrix

202. SAFE strategy has been developed for the control of:
    a. Onchocerciasis
    b. Trachoma
    c. Refractive error
    d. Ocular trauma

203. 'NIKSHAY' is a newly launched central government software. It is used for tracking:
    a. High risk newborns
    b. Malaria
    c. Tuberculosis
    d. High risk pregnancies

204. A screening test is applied for screening of liver cancer in a population of 500. The test shows positive result in 80 individuals and negative in remaining 420. Out of 80 positive individuals 60 confirmed to be diagnosed with liver cancer by diagnostic test and 20 were ruled out. Out of negative 420 individuals 40 had liver cancer. The sensitivity of the test is:
    a. 60%
    b. 80%
    c. 90%
    d. 95%

205. Hawthorne effect is seen in:
    a. Case-control study
    b. Cohort study
    c. Cross-sectional study
    d. Retrospective cohort study

206. All of the following are advantages of case control studies except:
    a. Useful in rare disease
    b. Relative risk can be calculated
    c. Odds ratio can be calculated
    d. Cost-effective and inexpensive

207. Efficacy of new drug A is compared with an existing drug B in:
    a. Clinical trial phase I
    b. Clinical trial phase II
    c. Clinical trial phase III
    d. Clinical trial phase IV

208. Which is NOT a benefit of Randomization?
    a. Reduction of bias in selection of groups
    b. Ensure comparability of both groups
    c. Facilitates blinding of treatment
    d. Increases external validity of study

209. Vaccine derived poliovirus outbreaks are mostly due to:
    a. Type-2 virus
    b. Type-3 virus
    c. Type-1 virus
    d. All of the above

210. Naltrexone is:
    a. Mu receptor agonist
    b. Delta receptor agonist
    c. Kappa receptor agonist
    d. Mu receptor antagonist

211. All of the following are used in management of acute severe bleeding due to warfarin overdose except:
    a. Withhold the anticoagulant
    b. Vitamin K1
    c. Protamine sulphate
    d. Fresh frozen plasma

FMGE Solutions Screening Examination

212. Suprarenal gland develops from:
    a. Metanephros
    b. Ureteric bud
    c. Neural crest
    d. Endoderm
213. All are true about brachial plexus EXCEPT:
    a. Lower trunk is formed by root C8 and T1
    b. Lateral cord is formed by upper and middle trunk
    c. Posterior cord is formed by posterior divisions of all three trunks
    d. C4 root is post fixed to plexus
214. Nerve supply to the perineum is
    a. Pudendal nerve
    b. Inferior rectal nerve
    c. Pelvic splanchnic nerves
    d. Hypogastric plexus
215. Sacral promontory is the landmark for
    a. Origin of superior mesenteric artery
    b. Termination of presacral nerve
    c. Origin of inferior mesenteric artery
    d. None of the above
216. What is the ideal time for doing quadruple test?
    a. 8–12 weeks
    b. 11–15 weeks
    c. 15–18 weeks
    d. 18–22 weeks
217. The best gas used for pneumoperitoneum laparoscopy is
    a. N_2
    b. O_2
    c. CO_2
    d. NO
218. Most common type of monozygotic twin pregnancy is:
    a. Monochorionic Monoamniotic twins with Siamese presentation
    b. Monochorionic Monoamniotic (MO-MO) twins
    c. Monochorionic Diamniotic twins (MO-DI)
    d. Dichorionic Diamniotic twins (DI-DI)
219. All are causes of primary amenorrhea EXCEPT
    a. MRKH syndrome
    b. Sheehan's syndrome
    c. Kallmann syndrome
    d. Turner's syndrome
220. GFR is increased by all of the following EXCEPT:
    a. Increased renal blood flow
    b. Efferent arteriolar constriction
    c. Renal stone in ureter
    d. Decreased oncotic pressure
221. Which of the following presents as nephritic syndrome?
    a. P.I.G.N
    b. Minimal change disease
    c. F.S.G.S
    d. Membranous Glomerulopathy

222. Following diagram represents which obstetric grips during palpation?

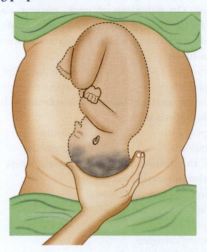

    a. First Leopold
    b. Second Leopold
    c. Third Leopold
    d. Fourth Leopold
223. The most common cause of tubal block in India is:
    a. Gonorrhea infection
    b. Chlamydia infection
    c. Tuberculosis
    d. Bacterial vaginosis
224. CA-125 is a marker antigen for the diagnosis of:
    a. Colon cancer
    b. Breast cancer
    c. Brain cancer
    d. Ovarian cancer
225. A 13-year-old young girl presents in the casualty with acute pain in the lower abdomen. She has history of cyclical pain for last 6 months and she has not attained her menarche yet. On local genital examination, a tense bulge in the region of hymen was seen. The most probable diagnosis is:
    a. Rokitansky Kuster Hauser syndrome
    b. Testicular feminization syndrome
    c. Imperforate hymen
    d. Asherman's syndrome
226. hCG is secreted by:
    a. Trophoblast cells
    b. Amniotic membrane
    c. Fetal yolk sac
    d. Hypothalamus
227. Which of the following IUCD has a life span of 10 years?
    a. Cu 380 A
    b. Cu 200
    c. LNG IUS
    d. Multiload
228. Nuchal translucency more than 3 mm at 14 weeks is suggestive of
    a. Down syndrome (Trisomy 21)
    b. Oesophageal atresia
    c. Edwards syndrome (Trisomy 18)
    d. Foregut duplication cyst
229. Late deaths in burns is due to:
    a. Sepsis
    b. Hypovolemia
    c. Contractures
    d. Neurogenic

230. Which of the following is true about Marjolin's ulcer?
    a. Ulcer over scar
    b. Rapid growth
    c. Rodent ulcer
    d. Painful
231. Characteristic feature of basal cell carcinoma is:
    a. Keratin pearls
    b. Foam cells
    c. Nuclear palisading
    d. Psammoma bodies
232. Spontaneous regression is seen in all except:
    a. Salmon patch
    b. Small cavernous hemangioma
    c. Portwine stain
    d. Strawberry angioma
233. Delayed wound healing is seen in all except:
    a. Malignancy
    b. Hypertension
    c. Diabetes
    d. Infection
234. Which of the following is marker for carcinoma?
    a. Cytokeratin
    b. Vimentin
    c. Calcitonin
    d. CD-45
235. Most common cause of skeletal metastasis is:
    a. Kidney
    b. Prostate
    c. Breast
    d. Thyroid
236. In which case spontaneous regression is not seen?
    a. Malignant melanoma
    b. Osteosarcoma
    c. Neuroblastoma
    d. Choriocarcinoma
237. The most common pure germ cell tumor of the ovary is:
    a. Choriocarcinoma
    b. Dysgerminoma
    c. Embryonal cell tumor
    d. Malignant Teratoma
238. The best way of diagnosing Trisomy-21 during second trimester of pregnancy is:
    a. Triple marker estimation
    b. Nuchal skin fold thickness measurement
    c. Chorionic villus sampling
    d. Amniocentesis
239. The shortest diameter in fetal head is:
    a. Biparietal diameter
    b. Bimastoid diameter
    c. Occipito frontal diameter
    d. Bitemporal Diameter
240. Not used as emergency contraception
    a. Intrauterine LNG system
    b. Mifepristone
    c. Oral LNG
    d. Copper intrauterine device
241. Pure gonadal dysgenesis will be diagnosed in the presence of:
    a. Bilateral streak gonads
    b. Bilateral dysgenetic gonads
    c. One side streak and other dysgenetic gonads
    d. One side streak and other normal looking gonad
242. Which of the following drug is not used for medical management of ectopic pregnancy?
    a. Potassium Chloride
    b. Methotrexate
    c. Actinomycin D
    d. Misoprostol
243. The following is always an indication of Caesarean section, except:
    a. Abruptio Placentae
    b. Untreated stage of II B Ca cervix
    c. Active genital herpes
    d. Type IV Placenta Previa (major previa)
244. Most common ovarian tumor to undergo torsion
    a. Benign cystic teratoma
    b. Dysgerminoma
    c. Serous adenoma
    d. Brenners tumour
245. Not true about Red degeneration of myomas:
    a. It occurs commonly during pregnancy
    b. Immediate surgical intervention is needed
    c. Due to interference with blood supply
    d. Treated with analgesics
246. Best parameter for estimation of fetal age by ultrasound in third trimester is:
    a. Femur length
    b. Biparietal diameter
    c. Abdominal circumference
    d. Inter-ocular distance
247. All of the following statements are true except:
    a. Oxytocin sensitivity is increased during delivery
    b. Prostaglandins may be given for inducing abortion during IInd trimester
    c. In lactating women genital stimulation enhances oxytocin release
    d. Oxytocin is used for inducing abortion in 1 st trimester
248. From what cm of cervical dilatation is partogram plotted in regular intervals?
    a. 4 cm
    b. 5 cm
    c. 6 cm
    d. 8 cm
249. Mirena has to be replaced after:
    a. 1 year
    b. 5 years
    c. 3 years
    d. 6 months
250. A 35-year-old mother of two children is suffering from amenorrhea for last 12 months. She has history of failure of lactation following 2nd delivery but remained asymptomatic thereafter. Skull X-ray shows "Empty sella". Most likely diagnosis is:
    a. Menopause
    b. Pituitary tumor
    c. Sheehan's syndrome
    d. Intraductal papilloma of breast
251. Pap smear is useful in the diagnosis of all, except
    a. Gonorrhoea
    b. Trichomonas vaginalis
    c. Human papilloma virus
    d. Inflammatory changes
252. Most Definitive test for evaluating Intracranial aneurysms is.
    a. CT
    b. MRI
    c. Angiography
    d. PET

FMGE Solutions Screening Examination

253. In myxedema, yellowish tint of the skin is due to:
    a. Increased levels (decreased elimination) of bilirubin
    b. Increased carotene in the skin
    c. Anaemia
    d. Increased cholesterol levels in plasma

254. In the development of an ovum, second meiotic division is completed:
    a. Just before ovulation   b. Just after ovulation
    c. Just before fertilization d. Just after fertilization

255. Oxygen saturation of blood in the umbilical artery is about:
    a. 40%
    b. 60%
    c. 75%
    d. 97%

256. The basic reason for "reperfusion injury" to the myocardium is:
    a. Generation of free radicals
    b. Extension of the ischemic zone
    c. Increased ICF [Ca++]
    d. Increased ECF [Ca++]

257. Bifid (or "M" shaped) P-wave on an ECG may be seen in:
    a. Mitral stenosis   b. Atrial flutter
    c. WPW syndrome   d. Sinus bradycardia

258. Clinical features of Kartegener's syndrome include
    a. Recurrent sinusitis   b. Bronchiectasis
    c. Situs inversus   d. All of the above

259. A 15-year-old boy presents with enophthalmos after trauma to face by cricket ball. CT Scan of face revealed following finding. What would be the most common orbital wall involved?

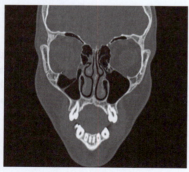

    a. Floor
    b. Medial wall
    c. Lateral wall
    d. Superior wall

260. Identify the type of septal fracture shown below & comment on fracture line.
    a. Chevallet Fracture
    b. Jarjaway Fracture
    c. Gurein fracture
    d. Lefort Fracture

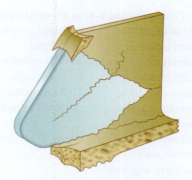

261. What is the ionic basis for after-depolarization in a record of an AP?
    a. Entry of Ca++ via slow channels.
    b. Late entry of Na+ via channels that have been activated.
    c. Altered gradient for K+ movement.
    d. Prolonged open state of K+ channels.

262. The image given below shows two scenarios (A and B) when 2 Kgs of weight is applied to the muscle in its relaxed state. Choose the correct statement regarding the scenarios:

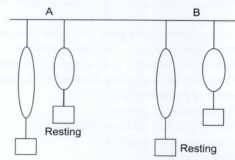

    a. B has done more work than A
    b. B has both preload and afterload added to it
    c. B has undergone maximum tension
    d. A has produced isometric tension

263. A 12-year-child, who has intellectual disability, is having large face, large jaw, large ear and macroorchidism. Diagnosis is
    a. Mc Cune Albright syndrome
    b. Down syndrome
    c. Cri-du chat syndrome
    d. Fragile X syndrome

264. Infraclavicular lesion of tuberculosis is known as:
    a. Ghon's focus   b. Puhl's focus
    c. Assmann's focus   d. Simon's focus

265. Unlawful abortion of a woman with her consent is punishable under
    a. 310 IPC
    b. 312 IPC
    c. 313 IPC
    d. 314 IPC

266. In camera trial of a rape case hearing is done under
    a. 376 IPC
    b. 327 (2) CrPC
    c. 53 CrPC
    d. 375 IPC
267. Pick out the cell seen in Rhinoscleroma
    a. Sarcoid bodies
    b. Asteroid bodies
    c. Mikulicz cells
    d. Langerhans cells
268. Histogram is used to describe
    a. Quantitative data of a group of patients
    b. Qualitative data of a group of patients
    c. Data collected on nominal scale
    d. Data collected on ordinal scale
269. For a given set of values, Mean = 20, Median = 24 & Mode = 26. The given distribution is:
    a. Symmetric
    b. Right-skewed
    c. Left-skewed
    d. Can be either symmetric or skewed
270. Which of these is not a Parametric test of significance?
    a. Z-test
    b. ANOVA
    c. Student 't-test'
    d. Chi-square test
271. While applying chi-square test to a contingency table of 4 rows and 4 columns, the degree of freedom would be:
    a. 1
    b. 4
    c. 9
    d. 8
272. Contraceptive efficacy is measured by:
    a. Pearl index only
    b. Pearl index and life table analysis
    c. Life table analysis and couple protection rate
    d. Pearl index and couple protection rate
273. All are included in Kangaroo Mother Care except:
    a. Skin to skin contact
    b. Early discharge and follow up
    c. Free nutritional supplements
    d. Exclusive Breast feeding
274. The Medical Termination Of Pregnancy Act does not protect act of termination of pregnancies after:
    a. 20 weeks
    b. 24 weeks
    c. 28 weeks
    d. 30 weeks
275. Lice are not the vector of:
    a. Relapsing fever
    b. Q fever
    c. Trench fever
    d. Epidemic typhus
276. Most common site of Otosclerotic focus is
    a. Fissula ante fenestram
    b. Fissula post fenestram
    c. Round window
    d. Stapes supra-structure
277. The vector for KFD is:
    a. Aedes aegypti
    b. Haemaphysalis
    c. Culex
    d. Xenopsylla
278. MCC of Cervical cancer in India is:
    a. HPV 31, 33
    b. HPV 6, 11
    c. HPV 16, 18
    d. HPV 31, 45

279. Disease not included in Vision 2020, India is:
    a. Cataract
    b. Glaucoma
    c. Diabetic retinopathy
    d. Onchocerciasis
280. Ideal Tuning fork to test hearing in normal adult is
    a. 125 Hz
    b. 256 Hz
    c. 512 Hz
    d. 1024 Hz
281. Organ of Corti is present on
    a. Reissner's membrane
    b. Basilar membrane
    c. Tectorial membrane
    d. Secondary Tympanic membrane
282. Triad of Meniere's disease includes all except
    a. Vertigo
    b. Hearing loss
    c. Tinnitus
    d. Diplopia
283. Phelp sign is seen in
    a. Otosclerosis
    b. Glomus tumors
    c. Meniere disease
    d. CSOM
284. All of the following should be avoided by a patient with lactose intolerance, except:
    a. Condensed milk
    b. Ice-cream
    c. Skimmed milk
    d. Yoghurt
285. According to MCI, medical records of patients must be maintained by a Practitioner for a minimum period of:
    a. 1 year
    b. 2 year
    c. 3 year
    d. 5 year
286. Illusion is:
    a. Misinterpretation of real objects
    b. False, firm belief
    c. Absence of sensory stimulus
    d. Hearing of voices
287. Pure Aryans have which type of skull:
    a. Mesaticephalic
    b. Brachycephalic
    c. Dolicocephalic
    d. None of the above
288. A child can make a tower of 6 cubes at the age of?
    a. 36 months
    b. 18 months
    c. 12 months
    d. 24 months
289. Earliest sign of puberty in females is?
    a. Growth spurt
    b. Pubarche
    c. Thelarche
    d. Menarche
290. Identify this skin lesion in a newborn seen in first week of life:

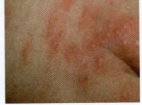

    a. Milia
    b. Stork bite
    c. Erythema toxicum
    d. Epstein pearls

FMGE Solutions Screening Examination

291. Conjugated hyperbilirubinemia in infancy is seen in:
    a. Gilbert syndrome
    b. Crigler Najjar syndrome
    c. Dubin Johnson syndrome
    d. Erythroblastosis fetalis

292. What is this device used by health workers to assess nutritional status of under-5 children?

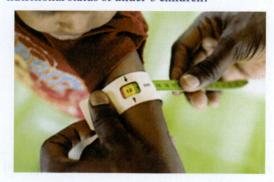

    a. Harpenden calipers   b. Shakir's tape
    c. Orchidometer   d. Infantometer

293. Which disease is this child suffering from?

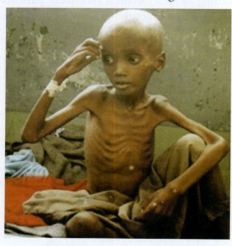

    a. Kwashiorkor   b. Marasmus
    c. Rickets   d. Achondroplasia

294. First clinical sign of vitamin A deficiency:
    a. Poor growth   b. Conjunctival xerosis
    c. Hydrocephalus   d. Phrynoderma

295. What is the most common underlying cause responsible for the disease in which this X ray finding is seen?

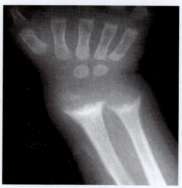

    a. Calcium deficiency   b. Phosphate deficiency
    c. Vit D deficiency   d. Vit C deficiency

296. Most common cardiac anomaly in Turner's Syndrome is?
    a. Coarctation of aorta b. Bicuspid aortic valve
    c. Ventricular septal defect d. Atrial septal defect

297. "Boot shaped" heart is seen in:
    a. Fallot's tetralogy
    b. Transposition of great vessels
    c. Ebstein's anomaly
    d. Ventricular septal defect

298. Severe hypothermia in a neonate refers to axillary temperature less than:
    a. 36.5 C   b. 36 C
    c. 34 C   d. 32 C

299. Definition of Extremely low birth weight neonate is?
    a. <2500 gm of birth weight
    b. <1500 gm of birth weight
    c. <1000 gm of birth weight
    d. <700 gm of birth weight

300. Most common cause of Bronchiolitis is:
    a. RSV   b. Adenovirus
    c. Hospitalize and treat d. Mycoplasma

Model Test Paper-II

Ans.

1. b.	2. b.	3. c.	4. d.	5. d.	6. b.	7. d.	8. c.	9. a.	10. d.	11. c
12. a.	13. c.	14. d.	15. a.	16. d.	17. b.	18. d.	19. a.	20. b.	21. c.	22. b.
23. b.	24. a.	25. a.	26. a.	27. a.	28. b.	29. d.	30. d.	31. d.	32. c.	33. c.
34. a.	35. d.	36. b.	37. c.	38. d.	39. d.	40. b.	41. b.	42. d.	43. d.	44. d.
45. d.	46. b.	47. b.	48. c.	49. a.	50. c.	51. d.	52. d.	53. c.	54. b.	55. a.
56. c.	57. b.	58. a.	59. a.	60. a.	61. d.	62. c.	63. b.	64. a.	65. a.	66. c.
67. d.	68. b.	69. d.	70. c.	71. a.	72. a.	73. d.	74. b.	75. a.	76. b.	77. a.
78. d.	79. b.	80. d.	81. c.	82. c.	83. d.	84. b.	85. b.	86. d.	87. d.	88. a.
89. c.	90. b.	91. d.	92. c.	93. c.	94. a.	95. c.	96. a.	97. c.	98. a.	99. b.
100. a.	101. d.	102. d.	103. b.	104. a.	105. a.	106. a.	107. d.	108. c.	109. a.	110. c.
111. a.	112. d.	113. d.	114. c.	115. a.	116. b.	117. b.	118. b.	119. d.	120. c.	121. a.
122. d.	123. b.	124. b.	125. b.	126. a.	127. b.	128. b.	129. c.	130. d.	131. d.	132. b.
133. c.	134. a.	135. c.	136. a.	137. a.	138. b.	139. d.	140. b.	141. b.	142. a.	143. d.
144. b.	145. a.	146. c.	147. c.	148. c.	149. a.	150. a.	151. a.	152. a.	153. a.	154. a.
155. c.	156. c.	157. c.	158. b.	159. a.	160. c.	161. b.	162. c.	163. c.	164. b.	165. a.
166. b.	167. b.	168. b.	169. b.	170. b.	171. c.	172. c.	173. b.	174. b.	175. c.	176. a.
177. c.	178. b.	179. a.	180. a.	181. b.	182. d.	183. a.	184. c.	185. a.	186. d.	187. d.
188. d.	189. c.	190. b.	191. c.	192. d.	193. d.	194. a.	195. a.	196. d.	197. c.	198. a.
199. b.	200. c.	201. d.	202. b.	203. c.	204. a.	205. a.	206. b.	207. c.	208. d.	209. a.
210. d.	211. c.	212. c.	213. d.	214. a.	215. b.	216. c.	217. c.	218. c.	219. b.	220. c.
221. a.	222. c.	223. b.	224. d.	225. c.	226. a.	227. a.	228. a.	229. a.	230. a.	231. c.
232. c.	233. b.	234. a.	235. c.	236. d.	237. b.	238. d.	239. b.	240. a.	241. a.	242. d.
243. a.	244. a.	245. b.	246. b.	247. d.	248. a.	249. b.	250. c.	251. a.	252. c.	253. b.
254. d.	255. b.	256. c.	257. a.	258. d.	259. a.	260. b.	261. c.	262. a.	263. d.	264. c.
265. b.	266. b.	267. c.	268. a.	269. c.	270. d.	271. c.	272. b.	273. c.	274. a.	275. b.
276. a.	277. b.	278. c.	279. d.	280. c.	281. b.	282. d.	283. b.	284. d.	285. c.	286. a.
287. c.	288. d.	289. c.	290. c.	291. c.	292. b.	293. b.	294. b.	295. c.	296. b.	297. a.
298. d.	299. c.	300. a.								

CBS Exam Books 2019-20
Subject Wise Books

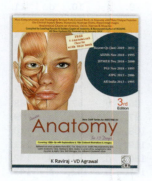
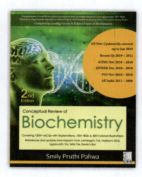
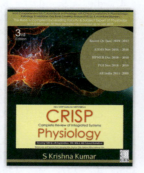
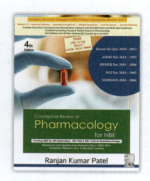
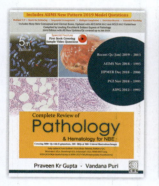
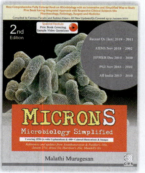
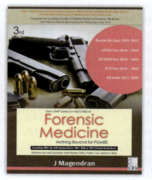
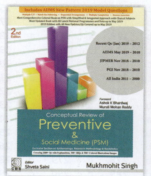
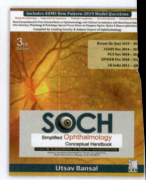
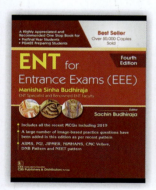
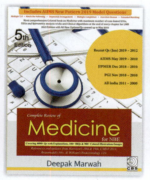
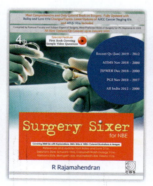
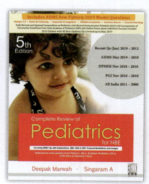
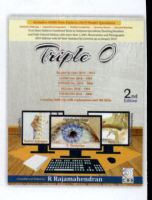
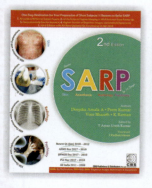
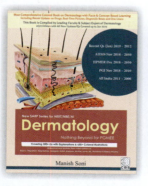
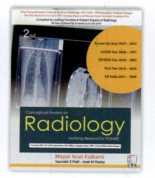
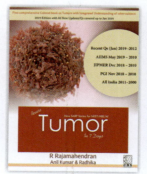
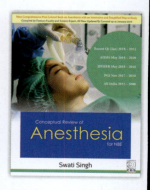

 CBS Publishers & Distributors Pvt. Ltd.
• New Delhi • Bengaluru • Chennai • Kochi • Kolkata • Mumbai • Pune • Hyderabad • Nagpur • Patna • Vijayawada

Above books available at **All Medical Book Stores of India**

Buy online   cbspd.co.in  amazon.in  Parasredkart.com flipkart

For any availability issue please contact : +91-955559018

CBS Exam Books 2019-20

Exam Wise Books

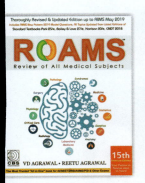 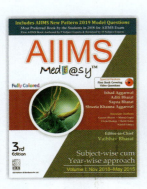 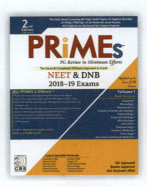 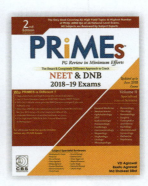 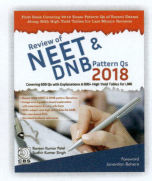

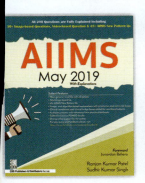 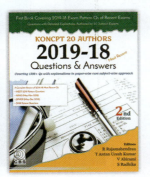 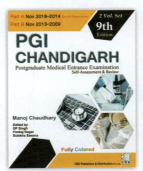 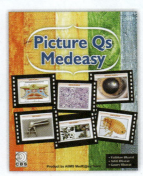 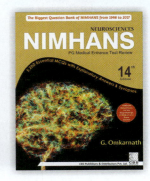

FMGE Series

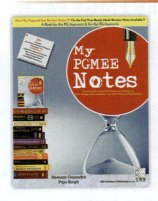 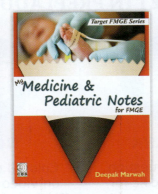 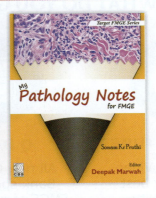

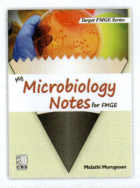 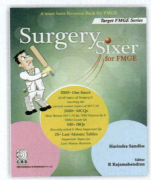 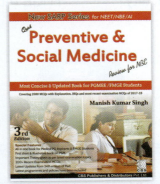

 CBS Publishers & Distributors Pvt. Ltd.
• New Delhi • Bengaluru • Chennai • Kochi • Kolkata • Mumbai • Pune • Hyderabad • Nagpur • Patna • Vijayawada

Above books available at **All Medical Book Stores of India**

Buy online  cbspd.co.in Parasredkart.com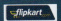

For any availability issue please contact : +91-9555590180

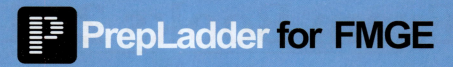

PrepLadder for FMGE

THE ONLY PACK CREATED SPECIALLY FOR FMGE BY

THE DREAM TEAM

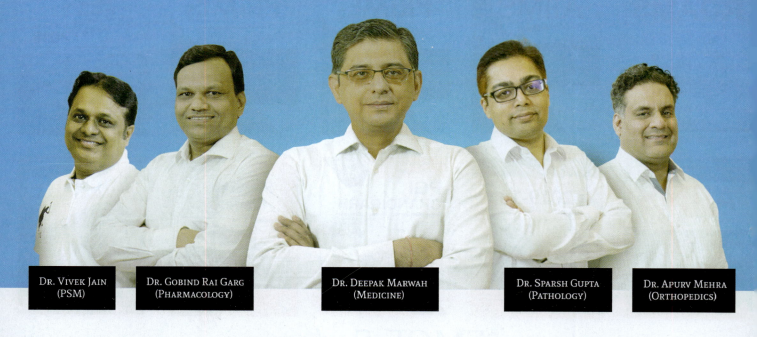

Dr. Vivek Jain (PSM) | Dr. Gobind Rai Garg (Pharmacology) | Dr. Deepak Marwah (Medicine) | Dr. Sparsh Gupta (Pathology) | Dr. Apurv Mehra (Orthopedics)

WHAT DO YOU GET IN PREPLADDER FMGE PACK?

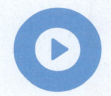   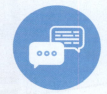

VIDEO LECTURES
Conceptual Video lectures by best FMGE faculty.

Q BANK
All new Question Bank specific for FMGE requirements.

NOTES
Colored notes based on video lectures for effective study & revision.

T&D
Select your own Test & Discussion schedule.

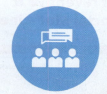 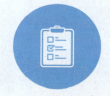 

EXAM DISCUSSION
Previous year Exam Discussion videos.

TEST SERIES
India's biggest test series.

DOUBT SUPPORT
Doubt support on app & through Premium club.

 medical@prepladder.com   www.prepladder.com